Cells, Tissues, and Disease

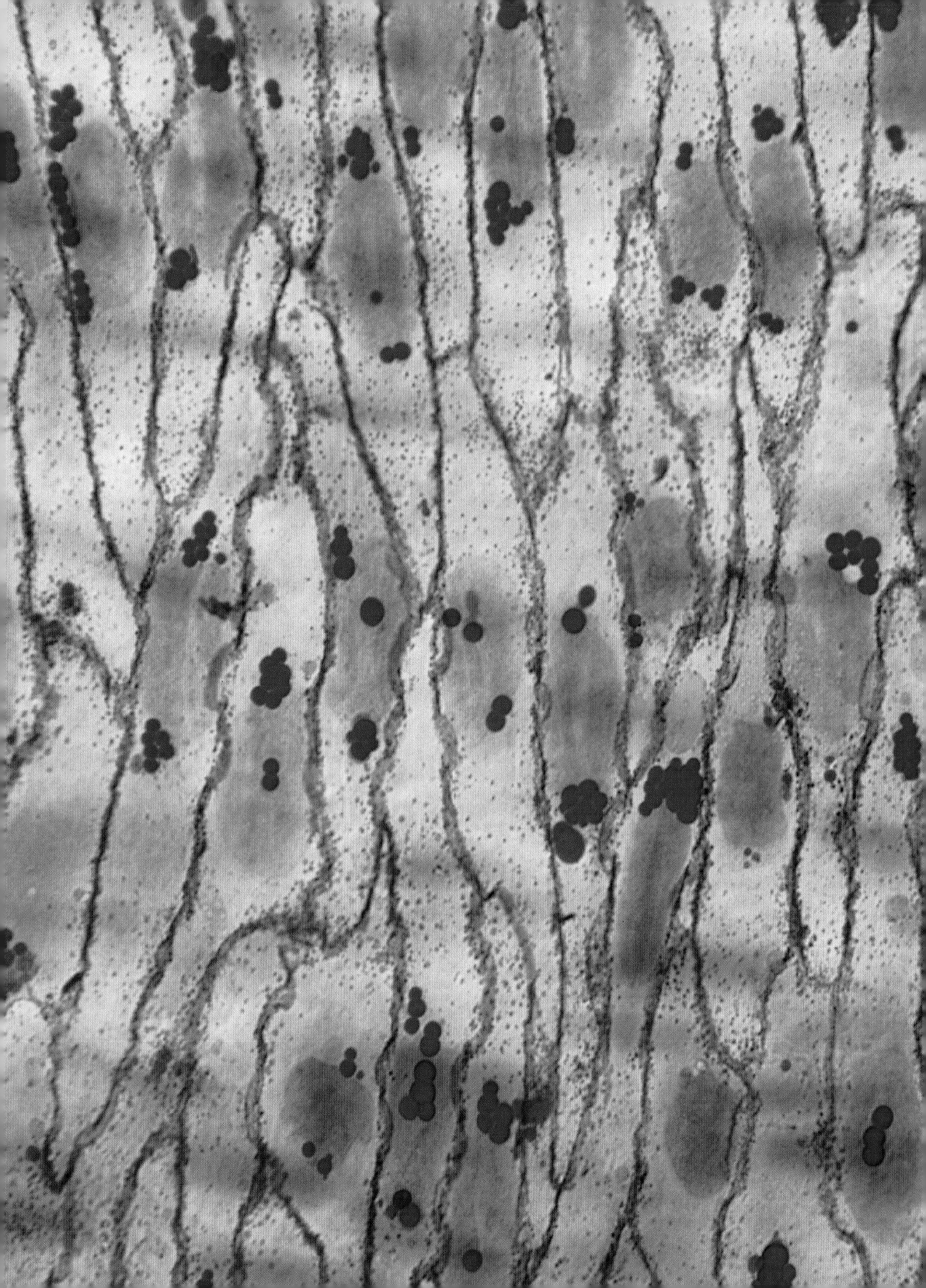

Cells, Tissues, and Disease

PRINCIPLES OF GENERAL PATHOLOGY

SECOND EDITION

Guido Majno, M.D.

Isabelle Joris, Ph.D.

New York   Oxford

OXFORD UNIVERSITY PRESS

2004

Oxford University Press

Oxford New York
Auckland Bangkok Buenos Aires Cape Town Chennai
Dar es Salaam Delhi Hong Kong Istanbul Karachi Kolkata
Kuala Lumpur Madrid Melbourne Mexico City Mumbai Nairobi
São Paulo Shanghai Singapore Taipei Tokyo Toronto

Published by Oxford University Press, Inc.,
198 Madison Avenue, New York, New York 10016
www.oup.com

Oxford is a registered trademark of Oxford University Press

Library of Congress Cataloging-in-Publication Data
Majno, Guido.
Cells, tissues, and disease: principles of general pathology / Guido Majno, Isabelle
Joris.—2nd ed.
p. ; cm.
Includes bibliographical references and index.
ISBN 0-19-514090-7
1. Pathology. I. Joris, Isabelle. II. Title.
[DNLM: 1. Histology. 2. Pathology. QZ 4 M233c 2004]
RB111.M265 2004
616.07—dc21   2003050657

Book design by Cathleen Bennett

Cover illustration: This illustration is a pun on the title of the book. It shows an *en face* view of the inner surface of the aorta of a hypercholesterolemic rat (experimental atherosclerosis), stained with silver nitrate (which outlines each endothelial cell in black) and with Oil red O (which stains fat droplets in red). Each unit of the flagstone pattern is a *cell;* the overall flagstone pattern of endothelium is a *tissue;* and the red droplets of fat represent *disease.*

9 8 7 6 5 4 3 2 1

Printed in China
on acid-free paper

This book is dedicated
to all patients
in all times and places
and to all those who helped us understand
the primal patient—
the cell

Preface to the Second Edition

For two people to self-inflict—for the second time—the production of a textbook as weighty and complex as this one, there must have been a powerful motivation. There were several. Oxford University Press offered to publish a new version in full color. The feedback had been encouraging. The book had been translated into Italian. And then, General Pathology is a captivating science; it is everywhere; it runs through all of biology, it explains how right things go wrong and wrong things go right. You cannot work, eat, run, cook, play the piano, lie in the sun, even sleep or sit through Wagner's Ring (it has to be the Ring) without running into General Pathology. Besides, learning to decipher disease through the light and electron microscope is intellectually as well as aesthetically exhilarating. We want to share this adventure not only with medical students but also with anyone who is conducting research or teaching in fields related to biology: *cell biology, anatomy, physiology, pharmocology, biochemistry, biophysics, bacteriology, immunology, molecular biology*—for a start.

This being said, we should take a look at the big picture. Pathology is the science of disease *par excellence*. Physicians and medical students are well aware of this, but Ph.D.'s and graduate students in the basic medical sciences are often not. In fact, they tend to recoil at the word "pathology". We looked into this strange phenomenon. It has a reason; not a scientific one, but a strong one, and very human. We reconstruct it as follows.

Think historically, Pathology about 1300 A.D. Think terrible smells, revolting sights. Presumed criminals getting hung, and their bodies stolen at night to keep the dissectors busy, year after year, for centuries. Autopsies done in the early universities with no rubber gloves, no running water, no refrigeration, no disinfection, at night, sometimes against the law of the State and the will of the Church. The pioneers, who became the heroes of pathology, projected an image that few could envy. Even for Harvey (1578–1657), dissection

meant "much nausea, loathing and foetor." Teaching had to be limited to the cold months. We have often fantasized about those great anatomists such as Vesalius (1514–1564) or Morgagni (1682–1771): surely when they returned home after a long day of dissection, they must have left quite an odorous trail. If by some miracle we could have today the privilege of shaking hands with some of them, we would feel unbelievably honored, but we would probably also wonder how many *Mycobacteria tuberculosis* we might have acquired with each handshake. Tradition maintains that Xavier Bichat, the great French physician-pathologist (1771–1802), died prematurely after he opened a specimen jar and was overwhelmed by the awful stench. Doctors of Philosophy (Ph.D.'s) in other subjects had little to gain by associating with these primordial physicians, and a gap slowly developed between the two worlds. They had different heroes.

And so it came to pass that pathology, with its unseemly birth, never came to be accepted as comparable to the other basic sciences; when it did become a basic science on its own, around 1850, it retained its special status even in academia, being perceived as hospital-bound, cadaverous, semi-illegal, descriptive, nonquantitative, and only half scientific. The historical reasons are so strong that it may take many more generations to overcome them. Only the physicians—who learned pathology—realize that this is the foundation of Medicine. Today, in the mind of the average taxpayer who supports us, our work is crime detection.

All of this, of course, matters little: what counts is what we really do. Today, pathology can be studied elegantly at eight levels (Figure P.1). To explain its role in relation to medicine, the metaphor of a tree works very well (Figure P.2). All researchers in the field of biology are perched in one or two places of this tree; those in the basic medical sciences (the roots) provide facts and concepts, which help understand the normal as well as the abnormal condition. Historically the task of synthesis ("what are the basic mechanisms of disease?") has been

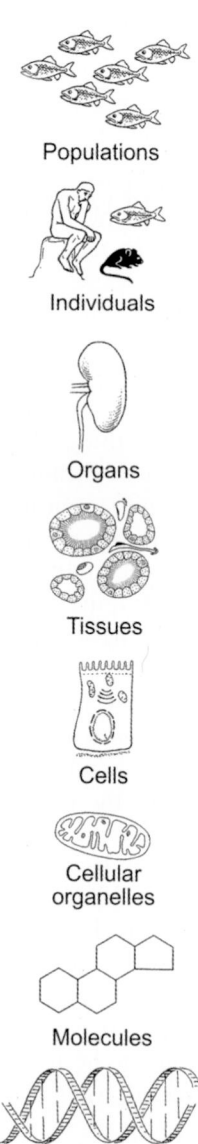

Populations

Individuals

Organs

Tissues

Cells

Cellular organelles

Molecules

Genes

FIGURE P.1 Disease can be studied at many levels: whole populations (epidemiology), individual patients (clinical medicine), individual organs (pathophysiology), tissues (histopathology), cells (cytology), single organelles (biochemistry), molecules (biophysics), and genes (molecular biology).

the calling of General Pathology (the tree trunk). The branches convey the same principles as applied to each medical specialty. Medicine is the crown of the tree.

And so, since we are all perched in the same tree, should we not try to understand each other, speak each other's language? Future physicians have to learn something about electrons and free radicals; faced with infarcts and thrombi, graduate students tend to feel lost. True, medical texts are often written in unfriendly

THE TREE OF MEDICINE

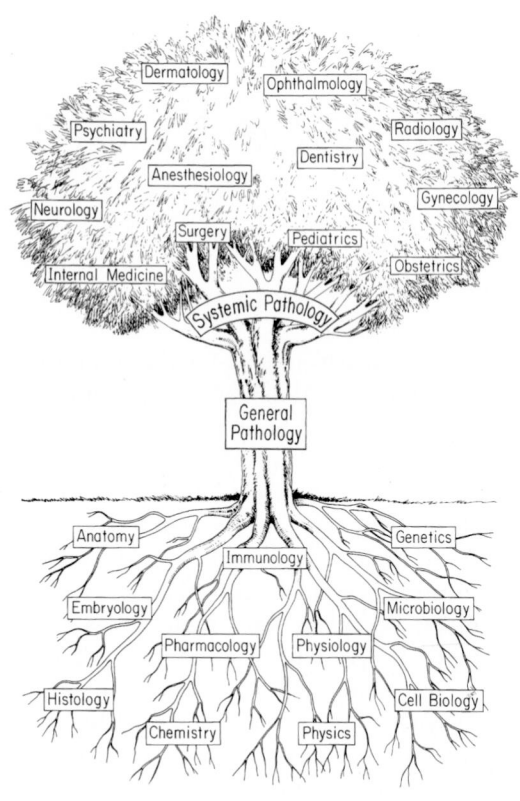

FIGURE P.2 The Tree of Medicine: the trunk is General Pathology, which draws from all the basic sciences, and divides into the many branches of Special Pathology; each one of these supports a specialized field of Medicine, the crown of the tree. (Courtesy of Dr. George Th. Diamandopoulos, Harvard Medical School, Boston, MA.)

jargon. This text may have an accent, but it was written in plain English.

To sum up, we are suggesting that experimenters in the field of biology would have a lot to gain if they had some basic, introductory training in General Pathology. We wrote this book, in part, to address this need.

How long does it take to learn enough general pathology to make a difference? In our medical school, the students learn it in 25 hours of lectures and about 50 hours of laboratory, mainly with microscopes. The time investment is not prohibitive.

We recognize an obstacle: not all Schools of Biomedical Sciences offer General Pathology courses for graduate students. One way to obtain some practical experience might be to coax a friendly pathologist into offering some time on a two-headed microscope as a tutor. The tutor might learn something too.

What is lost if this exchange does not occur? The loss comes in several forms. We do not want to sound presumptuous (surely there is no lack of errors in the pages of this book), but here is an example.

Sometimes, in disease, one kind of tissue is replaced by another; this event is called metaplasia, a well-chosen term that is about 150 years old and as alive as ever. A few years ago, the monster-word transdifferentiation appeared in the literature, ostensibly to mean the same as metaplasia, although the word was not clearly defined. We contacted some of the authors of papers on "transdifferentiation" and asked why they had chosen that new term. Some of the answers: (a) metaplasia was not a familiar term; (b) metaplasia is used by pathologists (!): (c) the two terms mean the same thing; and (d) the two terms mean different things. Now this has created real confusion in the field. Who will take the time to clean it up?

How This Book Was Written

(1) We chose to focus on the cell (level 5 in Figure P.1) because both injury and repair depend, ultimately, on what happens to the cells. The trend to "think cell" is also current in modern medicine. (2) We emphasized principles rather than the latest fact. Principles have a longer half-life than details. (3) We adopted the historical approach as often as possible. It is a part of the picture. The path to a discovery helps to understand it, and allows students to realize how the opportunity for discovery may present itself. (4) Our 1070 illustrations were selected, and explained, with special care, assuming that the reader needed some assistance in roaming through a microscopic field. (5) We tried to underscore that cellular disease can be found in all walks of life. There are references to fish markets, deer antlers, cooked meat, autumn leaves, oranges, wounded trees, branded cattle, linoleum, nettles and wasps, pâté de foie gras, sky and snow, dried insects, Japanese pearls, and many other subjects not usually encountered in this academic setting.

A note on the subject matter. As in the first edition, we assumed that the readers would be familiar with basic biology and immunology. We did retain a few topics in immunopathology, especially hypersensitivity, because they are an integral part of General Pathology. We left out genetics, usually covered in other courses, most of infection, and most of nutritional pathology, because the cellular responses to infectious agents and malnutrition can be understood in the light of the existing chapters.

We are acutely aware that every sentence and many illustrations could be improved, that someone else could write a whole textbook using references that we did not quote. All we can say is that we could not have tried harder. We hope that this book will help many readers discover the enjoyment of stealing secrets from the silent world of the cell.

Guido Majno
Isabelle Joris

Acknowledgments for the First Edition

One day, as we were attempting to calculate how many letters had been written for this book, Mrs. Linda Johnston, our precious secretary, quietly commented: "This book should have thousands of authors." She was absolutely right, and we should begin by acknowledging our secretarial help.

Secretaries. The roots of this book go back at least 20 years, when we enjoyed the assistance of Lise Karageorge and Karen Melia. Then, during 11 years, we were fortunate to have the extraordinary help of Jane M. Manzi, who typed as fast as we could speak, and took us from the age of the typewriter through that of the word processor to that of the computer. It is absurd to thank her in only a few words. Jane Manzi's tenure overlapped with that of Linda Johnston, who also helped us collect and file thousands of photographs, not to mention endless references and scores of bibliographic searches, and never lost her smile even when a key reference disappeared. Without her sense of perfection, her care, and her unfailing memory, this book would never have come to completion. Paula Dadian did a masterly job in gathering and keeping track of hundreds of permissions. Finally, we are indebted to Beryl Edney who took over with great enthusiasm and competence in the last, critical, and very demanding phase.

Illustrations. Most of our 1074 illustrations were obtained from all over the world, including Moscow when it was still behind the Iron Curtain. Many colleagues took the trouble of preparing new figures or sending us microscopic sections to photograph. Our warmest thanks go to all.

Having overheard the words "medical illustrator" in the crowd of a concert hall, we were fortunate to discover and then acquire the help of Anne B. Greene, whose exceptional skill is matched by her knowledge of biology and her sense of perfection. On many occasions Anne Greene pointed out inaccuracies in our sketches and miraculously turned our scribbles into beautiful drawings. The inimitable skills of Mr. J. B. Clark are also reflected in many illustrations. Beth H. Maynard of the Biomedical Media Service of this Medical Center designed almost all of our graphs and helped us assemble some of our most demanding illustrations, kindly and gracefully even in times of great pressure. In some of her drawings Beth was assisted by Themia A. Pappas-Fillmore and by George W. Jamieson. Credits for individual illustrations are listed below.

Photographers. Peter W. Healey was our first departmental photographer, and prepared gross and microscopic photographs in large numbers, while also setting the standards of excellence that were picked up by his followers. Christopher D. Hebert, aided by his background in biology, was a master in producing top-notch electron micrographs; he was also instrumental in setting up the messy but extremely effective technique of photographing gross specimens under water. We will never forget his patience while waiting until the last little bubble had disappeared, and the last floater had stopped moving. He was followed by Marie Picard-Craig; we especially appreciated her understanding of electron micrographs and her skill in converting color slides to black and white prints. Some of our earlier photographs were taken by Jean-Claude Rumbeli in Geneva. The patience and dedication of these wonderful artists is reflected throughout this volume. We are equally indebted to Jean M. Underwood and John J. Nunnari, who—in addition to their ordinary duties—laboriously navigated through our files, trimmed illustrations, calculated enlargements, and lettered photographs, while often pointing out to us ways to improve the final result.

Medical Students. Many medical students, mostly from the second year, worked with us during summers to collect references and prepare summaries on specific subjects. Their input contributed a great deal to our overall effort of synthesis. The list includes Jim A. Goldman, Rick J. Evans, Joseph E. Fuller, Reynaldo Cordero, Diane M. Pingeton (who drew also from her background as a nurse), Subhash C. Gumber (whose background in biochemistry allowed him to tackle some of the most intricate topics), Leslie A. O'Meara, a true expert in library research, Judy E. Tapper, who convinced us that matrix vesicles really exist, Stephen J. Barr, who provided some masterful orthopedic summaries, Matthew E. Cohen, who also produced some masterful summaries, and Deborah A. Vatcher who researched the history of oncogenes. A special place must be reserved for Charles R. Taylor, who spent a summer on the thankless task of counting the number of diseases (published here for the first time). To all these generous young people, and to any others whose names may have remained buried in our files, go our warmest thanks.

We should extend these thanks to include all the medical students who asked questions in class and in the lab—and forced us to think WHY.

Libraries. We are profoundly indebted to the staff of the Lamar Soutter Library at the University of Massachusetts Medical Center, especially to Dr. Donald J. Morton, Annanaomi Sams, Karen R. Cangello, Gael A. Evans, Linda M. Hayes, Paul H. Julian, Mary J. Markland, and Eileen M. Ritchie; once again, without them, this book could not have existed. Although we were perennially delinquent in returning books we were treated with great understanding, even when the computer coughed up threatening letters. Mme. Muriel Serodino, Director of the Library of the Faculty of Medicine in Geneva, kindly helped us track down the papers of Wilhelm Zahn, and as always, Richard Wolfe of the Rare Books division of Harvard University's Countway Library stood by to help us solve historical problems.

Help on Specific Topics. The input of experts has been essential in preventing us from making major blunders. However, let it be clear that we are entirely responsible for whatever blunders have slipped through the filter. One of the sections on Cellular Pathology returned from an expert consultant with an entire page crossed out, and the following notation in huge capital letters: NO WAY. We were a little shaken up, but to the horror of Linda Johnston we decided to keep that page anyway. This goes to say that our generous readers can be in "no way" responsible for whatever mistakes slipped through.

The section on Cellular Pathology was carefully read and annotated by Dr. George E. Palade, who took his precious time to make wonderful suggestions typically ranging from ATP to Zeus. The same section was also checked by Maya and Nicolae Simionescu in Bucharest, who remained our friends even after the arrival of a 40-pound package of manuscript and illustrations. The section on immunopathology was reviewed by Dr. Peter C. Kolbeck of the University of Nebraska. The section on vascular disturbances was reviewed by Dr. Henri F. Cuénoud, whose criticisms and contributions—including several illustrations— were absolutely essential. The section on tumors was read and criticized by Dr. Samuel M. Cohen of the University of Nebraska. Specific chapters or segments were further reviewed by specialists: the chapter on free radicals was reviewed by Dr. Steven D. Aust of Utah State University, the topic of molecular pathology was checked by Dr. James M. Pullman of our institution, the chapter on amyloid by Dr. Alan S. Cohen of Boston University, the chapter on calcification by Dr. Adele L. Boskey of Cornell University. Dr. Marie-Claude Badonnel was very helpful in guiding us through the HLA maze, and Dr. Parker A. Small, Jr. of the University of Florida checked our rendition of his influenza story.

We are also indebted to countless others whom we consulted on specific topics, often with the excuse of having lunch together. Here is a partial list, beginning with our Medical Center: Dr. Thomas W. Smith (an inexhaustible source of advice, slides and illustrations on the biology and pathology of nervous tissue), Dr. David A. Drachman (our wise neurologic consultant), Dr. Ashley Davidoff (a patient and thorough source of help on radiologic problems), Drs. Jag Bhawan, Rajwant Malhotra and Jeffrey D. Bernhard (our key consultants in matters of skin diseases), Dr. Thomas Zand (who stood by year after year and generously provided us with input on pediatric problems as well as on a variety of practical and philosophical problems), Dr. Armando Fraire (lung dilemmas), Dr. Bruce A. Woda and Marcia L. McFadden (lymphocyte dilemmas, cell sorting, lymphomas and immunology), Dr. Aldo A. Rossini (our guide through the complications of diabetes), Dr. Frank R. Reale and Joyce M. Compton (cytology, gynecologic pathology), Dr. Umberto De Girolami (muscle and nervous tissue), Dr. Arthur A. Like (experimental diabetes), Dr. Barbara F. Banner (kidney pathology, Dr. Ray M. Welsh (immunology), Dr. John J. Monahan (orthopedic problems), Dr. Gary V. Doern (bacterial problems), Dr. Irma O. Szymanski (red blood cells), Dr. H. Brownell Wheeler (wound healing), Dr. Harriet L. Robinson (viral infection). From other medical centers we should mention at least Dr. John W. Harshbarger of the Smithsonian Institution, who went to a great deal of trouble to provide us with information and illustrations on tumors in fish, oysters and other "lower animals", Dr. Bernie A. Ackerman (for cutaneous puzzles), Dr. Alan S. Cohen (amyloid), Dr. Stephen J. Galli (mast cells), Dr. Abul Abbas (delayed hypersensitivity), Dr. Victor E. Gould (neuroendocrine tumors and much else), Dr. Yusuf Kapanci (oxygen damage to the lungs, metastatic calcification), Drs. Linda M. McManus and R. Neal Pinckard (platelet activating factor), Dr. Michael A. Gimbrone (thrombosis), Dr. Pietro Gullino (experimental tumors), Dr. Henry C. Pitot ("what is a benign tumor?"), Dr. Gerald Nash (lung pathology), Dr. David L. Gang (gastroenterology), Dr. G. Fiore-Donno of Geneva (who should be an oral pathologist *honoris causa*), and Dr. Lelio Orci of Geneva and his pioneering team for various topics of cell biology. The friendship of Dr. Ruy Pérez Tamayo was always a stimulus and a source of wisdom. Special thanks are due to colleagues who wrote us personal accounts of their discoveries, such as a wonderful two-page letter from Dr. Björn Afzelius on the discovery of the immotile cilia syndrome, and a similar message from the late David Th. Purtilo on the discovery of XLP disease.

The pathogenesis of Japanese cultured pearls was unveiled to us thanks to Dr. Makoto Katori of Tokyo, who took us to the National Aquaculture Research Institute in Nansei, where Dr. Koji Wada guided us through that amazing biological process.

The title of this book is largely due to a conversation with a microbiologist, Dr. Jon D. Goguen, who told us that he would certainly buy a book on cellular disease—but not a book entitled "Pathology."

Former Collaborators, Friends, and Family. Much of the information presented in this book was derived from research that we accomplished with many collaborators. The first place must be reserved for Dr. Ramzi S. Cotran, who contributed in a major way not only as an investigator but also as a constant advisor; it was very important for us to have his blessing for our choice of an unusual title. Among our former collaborators we should also thank Dr. Gutta I. Schoefl, Dr. Renate Müller, Dr. Kaethe Kretchmer, Dr. Graeme B. Ryan (with whom the first few pages of this book were written), Dr. Giulio Gabbiani, Dr. Mark C. Kowala, Dr. Carl A. Boswell, Dr. John T. Doukas, as well as Monica Clowes and other marvelous research technicians, including Geneviève Leyvraz of Geneva, Claudia Froesch, Suzie Edwards, Jean M. Underwood, John J. Nunnari, and Anne H. Cutler. For our choice histologic sections we are indebted to Eva Moring, Laura S. Rooney, and Gail L. Bouliane.

Our friends and families also contributed in another way. A book such as this one should be the product of full-time work; because we could only give it part-time attention, we had to expand the work into nights and week-ends, thus stealing time from all those dear to us, who had to wait year after year for the completion of "The Book," and accept the fact that Inflammation could take priority over Christmas. They deserve special thanks for their patience, which amounted to a substantial and needed support.

Publishers. We are especially grateful to the team at Blackwell Science, Inc. for the enthusiasm with which our book was adopted after it had been dropped by another publisher. Rather than trying to explain why publication took the better part of 3 years, we prefer to thank the President, William L. Gibson, for taking the matter in his own hands and assigning to us the precious help of Karen M. Feeney, Ellen D. Samia, Heather Garrison, Irene Herlihy, and Lisa Flanagan. For the wise editing of the text we are indebted to Penny Hull, Yvonne Howell, and Glen Cochran.

Last, in the process of physically handling several tons of books, reprints, photocopies, and manuscript pages—just our first mailing to the publisher weighed 200 pounds—we are acutely aware that we have consumed vast amounts of cellulose. As a token of gratitude, upon the completion of this book, we planted 101 trees.

Guido Majno, M.D.
Isabelle Joris, Ph.D.

Credits for individual illustrations:

Anne B. Greene: 1.1, 2.9, 2.35, 2.58, 2.59, 2.63, 3.1, 3.7, 3.59, 3.60, 4.6, 4.18, 4.24, 4.33, 5.8, 5.11, 5.13, 5.29, 6.11, 8.1, 8.2, 8.15, 9.10, 9.15, 9.20, 9.28, 9.29, 10.5, 11.6, 11.7, 11.16, 11.24, 12.14, 13.16, 13.22, 13.42, 14.1, 14.2, 16.2, 17.1, 17.6, 17.13, 17.17, 17.22, 17.27, 17.39, 17.41, 17.45, 19.14, 21.15, 22.1, 22.23, 22.28, 22.34, 23.1, 23.5, 23.8, 23.31, 23.32, 23.36, 23.37, 23.42, 24.9, 24.29, 24.31, 26.51, 26.56, 26.71, 27.9, 27.16, 27.18, 27.19, 27.20, 27.28, 27.31, 27.33, 27.35, 27.41, 28.17, 28.44, 28.46, 31.6, 31.11, 33.3

Joshua B. Clark: 1.6, 2.11, 2.34, 3.17, 4.50, 7.9, 7.45, 22.13, 24.5

Dr. H.F. Cuénoud: 1.4, 2.28, 21.15, 21.16, 23.20, 30.2

Beth H. Maynard prepared the 204 remaining original charts and drawings.

Acknowledgments
for the Second Edition

A single event, human or other, may have many causes. To illustrate this concept as it applies to tumors construct we used the metaphor of a chain. With all of its links intact, the chain is a powerful tool; remove one link, and the whole falls apart. The paragraphs below contain the links of this book.

Secretarial Help. For 3 years the pillar of our system remained—to our great good fortune—Beryl Edney. The excellence of her work set the standards; her elegant style and gentle British accent added a touch of distinction to our office. When the Edneys moved to Colorado the whole endeavor threatened to capsize; we were rescued by the beautiful work, kindness, and good cheer of June M. Falcone, Christine M. Bibeault and Kathy V. Zelny; when their help ran out, we appreciated even more the significance of excellent secretarial backing.

Artists and Photographers. The second edition required the drawing of new illustrations, modifying the old ones, and converting hundreds of black and white photographs to full color. Ms. Anne B. Greene stood by with her well-known competence and a smile, even when a "final" drawing continued to bounce back for more changes. Her sketches helped us crystallize our thoughts. Anne Greene was the ideal collaborator. Another totally reliable and patient associate was Jackie Robinson; she was always ready to drop lunch for an urgent photograph if a skin reaction threatened to fade away, and always willing to try for a better print, while George W. Jamieson stood by and took over in emergencies. Arthur A. Hall scanned our documents with great skill and care. Dr. Henri F. Cuénoud remained, as always, an replaceable source of photographic marvels ranging from a rare thrombus to spiked rye growing along a fence in his garden.

Help on Special Topics. Besides the long list compiled for the first edition, we have special gratitude to many who were generous of their time. In no particular order, but beginning from the University of Massachusetts Medical School: Dr. Merrill K. Wolf (regeneration of neurons), Dr. Irma O. Szymanski (stem cells), Dr. Lawrence D. Recht (stem cells), Dr. Diane M. Savarese (review of Chapter 34), Dr. Michael Wertheimer (sentinel lymph node, a surgeon's view), Dr. Ashraf Khan (sentinel lymph node, a pathologist's view), Dr. Mark P. Callery (shock), Dr. Gary L. Stein (cell biology), Dr. David A. Drachman (problems of neurons and nervous tissue), and Dr. Aldo A. Rossini (our walking encyclopedia for diabetes and much else). Dr. Thomas W. Smith, whenever called upon, guided us patiently through the idiosyncrasies of neuropathology, such as the vacuoles of spongiform encephalopathies. Dr. Henri F. Cuénoud, the artist, must be thanked once again for his unequaled help in working out mechanisms of pathophysiology, cardiovascular or otherwise. Dr. German Pihan, whom we consulted pitilessly, must have regretted more than once the depth of his knowledge in almost every field of medical science, but he never gave signs of fatigue. We are deeply indebted to Paul R. Odgren for initiating us to the mysteries of microarray technology ("high throughput screening methods"), to Dr. Jeffrey D. Bernhard, Dr. Jag Bhawan of Boston University School of Medicine, and Dr. A. Bernard Ackerman of the Ackerman Academy of Dermatopathology (for never-ending subtle problems of skin diseases), to Dr. Victor E. Gould (of Rush-Presbyterian-St. Luke's Medical Center, Chicago) for advice on tumors *et alia*. Dr. Frederick Grinnell of the University of Texas was most helpful and kind whenever we called him about fibroblasts, Dr. Miguel J. Stadecker of Tufts University Medical School was equally kind and generous when we consulted him again and again about granulomas, Dr. Samuel M. Cohen was ever ready to answer without notice cancer-related questions, and Dr. Charles N. Serhan of

Harvard Medical School went miles out of his way to help us with the progeny of arachidonic acid (Figure 9.33). Dr. Alan S. Cohen of Boston University School of Medicine was our ultimate resource for amyloid, Dr. Arthur M. Dannenberg of Johns Hopkins University was incredibly helpful and read every word of our text on tuberculosis and granulomas (the remaining errors are strictly our own) and even asked us not to thank him, which we will gladly do. And what shall we say about Dr. Graeme B. Ryan, former collaborator, and later Dean of Melbourne Medical School? When called by telephone without warning (in Australia from North America) about an experiment done with us in Switzerland 31 years earlier, within minutes he pulled out the requested color slide of an unpublished rabbit. No wonder they made him dean.

As a last resort, it was a great privilege to know that we could always pick up the telephone and call Dr. George E. Palade, whose wisdom and advice are unique.

To the Italian translators of this book. We owe special gratitude to Professors Salvatore Ruggieri, Massimo Olivotto, and Gabriele Mugnai, of the University of Florence Medical School, Department of General Pathology, who undertook this heavy task on their own, thereby confirming that science—like music—is an international language. Their comments and corrections were very helpful for the present second English edition.

Books and References. Once again we acknowledge with deep gratitude the help, patience, and kindness of the employees of the Lamar Soutter Library, as represented by James F. Comes and Paul H. Julian. John J. Nunnari was a special case. During a chance encounter in a corridor, he correctly interpreted our somber "Hi, John" as a distress call of two overburdened textbook writers, volunteered to help for a month or so, and almost 2 years later was still working in the library during late night hours, churning out computer searches, photocopies and permissions, and finally copying twice and binding the huge pile of folders called The Manuscript. John, may long your chimney smoke.

Dr. Kenneth L. Rock, Chairman of our Pathology Department, contributed to this book in a decisive way by allowing his first two *Professores Emeriti* to retain a large office full of books and memorabilia where a grant-supported faculty member could have been settled.

Apologies, explanations, regrets, and thanks on a large scale is the least we owe to our beloved families and friends, in Switzerland, Italy, the United States, Canada, and elsewhere, who patiently waited for the completion of this manuscript. All we can offer as an excuse is that the time was just as long for us, if not longer.

Publishers. To begin, our warmest thanks go to Kirk Jensen, the former Acquisition Editor of Oxford University Press in New York. Without his vision of General Pathology, we would never have seen this textbook in full color. After his departure our book came under the wing of Nancy Wolitzer, Managing Editor, with Allison Esposito as Copy Editor, and Cathleen Bennett as Book Designer. We are deeply indebted to this team for making the transition so smooth. Eventually Nancy Wolitzer assigned the book to ICC (Interactive Composition Corporation in Portland, Oregon). The task of Production Editor fell to Rozi Harris, with Richard Curwen as Art Coordinator. The collaboration with both the New York and the Oregon groups has been a true pleasure. Nancy's gentle and firm touch, Rozi's instant e-mail responses to a stream of authors' questions, and her cheer will remain proverbial. To Louise Martin, who constructed the Index, go our heartfelt thanks.

And to all those mentioned above go our further heartfelt thanks for their moral support when *all our color slides—hundreds—were lost inexplicably* while in the hands of a national carrier of impeccable reputation. They all came back 62 very long days later. There was no explanation.

Guido Majno, M.D.
Isabelle Joris, Ph.D.

Contents

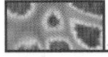

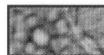 PART II INFLAMMATION

PART III IMMUNOPATHOLOGY

PART IV VASCULAR DISTURBANCES

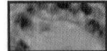

PART V TUMORS

Cells, Tissues, and Disease

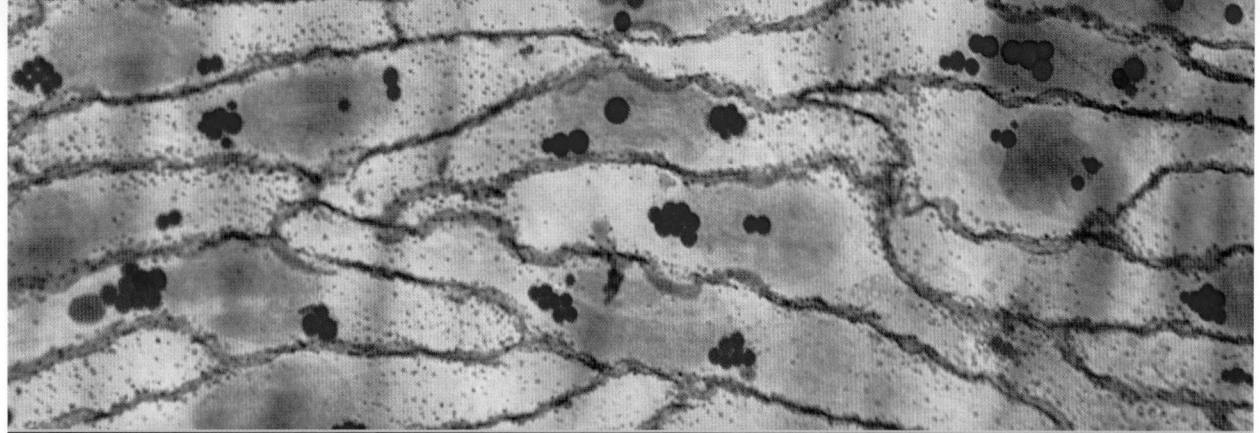

INTRODUCTION

What Is Disease?

As seen through the microscope or in a test tube, disease is fairly easy to define. For every tissue there are standards of form and function, with some allowance for acceptable variance; any deviation from those limits implies disease. Normal bronchi, for example, are lined by ciliated, mucus-secreting epithelium. If this is replaced by squamous stratified epithelium—as is often the case in smokers—the bronchus becomes pathologic; not only structurally, but also functionally, because ciliary motion and mucus secretion are lost.

Disease at the level of the individual is much more difficult to define because the boundaries between normal and abnormal are vague and shifting. But here is an old definition that we can use as a starting point:

> Disease is any condition of the body or mind that decreases the chances of survival of the individual or of the species.

This definition has some merit, but it can be challenged in several ways. First, the threatening condition must be qualified as intrinsic to the body or mind; otherwise flying in an airplane would be a disease. More important, if we base our definition of disease on the threat to survival, it will include two threatening conditions that seem perfectly normal: old age and childbirth. In fact, these two conditions do lie in a gray area. Old age does predispose to disease and death; and childbirth, even though it is the very mechanism for preserving the species, does imply a certain threat to the mother. There are lying-in *hospitals* where mothers are routinely referred to as *patients*.

Another flaw in this definition is that *some diseases can be assets and actually increase the chances of survival.* The best-known example is sickle cell anemia, which confers some protection against malaria (14). Then there is the peculiar case of the basset hound,

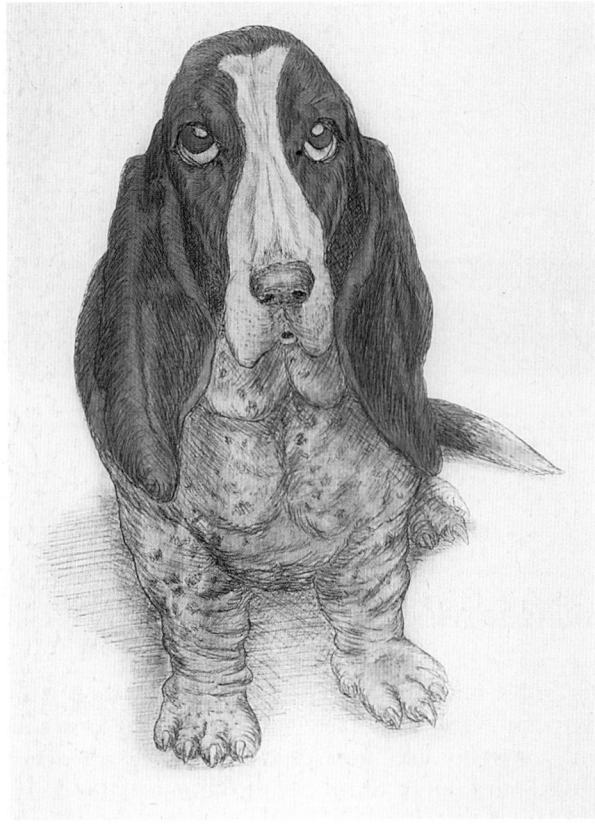

FIGURE I.1   A disease that favored the preservation of a species: the short legs of the basset hound are the result of an inborn defect, achondroplasia. (Etching by Martha Hinson.)

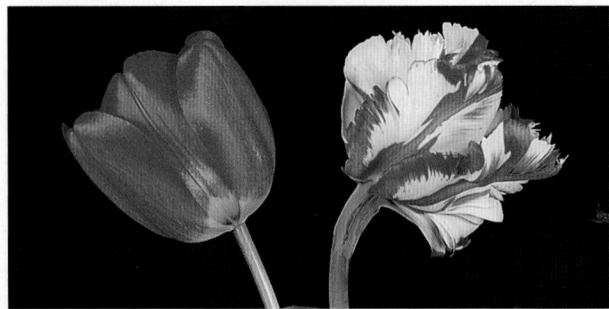

FIGURE I.2   Another disease that favored the preservation of a species: the tulip at the right is infected with a virus of the mosaic type. These Rembrandt or broken tulips are less hardy but much coveted; in Holland in the early 1600s they caused an outbreak of social tulipomania. Tiger lilies are a similar example of "beautiful disease."

which owes its existence to a congenital disease, **achondroplasia.** Dog fanciers decided thousands of years ago to perpetuate this defect, which must have sprung up in a family of hounds. In this condition, the growth of long bones is stopped prematurely, whereas flat bones such as those of the head are unaffected; this is why bassets are small but bright (Figure I.1). So were the medieval court jesters, history's most famous achondroplastics. Horticulturists have provided another example of selected disease: the attractive splotchy color of the so-called Rembrandt tulips is due to a viral infection (Figure I.2) (13).

Not all conditions that suppress reproduction (survival of the species) are diseases: consider celibacy. The case of homosexuality is more complex. For the ancient Greeks it was a godly way of life (Zeus himself fell in love with a human male, Ganymede, snatched him up and gave him a place among the gods). In the Christian world it became a sin, then a crime, and later a disease, which it still is in many countries. Then, in 1973, the American Psychiatric Association eliminated

homosexuality from its roster of diseases (35). Since then, several scientific reports suggested a link between homosexuality and genes (2, 17, 27) but the evidence did not go unchallenged (38). Anyway, if we consider homosexuality just from the standpoint of a "threat to the survival of the species," we should recall that in the most successful insect societies—ants and bees—some individuals are programmed to be sterile, and the species still thrive. It has also been argued that, in human evolution, putative "homosexuality genes" could have been preserved because certain societal roles of homosexuals may have outweighed their weak or negative role in reproduction (40).

Last, it can be argued that *disease in general helps the survival of species by eliminating the unfit.* In this view, disease is not just a curse; it is also a major driving force of evolution (41).

We must conclude that tying the definition of clinical disease to the notion of survival can be misleading. Perhaps we should side with the pessimists who argue that no final definition is possible and that *the clinical notion of disease is colored by the cultural, social, and political climate* (22, 23, 26). There is a great deal of truth in this statement. In our culture the loss of a tooth calls for medical attention; in other cultures teeth are knocked out for beauty. For a Navajo, the fact of having a car accident is the result of a disharmony with Nature (25). In the Soviet Union, opposition to the government was treated as a disease. If we look back into our own not-too-distant history, there are many examples of "diseases" related to the prevailing social climate. In the Napoleonic armies, *nostalgia* was listed as a dangerous contagious disease, and was treated by burying alive the first case to appear (32); during the American Civil

War nostalgia was an accepted complication of wounds. In 1851 the *New Orleans Medical and Surgical Journal* published a "Report on the Diseases/of the Negro Race" (7); one of these diseases was the tendency to run away. It was actually given a scientific name, *drapetomania* (from the Greek *drapetéuein,* "to run away"). Up to the late 1800s, masturbation was considered a dangerous disease; the appropriate therapy was thought to be "preventive" circumcision. Later, the purpose was forgotten but the operation persisted, which is how the United States has become the only country in the world in which nonreligious circumcision is still routinely practiced (16, 37). So here is a supposed mental disease that has left—quite unnecessarily—millions of physical scars.

There is much to be learned from diseases that have disappeared. Some vanished because they were truly eradicated; others vanished because they were a product of erroneous medical theories and faded away as knowledge advanced.

> Just before World War II, one of us (G.M.) received elaborate therapy for a disease that was very common at that time, "dropped stomach," also known as gastroptosis or Glénard's disease. The diagnosis was based on the radiologic misconception that the normal stomach lies in the same horizontal position as seen at autopsy. Now: if a patient standing behind a fluoroscopic screen is asked to swallow a cup of barium sulfate (*barium* means "heavy"), his or her stomach will tend to sag. This means that most people in a radiologist's clinic would be diagnosed as suffering from dropped stomach. As radiologic knowledge advanced, gastroptosis quietly disappeared, but it is a fair guess that we are still living with "diseases" of this kind.

All in all, we are obliged to conclude that the microcosm of individual diseases is related to the macrocosm of society: it depends on time, place, and culture. The same correlation is recognized in the definition of health adopted in 1946 by the World Health Organization (42):

> Health is the state of complete physical, mental, and social well-being, and not only the absence of disease or ailment.

If this is health, the World Health Organization is telling us that poverty, poor housing, and poor education are part of disease, which they certainly are, in the big picture.

Let all this be food for thought. For those who would like to learn what philosophers have to say, several sources are available (20, 27, 28, 29). This book will deal, more modestly, with mechanisms of physical disease within the microcosm of cells and tissues.

Life, Death, and Suspended Life

Anyone interested in disease would also want to know the meaning of life and death (6). We have no final answer, but we can offer a few facts drawn from biology and a few thoughts.

Up to the 1960s, it was safe to define death as *prolonged cessation of respiration and circulation.* Then, advances in technology made both criteria obsolete, and complicated the issue by making it possible to postpone the time of "death" almost indefinitely. So the focus shifted to the brain (5, 31, 34), and the concept of *brain death* was introduced, largely as a "social construct created for utilitarian purposes, primarily to permit organ transplantation" (34). In the United States and in most of Europe, it is agreed that when the electroencephalogram is irreversibly flat, brain death has occurred (Figure I.3); all functions of the brainstem must also be abolished (33): beyond circulation and respiration, these include several reflexes, such as the corneal and the cough reflex (39). However, does brain death coincide with death of the individual? Not

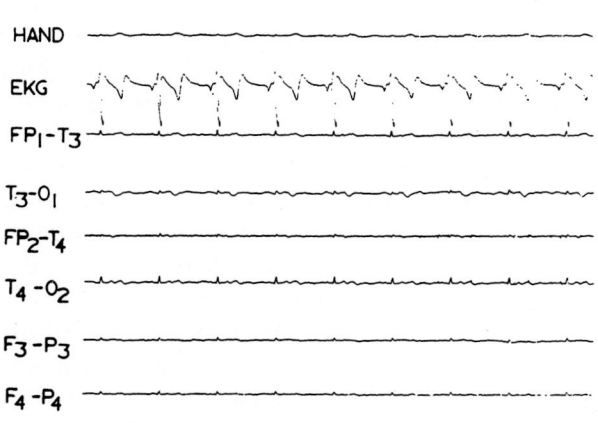

FIGURE I.3 Brain death ("electrocerebral silence") in a head-injured man. The first channel, taken from the back of the hand, is a control to show the baseline noise. The second is the electrocardiogram; the others refer to the brain and show no activity except artifacts correlated with the electrocardiogram. (From Walker AE. Cerebral death, 3rd ed. Baltimore: Urban & Schwarzenberg, 1985; reproduced with permission from [36].)

everywhere (18). In the United States, most states leave that decision to the parents or guardians, but some do not. As of 1990 the Supreme Court ruled 5 to 4 that Nancy Cruzan, who had been brain dead for 7 years, should be kept alive artificially if the State of Missouri so required (1); in that same year, it was estimated that 10,000 Americans were being maintained in irreversible coma because they had not left any clear instructions such as a "living will" (15).

At a purely biological level, cells can continue to live in the absence of both heart and brain, indeed in the absence of the entire body. This is the very principle of cell culture *in vitro:* Should we then accept the cell as the ultimate level of organized life? Probably so, because a key attribute of life as we know it is self-replication, and the cell is the smallest unit that can replicate independently (viruses and prions cannot). It is true that biochemists break up cells and study "surviving" mitochondria, until they, too, eventually die; however, mitochondria that are breathing oxygen in a test tube are alive only in a limited way, because they are unable to self-replicate (mitochondria do replicate *in vivo,* perhaps because they derive from archaic bacterial cells, but they are not known to replicate *in vitro*). So, for the time being, we can assume that there is no life below the level of cells.

While society struggles to fit all this into a new and acceptable definition of somatic death, we must tentatively conclude that *life can exist at several levels,* from the whole body to isolated organs to cells, and perhaps—in part—to subcellular particles. The next question, then, should be: what is the intrinsic difference between a live being and an inanimate object?

One answer could be metabolic processes. This sounds like a defensible proposition, except that *metabolism can be stopped without compromising life.* Scientists who use tissue cultures freeze their cells routinely and store them for as long as 20 years until they are ready to thaw them out and use them. This suggests that life, whatever it may be, can be suspended. So what are the mechanisms of suspended life?

One of the best models of suspended life is the dried food you buy in a pet store to feed aquarium fish: eggs of brine shrimp (Figure I.4). These microscopic eggs can be stored in the dry state for months or years. Placed in water they swell, and 16 hours later they hatch: instant shrimp. A variety of small animals are capable of suspended life in the dry state, including rotifers, nematodes and insects. "Instant insects" wait for the next flood in parched African soils (19). Some are endowed with a nervous system, a digestive tract, and muscle—all it takes to make a respectable multicel-

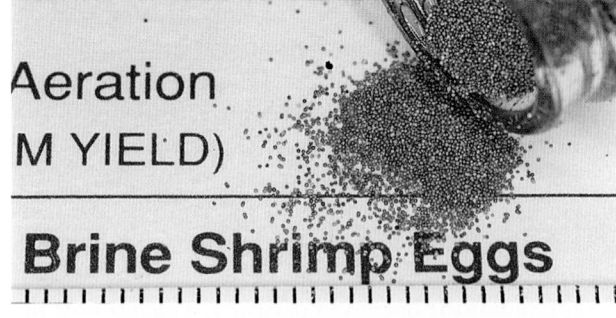

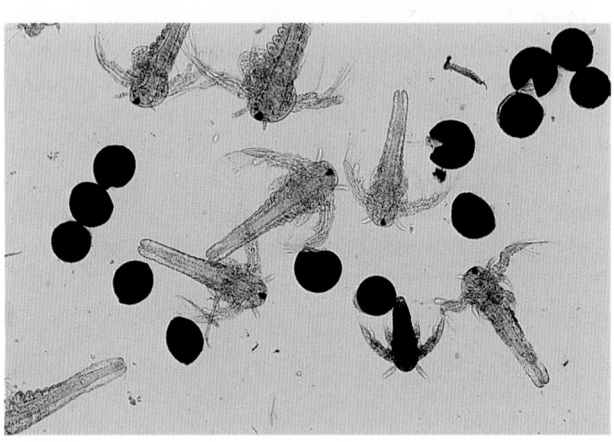

FIGURE I.4   Example of suspended life. *Top:* Commercial dried brine shrimp eggs. Scale in mm. *Bottom:* After 3 days in a suitable medium, the shrimp have hatched. (Courtesy of Dr. H. F. Cuénoud, University of Massachusetts Medical School Worcester, MA.)

lular creature, although usually smaller than one millimeter (8–12).

The first to marvel at "animalcules" that could survive drying was Leeuwenhoek in 1702, but his letter to the Royal Society of London was soon forgotten (10). In 1743 an English Jesuit working in France, John Turberville Needham, rediscovered these creatures in the microscopic eelworms of blighted wheat. He sent a little package of eelworms to the Royal Society, and his discovery was confirmed by Henry Baker, who wrote:

> We find an instance here that life may be suspended and seemingly destroyed; that by an Exhalation of the Fluids necessary to a living Animal, the Circulations may cease, all the Organs and Vessels of the Body may be shrunk up, dried and hardened, and yet, after a long while, Life may begin anew to actuate the same Body and all the animal Motions and Faculties may be restored, merely by replenishing the Organs and Vessels with a fresh supply of Fluid. . . . What life really is, seems as much too subtle for our Understanding to conceive or define, as for our senses to discern and examine. (10)

Needham's discovery was sensational. Was it resurrection? Voltaire attacked it viciously in prose and verse, as "providing weapons for atheistic philosophy" (30). In Italy, Lazzaro Spallanzani (1729–1799), an abbot and one of the greatest biologists of all time, joined Needham's camp. "The phenomenon," he wrote, "confounds the most accepted ideas of animality." While the "admirable resurrections" of nematodes became a form of entertainment in French society, the debate went on and flared up acrimoniously in the 1850s between two sharply divided camps, the resurrectionists and antiresurrectionists. The prestigious French Society of Biology was asked to arbitrate; it did so by nominating a Commission of Seven, presided over by no less than Paul Broca, the physician and anthropologist who discovered the speech center of the brain. The learned men spoke to both parties, met 42 times, dried rotifers as best they could (82 days in a vacuum, plus 30 minutes at 100°C at atmospheric pressure), and yet the creatures "revived in contact with water." Such was the essence of the 60,000-word report published in 1860. However, the group wisely refrained from discussing the metaphysical point: resurrection (10, 28).

Today the argument is avoided by using the new and conveniently ambiguous word *cryptobiosis* (hidden life). There are four subtypes, depending on the mechanism that suspends life: anhydrobiosis (dehydration), cryobiosis (cooling), anoxybiosis (lack of oxygen), and osmobiosis (high salt concentration) (10). As a prototype of cryptobiotic animals we propose the so-called water bears, or tardigrades (slow walkers) (Figure I.5), a name chosen by Spallanzani. These creatures can survive a vacuum of a millionth of a millimeter, heating to 151°C, cooling to near absolute zero (conditions not unlike those of outer space). The record is 120 years of suspended life in the moss of a museum collection; however, in the tardigrades recovered from this specimen, the revival lasted only a few minutes (28).

Cryptobiotic animals exist in all habitats, from the poles to the deserts to anybody's back yard. Leeuwenhoek took them from the lead gutter of his roof. Clearly they have developed their physiology as an adaptive strategy to favor dissemination, to survive hostile environments, and to time their existence with "good days." Their normal life span of a couple of months can be prolonged to something on the order of a century.

The secret of resuscitation from dryness, it is now clear, lies in drying slowly. As the creature on its way to cryptobiosis begins to lose water, it produces several chemicals that will be its passport to survival: especially small sugars, such as sucrose and trehalose, and glycerol,

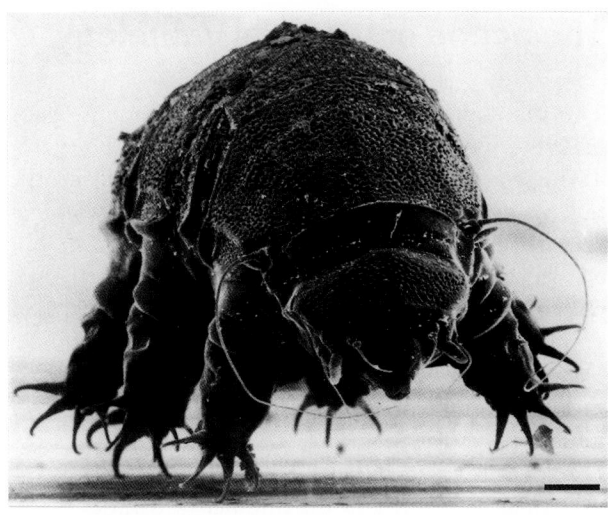

FIGURE I.5 One of the creatures that share the secret of death and resuscitation: a tardigrade, as seen by scanning electron microscopy. The name means "slow walker." **Bar** = 100 μm. (Reproduced by permission from [11].)

another small molecule. As the cellular organelles dry up, these molecules bond to the layers of shriveling proteins, keeping them separate and ready to reexpand (12, 21). In the end, the whole creature appears as if it were embedded in glass (*vitrification* [9]).

This secret, stolen from the tardigrades, has helped prolong the survival of stored human pancreatic islets (4). As to glycerol, it is surely no coincidence that it protects cells against another type of dehydration: freezing. We use it today to preserve frozen red blood cells.

For our purposes, *the most important aspect of cryptobiosis is that metabolism comes to a complete standstill (10).* It was once found that a small amount of oxygen is taken up by cryptobiotic animals kept in air (10), but it then turned out that this uptake indicates damage, not respiration. It is the equivalent of turning rancid by oxidation (11) (free radical injury, p. 196), which has nothing to do with metabolism. Potato chips can do it, too (28).

What does this tell us about life? The resuscitation of cryptobiotic animals suggests that *the critical requirement for life as we know it is a molecular arrangement; a structure that—in the presence of water—behaves like a machine.* Its function is called metabolism. If water is removed or frozen the machine can stop for a limited time; otherwise it grinds forth toward its basic goal, replication.

In essence, then, the message whispered by the tardigrades seems to be—*life is a molecular machine.*

The Scope of General Pathology

The number of possible diseases is enormous. Back in 1980, we asked a medical student, now Dr. C. S. Taylor, to count them. He spent several weeks on the task using mainly the *International Classification of Diseases* and came up with the figure of 8,294, but warned us that the true figure was probably greater, perhaps 30,000.

Then came molecular medicine and the Human Genome Project, and virtually all tumors turned out to be the result of hundreds and even thousands of mutations—suggesting that two tumors of the same histological type may never be exactly the same at the molecular level. Perhaps the number of diseases is uncountable, but this makes our point even more cogent. Clearly the parts—and the mechanisms—of the body can go wrong in an infinite number of ways, helped by thousands of genes, parasites, toxic agents, and other environmental causes. If each one of these agents caused a special type of disease, different from all others, learning medicine or pathology would be a hopeless task. Fortunately, this is not the case. Bacteria, for example, are of many types, but their ways of producing disease fall into a few categories: they all tend to elicit tissue reactions known as *inflammation* and *immune response*, and they all produce fever by similar pathways. *The purpose of general pathology is to work out these common pathways.*

And so it was learned, step by step, that the basic processes at work in disease can be grouped under five main headings, which are covered in the five parts of this book.

The Jargon of Pathology: A Few Key Terms

The reader will be well advised to absorb in advance the following few basic terms. They may sound empirical and imprecise, and so they are: some are at least 2500 years old. But they are practical.

The Topography of Disease

The following terms are illustrated in Figure I.6.

- **Focal** is said of a disease limited to a discrete, well-limited *focus* (e.g., a boil); the plural is *foci*. **Localized** means limited to a given part (e.g., a hand, a lobe of the lung).

- **Diffuse** means that the disease affects a large area (e.g., pneumonia can diffusely affect a whole lung) rather than forming discrete foci.
- **Disseminated** means scattered in many small foci.
- **Systemic** should be used to mean spread throughout a single system (like the nervous system). It is sometimes used loosely and improperly as a synonym of *generalized.*
- **Generalized** means spread through the entire body (e.g., an infection spread by the bloodstream).

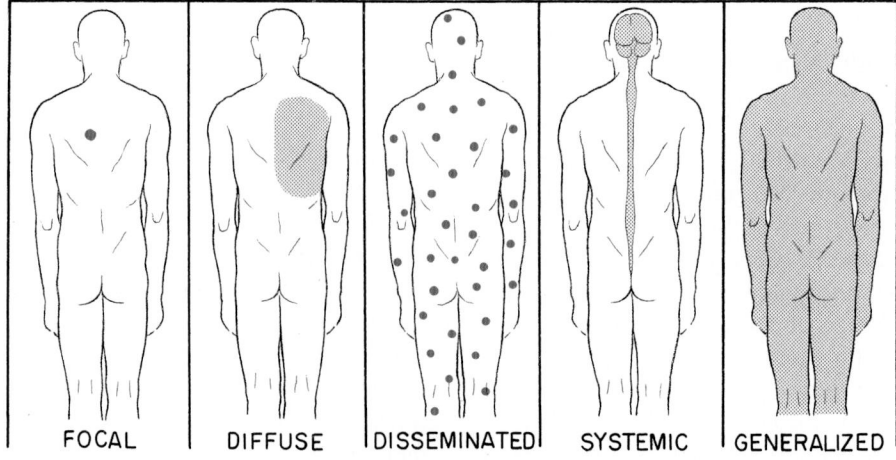

FOCAL   DIFFUSE   DISSEMINATED   SYSTEMIC   GENERALIZED

FIGURE I.6   Five terms referring to the topographic distribution of disease in the body.

The Time Course of Disease

- **Acute** means "coming sharply to a climax"; changes (good or bad) are occurring rapidly. It does not mean severe, although many acute diseases are severe. In terms of real time, acute can mean anything from minutes to a few days (e.g., acute appendicitis).
- **Chronic** means long-lasting. It usually refers to weeks, months, or years.
- **Subacute** means "not very acute," and **subchronic** means "not very chronic" (imprecision compounded by imprecision, but again very handy to describe clinical situations).

***

- **Pathogenesis** refers to the steps whereby an agent brings about disease. It concerns the mechanisms rather than the causes. For example, pollen is the cause of hay fever, but the pathogenesis of hay fever requires many steps: pollen proteins are picked up by macrophages, which pass them on to appropriate lymphocytes, which produce antibodies, which sensitize mast cells, which respond to the pollen antigens by releasing inflammatory agents.
- **Differential diagnosis** is the exercise of listing in orderly fashion all possible diagnoses of a given condition, usually from the most likely to the least likely (e.g., a lump on the head could be a mass of spilled blood, a tumor of the skin, a tumor of the skull, a metastatic tumor of an internal organ, an abscess, or a congenital defect).

Armed with these basic means of communication, we can now begin our trek through the world of disease.

References

1. Annas GJ. Nancy Cruzan and the right to die. N Engl J Med 1990;323:670–673.
2. Barinaga M. Is homosexuality biological? Science 1991; 253:956–957.
3. Bayer R. Homosexuality and American psychiatry. The politics of diagnosis. Princeton: Princeton University Press, 1987.
4. Beattie GM, Crowe JH, Lopez AD, Cirulli V, Ricordi C, Hayek A. Trehalose: a cryoprotectant that enhances recovery and preserves function of human pancreatic islets after long-term storage. Diabetes 1997;46:519–523.
5. Bernat JL. A defense of the whole-brain concept of death. Hastings Center Rep 1998;March-April:14–23.
6. Botkin JR, Post SG. Confusion in the determination of death: distinguishing philosophy from physiology. Perspect Biol Med 1992;36:129–138.
7. Cartwright SA. Report on the diseases and physical peculiarities of the Negro race. In: Caplan AL, Engelhardt HT Jr, McCartney JJ (eds). Concepts of health and disease. Interdisciplinary perspectives. Reading, MA: Addison-Wesley Publishing Company, 1981, pp. 305–325.
8. Clegg JS. Interrelationships between water and cellular metabolism in Artemia cysts. XI. Density measurements. Cell Biophys 1984;6:153–169.
9. Crowe JH, Carpenter JF, Crowe LM. The role of vitrification in anhydrobiosis. Annu Rev Physiol 1998;60:73–103.
10. Crowe JH, Clegg JS (eds). Anhydrobiosis. Stroudsberg: Dowden, Hutchinson & Ross, Inc., 1973, pp. 8–50.
11. Crowe JH, Cooper AF Jr. Cryptobiosis. Sci Am 1971;225: 30–36.
12. Crowe JH, Crowe LM. Induction of anhydrobiosis: membrane changes during drying. Cryobiology 1982;19:317–328.
13. Dubos RJ. Tulipomania and the benevolent virus. Perspect Virol 1959;1:291–299.
14. Eaton JW, Wood PA. Antimalarial red cells. Prog Clin Biol Res 1984;165:395–412.
15. Friedrich O. A limited right to die. *Time,* July 9, 1990, p. 59.
16. Gollaher DL. Circumcision: a history of the world's most controversial surgery. New York: Basic Books, 2000.
17. Hamer DH, Hu S, Magnuson VL, Hu N, Pattatucci AM. A linkage between DNA markers on the X chromosome and male sexual orientation. Science 1993;261:321–327.
18. Haupt WF, Rudolf J. European brain death codes: a comparison of national guidelines. J Neurol 1999;246:432–437.
19. Hinton HE. A new Chironomid from Africa. Proc Zool Soc 1951;121:371–380.
20. Humber JM, Almeder RF (eds). What is disease? Totowa, NJ: Humana Press, 1997.
21. Kandror O, DeLeon A, Goldberg AL. Trehalose synthesis is induced upon exposure of *Escherichia coli* to cold and is essential for viability at low temperatures. Proc Natl Acad Sci USA 2002;99:9727–9732.
22. King LS. What is disease? Phil Sci 1954;21:193–203.
23. King LS. Medical thinking. A historical preface. Princeton: Princeton University Press, 1982.
24. LeVay S. A difference in hypothalamic structure between heterosexual and homosexual men. Science 1991;253:1035–1037.
25. Majno G. The lost secret of ancient medicine. In: Bulger RJ (ed). In search of the modern Hippocrates. Iowa City: University of Iowa Press, 1987, pp. 146–155.
26. Pérez Tamayo R. El concepto de enfermedad, 2 volumes. Mexico: Fondo de Cultura Económica, 1988.
27. Pool R. Evidence for homosexuality gene. Science 1993;261: 291–292.
28. Rensberger B. Life in limbo. *Science 80,* November 1980, pp. 36–43.
29. Reznek L. The nature of disease. New York: Routledge & Kegan Paul, 1987.
30. Roe S. Voltaire versus Needham: atheism, materialism, and the generation of life. J Hist Ideas 1985;46:65–87.
31. Shewmon DA. "Brainstem death," "Brain death" and death: a critical re-evaluation of the purported equivalence. Issues Law Med 1998;14:125–145.
32. Starobinski J. The idea of nostalgia. Diogenes 1966;54: 92–115.
33. Sullivan J, Seem DL, Chabalewski F. Determining brain death. Crit Care Nurse 1999;19:37–46.

34. Taylor RM. Reexamining the definition and criteria of death. Semin Neurol 1997;17:265–270.

35. U.S. Dept. of Health and Human Services. The international classification of diseases, 9th revision. Clinical modification, volume I, diseases tabular list, 2nd edition, September 1980. DHHS publication No. (PHS) 80-1260, Washington, D.C.

36. Walker AE. Cerebral death, 3rd ed. Baltimore: Urban & Schwarzenberg, 1985.

37. Wallerstein E. Circumcision: an American health fallacy. New York: Springer Publishing Company, 1980.

38. Wickelgren I. Discovery of "gay gene" questioned. Science 1999;284:571.

39. Wijdicks EFM. The diagnosis of brain death. N Engl J Med 2001;344:1215–1221.

40. Wilson EO. Sociobiology. The new synthesis. Cambridge: Harvard University Press, 1975.

41. Wolbach SB. The glorious past, the doleful present and the uncertain future of pathology. Harvard Med Alumni Bull 1954;June:45–48.

42. World Health Organization. Constitution of the World Health Organization. New York: WHO Interim Commission, 1946.

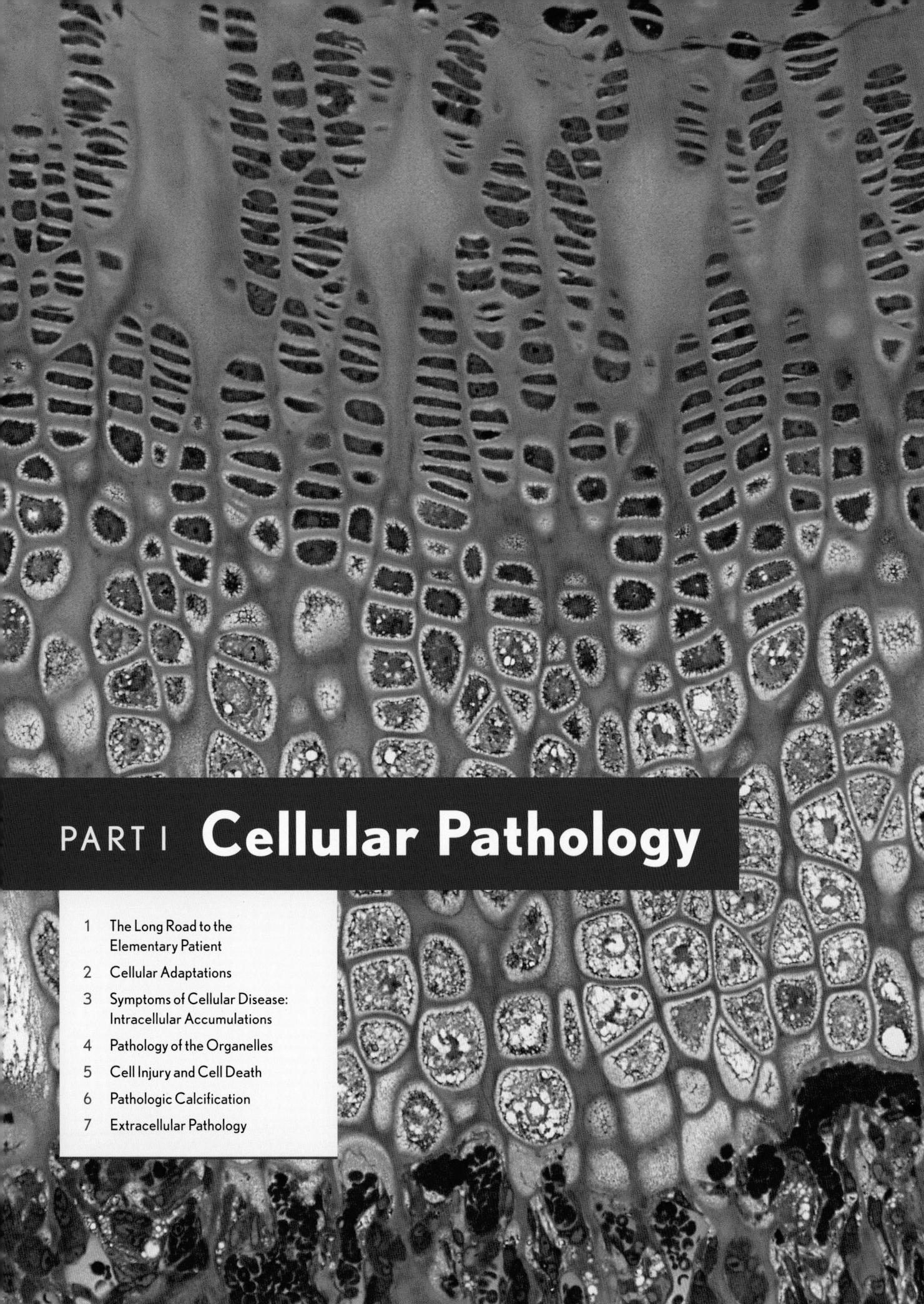

PART I Cellular Pathology

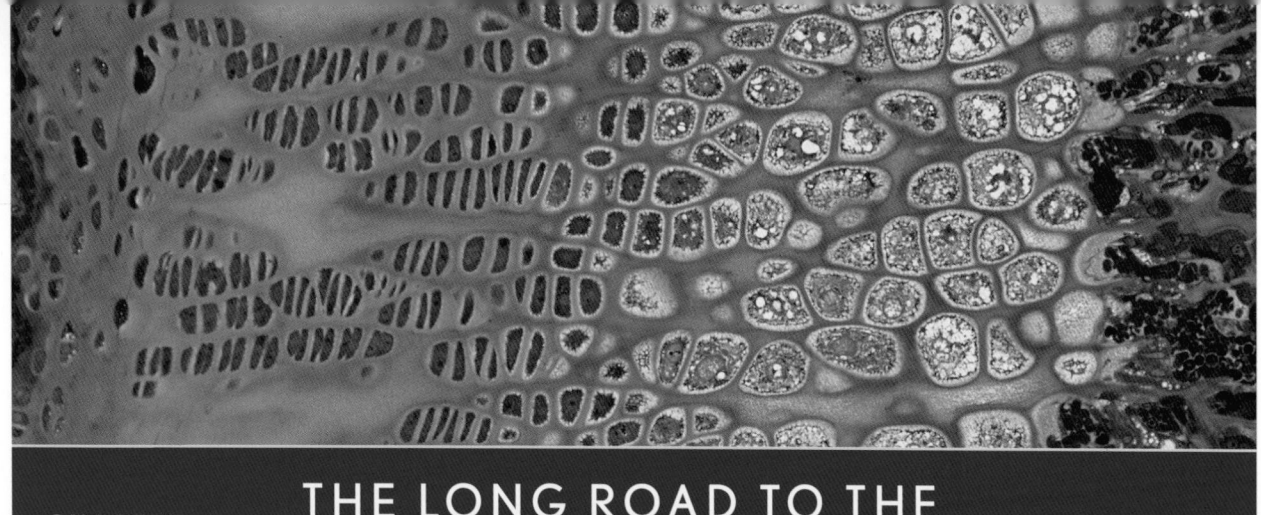

CHAPTER 1

THE LONG ROAD TO THE ELEMENTARY PATIENT

Every branch of science has its elementary unit; for physics it is the atom, for chemistry the molecule. *Medicine is both art and science; as an art, its elementary unit has always been the patient; as a science, its unit is the cell.*

Because they lacked this basic unit, our ancestors were obliged for thousands of years to struggle for some way to explain disease. Primal people blame several mechanisms; the most common are magic curses, intrusion of some extraneous object into the body, punishment, or even loss of the soul (Figure 1.1): the specific function of the shaman (a word of Siberian origin) is precisely to go and retrieve the patient's lost soul.

The ancient Greeks broke away from this pattern. Although they were a very religious people, they felt that the gods were not necessarily involved in disease. They blamed natural causes, such as a "breath" or "wind" (a similar thought also prevailed in China). According to the Hippocratic school (ca. 400 B.C.), the body was composed of four humors that were normally blended in a delicate fashion; any imbalance of the humors caused disease. The four humors were blood, phlegm, yellow bile, and black bile; exactly how they were chosen is not clear. Note that this theory focuses entirely on internal causes and leaves no space for infection. In fact, the ancient Greeks ignored infection entirely; they did not even have a word for it (*infection* comes from Latin).

The theory of the four humors was especially convenient because it implies that there is only one disease—an imbalance of humors—and correspondingly only one therapy: removing fluids in any possible way—by bleeding, purging, emptying the stomach by vomiting, and even sweating—in the hope of giving the humors a fresh start. The theory was so successful that it lasted into our own days: in his childhood, the senior author of this book was purged for every minor ailment (bleeding was already frowned upon); the younger author was treated for bronchitis with suction cups that were supposed to draw out bad humors. Even now we

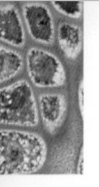

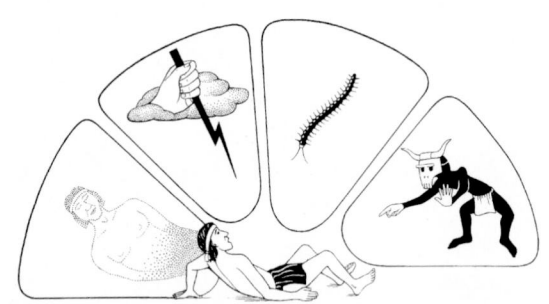

FIGURE 1.1   Four primal concepts of disease: loss of the soul, divine punishment, intrusion of a foreign body or creature, and a spell cast by a witch.

refer to the four humors when we speak of someone being phlegmatic, sanguine, choleric, or melancholic (from *mélas,* "black," and *cholé,* "bile").

The healers of antiquity did make some progress with regard to surgical wounds and fractures, but internal diseases remained a mystery: it is practically impossible to repair a machine without knowing how it is made and how it works. The first systematic approach to dissection in the Western world occurred at that magnificent, state-supported institution called the Museum ("Place of the Muses") in Alexandria of Egypt, around 300 B.C.; the names *prostate* and *duodenum* come from that time. Those Greeks working at Alexandria had no microscope, but they had what they called the "eye of the mind": they used it so well that two of our key microscopic concepts, **tissue** and **parenchyma,** were created then and there (4).

After these and many other great achievements, such as measuring the diameter of the earth, the flame of the Museum flickered out. Experimentation was revived in the second century A.D. by another Greek, Galen, who was born in Pergamon (Asia Minor) and studied at Alexandria but worked in Rome. Galen dissected animals, both dead and alive; it was by dissecting a live pig that he discovered the function of Galen's nerve, the recurrent laryngeal nerve (when he cut it, the squeal of the unfortunate pig became inaudible). Galen also observed the effects of partial and total section of the spinal cord and went as far as refuting one of the pet notions of antiquity: that arteries contain air. Again using a live animal, Galen proved beyond a doubt that arteries contained blood.

Later, the western Roman Empire collapsed and the turbulent conditions of Europe were no climate for scholarly efforts. Social conditions favorable to dissection finally appeared in Italy in the late thirteenth century; the first small textbook of anatomy was written around 1316 by Mondino de' Luzzi in Bologna (it had

39 editions). In those days it was a heroic enterprise to dissect a human corpse. As mentioned in the Preface, consider the realities of performing an autopsy on a partially decomposed body without rubber gloves, antiseptics, fixatives, running water, refrigeration, or notions of infection. Many an early dissector must have died of tuberculosis contracted at an autopsy. Furthermore, religion took a dim view of any such intrusion into the dead body. One of the Church's concerns was the removal of bodily parts, in view of future resurrection. It was specifically forbidden to boil dead bodies to produce "clean" skeletons, hence a complaint of Mondino de' Luzzi, who thought that he would have better understood the inner ear if he could have boiled the temporal bone: he refrained from doing so because it was a sin (*peccatum*).

As the first universities were born in the late Middle Ages, dissection became a major part of the medical curriculum, and chairs of anatomy were established. This means that the anatomists were also the first pathologists: inevitably, during their dissections, anatomists came across abnormal organs and provided us with the first descriptions of internal disease.

As the practice of "anatomies" continued—today we prefer to say autopsies—better and better descriptions of diseased organs were given. The most systematic came from the pen of Giovanni Battista Morgagni, Professor of Anatomy in Padua (1682–1771). His book, *On the Seats and Causes of Disease Investigated by Anatomy,* was published in 1761. For each case, Morgagni considered first the clinical history and then attempted to explain it by the autopsy, pioneering in what we now call clinicopathologic correlations. He used no illustrations, but as soon as color printing was invented, medical illustrations became a form of art. A spectacular collection of such illustrations is the huge atlas published in Paris by G. B. Cruveilhier (1829–1842). Torn out of their context, many of its plates now decorate the walls of pathologists' offices (Figure 1.2).

These masterpieces show both the achievements and the limitations of dissection. Some basic correlations could be established beyond a doubt. Perforations or obstructions of the intestine could easily explain disease and death; compression of the main bile duct by a tumor could easily be correlated with jaundice. But the ultimate mechanism of disease could not be worked out: it was fine to describe an internal abscess, but nobody knew what an abscess really was.

Without a framework of basic data, therapy could make no progress. By 1850, European medicine was grinding to a halt. Even surgery, potentially improved by

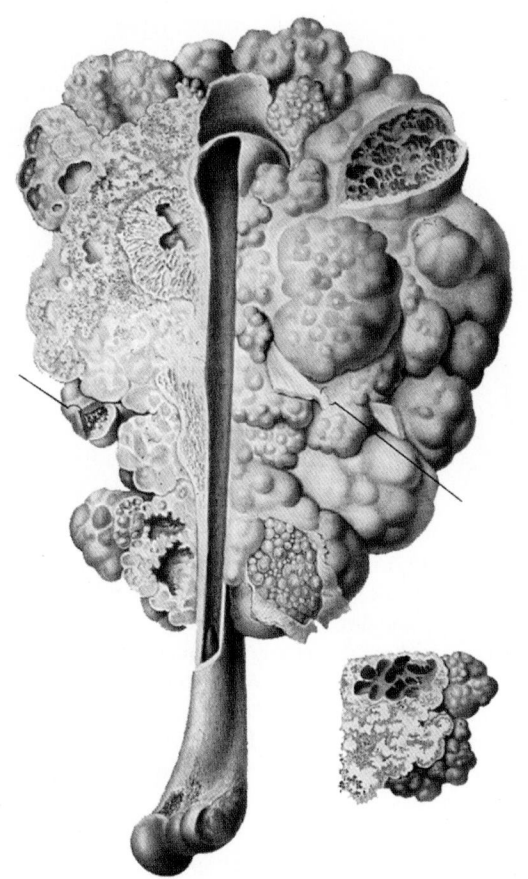

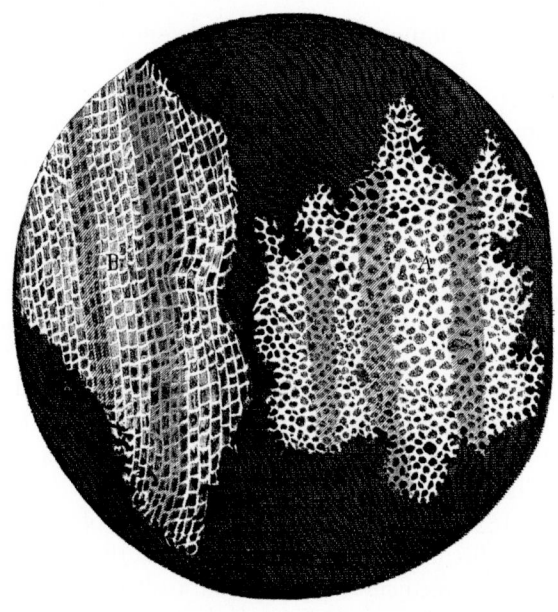

FIGURE 1.2   A plate from the famed atlas of Jean Cruveilhier (Anatomie pathologique du corps humain) (2) showing a malignant tumor of the femur. The physicians of that time had learned to describe beautifully what they saw, although they could not do much about it. (Tome II, Livraison 34, Plate 4.)

FIGURE 1.3   First illustration of cells by Robert Hooke in 1665 (3). The drawing represents a longitudinal and transversal section of cork. Writes Hooke (3, p. 116): "In several . . . Vegetables, . . . I have with my *Microscope,* plainly enough discover'd these Cells . . . [But regarding tissues of] Animals I have not hitherto been able to say anything positive. . . . Though, me thinks, it seems very probable, that Nature has in these passages, as well as in those of Animal bodies, very many appropriated Instruments and contrivances, whereby to bring her designs and end to pass, which 'tis not improbable, but that some diligent Observer, if help'd with better *Microscopes,* may in time detect."

a much better knowledge of anatomy, was paralyzed by infection. Internal medicine could offer some diagnoses, thanks to knowledge gained from autopsies, but practically no cures. It was clear to many that a new approach was needed. But what approach?

The answer was at hand. Today it seems obvious, but in the darkness nothing is obvious. The first clue came from botany: a whole new Promised Land could be reached through the microscope. The basic structure of plants (compared with that of the brain or the liver) is starkly simple: each cell is individually packaged in a box that retains its walls even after the cell is dead. In fact, the term **cell** was originally applied to the "empty boxes" of cork (Figure 1.3). In 1838, Matthias Jacob Schleiden, lawyer, botanist, and physician, published a momentous paper stating that plants are made of microscopic units, or cells. Then, one evening after dinner, Schleiden had a chat with a younger colleague named

Theodor Schwann (1810–1882). Schwann, a creative anatomist and physiologist, had recently discovered nucleated cells in animal tissues. Instantly, thanks to that conversation, he saw the light: *all plant and animal tissues are made of individual microscopic units.* The result was his famous book, published in 1839, entitled *Microscopic Researches on the Similarity in Structure and Function of Animals and Plants.* He was made professor of anatomy and physiology in Louvain (Belgium) and did little else thereafter, but he had hit on one of the most important generalizations in the history of biology. At long last biology had its elementary unit, the cell.

Plant and animal tissues could now be seen in a new light, and it became immediately obvious that the entire field of disease had to be restudied in the context of the cell. All revolutions have a hero, and the hero of cellular pathology is Rudolf Virchow (1821–1902), Professor of Pathology and Therapy in Berlin. He was a man of gigantic intellect, a statesman and an anthropologist as well as a physician and scientist (1). Despite

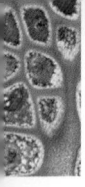

his overwhelming professional and political commitments, he found time to help Schliemann discover the treasures of ancient Troy and to edit three journals of anthropology as well as the prestigious *Archiv für pathologische Anatomie und Physiologie,* now known as *Virchow's Archiv.* Few medical journals can match its record of continuous publication since 1847. Virchow also realized that social conditions can create disease, fought for the rights of the underprivileged, even took to the barricades in 1848, lost his academic position, and had to leave Berlin. Eight years later, however, he was recalled with full honors, including the directorship of a "Pathological Institute" built for him. Eventually he became a member of the Prussian parliament, and as such he continued to press for social reform.

In 1858, just 19 years after the birth of the cell theory, Virchow gave a set of 20 lectures that changed the face of medicine. Collected in a small book entitled (in translation) *Cellular Pathology as Based upon Physiological and Pathological Histology* (5), these lectures conveyed a new point of view: *disease cannot be understood unless it is realized that the ultimate abnormality must lie in the cell.* The body, therefore, had to be understood as a cell-state in which every cell is a citizen; "a society of living cells, a tiny well-ordered state, with all the accessories—high officials and underlings, servants and masters. . . . The human individual is also a commonwealth" (6, pp. 130, 138). It was a revelation. So forceful was its impact that by the end of the century Virchow's word was gospel.

Virchow used the microscope but also drew the best he could from the chemistry and physiology of his time. As a matter of fact, we owe him a marvelous, functional definition of pathology: *pathology is physiology with obstacles* (6, p. 81).

Many of the terms we use today—thrombosis, leukemia, atrophy, hypertrophy, amyloid, myelin, teratoma—were created by Virchow. His feats are all the more astounding if we consider that in 1858 methods for embedding and for cutting thin sections of tissues were not available. His drawings show the effort of reproducing thick, three-dimensional structures as he saw them in slivers of fresh tissue cut by hand (Figure 1.4).

In essence, modern pathology is based squarely on Virchow's cellular pathology: this is why Part One of this book deals with the cell as the elementary patient. Modern cell biology makes this concept even more fitting because it portrays the cell as an individual little creature with a skeleton, a musculature, digestive organs, respiratory organs, a synthetic apparatus that functions like a microscopic liver, and of course a skin. Clinicians now think in terms of cellular receptors and organelles, and

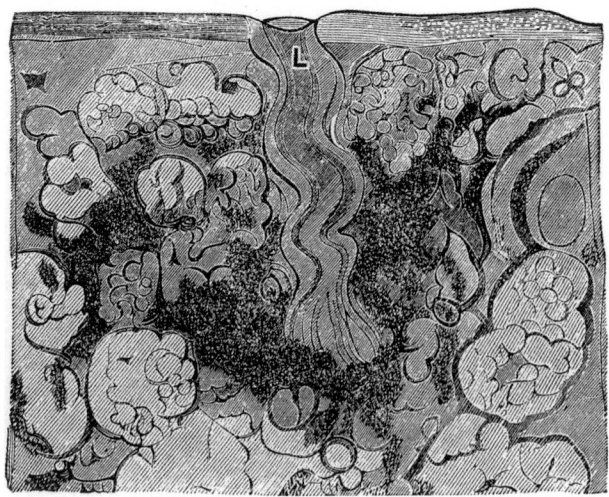

FIGURE 1.4   Illustration from Virchow's *Cellular Pathology* (1858) (5). It shows that microscope sections at that time were really slabs of tissue sliced with a razor and examined unstained; the thickness of the slice is clearly indicated by the perspective at the top. Shown here is a lymph node from the axilla of a tattooed sailor; the black mass in the center represents red pigment (cinnabar). The winding vessel (**L**) is a lymphatic. It is actually seen more clearly here than in modern thin sections.

they treat with drugs that select specific cellular targets. Even shock, the ultimate "total," whole body disease, is now recognized as a generalized cellular disease.

The last two decades have produced an even finer, "molecular" pathology, capable of revealing minute flaws in genes and their products. And yet, although we now can study disease at no less than eight levels of complexity, from populations to single genes (Figure P-1), at each level, *disease ultimately makes sense only in the context of the elementary patient—the cell.*

References

1. Ackerknecht EH. Rudolf Virchow: doctor, statesman, anthropologist. Madison: University of Wisconsin Press, 1953.
2. Cruveilhier J. Anatomie pathologique du corps humain, 2 vols. Paris: J.B. Baillière, 1829–1842.
3. Hooke R. Micrographia. London: John Martyn and Alleftry, 1665.
4. Majno G. The healing hand. Man and wound in the ancient world. Cambridge: Harvard University Press, 1975.
5. Virchow R. Cellular pathology as based upon physiological and pathological histology. (Translated from 2nd German ed. by B. Chance, 1859, reproduced by Dover Publications, New York, 1971.)
6. Virchow R. Disease, life and man. (Translated by L.J. Rather.) Stanford: Stanford University Press, 1958.

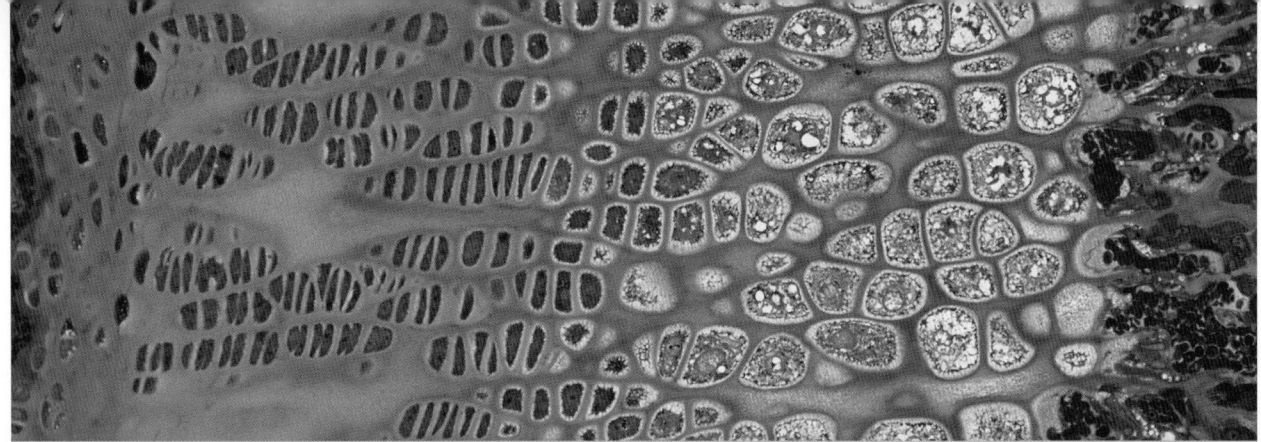

CHAPTER 2   CELLULAR ADAPTATIONS

Disease affects individual cells as it affects individual human beings: it causes changes in structure, function, and social behavior. The problem of diagnosing cellular disease is not as difficult as it may seem because, fortunately for pathologists, most cellular malfunctions are accompanied by structural changes, which are easier to identify. Furthermore, *structural changes guide us to the underlying functional problems.* For example, unusual droplets of a phospholipid point to a metabolic problem affecting phospholipids; hemoglobin escaping from red blood cells points to a defect in the red cell membrane.

Quite a few cellular changes are visible to the naked eye. Hypertrophic muscles in body builders can be seen without a microscope; droplets of fat in liver cells change the color of that organ from deep red to yellow, and grains of hemosiderin (a form of stored iron) change the color to a rusty brown. For this reason, *the naked eye is an important guide in searching for pathologic tissues.* After the microscope has provided its answers, the path is clear to countless histochemical, biochemical, functional, and molecular tests.

A powerful tool for cellular diagnosis is a computer-assisted device called **fluorescence-activated cell sorter** (FACS) (Figure 2.1), which can provide almost instantly quantitative answers regarding size, shape, or specific qualities of as few as 10,000 cells. Presently (2003), it can distinguish in human blood more than 100 subsets of lymphocytes (45a).

For cells, as for human beings, there are degrees, or "shades," of normality. An athlete may weigh three or four times as much as an ascetic monk, yet both are normal; they just differ in their adaptations to the calls of life, and both face certain hazards due to their adaptations. Similarly, cells can respond to various stimuli by adaptations that are not truly pathologic, although they may open the door to disease. They may

- Multiply to replace losses (regeneration)
- Increase in number above normal (hyperplasia)
- Increase in size (hypertrophy, polyploidy)

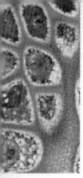

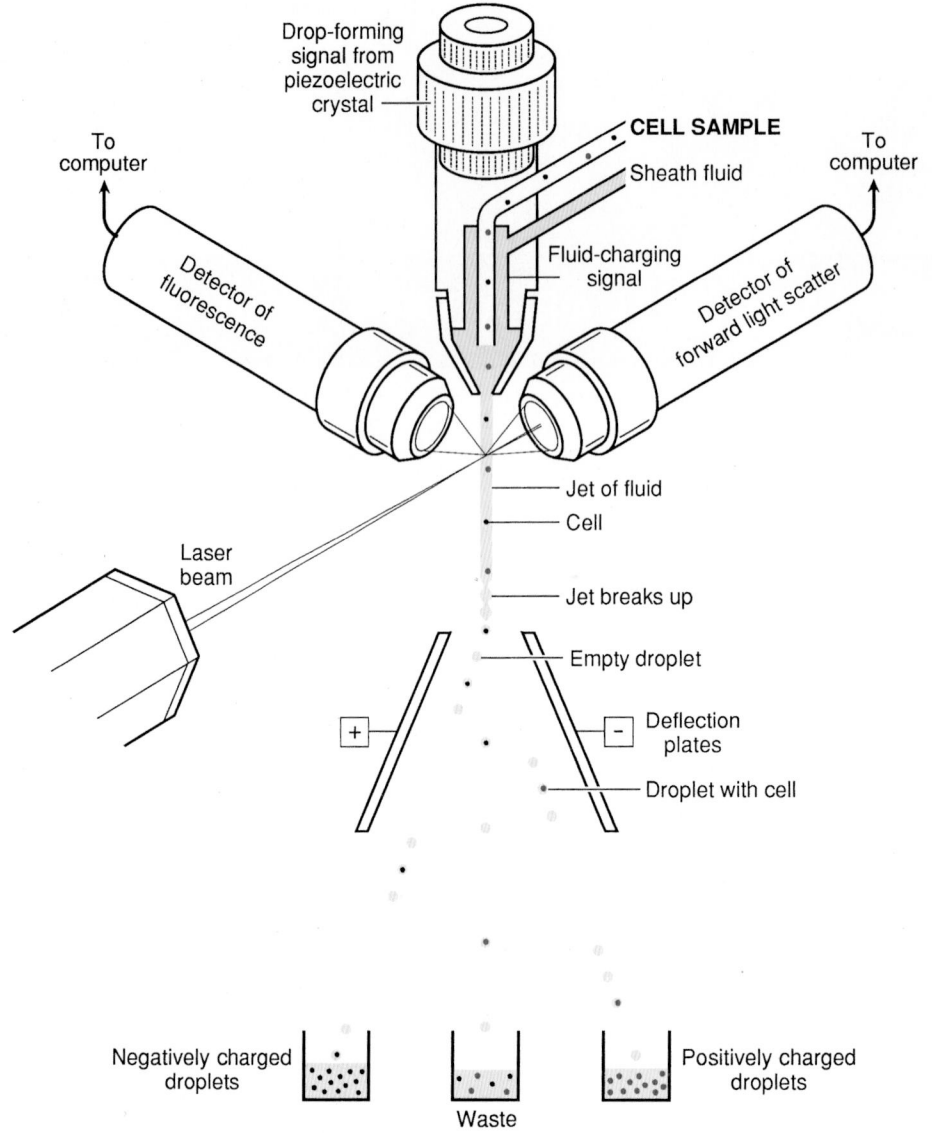

FIGURE 2.1   The principle of fluorescence-activated flow cytometry. In this example, two types of cells are fed into the cytometer (fluorescent and nonfluorescent, which will have to be sorted out by being assigned either a positive or a negative charge). The cells emerge from the nozzle in a threadlike stream; single cells flow in the axis of the stream, surrounded by a sheath of fluid. As each cell is individually hit by the laser beam, the cytometer senses whether it is fluorescent or not and advises the computer, which will then decide whether the cell should be charged positively or negatively. The charge is instantly applied to the stream, and as the stream breaks up into droplets, each droplet maintains the charge that the stream had. The droplets then pass between two charged plates, which deflect the droplets right or left depending on their charge. The flow is adjusted in such a manner that (ideally) one droplet containing a single cell is flanked by two empty droplets with the same charge. In some cases the computer's decision is aborted, and these droplets are collected as waste. (Adapted from [79].)

- Become smaller (atrophy)
- Modify their phenotype reversibly (modulation)
- Be replaced by different types of cells (metaplasia)
- Adapt their organelles (subcellular adaptations)

On this tremendous span of cellular adaptability hinges our capacity to meet the challenges of this dangerous world. We begin our trek through cellular pathology by reviewing these adaptations.

Regeneration: The Era of the Stem Cells

Any part of the body can be lost through accident or disease. If the individual survives, the part can *sometimes* be replaced; to know when and how we must learn the rules of the game, which are changing.

Two Levels of Regeneration

One rule that still holds is that *mammals can replace cells and tissues, but not organs or limbs* (29). This higher capacity is limited to "lower" animals, such as lizards, which can grow a new tail; it requires the coordinated regeneration of many tissues, a process once known as **reconstitution** (122), a very convenient term that somehow disappeared. Most mammals cannot replace ("reconstitute") even the root of a hair; if you have a scar, you may have noticed that it is hairless (48, 61).

This being said, there are some partial exceptions. There is one set of microscopic organs that even human beings unfailingly replace: small blood vessels (capillaries, arterioles, and venules). Without this exception, wound healing would be virtually impossible.

> It has also been reported that children under the age of 4 ½ years can reconstitute the tip of a finger if it has been cleanly severed and if the amputation falls beyond the distal phalangeal joint (47, 75, 76). Similar findings have been reported in mice (24). The published documents are not very convincing; they do show, however, that repair in young age is excellent. The most interesting conclusion of these studies is that optimal regeneration occurs if the raw surface is not occluded by a dressing, which inhibits growth.

Whatever regrowth does occur in these childrens' fingers, the average male deer would not be impressed. He is able to regrow a new set of antlers each year, a startling example of reconstitution (62) (Figure 2.2); antlers are complex organs made of bone, skin, nerves, and a large supply of blood vessels. There are other minor examples among mammals: rabbits and cats can repair holes punched into their ears but only up to a point. In fact, the expression *ear-marking* proves that notches or holes in mammalian ears—with a few exceptions (104)—tend to be permanent (63). It has been speculated that mammals never developed the ability to regenerate limbs because it could not confer a selective advantage: by the time a mammal could regenerate a whole limb, it would have succumbed to predators or to starvation (63).

The Old Dogma: Three Types of Cells

In 1894, an Italian professor of general pathology, Giulio Bizzózero, a pupil of Camillo Golgi, was looking for some basic law regarding regeneration. He noticed

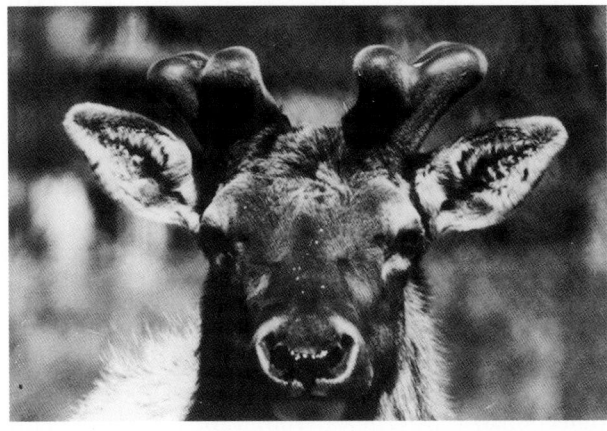

FIGURE 2.2 Antler buds are among the fastest-growing mammalian tissues. This wapiti's buds will elongate at the rate of about 17.5 mm/day. The regeneration of antlers is a rare example of organ reconstitution (as opposed to tissue regeneration) in mammals. (Reproduced from [62].)

that there was a link between the occurrence of mitoses in a given type of normal tissue and its capacity to regenerate (18) and concluded that all cells fall into one of three categories: *labile cells,* which show mitoses throughout life and regenerate incessantly (e.g., bone marrow, epidermis); *stable cells,* in which spontaneous mitoses are uncommon after birth but do occur in response to stimuli (e.g., connective tissue, liver cells); and *permanent* cells, which "never" show mitoses in the adult and do not regenerate (e.g., striated muscle and neurons; later additions were the cells of the crystalline lens, the Sertoli cells, the hair cells of the cochlea, and the glomerular podocytes [118, 154]). This three-fold classification soon acquired the status of dogma, because it fits neatly with daily experience. Some exceptions did show up, providing that in matters biological, "never" is almost never true: in striated muscle, for example, mitoses do occur after injury; but overall the rule still worked. Today, the notion of labile, stable, and "permanent" cells is still useful as an approximation, but experimental science has discovered a whole new panorama of regeneration.

The 1990s: Focus on Stem Cells and Their Niches

Bizzozero was a naturalist: he correctly described what he saw. Today's scientists are aggressive; they manipulate cells, grow them *in vitro,* prod them with growth factors, and change their genes. Thanks to these manipulations, they discovered that all tissues contain "stem cells" with a huge growth potential; this includes striated muscle, heart cells, and even the human brain.

What is a stem cell? The concept is as old as the cell theory, but to explain it we can only give a rather lame operative definition: *a stem cell is an undifferentiated cell capable throughout life of renewing itself as well as of generating one or more types of differentiated cells* (54, 70, 167, 171). Every adult cell has a "mother" (who may have parted from her years ago), and a line of ancestors—stem cells—of increasing potential. The ultimate stem cells are those of the early embryo, which can be considered as *totipotential;* farther down along the line—in the fetus, *and also in the adult*—we find *multipotential* (*pluripotential*) cells; those closer to final differentiation are called either *progenitor, committed,* or *transit* (or *transitional*) cells (70, 94, 108, 126, 127, 167). This nomenclature is still in a state of flux.

In ordinary histologic sections, the search for stem cells is easy only in lining epithelia, such as the epidermis, because the stem cells squat against the basement membrane; in other tissues the search is frustrating, because by definition stem cells look bland and undifferentiated. However, they can usually be recognized by immunohistochemistry, which reveals distinctive proteins (antigens) on their surface or in the cytoplasm. *The critical proof is to grow the putative stem cells in vitro and to make them differentiate by supplying them with appropriate growth factors.* When a stem cell replicates, its mitosis can be *symmetrical* (producing two stem cells) or *asymmetrical* (producing one stem cell and one progenitor or differentiated cell). The two patterns can alternate (Figure 2.3). In several models of stem cell asymmetric division, asymmetry between the two daughter cells (one remaining a stem cell, the other differentiating into a mature cell) was brought about by spindle orientation (178a) or by

molecules expressed on the stem cells or on cells of the niche (95a).

A model for studying stem cells was provided by the cells of the blood-forming line; knowledge in this field is so far advanced that therapeutic applications of stem cells are already standard medical practice in hematology (94, 97, 116, 139). This has happened in part because the blood's stem cells are relatively easy to find without resorting to the embryo. They have a distinctive marker, the surface protein CD34 (38); they can be harvested from adult blood, where they represent about 0.01 percent of the mononuclear cells (94) and from blood in the umbilical cord and placenta (neonatal blood), where they are more abundant and more prolific (139). After they have been expanded *ex vivo* (outside the body), they can be reinjected intravenously, because they know how to home right back into the bone marrow: exactly where they are needed when they are injected to repopulate a bone marrow destroyed by chemotherapy (94, 126).

This "sympathy" between blood stem cells and bone marrow runs deep, and it taught us something about stem cell biology in general. *In vitro,* blood stem cells totally deprived of a bone marrow–like environment will not survive very long: they need the company of endothelial cells, fat cells, fibroblasts, macrophages, osteoblasts, and even some matrix. This has led to speculate that normally, in the bone marrow, each hematopoietic stem cell lives in a microscopic "**niche**" of stromal cells that nurse it and provide it with the proper instructions, somewhat like worker bees nurse the queen bee in a hive (57, 97, 116, 144, 171). Stem cell niches (Figure 2.3) surely exist in other tissues (95a, 178a). In the hair follicles of the mouse it has been possible to pinpoint the area that could function as a niche for melanocytic stem cells (111).

The concept of niche, born of pure speculation, was confirmed in 2003 by elegant experiments *in vivo* (179a). In trabecular bone, each trabecula is covered with endosteal cells; among these are clusters of special SNO cells (Spindle-shaped N-cadherin$^+$ CD45$^-$ Osteoblastic cells), which are the key components of the niche; they hold in place hemopoietic stem cells by means of tight junctions containing N-cadherin and beta-catenin.

The technical difficulties involved in stem cell research are great and compounded by ethical and political issues. And so the key scientific problems have become a public concern: What can be expected of stem cells? How can they be instructed to differentiate into the required specialized cells? How can they be physically placed where they are needed? How long will they survive and perform? Will they generate tumors or

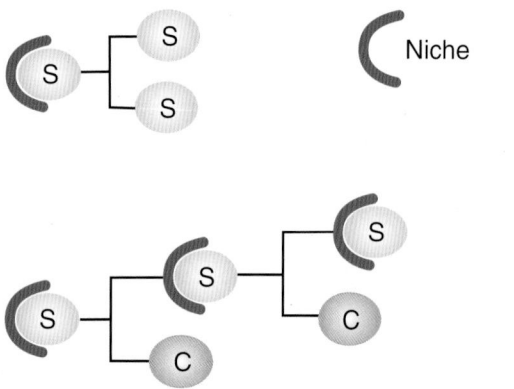

FIGURE 2.3   Symmetrical (*top*) versus asymmetrical cell division. **S** = stem cell, **C** = committed cell.

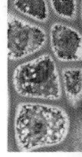

other problems? Can human embryonic stem cells be used? How do blood-derived stem cells compare with embryonic stem cells (125)? These are just some of the questions being asked in the press. The long-term hope is to produce spare parts for humans; most of these are still in the future, but some astonishing feats have already been accomplished, mainly in mice; enough to make Bizzozero giddy, and us as well.

The Acrobatics of Stem Cells: A Word of Caution

Lately, stem cells have been making the headlines, not only with regard to political or ethical issues but also on account of their reported feats: who would not be astonished to hear of blood-forming stem cells turning into liver (89, 124) or into striated muscle and heart (19) or of skin cells turning into neurons (161)? Yet, we must wait for the dust to settle (1, 7) and for a second look. A paper with the flamboyant title "Turning Brain into Blood" (brain stem cells into hematopoietic stem cells) (376) was not confirmed by others (43, 109). A more cautious view is that the so-called multipotent hematopoietic stem cells are a mixed group from the beginning (115). And then, in a new field, it is easy to fall into the trap of unexpected results. A 2002 report on stem cell research (entitled "Cell Fusion Raises Confusion") revealed that stem cells injected intravenously may fuse with cells of the host and generate cells that *look* like embryonic stem cells but have twice the number of chromosomes and are likely to be genetically unstable (74, 178).

A quick look back. Were there no prophets in the stem cell world? There were some, but working against dogma tends to be frowned upon. A classic example is the story of a few researchers who doggedly maintained that they could grow connective tissue from blood cells, a topic now considered as "hot." It should have been fairly simple to show that white blood cells could produce collagen; by the 1950s this was done several times and allegedly with success, but all these early studies were flawed and had to be dismissed: the experimenters failed to consider that skin fibroblasts could be picked up by the needles used, for example, to draw venous blood for the cultures. In 1960, a Swiss surgeon drew blood with the necessary precautions, and some of his blood cultures regularly produced collagen, but nobody listened. In 1965, a very expert team tried again, with flawless technique, and again some of the cultures produced collagen; but rather than accepting that they had proved a heresy to be true, they concluded that somehow their cultures were being contaminated with fibroblasts, and they gave up (407). Such is the power of dogma.

Regeneration of Epithelia

Epithelia regenerate very well, with the few exceptions mentioned above.

Surface epithelia. All surface epithelia are programmed to regenerate over denuded areas. They do so via an efficient two-phase operation, as described for the endothelium (see further). The most urgent task is to cover the exposed connective tissue surface, no matter how (the urgency here is to close the door to bacteria, not to platelets). Thus, the epithelial cells at the edge of the wound spread out a sheet of lamellipodia that glide over the denuded surface (169), whereas new epithelial cells are produced 1 or 2 millimeters behind the edge; it seems that cells will *either* move or multiply (153). The advancing cells can speed up their task by producing a single cable of actin fibrils that runs around the edge, acting as a purse-string (Figure 2.4) (77, 98, 101). After they have covered the gap, the undifferentiated cells mature into the required types, such as ciliated or mucus-secreting cells (60). Maturation may take a week or two, sometimes less. The gastric lining of the rat *stomach* repairs itself with incredible speed; after absolute alcohol has destroyed over 90 percent of the surface cells, 45 percent of the denuded surface is covered within *7 minutes* by flat cells emerging from the gastric pits and moving at the rate of 1 to 2 μm per minute; within 1 hour, 95 percent of the damage is repaired with near-normal columnar cells (88a). It must be an urgent matter to reline the stomach.

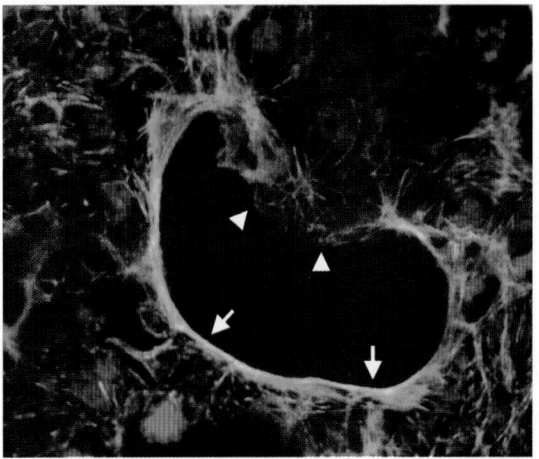

FIGURE 2.4　Wound in a monolayer of epithelial cells, healing by two characteristic methods—(1) *purse-stringing* (**arrows**): most of the leading-edge cells are being drawn forward by the contraction of a single actin cable running along the edge and continuous from cell to cell; and (2) lamellipodial crawling: a group of cells is crawling forward by extending veil-like lamellipodia (**arrowheads**). (**Green** = filamentous actin tagged with phalloidin stained with fluorescent isothiocyanate; **red** = nuclei.) (Reprinted by permission from Nature Cell Biology, Vol. 3, No. 5, pp. E117. Copyright © 2001 MacMillan Magazines Ltd. and by J. Brock and P. Martin [77].)

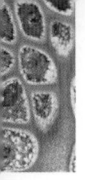
In most epithelia, the stem cells are spread along the basement membrane, but the cornea is an interesting exception (107, 148).

The outer cover of the cornea is a stratified, squamous, nonkeratinized epithelium; its cells are constantly sloughed off and must be replaced, *but the epithelium of the cornea itself contains no stem cells.* However, there is a narrow ring of stem cells at the *limbus,* that is, at the junction of the cornea and sclera. Normally, mitoses in these cells generate a slow stream of epithelium that creeps over the cornea, much as the epithelium of intestinal villi is maintained by cells that glide up from the crypts and eventually drop off (39). If the limbus is destroyed by trauma or disease, the cornea can be saved by a ring-shaped graft of limbus taken from a cadaver (163). Incidentally, the vast majority of corneal tumors arise from the limbus.

Melanocytes. These cells of neuroepithelial origin tend to regenerate rather capriciously: too little or too much. Often, especially after freezing (157), they fail to regenerate altogether, which is why most scars in pigmented skin are pale. This property is currently exploited for "freeze branding" cattle, a more humane procedure than fire branding (Figure 2.5).

Liver. Liver cells have great powers of regeneration, although not quite as great as the ancient Greeks assumed (Figure 2.6). Experimentally, it is easy to remove about 70 percent of a rat's liver; it will promptly regrow, and this can be done at least 12 times (106). Of course, if we cut off a liver lobe, we will not expect a new lobe to grow out of the stump like the tail of a lizard: new cells are added throughout the liver until the volume is restored (99).

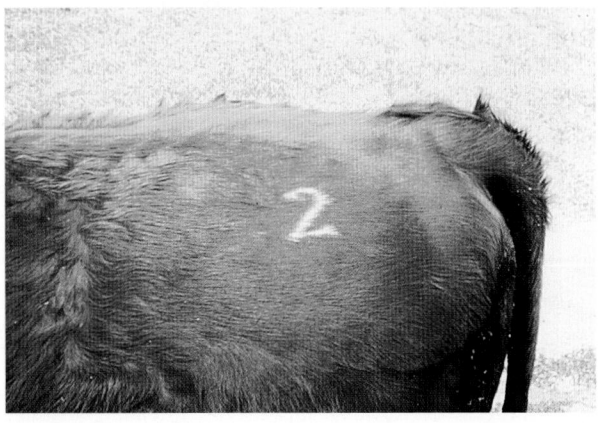

FIGURE 2.5 Freeze-branding of a cow: the procedure exploits the failure of melanocytes to regenerate after a freezing injury. (Courtesy of T. J. Steinhaus, Nasco International, Inc., Fort Atkinson, WI.)

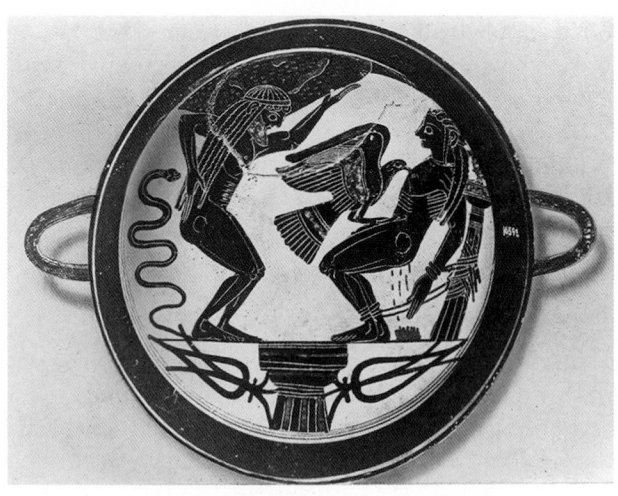

FIGURE 2.6 Liver regeneration as seen by the ancient Greeks. Because he had smuggled the gift of fire to humans, Prometheus was punished by Zeus. He was tied to a pole, and every day an eagle came to devour his liver, which continued to regenerate. Vase (Kylix) from 575–550 B.C. (Courtesy of the Vatican Museums.)

After partial hepatectomy in rats, minimal cellular changes are visible in 1–3 hours; after 6–12 hours the cells, nuclei, and nucleoli enlarge; mitoses begin after about 12 hours and peak at 30 hours. In 7 days, the original weight is restored. When partial hepatectomy is performed in humans to remove tumors, the response is more sluggish than in rats; the original weight is restored in about 6 months (29a).

There seems to be no specific need for stem cells: if every liver cell undergoes mitosis once or twice, the job is done. However, there is an exception: when the demand for new cells is overwhelming, as in extensive liver necrosis due to a poison, the "oval cells" take over. These cells are normally inserted in the wall of the fine interlobular bile ducts; in emergencies they appear to behave as facultative stem cells (3, 66) and they may even be supplied by the bone marrow (124). Indeed, *here is a real example of cell therapy: with an intravenous injection of bone marrow stem cells, it has been possible to save from death some mice with a lethal enzymatic deficiency* (Figure 2.7) (89).

The process of liver regeneration involves many growth factors and hormones including insulin, T3, and norepinephrine, as well as IL-6. The quest for liver growth factors—still ongoing (50)—has provided many surprises. There are regular growth factors and "primers"; the most potent factor, hepatocyte growth factor (HGF), is secreted by mesenchymal cells throughout the body, liver included, but NOT by hepatocytes (Figure 2.8); however, a large amount of

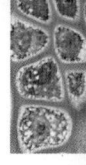

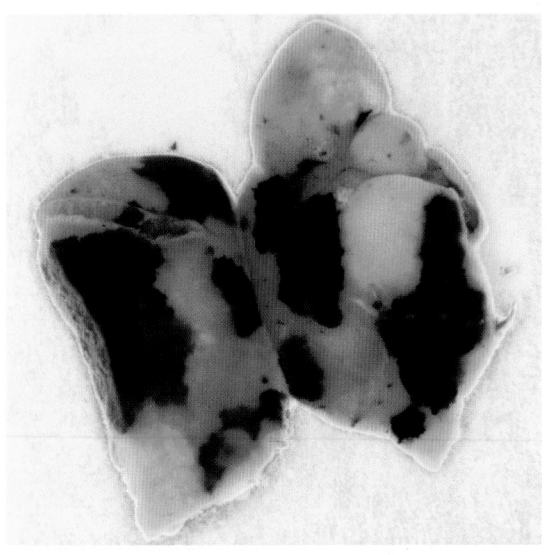

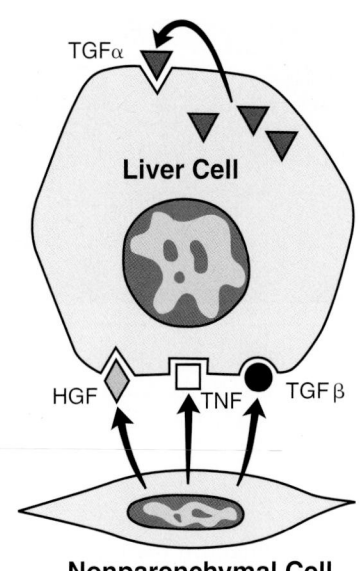

FIGURE 2.7   Proof that mouse hematopoietic cells can turn into liver cells. This liver belonged to a mouse that, if untreated, would have died of liver failure (from fatal hereditary tyrosinemia Type 1). Seven months earlier, it was rescued with an intravenous injection of hematopoietic cells from a mouse whose cells stain blue for the enzyme beta-galactosidase. *Light areas:* Natural liver tissue. *Dark areas:* Liver tissue produced by the rescuing cells. (Reproduced with permission from Lagasse E, Connors H, Al-Dhalimy, et al. Nat Med 2000; 6:1229–1234 [89].)

FIGURE 2.8   Main growth factors involved in liver regeneration, produced by the liver cells themselves and by nonepithelial cells. HGF = hepatic growth factor; TNF = tumor necrosis factor; TGFα, TGFβ = transforming growth factors. (Adapted from Fausto N. Hepatic regeneration. In: Bicher J, et al. (eds). Oxford textbook of clinical hepatology, 2nd edition. New York: Oxford University Press, 1999, pp. 189–201. Reprinted by permission from Oxford University Press [50].)

HGF is normally bound to the liver matrix and can be released by proteolysis. HGF is also classified among the so-called **scatter factors** because it can dissociate polarized epithelial cells (162). It appears in the blood within 1 hour of hepatectomy and stimulates mitosis in a variety of tissues. It rises in the blood also after the removal of one kidney (11), but its effect is organ-specific: after nephrectomy it induces mitoses in the remaining kidney, after partial hepatectomy in the remaining liver. Overall the biology of liver regeneration is extremely complicated, and so it comes as some relief to find at least one symmetry: as TGF-alpha, produced by liver cells, helps initiate the process, TGF-beta 1 (a mitogen inhibitor, produced by stromal cells) helps to close it (50). But we still have no clue as to an amazing phenomenon, well known to the surgeons who transplant livers: unlike other transplanted organs, such as the kidney, *the transplanted liver adjusts its volume to the weight of the host,* in a matter of weeks (Figure 2.9) (52).

Mesothelia. The sheets of flat cells that line the serosal cavities are definitely epithelial: they contain cytokeratin as well as—surprisingly—a surfactant similar to that produced by pulmonary alveolar epithelium (46). Being about as thin as endothelium they are very delicate; they can be destroyed over large areas just by mechanical handling or by drying, e.g., during abdominal surgery. It is crucial that they regenerate fast, because in their absence the viscera could stick together, creating *adhesions*—a complication very difficult to correct (p. 451). Indeed the mesothelial cells "reappear" at record speed: if the entire peritoneal lining of a rat is destroyed by drying with a jet of air, within 3–5 days a new mesothelium is in place (141). Electron microscopy shows that the denuded surfaces are quickly seeded with large round cells that look like macrophages, which flatten out, develop microvilli like peritoneal cells, join up, and become mesothelium. What cells are these? They could come from two sources: from the free mononuclear cells normally contained in the peritoneal cavity, or from the blood, possibly as stem cells. Whatever their origin, we can admire once again the wisdom of the healing process: if the regenerating cells had to crawl over from the edges of the denuded area, they might take weeks to cover the distance. Seeding the area with free cells, parachuted behind the lines, and instructed to flatten out, is the fastest solution.

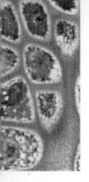
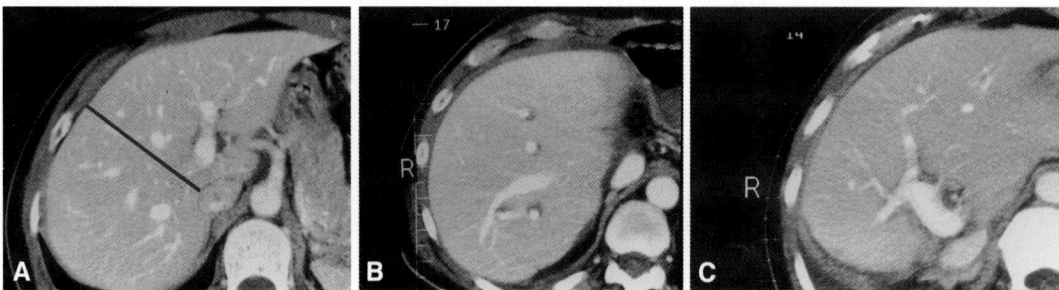

FIGURE 2.9   Computed tomography scans showing the adaptation in size of a human liver transplant. **A:** Donor's liver before surgery (black line = line of transection through the right liver). Total computed volume, 1230 ml. **B:** Transplanted liver 3 weeks after surgery; volume = 1503 ml. **C:** Residual liver of donor 3 weeks after surgery; volume 1070 ml. (Reproduced by permission from [99].)

Regeneration of Connective Tissues

All varieties of connective tissue cells can regenerate, but to different degrees.

Fibroblasts. Fibroblasts are typical stable cells. They regenerate promptly, in fact they are among the easiest cells to grow *in vitro;* they reproduce extensively *in vivo* in response to almost any kind of injury. This exuberant behavior might suggest that fibroblasts are especially prone to produce tumors, but the reverse is true (p. 855). The dermis contains mainly "fibroblasts," but hidden among them are multipotential stem cells which are capable of generating—depending on how they are fed—smooth muscle cells, fat cells, glia, and even neurons (PLEASE NOTE: *neurons from the skin*) (147, 161).

Endothelial cells. Endothelial cells belong to the "stable" group, like the fibroblasts, and they are just as ready to multiply, although it took much longer to find out how to grow them *in vitro* (126). In mice with myocardial infarcts, it was well proven that new endothelial cells can be supplied by circulating adult bone-marrow stem cells (78, 85, 117). In fact, we will see later (Chapter 18) that grafted organs become seeded with the donor's endothelial cells (129). Locally, endothelial cells regenerate somewhat differently depending on the setting. Those of the microcirculation are programmed to form a network of fine branching tubes; when new microvessels are needed, e.g., after injury, the endothelial cells of capillaries and venules in the surrounding tissues give rise to solid sprouts that connect with each other, become hollow tubes, and build a new capillary network: this is *angiogenesis,* a key process in inflammation and tumors (p. 774) (to be contrasted with *arteriogenesis,* Chapter 24). By contrast, in the large vessels, the endothelium forms extensive sheets. Now visualize a fine scratch produced inside a rat aorta with a stiff nylon thread; for the cells that surround this microscopic wound, the most urgent problem is to cover the exposed subendothelial surface before it interacts with the circulating blood and initiates a potentially dangerous thrombus (p. 646). So the endothelial cells spread over the denuded area without taking the time to undergo mitosis: a scratch 50 μm wide can be covered in 8 hours (Figure 2.10) (134). Mitosis will follow. The same sequence can be observed in a sheet of endothelial cells grown *in vitro:* if a single cell is plucked out, its neighbors spread over the gap in 30–45 minutes (174, 175); a nine-cell wound heals in the same way (Figure 2.11). This two-phase repair mechanism speeds up the healing process. Epithelia use it as well. This is how corneal scratches can heal within a day and gastric erosions can be covered in minutes, as we will see shortly.

Bone tissue. Stone hard as it is, bone tissue also regenerates beautifully, as might be predicted from the fact that osteoblasts and osteoclasts continue to perform their contrasting tasks throughout life. It is amazing that bone regenerates as fast as it does because its cells face two problems: they must regenerate themselves, while also rebuilding a complex extracellular scaffolding. Like a well-trained emergency repair team, they perform their task in two phases. First *the cells hurriedly make temporary bone* with thin, immature trabeculae in which the collagen fibers are woven haphazardly; this is woven bone (Figure 2.12), which is very similar to fetal bone. Later, *swarms of osteoclasts slowly remove this provisional bone and then osteoblasts replace it with better built, orderly lamellar bone.*

Bone tissue contains more polypeptide growth factors than any other tissue (71), perhaps reflecting the fact that it is constantly destroying and rebuilding itself, faster

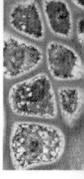

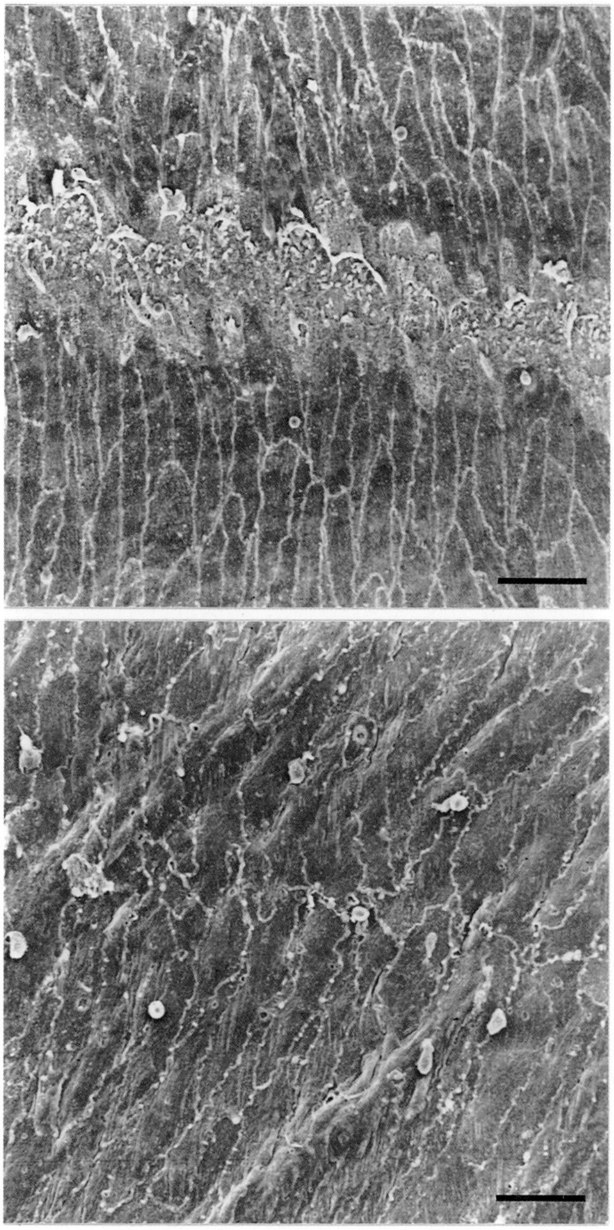

FIGURE 2.10 Scanning electron micrographs of rat aorta. *Top:* Immediately after a transverse scratch produced with a nylon thread, removing the endothelium. The white dots on the de-nuded area are platelets. *Bottom:* Eight hours later endothelial cells have glided over the scratch and covered it, without mi-toses. **Bars** = 25 μm. (Reproduced from [134] © by the U.S. and Canadian Academy of Pathology, Inc.)

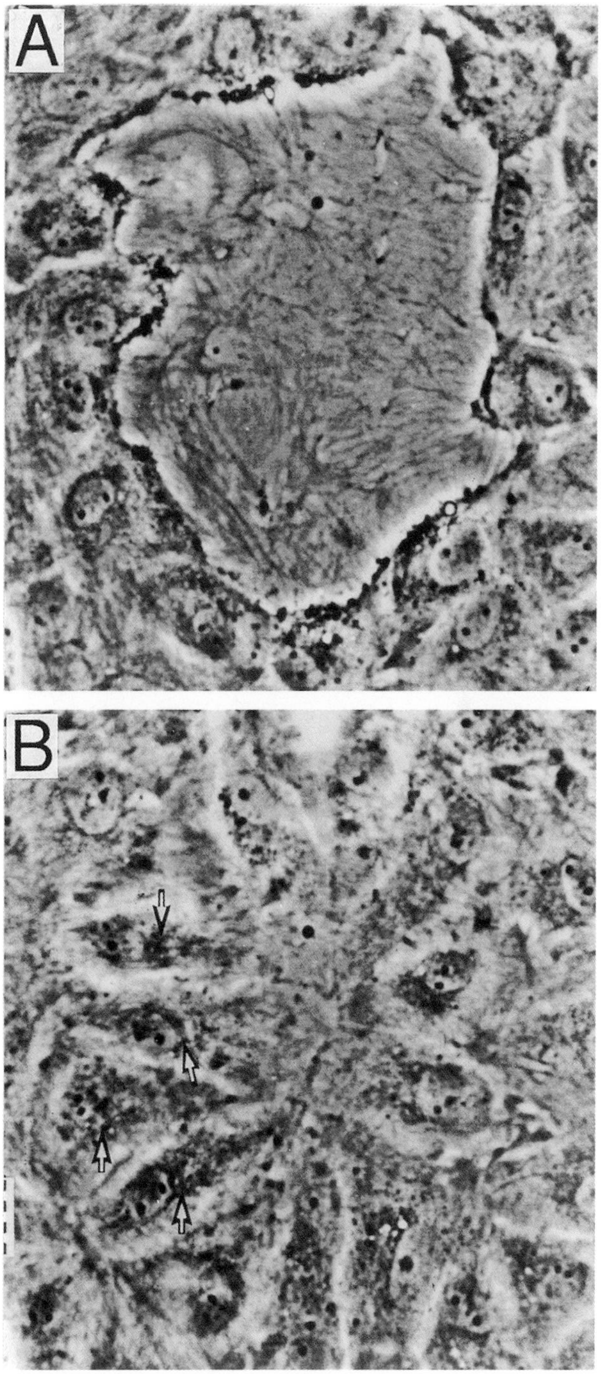

FIGURE 2.11 Healing of a microscopic, nine-cell wound in a sheet of endothelial cells growing *in vitro*. Phase contrast micrographs. **A:** Immediately after microsurgery. **B:** One hundred fifty minutes later, the wound has closed by expansion of the surrounding cells, without mitoses. (Reproduced from the **Journal of Cell Biology,** 1988;107:1777–1783 by copyright permission of the Rockefeller University Press [175].)

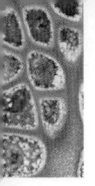

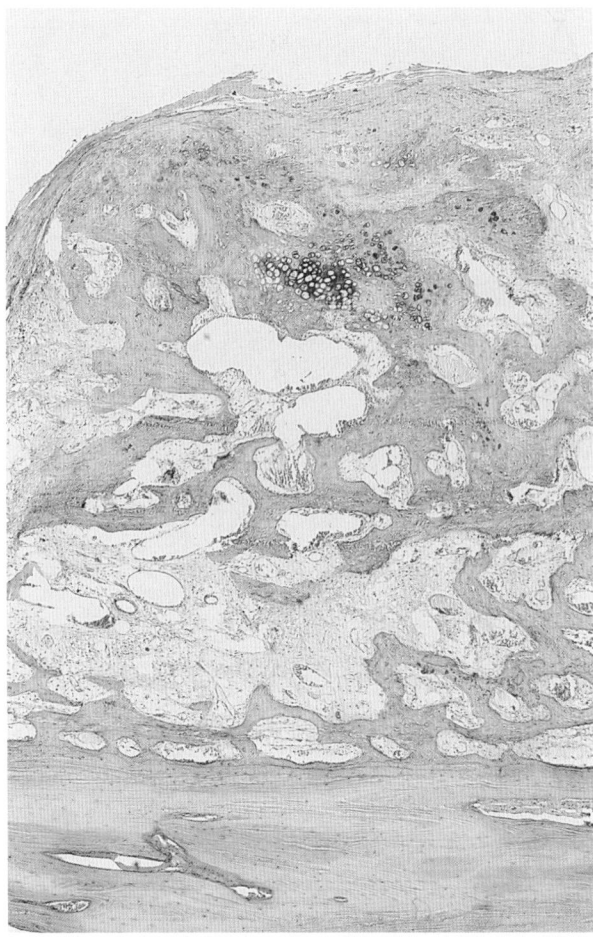

FIGURE 2.12   Regenerating bone (*callus*) near a tibial fracture in a rabbit. Bottom 1/5: compact bone of the tibia. Top margin: the thin fibrous layer = periosteum. The space between these two structures is filled with branching trabeculae of newly formed bone (*callus*) arising from the deep face of the periosteum. Small islands of cartilage (basophilic areas, near the top) are common in a callus.

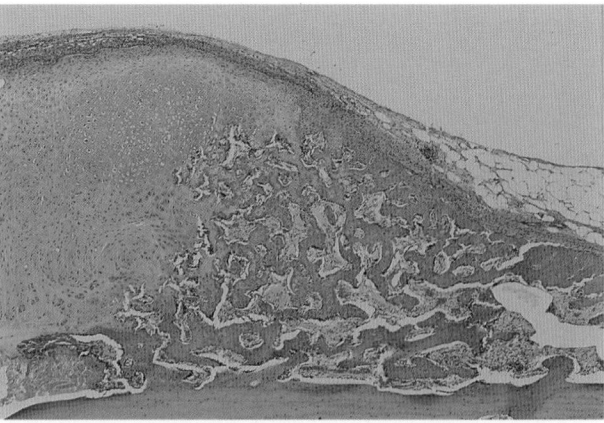

FIGURE 2.13   Fracture of the tibia, not immobilized, at 21 days (rabbit). Bottom margin: cortical bone of the tibia. Upper margin: periosteum. The space between the two structures is filled with newly formed bony trabeculae; toward the left the trabeculae blend into a mass of cartilage, which corresponds to the fracture site. Extensive development of cartilage instead of bone suggests that motion was occurring at the fracture site.

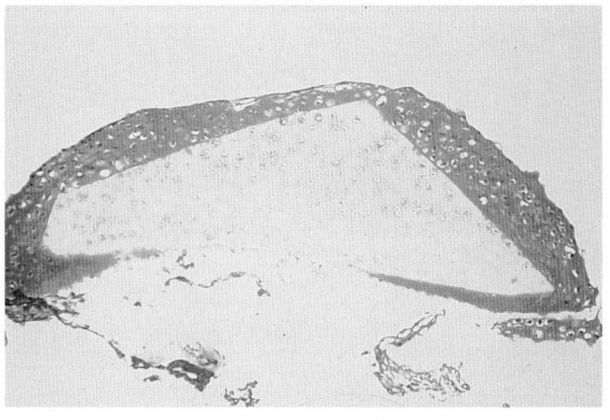

FIGURE 2.14   Regeneration of cartilage *in vitro*. Center: Sliver of cartilage (barely stained) taken from the knee joint of an adult rabbit and placed in culture; 32 days later, it is surrounded by a rim of regenerating chondrocytes five or six cells deep, emphasized by the stain (Safranin O, Fast Green). (Reproduced from [100] by permission of Gordon and Breach, Science Publishers.)

than any other tissue. These factors (30, 53, 80, 133, 136, 165, 179) are also involved in the genesis of cartilage. Physical conditions (30, 35) help determine which types of cell will ultimately differentiate (Figure 2.13). Here are some well-recognized associations (35):

High tensile strain	⟶	fibrous tissue
Compression	⟶	cartilage
Poor vascularity	⟶	cartilage
Motion	⟶	cartilage
Low stress/strain	⟶	bone

Articular cartilage. This tissue tells us two different stories. It is common knowledge that with age the layer of cartilage in the joints tends to wear down; the result is

osteoarthritis ("degenerative" arthritis). This suggests that its cells, the chondrocytes, are unable to regenerate; yet, nests of regenerating cells do develop in the worn-down cartilage, only they are too few and not effective. A sliver of joint cartilage grown *in vitro* produces an excellent outgrowth of cells (chondrocytes) (Figure 2.14) (100). All this suggests that the poor regeneration of cartilage *in vivo* is related at least in part to mechanical conditions: the cells may be having a hard time growing while exposed to the grinding effect of the joint. This more optimistic point of view has allowed orthopedic surgeons to devise a method for treating those cases of osteoarthritis in which the loss of cartilage is a deep, ulcer-like lesion. In a first operation a sliver of cartilage is taken from a normal-looking area and grown *in vitro* for 2–3 weeks; the cell culture is then transferred to the "ulcer" and covered with a strip of periosteum (27).

Of course, we must remember that the chondrocytes are buried in a mass of extracellular matrix, which they have produced, and which has its own pathology. Normally the matrix is built around fibers of Type 2 collagen; under pathologic conditions, e.g., in osteoarthritis, the chondrocytes can switch to making Type 1 fibers (56).

> *Joint mice.* If a piece of cartilage and bone is chipped off accidentally and allowed to move about in the joint, it behaves as if it were in tissue culture (13); it grows and gives rise to a rounded body consisting of a crust of cartilage over a core of dead bone tissue (the cartilage survives because it is nourished by diffusion) (Figure 2.15). The chip survives even better if it becomes attached to the synovium. The free bodies are called joint mice and can cause sudden blockage of the joint, especially in the knee.

Tendons. If severed, tendons heal slowly, which is understandable because they have few cells and few blood vessels. The tendon sheath sometimes participates in the healing process, but at the price of adhesions that impair the function of the tendon (6). Secondary rupture at the injured site is not uncommon. The search for artificial tendons is still going on (123).

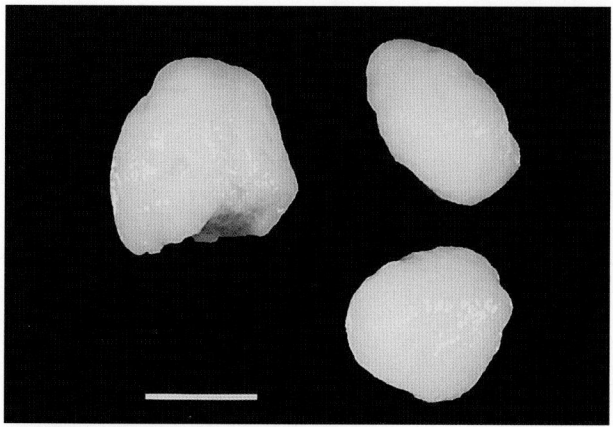

FIGURE 2.15 "Joint mice": fragments of cartilage growing freely in the knee joint of a 55-year-old man with osteoarthritis. **Bar** = 1 cm.

Adult fat cells (adipocytes). This type of connective tissue cell cannot duplicate itself at all; we might even consider including it among the permanent cells. Actually, it is hard to imagine how a fat cell could partition its fat droplet between two daughter cells. However, everyone knows that fat tissue can very definitely expand; this happens because new fat cells develop from undifferentiated but committed *precursor* cells (called lipoblasts, adipoblasts, or preadipocytes) that lie among the mature fat cells; they look like fibroblasts or macrophages (20, 41). We will discuss them in relation to hypertrophy.

Bone marrow. Bone marrow cells belong to the labile category and therefore regenerate all the time, but experimentally they can do much more than that (see later). It has been possible to isolate from the bone marrow of adult human volunteers stem cells of truly mesenchymal potential (strictly speaking, *mesenchyme* refers to embryonic connective tissue, which generates—besides connective tissues—also contractile tissues). Grown with different sets of nutrients and factors these stem cells differentiated into bone, cartilage, fat, tendon, and muscle (125).

Regeneration of Muscular Tissues

Smooth muscle cells regenerate very well (105); for example, during wound healing, when new microscopic blood vessels develop, the arteries acquire a new coat of smooth muscle cells supplied by the media of the preexisting vessels. The so-called *plaques* on the intima of atherosclerotic arteries consist largely of medial smooth muscle cells; it was assumed that these cells had crept up from the media, which may well be true, but recent work on mice shows that they can also arise from circulating progenitor cells (142).

Striated muscle has been traditionally maligned as a permanent tissue, incapable of regeneration. It is true that a muscle surgically amputated does not grow back, but at the biological level some potential for regeneration is obvious (32, 33, 48a, 170). If striated muscle cells, which are several centimeters long, are cut across, the ends retract immediately and form "retraction clots", masses of tangled filaments that probably protect the cell from the influx of extracellular calcium. Then a crowd of cells appears over and around each stump (Figure 2.16), including cells with many nuclei (*myotubes,* Figure 2.17). This was long interpreted as a futile attempt of the fiber's myonuclei to regenerate. It is now thought that most of the nuclei belong to **satellite cells,** i.e., stem cells that normally lie dormant within a pocket of the basement membrane

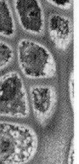

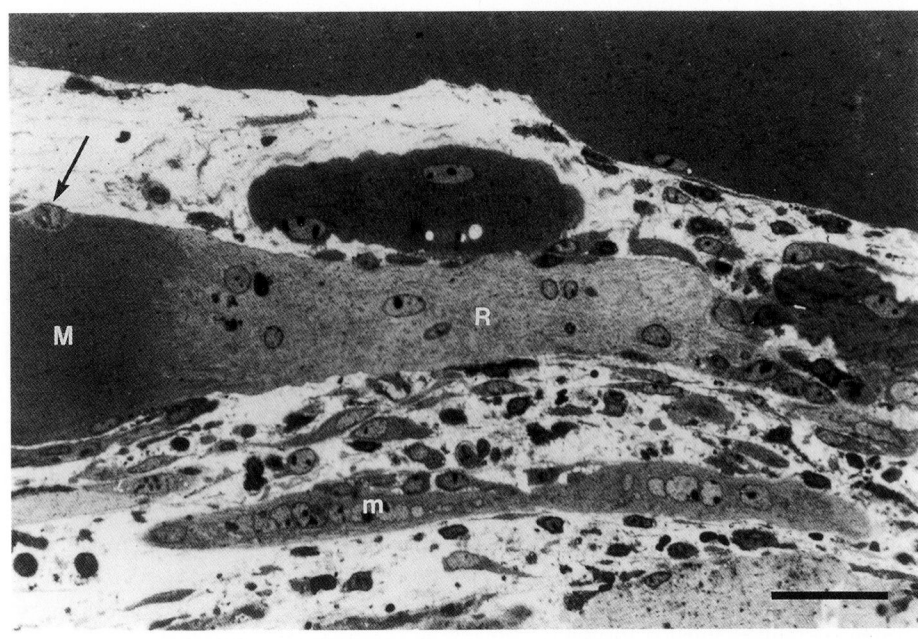

FIGURE 2.16   Regenerating striated muscle of an adult mouse 10 days after a crush injury. **M:** Striated muscle fiber; **arrow:** satellite cell; **R:** regenerating sprout (most of its nuclei probably derive from satellite cells); **m:** "myotube," which may later fuse with a regenerating sprout. Myotubes derive from sprouts and perhaps also from interstitial cells with myogenic potential. **Bar** = 25 μm. (Courtesy of Mr. T. A. Robertson and Dr. M. D. Grounds, Department of Pathology, University of Western Australia, Nedlands, Western Australia.)

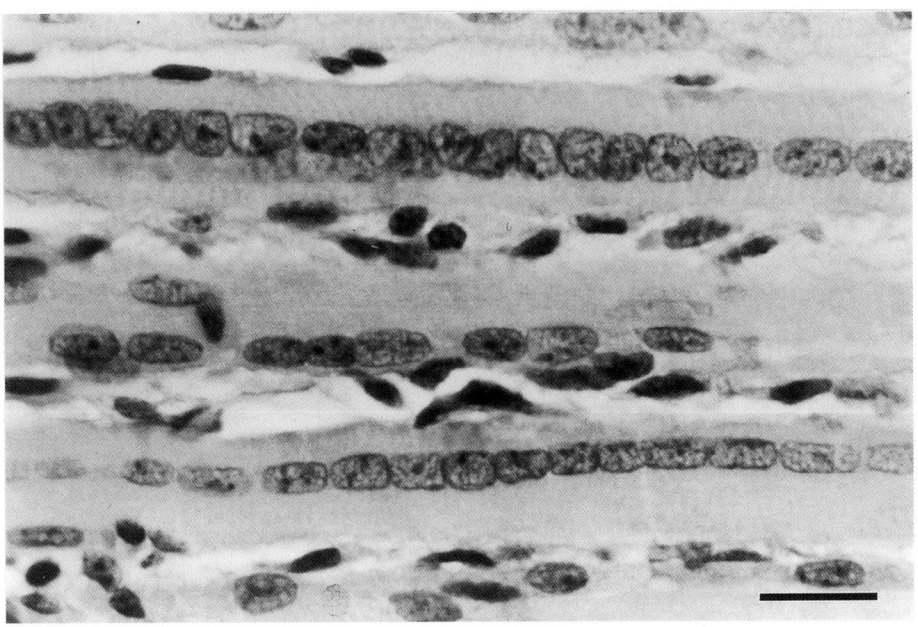

FIGURE 2.17   Longitudinal section of several myotubes containing arrays of centrally placed nuclei. From a striated muscle of an adult mouse, 10 days after a crush injury. **Bar** = 25 μm. (Courtesy of Dr. M. D. Grounds, Department of Pathology, University of Western Australia, Nedlands, Western Australia.)

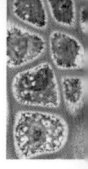

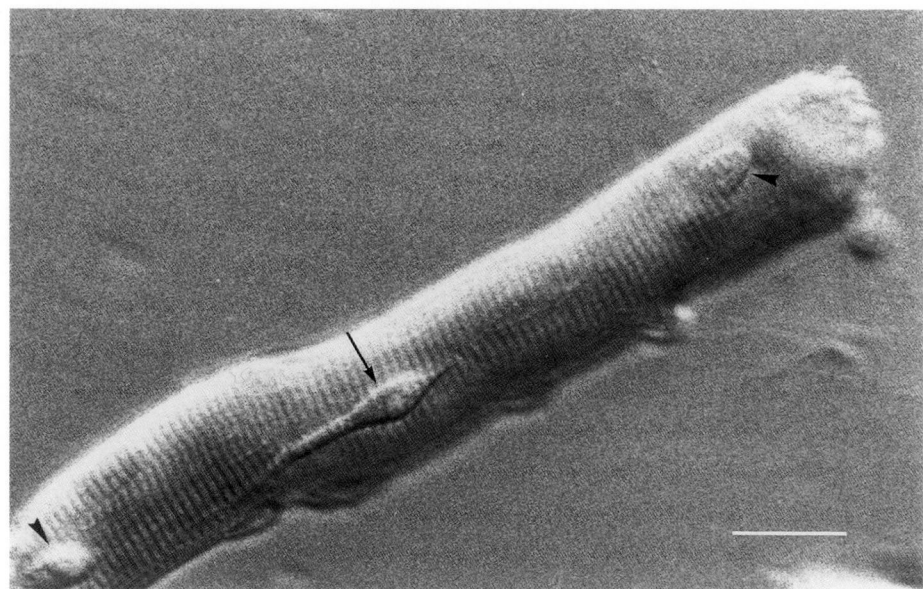

FIGURE 2.18 Satellite cell (*arrow*), attached to a dissociated striated muscle cell fiber of a rat. Satellite cells are enclosed in the basement membrane wrapping of a muscle cell; they take part in the regeneration of damaged muscle. **Arrowheads:** Muscle nuclei. **Bar** = 50 μm. (Reproduced from [10].)

(Figure 2.18) (102, 103). Elegant experiments *in vitro* have shown that a gap in a muscle fiber is rebuilt by satellite cells—not by the myonuclei—as long as the tube of basement membrane surrounding the fiber is intact (Figure 2.19) (17). After injury *in vivo,* the sequence seems to be the following (170): the satellite cells "wake up" and turn into myoblasts, which fuse (within 2–3 days) to form myotubes. The myotubes fuse with the stump and can differentiate into mature fibers. It may be that satellite cells from neighboring fibers join the effort, as well as muscle precursor cells thought to lie in the interstitium (29, 67, 68, 137).

There is one more source of regenerating muscle, but the experiment that proved it still bears the mark of the unthinkable: *muscle cells can be seeded by the bone marrow.* These stem cells truly accomplished a "fantastic voyage" (51, 119).

> The experiment consisted in producing a leg muscle injury in mice with a genetically marked bone marrow. When the damaged, regenerating muscle fibers were examined, it was found that a few had fused with bone marrow cells, obviously recruited from the blood (51, 119). This means that bone marrow cells know how to help an injured muscle and also know how to find it.

In these high-tech experiments, the rate of success was not sufficient for a therapeutic effect, but a new road is now open.

In the reality of today's surgery, striated muscles, however carefully sutured, usually fail to regenerate, because the stumps retract too far apart; the gap is filled by clotted blood and eventually by a scar. However, in experimental animals, if the gap between the stumps is bridged by a graft of striated muscle, the cells of the graft die but their cylindrical wrappings of basal lamina remain as guides for the regenerating muscle fibers (34). Similarly, if part of a striated muscle is *not cut, but is crushed or frozen,* the remaining basal laminae guide the young sprouts to successful regeneration (149). The same is true when the muscle cells are killed by injection of a local anesthetic (14). These examples are among the best for illustrating the role of basement membrane in regeneration (p. 34).

Heart muscle does not have satellite cells and was traditionally thought to be incapable of mitosis, but all this has changed (15). Confocal microscopy has shown unquestionable mitoses, especially near infarcts (117), frequent enough to offset the slow dropout of heart cells related to aging. Even more surprisingly, by looking for Y chromosomes in female hearts transplanted into males, it was found that nearly one fifth of the heart cells had been supplied by the host in an average time of 53 days (23, 129). In mice, mobilizing the stem cells by intravenous injection of stem cell factor (SCF) and granulocyte colony-stimulating factor (G-CSF) accelerated the healing process of infarcts (117).

And finally, with sophisticated immunohistochemical methods, beautiful stem cells were found in normal rat hearts (14a). Injected in rat ischemic hearts they took part in the healing process; in cultures they differentiated into heart cells, smooth muscle cells and endothelium. What is the role of these cells, versus circulating stem cells, in human healing myocardial infarcts? This remains an open question.

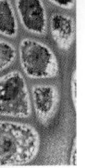

FIGURE 2.19   Regeneration of a striated fiber *in vitro. Top:* Muscle fiber that broke accidentally during dissection; the two stumps retracted within the basement membrane to form "retraction clots" (**C**). A satellite cell is present in the intervening space. The subsequent stages show that this space becomes filled with myoblasts, which probably derived from one or more satellite cells. *Bottom:* After 6 days most of the myoblasts have fused to form striated myotubes. **Bar** = 50 μm. (Reproduced from [17] Copyright © 1975 by the Wistar Institute Press. Reprinted by permission of Wiley-Liss, a division of John Wiley and Sons, Inc.)

Regeneration of Peripheral Nerves

Peripheral nerves can regenerate, although not very effectively (160). If a nerve is severed, downstream from the cut the axons and the myelin break down into oval droplets and are removed by the Schwann cells assisted by macrophages (Figure 2.20). While this happens, the continuity of the basement membrane in which each fiber was wrapped is not disturbed. Therefore, after about 30 days, the nerve has become a bundle of basement membrane tubes, each one filled with a chain of Schwann cells (*Büngner bands,* Figure 2.20)

> NOTE: Central axons have no Schwann cell covering, which means that if they are severed, Büngner bands do not develop.

This process is known as Wallerian degeneration, from the British physiologist Augustus Waller who described it briefly in 1850. In the meantime regeneration has started: within 3–5 hours, sprouts emerge from the proximal stump and seem to feel their way toward the distal stump, guided (and more often misguided, as we will see) by those tiny mysterious feelers called *growth cones* (Figure 2.21).

The axons that reach the distal stump proceed to grow inside a Büngner band. Each growing fiber advances between the Schwann cell and the basement membrane, probably utilizing adhesion molecules on the latter. Axon guidance is an intricate process (159, 160); the growth cones are guided by molecules that are either free or bound to surfaces, and either attract or repel; the five families of *semaphorins,* for example, function as repellents or inhibitors (42, 44, 159). Other molecules involved are *insulin-like growth factors (IGFs) I and II,* secreted by the liver; if the sciatic nerve of a rat is severed, IGF-1 accumulates in and around the Schwann cells of the proximal stump, and local infusion of more IGF-1 speeds up the process (110). The regenerating axons are said to grow about 1 mm per day (160a), about the same as hair (168). All this is biologically beautiful, but there

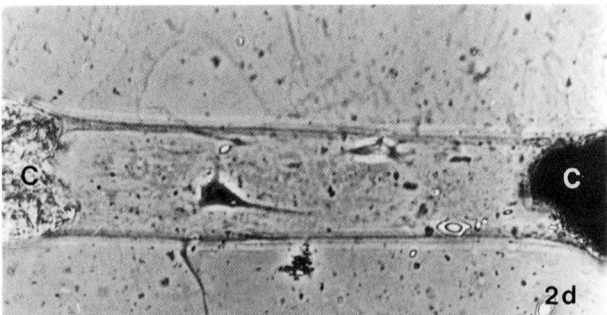

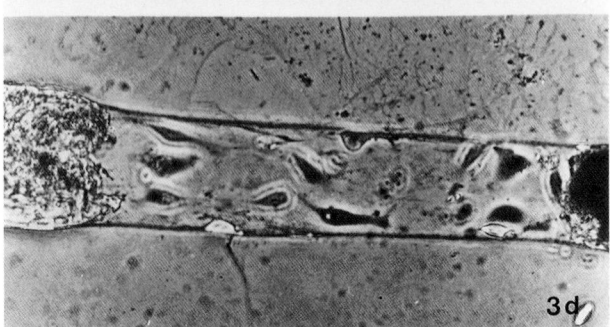

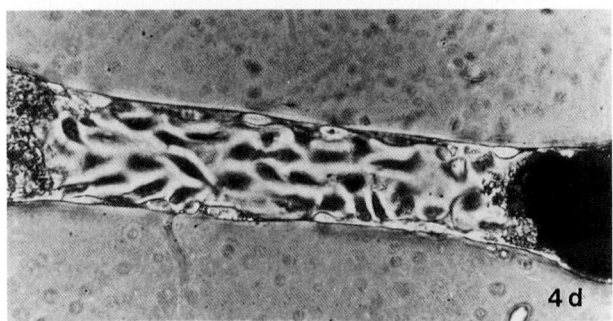

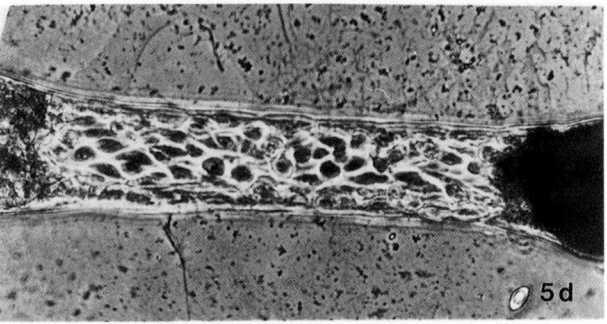

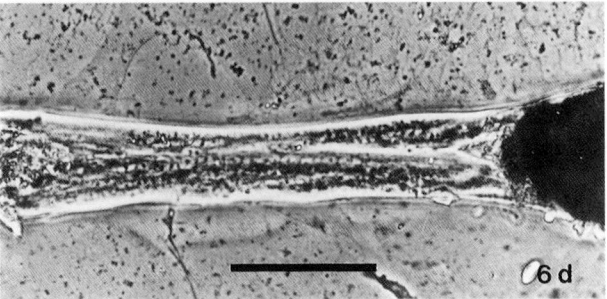

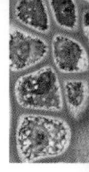

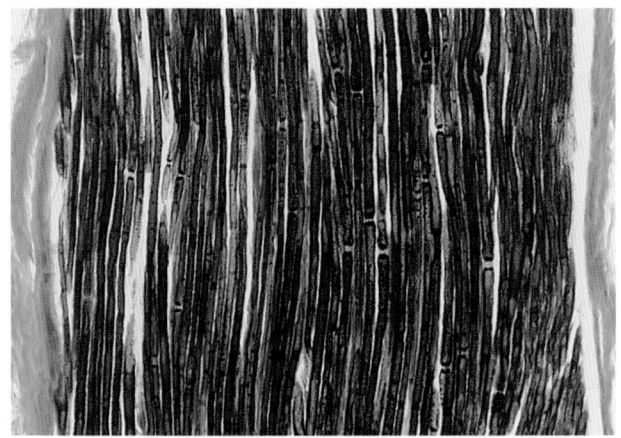

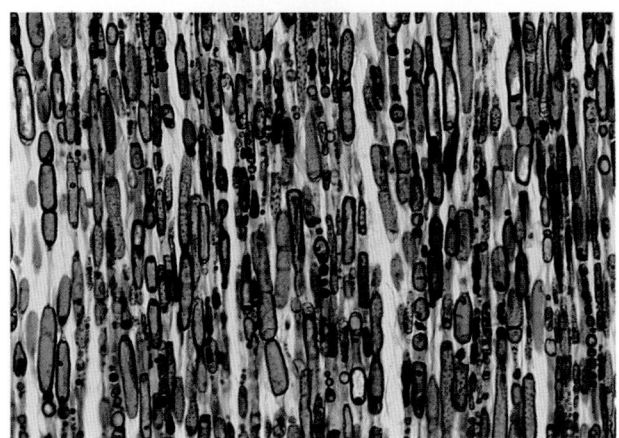

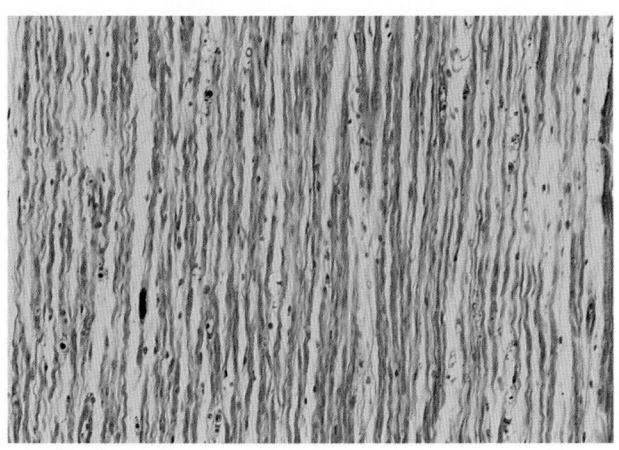

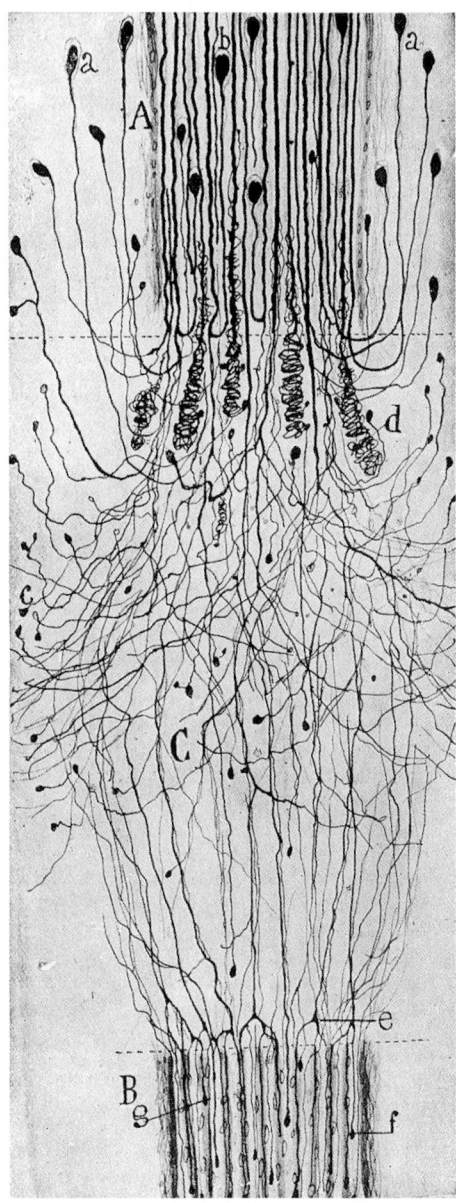

FIGURE 2.21 Pattern of axonal regeneration when a nerve is transsected and the stumps are only slightly separated. Some axons reach the distal stump and grow into it, others wander at random and eventually form a purposeless tangle—an extreme case being the "amputation neuroma." (Reproduced from [31].)

FIGURE 2.20 Wallerian degeneration in the severed sciatic nerve of a rat. *Top:* Normal sciatic nerve. *Center:* After 4 days, the myelin sheaths have broken down into oval bodies. *Bottom:* After 49 days, the debris of the myelin sheets have been removed; all that remains is a bundle of cords representing interconnected Schwann cells (osmium fixation, hematoxylin-eosin stain).

is a hitch. Most nerves contain different types of fibers. There are "motor" fibers that convey orders from the brain to make muscles contract, sensory fibers that run the other way and bring pain stimuli to the brain, sympathetic fibers that bring orders to blood vessels, and so on. When a nerve is severed, it is crucial that the new connections be made according to the original plan, but there is no arrangement for this to occur, except for a

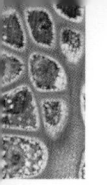
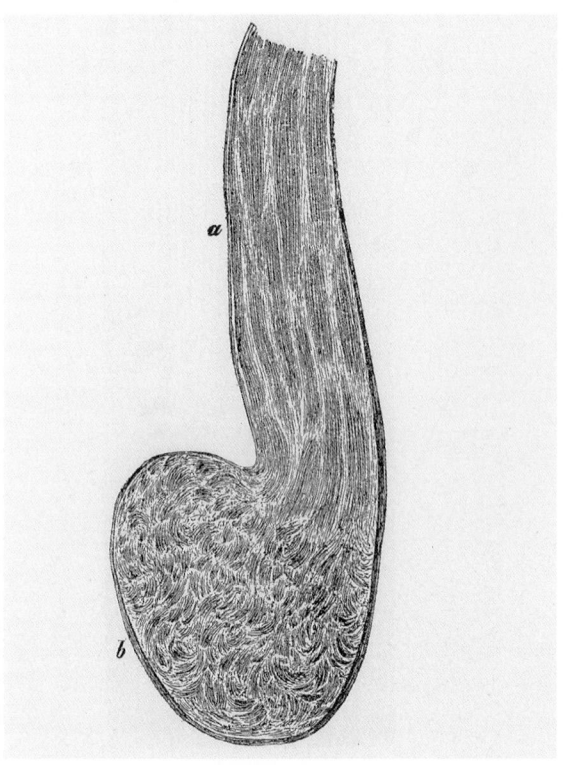

FIGURE 2.22 Amputation neuroma of the sciatic nerve, 9 years after amputation. **a:** Nerve, **b:** neuroma. Enlarged × 3–4. Drawing from circa 1900. (Reproduced from [180].)

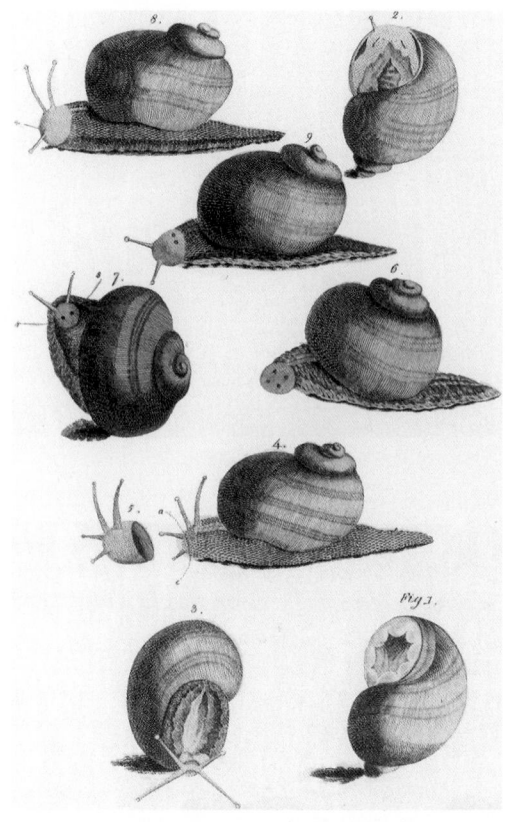

FIGURE 2.23 Some of the 145 snails that Spallanzani decapitated, fully or partially, circa 1766; heads regenerated in 219 snails. (Reproduced from [151].)

tendency for motor fibers to grow back into the Büngner bands of motor fibers (155). Alas, this is not good enough. The common result is *aberrant* or *misdirected regeneration,* meaning that regenerating axons have chosen the wrong pathway and have innervated the wrong target. This is an irreversible event; the brain makes no correction for it, and the end result may be quite disabling. Such is the symptom of "crocodile tears" due to an injury to the facial nerve, whereby the patient sheds tears instead of secreting saliva at the sight of food (143, 155).

When the gap between proximal and distal stump of the nerve is too wide, the axons form a disorderly tangle, which can become clinically evident as a painful **amputation neuroma** (Figure 2.22) (152). It is not known why amputation neuromas develop in some patients and not in others, why they may recur after removal, or why they eventually stop growing.

Regeneration in the Central Nervous Tissue

The first scientific study in this field came very early, in the 1700s, and it produced startling results. It was the work of two men of the Church, the Jesuit J. T. Needham in Paris and the Abbot L. Spallanzani in

Pavia, Italy; neither could know about neurons but both had a vested interest in the seat of the soul. They found that decapitated snails could survive and regenerate new heads (Figure 2.23). This caused "from novelty and singularity, a great noise" (151) because survival after decapitation was not compatible with the notion that the soul is in the head. In retrospect, we note that Spallanzani's 745 decapitated snails must have been cut rather high up because it is now known that they can regenerate only half of their brain (128).

Modern neuropathology was born in Spain with Santiago Ramón y Cajal (1852–1934), a scientist of legendary stature.

One day about 1885, Cajal—then professor of anatomy—was shown a slide of brain prepared by Golgi's silver method, which visualized some of the brain structures. That night he could not sleep. Back in the laboratory, he worked on Golgi's method, modified it, used it for years, and created the notion of neuron. In 1906 he was awarded the Nobel prize together with Golgi. At the Stockholm ceremony Cajal was extremely gracious toward Golgi; the reverse, alas, was not the case.

Cajal and his pupils studied regeneration in peripheral nerves (Figure 2.21 was drawn by Cajal, who was also a fine artist) as well as in the central nervous system. Regarding the latter, the Cajal team did notice that severed axons could perform "abortive attempts" to regenerate, but their conclusions were somewhat ambiguous: they could be quoted as supporting, or refuting, the possibility of regeneration. Posterity chose to adopt the negative view, and thus another medical dogma was born: *in the central nervous system of mammals axons do not regenerate.* Or, more broadly, *there is no regeneration in the central nervous system of mammals* (164).

Years passed and exceptions did turn up, but a medical dogma is not particularly sensitive to exceptions. Still, it was difficult to dismiss the startling news that came from Rockefeller University in 1983 (5). S. A. Goldman and F. Nottebohm had chosen a topic that might appear frivolous: bird songs. Having taped the songs of male canaries, they identified the part of the brain from which they originated. They then discovered that this center swells and shrinks with the coming and going of the singing season (Figure 2.24). The swelling is due to the formation of 30,000–40,000 new neurons, which are destroyed when the season is over. The stimulus is testosterone. Female canaries do not sing but their brain undergoes the same testosterone-driven cycle, presumably because they have to recognize the songs (59, 112, 113, 121).

This story from Nottebohm's laboratory met at first with little enthusiasm; it was easy to retort that birds are not people (we shall run into this argument again).

However, the exceptions to the dogma about "no regeneration in the central nervous system" began to coalesce into a defensible position. *It became quietly accepted that in the forebrain of vertebrates a zone around the lateral ventricles and another in the hippocampus produced new cells, but the progeny was believed by most to be "just glia"* (8, 88, 95, 138). In 1992 stem cells were grown *in vitro* from rodent brains (12) and a few years later from biopsy samples of adult human brains (88, 138).

In 1999, an exciting paper on the adult macaque (64) reported that neurons had been caught in the act of migrating from the paraventricular zone into the neocortex, an area connected with learning and memory. In 2001 another laboratory concluded, alas, that the traveling cells were not neurons (87). We must wait for a final judgment.

Finally, there came an experiment that we believe is definitive: in 1999, G. J. Brewer of Southern Illinois University (26, 131) took slices of brain from adult rats, released their cells by mild digestion with papain, maintained them in a medium containing fibroblast growth factor 2 (FGF2), and found that *most of the neurons began to proliferate;* they even expressed the intermediate filament marker *nestin* typical of embryonic neurons (92, 181) (*nestin* stands for NEuroepithelial STem cell). This was tangible (visible) proof that fully differentiated neurons—and probably other cells—can divide: the reader can judge (Figure 2.25) (131). As to the dogma that *axons* in the central nervous system do not regenerate, it was challenged from many sources. Studies in this field focussed mainly on repairing spinal

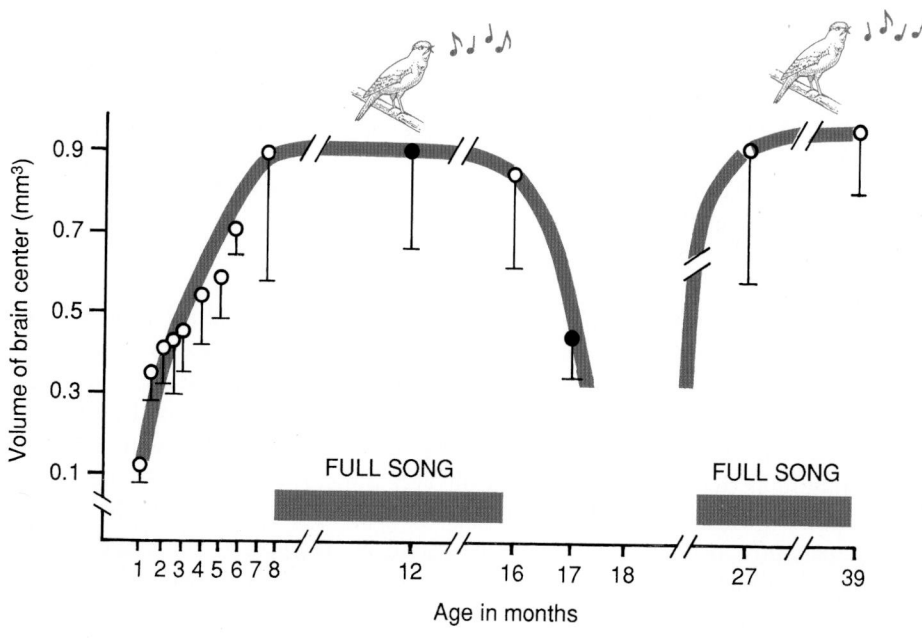

FIGURE 2.24 Correlation—in canaries—between the season of "full song" and the volume of the brain nucleus where the song originates. The fall and rise of the curve corresponds to death and regeneration of nerve cells. (Reproduced from [112].)

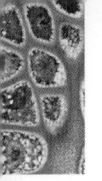

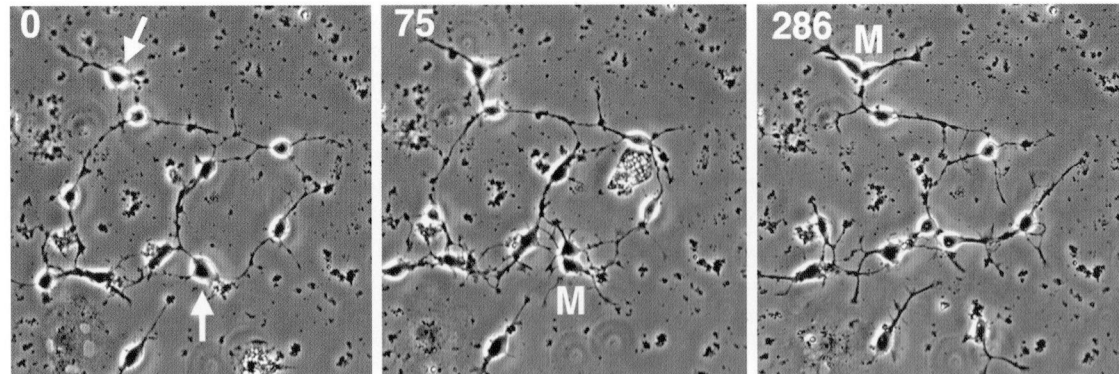

FIGURE 2.25   Regeneration of mammalian neurons. Hippocampal tissue from a 36-month-old rat grown in culture for 4 days with fibroblast growth factor. *Top left corners* = minutes. Cells with neuron morphology (**arrows**) undergo unquestionable mitosis (in the original paper, the cell indicated in panel *O* is aptly described as having a "pregnant appearance"). (Figure from "Regeneration and Proliferation of Embryonic and Adult Rat Hippocampal Neurons in Culture" by G. J. Brewer in Experimental Neurology, Volume 159:237–247, copyright © 1999 by Academic Press, reproduced by permission of the publisher [26].)

cord injury (145), which affects 2 million people worldwide (82, 164). It soon became apparent that in the central nervous system severed axons do regenerate over 1–2 mm, but then they stop. Why so? This failure is unlikely to depend on a property of the neuron itself, because the motor neurons in the spinal cord have an axon of each kind—one central, one peripheral—and the peripheral axon regenerates perfectly well, whereas the central axon does not. One clearcut difference between peripheral and central axons is that the central axons lack a Schwann cell wrapping; "wallerian" degeneration takes 3 times longer than in peripheral nerves (90 versus 30 days [164]). To test whether the lack of Schwann cells is involved, A. Aguayo of McGill University performed a series of experiments based on earlier work of Cajal's group (31, 168). The basic procedure was to take a segment of sciatic nerve from an adult rat and plug it into the central nervous system of the same rat, in one of various configurations (Figure 2.26) (2, 135). Result: a central axon can be induced to grow *into* a peripheral nerve, proving that *central axons can indeed regenerate,* if they find the right environment.

These clever experiments prove beyond doubt that central axons can be coaxed to grow *out* of the central nervous system, but alas, it is much more difficult to make them grow back into it. *Most of the central axons that grow into a bridge of nerve stop as soon as they confront central nervous tissue.* Current thinking is that the obstacles are many, structural and biochemical; they include (a) a myelin-related molecule aptly named Nogo expressed on the surface of oligodendrocytes; it can be overcome by means of an antibody (145) or by saturating its receptor NgR with a fragment of Nogo

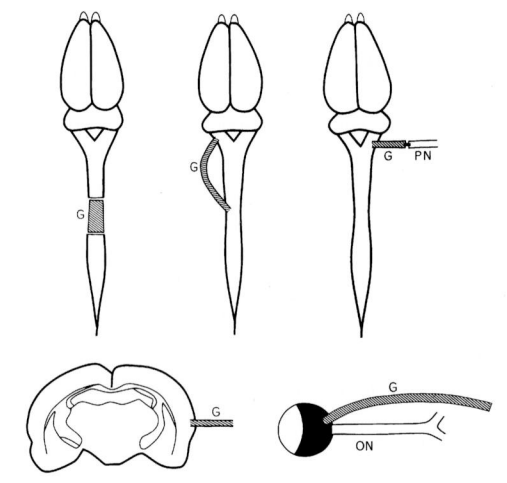

FIGURE 2.26   Experiments on rats proving that axons can be made to grow out of the central nervous system into peripheral nerve tissue. The basic method is to insert a free segment of rat peripheral nerve (stippled, **G**) into central nervous tissue; axons grow into it. **ON:** optic nerve; **PN:** peripheral nerve. (Reproduced with permission from [2].)

(65, 176); and (b) chondroitin sulfate proteoglycan, which can be overcome with bacterial chondroitinase (114). In the "bridge" experiments just mentioned, the myelin-related obstacle can be overcome by plugging the bridge into gray matter rather than white; a clever but technically very difficult task (164). At the time of this writing, the dogma of no regeneration in the central nervous system is obviously dead, but the axons growing across gaps—however assisted by growth factors, support molecules, or cultured stem cells—are few. Another worry, born of experience with peripheral nerves, is that even those few may fall into the trap of misguided regeneration.

The victims of spinal cord injury—about 11,000 new cases per year in the United States—will have to wait; but they may find some comfort in the fact that neural stem cells from many sources, humans included, are growing in several laboratories (54, 156, 158, 166, 167).

Plasticity and Regeneration in the Nervous System

The dismal performance of spontaneous regeneration in the central nervous system might lead us to conclude that recovery from massive brain lesions should be practically impossible. The facts speak otherwise. Patients who have suffered from hemiplegia due to a stroke can—over months—make significant recoveries. What is the mechanism if axon regeneration is so restricted? The answer is plasticity, a vague term denoting *the ability of the central nervous system to establish alternative pathways.* Axonal sprouting could lead to the formation of new circuits. Morphologic proof of this mechanism is very difficult to obtain, but some evidence exists (16, 58, 132, 168). For example, injury to a peripheral nerve causes sprouting in the central nervous system (152a). Plasticity seems to be the central nervous system's secret way of regenerating. Once again, structure and function are both cause and effect.

Are the Regenerated Cells As Good As the Old Ones?

The answer is *usually yes, but not always and not immediately.* In general, the new cells—whatever their type—look undifferentiated and take some time to reach full maturity, as shown by their enzymatic activities (9, 55). For example, if the kidneys of a rat are acutely poisoned with mercuric chloride, the epithelial cells of the tubules quickly regenerate, but they are low, almost flat, and partly undifferentiated. The functional result is an excess of urine outflow (polyuria) because the cells are still unable to reabsorb water and solutes as they should. Biochemically, there is a return to anaerobic glycolysis (9), which is, interestingly, a characteristic of embryonic cells. A return to normal metabolism requires 2–3 weeks. The same shift occurs in the regenerating liver, perhaps explaining the accumulation of unoxidized triglycerides in this condition (p. 92). It has been reported that regenerated endothelium in pig coronary arteries gives inappropriate functional responses for up to 6 months (146) and that *regenerated axons may show abnormal reactions for as long as 2 years* (86) (regenerated nerves, as we have seen, are a special case).

Occasionally, slow recovery can be an advantage. Precisely because regenerating cells are immature, they may be insensitive to certain toxic effects (p. 144).

Similarly, influenza virus kills the epithelial cells of the upper respiratory tract but spares the regenerating cells that follow because they do not yet have receptors for influenza virus (p. 608).

Telomeres and the Limit to Regeneration

The unfortunate lizards whose tails Spallanzani amputated over and over again two centuries ago proved that *cells can regenerate many times.* But how many times? In 1961, Hayflick and Moorhead asked the question by letting human fibroblasts grow *in vitro* for as long as they would last, and found that after about 50–100 divisions all mitotic activity stopped (72, 73). In other animals this "Hayflick number"—as it came to be called—was found to be greater or smaller, depending on the maximum life-span of the species (Table 2.1) (128). This correlation implies that there must be a mitotic timekeeper, and when the telomeres were discovered, they were hailed as the perfect candidates (21, 22, 40, 49).

The telomeres and their companion enzyme telomerase would deserve several pages of their own. In essence: the telomere is a strip of *noncoded* DNA tagged on at each end of every linear chromosome. It is needed, because the enzyme that duplicates the DNA is unable to read the 5′ tip of the DNA strand; if this defect were not corrected, *at every mitosis both ends of every chromosome would lose some DNA,* roughly 100 kilobases in humans (36). Almost all bacteria cope with this threat most ingeniously by adopting circular chromosomes. Eukaryotes responded by capping the chromosomes with telomeres, whereby at each mitosis a little segment of spare DNA is lost, with no loss of genes. In the absence of telomeres, the exposed tips of the chromosomes would tend to join end-to-end or develop other pathologic connections, ultimately incompatible with life.

Table 2.1 Correlation Between Life-Span of Species and Hayflick Number[a]

Species	Maximum Life-span (Yr)	Mean No. of Cell Population Doublings
Mouse	2	9.2
Rat	3.5	12.8
Kangaroo rat	7	12.8
Mink	10	25.0
Rabbit	13	22.5
Bat	14	18.0
Chicken	30	25
Horse	46	28.8
Human	110	61.3
Galapagos tortoise	150+	120

[a]Number of potential fibroblast divisions (*in vitro*).

Reprinted from [84] with permission of Cambridge University Press.

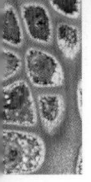

The other half of the telomere story, the synthetic enzyme *telomerase,* is also relevant to regeneration. The function of telomerase is to rebuild the shrinking telomere (91) whereby it earned the title of "enzyme of immortality." It is not expressed in most somatic cells, but it is present in germ cells, in activated T cells, in malignant tumors (p. 752), and *in the stem cells of several tissues* (91, 140), which suggests that these stem cells would be unable to perform their task within the limits of the Hayflick number (50–100 mitoses).

> Mice lacking the telomerase gene can live for two generations without apparent trouble; generations 3–6 develop defects typical of aging, such as gray hair, sluggish wound healing, and increased incidence of cancer (140).

Clearly, the telomeres, which are clipped shorter at each mitosis, seem ideally set up to function as a life-clock, and a great deal of evidence supports this view (81): but as of 2002 several ugly facts have distorted the beauty of the picture (177). The rule "long life, long telomeres; short life, short telomeres" does not fit the mice: their life is 30 times shorter than ours, but their telomeres are at last 3 times longer (45, 83). Also, the Schwann cells of rodents are able to divide without apparent limit, while fibroblasts from the same nerves stop growing after less than 10 doublings (96). Furthermore,

if rodent Schwann cells are fed higher concentrations of serum, they stop growing (could this be oxidative damage from higher metabolism? [96]). We must conclude that rodents have a different time clock, which we do not yet understand (96), and that cell longevity is decided not only by genes but also by external factors (96).

How Do Regenerating Cells Know Where to Go?

In the course of regeneration, cells that are normally supported by basement membranes (e.g., epithelial or endothelial cells) can find their way by gliding over their basement membranes, if they have remained intact (Figures 2.27, 2.28). It is quite another matter for cells circulating in the bloodstream to settle in any particular tissue. This will be a critical issue for intravenous cell therapy with stem cells. Bone marrow cells are at present the only "easy" case: grown in culture and reinjected, they find their way to the bone marrow thanks to *homing molecules* on their own surface and on the endothelium (126, 130). They can also home to *injured striated muscles,* as we have seen earlier; presumably this happens because the local injury induces vascular adhesion molecules. Oddly enough the homing to muscles occurs also in mice with congenital dystrophies, such as Duchenne's muscular dystrophy, in which the muscle fibers are all congenitally abnormal (lacking dystrophin)

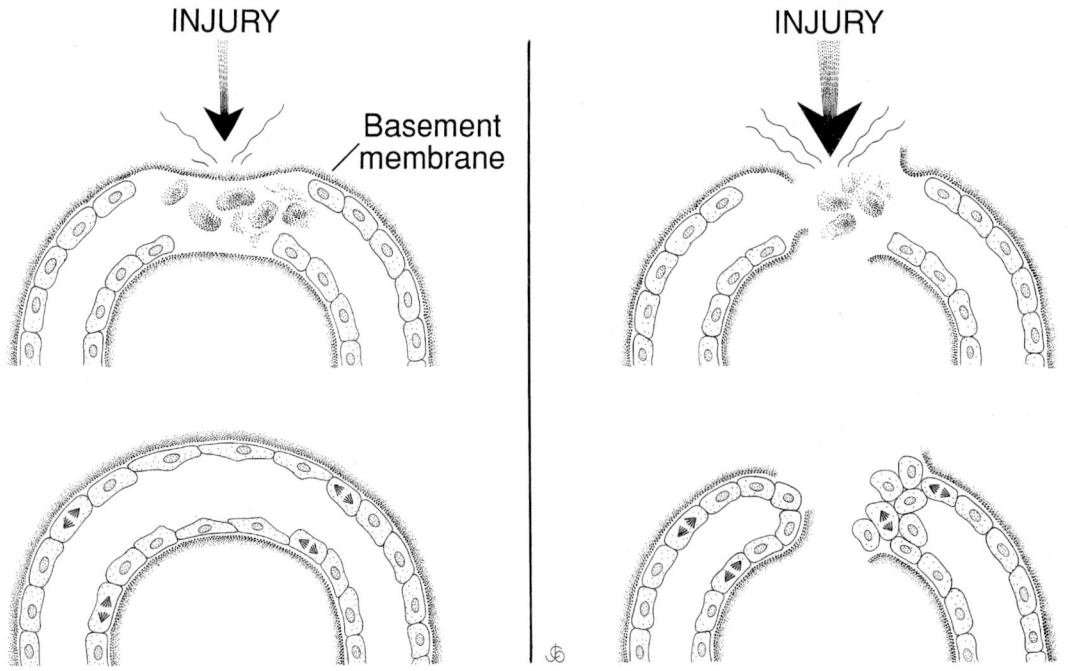

FIGURE 2.27　Guiding role of the basement membrane illustrated in a hypothetical epithelial tubule. *Left:* Mild injury to the tubule destroys some epithelial cells but not the basement membrane; the basement membrane remains as a guide to the regenerating epithelial cells, which crawl along it. *Right:* If the endothelial membrane is destroyed together with the epithelial cells, the latter regenerate at random, and the continuity of the tubule is lost.

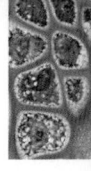

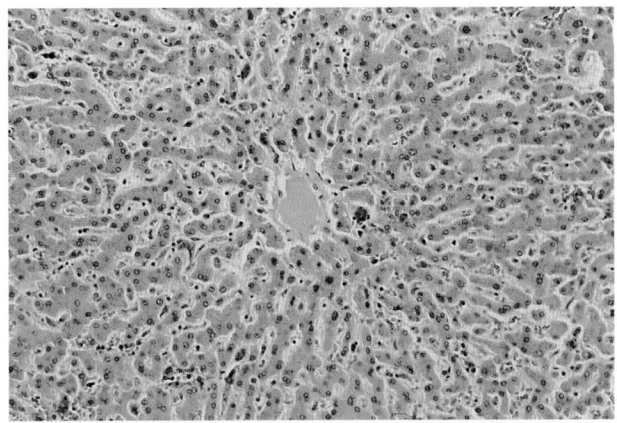

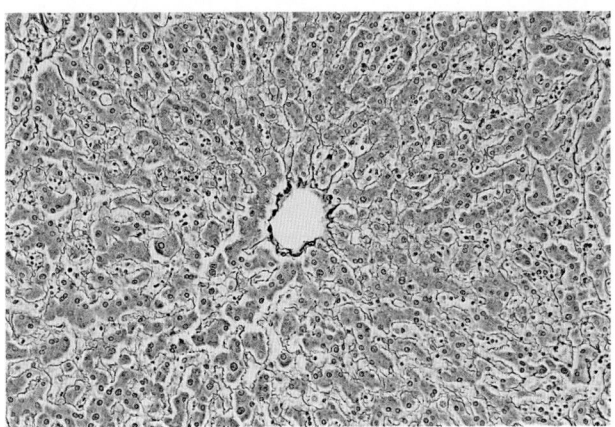

FIGURE 2.28 Liver tissue. *Top:* Normal liver parenchyma (hematoxylin-eosin stain). *Bottom:* The black reticular framework represents basement membranes that may provide liver with a framework for regeneration (silver stain and eosin).

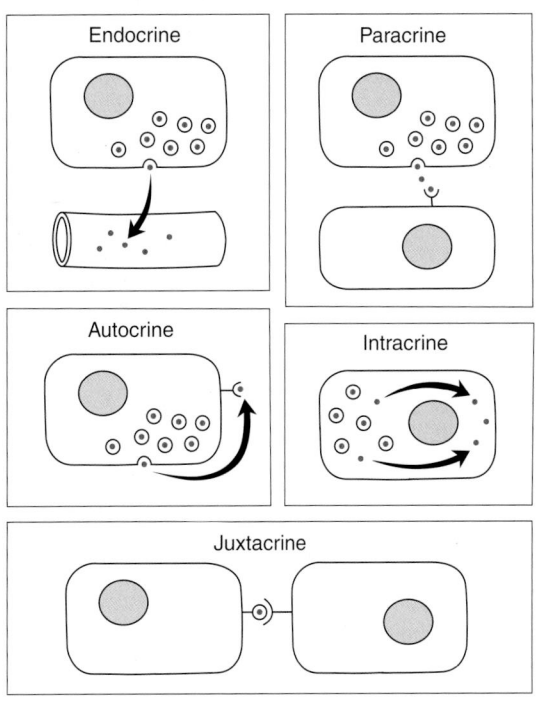

FIGURE 2.29 What was once called internal secretion is now subdivided into 5 subtypes, depending on the location and distance of the target.

but without an overt "injury." Twelve weeks after intravenous "cell therapy" with bone marrow cells, 4 percent of the fibers contain dystrophin (69). This is probably explained by the fact that dystrophic muscles are in a slow, constant state of repair, as if trying to heal themselves.

What Makes Cells Regenerate?

Something must be telling cells that they must turn on their replication program. As far as we know, the news could reach the cells in four ways: (a) principally by growth factors, and to a lesser extent by (b) electric currents, (c) cell-to-cell communication, and (d) nervous stimuli.

Growth factors. Growth factors are one of the busiest fields of research (173), not only because of their enormous therapeutic potential but also because the same genes that are responsible for cell proliferation are also involved in carcinogenesis. There are so many growth factors and they are so varied in their effects that we

cannot begin to describe them here; we will limit ourselves to a few generalizations and discuss individual growth factors in more detail as needed.

Growth factors are polypeptides with a molecular weight between 5000 and 30,000 kD that act on specific surface receptors. Unlike the hormones of the endocrine organs, which reach their targets via the bloodstream, growth factors behave mainly as local hormones, acting over a short distance or on the secreting cell itself (paracrine, juxtacrine, autocrine, and intracrine secretion) (Figure 2.29). They can be extracted from growing tissues, from tumors and from normal tissues.

Growth factors are multifunctional (Table 2.2); they can inhibit as well as stimulate. *They modulate each other,* which means that their effects depend on the presence or absence of other factors. It has been suggested that they function together like letters of an alphabet, from which the cells synthesize the ultimate message (152a).

The biology of the growth factors puts a severe strain on the memory of the nonexpert, who is endowed with a brain and not with a computer. Here is a partial list of effects:

- Cell growth
- Cell proliferation or inhibition
- Cell differentiation

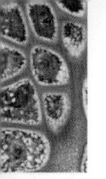

Table 2.2 Peptide Growth Factors Are Multifunctional

Growth Factor	Proliferative Effects	Antiproliferative Effects	Effects Unrelated to Proliferation
Epidermal growth factor	Keratinocytes, fibroblasts	Hair follicle cells	Suppression of gastric acid secretion
Fibroblast growth factor (basic)	Many mesenchymal cells, especially endothelial cells	Ewing's sarcoma cells, other tumor cells	Regulation of pituitary and ovarian cell function
Transforming growth factor-beta	Fibroblasts, osteoblasts	Fibroblasts, epithelial cells, T-lymphocytes, osteoblasts	Suppression of immunoglobulin secretion and adrenal steroidogenesis
Interleukin-1	Lymphocytes, keratinocytes, fibroblasts	Breast cancer cells	Endogenous pyrogen, bone resorption
Interleukin-2	T- and B-lymphocytes, oligodendrocytes	T-lymphocytes, oligodendrocytes	Increased cytotoxic activity of monocytes
Interleukin-6	Hybridoma, plasmacytoma cell lines	Breast cancer cells	Increased expression of cell surface antigens and secretion of immunoglobulins
Tumor necrosis factor-alpha	Diploid fibroblasts, epithelial cells	Many tumor cells	Inhibition of lipoprotein lipase, stimulation of collagenase

Adapted and reprinted with permission from Sporn MB and Roberts AB. Peptide growth factors are multifunctional. Nature 1988;332:217–219. Copyright 1988 Macmillan Magazines Limited.

- Cell activation
- Secretion
- Chemotaxis
- Other effects, such as vasoconstriction by platelet-derived growth factor (PDGF)

A further strain for the nonexpert is that most of the growth factors are plagued by names that are either obsolete, misleading, or not informative. We are particularly distressed by the "transforming growth factors," which do not transform at all (p. 748). Yet, appropriate names would be hard to find because each factor has so many effects. It would be like naming Harlequin from a single one of his colors. We will slowly become acquainted with them as we meet them.

The first growth factor to be discovered was nerve growth factor (NGF). Rita Levi-Montalcini noticed in 1948 that fragments of a mouse sarcoma, implanted into the body wall of a 3-day-old chick embryo, caused an outgrowth of sensory and sympathetic fibers; a similar effect was produced (an accidental discovery) by snake venom and by an extract of mouse salivary glands, tested as potentially homologous to snake venom glands (93). NGF was then extracted with the help of chemist Stanley Cohen. Tested *in vitro* on sympathetic ganglia, it produced the now-classic halo of sprouting fibers (Figure 2.30). Later, Cohen tested the effect of various preparations of NGF injected into newborn mice. A sharp biologist as well as a chemist, he noticed two epithelium-related events that could be obtained only with impure extracts: the teeth erupted faster, and the eyelids, normally closed at birth,

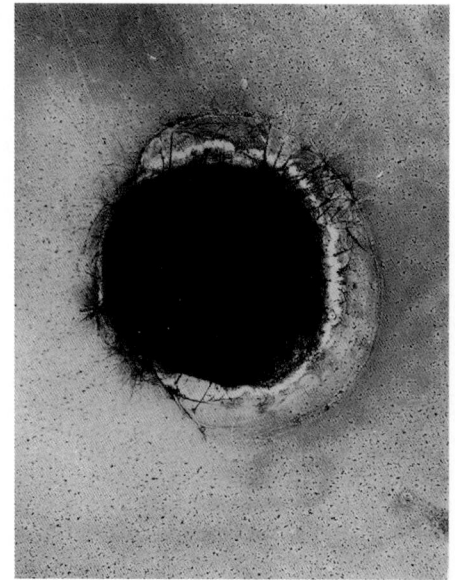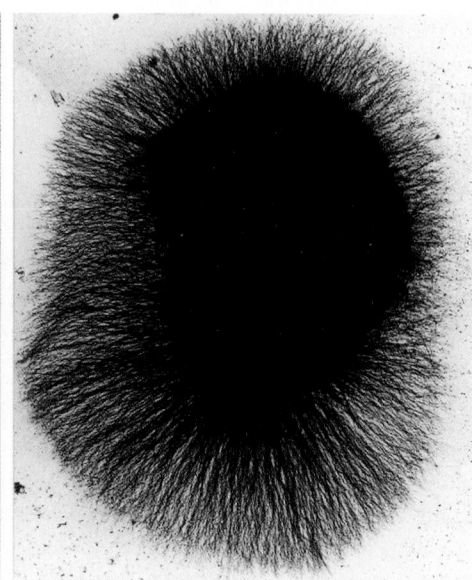

FIGURE 2.30 The famous halo effect that enabled Rita Levi-Montalcini to confirm the existence of the nerve growth factor (NGF). Low-power photomicrographs of two sensory ganglia from an 8-day chick embryo. *Left:* Ganglion grown in ordinary medium. *Right:* Ganglion grown in a medium enriched with NGF. The halo is due to the outgrowth of axons. (Courtesy of Dr. R. Levi-Montalcini, Istituto Superiore di Sanità, Rome, Italy.)

separated earlier. The active agent turned out to be an impurity, which was named epithelium growth factor (EGF). Rita Levi-Montalcini and Stanley Cohen shared the Nobel prize in 1986.

Other factors involved in regeneration. Mechanical stimuli, as we have seen, are important in the regeneration of bone, cartilage, and fibrous tissue. Electric currents are produced by injury (pp. 193, 370). Mild currents have been used successfully for many years to encourage bone healing; new bone forms at the anode, whereas osteoclasts get to work at the cathode. There are good data to show that electric currents play a role in the regeneration of limbs in amphibians. Beyond these facts and a few others on wound healing, the literature is meager (25). Cells connected by communicating junctions (also called gap junctions) should be able to pass along the news of a local injury; some do so *in vitro* (90), but the importance of this mechanism is not known. Nerves assist the regeneration of limbs in amphibians and of fins in fish (146a), perhaps by supplying mitogenic factors

(28). Nothing similar is known for mammals with one peculiar exception: in rats, the submandibular salivary gland fails to grow if the corresponding sympathetic ganglion is removed; it shrinks with adrenergic blocking agents and swells with sympathicomimetics (172).

> **TO SUM UP:** The new focus on regeneration and stem cells has led to the demise of two dogmas previously held to be among those medical truths that are self-evident: *neurons cannot duplicate, central axons cannot regenerate.* Now that we know that neurons do have these powers, we need to find out why they normally fail to apply them. A nagging thought: what if it turned out that it is better for the patient if axons in the central nervous system do not regenerate? They might get lost in the maze of fibers and make the wrong connections. Maybe so; but pessimism is not a guiding light in research.

Hypertrophy, Hyperplasia, and Polyploidy

Regeneration, as we described it, refers to the replacement of lost parts. Now we will see how cells and tissues respond to the need to become larger.

Hypertrophy defines an *acquired increase in the size of a cell, tissue, or organ.* When a part of the body is called on to increase its size, it can do so by increasing the volume of its cells (hypertrophy), their number (hyperplasia), and often both. The type of response depends on the tissue and on the causal agent: cells that can enlarge *or* multiply usually favor one pathway (249). Hyperplasia is similar to regeneration, except that it leads to an increase in size of the organ. When an organ appears grossly enlarged, it is of course impossible to distinguish with the naked eye the relative contributions of hypertrophy versus hyperplasia; hence the colloquial use of "hypertrophy" for both. Biologically, however, the type of process involved does make a difference.

Cells that are undergoing either hypertrophy or hyperplasia are synthesizing more cytoplasm, i.e., more protein. Therefore we can expect that their cytoplasm, seen by light microscopy, will be more basophilic than usual because the number of ribosomes is increased. The nucleolus enlarges because it is synthesizing more ribosomes; as for the nucleus, it will also be enlarged but *less* basophilic (!) because its chromatin is dispersed, reflecting enhanced DNA transcription.

> **NOTE:** If a cell appears much larger than normal and its nucleus is also very large, it is reasonable to suspect more than hypertrophy, namely polyploidy (p. 41).

Pathways to Hypertrophy and Hyperplasia

The mechanisms that lead to hypertrophy and hyperplasia fall into five groups, which we will now examine.

(1) Increased Functional Demand

Kidneys. A simple way to study the effects of functional stress is to remove one of two paired organs; if one kidney is removed (nephrectomy) the other enlarges. This is called compensatory hypertrophy. Compensatory hypertrophy of the kidney is said to be a combination of hypertrophy and hyperplasia (Figure 2.31) (200, 215) but mainly hypertrophy (229, 249). Interestingly, *renal hypertrophy (as opposed to hyperplasia) is thought to be a maladaptive process that fosters gradual loss of renal function* (259). The glomeruli enlarge and their capillaries multiply (233) and become longer (233, 251), but there are no new glomeruli or new tubules. The podocytes, recall, behave *in vivo* as permanent cells, which further limits glomerular enlargement. The

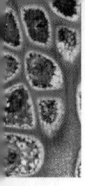

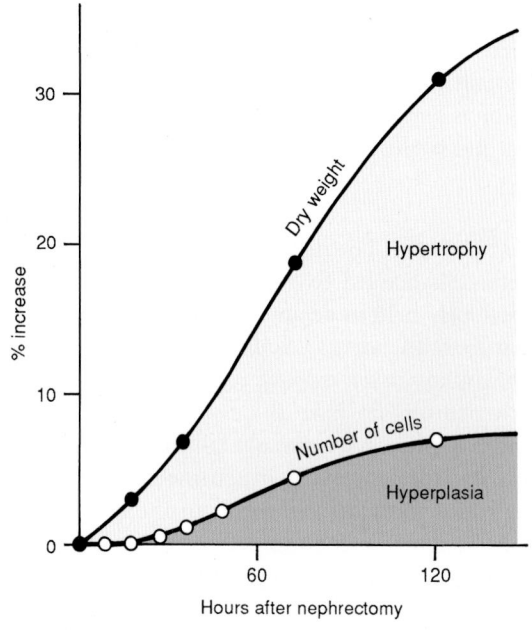

FIGURE 2.31   Relative extents of hyperplasia and hypertrophy of a mouse kidney after contralateral nephrectomy. The space between the two curves (dry weight, number of cells) reflects cellular hypertrophy. (Adapted with permission from [224], © American Society for Investigative Pathology.)

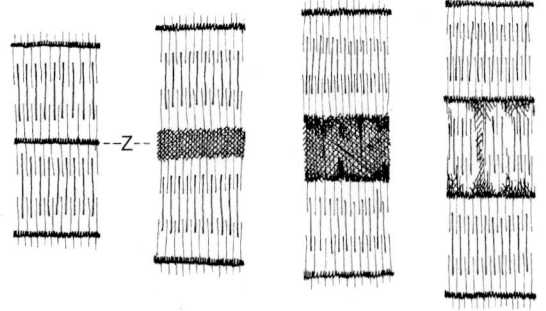

FIGURE 2.32   New sarcomeres can develop (during myocardial hypertrophy) by broadening and splitting of the Z lines. (Courtesy of Dr. H. F. Cuénoud, University of Massachusetts Medical School, Worcester, MA.)

cellular response to unilateral nephrectomy is somewhat sluggish because the remaining kidney can increase its function almost instantly by vascular adjustments (208). In dogs, the glomerular filtration rate can increase up to 100 percent within minutes. In rats, the weight of the remaining kidney increases by 30 percent in 1 week; it never doubles.

Striated muscle. Increased functional demand on striated muscles has dramatic cellular effects. Clearly, the cells know what they are doing because they adapt their response to the type of challenge. *In response to endurance exercise, they increase the number and volume of the mitochondria, whereas heavy resistance training induces mainly hypertrophy of the contractile apparatus* (186) and probably also an increase in fiber number (185). The capillary network increases too (226).

Smooth muscle. Enlargements of smooth muscle tissue are usually due to a combination of hypertrophy, polyploidy, and hyperplasia (223, 244). For instance, in pregnancy the body of the uterus enlarges about 70-fold by these mechanisms. It is common to observe smooth muscle thickening upstream from an intestinal stenosis, due to the effort of pumping the content through the stricture; a 10-fold increase in mass can be

measured experimentally in 3–5 weeks (210, 223). In hypertensive rats, the aortic media acquires more cells, larger cells, thicker elastic fibers, and more collagen—changes that are only partly reversible (244).

Heart. Increased effort due to exercise, hypertension, or a valvular defect translates into increased mass of the heart muscle. Athletic exertion alone can increase the human heart weight to 500 g (300 g is normal for men and 250 g for women) (222). Occasionally, the heart of a patient with long-standing valvular disease can exceed 2 kg; such enormous increases are not seen in other animals (206). The cells expand their contractile machinery by adding sarcomeres; depending on the functional demands, the new sarcomeres are added *in parallel* with the old ones (i.e., side by side) or *in series* (end to end) by the peculiar mechanism of Z-band splitting (Figure 2.32) (206, 234). In the "physiologic" hypertrophy of athletes, there is a proportionate increase in length and width (221).

Although the heart cells (myocardiocytes) were long thought to be incapable of dividing, the facts are different. Shortly after birth, human myocardiocytes cease to multiply and then enlarge 30–40 times (hypertrophic growth) (243). Later, between 5 and 9 years of age, they begin to become polyploid and continue to do so through life; in adults two thirds of these cells are polyploid (up to 16N) and about one fifth of them are binucleated (206, 247). If the heart is submitted to functional strain, polyploidization increases (Figure 2.33) (183), and in human adults, gigantic nuclei appear (Figure 2.34). Because the size of the cells ceases to increase after a critical heart weight is reached, an increase in cell number must take place; this is today an accepted fact, as we have seen (189).

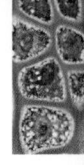

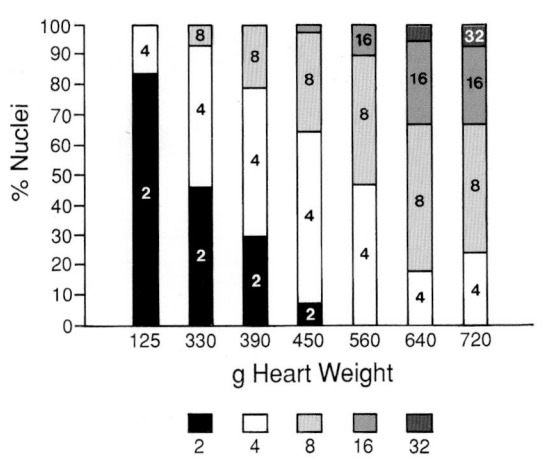

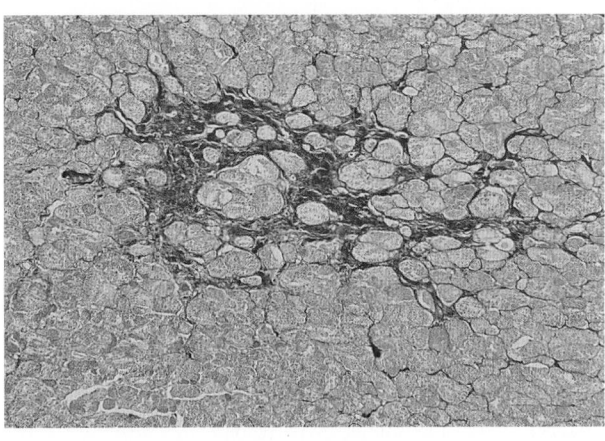

FIGURE 2.33   With increasing heart weight there is a progressive increase in ploidy of myocardial cells (indicated by the figures on the bars). The 125-g heart came from an 8-year-old child. (Adapted from [183].)

FIGURE 2.35   Hypertrophic human hearts tend to develop fibrosis, as well shown with this trichrome method: collagen is stained blue. Note the infiltration of connective tissue strands between individual myocardial fibers. (Preparation courtesy of Dr. F. J. Schoen, Brigham and Women's Hospital, Boston, MA.)

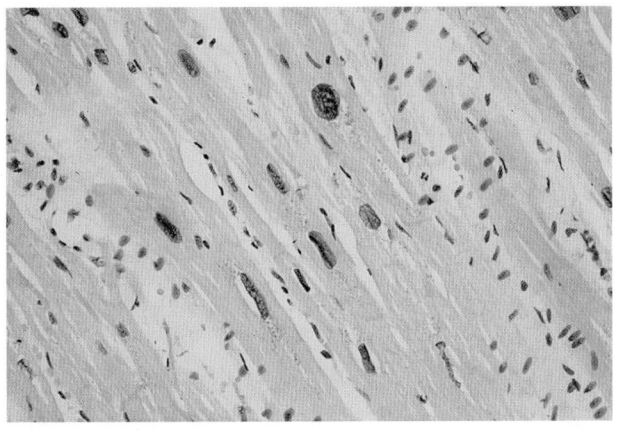

FIGURE 2.34   Human myocardium with hypertrophic and polyploid nuclei. Note the gigantic nucleus at *top center;* compare with normal nuclei in *bottom left corner.*

As myocardial hypertrophy progresses, a worrisome development takes place in the extracellular spaces. The connective tissue stroma increases in excess of the apparent need (Figure 2.35) (182). This fibrosis stiffens the myocardium and decreases its compliance. Why fibrosis develops is unclear; perhaps it is a response to cellular damage (252). To this day it is not treatable. At the same time, the number of capillaries increases but does not keep pace with the muscular mass, leading to relative anoxia (188, 190, 230). Furthermore, as the myocardial cells continue to enlarge, they develop pathologic features (206, 234) such as abnormal aggregates of sarcotubules, masses of abnormal mitochondria

and myelin figures, excessive amounts of glycogen (including intramitochondrial glycogen), bizarre nuclear infoldings (207), and eventually loss of contractile elements and of specialized intercellular junctions.

We have now partially answered a critical question: is myocardial hypertrophy pathologic? The many structural changes that occur in progressive hypertrophy lead eventually to myocardial "exhaustion." It should be clear, however, that an athlete's heart does not fit this category; it may have a reduced reserve, but it is not intrinsically diseased (222). Notice also that an athlete's heart (unlike that of a patient with a valvular defect) is placed under strain for a few hours at a time, after which it has the rest of the day to recover.

Is myocardial hypertrophy reversible? Initially, it is. However, it has been shown experimentally that if the cause of the hypertrophy is removed, the muscle mass and the RNA return to normal, but the DNA and the interstitial collagen do not (202). This leads to the bizarre situation of huge polyploid nuclei in fibers of normal size.

The brain and mental activity.   How does the brain respond to chronic stimulation? Nobody has ever taken brain biopsies from students before and after exams, but the basic question can be approached by "non-invasive" means. Here is a beginning: a well-controlled study in 2003 has shown that the risk of dementia is reduced by leisure activities requiring mental effort such as playing board games, musical instruments, dancing and reading (201a, 257a). We shall return to this question in relation to "atrophy of disuse."

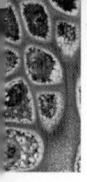

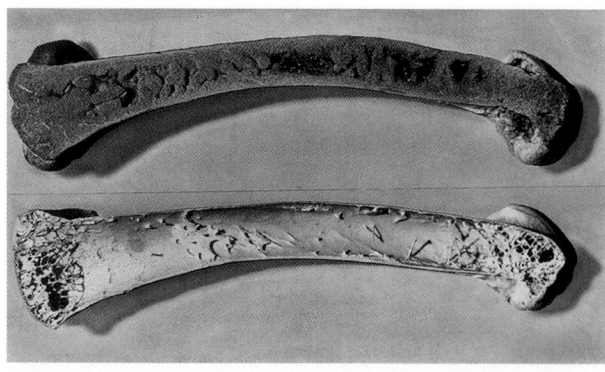

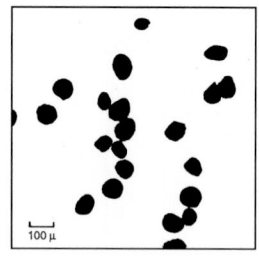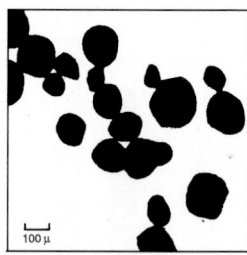

FIGURE 2.37 Microphotograph of fat cells from a normal child (*left*) and from an obese child (*right*). The cells are black because they have been fixed with osmium tetroxide (194.)

FIGURE 2.36 Physiologic hypertrophy and atrophy of the femur in hens. *Top:* The bone of a laying bird is filled with medullary bone as a source of calcium. *Bottom:* In a nonlaying bird the bone is hollow. (Reproduced from [257].)

(2) Endocrine Stimulation

The enlargement of the uterus due to estrogen (216) is a classic example of endocrine stimulation. The result is hypertrophy as well as hyperplasia. Another example is the estrogen-induced hypertrophy of bone in egg-laying hens (Figure 2.36) (257).

> An oddity: isoproterenol, a beta-adrenergic agonist, mysteriously induces hypertrophy of the salivary glands in rats and mice (192).

(3) Excessive Nutrition

Excess nutrition leads to an increase, as everyone knows, of fat tissue; it is less known that it also leads to a 50 percent increase in protein synthesis throughout the body (235). In other words, the overfed Sumo wrestlers do not accumulate fat only.

An increase in fat beyond a certain limit has a name: **obesity.** At the cellular level it involves an interplay between hypertrophy and hyperplasia; the details are still controversial, but there is some consensus, as follows (187, 194, 242). During the first year of life, the fat cells enlarge and by 12 months they reach adult size; *from then on, the increase in fat tissue mass is mainly due to an increase in fat cell number.* In adults, excess calories are stored at first in preexisting fat cells, which become larger (hypertrophy), but prolonged overnutrition can eventually induce an increase in fat cell number. This means that *obese individuals have more and bigger fat cells* (Figure 2.37) (194).

It seems that fat cells can enlarge up to a certain critical size; at that point they transmit a signal to the preadipocytes, which differentiate into new fat cells. It is thought that once new fat cells are formed, they can

be made to shrink, but they never disappear (205). We just said never, a word never to be used in a medical context. The fact is that *under conditions of extreme starvation, all traces of adipose tissue do disappear.*

Because getting rid of fat cells is so difficult, it is particularly bad for obesity to develop in children. *Fat cells acquired at an early age will be there for life.* Adult-onset obesity seems to imply mainly hypertrophy, which can be reversible. In this regard we can only wish that we could be more like the woodchuck (205). Before hibernation the woodchuck goes through a phase of overeating in order to store fat; if its fat cells had to undergo a wave of hyperplasia every year, it would soon become obese and unfit to survive. Thus, the woodchuck has a built-in mechanism that allows fat cells to undergo hypertrophy but not hyperplasia.

> There seems to be a peculiar correlation between fat cell size and the brain. If adult rats are submitted to lipectomy (removal of about 25 percent of their adipose tissue, which reduces the fat storage capacity), their appetite drops (204). Also, if fat cells are depleted beyond a certain point by a severely restricted diet, symptoms of depression and hormonal changes ensue (205), as if the fat cells were signaling that fat reserves are too low. This is another reason that makes it very difficult for obese people to return to normal weight.

We can now ask the same question we asked about hypertrophy of the heart: *is excess fat a disease?* Obesity was indeed declared a disease in 1985 (218a, 225). It causes about 300,000 deaths per year in the United States alone (184) and has become a world-wide epidemic (248). It is such a threat to health that we feel obliged to offer some detail, as general pathology of the world at wide.

The threat of obesity is largely due to its complications, which are many and diverse (239, 240): osteoarthritis due to the weight on the joints, hypertension, a higher risk of coronary heart disease, atherosclerosis, stroke, cancer of the colon, endometrium, breast and

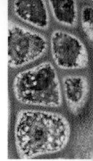

prostate, diabetes Type 2, gout (237), gallstones, stress incontinence, sleep apnea, increased mortality from all causes, social discrimination, and even poverty (214).

> Some of these complications can be explained. Fat cells are depots of cholesterol dissolved in the triacylglycerols; cholesterol is excreted through the bile, and a chain of events correlates obesity and gall stone formation (196). Fat cells are also able to aromatize androgens to estrogens; in fact they are the major source of extragenital estrogen synthesis in postmenopausal women. This is the link between obesity and cancer of the endometrium (203, 256).

Diabetes Type 2 needs special emphasis, because it occurs in about 10 percent of the obese. Just decades ago it was a disease of minor significance; it is now riding on the wave of obesity as another major threat to public health, for which the name **diabesity** was suggested (260). According to a report from Cincinnati, between 1982 and 1994, as obesity increased, the incidence of diabetes Type 2 rose almost tenfold (254). When we say that diabetes Type 2 arises as a complication of obesity, we must remember that diabetes itself is a source of nasty complications, including generalized microvascular disease leading to blindness, renal failure, neuropathies, impotence, and acceleration of atherosclerosis with its own complications.

How does diabetes Type 2 (non–insulin dependent) develop from obesity? An answer is urgently needed. We shall return to this topic in relation to lipid storage (p. 91).

(4) Increased Blood Flow

Vascular tumors of a limb can cause that limb to become longer. A similar overgrowth is sometimes seen in children after fracture or infection of a long bone (osteomyelitis). These effects are usually attributed to increased blood flow, but a local flooding with growth factors should also be considered.

(5) Mechanical Factors

In long bones, mechanical load stimulates the osteoblasts, leading to hypertrophy; lack of mechanical load causes bone atrophy. In the skin, it is *traction* that induces hypertrophy. When plastic surgeons need to cover a skin defect but the surrounding skin cannot be stretched over it, they use a method known as tissue expansion. A balloonlike device is slipped under the skin and slowly inflated over several weeks, until the overlying skin expands enough for the purpose (198). This stretching mechanism was known thousands of years ago and exploited for cosmetic and even surgical purposes. Even today, in several parts of the world, earlobes and lips are stretched with weights or other devices; Buddha is usually represented with stretched earlobes (232). Somehow the cells transduce a pull to hyperplasia.

Can Any Cell Be Stimulated to Exhaustion?

The hypertrophic heart is the best example; there are hints that exhaustion can occur also in other systems. Renal glomeruli can be overstrained; by removing five sixths of a rat's kidney tissue, the remaining portion (called *remnant kidney*) shows glomerular damage that has been ascribed to hyperfiltration (197), and the damage is more severe if the rat is kept on a high protein diet (219, 220), which is itself a stimulus to renal hypertrophy. The glomerular exhaustion may be due to the fact that the glomerular epithelial cells (podocytes) do not regenerate and therefore cannot keep up with the increased functional demands (209). It is often mentioned that pancreatic beta cells overstimulated by chronic hyperglycemia develop "metabolic exhaustion" (228), but the distinction between chronic glucose toxicity and beta-cell exhaustion is not clear (253).

Finally, we offer two teasers:

- *High altitude anoxia causes hypertrophy of the myocardium.* How could lack of oxygen increase the size of the heart? Here is the most obvious reason: if the supply of atmospheric oxygen is low, the heart has to pump harder to maintain a normal oxygen supply to all the tissues (231). However, there is an additional factor: the heart must also pump harder because anoxia, strangely enough, causes the pulmonary arteries to constrict (236).
- *Why is myocardial hypertrophy sometimes seen after a large myocardial infarct?* Infarcts destroy heart tissue and leave scars, and therefore oblige the rest of the ventricular myocardium to undergo compensatory hypertrophy.

The Biology of Polyploidy

At long last we have an answer to the meaning of polyploidy in animal tissues.

Polyploidy (Figure 2.38) my accompany hypertrophy, as discussed earlier, but polyploid cells—recognized by their large nuclei and overall large size—are also found in many normal tissues, *in numbers that increase with age* (213): especially in the liver, but also in the salivary glands, pancreas, epidermis, and other organs (191, 193, 195, 199, 261). If it is true that some brain cells are polyploid, a relatively old observation (227), it would be interesting to find out at what stage of development these cells—so reluctant to divide—have duplicated their DNA. The megakaryocyte is a special case in that it is an obligate polyploid (261). Its chromosomal

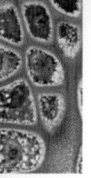

FIGURE 2.38   Steps leading from a diploid to a polyploid cell. (Adapted from [238].)

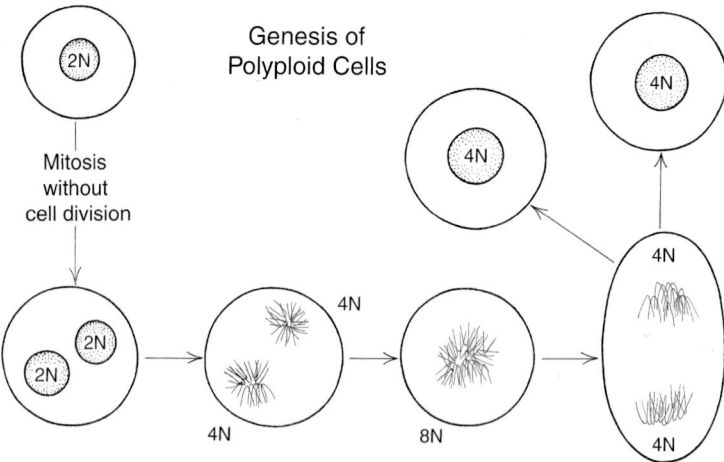

endowment ranges from 4N to 64N (241, 245, 246), and it clearly relates to function, since *the megakaryocyte does not begin to make platelets until it is octoploid* (199). From then on, the platelets increase in size slightly with the degree of ploidy of the parent cell (261).

What could be the advantage of polyploidy for animal cells? The standard explanation used to be that having several copies of the same gene is an insurance against gene damage, e.g., by radiation or aging (211). Indeed, there is a species of wasp, *Habrobracon,* that comes in two variants: haploid and diploid; radiation damage, as measured by survival, is markedly more severe in haploids (201). This makes sense, but there must be a deeper reason for polyploidy, and one was found in 1999 by studying the yeast that produces beer, *Saccharomyces cerevisae* (212, 218). *Yeast cells with identical DNA can be quite different in regard to structure, function, and behavior if they differ with regard to ploidy.* In other words, there are things cells can do only if they are polyploid: megakaryocytes are what they are for professional purposes—not just for fear of radiation damage. In the world of botany, polyploidy has a further significance: it is a major mechanism for the development of new species. Almost half of the existing 300,000 plant species have a polyploid origin (250). Famous polyploids include the chrysanthemum, the potato (here the advantage of larger cell size is obvious at least for the farmer), wheat, tobacco, and sugar cane.

In plants, polyploidy is a major evolutionary mechanism. The effect of polyploidy on the plant varies, but it is often associated with greater size and vigor (250). Because polyploid plants usually cannot produce fertile offspring with diploid plants, the new hybrids are reproductively isolated from the parental strains and become new species. Polyploid animals are very rare (258); triploid infants live just a few weeks (217).

Unlike animals, plants live in a cloud of potentially fertilizing pollen. In most cases nothing comes of it, but if hybridization does occur, the two sets of chromosomes may be so different that at the time of meiosis the chromosomes cannot pair off acceptably and no fertile gamete develops. However, if a "mistake" occurs at meiosis, such that the chromosomes double but the cell fails to divide, a tetraploid cell results. Meiosis at this stage can produce two fertile tetraploid gametes (255).

TO SUM UP: We have learned that cells respond to a variety of stimuli by becoming larger; when these stimuli disappear the cells usually return to their standard size, but in some cases they can make the enlargement permanent by becoming polyploid. Polyploidy *per se* has important genetic functions. We have also learned that hypertrophic cells, tissues, and organs may have built-in liabilities: bigger is not necessarily better.

Atrophy

Atrophy is *an acquired decrease in size of cells, tissues, or organs.* In ancient Greece, *a-trophia* meant "lack of food." Starvation is indeed the most obvious cause of atrophy, but there are at least 10 others (Table 2.3).

Some bits of necessary jargon: if an organ or tissue is congenitally underdeveloped, the proper term is **hypoplasia. Aplasia** means that an organ has never developed at all (e.g., aplasia of the left kidney) or that its cells

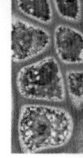

Table 2.3 **Causes of Atrophy**

Decreased function
Starvation
Reduced blood flow
Local pressure
Occlusion of secretory ducts
Hormonal effects
Old age
Space flight
Denervation
Toxic agents, drugs
X-rays
Immunologic mechanisms
Germ-free condition

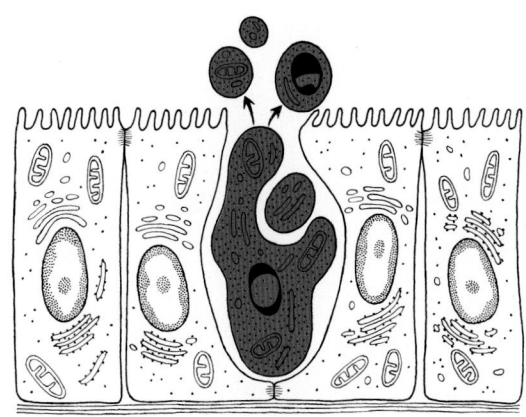

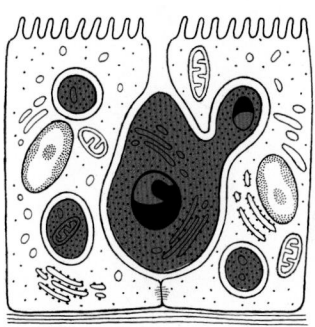

FIGURE 2.39 Apoptosis in an epithelium: a single cell dies and becomes detached from its neighbors; its rounded fragments (apoptotic bodies) can be actively extruded to the lumen (*top*), or phagocytized by neighboring cells (*bottom*). (Adapted from [370].)

have ceased to multiply (e.g., aplasia of the bone marrow in aplastic anemia). Do not confuse atrophy with **atresia,** "no-orifice," which refers to congenital imperforation (e.g., atresia of the anus or vagina). The term **involution** overlaps atrophy; it applies to the normal, programmed shrinkage of certain organs such as the uterus after childbirth, the thymus in early life, or temporary fetal organs such as the pro- and mesonephros.

The follicles of all our hair are programmed to repeat, throughout life, a cycle subdivided into three phases: **growth (anagen), rest (telogen) and involution (catagen).** In the human scalp these phases last respectively about 100 days, 1000 days, and a few days (340), which sums up to years, but for the eyebrows, a few weeks are enough (319).

Mechanisms of Atrophy

Two options are available to an organ that must shrink; it can reduce the *number* of its cells by cell deletion, or their *size* by shrinkage. The modality depends mainly on the type of tissue.

Cell Deletion

Deletion is indeed a peculiar phenomenon. Certain cells are somehow picked out as obsolete or dispensable, and are induced to commit suicide. Virchow, who considered the body as a democratic cell-state in which each individual has its function, might have had some difficulty in justifying this ruthless arrangement, which occurs also physiologically as **programmed cell death** (p. 217). Histologically, in an organ undergoing atrophy, cell deletion requires attentive searching because the cells disappear quickly and without fanfare. They shrink and break up, and so do their nuclei, according to a ritual known as **apoptosis** (p. 210). If they line a free surface, their remains are cast off as apoptotic bodies; otherwise they are swiftly removed by macrophages

or by the very cells that hours before were friendly neighbors (Figure 2.39).

The death sentence—more correctly, the order to commit suicide—is somehow delivered to the various types of cells according to hierarchy: in a gland, for example, the most specialized cells (the secretory cells) disappear before those of the ducts. The stroma, however, is relatively spared, so in the end an atrophic organ may appear to contain too much connective tissue.

Cell Shrinkage

The second option available to an organ that must decrease its size is to make each one of its cells shrink. This mechanism has its limits because most cellular organelles are essential for survival; however, some can be trimmed down. This is best seen in striated muscle; its huge cells contain a vast amount of fibrillar material, some of which can be sacrificed.

The "flesh and bones" of the cell are proteins; therefore, to reduce its volume, the cell must resort to proteolysis. Intracellular proteins can be digested by two

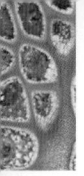

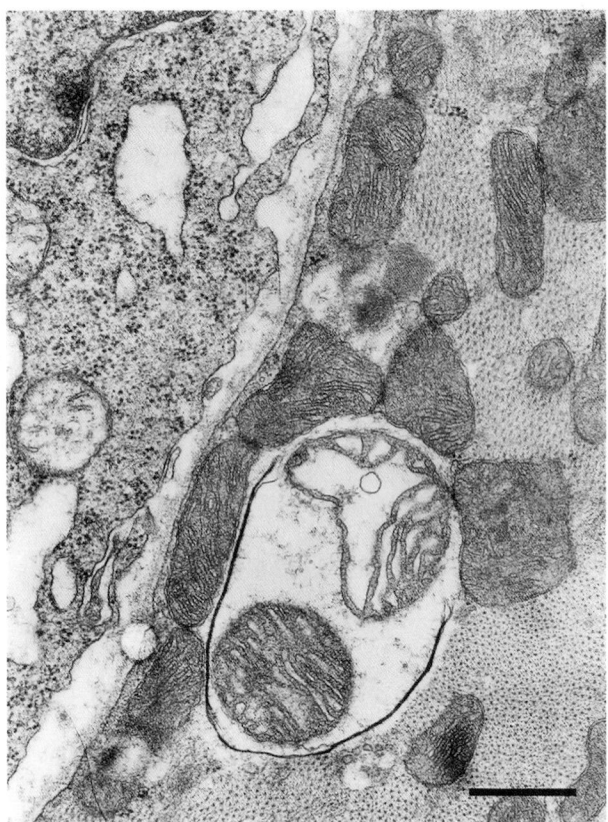

FIGURE 2.40   Autophagic vacuole in the leg muscle of a mouse 5 days after strenuous exercise (9 hours of running). **Bar** = 0.5 μm. (Reproduced from [328].)

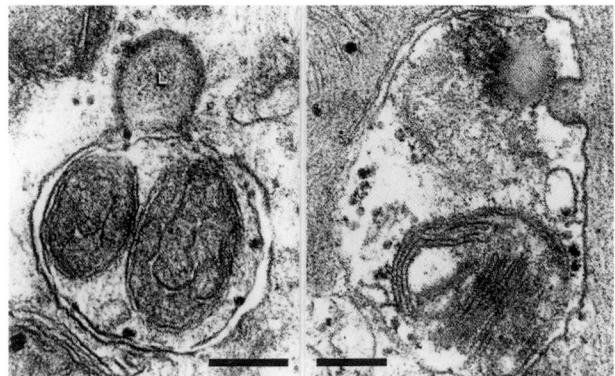

FIGURE 2.41   Autophagic vacuoles in rat myocardium. *Left:* Two mitochondria have been segregated for destruction; at the top, a lysosome (**L**) fusing with the autophagosome. *Right:* More advanced stage of digestion. The content includes a semidigested mitochondrion. **Bars** = 0.2 μm. (Reproduced from [287], by permission of Dr. U. Pfeifer.)

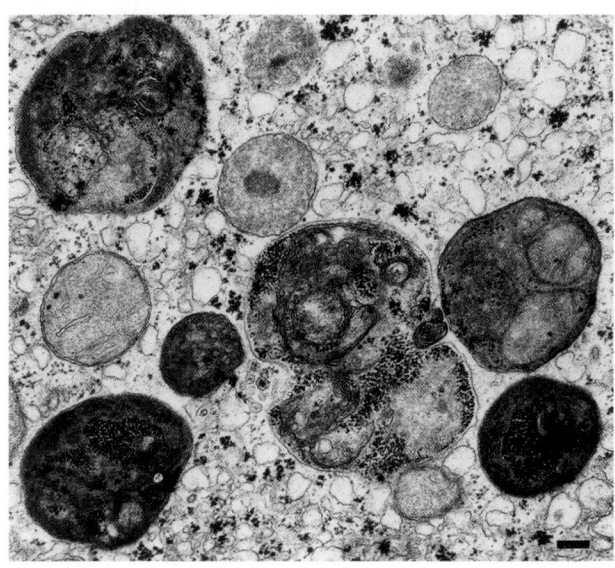

FIGURE 2.42   Autophagic vacuoles and residual bodies rapidly forming in a liver cell during acute atrophy induced by ligation of a branch of the portal vein. The recognizable content of the vacuoles includes glycogen and mitochondria. **Bar** = 0.2 μm. (Reproduced from [329], by permission of Dr. U. Pfeifer.)

main pathways: the phagosome-lysosome pathway (*autophagocytosis*) and the ATP-dependent proteasome pathway.

Autophagic vacuoles. These busy little bodies were discovered in 1962 (266) in liver cells, where they are prominent also under normal circumstances; they exist in animals, plants, and fungi (306a, 307). They are membrane bound and usually contain one or more semidigested cellular organelles. They can form amazingly fast, within 5 minutes or so (330). A spoon-shaped double membrane seems to arise out of nowhere (but probably from the endoplasmic reticulum [324, 337]), curves spoonlike around a little island of cytoplasm, surrounding it completely, and imprisons whatever organelles happen to be within (Figure 2.40) (290, 346, 356). Primary lysosomes are sometimes seen fusing with autophagic vacuoles (Figure 2.41).

As autodigestion advances, the content of the vacuole is dissolved and presumably reutilized. However, some of the lipid seems to be difficult to digest; it becomes denser and darker and eventually forms brownish granules called **lipofuscin** (p. 102). The few

autophagic vacuoles that are condemned to remain stuffed with this undigestible material are called **residual bodies:** spent autophagosomes containing the remains of spent organelles. Residual bodies seem to be the internal garbage cans in which cells dump all the material that they are unable to digest or excrete (Figure 2.42). They can be numerous enough to give an atrophic organ a brownish hue, especially in the liver

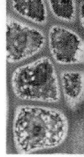

and heart, hence the term **brown atrophy.** The same faint discoloration can be induced at a slower rate by the normal process of aging.

Single electron micrographs cannot do justice to the extraordinarily active behavior of autophagic vacuoles in their normal task of organelle turnover. They may account for as much as 50 percent of mitochondrial turnover in the liver. Considering that a liver cell has some 2000 mitochondria and that about 5 percent per day are taken in by autophagic vacuoles, we can say that about four mitochondria have to be digested per cell per hour. The job is performed very fast: the half-life of the autophagic vacuoles is in the order of 8 or 9 minutes, with some difference according to the organelle engulfed (327, 331). Clearly there is plenty of work for the autophagic vacuoles even in the absence of atrophy.

Several mysteries remain about autophagic vacuoles. For example, what makes them entrap this or that organelle and never the nucleus? They certainly have no horror of DNA because there is some in the mitochondria that they happily devour. Incidentally, no genetic harm is done by destroying some of the mitochondria, because the DNA is identical in each mitochondrion, as it is in each bacterium of a given species.

> Autophagic vacuoles increase in number in muscle after strenuous exercise (Figure 2.40) (342). Experimentally they can be rapidly induced in the liver by glucagon, a catabolic agent (266, 346); by isoproterenol, a beta-adrenergic stimulant (330); and by antimicrotubule agents such as vinblastine and colchicine (337). In the liver they can be produced in such numbers that they can be isolated by cell fractionation (275). Their number is reduced by insulin, an anticatabolic hormone (330, 331); for reasons unknown, they have a circadian rhythm (328).

The second mechanism of cell shrinkage by proteolysis is provided by the **26S proteasome,** an astonishing molecular construct roughly in the shape of a cylinder with a lid at each end, about 200 Å in height and therefore visible by high-power electron microscopy. Proteins that have to be removed must first be covalently bound to a small protein, *ubiquitin,* free in the cytosol; thus labeled they are recognized and captured by the "lids" and then shoved into the cylinder, where they are broken down. These operations require ATP (263).

The pathophysiology of the 26S proteasome (so named in 1988) is just being worked out. For lack of space we can say no more, but *beware of considering it as just another protease.* By its controlled destruction of growth factors (such as cyclins), it becomes, in turn, an important factor in regeneration, apoptosis, cancer, and even neurogenerative diseases (323), not to mention inflammation (345), the immune response and autoimmune disease (300).

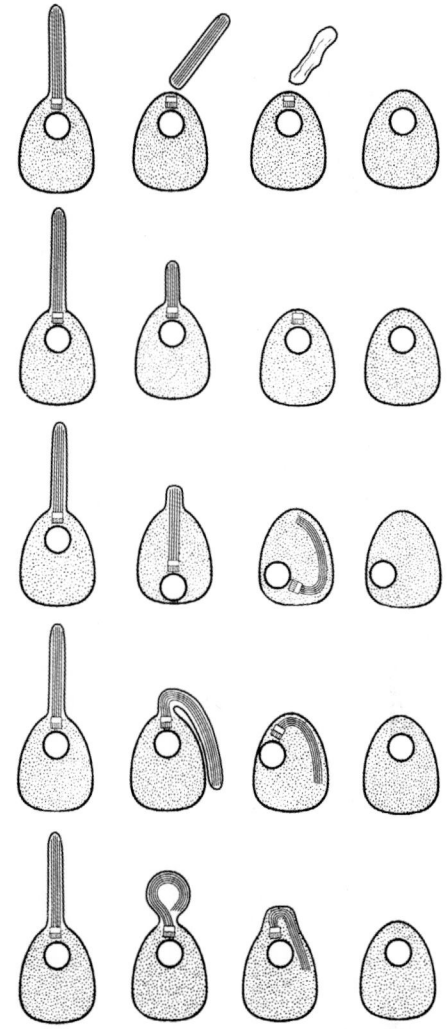

FIGURE 2.43 Cilia can disappear by several mechanisms; this table summarizes data from protozoa, algae, and fungi. A comparative study on mammals does not yet exist. (Reproduced from [277]. Reprinted by permission of The Faculty Press, Cambridge, England.)

Although autophagosomes and proteasomes explain the major steps of atrophy, not all the steps are understood. Figure 2.43 illustrates the surprising variety of mechanisms whereby cilia are lost in lower organisms (277). Their disappearance has been studied extensively in protozoa and other lower organisms, but little is known for humans, although the loss of cilia from bronchial epithelium affects millions of smokers.

> In general, the enzymes of an atrophic cell tend to decrease (Figure 2.44) (362); however, while striated muscle undergoes atrophy, acid phosphatase increases (339). This is not a contradiction: acid phosphatase is the hallmark of lysosomes, which become temporarily more active in a self-digesting cell.

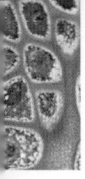

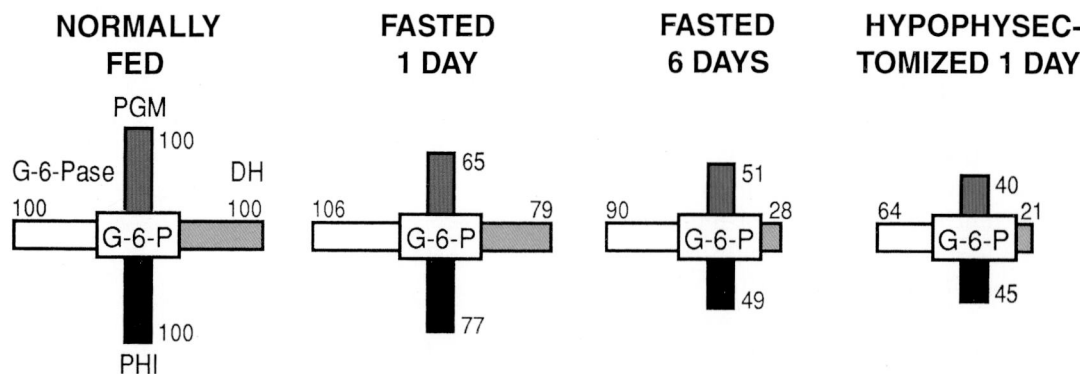

FIGURE 2.44   Atrophy at the level of enzymes: reduced activity of four enzymes involved in the utilization of glucose-6-phosphate (G-6-P) under various conditions (expressed as percent of normal). **G-6-Pase:** Glucose-6-phosphatase; **PHI:** phospho-hexose-isomerase; **DH:** glucose-6-phosphate dehydrogenase; **PGM:** phosphoglucomutase. (Reproduced by permission from [362].)

Atrophy and the Extracellular Materials

Extracellular materials are not spared by atrophy because they depend in part on cellular metabolism. For example, in immobilized limbs the articular cartilage tends to lose its proteoglycans (p. 282); even the ligaments lose strength and may take months to recover (264, 325). The most dramatic changes occur in bone because its extracellular materials are being perpetually remodeled. If the balance between osteogenesis and osteolysis is upset, the amount of tissue can increase or decrease strikingly.

Bone atrophy, commonly known as **osteoporosis** or **osteopenia,** is an enormous public health problem in the United States (at least 1.2 million fractures per year) (Figure 2.45). The slow, age-related osteoporosis is due to reduced bone formation, and the post-menopausal accelerated osteoporosis is due to increased bone destruction (312). In a heroic 36-week experiment on bedridden volunteers, the total calcium loss amounted to 4.2 percent of the body's store (289).

Remember, however, that *there is no such thing as bone decalcification,* although the expression still recurs in the language of radiologists. No matter how atrophic, bone never loses its calcium; the loss of opacity to X-rays represents loss of bone mass.

Causes of Atrophy

Cells and tissues can be induced to shrink by a surprising variety of agents; 12 are discussed here.

(1) Decreased Function

As everyone knows, decreased function causes organs to atrophy. The process can occur very fast. When a fractured limb is placed in a plaster cast, for example, the muscles shrink in a matter of days. However, this atrophy has two components: inactivity and trauma (267). Inactivity accelerates protein catabolism; in a striated muscle isolated *in vitro,* protein breakdown can be reduced by passive mechanical stretching and by electrical stimulation (294)—facts that are clinically applied in physiotherapy. The trauma itself—more precisely, the very fact of having sustained an injury—brings about a general reaction that speeds up the catabolism of muscle (p. 511).

> Experiments on three volunteers with both lower limbs immobilized in plaster casts showed that a negative nitrogen balance appeared (despite an adequate diet) after 5 days (344). The data suggest that protein synthesis was reduced while breakdown continued. Space travel has the same effect (357).

The popular notion that the function makes the organ ("use it or lose it") has been strikingly demonstrated by experiments on the eye. If one eyelid of a kitten is kept closed for the first 3–4 months of its life, the central visual pathways do not develop properly (in this case, however, we are dealing with hypoplasia rather than atrophy) (347, 349). That darkness should affect the visual cortex is perhaps not too surprising, but it is somewhat startling that in hamsters it should cause atrophy of the *testes.* The mechanism is hormonal and operates through the hypophysis. But male readers need not worry. This happens, it seems, only in hamsters (296).

(2) Starvation

This topic echoes grim circumstances (Table 2.4). Compared with other organs the brain is the least susceptible to atrophy, as measured by changes in weight (352, 369). This means only that the nutritionally starved adult brain is protected from gross atrophy;

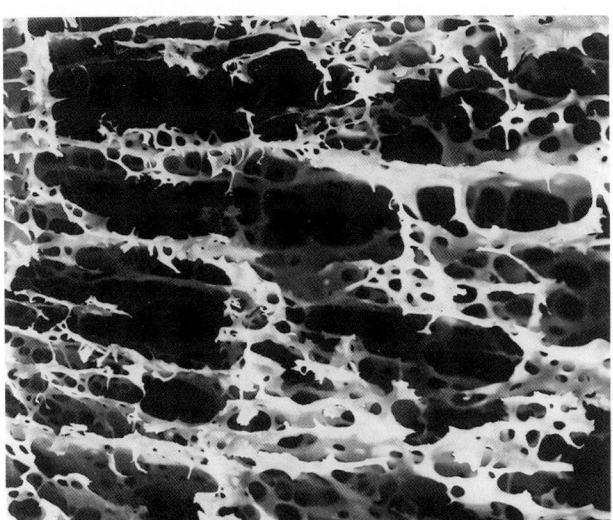

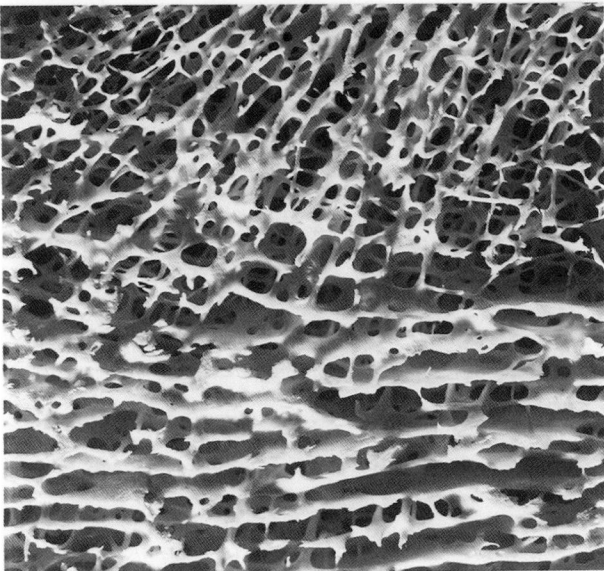

FIGURE 2.45 *Top:* Atrophic (osteopenic) and (*bottom*) normal human bone. Slices of vertebrae, washed clean of bone marrow, bleached and dried. (Courtesy of Dr. C. Hedinger, Kantonsspital, Zurich, Switzerland.)

Table 2.4 Human Hunger Disease

Organ	Weight Recorded[a]	Normal Value[b]
Brain	1309	1310
Heart	220	275
Liver	865	1500–2000
Kidneys	226	305
Spleen	103	150–250

[a]Values in grams from 492 autopsies recorded at the Jewish Hospital in Warsaw during the 2½ years before the ghetto was overrun. The work was performed under heroic conditions; the manuscript survived because it was buried.
[b]Normal values quoted by the authors refer to a contemporary source; present values in grams would be: heart 300–350, liver 1500, and spleen 150.
(Slightly simplified from: Pathological anatomy of hunger disease, Stein J, Fenigsten H in: Hunger Disease, Winick M (ed.). Copyright © 1979 John Wiley & Sons, Inc. Reprinted by permission of John Wiley & Sons, Inc.)

type—e.g., fibroblasts—are not identical throughout the body. Regional differences in the lipid content and behavior of adipocytes are well known (265).

Caloric restriction and the prolongation of life. Here we run into one of the paradoxes of pathology. Among the mechanisms of atrophy, the most logical should be starvation, and so it is. But starvation has also a contrasting virtue: *a moderate degree of food restriction can increase the life-span by about 50 percent* (298, 363, 365). This is the only known method for extending the life-span of warm-blooded animals (286, 371). It works even for spiders (Figure 2.47) (268), for paramecia (341), and in fact for all the creatures that have been tested (310a, 314, 332), including genetically long-lived dwarf flies (285). Experimentally it delays many conditions associated with aging, such as skin problems, loss of fertility (274), many chronic diseases (318), senile cataracts

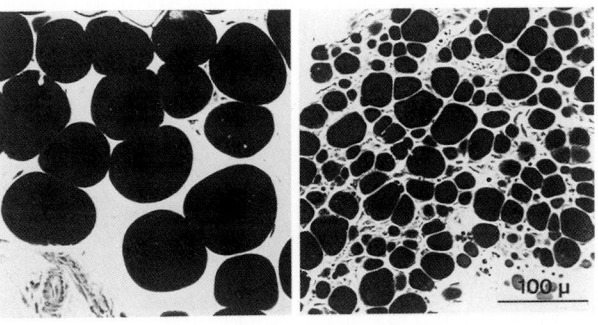

FIGURE 2.46 Atrophy of fat cells in acute experimental diabetes. *Left:* Control adipose tissue, blackened with osmium tetroxide (OsO_4). *Right:* 6 days after an intravenous injection of streptozotocin, which destroys the pancreatic beta cells: dramatic atrophy of the adipocytes. A similar result is produced by fasting. (Reproduced from the **Journal of Cell Biology,** 1977;72,104–117, by copyright permission of The Rockefeller University Press [283].)

however, biochemical changes do occur (350), and starvation during growth can lead to permanent brain damage (271, 333, 336).

In contrast, the effects of starvation on the adipocytes (energy-storing cells) are great. As triglycerides are depleted, the cells shrink drastically (368); the same can happen during the ketotic phase of diabetes (Figure 2.46) (281, 283). Oddly enough, the fat cells in some areas are affected more than others; the mechanism is not known, but this is merely one of the many examples showing that *cells of a given*

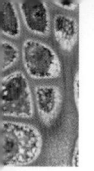

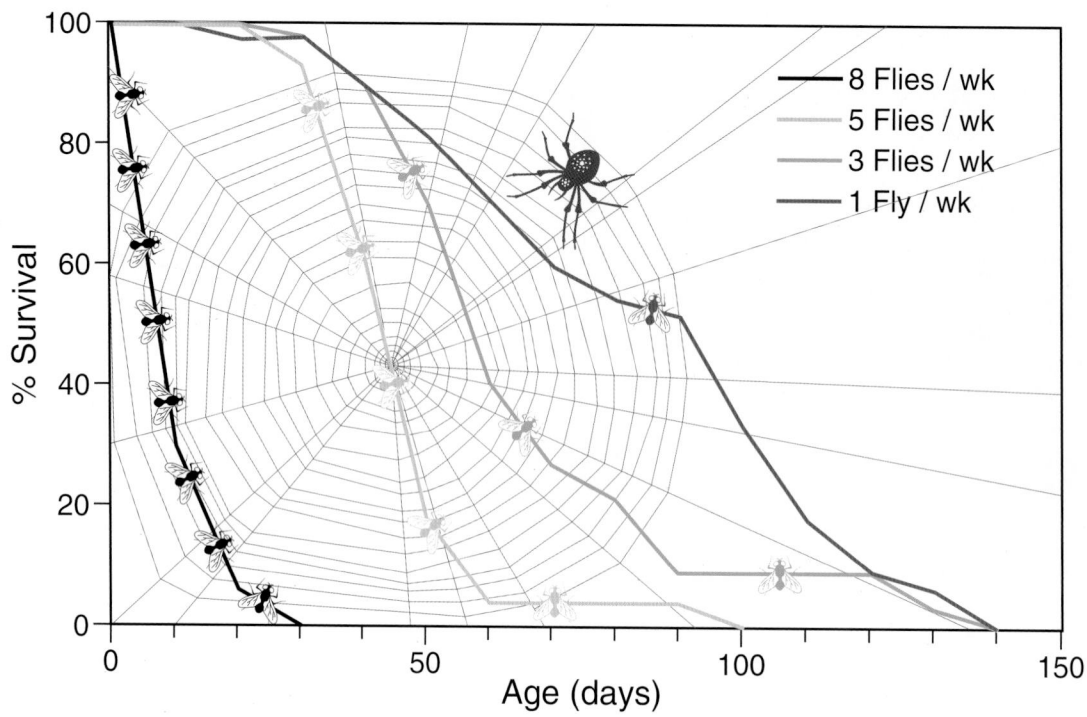

FIGURE 2.47 The prolongation of life by dietary restriction applies also to the spider *Frontinella pyramitela*. In free-living spiders on a rich diet of eight flies per week, the average life-span is 30 days. In captured spiders on an austerity diet of one to three flies per week, the life-span increases to 140 days. (Adapted from [268], copyright 1989, with permission from Elsevier.)

(354), cancers, and the decline of T-lymphocyte function (366). It also protects rats against kidney damage (315) and against many manifestations of stress (297, 298, 343), and rabbits against myocardial infarcts (288). The basic premise, let this be clear, is that we are dealing with *undernutrition but without malnutrition.*

It remains to be seen why undernutrition should be so beneficial. The latest theory, laid forth in *Nature,* sounds like a major breakthrough, although the authors play very cool (303a). May the reader decide.

> Starvation increases protein turnover, with activation of protein deacetylases called **sirtuins.** Now Howitz et al. discovered three classes of small molecules that activate sirtuins directly, in the absence of caloric restriction. One of these is resveratrol, a polyphenol found in red wine "that is associated with a surprising number of health benefits." It prolonged the life of yeast by 70 percent, and increased DNA stability. It was previously known to mitigate age-related diseases, including neurodegeneration, carcinogenesis, and atherosclerosis. The sertuins, by the way, increase cell survival by inhibiting p53 (p. 887) thereby delaying apoptosis: this gives damaged cells more time to repair themselves and avoid unnecessary death (303a).

"Reduced use of the genetic code" has also been suggested (272), and recent work shows that caloric restriction leads to a very different gene expression, with emphasis on increased protein turnover and reduced macromolecular damage (308). A study on undernourished rats found that the release of toxic free radicals (p. 196) in the liver was reduced, while protective antioxidant enzymes were increased (297, 298). So far there have been no experiments on volunteer humans, but all indications are that the principle should work (365). The residents of Okinawa, who live on a typical low-calorie diet, have a 40-fold greater chance of becoming centenarians (358).

The argument in favor of undernutrition can be stretched even further. Famine can have protective effects, which are abolished by feeding (322). A study among natives of Niger has shown that cerebral malaria selected undernourished children *after they were refed.* The protective mechanism of starvation may be related to iron deficiency, since many parasites, including those of malaria, thrive in an excess of free iron (295). One of the body's standard protective responses to injury is to make iron *less* available (p. 116). Evolution may have preserved this response to starvation as a protection against infectious agents during hard times.

> Some marine iguanas from the Galapagos Islands have developed a special adaptation to shrinking food supplies: they shrink in length up to 20 percent (367).

FIGURE 2.48 Cross sections of four rat kidneys showing progressive renal atrophy after complete obstruction of the ureter. Numbers indicate weeks after surgery. **Bar** = 5 μm. (Reproduced from [293], © by the U.S. and Canadian Academy of Pathology, Inc.)

(3) Prolonged Inadequacy of Blood Flow

Chronic ischemia leads to atrophy of the blood-starved areas. Note the difference between a sudden stoppage of flow, which promptly kills the blood-starved tissue, and a partial but prolonged inadequacy of flow, which leads to tissue atrophy. A classic example is the kidneys of people who suffer from sclerosis (hardening) of the renal arterioles. The nephrons supplied by these arterioles slowly shrink, leaving a shallow depression on the surface of the kidney; the presence of many such areas gives the surface a granular aspect.

(4) Local Pressure

Growing tumors or other swellings can cause local pressure. The surface of a cerebral hemisphere may become deeply indented by a slow-growing meningeal tumor, leading to the atrophy of a large mass of brain tissue. The mechanism is certainly due (in part) to reduced blood flow. Mild, persistent pressure on a bone can cause its surface to recede as if it were made of a soft plastic material. Before the days of thoracic surgery, an aneurysm of the thoracic aorta (an outpouching that develops when the aortic wall is weakened) could press against the sternum, gnaw its way through it, and appear beneath the skin as a pulsating mass.

> Bone does behave like a malleable material, but this plasticity must be understood in a biological, rather than physical sense; it occurs over weeks and months by a slow process of remodeling. Constant local pressure stimulates the osteoclasts. Pressure from a tumor acts in this fashion; prostaglandin E_2 secreted by tumor cells may be the chemical mediator (335).

(5) Occlusion of a Duct

In exocrine glands, occlusion causes the glandular cells to stop secreting; ultimately they commit suicide and disappear by apoptosis. For example, if one ureter is occluded, the kidney continues to produce urine for a short time (hours, days); urinary pressure rises, and there is a great dilation of the urinary pathways above the occlusion, while the kidney itself becomes atrophic and eventually becomes almost paper-thin (Figure 2.48) (293). In mouse kidneys, the tubules may disappear in 12 weeks (280). The tubular epithelial cells

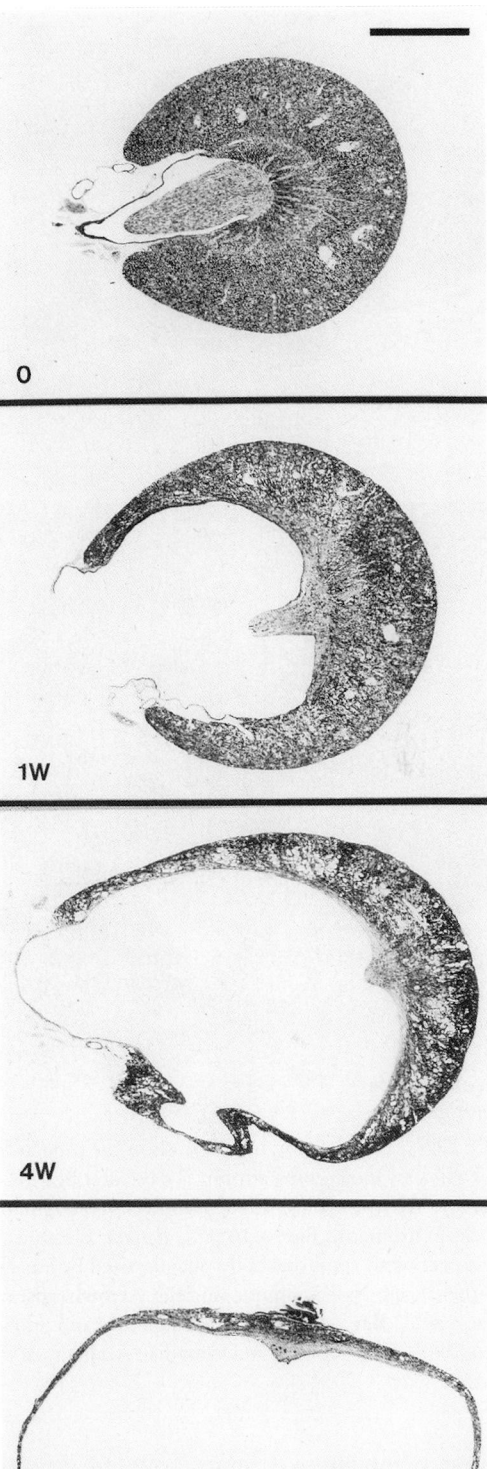

0

1W

4W

12W

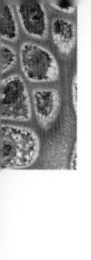

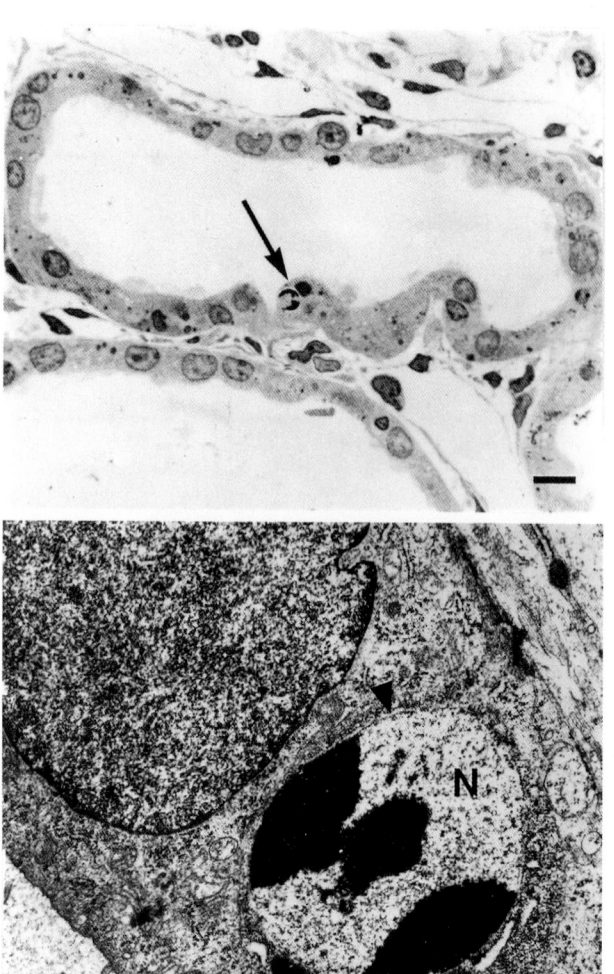

FIGURE 2.49 Cell deletion by apoptosis in the tubular epithelium of a kidney undergoing atrophy 7 days after ligation of the ureter. *Top:* **Arrow:** typical condensation and margination of the nuclear chromatin. **Bar** = 10 μm. *Bottom:* Electron microscopic aspect of an apoptotic body phagocytized by a neighboring epithelial cell. **N** = apoptotic nucleus. **Arrowheads:** margin of phagosome. **Bar** = 1 μm (Reproduced from Gobé and Axelsen [293], © by the U.S. and Canadian Academy of Pathology, Inc.)

disappear by apoptosis (Figure 2.49). In general, the pressure within occluded ducts rises and then falls; the longer the period of obstruction, the greater are the effects. *The testis may be a partial exception* (Figure 2.50) (304): after ligation of the vas deferens in men (but not in rats [316]), atrophy is slight. Procreation was possible for about 50 percent of men reoperated (an operation called vasovasostomy) 8–15 years after vasectomy (302, 306). How these facts fit together is presently not clear.

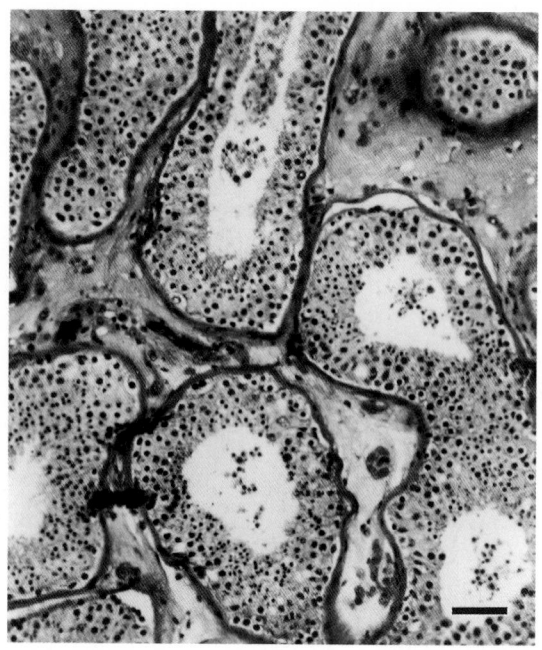

FIGURE 2.50 Biopsy of a human testis 10 years after vasectomy in a 35-year-old man. Spermatogenesis is reduced, but all the various cellular elements in the tubular wall are preserved. This lack of atrophy after ligation of the secretory duct is characteristic of the testes. **Bar** = 50 μm. (Reprinted, by permission of the New England Journal of Medicine 313; 1252, 1985. [304].)

Exocrine glands in general are very sensitive to duct ligation (Figure 2.51). In the rat, 31 days after the duct of the submaxillary gland is occluded, the secretory cells have become atrophic and stop secreting; they retain the capacity to regenerate if the occlusion is removed, although after 180 days they have not yet fully recovered (353). In this model, the changes induced by ligation resemble those brought on by starvation. *In the pancreas, ligation of the main duct leads to the slow disappearance of the exocrine component alone,* by cell deletion (359). In the end the pancreas becomes a mass of connective tissue containing the larger ducts and intact islets of Langerhans (Figure 2.52). This sequence led to the discovery of insulin.

One evening in 1920 in London, Ontario, while preparing a lecture for medical students, F. G. Banting came across a paper reporting that a pancreatic stone in a patient had blocked the main duct, causing atrophy of the exocrine pancreas but sparing the islets. Suddenly he saw an answer to his problem: he was trying to obtain a pure preparation of islets, to extract their endocrine secretion. He promptly tried ligating the pancreatic duct in dogs, and it worked. Later it turned out that the ligation was unnecessary, but he won the Nobel prize anyway (276).

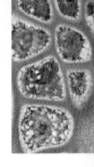

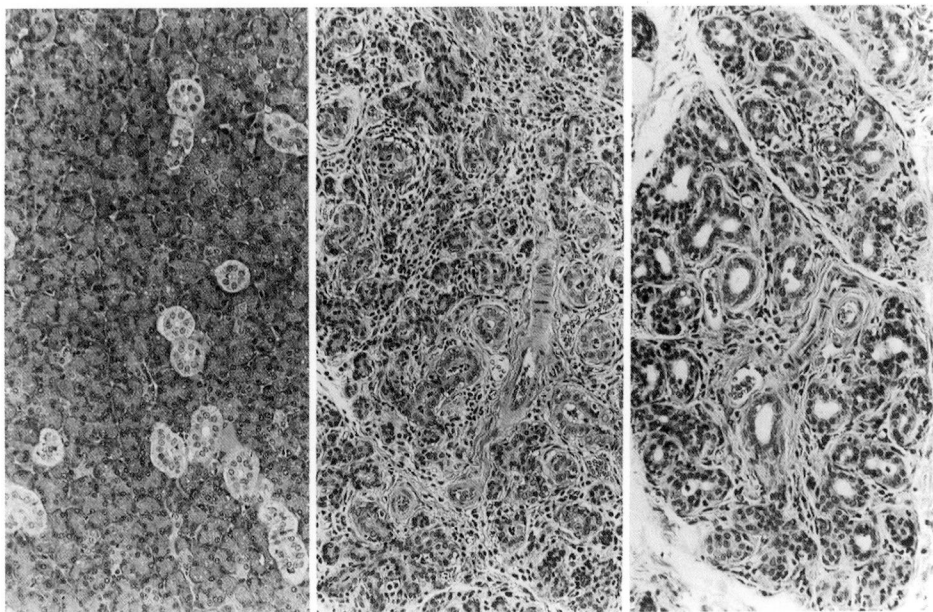

FIGURE 2.51 Effect of obstructing the duct of a parotid gland in the rat. *Left:* Normal control. *Center:* One week after obstruction there is significant loss of acinar cells. *Right:* Four weeks after obstruction, the acini have disappeared; the gland is reduced to collecting ducts in a bed of connective tissue. These changes are accompanied by a reduction in the capillary bed. (Reproduced from [360]. Reprinted by permission of John Wiley & Sons, Ltd.)

(6) Hormones

Hormones are a common cause of atrophy, despite their name, which means "stimulators." Common targets of hormonal atrophy are the endocrine glands themselves. *The best way to shut down and to atrophy an endocrine gland is to supply it with its own hormone.* This fact can be put to practical use. For example, some people are at an increased risk of developing cancer of the thyroid because their thyroid was irradiated "incidentally" in childhood: it was fashionable at one time to prescribe X-rays on the neck for enlarged tonsils, whooping cough, and other conditions. The best way to reduce the proliferative activity of the thyroid follicles in such cases is to administer small doses of L-thyroxine (321).

Another mechanism of endocrine-induced atrophy is the absence of a trophic hormone. Hypophysectomy leads to adrenal atrophy, which can be reversed, up to a point, with ACTH (355). Leptin, a hormone secreted by fat cells, has an anorectic effect; it also inhibits fatty acid synthesis, but its action is very complex (285a, 326).

(7) Old Age

Aging is, of course, a much broader problem than atrophy, but it does include atrophy at many levels. There is a total decrease in body mass after the age of 45–55 years, with a relative increase of body fat and a well-documented decrease in weight of the brain, liver, kidneys, and spleen (279). The immune system becomes less responsive (364).

Why does life lead to old age? There is no dearth of theories (343). The notion of a limit to life brings to

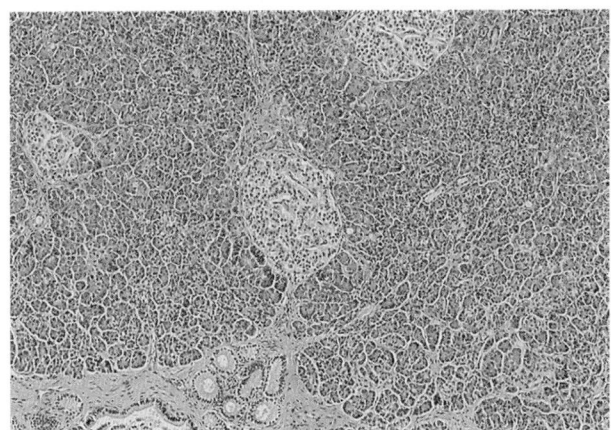

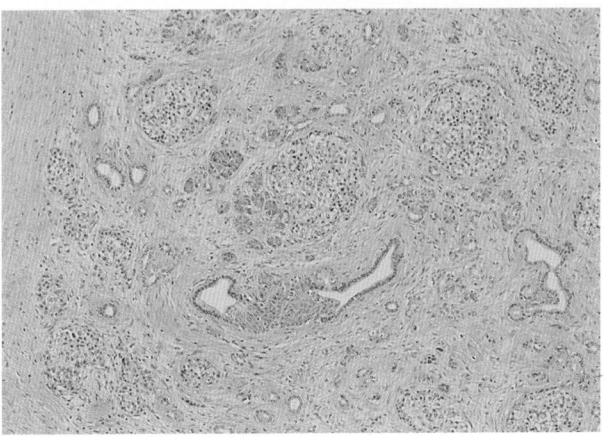

FIGURE 2.52 *Top:* Normal human pancreas: Islet of Langerhans. *Bottom:* Atrophic human pancreas after long-standing obliteration of the main duct. The exocrine pancreas has largely disappeared; the islets have survived and appear closer together.

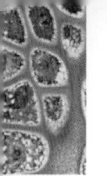

mind the Hayflick number and the shortening telomeres (p. 33), but there is more to old age than running out of mitoses. One theory blames the DNA: a daily dose of somatic mutations results in a progressive accumulation of errors until the system can no longer function (309). The errors could be due to free radical damage (299). The free radical theory is supported by many facts; for example, antioxidants increase the lifespans of many species, from yeast, worms, and mosquitoes (338) to mice, rats, and guinea pigs. Recent studies on senescent human fibroblasts showed a progressive shift in gene expression, including the repression of c-fos, which is essential for proliferation; it follows that cellular senescence could be a process of *terminal differentiation.* In other words, senescence would not be the result of accidents or errors but of programming.

Much remains to be done on very old humans. A recent study on 213 Ashkenazi Jews with exceptional longevity (98.2 years) showed that they and their offspring had significantly larger HDL and LDL particle sizes (272a). It has been pointed out that if we truly descend from short-lived unicellular ancestors, evolution has stretched our life span more than 1000 times (265a).

Although *space travel* is not an immediate concern for most of us, it should be mentioned here because it has effects comparable to those of age (361): atrophy of bone and muscle. Experiments with isolated muscle preparations have shown that microgravity has a *direct* effect on muscle cells, decreasing protein synthesis (313, 357).

The lesson of progeria. Imagine a child shaped as a withered little man, arthritic, bald, and with the wrinkled skin of old age. Actually he is 10, but he was born with progeria, a rare congenital disease (less than 100 cases worldwide) which leads to greatly accelerated aging. The brain is spared; life expectancy is about 13 years. The genetic mechanism was just worked out, in part by a married couple of scientists whose son was born with this disease (290a, 357a): *a point mutation on chromosome 1 affects the gene that codes for lamin A,* a fibrillar protein previously known to provide mechanical support to the nucleus. Lack of lamin leads to nuclear deformations that may be involved in the pathogenesis of progeria—and there is reason to hope that this molecular mechanism may lead to a better understanding of the normal aging process.

(8) Denervation

Removal of the nerve supply has different effects depending on the type of nerve and end organ. **Motor nerve denervation** has drastic effects on striated muscle

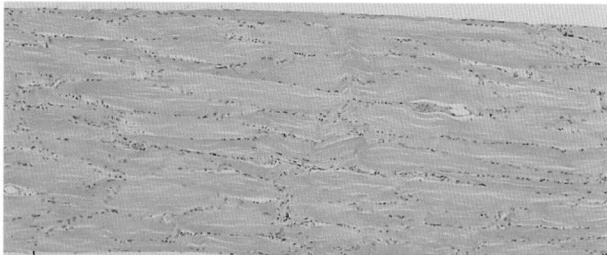

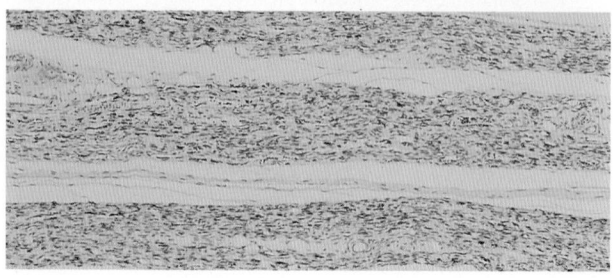

FIGURE 2.53   *Top:* Single bundle of normal human striated muscle fibers (control). *Bottom:* Extreme atrophy of striated muscle in a long-standing paraplegic. Each of the 3 bundles shown was originally about the size of the control.

(Figure 2.53). Apparently the nerves supply their target organs with some trophic material; its nature is not clear, but the trophic interaction may be mutual (334). As to **sensory nerve denervation,** for reasons unknown the effects are pronounced only on the hand and to a lesser degree on the foot; the mitotic rate of the epidermis drops, the skin becomes thinner (atrophic) and scaly, and the nails become coarse and brittle (348). An intriguing observation is that in paraplegic and tetraplegic patients, wounds below the level of spinal denervation do have more complications than expected (273).

Complete sympathetic denervation can be obtained by chemically treating newborn animals with 6-hydroxydopamine. It has been said that such denervation has metabolic effects on arteries (291). The surgical sympathetic denervation of arteries, a procedure used to obtain vasodilatation and thus increased flow, leads to structural changes in the arterial wall that mimic, interestingly, those of old age (292). Sympathetic denervation of the major salivary glands induces atrophy; in perirenal fat it does not cause atrophy but leads, surprisingly, to metaplasia from yellow to brown fat (p. 58). The classic but puzzling bladder hypertrophy by denervation (**neurogenic bladder**) occurs in paraplegics because the connections between the bladder and the brain are interrupted; the bladder becomes overfilled, but the sphincter receives no message to relax. Evacuation occurs only by overflow. Under such conditions the smooth muscle is stretched and becomes hypertrophic.

(9) Toxic Agents and Drugs

Specific tissues, such as the testis, are induced to atrophy by specific substances (305). Bone marrow is a sensitive and frequent target (311). Some drugs induce atrophy by causing selected cells to undergo apoptosis.

> For readers who enjoy puzzles: chronic intoxication of rats with selenium was said to cause atrophy of the left liver lobe and hypertrophy of the right liver lobe (282). Bizarre as this may be, there is a plausible explanation. Selenium is absorbed by the gut in such a way that it drains preferentially into the left lobe, which shrinks, while the right lobe increases by compensatory hypertrophy.

(10) X-Rays

X-rays induce atrophy of many tissues, but at the level of cells their effects are complicated, a mixture of direct cellular damage, including cell death, and indirect effects by microcirculatory damage (Figure 2.54) (284, 303, 351). Another peculiar effect has been called reproductive cell death, in which the cells survive but lose their ability to divide; sometimes they form multi-nucleated giant cells (p. 220).

(11) Immunologic Mechanisms

In pernicious anemia, the gastric mucosa becomes atrophic. The loss of parietal cells in this typical atrophic gastritis is attributed to an autoimmune attack, and autoantibodies against parietal cells can often be demonstrated. Another mechanism of immunologic atrophy is the overactivation of suppressor T lymphocytes; aplastic anemia can arise in this manner (372).

(12) The Germ-Free Condition

We kept this for the end because it raises an unusual question. Look at Figure 2.55; it shows two sections of mouse small intestine. Which one is normal? If you know your histology, you will choose the top one; its villi are more plump and contain many more cells. This is what textbooks teach us to call normal. The gut in the bottom panel has short, stunted villi, with few cells in their connective tissue. This is the picture of *mucosal atrophy*. Yet this gut comes from a germ-free mouse. The cells in the villi in the top panel are "inflammatory" cells, gathered there in response to bacterial products. In other words, *part of our structure is determined by our bacterial guests* (278, 301).

Is Atrophy Reversible?

It has been suggested that protease inhibitors, by decreasing protein catabolism, might slow down the pace of

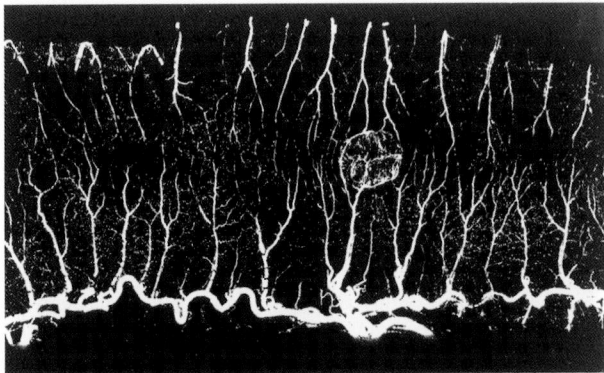
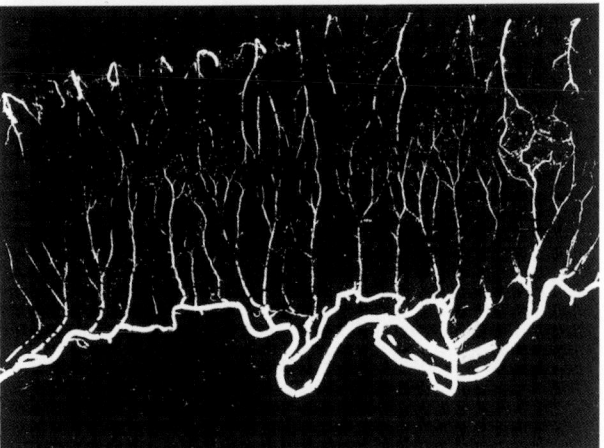
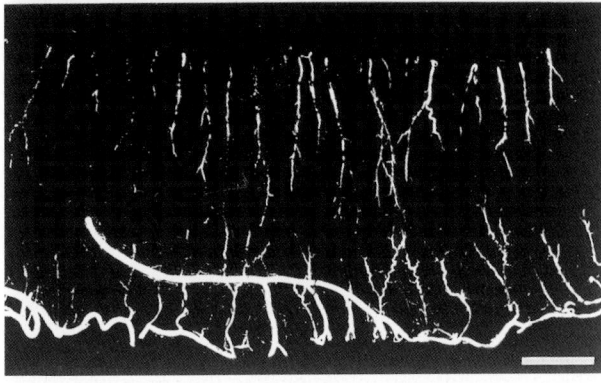

FIGURE 2.54 Effect of X-rays on the microcirculation. Microangiographs of rat duodenum 1 day after various X-ray exposures. *Top:* No exposure (control). *Center:* After exposure to 1000 R. *Bottom:* After exposure to 1460 R. Note the progressively decreased filling of the finer vessels. **Bar** = 100 μm. (Reprinted from Casarett, G. W. *Radiation Histopathology,* vol. I. Copyright © 1981 CRC Press, Inc., Boca Raton, FL. [284].)

atrophy (310). Overall, the reversibility of atrophy depends on the tissue. Starvation atrophy of adipose tissue remains reversible even after years. Fibers of striated muscle can recover from denervation atrophy if the nerve is repaired within 3–5 weeks; longer intervals imply loss of function, and after 20–24 months nerve repair is useless

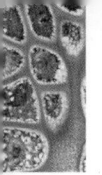

FIGURE 2.55 The structure and function of the normal intestinal mucosa depend in part on the presence of bacteria in the lumen. *Top:* Ileum of a normal mouse 48 hours after administration of tritiated thymidine. The regenerating, labeled epithelial cells (black) have almost reached the tip of the villi. *Bottom:* Ileum of a germ-free mouse under similar conditions. The villi are shorter and thinner, and the crypts are shallow. The labeled epithelium extends only halfway up the villi. Autoradiographs; hematoxylin. **Bars** = 100 μm. (Reproduced from [262]. © by the U.S. and Canadian Academy of Pathology, Inc.)

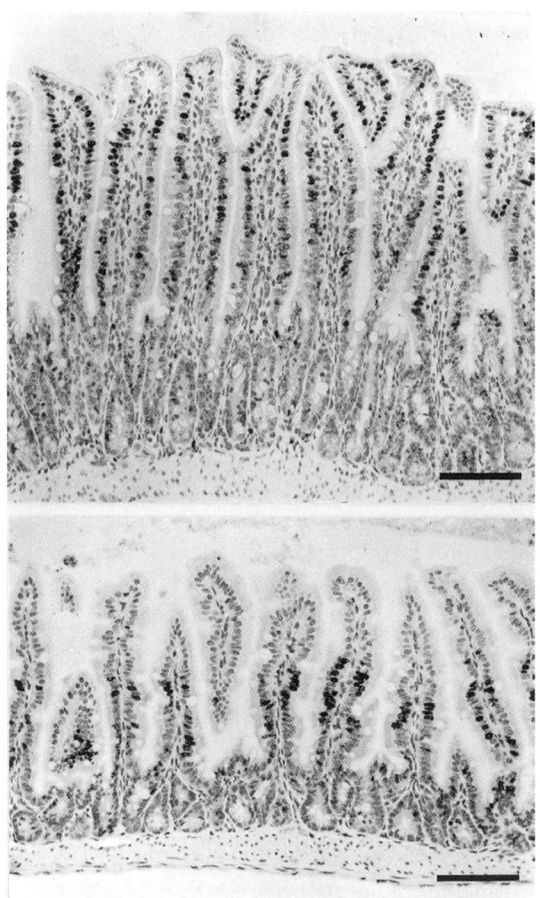

because the fibers are atrophied almost beyond recognition (Figure 2.53). Ultimately, in advanced atrophy, the parenchymal cells tend to disappear and to be replaced by connective tissue (or by astrocytes in the brain).

TO SUM UP: Atrophy, more often than hypertrophy, is linked with disease; it is also linked with senescence. In recent times the study of atrophy has taught us three valuable lessons about "shrinking". At the whole-body level it has revealed that leanness is an excellent survival formula, as the Spartans seem to have known. At the cellular level, it taught us that cells can shrink by the strange phenomenon of autophagocytosis. It also taught us that organs forced to shrink beyond a certain point do so by deleting some of their cells, and this led to the discovery of apoptosis, a modality of cell death now hailed as a biological phenomenon of major significance (p. 210).

Modulation and Metaplasia

Phenotypic changes in response to the environment are common in people as well as in cells. Human beings can adapt reversibly by developing a suntan, changing the haircut, or switching to a new profession; cells can turn genes on and off, change shape, alter their function. These cellular adaptations are just beginning to be studied at the level of gene expression.

What type of changes can occur and how do they occur? Two degrees are recognized: *modulation,* a term introduced by cell biologists, refers to mild, reversible phenotypic changes; and *metaplasia,* a term coined by Virchow, which means *the replacement of cells of one type with cells of another type;* it is also (potentially) reversible. There is some overlap between these two concepts: for example, a reversible change between

alveolar cells Types 1 and 2 (384) could belong to either group.

Biologists unfamiliar with pathology rediscovered metaplasia in the 1990s (there is an unfortunate gulf between biology and pathology) and called it *transdifferentiation* (374, 410). There was no need for this ill-defined, confusing seven-syllable monster. Wherever it is used, just read *metaplasia* (421).

Modulation

Modulation as we defined it can occur in any kind of cell in a matter of hours and does not require cell division. Modulated cells are not pathologic; they are temporarily adapted to different needs or to different stimuli, *and* they remain recognizable as members of their cell type. Smooth muscle cells, for example, are specialized for contraction, but they also manufacture collagen, elastin and glycosaminoglycans. In culture, with a small change in the medium (e.g., by adding heparin) they can be made to emphasize reversibly their synthetic apparatus; that is, to swing from the *contractile mode* to the *synthetic mode* (381, 406). *Fibroblasts* are in some way a mirror image of smooth muscle cells: they are specialized for matrix synthesis, but they also contain a contractile machinery and can be induced to emphasize it, whereby they become *myofibroblasts* (p. 485). Endothelial cells can change from fenestrated to continuous.

These modulations can be seen or guessed in histologic sections, but they are best observed under the dynamic conditions of cell culture. Endothelial cells offer some classic examples (126, 401, 426). These cells are naturally programmed either to cover large surfaces (as in the aorta) or to form little tubes (as in capillaries). If they are grown *in vitro* on a surface coated with collagen, they form a continuous sheet; if at that point they are sandwiched beneath another layer of collagen, they modulate into branching little tubes (Figure 2.56) (415). Studies of this kind are teaching a great deal about the mechanisms of morphogenesis: *cells modulate in response to soluble factors (e.g., vitamins, cytokines) and to the nature of the substrate* (387, 402, 411, 416).

Metaplasia

Metaplasia is a common event, diagnosed microscopically but often accessible to the naked eye: *a patch of differentiated cells of one kind is replaced by a patch of differentiated cells of a different kind,* often as a result of chronic irritation (404). Theoretically, the possibilities of metaplasia may seem almost infinite, because every cell has a full complement of genetic information, and any repressed gene could conceivably be derepressed (386). In real life, however, the rules of the game are more strict: in adult mammals *metaplasia occurs mostly (although not only) within varieties of epithelium and within varieties of mesenchyme* (connective tissues and muscle). Let us first take a look at the evidence.

Examples of Metaplasia

Metaplasia occurs in cells that replicate: a strong argument for the theory that metaplasia is a form of abnormal regeneration. It is not known to occur in adult striated muscle cells and in neurons (but do remember that "brain has been turned into blood").

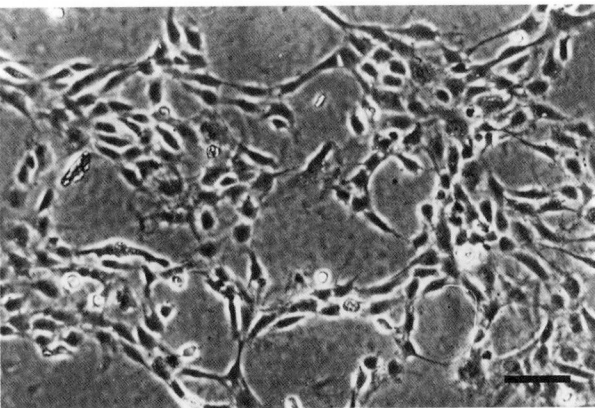
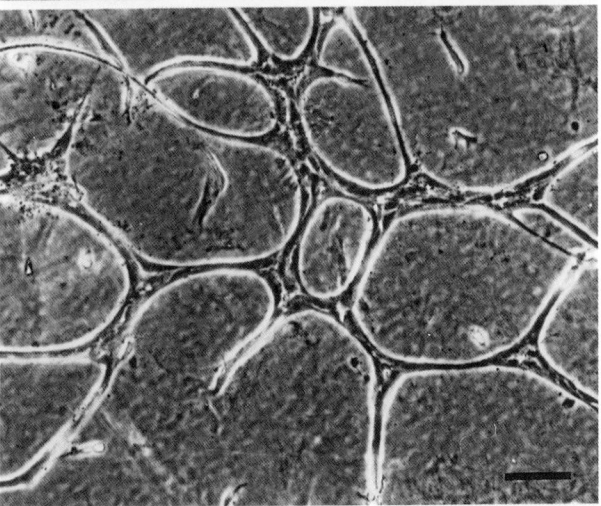

FIGURE 2.56 Example of modulation. *Top:* Capillary endothelial cells grown on the surface of a collagen gel form a subconfluent monolayer. *Bottom:* The same culture, 2 days after it has been covered with a second layer of collagen. The cells have now formed a network of interconnected cords; some of these are hollow suggesting early capillary formation. (Phase contrast microscopy) **Bars** = 100 μm. (Reproduced from the **Journal of Cell Biology,** 1983;97:1648–1652, by copyright permission of The Rockefeller University Press [415].)

Epithelial Metaplasia

Typically, a single-cell epithelium is replaced by squamous stratified or by glandular epithelium, or vice versa. For example, in the bronchi of a smoker, patches of normal columnar ciliated epithelium may be replaced by a squamous stratified epithelium (squamous metaplasia), sometimes even keratinized (epidermoid metaplasia) (Figure 2.57) (409). If the left nostril of a rabbit is closed by a suture, the respiratory epithelium on the right side will undergo metaplasia to stratified squamous; on the left it becomes mucus secreting (394).

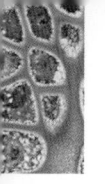

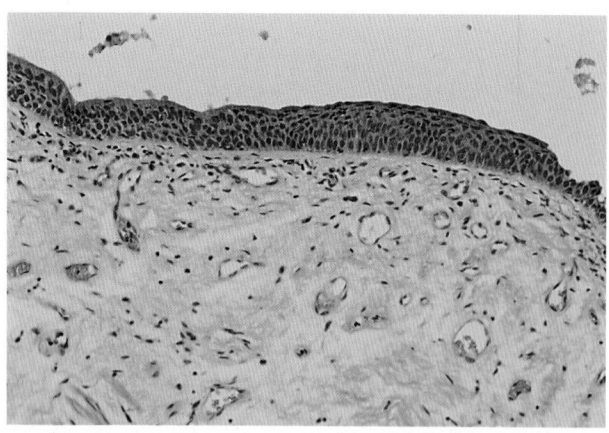

FIGURE 2.57 Squamous metaplasia in the bronchus of a smoker: the normal cylindrical, ciliated epithelium is replaced by a multilayered epithelium resembling the epidermis. The lack of cilia interrupts the outflow of mucus.

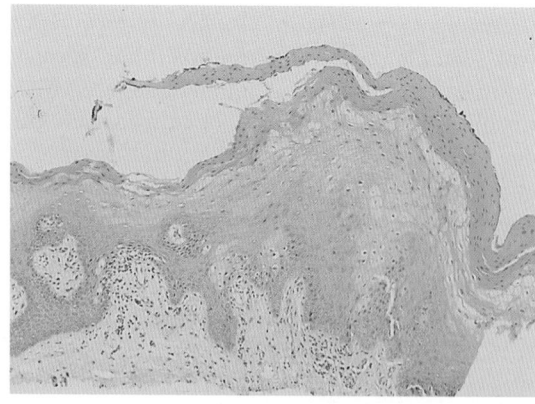

FIGURE 2.59 Histological aspect of leukoplakia. The superficial cells have become keratinized but retain their nuclei, a pathologic feature called *parakeratosis*. (Courtesy of M. J. Imber, Dermatopathology Division, Massachusetts General Hospital, Boston, MA.)

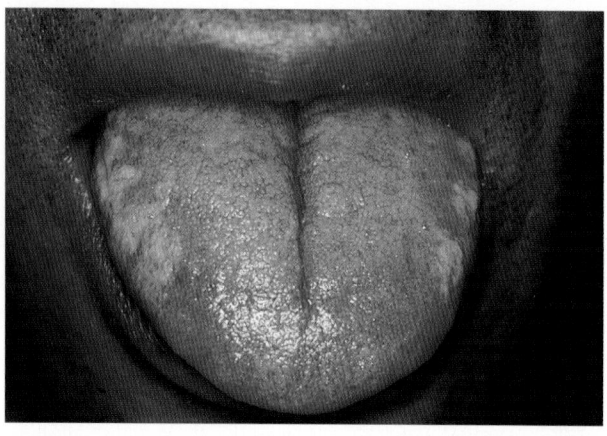

FIGURE 2.58 Patches of leukoplakia on the margin of the tongue in a heavy smoker. (Courtesy of Dr. R. Johnson, Department of Dermatology, Harvard Community Health Plan, Cambridge, MA.)

One type of epithelial metaplasia became deservedly famous because it was worked out in the laboratory to the point of producing a cure: squamous stratified metaplasia due to lack of Vitamin A (retinoic acid).

The first step was a classic paper by Wolbach and Howe in 1928 showing squamous stratified metaplasia in guinea pigs deficient in vitamin A (Figure 2.60) (430). Then, in 1953 metaplasia by vitamin A was produced *in vitro*. This experiment too became a classic because it explained the cellular mechanism of metaplastic cell replacement. In Cambridge, England, Dame Honor B. Fell and E. Mellanby (387) found that chick embryo ectoderm, maintained in organ culture with normal medium, produces normal skin epithelium (stratified, squamous, keratinizing). If excess vitamin A is added, keratinization is suppressed, and the basal cells give rise to a layer of mucus-secreting or ciliated cells. If the medium is changed again to normal, the basal cells produce a new layer of flat cells that undermine the columnar cells and eventually replace them. This has been confirmed many times (383, 397). Correspondingly, *in vivo,* vitamin A deficiency causes diffuse squamous metaplasia (424) and retinoic acid is used successfully for treating leukoplakia (395), although the mechanism is not understood (427). Estrogen, by the way, produced epidermoid metaplasia in the prostate (413).

Readers accustomed to inhale smog may be interested in knowing that chronic exposure to ozone causes the nasal epithelium (of rats) to become mucus-secreting (391). Gland ducts can also undergo epidermoid metaplasia, especially in the pancreas; the stimulus may be chronic inflammation or vitamin A deficiency. On the tongue and in the esophagus of a smoker, the epithelium may become thicker and excessively keratinized, forming whitish plaques quite obvious to the naked eye; this is leukoplakia (Figure 2.58), equivalent to the smoker's patches described in 1870 by James Paget. Similar patches—but not related to smoking—are common in the cervix. The histology of leukoplakia is shown in Figure 2.59.

Sometimes a flat, nonsecreting epithelium is replaced by a secreting epithelium or by glands. This can occur in the ureters and bladder (403), but the commonest example is found in the lower esophagus: through a malfunction of the cardia, gastric juice may flow back into the esophagus. In the long run, erosions develop and become lined by metaplastic epithelium of the gastric or intestinal type. These metaplastic patches are commonly known as Barrett's epithelium (p. 898) (390).

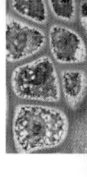

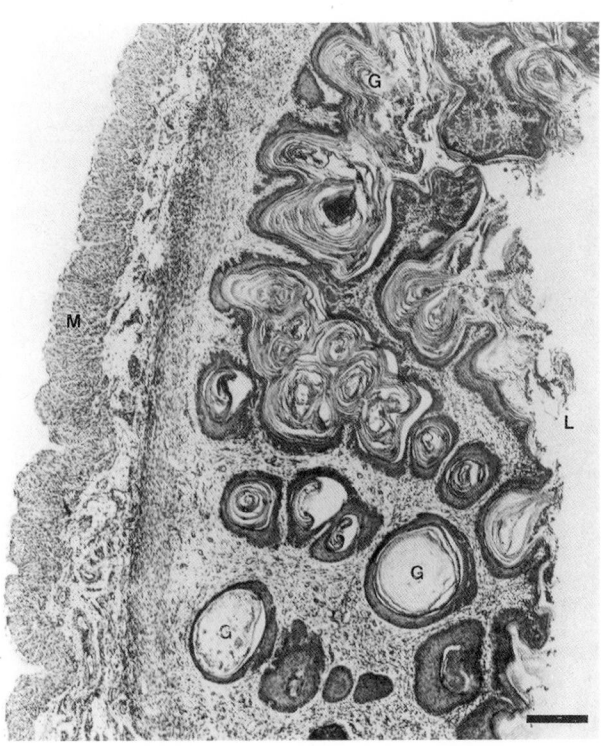

FIGURE 2.60   Severe squamous stratified metaplasia of the guinea pig uterus due to vitamin A deficiency. **M:** Muscular layer; **L:** lumen. The endometrial glands (**G**) are altered beyond recognition. Such uteri may be filled with a white pasty mass of desquamated cornified cells, just as in an epidermal cyst. **Bar** = 250 μm. (Reproduced by permission from Arch. Pathol. 1928,5:239–253. Copyright 1928, American Medical Association [430].)

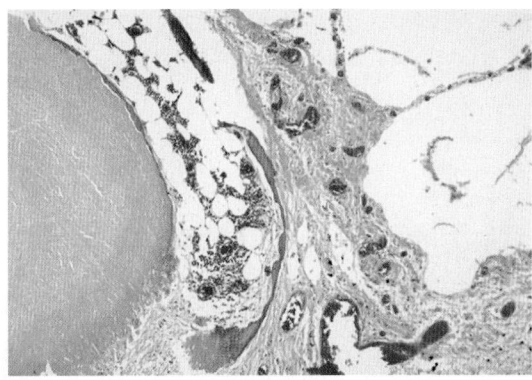

FIGURE 2.61   Induction of bone by a calcification, in the lung. *Left:* The rounded, magenta-colored mass bulging to the right is a pathologic calcification, probably tuberculous. Its top half is covered by a thin, uneven pink line: this is bone tissue. Farther to the right is a mixed layer of adipose tissue and hematopoietic bone marrow. *Low center:* The thin pink line forming an inverted C is a "trabecula" of bone.

The digestive tract, with its many varieties of epithelium and its propensity to become eroded and to regenerate quickly, is a favorite site of metaplasia. In the stomach, patches of epithelium with the features of intestinal lining (intestinal metaplasia) are common (405); they include endocrine cells typical of the small intestine (378).

Finally, there have been several reports of *metaplastic liver cells appearing in the pancreas,* in the course of pancreatic regeneration (408, 421) or after prolonged treatment with cadmium chloride (399). This phenomenon has been reproduced *in vitro* with a cortocoid, dexamethasone, and it involved the transcription factor C/EBP beta (425).

Connective Tissue Metaplasia

This type of metaplasia offers some striking examples.

Metaplasia of connective tissue to bone.   This is commonplace in atherosclerotic arteries as part of a sequence: calcification → ossification → bone marrow formation

(Figure 2.61) (p. 258). Metaplastic bone often develops in the connective tissue of muscles as a result of trauma (*traumatic myositis ossificans*), especially in young people, as athletes well know. A classic setting is that of a muscle bruised, for example, by the kick of a horse; a stone-hard mass develops under the bruise, visible in X-ray. Fortunately, such masses tend to disappear spontaneously by metaplasia in the reverse direction. For reasons totally unknown, metaplastic bone tends to form around the joints of some paraplegic patients (398); a bony shell can form around the knees in a few weeks. Metaplastic bone sometimes develops in scars, with a peculiar preference for scars of midline abdominal operations (385); this could be the result of a cytokine, BMP-2, acting on fibroblasts or on connective tissue stem cells (389).

Chondroid (cartilaginous) metaplasia.   When a long bone is broken and immobilized, it heals with an exuberant mass (called a *callus*) of bone tissue containing occasional islands of cartilage; if the bone is not immobilized, the predominant tissue will be cartilage (Figure 2.13). Cartilage (xiphoid bone of neborn rats) maintained *in vitro* slowly changes to adipose tissue (393).

Myxoid metaplasia.   In the heart valves, the fibrous tissue can turn into myxoid (meaning mucoid) connective tissue of the embryonic type. This is usually and incorrectly referred to as myxoid degeneration. Nothing at all is degenerating: there is just a change in cell type and cell secretion. This may be, in fact, an adaptive response to abnormal shear forces in the valve: we have seen myxoid metaplasia also in the so-called singer's

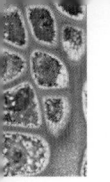

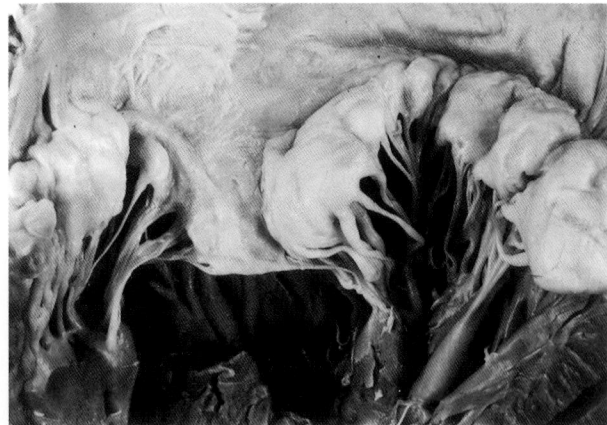

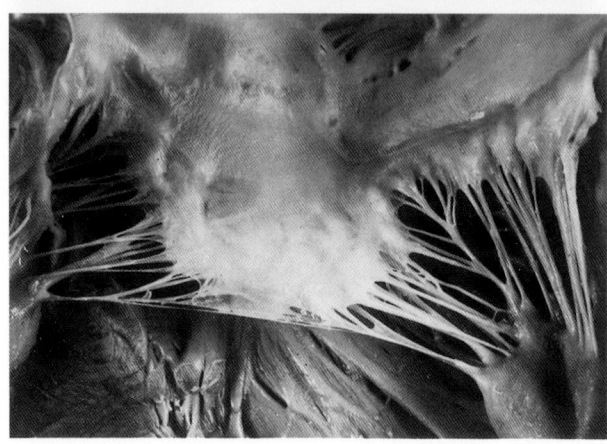

FIGURE 2.62   Result of myxoid metaplasia (incorrectly called myxoid degeneration) of the mitral valve. *Top:* The leaflets of the valve give way under functional strain and tend to protrude, recalling the shape of a parachute (floppy valve syndrome). This anatomical prolapse of the valve results in functional insufficiency. *Bottom:* Normal mitral valve of a 22-year-old man. (Courtesy of Dr. W. D. Edwards, Mayo Clinic, Rochester, MN.)

nodules, which arise on vocal cords perhaps as a result of another type of shear: forced vibration. Heart valves with myxoid metaplasia soften and tend to expand, so the cusps come to be shaped like parachutes (Figure 2.62).

Adipose tissue metaplasia. The metaplasia of adipose tissue into brown fat may be hiding a jackpot of enormous dimensions. Here is a tale for entrepreneurial biologists.

The type of adipose tissue called brown fat is made of cells filled with a special variety of mitochondria and small droplets of fat; these mitochondria are able to consume energy to produce heat. They can do this thanks to a

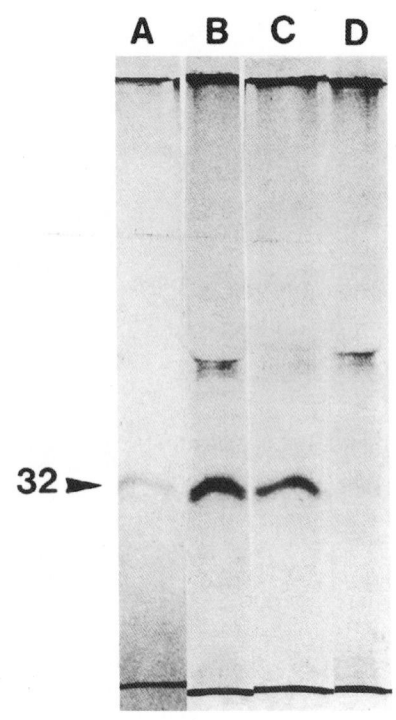

FIGURE 2.63   Gel demonstrating the presence of the 32-kD *uncoupling protein* of brown adipose tissue in control rats (lane **A**), in the brown fat of cold-exposed animals (lane **B**), and in brown fat of animals bearing a pheochromocytoma (lane **C**). Lane **D:** Control. (Reproduced from [380].)

specific mitochondrial uncoupling protein (422, 423), which uncouples oxidative phosphorylation and allows the respiring brown fat to become a "heat gland." As may be expected in rats, this protein is produced in greater amount by exposure to the cold (Figure 2.63) (380). Now, brown fat is richly supplied with sympathetic nerves. If these nerves are severed, the brown fat turns into white fat; conversely, in patients bearing a pheochromocytoma (a tumor that secretes epinephrine and other catecholamines), the perirenal fat may turn from white to brown (400, 412). The same effects have been observed in rats (422, 423). The change from white to brown fat is accompanied by the appearance of the typical uncoupling protein in the inner mitochondrial membrane. This seemingly academic observation did not escape the pharmacologists (431). Imagine what would happen in overfed countries if someone discovered a harmless analog of epinephrine that would cause excess dietary calories to be burned up and released as heat rather than stored as fat.

Mechanisms of Metaplasia

When a patch of "inappropriate" cells, say of type B, appears where we would normally expect cells of type A, the metaplasia can be explained in one of two ways:

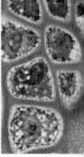

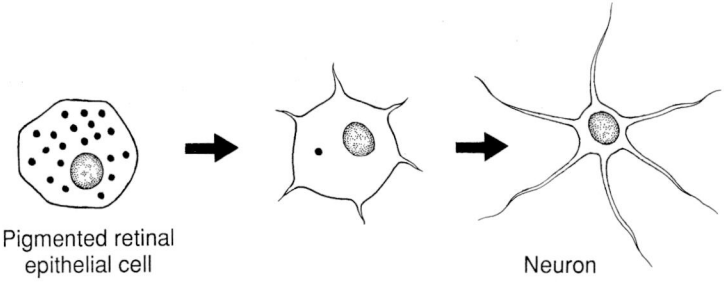

Pigmented retinal epithelial cell   Neuron

FIGURE 2.64   Direct metaplasia: a cell of a given type turns into a cell of a different type, without an intervening mitosis (in essence, the cell undergoes a metamorphosis). Direct metaplasia was thought to be extremely rare in adult mammals, but see Figure 2.65.

(1) Direct Metaplasia: Type A Cells Change into Type B Cells (Figure 2.64) which Amounts to Metamorphosis

This behavior is thought to be extremely rare in mammalian cells, although it is—ironically—the mechanism that Virchow had in mind when he coined the term "metaplasia," from the Greek *metaplássein,* "to cast into a new mold, to counterfeit" (404). However, some examples do exist. The most spectacular known to us is shown in Figure 2.65 (414): within 16–36 hours, a cytokine—TGF beta—changes mammary epithelial cells (reversibly) into cells that any unbiased observer would call fibroblasts (375). *Epithelial cells turning into fibroblasts?* We know very few pathologists who would accept this possibility, but Figure 2.65 speaks for itself. A number of papers have been reporting that this happens all the time in renal fibrosis (417, 428, 429) and in embryonic development (392, 432). After all, there is nothing extraordinary about epithelial cells turning to produce fibers of collagen Type 1; they constantly produce collagen Type 4 for their own basement membrane. In the kidney the metaplasia from epithelium to fibroblasts may perhaps echo the distant fact that the tubules derive from the mesoderm. There is also a rat carcinoma cell line that becomes "fibroblastoid" with fibroblast growth factor 1 (FGF-1) (377). Definitive proof should be forthcoming soon for this and other heresies.

> Examples of direct metaplasia *in vivo:* Aloe and Levi-Montalcini have shown that chromaffin cells of the neonatal rat adrenal medulla can be induced to sprout axons and to turn into neural cells; this was done by injecting nerve growth factor into pregnant rats, and then again for 10 days into the newborn rats (373). The same result was obtained *in vitro* (418a). Also: in the rat, if the aorta is partially constricted, the smooth muscle cells in the small arteries of the kidney were said to turn into endocrine cells of the juxtaglomerular type (382).

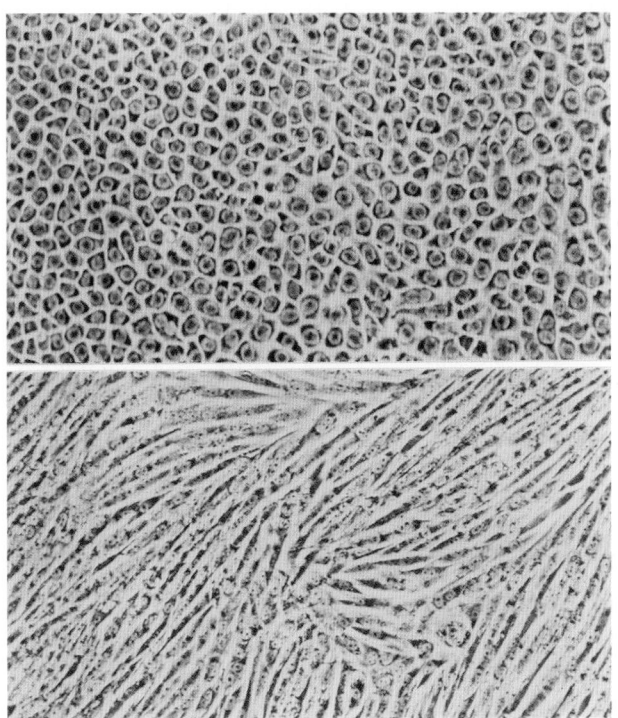

FIGURE 2.65   A spectacular example of direct metaplasia. *Top:* Culture of mammary epithelial cells. *Bottom:* After a 36 hour treatment with TGF beta, the cells undergo a reversible "fibroblastic transition." (Reproduced from **The Journal of Cell Biology,** 1994;127:2021–2036 by copyright permission of the Rockefeller University Press [414].)

Cell "metamorphosis" has been said to occur in *larval* frogs and *embryonic* chicks: using tissue cultures of the eye (in which it is easy to distinguish the cornea, the lens, the retina, and the pigmented epithelium) it can be shown that tissues as diverse as those mentioned can change into each other by varying the culture conditions. If a mitotic poison such as colchicine is present in the medium, the change from one cell type to another can not occur by cell division, only by the process that we have called metamorphosis (379, 396, 419). *However, experiments on such embryonic, immature and pluripotential cells concern differentiation of immature cells; they can tell us little about metaplasia in adult tissues.*

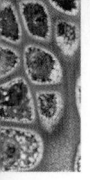
FIGURE 2.66 A mechanism of metaplasia well proven in epithelia. Reserve cells (stem cells) multiply, and differentiate into a new phenotype which displaces the old one. In essence, this is "abnormal regeneration."

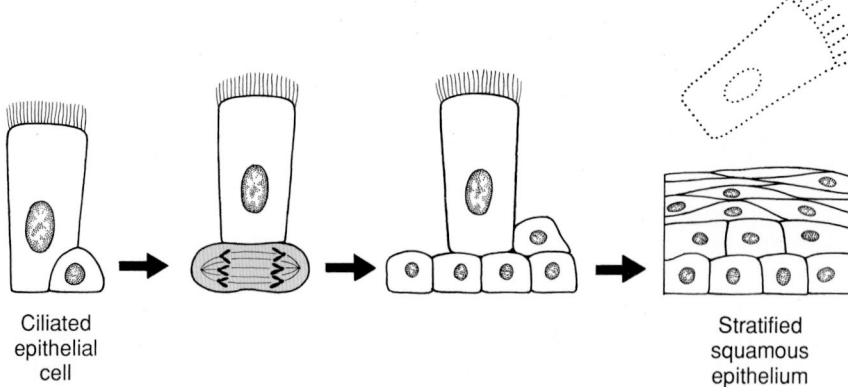

Ciliated epithelial cell

Stratified squamous epithelium

(2) Indirect Metaplasia: Progenitor Cells Stop Producing Type A Cells and Switch to Producing Type B Cells

This is thought to be the most common mechanism for metaplasia in mammals (Figure 2.66). It is especially obvious when metaplasia occurs in the course of regeneration: for example, in copper-deficient rats, the acini of the exocrine pancreas are destroyed; refeeding after 10 weeks causes intense regeneration of the acini, interspersed with patches of liver cells (421).

Biological Significance of Metaplasia

Occasionally metaplasia is adaptive and useful. When bone marrow is destroyed by disease, the metaplasia of spleen tissue to bone marrow (myeloid metaplasia) is a helpful response. Similarly, the squamous stratified epithelium that forms in the renal pelvis around a ragged kidney stone is presumably more resistant to mechanical abrasion.

In most situations, metaplasia is of no apparent use and may even be a hazard. Epidermoid metaplasia of the pancreatic ducts has been listed among the possible causes of obstruction, because the new epithelium is much thicker. In the bronchi of smokers, squamous metaplasia interrupts the cleansing flow of mucus, which is produced by mucus-secreting cells and whipped along by ciliated cells (epidermal cells produce no mucus and have no cilia). Worse yet, it is well established that several types of epithelial metaplasia predispose to malignant epithelial tumors; leukoplakia, Barrett's epithelium, and intestinal metaplasia of the stomach are classic examples. The reason: wherever epithelial metaplasia occurs a chemical or physical irritant is at work, usually a chronic stimulus that produces damage and regeneration. Seen in this light, *metaplasia amounts to abnormal regeneration,* and the link between metaplasia and cancer becomes obvious (p. 898). However, all that metaplasia contributes to cancer is the predisposing phenomenon of chronic regeneration: metaplasia itself is NOT a tumor—it is not a monoclonal lesion (418).

At a molecular level, of course, the meaning of metaplasia and modulation lies in altered gene expression. The curtain over this field is just beginning to rise.

Genetic engineering as "artificial metaplasia." If metaplasia is due to altered gene expression, then we can understand genetically engineered animals as the result of an artificial, functional, irreversible form of metaplasia. An example: we just mentioned pancreas-to-liver metaplasia; a team in Israel has been able to produce transgenic mice in which the liver expresses a gene (*PDX-1*) normally expressed only in the pancreas and provides partial protection against diabetes (streptozotocin-induced hyperglycemia) (388).

Activation

It may seem obvious now that cells, like people, can exist at several levels of activity, but this concept emerged very slowly, through studies of leukocytes. Metchnikoff himself, who discovered and named the macrophages, noticed that those from an infected animal were better able to phagocytize bacteria (437). Almost a century later the "angry macrophage" was described (p. 340). All the cells involved in inflammation need to be activated before they can perform their defensive functions (Figure 2.67). *Activation means that the cell acquires the ability to perform one or more new functions or to perform normal function(s) at a higher rate*

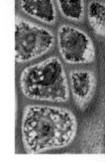

Resting　　　　　Activated

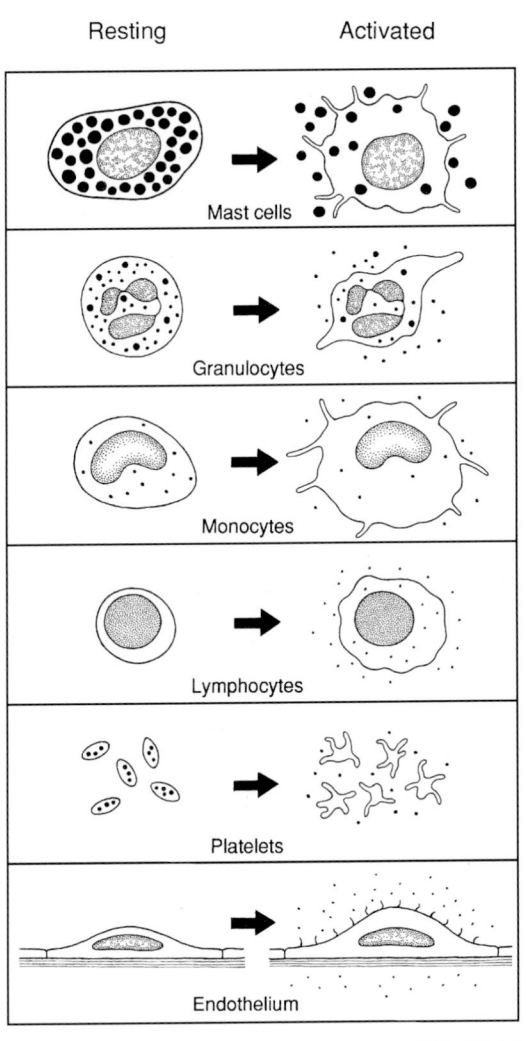

Mast cells

Granulocytes

Monocytes

Lymphocytes

Platelets

Endothelium

FIGURE 2.67 Six cell types that can be activated from their resting state. Note that they are all participants of the inflammatory reaction.

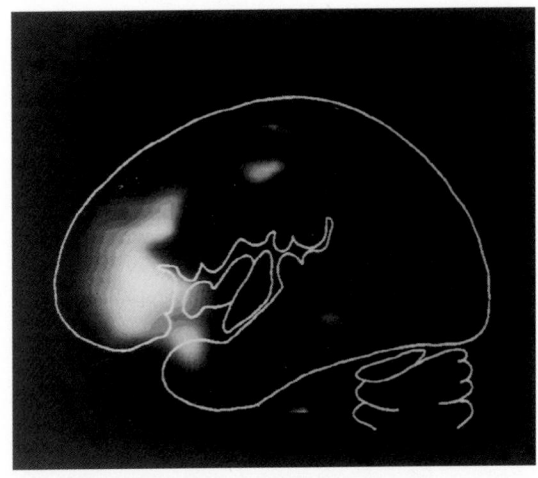

FIGURE 2.68 Evidence of activation in brain cells, as a mechanism of disease (depression). This type of image is obtained by positron emission tomography, which actually measures the blood flow in specific areas of the brain after an intravenous injection of radioactive water ($H_2^{15}O$). The area shown in graded white in the left ventrolateral prefrontal cortex shows the computed *difference* in regional blood flow between a normal series of individuals ($n = 33$) and a series affected by familial depressive disease ($n = 13$). Although the method reveals blood flow rather than neuronal activity, it is safe to assume that increased flow reflects increased local activity of neurons. (Courtesy of Dr. M. E. Raichle, Mallinckrodt Institute of Radiology, Washington University School of Medicine, St. Louis, MO.)

(263). For example, a macrophage can be induced to secrete a given protein in quantities 800 times greater than normal. For those who study cells *in vitro,* it is important to know whether the cells are in a quiescent or activated state.

An activated cell undergoes subtle changes in structure and function that may require seconds, minutes, or days. In some cells activation is a multistep process that begins with priming, a condition recalling a state of alert with no visible changes. For the endothelium, as we will see, *at least two levels of activation* can be defined.

Neurons are activated faster than any other cell type; their state of activation can be demonstrated indirectly, by its effect on blood flow. Studies by positron emission tomography show that individuals asked to think sad thoughts activate almost instantly a certain center in the left frontal lobe; in clinically depressed individuals the same center is chronically activated (Figure 2.68) (436).

To activate cells, biologists can use many devices, but the most effective is a derivative of phorbol, namely tetradecanoyl phorbol acetate better known as TPA. Why this esoteric substance?

For thousands of years, on the west coast of India, an irritating oil of incredible potency was extracted from the seeds of *Croton tiglium* (Figure 2.69) (434). Tiny amounts on the skin produced blisters; taken by mouth they induced vomiting and a bloody diarrhea. Because the effects were so drastic, medical uses faded away in the 1800s, but the oil remained in use for producing experimental inflammation; then it also became the standard tumor promotor (p. 780). Eventually, its active principle was isolated: this is how TPA was discovered and came to be used as an all-purpose cellular activator. The secret of its power is now known: TPA activates protein kinase C, for which the physiologic activators are diacylglycerols; in this way, TPA inserts itself as a link in the transduction of signals from the cell surface to effectors in the cytoplasm (Figure 2.70) (435). Modern cell biologists stand on the shoulders of ancient healers.

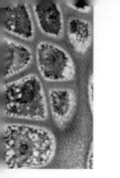

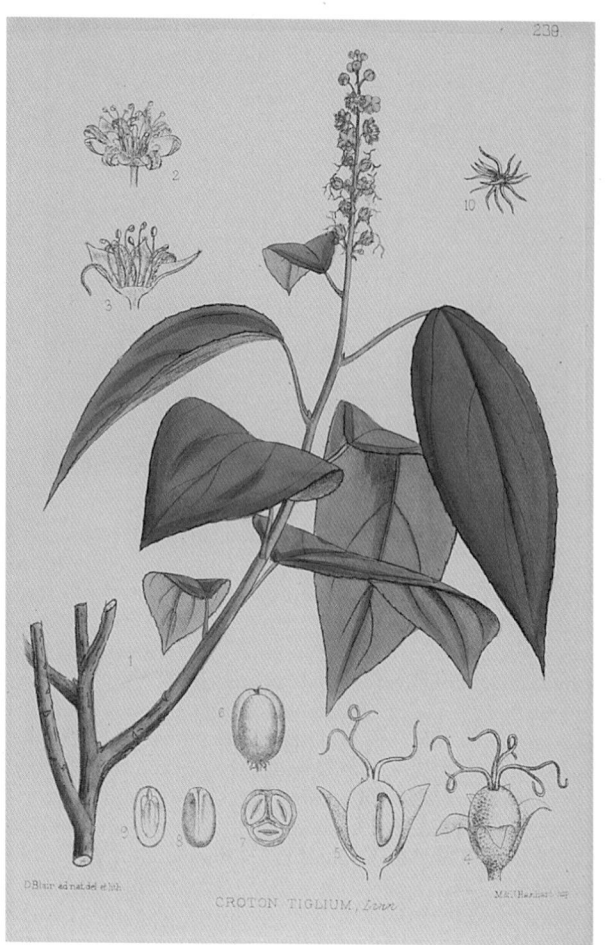

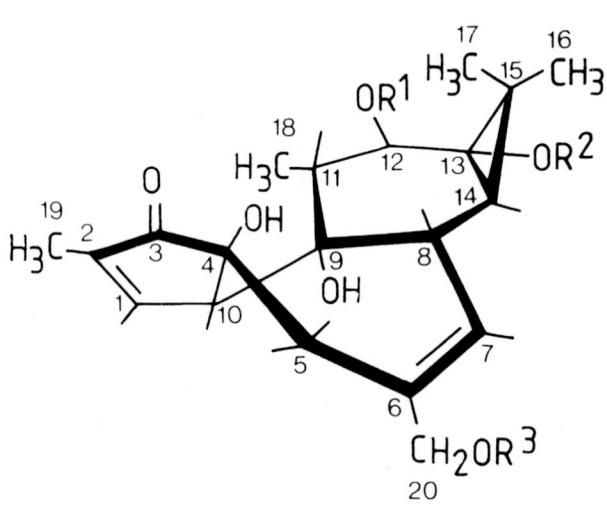

FIGURE 2.69 *Left: Croton tiglium,* the source of croton oil and of phorbol esters. (Reproduced from [434].) *Right:* Chemical formula of phorbol. ([433] Copyright © 1986 CRC Press, Inc., Boca Raton, FL.)

FIGURE 2.70   The secret of phorbol esters as cell activators: they activate protein kinase C in the place of diacylglycerol. (Copyright 2002. From Molecular Biology of the Cell, 4th ed. Alberts B, Johnson A, Lewis J, et al. [eds]. Reproduced by permission of Routledge, Inc., part of The Taylor & Francis Group. [263].)

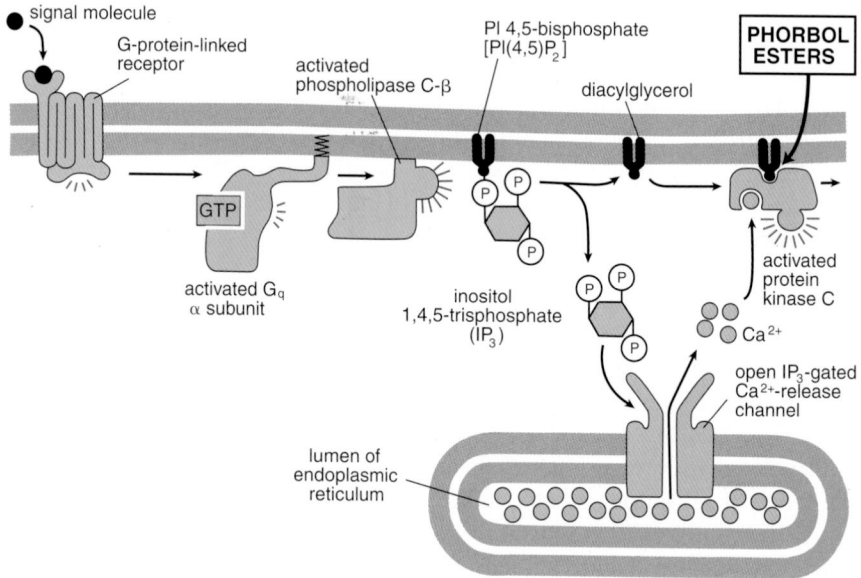

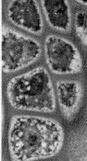

References

Regeneration

1. Abkowitz JL. Can human hematopoietic stem cells become skin, gut or liver cells? N Engl J Med 2002;346:770–772.

2. Aguayo AJ. Axonal regeneration from injured neurons in the adult mammalian central nervous system. In: Cotman CW (ed). Synaptic plasticity. New York: Guilford Press, 1985, pp. 457–484.

3. Alison M, Golding M, Lalani E-N, et al. Wholesale hepatocytic differentiation in the rat from ductular oval cells, the progeny of biliary stem cells. J Hepatol 1997;26:343–352.

4. Allsopp RC, Chang E, Kashefi-Aazam M, et al. Telomere shortening is associated with cell division in vitro and in vivo. Exp Cell Res 1995;220:194–200.

5. Alvarez-Buylla A. Kirn JR. Birth, migration, incorporation, and death of vocal control neurons in adult songbirds. J Neurobiol 1997;33:585–601.

6. Amadio PC. Tendon and ligament. In: Cohen IK, Diegelmann RF, Lindblad WJ (eds). Wound healing: biochemical & clinical aspects. Philadelphia: WB Saunders Company, 1992, pp. 384–395.

7. Anderson DJ, Gage FH, Weissman IL. Can stem cells cross lineage boundaries? Nat Med 2001;7:393–395.

8. Antel JP, Nalbantoglu J, Olivier A. Neuronal progenitors-learning from the hippocampus. Nat Med 2000;6:249–250.

9. Ash SR, Cuppage FE. Shift toward anaerobic glycolysis in the regenerating rat kidney. Am J Pathol 1970;60:385–402.

10. Bader CR, Bertrand D, Cooper E, Mauro A. Membrane currents of rat satellite cells attached to intact skeletal muscle fibers. Neuron 1988;1:237–240.

11. Balkovetz DF, Lipschultz JH. Hepatocyte growth factor and the kidney: it is not just for the liver. Int Rev Cytol 1999;186:225–260.

12. Barinaga M. Challenging the "no new neurons" dogma. Science 1992;255:1646.

13. Barrie HJ. Intra-articular loose bodies regarded as organ cultures in vivo. J Pathol 1978;125:163–169.

14. Basson MC, Carlson BM. Myotoxicity of single and repeated injections of mepivacaine (carbocaine) in the rat. Anesth Analg 1980;59:275–282.

14a. Beltrami AP, Barlucchi L, Torella D. et al. Adult cardiac stem cells are multipotent and support myocardial regeneration. Cell 2003;114:763–776.

15. Beltrami AP, Urbanek K, Kajstura J, et al. Evidence that human cardiac myocytes divide after myocardial infarction. N Engl J Med 2001;344:1750–1757.

16. Bernstein JJ, Bernstein ME. Plasticity in the damaged spinal cord. In: Windle WF (ed). The spinal cord and its reaction to traumatic injury. New York Basel: Marcel Dekker, Inc., 1980, pp. 237–247.

17. Bischoff R. Regeneration of single skeletal muscle fibers in vitro. Anat Rec 1975;182:215–236.

18. Bizzozero G. An address on the growth and regeneration of the organism. Br Med J 1894;1:728–732.

19. Bittner RE, Schöfer C, Weipoltshammer K, et al. Recruitment of bone-marrow-derived cells by skeletal and cardiac muscle in adult dystrophic *mdx* mice. Anat Embryol 1999;199:391–396.

20. Björntorp P. Adipocyte precursor cells. In: Björntorp P, Cairella M, Howard AN (eds). Recent advances in obesity research: III. London: John Libbey, 1981, pp. 58–69.

21. Blackburn EH, Greider CW (eds). Telomeres. New York: Cold Spring Harbor Laboratory Press, 1995.

22. Bodnar AG, Ouellette M, Frolkis M, Holt SE, Chiu C-P, Morin GB, Harley CB, Shay JW, Lichtsteiner S, Wright WE. Extension of life-span by introduction of telomerase into normal human cells. Science 1998;279:349–352.

23. Bolli R. Regeneration of the human heart—no chimera? N Engl J Med 2002;346:55–56.

24. Borgens RB. Mice regrow the tips of their foretoes. Science 1982a;217:747–750.

25. Borgens RB, Robinson KR, Vanable JW Jr, McGinnis ME, McCaig CD. Electric fields in vertebrate repair. New York: Alan R. Liss, Inc., 1989.

26. Brewer GJ. Regeneration and proliferation of embryonic and adult rat hippocampal nurons in culture. Exp Neurol 1999;159:237–247.

27. Brittberg M, Lindahl A, Nilsson A, et al. Treatment of deep cartilage defects in the knee with autologous chondrocyte transplantation. N Engl J Med 1994;331:889–895.

28. Brockes JP. Mitogenic growth factors and nerve dependence of limb regeneration. Science 1984;225:1280–1287.

29. Brockes JP, Kumar A. Plasticity and reprogramming of differentiated cells in amphibian regeneration. Nat Rev Mol Cell Biol 2002;3:566–574.

29a. Bucher NLR, Malt RA. Regeneration of liver and kidney. Boston: Little, Brown & Co., 1971.

30. Burger EH, Klein-Nulend J. Mechanotransduction in bone—role of the lacuno-canalicular network. FASEB J 1999;13(Suppl.):S101–S112.

31. Cajal SR. Degeneration and regeneration of the nervous system, Vol. 1. London: Oxford University Press, 1928.

32. Carlson BM. The regeneration of skeletal muscle—A review. Am J Anat 1973;137:119–150.

33. Carlson BM. Regeneration of entire skeletal muscles. Fed Proc 1986;45:1456–1460.

34. Carlson BM, Gutmann E. Regeneration in grafts of normal and denervated rat muscles. Pflügers Arch 1975;353:215–225.

35. Carter DR, Beaupré GS, Giori NJ, Helms JA. Mechanobiology of skeletal regeneration. Clin Orthop Rel Res 1998;355S:S41–S55.

36. Chiu C-P, Harley CB. Replicative senescence and cell immortality: the role of telomeres and telomerase. PSEBM 1997;214:99–106.

37. Cohen IK, Diegelmann RF, Crossland, MC. Wound care and wound healing. In: Swartz SI. Principles of surgery. New York: McGraw Hill, Inc., 1994, pp. 279–303.

38. Collins RH Jr. CD34+ selected cells in clinical transplantation. Stem Cells 1993;12:577–585.

39. Cotsarelis G, Cheng S-Z, Dong G, Sun T-T, Lavker RM. Existence of slow-cycling limbal epithelial basal cells that can be preferentially stimulated to proliferate: implications on epithelial stem cells. Cell 1989;57:201–209.

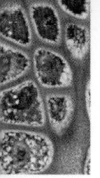

40. Counter CM. The roles of telomeres and telomerase in cell life span. Mutat Res 1996;366:45–63.

41. Cousin B, Munoz O, Andre M, et al. A role for preadipocytes as macrophage-like cells. FASEB J 1999;13:305–312.

42. Culotti JG, Kolodkin AL. Functions of netrins and semaphorins in axon guidance. Curr Opin Neurobiol 1996; 6:81–88.

43. D'Amour KA, Gage FH. Are somatic stem cells pluripotent or lineage-restricted? Nat Med 2002;8:213–214.

44. De Castro F, Hu L, Drabkin H, Sotelo C, Chédotal A. Chemoattraction and chemorepulsion of olfactory bulb axons by different secreted semaphorins. J Neurosci 1999; 19:4428–4436.

45. de Lange T. Telomeres and senescence: ending the debate. Science 1998;279:334–335.

45a. De Rosa SC, Brenchley JM, Roederer M. Beyond six colors: a new era in flow cytometry. Nat Med 2003;9:112–117.

46. Dobbie JW. New concepts in molecular biology and ultrastructural pathology of the peritoneum: their significance for peritoneal dialysis. Am J Kidney Dis 1990;15:97–109.

47. Douglas BS. Conservative management of guillotine amputation of the finger in children. Aust Paediatr J 1972; 8:86–89.

48. Elder D. Why is regenerative capacity restricted in higher organisms? J Theor Biol 1979;81:563–568.

48a. Engel AG, Franzini-Armstrong C. Myology, 2nd edition. New York: McGraw-Hill Inc., 1994.

49. Engelhardt M, Martens UM. The implication of telomerase activity and telomere stability for replicative aging and cellular immortality. Oncol Rep 1998;15:1043–1052.

50. Fausto N. Hepatic regeneration. In: Bircher J, Benhamou J-P, McIntyre N, Rizzetto M, Rodés J (eds). Oxford Textbook of Clinical Hepatology, 2nd ed, vol. I. New York: Oxford University Press, 1999, pp. 189–201.

51. Ferrari G, Cusella-De Angelis G, Coletta M, et al. Muscle regeneration by bone marrow-derived myogenic progenitors. Science 1998;279:1528–1530.

52. Francavilla A, Ove P, Polimeno L, et al. Regulation of liver size and regeneration: importance in liver transplantation. Transplant Proc 1988;20:494–497.

53. Fujii M, Takeda K, Imamura T, et al. Roles of bone morphogenetic protein type I receptors and smad proteins in osteoblast and chondroblast differentiation. Mol Biol Cell 1999; 10:3801–3813.

54. Gage FH. Mammalian neural stem cells. Science 2000; 287:1433–1446.

55. Galjaard H, Bootsma D. The regulation of cell proliferation and differentiation in intestinal epithelium. Exp Cell Res 1969;58:79–92.

56. Gay S, Rhodes RK. Immunohistologic demonstration of distinct collagens in normal and osteoarthritic joints. Semin Arthritis Rheum 1982;11:43–44.

57. Gimble JM, Robinson CE, Wu X, Kelly KA. The function of adipocytes in the bone marrow stroma: an update. Bone 1996;19:421–428.

58. Goldberger ME, Murray M. Patterns of sprouting and implications for recovery of function. Adv Neurol 1988;47: 361–385.

59. Goldman SA, Nottebohm F. Neuronal production, migration, and differentiation in a vocal control nucleus of the adult female canary brain. Proc Natl Acad Sci USA 1983;80: 2390–2394.

60. Gordon RE, Lane BP. Wound repair in rat tracheal epithelium. Lab Invest 1980;42:616–621.

61. Goss RJ. Prospects for regeneration in man. Clin Orthop 1980;151:270–282.

62. Goss RJ. Deer antlers. Regeneration, function, and evolution. New York: Academic Press, 1983.

63. Goss, RJ. Why mammals don't regenerate—or do they? News Physiol Sci 1987;2:112–115.

64. Gould E, Reeves AJ, Graziano MSA, Gross CG. Neurogenesis in the neocortex of adult primates. Science 1999;286: 548–552.

65. GrandPré T, Li S, Strittmatter SM. Nogo-66 receptor antagonist peptide promotes axonal regeneration. Nature 2002; 417:547–551.

66. Grisham JW, Thorgeirsson SS. Liver stem cells. In: Potten CS (ed.) Stem Cells. London: Academic Press Ltd, 1997, pp. 233–282.

67. Grounds MD. Towards understanding skeletal muscle regeneration. Pathol Res Pract 1991;187:1–22.

68. Grounds MD, Garrett KL, Lai MC, Wright WE, Beilharz MW. Identification of skeletal muscle precursor cells in vivo by use of MyoD1 and myogenin probes. Cell Tissue Res 1992;267:99–104.

69. Gussoni E, Blau HM, Kunkel LM. The fate of individual myoblasts after transplantation into muscles of DMD patients. Nat Med 1997;3:970–977.

70. Hall PA, Watt FM. Stem cells: the generation and maintenance of cellular diversity. Development 1989;106:619–633.

71. Hauschka PV, Mavrakos AE, Iafrati MD, Doleman SE, Klagsbrun M. Growth factors in bone matrix. J Biol Chem 1986;261:12665–12674.

72. Hayflick L. The biology of human aging. Am J Med Sci 1973; 265:432–445.

73. Hayflick L. Recent advances in the cell biology of aging. Mech Aging Dev 1980;14:59–79.

74. Holden C, Vogel G. Plasticity: time for a reappraisal? Science 2002;296:2126–2129.

75. Illingworth CM. Trapped fingers and amputated finger tips in children. J Pediatr Surg 1974;9:853–857.

76. Illingworth CM, Barker AT. Measurement of electrical currents emerging during the regeneration of amputated finger tips in children. Clin Phys Physiol Meas 1980;1:87–89.

77. Jacinto A, Martinez-Arias A, Martin P. Mechanisms of epithelial fusion and repair. Nat Cell Biol 2001;3:E117–E123.

78. Jackson KA, Majka SM, Wang H, et al. Regeneration of ischemic cardiac muscle and vascular endothelium by adult stem cells. J Clin Invest 2001;107:1395–1402.

79. Jones S. Flow cytometry: applications in research and medicine. Immunochemica 1989;3:1–4.

80. Kale AA, Di Cesare PE. Osteoinductive agents. Basic science and clinical applications. Am J Orthop 1995;24:752–761.

81. Kajstura J, Pertoldi B, Leri A, et al. Telomere shortening is an in vivo marker of myocyte replication and aging. Am J Pathol 2000;156:813–819.

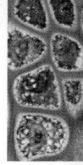

82. Kalb RG, Strittmatter SM (eds). Neurobiology of spinal cord injury. Totowa, NJ: Humana Press, 2000.

83. Kipling D, Cooke HJ. Hypervariable ultra-long telomeres in mice. Nature 1990;347:400–402.

84. Kirkwood TBL. In vitro ageing of animal cells. In: Davies I, Sigee DC (eds). Cell ageing and cell death. Cambridge: Cambridge University Press, 1984, pp. 55–72.

85. Kocher AA, Schuster MD, Szabolcs MJ, et al. Neovascularization of ischemic myocardium by human bone-marrow-derived angioblasts prevents cardiomyocyte apoptosis, reduces remodeling and improves cardiac function. Nat Med 2001;7:430–436.

86. Kocsis JD, Waxman SG. Membrane organization and myelin remodeling in regenerating axons. Adv Neurol 1988;47:31–50.

87. Kornack DR, Rakic P. Cell proliferation without neurogenesis in adult primate neocortex. Science 2001;294:2127–2130.

88. Kukekov VG, Laywell ED, Suslov O, et al. Multipotent stem/progenitor cells with similar properties arise from two neurogenic regions of adult human brain. Exp Neurol 1999; 156:333–344.

88a. Lacy ER, Ito S. Rapid epithelial restitution of the rat gastric mucosa after ethanol injury. Lab Invest 1984;51:573–583.

89. Lagasse E, Connors H, Al-Dhalimy M, et al. Purified hematopoietic stem cells can differentiate into hepatocytes in vivo. Nat Med 2000;6:1229–1234.

90. Larson DM, Haudenschild CC. Junctional transfer in wounded cultures of bovine aortic endothelial cells. Lab Invest 1988;59:373–379.

91. Lee H-W, Blasco MA, Gottlieb GJ, Horner II JW, Greider CW. Essential role of mouse telomerase in highly proliferative organs. Nature 1998;392:569–574.

92. Lenddahl U, Zimmerman LB, McKay RDG. CNS stem cells express a new class of intermediate filament protein. Cell 1990;60:585–595.

93. Levi-Montalcini R. The nerve growth factor 35 years later. Science 1987;237:1154–1162.

94. Levitt D, Mertelsmann R (eds). Hematopoietic Stem Cells. New York: Marcel Dekker, Inc., 1995.

95. Lim DA, Alvarez-Buylla A. Interaction between astrocytes and adult subventricular zone precursors stimulates neurogenesis. Proc Natl Acad Sci USA 1999;96:7526–7531.

95a. Lin H. To be or not to be. Nature 2003;425:353–355.

96. Lloyd AC. Limit to lifespan. Nat Cell Biol 2002;4:E25–E27.

97. Lord BI. Biology of the haemopoietic stem cell. In: Potten CS (ed). Stem cells. London: Academic Press Ltd, 1997, pp. 401–422.

98. Lotz MM, Rabinovitz I, Mercurio AM. Intestinal restitution: progression of actin cytoskeleton rearrangements and integrin function in a model of epithelial wound healing. Am J Pathol 2000;156:985–996.

99. Majno P, Morel P, Giostra E, Hadengue A, Mentha G. Transplantation du foie: pourquoi a-t-on recours au donneur vivant? Med Hyg 2001;59:266–272.

100. Malemud CJ, Norby DP, Sokoloff L. Explant culture of human and rabbit articular chondrocytes. Connect Tissue Res 1978;6:171–179.

101. Martin P, Lewis J. Actin cables and epidermal movement in embryonic wound healing. Nature 1992;360:179–183.

102. Mauro A. Satellite cell of skeletal muscle fibers. J Biophys Biochem Cytol 1961;9:493–495.

103. Mazanet R, Franzini-Armstrong C. The satellite cell. In: Engel AG, Banker BQ (eds). Myology: basic and clinical. New York: McGraw-Hill Book Company, 1986 pp. 285–307.

104. McBrearty BA, Clark LD, Zhang X-M, Blaaankenhorn EP, Heber-Katz E. Genetic analysis of a mammalian wound-healing trait. Proc Natl Acad Sci USA 1998;95: 11792–11797.

105. McGeachie JK. Smooth muscle regeneration. Monogr Dev Biol 1975;9:1–90.

106. Michalopoulos GK. Liver regeneration: molecular mechanisms of growth control. FASEB J 1990;4:176–187.

107. Miller SJ, Lavker RM, Sun T-T. Keratinocyte stem cells of cornea, skin and hair follicles. In: Potten CS (ed). Stem cells. London: Academic Press Ltd, 1997, pp. 331–362.

108. Morrison SJ, Shah NM, Anderson DJ. Regulatory mechanisms in stem cell biology. Cell 1997;88:287–298.

109. Morshead CM, Benveniste P, Iscove NN, van der Kooy D. Hematopoietic competence is a rare property of neural stem cells that may depend on genetic and epigenetic alterations. Nat Med 2002;8:268–273.

110. Nachemson AK, Lundborg G, Hansson H-A. Insulin-like growth factor I promotes nerve regeneration: an experimental study on rat sciatic nerve. Growth Factors 1990;3: 309–314.

111. Nishimura EK, Jordan SA, Oshima H, et al. Dominant role of the niche in melanocyte stem-cell fate determination. Nature 2002;416:854–859.

112. Nottebohm F. Birdsong as a model in which to study brain processes related to learning. The Condor 1984a;86: 227–236.

113. Nottebohm F. From bird song to neurogenesis. Sci Am 1989; 260:74–79.

114. Olson L. Clearing a path for nerve growth. Nature 2002;416: 589–590.

115. Orkin SH, Zon LI. Hematopoiesis and stem cells: plasticity versus developmental heterogeneity. Nat Immunol 2002;3: 323–328.

116. Orlic D, Bock TA, Kanz L (eds). Hematopoietic stem cells. Biology and transplantation. New York: The New York Academy of Sciences, 1999.

117. Orlic D, Kajstura J, Chimenti S, et al. Mobilized bone marrow cells repair the infarcted heart, improving function and survival. Proc Natl Acad Sci USA 2001;98:10344–10349.

118. Pabst R, Sterzel RB. Cell renewal of glomerular cell types in normal rats. An autoradiographic analysis. Kidney Int 1983; 24:626–631.

119. Partridge T. The "Fantastic Voyage" of muscle progenitor cells. Nat Med 1998;4:554–555.

120. Partridge TA. Invited review: myoblast transfer: a possible therapy for inherited myopathies? Muscle Nerve 1991;14: 197–212.

121. Paton JA, Nottebohm F. Neurons generated in the adult brain are recruited into functional circuits. Science 1984; 225:1046–1048.

122. Payling Wright G. Introduction to pathology. Boston: Little, Brown, & Co., 1958.

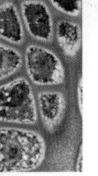

123. Pennisi E. Tending tender tendons. Science 2002;295:101.

124. Petersen BE, Bowen WC, Patrene KD, et al. Bone marrow as a potential source of hepatic oval cells. Science 1999;284: 1168–1170.

125. Pittenger MF, Mackay AM, Beck SC, et al. Multilineage potential of adult human mesenchymal stem cells. Science 1999;284:143–147.

126. Potten CS (ed). Stem cells. London: Academic Press, 1997.

127. Potten CS, Loeffler M. Stem cells: attributes, cycles, spirals, pitfalls and uncertainties. Lessons for and from the crypt. Development 1990;110:1001–1020.

128. Price CH. Regeneration in the central nervous system of a pulmonate mollusc, Melampus. Cell Tissue Res 1977;180: 529–536.

129. Quaini F, Urbanek K, Beltrami AP, et al. Chimerism of the transplanted heart. N Engl J Med 2002;346:5–15.

130. Quesenbery PJ, Becker PS. Stem cell homing: rolling, crawling, and nesting. Proc Natl Acad Sci USA 1998;95: 15155–15157.

131. Raina AK, Takeda A, Smith MA. Mitotic neurons: a dogma succumbs. Exp Neurol 1999;159:248–249.

132. Raisman G. Neuronal plasticity in the septal nuclei of the adult rat. Brain Res 1969;14:25–48.

133. Reddi AH. Cartilage-derived morphogenetic proteins and carilage morphogenesis. Microsc Res Tech 1998;34:131–136.

134. Reidy MA, Schwartz SM. Endothelial regeneration. III. Time course of intimal changes after small defined injury to rat aortic endothelium. Lab Invest 1981;44:301–308.

135. Richardson PM, McGuinness UM, Aguayo AJ. Axons from CNS neurones regenerate into PNS grafts. Nature 1980; 284:264–265.

136. Riley EH, Lane JM, Urist MR, Lyons KM, Lieberman JR. Bone morphogenetic protein-2. Clin Orthop 1996; 324:39–46.

137. Robertson TA, Grounds MD, Mitchell CA, Papadimitriou JM. Fusion between myogenic cells in vivo: an ultrastructural study in regenerating murine skeletal muscle. J Struct Biol 1990;105:170–182.

138. Roy NS, Wang S, Jiang L, Kang J, Benraiss A, Harrison-Restelli C, Fraser RAR, Couldwell WT, Kawaguchi A, Okano H, Nedergaard M, Goldman SA. In vitro neurogenesis by progenitor cells isolated from the adult human hippocampus. Nat Med 2000;6:271–277.

139. Rubinstein P, Carrier C, Scaradavou A, et al. Outcomes among 562 recipients of placental-blood transplants from unrelated donors. N Engl J Med 1998;339:1565–1577.

140. Rudolph KL, Chang S, Lee H-W, et al. Longevity, stress response, and cancer in aging telomerase-deficient mice. Cell 1999;96:701–712.

141. Ryan GB, Grobéty J, Majno G. Mesothelial injury and recovery. Am J Pathol 1973;71:93–112.

142. Saiura A, Sata M, Hirata Y, Nagai R, Makuuchi M. Circulating smooth muscle progenitor cells contribute to atherosclerosis. Nat Med 2001;7:382–383.

143. Schaumburg HH, Berger AR, Thomas PK, (eds). Disorders of peripheral nerves. 2nd ed. Philadelphia: F.A. Davis Company, 1992.

144. Schofield R. The relationship between the spleen colony-forming cell and the haemopoietic stem cell. Blood Cells 1978;4:7–25.

145. Schwab ME. Repairing the injured spinal cord. Science 2002;295:1029–1031.

146. Shimokawa H, Flavahan NA, Vanhoutte PM. Natural course of the impairment of endothelium-dependent relaxations after balloon endothelium removal in porcine coronary arteries. Possible dysfunction of a pertussis toxin-sensitive G protein. Circ Res 1989;65:740–753.

146a. Singer M, Géraudie J. An overview of the historical origin of the nerve influence on limb regeneration. In: Kiortsis V, Koussoulakos S, Wallace H (eds). Recent trends in regeneration research. New York: Plenum Press 1989, pp. 1–5.

147. Slack J. Skinny dipping for stem cells. Nature Cell Biol 2001;3:E205–E206.

148. Slack JMW. Stem cells in epithelial tissues. Science 2000; 287:1431–1433.

149. Sloper JC, Pegrum GD. Regeneration of crushed mammalian skeletal muscle and effects of steroids. J Pathol Bacteriol 1967;93:47–63.

150. Song X, Zhu C-H, Doan C, Xie T. Germline stem cells anchored by adherens junctions in the Drosophila ovary niches. Science 2002;296:1855–1857.

151. Spallanzani L. Tracts on the natural history of animals and vegetables, 2nd ed., vol. II. (Translated from the original Italian edition by John Graham Dalyell.) Edinburgh: W. Creech and A. Constable, 1803.

152. Spencer PS. The traumatic neuroma and proximal stump. Bull Hosp Joint Dis 1974;35:85–102.

152a. Sporn MB, Roberts AB. Peptide growth factors are multifunctional. Nature 1988;332:217–219.

153. Stenn KS, DePalma L. Re-epithelialization. In: Clark RAF, Henson PM (eds). The molecular and cellular biology of wound repair. New York: Plenum Press, 1988, pp. 321–335.

154. Striker LJ, Tannen RL, Lange MA, Striker GE. The contribution of cell culture to the study of renal diseases. Int Rev Exp Pathol 1988;30:55–105.

155. Sumner AJ. Aberrant reinnervation. Muscle Nerve 1990;13: 801–803.

156. Svendsen CN, Smith AG. New prospects for human stem-cell therapy in the nervous system. Trends Neurosci 1999;22: 357–364.

157. Taylor AC. Survival of rat skin and changes in hair pigmentation following freezing. J Exp Zool 1949;110:77–111.

158. Temple S, Alvarez-Buylla A. Stem cells in the adult mammalian central nervous system. Curr Opin Neurobiol 1999;9:135–141.

159. Tessier-Lavigne M, Goodman CS. The molecular biology of axon guidance. Science 1996;274:1123–1133.

160. Thanos PK, Okajima S, Terzis JK. Ultrastructure and cellular biology of nerve regeneration. J Reconstr Microsurg 1998;14:423–436.

160a. Thomas PK. Clinical aspects of PNS regeneration. Adv Neurol 1988;47:9–29.

161. Toma JG, Akhavan M, Fernandes KJL, et al. Isolation of multipotent adult stem cells from the dermis of mammalian skin. Nat Cell Biol 2001;3:778–784.

162. Trusolino L, Pugliese L, Comoglio PM. Interactions between scatter factors and their receptors: hints for therapeutic applications. FASEB J 1998;12:1267–1280.

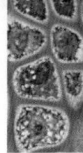

163. Tsubota K, Satake Y, Kaido M, et al. Treatment of severe ocular-surface disorders with corneal epithelial stem-cell transplantation. N Engl J Med 1999;340:1697–1703.

164. Tuszynski MH, Kordower JH (eds). CNS regeneration. Basic science and clinical advances. San Diego: Academic Press, 1999.

165. Urist MR, DeLange RJ, Finerman GAM. Bone cell differentiation and growth factors. Science 1983;220: 680–686.

166. van Praag H, Schinder AF, Christie BR, et al. Functional neurogenesis in the adult hippocampus. Nature 2002; 415:1030–1034.

167. Vescovi AL, Snyder EY. Establishment and properties of neural stem cell clones:plasticity in vitro and in vivo. Brain Pathol 1999;9:569–598.

168. Vikhanski L. In search of the lost cord. Solving the mystery of spinal cord regeneration. Washington, DC: Joseph Henry Press, 2001.

169. Watanabe N, Mitchison TJ. Single-molecule speckle analysis of actin filament turnover in lamellipodia. Science 2002; 295:1083–1086.

170. Watt DJ, Jones GE. Skeletal muscle stem cells: function and potential role in therapy. In: Potten CS (ed.) Stem Cells. London: Academic Press Ltd, 1997, pp. 75–98.

171. Watt FM, Hogan BLM. Out of Eden: stem cells and their niches. Science 2000;287:1427–1430.

172. Wells H, Handelman C, Milgram E. Regulation by sympathetic nervous system of accelerated growth of salivary glands of rats. Am J Physiol 1961;201:707–710.

173. Westermark B, Betsholtz C, Hookfelt B (eds). Growth factors in health and disease: basic and clinical Aspects (International Congress Series No. 925). Amsterdam: Excerpta Medica, 1990.

174. Wong MKK, Gotlieb AI. In vitro reendothelialization of a single-cell wound. Role of microfilament bundles in rapid lamellipodia-mediated wound closure. Lab Invest 1984;51: 75–81.

175. Wong MKK, Gotlieb AI. The reorganization of microfilaments, centrosomes, and microtubules during in vitro small would reendothelialization. J Cell Biol 1988;107: 1777–1783.

176. Woolf CJ, Bloechlinger S. It takes more than two to nogo. Science 2002;297:1132–1134.

177. Wright WE, Shay JW. Historical claims and current interpretations of replicative aging. Nat Biotech 2002;20: 682–688.

178. Wurmser AE, Gage FH. Cell fusion causes confusion. Nature 2002;416:485–487.

178a. Yamashita YM, Jones DL, Fuller MT. Orientation of asymmetric stem cell division by APC tumor suppressor and centrosome. Science 2003;301:1547–1550.

179. Yonemori K, Imamura T, Ishidou Y, et al. Bone morphogenetic protein receptors and activin receptors are highly expressed in ossified ligament tissues of patients with ossification of the posterior longitudinal ligament. Am J Pathol 1997;150:1335–1347.

179a. Zhang J, Niu C, Huan H, et al. Identification of the haematopoietic stem cell niche and control of the niche size. Nature 2003;425:836–841.

180. Ziegler E. General pathology. New York: William Wood and Company, 1908.

181. Zimmerman L, Lendahl U, Cunningham M, McKay R, Parr B, Gavin B, Mann J, Vassileva G, McMahon A. Independent regulatory elements in the nestin gene direct transgene expression to neural stem cells or muscle precursors. Neuron 1994;12:11–24.

Hypertrophy and Hyperplasia

182. Abrahams C, Janicki JS, Weber KT. Myocardial hypertrophy in Macaca fascicularis. Structural remodeling of the collagen matrix. Lab Invest 1987;56:676–683.

183. Adler CP, Sandritter W. Numerische Hyperplasie der Herzmuskelzellen bei Herzhypertrophie. Dtsch Med Wochenschr 1971;48:1895–1897.

184. Allison DB, Fontaine KR, Manson JE, Stevens J, VanItallie TB. Annual deaths attributable to obesity in the United States. JAMA 1999;282:1530–1538.

185. Alway SE, Grumbt WH, Gonyea WJ, Stray-Gundersen J. Contrasts in muscle and myofibers of elite male and female bodybuilders. J Appl Physiol 1989;67:24–31.

186. Alway SE, MacDougall JD, Sale DG, Sutton JR, McComas AJ. Functional and structural adaptations in skeletal muscle of trained athletes. J Appl Physiol 1988;64:1114–1120.

187. Angel A, Hollenberg CH, Roncari DAK. The Adipocyte and obesity: cellular and molecular mechanisms. New York: Raven Press, 1983.

188. Anversa P, Beghi C, McDonald SL, Levicky V, Kikkawa Y, Olivetti G. Morphometry of right ventricular hypertrophy induced by myocardial infarction in the rat. Am J Pathol 1984;116:504–513.

189. Anversa P, Nadal-Ginard B. Myocyte renewal and ventricular remodelling. Nature 2002;415:240–243.

190. Astorri E, Bolognesi R, Colla B, Chizzola A, Visioli O. Left ventricular hypertrophy: a cytometric study on 42 human hearts. J Mol Cell Cardiol 1977;9:763–775.

191. Baatout S. Molecular basis to understand polyploidy. Hematol Cell Ther 1999;41:169–170.

192. Barka T, Yagil C, van der Noen H, Naito Y. Induction of the synthesis of a specific protein in rat submandibular gland by isoproterenol. Lab Invest 1986;54:165–171.

193. Barrett TB, Sampson P, Owens GK, Schwartz SM, Benditt EP. Polyploid nuclei in human artery wall smooth muscle cells. Proc Natl Acad Sci USA 1983;80:882–885.

194. Bonnet F, Gosselin L, Chantraine J, Senteree J. Adipose cell number and size in normal and obese children. Rev Eur Etud Clin Biol 1970;25:1101–1104.

195. Bowen RE, Swartz FJ. The ultrastructure of polyploid B-cells in the islets of normal mice. Diabetologia 1976;12:171–180.

196. Bray GA. Obesity: what comes first. In: Angel A, Hollenberg, CH, Roncari DAK (eds). The adipocyte and obesity: cellular and molecular mechanisms. New York: Raven Press, 1983, pp. 19–27.

197. Brenner BM, Lawler EV, Mackenzie HS. The hyperfiltration theory: a paradigm shift in nephrology. Kidney Int 1996; 49:1774–1777.

198. Brent B, Brent BP. The artistry of reconstructive surgery. St. Louis: The CV Mosby Company, 1987.

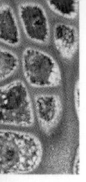

199. Brodsky WY, Uryvaeva IV. Cell polyploidy: its relation to tissue growth and function. Int Rev Cytol 1977;50:275–332.

200. Bucher NLR, Malt RA. Regeneration of liver and kidney. Boston: Little Brown and Company, 1971.

201. Clark AM, Rubin MA. The modification by X-irradiation of the life span of haploids and diploids of the wasp, Habrobracon SP. Radiat Res 1961;15:244–253.

201a. Coyle JT. Use it or lose it—Do effortful mental activities protect against dementia? N Engl J Med 2003;348: 2489–2490.

202. Cutilletta AF, Dowell RT, Rudnik M, Arcilla RA, Zak R. Regression of myocardial hypertrophy. I. Experimental model, changes in heart weight, nucleic acids and collagen. J Mol Cell Cardiol 1975;7:767–781.

203. Enriori CL, Reforzo-Membrives J. Peripheral aromatization as a risk factor for breast and endometrial cancer in postmenopausal women: a review. Gynecol Oncol 1984;17:1–21.

204. Faust IM, Johnson PR, Hirsch J. Surgical removal of adipose tissue alters feeding behavior and the development of obesity in rats. Science 1977;197:393–396.

205. Faust IM, Miller WH Jr. Hyperplastic growth of adipose tissue in obesity. In: Angel A, Hollenberg CH, Roncari DAK (eds). The adipocyte and obesity: cellular and molecular mechanisms. New York: Raven Press, 1983, pp. 41–51.

206. Ferrans VJ. Cardiac hypertrophy: morphological aspects. In: Zak R (ed). Growth of the heart in health and disease. New York: Raven Press, 1984, pp. 187–239.

207. Ferrans VJ, Jones M, Maron BJ, Roberts WC. The nuclear membranes in hypertrophied human cardiac muscle cells. Am J Pathol 1975;78:427–446.

208. Fleck C, Bräunlich H. Kidney function after unilateral nephrectomy. Exp Pathol 1984;25:3–18.

209. Fries JWU, Sandstrom DJ, Meyer TW, Rennke HG. Glomerular hypertrophy and epithelial cell injury modulate progressive glomerulosclerosis in the rat. Lab Invest 1989; 60:205–218.

210. Gabella G. Hypertrophic smooth muscle. Cell Tissue Res 1979;201:63–78.

211. Gahan PB. Increased levels of euploidy as a strategy against rapid ageing in diploid mammalian systems: an hypothesis. Exp Gerontol 1977;12:133–136.

212. Galitski T, Saldanha AJ, Styles CA, Lander ES, Fink GR. Ploidy regulation of gene expression. Science 1999;285: 251–254.

213. Goldberg ID, Shapiro H, Stemerman MB, et al. Frequency of tetraploid nuclei in the rat aorta increases with age. Ann N Y Acad Sci 1984;435:422–424.

214. Gortmaker SL, Must A, Perrin JM, Sobol AM, Dietz WH. Social and economic consequences of overweight in adolescence and young adulthood. N Engl J Med 1993;329: 1008–1012.

215. Goss RJ, Dittmer JE. Compensatory renal hypertrophy: problems and prospects. In: Nowinski WW, Goss RJ (eds). Compensatory renal hypertrophy. New York: Academic Press, 1969, pp. 299–307.

216. Greene GL, Press MF: I. Steroid receptor structure (including monoclonal antibodies and new methods of determination). Structure and dynamics of the estrogen receptor. J Steroid Biochem 1986;24:1–7.

217. Hasegawa T, Harada N, Ikeda K, et al. Digynic triploid infant surviving for 46 days. Am J Genet 1999;87:306–310.

218. Hieter P, Griffiths T. Polyploidy-more is more or less. Science 1999;285:210–211.

218a. Hill JO, Wyatt HR, Reed GW, Peters JC. Obesity and the environment: where do we go from here? Science 2003; 299:853–855.

219. Hostetter TH, Meyer TW, Rennke HG, et al. Chronic effects of dietary protein in the rat with intact and reduced renal mass. Kidney Int 1986;30:509–517.

220. Hostetter TH, Olson JL, Rennke HG, Venkatachalam MA, Brenner BM. Hyperfiltration in remnant nephrons: a potentially adverse response to renal ablation. Am J Physiol 1981;241:F85–F93.

221. Hunter JJ, Chien KR. Signaling pathways for cardiac hypertrophy and failure. N Engl J Med 1999;341: 1276–1283.

222. Huston TP, Puffer JC, Rodney WM. The athletic heart syndrome. N Engl J Med 1985;313:24–32.

223. Johansson B. Different types of smooth muscle hypertrophy. Hypertension 1984;6(suppl. III):64–68.

224. Johnson HA, Vera Roman JM. Compensatory renal enlargement. Hypertrophy versus hyperplasia. Am J Pathol 1966; 49:1–13.

225. Kolata G. Obesity declared a disease. Science 1985;227: 1019–1020.

226. Kuzon WM Jr, Rosenblatt JD, Huebel SC, et al. Skeletal muscle fiber type, fiber size, and capillary supply in elite soccer players. Int J Sports Med 1990;11:99–102.

227. Lapham LW. Tetraploid DNA content of Purkinje neurons of human cerebellar cortex. Science 1968;159:310–312.

228. Leiter EH. Genetics of β-cell abnormalities in rodents. In: Hanahan D, McDevitt HO, Cahill GF Jr (eds). Perspectives on the molecular biology and immunology of the pancreatic β cell. Cold Spring Harbor: Cold Spring Harbor Laboratory, 1989, pp. 69–79.

229. Levine E. Compensatory renal hypertrophy. Abdom Imaging 1995;20:181.

230. Loud AV, Beghi C, Olivetti G, Anversa P. Morphometry of right and left ventricular myocardium after strenuous exercise in preconditioned rats. Lab Invest 1984;51:104–111.

231. Lund DD, Tomanek RJ. The effects of chronic hypoxia on the myocardial cell of normotensive and hypertensive rats. Anat Rec 1980;196:421–430.

232. Majno G. The healing hand: man and wound in the ancient world. Cambridge: Harvard University Press 1975.

233. Marcussen N, Nyengaard JR, Christensen S. Compensatory growth of glomeruli is accomplished by an increased number of glomerular capillaries. Lab Invest 1994;70:868–874.

234. Maron BJ, Ferrans VJ. Ultrastructural features of hypertrophied human ventricular myocardium. Prog Cardiovasc Dis 1978;21:207–238.

235. McNurlan MA, McHardy KC, Broom J, et al. The effect of indomethacin on the response of protein synthesis to feeding in rats and man. Clin Sci 1987;73:69–75.

236. Meyrick B, Reid L. The effect of continued hypoxia on rat pulmonary arterial circulation. An ultrastructural study. Lab Invest 1978;38:188–200.

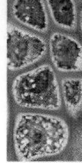

237. Must A, Jacques PF, Dallal GE, Bajema CJ, Dietz WH. Long-term morbidity and mortality of overweight adolescents. N Engl J Med 1992;327:1350–1355.

238. Nadal C, Zajdela F. Polyploïdie somatique dans le foie de rat. I. Le rôle des cellules binucléées dans la genèse des cellules polyploïdes. Exp Cell Res 1966;42:99–116.

239. NHLBI Obesity Education Initiative. Clinical guidelines on the identification, evaluation, and treatment of overweight and obesity in adults: the evidence report. U.S. Department of Health and Human Services, NIH Publication No. 98-4083, 1998.

240. NHLBI Obesity Education Initiative. The practical guide. Identification, evaluation and treatment of overweight and obesity in adults. U.S. Department of Health and Human Services, NIH Publication No. 00-4084, 2000.

241. Odell TT Jr, Jackson CW, Friday TJ. Megakaryo-cytopoiesis in rats with special reference to polyploidy. Blood 1970;35:775–782.

242. Olivecrona T, Bengtsson G. Lipoprotein lipase. In: Angel A, Hollenberg CH, Roncari DAK (eds). The adipocyte and obesity: cellular and molecular mechanisms. New York: Raven Press, 1983, pp. 117–126.

243. Oparil S, Bishop SP, Clubb FJ. Myocardial cell hypertrophy or hyperplasia. Hypertension 1984;6(suppl. III):38–43.

244. Owens GK. Growth response of aortic smooth muscle cells in hypertension. In: Lee RMKW (ed). Blood vessel changes in hypertension: structure and function, vol. 1. Boca Raton: CRC Press, Inc., 1989, pp. 45–63.

245. Penington DG. The cellular biology of megakaryocytes. Blood Cells 1979;5:5–10.

246. Penington DG, Streatfield K, Roxburgh AE. Megakaryocytes and the heterogeneity of circulating platelets. Br J Haematol 1976;34:639–653.

247. Pfitzer P, Capurso A. Der DNS-Gehalt der Zellkerne im Herzohr des Menschen. Virchows Arch B Zellpathol 1970;5:254–267.

248. Popkin BM, Doak CM. The obesity epidemic is a worldwide phenomenon. Nutr Rev 1998;56:106–114.

249. Preisig P. What makes cells grow larger and how do they do it? Renal hypertrophy revisited. Exp Nephrol 1999;7:273–283.

250. Raven PH, Curtis H. Biology of plants. New York: Worth Publishers, Inc., 1971.

251. Rennke HG. Glomerular adaptations to renal injury or ablation. Blood Purif 1988;6:230–239.

252. Revis NW, Cameron AJV. Association of myocardial cell necrosis with experimental cardiac hypertrophy. J Pathol 1979;128:193–202.

253. Robertson RP, Harmon J, Tanaka Y, et al. Glucose toxicity of the β-cell: cellular and molecular mechanisms. In: LeRoith D, Taylor SI, Olefsky JM (eds). Diabetes Mellitus. A fundamental and clinical text. Philadelphia: Lippincott Williams & Wilkins, 2000, pp. 125–132.

254. Rocchini AP. Childhood obesity and a diabetes epidemic. N Engl J Med 2002;346:854–855.

255. Rost TL, Barbour MG, Thornton RM, Weier TE, Stocking CR. Botany. 2nd ed. New York: John Wiley & Sons, 1984.

256. Siiteri PK, Schwarz BE, MacDonald PC. Estrogen receptors and the estrone hypothesis in relation to endometrial and breast cancer. Gynecol Oncol 1974;2:228–238.

257. Taylor TG. How an eggshell is made. Sci Am 1970;222:89–95.

257a. Verghese J, Lipton RB, Katz MJ, et al. Leisure activities and the risk of dementia in the elderly. N Engl J Med 2003;348,2508–2516.

258. Weisz PB, Keogh RN. The Science of Biology, 5th ed. New York: McGraw-Hill Book Company, 1982.

259. Wolf G. Molecular mechanisms of renal hypertrophy: role of p27Kip1. Kidney Int 1999;56:1262–1265.

260. Zimmet P, Alberti KGMM, Shaw J. Global and societal implications of the diabetes epidemic. Nature 2001;414:782–787.

261. Zimmet J, Ravid K. Polyploidy: occurrence in nature, mechanisms, and significance for the megakaryocyte-platelet system. Exp Hematol 2000;28:3–16.

Atrophy

262. Abrams GD, Bauer H, Sprinz H. Influence of the normal flora on mucosal morphology and cellular renewal in the ileum. A comparison of germ-free and conventional mice. Lab Invest 1963;12:355–364.

263. Alberts B, Johnson A, Lewis J, Raff M, Roberts K, Walter P (eds). Molecular biology of the cell. 4th ed. New York: Garland Science, 2002.

264. Amiel D, Woo S L-Y, Harwood FL, Akeson WH. The effect of immobilization on collagen turnover in connective tissue: a biochemical-biomechanical correlation. Acta Orthop Scand 1982;53:325–332.

265. Angel A, Hollenberg CH, Roncari DAK (eds). The adipocyte and obesity: cellular and molecular mechanisms. New York: Raven Press, 1983.

265a. Arantes-Oliveira N, Berman JR, Kenyon C. Healthy animals with extreme longevity. Science 2003;302:611.

266. Ashford TP, Porter KR. Cytoplasmic components in hepatic cell lysosomes. J Cell Biol 1962;12:198–202.

267. Askanazi J, Elwyn DH, Kinney JM, et al. Muscle and plasma amino acids after injury: the role of inactivity. Ann Surg 1978;188:797–803.

268. Austad SN. Life extension by dietary restriction in the bowl and doily spider, Frontinella pyramitela. Exp Gerontol 1989;24:83–92.

269. Bachmair A, Finley D, Varshavsky A. In vivo half-life of a protein is a function of its amino-terminal residue. Science 1986;234:179–186.

271. Barnes RH. Nutrition and man's intellect and behavior. Fed Proc 1971;30:1429–1433.

272. Barrows CH Jr, Kokkonen GC. Diet and life extension in animal model systems. Age 1978;1:131–143.

272a. Barzilai N, Atzmon G, Schechter C, et al. Unique lipoprotein phenotype and genotype associated with exceptional longevity. JAMA 2003;290:2003–2040.

273. Basson MD, Burney RE. Defective wound healing in patients with paraplegia and quadriplegia. Surg Gynecol Obstet 1982;155:9–12.

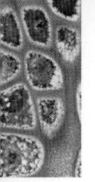

274. Bellamy D. Cell death in the context of ageing. In: Davies I, Sigee DC (eds). Cell ageing and cell death. Cambridge: Cambridge University Press, 1984, pp. 105–121.

275. Berkenstam A, Ahlberg J, Glaumann H. Isolation and characterization of autophagic vacuoles from rat kidney cortex. Virchows Arch B Cell Pathol 1983;44:275–286.

276. Bliss M. The discovery of insulin: how it really happened. In: Hollenberg MD (ed). Insulin: its receptor and diabetes. New York: Marcel Dekker, Inc., 1985, pp. 7–19.

277. Bloodgood RA. Resorption of organelles containing microtubules. Cytobios 1974;9:143–161.

278. Bocci V. The neglected organ: bacterial flora has a crucial immunostimulatory role. Perspect Biol Med 1992;35:251–260.

279. Buetow DE. Cell numbers vs. age in mammalian tissues and organs. In: Cristofalo VJ (ed). CRC handbook of cell biology of aging. Boca Raton: CRC Press, Inc., 1985, pp. 1–115.

280. Bührle CP, Hackenthal E, Helmchen U, et al. The hydronephrotic kidney of the mouse as a tool for intravital microscopy and in vitro electrophysiological studies of renin-containing cells. Lab Invest 1986;54:462–472.

281. Cahill GF. President's address: starvation. Trans Am Clin Climatol Assoc 1982;94:1–21.

282. Cameron GR. Liver atrophy produced by chronic selenium intoxication. J Pathol Bacteriol 1947;59:539–545.

283. Carpentier J-L, Perrelet A, Orci L. Morphological changes of the adipose cell plasma membrane during lipolysis. J Cell Biol 1977;72:104–117.

284. Casarett GW. Radiation histopathology, vol. I. Boca Raton: CRC Press, Inc., 1981.

285. Clancy DJ, Gems D, Hafen E, Leevers SJ, Partridge L. Dietary restriction in long-lived dwarf flies. Science 2002;296:319.

285a. Cohen P, Miyazaki M, Socci ND, et al. Role for stearoyl-CoA desaturase-1 in leptin-mediated weight loss. Science 2002; 297:240–243.

286. Cristofalo VJ. Perspectives in the biology of aging. In: Bates SR, Gangloff EC (eds). Atherogenesis and aging. New York: Springer-Verlag, 1987, pp. 48–56.

287. Dämmrich J, Pfeifer U. Cardiac hypertrophy in rats after supravalvular aortic constriction. II. Inhibition of cellular autophagy in hypertrophying cardiomyocytes. Virchows Arch B Cell Pathol 1983;43:287–307.

288. Decker RS, Crie JS, Poole AR, Dingle JT, Wildenthal K. Resistance to ischemic damage in hearts of starved rabbits. Correlation with lysosomal alterations and delayed release of cathepsin d. Lab Invest 1980;43:197–207.

289. Donaldson CL, Hulley SB, Vogel JM, Hattner R, Bayers JH, McMillan DE. Effect of prolonged bed rest on bone mineral. Metabolism 1970;19:1071–1084.

290. Ericsson JLE, Trump BF, Weibel J. Electron microscopic studies of the proximal tubule of the rat kidney. II. Cytosegresomes and cytosomes: their relationship to each other and to the lysosome concept. Lab Invest 1965;14:1341–1365.

290a. Eriksson M, Brown WT, Gordon LB, et al. Recurrent de novo point mutations in lamin A cause Hutchinson-Gilford progeria syndrome. Nature 2003;423:293–298.

291. Fronek K. Trophic influence of the sympathetic nervous system on the arterial wall. In: Gaehtgens P (ed). Bibliotheca anatomica, No. 20, Basel S. Karger, 1981, p. 414–417.

292. Fronek K, Bloor CM, Amiel D, Chvapil M. Effect of long-term sympathectomy on the arterial wall in rabbits and rats. Exp Mol Pathol 1978;28:279–289.

293. Gobé GC, Axelsen RA. Genesis of renal tubular atrophy in experimental hydronephrosis in the rat. Role of apoptosis. Lab Invest 1987;56:273–281.

294. Goldberg AL, Etlinger JD, Goldspink DF, Jablecki C. Mechanism of work-induced hypertrophy of skeletal muscle. Med Sci Sports 1975;7:248–261.

295. Gordeuk V, Thuma P, Brittenham G, McLaren C, Parry D, Backenstose A, et al. Effect of iron chelation therapy on recovery from deep coma in children with cerebral malaria. N Engl J Med 1992;327:1473–1477.

296. Gravis CJ, Weaker FJ. Testicular involution following optic enucleation. An ultrastructural and cytochemical study. Cell Tissue Res 1977;184:67–77.

297. Gredilla R, Sanz A, Lopez-Torres M, Barja G. Caloric restriction decreases mitochondrial free radical generation at complex I and lowers oxidative damage to mitochondrial DNA in the rat heart. FASEB J 2001;15:1589–1591.

298. Hall DM, Oberley TD, Moseley PM, et al. Caloric restriction improves thermotolerance and reduces hyperthermia-induced cellular damage in old rats. FASEB J 2000;14: 87–86.

299. Harman D. Free radical theory of aging: the "free radical" diseases. Age 1984;7:111–131.

300. Hayashi T, Faustman, D. The role of proteasome in autoimmunity. Diabetes Metab Res Rev 2000;16:325–337.

301. Heneghan JB. Alimentary tract physiology: interactions between the host and its microbial flora. In: Rowland IR (ed). Role of the gut flora in toxicity and cancer. London:Academic Press, 1988, pp. 39–77.

302. Holman CDJ, Wisniewski ZS, Semmens JB, Rouse IL, Bass AJ. Population-based outcomes after 28 246 in-hospital vasectomies and 1902 vasovasostomies in Western Australia. BJU Int 2000;86:1043–1049.

303. Hopewell JW, Young CMA. Changes in the microcirculation of normal tissues after irradiation. Int J Radiat Oncol Biol Phys 1978;4:53–58.

303a. Howitz KT, Bitterman KJ, Cohen HY, et al. Small molecules activators of sirtuins extend Saccharomyces cerevisiae lifespan. Nature 2003;425:191–196.

304. Jarow JP, Budin RE, Dym M, et al. Quantitative pathologic changes in the human testis after vasectomy. A controlled study. N Engl J Med 1985; 313:1252–1256.

305. Jaweed MM, Alleva FR, Herbison GJ, Ditunno JF, Balazs T. Muscle atrophy and histopathology of the soleus in 6-mercaptopurine-treated rats. Exp Mol Pathol 1985;43: 74–81.

306. Jokelainen OS, Rintala E, Koskimies AI, Rannikko S. Vaso-vasostomy—a 15-year experience. Scand J Urol Nephrol 2001;35:132–135.

306a. Kim J, Klionsky DJ. Autophagy, cytoplasm-to-vacuole targeting pathway, and pexophagy in yeast and mammalian cells. Ann Rev Biochem 2000;69:303–342.

307. Klionsky DJ, Emr SD. Autophagy as a regulated pathway of cellular degradation. Science 2000;290:1717–1721.

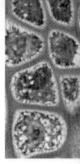

308. Lee, C-K, Klopp RG, Weindruch R, Prolla TA. Gene expression profile of aging and its retardation by caloric restriction. Science 1999;285:1390–1393.

309. Lewis CM, Tarrant GM. Error theory and aging in human diploid fibroblasts. Nature 1972;239:316–318.

310. Libby P, Goldberg AL. Leupeptin, a protease inhibitor, decreases protein degradation in normal and diseases muscles. Science 1978;199:534–536.

310a. Mair W, Goymer P, Pletcher SD, Partridge L. Demography of dietary restriction on death in *Drosophila*. Science 2003; 301:1731–1733.

311. Mamus SW, Burton JD, Groat JD, et al. Ibuprofen-associated pure white-cell aplasia. N Engl J Med 1986;314: 624–625.

312. Manolagas SC, Jilka RL. Bone marrow, cytokines, and bone remodeling. N Engl J Med 1995;332:305–311.

313. Martin GA. Space medicine. In: Flight surgeon's guide, Ch. 25. Air Force pamphlet No. 161-18. Washington, DC; Dept of the Air Force, 1968.

314. Masoro EJ. Caloric restriction and aging: an update. Exp Gerontol 2000;35:299–305.

315. Masoro EJ, Yu BP. Diet and nephropathy. Lab Invest 1989; 60:165–167.

316. McDonald SW, Lockhart A, Gormal D, Bennett NK. Changes in the testes following vasectomy in the rat. Clin Anat 1996;9:296–301.

317. Mellgren RL. Calcium-dependent proteases: an enzyme system active at cellular membranes? FASEB J 1987;1: 110–115.

318. Merry BJ, Holehan AM. Serum profiles of LH, FSH, testosterone and 5α-DHT from 21 to 1000 days of age in ad libitum fed and dietary restricted rats. Exp Gerontol 1981;16: 431–444.

319. Messenger AG. Hair follicles: kinetic concepts and human disease. Hosp Med 1998;59:393–397.

320. Munkres KD. Biochemical genetics of aging of Neurospora crassa and Podospora anserina: a review. In: Sohal RS (ed). Age pigments. Amsterdam: Elsevier/North-Holland Biomedical Press, 1981, pp. 83–100.

321. Murphy ED, Scanlon EF, Garces RM, Khandekar JD, Bailey L. Thyroid hormone administration in irradiated patients. J Surg Oncol 1986;31:214–217.

322. Murray J, Murray A. Suppression of infection by famine and its activation by refeeding—a paradox? Perspect Biol Med 1977;20:471–483.

323. Naujokat C, Hoffman S. Role and function of the 26S proteasome in proliferation and apoptosis. Lab Invest 2002;82: 965–980.

324. Novikoff AB, Shin WY. Endoplasmic reticulum and autophagy in rat hepatocytes. Proc Natl Acad Sci USA 1978; 75:5039–5042.

325. Noyes FR. Functional properties of knee ligaments and alterations induced by immobilization. Clin Orthop 1977; 123:210–242.

326. Ntambi JM, Miyazaki M, Stoehr JP, et al. Loss of stearoyl-CoA desaturase-1 function protects mice against adiposity. Proc Natl Acad Sci USA 2002;99:11482–11486.

327. Papadopoulos T, Pfeifer U. Regression of rat liver autophagic vacuoles by locally applied cycloheximide. Lab Invest 1986;54:100–107.

328. Pfeifer U. Cellular autophagy and cell atrophy in the rat liver during long-term starvation. A quantitative morphological study with regard to diurnal variations. Virchows Arch Abt B Zellpathol 1973;12:195–211.

329. Pfeifer U. Kinetic and subcellular aspects of hypertrophy and atrophy. Int Rev Exp Pathol 1982;23:1–45.

330. Pfeifer U. Application of test substances to the surface of rat liver in situ: opposite effects of insulin and isoproterenol on cellular autophagy. Lab Invest 1984;50:348–354.

331. Pfeifer U, Werder E, Bergeest H. Inhibition by insulin of the formation of autophagic vacuoles in rat liver. A morphometric approach to the kinetics of intracellular degradation by autophagy. J Cell Biol 1978;78:152–167.

332. Pierpaoli W, Fabris N. Physiological senescence and its postponement: Theoretical approaches and rational interventions. (Ann N Y Acad Sci, vol. 621). New York: The New York Academy of Sciences, 1991.

333. Pryor G. Malnutrition and the "critical period" hypothesis. In: Prescott JW, Read MS, Coursin DB (eds). Brain function and malnutrition. New York: John Wiley & Sons, 1975, pp. 103–112.

334. Purves D, Snider WD, Voyvodic JT. Trophic regulation of nerve cell morphology and innervation in the autonomic nervous system. Nature 1988;336:123–128.

335. Raisz LG. What marrow does to bone. N Engl J Med 1981;304:1485–1486.

336. Read MS. Malnutrition and behavior. Appl Res Mental Retard 1982;3:279–291.

337. Reunanen H, Hirsimaki P. Studies on vinblastine-induced autophagocytosis in mouse liver. IV. Origin of membranes. Histochemistry 1983;79:59–67.

338. Richie JP Jr, Mills BJ, Lang CA. Dietary nordi-hydroguaiaretic acid increases the life span of the mosquito. Proc Soc Exp Biol Med 1986;183:81–85.

339. Romanul FCA, Hogan EL. Enzymatic changes in denervated muscle. I. Histochemical studies. Arch Neurol 1965; 13:263–273.

340. Rook A, Dawber R. (eds). Diseases of the hair and scalp. 2nd ed. Oxford: Blackwell Scientific Publications, 1991.

341. Rudzinska MA. The use of a protozoan for studies on ageing. III. Similarities between young overfed and old normally fed Tokophrya infusionum: A light and electron microscope study. Gerontologia 1962;6:206–226.

342. Salminen A, Vihko V. Autophagic response to strenuous exercise in mouse skeletal muscle fibers. Virchows Arch B Cell Pathol 1984;45:97–106.

343. Schneider EL, Rowe JW (eds). Handbook of the biology of aging. 4th ed. San Diego: Academic Press, 1996.

344. Schonheyder F, Heilskov NSC, Olesen K. Isotopic studies on the mechanism of negative nitrogen balance produced by immobilization. Scand J Clin Lab Invest 1954;6:178–188.

345. Schwartz AL, Ciechanover A. The ubiquitin-proteasome pathway and pathogenesis of human diseases. Annu Rev Med 1999;50:57–74.

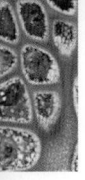
346. Shelburne JD, Arstila AU, Trump BF. Studies on cellular autophagocytosis. The relationship of autophagocytosis to protein synthesis and to energy metabolism in rat liver and flounder kidney tabules in vitro. Am J Pathol 1973;73: 641–662.

347. Sherman SM, Spear PD. neural development of cats raised with deprivation of visual patterns. In: Rosenberg RN (ed). The clinical neurosciences. New York: Churchill Livingstone, 1983, pp. V:385–V:434.

348. Sinclair D. Motor nerves and reflexes. In: Jarrett A (ed). The physiology and pathophysiology of the skin. New York: Academic Press, 1973, p. 475–573.

349. Smith DC. Functional restoration of vision in the cat after long-term monocular deprivation. Science 1981;213: 1137–1139.

350. Smith ME. The effect of fasting on lipid metabolism of the central nervous system of the rat. J Neurochem 1963; 10:531–536.

351. Stearner SP, Christian EJB. Long-term vascular effects of ionizing radiations in the mouse: capillary blood flow. Radiat Res 1978;73:553–567.

352. Stein J, Fenigstein H. Pathological anatomy of hunger disease. In: Winick M (ed). Hunger disease. New York: John Wiley & Sons, 1979, p. 220.

353. Tamarin A. Submaxillary gland recovery from obstruction. I. Overall changes and electron microscopic alterations of granular duct cells. J Ultrastruct Res 1971;34:276–287.

354. Taylor A, Zuliani AM, Hopkins RE, et al. Moderate caloric restriction delays cataract formation in the Emory mouse. FASEB J 1989;3:1741–1746.

355. Tchen TT, Chan SW, Kuo TH, Mostafapour KM, Dezewiecki VH. Studies on the adrenal cortex of hypophysectomized rats: A model for abnormal cellular atrophy and death. Mol Cell Biochem 1977;15:79–87.

356. Trump BF, Bulger RE. Studies of cellular injury in isolated flounder tubules. I. Correlation between morphology and function of control tubules and observations of autophagocytosis and mechanical cell damage. Lab Invest 1967; 16:453–482.

357. Vandenburgh H, Chromiak J, Shansky J, Del Tatto M, Lemaire J. Space travel directly induces skeletal muscle atrophy. FASEB J 1999;13:1031–1038.

357a. Vastag B. Cause of progeria's premature aging found: expected to provide insight into normal aging process. JAMA 2003;289:2481–2482.

358. Vojta CL, Fraga PD, Forciea MA, Lavizzo-Mourey R. Anti-aging therapy: an overview. Hosp Pract 2001;36:43–56.

359. Walker NI. Ultrastructure of the rat pancreas after experimental duct ligation. I. The role of apoptosis and intraepithelial macrophages in acinar cell deletion. Am J Pathol 1987;126:439–451.

360. Walker NI, Gobé GC. Cell death and cell proliferation during atrophy of the rat parotid gland induced by duct obstruction. J Pathol 1987;153:333–344.

361. Wang E. Age-dependent atrophy and microgravity travel: what do they have in common? FASEB J 1999;13 Suppl: S167–S174.

362. Weber G. Pathology of glucose-6-phosphate metabolism. A study in enzyme pathology. Rev Can Biol 1959;18:245–282.

363. Weindruch R. Caloric restriction and aging. Sci Am 1996; 274:46–52.

364. Weindruch RH, Walford RL. Aging and functions of the RES. In: Cohen N, Sigel MM (eds). The reticulo-endothelial system: a comprehensive treatise, vol. 3. New York: Plenum Press, 1982, pp. 713–748.

365. Weindruch R, Walford RL. The retardation of aging and disease by dietary restriction. Springfield: Charles C Thomas, 1988.

366. Weindruch R, Walford RL, Fligiel S, Guthrie D. The retardation of aging in mice by dietary restriction: longevity, cancer, immunity and lifetime energy intake. J Nutrition 1986; 116:641–654.

367. Wikelski M, Thom C. Marine iguanas shrink to survive El Niño. Nature 2000;403:37–38.

368. Williamson JR. Adipose tissue. Morphological changes associated with lipid mobilization. J Cell Biol 1964;20:57–74.

369. Winick M (ed). Hunger disease. New York: John Wiley & Sons, 1979.

370. Wyllie AH, Kerr JFR, Currie AR. Cell death: the significance of apoptosis. Int Rev Cytol 1980;68:251–306.

371. Yu BP. Recent advances in dietary restriction and aging. In: Rothstein M (ed). Review of biological research in aging, vol. 2. New York: Alan R. Liss, Inc., 1985, pp. 435–443.

372. Zoumbos NC, Gascón P, Djeu JY, Trost SR, Young NS. Circulating activated suppressor T lymphocytes in aplastic anemia. N Engl J Med 1985;312:257–265.

Modulation, Metaplasia

373. Aloe L, Levi-Montalcini R. Nerve growth factor-induced transformation of immature chromaffin cells in vivo into sympathetic neurons: effect of antiserum to nerve growth factor. Proc Natl Acad Sci USA 1979;76:1246–1250.

374. Beresford WA. Transdifferentiation and the vascular wall. In: Zilla P, Greisler HP (eds). Tissue engineering of prosthetic vascular grafts. Georgetown, TX: RG Landes, 1998, pp. 399–412.

375. Bhowmick NA, Ghiassi M, Bakin A, et al. Transforming growth factor-β1 mediates epithelial to mesenchymal transdifferentiation through a RhoA-dependent mechanism. Mol Biol Cell 2001;12:27–36.

376. Bjornson CRR, Rietze RL, Reynolds BA, Magli MC, Vescovi AL. Turning brain into blood: a hematopoietic fate adopted by adult neural stem cells in vivo. Science 1999;283: 534–537.

377. Bonneton C, Sibarita JB, Thiery JP. Relationship between cell migration and cell cycle during the initiation of epithelial to fibrobalstoid transition. Cell Motil Cytoskeleton 1999;43: 288–295.

378. Bordi C, Ravazzola M. Endocrine cells in the intestinal metaplasia of gastric mucosa. Am J Pathol 1979;96:391–398.

379. Bosco L, Venturini G, Willems D. In vitro lens transdifferentiation of Xenopus laevis outer cornea induced by fibroblast growth factor (FGF). Development 1997;124:421–428.

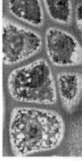

380. Bouillaud F, Ricquier D, Mory G, Thibault J. Increased level of mRNA for the uncoupling protein in brown adipose tissue of rats during thermogenesis induced by cold exposure or norepinephrine infusion. J Biol Chem 1984;259:11583–11586.

381. Campbell GR, Campbell JH. Smooth muscle phenotypic changes in arterial wall homeostasis: implications for the pathogenesis of atherosclerosis. Exp Mol Pathol 1985;42:139–162.

382. Cantin M, Araujo-Nascimento MD, Benchimol S, Desormeaux Y. Metaplasia of smooth muscle cells into juxtaglomerular cells in the juxtaglomerular apparatus, arteries, and arterioles of the ischemic (endocrine) kidney. Am J Pathol 1977;87:581–602.

383. Chopra DP. Squamous metaplasia in organ cultures of vitamin A-deficient hamster trachea: cytokinetic and ultrastructural alterations. J Natl Cancer Inst 1982;69:895–905.

384. Danto SI, Shannon JM, Borok Z, Zabski SM, Crandall ED. Reversible transdifferentiation of alveolar epithelial cells. Am J Respir Cell Mol Biol 1995;12:497–502.

385. Daoud RA, Watkins MJ, Brown G, Carr N. Mature bone metaplasia in abdominal wall scar. Postgrad Med J 1999;75:226–227.

386. DiBerardino MA, Hoffner NJ, Etkin LD. Activation of dormant genes in specialized cells. Science 1984;224:946–952.

387. Fell HB, Mellanby E. Metaplasia produced in cultures of chick ectoderm by high vitamin A. J Physiol 1953;119:470–488.

388. Ferber S. Can we create new organs from our own tissues? Isr Med Assoc J 2000;2(Suppl):32–36.

389. Grimaldi PA, Teboul L, Inadera H, Gaillard D, Amri EZ. Transdifferentiation of myoblasts to adipoblasts: triggering effects of fatty acids and thiazolidinediones. Prostaglandins, Leukotrienes and Essential Fatty Acids 1997;57:71–75.

390. Hamilton SR. Pathogenesis of columnar cell-lined (Barrett's) esophagus. In: Spechler SJ, Goyal RK (eds). Barrett's esophagus: pathophysiology, diagnosis and management. New York: Elsevier, 1985, pp. 29–37.

391. Harkema JR, Barr EB, Hotchkiss JA. Responses of rat nasal epithelium to short-and long-term exposures of ozone: image analysis of epithelial injury, adaptation and repair. Microsc Res Tech 1997;36:276–286.

392. Hay ED, Zuk A. Transformations between epithelium and mesenchyme: normal, pathological, and experimentally induced. Am J Kidney Dis 1995;26:678–690.

393. Heermeier K, Strauss PG, Erfle V, Schmidt J. Adipose differentiation of cartilage in vitro. Differentiation 1994;56:45–53.

394. Hilding A. Experimental surgery of the nose and sinuses. I. Changes in the morphology of the epithelium following variations in ventilation. Arch Otolaryngol 1932;15:9–18.

395. Hong WK, Endicott J, Itri LM, et al. 13-cis-retinoic acid in the treatment of oral leukoplakia. N Engl J Med 1986;315:1501–1505.

396. Itoh Y, Eguchi G. In vitro analysis of cellular metaplasia from pigmented epithelial cells to lens phenotypes: a unique model system for studying cellular and molecular mechanisms of "transdifferentiation." Dev Biol 1986;115:353–362.

397. Jetten AM, Brody AR, Deas MA, et al. Retinoic acid and substratum regulate the differentiation of rabbit tracheal epithelial cells into squamous and secretory phenotype. Morphological and biochemical characterization. Lab Invest 1987;56:654–664.

398. Kim SW, Charter RA, Chai CJ, Kim SK, Kim ES. Serum alkaline phosphatase and inorganic phosphorus values in spinal cord injury patients with heterotopic ossification. Paraplegia 1990;28:441–447.

399. Konishi N, Ward JM, Waalkes MP. Pancreatic hepatocytes in Fischer and Wistar rats induced by repeated injections of cadmium chloride. Toxicol App Pharmacol 1990;104:149–156.

400. Lean MEJ, James WPT, Jennings G, Trayhurn P. Brown adipose tissue in patients with phaeochromocytoma. Int J Obesity 1986;10:219–227.

401. Lombardi T, Montesano R, Furie MB, Silverstein SC, Orci L. Endothelial diaphragmed fenestrae: In vitro modulation by phorbol myristate acetate. J Cell Biol 1986;102:1965–1970.

402. Lombardi T, Montesano R, Furie MB, Silverstein SC, Orci L. In vitro modulation of endothelial fenestrae: opposing effects of retinoic acid and transforming growth factor β. J Cell Sci 1988;91:313–318.

403. Lugo M, Petersen RO, Elfenbein IB, Stein BS, Duker NJ. Nephrogenic metaplasia of the ureter. Am J Clin Pathol 1983;80:92–97.

404. Lugo M, Putong PB. Metaplasia. An overview. Arch Pathol Lab Med 1984;108:185–189.

405. Ma J, De Boer WGRM, Nayman J. Intestinal mucinous substances in gastric intestinal metaplasia and carcinoma studied by immunofluorescence. Cancer 1982;49:1664–1667.

406. Majack RA, Bornstein P. Heparin regulates the collagen phenotype of vascular smooth muscle cells: Induced synthesis of an M_r 60,000 collagen. J Cell Biol 1985;100:613–619.

407. Majno G. Chronic Inflammation. Links with angiogenesis and wound healing. Am J Pathol 1998;153:1035–1039.

408. Makino T, Usuda N, Rao S, Reddy JK, Scarpelli DG. Transdifferentiation of ductular cells into hepatocytes in regenerating hamster pancreas. Lab Invest 1990;62:552–561.

409. McCarthy PL, Shklar G. Diseases of the oral mucosa, 2nd ed. Philadelphia: Lea & Febiger, 1980.

410. McDevitt DS. Transdifferentiation in animals. A model for differentiation control. Dev Biol (NY 1985) 1989;6:149–173.

411. McGuire PG, Orkin RW. Isolation of rat aortic endothelial cells by primary explant techniques and their phenotypic modulation by defined substrata. Lab Invest 1987;57:94–105.

412. Melicow MM. Hibernating fat and pheochromocytoma. Arch Pathol 1957;63:367–372.

413. Merk FB, Warhol MJ, Kwan PW-L, et al. Multiple phenotypes of prostatic glandular cells in castrated dogs after individual or combined treatment with androgen and estrogen. Morphometric, ultrastructural, and cytochemical distinctions. Lab Invest 1986;54:442–456.

414. Miettinen PJ, Ebner R, Lopez AR, Derynck R. TGF-β induced transdifferentiation of mammary epithelial cells to mesenchymal cells: involvement of type I receptors. J Cell Biol 1994;127:2021–2036.

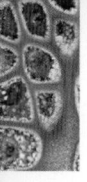
415. Montesano R, Orci L, Vassalli P. In vitro rapid organization of endothelial cells into capillary-like networks is promoted by collagen matrices. J Cell Biol 1983;97:1648–1652.

416. Montesano R, Orci L, Vassalli P. Human endothelial cell cultures: phenotypic modulation by leukocyte interleukins. J Cell Physiol 1985;122:424–434.

417. Ng Y-Y, Huang T-P, Yang W-C, et al. Tubular epithelial-myofibroblast transdifferentiation in progressive tubulointerstitial fibrosis in 5/6 nephrectomized rats. Kidney Int 1998;54:864–876.

418. Nomura S, Kaminishi M, Sugiyama K, Oohara T, Esumi H. Clonal analysis of isolated intestinal metaplastic glands of stomach using X linked polymorphism. Gut 1998;42: 663–668.

418a. Ogawa M, Ishikawa T, Ohta H. Transdifferentiation of endocrine chromaffin cells into neuronal cells. Curr Top Dev Biol 1986;20:99–110.

419. Opas M, Dziak E. Direct transdifferentiation in the vertebrate retina. Int J Dev Biol 1998;42:199–208.

420. Petersen BE, Bowen WC, Patrene KD, et al. Bone marrow as a potential source of hepatic oval cells. Science 1999;284: 1168–1170.

421. Rao MS, Reddy JK. Hepatic transdifferentiation in the pancreas. Semin Cell Biol 1995;6:151–156.

422. Ricquier D, Mory G, Bouillaud F, Combes-George M, Thibault J. Factors controlling brown adipose tissue development. Reprod Nutr Dev 1985;25:175–181.

423. Ricquier D, Mory G, Nechad M, Combes-George M, Thibault J. Development and activation of brown fat in rats with pheochromocytoma PC 12 tumors. Am J Physiol 1983; 245:C172–C177.

424. Salley JJ. Bryson WF. Vitamin A deficiency in the hamster. J Dent Res 1957;36:935–944.

425. Shen C-N, Slack JMW, Tosh D. Molecular basis of transdifferentiation of pancreas to liver. Nat Cell Biol 2000;2: 879–887.

426. Schor AM, Schor SL, Arciniegas E. Phenotypic diversity and lineage relationships in vascular endothelial cells. In: Potten CS (ed). Stem cells. London: Academic Press, 1997, pp. 119–146.

427. Shklar G. Oral leukoplakia. N Engl J Med 1986;315: 1544–1546.

428. Strutz F, Müller GA, Neilson EG. Transdifferentiation: a new angle on renal fibrosis. Exp Nephrol 1996;4:267–270.

429. Suzuki T, Kimura M, Asano M, Fujigaki Y, Hishida A. Role of atrophic tubules in development of interstitial fibrosis in microembolism-induced renal failure in rat. Am J Pathol 2001;158:75–85.

430. Wolbach SB, Howe PR. Vitamin A deficiency in the guinea-pig. Arch Pathol 1928;5:239–253.

431. Yoshida T, Umekawa T, Wakabayashi Y, Sakane N, Kondo M. Mechanism of anti-obesity action of benidipine hydrochloride in mice. Int J Obes 1994;18:776–779.

432. Zuk A, Matlin KS, Hay ED. Type I collagen gel induces Madin-Darby canine kidney cells to become fusiform in shape and lose apical-basal polarity. J Cell Biol 1989;108: 903–919.

Cell Activation and Priming

433. Aitken A. The biochemical mechanism of action of phorbol esters. In: Evans FJ (ed). Naturally occurring phorbol esters. Boca Raton: CRC Press, Inc., 1986, pp. 271–288.

434. Bentley R, Trimen H. Medicinal plants, vol. 4. London: Churchill, 1880.

435. Chiu R, Imagawa M, Imbra RJ, Bockoven JR, Karin M. Multiple cis- and trans-acting elements mediate the transcriptional response to phorbol esters. Nature 1987;329: 648–651.

436. Drevets WC, Videen TO, Price JL, et al. A functional anatomical study of unipolar depression. J Neurosci 1992;12: 3628–3641.

437. Metchnikoff E. L'immunité dans les maladies infectieuses. Paris: Masson & Co., 1901.

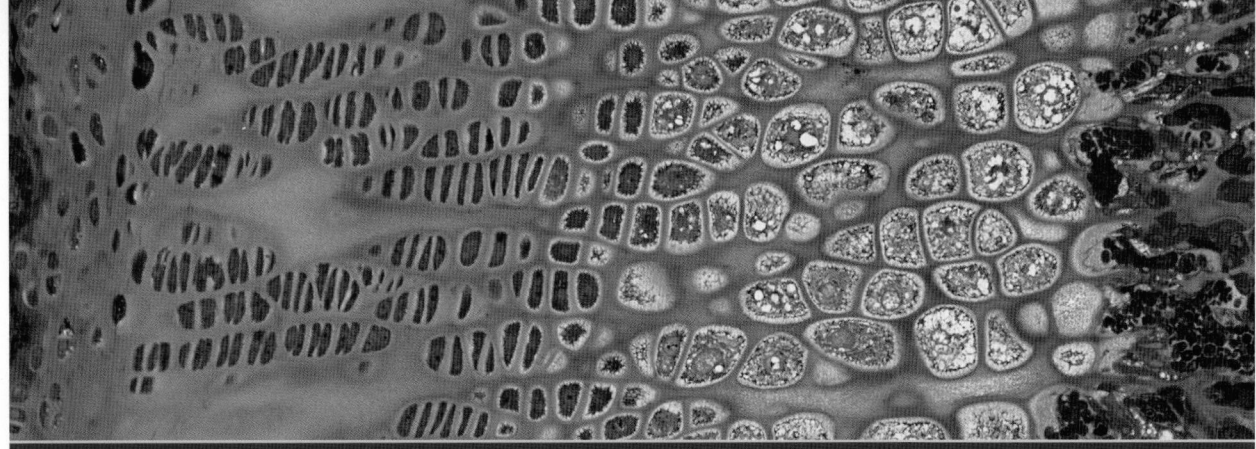

SYMPTOMS OF CELLULAR DISEASE: INTRACELLULAR ACCUMULATIONS

Up to this point we have discussed cellular adaptations such as increases or decreases in cell size or number. Now we can proceed to examine true symptoms of cellular disease. To begin, we can assume that something is wrong with a cell if it contains unusual intracellular granules or droplets (vacuoles). The hoarded material may be derived from the cell's own metabolism, from the extracellular space (such as spilled blood), or from the outer environment (such as dust). Whatever its nature, this material always carries a message, which may be good, bad, or indifferent regarding the health of the cell and of the body as a whole.

It is convenient to classify abnormal intracellular content by its chemical nature. If we exclude rare congenital storage diseases, in which special macromolecules are hoarded (p. 148), there are five main groups:

- Water and electrolytes
- Lipids
- Carbohydrates
- Proteins
- A motley group of "pigments"

Accumulation of Fluid

Excess fluid can appear in the cell as discrete droplets (*vacuoles*) or as diffuse waterlogging of the entire cell, which results in cellular swelling, sometimes called **hydropic swelling.**

Vacuoles

Droplets of fluid in cells are very common; under the microscope they appear as empty little spheres, hence their name (*vacu-olus* is Latin for "empty-small"). In plant cells, but not in animal cells, a large vacuole called a **tonoplast** is a normal and important

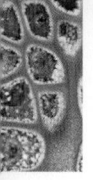

FIGURE 3.1 Mechanisms that lead to the formation of vacuoles.

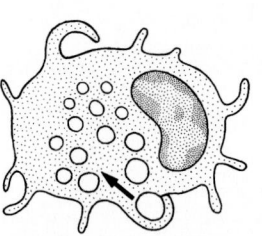 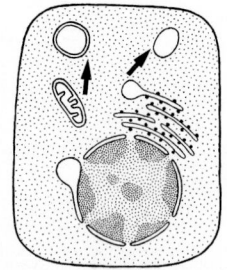 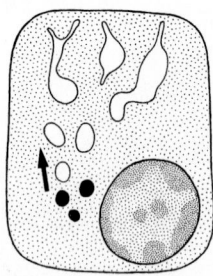

1   By pinocytosis

2   From mitochondria or endoplasmic reticulum

3   From lysosomes

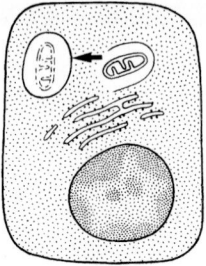 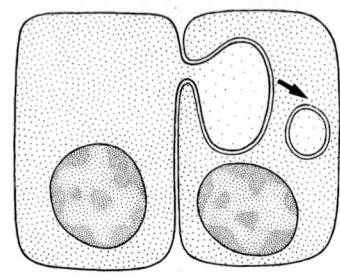 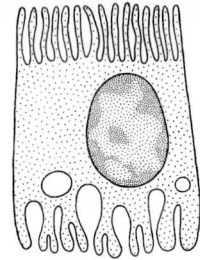

4   By (auto)phagocytosis

5   By herniation

6   By cell membrane infolding

cellular organelle that contributes to the cell's turgor (9, 29). If the tonoplasts of a leaf collapse, the whole leaf collapses; this is why plants wilt and animals do not—we have no tonoplasts.

Simple as they may look, vacuoles can form in many ways: by pinocytosis, by phagocytosis, by swelling of one organelle or another, and by herniation—plus a bizarre type of extracellular vacuole specific to the kidney tubules. One cell may contain vacuoles of different kinds (Figure 3.1).

Vacuoles due to Pinocytosis

Some cells drink more than others. The champions are the activated macrophages, which pinocytize so frantically that every hour they can take in one quarter of their volume of fluid (12, 32). Of course, most of the fluid taken in is promptly returned to the outside. Vacuoles generated in this manner are of little or no pathologic significance, except that they point to heavy drinking. Now, *if the extracellular medium happens to contain a soluble molecule that the macrophages cannot digest, such as sucrose, the macrophage can still expel the fluid—but not the sucrose, which is retained.* If this is happening *in vitro,* the overloaded macrophage can be put out of its misery by adding the appropriate enzyme to the medium (Figure 3.2) (13).

Osmotic nephrosis. There is an *in vivo* counterpart to this sucrose indigestion. In the 1940s it was noticed

that patients who had been given intravenous injections of hypertonic sucrose solutions (an attempt to promote diuresis) developed extensive vacuolization of the renal convoluted tubules (27). The epithelium had reabsorbed tubular fluid loaded with sucrose. The resulting vacuoles correspond to watery phagosomes, and the tubular change that follows is known as *sucrose nephrosis* or *osmotic nephrosis* (22, 24, 34).

Vacuoles due to Organelle Swelling

Three organelles are prone to pathologic swelling: *the mitochondria, the endoplasmic reticulum, and the lysosomes.* The mechanisms are not understood. Even with the electron microscope it can be difficult to find out how a vacuole developed; however, if a vacuole contains acid phosphatase, it can be assumed to derive from a lysosome.

In suffering cells, *mitochondria are apt to swell to the point of appearing like vacuoles;* this change is extremely common and extremely fast (minutes), and almost unfailingly develops as an artefact in tissue samples if fixation is not immediate, because cells have time to suffer from asphyxia or from slow poisoning by the fixative. Mitochondrial swelling is therefore a curse for the electron microscopist; it is not always easy to decide whether it represents artefact or disease.

Other vacuoles represent expanded cisternae of the endoplasmic reticulum (4, 5). For reasons unknown, the

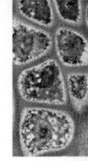

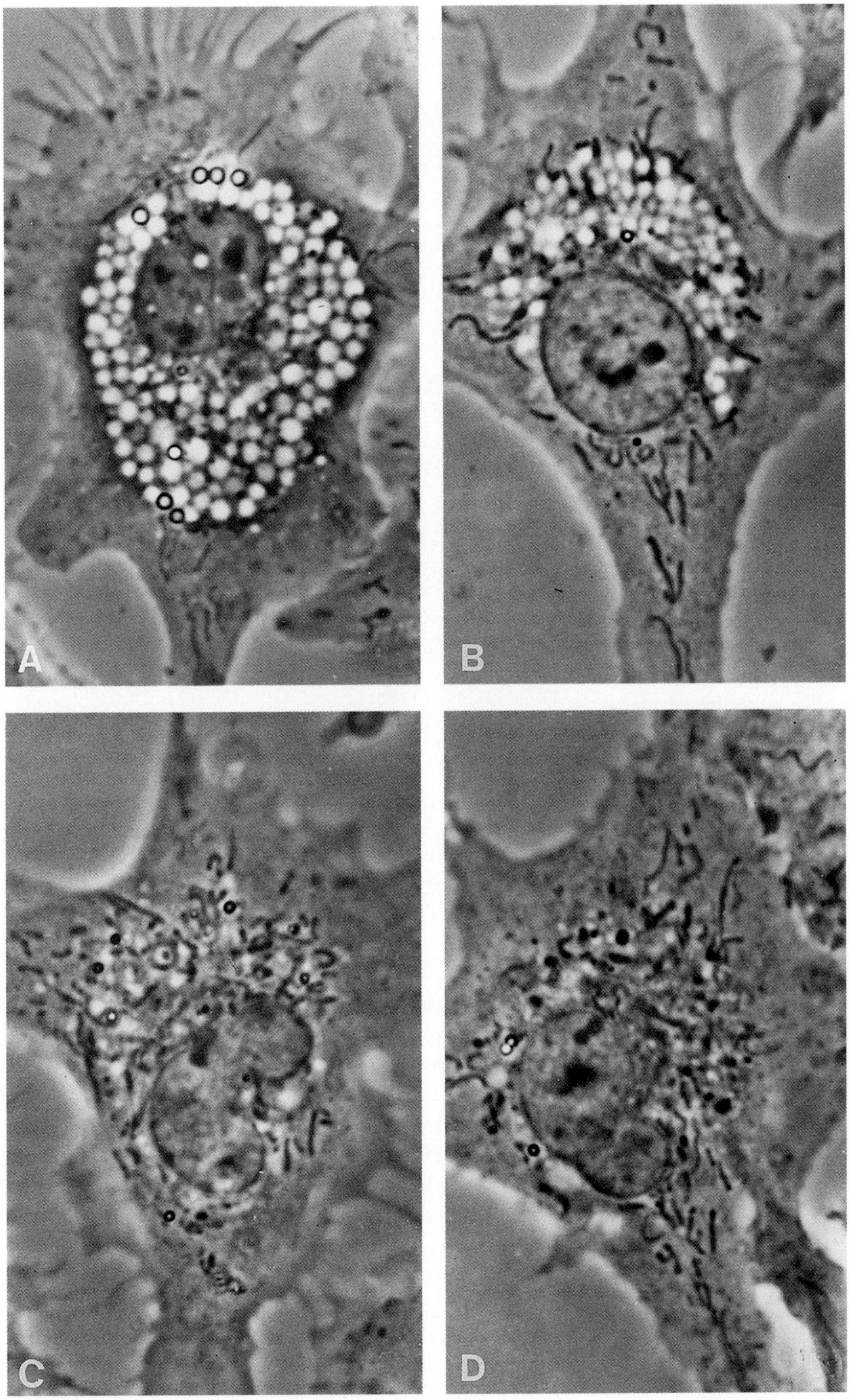

FIGURE 3.2 Cellular indigestion and its treatment. **A:** Vacuolization of a mouse macrophage *in vitro* after 24-hour exposure to an undigestible sugar (sucrose). **B:** 30 minutes after the addition of invertase. **C:** 75 minutes after invertase. **D:** 120 minutes after invertase. The vacuoles disappear, leaving a residue of small dense granules. (2,500x) (Reproduced from the **Journal of Experimental Medicine,** 1969;129:201–225 by copyright permission of the Rockefeller University Press [13].)

perinuclear cisterna is especially prone to swell; and when it does so, this is a reliable sign of cellular distress.

Genesis of vacuoles from cisternae of the endoplasmic reticulum was proven by a technical tour de force by a determined Australian pathologist, Ian Buckley (5). Although single cisternae should not be visible by light microscopy, Buckley (working in the laboratory of Keith Porter) managed to see them in very thin expansions of cells grown *in vitro,* the same biological model that had

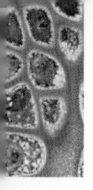

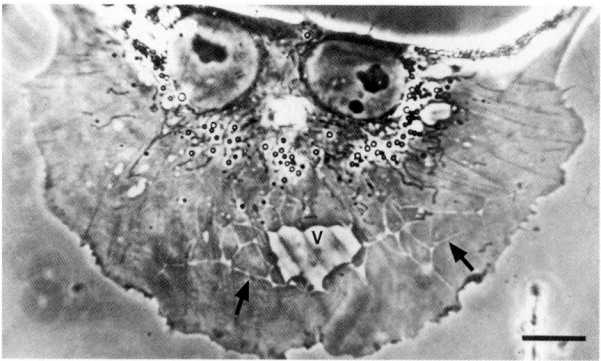

FIGURE 3.3   Development of vacuoles from the endoplasmic reticulum. This live, cultured chick embryo cell contains a reticular network (**arrows**) that appears white by phase contrast microscopy: the endoplasmic reticulum. **V:** vacuole arising within it. As seen *in vivo* the size and shape of such ER vacuoles continue to change. **Bar** = 10 μm. (Reproduced with permission from [4].)

allowed Porter to discover the endoplasmic reticulum (p. 144). In asphyxiated fibroblasts, Buckley saw swellings appear here and there in the endoplasmic reticulum, running up and down a cisterna like beads on a string, as documented by an excellent movie (Figure 3.3).

The third organelle that is prone to swell is the lysosome. The primal studies are due again to Ian Buckley (6), who examined living cultured cells that either were undergoing spontaneous aging or were mildly injured by cooling to 25°C. The lysosomes swelled into vacuoles; then their membranes began to emit and retract thin tubular extensions, which could also anastomose and form a network that was very difficult to distinguish from the endoplasmic reticulum network just described. The tentacles of the swollen lysosomes seemed to be probing the cytoplasm for material to digest. If this optimistic interpretation is correct, we would have an instance of "helpful" vacuoles.

Vacuoles that Represent Cellular Herniae

This strange microscopic accident happens when a cell gives rise to a process that pokes into a neighboring cell (18) (Figure 3.4). Dictionaries define hernia as *the protrusion of a bodily structure through the wall that normally contains it.* It must be understood that the retaining wall of a hernia is weakened but not broken, so that the herniating structure becomes contained in a thin sac called a *hernia sac.*

Most commonly cellular herniation occurs between contracting smooth muscle cells. As the cell shortens, its surface gives rise to bulges that can be firm enough

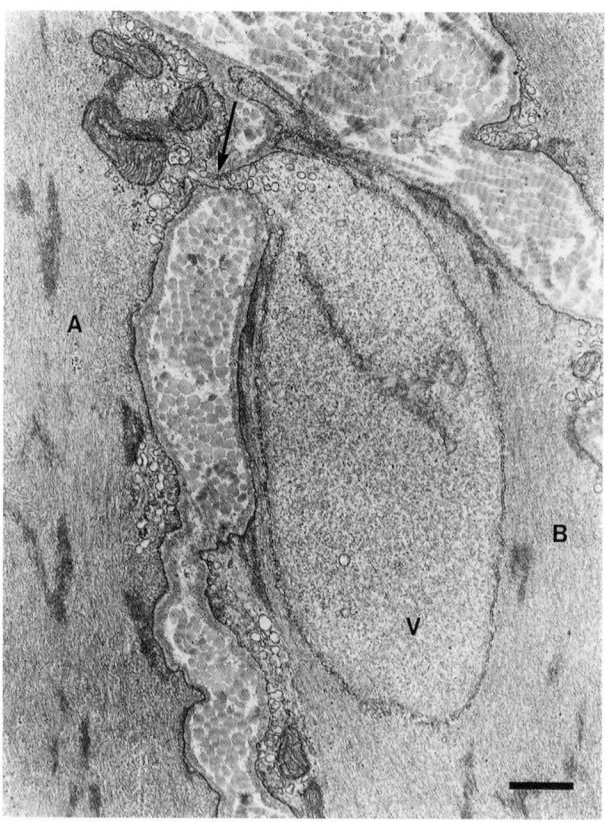

FIGURE 3.4   Special type of vacuole (**v**) caused by herniation of one smooth muscle cell into another in the wall of a contracting artery. Cell **A** is herniating into its neighbor **B**. The stalk of the hernia is indicated by the **arrow. Bar** = 0.5 μm. (Reproduced with permission from [18], © American Society for Investigative Pathology.)

to push their way into the neighbor cell, usually at points of close contact where the basement membrane is absent. During relaxation the bulges can retract, but some break off and remain inside the "host" cell, where they tend to swell and become vacuoles. We call these bizarre structures **cell-to-cell herniae.** They are interesting because, in the media of arteries, they tell us that an intense contraction (*spasm*) has occurred (18) and because, in a more general way, they mean that a smooth muscle cell can be damaged in the course of its physiologic function. The hallmark of these special vacuoles, as shown by electron microscopy, is that they are limited by two cell membranes: the inner from the herniating cell and the outer (hernia sac) from the host cell.

Similar herniae can occur when a medial smooth muscle cell pokes into an endothelial cell (myoendothelial herniae) (33) or when a myocardial cell protrudes into its neighbor across the intercalated disc. Why the cell-to-cell herniae tend to swell is not clear. The term **extracellular vacuoles** sounds like a contradiction, but in renal convoluted tubules the following can happen, thanks to the unique arrangement of the basal part of the cells. Deep infoldings of the basal cell membrane create a succession of thin cytoplasmic sheets and virtual extracellular spaces. If the latter swell, the fluid is anatomically outside the cell wall, but with the light microscope it appears as a basal vacuole (*subbasilar vacuolation*) (Figure 3.1) (3). This lesion was once thought to be specific for low-plasma potassium (hypokalemia), such as may occur with chronic diarrhea or vomiting; actually it has a variety of causes that presumably affect the function of the basilar cell membrane. Even an overload of intravenous saline can produce it (26).

Vacuoles in the Central Nervous System

Myriads of vacuoles in the gray matter are the hallmark of **spongiform encephalopathy** (seen in victims of prion diseases [22a]) and of **vacuolar myelopathy** (seen in the white matter of the spinal cord in victims of AIDS [2]). The microscopic picture is striking; it is just beginning to be deciphered (p. 165).

Cellular Swelling

Besides suffering from fluid-filled vacuoles, cells can also become waterlogged as a whole, as a result of an osmotic disturbance (23). In this condition they are enlarged but not hypertrophic. Typically, this disturbance occurs in an acute setting, in a matter of minutes and hours. There is also a chronic form of osmotic swelling that occurs in diabetes, over weeks, months, and years. Whether chronically swollen cells may adapt by becoming hypertrophic is not known.

Acute Cellular Swelling

Some cells rapidly become bloated—**hydropic** is the traditional term—if the ionic pumps in the cell membrane fail (23). This happens when the cell's energy supplies are cut off, either by failure of the blood supply or by a metabolic poison. Sodium ions seep in, taking water with them; the cell swells. We will return to this topic in discussing cellular injury (p. 203).

Acute cellular swelling is an indication of severe cellular distress, but it may become the cause of further problems by the very fact that it takes up space and may therefore impair blood flow. This is especially critical in the brain, where there is no room for expansion. The impairment of blood flow by acute cellular swelling was first demonstrated in rat liver by an ingenious experiment. The liver was acutely poisoned by means of carbon tetrachloride; four hours later it had become so swollen that India ink

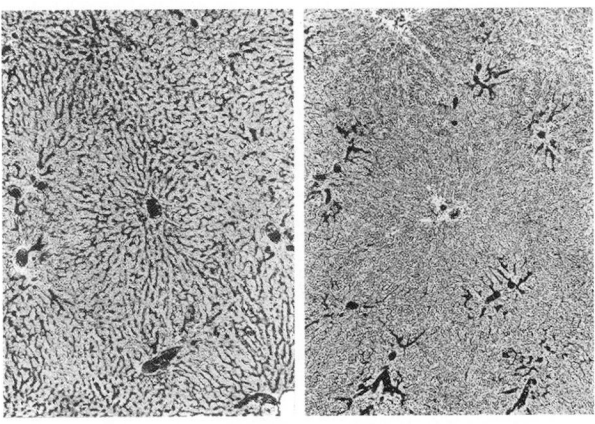

FIGURE 3.5   Impaired circulation in the liver lobule due to cellular swelling. India ink was injected into the portal circulation just prior to sacrifice. *Left:* Normal rat liver; the sinusoids are completely filled with India ink. *Right:* 2 hours after carbon tetrachloride injection (0.2 ml/100 g) the India ink is present at the periphery of the lobule but has difficulty in penetrating toward the central vein. (~35x) (Reproduced with permission from [15].)

injected into the portal blood could not flow through the lobules (Figure 3.5) (15). A similar circulatory problem arises if the liver cells are bloated with fat (p. 84).

Another example of flow impaired by swollen cells is provided by the toxemia of pregnancy, or **eclampsia,** a serious complication of pregnancy characterized by hypertension, proteinuria, and edema. In this case the endothelial cells of the glomeruli swell and reduce blood flow through the kidney (ischemia), causing hypertension.

> Renal ischemia causes hypertension because it stimulates the juxtaglomerular cells to secrete more renin, which acts on angiotensinogen to produce angiotensin I, which is converted in the lung to the potent vasoconstrictor angiotensin II. The plasma of these patients contains material that is toxic for cultured endothelial cells (30), probably released by the placenta during bouts of ischemia and reperfusion (28).

Chronic Cellular Swelling: A Misdeed of Sugars

Chronic cellular swelling was discovered by studying the complications of diabetes, especially the cataract and the nerve changes (neuropathies). Despite many open ends, the basic mechanism is clear. Some types of cells, such as those of the lens and the Schwann cells of nerve sheaths, allow glucose to penetrate the cell membrane independent of insulin control (by contrast with

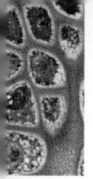

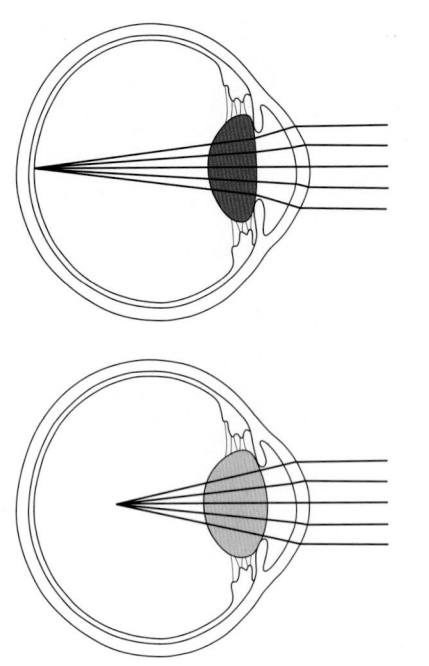

FIGURE 3.6   Osmotic swelling of the lens causing sudden myopia: this may be the first manifestation of diabetes.

fat and muscle cells, in which the entry of glucose is regulated by insulin). This means that if the blood glucose rises, the cells become overloaded with glucose. Then the trouble begins: some of the excess glucose is reduced to sorbitol by the enzyme aldose reductase, and some of the sorbitol is converted to fructose. Both sorbitol and fructose are retained within the cell, and being osmotically active, they cause the cell to swell. *The lens is especially vulnerable because its ability to metabolize glucose is very low* (35). As the lens swells, its converging power increases, and the patient suddenly becomes short-sighted: it is not uncommon for diabetes to manifest itself for the first time in this manner (Figure 3.6).

Eventually the swollen cells develop leaky plasma membranes and die; for the lens, this means developing a cataract (p. 207). The crowning proof of this mechanism is that, in hyperglycemic animals, inhibitors of aldose reductase prevent the cataract (20).

As related to experimental cataracts the sorbitol mechanism seems to fit like a glove, but when applied to other tissues and to human diabetes the fit is not as tight (7, 8, 11, 14, 21). In diabetic neuropathies, for example, sorbitol in degenerated nerves is not always increased. The preventive or curative effect of aldose reductase (19) has many exceptions, and besides, in humans both cataract and neuropathies develop so slowly that the effects of therapy are difficult to evaluate. Furthermore, another

metabolic mechanism seems to intervene, namely a drop in myo-inositol. This is a six-carbon cyclic hexanol sterically similar to glucose that is ubiquitous in animal and plant cells, often in millimolar concentrations—yet its functions are not well understood (16). Cells obtain it from nutritional sources and by synthesis. Somehow, in hyperglycemia the intracellular myo-inositol drops; this leads to metabolic disturbances in the membrane phospholipids and thereby to defects in membrane function leading to cell death. Alas, the neat sorbitol-related cell swelling has grown into a gigantic puzzle—but one that promises to be important for understanding some of the complications of diabetes.

Cellular shrinkage may also occur. Whereas tardigrades and other small creatures can survive the loss of virtually all their water, most animal cells cannot afford to lose more than roughly 50 percent (10). Possible causes of cell death by dehydration include damage to the plasma membrane, to the cytoplasmic proteins, to the cytoskeleton, and even to the microtrabecular lattice (MTL; p. 162) (10, 17). To our knowledge, this is the only suggested role for the MTL in cellular pathology. Dehydration of the intestinal mucosa for one minute with a hypertonic solution produces severe changes (Figure 3.7) (25), and dehydration of the body as a whole leads to damage to the renal medulla (31), where—interestingly—the interstitium is normally hypertonic. This topic needs further study.

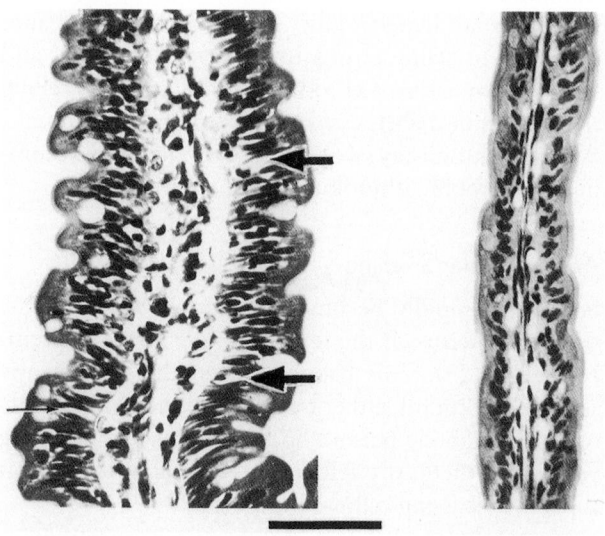

FIGURE 3.7   Effect of dehydration on the intestinal mucosa. *Left:* Control; normal villus incubated for 1 minute with 150 mM saline solution. Some dilatation of intercellular spaces (**arrows**) appears in the epithelium. *Right:* Villus of the same animal after 1-minute exposure to 780 mOsm/kg solution (a 50 percent solution of the hypertonic radiographic contrast medium Hypaque). **Bar** = 50 μm. (Reproduced with permission from [25], © American Society for Investigative Pathology.)

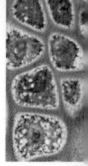

Accumulation of Lipids

Lipid droplets are part of life, but when they are of the wrong kind in the wrong place or in the wrong amount, they mean cellular disease. Microscopically they can be identified by means of lipid-soluble stains. The lipids that can be found in abnormal deposits belong, understandably, to the types of lipid normally found in the body (Figure 3.8). The most common are:

- **Triglycerides** (the main lipids of fat cells, also called **triacylglycerols**) are such frequent offenders in liver cells that this cellular storage has earned its own special name, **steatosis** (from the Greek *stéar,* "fat").
- **Fatty acids,** dangerous guests for the cells that hoard them.
- **Cholesterol** and its esters are chemically ubiquitous, but abnormal deposits occur preferentially in three cell types: macrophages, arterial endothelium and arterial smooth muscle cells. The context most common is an atherosclerotic artery (p. 674).
- **Phospholipids,** the ubiquitous components of cell membranes, tend to form abnormal membranous structures called **myelin figures,** either within the cells or in the tissue spaces (p. 223).
- **Lipofuscin,** a special category of heavily oxidized, indigestible, brownish, leftover intracellular lipids, will be considered among the pigments (p. 102).

A technical parenthesis: how are lipids identified? This is not a small problem, because lipids are microscopically elusive, compared with the thousands of different proteins that can be identified by antibody methods. Triglycerides (triacylglycerols) and cholesteryl esters, collectively called **neutral fats,** are lost forever during paraffin embedding, which requires soaking the tissues in fat solvents (ethyl alcohol, xylene). Therefore, to search for neutral fats, unprocessed tissue must be cut in the frozen state (with or without previous fixation) using a special type of microtome; the sections are then treated with a fat stain. Fat stains are simply dyes that are indiscriminately soluble in neutral fats. Thus, a stained droplet tells us, "This is triglyceride, cholesteryl ester, or a mixture of both," which enables us to rule out proteins and water-soluble materials; but we still do not know which type of neutral fat is present. *There are no specific stains for triglycerides,* so the best approach is to rule out cholesterol ester by study in polarized light. If the droplet is birefringent—that is, it produces the typical "maltese cross"—it should contain cholesteryl ester. In highly specialized laboratories the lipid droplet can be diagnosed by studying its melting point on a heating stage (102). However, remember that **lipids tend to dissolve into each other;** therefore, in practice, **all lipid droplets are likely to contain a mixture of lipids.** Definitive identification must rest on fractionation and chemical analysis. This means that a microscopic diagnosis of "fat droplet," strictly speaking, is always circumstantial. On paraffin sections, neutral fat cannot be diagnosed at all, because the lipid has disappeared altogether, leaving a hole. The meaning of this hole can only be a guess based on cell type, circumstances, size and number of droplets, and personal experience. Phospholipids are not extracted by histological processing, in part because they are bound to cell proteins as structural components of all membranes.

In tissues processed for electron microscopy and fixed with osmium tetroxide, small droplets of neutral fats are usually preserved as a homogeneous mass (Figure 3.9); the diagnosis of lipid is again circumstantial.

LIVER CELL   LIVER CELL   MACROPHAGE   INJURED CELL

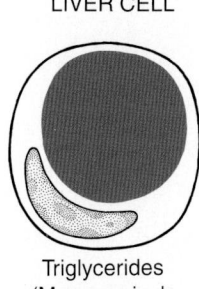 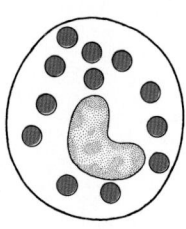 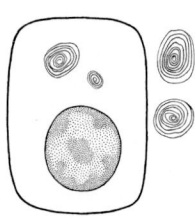

Triglycerides (Macrovesicular Steatosis)   Triglycerides + (?) Fatty Acids (Microvesicular Steatosis)   Cholesteryl esters   Phospholipids ("myelin figures")

FIGURE 3.8   Common types of abnormal lipid deposits. **Triglycerides:** droplets, usually single, not bound by a membrane. Triglycerides **mixed with? toxic fatty acids** in the liver: small uniform droplets that do not fuse. **Cholesteryl esters** in macrophages: small, uniform droplets, mainly intralysosomal. **Phospholipids:** irregular **myelin figures,** intra- and extracellular.

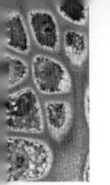

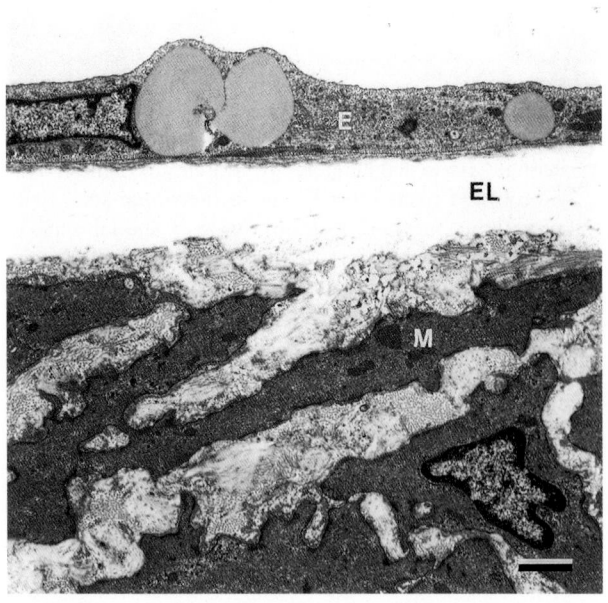

FIGURE 3.9   Droplets of lipid (cholesteryl esters) in the aortic endothelium of a hypercholesterolemic rat. **E:** endothelium. **EL:** internal elastic lamina. **M:** smooth muscle cells. **Bar** = 1 μm.

Steatosis: Accumulation of Triglycerides and/or Fatty Acids

The standard definition of steatosis is "abnormal accumulation of TRIGLYCERIDES in cells other than adipocytes." We must change this to TRIGLYCERIDES AND/OR FATTY ACIDS, because histologic and biochemical studies on the liver have shown that there are (in that organ) two overlapping varieties of intracellular fat deposits, of vastly different significance: large droplets containing mainly triglycerides, and small droplets containing mainly fatty acids (Figure 3.10) (40, 68, 77). The two varieties are referred to as **macrovesicular** and **microvesicular.** For other organs undergoing lipid storage chemical analysis is still lacking, so we can only define them by the noncommittal histologic term "steatosis." What is the biological difference between the two types of lipid? Fatty acids can destroy cell membranes (p. 133); triglycerides cannot. However, *there is now a tendency to play down the innocuous behavior of triglycerides.*

> Steatosis is also called *fatty change;* this awkward name was created as a reaction against the ancient term *fatty degeneration* (still used), which implied—wrongly—that the fat was the result of some obscure "degenerative" process.

Cellular Pathology of Steatosis

Normally, droplets of triglycerides are present in a few types of cells (besides adipose tissue): especially in the liver, heart, muscle, and, strangely enough, in the chondrocytes (88). It was once believed that steatosis could occur in any type of cell, and it may be true, but as far as we know it has been chemically confirmed only in four organs: *liver, heart, muscle,* and *kidney.* It is surely no accident that these four organs can derive all or almost all their energy from the oxidation of fatty acids (42, 78, 101), the principal building blocks of triglycerides. In practice, steatosis is a significant problem

FIGURE 3.10   Contrasting two types of fatty liver. *Left:* **Macrovesicular steatosis** in an alcoholic. Liver cells distended by a single droplet of fat resemble adipocytes; the nucleus is pushed to the periphery. *Right:* **Microvesicular steatosis.** The nucleus retains its central position (see also Figure 3.23). (Needle liver specimen taken shortly after death from an HIV-positive young man, in whom liver failure developed after treatment with an antiretrovirus drug, a nucleoside analog. Courtesy of Dr. B. Portmann, King's College School of Medicine and Dentistry, London, UK.)

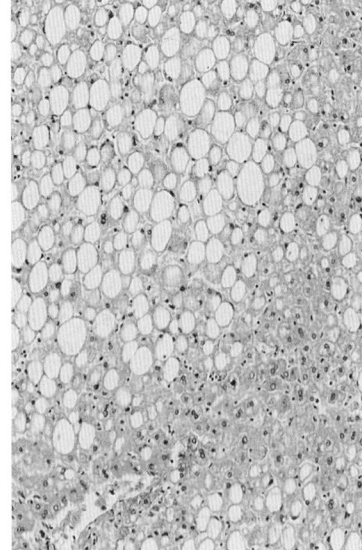

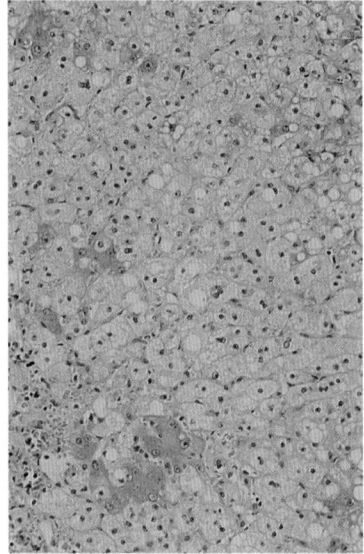

only for the liver, which is, after adipose tissue, the principal organ of triglyceride biosynthesis.

In the liver *macro*vesicular steatosis indicates that the fat in the cell tends to coalesce into a single droplet, which pushes the nucleus to one side, producing the so-called *signet ring* pattern typical of adipocytes (Figure 3.10). This change develops slowly, over weeks, months, years; its main causes—as we will see—are overfeeding, diabetes, obesity, starvation, toxic agents, and anoxia. Liver steatosis has long been in the limelight because it can be recognized with the naked eye (Figure 3.11). Furthermore, it has the singular privilege of being one of the few diseases that are eaten: *foie gras* is the sick, fatty liver of artificially overfed geese.

> This ancient delicacy has even left a trace in the Italian language: *fégato,* "liver," comes from the Latin *hepar ficatum,* "figged liver," recording the fact that Romans liked the taste of the (presumably fatty) liver of pigs kept on a fig diet.

To the naked eye, a pale liver, heart, or kidney always suggests steatosis, especially *if the organ has a yellowish hue* (paleness alone can also mean reduced blood content). It is surprising that tiny intracellular droplets of lipid can lead to such a difference in the gross color. Triglycerides are actually white; the pigmentation is due to carotenoids dissolved in the droplets (86).

> There has been a language mixup about **cirrhosis.** It was the yellowness of the liver in chronic alcoholics that first impressed Laennec in 1819, when he coined the name cirrhosis from the Greek *kirrhós,* "yellow." Posterity then decided that the fibrosis of these livers is more impressive than the color, so we now use the name cirrhosis to mean "severe fibrosis." Cirrhosis has therefore lost all connections with yellowness. Laennec would be horrified.

Advanced macrovesicular steatosis increases the size of the liver, which can double its normal weight of 1500 g. The change in liver texture can be great enough to be picked up by computer tomography (CT) scanning, ultrasonography, and magnetic resonance imaging; radiologists use the density of the spleen for comparison. At autopsy, livers with severe steatosis feel softer, and the knife that cuts them becomes greasy. The yellow color may show special patterns, because the lipid is not evenly distributed in the liver lobules. For example, in cases of severe anemia, fatty hepatocytes prevail in the central part of the lobule, which receives the least amount of oxygen: this is *anemic anoxia* (remember that, in the lobule, blood flows from the periphery to the center). The same pattern is produced if the oxygen-carrying capacity of hemoglobin is impaired (*toxic anoxia*) (Figure 3.12).

> Triglyceride storage is common around recent myocardial infarcts: we can rationalize that the bulk of the infarct consists of cells that receive no oxygen, whereas the cells at the periphery are surviving on a minimal supply (43). Severely anemic hearts sometimes show a strange patch of fine, parallel, yellowish stripes known as **thrush-breast heart** or **tabby-cat heart** (*coeur tigré* in French). Despite the zoological flurry, no study has been made to explain it, but the yellow stripes probably represent perivenular zones of poor oxygenation.

In severe steatosis, some liver cells may burst, releasing their fatty droplets, which create a small cyst (58, 59); later this will induce a chronic inflammatory reaction called a *granuloma.* The spilled fat can also find its way into the bloodstream and then to the lung, where it will become impacted (p. 668) (74).

Seen by electron microscopy, the triglyceride droplets have no limiting membrane, even though their rim may appear slightly darker (79). That fat droplets may be allowed to float naked and free in the cytosol should not surprise because, presumably, the enzymes that assemble and break down the triglycerides are also available in the cytosol. The same is true for glycogen; it makes sense that fuels such as fat or glycogen should be freely available and not barricaded behind membranes. *The lack of a limiting membrane probably explains the tendency of the droplets to coalesce,* like drops of fat floating on a broth. Mitochondria are often apposed to the droplets, which they are probably oxidizing (75, 82).

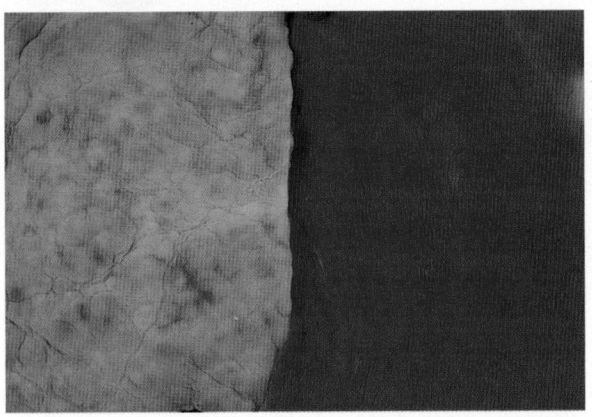

FIGURE 3.11 Close-up view of two livers, placed next to each other and reproduced here in natural size. *Left:* Fatty liver with early cirrhosis in an alcoholic. *Right:* Normal liver as a control.

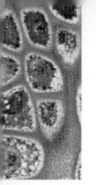

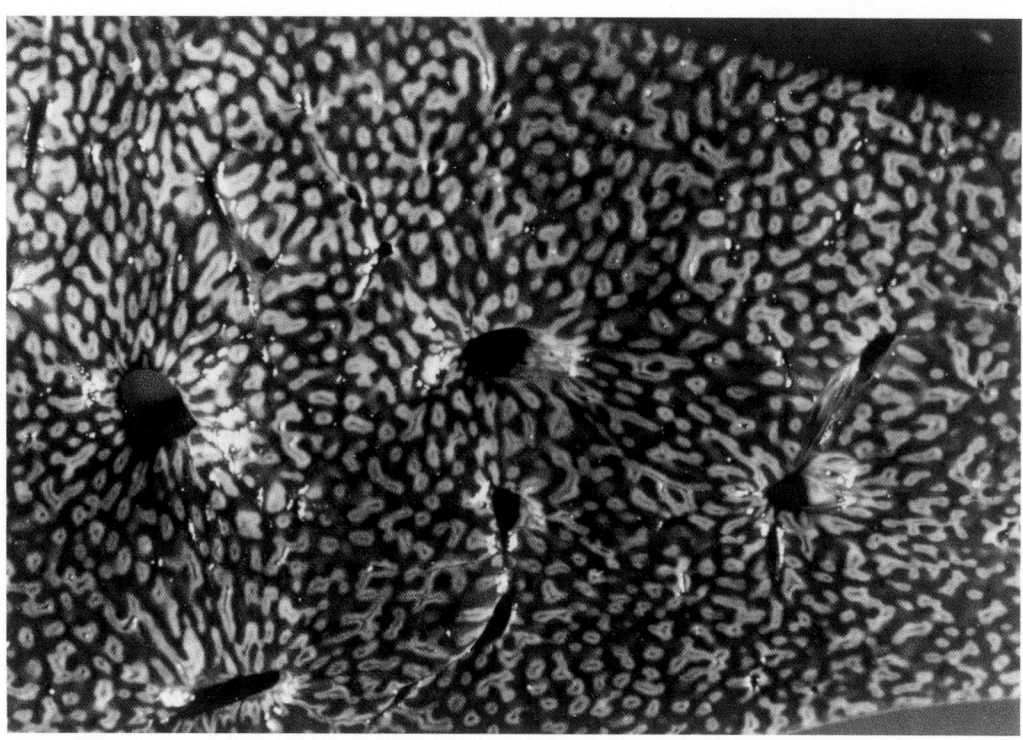

FIGURE 3.12   Centrolobular fatty change from anoxia in the liver of a horse, which died of methemoglobinemia from eating red maple leaves off the ground in the fall. The central cells of each liver lobule are oxygen-starved because methemoglobin does not carry oxygen. (Reproduced by permission from Slauson, David O, and Cooper, Barry J: Mechanisms of disease, ed. 2, Baltimore, 1990, Williams & Wilkins Co.; copyrighted by Mosby-Year Book, Inc., St. Louis.)

When steatosis develops in myocardial or striated muscle cells, where the cytoplasm is crowded with fibrils, the lipid droplets remain quite small; they are neatly strung like beads along the rows of mitochondria (Figure 3.13).

Does macrovesicular steatosis cause damage? Triglycerides have the reputation of being innocuous (perhaps because fat in general is so sedentary) and in the short typically this is true: this type of steatosis is run asymptomatic and clinically reversible. Everyday clinical experience shows that a mild alcoholic fatty liver confirmed by biopsy can be reversed in about 10 days (1–6 weeks) provided that alcohol supplies are out of reach. Clinical tests of liver function show little change (84, 85); perhaps some liver function tests on the geese used to produce *foie gras* would be illuminating.

On the other hand, we must not forget that liver steatosis, in the long run, is the prelude to cirrhosis. Experimentally, it can be shown that triglycerides are susceptible to peroxidation, with release of free radicals and secondary damage to the liver cells (70). A chronic, low-key effect of fatty acids is another possibility: it has been long known that in alcoholic liver disease and in

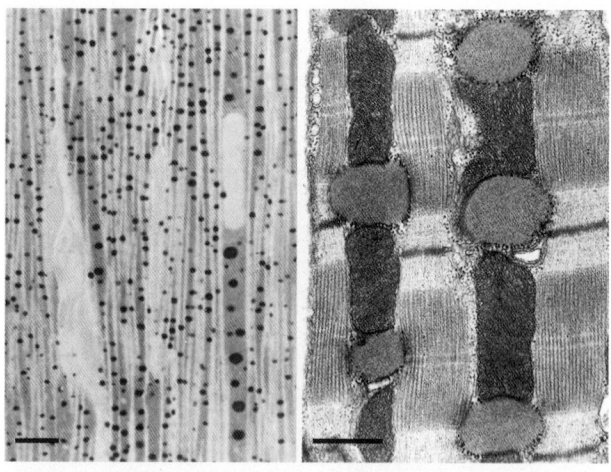

FIGURE 3.13   Steatosis of the myocardium in a rat, after treatment with clofibrate (clinically used as a hypolipemic agent). *Left:* Staining with Sudan black to demonstrate lipid. **Bar** = 10 μm. *Right:* Electron microscopy shows the close association between lipid droplets and mitochondria. This steatosis may be due to an inhibitory effect of the drug on mitochondrial oxidation. **Bar** = 0.5 μm. (Reproduced with permission from [49].)

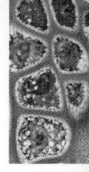

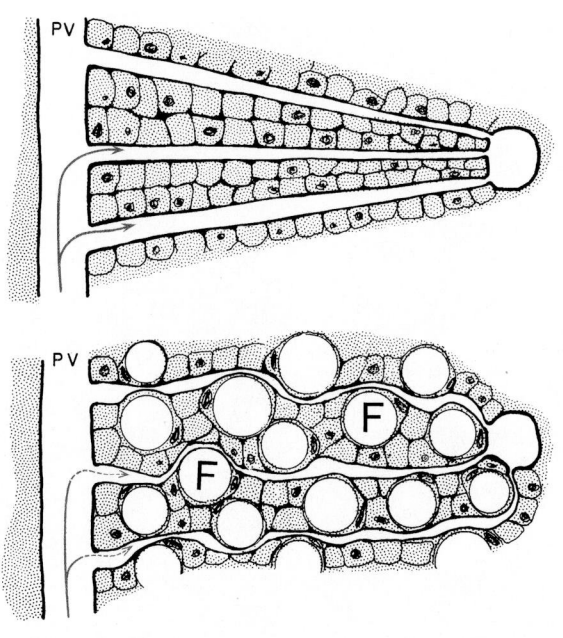

FIGURE 3.14 Compression of sinusoids in liver lobules in severe steatosis. Blood flow is from left to right (**PV:** portal vein). *Top:* Normal liver. *Bottom:* Liver cells bloated with fat (**F**) impair flow and can lead to increased pressure in the portal vein (portal hypertension). (Modified from [87], by courtesy of Marcel Dekker, Inc.)

Bovine serum albumin

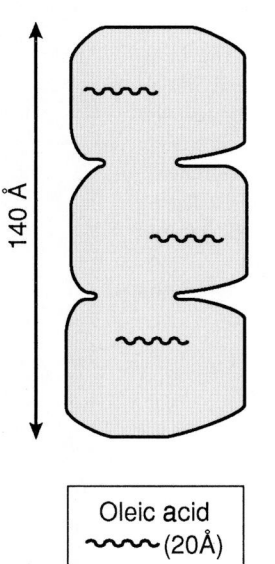

FIGURE 3.15 Serum albumin acts as a carrier for fatty acids and for many other small molecules that have a low water solubility. It can carry up to 10 fatty acid molecules (J. A. Hamilton, personal communication) and in this sense it can be considered as a lipoprotein. (Adapted from [96], by courtesy of Marcel Dekker, Inc.)

morbid obesity, the fatty acid content is increased about 10-fold (76). Another possible mechanism of liver damage by extreme steatosis is the compression of the sinusoids by hepatocytes bulging with fat (Figure 3.14). This mechanical effect has been well demonstrated after acute, toxic hepatocellular swelling (see Figure 3.5).

Biochemical Mechanisms of Steatosis

The biochemical mechanisms of steatosis (both macrovesicular and microvesicular) have been studied almost exclusively in the liver (46), not only because this organ is so well suited for chemical analysis but also because, historically, many of the toxic agents that were in vogue at a given time—for reasons industrial, medical, or cultural—were found to induce a fatty liver (remember that the liver is the principal site of detoxification). Classic examples are chloroform in the early days of anesthesia; yellow phosphorus, once used in matches and also for suicidal purposes; and especially carbon tetrachloride, a deadly fat solvent used until recently for many industrial and household purposes, for cleaning fluids, paints, and detergents, and even in bulk in fire extinguishers, which were about as dangerous as the fire itself (73). Today fatty liver is still a social

problem, being the first stage of the liver disease induced by the most common poison of our day, alcohol.

Triglyceride storage requires a supply of fatty acids from other tissues, so it will be useful to summarize the key facts about fatty acid physiology. Fatty acids can arise from three sources.

- **Dietary fat,** which enters the circulation packaged into droplets of triglycerides (chylomicrons).
- **Fat mobilized** from stores in adipose tissue. Here the triglycerides are broken down and reach the bloodstream as free fatty acids (FFA) transported by albumin molecules, which have special hydrophobic domains for this purpose (Figure 3.15). The release of fatty acids from fat cells is induced by hormones (epinephrine, norepinephrine, cortisol, ACTH, some prostaglandins) and drugs (caffeine, theophylline) (46). Steatosis of liver and muscles has been induced experimentally with some of these agents (69) (Figure 3.16).
- **New synthesis** from acetate, a lesser source.

Circulating free fatty acids (FFA) are taken up mainly by the liver (30 percent) and by muscle; chylomicrons are

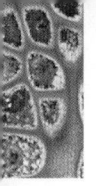

FIGURE 3.16 Catecholamines increase the mobilization of free fatty acids. *Right:* Lipid droplets are packed between the mitochondria in a striated muscle fiber of a dog, 8 hours after infusion of noradrenaline. *Left:* An adjacent fiber is completely spared, presumably reflecting functional differences between muscle fibers. **Bars** = 2 μm. (Reproduced with permission from [75].)

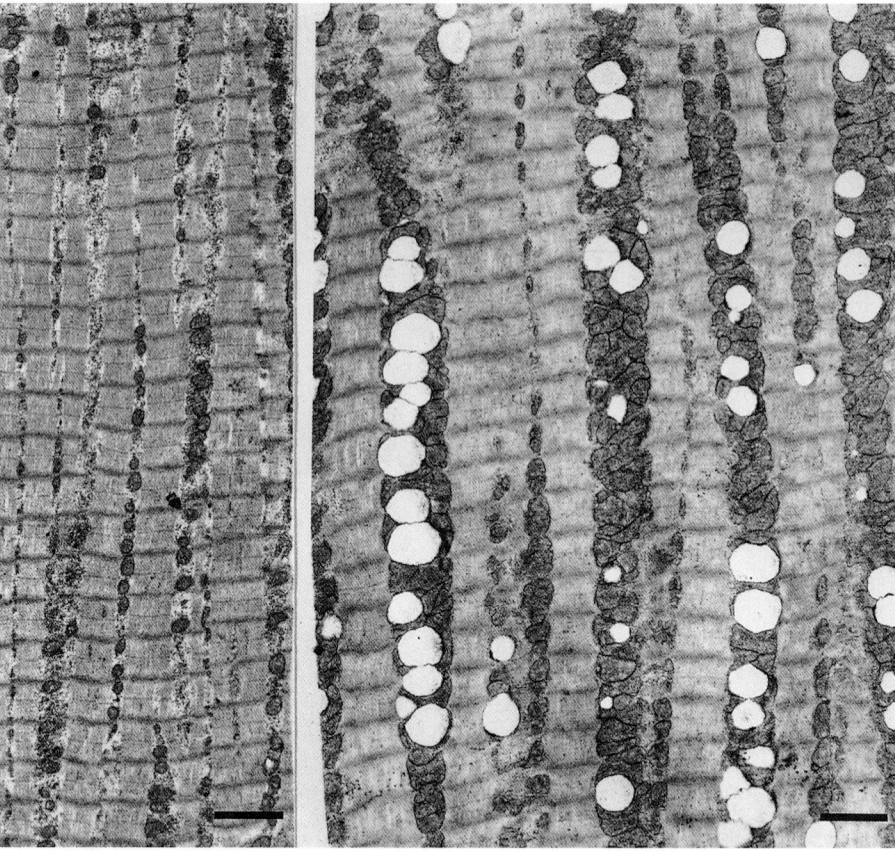

taken up by the liver (30 percent), adipose tissue (40 percent), and other tissues. Chylomicrons in the liver cell are hydrolyzed by lysosomes, and the resulting fatty acids join the FFA intracellular pool.

The simplified metabolic diagram of Figure 3.17 was conceived for the liver and therefore includes lipoprotein synthesis; but if the latter part of the scheme is left out, the remaining pathways should be applicable to other cell types. The diagram shows that free fatty acids supplied by the bloodstream find their way to a FFA pool inside the liver cell. The main point for our purpose is that *fatty acids are used to form triglycerides, but they can also be processed in at least three ways:*

- They can combine with glycerol and give rise to triglycerides.
- They can be oxidized by mitochondria and/or burned as fuel.
- They can be combined with glycerol, plus choline and phosphate, giving rise to phospholipids.

To be exported out of the liver cell, the triglycerides need to be assembled into a particle summarily called a **lipoprotein,** actually a globule filled with molecules of cholesteryl esters and free cholesterol, wrapped in a membrane of phospholipids and held together by a winding molecule of apoprotein (Figure 3.18). *The key point is that without the apoprotein, the lipoprotein cannot be built and its lipid components cannot be exported from the cell.* This helps to understand why steatosis can be induced by inhibitors of protein synthesis. One of the favorite experimental models of fatty liver (ethionine poisoning) exploits this mechanism.

With the preceding facts in mind we can begin to unravel what happens in individual situations. The innumerable causes of steatosis fall into three groups: lack of oxygen, nutritional disturbances, and toxic and hormonal effects.

Lack of oxygen. If fewer molecules of fatty acids are oxidized, more should remain available for triglyceride synthesis. In practice, this is seen in anemia and in some intoxications; data are available only for the liver.

Regarding failure of oxygen supply, consider the long path that atmospheric oxygen must travel to reach the mitochondria where it will be used. This means that there

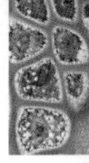

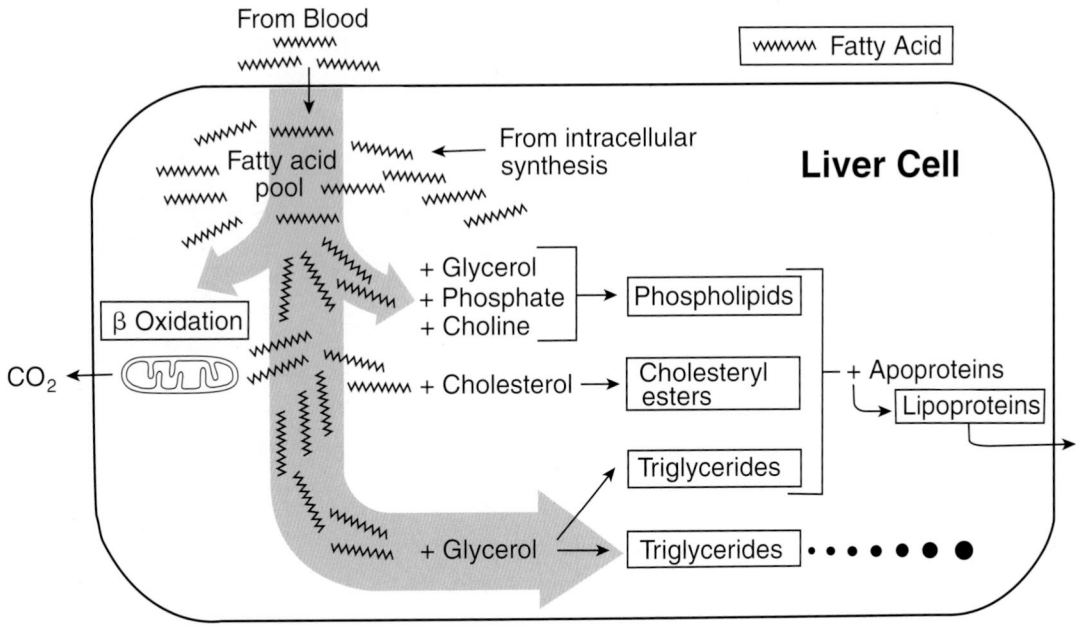

FIGURE 3.17   Fatty acid metabolism in a liver cell. The large pink arrow emphasizes 3 pathways leading to triglyceride overload (4 in rodents): (a) Increased input of fatty acids (e.g., overfeeding); (b) decreased oxidation (e.g., anoxia); and (c) inhibition of (apo)protein synthesis; (4) choline deficiency (experimentally). See text.

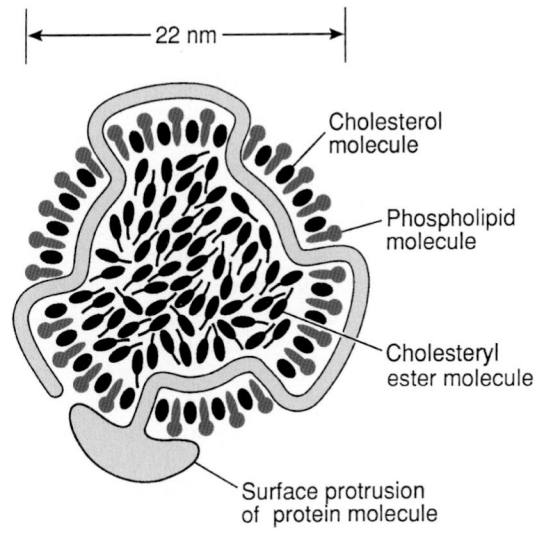

FIGURE 3.18   Cross section of a low-density lipoprotein (LDL) particle. A core of about 1500 cholesterol molecules, esterified to long-chain fatty acids, is surrounded by a lipid monolayer. A single large protein molecule organizes the particle. (Adapted from [1].)

must also be a long list of possible mechanisms for causing the supply to run short:

- Drop in atmospheric oxygen (**anoxic anoxia**) (thus high altitude can cause steatosis, and so can hypoxia in tissue cultures) (54, 55, 56)

- Obstacle in the bronchial tree
- Defect in the alveolar membrane
- Defect in the transport system due to inadequate blood flow, inadequate number of red blood cells (**anemic anoxia**), or a defect in the hemoglobin (carboxyhemoglobin, i.e., hemoglobin combined with CO, can no longer carry oxygen)
- Toxic effect on the cell's oxidative metabolism, called **toxic anoxia** (when diphtheria was prevalent, steatosis of the heart was an expected finding: diphtheria toxin depresses the oxidation of long-chain fatty acids by inducing a deficiency of carnitine, which is required for that step) (104, 105)
- Vitamin deficiencies affecting the respiratory chain (niacin, riboflavin, etc.)

Nutritional disturbances. Before the 1960s, malnutrition was thought to be the main cause of steatosis, hence the persistent and complacent legend that a hearty meal could prevent liver damage by alcohol.

This legend, which maintained that alcoholics developed fatty livers simply because they were malnourished, was hard to extirpate even after the evidence of alcohol toxicity became overwhelming in 1974 (93). The belief stemmed in part from experiments with rodents kept on a diet deficient in choline and methionine, ingredients essential for phospholipid synthesis; the animals acquired typical fatty livers. However, this mechanism appears to have little or no relevance for humans.

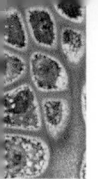

Imbalanced nutrition can work in several ways. **Overfeeding** causes liver steatosis (including the commercial *foie gras*) by oversupplying the cells with fatty acids. Paradoxically, **starvation** also causes a steatosis of the liver and heart (104, 105). This is not so surprising when it is realized that in laboratory rodents starved for 2–3 days the peripheral fat stores (adipose tissue) are mobilized so rapidly that the plasma appears milky. A sorry example of chronic starvation is offered by **kwashiorkor,** a Ghanian name that means "the-disease-that-the-older-one-gets-when-the-second-one-is-born" (98, 101). When the second child is born, the older one is taken off the breast and fed a meager cereal diet that leads to protein-calorie starvation; despite emaciation the liver is usually enlarged and fatty (Figures 3.19, 3.20). Presumably, *lack of protein synthesis blocks the synthesis and export of lipoproteins, with retention of the lipid components* as explained in Figure 3.17.

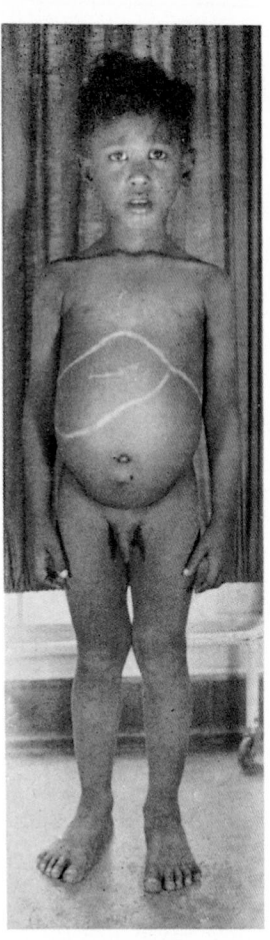

FIGURE 3.19   Kwashiorkor in a 5½-year-old child. Note the distended abdomen and enlarged liver (margin outlined with chalk) contrasting with an otherwise fair nutritional state. (Reproduced with permission from [101].)

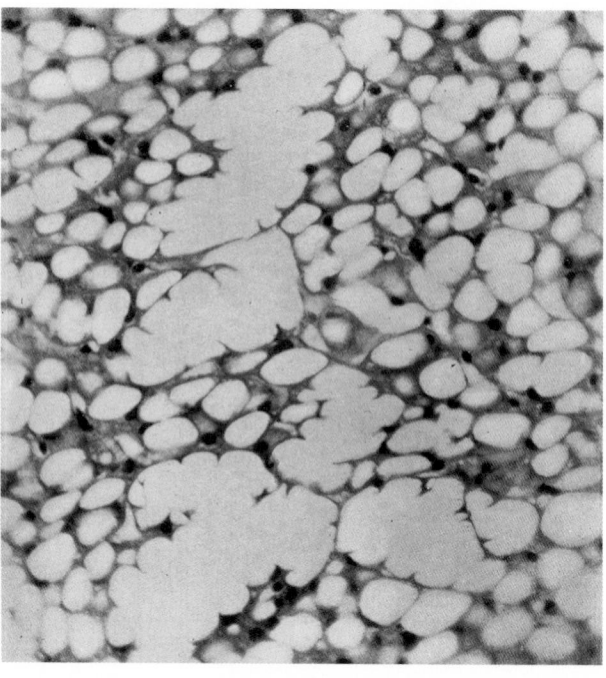

FIGURE 3.20   Fatty liver in a case of kwashiorkor. Note the confluence of fat droplets from adjacent liver cells. (Reproduced with permission from [101].)

So goes the standard theory, but the picture is probably more complicated. Some children affected by kwashiorkor are breast-fed and even well nourished: aflatoxin intoxication seems to be a complicating factor (60, 62).

Nutritional imbalance is well demonstrated in genetically obese Zucker rats, which are also hyperlipemic, hyperinsulinemic, but normoglycemic: a diet enriched in sucrose rapidly induces a fatty liver (80). A similar mechanism probably underlies the fatty livers typical of very obese humans consuming a low-protein, high-carbohydrate diet (63); however, morbid obesity and fatty liver are not always associated (36).

In birds, malnutrition can produce a severe steatosis of the liver and kidney known as **fatty liver and kidney syndrome** (FLKS), which has troubled not only wild birds but also the poultry industry (38, 83).

Toxic and hormonal effects. Toxic agents can induce steatosis by a bewildering variety of mechanisms (50) because they may disrupt any conceivable link in lipid, protein, and energy metabolism. In the liver, the most common mechanism by far is *decreased synthesis of lipoproteins.* This can be proven experimentally with inhibitors of protein synthesis.

Ethionine depresses protein synthesis primarily by sequestering ATP and thus preventing the activation of amino acids (46). Puromycin is another inhibitor, so is tetracycline (44), and so is a toxin of the highly poisonous

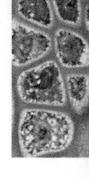

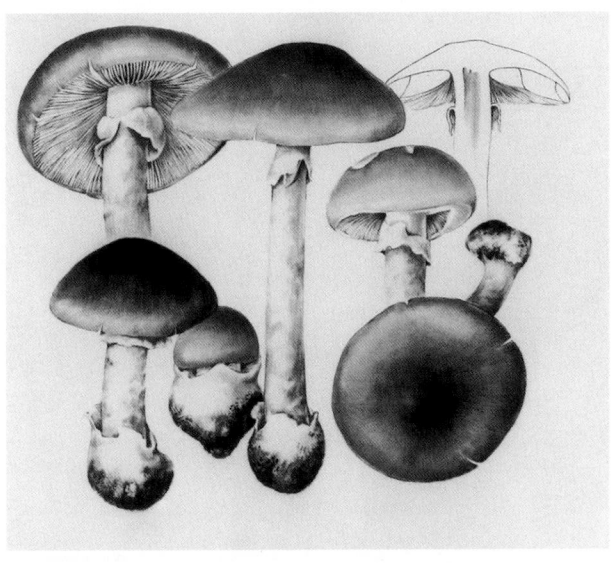

FIGURE 3.21 Phalloidin is produced by this mushroom, *Amanita phalloides,* deadly even if cooked. (Reproduced from [89].)

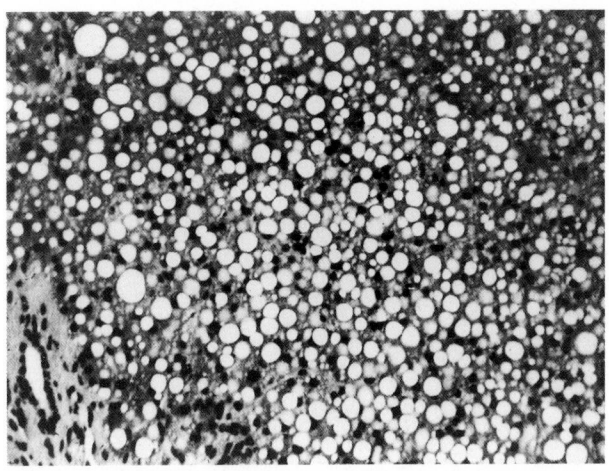

FIGURE 3.22 Alcoholic fatty liver without drunkenness. This patient (an alcoholic) was hospitalized long enough to develop a histologically normal liver. She then received alcohol in fruit juice, about half the daily amount she would previously absorb (86 proof whiskey, 8 oz/day for 2 days; then 12 oz/day for 2 days; then 16 oz/day for 3 days). The patient was never drunk. (Courtesy of Dr. E. Rubin, Thomas Jefferson University Medical Center, Philadelphia, PA.)

mushroom *Amanita phalloides* (Figure 3.21), alpha-amanitin, a specific inhibitor of RNA polymerase II, the enzyme synthesizing RNA (46).

It is satisfying to pinpoint simple biochemical mechanisms, but beware: *a toxic agent can act in many different ways by disrupting different metabolic pathways* (92).

Anyone who needs to be cured of wanting to know the mechanism of toxic steatosis should look into carbon tetrachloride intoxication of the liver, which has been studied for decades because industrial and household exposure to inhalation of CCl_4 vapors was a common accident. The principal effect is decreased export of lipoproteins from the liver, but a variety of mechanisms are possible: a decrease of lipoprotein export by blockage of tubulin and possibly by a direct denaturation of lipoproteins; a block in protein synthesis by free radical damage to the ER membranes (p. 199); a decrease of FFA oxidation by the mitochondria; and stress, which increases lipolysis (p. 199) and thus leads to an increased supply of FFA (46).

Ethanol intoxication is just as complicated as CCl_4 intoxication (51, 71, 97): the mechanisms of steatosis include increased synthesis of glycerol as well as of fatty acids, decreased oxidation of FFA due to mitochondrial damage, possibly decreased lipoprotein secretion, and increased lipolysis in adipose tissue (71, 93). An interesting point—more important to remember—is that ethanol can lead to steatosis after a weekend of heavy

social drinking without drunkenness (Figure 3.22) (93). However, it should not be forgotten that liver damage by ethanol includes more than steatosis (71).

Steatosis due to Fatty Acids

Again, the picture is dominated by the liver, but there is beginning evidence of toxic effects in other organs.

Clinically, in sharp contrast with the mild nature of triglyceride overload, the toxic effect of fatty acids on the liver manifests itself as an acute, life-threatening event that may lead to liver failure. The episode can be triggered by many common drugs: tetracycline, antiviral agents (usually for HIV infection), valproic acid (an antiepileptic fatty acid), amiodarone (an antiarrhythmic), and even an overdose of aspirin (52, 53). All of these drugs share the property of *inhibiting the beta-oxidation of fatty acids by the mitochondria.* According to the diagram in Figure 3.17, this metabolic obstacle should lead to a backup of fatty acids; some may indeed be diverted into the triglyceride pathway, but the bulk will probably pile up in the cytoplasm and cause toxic trouble by the products of fatty acid metabolism via the non–beta-oxidative pathway (100). Microscopically, the picture is microvesicular steatosis (Figure 3.23); the liver is usually enlarged, but it can be shrunken if the toxic agent has killed many liver cells, hence the old, inappropriate name of *acute yellow "atrophy"* (47). Two

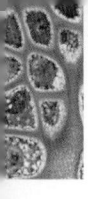

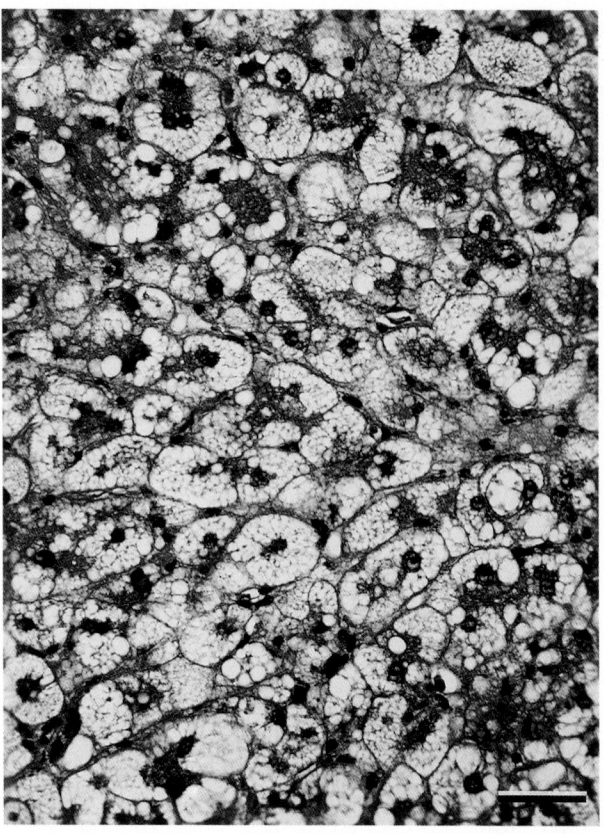

FIGURE 3.23 Fatty liver of pregnancy: typical microvesicular pattern (see also Figure 3.10). **Bar** = 50 μm. (Courtesy of Dr. K. G. Ishak, Armed Forces Institute of Pathology, photograph No. 79-11084.)

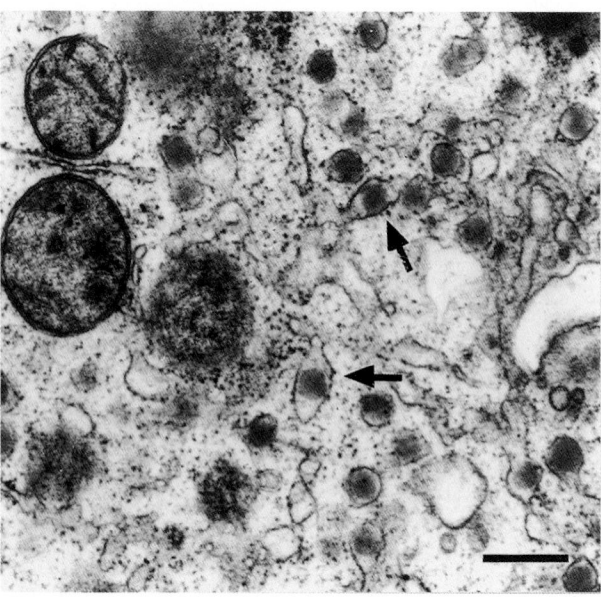

FIGURE 3.24 Rat liver 5 hours after ethionine poisoning. **Arrows:** Lipid droplets within the endoplasmic reticulum. **Bar:** 0.5 μm. (Reproduced by permission from [94], © by The US & Canadian Academy of Pathology, Inc.)

questions come to mind: *What are the droplets made of? Why do they remain small and do not fuse?*

Surprisingly, the answers are skimpy. The droplets, on frozen sections, stain positively for fat and surely contain some triglycerides, but their main content probably consists of fatty acids. Histochemical proof is still wanting. Fatty acids disrupt cell membranes and therefore are very toxic (47), which would fit with the poor prognosis of microvesicular steatosis. The other question—why do the droplets fail to fuse?—is even less understood. Some liver poisons cause "liposomes" to develop within the endoplasmic reticulum (Figure 3.24) (72, 94), but the ultimate fate of these droplets is not known. It was proposed in 1995 that *the microvesicular pattern might be explained by the presence of fatty acids:* these amphiphilic molecules could emulsify the lipid droplets by surrounding them, with the lipophilic end embedded in the lipid core of triglyceride, and the hydrophilic pole facing the cytoplasm (52, 53). Electron microscopy of the liver has shown fat droplets and mitochondrial changes, including swelling

and occasional crystalline inclusions (42a). More work is sorely needed.

This overall picture of microvesicular steatosis has been further clarified by two rare diseases, which are essentially experiments of Nature; one of them links steatosis to pregnancy, and the other to aspirin.

The acute fatty liver of pregnancy. This occurs in about 1 of 13,000 pregnancies (68) and is only beginning to be understood (61, 90). It is a fearful event, although the mortality rate has been reduced to less than 20 percent for both mother and fetus (64). Late in pregnancy, an expectant mother suddenly experiences nausea, vomiting, headaches, jaundice, and abdominal pain; these symptoms may be the prelude to hepatic coma. This nasty turn of events is explained by the fact that the woman suffers—unknowingly—from a latent genetic disorder: an approximately *50 percent deficiency of the mitochondrial enzyme responsible for the last step in the beta-oxidation of fatty acids* (long-chain 3-hydroxyacyl coenzyme A dehydrogenase). The fetus has the same problem. Not all of the details are clear, but it seems that the woman has just enough enzyme to deal with the output of fatty acids from her own liver; late in pregnancy, an extra dose coming from the fetus upsets the balance. Her liver shows classic microvesicular steatosis (Figure 3.23); for once we have the support of chemical analysis: a semiforgotten 1955 paper by two distinguished Boston pathologists reported that a fatty

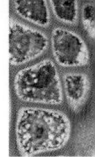

liver of pregnancy contained a large amount of fatty acids (47, 81).

Microvesicular steatosis and aspirin: Reye's syndrome. Reye's syndrome is a rare and usually pediatric disorder with a mortality rate of about 30 percent (40, 68). In the typical setting, an apparently benign febrile illness in a child had been treated with aspirin; suddenly, severe neurologic symptoms developed, due to cerebral edema: lethargy, delirium, and seizures. The liver showed microvesicular steatosis and mitochondrial damage. Happily, because the public was warned not to give aspirin indiscriminately to feverish children, Reye's disease has almost disappeared. *The few cases still seen may be due to a latent mitochondrial beta-oxidation defect* (68).

> We have emphasized the differences between two types of intracellular lipid deposition (triglyceride and fatty acids), but there is some overlap, e.g., by different doses of the same toxic agent. Mice given high doses of alcohol over a short time will develop microvesicular steatosis; alcohol in drinking water for 6 months will produce macrovesicular steatosis (70).

Lipotoxic Diseases: A Growing Threat

The rise of obesity on the world scene, in association with diabetes Type 2 and hyperlipidemia, has created a new syndrome known in humans as *nonalcoholic fatty liver disease, diabetes hepatitis,* or **nonalcoholic steatohepatitis** (NASH). It affects all ages, and 57 to 74 percent of obese individuals (37). In one study, 100 percent of diabetic obese persons had at least mild steatosis; 50 percent had steatohepatitis (37). It is not understood why in some patients steatosis remains as such, whereas in others it progresses to steatohepatitis, cirrhosis, and liver failure. A likely sequence is that insulin resistance causes steatosis, and reactive oxygen species arising from the mitochondria induce lipid peroxidation and further cell damage (37).

An experimental model for this condition is the diabetic and (very) obese Zucker rat. Using this model, R. H. Unger, L. Orci, and colleagues have proposed a pathogenesis based on the notion of **lipotoxicity** (99, 100).

> In summary: when overnutrition occurs, the hormone **leptin** rises so as to prevent the deposition of triglycerides in nonadipose tissues (which are not equipped for such storage). If leptin fails, triglycerides deposit in the "wrong" cells and cause a syndrome of lipotoxicity, including **"lipoapoptosis"** of the affected cells. At present, only three types of cells are demonstrably involved: pancreatic beta cells, leading to diabetes Type 2; cardiomyocytes, leading to cardiomyopathy; and striated muscle, leading to insulin resistance.

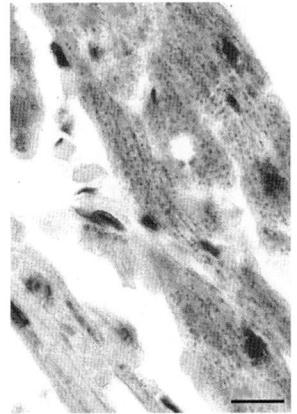 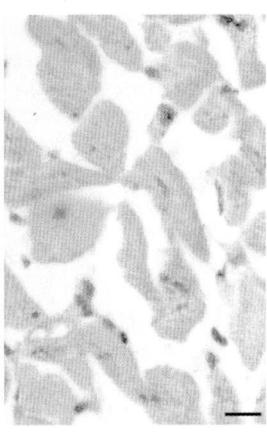

FIGURE 3.25 Cardiac lipotoxicity. Note the accumulation of lipid droplets in the cardiac muscle from (*left*) an obese man (with a body mass index [BMI] = 42) compared with the cardiac muscle of a lean man (BMI = 28) (*right*). (Frozen sections, Oil red O stain and hematoxylin.) **Bars** = 10 μm. (Reproduced from Unger RH, Orci L. FASEB J. with permission of Federation of American Societies for Experimental Biology. Copyright 2001 by Federation of American Societies for Experimental Biology. In the format Textbook via Copyright Clearance Center [100].)

Time will tell whether this attractive hypothesis fits all of the aspects of the human condition; certainly the steatosis of myocardial cells can be impressive (Figure 3.25).

Some unusual forms of steatosis

- Triglycerides can accumulate by congenital **deficiency of acid lipase** (Wolman's disease of infants and an adult form called **cholesteryl ester storage** disease) (66). In this rare condition, both triglycerides and cholesterol esters accumulate in lysosomes, as occurs in other storage diseases due to enzyme deficiencies (p. 148). The deposits occur in most tissues, even in lymphocytes. A similar condition can be reproduced in only 4 hours by feeding egg yolk to rats (67).
- There is also a rare lipid-storage myopathy due to a defect in oxidative metabolism leading to **carnitine deficiency** (48). You will notice here an overlap with the effect of diphtheria toxin mentioned earlier.
- In the triglyceride-laden heart of diabetic mice a similar oxidation defect was found (65).

Some conditions akin to steatosis:

- ***Triglyceride load as a normal condition.***
  Strangely, the tubules in the renal cortex of the cat and other carnivores always contain lipid droplets (39).
- ***Phagocytosis leading to the accumulation of fat.***
  In the convoluted tubules of the kidney, there is no

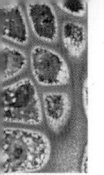

doubt that true steatosis can develop as a result of metabolic disturbances (75, 83, 103); however, in those diseases that imply leakage of plasma proteins through the glomerulus (lipoid nephrosis), the mechanism of lipid storage in the tubules is phagocytosis. The tubular epithelium reabsorbs lipoproteins from the lumen and accumulates droplets containing triglycerides, cholesterol, and phospholipids, as leftovers from digestion of the lipoproteins (39).

- *Lipid droplets in regenerating cells* are common (41). There is no documented explanation; however, it is a fact that the respiratory metabolism of young cells and fetal cells depends more heavily on anaerobic glycolysis, which may make the cell less able to oxidize fatty acids.
- *Lipid accumulation in cultured cells* is another well-known phenomenon (91). True steatosis can result from anoxia, but most of the lipid is phospholipid from autophagocytosis (54, 55) and probably also from "overfeeding" with plasma loaded with lipoproteins.
- *Renal cell carcinoma,* which derives from the renal tubules, typically accumulates so much triglyceride that the tumor appears yellow. This is quite surprising because normal tubular cells of the human kidney contain few or no fat droplets .

TO SUM UP: Steatosis has been long defined as the intracellular accumulation of *triglycerides,* a supposedly innocuous type of lipid. Now we have learned that even the peaceful triglycerides, in the long run, can release dangerous fatty acids, or become oxidized, generate free radicals, and cause liver damage. Perhaps the liver cells should take a lesson from the fat cells—on how to live with this ambivalent intracellular lipid. We have also learned that a common type of steatosis (microvesicular steatosis of the liver) is dangerous because the fat droplets contain a large proportion of fatty acids.

Accumulation of Cholesteryl Esters

Continuing our search for symptoms of cellular disease, we now turn to the hoarding of cholesteryl esters. *This particular form of excess storage is a true case of cellular indigestion.* All cells need cholesterol as a building block for their membranes, but when the supply exceeds the demand, the cells store the excess ester in the form of droplets, mostly in lysosomes (Figure 3.26). The extreme but common example of this storage is offered by macrophages, whose uncontrolled appetite may lead

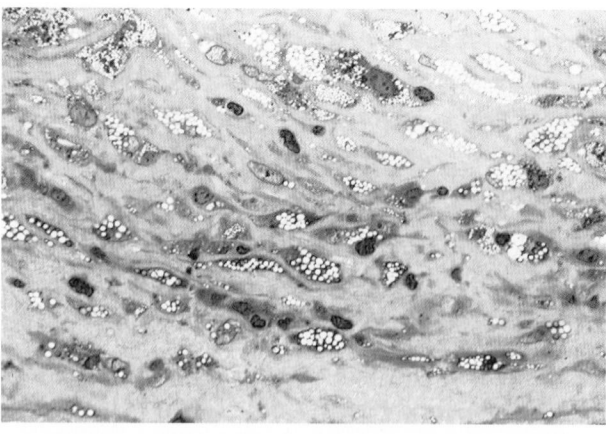

FIGURE 3.26   Foam cells in the intima of a human atherosclerotic artery. The cytoplasm appears foamy because it is packed with droplets of cholesteryl esters. The larger foam cells are macrophage-derived; some of the smaller ones derive from smooth muscle cells. (1-μm section; toluidine blue stain.)

them to swell enormously and to become bags of lipid droplets; in this bloated condition they are known internationally as **foam cells.** Bloated is an understatement: a foam cell may attain a diameter of 40–50 μm (124), which is 4–5 times above normal; the volume is therefore increased by a factor of 64–125.

To identify droplets of cholesteryl esters, the method of choice is polarized light on sections of fresh tissue, as mentioned earlier; cholesteryl esters are birefringent (113). Normally such droplets are present in adrenal glands and in neural tissue prior to myelinization.

Mammalian cells obtain their cholesterol mainly from two sources: *synthesis* within the cell, which needs to be supplemented by *uptake of low-density lipoproteins* (LDL) via a receptor mechanism (Figure 3.27). The LDL particles are assembled in the liver and can be considered as a door-to-door delivery system of cholesteryl ester. The cells then obtain cholesterol by hydrolyzing the ester. For phagocytic cells, there is a third source of cholesterol, namely *phagocytosis*. Macrophages are especially prone to obtain cholesterol by this mechanism because, as scavengers, they are often called upon to ingest cell debris, a rich source of membrane cholesterol. (Recall that in red cell membranes the cholesterol/phospholipid ratio is close to 1:1.)

The Cell's Problems in Dealing with Cholesterol

A cell overloaded with cholesterol faces a difficult challenge: cholesterol is one of the few molecules that

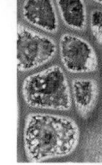

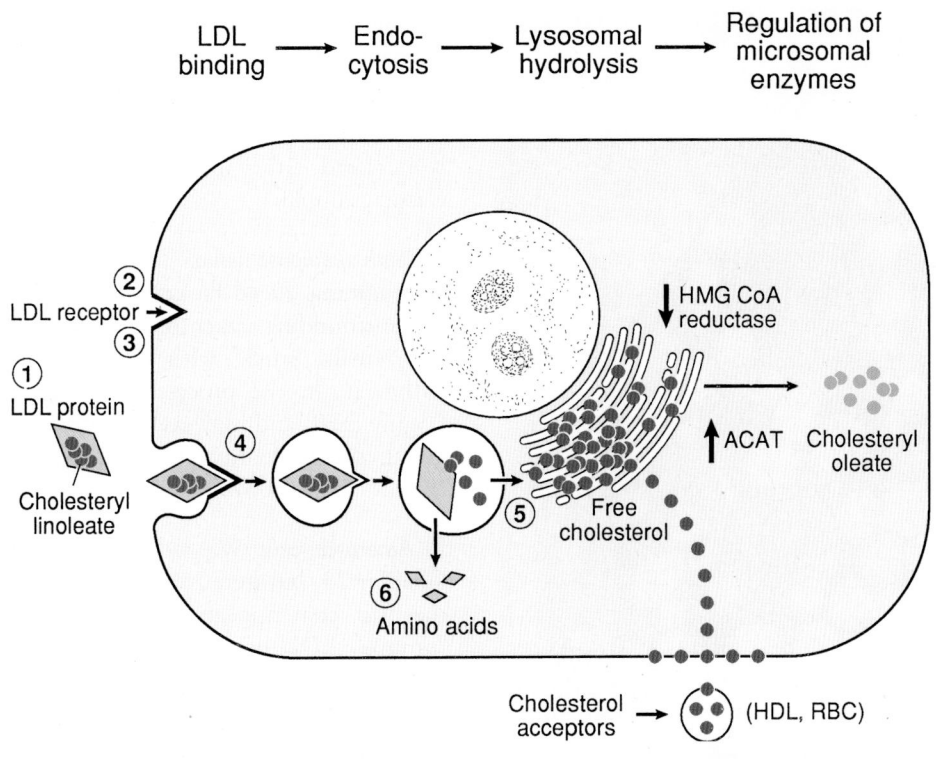

FIGURE 3.27   Steps in LDL uptake and breakdown by human macrophages and fibroblasts. Some of the cholesterol released is recycled to the cell membrane and then taken away by acceptors such as high-density lipoproteins (HDL) or red blood cells. Sites at which mutations have been identified, leading to congenital defects, are: (**1**) abetalipoproteinemia, (**2**) familial hypercholesterolemia (FH), receptor-negative, (**3**) FH, receptor-defective, (**4**) FH, internalization defect, (**5**) Wolman syndrome, (**6**) cholesteryl ester storage disease. (**HMG CoA reductase** = 3-hydroxy-3-methylglutaryl coenzyme A reductase. **ACAT** = acyl-coenzyme A:cholesterol acyl-transferase). (Modified from [114].)

cannot be broken down in the body; it is also insoluble. It can be eliminated only through the liver, which incorporates it into micelles containing bile acids and lecithin (119). These being the facts, any cell that takes up an excess of cholesterol (be it from LDL or from phagocytized debris) does not have the option of breaking it down; it can use a limited amount for its own membranes, but the rest must be esterified and stored in membrane-bound droplets. This mechanism is now well understood, thanks to the work of Michael Brown and Joseph Goldstein (107), who were awarded the Nobel Prize in 1985. A look at Figure 3.27 shows that the overloaded cell has, in fact, a safeguard. Some of the excess cholesterol can be carried to the cell surface and "offered" to any willing cholesterol acceptor that may be passing by. One such benefactor is known, namely high density lipoprotein (HDL) (108, 115). The details of this last and critical step, whereby a cell transfers its cholesterol to a passer-by, are not yet clear. For the time being, we may visualize an HDL particle bumping into

the surface of the overloaded cell, picking up a few cholesterol molecules, incorporating them into its cholesterol-rich core, and floating away with them.

Foam cells are striking to behold but not fully understood. Why, for example, are all the droplets the same size (Figure 3.28)? Why do they fail to fuse into one large droplet, as triglycerides do? Why do some droplets have membranes and others not? And why are they sometimes oval? No expert could give us answers, except for speculating that the molecular arrangement of the esters within the droplet must impose a certain shape; the droplets are in fact liquid crystals, as shown by their birefringency.

There is an alternative form of intracellular cholesterol storage: rhomboid crystals of pure cholesterol free in the cytosol, occasionally found in living foam cells and in the endothelium of hypercholesterolemic rats, presumably as an indication of extreme cholesterol overload. The cells containing such crystals appear to be in fine shape despite the sharp object developing within them.

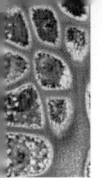

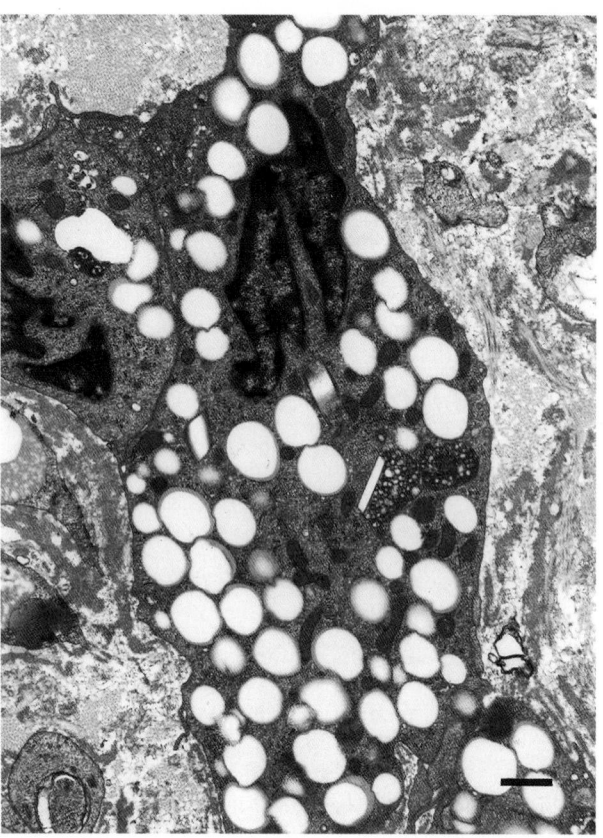

FIGURE 3.28   Foam cell derived from a smooth muscle cell, in a human atherosclerotic plaque. *Center:* Small cholesterol crystal in a lysosome. **Bar** = 1 μm.

Conditions that Favor the Development of Foam Cells

From what we have said, to find foam cells we will have to look for situations in which the supply of cholesterol is increased, either locally or generally. Here are some classic examples.

1) Death of adipose tissue. This may occur, for example, after trauma. Dead fat cells release their content, and the surrounding macrophages digest the triglyceride and remain "stuck" with all the cholesterol dissolved within it. In the process they turn into foam cells (Figure 3.29) and may even fuse, as we will see shortly, giving rise to foamy giant cells called **Touton cells** (Figure 3.30) (106).

2) Atherosclerosis. We will summarize this topic in Chapter 23, but here is the essence. In atherosclerosis, the first step appears to be that the endothelium "pumps" LDL lipoproteins into the arterial intima; monocytes then migrate from the blood into the intima, pick up the lipid, and become foam cells.

In view of these well-established facts, it came as an utter surprise to discover that *macrophages or monocytes incubated with particles of LDL refuse to phagocytize them.* Later it was found that macrophages exposed to LDL down-regulate their surface receptors for LDL; they only take up LDL particles that have been "modified" (oxidized) by the endothelium, a process that may

FIGURE 3.29   The lipid contained in necrotic fat cells (**N**) is taken up by macrophages, which become foam cells (**arrows**).

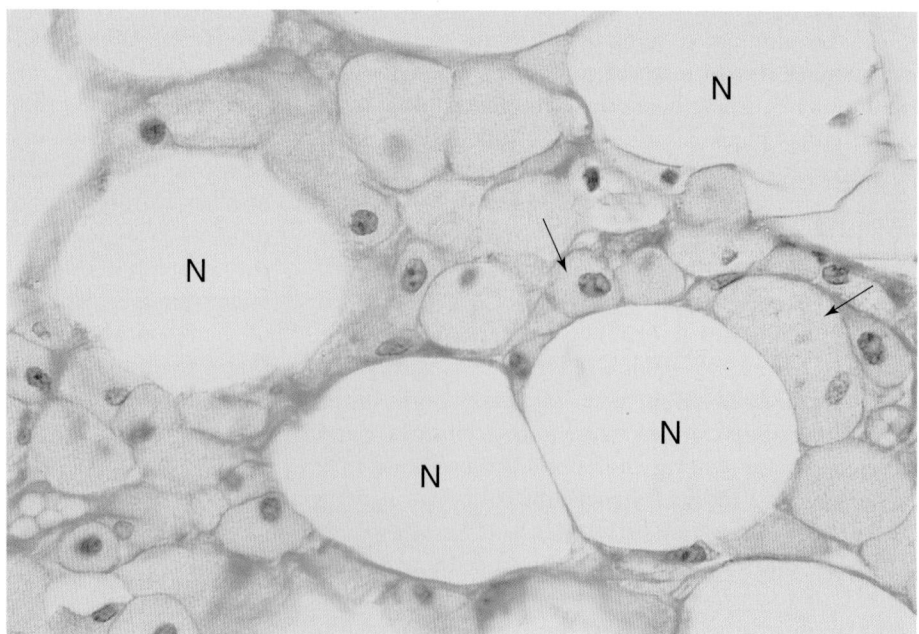

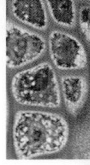

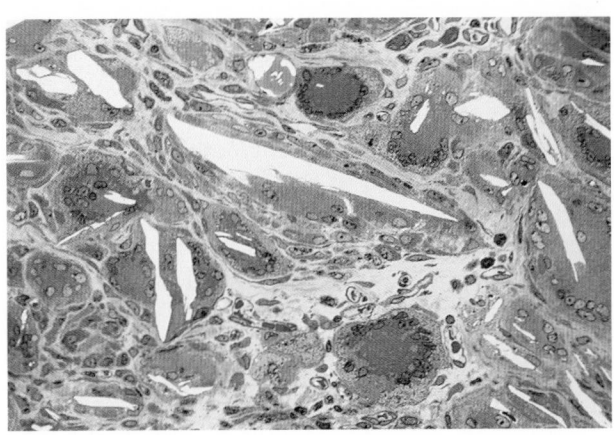

FIGURE 3.30 Touton cells, multinucleated giant cells that develop by fusion of foam cells. The nuclei are in the center, surrounded by cholesteryl ester droplets. The intracellular crystals probably correspond to pure cholesterol. (These Touton cells were obtained experimentally by injecting a cholesteryl ester [N-nonanoate] in corn oil subcutaneously into the rat; the tissue was fixed 2 weeks later.) (1-μm section; toluidine blue stain.)

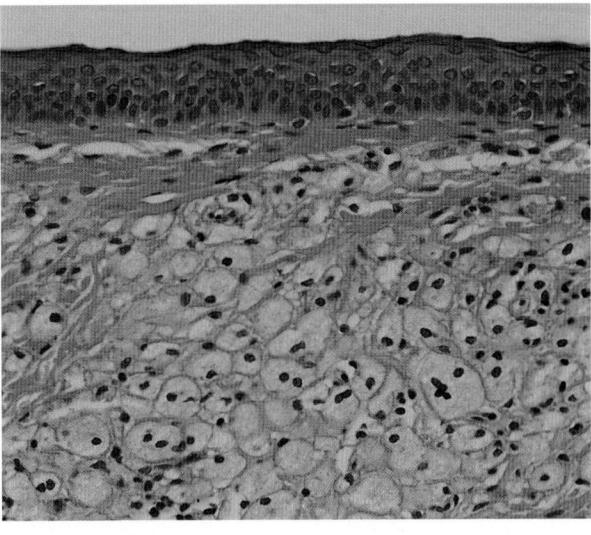

FIGURE 3.31 Macrophages loaded with lipid (foam cells). From a xanthelasma (a little yellow spot on an eyelid) that was removed for cosmetic reasons.

involve free radicals (120, 121). This is not an academic detail: it suggested the idea of trying to treat atherosclerosis with antioxidants (123)—a good idea but still unproven.

> From atherosclerotic lesions, the foam cells can be isolated, studied, and even analyzed with the cell sorter (p. 15); this method helped to establish that some arterial "foam cells" (not quite as filled with lipid) derive from smooth muscle cells (111).

3) Housekeeping in the lung.

The pulmonary alveoli and the small bronchi contain macrophages apparently adapted to live in the air. These cells work as scavengers: they keep the place clean, and for this deed they are rewarded by being coughed out or swallowed (p. 316). Their normal diet is mainly dust, but they are ready to take up also dead cells, surfactant, and lipoproteins that may have leaked into the alveoli. In so doing they turn into foam cells, whose presence in lower respiratory secretions can be considered a nonspecific marker of lung disease (109). When the bronchi are obstructed these free macrophages become numerous enough to produce a pattern called **lipid pneumonia** (122).

4) Xanthomas.

Xanthomas are yellow, tumorlike lumps of foam cells commonly found as a complication of hypercholesterolemia; the name xanthoma literally means "yellowma." The reader may ask why xanthomas develop locally, whereas hypercholesterolemia is a generalized condition. There is no good answer, except

that many xanthomas develop in areas more exposed to trauma, such as the skin of the elbows. Some localizations remain mysterious: **xanthelasmas,** for example, are little yellow lumps that develop on the eyelid or at the nasal corner of the eye. Why should foam cells develop there (Figure 3.31)?

5) Cholesterolosis of the gallbladder.

Occasionally, an excess of cholesterol is deposited in the mucosa of the gallbladder (Figure 3.32).

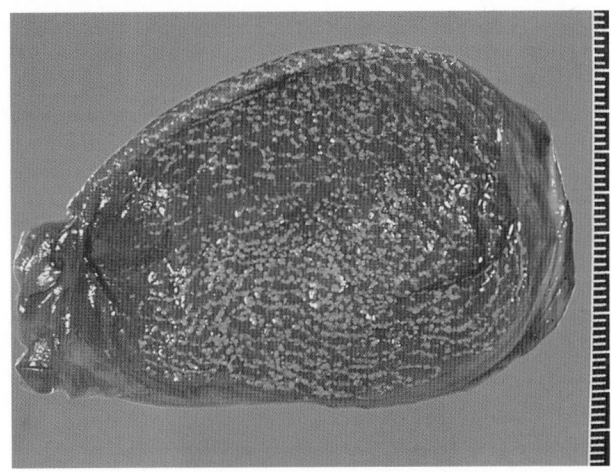

FIGURE 3.32 Cholesterolosis of the gallbladder ("strawberry gallbladder"), a striking but innocuous change. The yellowish lumps and ridges are submucosal clusters of foam cells. **Scale** in millimeter.

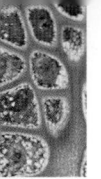

Fibroblasts have LDL receptors, and, in fact, cultured fibroblasts were first used by Brown and Goldstein in their masterly studies. Thus, it is not too surprising to see long, thin, but foamy cells in inflamed tissues. This property of fibroblasts may also help understand the peculiar localization of xanthomas in tendons (118). A special variety of lipid-storing fibroblasts are the so-called Ito cells of the liver, which act as a reservoir of the fat-soluble vitamin A; their droplets contain cholesteryl esters and about 25 percent of triglycerides (112). Lipid-storing fibroblasts exist also in the lung (117).

TO SUM UP: The pathology of cholesteryl esters is largely the pathology of foam cells. Long a favorite of microscopists, these distinctive little creatures are a flag for certain local or general disturbances that lead to cholesteryl ester overload. However, we should remind the reader that cholesterol does more, in pathology, than creating storage problems; it is also involved in diseases of cell membranes (p. 132). Last, we said that cholesterol cannot be broken down: then why is it that the world did not long ago become a vast, greasy dump of cholesterol crystals? Obviously because there are bacteria that can deal with it (110, 116).

Accumulation of Glycogen and Related Materials

Intracellular glycogen is a readily available, water-soluble store of energy. As one would expect of fuel that must be at hand, most of it is free in the cytosol and is catabolized there; we made the same remark about triglyceride droplets.

An easy histochemical stain for glycogen is the PAS method (for periodic-acid–Schiff), based on the reactivity of aldehyde groups, which yields a red color. Other carbohydrate-containing macromolecules also give this reaction, but a simple test can help to identify them: glycogen can be removed by placing the unstained section in a dilute solution of "diastase" (in practice, saliva). By electron microscopy, glycogen appears in the form of aggregated alpha or isolated beta granules 150–300 Å in diameter, not always easy to distinguish from ribosomes; impregnation of glycogen with silver proteinate is helpful (p. 336). At very high powers, the beta particles appear to be composed of filaments 30 Å in diameter and up to 200 Å long, known as gamma particles. Occasionally, glycogen particles can be found in almost any organelle (125).

A persistent legend about glycogen is that it is dissolved by ordinary fixatives. Actually, no glycogen seems to be lost by the ordinary 3 percent glutaraldehyde solution used for electron microscopy. Some is lost, however, during the staining of histologic sections. This is why the cytoplasm of rat liver cells looks so ragged in histologic sections; the "empty" spaces correspond to glycogen deposits. This also explains a paradox: liver cells in sections of human liver taken postmortem look more compact and "nicer" than cells from liver biopsies (Figure 3.33). They are not nicer at all. They appear compact only because their glycogen stores were burned up during the agonal period.

Our knowledge of the cellular pathology of glycogen accumulation consists, so far, of a collection of interesting but isolated facts.

- *Young cells,* which lean more heavily on anaerobic glycolysis, *contain more glycogen than mature cells;* so do many tumor cells, which share many characteristics with young cells.

- *Anoxia is sometimes associated with excessive amounts of intracellular glycogen,* presumably because the cell is on the brink of death and can no longer metabolize its substrates. The mechanism probably underlies the appearance of glycogen and of triglycerides in cells around myocardial infarcts.

- *Diabetes can increase intracellular glycogen* (130). In untreated diabetes, tissues that depend on insulin for their glucose supply, such as liver and muscle, become glucose-starved and thus glycogen-depleted, whereas tissues insensitive to insulin become overloaded with glycogen; thus in rats with alloxan-induced diabetes, glycogen is reduced in the liver and increased in the brain. Large deposits of glycogen occur also in the kidney, in the straight portion of the proximal tubules, as can be demonstrated by microdissection (132); they are probably a consequence of glucose overload. Electron microscopy shows the glycogen both free and enclosed within large autophagocytic vacuoles called glycogenosomes (Figure 3.34) (129).

- *Glycogenic nuclei* are still a cytologic puzzle. While studying diabetic tissues as long ago as 1883, Paul Ehrlich noticed glycogen in the nuclei of liver cells, a surprising observation because the nucleus rarely accumulates abnormal materials. However, this discovery turned out to be a disappointment because glycogenic nuclei are present also in normal livers

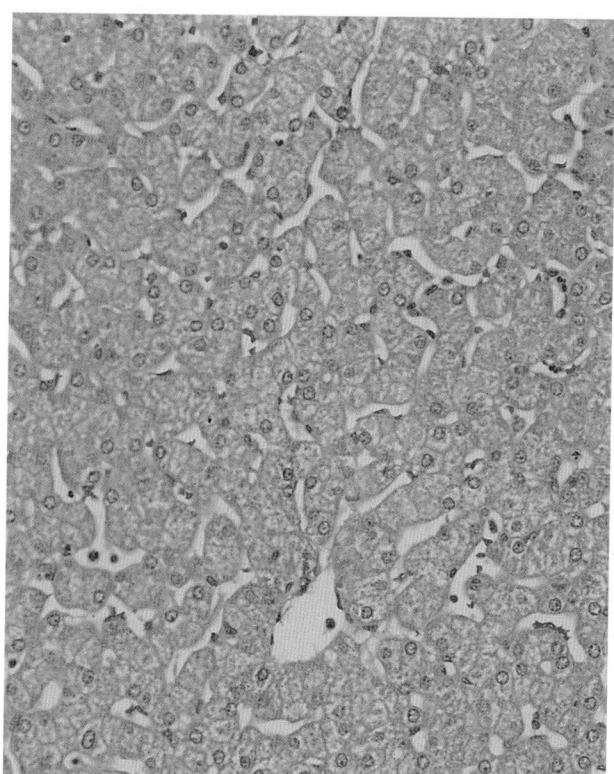

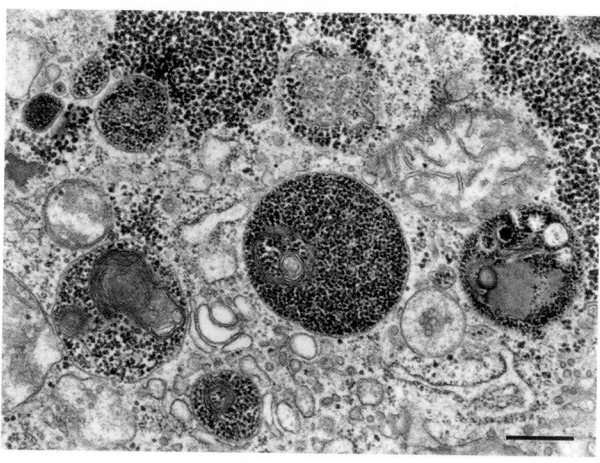

FIGURE 3.34   Accumulation of glycogen in a renal tubular cell of a rat made diabetic with streptozotocin (which kills pancreatic beta cells selectively). Many glycogen particles are free in the cytoplasm; others are contained in glycogenosomes as a result of autophagocytosis. **Bar** = 0.5 µm. (Reproduced from [129] with permission of Taylor and Francis Ltd.)

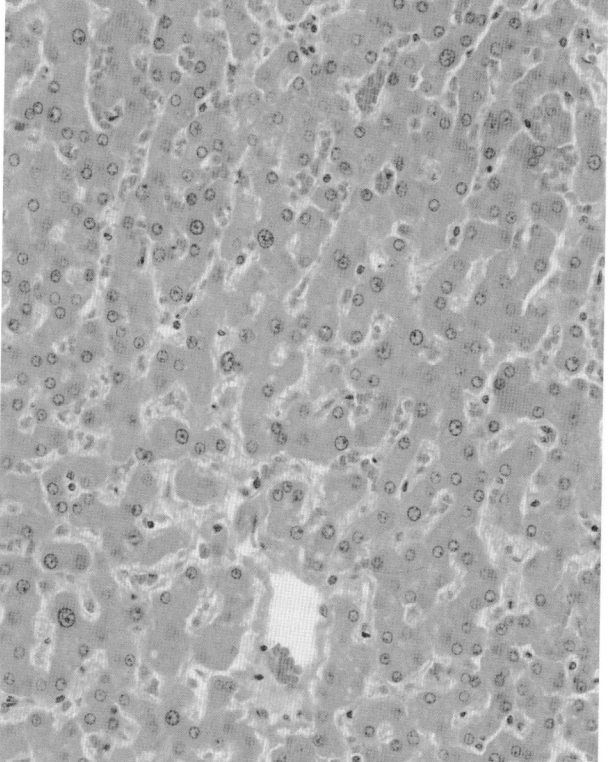

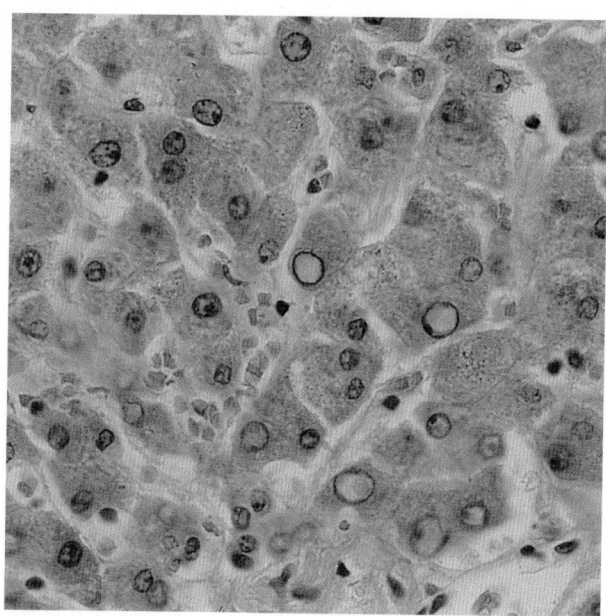

FIGURE 3.35   Normal human liver with glycogen-filled nuclei (large, empty-looking nuclei). The brown pigment is lipofuscin.

FIGURE 3.33   Two aspects of "normal" liver, obtained by biopsy (*top*) and at autopsy (*bottom*). In the biopsy, the liver cells are filled with glycogen, which has virtually disappeared from the autopsy liver.

(Figure 3.35), in the human myocardium, and in a variety of tumor cells (126). There is some evidence that nuclear glycogen is actually synthesized in the nucleus (127).

- *Lysosomal diseases offer the most striking pictures of intracellular glycogen storage,* due to the lack of a lysosomal enzyme (many glycogen-related enzymatic defects have been described) (p. 148).

The buildup of glycogen *in lysosomes* is rather peculiar because cell biology tells us that glycogen should be degradable in the cytoplasm. The answer may be that, no matter how fast the cytoplasmic glycogen is degraded, whatever amount reaches the lysosomes is bound to remain undigested and to lead, over the years, to massive storage.

- *Corpora amylacea and Lafora bodies* are spherical bodies of neuropathologic interest; *both are glucose polymers* (polyglycosans) *and thus related to glycogen.* One may wonder why the central nervous system should develop such a wealth of glucose polymers. Brain tissue is absolutely dependent on glucose as a source of energy; perhaps the spherical bodies are the neuropathologic way to deal with an oversupply of glucose (130, 134).

The **corpora amylacea** have nothing to do with amyloid; the name means that they show concentric lines like starch granules (*ámylon* is Greek for starch) (Figure 3.36). They are extremely common and, it seems, totally harmless. In the grey matter, strangely enough, they arise in the branches of fibrous astrocytes, causing them to swell enormously; thus, in a single section, they will appear to be extracellular. They can be found also in nerves. By electron microscopy they are fibrillar (131). Chemically they consist of a glycogenlike material (~80 percent) with phosphate and sulphate groups attached (135).

Lafora bodies are structurally similar but are pathologically far more significant. They were discovered in 1911 in the neurons in a case of myoclonic epilepsy and since then have been seen in other neurologic conditions. They may well represent a generalized metabolic

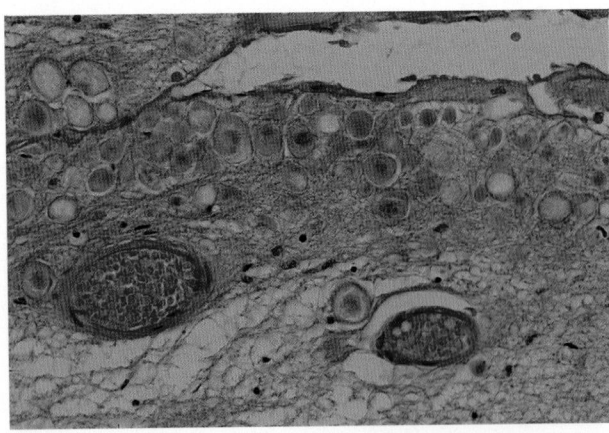

FIGURE 3.36 Cluster of corpora amylacea around a lateral ventricle a human brain. These structures, which increase in number with age, are not associated with any known pathology. (Courtesy of Dr. T. W. Smith, University of Massachusetts Medical School, Worcester, Mass.)

disease because they are found in many tissues including the liver and skin. They can be degraded *in vitro* by amylase (130). Similar bodies can be seen to arise in the axons of diabetic rats (130).

Basophilic degeneration of the myocardium is a bizarre but not uncommon, age-dependent cellular change related to glycogen metabolism, in which a basophilic mass appears in many myocardial fibers. Chemical, enzymatic, and spectroscopic studies indicate that this material is related to glycogen (128, 133). By electron microscopy it is mostly fibrillar, like the corpora amylacea.

Accumulation of Pigments

It may sound too simple to be scientific, but a change in color may be the first clue that something is wrong with a given tissue. The change may be obvious to the naked eye, or it may be apparent only through the microscope. Most of the coloring materials come from within the body, though some are environmental (167); they may be intracellular or extracellular. Chemically, they may be as different as soot and hemoglobin, but it is convenient to consider them as a group because they all convey the same general message: "*Abnormal color—something may be wrong.*" Each pigment, of course, has its own particular significance.

We will never forget the case of a 52-year-old man with a round mass in his lung, discovered accidentally on an X-ray. A needle biopsy yielded some nondescript cells, plus one cell containing a few brown granules. We hoped they would represent an innocuous blood-derived pigment, but they gave the reactions of melanin. The presence of melanin in a mass within the lung makes it almost certain that a malignant melanoma has metastasized to the lung. This proved to be the case; a small melanoma of the back had escaped attention.

Coloring material is also a versatile tool in experimental pathology, for staining sections and for studies *in vivo*.

Although the term pigment is often used interchangeably with the term dye for any coloring material, we will follow the proper tradition and use **dye** for colors (usually artificial) that form solutions, and **pigment** for particulate, insoluble colors that form suspensions. Ordinary ink is a dye whereas India ink (a suspension of

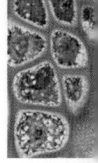

carbon black particles) and melanin are pigments. The distinction is important biologically because *exogenous dyes and pigments introduced into the body meet different fates.* We will return to this topic in the chapter on inflammation (p. 314).

Exogenous Pigments in Everyday Life: Some Examples

The prototype of exogenous pigments is carbon black, a polite name for soot. This homely topic has taught us some major biologic lessons, due to two of its properties: it is virtually harmless, and it is so black that even minuscule grains are visible under the microscope. In other words, it is an ideal tracer.

Our Daily Dose of Soot

City dwellers are condemned to breathe soot, which discolors the lungs for life. This blackening is called **anthracosis** (from Greek *ánthrax,* charcoal, in the lung, anthracosis is an example of **pneumoconiosis,** "lung-dust disease"). Any inhaled particles that measure less than 0.5 μm (138) can reach the alveolus, where they are engulfed by the resident alveolar macrophages. After this feat these macrophages acquire a new name, **dust cells** (Figure 3.37). Obviously they cannot remain in the alveolus, or the air spaces would soon be clogged. Most of them escape along the bronchial tree, whence they are swept out by the cilia and then swallowed or coughed out. In the mouse this cycle takes about 27 days (163).

> Surprise! Some of the swallowed carbon black can be picked up again in the gut (162). Dust particles have been found in Peyer's patches, where they are picked up by the M cells, phagocytic epithelial cells specialized in taking up macromolecules and even bacteria (p. 535). Another possible route from the lungs to the gut would be via the bloodstream, with leakage out of the venules in Peyer's patches (p. 317).

Despite the efforts of the dust cells, some carbon finds its way into the connective tissue spaces of the lung, which become loaded with blackened macrophages. The particles are carried across the alveolar barrier by two mechanisms: some are picked up and transcytosed by the flat epithelial cells lining the alveolus (Type 1 pneumocytes); experimentally, this can happen within 2 hours (57). More carbon is carried across by macrophages, which can also carry it back out, because miners continue to cough up black macrophages years after they leave the mine (57). Another batch of macrophages will carry some carbon via the lymphatics to the lymph nodes. But in the end, most of the carbon will remain trapped in the lung and in its lymph nodes until the host dies.

Macrophages do not live for a human lifetime. Exactly how long they live nobody knows; our guess is months or even years. When they die, another macrophage picks up the pigment released by the dead colleague and holds it until it is its turn to pass on. So the cycle continues. A few loaded macrophages may escape from a blackened lymph node, reach the thoracic duct, and plunge into the bloodstream. Some of these escapees may settle in the spleen, but most probably circulate until they die, at which time their load of pigment will be picked up by the littoral phagocytes (p. 316).

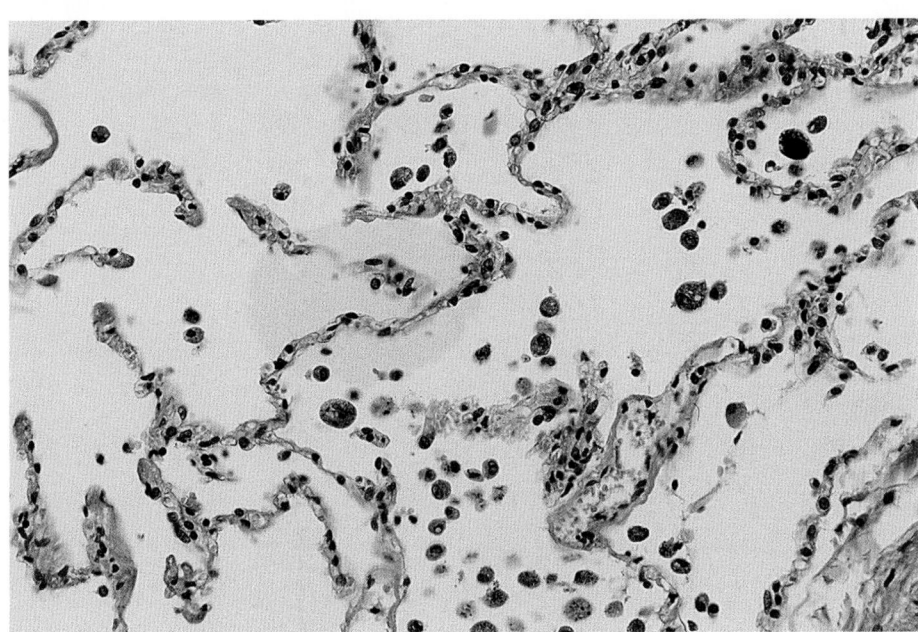

FIGURE 3.37 "Dust cells" in a human lung: large, oval cells in the alveolar spaces loaded with granules of carbon black, i.e., soot (top right). The dust cells as well as other macrophages in the alveolar spaces contain also brown granules of hemosiderin, possibly from an episode of bleeding in the lung. (180x)

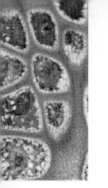

Soot is not an unusual sight in the human liver and spleen (149). This is a dead end for undigestible particles; which may seem inappropriate, but in the course of evolution there was little need to evolve a disposal route for circulating soot. Cities are a fairly recent development, and soot, after all, is messy but almost harmless.

Coal Miner's Lung

We mention here this condition to make the point that even "inert" coal dust—another black pigment—can

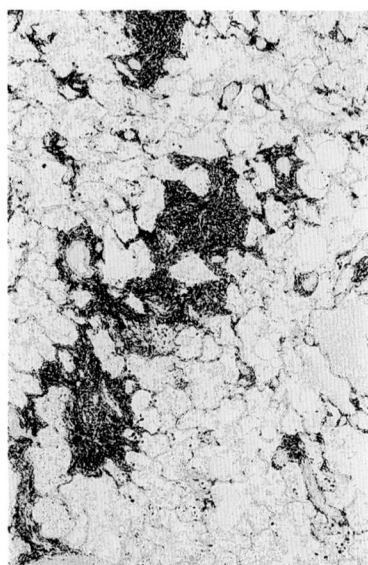

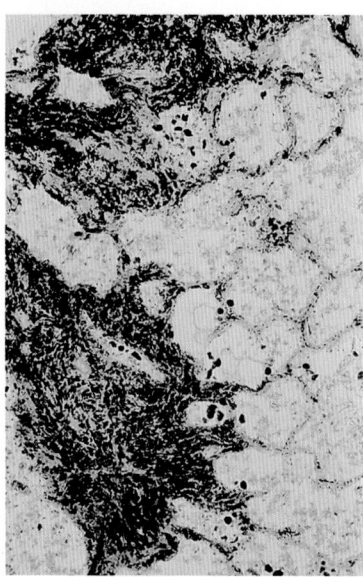

FIGURE 3.38   Sections of a miner's lung, lightly stained. The black material is carbon (coal), but these are early lesions: advanced lesions from the same lung would appear microscopically as solid black. The round, black dots free in the alveoli are single macrophages loaded with carbon.

kill (Figure 3.38). It destroys the lung, creating cavities filled with black fluid; the first paper on coal miner's lung was written in part with this fluid coughed up by a miner (140). Exactly why the lung tissue is broken down is not understood; the enzymes may be released by activated or dead macrophages, neutrophils, and/or bacteria. The sad story of coal miners' lung should be read; it did not end until 1969 (140).

Tattoos

Tattooing is another cultural exposure to carbon black and more colorful pigments. After the particles are pricked into the skin, they are taken up by the local macrophages, aided by a few monocytes attracted out of the blood stream by the irritation; but *the macrophages of the skin remain where they are,* unlike those of the lung. Tattoo artists exploit this provincial attitude of skin macrophages, which, if undisturbed, tend to live out their long lives in the same place (Figure 3.39).

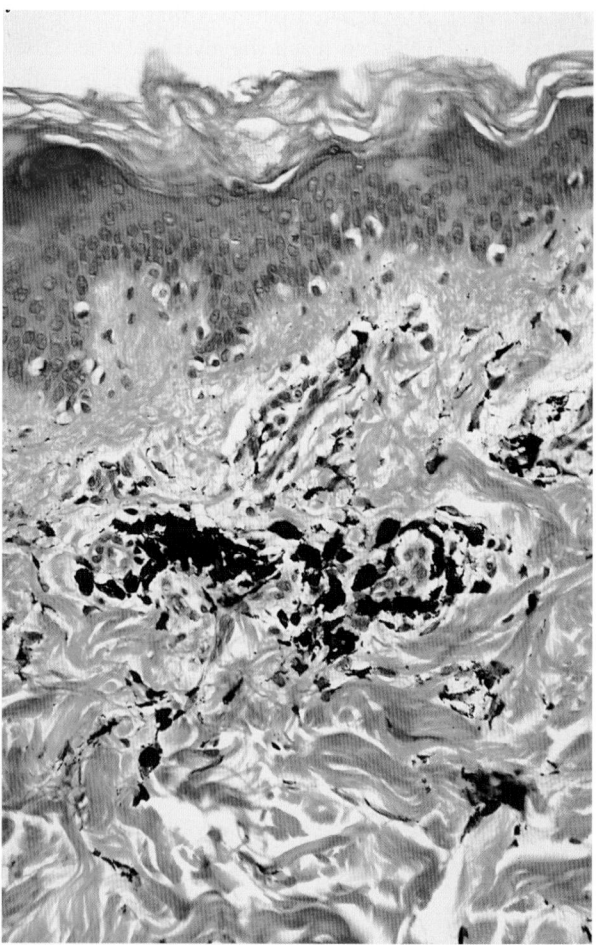

FIGURE 3.39   Tattooed human skin. The pigment is contained in clusters of black macrophages.

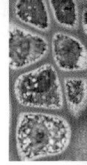

At the time of the tattooing operation, however, the skin becomes inflamed and swollen. The lymphatics come into action and gradually pump away the fluid, including some particles of pigment. As soon as the particles reach a lymph node, they are trapped because lymph nodes act as filters. Perhaps, over the years, a few more particles—either free or in macrophages—will reach the node (tattoos do tend to fade with time), but the vast majority of pigment-laden macrophages will hold their position in the skin.

Should the tattooed area become inflamed again in later years, the macrophages will rise to the call, move around, multiply, and pick up bacteria or other extraneous matter. Thereafter, many will be drained away by the lymphatics, oblivious of their artistic role. The tattoo will be smudged or partially erased (Figure 3.40) (155).

Historically, the filtering function of the lymph nodes was discovered by Virchow through the autopsy of a soldier whose arm had been tattooed 50 years earlier. The red pigment of the tattoo, cinnabar, was also present in the nodes of the axilla (164) (see Figure 1.4). This mechanism is biologically important because the lymph nodes are called to filter many unwanted particles, such as bacteria from foci of infection, and metastatic cells from malignant tumors.

Drug-Induced Discolorations

Several drugs lead to abnormal colorations even though the drug itself is not necessarily colored. **Tetracycline** is well known for its property of becoming deposited in calcifying tissues, where it can be recognized by its yellow color and its golden fluorescence (136). The antibiotic is incorporated in the enamel as well as in the dentin (136). If tetracycline is administered to a pregnant woman, it becomes deposited in the growing teeth of the baby; the result is an unsightly discoloration of

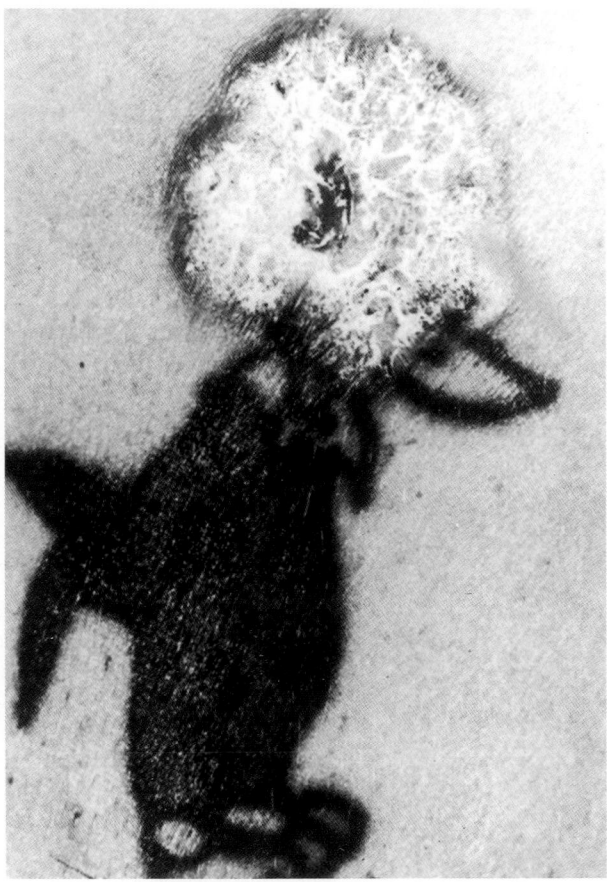

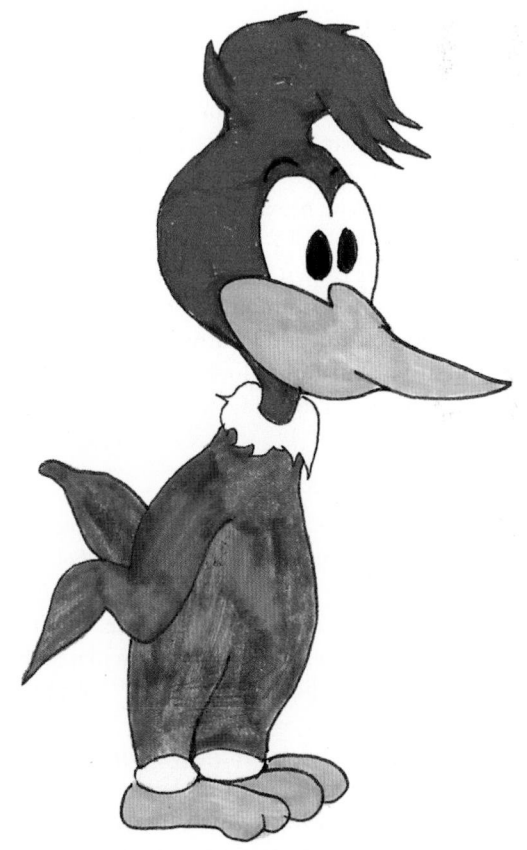

FIGURE 3.40 Macrophages become mobilized in inflammation. *Left:* Tattoo in the shape of Woody Woodpecker. At the top an accidental inflammatory reaction (dermatitis) has mobilized the macrophages, hence the drawing is scattered. *Right:* Control drawing for readers not familiar with Woody Woodpecker. [Reproduced with permission from Abel EA, Silberberg I, Queen D. Studies of chronic inflammation in a red tattoo by electron microscopy and histochemistry. Acta Dermatol (Stock) 1972;52:453–461.] (Drawing courtesy of William Silberberg.)

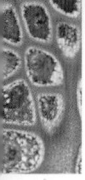

Table 3.1 Endogenous Brown Pigments

	Nature	Significance
Melanin	Polymer of hydroxyaromatics	In the skin: light protection Elsewhere: free-radical sink?
Lipofuscin	Polymer of oxidized lipids	Present in long-lived cells, index of aging, no "use" proven
Ferritin	Ferric oxyhydroxide (FeOOH) stored inside a protein hull	Principal storage form of iron
Hemosiderin	Denatured, partially digested ferritin	Present in secondary lysosomes when ferritin is stored in excess

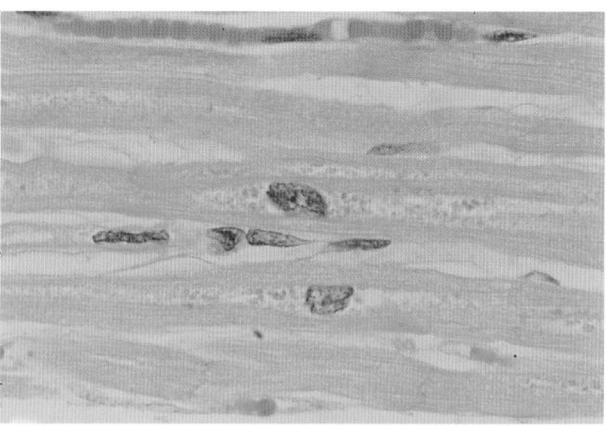

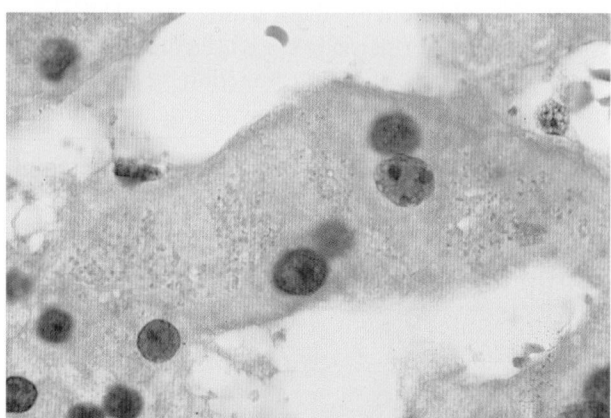

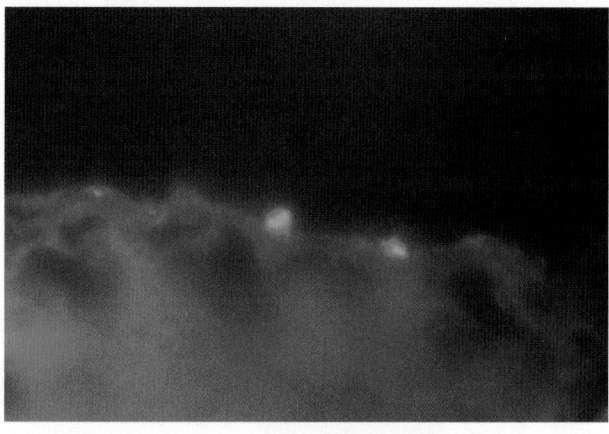

the deciduous teeth, and the development of the enamel is inhibited (**enamel dysplasia**). We once saw the jaw of a slaughtered cow stained bright yellow by a mistake in the commercial feed: a huge overdose of tetracycline. Silver nitrate intake causes a generalized pigmentation (**argyria**), described on page 279.

Endogenous Pigments

The gamut of colors available to mammalian tissues includes hues of yellow, brown, orange, red, and black; bile green is also available. Blue is underrepresented because the blue plasma protein ceruloplasmin is always too dilute to show up. The blue color of the iris and the sexual skin of certain monkeys is due to interference phenomena, not to a sky-colored pigment. Monkey "blue skin" appears brown if transilluminated.

The three most common endogenous pigments are lipofuscin, melanin, and ferritin/hemosiderin. Being brown and intracellular, they look deceptively similar in histologic sections (Table 3.1).

Lipofuscin

Lipofuscin, also known as age pigment or wear-and-tear pigment, is a very common, brown, granular, lipidic, intracellular material found in all animals, including worms and flies; even fungi have some. Because it increases in amount with age, it has fascinated biologists ever since it was discovered in 1842 (Figure 3.41) (150, 157, 167).

Lipofuscin is a reminder that living matter is transient. Life depends on oxygen, and cellular lipids are prone to peroxidation (p. 196), which makes them not only useless, but resistant to enzymatic breakdown. In cells, peroxidized lipids may come from two sources: (a) *Membrane phospholipids.* Mitochondria, the prime site of oxidative metabolism, are most exposed to oxidative damage. Cellular organelles are constantly recycled by autophagocytosis, but cross-linked lipids

FIGURE 3.41 Three aspects of lipofuscin. *Top:* Human myocardium; lipofuscin granules occupy the only space available, near the nucleus (hematoxylin and eosin stain). *Center:* Human liver cells (hematoxylin and eosin stain). *Bottom:* Two autofluorescent granules of lipofuscin, bulging from the endothelium of a human coronary artery (frozen section, examined by UV light). (Reprinted from Joris et al. Lipofuscin and lipid oxidation in human coronary endothelium. 1998;7:75–85. Copyright 1998, with permission from Elsevier Science.)

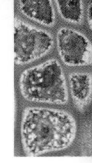

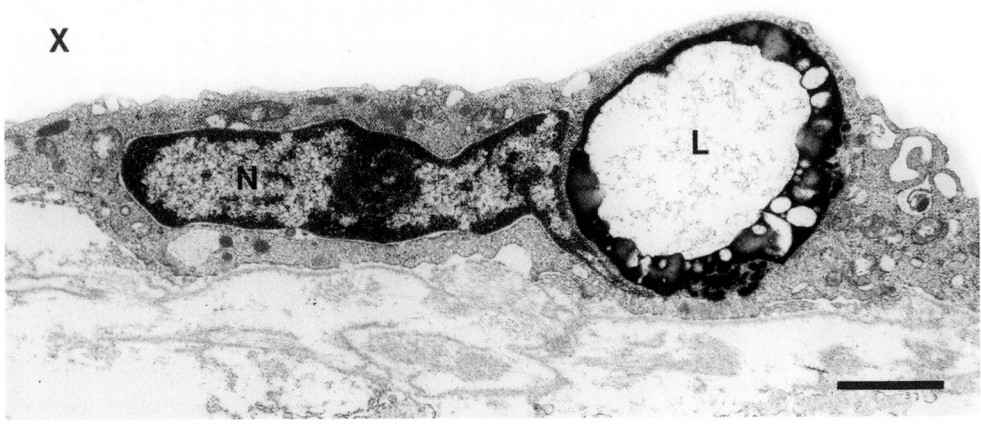

FIGURE 3.42 Lipofuscin in the endothelium of a human coronary artery, as seen by electron microscopy. **X** = arterial lumen. **N** = nucleus of endothelial cell. **L** = lipofuscin, derived from the oxidation of a lipid droplet (the central part was extracted during processing). **Bar** = 1 μm.

remain undigested; therefore every round of autophagocytosis will lead to an ever-increasing residue. (b) *Neutral fat* (triglycerides and cholesteryl esters). Droplets of neutral fat are present in normal human arterial endothelium (146), where they presumably arise by pinocytosis of lipoproteins (Figure 3.42). In these endothelial cells, it is easy to follow the slow peroxidation of the lipid droplets, proceeding from the periphery to the center.

A good way to understand lipofuscin is to compare it with linoleum. Linoleum, as its name implies, is obtained from linseed oil. The British citizen who invented it around 1860 discovered that if linseed oil is heated long enough in the presence of oxygen, it becomes darker and darker, less and less oily, and eventually turns into a solid. In more general terms, *if long-chain fatty acids are progressively oxidized, they gradually lose the typical properties of lipids. As their color slowly shifts from white to yellow to brown (Figure 3.43), they become less and less soluble in fat solvents, more and more cross-linked, and eventually turn into a solid mass.* The

hardening of oil-based paints is based on the same process (142).

The progressive "maturation" of lipofuscin explains one of its singular properties: it can be stained with fat stains even on paraffin sections, although lipids are supposed to be extracted during the paraffin embedding. Obviously, solvents such as xylene are not able to extract highly oxidized lipids.

By electron microscopy the granules of phospholipid-derived lipofuscin, such as in neurons or in the liver, are seen to lie in the so-called **residual bodies** (Figure 3.44) (p. 147), usually in the company of lipid

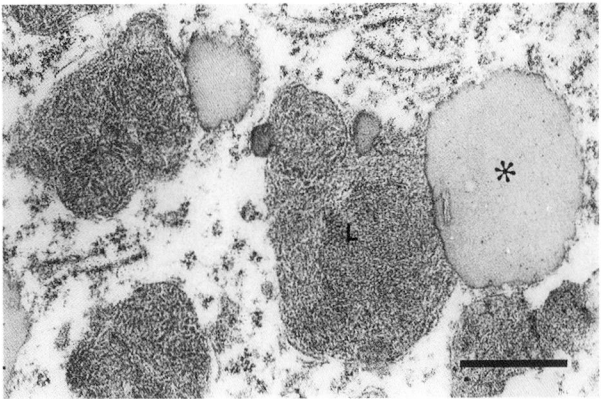

FIGURE 3.44 Granules of lipofuscin in a neuron of the human cortex, biopsied in the course of surgery for a brain tumor. The lipofuscin (**L**) here appears filamentous; it is contained in residual bodies that also include droplets of lipid (∗). **Bar** = 0.5 μm. (Courtesy of Dr. J. W. Boellaard, University of Tübingen, Germany.)

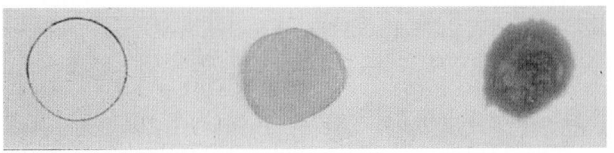

FIGURE 3.43 Progressive autooxidation of unsaturated fatty acids on filter paper. *Left circle:* Contains colorless fatty acids. *Center:* Same after 8 months' incubation at 37°C in room air; the spot begins to turn brown. *Right:* After 18 months. (Reproduced with permission from [143].)

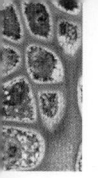

droplets, proteins, "fingerprint structures" (remnants of phospholipid membranes), and other poorly digestible materials, including melanin, as well as iron pigments (ferritin, hemosiderin), which may contribute to the further oxidation of the original lipid. The droplets of lipofuscin derived from neutral fat are not membrane bound (146).

Histologically, the best way to identify lipofuscin is to examine fixed frozen tissue under UV light: it becomes strikingly **autofluorescent,** usually gold or orange and, sometimes green (Figure 3.41c).

> The genesis of lipofuscin tells us that we cannot expect it to be a single, chemically defined compound. It is best conceived as a random polymer, in which other types of molecules are trapped or copolymerized (139). Histochemically, lipofuscin is basophilic and PAS positive; it can also be stained with acid fuchsin by the same acid-fast method used for *Mycobacterium tuberculosis,* probably because its lipid behaves much like the lipid of that bacterium (142). If treated with H_2O_2 it becomes further oxidized and thus even more autofluorescent; this helps to distinguish it from melanin, another brown endogenous pigment, that is bleached by the same treatment. Lipofuscin can be extracted with a powerful lipid solvent, chloroform-methanol (157).

Lipofuscin is abundant in neurons and myocardial cells, which can continue to accumulate oxidized lipids for as long as the individual survives. In the heart, the amount of lipofuscin increases progressively with age

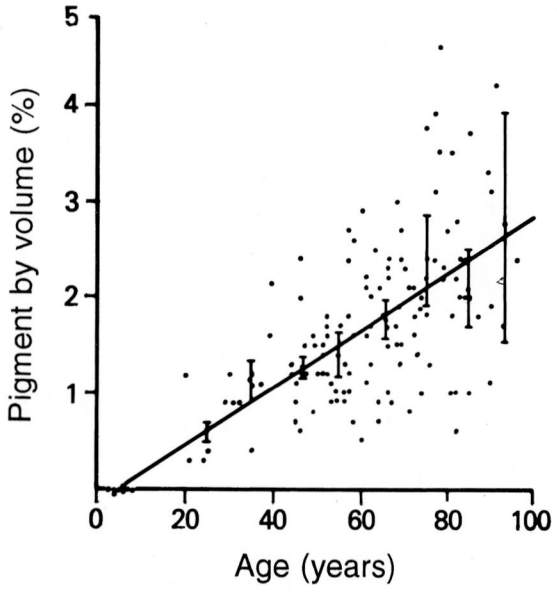

FIGURE 3.45 Progressive accumulation of lipofuscin in the human myocardium. (Reproduced with permission from [160].)

(Figure 3.45). Liver cells also contain a great deal of lipofuscin due to their long lives and high rate of autophagocytosis (a liver cell turns over all its organelles in less than a week [141]). Labile cells such as those of the intestinal epithelium, with a life-span of about two days, do not have a chance to accumulate metabolic wastes. However, there is lipofuscin in fruit flies, which live only 40 days or so, and in dogs it develops 5.5 times faster than in man. This rate is proportional to the shorter life-span of the dog, suggesting that lipofuscin is a marker not only of age but of physiologic or "relative" age (157).

Besides age, another factor enhancing lipofuscin deposition is a high metabolic rate. This was shown in nerve cells (137) and even in houseflies, which were cleverly kept at various levels of activity (158, 168). The very busy eye muscles of mammals are also particularly rich in lipofuscin.

What does lipofuscin mean to the cell? It is often stated that lipofuscin increases with age but does not *cause* aging. Yet, several theories of "lipofuscin damage" have been proposed (148); a recent study on cultured fibroblasts showed that proteasome activity was inhibited by added artificial lipofuscin (156). If lipofuscin does affect cell metabolism, it is probably a very sluggish effect.

Lipofuscin is involved in a few pathologic processes. The brownish color of atrophic organs, especially heart and liver, is due to abundant lipofuscin, which increases both relatively (atrophic cells shrink) and absolutely (atrophy involves autophagocytosis, which produces more lipofuscin); hence the term **brown atrophy.** *Deficiency of vitamin E leads to excessive deposition of lipofuscin in several organs* (154, 157). This is understandable because lipofuscin is generated by oxidation, and nutritional lack of vitamin E means lack of an antioxidant. The pigment accumulates especially (for reasons unknown) in the smooth muscle cells of the uterus and of the gut. Here is one scenario that may occur in chronic pancreatic disease: pancreatic insufficiency → malabsorption of fat → lost fat carries with it the fat-soluble vitamin E → avitaminosis E with deposition of lipofuscin in the muscularis of the gut → "*brown bowel syndrome*" (168).

Melanosis coli has nothing to do with melanin. It is a visually striking but harmless condition in which the mucosa of the entire colon (or sometimes just a segment) is uniformly black, with a sharp limit toward the small intestine. The pigment—a variety of lipofuscin—is contained in macrophages in the mucosa; its presence is associated with the prolonged use of cathartics of the anthracene group (cascara sagrada, senna, aloe, rhubarb)

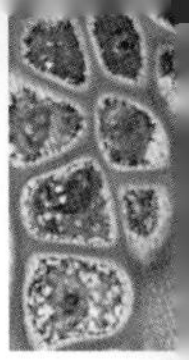

(159). An experimental study in guinea pigs suggests the following mechanism: intake of a given purgative → wave of cell death (apoptosis, p. 210) in the mucosal epithelium → phagocytosis of these dead cells by macrophages → loading of the macrophages with undigested lipid (165).

A rare group of inborn diseases of the nervous system, named **ceroid lipofuscinoses** (166), are hereditary encephalopathies in which brain cells and many peripheral cells store abnormally large amounts of lipofuscin; some pigment can be found even in the urine.

"Ceroid" versus lipofuscin. Ceroid is a confusing term that has probably outlived its usefulness (142) although not everybody agrees (151, 152, 153). The name was used in 1942 by Lillie to define a brown pigment seen in the liver of nutritionally deficient rats (139). Some experts then proposed that ceroid be applied to oxidized lipids of exogenous origin, and lipofuscin to oxidized endogenous lipids (147). Microscopically the two are not distinguishable and so the distinction is rather academic. It is useful, however, to remember that *exogenous lipids may also become oxidized and turn into brown residues* as they do *in vitro*. Such is the brown pigment found in the sinusoidal phagocytes (p. 316) of patients fed intravenously with a fat emulsion (161). Unsaturated fatty acids injected into the skin of a rat can be found a whole year later in the local macrophages as brownish granules (144). At that time some of the lipid is still extracellular; it has also become oxidized as a brownish mass, proving that the oxidation also can take place outside cells.

Melanins

Brown granules inside a cell could belong to one of three main families: lipofuscin, melanin or iron pigments. There are several varieties of melanin; all are random polymers of hydroxyaromatics. They are very ancient molecules and extremely stable: melanin was found in the ink sacs of a fossilized squid that died 180 million years ago (177, 179). Although melanin comes from the Greek *mélas*, "black," not all melanins are black. In mammals the prevailing type is the dark brown **eumelanin** (roughly "melanin proper"); a subtype of eumelanin is neuromelanin, found in the nervous system. **Phaeomelanin** is yellow or red (*phaiós* is Greek for grey; the ancient Greeks had no word for brown).

Eumelanin and phaeomelanin. Eumelanin is the brown-black pigment of the skin (174, 176, 177, 188, 189); for this reason the main impact of melanin on humankind has been, alas, in the form of social pathology. Eumelanin is present not only in the skin and hair but also in the pigmented epithelium of the eye and in the meninges (where melanomas occasionally arise), in a row of nuclei along the brain stem (the substantia nigra and the bluish-black locus coeruleus owe their color and their names to melanin), in the chromaffin system (adrenal medulla, sympathetic ganglia), and in a few other sites.

The reader may have enough recollection of embryology to remember that *the melanin-containing organs just listed are all of ectodermal origin, like the nervous system.* The pathophysiology of melanin includes many links between the nervous system, adrenals, and skin. Just consider some of melanin's precursors: epinephrine, norepinephrine, and adrenochrome (Figure 3.46). We must also admit that these links are not self-evident; the skin, after all, could not be farther removed from the central nervous system. However, if there are still any skeptics who find it hard to believe that the melanocytes of the skin really have their ancestors in the central nervous system, Figure 3.47 provides final proof. This two-tone chick, which would normally be white, was born after an amazing feat of microsurgery by Nicole Le Douarin (180, 181). When it was still an embryo, a segment of its neural crest was replaced with a segment of neural crest from the embryo of a quail.

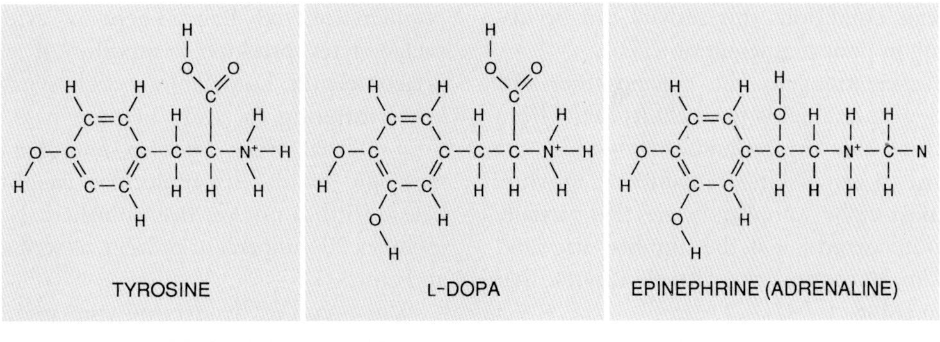

TYROSINE   L-DOPA   EPINEPHRINE (ADRENALINE)

FIGURE 3.46   Melanin, as inert as it is, has some very dynamic predecessors, namely neurotransmitters derived from tyrosine (dopamine, norepinephrine, epinephrine.) (Adapted with permission from [190].)

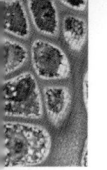

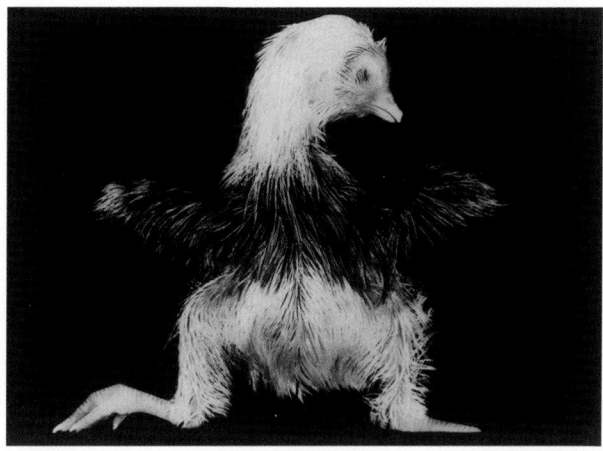

FIGURE 3.47   Proving the neural origin of melanocytes. When this white chick was an embryo, a segment of brown quail neural tube was grafted into its own neural tube, which resulted in a transverse stripe of brown quail color. (Reproduced with permission from [180].)

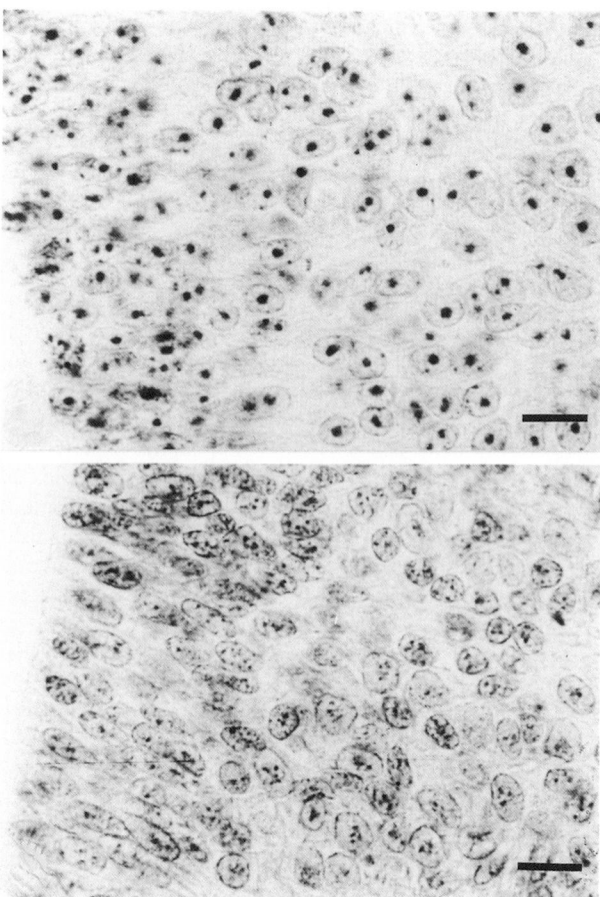

FIGURE 3.48   Distinctive appearance of heterochromatin in embryonic neuroblasts of two species of birds. *Top:* **Quail.** The heterochromatin forms a large centronuclear mass. *Bottom:* **Chick.** The heterochromatin is broken up in small scattered clumps. This difference makes it possible to follow the behavior and migrations of embryonic quail cells grafted into a chick. **Bar** = 10 μm. (Reproduced with permission from [180].)

Following its inborn schedule, the graft sent out cells that migrated to the skin, where they became melanocytes. The migrating cells can actually be traced in microscopic sections because quail cell nuclei have distinctive nucleoli (Figure 3.48). The grafted chick hatched normally but with a transverse band of brown, quail-type feathers; this zone had been colonized by swarms of melanin-forming cells that wandered out from the segment of quail neural crest.

The pigment in skin is produced by the melanocytes and packed in granules (**melanosomes**) which, by electron microscopy, are membrane-bound and have a characteristic structure (Figure 3.49). These granules are transmitted to the surrounding epithelial cells (**keratinocytes**) in a manner that may be unique in biology: *each melanocyte actively implants its granules into the body of the cells close to it* (Figure 3.50) (171). Under pathologic conditions this activity can be disturbed, resulting in poor pigmentation (176).

Once in the keratinocyte, the melanosomes surround the nucleus, presumably to shield its DNA from radiation. In black skin the melanosomes—which are larger than those in white skin—remain free; in white skin they are taken up by autophagosomes and partially degraded. In other words, it is the number, size, and distribution of melanosomes, not of melanocytes, that determines skin color.

Chemically, eumelanin is an insoluble polymer of tyrosine, and phaeomelanin is an alkali-soluble polymer of tyrosine and cysteine. The latter is the typical pigment of red hair. There is evidence that all melanocytes produce a mixture of eumelanin and phaeomelanin. Eumelanin is easily synthesized *in vitro* but frustrating to study because it is insoluble, has little internal order, and has few characteristic spectroscopic bands. Its molecular weight is unknown because it has not yet been purified. Natural melanin includes 20–50 percent protein, as well as copper, iron, and zinc.

When studied by electron spin resonance, melanin gives a signal characteristic of organic free radicals. It has been proposed that the free radical nature of eumelanin

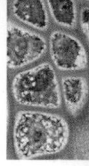

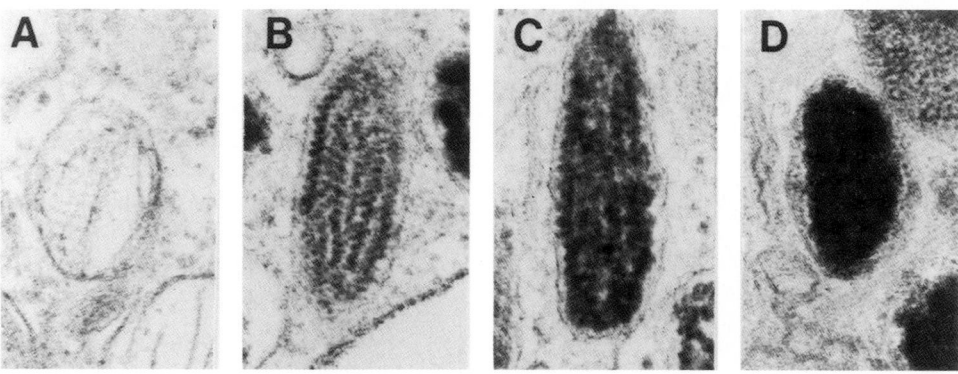

FIGURE 3.49   Four stages of melanosome development as seen by electron microscopy in cultured human melanocytes. The electron-dense material represents eumelanin. (~80,000x) (Reproduced by permission from J Am Acad Dermatol. Bolognia JL, Pawelek JM: Biology of hypopigmentation. 19:217–255,1988.)

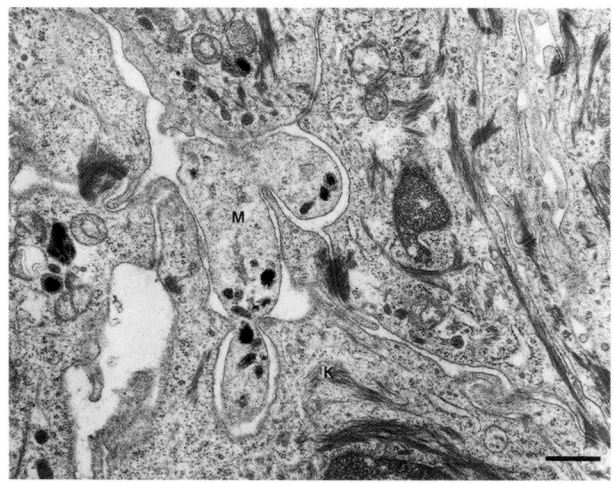

FIGURE 3.50   A natural autograft: a pseudopod of a melanocyte (**M**) containing melanosomes is being implanted into a keratinocyte. **K** = keratinocyte. In this particular case the grafting process is demonstrated in a basal cell carcinoma. **Bar** = 0.5 μm. (Reproduced by permission from [171] and S. Karger AG, Basel.)

is due to a quinone/hydroquinone/semiquinone equilibrium (174):

$$\text{OH} + \text{O} \rightleftharpoons 2 \text{O} + 2H^+$$

The redox properties of melanin have long been exploited in histochemistry. At pH 4, melanin granules reduce silver nitrate to metallic silver. This is the classic method for the histochemical detection of melanin (**Fontana reaction**), now being replaced by more specific but more expensive monoclonal antibodies.

Plant melanins are catechol melanins, unlike mammalian melanins, which are indole melanins (177). The blackening reaction of plants, as seen on a banana or a slice of apple, does not necessarily produce a polymer, but it does have links with melanin. Normally in plants, polyphenols and phenol oxidases are segregated in different compartments; when mixed as a result of damage, the oxidases turn the polyphenols into quinones, which are powerful oxidants and therefore antibacterial. As such, this reaction might be useful not only in plants (191) but possibly also in insects (192); nothing comparable is proven for mammals.

Neuromelanin, the melanin of the nervous system, is chemically a brown-black eumelanin like that of the skin. However, when studied by electron microscopy, it has no specific ultrastructure. *It is not segregated in specific pigment cells such as melanocytes but resides in neurons* where it is contained in residual bodies (Figure 3.51) together with lipofuscin (169). It is present in a row of nuclei along the brainstem; the total amount of neuromelanin tends to decrease with age (157, 170) because the neuromelanin-containing neurons decrease in number. The distribution of neuromelanin- and catecholamine-containing neurons is very similar (183); it is tempting to conclude that neuromelanin has the purpose of detoxifying some molecule of the catecholamine family. Catecholamines are derivatives of tyrosine, the basic monomer of skin melanin (see Figure 3.46). Other interesting facts: albinos do have neuromelanin, although they have little or no melanin in the skin and in the eye (they have eyesight problems);

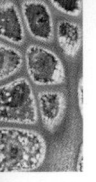

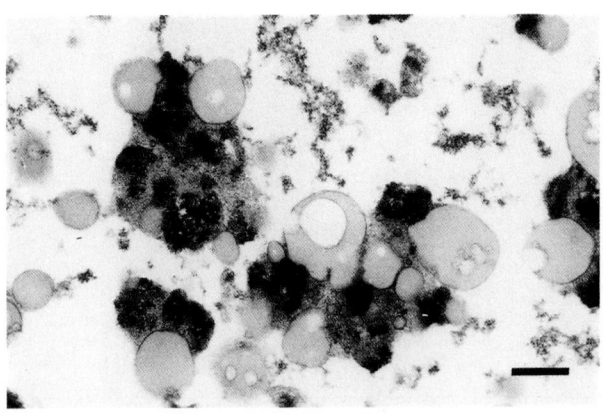

FIGURE 3.51 Residual bodies of human substantia nigra obtained at autopsy. The dark, electron-dense material is neuromelanin. **Bar** = 0.5 μm. (Courtesy of Dr. J. W. Boellaard, University of Tübingen, Germany.)

carnivores, including man, have the largest amount of neuromelanin; rodents have none (170).

Melanin and lipofuscin can be associated. About 70 percent of the brown pigment in the myocardium is lipofuscin; 30 percent is melanin. The two pigments are associated also in the nerve cells (169), the liver, and possibly other organs (178, 184). What this correlation means is not clear, but there are similarities between the two pigments. Both are polymers resulting from the oxidative attack of certain substrates (amines and amino acids for melanin, unsaturated lipids for lipofuscin); the two processes might sometimes occur together and produce a mixed polymer (193).

The known functions of eumelanin are three:

- *Light absorption.* Eumelanin absorbs throughout the ultraviolet and visible regions of the spectrum;

it converts light to heat and in the process becomes oxidized and darker (188). In essence, black skin proves to be a sunscreen rated at 13.4 (177). The sunscreen effect is beneficial because ultraviolet rays are carcinogenic. Dark-skinned people are much less susceptible to melanoma and to epidermal cancers than whites. Damage to the dermis is also reduced: solar elastosis (p. 277) is much more prevalent in the skin of blond and red-haired individuals.

Suntan and sunburn result from ultraviolet (UV) radiation. UV rays are classified as UV-A, the longest (400–315 nm), which cause suntanning and very weak inflammation; UV-B (315–280 nm), which also tan but cause sunburn; and UV-C (280–200 nm), which are germicidal but do not reach the earth's surface (Figure 3.52) (177). Suntanning occurs in two phases: (1) within minutes of exposure to UV rays there is an immediate darkening due to oxidation of melanin; (2) this fades in 6–8 hours and is followed by increased production and transfer of melanosomes from melanocytes to keratinocytes, evident after 2 days (175).

- *Free-radical sink.* A great deal of speculation has grown around this property of melanin. There is a free-radical theory of aging: does this imply that melanin could prolong life? The answer appears to be no, but it is certainly true that black skin ages better than white. Oddly enough, eumelanin produces potentially damaging free radicals when exposed to light (188).

- *Ion-exchange resin.* Melanin granules do behave as lumps of ion-exchange material, but whether this amounts to a useful function is not clear. In practice, melanin, as an electron acceptor, binds many drugs, which act as electron donors. Among these are cocaine, epinephrine, the antidepressant phenothiazines (which block dopamine receptors) and especially chlorpromazine, an antidepressant used in

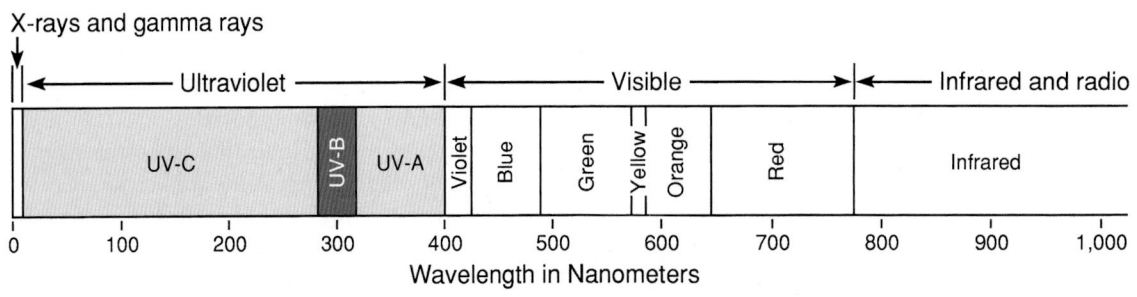

FIGURE 3.52 Electromagnetic spectrum, emphasizing the ultraviolet range. The wavelength band responsible for the most severe photobiologic effects is UV-B. The UV-A band contributes to tanning, and the UV-C band is germicidal. (Adapted from [187].)

the treatment of amphetamine poisoning. Patients treated with phenothiazines can develop an increased photosensitivity (176) and even a peculiar skin color ("purple people") (185).

Self-destruction of the melanocytes can be induced with certain drugs, which can therefore be applied locally to attenuate overpigmented areas. Among these is hydroxyanisole, a substituted phenol. Apparently the melanosomes accept it as a substrate for melanogenesis, whereby tyrosinase converts it to damaging free radicals that kill the melanocyte (186).

Pathology of melanin. *The pathology of melanin is largely a matter of increased or decreased pigmentation* (176, 177). In either case, many chemical agents are involved; the defect may be a side effect of a drug (such as a chemotherapeutic agent against cancer) or the result of industrial exposure (182), and it may be permanent. Not all the mechanisms are known.

The best understood mechanism of depigmentation (172) is the autoimmune destruction of the melanocytes. Compared with other epidermal cells, such as keratinocytes, the melanocytes are unusually susceptible to immune damage. The white patches of depigmented skin known as **vitiligo** (an ancient Latin name of unknown origin) are thought to arise by such a mechanism (p. 593).

Albinism, due to a congenital partial or total absence of melanin, is found in man and many animals including rodents, birds, fish, and reptiles; it is basically due to lack of tyrosinase.

Patches of increased pigmentation appear when the adrenals are destroyed (Addison's disease). The pituitary responds to the drop in adrenal cortical hormones by increasing its adrenotropic output, which includes two melanizing hormones: ACTH, primarily a cortical stimulant (which also happens to stimulate melanocytes), and MSH, primarily a *m*elanocyte *s*timulating *h*ormone (which is also a weak adrenal stimulant).

Melanomas are tumors of melanocytes; typically they retain their ability to make melanosomes and therefore appear as brown-black masses in man and other animals (Figure 3.53). At times, however, they contain so little melanin that they appear colorless and diagnosis is difficult unless special methods are used to detect a few telltale melanosomes (electron microscopy or histochemistry). If patches of vitiliginous skin are associated with melanoma, the prognosis of the melanoma is better (173): the reason should be obvious.

> **TO SUM UP:** Melanins are biologically important but little understood. Their physicochemical properties are frustrating. Much remains to be learned.

Ferritin and Hemosiderin

The rusty color of the two closely related intracellular pigments, ferritin and hemosiderin, reflects their vital function: iron storage.

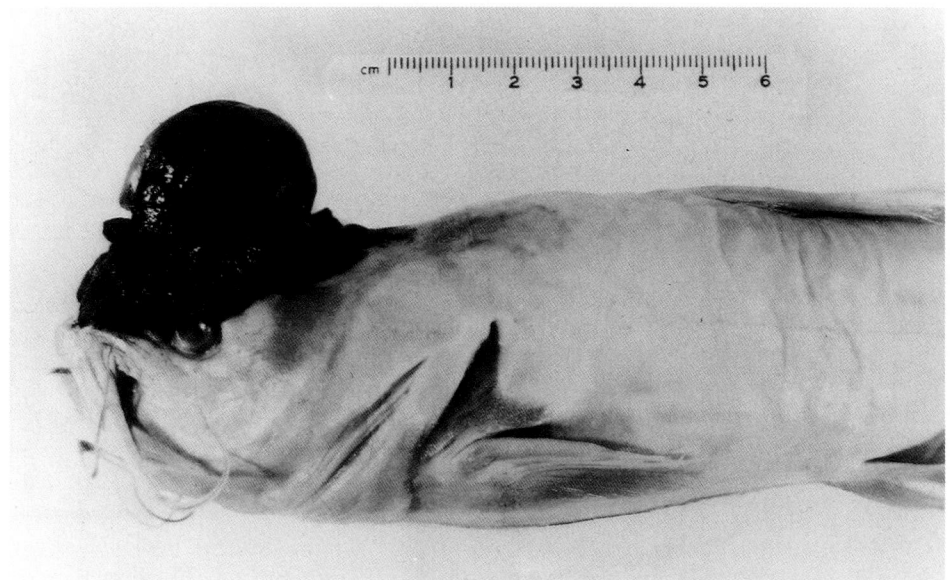

FIGURE 3.53 Brown bullhead with a primary melanoma of the head. (Courtesy of Dr. J. C. Harshbarger, Smithsonian Institution, Washington, D.C.)

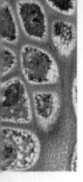

FIGURE 3.54 Economy of iron in the human adult. It involves balancing about 4000 milligrams in men and 3500 milligrams in women. Red blood cells carry 2000 milligrams and other cells about 1000 milligrams. The rest is stored in the liver, spleen, and bone marrow as ferritin and hemosiderin. Dietary absorption compensates for losses. It is assumed that there are exchanges between storage compartments and active compartments. (Adapted by permission from Nancy Lou Makris and from [203].)

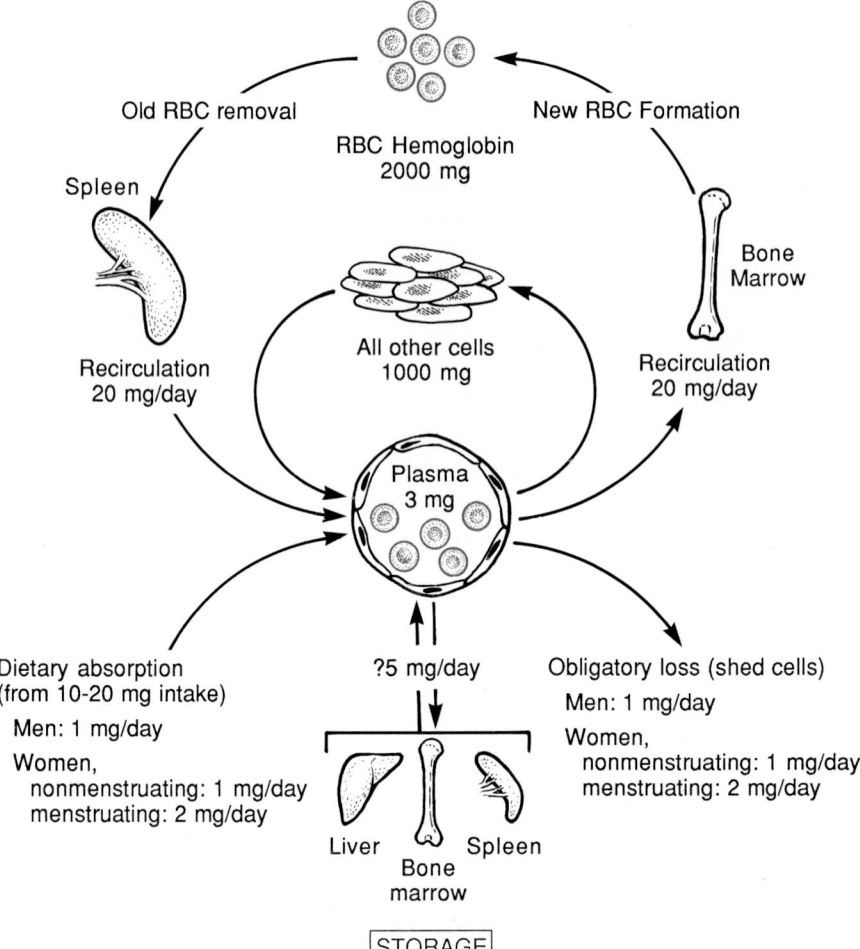

A glance at Figure 3.54 gives us some basic facts about iron metabolism. Note the tiny daily uptake: 1–2 millgram, balanced by an equally tiny loss. This means that *there is no major way out for iron,* beyond the traces lost by cellular desquamation (195, 207, 216, 223, 248). It also means that an iron reserve is essential to compensate for blood loss: the standard blood donation of 450–500 millimeter contains 200–250 milligram of iron (195, 226); if the donor had to depend on food for restoring the balance, at the rate of 1–2 milligram per day, recovery would be very slow. So we need an easily accessible store of iron: no simple matter, because iron, although essential, is extremely toxic (212, 235, 238) (p. 194). Nature solved this storage problem by creating a beautiful protein molecule shaped like a hollow bead, **apoferritin,** in which iron atoms can be safely stockpiled in the nearly insoluble trivalent form, yielding **ferritin** (Figure 3.55). This brilliant solution is so ancient that apoferritin can be produced by virtually all cells in animals and plants, in the latter as **phytoferritin** (202, 203, 208, 230).

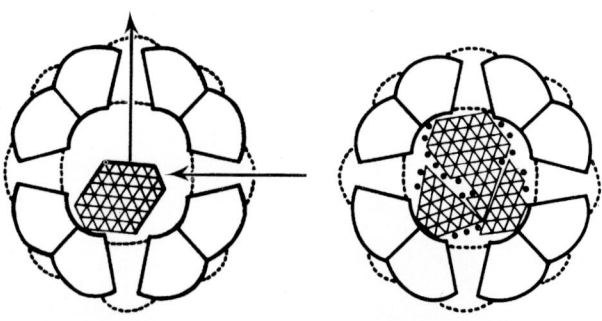

FIGURE 3.55 Cross section of two molecules of ferritin. *Left:* Molecule containing a single crystal of ferric oxyhydroxide. *Right:* Inner space nearly filled with crystals. Dots represent phosphate and other ions bound to the crystal surface. (Reproduced by permission from The Ciba Foundation (Iron metabolism; vol 51) and Elsevier/Excerpta Medica/North-Holland, Amsterdam [217].)

In a test tube and in dense intracellular deposits ferritin is brown. Fine deposits are invisible by light microscopy (unless stained histochemically for iron). The brown granules of iron-storing cells are autophagosomes loaded

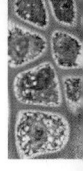

with semidigested ferritin; this material is called **hemosiderin,** a name chosen by Virchow. *Both ferritin and hemosiderin are normal products, but they can be present in excessive amounts* (230).

The ferritin molecule recalls certain viruses. It consists of 24 very similar cylindrical subunits assembled to form a box 130 Å in diameter with rounded corners and an internal chamber of about 70 Å (see Figure 3.55). On each face there are four subunits and a pore about 10 Å in diameter. Ferrous ions diffuse through the pores into the hollow core where they assemble in crystals of ferric oxyhydroxide (FeOOH) (196, 211, 217). Ferrous ions, however, cannot fit into the crystal lattice; thus *the Fe^{++} ions that diffuse into the pores are somehow oxidized to Fe^{3+} as they pass.* The reverse occurs when iron is extracted; this means that the reducing agents—whatever they may be— must diffuse into the pores and reach the surface of the crystal (Figure 3.55) (208). Iron can be mobilized from ferritin by superoxide from activated leukocytes (198).

The molecular weight of apoferritin is 441,000 daltons. The maximal loading capacity is about 4300 units of FeOOH (ferric oxyhydroxide), and the average ferritin molecule contains about 2000 of them. One or more crystals of FeOOH can be in the core; they also contain phosphate, perhaps as impurity. The protein subunits of apoferritin are of two kinds, H (for heart, or heavy) and L (for liver, or light); they are present in different proportions, which may explain the existence of several isoferritins (205).

By electron microscopy at very high powers, the protein shell of the ferritin molecules can be outlined by the procedure known as **negative staining** (Figure 3.56) (227). In ordinary transmission electron

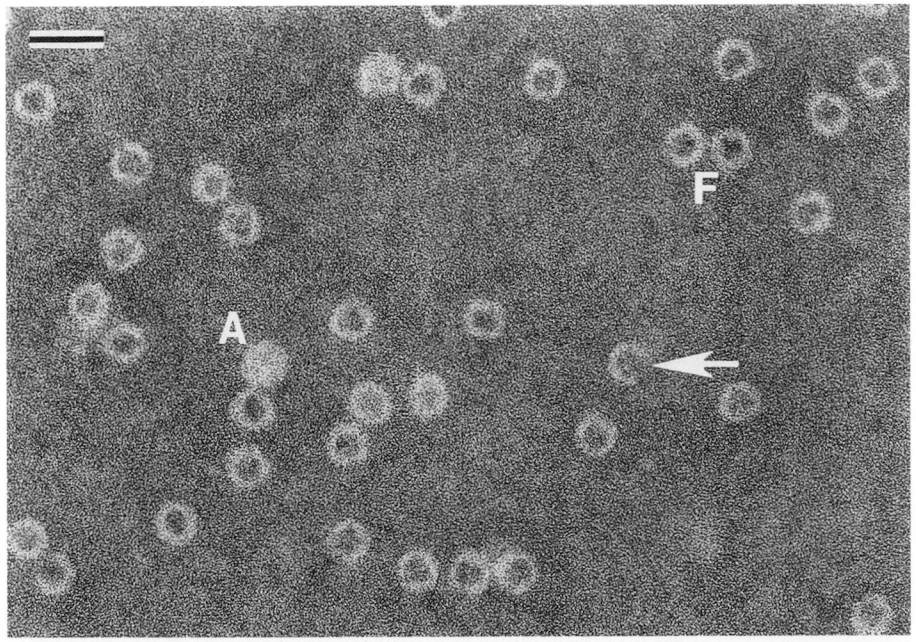

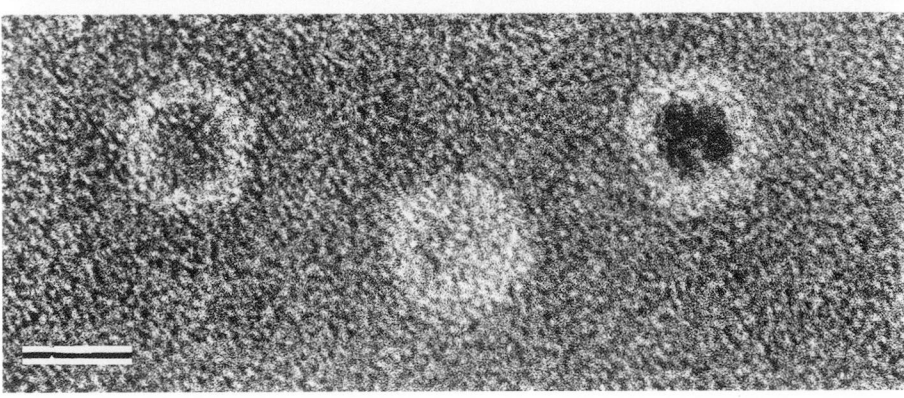

FIGURE 3.56 Ferritin molecules, negatively stained and seen by high-power electron microscopy. *Top:* The light rings represent the protein shell. **Arrow** points to a broken shell. **F:** Molecules loaded with iron. **A:** Molecule free of iron or not penetrated by the contrast medium. **Bar** = 200 Å. *Bottom:* The dense core at the left represents either a moderate iron load or penetration of the contrast medium. In the center is an apoferritin molecule without contrast. At the right, ferritin is heavily loaded with iron. **Bar** = 100 Å. (Reproduced with permission from [227].)

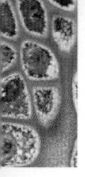

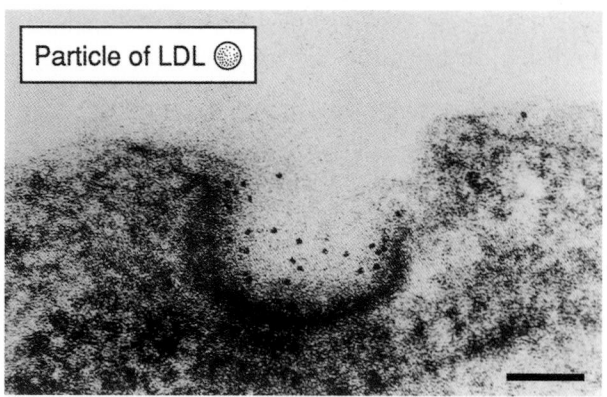

FIGURE 3.57   Ferritin as an electron microscopic label for invisible macromolecules. A pit in the membrane of a human fibroblast is picking up LDL particles, the size of which is indicated in the inset. The particles themselves are invisible, but the ferritin label indicates that they are present. **Bar** = 0.1 μm. (Reproduced with permission from [236].)

micrographs the shell is too transparent to create an image, but the iron core stands out as a tiny dot, which makes it one of the few molecules directly identifiable by electron microscopy. This property is exploited experimentally; when it is necessary to visualize macromolecules that are invisible by themselves, a standard trick is to bind them to ferritin molecules (Figure 3.57).

Histochemical reactions. Both ferritin and hemosiderin react positively to the histochemical test for iron. With ferric ferrocyanide they yield the beautiful Prussian blue (Figure 3.58). Red blood cells, however, remain red because the iron of hemoglobin is tightly bound within the heme and not available for the Prussian blue reaction (Figure 3.59).

> There is no histochemical difference between ferritin and hemosiderin; however, by light microscopy, a diffuse blue stain of the cytoplasm suggests free ferritin, whereas hemosiderin is present as granules, which correspond to phagosomes.

At autopsy, if the rusty color of an organ suggests the presence of excess iron pigment, it is easy to perform the Prussian blue test; a positive test can be quite spectacular (Figure 3.60). An even simpler but malodorous procedure is to wipe the surface of the tissue with ammonium sulfide: histochemically reactable iron instantly turns black due to the formation of iron sulfide. Both these color reactions date from the mid-1800s (231). Iron sulfide is also responsible for the black discoloration seen especially on the underside of the liver at autopsy. In this case H_2S is provided by colonic bacteria.

Pathology of Iron Overload
Local Iron Overload

When red blood cells are spilled into the collagen jungle of the tissues, they survive for some time: a few hours up to a few days. The local macrophages (seen by electron microscopy) do not seem particularly eager to attack these intruders, presumably because they emit few, if any, "eat me" signals (some do hemolyze). Each macrophage can take in several red blood cells. As the phagosomes digest the hemoglobin, electron

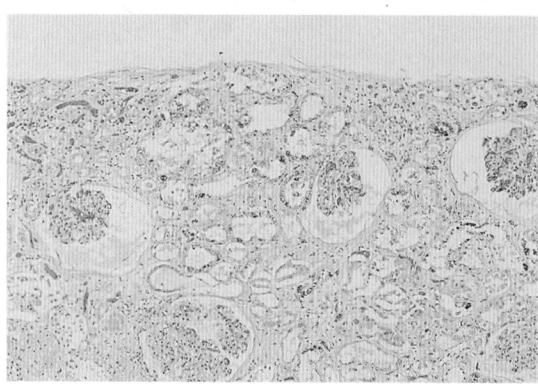
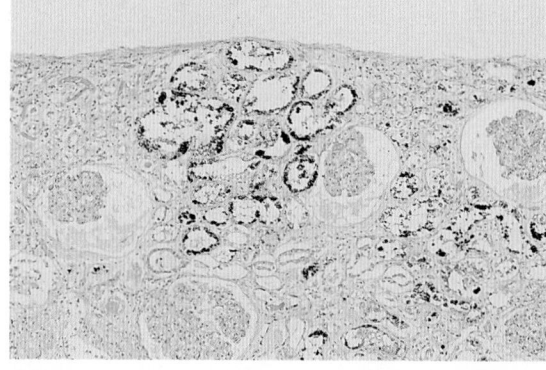

FIGURE 3.58   Hemosiderin in a human kidney due to chronic, low-grade hemolysis caused by a metallic prosthetic aortic valve (St. Jude valve). *Left:* The brown deposit in the tubules is hemosiderin derived from reabsorbed hemoglobin. (Hematoxylin and eosin stain). *Right:* Similar section stained for iron (Perls Prussian blue reaction.)

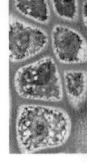

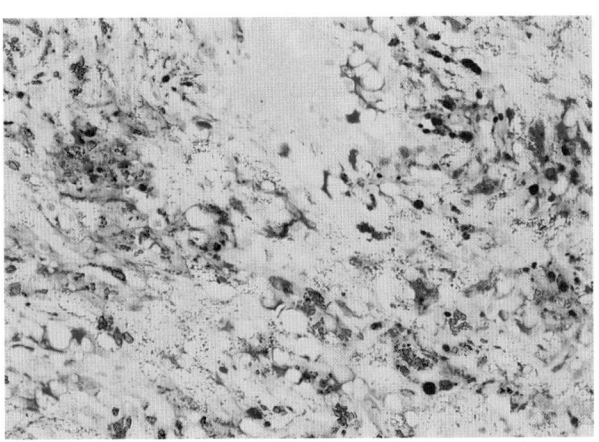

FIGURE 3.59 Human granulation tissue at the site of a hemorrhage (age unknown, probably weeks) (Perls Prussian blue reaction). The blue dots and streaks are macrophages loaded with hemosiderin. The clusters of yellowish grains are bilirubin, unstained because it contains no iron. *Top:* Red blood cells in a vessel fail to stain, because the iron of hemoglobin is tightly bound and unavailable to the histochemical reaction.

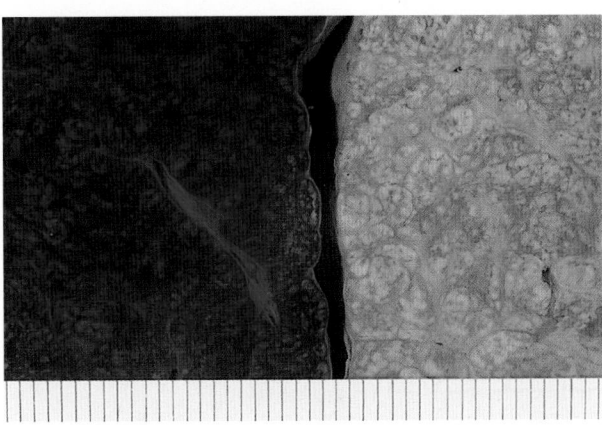

FIGURE 3.60 Two slices of the same cirrhotic liver, from a case of hemochromatosis. *Right:* Fresh, untreated tissue. The rusty color betrays the presence of iron pigments (hemosiderin, ferritin). Lighter dots represent areas of regenerating liver. *Left:* Similar slice after a histochemical reaction for iron. The resulting Prussian blue shows that iron is everywhere, in the stroma as well as in the liver cells. **Scale** in millimeters.

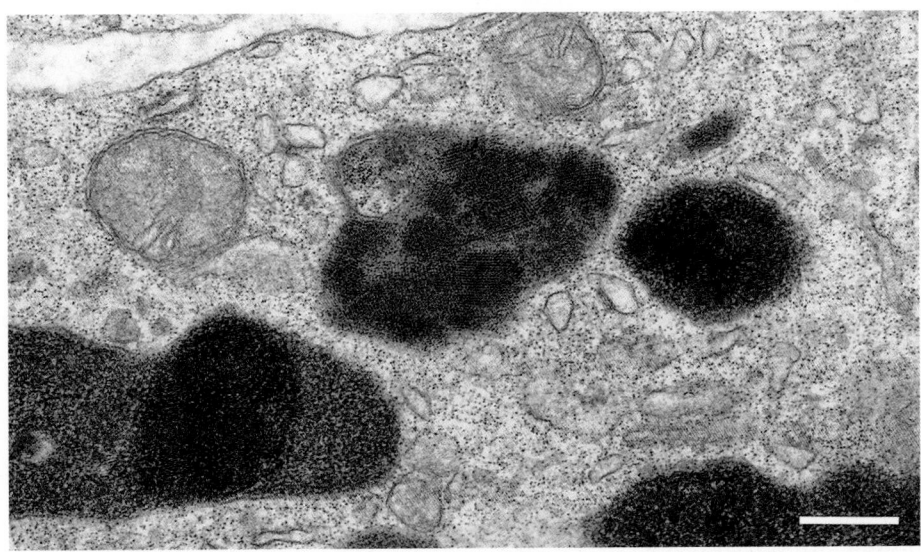

FIGURE 3.61 Part of a macrophage in the synovium of a human knee joint subjected to constant bleeding. Several siderosomes are shown, one containing crystalline masses of ferritin. No ferritin is recognizable in the others; it was presumably transformed into hemosiderin. Many of the small dots in the cytosol correspond to free ferritin particles; they are more electron dense than the ribosomes. **Bar** = 0.3 μm. (Courtesy of Dr. J. Bhawan, Boston University School of Medicine, Boston, MA.)

microscopy shows tiny black dots of ferritin crowding the cytosol of the macrophage (Figure 3.61): clearly the endoplasmic reticulum is responding by pouring out new molecules of apoferritin, which are capturing iron atoms as fast as they are removed from the hemoglobin (197). This response of the macrophage is very quick: experimentally, macrophages surrounding a mass of injected particles of iron oxide show cytoplasmic ferritin molecules within 4 hours (234); in tissue culture, the delay shrinks to minutes (204).

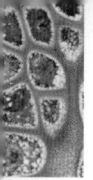
Now **autophagocytosis** sets in: here and there the endoplasmic reticulum of the macrophage sprouts a double membrane that surrounds a parcel of cytoplasm filled with ferritin molecules and sequesters it to form a typical autophagosome, also called a **siderosome** (234). The iron-loaded ferritin molecules are being strained out and condensed into brown granules of hemosiderin. By electron microscopy the siderosomes contain some recognizable molecules of ferritin, sometimes even crystallized, mixed with dense debris of partially digested ferritin and loose iron cores of ferric hydrohydroxide, FeOOH (Figure 3.61).

Ferritin and the siderosomes represent the iron store, which contains 20–25 percent of the total body iron (see Figure 3.54). A busy molecule, **transferrin** (214, 219), acts as a shuttle between the sources of iron and cells that need it: iron absorbed from the gut passes into the blood, where it is taken up by transferrin.

> Compared with ferritin (which can hoard a "truckload" of iron, up to 450,000 atoms), transferrin is rather like a bicycle: it can carry only two atoms. Cells that need iron for their own use bind transferrin to their membrane by means of specific receptors, the receptor complex is internalized, the iron is released, and the transferrin is returned to the surface for recycling.

How long does it take for ferritin and hemosiderin to develop from spilled blood? The question could be of medicolegal importance in determining the age of an injury (221). Experimentally, after an injection of blood into the skin, a positive Prussian blue reaction was found after 24 hours in rats and mice (229) but not in rabbits (225). In humans, the first histochemically detectable traces were found after 50–72 hours (239). *At the biochemical level,* as we mentioned earlier, the time required for apoferritin synthesis is on the order of minutes. We can conclude that the delay between bleeding and the appearance of histochemically demonstrable iron depends on the sensitivity of the method. With routine stains, it lies somewhere around 24–48 hours.

> NOTE: *The macrophages at a site of injury do not retain their hemosiderin forever;* it slowly disappears—over months—presumably because the iron is slowly transferred to the macrophages of the bone marrow and spleen, the appointed custodians of the iron bank. How this transfer of capital between macrophages is organized is not known.

The "pathology of the black eye" due to hemoglobin breakdown makes one wonder whether the beautiful display of leaf colors in autumn may be due to a comparable *chlorophyll breakdown.* The answer is yes and no: the yellows and oranges are due mainly to carotenoids, normally present in the leaves but masked by the chlorophyll, and to phaeophytins consisting of chlorophyll that lost its magnesium. Some trees synthesize blue pigments (anthocyanins), possibly as a sunscreen to prevent chlorophyll from generating injurious free radicals (209).

Systemic Iron Overload

This serious affliction can be either congenital (**genetic hemochromatosis**) or accidental (**secondary hemochromatosis,** formerly called hemosiderosis) (195, 203, 218, 226, 233, 237, 238). In either case the same organs are affected, but the damage is more severe in the congenital form.

Genetic hemochromatosis, an autosomal recessive disease, is widely thought to be rare, but in fact *it is the most common genetic disturbance;* its prevalence is about 1:300. Heterozygotes are not affected, but their prevalence is 1:20 (237). Hemochromatosis patients (9:1 males/females) absorb every day, for reasons unknown, 1–3 extra milligrams of iron; over the years this excess leads to deposits of hemosiderin—and corresponding damage—in many tissues, especially in the joints (hence joint pains), liver (cirrhosis, see Figure 3.60), heart (fibrosis), endocrine glands (diabetes, hypothyroidism), and skin (a brownish discoloration, due to hemosiderin and melanin). The combination of diabetes and darkened skin has given this disease the surname of **"bronze diabetes."** This is unfortunate, because in many cases an early symptom is **joint pain,** and by the time the "bronze" and the diabetes appear, the articular cartilages are badly damaged. Future physicians beware.

> The mechanism of articular damage: iron inhibits the joint enzyme pyrophosphatase; this allows crystals of pyrophosphate to develop, leading to chondrocalcinosis (p. 260). Mechanisms of damage in other tissues include iron-induced peroxidation of membrane lipids, impairing the function of mitochondria (212), lysosomes, and other organelles (194, 232). Fibrosis is attributed to iron-induced stimulation of collagen synthesis (237).

In the early stages, the treatment is fairly straightforward; in fact, it is based on the classic Hippocratic method: repeated bloodletting, to remove the excess iron (195, 226).

Secondary hemochromatosis occurs most frequently as a result of repeated blood transfusions. Imagine a patient with a chronic form of anemia that

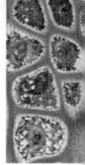

requires repeated transfusions; and remember that iron has no way to leave the body—except in minimal amounts. Each transfusion provides 200–250 milligram of additional iron; as a result, deposits of hemosiderin develop throughout the body, as in the congenital form, with slight differences (e.g., in the liver, most of the hemosiderin is in the Kupffer cells rather than in the liver cells) (195, 226).

Iron, Hemolysis, and Infection

Intravascular hemolysis occurs in many settings and involves much more than iron overload, but we should briefly mention it here because it shows very clearly the countermeasures of the body: (a) retrieval of the hemoglobin for the amino acid pool and (b) retrieval and recycling of the iron atoms. Follow the diagram of Figure 3.62.

(a) *Retrieval of hemoglobin.* If many red blood cells are lost by intravascular hemolysis, some of the hemoglobin dissolved in the plasma inevitably escapes through the glomeruli (remember that the glomerular filter is permeable to molecules smaller than ~60–70 kilodaltons, and hemoglobin is about 40 kilodaltons). However, on its way out along the kidney tubules, some of the hemoglobin is recovered by endocytosis (Figures 3.58, 3.62).

In the meantime, any hemoglobin that circulates free in the plasma is captured by a special protein, **haptoglobin** (*hápto* is Greek for "I bind"). The complex ends up in the liver, where it is recycled. If a great deal of free hemoglobin is present in the plasma, some of it is oxidized to **methemoglobin** (ferrihemoglobin), a chocolate-colored compound in which the four iron atoms are trivalent. Finally, some of the free hemoglobin will lose its hemes, but these too can be promptly captured by albumin and by the protein **hemopexin,** and again the complexes are recovered by the Kupffer cells.

Methemoglobin, when it is formed inside red blood cells, can be easily reduced to hemoglobin (220). When it develops in spilled blood it is presumably catabolized like hemoglobin. It is not recognizable microscopically. Lately it has become important in radiology due to its magnetic properties: recent brain hemorrhages are visible by nuclear magnetic resonance due to the contrast provided by their content of methemoglobin (199).

(b) *Retrieval of iron.* Now let us see what happens to the hemes, the custodians of the iron (Figure 3.63). It so happens that the four hemes carried by each hemoglobin molecule can be detached fairly easily from the globin.

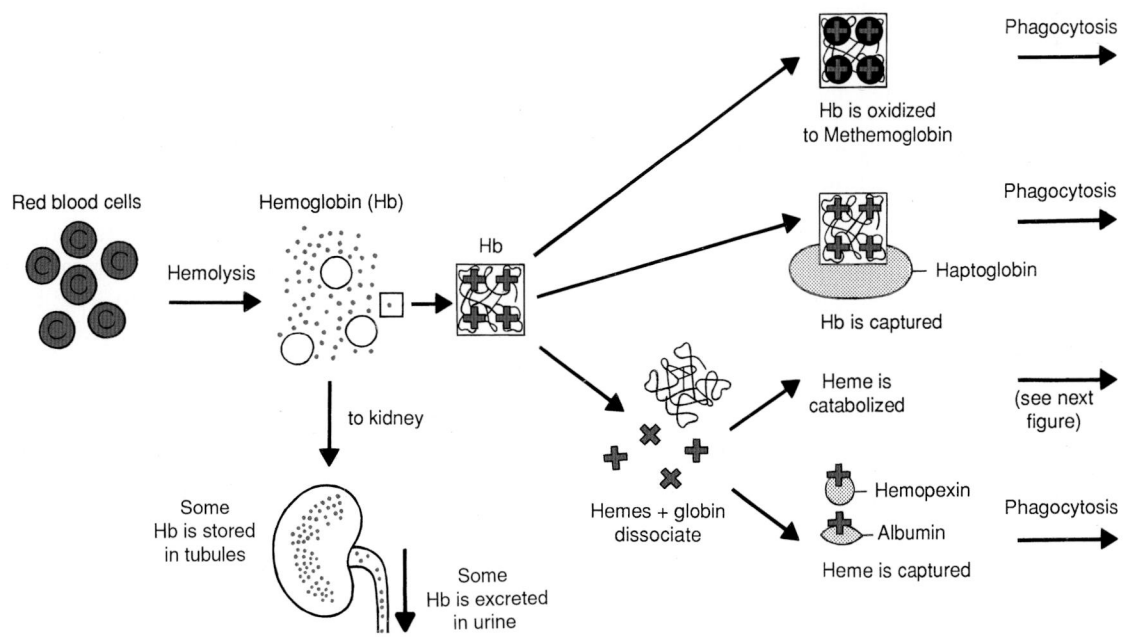

FIGURE 3.62 Possible fates of hemoglobin released by red blood cells. Any of the iron-containing molecules can be phagocytized. Phagocytosis (extreme right) is performed by the littoral or tissue macrophages.

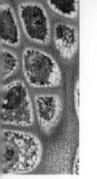

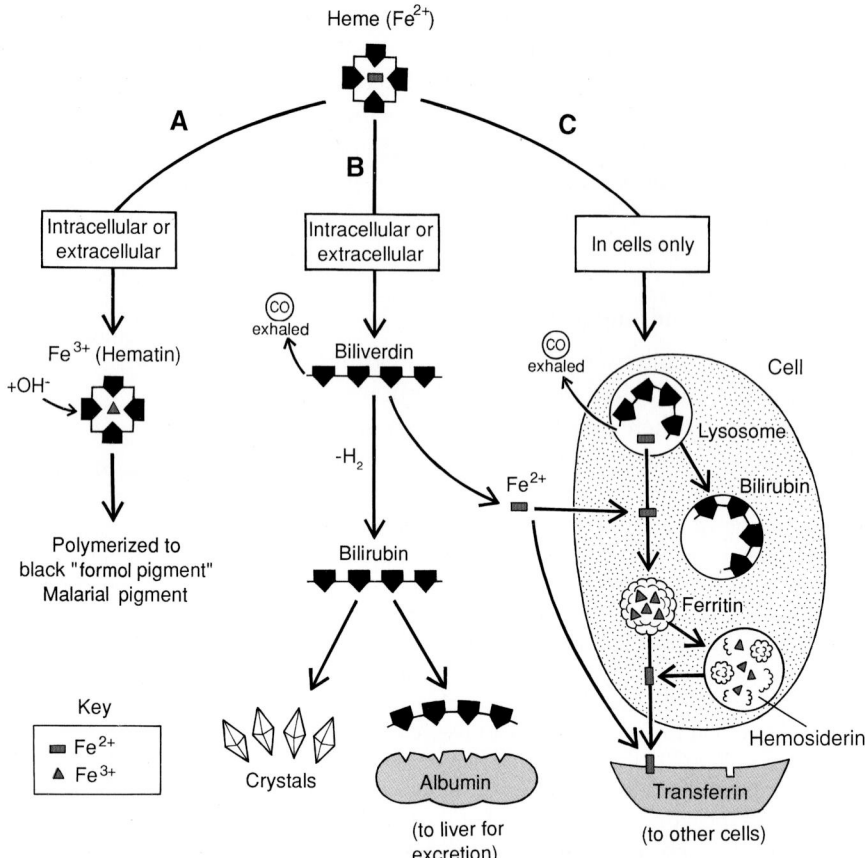

FIGURE 3.63 Three pathways contribute to the disposal of the heme molecule. **A:** The heme ring remains intact and polymerizes to black pigment. **B:** The heme ring is broken open and loses the iron; bilirubin is formed. **C:** The iron is incorporated into ferritin and recycled by transferrin.

Once they have left the globin, the hemes break open and the iron atom is freed. From then on, *the two parts of the original heme follow separate routes;* the broken ring gives rise to bilirubin (p. 117), and the iron finds its way into the surrounding cells, presumably by hitching a ride on transferrin molecules floating around.

One feature that runs throughout iron metabolism is the astonishing cascade of molecular traps set for catching free iron and iron-containing molecules (224). In summary:

- Free hemoglobin is bound by **haptoglobin** (1:1).
- Heme is captured by **hemopexin** (1:1).
- Excess heme is bound by **albumin** (2:1).
- Free iron in plasma is captured by **transferrin** (2:1).
- Free iron in secretions is captured by **lactoferrin** (2:1).
- Free iron is stored in **apoferritin** (about 4000:1).

What evolutionary pressures could have produced these trapping mechanisms? An obvious reason is the conservation of iron, but a strong case can be made also for the defense against infection (201).

Iron is so important for bacterial growth that it can be considered a virulence factor (200). When bacteria invade tissues, they find themselves in a world in which almost all the iron is hidden inside cells; there is some in the interstitial fluids, but it is almost entirely bound to transport proteins. What is left is far too little to support bacterial growth (215). Interestingly, transferrin was known as a bacteriostatic protein long before its role was understood. When it was added to bacterial cultures, it inhibited bacterial growth. Now we know that it did so by sequestering iron. To survive in such inhospitable juices, bacteria have elaborated complex iron-snatching mechanisms. Their main strategy is to secrete molecules called **siderophores** that have strong affinity for iron.

There is plenty of evidence that iron favors infection (240). In rats, a nonlethal dose of *Escherichia coli* injected into the peritoneum becomes lethal if accompanied by just 20 milligram of hemoglobin (Figure 3.64) (206). *Extensive hemolysis is associated with infection,*

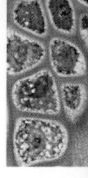

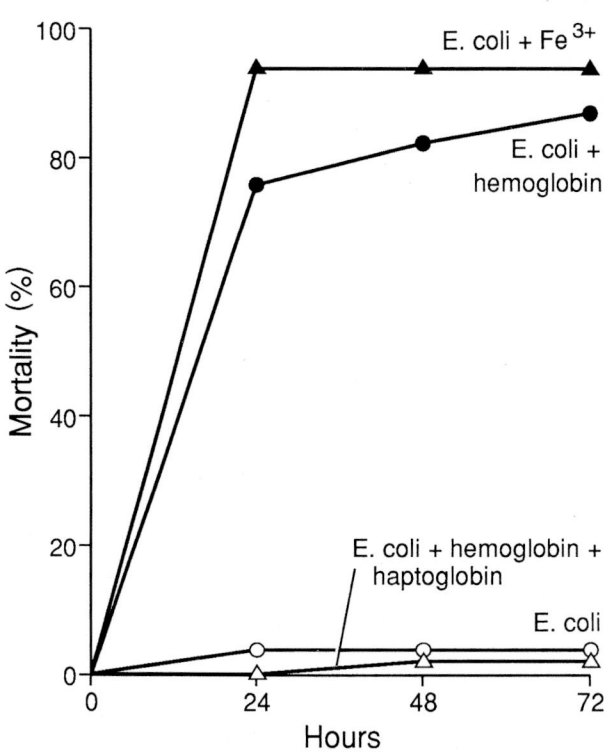

FIGURE 3.64 Iron favors infection. *Top two curves:* High mortality rate in rats inoculated intraperitoneally with 10^7 *Escherichia coli,* mixed with either Fe^{3+} or hemoglobin. *Two bottom curves: E. coli* injected alone, or with hemoglobin + haptoglobin, induces a very mild infection (no mortality). (Adapted by permission from [206]. Copyright 1982 by the American Association for the Advancement of Science.)

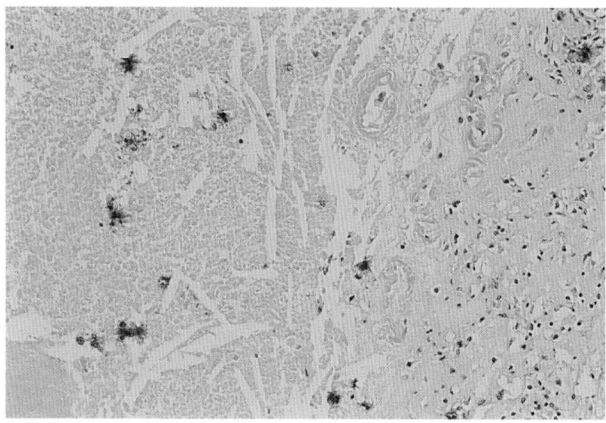

FIGURE 3.65 Clusters of yellow-brown bilirubin crystals at the edge of a spleen infarct (*left*). The empty "cracks" are the negative images of cholesterol crystals, often seen in necrotic tissue. The nuclei at right belong mainly to macrophages surrounding the infarct.

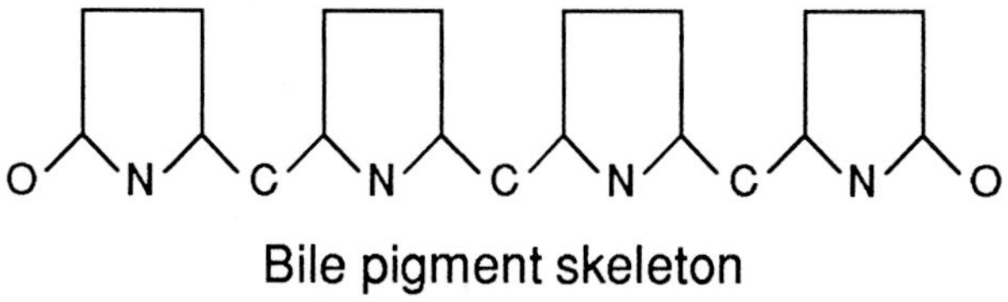

Bile pigment skeleton

FIGURE 3.66 Skeleton of bile pigments. The porphyrin ring is broken open and the iron atom is lost. (From Hematin compounds and bile pigments, Lemberg R, Legge JW (eds) [250]. Copyright © 1949 John Wiley & Sons. Reprinted by permission of John Wiley & Sons, Inc.)

especially in the peritoneum: a classic setting is the seepage of blood and bacteria into the peritoneal cavity from a strangulated loop of intestine (224). "Iron sepsis" can occur after an overdose of iron (228) and in infants even after therapeutic doses (206). A similar irony is that the well-meant refeeding of starved populations with low plasma transferrin levels may lead to saturation of transferrin and to increased attacks of malaria, suggesting that protozoan infections are also enhanced by iron (224). Hypoferremia may be an adaptation in parts of the world where infections are prevalent (222).

Once again, more is not necessarily better.

Bilirubin

If melanin influenced the course of history, bilirubin did so too, in a different way. As the name implies, bilirubin

is the pigment of mammalian bile. Its bright yellow color (Figures 3.59, 3.65) struck the imagination of the Greeks and the Hindus so strongly that they considered "yellow bile" to be one of the four basic components of the human body. We still refer to this theory when we accuse someone of being bilious (252).

Bilirubin (249) *is a stack of porphyrin rings that broke open and lost their iron* (Figure 3.66). Once broken, the beautiful porphyrin ring can never be mended and must be eliminated through the bile (Figure 3.63). When this exit is obstructed or overwhelmed, bilirubin levels in the blood rise and cause jaundice.

Genesis of bilirubin. Bilirubin can be formed anywhere in the body. It has been difficult to eradicate the erroneous belief that bile pigments are formed only in the liver—even Virchow knew better (256). The pathway from heme to bilirubin implies two major steps (244, 245, 247, 250):

1. *Breaking open the heme ring,* an oxidative reaction. In the process, the iron atom drops off, and the resulting molecule is **biliverdin.** The broken methene bridge is lost as carbon monoxide (CO). This CO is partly eliminated by the breath, so expired CO can be used as a measure of hemoglobin breakdown.

2. *Reducing biliverdin to bilirubin.* Because all cells contain heme proteins as cytochromes, any cell type can form bilirubin during the catabolism of these particular proteins. Macrophages, however, produce bilirubin from heme on a much larger scale when they digest red blood cells; this is why intracellular and extracellular bilirubin always appear—in due time—around spilled blood (Figures 3.59, 3.65).

Virchow noticed its colorful crystals and reasoned that they were probably bilirubin; however, he was not absolutely sure, so he called it **hematoidin** (the name is now being dropped). He was quite carried away by its color (257).

Hematoidin is one of the most beautiful crystals we are acquainted with. . . . When a young woman menstruates, and the cavity of the Graafian vesicle, from which the ovum has been extruded, becomes filled with coagulated blood, the haematine [hemoglobin] is gradually converted to haematoidine, and we afterwards find at the spot where the ovum had lain the beautiful deep-red colour of the haematoidine crystals, which remain as the last memorials of this episode.

NOTE: Bilirubin is orange-red when very concentrated: bilirubin stands for "bile red".

A yellow rim of bilirubin is commonly seen grossly in masses of necrotic tissue such as recent infarcts, 1–2 millimeter within the edge. This is not easily explained because heme breakdown is commonly described as an enzymatic intracellular process, and as such it should not occur in dead tissue. We propose to reconcile the facts as follows. The initial oxidative opening of the heme ring can be obtained also *in vitro;* it requires molecular oxygen and a reductant (so-called coupled oxidation) (254). The next, reducing step does require an enzyme, but enzymes might still be floating around in an area of cells that just died, and the proper combination of oxidation and reduction might well exist precisely at the periphery of an infarct.

Light microscopic appearance. The diagnosis of bilirubin is suggested by extracellular golden needles and rhomboids around a not-so-recent hemorrhage. Tiny, yellowish granules or crystals in macrophages can be distinguished from ferritin and hemosiderin if an iron reaction is negative: of course, bilirubin contains no iron (see Figures 3.59, 3.66). Still used is the Gmelin reaction with nitric acid proposed in 1826 by the German chemist Gmelin, who also invented the terms *ester* and *ketone.*

There is a peculiar discrepancy in the behavior of bilirubin. Around a mass of spilled blood one would expect that the two heme-derived pigments, ferritin and bilirubin, would appear in roughly similar amounts and at the same time. They do not. In tissue sections, bilirubin appears late, in small amounts, and sometimes not at all. Perhaps it is easily carried away by albumin, or perhaps it does form (we do see a lot of yellow in a bruise) but being fat-soluble it is dissolved out of the tissue during the embedding procedure. Bilirubin can indeed be extracted from tissues with chloroform (256).

Toxicity. Bilirubin is very toxic. Oddly enough, its precursor biliverdin is harmless. Birds and reptiles wisely stop the heme breakdown at that point and simply eliminate the green pigment in the bile, but mammals take the trouble of actively converting the innocuous biliverdin into a toxic compound by adding two hydrogen atoms.

This oddity is perhaps explained by a problem introduced by the placenta. The fetus must get rid of its bile pigment by transferring it to the mother; the placenta, however, is impermeable to biliverdin but not to bilirubin (248).

Being fat-soluble, bilirubin can cross cell membranes and kill cells, perhaps by a toxic effect on mitochondria (253). Fortunately, to reach any cell the bilirubin must float through extracellular water. Because its solubility in water is very low, toxic effects are usually avoided. Furthermore, what little does dissolve in water is promptly taken up by that all-purpose carrier molecule, albumin (p. 85). Only about 1 percent of bilirubin remains free. Albumin deposits its load of bilirubin in the liver, which conjugates it with glucuronic acid and excretes it in the bile. This mechanism protects us from bilirubin poisoning in all but the most severe cases of jaundice.

The toxicity of free bilirubin is well demonstrated in a strain of rats called Gunn rats, in which liver conjugation of bilirubin is deficient; bilirubin accumulates in the interstitium of the renal papillae, which becomes necrotic (Figure 3.67) (242, 243).

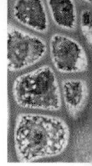

can cause damage in the central nervous system wherever the blood–brain barrier is not yet fully developed. Bilirubin seeps out of the capillaries and into cells of the gray matter, especially in basal nuclei, in amounts large enough to stain them yellow. Hence the German name **Kernicterus,** jaundice of nuclei. The condition is rare in our day; it results in death or brain damage (241, 255). One risk factor for kernicterus are drugs such as certain antibiotics that compete for albumin as a carrier (see Figure 3.15).

The preventive treatment used in years past was a marvel of applied cell biology. Infants at risk for bilirubin toxicity were given phenobarbital in order to stimulate the formation in the liver of smooth endoplasmic reticulum and thus of P-450, which helps conjugate the bilirubin (p. 142). Today jaundiced neonates are exposed to bright light; this converts bilirubin to photoisomers (photobilirubin), which can be excreted in the bile even without conjugation (248, 251). Unfortunately, prolonged exposure to bright light (**phototherapy**) injured the tender retina of many newborns before this unexpected danger was discovered and the eyes were covered (246).

Hematin

Hematin is a black pigment derived from hemoglobin. It is made of intact porphyrin rings that have been shed by the globin molecule (Figure 3.68); their iron is oxidized to trivalent, firmly bound, and histochemically not reactive (250). It does not give the Prussian blue reaction typical of hemosiderin and ferritin.

Hematin in pathology occurs largely as a nuisance, but it is interesting on several accounts.

- *Hematin is a nuisance pigment.* Hematin, alas, develops artefactually in tissues that are being fixed in nonbuffered, *acid* formalin. The red blood cells shed their hemes and become peppered with black granules of hematin, to the dismay of aesthetically minded pathologists and to the confusion of medical students (Figure 3.69). This common artefact should not be misleading because it would be unlikely for any black pigment to be riding piggyback on red blood cells; in malaria it would be *inside* the red blood cells. The lesson is that tissues should be fixed in buffered formalin at pH 6.9–7.5 (263).

- *Hematin develops in vivo in hematomas* (i.e., in blood spilled in the tissues). This is our own belief, based on microscopic experience; the literature is silent on the subject. The significance and fate of hematin in spilled blood are unknown.

- *Malarial pigment is a variety of hematin.* The malarial parasite *Plasmodium,* living inside a red blood

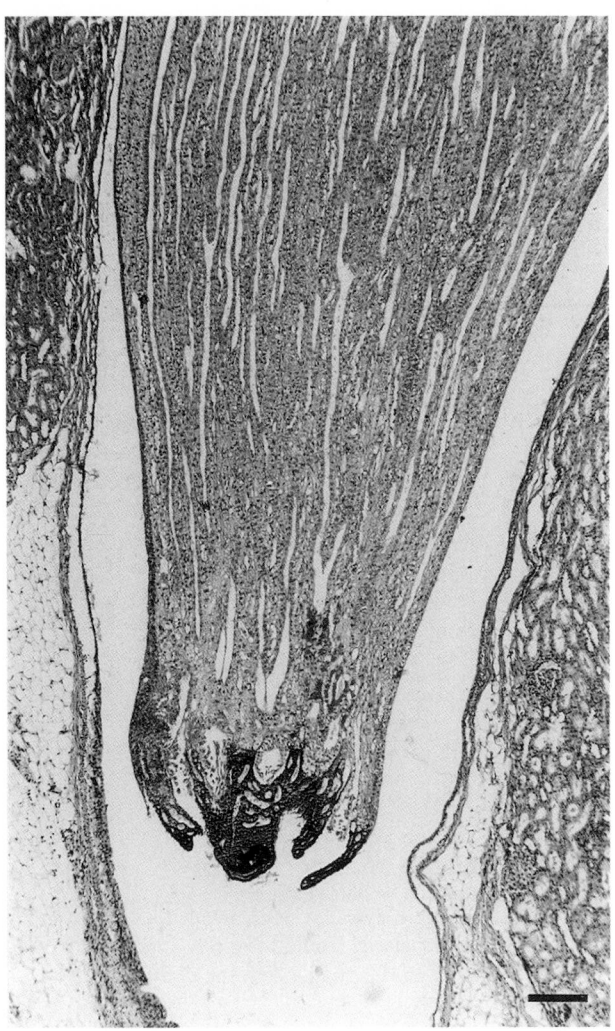

FIGURE 3.67 Toxicity of bilirubin. Renal papilla in a Gunn rat. These rats suffer from a congenital defect in the conjugation of bilirubin and become jaundiced; bilirubin is concentrated at the tip of the papilla. The papilla is necrotic and appears dark due to the heavy concentration of bilirubin. **Bar** = 100 μm. (Reproduced with permission from [242].)

In the fetus and the newborn, however, liver conjugation of bilirubin is low because the necessary enzyme system (cytochrome P-450) is not yet fully developed. Danger can arise if the baby develops severe jaundice. This can happen either *in utero* by Rh or ABO incompatibility with the mother's blood, or after birth when the newborn normally eliminates its excess of red blood cells, which are no longer needed because oxygen transport from the lungs is much more efficient than across the placenta. Whatever the cause of the jaundice in the newborn, the small amount of unconjugated bilirubin

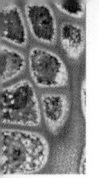

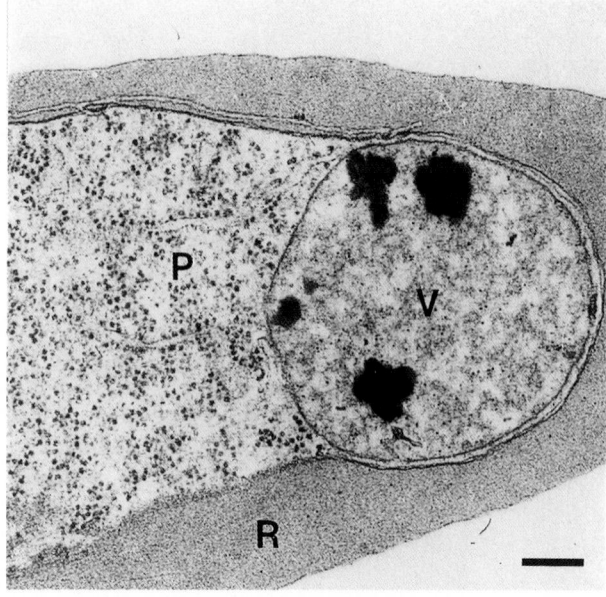

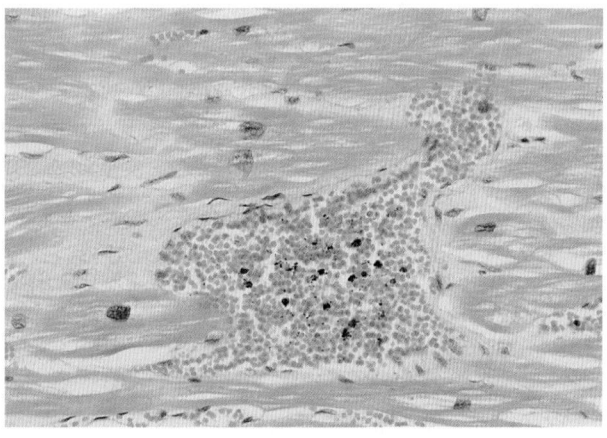

FIGURE 3.68 Hematin, the building block of several black pigments. The porphyrin ring is intact; the oxidized iron is not available for histochemical reaction. (From Budavari S et al. (eds): The Merck Index: An encyclopedia of chemicals, drugs, and biologicals, 11th ed. Rahway, NJ, Merck & Co., Inc., 1989, p. 723.)

FIGURE 3.70 Malarial pigment (*hemozoin,* akin to hematin) in the food vacuole (**V**) of the malarial parasite *Plasmodium gallinaceum* (**P**) inside a red blood cell (**R**). **Bar** = 0.2 μm. (Reproduced with permission from [258].)

FIGURE 3.69 The blood in this myocardial venule contains a black pigment. This is hematin, an obvious artefact, but the tendency of the hematin to precipitate on monocytes/macrophages is unexplained. Perhaps these cells have surface receptors for hematin?

cell, digests the hemoglobin and protects itself from the toxic heme products by polymerizing them into *hemozoin* (Figure 3.70) (258, 260, 262). The antimalarial chloroquine works precisely by inhibiting this polymerization (264). When the parasitized red blood cells die, their black pigment ends up in the sinusoidal phagocytes (p. 316), hence the dusky color of the malarial liver and spleen. Once it is tucked away in the phagocytes, the pigment is harmless.

The only saving feature of hematin is that it can be used for the therapy of porphyrias, disorders of heme synthesis (261). Even there it is toxic.

TO SUM UP: The three main types of endogenous brown pigments (lipofuscin, melanin, blood-derived pigments) are biologically similar in that they are all part of normal life. However, *blood-derived pigments are unique in that they can be toxic;* iron itself is a dangerous atom, hematin and heme-derived pigments are also toxic, and so is the iron-free bilirubin. Correspondingly, there are diseases caused by *blood-related* pigments (e.g., hemochromatosis, jaundice, porphyrias due to mistakes in heme biosynthesis) whereas there is no example of disease due to an effect of lipofuscin or melanin; indeed, melanin may be a detoxifying polymer.

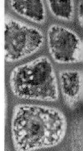

References

Vacuoles

1. Alberts B, Bray D, Lewis J, Raff M, Roberts K, Watson JD. Molecular biology of the cell, 2nd ed. New York: Garland Publishing, Inc., 1989.
2. Artigas J, Grosse G, Niedobitek F. Vacuolar myelopathy in AIDS. A morphological analysis. Pathol Res Pract 1990; 86:228–237.
3. Biava CG, Dyrda I, Genest J, Bencosme SA. Kaliopenic nephropathy. A correlated light and electron microscopic study. Lab Invest 1963;12:443–453.
4. Buckley IK. Cellular injury in vitro: phase contrast studies on injured cytoplasm. J Cell Biol 1962;14:40–420.
5. Buckley IK. Phase contrast observations on the endoplasmic reticulum of living cells in culture. Protoplasma 1965; 59:569–588.
6. Buckley IK. The lysosomes of cultured chick embryo cells. A correlated light and electron microscopic study. Lab Invest 1973;29:411–421.
7. Burg MB. Role of aldose reductase and sorbitol in maintaining the medullary intracellular milieu. Kidney Int 1988; 33:35–641.
8. Burg MD, Kador PF. Sorbitol, osmoregulation, and the complications of diabetes. J Clin Invest 1988;81:635–640.
9. Buvat R. Origin and continuity of cell vacuoles. In: Reinert J, Ursprung H (eds). Origin and continuity of cell organelles. New York: Springer-Verlag, 1971, pp. 127–157.
10. Clegg JS, Seitz P, Seitz W, Hazlewood CF. Cellular responses to extreme water loss: the water-replacement hypothesis. Cryobiology 1982;19:306–316.
11. Clements RS Jr. The polyol pathway. A historical review. Drugs 1986;32(Suppl 2):3–5.
12. Cohn ZA, Benson B. The in vitro differentiation of mononuclear phagocytes. II. The influence of serum on granule formation, hydrolase production, and pino-cytosis. J Exp Med 1965;121:835–848.
13. Cohn ZA, Ehrenreich BA. The uptake, storage and intracellular hydrolysis of carbohydrates by macrophages. J Exp Med 1969;129:30–225.
14. Dyck PJ. Resolvable problems in diabetic neuropathy. J NIH Res 1990;2:57–62.
15. Glynn LE, Himsworth HP. The intralobular circulation in acute liver injury by carbon tetrachloride. Clin Sci 1948; 6:235–245.
16. Greene DA, Lattimer SA. Altered myo-inositol metabolism in diabetic nerve. In: Dyck PJ, Thomas PK, Asbury AK, Winegrad AI, Porte D Jr (eds). Diabetic neuropathy. Philadelphia: WB Saunders Company, 1987, pp. 289–298.
17. Griffiths JB. Effect of hypertonic stress on mammalian cell lines and its relevance to freeze-thaw injury. Cryobiology 1978; 15:517–529.
18. Joris I, Majno G. Cell-to-cell herniae in the arterial wall. Am J Pathol 1977;87:375–398.
19. Judzewitsch RG, Jaspan JB, Polonsky KS, et al. Aldose reductase inhibition improves nerve conduction velocity in diabetic patients. N Engl J Med 1983;308:119–125.

20. Kirchain WR, Rendell MS. Aldose reductase inhibitors. Pharmacotherapy 1990;10:326–336.
21. Kohner EM, Porta M, Hyer SL. The pathogenesis of diabetic retinopathy and cataract. In: Pickup JC, Williams G (eds). Textbook of diabetes, vol. 2. Oxford: Blackwell Scientific Publications, 1991, pp. 564–574.
22. Li MK, Kavanagh JP, Prendiville V, et al. Does sucrose damage kidneys? Br J Urol 1986;58:353–357.
22a. Masters CL, Richardson Jr. E.P. Subacute spongiform encephalopathy (Creutzfeld-Jakob disease). The nature and progression of spongiform change. Brain 1978;101:333–344.
23. McManus ML, Churchwell KB, Strange K. Mechanisms of disease: regulation of cell volume in health and disease. N Engl J Med 1995;333:1260–1266.
24. Monserrat AJ, Chandler AE. Effects of repeated injections of sucrose on the kidney. Histologic, cytochemical and functional studies in an animal model. Virchows Arch [B] 1975; 19:77–91.
25. Norris HT. Response of the small intestine to the application of a hypertonic solution. Am J Pathol 1973;73:747–764.
26. Riemenschneider T, Bohle A. Morphologic aspects of low-potassium and low-sodium nephropathy. Clin Nephrol 1983;19:271–279.
27. Rigdon RH, Cardwell ES. Renal lesions following the intravenous injection of a hypertonic solution of sucrose. A clinical and experimental study. Arch Intern Med 1942;69:670–690.
28. Roberts JM. Preeclampsia: what we know and what we do not know. Semin Perinatol 2000;24:24–28.
29. Robinson DG. Plant membranes. New York: John Wiley & Sons, 1985.
30. Rodgers GM, Taylor RN, Roberts JM. Preeclampsia is associated with a serum factor cytotoxic to human endothelial cells. Am J Obstet Gynecol 1988;159:908–914.
31. Shimamura T, Trojanowski S. Effects of repeated deprivation of drinking water on the structure of renal medulla of rats. Am J Pathol 1976;84:87–92.
32. Steinman RM, Brodie SE, Cohn ZA. Membrane flow during pinocytosis. A stereologic analysis. J Cell Biol 1976; 68:665–687.
33. Stetz EM, Majno G, Joris I. Cellular pathology of the rat. Virchows Arch A Pathol Anat Histol 1979;383:135–148.
34. Trump BF, Janigan DT. The pathogenesis of cytologic vacuolization in sucrose nephrosis. An electron microscopic and histochemical study. Lab Invest 1962;11:395–411.
35. Zimmerman BR. Aldose reductase inhibitors. In: Dyck PJ, Thomas PK, Asbury AK, Winegrad AI, Porte D Jr (eds). Diabetic neuropathy. Philadelphia: WB Saunders Co, 1987, pp. 190–193.

Steatosis

36. Andersen T, Gluud C. Liver morphology in morbid obesity: a literature study. Int J Obesity 1984;8:97–106.
37. Angulo P. Nonalcoholic fatty liver disease. N Engl J Med 2002;346:1221–1231.
38. Bannister DW. Recent advances in avian biochemistry: The fatty liver and kidney syndrome. Int J Biochem 1979;10: 193–199.

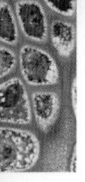

39. Bargmann W, Krisch B, Leonhardt H. Lipids in the proximal convoluted tubule of the cat kidney and the reabsorption of cholesterol. Cell Tissue Res 1977;177:523–538.

40. Bircher J, Benhamou J-P, McIntyre N, Rizzetto M, Rodés J (eds). Oxford textbook of clinical hepatology, 2nd ed. Oxford: Oxford University Press, 1999.

41. Bucher NLR, Malt RA. Regeneration of liver and kidney. Boston: Little, Brown and Company, 1971.

42. Cahill GF, Owen OE. Body fuels and starvation. Int Psychiatry Clin 1970;7:25–36.

42a. Caldwell SH, Swerdlow RH, Khan EM, et al. Mitochondrial abnormalities in non-alcoholic steatohepatits. J Hepatol 1999;31:430–434.

43. Chien KR, Bellary A, Nicar M, Mukherjee A, Buja M. Induction of a reversible cardiac lipidosis by a dietary long-chain fatty acid (erucic acid). Am J Pathol 1983;112:68–77.

44. Combes B, Whalley PJ, Adams RH. Tetracycline and the liver. Prog Liver Dis 1972;4:589–596.

45. Derickson A. Black lung: anatomy of a public health disaster. Ithaca: Cornell University Press, 1998.

46. Dianzani MU. Reactions of the liver to injury: fatty liver. In: Farber E, Fisher MM (eds). Toxic injury of the liver, part A. New York: Marcel Dekker, Inc., 1979, pp. 281–331.

47. Eisele JW, Barker EA, Smuckler EA. Lipid content in the liver of fatty metamorphosis of pregnancy. Am J Pathol 1975; 81:545–560.

48. Engel AG, Angelini C. Carnitine deficiency of human skeletal muscle with associated lipid storage myopathy: a new syndrome. Science 1973;179:899–901.

49. Fahimi HD, Kalmbach P, Stegmeier K, Stork H. Comparison between the effects of clofibrate and bezafibrate upon the ultrastructure of rat heart and liver. In: Greten H, Lang PD, Schettler G (eds). Lipoproteins and coronary heart disease. New York: Gerhard Witzstrock Publishing House, 1980, pp. 64–75.

50. Farber E, Fisher MM (eds). Toxic injury of the liver, parts A and B. New York: Marcel Dekker, Inc., 1979.

51. Flatt JP. Body weight, fat storage, and alcohol metabolism. Nutr Rev 1992;50:267–270.

52. Fromenty B, Berson A, Pessayre D. Microvesicular steatosis and steatohepatitis: role of mitochondrial dysfunction and lipid peroxidation. J Hepatol 1997;26:13–22.

53. Fromenty B, Pessayre D. Inhibition of mitochondrial beta-oxidation as a mechanism of hepatotoxicity. Pharmac Ther 1995;67:101–154.

54. Gordon GB. Saturated free fatty acid toxicity. II. Lipid accumulation, ultrastructural alterations, and toxicity in mammalian cells in culture. Exp Mol Pathol 1977;27:262–276.

55. Gordon GB. Lipid accumulation in the stationary phase of strain L cells in suspension culture. Lab Invest 1977;36:114–121.

56. Gordon GB, Barcza MA, Bush ME. Lipid accumulation in hypoxic tissue culture cells. Am J Pathol 1977;88:663–678.

57. Green FH, Laqueur WA. Coal workers' pneumoconiosis. Pathol Annu 1980;15(Pt 2):333–410.

58. Hartroft WS. The escape of lipid from fatty cysts in experimental dietary cirrhosis. In: Hoffbauer FW (ed). Conference on liver injury: liver injury; transactions. New York: Josiah Macy, Jr Foundation, 1950, pp. 109–150.

59. Hartroft WS. The sequence of pathologic events in the development of experimental fatty liver and cirrhosis. Ann NY Acad Sci 1954;57:633–645.

60. Hendrickse RG. Kwashiorkor: the hypothesis that incriminates aflatoxins. Pediatrics 1991;88:376–379.

61. Ibdah JA, Bennett MJ, Rinaldo P, et al. A fetal fatty-acid oxidation disorder as a cause of liver disease in pregnant women. N Engl J Med 1999;340:1723–1731.

62. Jelliffe DB, Jelliffe EFP. Causation of kwashiorkor: toward a multifactorial consensus. Pediatrics 1992;90:110–113.

63. Kern WH, Heger AH, Payne JH, DeWind LT. Fatty metamorphosis of the liver in morbid obesity. Arch Pathol 1973; 96:342–346.

64. Knox TA, Olans LB. Liver disease in pregnancy. N Engl J Med 1996;335:569–576.

65. Kuo TH, Moore KH, Giacomelli F, Wiener J. Defective metabolism of heart mitochondria from genetically diabetic mice. Diabetes 1983;32:781–787.

66. Lake BD, Patrick AD. Wolman's disease: deficiency of E600-resistant acid esterase activity with storage of lipids in lysosomes. J Pediatr 1970;76:262–266.

67. Lee M, Hatyashi H, Kato S, Sameshima Y, Hotta Y. Egg yolk-induced lipolysosome proliferation and fat infiltration of rat liver. Lab Invest 1982;47:194–197.

68. Lee RG. Fatty change and steatohepatitis. In: Diagnostic liver pathology. St. Louis: Mosby, 1994, pp. 167–194.

69. Leevy C. Fatty liver: a study of 270 patients with biopsy proven fatty liver and a review of the literature. Medicine 1962;41:249–276.

70. Lettéron P, Fromenty B, Terris B, Degott C, Pessayre D. Acute and chronic hepatic steatosis lead to *in vivo* lipid peroxidation in mice. J Hepatol 1996;24:200–208.

71. Lieber CS. Biochemical and molecular basis of alcohol-induced injury to liver and other tissues. N Engl J Med 1988; 319:1639–1650.

72. Lombardi B. Considerations on the pathogenesis of fatty liver. Lab Invest 1966;15:1–20.

73. Luse SA, Wood WG. The brain in fatal carbon tetrachloride poisoning. Arch Neurol 1967;17:304–312.

74. MacMahon HE, Weiss S. Carbon tetrachloride poisoning with macroscopic fat in the pulmonary artery. Am J Pathol 1929;5:623–630.

75. Maunsbach AB, Wirsén C. Ultrastructural changes in kidney, myocardium and skeletal muscle of the dog during excessive mobilization of free fatty acids. J Ultrastruct Res 1966; 16:35–54.

76. Mavrelis PG, Ammon HV, Gleysteen JJ, Komorowski RA, Charaf UK. Hepatic free fatty acids in alcoholic liver disease and morbid obesity. Hepatology 1983;3:226–231.

77. Murray M. Role of the liver in drug metabolism. In: Farrell GC. Drug-induced liver disease. Edinburgh: Churchill Livingstone, 1994, pp. 3–21.

78. Nieth H, Schollmeyer P. Substrate-utilization of the human kidney. Nature 1966;209:1244–1245.

79. Novikoff PM. Intracellular organelles and lipoprotein metabolism in normal and fatty livers. In: Arias I, Popper H, Schachter D, Shafritz DA (eds). The liver: biology and patholobiology. New York: Raven Press, 1982, pp. 143–167.

80. Novikoff PM, Roheim PS, Novikoff AB, Edelstein D. Production and prevention of fatty liver in rats fed clofibrate and orotic acid diets containing sucrose. Lab Invest 1974; 30:732–750.

81. Ober WB, LeCompte PM. Acute fatty metamorphosis of the liver associated with pregnancy: a distinctive lesion. Am J Med 1955;19:743–758.

82. Palade GE. Functional changes in the structure of cell components. In: Hayashi T (ed). Subcellular particles. New York: The Ronald Press Company, 1959, pp. 64–83.

83. Perry MM, Siller WG. Incorporation of ^{3}H-oleic acid by the proximal convoluted tubule cells of the chick (gallus domesticus). Cell Tissue Res 1980;210:447–459.

84. Pessayre D, Larrey D, Biour M. Drug-induced liver injury. In: Bircher J, Benhamou JP, McIntyre N, Rizzetto M, Rodés J. Oxford textbook of clinical hepatology, 2nd ed. Oxford: Oxford University Press, 1999, pp. 1261–1315.

85. Pessayre D, Mansouri A, Haouzi D, Fromenty B. Hepatotoxicity due to mitochondrial dysfunction. Cell Biol Toxicol 1999;15:367–373.

86. Popper H, Thung SN, Gerber MA. Pathology of alcoholic liver diseases. Semin Liver Dis 1981;1:203–216.

87. Rappaport AM. Physioanatomical basis of toxic liver injury. In: Farber E, Fisher MM (eds). Toxic injury of the liver, part A. New York: Marcel Dekker, Inc., 1979, pp. 1–57.

88. Rhodin JAG. Histology. A text and atlas. New York: Oxford University Press, 1974.

89. Rinaldi A, Tyndalo V. The complete book of mushrooms. New York: Crown Publishers, Inc., 1974.

90. Rolfes DB, Ishak KG. Acute fatty liver of pregnancy: a clinicopathologic study of 35 cases. Hepatology 1985; 5:1149–1158.

91. Rothblat GH, Kritchevsky D. Lipid metabolism in tissue culture cells. Philadelphia: Wistar Institute Press, 1967.

92. Rubin E (ed). Alcohol and the cell. (Ann NY Acad Sci, vol. 492.) New York: New York Academy of Sciences, 1987.

93. Rubin E, Lieber CS. Fatty liver, alcoholic hepatitis and cirrhosis produced by alcohol in primates. N Engl J Med 1974; 290:128–135.

94. Schlunk FF, Lombardi B. Liver liposomes. I. Isolation and chemical characterization. Lab Invest 1967;17:30–38.

95. Slauson DO, Cooper BJ. Mechanisms of disease. Baltimore: Williams & Wilkins, 1982.

96. Spector AA. Plasma albumin as a lipoprotein. In: Scanu AM, Spector AA(eds). Biochemistry and biology of plasma lipoproteins. New York: Marcel Dekker, Inc., 1986, pp. 247–280.

97. Suter PM, Schutz Y, Jequier E. The effect of ethanol on fat storage in healthy subjects. N Engl J Med 1992; 326:983–987.

98. Trowell HC, Davies JNP, Dean RFA. Kwashiorkor. New York: Academic Press, 1982.

99. Unger RH. Lipotoxic diseases. Annu Rev Med 2002; 53:319–336.

100. Unger RH, Orci L. Diseases of liporegulation: new perspective on obesity and related disorders. FASEB J 2001;15:312–321.

101. Waterlow JC (ed). Protein malnutrition. Cambridge: Cambridge University Press, 1955.

102. Waugh DA, Small DM. Identification and detection of in situ cellular and regional differences of lipid composition and class in lipid-rich tissue using hot stage polarizing light microscopy. Lab Invest 1984;51:702–714.

103. Wirthensohn G, Guder WG. Triacyglycerol metabolism in isolated rat kidney cortex tubules. Biochem J 1980;186:317–324.

104. Wittels B, Bressler R. Biochemical lesion of diphtheria toxin in the heart. J Clin Invest 1964a;43:630–637.

105. Wittels B, Bressler R. Lipid metabolism in the heart during fasting. Lab Invest 1964b;13:794–799.

Cholesterol

106. Aterman K, Remmele W, Smith M. Karl Touton and his "xanthelasmatic giant cell." A selective review of multinucleated giant cells. Am J Dermatopathol 1988;10:257–269.

107. Brown MS, Goldstein JL. Lipoprotein metabolism in the macrophage: implications for cholesterol deposition in atherosclerosis. Annu Rev Biochem 1983;52:223–261.

108. Brown MS, Ho YK, Goldstein JL. The cholesteryl ester cycle in macrophage foam cells: continual hydrolysis and reesterification of cytoplasmic cholesteryl esters. J Biol Chem 1980; 255:9344–9352.

109. Corwin RW, Irwin RS. The lipid-laden alveolar macrophage as a marker of aspiration in parenchymal lung disease. Am Rev Respir Dis 1985;132:576–581.

110. Druilhet RE, Traxler RW, Sobek JM. Bacterial utilization of cholesterol. Antonie van Leeuwenhoek 1968;34:315–325.

111. Fowler S, Shio H, Haley NJ. Characterization of lipidladen aortic cells from cholesterol-fed rabbits. IV. Investigation of macrophage-like properties of aortic cell populations. Lab Invest 1979;41:372–378.

112. French SW, Miyamoto K, Wong K, Jui L, Briere L. Role of the Ito cell in liver parenchymal fibrosis in rats fed alcohol and a high fat-low protein diet. Am J Pathol 1988;132:73–85.

113. Ginsburg GS, Atkinson D, Small DM. Physical properties of cholesteryl esters. Prog Lipid Res 1984;23:135–167.

114. Goldstein JL, Brown MS. Familiar hypercholesterolemia: pathogeneses of a receptor disease. Johns Hopkins Med J 1978;143:8–16.

115. Ho YK, Brown MS, Goldstein JL. Hydrolysis and excretion of cytoplasmic cholesteryl esters by macrophages: stimulation by high density lipoprotein and other agents. J Lipid Res 1980; 21:391–398.

116. Imshenetskii AA, Nikitin LE, Nazarova TS, Efimochkina EF. Activities of cholesterol degrading microorganisms. Mikrobiologiya 1975;44:210–213.

117. Kaplan NB, Grant MM, Brody JS. The lipid interstitial cell of the pulmonary alveolus. Age and species differences. Am Rev Respir Dis 1985;132:1307–1312.

118. Kruth HS. Lipid deposition in human tendon xanthoma. Am J Pathol 1985;121:311–315.

119. Sedaghat A, Grundy SM. Cholesterol crystals and the formation of cholesterol gallstones. N Engl J Med 1980;302:1274–1277.

120. Steinberg D. Lipoproteins and atherosclerosis. A look back and a look ahead. Arteriosclerosis 1983;3:283–301.

121. Steinbrecher UP, Parthasarathy S, Leake DS, Witztum JL, Steinberg D. Modification of low density lipoprotein by endothelial cells involves lipid peroxidation and degradation of low density lipoprotein phospholipids. Proc Natl Acad Sci USA 1984;81:3883–3887.

122. Wright BA, Jeffrey PH. Lipoid pneumonia. Semin Respir Infect 1990;5:314–321.

123. Zimetbaum P, Eder H, Frishman W. Probucol: pharmacology and clinical application. J Clin Pharmacol 1990;30:3–9.

124. Zucker-Franklin D, Grusky G, Marcus A. Transformation of monocytes into "fat" cells. Lab Invest 1978;38:620–628.

Accumulation of Glycogen and Related Materials

125. Buja LM, Ferrans VJ, Levitsky S. Occurrence of intramitochondrial glycogen in canine myocardium after prolonged anoxic cardiac arrest. J Mol Cell Cardiol 1972;4:237–254.

126. Ghadially PN. Ultrastructural pathology of the cell and matrix, 2nd ed. London: Butterworths, 1982.

127. Karasaki S. Cytoplasmic and nuclear glycogen synthesis in Novikoff ascites hepatoma cells. J Ultrastruct Res 1971;35:181–196.

128. Kosek JC, Angell W. Fine structure of basophilic myocardial degeneration. Arch Pathol 1970;89:491–499.

129. Orci L, Stauffacher W. Glycogenosomes in renal tubular cells of diabetic animals. J Ultrastruct Res 1971;36:499–503. http://www.tandf.co.uk/journals

130. Powell HC, Ward HW, Garrett RS, Orloff MJ, Lampert PW. Glycogen accumulation in the nerves and kidneys of chronically diabetic rats. A quantitative electron microscopic study. J Neuropathol Exp Neurol 1979;38:114–127.

131. Ramsey HJ. Ultrastructure of corpora amylacea. J Neuropathol Exp Neurol 1965;24:25–39.

132. Ritchie S, Waugh D. The pathology of Armanni-Ebstein diabetic nephropathy. Am J Pathol 1957;33:1035–1057.

133. Rosai J, Lascano EF. Basophilic (mucoid) degeneration of myocardium. A disorder of glycogen metabolism. Am J Pathol 1970;61:99–112.

134. Schwalbe H-P, Quadbeck G. Die Corpora amylacea immenschlichen Gihirn. Virchows Arch [A] 1975;366:305–311.

135. Stam FC, Roukema PA. Histochemical and biochemical aspects of corpora amylacea. Acta Neuropathol 1973;25:95–102.

Pigments: Soot and Carbon; Lipofuscin

136. Bevelander G, Nakahara H. The effect of diverse amounts of tetracycline on fluorescence and coloration of teeth. J Pediatr 1966;68:114–120.

137. Brizzee KR, Ordy JM. Cellular features, regional accumulation, and prospects of modification of age pigments in mammals. In: Sohal RS (ed). Age pigments. Amsterdam: Elsevier/North-Holland Biomedical Press, 1981, pp. 101–154.

138. Cadle RD. Particle size. Theory and industrial applications. New York: Reinhold Publishing Corporation, 1965.

139. Casselman WGB. The in vitro preparation and histochemical properties of substances resembling ceroid. J Exp Med 1951; 94:549–562.

140. Derickson A. Black lung. Anatomy of a public disaster. Ithaca: Cornell University Press, 1998.

141. de Duve C. A guided tour of the living cell, vol. 1. New York: Scientific American Books, Inc., 1984.

142. Elleder M. Chemical characterization of age pigments. In: Sohal RS (ed). Age pigments. Amsterdam: Elsevier/North-Holland Biomedical Press, 1981, pp. 203–241.

143. Gedigk P, Pioch W. Über die formale Genese lipogener Pigmente. Untersuchungen mit Estern hochungesättigter Fettsäuren. Virchows Arch [Pathol Anat] 1965;339:100–135.

144. Gedigk P, Totovic V. 4. Lysosomen und Pigmente. Verh Dtsch Ges Pathol 1976;60:64–94.

145. Green FH, Laqueur WA. Coal workers' pneumoconiosis. Pathol Annu 1980;15:333–410.

146. Joris I, Billingham ME, Underwood JM, Majno G. Lipofuscin and lipid oxidation in human coronary endothelium. Cardiovasc Pathol 1998;7:75–85.

147. Kajihara H, Totovic V, Gedigk P. Zur Ultrastruktur und Morphogenese des Ceroidpigmentes. II. Spätveränderungen der Lysosomen in Kuppferschen Sternzellen der Rattenleber nach Phagozytose hochungesättigter Lipide. Virchows Arch B Cell Pathol 1975;19:239–254.

148. Koobs DH, Schultz RL, Jutzy RV. The origin of lipofuscin and possible consequences to the myocardium. Arch Pathol Lab Med 1978;102:66–68.

149. LeFevre ME, Green FHY, Joel DD, Laqueur W. Frequency of black pigment in livers and spleens of coal workers: correlation with pulmonary pathology and occupational information. Hum Pathol 1982;13:1121–1126.

150. Miquel J, Oro J, Bensch KG, Johnson JE Jr. Lipofuscin: fine-structural and biochemical studies. In: Pryor WA (ed). Free radicals in biology, vol. III. New York: Academic Press, 1977, pp. 133–182.

151. Porta E, Llesuy S, Monserrat AJ, Benavides S, Travacio M. Changes in cathepsin B and lipofuscin during development and aging rat brain and heart. Gerontology 1995; 41(Suppl 2):81–89.

152. Porta EA. Advances in age pigment research. Arch Gerontol Geriatr 1991;12:303–320.

153. Porta EA. Is lipofuscin a proven marker of oxidative stress? Oxygen Club of Calif, 1999;(abstract).

154. Raychaudhuri C, Desai ID. Ceroid pigment formation and irreversible sterility in vitamin E deficiency. Science 1971; 173:1028–1029.

155. Silberberg I, Leider M. Studies on a red tattoo. Arch Dermatol 1970;101:299–304.

156. Sitte N, Huber M, Grune T, et al. Proteasome inhibition by lipofuscin/ceroid during postmitotic aging of fibroblasts. FASEB J 2000;14:1490–1498.

157. Sohal RS. Metabolic rate, aging, and lipofuscin accumulation. In: Sohal RS (ed). Age pigments. Amsterdam: Elsevier/North-Holland Biomedical Press, 1981, pp. 303–316.

158. Sohal RS, Donato H Jr. Effect of experimental prolongation of life span on lipofuscin content and lysosomal enzyme activity in the brain of the housefly, Musca domestica. J Gerontol 1979;34:489–496.

159. Steer HW, Colin-Jones DG. Melanosis coli: studies of the toxic effects of irritant purgatives. J Pathol 1975;155:199–205.

160. Strehler BL, Mark DD, Mildvan AS, Gee MV. Rate and magnitude of age pigment accumulation in the human myocardium. J Gerontol 1959;14:430–439.

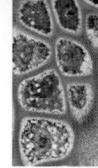

161. Thompson SW II. Lipogenic pigments related to treatment with exogenous lipid. In: Wolman M (ed). Pigments in pathology. New York: Academic Press, 1969, pp. 237–286.

162. Urbanski SJ, Arsenault AL, Green FHY, Haber G. Pigment resembling atmospheric dust in Peyer's patches. Mod Pathol 1989;2:222–226.

163. van Oud Alblas AB, van Furth R. Origin, kinetics, and characteristics of pulmonary macrophages in the normal steady state. J Exp Med 1979;149:1504–1518.

164. Virchow R. Cellular pathology as based upon physiological and pathological histology (translated from the second German edition by Britton Chance, 1859). New York: Dover Publications, 1971.

165. Walker NI, Bennett RE, Axelsen RA. Melanosis coli. A consequence of anthraquinone-induced apoptosis of colonic epithelial cells. Am J Pathol 1988;131:465–476.

166. Wolfe LS, Ng Ying Kin NMK, Baker RR. Batten disease and related disorders: new findings on the chemistry of the storage material. In: Callahan JW, Lowden JA (eds). Lysosomes and lysosomal storage diseases. New York: Raven Press, 1981, pp. 315–330.

167. Wolman M. Pigments in pathology. New York: Academic Press, 1969.

168. Wolman M. Factors affecting lipid pigment formation. In: Sohal RS (ed). Age pigments. Amsterdam: Elsevier/North-Holland Biomedical Press, 1981, pp. 265–281.

Melanin

169. Barden H. Further histochemical studies characterizing the lipofuscin component of human neuromelanin. J Neuropathol Exp Neurol 1978;37:437–451.

170. Barden H. The biology and chemistry of neuromelanin. In: Sohal RS (ed). Age pigments. Amsterdam: Elsevier/North-Holland Biomedical Press, 1981, pp. 155–180.

171. Bhawan J. Ultrastructure of melanocyte-keratinocyte interactions in pigmented basal cell carcinoma. Pigment Cell 1979; 5:38–47.

172. Bolognia JL, Pawelek JM. Biology of hypopigmentation. J Am Acad Dermatol 1988;19:217–255.

173. Bystryn J-C, Pfeffer S. Vitiligo and antibodies to melanocytes. Prog Clin Biol Res 1988;256:195–206.

174. Chedekel MR. Photochemistry and photobiology of epidermal melanins. Photochem Photobiol 1982;35:881–885.

175. Edelstein LM. Melanin: a unique biopolymer. Pathobiol Annu 1971;1:309–324.

176. Fitzpatrick TB, Soter NA. Pathophysiology of skin. In: Smith LH, Thier SO (eds). Pathophysiology. The biological principles of disease. Philadelphia: WB Saunders Co., 1981, pp. 1745–1795.

177. Fitzpatrick TB, Szabó, Wick MM. Biochemistry and physiology of melanin pigmentation. In: Goldsmith LA (ed). Biochemistry and physiology of the skin. New York: Oxford University Press, 1983, pp. 687–712.

178. Gedigk P, Totovic V. Lysosomes and pigments. Verh Dtsch Ges Pathol 1976;60:64–94.

179. Goldsmith LA. Biochemistry and physiology of the skin. New York: Oxford University Press, 1983.

180. Le Douarin N. The neural crest. Cambridge: Cambridge University Press, 1982.

181. Le Douarin NM. Ontogeny of the peripheral nervous system from the neural crest and the placodes. A developmental model studied on the basis of the quail-chick chimaera system. Harvey Lect 1986;80:137–186.

182. Lerner EA, Sober AJ. Chemical and pharmacologic agents that cause hyperpigmentation or hypopigmentation of the skin. Dermatol Clin 1988;6:327–337.

183. Marsden CD. Brain melanin. In: Wolman M (ed). Pigments in pathology. New York: Academic Press, 1969, pp. 395–420.

184. Miquel J, Oro J, Bensch KG, Johnson JE Jr. Lipofuscin: fine-structural and biochemical studies. In: Pryor WA (ed). Free radicals in biology, Vol. III. New York: Academic Press, 1977, pp. 133–182.

185. Nahum LH. The purple-people syndrome. Conn Med 1965; 29:332.

186. Riley PA. Mechanism of pigment-cell toxicity produced by hydroxyanisole. J Pathol 1970;101:163–169.

187. Scotto J, Fears TR, Fraumeni JF Jr. Solar radiation. In: Schottenfeld D, Fraumeni JF Jr (eds). Cancer epidemiology and prevention. Philadelphia: WB Saunders Company, 1982, pp. 254–276.

188. Sealy RC, Felix CC, Hyde JS, Swartz HM. Structure and reactivity of melanins: influence of free radicals and metal ions. In: Pryor WA (ed). Free radicals in biology, vol. IV. New York: Academic Press, 1980, pp. 209–259.

189. Smith LH Jr, Thier SO. Pathophysiology. The biological principles of disease. Philadelphia: WB Saunders Company, 1981.

190. Snyder SH. The molecular basis of communication between cells. Sci Am 1985;253:132–141.

191. Szent-Györgyi A. Bioelectronics. Science 1968;161:988–990.

192. Taylor RL. A suggested role for the polyphenol-phenoloxidase system in invertebrate immunity. J Invert Pathol 1969;14: 427–428.

193. Wolman M. Factors affecting lipid pigment formation. In: Sohal RS (ed). Age pigments. Amsterdam: Elsevier/North-Holland Biomedical Press, 1981, pp. 265–281.

Ferritin and Hemosiderin

194. Abok K, Hirth T, Ericsson JLE, Brunk U. Effect of iron on the stability of macrophage lysosomes. Virchows Arch B Cell Pathol 1983;43:85–101.

195. Andrews NC. Disorders of iron metabolism. N Engl J Med 1999;341:1986–1995.

196. Banyard SH, Stammers DK, Harrison PM. Electron density map of apoferritin at 2.8-A resolution. Nature 1978; 271:282–284.

197. Bhawan J, Joris I, Cohen N, Majno G. Microcirculatory changes in posttraumatic pigmented villonodular synovitis. Arch Pathol Lab Med 1980;104:328–332.

198. Biemond P, van Eijk HG, Swaak AJG, Koster JF. Iron mobilization from ferritin by superoxide derived from stimulated polymorphonuclear leukocytes. Possible mechanism in inflammation diseases. J Clin Invest 1984;73: 1576–1579.

199. Bradley WG Jr. MRI of hemorrhage and iron in the brain. In: Stark DD, Bradley WG Jr (eds). Magnetic resonance imaging. St. Louis: The CV Mosby Co., 1988, pp. 359–374.

200. Braun V. Iron supply as a virulence factor. In: Jackson GG, Thomas H (eds). The pathogenesis of bacterial infections. Berlin: Springer-Verlag, 1985, pp. 168–176.

201. Bullen JJ, Griffiths E (eds). Iron and infection. Chichester: John Wiley & Sons, 1987.

202. Crichton RR. Ferritin: structure, synthesis and function. N Engl J Med 1971;284:1413–1422.

203. Crosby WH. Hemochromatosis: current concepts and management. Hosp Pract 1987;22:173–192.

204. Doolittle RL, Richter GW. Isoferritins in rat Kupffer cells, hepatocytes, and extrahepatic macrophages. Biosynthesis in cell suspensions and cultures in response to iron. Lab Invest 1981;45:567–574.

205. Drysdale JW. Ferritin phenotypes: structure and metabolism. Ciba Found Symp 1977;51:41–67.

206. Eaton JW, Brandt P, Mahoney JR, Lee JT Jr. Haptoglobin: a natural bacteriostat. Science 1982;215:691–693.

207. Emery T. Iron metabolism in humans and plants. Am Sci 1982;70:626–632.

208. Fairbanks VF, Klee GG. Ferritin. Prog Clin Pathol 1981; 8:175–203.

209. Feild TS, Lee DW, Holbrook NM. Why leaves turn red in autumn. The role of anthocyanins in senescing leaves of red-osier dogwood. Plant Physiol 2001;127:566–574.

210. Finch CA, Huebers H. Perspectives in iron metabolism. N Engl J Med 1982;306:1520–1528.

211. Ford GC, Harrison PM, Rice DW, et al. Ferritin: design and formation of an iron-storage molecule. Philos Trans R Soc Lond [Biol] 1984;304:551–565.

212. Ganote CE, Nahara G. Acute ferrous sulfate hepatotoxicity in rats. An electron microscopic and biochemical study. Lab Invest 1973;28:426–436.

213. Ghadially FN. Haemorrhage and hemosiderin. J Submicrosc Cytol 1979;11:271–291.

214. Gorinsky B. Transferrin: structure and function. In: Weatherall DJ, Fiorelli G, Gorini S (eds). Advances in red cell biology. New York: Raven Press, 1982, pp. 7–17.

215. Griffiths E. The iron-uptake systems of pathogenic bacteria. In: Bullen JJ, Griffiths E (eds). Iron and infection. Chichester: John Wiley & Sons, 1987, pp. 69–137.

216. Harding C, Heuser J, Stahl P. Receptor-mediated endocytosis of transferrin and recycling of the transferrin receptor in rat reticulocytes. J Cell Biol 1983;97:329–339.

217. Harrison PM, Banyard SH, Hoare RJ, Russell SM, Treffry A. The structure and function of ferritin. Ciba Found Symp 1977;51:19–40.

218. Hennigar GR, Greene WB, Walker EM, deSaussure C. Hemochromatosis caused by excessive vitamin iron intake. Am J Pathol 1979;96:611–624.

219. Huebers HA, Huebers E, Csiba E, Rummel W, Finch CA. The significance of transferrin for intestinal iron absorption. Blood 1983;61;283–290.

220. Jandl JH. Blood: Textbook of hematology. Boston: Little, Brown and Company, 1987.

221. Janssen W. Forensic histopathology. Berlin: Springer-Verlag, 1984.

222. Kent S, Weinberg E. Hypoferremia: adaptation to disease? N Engl J Med 1989;320:672.

223. Kimber RJ, Rudzki Z, Blunden RW. Clinching the diagnosis: 1. Iron deficiency and iron overload: serum ferritin and serum iron in clinical medicine. Pathology 1983;15:497–503.

224. Kluger MJ, Bullen JJ. Clinical and physiological aspects. In: Bullen JJ, Griffiths E (eds). Iron and infection. Chichester: John Wiley & Sons, 1987, pp. 243–282.

225. Lalonde J-MA, Ghadially FN. Ultrastructure of experimentally produced subcutaneous haematomas in the rabbit. Virchows Arch B Cell Pathol 1977;25:221–232.

226. Lambert RE. Iron storage disease. In: Ruddy S, Harris ED Jr, Sledge CB, Budd RC, Sergent JS (eds). Kelley's textbook of rheumatology, 6th ed. Philadelphia: WB Saunders Co., 2001, pp. 1559–1566.

227. Massover WH. The ultrastructure of ferritin macromolecules. III. Mineralized iron in ferritin is attached to the protein shell. J Mol Biol 1978;123:721–726.

228. Mofenson HC, Caraccio TR, Sharieff N. Iron sepsis: Versinia enterocolitica septicemia possibly caused by an overdose of iron. N Engl J Med 1987;316:1092–1093.

229. Muir R, Niven JSF. The local formation of blood pigments. J Pathol Bacteriol 1935;41:183–197.

230. Munro HN, Linder MC. Ferritin: structure, biosynthesis, and role in iron metabolism. Physiol Rev 1978;58:317–396.

231. Neumann E. Beiträge zur Kenntniss der pathologischen Pigmente. Virchows Arch Pathol Anat. Physiol Klin Med 1888;111:25–47.

232. O'Connell MJ, Ward RJ, Baum H, Peters TJ. Iron overload, lysosomes and free radicals. In: Reid E, Cook GMW, Luzio JP (eds). Cells, membranes, and disease, including renal. New York: Plenum Press, 1987, pp. 109–112.

233. Powell LW, Bassett ML, Halliday JW. Hemochromatosis: 1980 update. Gastroenterology 1980;78:374–381.

234. Richter GW. The cellular transformation of injected colloidal iron complexes into ferritin and hemosiderin in experimental animals. J Exp Med 1959;109:197–216.

235. Robotham JL, Lietman PS. Acute iron poisoning. A review. Am J Dis Child 1980;134:875–879.

236. Rubenstein E. Diseases caused by impaired communication among cells. Sci Am 1980;242:102–121.

237. Ruiz J, Wu GY. Inherited liver disease. In: Jameson JL (ed). Principles of molecular medicine. Totowa, NJ: Humana Press Inc., 1998, pp. 375–386.

238. Schafer AI, Cheron RG, Dluhy R, et al. Clinical consequences of acquired transfusional iron overload in adults. N Engl J Med 1981;304:319–324.

239. Sherman JM, Winnie G, Thomassen MJ, Abdul-Karim FW, Boat TF. Time course of hemosiderin production and clearance by human pulmonary macrophages. Chest 1984;86:409–411.

240 Weinberg ED. The development of awareness of iron-withholding defense. Perspect Biol Med 1993;36:215–221.

Bilirubin

241. Avery ME, Taeusch HW Jr (eds). Schaffer's diseases of the newborn, 5th ed. Philadelphia: WB Saunders Co., 1984.

242. Axelsen RA. Spontaneous renal papillary necrosis in the Gunn rat. Pathology 1973;5:43–50.

243. Axelsen RA, Burry AF. Bilirubin-associated renal papillary necrosis in the homozygous Gunn rat: light- and electron-microscopic observations. J Pathol 1976;120:165–175.

244. Berk PD, Berlin NI. Chemistry and physiology of bile pigments, Fogarty International Center proceedings, No. 35. DHEW Publication No. (NIH) 77-1100, U.S. Department of Health, Education, and Welfare. Public Health Service, National Institutes of Health, 1977.

245. Brown SB, Troxler RF. Heme degradation and bilirubin formation. In: Heirwegh KPM, Brown SB (eds). Bilirubin, vol. II. Boca Raton: CRC Press, 1982, pp. 1–38.

246. Glass P, Avery GB, Subramanian KNS, et al. Effect of bright light in the hospital nursery on the incidence of retinopathy of prematurity. N Engl J Med 1985;313:401–404.

247. Gollan JL, Knapp AB. Bilirubin metabolism and congenital jaundice. Hosp Pract 1985;20:83–106.

248. Gollan JL, Schmid R. Bilirubin update: formation, transport, and metabolism. Prog Liver Dis 1982;8:261–283.

249. Heirwegh KPM, Brown SB (eds). Bilirubin, 2 vols. Boca Raton: CRC Press, Inc., 1982.

250. Lemberg R, Legge JW. Hematin compounds and bile pigments. New York: Interscience Publishers, 1949.

251. Lightner DA. Structure, photochemistry, and organic chemistry of bilirubin. In: Heirwegh KPM, Brown SB (eds). Bilirubin, vol. I. Chemistry. Boca Raton: CRC Press, 1982, pp. 1–58.

252. Majno G. The healing hand. Man and wound in the ancient world. Cambridge: Harvard University Press, 1975.

253. Mustafa MG, King TE. Binding of bilirubin with lipid. A possible mechanism of its toxic reactions in mitochondria. J Biol Chem 1970;245:1084–1089.

254. O'Carra P, Colleran E. Nonenzymatic and quasienzymatic models for catabolic heme cleavage. In: Berk PD, Berlin NI (eds). International symposium on chemistry and physiology of bile pigments, Fogarty International Center proceedings, No. 35. DHEW Publication No. (NIH) 77-1100. U.S. Department of Health, Education, and Welfare. Bethesda: National Institutes of Health, 1977, p. 26.

255. Oski FA. Kernicterus. In: Avery ME, Taeusch HW Jr (eds). Schaffer's diseases of the newborn, 5th ed. Philadelphia: WB Saunders Co., 1984, pp. 633–635.

256. Rich AR, Bumstead JH. On the identity of haematoidin and bilirubin. Bull Johns Hopkins Hosp 1925;36:225–232.

257. Virchow R. Cellular pathology (translated from the second German edition by B. Chance), 1859, Reproduced by Dover Publications, New York: 1971.

Hematin

258. Aikawa M, Huff CG, Sprinz H. Comparative feeding mechanisms of avian and primate malarial parasites. Milit Med 1966;131(suppl):969–983.

259. Budavari S, O'Neil MJ, Smith A, Heckelman PE (eds). The Merck index: An encyclopedia of chemicals, drugs, and biologicals, 11th ed. Rahway, NJ: Merck & Co., Inc., 1989, p. 732.

260. Fulton JD, Rimington C. The pigment of the malaria parasite Plasmodium berghei. J Gen Microbiol 1953;8:157–159.

261. Glueck R, Green D, Cohen I, Ts'ao C-h. Hematin: unique effects on hemostasis. Blood 1983;61:243–249.

262. Olliaro P. Phagocytosis of hemozoin (native and synthetic malaria pigment), and *Plasmodium falciparum* intraerythrocyte-stage parasites by human and mouse phagocytes. Ultrastruct Pathol 2000;24:9–13.

263. Pizzolato P. Formalin pigment (acid hematin) and related pigments. Am J Med Technol 1976;42:446–439.

264. Wellems TE. How chloroquine works. Nature 1992;355:108–109.

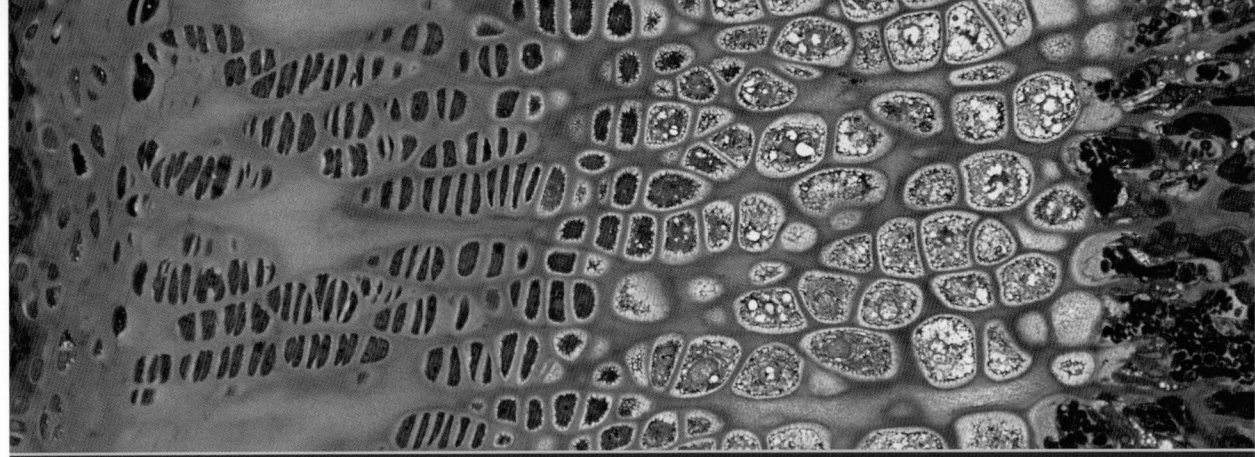

There are many ways to recognize cellular disease. In Chapter 3 we used the presence of abnormal cellular contents. We will now see what we can learn by studying individual cellular organelles.

Prelude: A New Category of Disease, Protein Misfolding

As we review the pathologic changes of each cellular organelle, we must acknowledge a basic, molecular mechanism of disease that was fully recognized in the late 1990s (2): **protein misfolding,** which underlies a great deal of intracellular and extracellular pathology. The misfolding is usually followed by **aggregation,** because the misshaped proteins expose some of their inner hydrophobic domains, which are sticky and lead the molecules to assemble into fibrils or clusters. These aggregates tend to cause trouble both inside and outside the cells (3). It has been argued that under certain circumstances their presence may be protective, but this can be only a rare exception.

To understand this group of diseases, it will help to understand how they were discovered (3). Between the 1850s and the 1980s, the medical world struggled to explain a group of chronic diseases in which a strange, fibrillar, proteinaceous material (*amyloid*) was deposited in the tissues, overwhelmingly *outside the cells.* It was understood that chemically there were many different kinds of amyloid proteins. In the 1990s, the mystery was solved: great strides had been made in the field of protein structure and folding, and amyloids turned out to be typical misfolded proteins, consisting largely of filaments (ribbons) made from known precursors. Armed with this knowledge, pathologists in recent years searched for other protein masses that might fit in the constellation of

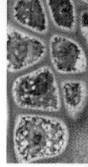

amyloid; several well known but apparently unrelated **intracellular bodies** suddenly turned out to be amyloid-like, e.g., the Mallory bodies in the liver of alcoholics, the Lewy bodies of neurons in Parkinson's disease, the plaques of Alzheimer's disease. For these relatively recent discoveries, we are greatly indebted to the pioneering work of the early "amyloid" crowd, consisting largely of pathologists. However, without the insight provided through modern protein science, this field of cellular pathology would not have been a field at all but rather a patchwork of unrelated observations.

Each cell, as we now understand it, faces the mind-boggling task of looking after its own 2 billion molecules, of perhaps 10,000 or 20,000 kinds (1). These molecules are not floating around as in a soup but instead are crowded like a dense jelly in which they occupy 20–30 percent of the space (4, 6). Up to a point this crowding helps the individual molecule to fold as required, but it can also have the opposite result, whereby as many as 30 percent of the molecules generated are misfolded and must be corrected or destroyed (5). To this effect, the endoplasmic reticulum (ER) is equipped with a *quality control apparatus:* the faulty proteins are labeled with ubiquitin, massaged by stress proteins (Chapter 5), and corrected, or directed to the proteasomes for destruction. If the proteasomes are overwhelmed or are inhibited by some toxic agent, the dire effects of misfolding are accelerated and multiplied, as we will see.

This chapter will include the effects of misfolded proteins *inside the cells,* and the amazing story of the **prions.** The interstitial deposition of misfolded proteins (classic amyloid) will be discussed in Chapter 7 along with extracellular pathology.

Pathology of the Cell Membrane

The skin of the cell—our elementary patient—is such a complex organ that we should briefly depict it before we explore its pathology.

In an evolutionary sense, the cell membrane is the oldest organelle: by enclosing a space it created a premise for life. Although it has a superficial analogy with the skin, it performs many more functions than the skin, being a physical boundary as well as an organ of contact, recognition, adhesion, communication, exchange, respiration, and even digestion. It should be visualized as a shifting, squirming carpet, studded with specialized domains—junctions, microvilli, caveolae, "lipid rafts," channels of all sorts (8)—hidden beneath an outer fluffy layer that coats a thinner sheet of soap-bubble texture, the bimolecular phospholipid leaflet. This sheet, actually a fluid (58), hangs together even though its molecules are not linked by covalent bonds. There are about 5 million lipid molecules per square micrometer (μm) (1), constantly dancing about and rotating, stabilized by cholesterol molecules spaced between them. The cholesterol molecules themselves are so free that they can pop in and out of the sheet, changing places with cholesterol in the surroundings. Protein molecules float in this lipid layer; their deep end is sometimes anchored by ropelike elements of the cytoskeleton, conferring some stability to that patch of the membrane. The fluffy overlay, the **glycocalyx** ("sweet cover"), is made of protein and carbohydrate molecules; it is actually more acid than sweet because enough H^+ ions can surround the cell to create an environment of pH 5 or lower (57). Chemically the glycocalyx may look relatively simple, but it is in fact extremely sophisticated. *The glycocalyx carries a code that is perhaps as important as the genetic code,* being in charge of the myriad recognition functions on which cell life depends (51).

The possibilities of malfunction in such a complex system are enormous (9, 11, 15, 16, 61, 65, 70, 71). Many of the cell membrane disorders are congenital, but none affects all cells: that would probably be lethal. Only one (blebbing) is visible by light microscopy; the vast majority lie even beyond the range of electron microscopy. A general classification does not yet exist; Figure 4.1 offers a bird's eye view of the main types. We will comment on a few.

Trauma: Healing of Cell Wounds

This topic is discussed in Chapter 5 (p. 191).

Blebbing

Blebbing is the most common symptom of acute cellular disease. Almost any type of insult will cause cells to develop protrusions, called **blebs,** shaped like blisters or balloons attached to the cell by a narrow neck (Figure 4.2). Blebs are very much like blisters; they contain fluid with few cytoplasmic organelles or none at all (66). Some blebs pinch off and float away, as has

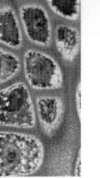

FIGURE 4.1 Disturbances of the cell membrane: a diagram of the 16 most common types.

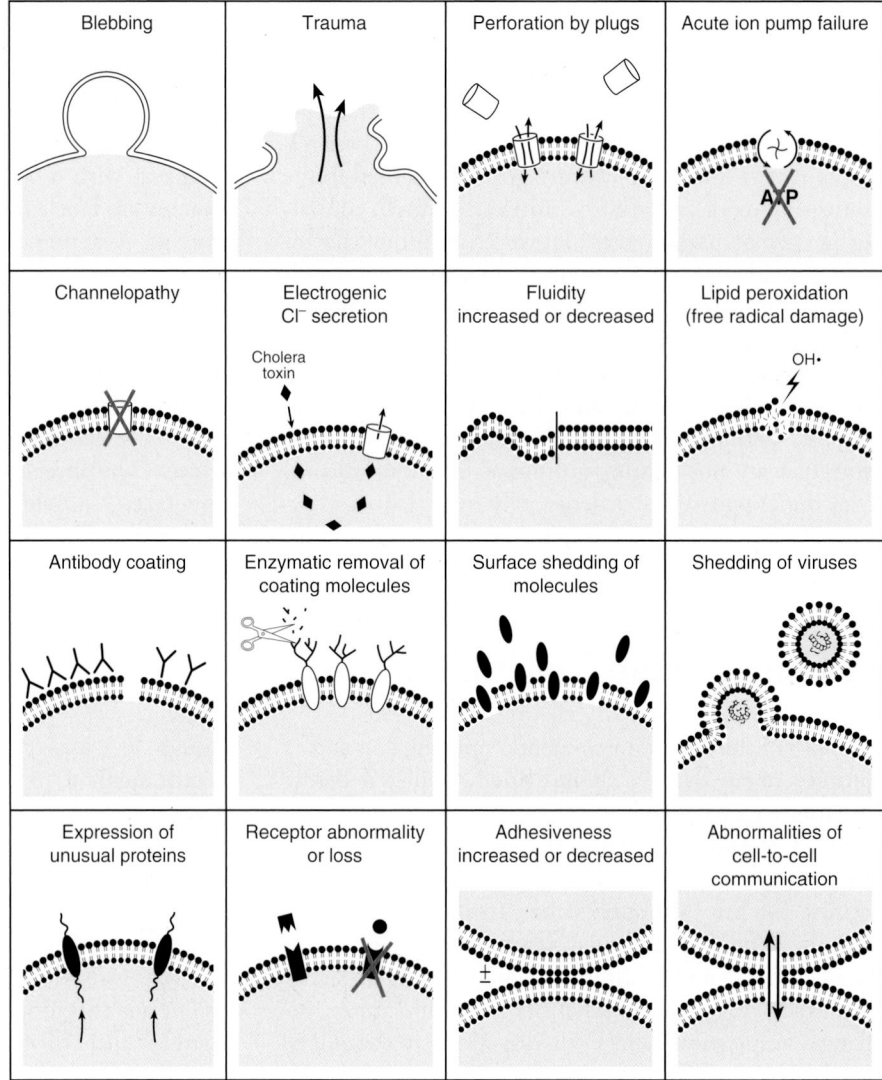

been observed *in vivo* (21); small ones can retract; some may ultimately explode. Blebbing occurs so quickly after cell damage, in seconds or minutes, that it has become (along with mitochondrial swelling) a very sensitive indicator of cellular suffering. However, if you see blebs on a published electron micrograph, beware; like swollen mitochondria, blebs can develop also as a result of poor fixation (33). It can be difficult to decide whether they are significant or artefactual. Specimens for ordinary histology are fixed with less rigorous standards than those required for electron microscopy, which means that paraffin sections are riddled with blebs. Fortunately, they are so tenuous that they are practically invisible; only the worried electron microscopist suspects them everywhere.

Blebbing is not necessarily a threatening event for the cell. Controlled experiments (54) show that some blebs are reversible (p. 698). On the other hand, the bursting of a bleb in anoxic liver cells can be the final blow for a cell by causing a gash in the plasma membrane (31, 36).

By light microscopy, a bleb can be clearly seen only when it is surrounded by a denser medium such as plasma, rather like an air bubble can be seen in water. The round holes so common in the plasma of blood vessels are nothing but blebs arising from poorly fixed endothelial cells or leukocytes (Figure 4.3). The thyroid is a special (unsolved) case. Many pathologists believe that the epithelium of the normal follicle may or may not carry blebs (Figure 4.4) (43a, 47a); they interpret some blebs as "reabsorption droplets," rather as if the

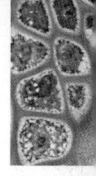

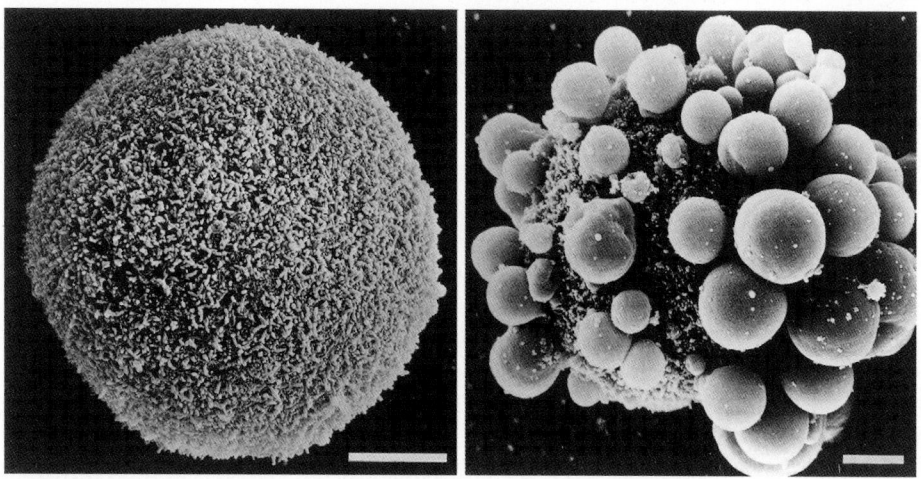

FIGURE 4.2   *Left:* Normal rat liver cell incubated in buffer. *Right:* Similar cell that is blebbing after 30 minutes' incubation with two toxic agents (dicoumarol and menadione). The formation of blebs appears to reflect the inability of the cell to maintain normal links between cytoskeleton and surface membrane. Scanning electron micrographs. **Bars** = 3 μm. (Reproduced with permission from [32]. Copyright 1982 by the American Association for the Advancement of Science.)

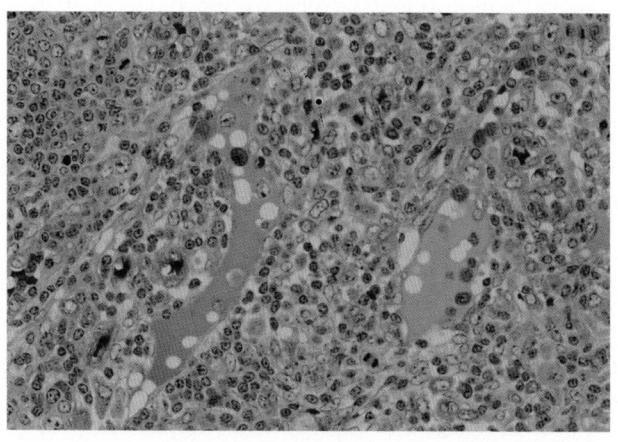

FIGURE 4.3   Blebs as fixation artefact in a lymph node. Blebs arising from endothelial cells are seen as punched-out holes in the plasma. Blebs arising in the interstitium are not easily detected by light microscopy (1-μm section; toluidine blue stain).

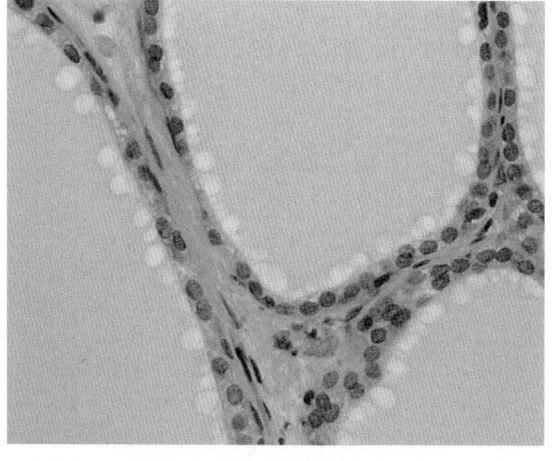

FIGURE 4.4   Blebbing of epithelial cells in the follicles of a human thyroid. The blebs are made visible by the colloid that fills the follicle. Artefact, significant change, or some of each?

epithelium had taken a bite out of the colloid. So, are we dealing with poorly fixed or with hyperactive epithelium? It is high time for someone to perform a well-controlled experiment to settle this issue.

Mechanism of Blebbing

A bleb develops where a patch of the cell membrane has become disconnected from its lining of cytoskeleton (23); by electron microscopy this is the distinctive feature of blebs. Having lost its support, the cell membrane bulges outward, showing that it is under pressure: either hydrostatic pressure generated by contraction of the actin-myosin system of the whole cell (55), osmotic pressure (23), or both. This pathogenesis would explain the curious phenomenon that we like to call **retroblebbing:** in some epithelia, under the stress of

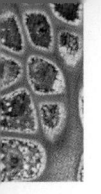

ischemia (68, 69) or toxic agents such as ethanol (13), blebs develop very rapidly *from the basal surface* of the epithelial cells. As a result, histologically a clear space develops between the epithelial cells and the basement membrane. Eventually, the whole epithelial sheet can be lifted off. The likely mechanism: blebs cannot easily squeeze out at the apex of the cell, which is covered by a dense forest of microvilli.

> In heart fibers, which are wrapped in sarcolemma, blebs caused by ischemia remain "squeezed" beneath the sarcolemma (50).
>
> Red blood cells rarely form blebs because their membranes are firmly anchored to their cytoskeletons, presumably a safety measure in view of their turbulent life. However, they do shed submicroscopic vesicles *in vitro* if they are depleted of ATP (59).

A practical use for blebbing. Ingenious cell biologists have turned blebbing into an experimentally useful tool. Chemically induced blebbing, followed by shedding of the blebs, has been used as a source of pure cell membranes (43). Ironically, the best method for obtaining such reproducible blebbing is to treat cells with formaldehyde, the standard fixative. It is no wonder that histologic sections are full of blebs.

Failure of the Membrane Pumps (Acute Cellular Swelling)

Physiology teaches that most cells spend over 30 percent of their energy to keep their sodium pumps working (1). If energy supplies suddenly fail (e.g., because the blood supply is cut off), the pumps will fail (p. 79). Nobody can *see* a defective ion pump, but the result of its failure is dramatic and predictable—acute cellular swelling—a perfect example of Virchow's statement that pathology is physiology with obstacles. From these premises it should be obvious that *cellular swelling is common and can develop very rapidly and (up to a point) reversibly* (35).

If challenged beyond the point of no return, the swollen cell dies (by *oncosis,* p. 203). Its internal organelles often participate in the swelling, especially the mitochondria.

> NOTE: We have never seen a swollen fibroblast in anoxic tissue, yet fibroblasts can swell reversibly in a hypotonic medium (24). We have no explanation. Red blood cells, too, do not visibly swell in ischemic tissues, although they do have sodium

pumps. This is fortunate because red blood cells have to squeeze through capillaries; if they ever became bloated, they would block the passage altogether. (Perhaps they swell just a little. The hematocrit of venous blood is 1–2 percent higher than in arterial blood, which would amount to a 2.5–5 percent swelling.) *It is likely that factors besides the sodium pump intervene in the pathogenesis of acute cellular swelling, such as the rigidity of internal structures.*

Only extreme examples of swelling are easy to recognize in histologic sections: the affected cells appear larger, vacuolated, and more transparent, as if an excess of water had diluted the cytoplasm; the obsolete term "hydropic degeneration" portrayed this aspect. Milder degrees of swelling are difficult to detect because a doubling of the volume implies only a 26 percent increase in diameter, which can easily escape notice (41).

What are the dangers of cellular swelling? First, *the distended membrane may become leaky and/or burst.* This can be demonstrated by placing red blood cells in a hypotonic solution: they swell, eventually allowing the hemoglobin to escape. With the same experiment one can show that the holes in the membrane are reversible (56). Second, cellular swelling can be dangerous indirectly because it occupies space. Swollen cells can compress capillaries and inhibit blood flow, with catastrophic results, especially in the brain (p. 712); a similar complication can arise in the liver if the hepatocytes are bloated with water (Figure 3.5) or with fat (Figure 3.14).

> NOTE: Cells can also swell, despite normal membrane function, by an increase in internal osmotic pressure (the sorbitol mechanism, p. 79). This type of swelling develops much more slowly.

Changes in Fluidity of the Cell Membrane

Under the microscope we cannot hope to see chemical defects in the cell membrane, but we can see their effects. Especially interesting are the chemical defects that lead to *changes in membrane fluidity.*

Excess cholesterol. Remember that cholesterol molecules are inserted into the cell membrane as stabilizers and that they can move in and out, exchanging with cholesterol in the surrounding fluid. In red blood cells

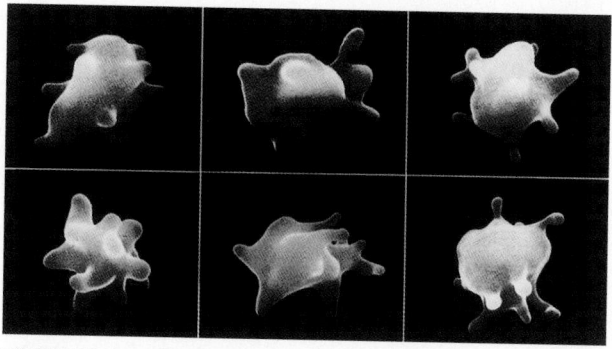

FIGURE 4.5 Scanning electron micrographs of acanthocytes, spiny red blood cells deformed by an excess of cholesterol in their membranes. (Reproduced with permission from [14], copyright 1973 by Springer-Verlag.)

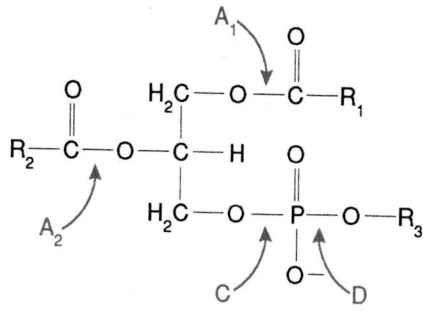

FIGURE 4.6 Structure of a phospholipid molecule. **Arrows:** Bonds attacked by phospholipases A₁, A₂, C, or D. (Reproduced with permission [60].)

their number is equal to that of the phospholipid molecules. If the plasma carries too much cholesterol, this excess equilibrates with the membranes of red blood cells, which become overloaded (25–65 percent) and stiffened (44). This causes the red blood cells to develop odd prickly shapes (Figure 4.5). These abnormal cells (acanthocytes, from *ácantha,* thorn) are removed by the spleen. This sequence can be produced experimentally, but it happens naturally in alcoholics with liver cirrhosis, who have an exces of cholesterol in their low-density lipoproteins (62).

The effect of alcohol. Alcohol is a mild anesthetic, and it acts on membranes much like other anesthetics. In acute alcoholic intoxication it has a "disordering" or "fluidifying" effect, which could explain the increased sensitivity to drugs of acutely intoxicated individuals (63). In chronic alcoholic intoxication the effect is opposite; an adaptive mechanism makes the membranes more rigid and less sensitive to drugs. This adaptation could well be linked with addiction (29).

Multiple Perforations of the Cell Membrane

One of the hazards to which cells are exposed is damage to the plasma membrane by agents that cause extensive perforations, severe enough to suggest the comparison with a sieve. These agents may target a particular component of the cell membrane (phospholipids, cholesterol) or the membrane as a whole.

Target: the phospholipids. Phospholipases include enzymes important in lipid metabolism (Figure 4.6); they are associated with plasma membranes and lysosomes,

probably in all cells. Large amounts are secreted by the pancreatic juice, and when spilled (as in acute pancreatitis), they cause great damage. This catastrophic event explains why phospholipases are a component of nearly all snake poisons (19, 20, 67). These enzymes are dangerous in two ways: they can digest the cell membranes directly, and they turn the phospholipid molecule into a detergent, that is, into a further membrane-destroying device, by snipping off one of its fatty acids. This works as follows. A phospholipid molecule such as lecithin is two-legged and roughly cylindrical; amputation of one of its legs makes it wedge shaped (Figure 4.7). This wedge is called **lysolecithin** because it lyses red blood cells. It is easy to understand that the sheet of cell membrane phospholipids will tend to reassemble into spherical micelles (Figure 4.7). Via this mechanism, cell membranes are perforated or destroyed.

Target: membrane cholesterol. Saponins are plant and echinoderm poisons that disrupt the cell membrane by combining with cholesterol. The principle is very effective (Figure 4.8). Basically, these agents function as detergents (*saponin* means "soap-like"). Primal people have known for millennia that saponins can be used not only as soap but also for catching fish. Dissolved in water, they destroy the function of the gills, and the fish turn belly up (64).

Target: the whole cell membrane. A more descriptive title for this aggressive cell-perforating strategy widely used in nature would be **weaponized pores.** It consists of spraying the surface of the target cell with short, stiff microscopic tubes or with proteins that will assemble within the cell membrane and generate such tubes. The

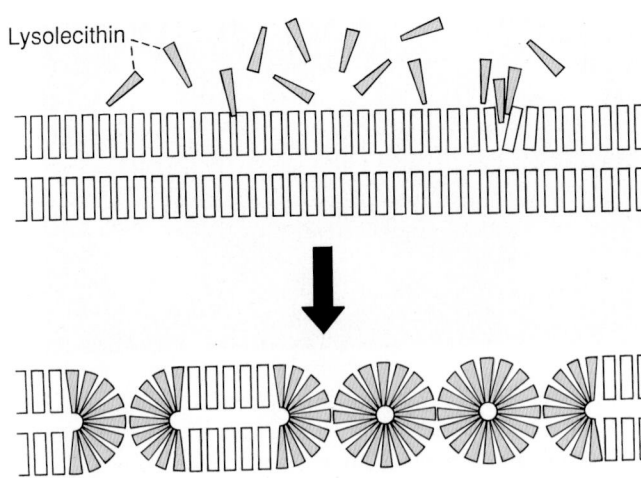

FIGURE 4.7 Disruption of cell membranes by lysolecithin. Lecithin is a normal component of cell membranes; when a phospholipase splits off one of its fatty-acid legs, it becomes lysolecithin, a wedge-shaped molecule that can break up lipid bilayers into micelles. (Modified [40].)

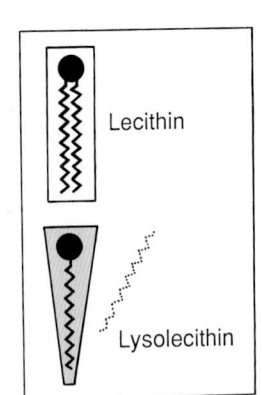

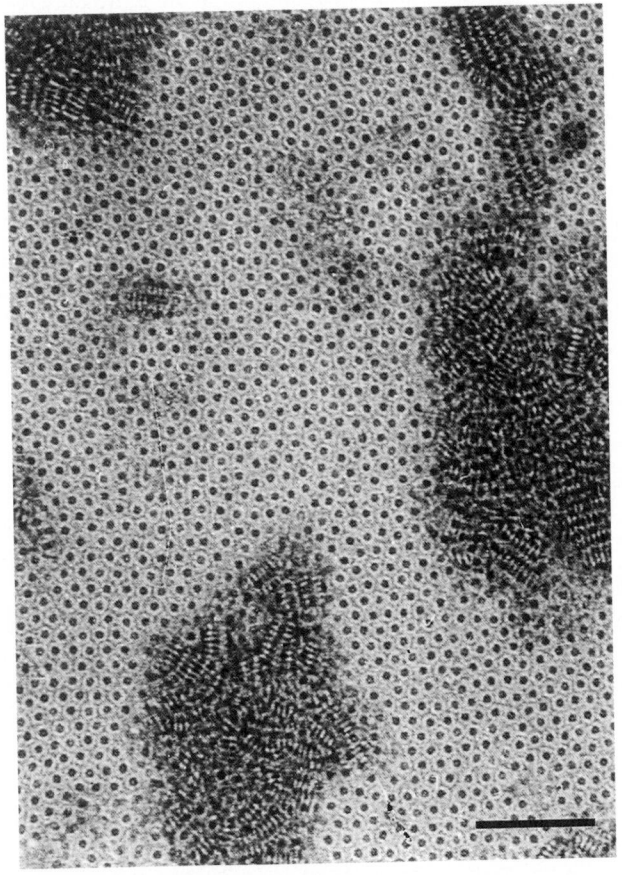

FIGURE 4.8 Perforations produced by saponin in an artificial lipid membrane, a mixture of lecithin and cholesterol. Saponin binds with cholesterol and produces a disturbance in the cell membrane comparable to that produced by lysolecithin (Figure 4.7). **Bar** = 0.1 μm. (Courtesy of Dr. A. D. Bangham, Cambridge, England.)

obvious plan is to create a myriad of circular wounds *and to keep them open.* The reason for this elaborate and somewhat gruesome procedure: a wounded cell does not "bleed" profusely like a wounded animal. A single cell wound closes in seconds (p. 191); hence the need for multiple wounds and for a device to keep them open so that they may drain vital ions. To this end, the cell uses molecular assemblies similar to those of normal membrane channels but "weaponized," that is, jammed in the "open" position. Details on the construction of these pores will be given later in discussing complement (p. 353).

This elaborate killing strategy is used in nature on many occasions: (1) by the **perforins** of killer lymphocytes, (2) by plasma, which contains some 20 proteins capable of assembling in seconds to create a cell- or bacteria-perforating machine called **complement** (p. 353); and (3) by **defensins,** antibacterial molecules secreted by some intestinal cells; macrophages and neutrophils also use defensins, but they secrete them only into phagocytic vacuoles. Defensins are used also by plants. (4) **Magainins** are secreted by the skin of an African toad (they were discovered because the toads did not become infected after nonaseptic surgery). (5) Also, many **bacterial toxins** are involved, such as the colicins of *Escherichia coli* and alpha-hemolysin of *Staphylococcus aureus* (the pores, of course, explain the hemolysis), as well as several **antibiotics** and **antifungal agents** (11). The weaponized pore design was clearly not patented.

Disorders of Membrane Receptors

Woven into the cell membrane are myriads of receptors that can malfunction in many ways. The ills of these membrane receptors have also been called diseases of cell communication (48). A few examples follow.

Acquired Disorders

Overstimulation of a receptor by a toxin. The classic example is overstimulation by cholera toxin. People infected with *Vibrio cholerae* have only one problem, phenomenal loss of fluid by the intestine, the so-called rice water diarrhea. This loss can amount to 20–30 liters in one day. And yet, intestinal biopsies show that the intestinal mucosa is intact; there is no lesion or inflammatory reaction whatsoever. What happens is that the molecule of cholera toxin becomes attached to a specific glycolipid in the cell membrane, which acts as a receptor. Then the complex penetrates into the cell, undergoes a change in the ER, and moves to the cell surface where it leads to a permanent stimulation of adenylyl cyclase and thereby to a steady secretion of chloride and water (37). The whole drama of cholera, therefore, boils down to excessive cell stimulation. The patient can be treated with the simple device of fluid intake (46) until the vibrio washes away. Other toxins, such as one from *E. coli*, act in a similar fashion (26).

Binding of anti-receptor antibodies. In autoimmune diseases, antibodies may develop against receptors, such as receptors for a given hormone. The result, as we will see, may be either stimulation or destruction of the receptor (Chapter 19).

Unmasking of a hidden receptor. A receptor can be present but hidden by proteins. For example, endothelial cells exposed to leukocytic enzymes can reveal previously masked receptors for the Fc segment (the tail end) of immunoglobulin G (49). The unmasked receptors give endothelial cells the capacity to bind antigen–antibody complexes, which bristle with Fc segments. But complexes are dangerous. For the endothelial cell the ability to bind complexes is like catching a tiger by the tail (p. 543).

Attachment of lectins to membrane components and the "capping" phenomenon. Lectins are, to a large extent, laboratory tools (39). These molecules, derived mostly from plants (but also from bacteria and animals), were empirically found to have the property of combining specifically with carbohydrate components (ligands) of the cell surface (25, 30). Commercial catalogs of

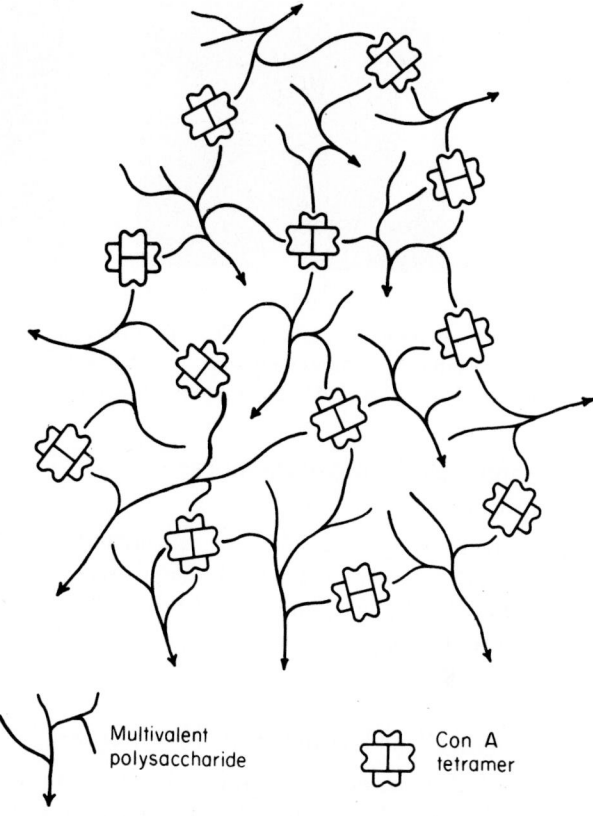

Multivalent polysaccharide

Con A tetramer

FIGURE 4.9 The chain-end mechanism, whereby tetravalent concanavalin A is thought to aggregate and precipitate polysaccharides or glycoproteins. (Reproduced with permission [30].)

chemicals list them by the dozen, each with a different specificity; as such they are precious for experimental purposes, for example, as devices for identifying a given cell type *in vitro*. Some are potent cell-agglutinators (phytohemagglutinins); others are used as mitogens, and that may be one of their functions in plants (30).

A widely used lectin is concanavalin A (Con A), extracted from the jack bean, which combines with specific carbohydrate groupings on chain ends (Figure 4.9). When lymphocytes are exposed to this lectin, at first a diffuse bonding of Con A molecules occurs all over the cell surface. Then, as the cell moves about, it gathers all the binding sites to one spot, or **cap,** corresponding to its tail end (uropige). Ultimately, it internalizes the cap into a phagosome (Figure 4.10). The capping sequence has been studied extensively in relation to antibody binding (53).

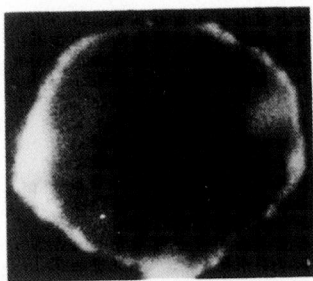 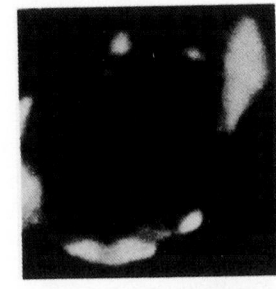 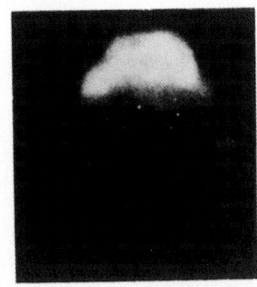

FIGURE 4.10   Capping phenomenon demonstrated in mouse lymphocytes. *Left:* Mouse lymphocyte incubated with the ligand Con A and photographed by immunofluorescence. The ligand is bound over most of the surface. *Center:* After further incubation, the ligand–receptor complex is aggregated into patches. *Right:* Later, a single cap is formed. (Reproduced with permission [17].)

Congenital Disorders of Membrane Receptors

Lack of a receptor. An example: The cell membranes of patients with familial hypercholesterolemia have virtually no low-density lipoprotein (LDL) receptors. Thus, cholesterol-bearing particles are forced to accumulate in the blood (18).

Congenital Disorders of the Cell Membrane

Diseases linked to defects in the cell membrane are many but are poorly understood at the molecular level. One of these, lactase deficiency, is extremely common; the others are rather rare. Fortunately, even the most severe are not in themselves lethal.

Brush Border Diseases

A large group of membrane disorders affect the epithelium of the gut and of the proximal convoluted tubules of the kidney—mesodermal derivatives that are structurally and functionally very similar: both have microvilli and are specialized for absorption. Congenital defects arise through deficiency or lack of a protein component in the membrane (22).

> NOTE: There is evidence that *the brush borders can be affected also secondarily,* that is, during the regeneration of intestinal cells, e.g., after an episode of acute inflammation.

Deficiency of lactase in the gut. This deficiency leads to **lactose intolerance,** that is, to gastrointestinal disturbances after ingestion of milk and its products (except butter). Because northern Europeans and their North American descendants are generally spared, medical textbooks written in these regions have nearly ignored this condition. Actually, lactase deficiency is so common that it raises a philosophical problem: because it affects most of humanity, perhaps it should not be considered a disease at all. It is the biologically sensible condition whereby the enzyme for digesting lactose disappears after the infant is weaned and milk ceases to be a natural food. In human history milk products are a recent acquisition, not shared by large parts of Asia and Africa. Evolution has not yet had the time to fully acknowledge the use of milk by adults. It could be argued that **lactase persistence** is the disease (34).

Cystinuria. Cystinuria is a rare defect in intestinal and renal reabsorption of dibasic amino acids and cystine. As in other conditions of this group, the brush border appears normal by electron microscopy. Clinically, the *intestinal* defect itself is of no consequence, but cystine is poorly soluble, and because the kidney tubules fail to reabsorb it, it precipitates as stones in the urinary pathways, causing all the complications of urolithiasis: infections and even renal failure and death.

Muscular Dystrophy

A condition that represents a widespread membrane defect is muscular dystrophy, in which the dominating clinical defect concerns striated muscles, but membrane defects have been described in blood cells and other tissues (52). It has been reported that about 5 percent of a patient's muscle fibers show missing patches of plasma membrane, which could account for a clinical sign: high blood levels of creatine phosphokinase, a muscular enzyme (42). However, this structural membrane defect may be secondary to muscular breakdown. Muscular dystrophy was shown to reflect the absence of a protein, dystrophin, that may strengthen the plasmalemma by anchoring elements of the cytoskeleton to the surface membrane (10, 27, 72).

Channelopathies: Congenital and Acquired

This term, quite young in the new millennium, refers to diseases of ion channels (11). They may be acquired (usually toxic) or congenital; because channels are made of proteins, mutations account for much of their pathology.

Cystic fibrosis is due to a defect in a chloride channel present in many epithelia, especially of the gut, lung, pancreatic ducts, and sweat glands (7, 11). As a result, the mucus in the ducts of these organs becomes abnormally viscous, leading to obstructions, infection, inflammation, tissue destruction, and scarring (fibrosis). This common channelopathy (1 in 2000–2500 people in the United States) illustrates the chain of diverse complications that can follow a minuscule molecular fault in a single protein. The single clinical sign that suggests a very specific molecular defect is sometimes reported by mothers: when kissed good night, a child "tastes salty."

Toxic channelopathies. Tetrodotoxin, the powerful poison of the puffer fish (Figure 4.11), blocks the sodium channels. When you order *fugu* in a Japanese restaurant, you depend on the chef's ability to dissect out the toxic liver and ovaries (38, 45). People of the Colombian forest

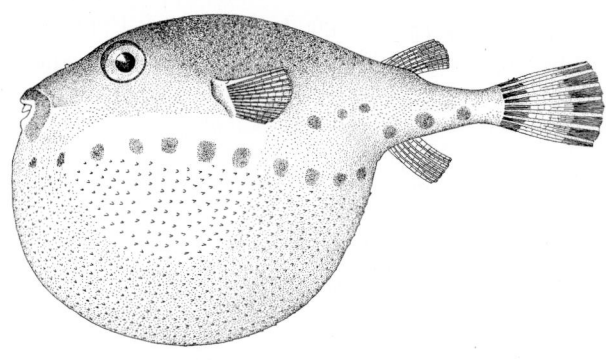

FIGURE 4.11 An enemy of sodium channels. Appropriately prepared, the puffer fish (*Spheroides spengleri*) is a delicacy of Japanese restaurants. The toxin produced by this fish (tetrodotoxin) is also present in the totally unrelated California newt. (Reproduced with permission [28].)

poison their blowdarts with the secretion of a frog that is laced with **batrachotoxin,** which has the opposite effect: it kills cells by keeping sodium channels open (45). Countless other toxins affect the membranes of nerve endings.

Pathology of the Mitochondria

Until 1962, nothing could be said about the pathology of mitochondria. They were the busy powerhouse of the cell, not even known to have their own DNA and not known to misbehave. The notion that they probably derived from bacteria could not yet be mentioned "in polite biological society" (87). Today there is a complex mitochondrial pathology with a clinical counterpart: (86, 95): some highlights follow.

Dramatic Beginning: The Sweaty Patient

The very sick young woman who sought help at the Karolinska Hospital in Stockholm in 1946 did indeed open the door to a new mitochondrial medicine (84), but 16 years later, when her case was published, her own final impression must have been one of total therapeutic failure.

> Her case, when first seen, was beyond available knowledge. She had been tired and feverish for as long as she could remember; she was in a constant, terrible sweat without exercising, to the point of having to change clothes several times a day; she ate and drank a lot but could not gain weight; and her basal metabolic rate was about 200 percent (86). She was treated at first as a hyperthyroid patient, but it did not help.

In 1959 a large muscle biopsy sample was taken; biochemists isolated the mitochondria, and found that oxidation and phosphorylation were not coupled; electron microscopic examination showed abnormal mitochondria, packed as tightly as in the muscle of a humming bird (74). Fortunately, this disease (*mitochondrial myopathy* or Luft's disease) is extremely rare.

Mitochondrial DNA

All the mitochondria are thought to be derived from the mother, because there is little space for mitochondria in the head of a sperm (but a single case of paternally inherited mitochondrial disease was found in 2002 [93]). Each mitochondrion has 2–10 rings of double-stranded DNA, encoding 13 proteins (79, 94). This is minuscule compared with the nucleus, but the number of muscular diseases based on mitochondrial biochemistry has reached 120 [86]). Because every cell contains many mitochondria (about 800 in a liver cell), when a mutation strikes, it will affect only one mitochondrion; the mutation will then slowly spread as mitochondria divide (much as bacteria). It follows that normal and mutated mitochondria can coexist (*heteroplasmy*), but eventually some cells may reach a condition of

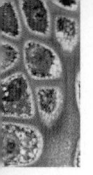

predominantly mutant DNA (*homoplasmy*). This explains why the genetic traits inherited from mitochondrial DNA are not expressed as predictably as are those transmitted by nuclear DNA.

> Incidentally, mitochondrial DNA is especially useful for identifying human remains such as those of a Russian czar's family (73). One of its advantages is that it can be extracted from skeletal parts under conditions that interfere with the availability of nuclear DNA.

Mitochondrial Encephalomyopathies

Genetic diseases caused by mitochondrial mutations tend to affect organs with a high metabolic rate, especially the brain and the muscles, hence the name encephalo-*myo*-pathies. The pattern of inheritance is quite bewildering: maternal, mendelian, or mixed (99). In a given family, all children—female or male—may inherit the disease from the mother (never from the father), but not necessarily with the same degree or severity. The onset is usually delayed and the course progressive, perhaps because of a slow decline in mitochondrial function. The diagnosis is difficult (94); a muscle biopsy can help ("ragged red fibers" as seen with the Gomori stain represent clusters of abnormal mitochondria); symptoms may point to virtually any organ. Severe exercise intolerance may be a hint (75). Alas, there is no cure.

Mitochondria and Aging

This is the latest and widely accepted theory of aging (77, 82, 89). It is based on the notion that life depends on energy (ATP); mitochondria are the major source of ATP, and with time they become damaged and inefficient. The progressive damage is explained by several features of mitochondrial structure: (1) mitochondrial DNA lacks histones, which protect against free radical damage; (2) it lacks an adequate repair system, such as repairs the nuclear DNA; (3) it has few noncoding sequences, hence a mutating event is more likely to hit a gene; and (4) the five sets of enzymes that perform oxidative phosphorylation are set on the inner mitochondria membrane, together with the mitochondrial DNA; this means that reactive oxygen species (generated by stray electrons from the respiratory chain) are likely to hit the DNA; and (5) to make matters worse, all of the proteins encoded by mitochondrial DNA take part in energy production (81).

All this explains why mutations occur 10–12 times faster in mitochondrial as opposed to nuclear DNA (89). In more dramatic terms, the symbiont mitochondria gradually turn into parasites (82).

Will this interpretation hold? We suspect that there will be, as usual, some truth in most of the theories of aging (we have some difficulty in believing that there have been over 300 such theories [82]).

Mitochondria and Cell Death

We will see in the next chapter that mitochondria take an active part in apoptosis (cell suicide) as well as in massive cell death (83, 80).

Mitochondria and Lipid Metabolism

Because the mitochondria are also the factories of fatty acid beta-oxidation, they are very much involved in the pathophysiology of fatty acids (76, 90) with ramifications in fatty livers, cirrhosis, aspirin toxicity, and sudden infant death, as we saw in Chapter 3.

Ultrastructural Anomalies of the Mitochondria

There are enough of these to fill a monograph (78). A common change is swelling, due to anoxia/ischemia as well as to toxic agents (Figure 4.12). Giant mitochondria are often found in the heart and striated muscle (78), and many bizarre patterns can be found in mitochondrial encephalomyopathies, including the bizarre "parking lot mitochondria" (Figure 4.13). Especially intriguing is the following tumor-like behavior.

Mitochondriomas. Mitochondria replicate within the cell much like bacteria; sometimes they do so in excess, filling up the cell and crowding the other organelles.

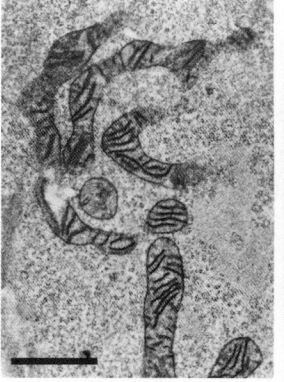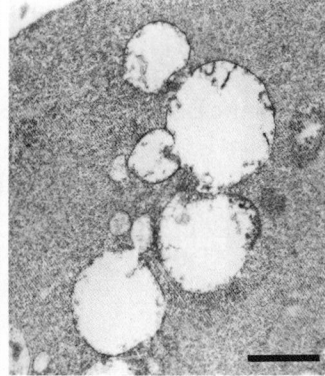

FIGURE 4.12 Example of toxic mitochondrial damage. *Left:* Normal mitochondria of Sertoli cell. *Right:* Mitochondrial swelling induced by gossypol, a disesquiterpene found in cottonseed, which has been used as a male contraceptive in China. **Bars** = 1 μm. (Reproduced with permission from [92], © American Society for Investigative Pathology.)

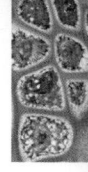

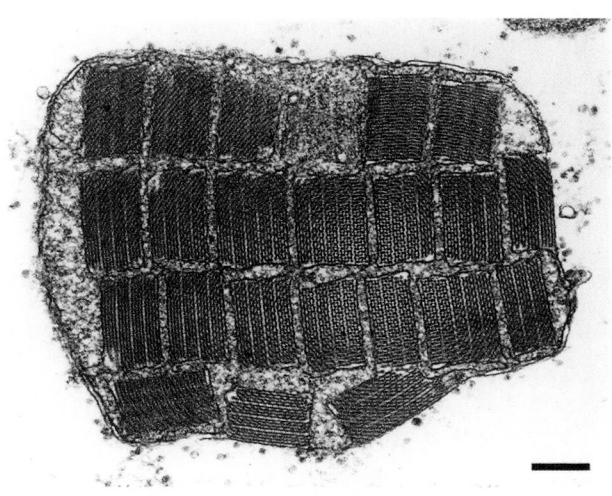

FIGURE 4.13 The astonishing "parking lot mitochondrion." These paracrystalline inclusions are one of many mitochondrial changes found in congenital myopathies. Their significance is unknown. (Reprinted from [88], Copyright 1982, with permission from Elsevier. Electron micrograph by Dr. D. L. Landon.)

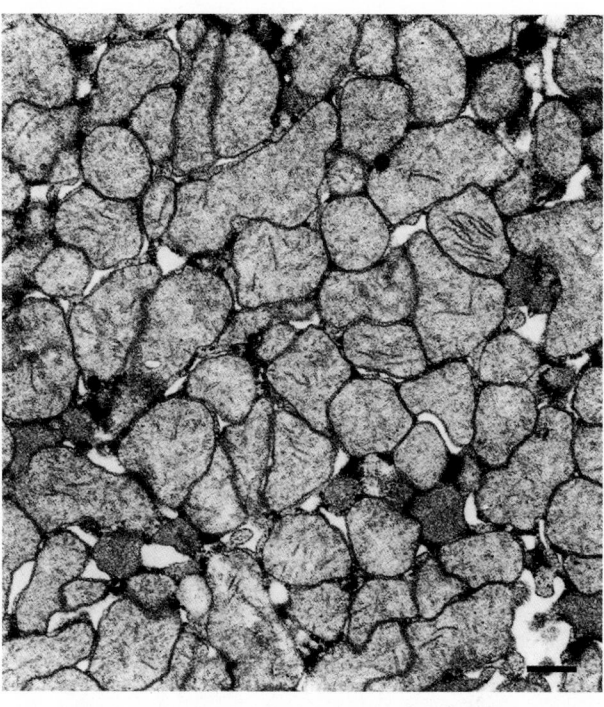

FIGURE 4.14 Abnormal crowding of mitochondria in a liver cell, possibly representing a "benign tumor" of mitochondria. This example was an accidental finding in a case of biliary cirrhosis. **Bar** = 0.5 μm. (Reproduced with permission [91].)

For reasons unknown, this happens characteristically in two tumors of the salivary glands, called Warthin's tumor and oncocytoma (96, 97, 98) and occasionally in other cells, such as in the liver (Figure 4.14) (91). In every case, histologically, the cell body stains strongly with eosin; only the electron microscope can show the real reason for this unusual feature: the cytoplasm is largely replaced by a compact mass of mitochondria. It has been proposed that this phenomenon should be interpreted as a benign tumor of the mitochondria, or mitochondrioma. Real bacteria, incidentally, are not known to form "tumors" (p. 736).

Pathology of the Endoplasmic Reticulum and Golgi Apparatus

The ER consists of cisternae and ribosomes, both of which were discovered in the late 1940s by the pioneer cell biologists/electron microscopists Keith R. Porter and George E. Palade. Neither structure is recognizable by light microscopy, but a few ER-related changes can be seen. For example, pathologists had long learned to associate increased cytoplasmic basophilia with "busy cells"—busy producing protein—but they could not possibly guess that the basophilia was due to the nucleic acids of protein-building machines, the ribosomes. Fluid-filled vacuoles often correspond to dilated cisternae of the ER (p. 76) (103); for reasons unknown, the perinuclear cisterna in dying cells is especially prone to swell and to create a clear halo hugging the nucleus (Figure 4.15) (100).

The ER has two different tasks: (a) protein synthesis (including quality control), carried out in the rough ER, and (b) detoxification, carried out in the smooth ER. Correspondingly, we find two types of pathologic changes.

Endoplasmic Reticulum Pathology Related to Protein Synthesis

As of 2002 there is no significant pathology of the ribosomes, but a few interesting anomalies can be seen by electron microscopy.

Some toxic agents cause polysomes to disperse as free ribosomes (Figure 4.16) (124) or cause the ribosomes to become detached from the cisternae (p. 199). The

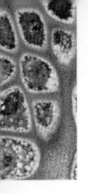

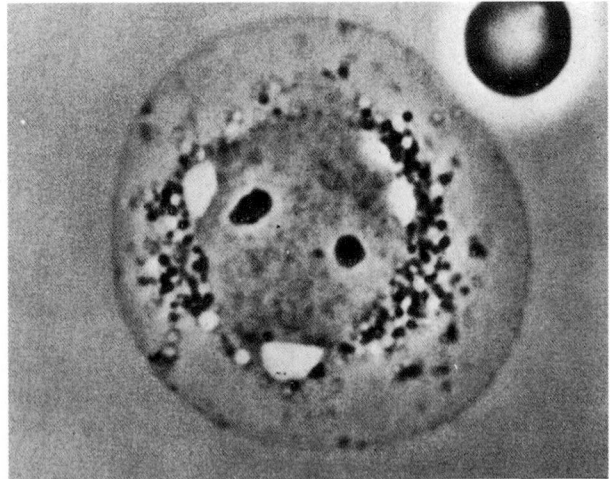

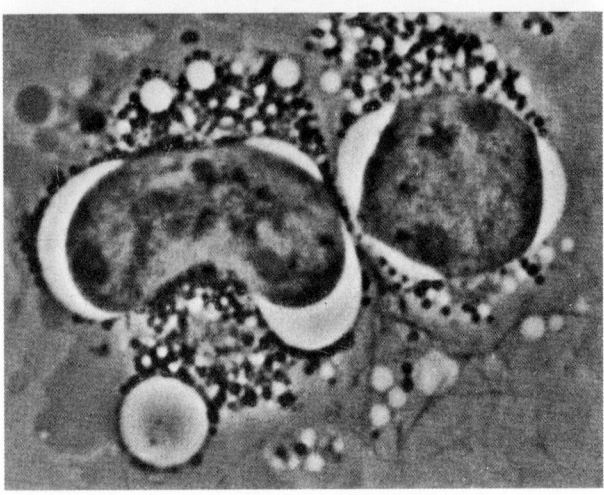

FIGURE 4.15   Vacuoles arising in the perinuclear cisterna. This common expression of cellular suffering is shown here in dying leukocytes. *Top:* Early stage. *Bottom:* Advanced stage. (2,300x) (Reproduced by permission from TRIANGLE, Sandoz Journal of Medical Science, Vol. 9 No. 6, pp. 191–199, Copyright Sandoz Pharma Ltd, Basle, Switzerland [14].)

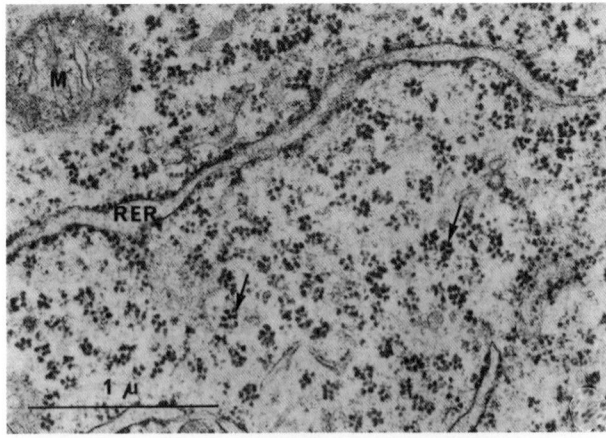

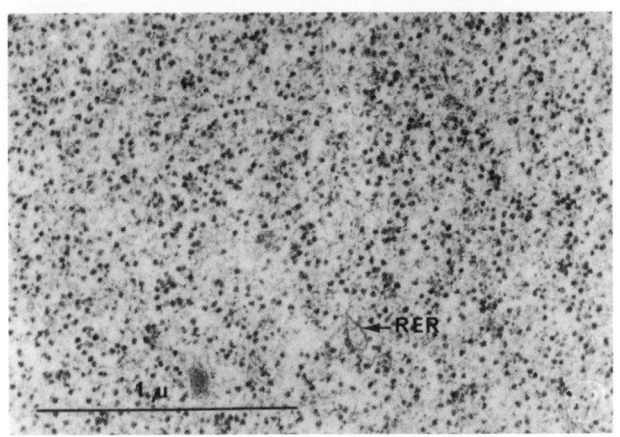

FIGURE 4.16   A subtle symptom of cellular disease: the dispersal of polysomes (*top*), which become free ribosomes (*bottom*). Mouse embryo cells 2 hours after treatment with an inhibitor of DNA synthesis, fluorodeoxyuridine. The other organelles remained normal. **Bars** = 1 μm. (Reproduced from Teratology 17:229–270, 1978, Langman J, Cardell EL. [124]. Copyright © 1978 John Wiley & Sons. Reprinted by permission of John Wiley & Sons, Inc.)

ribosomes can also aggregate into orderly crystals; this has been shown under conditions that imply a shut-down of protein synthesis, such as may occur with cooling or in the course of programmed cell death (p. 219).

Because the ER is *par excellence* the site of protein synthesis and folding, it is also the favorite site for hoarding misfolded proteins. Cell biologists teach us that the ER contains a *quality control* apparatus that recognizes the flawed molecules, attempts to correct them by a sort of massage administered by "chaperone" proteins, and destroys the hopeless molecules by addressing them to the proteasomes (115, 119, 120, 139). *The tell-tale cellular sign of ER disease based on hoarding misfolded proteins is the presence of greatly dilated cisternae*

filled with proteinaceous material; for this reason, the term ER storage disease is often used. A classic and common example is alpha-1-antitrypsin deficiency (Figure 4.17) (107, 123).

Alpha-1-Antitrypsin Deficiency

The best-known example of ER storage diseases is alpha-1-antitrypsin deficiency. This very technical name covers a fascinating story (112). The liver normally synthesizes and secretes into the plasma a protein that has the property of inhibiting trypsinlike enzymes, hence its name: alpha-1-*antitrypsin*. Why is it made? Normally many granulocytes end their short lives by breaking up in the narrow capillaries of the lungs. In so doing they spill dangerous enzymes that must be neutralized immediately. Especially dangerous is elastase, a

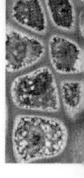

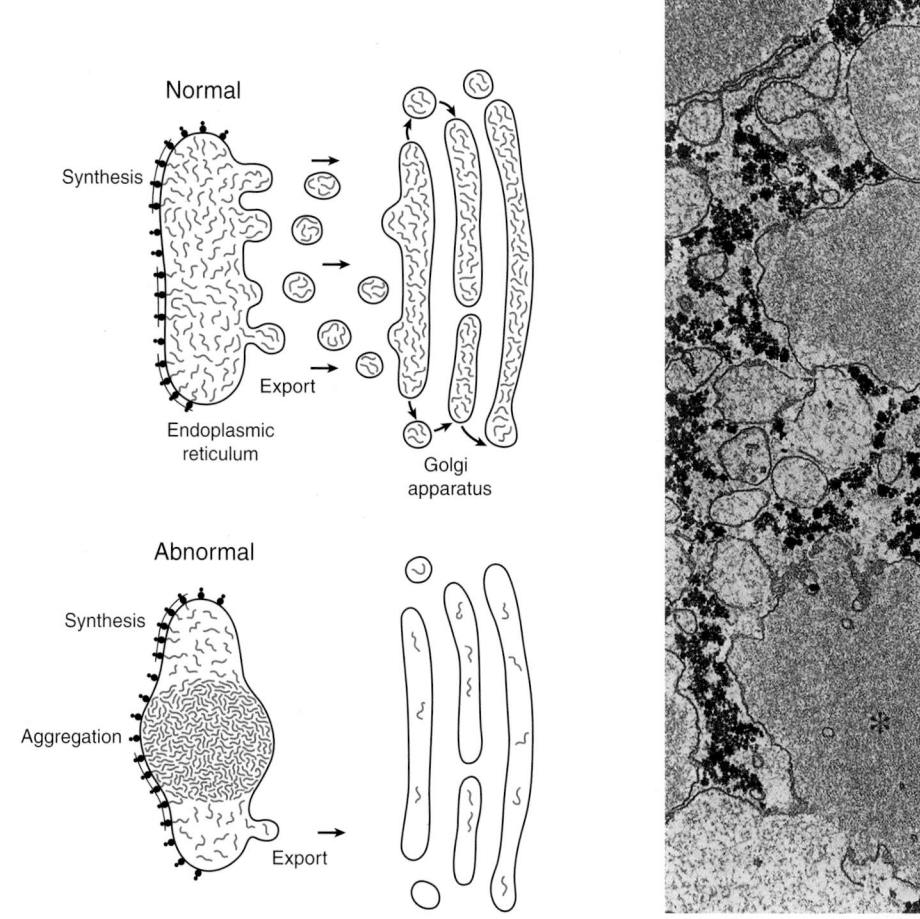

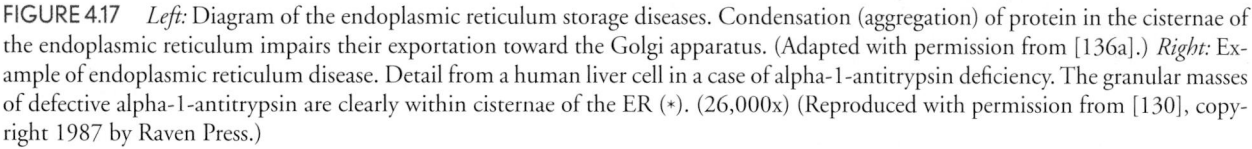

FIGURE 4.17 *Left:* Diagram of the endoplasmic reticulum storage diseases. Condensation (aggregation) of protein in the cisternae of the endoplasmic reticulum impairs their exportation toward the Golgi apparatus. (Adapted with permission from [136a].) *Right:* Example of endoplasmic reticulum disease. Detail from a human liver cell in a case of alpha-1-antitrypsin deficiency. The granular masses of defective alpha-1-antitrypsin are clearly within cisternae of the ER (*). (26,000x) (Reproduced with permission from [130], copyright 1987 by Raven Press.)

direct threat to the elastic framework of the lung. Now, *alpha-1-antitrypsin is also a potent elastase inhibitor,* and individuals with low plasma levels of this protein develop emphysema, a breakdown of the pulmonary alveolar structure.

The liver cells of some individuals do manufacture the inhibitor protein but cannot secrete it because it is defective by a single amino-acid substitution (102). As a result, the protein becomes compacted in the ER, especially in the liver cells, where the little lumps can easily be seen histologically (Figure 4.18). Although the connection is easy to see now, we are impressed with the insight of those who originally connected tiny granules in liver cells with a problem in the lungs (111).

Similar granules have been found in many other tissues by using alpha-1-antitrypsin antibodies (106). The prognosis

of emphysema in alpha-1-antitrypsin deficiency is far worse for smokers, another good reason for not smoking (112).

Many students are confused by the paradox of excess storage associated with deficiency, but the paradox is only apparent: the *amount of circulating protein is too low precisely because most of the product is being hoarded.*

Alpha-1-antitrypsin deficiency, a Swedish discovery (111), is common and has many variants of different severity; the homozygous state is found in 1:1750 individuals, the heterozygous in 1:20 (125). It can be reproduced experimentally in rats by treatment with galactosamine (102), as well as in transgenic mice who have received the defective human gene (Figure 4.19) (105).

Nature played a peculiar trick on turkeys: they too can be afflicted by an alpha-1-antitrypsin deficiency, but as a

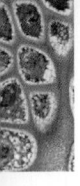

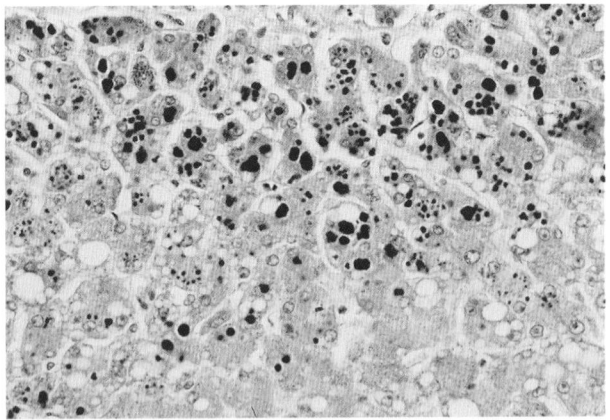

FIGURE 4.18 Liver of a patient suffering from alpha-1-antitrypsin deficiency. Periodic acid–Schiff stain, whereby glycoproteins are stained deep red (on sections stained with hematoxylin and eosin, the granules are easily missed). Initially the granules are mainly periportal. The liver cells in the lower part of the field contain fat droplets, not a known effect of this disease: the patient became depressed and resorted to alcohol abuse.

lysosomal storage disease: presumably the enzyme is sent to the wrong address (104).

 Cystic fibrosis was mentioned earlier in this chapter as a typical *channelopathy* affecting the cell membrane of certain epithelia: a single amino acid substitution in the gene for the chloride transporter (CFTR) is sufficient to prevent it from being carried to the surface of the cell. This makes the disease a channelopathy. Being misfolded, the protein of the chloride transporter is retained and degraded in the ER, which makes it possible to classify cystic fibrosis also as an ER storage disease. Ultimately, of course, the site of any congenital disease is the gene.

 Few other ER "storage" diseases are known; in one the protein affected is alpha-1-*chymo*trypsin, in another it is fibrinogen (Figure 4.20) (129). In a few cases the ER overstorage is incidental: such is the case of the **Russell bodies** in plasma cells (see below) and the **"ground glass" hepatocytes** in hepatitis B: the peculiar aspect of these hepatocytes is produced by dilated ER cisternae packed with a filamentous viral antigen (135).

Endoplasmic Reticulum Pathology Related to Detoxification

This is a strange phenomenon. The endoplasmic reticulum is equipped with an oxidase called **cytochrome P-450,** which has the role of metabolizing and inactivating certain toxic substrates. Sometimes, instead of producing inactive molecules, the P-450 oxidase produces free radicals, which can injure and even kill the cell.

 The liver is the principal site of detoxification and therefore the richest store of cytochrome P-450. Most toxic

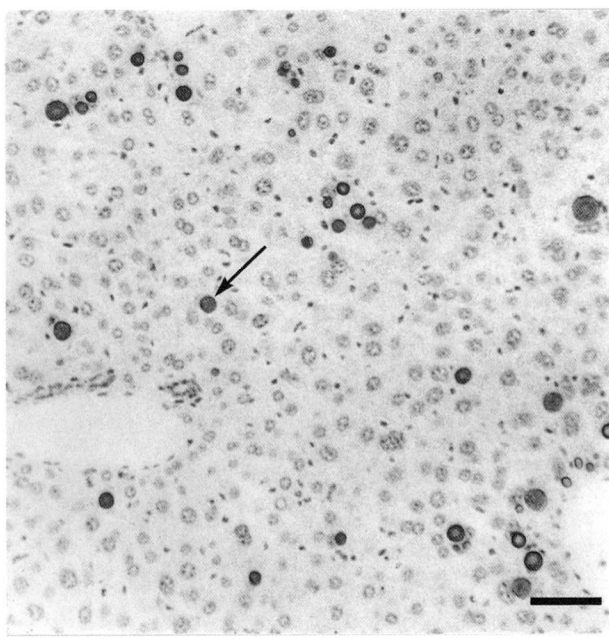

FIGURE 4.19 Globules of human alpha-1-antitrypsin in the liver of a transgenic mouse carrying a human gene for defective alpha-1-antitrypsin. The globules (**arrow**) are stained brown with an antibody against alpha-1-antitrypsin conjugated to peroxidase. **Bar** = 50 μm. (Courtesy of Dr. M. J. Finegold, Texas Children's Hospital.)

agents are taken in by mouth, and the gut is a very poor protective barrier against them (134). Thus, toxic agents are massively absorbed and transported directly to the liver. However, most, if not all, cell types contain some P-450, which explains how endothelial damage by the ER "detoxyfying" mechanism can occur also in the lung (110).

 Cytochrome P-450 (so named after its maximum spectrophotometric absorption, which is close to 450 nm) is built into the membrane of the smooth and rough ER in most (probably all) organs (137, 143). Slightly different varieties are found in mitochondria and, not surprisingly, in bacteria (128). There are many isozymes of P-450 (127), but not all are "dangerous": in some organs they are involved in the metabolism of *endogenous* substrates (122), such as steroid hormones, which are not known to create toxic products. However, in the liver, P-450 enzymes are specialized for metabolizing *exogenous* lipid-soluble substrates ("xenobiotics"), which happen to include a number of drugs and pollutants. This particular set of enzymes is **inducible,** that is, it is synthesized in response to toxic substrates.

 This potentially suicidal mechanism was discovered around 1960 as a result of efforts to understand the fatty liver caused by carbon tetrachloride, an industrial

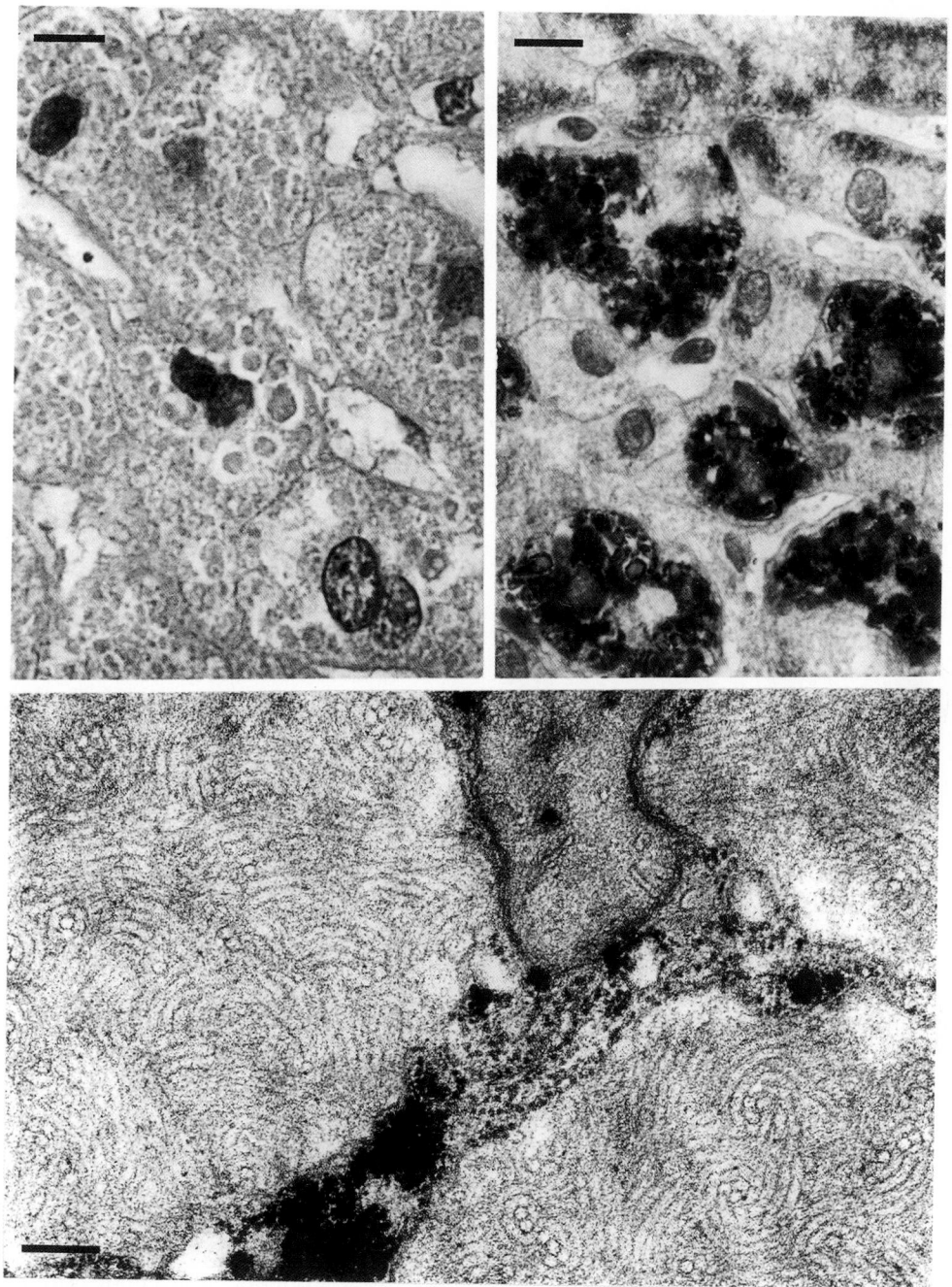

FIGURE 4.20   Fibrinogen storage disease, a newly discovered ER storage disease. *Top left:* Histological aspect of liver cells (note the large granules). **Bar** = 10 μm. *Top right:* Dark stain corresponds to specific antibody staining, identifying the material as fibrinogen. **Bar** = 10 μm. *Bottom:* Electron micrograph of the granule content. **Bar** = 0.2 μm. (Courtesy of Dr. U. Pfeifer, University of Würzburg, Germany.)

lipid solvent (133, 134) (p. 199). R. O. Recknagel, a biochemist and toxicologist, proposed that the CCl₄ molecule gave rise to highly toxic free radicals while being "detoxified" in the liver. This concept fit very well with electron microscopic studies of the liver after CCl₄ poisoning: they showed clear-cut damage to the ER evidenced by detachment of the ribosomes and "collapse" (flattening) of the cisternae (113, 138). These events are more fully analyzed in the section on free radical pathology (p. 196).

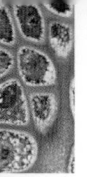

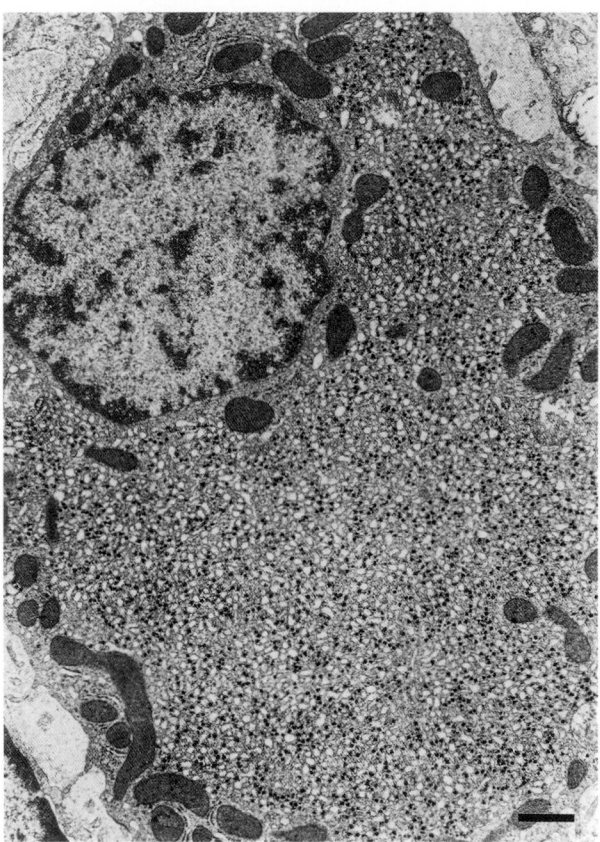

FIGURE 4.21   Hyperplasia of the smooth ER in a hepatocyte. All other organelles are displaced toward the periphery. By light microscopy the cytoplasm of such cells has an eosinophilic "ground glass" appearance. From a 53-year-old man on long-term prednisone treatment for chronic active hepatitis. **Bar** = 1.0 μm. (Reproduced with permission from [130], copyright 1987 by Raven Press.)

Today it is clear that, when challenged with fat-soluble drugs or toxic agents, the ER responds in one of two ways: hyperplasia or self-destruction, as just noted. The hyperplasia can be demonstrated in rats with therapeutic doses of barbiturates: the smooth ER expands greatly in a matter of days. Similar abnormalities are found in human liver (Figure 4.21). When examined by cell fractionation, the hypertrophic ER is found to contain large amounts of cytochrome P-450. This means that the enzyme has been induced: in some cases the normal P-450 enzyme is being synthesized more actively, and in other cases a new variety of P-450 is generated.

Now, supposing that a liver contains a great deal of hyperplastic ER produced in response to a given xenobiotic agent, will it be protected if it is exposed to a second agent? The answer is "It depends."

- *One poison followed by another may make the second more—or less—dangerous depending on the interplay between them at the level of the P-450,* as shown in the following examples.
- *Heavy smokers require higher doses of certain drugs* because their liver ER, having become hyperplastic by detoxifying nicotine, destroys them at a faster rate. The drugs include caffeine (121) (heavy smokers need more coffee for the same effect), beta blockers, and theophylline (126). In other words, if the effects of ER hyperplasia are not taken into account, heavy smokers who fall ill run the risk of inadequate therapy.
- *Insomniacs become distressingly tolerant to barbiturates:* they have developed so much smooth ER that the barbiturate is destroyed before it can induce sleep.
- *A small dose of CCl$_4$ protects a rat against a second lethal dose (for about 3 days)* (141). The reason: much of the liver ER is destroyed, which removes the source of the cytochrome P-450. By the same token, CCl$_4$ protects against a lethal dose of the mushroom poison phalloidin (116).
- *Removing two-thirds of the liver 4 days before a dose of CCl$_4$ protects rats from its lethal effect* (140): regenerating liver cells have an inefficient or immature P-450.
- *Newborn rats are insensitive to CCl$_4$* (109). The reason: much like regenerating liver, the liver of baby rats does not yet have enough P-450.

Why has the endoplasmic reticulum developed this dangerous set of enzymes? The answer is that *the mechanism evolved for processing internal or natural molecules;* the enormous output of synthetic chemicals by our society was not anticipated by evolution.

Another important practical aspect of P-450 biology is that *the response of any single patient to certain drugs and even to certain carcinogens depends on his or her enzymatic make-up,* which is genetically determined: hence the new field of pharmacogenetics (142).

In closing, the reader might be interested to know how the ER received its name, because the ER as we now see it is not obviously endoplasmic or reticular.

In 1944 the electron microscope existed but could not be used for the study of cells and tissues: there was no method for cutting tissue sections thin enough to be traversed by the electron beam. Then, Dr. Keith R. Porter, later the inventor of the Porter–Blum ultramicrotome, came upon the idea of preparing cultures of fibroblasts on cellophane. When grown in this manner, fibroblasts spread out and develop extremely thin, veil-like expansions. There was reason to hope that these expansions might be thin enough to allow the passage of electrons. So they were; their outer, thinner parts were empty, but a little closer to the cell center they contained a peculiar

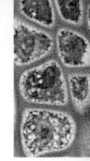

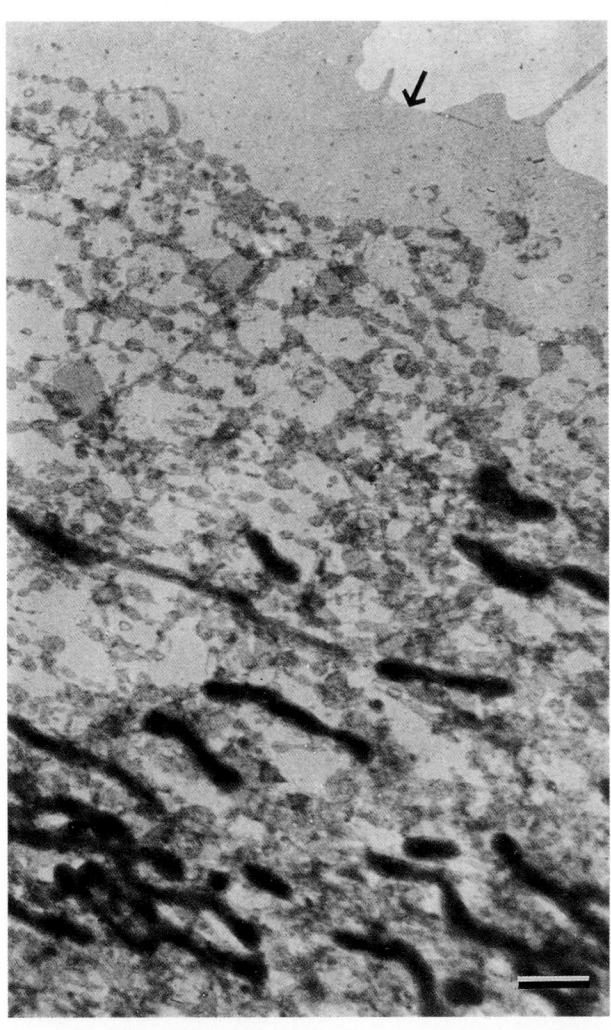

FIGURE 4.22   How the endoplasmic reticulum got its name. In the thin expansions of cultured cells, viewed by electron microscopy, it appears like a "reticulum" limited to the "endoplasm." **Arrow:** Ectoplasm. **Bar** = 1 μm. (Courtesy of Dr. K. R. Porter, University of Pennsylvania, Philadelphia, PA.)

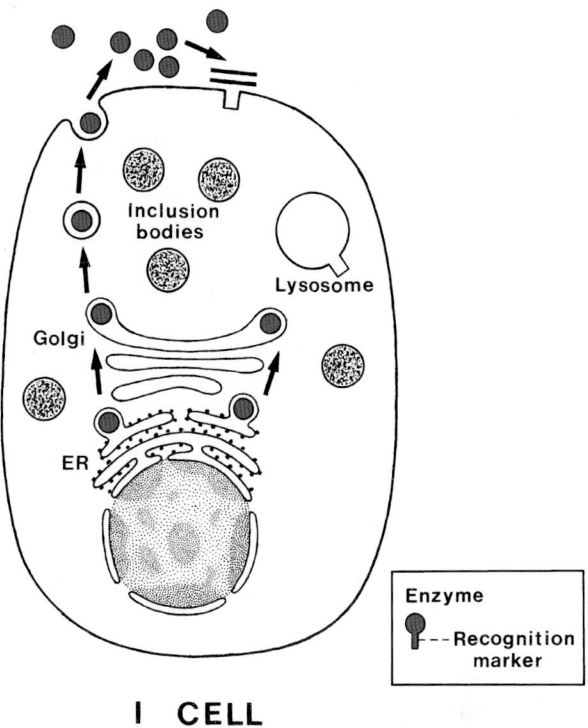

I CELL

FIGURE 4.23   Cellular disturbance in I-cell disease (compare with Figure 4.32). In I-cell disease the cells are unable to produce the enzyme recognition marker, which is essential for the intracellular transport of enzymes to the lysosomes as well as for the extracellular pathway. As a result, the hydrolytic enzymes cannot complete either pathway.

network of interconnected cords. Today we know that this surprising arrangement was due to the very special condition of the cells. The ER as seen in modern ultrathin sections appears as a stack of interconnected *pancakes.* Somehow, as they were squeezed in the expansions of Porter's very flat cells, the ER pancakes assumed the aspect of a network—such as no contemporary electron microscopist has ever seen. In any event, the network that Porter saw occupied the inner portion of the cytoplasm without reaching the edge of the cell: so it was a reticulum and it was endo-plasmic (Figure 4.22) (131, 132).

Pathology of the Golgi Apparatus

To the relief of many a student, the Golgi apparatus contributes little to pathology, at least in comparison

with other organelles (138a, 108, 117). If sustained it is practically invisible by light microscopy except in plasma cells: the typical half-moon of clear cytoplasm separating the nuclei of plasma cells from the basophilic cytoplasm is nothing but the negative image of the Golgi apparatus, enlarged in relation to the level of globulin synthesis. Electron microscopy helped to work out its intricate physiology (136) but the structural changes found are minor: e.g., the Golgi cisternae can swell or break up (108).

However, where there is function, there is malfunction. The basic task of the Golgi apparatus is to sort the proteins supplied by the endoplasmic reticulum and address them to various destinations: lysosomes, secretory granules, or the cell surface. In rare cases this function is flawed: *the lysosomal enzymes are secreted but deprived of their proper address. So their undigested substrates pile up as large cellular inclusions;* hence the name **I-cell disease** (Figure 4.23) (1). We will return to this disease in relation to lysosomes.

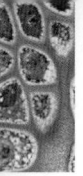

The Golgi apparatus attaches "address labels" to proteins and lipids by means of specific glycosylation reactions. It so happens that all the lysosomal enzymes are provided with the same label or "recognition marker" (mannose-6-phosphate) (114), which means that a single defect in the "addressing" enzymes can affect *all* the lysosomal hydrolases. In I-cell disease most hydrolytic enzymes missing in the lysosomes themselves are present in the extracellular fluid: this indicates a defect in the addressing system. For reasons unknown, not all cell types are affected.

The rather limited field of Golgi pathology recently made some connections that might lead to new developments; notably with Alzheimer's disease and with ricin intoxication (118). Also, two patients found to have anti-Golgi antibodies developed autoimmune disease 5 years later (101).

> **TO SUM UP:** The pathology of the ER concerns mainly the liver, because evolution concentrated in that organ two very different functions: detoxification of fat-soluble poisons, and protein synthesis. This explains the disparate nature—at the cellular and clinical level—of CC14 poisoning and alpha-1-antitrypsin deficiency. By comparison, the pathology of the Golgi apparatus is meager. The functions of this organelle are so basic that a body-wide dysfunction would probably be lethal.

Pathology of the Lysosomes and Peroxisomes

As the cell's principal digestive organs, the lysosomes are involved in most diseases, but in addition, they have over 50 diseases of their own (158, 159, 164, 165, 181, 205). After they were formally identified and described in 1955, it turned out (as is usual in such discoveries) that they had been seen before (147). But their rediscovery is unique in one respect: like the planet Neptune, they were predicted before they were seen.

About 1955, Christian DeDuve and collaborators were studying the distribution of enzymes in various fractions of liver-cell homogenates that had been separated by ultracentrifugation. From this analysis they predicted that acid phosphatase would be found to be contained in special granules, distinct from all other known organelles. A histochemical method for acid phosphatase then enabled Alex Novikoff to see the granules: almost overnight the lysosomes ceased to be a "concept" and became established as real organelles. Soon thereafter it was realized, to everyone's delight, that the unexplained granules of the blood-borne granulocytes were nothing but special varieties of lysosomes (155). Comparable organelles were later found in plants.

At least 50 lysosomal enzymes have been identified. Presumably not all are present in all cells, but acid phosphatase is always present. It has therefore retained its key function as a marker enzyme: *the standard procedure for proving, by light or electron microscopy, that an unknown organelle is a lysosome is to react it for acid phosphatase* (Figure 4.24).

The lysosome family is an untidy-looking group under the electron microscope (161). Unlike the highly stylized mitochondria, lysosomes vary in shape, size, and content because of their diversified and adventurous life cycle. Born as small **primary lysosomes** that bud off the Golgi apparatus, they sooner or later fuse with other vesicles, into which they pour their enzyme-rich contents. These other vesicles may have arisen from phagocytosis (phagosomes), pinocytosis (pinosomes),

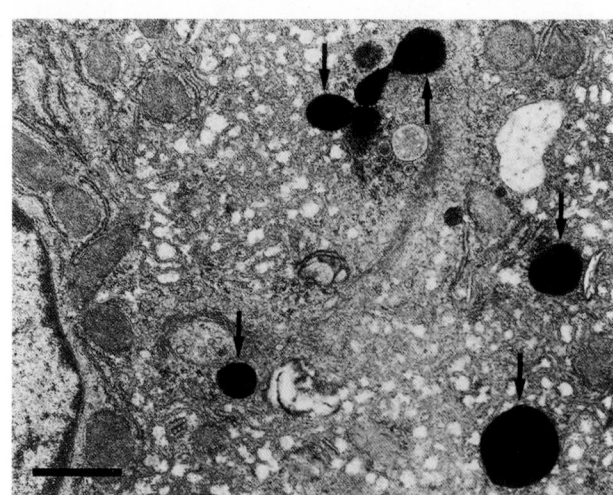

FIGURE 4.24   Demonstration of acid phosphatase in the lysosomes (**arrows**) of a liver cell in the guinea pig. The histochemical reaction is based on capturing, by means of cerium ions, the inorganic phosphate released during the enzymatic hydrolysis of phosphate-containing substrates. **Bar** = 1 μm. (Reproduced, with permission, from Robinson JM, Karnovsky MJ. Ultrastructural localization of several phosphatases with cerium. J Histochem Cytochem 31:1197, 1983 [213].)

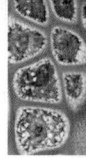

or autophagocytosis (p. 44). The result of any of these fusions is a **secondary lysosome.**

Micropinocytic vesicles, which are much smaller than primary lysosomes, also find their way into the primary lysosomes, where their membranes are recycled. This amounts to saying that lysosomes are a major site of phospholipid recycling: a property that lies at the root of many lysosomal diseases.

Whatever the lysosomes are unable to digest they simply retain; these leftovers may be foreign particles, heavily oxidized lipids from the cells' own catabolism (lipofuscin), or molecules not degraded by available enzymes. Lysosomes stuffed with such residues have been called **residual bodies** or *tertiary lysosomes* (205), but some electron microscopists refer to them irreverently as the garbage cans of the cell. As the stuffing continues, lysosomes may swell, up to several microns under extreme conditions (181). Incidentally, how the lysosomes manage not to digest themselves is not clear.

Garbage disposal, for metazoan cells, is a problem. The option of simply hoarding the wastes is only a short-term solution. Protozoans are much more effective: they get rid of bulky residues by a process referred to as defecation (biologists push anthropomorphism to the point of placing a little bottom [or cytopige] at the "rear end" of protozoans) (196). The trouble with our own metazoan cells is that they live on such refined foods and fuels (amino acids, glucose) that they are rarely faced with the need to evacuate solid residues; as a result, they have developed almost no ability to do so. It can also be that evolution downplayed evacuation of residues in metazoans because dumping the lysosomal enzymes into the tissue spaces would be dangerous to the surrounding cells (159). Whether mammalian cells ever "defecate" has been much debated (205). However, movies have documented beyond doubt that human leukocytes eject phagocytized bacteria. Exocytosis, of course, is routinely performed by mammalian cells as secretion.

> In plants the problem of getting rid of cellular leftovers is especially complex, because plants have no guts and no kidneys. Therefore, the cells dump some of their catabolites in the extracellular space, where they are polymerized and stored as resin.

Much of what we know about the pathology of lysosomes has been gleaned from studies of granulocytes, simply because they are such a convenient source of "granules." We have learned that lysosomes contribute to cellular pathology in several ways:

- Massive release of enzymes into the cell itself
- Massive release of enzymes to the extracellular spaces

- Failure of the lysosomes to fuse with phagosomes
- Failure of the lysosomes to digest.

Massive Release of Lysosomal Enzymes into the Cell

It does not take much imagination to realize that a collection of little enzyme bombs sitting in the cytoplasm could represent a hazard for the cell. At the whole-body scale, we are reminded of the pancreas, another time bomb full of enzymes that poses a threat to the individual (p. 230). Indeed, soon after lysosomes were discovered, a colorful theory was proposed: lysosomes might act as "suicide bags" in giving a dying cell the *coup de grâce* (205). Studies on cell death showed that this event is the exception, not the rule (p. 208). Though it turns out to be true that cells *can* commit suicide, they do so without firing off their lysosomes (p. 210).

On the other hand, we must briefly dwell on the exception: the lysosomes may become a hazard to the cell if they are broken open from inside. Imagine a situation in which a phagocytic cell takes in a microscopic crystal. The result may be as dangerous to the cell as swallowing a razor blade: the phagosome breaks open. The razor blade analogy is not quite exact, because breaking open the phagosome may occur not by a simple puncture but by a physicochemical interaction between the surface of the crystal and the phagosomal membrane (220). Because phagosomes are full of lysosomal enzymes, the cell can die of this accident. The victim is usually a phagocyte; the crystals can be of several sorts (154). The so-called **crystal-induced diseases** include gout (220), silicosis (144, 190), and pseudogout or **crystal arthropathy** a form of arthritis caused by microscopic crystals of calcium pyrophosphate (p. 260) (201). In this group of diseases the lysosomes are not giving the *coup de grâce* to dying cells; they are killing healthy ones outright.

Massive Release of Lysosomal Enzymes to the Extracellular Space

Spillage of enzymes into extracellular space occurs in two very different circumstances. In *inflammation,* leukocytes spill enzymes while they phagocytize and when they die; the result may or may not be an advantage. *Massive cell death* due to ischemia is usually accompanied by massive release of lysosomal enzymes into the blood: the advantage is purely diagnostic, as a signal of cell death (see Chapter 5).

Lysosomes Versus Parasites: Functional Failures

One of the major functions of lysosomes is to provide chemical agents for killing parasites. As expected, the

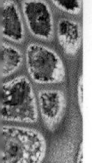

parasites have learned to fight back and inactivate the defenses; their many strategies are worthy of expert cell biologists. We will mention only four. (1) One is to *prevent the fusion of lysosomes with the phagosome* (146, 175, 176, 187). Imagine a *Mycobacterium tuberculosis* trapped in the phagosome of a macrophage. Phagosomes obtain their chemical weapons by fusing with lysosomes; mycobacteria prevent this fusion by secreting sulfatides, strongly acidic glycolipids (Figure 4.25) (174, 176, 201a). This was discovered thanks to a clue provided by the mycobacteria themselves: their virulence correlated with the production of sulfatides. (2) Mycobacteria, showered with toxic NO, switch their metabolism from an active to a dormant state, in which they do not multiply and resist chemical attacks (201a). (3) *Shigella* and *Listeria* avoid being soaked with lethal chemicals very simply: they escape from the phagosome into the cytoplasm (201a). (4) In our view, the prize goes to a protozoan, *Toxoplasma gondii,* because it shows last-minute foresight (185, 188). While it is being eaten, it manages to modify the patch of cell membrane that is entrapping it, by making it unable to fuse with lysosomes (Figure 4.26) (186).

Congenitally Abnormal Lysosomes (Lysosomal Storage Diseases)

There is a group of about 40 diseases—individually rare but collectively fairly common—characterized by the lack or malfunction of a lysosomal enzyme. They are inherited in a mendelian autosomal recessive pattern and are often fatal, whether they occur in humans, cats, dogs, or other animals (173, 193, 194, 217). The enzymatic defect leads primarily to stuffing of the lysosomes with the substrate of the affected enzyme, in some cell types more than in others, depending on the disease; the cells become bloated with huge lysosomes and eventually may even die.

These disorders are classified according to the nature of the material stored (178).

> Most commonly the enzymatic deficiency is due to the fact that a lysosomal enzyme is missing, but *at least five other genetic and one acquired mechanisms can lead to the same result* (145): (1) the enzyme may be present but inactive; (2) it may be synthesized but fail to reach the lysosomes; (3) it may be unstable at the acid lysosomal pH; (4) an activator protein can be missing; or (5) there may be a defect in the transport of the degradation product. (6) An acquired mechanism: the enzyme may be blocked by an inhibitor, such as a drug (this is **iatrogenic lysosomal disease,** see later). It follows that the same disease may be produced by several mechanisms.

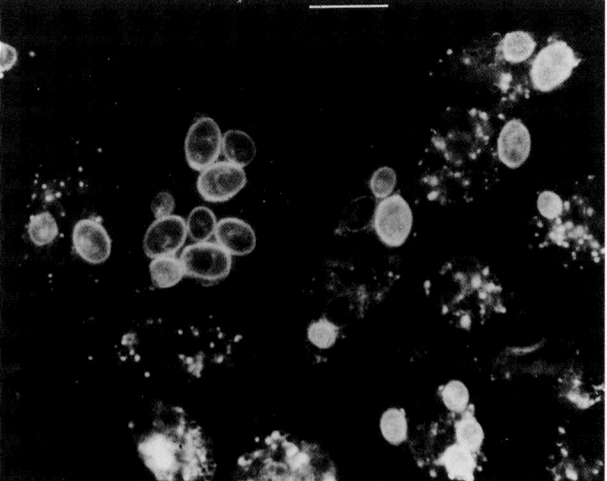

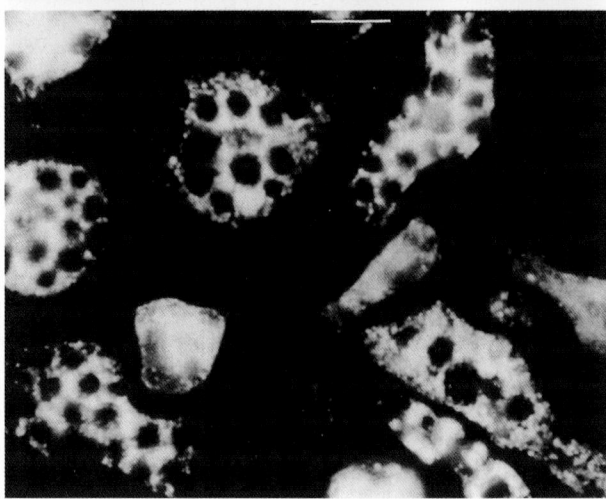

FIGURE 4.25   Prevention of fusion between phagosome and lysosome in cultured macrophages by sulfatides of *Mycobacterium tuberculosis*. *Top:* Live macrophages after 45 minutes incubation with live yeasts; staining of lysosomes with acridine orange and examination in fluorescent light. Phagocytized yeasts are fluorescent because the marker dye of the lysosomes has emptied itself into the phagosomes. This is the normal response. *Bottom:* These macrophages were pretreated with sulfatide for 18 hours, then stained with acridine and incubated with live yeasts for 2 hours. The macrophages are filled with packed lysosomes surrounding dark spaces, which represent unstained yeasts inside nonfused phagosomes. **Bars** = 10 μm. (Reproduced with permission [174].)

The lysosomal storage diseases are usually classified on the basis of the substrate that accumulates. The main groups are glycogen and glycoproteins, mucopolysaccharides, sphingolipids, lipids (triglycerides and cholesteryl esters), and mucolipids (Table 4.1).

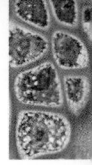

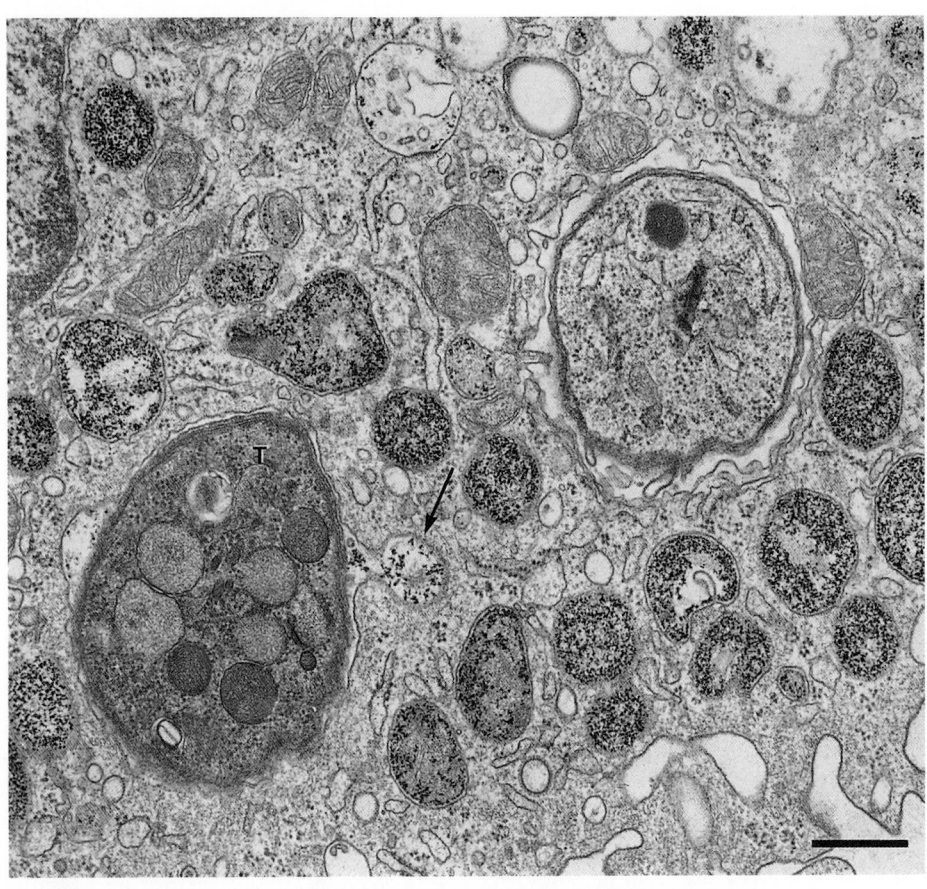

FIGURE 4.26 Inhibition of phagosome–lysosome fusion in a macrophage that phagocytized live Toxoplasma, as well as dead, glutaraldehyde-fixed Toxoplasma as control. The lysosomes of this macrophage were previously labeled with particles of thorotrast (**black dots**); then the macrophage was exposed to Toxoplasma and fixed 1 hour later. At lower left, a dead *Toxoplasma* (**T**), recognizable by its increased electron density, lies tightly wrapped in a phagosomal membrane that contains thorotrast particles; a lysosome loaded with thorotrast particles is just fusing with it (**arrow**). At top right, a living *Toxoplasma* is also wrapped in a phagosomal membrane, but there are no thorotrast particles in the phagosome and no lysosomes are fusing with it. **Bar** = 0.5 μm. (Reproduced from the **Journal of Experimental Medicine,** 1972;136:1173–1194, by copyright permission of The Rockefeller University Press [187].)

Being experiments of nature, these diseases have shed much light on lysosomal function. Without attempting to review them, we will choose some examples to show how lysosomal diseases work.

How do storage diseases reveal themselves? Pediatricians see most cases, for obvious reasons. Typically, the child is normal at birth but fails to thrive. Neurological symptoms and/or a large liver and spleen may be present. A liver biopsy may suggest the diagnosis (Figure 4.27) (208). Occasionally, the child has a particular facies; hence, for example, the alternative name *gargoylism* for Hurler disease, a mucopolysaccharidosis (Figure 4.28). (Gargoyles are the grotesque figures used as water spouts on Gothic cathedrals; see Figure 4.29).

Other physical signs vary, but a few themes predominate: stunted growth, mental retardation, blindness, deafness, heart and muscle dysfunction, a clouded cornea due to large, light-diffracting lysosomes in corneal cells. Yet some lysosomal disorders can appear in adult life; this is possible because the enzyme activity is not necessarily missing; it may be simply reduced.

What organs or tissues are affected? We would expect some degree of substrate backup in all or most cells, and extreme overloading in those tissues where the metabolism of that substrate is most active; for example, we would expect the glycogenoses (due to lack of one of the many enzymes of glycogen metabolism) to affect

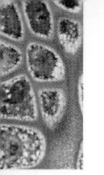

Table 4.1 Selected Lysosomal Storage Diseases

Disorder	Enzyme Deficiency	Stored Material	Unique Manifestations
Mucopolysaccharidoses (MPS)			
MPS I, Hurler	α-L-Iduronidase	Dermatan sulfate, heparan sulfate	Coarse facies, cardiovascular involvement, joint stiffness
GM₂ Gangliosidoses			
Tay-Sachs disease	β-Hexosaminidase A	GM₂ gangliosides	Macrocephaly, hyperacusis in infantile form
Neutral Glycosphingolipidoses			
Fabry disease	α-Galactosidase A	Globotriaosylceramide	Cutaneous angiokeratomas, hypohydrosis
Gaucher disease	Acid β-glucosidase	Glucosylceramide	Adult form highly variable, Gaucher cells in bone marrow, cytopenia
Niemann-Pick disease A and B	Sphingomyelinase	Sphingomyelin	(A) Pulmonary infiltrates (B) Lung failure
Glycoproteinoses			
α-Mannosidosis	α-Mannosidase	Oligosaccharides	Coarse facies, enlarged tongue
Mucolipidoses (ML)			
ML-II, I-cell disease	UDP-*N*-acetylglucosamine-1-phosphotransferase	Glycoprotein, glycolipids	Coarse facies, absence of mucopolysacchariduria, gingival hypoplasia
Leukodytophies			
Krabbe's disease	Galactosylceramidase	Galactosylceramide, Galactosyl sphingosine	White matter globoid cells
Disorders of Neutral Lipids			
Cholesteryl ester storage disease	Acid lysosomal lipase	Cholesteryl esters	Cirrhosis

Source: (Adapted from Grabowski GG. Lysosomal storage diseases. In: Braunwald E, et al. (eds). Harrison's Principles of Internal Medicine, 15th ed. New York: McGraw-Hill, 2001, pp. 2276–2281. With permission of The McGraw-Hill Companies.)

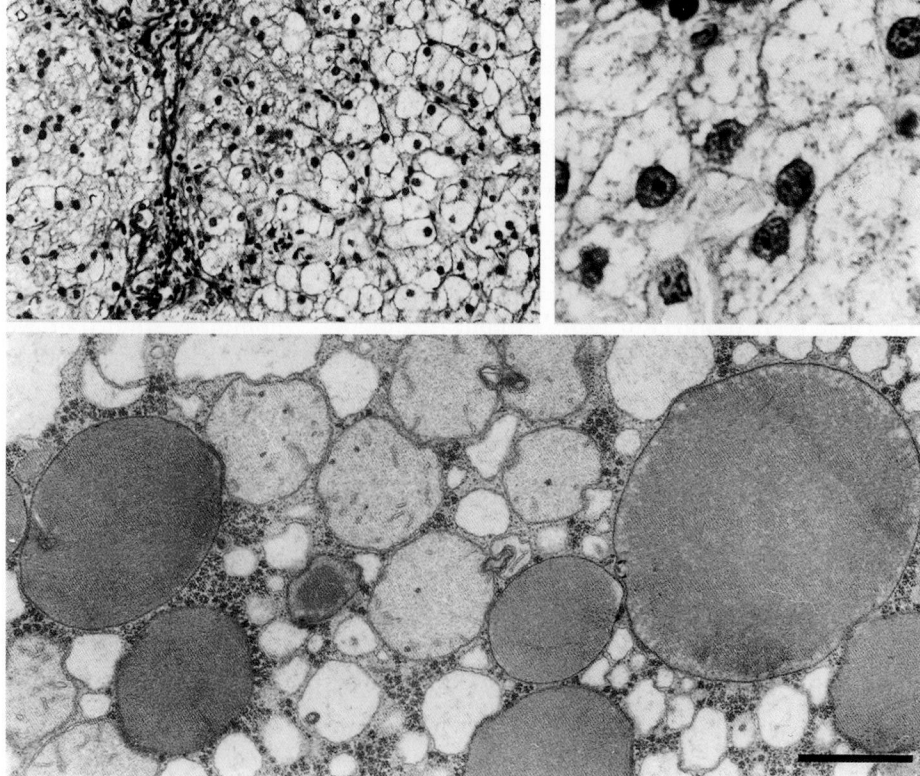

FIGURE 4.27 Cholesteryl ester storage disease. *Top left:* Histologic aspect of the liver. **Bar** = 25 μm. *Top right:* Detail, showing foamy aspect of liver cells. **Bar** = 25 μm. *Bottom:* Electron microscopy shows membrane-bound granules filled with lipid material. **Bar** = 1 μm. (Courtesy of Dr. U. Pfeifer, University of Würzburg, Germany.)

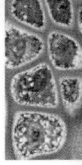

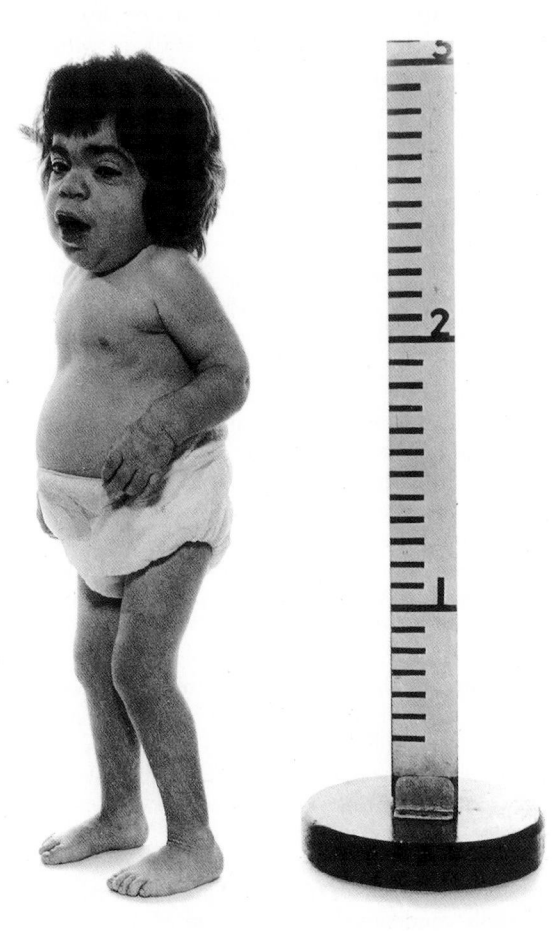

FIGURE 4.29   Gargoyle on the Parish Church of St. Peter and St. Paul, Tring, Hertfordshire, England. The depressed nasal bridge, wide nostrils, thick lips, and irregular teeth recall the features of children with Hurler's disease (gargoylism). (Courtesy of Professor D. Robinson, Queen Elizabeth College, University of London. Reproduced with permission [149].)

FIGURE 4.28   Five-year-old girl with a lysosomal disease, mucopolysaccharidosis Type 1 (also called Hurler disease or gargoylism). Scale in feet shows stunted growth (height appropriate for a 3-year-old). (Reproduced from [152] by permission of Oxford University Press.)

mainly the liver and muscle. These organs are indeed affected, but so are also the spleen and bone marrow. Now, the liver, spleen and bone marrow are the organs that contain *littoral phagocytes* (p. 314): this means that they have *two sources of undigestible material:* (a) their own cells (e.g., the hepatocytes), which cannot cope with undigestible substrates arising from their metabolism, and (b) the debris of cells that may have died in the bloodstream and need to be cleared out by the phagocytes of the RES (p. 314).

What happens to the overloaded cells? Signs of cell dysfunction are obvious in the central nervous system: the abnormal storage occurs in the cell body of the neurons—in the grey matter—but myelin development is impaired in the axons, in the white matter (191).

Oddly enough, there can also be signs of general lysosomal *overactivity* (198), perhaps reflecting increased compensatory manufacture of new but ineffective lysosomes. Also, the overstuffed lysosomes may be unable to fulfill other functions and show signs of secondary disturbances (160, 206) (Figure 4.30). Finally, in one group of lysosomal storage diseases, the sphingolipidoses, it was found that protein kinase C was inhibited, an event that could lead to general impairment of signal transduction within the cell (179).

Secondary effects of storage. The "garbage overload" has space-occupying effects. In Gaucher disease, for example, the population of macrophages in the marrow of the long bones expands, causing the bone cortex to undergo pressure atrophy and often to break. The spleen has been

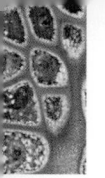

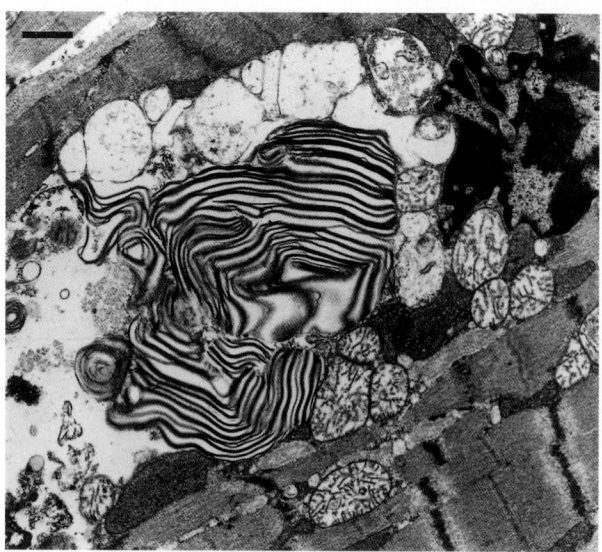

FIGURE 4.30 Zebra bodies: A manifestation of cellular disease in gargoylism, a lysosomal disorder characterized by the generalized accumulation of glycosaminoglycans. The zebra bodies represent the accumulation of phospholipids, which may be the consequence of a secondary lysosomal disturbance and may contribute to cardiac failure in these patients. (Myocardium of a 23-year-old man; tissue obtained at autopsy.) **Bar** = 1 μm. (Reproduced with permission [206].)

known to increase its volume by *more than 100 times,* creating considerable mechanical discomfort. Splenectomy relieves the discomfort, but sets the stage for more fractures (156) (the mechanism: splenectomy removes a major province of the littoral macrophages; the bone marrow has to take over some of the phagocytic function of the spleen; it expands, and leads to fractures as explained above). In the liver, deposits of undigested substrate can lead to pressure atrophy of liver cords. However, mechanical pressure is not the only factor. The reader may recall that an enlarged spleen—whatever the cause of the enlargement—increases its function, leading to *hypersplenism;* by destroying excessive amounts of platelets and red blood cells it leads to bleeding and anemia (p. 620). The enlarged liver may suggest that the excess weight is "garbage," undigested substrate but measurements in Gaucher disease found that the undigested substrate accounts for less than 2 percent of the excess weight (156). So, the extra weight must be due to a chronic, low-grade inflammatory response: phagocytizing macrophages are activated and therefore secrete many inflammatory cytokines (153) (see Chapter 11).

An example: Gaucher disease. To better appreciate the sequence and manifestations of lysosomal storage diseases

it will help to follow them in Gaucher disease (pronounced "go-shay") (151, 156, 200) in which the stored metabolite is a glucocerebroside, a normal intermediate in the lipid metabolism of cell membranes (156, 207). We chose Gaucher disease because it was the first lysosomal disease to be treated by enzyme replacement with spectacular results (148, 163, 200).

The disease is prevalent among eastern European Jews, with an incidence of about 1:450 and a carrier frequency as high as 1:10 (1:100 in the general population).

The adult form (Type 1) of Gaucher disease is more common and much less severe than the infantile form; it is characterized by splenomegaly, hepatomegaly, anemia, thrombocytopenia, and erosion of the inner cortex of the long bones. Typically, there are no neuropathic symptoms (perhaps because enough enzymatic activity is present in the nervous system). The clinical severity varies; some patients are devastated in their twenties whereas others, who may have up to 40 percent of the normal level of the critical enzyme, β-glucocerebrosidase, live fairly symptom-free into their seventies.

Regarding the pathogenesis, **obsolete leukocytes** are the most important source of glucocerebroside, quantitatively followed by red cells and neural tissue. Knowing this, the result can be predicted. Leukocytes and red cells are normally broken down and their products recycled by the phagocytic cells of the liver, spleen, and bone marrow, the three main locations of sinusoidal macrophages (littoral) (p. 316). Thus, in the adult disease the cells condemned to become most overloaded with glucocerebroside are the macrophages exposed to the blood stream. As more of them become filled up, some die and some divide; the new cells pick up and inherit the content of the old ones, and so the cycle continues. Liver, spleen, and bone marrow become massively filled with stuffed phagocytes, also called Gaucher cells (Figure 4.31). Secondary problems then arise. The blood-forming bone marrow is crowded out by Gaucher cells, leading to anemia and thrombocytopenia. The bone itself, compressed from inside, becomes thinner and may fracture (Miss Wheelchair America for 1987 was a Gaucher patient); the liver cells are also compressed but usually without major consequence because mammals can get by on about half of their liver mass. The spleen enlarges, leading to a syndrome of excessive splenic function (p. 620) *(spleens of 12 kg* have been recorded, and splenectomy can be of some relief).

The infantile form (Type 2) is deservedly called acute neuropathic or malignant. Typically, the baby looks normal at delivery. The problems begin at about 3 months, due to Gaucher cells infiltrating the central nervous system or the peripheral tissues: failure to thrive, difficult feeding, neuromuscular symptoms, large liver and spleen, spasticity, strabismus, and persistent retroflexion of the head. Death occurs within 2 years, often as a result of infection superimposed onto lungs filled with Gaucher cells.

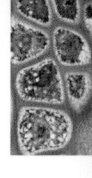

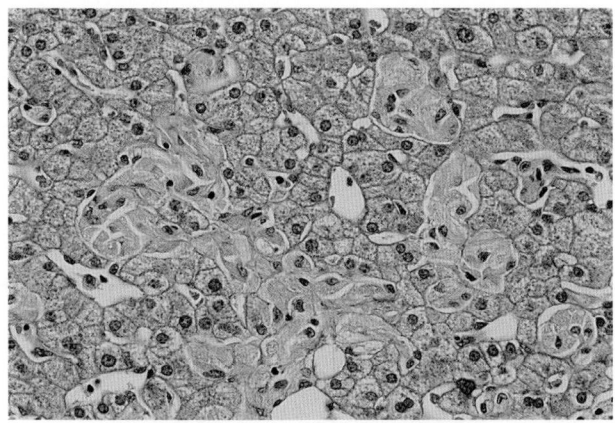

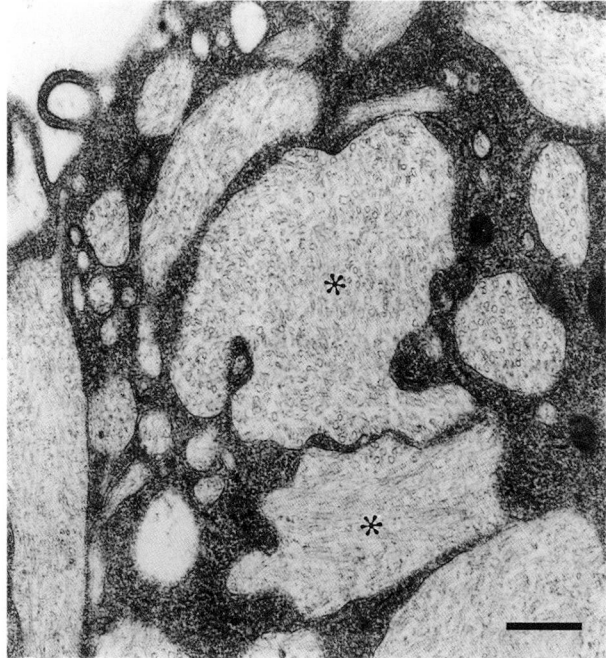

FIGURE 4.31 Liver in Gaucher disease. *Top:* Liver structure distorted by masses of swollen macrophages (bluish) filling most of the sinusoids. (Specimen courtesy of Geneviève Leyvraz, Department of Pathology, University of Geneva, Switzerland.) *Bottom:* An electron microscopic view. Part of a Gaucher cell from the bone marrow. Retained phospholipid (*) appears as a tangle of thin-walled, twisted tubules 300–600 Å in diameter. **Bar** = 0.5 μm. (Reproduced from Iancu TC. The ultrastructural spectrum of lysosomal storage diseases. Ultrastruct Pathol 16:231–244,1992 by permission of Hemisphere Publishing.)

Diagnosis and therapy of lysosomal storage diseases. The disease is first suspected clinically, then confirmed by biopsy. In a pregnant woman, the diagnosis of fetal disease can be made by amniocentesis between the second and third month of pregnancy; specialized laboratories can then test the fluid for the expected defect (reduced enzyme, excess substrate) or provide cells that can be cultured and tested in similar fashion. A first-trimester biopsy of the chorionic villi (by passing an ultrasound-directed catheter through the cervix) can yield enough cells for chromosomal, biochemical, and DNA studies and has the advantage of speed. Because it takes 2–4 weeks for the cells to grow, the pregnancy can be interrupted earlier (157, 184, 192).

Therapy entered a new era in 1991 with the intravenous administration of the missing enzyme: the choice fell to Gaucher disease, the most common (<1 : 40,000 births). The results have been spectacular: within 6 months the liver and spleen are demonstrably smaller, and the quality of life is vastly improved (148, 156, 163, 167, 200).

The enzyme, glucocerebrosidase, was at first extracted from human placentas with enormous effort: imagine *12 tons of placentas per year per patient* (177). Currently it is made by recombinant methodology (*Cerezyme®*); its preparation includes an enzymatic procedure to expose a mannose residue, whereby the molecule is targeted to the mannose receptor of the macrophages: precisely the cells that most need the treatment. This was a critical step (177).

The enzyme is infused intravenously on varying schedules, e.g., 1–3 times a week. The total amount of recombinant enzyme available during the year 2000 was sufficient for about 1500 patients, of 5000–10,000 patients worldwide; the yearly expense for a 30-kg child, given 2.5 U/kg three times weekly at a wholesale price of $3.95/U was on the order of $50,000. What about all the Gaucher patients left out? And what about all the other enzyme deficiencies? (Enzyme replacement is already being tested or developed for other selected lysosomal diseases [189, 209]). Fine topics for an ethics seminar.

Another breakthrough came from liver transplantation for Type 4 glycogen storage disease and Gaucher disease: liver function improved, as expected; in addition, *the abnormal deposits throughout the body regressed,* whereas the team that carried out this study had assumed that the disease would continue its relentless course (218). We invite our readers to explain this happy turn of events.

As for the therapeutic effect of normal liver transplants: the cells of the normal, implanted liver secrete lysosomal enzymes that circulate in the blood stream and are picked up by the enzyme-starved cells of the patient. Furthermore, in this study it was found that Kupffer cells emigrated from the implanted liver, settled elsewhere in the body, and presumably continued to produce their normal enzymes (10–15 percent of liver cells are Kupffer cells).

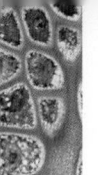

A lesson in cell biology from lysosomal storage diseases: lysosomal enzymes are normally secreted and then recaptured. This bizarre but important fact of normal cell biology was learned by culturing cells from patients with lysosomal storage diseases. These cultured cells, by the way, continue to manifest the abnormality and develop "granules" (stuffed lysosomes). Using fibroblasts cultured from various patients, Elizabeth Neufeld and her group at the National Institutes of Health made a surprising observation (203, 204). If cells from a storage disease are cultured *together with normal fibroblasts,* the diseased cells are cured and the storage granules reabsorbed. It was therefore assumed, at first, that the normal cells secreted some unknown "**correcting factor**": later it turned out that the factor was simply the missing enzyme, supplied by the normal cells present in the culture. This made it possible to understand an even more surprising result: *cells with two different storage diseases cured each other!* Clearly this happened because each cell type lacked an enzyme that was present in the other cell type. This result meant that a certain amount of lysosomal enzymes must normally be secreted by the cells. Following this lead, a new facet of normal lysosomal physiology was discovered. *The cells supply their lysosomes with enzymes by two pathways: one runs from the Golgi apparatus to the lysosome, the other leads to the cell surface. Thus, the enzyme is secreted and then*

recaptured, with some loss, and carried back to the lysosome (Figure 4.32). Now we can also understand, at long last, why in all normal people small amounts of lysosomal enzymes from many organs are present in the blood.

At this point we can return to the I-cell disease mentioned in relation to the Golgi apparatus. In this disease all the enzymes synthesized for the lysosomes are defective because they all lack the label addressing them to the lysosomes (Figure 4.24). The same label is required for recapture after secretion; therefore, if I-cells are cultured with cells of any lysosomal disease, the I-cells are unable to perform a cure on any of them because none of the enzyme molecules that an I-cell secretes can be recaptured.

Drug-Induced (Iatrogenic) Lysosomal Diseases

Strange but true: lysosomes can be disturbed by therapeutic agents, in fact by a number of *lysosomotropic molecules,* some of which are otherwise harmless dyes.

Biologists have long known that the so-called neutral red given *in vivo* will stain the macrophages, especially if they are very busy phagocytizing (Figure 5.37). This can now be explained: the red dye accumulates in the lysosomes. Another cationic dye, acridine orange (which has a beautiful fluorescence), gives striking pictures of primary and secondary lysosomes (Figure 4.25).

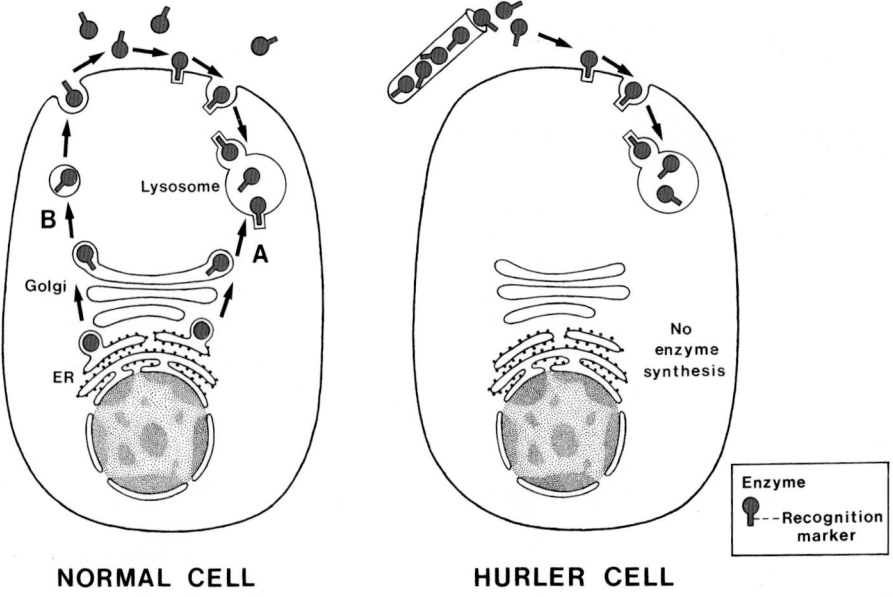

NORMAL CELL   **HURLER CELL**

FIGURE 4.32   The roundabout ways of normal lysosomal enzymes. *Left:* The normal condition. As soon as the molecules are synthesized, some migrate directly to the lysosomes (**A**) and some leave the cell and are recaptured (**B**). This odd mechanism was discovered by studying lysosomal disease. *Right:* Cells from a case of Hurler disease are incapable of synthesizing one enzyme (alpha-L-iduronidase) but can still pick it up and store it in their lysosomes if it is supplied from the outside. *This is a general rule for lysosomal storage diseases.*

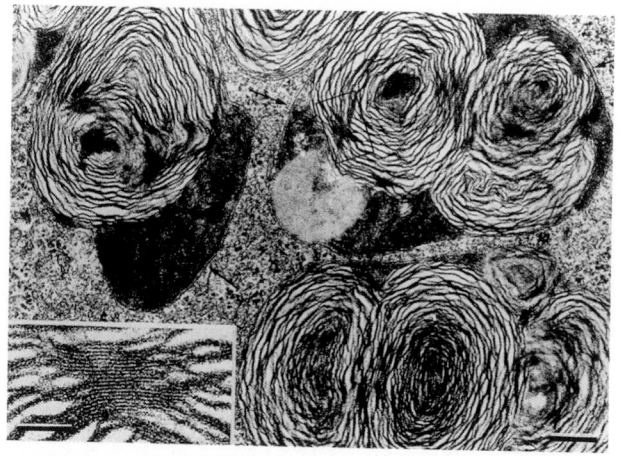

FIGURE 4.33 Drug-induced lysosomal disease: lamellated inclusion bodies in the liver cell of a guinea pig treated with chlorphentermine, an appetite suppressant, for 2 weeks. **Arrows:** membrane belonging to the remnants of a lysosome. **Bar** = 0.3 μm. *Inset:* Periodicity of the lamellar material (40–50 Å). **Bar** = 0.1 μm. (Reproduced with permission [197].)

There are many lysosomotropic drugs, which diffuse through the plasma membrane and into the lysosome. Like the dyes, they are cationic as well as amphipathic; that is, their polar end makes them water soluble, and their nonpolar end enables them to penetrate cell membranes. Once a drug is inside the lysosome, the acid environment modifies it in such a way that it is trapped and produces a "storage disease" (198, 216). A classic drug of this type is **chloroquine,** which happens to be an antimalarial drug; it also has the property of raising the internal pH of the lysosome, thus inactivating its enzymes. For this reason it has become a standard tool in lysosome research. Now we can explain the demise of the malarial parasite. Its aggressive strategy is based on invading the red blood cell, which is devoid of lysosomes and therefore defenseless. When the chloroquine comes along, it stops digestion also within the lysosomes *of the parasite,* and the creature starves to death (195).

Obviously, lysosomotropic drugs can be useful, but there is the other side of the coin: they can create iatrogenic lysosomal diseases. Once inside the lysosomes the drugs can combine with molecules that are to be processed, usually phospholipids, and make them resistant to breakdown. The result, seen under the electron microscope, is a typical storage disease (Figure 4.33) (182, 185). Clinical symptoms include muscular weakness, tremor, and mild clouding of the cornea, as seen in congenital lysosomal diseases (180). Fortunately, these changes, which are seen after months of drug use, are reversible. Chloroquine myopathy is a fine example (Figure 4.34) (199).

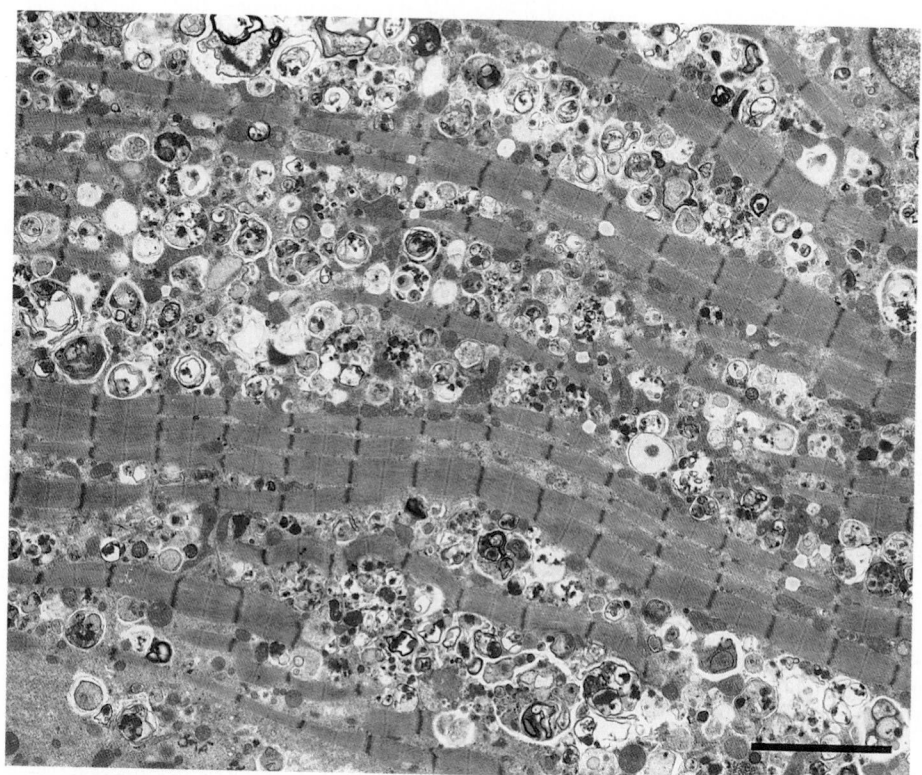

FIGURE 4.34 A drug-induced lysosomal disease: chloroquine myopathy. The patient, a 79-year-old lady with rheumatoid arthritis, had taken hydroxychloroquine for 6 years. During the last 3 months she developed weakness and fatigue. This muscle biopsy shows part of a striated muscle cell in which the bundles of fibrils are dissociated by myriads of myelin figures (phospholipids) some of which are clearly inside lysosomes. **Bar** = 5 μm. (Courtesy of Dr. U. De Girolami, Brigham and Women's Hospital, Boston, MA.)

Drugs that cause lysosomal storage diseases include antidepressants, inhibitors of cholesterol biosynthesis, vasodilators, antihistamines, anticancer agents, antibiotics (198), and the antiarrhythmic drug amiodarone. Cells affected, besides the cornea, include spleen phagocytes, which normally degrade blood cells; Sertoli cells, which normally degrade residues shed by spermatids; alveolar macrophages, which normally degrade surfactant; and retinal pigment epithelium, which normally renews visual cell membranes. In the retinal pigment epithelium cells, the outer segment of each rod contains a large stack of membranes which, in the rat, is totally renewed every 9 days. For the drug-induced storage effects to occur, chronic administration is required. Note the difference from congenital lysosomal disorders: in the drug-induced conditions just listed the lysosomes are only frustrated by adulteration of their substrate by a drug; there is no depletion or inhibition of their enzymes. An experimental model closer to the congenital condition would require a drug that reduces or inhibits a specific lysosomal enzyme. This has been achieved for Niemann-Pick's disease (215).

Pathology of the Peroxisomes

In our cholesterol-conscious culture, the peroxisomes attracted considerable interest when it was found that various hypolipidemic drugs, as well as aspirin, caused the number of these organelles to increase in the liver (Figures 4.35, 4.36) (150, 166, 168, 171, 183, 211).

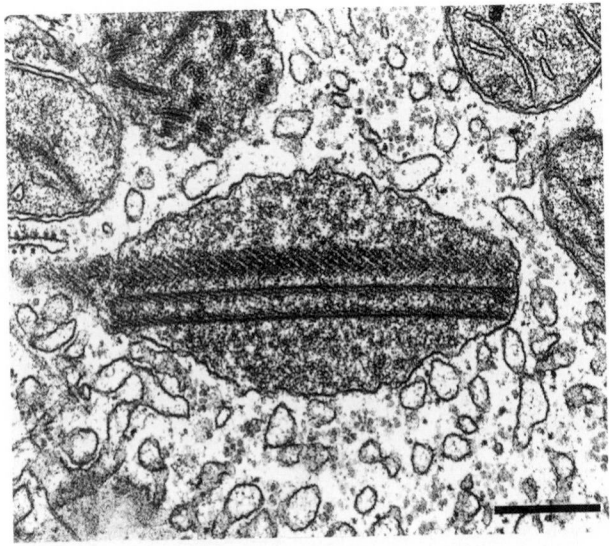

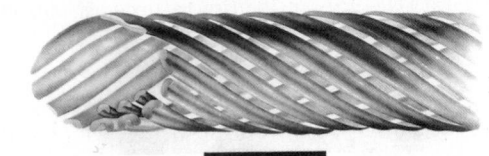

FIGURE 4.36　Effect of aspirin on peroxisomes in rat liver. *Top:* The treatment induces the appearance of rigid tubules, which are probably crystals of enzyme molecules. **Bar** = 0.4 μm. *Bottom:* Reconstructed model of the crystal. **Bar** = 110 nm. (Reproduced by permission from [183], © by The US & Canadian Academy of Pathology, Inc.)

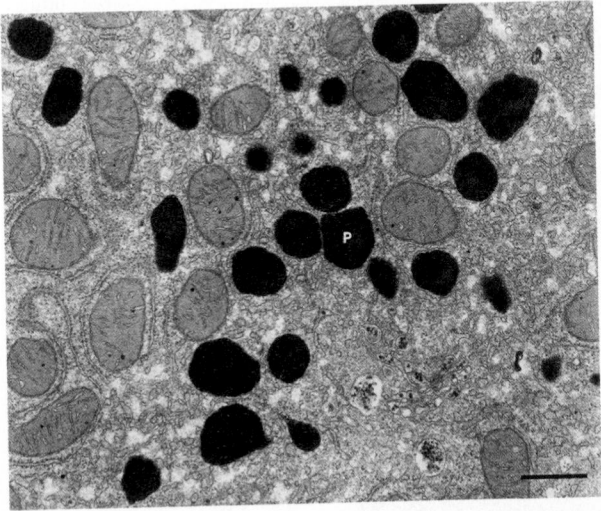

FIGURE 4.35　Increased number of peroxisomes in rat liver cells after administration of a hypocholesterolemic agent. Normally, the number of peroxisomes is about half the number of mitochondria; here they are more numerous. **Bar** = 0.5 μm. (Reproduced by permission from [150], © by The US & Canadian Academy of Pathology, Inc.)

This is still a puzzle, and so is the observation that these disparate peroxisome proliferators are also carcinogenic for the liver (210, 214).

Peroxisomes are ubiquitous organelles that are also present in protozoa and plants; they are small (0.5 μm or less) and numerous, about 1000 per liver cell and account for about one-fifth of the oxygen uptake of the liver (212). Their 15 (or so) enzymes include oxidases producing H_2O_2 and catalases destroying it. *They are specialized in the beta-oxidation of long-chain fatty acids* (C24–26) in contrast with the mitochondria, whose appetite is directed to shorter chains. They also synthesize plasmalogens, a unique category of phospholipids present in myelin and in platelet activating factor (202) (p. 362). Other possible roles include protecting the cell against buildup of H_2O_2, degrading bacterial walls, and providing an accessory pathway for the oxidation of lipids.

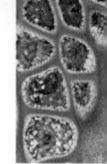

The 17 known and very rare congenital diseases of the peroxisomes (169, 211) have been classified by the number of functions involved (single, multiple, total [219]); the prototype of the latter is **Zellweger syndrome,** or cerebrohepatorenal syndrome. Multiple organs are affected because the functions of the peroxisomes are so basic. The diagnosis of these diseases is helped by one constant laboratory finding: *the very long chain fatty acids are always elevated* (219).

Pathology of the Cytoskeleton

Cells contain three kinds of thready structures, collectively called *cytoskeleton:* **thin filaments** (~60 Å), made of actin, a component of the muscle contractile system; **intermediate filaments** (~80–100 Å), a huge superfamily of about 50 molecules, of which ~30 are keratins, all rope-like and not contractile; and the stiff **microtubules** (~240 Å), associated with important proteins and capable of highly dynamic feats as we will see shortly. Because the cyto*skeleton* has mechanical as well as dynamic properties, its pathology will include static lumps (e.g., the Mallory bodies) as well as motion disorders (concerning the cilia).

> NOTE: *Many toxins produced by plants, including the most notorious poisonous mushrooms, are targeted at the cytoskeleton,* and for a good reason: plants do not like to be eaten, and not being able to run away they have taken this evolutionary path: animal cells cannot survive without their smoothly-running cytoskeleton (1). Nor can they live without protein synthesis: ricin, produced by the castor oil plant, is an extremely powerful ribosome poison.

Pathology of the Thin Filaments

The thin filaments (actin) are maximally developed in muscle cells and as such have a pathology specific to those cells. Here we will deal only with abnormalities of more general interest.

Rigor mortis. Rigor, that archetypal expression of death, occurs when myosin heads become locked to the actin filaments (Figure 4.37). This tight bond is due to the lack of ATP and can be released by ATP unless rigor is advanced (225). Despite its name, rigor "mortis" can develop also in the living body, for example in a recent myocardial infarct (238) or in a limb suddenly deprived of its blood supply. It may come as a shock to learn that rigor mortis has been studied extensively by the meat industry, the reason being that nobody would choose to buy a steak in rigor.

The essentials of the onset of rigor are as follows. If muscles are rich in glycogen, like those of well-fed nonexercised animals, glycolysis after death causes a sharp drop in pH to ~5.6. This is the setting of **acid rigor,** in which the contracture appears late (e.g., 11 hours at 17°C) and resolves by itself relatively fast, perhaps because the attached myosin heads are denatured and lose their grip. If muscles have little glycogen, like those of an animal that has been hunted down or a steer that struggled before death, the pH remains around 7.1–7.2; rigor sets in very rapidly, often with some shortening of the muscle, and may never resolve until putrefaction sets in. This is **alkaline rigor.** The alkaline pH gives the flesh its dark red color (225).

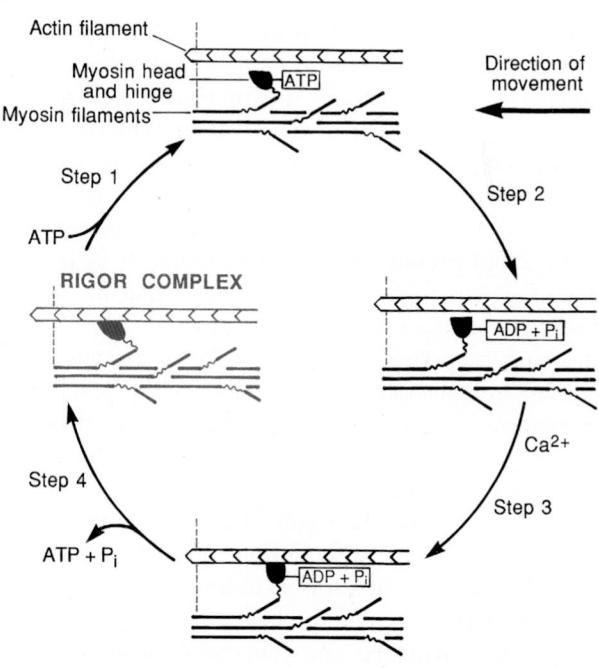

FIGURE 4.37 Genesis of rigor mortis: myosin-ATPase cycle during muscle contraction. If the supply of ATP runs out, the myosin head remains locked to the thin filament, in the so-called rigor complex (Step 4). Normally this lock is released by the binding of ATP to the myosin head, as shown in the next step of the cycle. (Adapted [231].)

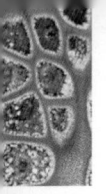

FIGURE 4.38 Disruption of actin-containing fibers (stress fibers) by cytochalasin D in cultured cells. The stress fibers are demonstrated by fluorescence microscopy, utilizing a fluorescent molecule (rhodamine) linked to phalloidin, which has a high affinity for actin. *Left:* Normal cell. *Right:* Cell after 10 minutes of exposure to cytochalasin D; most of the stress fibers have disappeared. (Courtesy of M. Schliwa, University of California, Berkeley, CA.)

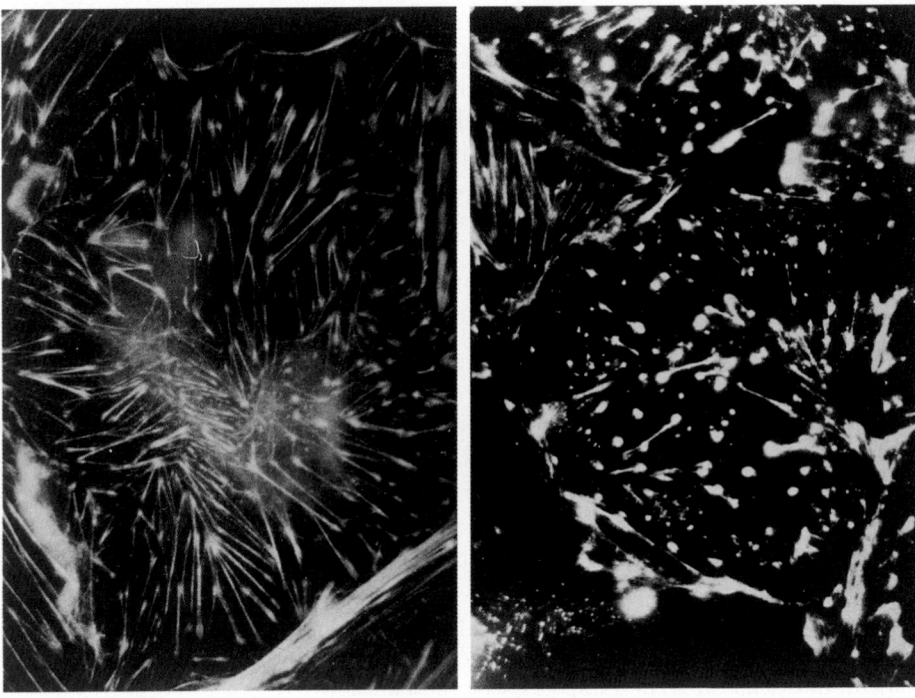

Drug-induced abnormalities. Beyond this macabre involvement with rigor mortis, *actin filaments are the target of several drugs and potent toxins* (229). *Phalloidin,* a toxin of the deadly mushroom *Amanita phalloides* (Figure 3.21), binds specifically to actin filaments (253); this gives it a practical use: it can be chemically bound to fluorescent dyes and used very effectively for the microscopic demonstration of actin by UV light (Figure 4.38). *Cytochalasin B* (extracted from Kodo millet, a grain crop) prevents the polymerization of actin filaments (Figure 4.38); it is so poisonous that in ancient India it was used to kill tigers (251). It also has the amazing properties of causing cells to extrude their nuclei (248) and of preventing cellular cleavage without preventing mitosis (227). *Cytochalasins,* incidentally, are a group of compounds that relax cells (from *khalásis,* slackening).

Jaundice can be the result of a cytoskeletal disturbance in the liver. The finest roots of the bile ducts are encircled by a coat of fibrils including actin. Drugs that interfere with actin, such as phalloidin and cytochalasin B, produce structural and functional changes in the canaliculi, as well as jaundice (244, 245).

Pathology of the Intermediate Filaments

The intermediate filaments are a superfamily of nearly 50 proteins (234, 239). They are subdivided into five classes, each typical (within limits) of a particular type of cell:

- **Keratins,** typical of epithelia
- **Vimentin,** most abundant in connective tissue cells
- **Desmin,** most abundant in muscle
- **Glial filaments,** typical of glial cells
- **Neurofibrils,** typical of neurons

This list is a challenge to the newcomer's memory, but in the practice of medicine it is useful because it helps trace the ancestry of bizarre tumor cells when all other criteria fail (p. 957). Only the cytokeratin filaments and the neurofilaments are known to have a significant pathology, and will be discussed below.

Pathology of keratin filaments. Keratin is by far the largest family, supported by at least 30 genes (235). Its functions are largely mechanical; the stiffness of hair is due to keratins. Lumps of keratin develop in the liver cells of alcoholics: these are the famous Mallory bodies, to be dealt with shortly under "Inclusion Bodies." Congenital diseases of keratin were not recognized as such until transgenic mice came along: by knocking out the appropriate genes ("reverse genetics"), it was found that mice developed the equivalent of the human **epidermolysis bullosa simplex,** a devastating disease whereby the skin responds with blisters to the slightest trauma (228). The mechanism: the basal cells, not supported by their normal cytokeratin skeleton, break up leaving an intraepithelial cleavage plane (236). Many more human diseases are expected to find an explanation with the **help of transgenic mice.**

Pathology of the Microtubules

Microtubules were discovered by electron microscopy in the 1960s; before then, electron microscopists, who always worry about artefacts, fixed their specimens with osmium tetroxide and in the cold—which just happens to create an artefact of its own by disassembling the microtubules. Eventually, fixation at room temperature—and with glutaraldehyde—in Keith Porter's laboratory opened the door to a new cellular structure.

> Microtubules are naturally unstable structures made from tubulin units free in the cytoplasm. They are constantly disassembled and reassembled, and may grow at one end while dissolving at the other. They provide rigidity and polarity to the cell, but also exert a more sophisticated function by means of proteins that come to settle on their surface and act as molecular cilia. Thanks to this arrangement, microtubules placed on a glass surface propel themselves in a straight line as if driven by an invisible force (224). By the same mechanism, microtubules inside a living cell act as engines that propel microvesicles, secretory granules, and other organelles from one part of the cell to another. *Microtubules are essential during mitosis and also represent the skeleton of cilia and of eukaryotic flagella.* Therefore, interfering with the structure and function of the microtubules can be disastrous to the cell and to the whole organism.

Antitubular drugs. Microtubules are the targets of many drugs, which have in common the property of binding to molecules of **tubulin,** the building blocks of microtubules, thereby preventing their assembly. *Because a spindle of tubules is essential for the cellular ritual of mitosis, these drugs can behave as antimitotic poisons, and therefore as antitumor agents.*

The prototype of the group is colchicine, obtained from the meadow saffron (Figure 4.39), one of the oldest specific drugs, which was used for the treatment of gout as early as the sixth century (230). Unfortunately, colchicine is very toxic. Given orally it causes diarrhea because, being an antimitotic, it stops mitoses in metaphase in the rapidly regenerating intestinal epithelium, just as X-rays do.

> An acute attack of gout occurs when a wave of neutrophils massively phagocytizes crystals of urate in a joint (p. 324). This extremely painful episode can be dramatically interrupted by colchicine taken by mouth. The effect of

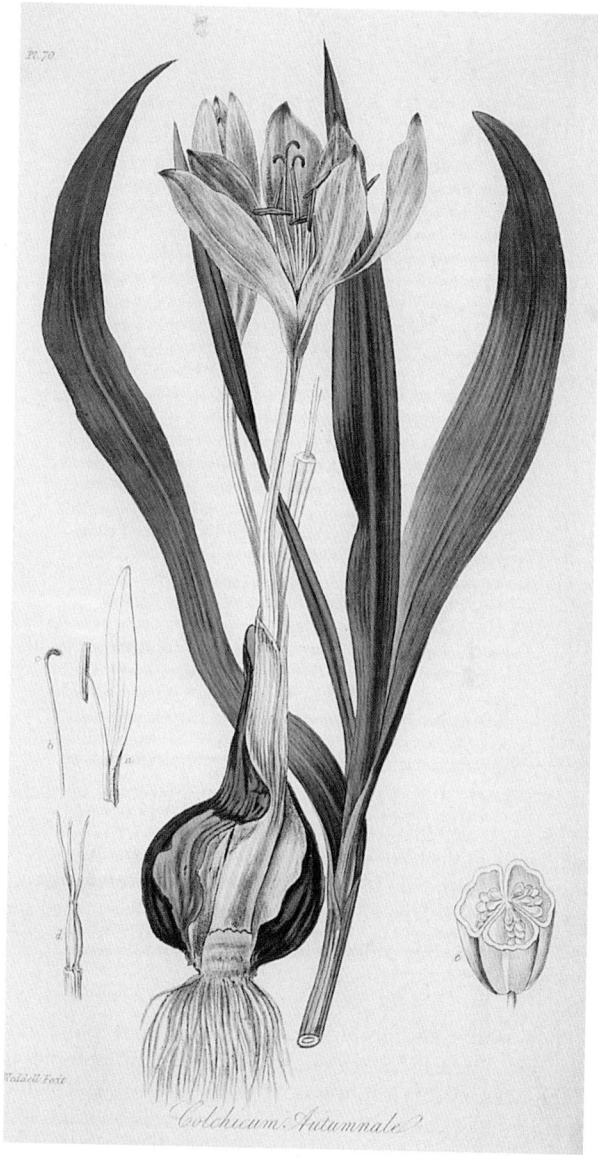

FIGURE 4.39   The source of colchicine, *Colchicum autumnale,* the meadow saffron. (Reproduced with permission [246a].)

colchicine is probably antileukocytic; that is, the disassembly of microtubules prevents the leukocytes from running to the scene and phagocytizing the crystals of urate. Other antitubule agents share this antigout effect. Intravenous colchicine is still used for gout, but it has a very low benefit-to-toxicity ratio (249).

In the 1800s, frequent cases of colchicine poisoning (some occurred during the treatment of gout) led to the study of its effects in experimental animals and to the discovery that colchicine arrested mitoses (Figure 4.40). In 1937 it was found that colchicine increases the number of chromosomes in plants; since then it has been a major

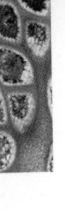

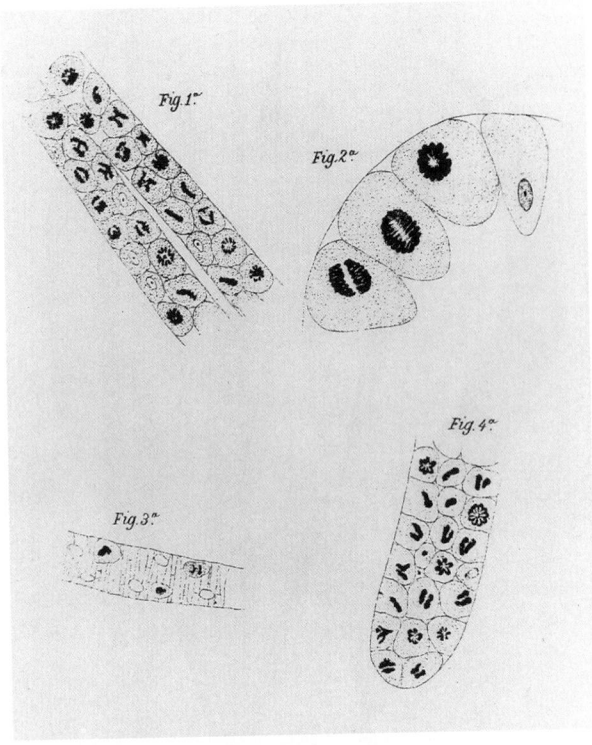

FIGURE 4.40   Effect of colchicine poisoning on the epithelial lining of the stomach and intestines, as seen by B. Pernice in 1889, in dogs that 24–48 hours previously were given a dose of tincture of colchicine by mouth. Pernice's conclusion was not that mitoses were arrested but that the cells were "stimulated and excited" by the colchicine. (Reproduced from [243].)

botanical tool for producing experimental polyploids (232). Until 1956, the exact number of chromosomes in humans was unclear; it was set at 46 thanks to colchicine. Eventually, colchicine also led to the discovery of tubulin, to which it binds stoichiometrically (232).

The antitubulin poisons include the **vinca alkaloids,** derived from the Madagascar periwinkle, which today are an essential weapon against cancer; **podophyllo-toxin,** obtained from the root of the May apple (*Podophyllum*), once used by the Penobscot tribe to treat warts (252); and **griseofulvin,** isolated from *Penicillium griseofulvum,* a fungistatic (Figure 4.41) (254). Colchicine, incidentally, is too toxic for use as an antitumor agent.

The cellular effect of these drugs, as observed on isolated cells, is no less than spectacular: the microtubules break up or disappear entirely (Figure 4.41). Most of the therapeutic effects can be explained by this mechanism. However, the blockage of mitoses does not tell the whole story. Colchicine, for instance, is 1000 times

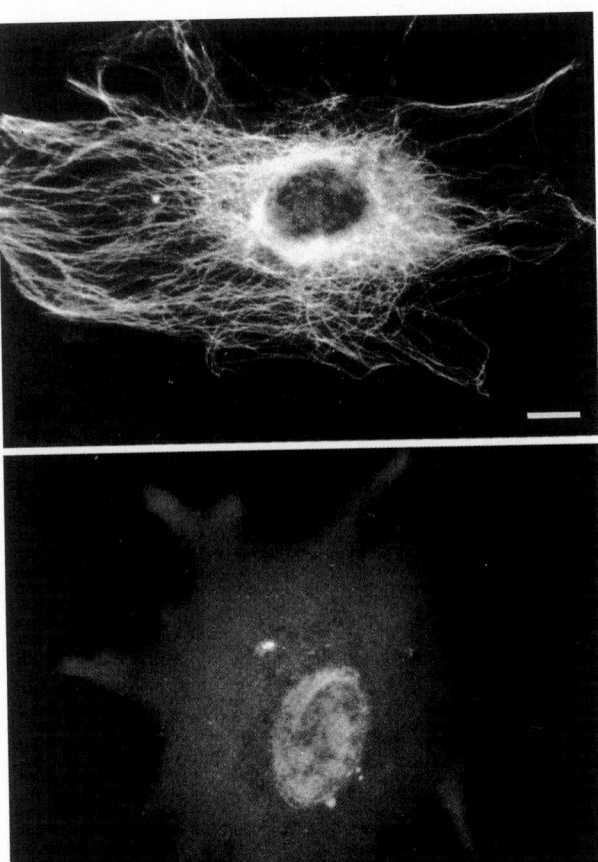

FIGURE 4.41   Disruption of microtubules by griseofulvin, a mold metabolite of the genus *Penicillium,* used as a fungi-static. *Top:* Normal cultured cell (mouse 3T3 cell). *Bottom:* Similar cell after 18 hours of exposure to griseofulvin. Comparable effects are induced by colchicine and by vinblastine, which also bind to tubulin. **Bars** = 5 μm. (Reproduced with permission [254].)

more toxic to the lymphocytes of lymphatic leukemia than to normal lymphocytes, a property that was proposed as a diagnostic test (250).

Pathology of the Cilia

Cilia are highly specialized assemblies of microtubules and other proteins. Sperm tails are essentially the same as cilia, only longer (Figure 4.42). Cilia can be damaged by infection and, in the upper airways, by smoke, hay fever, or the common cold (222); they can fall off or disappear by several different mechanisms (Figure 2.43) (226). *The best-known ciliary defects are congenital.*

Primary ciliary dyskinesia. The first example of congenitally abnormal cilia was reported in the 1950s: Ralph

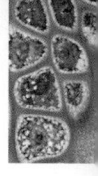

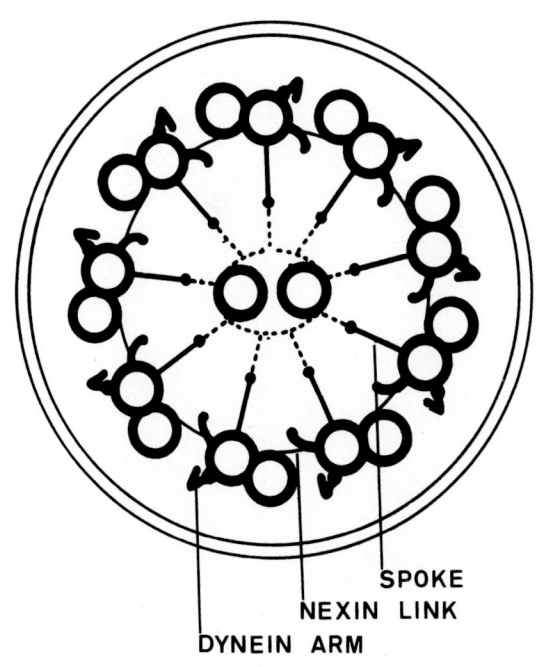

FIGURE 4.42 Diagram of the cross-section of a cilium or of the central portion of a spermatozoon's tail. The 9 + 2 microtubules are held together by three kinds of connections as indicated; the dynein arms are believed to be responsible for the motility. (Reprinted, by permission of the New England Journal of Medicine 297:1–6, 1977 [232a].)

Lewin at the Scripps Institution of Oceanography discovered a mutant strain of unicellular algae that could not swim because their two flagella (i.e., cilia) were motionless (221). Then, in 1975, a paper appeared describing the condition of a man whose spermatozoa were motionless (242). A Swedish cell biologist and expert on cilia, Björn Afzelius, confirmed the existence of this disease in a fertility clinic in Stockholm—but he went one step further: cilia are cilia, he thought, wherever they may be; perhaps the patients with immotile spermatozoa also suffered from immotile cilia in the bronchi? A quick look at some patients' files proved him right: immotile spermatozoa went along with chronic bronchitis and sinusitis (223). Thus was born the immotile Cilia Syndrome, now called Primary Ciliary Dyskinesia (237).

Afzelius was well qualified to discover this syndrome. Back in 1959, on a sunny day, while studying his electron micrographs on the beach, he had discovered the dynein arms, the engine that drives the cilia. It is missing in some cases of immotile cilia syndrome (Figure 4.43) (223).

After this syndrome was recognized, it turned out that some of the patients suffered from a triad of conditions long known as the utterly mysterious Kartagener syndrome: **bronchiectasis** (bronchial dilatations), **chronic sinusitis,** and **situs inversus viscerum** (heart

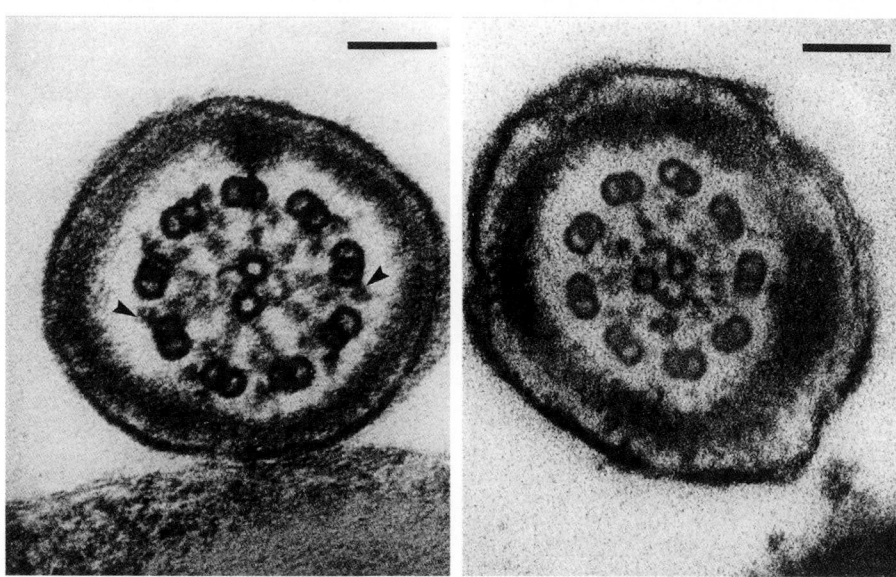

FIGURE 4.43 A classic cytoskeletal disease, primary ciliary dyskinesia, formerly known as the immotile cilia syndrome. *Left:* Cross section of the tail of a normal human spermatozoon; it is essentially a cilium. **Arrowheads:** Dynein arms. *Right:* Cross section through the tail of a spermatozoon from a patient with the immotile cilia syndrome. The dynein arms are missing. Lacking the dynein molecule, the spermatozoa are motionless; hence these individuals are sterile. **Bars** = 0.1 μm. (Courtesy of Dr. B. A. Afzelius, University of Stockholm, Stockholm, Sweden.)

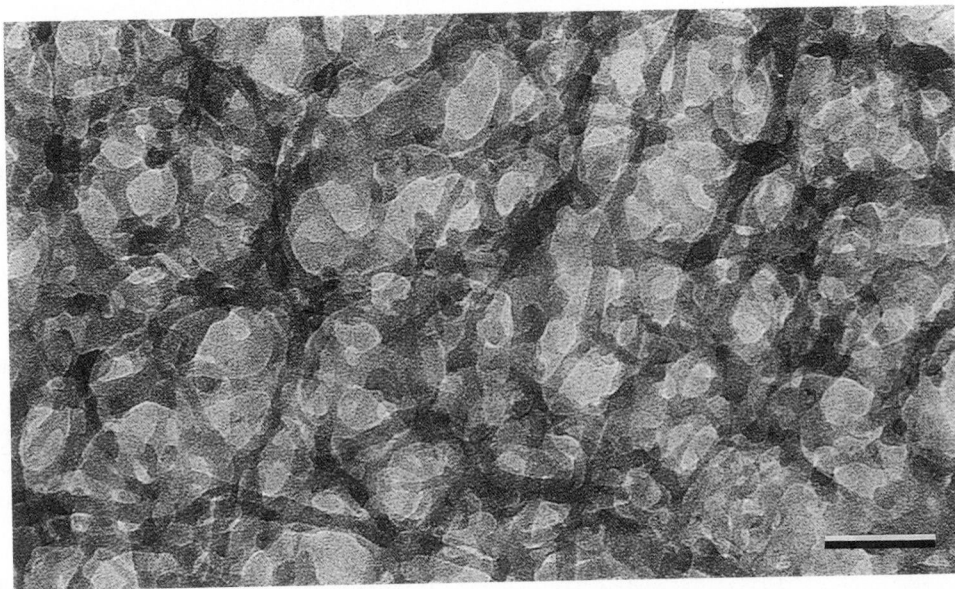

FIGURE 4.44   A high-voltage electron micrograph showing the ultimate structure of the cell, described by K. R. Porter et al. as "microtrabecular lattice" (247). It has been suggested that each trabecula may contain a central filament of F-actin (227). The three-dimensional effect is due to the depth of focus of the million-volt electron microscope. **Bar** = 0.1 μm. (Courtesy of Dr. K. R. Porter, University of Pennsylvania, Philadelphia, PA.)

on the right, liver on the left, etc.). Now the first two components of the triad are easy to understand. As for the situs inversus, it is also explained by a ciliary problem in very early embryologic development (241). Female infertility also may occur (there are cilia in the Fallopian tubes) but not in all cases. Today, 20 types of abnormal cilia are known; the incidence of such defects is about 1 per 15,000 births. Dogs and mice are also affected.

The most amazing part of this story is that several major and apparently unrelated problems, such as male and female infertility, a chronic cough, and even a right-sided heart, could be due to one molecular defect.

Microtrabecular lattice. In closing this review of cytoskeletal pathology, we should mention that in 1982–1984, Keith Porter and collaborators described what they understood to be the ultimate cytoskeletal component; it occupied 20 percent of the cell's volume. They called it *microtrabecular lattice.* Using the 1 million V electron microscope, which can see through tissue specimens much thicker than the conventional electron microscope, they saw an extremely fine three-dimensional network of fibrils (Figure 4.44). It looks very much like a tangle of gelatinous worms. We belatedly wonder whether they were seeing something else: the cell's proteins being shaped, folded, corrected, and forwarded—or condemned—by their chaperones, as we will now describe.

From Inclusion Bodies to Prions

Inclusion bodies are abnormal lumps of intracellular protein found under certain pathologic conditions. As such they do not belong in a list of intracellular organelles; we included them anyway, because they are built via a normal, planned cellular process, and contain parts of normal organelles.

"Aggresomes"

Inclusion bodies are usually single, located in the cytoplasm, occasionally in the nucleus. For reasons that are unclear, they are prone to arise especially in neurons and in liver cells. Until recently their main virtue was to

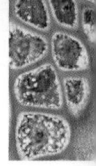

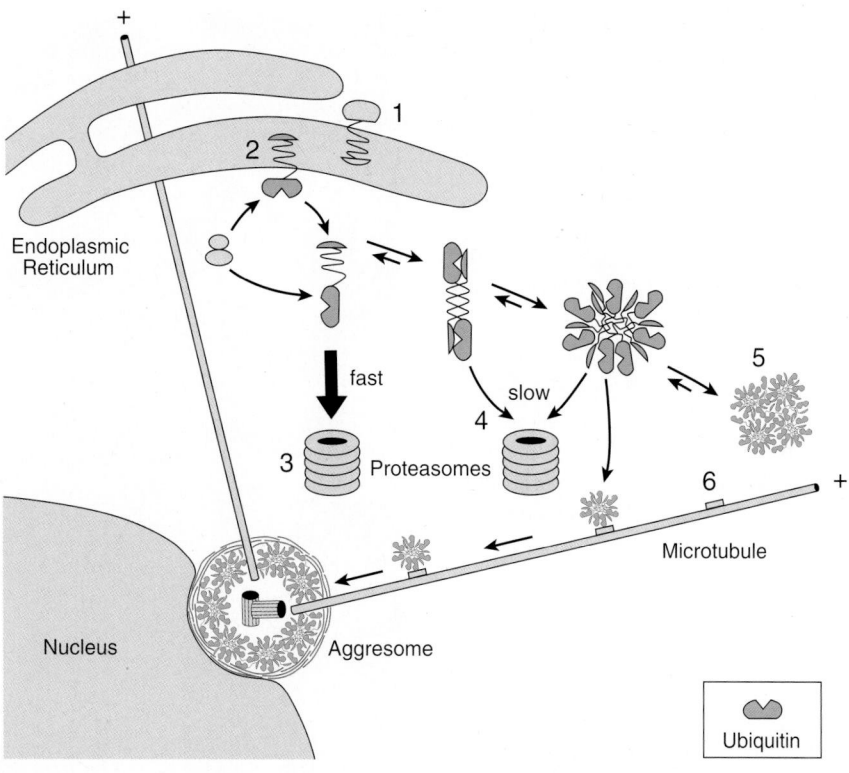

FIGURE 4.45   Model for aggresome formation. *Top:* Cisterna of endoplasmic reticulum. (**1**) Normal protein inserted in a membrane of the cisterna. (**2**) Misfolded protein, with a molecule of ubiquitin attached. (**3**) Quick digestion of the ubiquitinated protein by a proteasome. (**4**) The complex has grown, and is presumably degraded more slowly. (**5**) In the absence of microtubules, aggregates of ubiquitinated proteins remain dispersed in the cytoplasm. (**6**) Presumed motor protein transports aggregates to the microtubule organization center (MTOC), where they become entangled with intermediate filaments. (+) = Orientation of the microtubule in the cell. (Reproduced from the **Journal of Cell Biology,** 1998;143:1883–1898, by copyright permission of The Rockefeller University Press [267].)

help the diagnostic process; around 2000, they climbed up a notch or two in respectability by being assigned to the new "cutting edge" category of disease: *protein misfolding,* and also by acquiring a generic name as **aggresomes,** attractive conceptually if not linguistically (267, 270).

The theory of "aggresomes" (Figure 4.45) applies to those situations in which the production of aggregation-prone misfolded proteins within the cell exceeds the clearing capacity of the proteasome pathway, and generates **inclusion bodies.** These were previously thought to arise from the random collision of denatured proteins. The authors propose an alternate pathway, namely an orderly collection of the denatured proteins. A bunch of microtubules fans out from a point marked by an indentation of the nucleus, the MicroTubule Organization Center (MTOC); the microtubules gently sway through the cytoplasm, collect abnormal, "sticky" proteins, and convey them toward the MTOC thanks to one of the many motor proteins

attached to the microtubules (1). Besides the denatured proteins, the "aggresome" contain ubiquitin, stress proteins, bits of mitochondria and lysosomes, and a wrapping of intermediate filaments (vimentin). The purpose of this microtubular labor could be to concentrate an excess of cellular garbage in a single place for easier removal by autophagy.

This scenario (Figure 4.45) is well supported experimentally; for example, drugs that break up the microtubules inhibit the collection of misfolded proteins. Our guess is that this concept is here to stay, although it deserves a better name (*aggregosomes* would be more correct, although not more elegant—mixtures of Latin and Greek tend to be dissonant). As to the significance of inclusion bodies as a whole, there is no question that they arise under pathologic conditions, but in some cases a protective role has been suggested. The most important inclusion bodies and associated diseases are listed below.

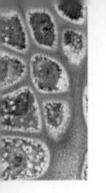

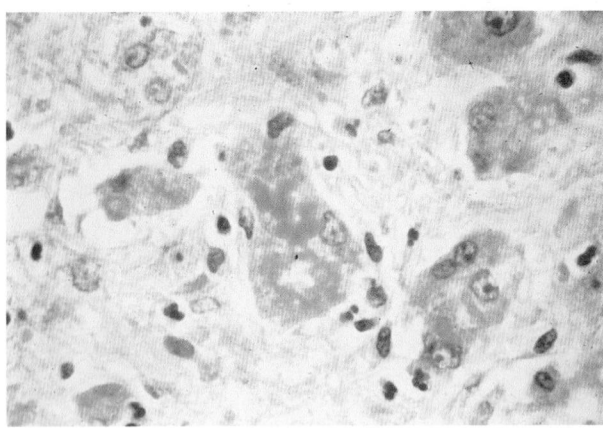

FIGURE 4.46 Clusters of Mallory bodies (purplish, fluffy masses) in the liver cells of a chronic alcoholic. (Courtesy of Dr. B. Banner, University of Massachusetts Medical School, Worcester, MA.)

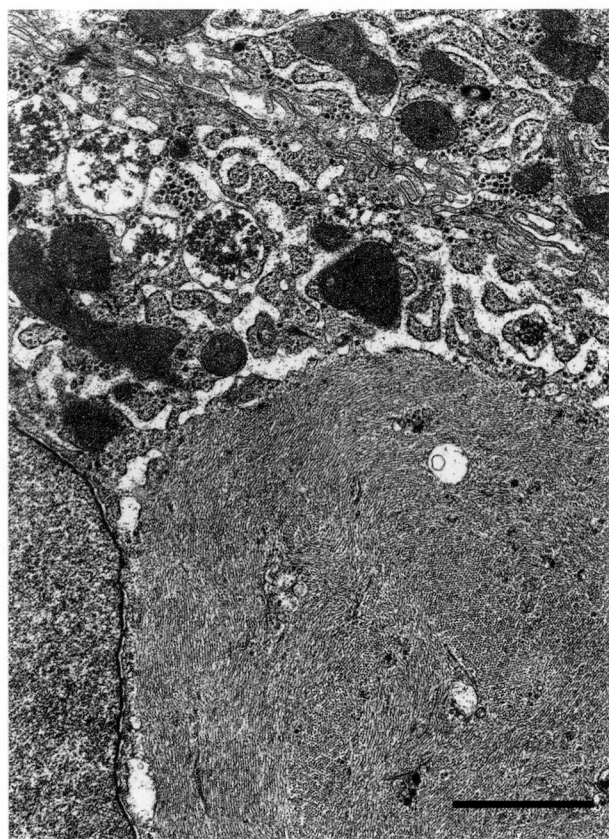

FIGURE 4.47 Typical Mallory body (Type 1) in alcoholic liver disease: electron microscopy. **Bar** = 5 μm. (Reproduced with permission from [246], copyright 1987 by Raven Press.)

Mallory bodies. In 1911, Frank B. Mallory noticed lumps of pale, hyalin ("glassy") material in the liver cells of chronic alcoholics (Figure 4.46). He had good reason to call them "*alcoholic* hyalin," considering the patient population typical of the Boston City Hospital. Today, however, it is best to call them Mallory bodies, because they develop in many other conditions unrelated to alcoholism; not only in the liver, but also in the pulmonary epithelium in asbestosis and in some tumors of the liver and lung (233). By electron microscopy they are fibrillar (Figures 4.47 and 4.48) with three predominant patterns (231). The fibrils are mainly cytokeratins 8 and 18 (277, 289), intermixed with representatives of the "protein emergency team," such as chaperonins and ubiquitin (260) and vimentin.

Mallory bodies are easily reproduced experimentally, e.g., with the drug griseofulvin (288), and oddly enough, also with anti*tubulin* drugs (232). When the toxic agent is discontinued the Mallory bodies disappear in 3–4 weeks, but if the intoxication is started again, the Mallory bodies reappear much faster (2–3 days), implying a sort of "toxic memory" (260). It is possible to prime the liver with a given drug, so that further challenge with other drugs will greatly facilitate the genesis of Mallory bodies (261). An interesting development is that Mallory bodies, and inclusion bodies in general, can develop via two complementary mechanisms: *by overwhelming the proteasome pathway,* and/or *by inhibiting it* (260, 261); it is no surprise to learn that alcohol inhibits the proteasome pathway.

Do the Mallory bodies *cause* damage? The cells in which they lie are often ballooned, i.e., full of fluid, not of fat. This may represent damage; however, knockout mice lacking cytokeratin 8 do not develop Mallory bodies and are more sensitive to toxic injury, suggesting that cytokeratin and the Mallory bodies may have a protective effect (289).

Russell bodies. In clusters of plasma cells it is common to encounter an occasional cell containing a spherical droplet of retained protein. Electron microscopy has shown these inclusions to be immunoglobulin retained within a dilated cisterna of the ER (276, 280, 286). Similar droplets have been produced in light chain myeloma cell lines transfected with a mutant heavy chain gene; some of the mutant immunoglobulin is degraded, and the remainder becomes an insoluble aggregate and is retained within the ER (285). Clearly this is another example of "aggresome" (270). (Incidentally, we checked Dr. W. Russell's paper from 1890 [278]. Whatever he saw had nothing at all to do with what we now call Russell bodies. Was the eponym a joke?)

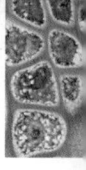

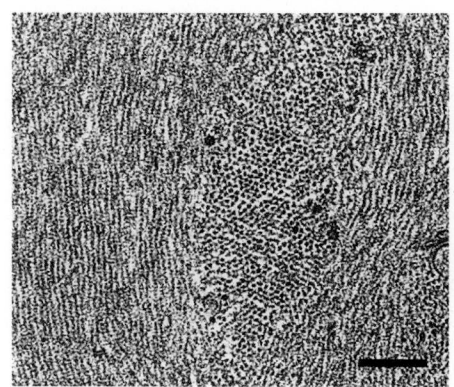 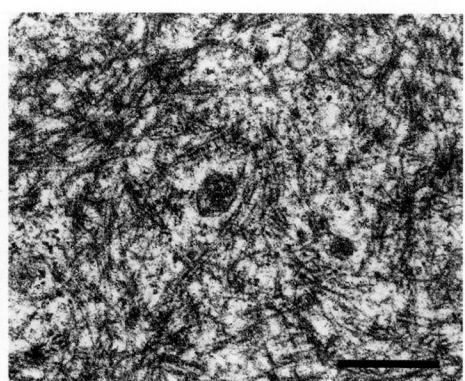

FIGURE 4.48 Fine structure of Mallory bodies. Type 1 (*left*) and Type 2 (*right*) in alcoholic liver disease. Type 3 Mallory bodies are extremely electron dense and structureless. **Bars:** left = 1 μm, right = 0.5 μm. (Reproduced with permission from [246], copyright 1987 by Raven Press.)

Crooke's hyalin, another type of intracellular hyalin, develops in the pituitary basophil cells (which secrete the adrenal cortical stimulant ACTH) as a response to excessive plasma levels of ACTH or glucocorticoids. Like the Mallory bodies, Crooke's hyalin consists of cytokeratin filaments. Apparently, the basophil cells, inhibited from secreting ACTH, produce excess cytokeratin. The hormonal imbalance may be due, for example, to an adrenal tumor or adrenal hyperplasia (Cushing's syndrome), or even to therapeutic doses of ACTH or corticoids (240).

Inclusion Bodies in "Neurodegenerative" Diseases

Degenerative? In modern pathology there is no category of disease labeled "degeneration" (on the level, say, of "inflammation" or "atrophy"). Degeneration was a catch-all term much used in the 1800s, when there was no better way to express "something going wrong with the tissues." The last of this kind to disappear was "fatty degeneration," which became the biochemically explainable steatosis. "Degenerative arthritis" may be accepted as referring to the extracellular breakdown of cartilage; occasional lapses such as "mucoid degeneration" are still to be read in modern papers. However, neuropathologists and neurologists still cling to **neurodegenerative diseases** as a major category.

There is a good reason. Until recently, these diseases simply did not seem to fit into the available categories. Neurons and neurites slowly shrivel up and die. Myriads of vacuoles develop in the gray matter (the term "spongiform encephalopathy" is very appropriate) (Figure 4.49) and the glial cells react, yet no mechanism is histologically apparent (265a). The patient's quality of life also "degenerates," adding more descriptive power to the term.

However, the third millennium is opening onto a new perspective. **A vast amount of evidence shows that**

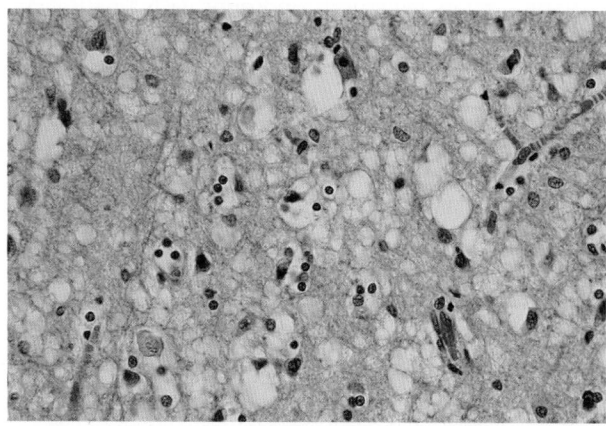

FIGURE 4.49 Gray matter from the brain of a patient who died of Creutzfeldt-Jacob disease. Note the large number of vacuoles, which suggested the name *spongiform encephalopathy*. The inflammatory infiltrate is very mild. (Courtesy of Dr. T. W. Smith, University of Massachusetts Medical School, Worcester, MA.)

these mysterious diseases hinge on abnormal processing of proteins (275) and especially on misfolding: soluble intracellular proteins turn into insoluble fibrils, not compatible with the survival of the cell. Why the fibrillization occurs is far from clear, but there is a reference point: virtually all of these "neurodegenerative" diseases have a rare familial, genetically transmitted variety. In the brain of individuals who inherited the disease, a mutant protein is found, and this mutation favors aggregation. This helps to find the corresponding pathologic protein of the wild type, but what causes it to misbehave if it is not mutated? Of the many critical questions, this one is perhaps the most critical.

We will begin by sketching the most important neurodegenerative diseases accompanied by inclusion bodies.

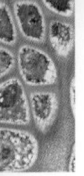

Lewy bodies, Parkinson's disease, and the alpha-synucleinopathies. Parkinson's disease is characterized by rigidity, tremor, and difficulty to initiate voluntary movement; anatomically, it is based on the progressive death of dopamine neurons in a part of the brain named *substantia nigra*. In the inherited variety of Parkinson's disease, **alpha-synuclein** (function unknown) was identified as mutant protein, and fibrillization of this protein makes it toxic (265). An important step in making it prone to aggregate is phosphorylation (262), a mechanism that also applies to Mallory bodies. Many of the affected neurons contain Lewy bodies, large, single inclusions containing mainly alpha-synuclein, ubiquitin, and parkin (Figure 4.50) (279). The term "synucleinopathy" refers to clinical conditions with a pathogenesis similar to Parkinson's disease (268, 287, 290).

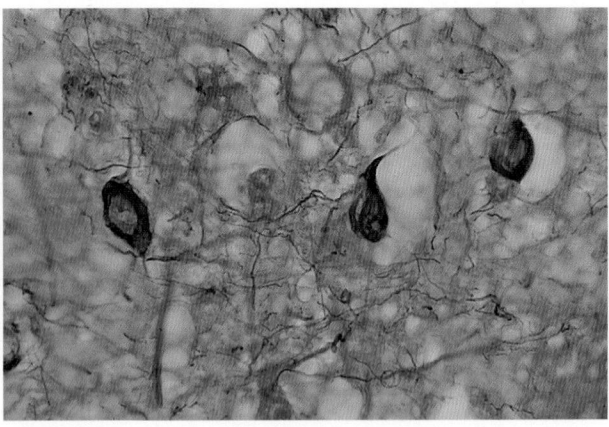

FIGURE 4.51 Three neurofibrillary tangles stained black with Bielschowski's silver technique. They consist of fibrillar aggregates of tau protein and can fill the neuron's body, hence the shape of a drop. See text. (Courtesy of Dr. T. W. Smith, University of Massachusetts Medical School, Worcester, MA.)

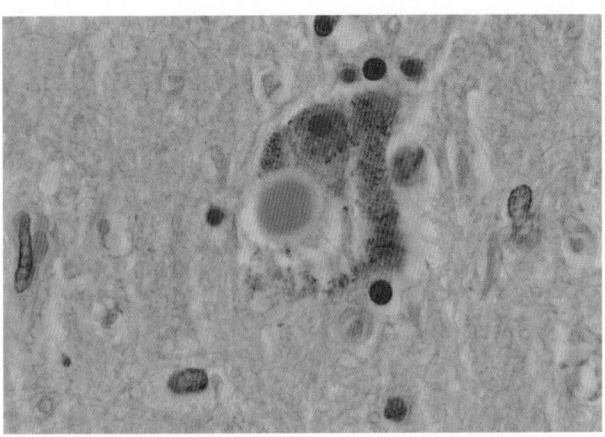

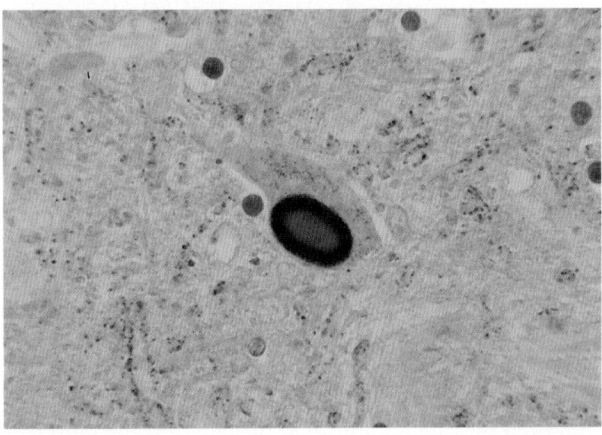

FIGURE 4.50 Lewy bodies in neurons of the *substantia nigra* in Parkinson's disease. *Top:* Single, rounded Lewy body; the nucleus of the neuron is not included at this level. Neuromelanin granules are present in the cytoplasm (hematoxylin-eosin stain). *Bottom:* Similar Lewy body stained with antibody against alpha-synuclein. (Courtesy of Dr. T. W. Smith, University of Massachusetts Medical School, Worcester, MA.)

There are new, exciting, and even hopeful twists to the Parkinson story, involving mitochondria and oxygen stress (259a).

Alzheimer's disease and the tauopathies. Regarding the pathogenesis of Alzheimer's disease, there are, as mentioned earlier, two views: the majority blame it on extracellular amyloid beta; a forceful minority blame it on the intracellular neurofibrillary tangles (Figure 4.51) (283) consisting of paired helical filaments and straight filaments. Both are made of **tau,** a phosphoprotein that is normally bound to the microtubules and helps them to assemble; in Alzheimer's disease and other dementing tauopathies it is hyperphosphorylated, unable to bind to the tubules, and it becomes fibrillar (264). When the neuron dies the fibrils may remain free in the extracellular space as "ghost tangles." The number of tangles correlates with dementia better than the amyloid plaques; still, the tangles are identical to those found in old age—which cause no known trouble.

> The latest Alzheimer news takes a wholly new direction, hence the small print: the brains of patients with Alzheimer's disease, *hereditary or not,* contain a mutant form of ubiquitin that becomes itself ubiquitinated, forming polyubiquitin chains that are highly resistant to proteasome digestion (272). Once again, time will tell.

Huntington's disease and the polyglutamine disorders. Huntington's disease (HD) is a late-onset, slowly progressive, and fatal neurodegenerative disorder based on a well-defined genetic error: *CAG triplet repeat expansions encode expanded polyglutamine repeats in the*

N *terminus of a single protein, huntingtin.* When the number of glutamines in a repeat exceeds 37–41, the molecules of huntingtin begin to stick to each other and form beta-pleated sheets (2). This leads to malfunction of the neurons and to the formation of inclusion bodies, typically in the nucleus (257). Are nuclear bodies toxic to the nucleus? Opinions are divided (259, 273). At least 14 diseases are based on this molecular model (2, 277a.).

The function of normal huntingtin is still unclear. *Aggregates of mutated huntingtin appear in the cytoplasm and/or in the nucleus of neurons in specific areas of the brain* (269); however, one leading research group warns that the single "aggregation" model may not hold for HD (255). Other disturbances in which the molecule of huntingtin may be involved include proteolysis, altered protein interactions, and activation of the endosomal–lysosomal system, which contributes to the autolysis of huntingtin, leading to an "autophagocytic process of neuronal cell death" (255, 269). We are reminded once again that single paradigms tend to be traps.

The ultimate protein misfolding disorder: the prion saga. This amazing tale actually began in true saga-land, Iceland. In the 1950s, a group of Icelandic pathologists studied two unexplained diseases of the local sheep and goats, visna and scrapie (so named because the ataxic sheep scraped off their wool by rubbing against the fence), and proposed that they were caused by invisible "slow viruses" (281, 282). Typical features were a long incubation (months to decades), a short clinical course leading to death, and strange, noninflammatory ("neurodegenerative") changes in the central nervous system. Similar diseases were known in humans, notably *Creutzfeldt-Jacob disease* (CJ) and *kuru;* the latter became widely known because it was originally transmitted by cannibalism in New Guinea (263). The infectious agents in all four diseases were presumed to be viruses. Visna did turn out to be due to a retrovirus, but no infectious agent was found for the other three. Then a neurologist, Stanley B. Prusiner, joined the search. Working on the brains of guinea pigs infected with scrapie, he came up—beginning in 1982—with startling results: the agent was an infectious particle of a new kind. It was a single, protease-resistant protein, smaller than a virus, and *the isoform of a host protein, encoded by a normal gene.* The particle was named PRION, which is supposed to echo PROTEIN INFECTIOUS PARTICLE; the infectious isoform was labeled PrP^{Sc} (scrapie-specific) as opposed to the normal, protease-sensitive cellular isoform, PrP^{C} (275, 284).

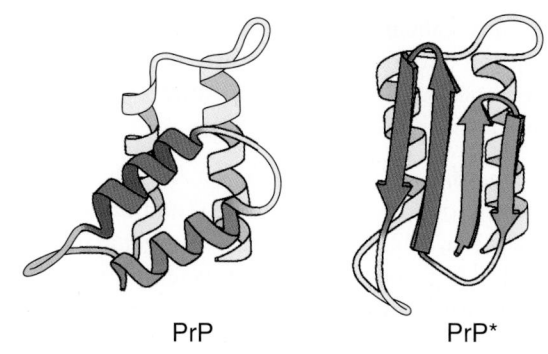

PrP   PrP*

FIGURE 4.52   One of several possible models to explain the conversion of PrP to PrP*, an infectious particle. This model requires the switch from two alpha-helices to four beta-pleated sheets. (Copyright 2002, from Molecular Biology of the Cell, 4th ed. Alberts B, Johnson A, Lewis J, et al. [eds]. Reproduced by permission of Routledge, Inc., part of Taylor & Francis Group and from Trends Biochem Sci 21, Prusiner SB. Molecular biology and pathogenesis of prion diseases, pp. 482–487, Copyright 1996, with permission from Elsevier Science.)

The first, burning question, of course, is how a normal protein can be induced to behave as an infectious particle. The process has been called "conformational contagion." One might envision the first infectious prion acting as a template to change the shape of the nearest normal prion protein. But how does the first one develop? Possibly with the help of a special chaperone, provisionally named "protein X." The conversion from PrP^{C} to PrP^{Sc} involved a reduction of alpha helix structures and an increase in beta pleated sheet component (Figure 4.52); no other differences, chemical or other, were found. Knockout mice for the PrP^{C} gene survive, suggesting that the normal prion protein is not vital; these mice are also immune to infection by prion particles, presumably because the infectious particles find no molecules to "convert" (256). The prion concept has the merit of explaining how the same disease can present as contagious, hereditary or sporadic; no other agent can do so (275).

To top it all, PrP^{Sc} can be made to crystallize into fibrils with all the properties of amyloid (Figure 4.53). It took a lot of courage to suggest that some type of amyloid (p. 286) may consist of infectious particles.

Needless to say, a huge controversy arose. Who could believe that a normal protein could be made to flip over into the shape and behavior of a virus, and multiply—in the absence of nucleic acids? To this day there are nonbelievers. Recent work proposes that vertebrate single-stranded RNA is required for the amplification of the PrP^{Sc} *in vitro* possibly as cofactor (256a): but this does not invalidate the protein-only prion hypothesis. Anti-prion antibodies and therapy are high on the list of priorities (266). In 1987 Prusiner was awarded a highly deserved Nobel prize (258).

Prion breakthrough Until 2003, no human or animal had survived a prion disease. Then, in a London laboratory (258a, 272a), two different transgenic mice were crossed; this generated mice that were normal at birth, but at 12 weeks they produced an enzyme that disabled the PrP gene—only in the neurons. If mice of this strain were injected with prions shortly after birth, at 12 weeks their brain showed the classic spongiform disease—yet without symptoms and they survived for over a year. At that time the spongiosis had disappeared and only glial cells contained prions. The implications are momentous. We cannot give more details here, but we did want our readers to see once again the path that can be followed for breaking a dogma.

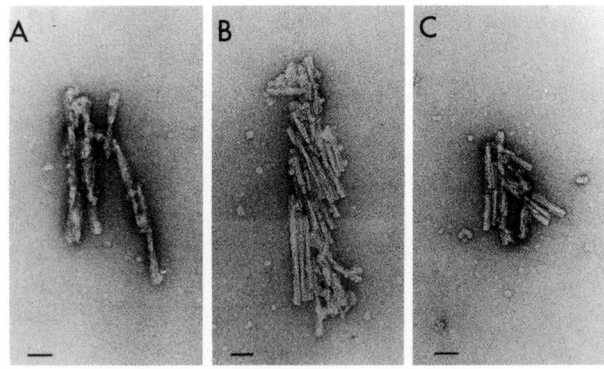

FIGURE 4.53   Electron microscopy of purified prion amyloid. **A:** Amyloid extracted from the brain of a scrapie-infected sheep. **B, C:** Amyloid obtained from human brains affected by Creutzfeldt–Jakob disease. **Bars** = 500 Å. (Reprinted by permission of the New England Journal of Medicine 317: 1571–1581,1987.)

Pathology of the Nucleus

Unlike any other organelle, the nucleus can be studied in several totally different ways; correspondingly, there are different types (or levels) of nuclear pathology. Basically, the nucleus is the custodian of an enormous treasure, the genome: It has been calculated that the DNA of a single human sperm or ovum contains 3×10^9 base pairs, more than 100 times the number of letters and punctuation marks in a set of the *Encyclopaedia Britannica*. This mind-boggling system is under constant repair by a maintenance crew of at least 30 specialized enzymes, without which we would die much sooner from DNA damage (294). This crew, of course, has its own set of disturbances, some of which predispose to cancer, and will be dealt with in Chapter 29. We might conclude that just *looking* at the nucleus is rather like staring at a textbook of genetics, closed. Indeed, if we only study the nucleus under the microscope, and follow its visible changes in disease, we will gather very little information. The nucleus by its very nature must be extremely stable; it cannot afford great variations in structure. Thus, before the DNA revolution, the nucleus held the reputation of being microscopically a rather dull structure.

Things began to change in 1949 when it was discovered, quite accidentally, that "just by *looking*" at a nucleus one could tell the sex of its owner (1). The scientific community was shocked; we recall an eminent anatomist muttering "I can't face it." Yet today sex chromatin belongs to basic biology. Then came the microscopic study of chromosomes, which grew into science of its own, cytogenetics. In the 1980s molecular biology appeared on the scene. Suddenly it became possible to isolate genes, to insert them into bacteria, and to create transgenic animals by the methodology of recombinant DNA. An offshoot of this science is *molecular pathology*, which aims at correlating DNA and disease. Parallel to these developments, the traditional morphology of the nucleus has progressed, in quality as well as in range, by the use of the fluorescence-activated cell-sorter, or FACS (p. 15).

Genetics used to be the only tool for exploring the genome. Today, the nucleus and its DNA can be studied in many other ways, requiring various specializations:

- Biochemistry
- Morphology of the intact nucleus (including the FACS)
- Morphology of the chromosomes (cytogenetics)
- Molecular biology (including transgenic animals)
- Molecular pathology
- Biology of DNA repair
- Microarrays

We will review the essentials of nuclear morphology, and provide a bird's eye view of other approaches.

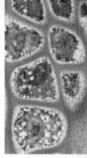

Microscopy of the Nucleus

In searching for signs of cellular disease, we can learn a lot by using the microscope simply to examine the size, shape, and structure of the nucleus. Tumor diagnosis hinges very much on such considerations.

Nuclear size can increase tremendously when quiescent cells are suddenly activated to a high level of protein synthesis, as best demonstrated by fibroblasts around a focus of injury (Figure 4.54). At the same time the heterochromatin becomes dispersed, and the nucleolus enlarges. A large nucleolus is the hallmark of heightened protein synthesis.

In most cells about 90 percent of the chromatin is thought to be transcriptionally inactive (292) and appears as dense masses of heterochromatin. A small fraction of the heterochromatin is permanently "turned off"; that is, it is never transcribed (*constitutive heterochromatin*). The rest is *facultative heterochromatin,* which probably reflects the level of transcriptional activity in various cell types: embryonic cells have very little of it, highly specialized cells such as lymphocytes have a great deal.

Nuclear size can also reflect nuclear ploidy, which represents another vital concern in tumor diagnosis. In practice, (a) a large, *pale* nucleus suggests an active transcriptional state; (b) a large and *very basophilic* nucleus suggests excessive DNA content; (c) a small and very basophilic nucleus suggests a low level of activity (transcription turned off).

In contractile cells, *the oblong nucleus becomes wrinkled like an accordion when the cell contracts* (Figure 4.55). This phenomenon gave the first hint that endothelial cells are contractile; it also helped identify the contractile modulation of fibroblasts (p. 485). *Grotesque nuclear shapes are typical of malignant tumors.*

The rock bottom of nuclear pathology is that *if the nucleus has disappeared, the cell must have been dead for a long time* (about a day or longer). This notion, however rudimentary, is very practical in histopathology: an area without nuclei is (usually) a cemetery of cells. The nucleus can break down in three ways: it can slowly lose its affinity for basic dyes and fade away (**karyolysis,** typical of ischemic cell death); conversely, it can shrivel into a dense, highly basophilic mass (**pyknosis,** from *pyknós,* dense); or it can become pyknotic and then break up into small pieces

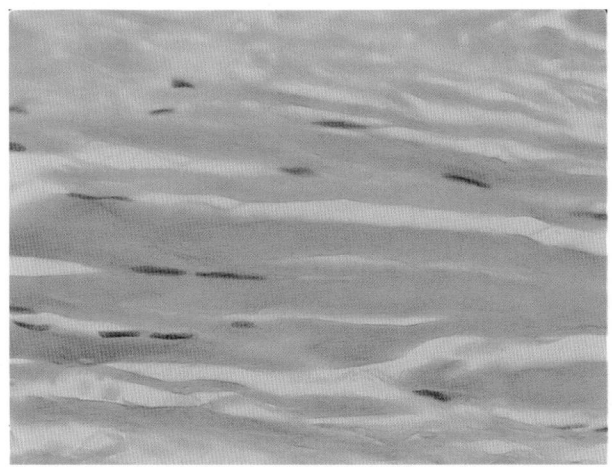

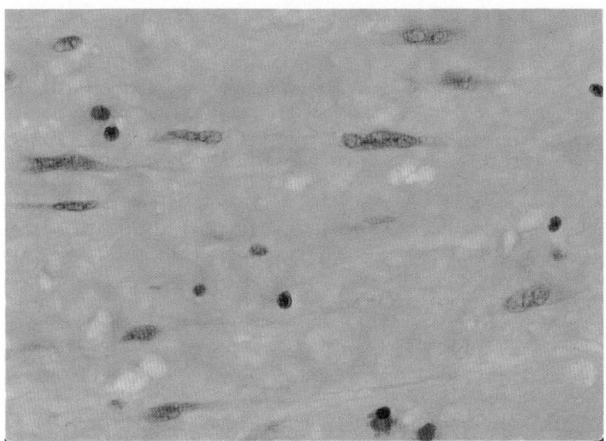

FIGURE 4.54   Effect of cellular activation on the nucleus. *Top:* Quiescent fibroblasts among collagen fibers of the skin. *Bottom:* Activated fibroblasts in a swollen nasal mucosa, slightly inflamed (as indicated by scattered lymphocytes).

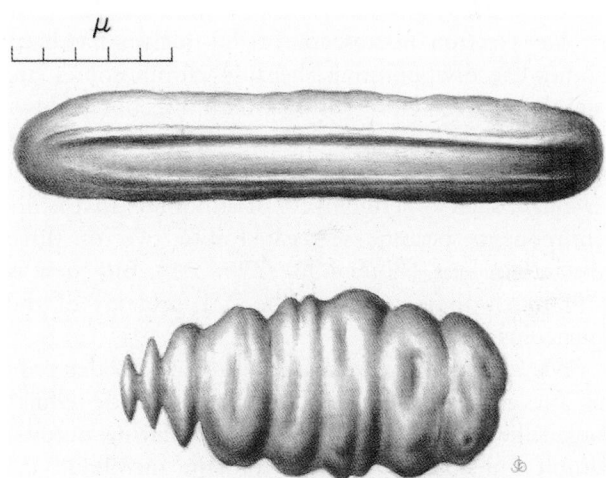

FIGURE 4.55   Deformation of myocardial nuclei by myocardial contraction: an artist's view. *Top:* Relaxed condition. *Bottom:* Contracted condition. (Adapted from [293] by permission of the American Heart Association, Inc.)

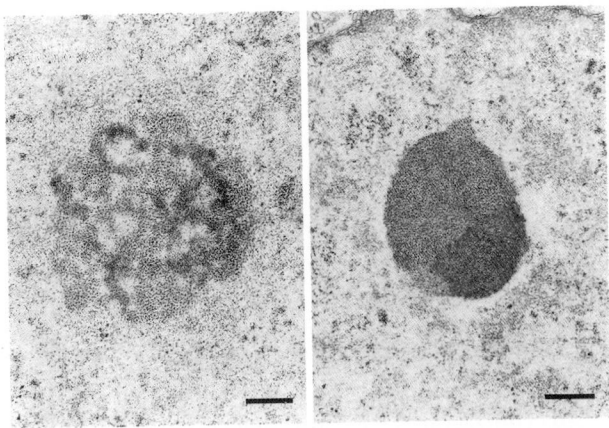

FIGURE 4.56   Effect of a protein synthesis inhibitor, actino-mycin D, on the nucleolus of liver cells (rat). *Left:* Normal liver nucleolus, showing the typical lacy structure. *Right:* Nucleolus 2 hours after actinomycin (1 μg/g body weight). Nucleolar components have separated out into two and possibly three masses. **Bars** = 0.5 μm. (Reproduced, with permission, from the Annual Review of Pharmacology, Vol. 11, © 1971 by Annual Reviews Inc. [296].)

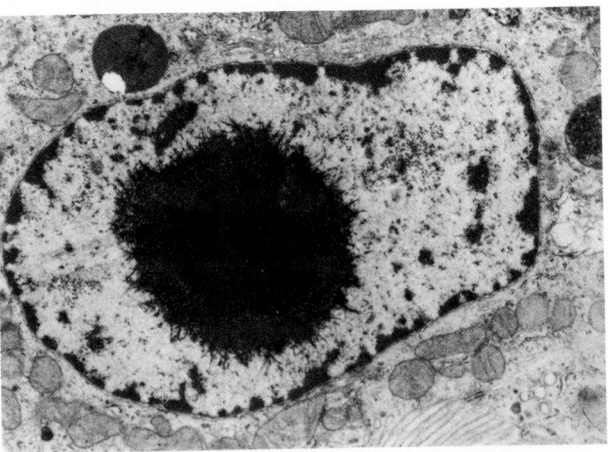

FIGURE 4.57   Lead inclusion body (dense mass) in a nucleus: electron microscopy. From the proximal convoluted tubule of a man professionally exposed to lead. (Reproduced with permission [302].)

(**karyorhexis**). Pyknosis and karyorhexis are important because they suggest that the cell has committed suicide (apoptosis, p. 210).

> The nucleus is the only cellular organelle to suffer the indignity of being expelled from the cytoplasm, such as during the maturation of erythrocytes (307). With cytochalasin it is possible to produce this phenomenon at will in other cells. An enucleated cell is called a **cytoplast.**

The electron microscopy of the nucleus has been somewhat disappointing, because chromosomes are simply not visible on routine ultrathin sections. However, *the nucleolus shows characteristic ultrastructural changes under the influence of inhibitors of protein synthesis,* such as actinomycin or ethionine; that is, its components become segregated into two or three discrete masses (Figure 4.56) (296, 319). But there is still much to learn about the 271 proteins of the nucleolus (291).

Nuclear inclusions listed to date are so many that only an atlas can do them justice (300): they include cellular organelles that were perhaps trapped during mitosis, droplets of lipid, glycogen, or protein, membrane infoldings, viruses, fibrils, crystals, and tubules; most are unexplained and visible only by electron microscopy. Easily seen by light and electron microscopy are the *lead inclusion bodies* found in epithelial cells of the renal convoluted tubules and in liver cells as a result of

chronic lead intoxication (Figure 4.57) (302, 313, 323). The fact that lead would choose to precipitate in the nuclei of just those two tissues is another example of the myriad of unexplained specificities of drugs and toxic agents. Cells with lead inclusion bodies look remarkably unaffected, possibly because the toxic lead is safely sequestered in the mass. Lead inclusion bodies have turned up in plants growing by the roadside, another sign of environmental pollution (321). The fascinating correlation between nuclear lamin A and progeria was discussed on p. 52.

The Study of Chromosomes: Cytogenetics

A great deal can be learned from the direct microscopic study of chromosomes, which can be visualized only in dividing cells. The basic principle is to start with a cell culture (e.g., white blood cells) and to treat it with colchicine, which arrests the mitoses in metaphase (p. 159). At this stage, using a nuclear stain, the chromosomes are visible—but clustered and not individually recognizable. By a fortunate accident (p. 894) it was discovered that distilled water swells the mitotic cells; using this trick it is possible to obtain "spreads" of the metaphase chromosomes. With some luck, one or more of the spreads will be perfect, with all the chromosomes separated. The best mitoses are then photographed and suitable enlargements are printed. The next step is very empirical but it works: from one such enlargement, all the images of chromosomes are cut out with scissors, identified by size and shape, paired, and pasted on a

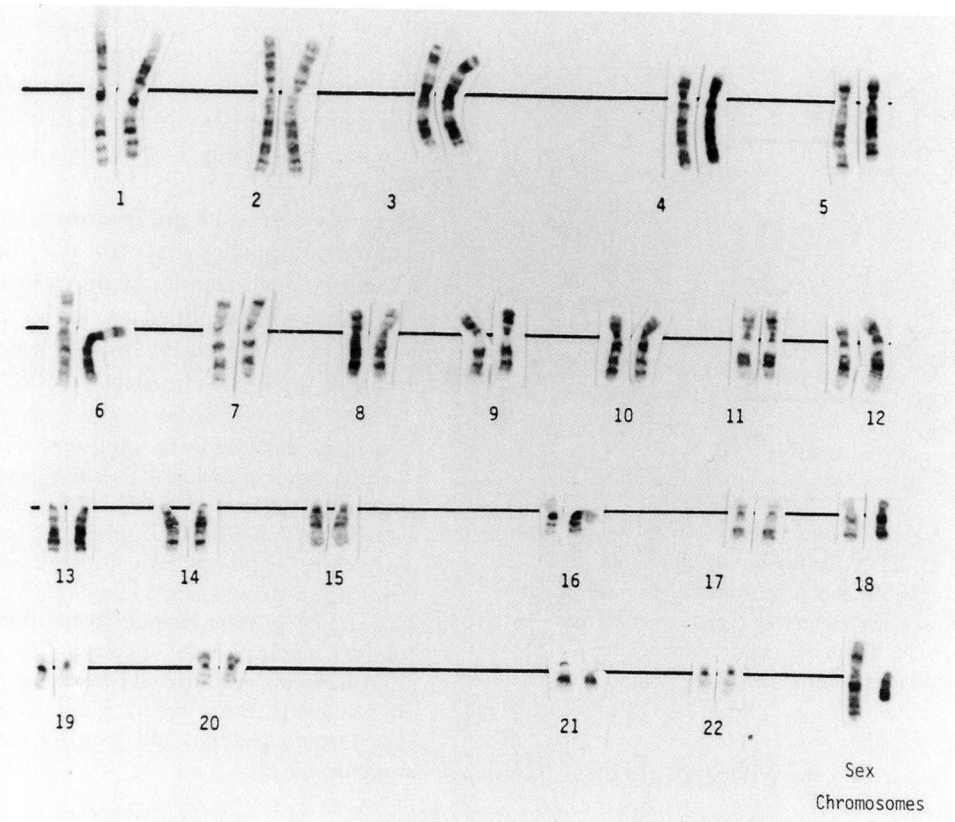

FIGURE 4.58 Normal human karyotype (male), displayed in the standard manner. The bands on the chromosomes were obtained by treatment with trypsin followed by Giemsa stain. (Courtesy of Dr. P. L. Townes, University of Massachusetts Medical School, Worcester, MA.)

sheet in a standard order. This display is called a **kary-otype** (Figure 4.58): in humans it consists of 22 pairs of autosomes, plus two sex chromosomes, XX in females and XY in males. Some applications of this technique are discussed in Chapter 29.

Molecular Biology: Transgenic Animals

Transgenic mice appeared on the scene in 1980. The term transgenic, as our readers surely know, means that these creatures carry sequences in their genome that have been inserted by laboratory techniques (306, 318, 324); *knockout* animals have undergone the opposite change: they have lost genomic sequences (310, 312, 315, 322). Another method for producing mutants is to feed *N*-ethyl-*N*-nitrosourea (ENU) to male mice, whereby mutations occur in their sperm. This is, of course, a random method, but it is also faster and cheaper (308). The resulting flow of genetic information is huge, and so is the housing problem for the

mice. Most of the strains are kept for future reference; in 2001 the number of knockout strains was about 3000 and growing ever faster, but nobody likes to pay housing bills for "just in case" mice. We are reminded of the old bacteriological quip: if *Escherichia coli* were allowed to grow unhindered, in a few days they would create a mass as big as the planet Earth. They do not, because they run out of substrate. For science, a key substrate is money.

Molecular Genetics: Methods of Molecular Pathology

Although the topic of molecular genetics is beyond the scope of our book, the reader should be aware of recent techniques that have had an enormous impact on medical science (297, 298, 304, 306, 309). When applied to problems of pathology these methods are known as molecular pathology. This term is here to stay, but it is an obvious misnomer. It seems to imply the study of pathology at the level of all molecules,

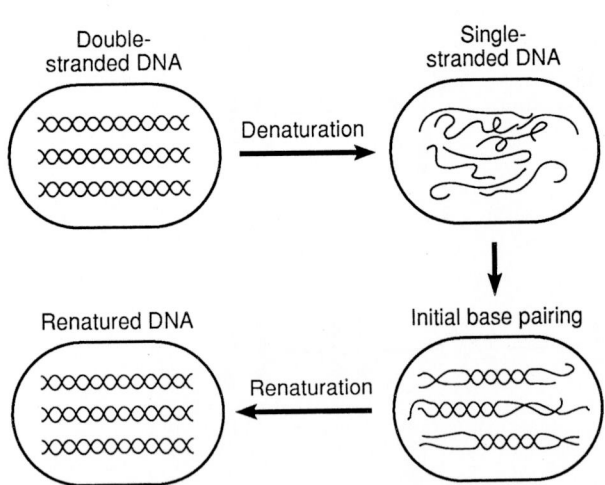

FIGURE 4.59   A basic procedure of molecular biology: denaturation (melting) and renaturation (reannealing) of DNA. Gentle heating causes the double-stranded DNA to unwind into two single strands; upon cooling, the single strands "find" each other and reanneal in the same sequence as in the original DNA. (Reproduced by permission from [297].)

whereas it is focused on the pathology of DNA, RNA and their products.

The techniques that we will sketch here are derived from the same DNA wizardry that led to transgenic animals, but all are *in vitro* methods. They all rely on the same basic principle: the DNA molecule is made of two parallel and complementary strands held together by hydrogen bonds. If the DNA molecule is gently heated (i.e., heat denatured), the two strands come apart; then if they are brought into proximity, they show the uncanny ability to reanneal exactly in the same position (Figure 4.59). This means that a short piece of artificially prepared single-stranded DNA, mixed with single-stranded DNA, will anneal or **bybridize** with the complementary segment of DNA—if any such segment is present. These short pieces of artificially prepared DNA, called **probes,** will hybridize whether the complementary DNA is in solution or in the nuclei of histologic sections.

The same principles apply to RNA. Thus, hybridization may occur as DNA/DNA, RNA/RNA, or DNA/RNA.

> Hybridization is not to be confused with recombination, which refers to the end-to-end attachment of double-stranded DNA fragments, which have "sticky ends."

The scientific applications of hybridization are limitless as long as the necessary DNA and RNA probes are at hand. These probes are obtained commercially, and producing them is part of this new science (they are prepared by cloning genes or cDNA fragments in bacterial cells; they can also be produced by amplification using the polymerase chain reaction, PCR) (304).

The **polymerase chain reaction** is a magnificent trick for multiplying enzymatically the amount of DNA in very small samples; within a matter of hours a tiny sample can be amplified a million times. So important is this method that polymerase was nominated as Molecule of the Year—the first—in 1989 (305).

> This methodology can be applied to tissue sections or to tissue extracts; each has its advantages. *In **histologic sections,** DNA or RNA probes can be made visible by any one of the methods shown in Figure 4.60.* The beauty of this microscopic method is its sensitivity; even a single cell shows up if it contains the specific DNA (Figure 4.61), whereas the *in vitro* method to be described later, the Southern blot, requires about one million cells (297). The DNA molecule is so resistant to change that the probes can be used on tissues that have been long since fixed and embedded in paraffin, and even on tissues of ancient mummies (314).

Here are two of the questions that can be answered by using probes on histologic sections. Is viral genome present in the cells? Is a given gene activated? The latter very subtle question can be answered by searching for the appropriate mRNA; it can also be answered by looking for the gene product, if the specific antibody is available.

*The standard method for examining the DNA in **tissue extracts*** *is the so-called* **Southern blot,** named after Dr. Edward M. Southern of Dallas, Texas. The basic principle of the Southern blot is shown in Figure 4.62.

> The DNA, obtained from a cell lysate, is digested into segments using an appropriate restriction endonuclease (an enzyme that recognizes a particular base sequence and cuts the DNA molecule only at the sites where that sequence occurs). The digest is then drawn electrophoretically along a plate of agarose gel; the shorter segments migrate farther, and to assess their molecular weight, standard molecules of known molecular weight are run alongside. Then the agarose gel is soaked in alkali to denature the DNA. Next, the whole mass of electrophoresed fragments is transferred to another gel (usually a sheet of nitrocellulose) that is more suitable for the following step of the procedure. To accomplish the transfer the sheet of nitrocellulose is placed over the agarose and covered with a stack of absorbent paper, which acts as a wick, drawing water and DNA from one gel into the other. In the end,

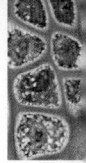

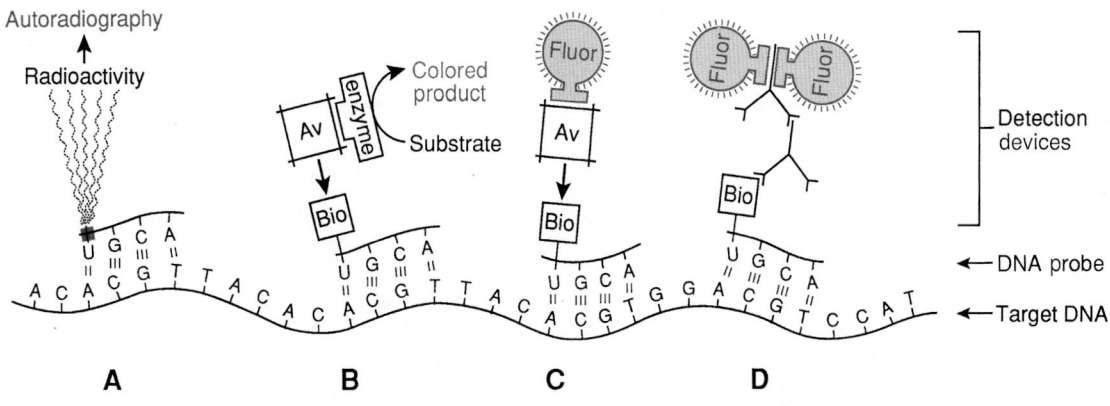

FIGURE 4.60 Basic principle of *in situ* hybridization, aimed at identifying specific sequences in nuclear DNA (target DNA). The key is to have a specific DNA probe (here labeled UGCA) that hybridizes with the DNA sequence that is to be identified. Once hybridized, the probe is made visible—in tissue sections—by one of four methods. **A:** With a radioactive label, to be detected by autoradiography. **B:** By enzyme histochemistry; the probe is labeled with biotin, and then the biotin is bound to avidin, a protein, which in turn carries an enzyme capable of producing a colored product. **C:** A variant of **B** in which the avidin carrier is bound to a fluorescent molecule. **D:** Double-antibody method, also based on fluorescence. (Reproduced by permission from [304], © Williams & Wilkins 1989.)

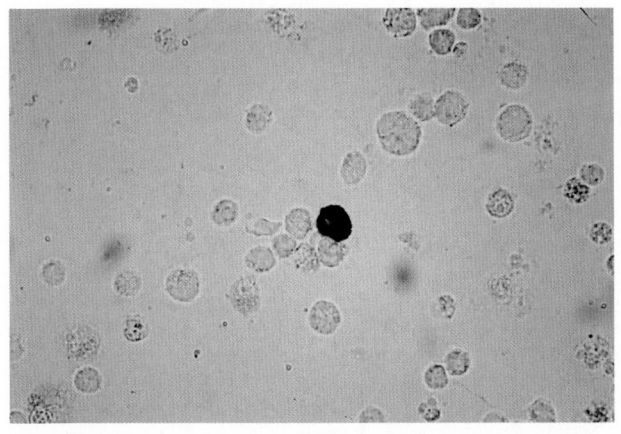

FIGURE 4.61 Detection of HIV-1–infected lymphocytes by means of *in situ* hybridization, in the peripheral blood of a hemophilic patient infected with HIV-1 by treatment with contaminated factor VIII. During the early symptom-free interval, lymphocytes were obtained by centrifugation and placed on a slide. A biotinated HIV genomic probe was hybridized to the cells and detected by alkaline phosphatase linked to streptavidin. The histochemical reaction for alkaline phosphatase produced a dark brown deposit (black cell in center). This positive reaction indicates the presence of viral RNA. Note that only one of many lymphocytes expresses HIV RNA. This is typical for this phase of the disease: 1/1000−1/10,000 of the blood lymphocytes are usually positive. (Courtesy of Dr. R. H. Singer, University of Massachusetts Medical School, Worcester, MA.)

the DNA fragments are distributed in the same way in the nitrocellulose gel as they were in the agarose. The nitrocellulose sheet is then immersed in a solution containing a radioactive probe, selected according to the purpose of the test. The probe hybridizes with the complementary DNA, and its location is determined by autoradiography. The final product is an autoradiograph.

Northern blots (a pun on the name of Dr. Southern) are the RNA equivalent of Southern blots. The joke has been extended to **Western blots,** used for sizing polypeptides by gel electrophoresis. The **dot-blot** is a simpler and faster variety of hybridization in which a known amount of DNA or RNA is dripped onto a membrane as a 4-mm dot and is then denatured and hybridized; the intensity of the radioactive dot is compared with that of dots prepared with known standards.

Restriction fragment length polymorphisms or RFLP (we agree that the name is repulsive) are harmless but useful oddities of the DNA molecule that can be brought out by Southern blots. Let us first clarify the name. An RFLP is a change in the length of the DNA fragments that are produced by restriction enzymes. DNA polymorphisms represent variations in genetic material between individuals; they occur every 200–500 base pairs (297). Some polymorphisms occur in or near genes and may be associated with phenotypic changes and disease. Others occur in noncoding DNA and may have no obvious effect on the phenotype; however, they are of interest for two reasons: (1) they represent an individual (innocuous) trait that can be used for "molecular fingerprinting,"

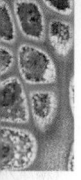

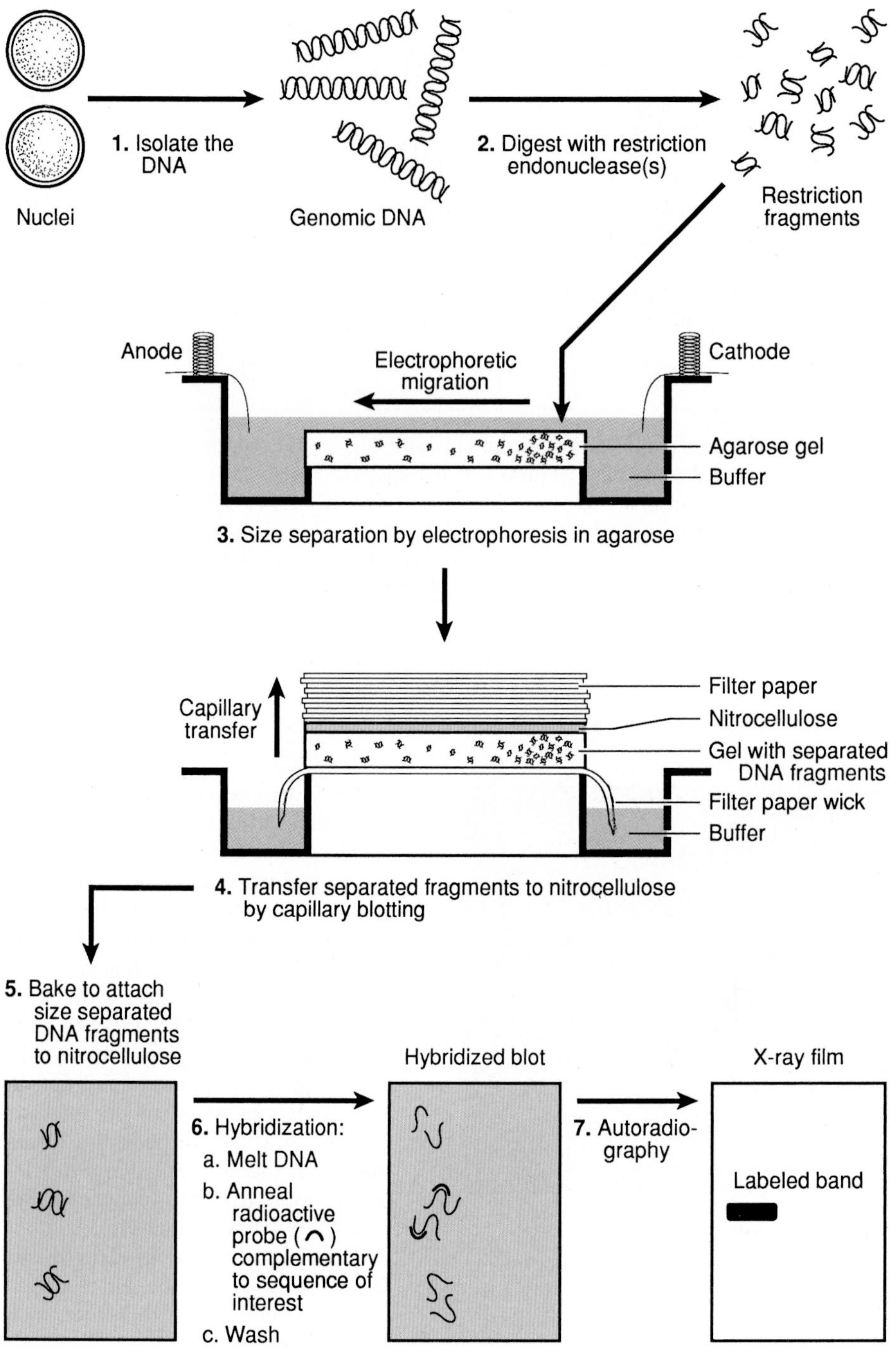

1. Isolate the DNA

Nuclei

Genomic DNA

2. Digest with restriction endonuclease(s)

Restriction fragments

Anode   Cathode

Electrophoretic migration

Agarose gel
Buffer

3. Size separation by electrophoresis in agarose

Capillary transfer

Filter paper
Nitrocellulose
Gel with separated DNA fragments
Filter paper wick
Buffer

4. Transfer separated fragments to nitrocellulose by capillary blotting

5. Bake to attach size separated DNA fragments to nitrocellulose

6. Hybridization:
a. Melt DNA
b. Anneal radioactive probe (⌒) complementary to sequence of interest
c. Wash

Hybridized blot

7. Autoradio-graphy

X-ray film

Labeled band

FIGURE 4.62   Southern blot hybridization: a method used for characterizing the organization of DNA that surrounds a specific nucleic acid sequence, e.g., a particular gene. (Adapted with permission from Abbas AK, Lichtman AH, Prober JS. Cellular and molecular immunology. Philadelphia: W.B. Saunders Company, 1991, p. 73.)

which is of great value in forensic medicine; (2) for reasons unknown, polymorphisms may be linked with a specific abnormal trait; if the trait is recessive, an RFLP may be present to indicate that the individual carries the gene. Carriers of the gene can therefore be identified.

Polymorphisms can be detected on Southern blots. After digestion of the DNA with a particular restriction enzyme, the pattern of bands on a Southern blot depends on the size of the fragments. Suppose that a deletion in an intron has deleted precisely a base sequence recognized by

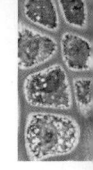

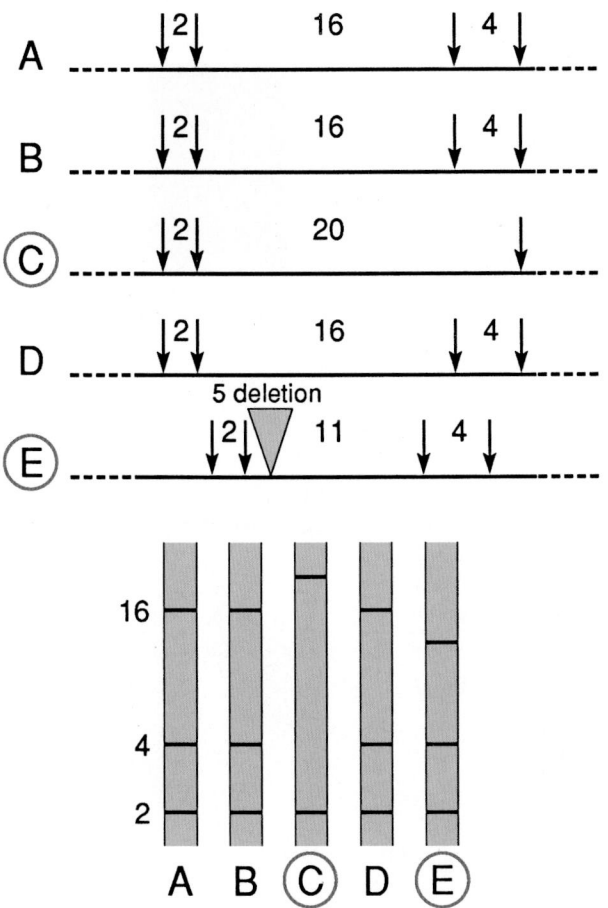

FIGURE 4.63 Hypothetical restriction map of part of the X chromosome from five males. *Top:* Horizontal lines represent DNA molecules cut by a restriction enzyme at certain points (**arrows**). Numbers represent lengths of restriction fragments in kilobases. Individuals **A**, **B**, and **D** have identical restriction maps with this enzyme. **C** and **E** illustrate restriction fragment length polymorphisms: **C** due to a point mutation that abolishes one of the restriction sites and **E** due to a deletion in the largest fragment between two adjacent restriction sites. *Bottom:* Agarose gel and electrophoresis of restriction fragments illustrated above. The polymorphism between individuals is obvious. (Reprinted from [301], Copyright 1989, with permission from Elsevier.)

the restriction enzyme: no cut will be made at that spot, and the result will be a larger and slower-moving DNA fragment (Figure 4.63).

Enter the Microarrays

In the world of genomics—which sees biology as a manifestation of genes—one of the goals is to know

ALL the genes that are involved in a given disease, including cancer. In this regard histochemistry cannot help; its role is to estimate the level of activation of a given gene—IF we already know the gene product AND have an antibody against it. To meet this need, a new approach was conceived: the so-called microarray technology (Figure 4.64). It is barely beginning to affect therapy, yet the competition to provide the hardware is intense. Here is, in a nutshell, the principle of this technique (299, 317, 320).

> Suppose that we want to know which genes are activated in a given case of breast cancer. Any gene that is activated must be synthesizing mRNA; so we must find out which genes are doing so. To this effect we extract the mRNA from a sample of the cancer, convert it to DNA by reverse transcriptase, and stain this DNA with a fluorescent dye. We than repeat the procedure with a control tissue, e.g., normal mammary gland, and stain this control DNA with a different dye. (These two sets of samples are called the **targets.**) Next, we hybridize both targets to a large collection of known genes—or fragments of genes—as many as possible (these are called **probes**). The probes are applied robotically, in neat **arrays,** and of course in a precise order, to a suitable surface (e.g., glass slide); they may be tiny spots of oligonucleotides (~10–20 μm) and at the other extreme they may be punched out of tissue sections (~300 μm). Arrays of probes are commercially available. Two laser beams of different wave lengths, aided by a computer, scan the array and read out the results (a common combination of colors: green = overrepresented, red = underrepresented, yellow = unchanged).

The results of such a method may amount to millions of data. More than 10,000 genes can be spotted on a single array. Paradoxically, for these very reasons the results can lack statistical significance, because a huge number of data is based on a relatively small number of biological samples ("targets"); also, the method itself needs to be refined (295). However, it has been received with enthusiasm. As pathologists we are curious to find out how the current classification of tumors, based on their microscopic features, will compare with a classification based on activated genes.

What next? After the gene come the proteins: **proteomics** (the science of cellular protein interactions) is now being born. "While DNA has the information," writes Dr. Lance Liotta of the NIH, "the proteins do all the work. The cause of most human disease lies in the functional dysregulation of protein interaction" (311). This means creating a whole new level of technology—and pathology.

It may be, then, that the next steps of molecular medicine will take us through the intricacies of proteomics.

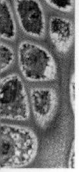

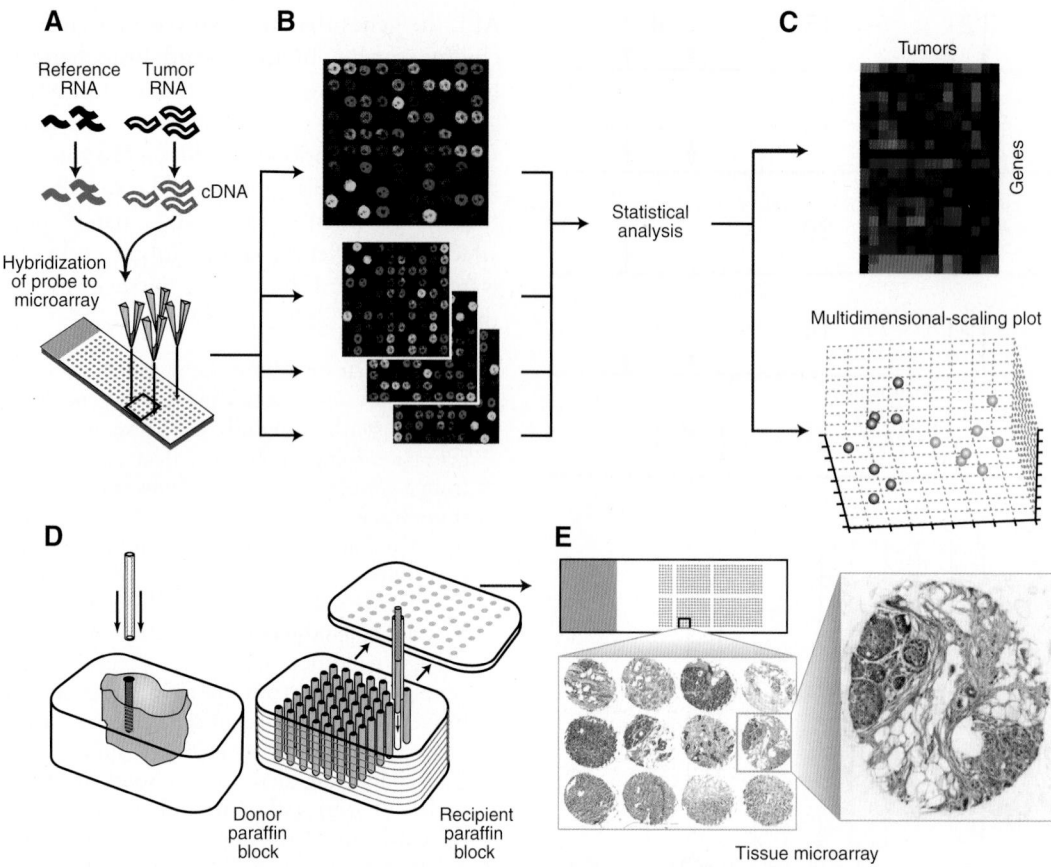

FIGURE 4.64 Preparation and analysis of microarrays of complementary DNA (cDNA) and breast tumor tissue. **A:** Reference and tumor RNA are submitted to reverse transcription, labeled with fluorescent dyes (green = reference cells, red = tumor cells), and hybridized to a cDNA microarray containing robotically printed cDNA clones. **B:** The slides are scanned with a confocal laser scanning microscope; color images are generated for each hybridization: genes upregulated in the tumors appear red, genes with decreased expression appear green, and genes with similar level of expression in the two samples appear yellow.

Genes of interest are selected on the basis of the differences in the level of expression of known tumor classes, and results are statistically controlled. **C:** Differences in the pattern of gene expression between tumor classes can be portrayed as a multidimensional scaling plot. Tumors with similar gene-expression profiles tend to cluster close to one another in the multidimensional scaling plot. **D:** Particular genes of interest can be further studied by using a large number of arrayed, paraffin-embedded tumor specimens (**tissue microarrays**). **E:** To extend the microarray findings even further, it is possible to perform immunohistochemical analysis of hundreds— or thousands—of arrayed tissue specimens (Reproduced with permission from Hedenfalk I, et al. Gene-expression profiles in hereditary breast cancer, N Engl J Med 2001;344:539–548. Copyright © 2001 Massachusetts Medical Society. All rights reserved.)

Wherever that path may lead, we should not forget its unlikely beginnings.

The forgotten hero of this epic is Frederick Griffith, a British medical officer so dedicated to his work that he was killed in his laboratory during an air raid over London in 1941 (303, 316). In 1928 he made a critical observation. Having noticed some unexplained shifts in the types of pneumococci in the population of his district, he tried to find out whether one type of pneumococcus could be turned into another. He did so *in vivo* by injecting mice with live pneumococci of a nonvirulent strain, together with dead pneumococci from a virulent strain: the mice died of infection with the virulent strain. Griffith concluded that something coming from the dead virulent bacteria had transformed the nonvirulent bacteria; in 1944 that "something" was identified as DNA by Avery, MacLeod, and McCarty at the Rockefeller Institute (Figure 4.65) (292).

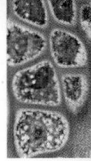

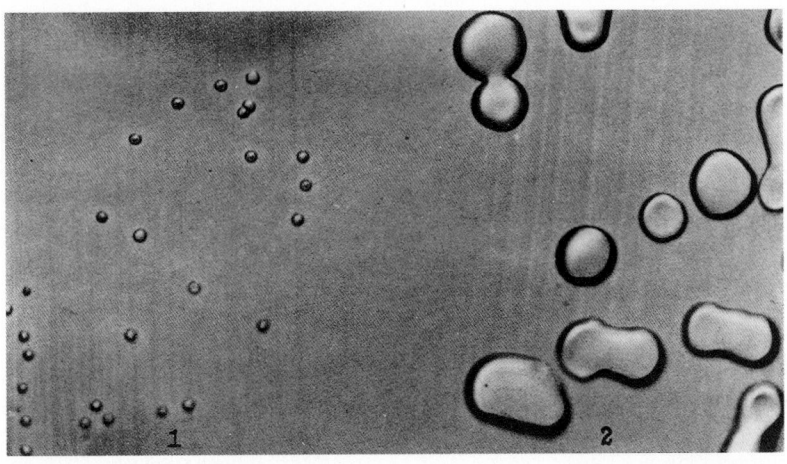

FIGURE 4.65   The classic transformation experiment by Avery et al. in 1944. At left, small colonies of pneumococcus Type 2, "rough" variant, are growing on agar. At right, colonies of the *same* pneumococcus grown in the presence of "transforming principle" (DNA) obtained from Type 3 pneumococci. The smooth, glistening, mucoid colonies are typical of pneumococcus Type 3. The conclusion is that exogenous DNA has been able to transform pneumococci Type 2 into Type 3. (Reproduced from the **Journal of Experimental Medicine,** 1944;79:137–158, by copyright permission of The Rockefeller University Press [292].)

References

Prelude: Protein Misfolding

1. Alberts B, Johnson A, Lewis J, et al. (eds). Molecular biology of the cell. 4th edition. New York: Garland Science, 2002.
2. Carrell RW, Lomas DA. Conformational disease. Lancet 1997; 350:134–138.
3. Dobson CM. Getting out of shape. Nature 2002;418:729–730.
4. Ellis RJ. Macromolecular crowding: obvious but underappreciated. Trends Biochem Sci 2001;26:597–604.
5. Kopito RR. ER quality control: the cytoplasmic connection. Cell 1997;88:427–430.
6. Minton AP. Implications of macromolecular crowding for protein assembly. Curr Opin Struct Biol 2000;10:34–39.

Pathology of the Cell Membrane

7. Ackerman MJ, Clapham DE. Ion channels—basic science and clinical disease. N Engl J Med 1997;336:1575–1586.
8. Anderson RGW, Jacobson K. A role for lipid shells in targeting proteins to caveolae, rafts, and other lipid domains. Science 2002;296:1821–1825.
9. Andreoli TE, Hoffman JF, Fanestil DD (eds). Physiology of membrane disorders. New York and London: Plenum Medical Book Co., 1978.
10. Arahata K, Ishiura S, Ishiguro T, et al. Immunostaining of skeletal and cardiac muscle surface membrane with antibody against Duchenne muscular dystrophy peptide. Nature 1988; 333:861–863.
11. Ashcroft FM. Ion channels and disease. Channelopathies. San Diego: Academic Press, 2000.
12. Bangham AD, Horne RW. Negative staining of phospholipids and their structural modification by surface-active agents as observed in the electron microscope. J Mol Biol 1964;8:660–668.
13. Beck IT, Dinda PK. Acute exposure of small intestine to ethanol: effects on morphology and function. Dig Dis Sci 1981;26:817–838.
14. Bessis M. Living blood cells and their ultrastructure. Berlin: Springer-Verlag, 1973.
15. Bianchi G, Carafoli E, Scarpa A (eds). Membrane pathology. (Ann NY Acad Sci, Vol 488). New York: The New York Academy of Sciences, 1986.
16. Bolis L, Hoffman JF, Leaf A (eds). Membranes and disease. New York: Raven Press, 1976.
17. Bourguignon LYW, Bourguignon GJ. Capping and the cytoskeleton. Int Rev Cytol 1984;47:195–224.
18. Brown MS, Goldstein JL. Familial hypercholesterolemia: defective binding of lipoproteins to cultured fibroblast associated with impaired regulation of 3-hydroxy-3-methylglutaryl coenzyme A reductase activity. Proc Natl Acad Sci USA 1974;71:788–792.
19. Bücherl W, Buckley E (eds). Venomous animals and their venoms. Volume II. Venomous vertebrates. New York: Academic Press, 1971.
20. Bücherl W, Buckley EE, Deulofeu V (eds). Venomous animals and their venoms. Volume I. Venomous vertebrates. New York: Academic Press, 1968.
21. Buckley IK. Tissue injury by high frequency electric current: observations with the Sandison-Clark ear chamber. Aust J Exp Biol Med Sci 1960;38:211–226.
22. Crane RK, Menard D, Preiser H, Cerda J. The molecular basis of brush-border membrane disease. In: Bolis L, Hoffman JF, Leaf A (eds). Membranes and disease. New York: Raven Press, 1976, pp. 229–241.

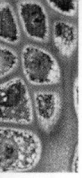

23. Dai J, Sheetz MP. Membrane tether formation from blebbing cells. Biophys J 1999;77:3363–3370.

24. Dall'Asta V, Rossi PA, Bussolati O, Gazzola GC. Regulatory volume decrease of cultured human fibroblasts involves changes in intracellular amino-acid pool. Biochim Biophys Acta 1994;1220:139–145.

25. Damjanov I. Lectin cytochemistry and histochemistry. Lab Invest 1987;57:5–20.

26. Eidels L, Proia RL, Hart DA. Membrane receptors for bacterial toxins. Microbiol Rev 1983;47:596–620.

27. England SB, Nicholson LVB, Johnson MA, et al. Very mild muscular dystrophy associated with the deletion of 46% of dystrophin. Nature 1990;343:180–182.

28. Fuhrman FA. Tetrodotoxin. Sci Am 1967;217:60–71.

29. Goldstein DB. The effects of drugs on membrane fluidity. Annu Rev Pharmacol Toxicol 1984;24:43–64.

30. Goldstein IJ, Poretz RD. Isolation, physicochemical characterization, and carbohydrate-binding specificity of lectins. In: Liener IE, Sharon N, Goldstein IJ (eds). The lectins: properties, functions, and applications in biology and medicine. Orlando: Academic Press, Inc., 1986, pp. 33–247.

31. Herman B, Nieminen AL, Gores GJ, Lemasters JJ. Irreversible injury in anoxic hepatocytes precipitated by an abrupt increase in plasma membrane permeability. FASEB J 1988;2:146–151.

32. Jewell SA, Bellomo G, Thor H, Orrenius S, Smith MT. Bleb formation in hepatocytes during drug metabolism is caused by disturbances in thiol and calcium ion homeostasis. Science 1982;217:1257–1259.

33. Johnston WH, Latta H, Osvaldo L. Variations in glomerular ultrastructure in rat kidneys fixed by perfusion. J Ultrastruct Res 1973;45:149–167.

34. Kretchmer N. Memorial Lecture: lactose and lactase—a historical perspective. Gastroenterology 1971;61:805–813.

35. Leaf A, Macknight ADC. Ischemia and disturbances in cell volume regulation. In: Andreoli TE, Hoffman JF, Fanestil DD (eds). Physiology of membrane disorders. New York: Plenum Medical Book Company, 1978, pp. 1093–1100.

36. Lemasters JJ, DiGuiseppi J, Nieminen A-L, Herman B. Blebbing, free Ca^{++} and mitochondrial membrane potential preceding cell death in hepatocytes. Nature 1987;325:78–81.

37. Lencer WI. Microbes and microbial toxins: paradigms for microbial-mucosal interactions V. Cholera: invasion of the intestinal epithelial barrier by a stably folded protein toxin. Am J Physiol Gastrointest Liver Physiol 2001;280:G781–G786.

38. Lewis R. Pufferfish genomes probe human genes. Scientist 2002;16:22–23.

39. Liener IE, Sharon N, Goldstein IJ (eds). The lectins: properties, functions, and applications in biology and medicine. Orlando: Academic Press, Inc., 1986.

40. Lucy JA. The fusion of cell membranes. In: Weissmann G, Claiborne R (eds). Cell membranes: biochemistry, cell biology & pathology. New York: HP Publishing Co., Inc., 1975, pp. 75–83.

41. Majno G, La Gattuta M, Thompson TE. Cellular death and necrosis: chemical, physical and morphologic changes in rat liver. Virchows Arch Pathol Anat 1960;333:421–465.

42. Mokri B, Engel AG. Duchenne dystrophy: electron microscopic findings pointing to a basic or early abnormality in the plasma membrane of the muscle fiber. Neurology 1975;25:1111–1120.

43. Moldovan NI, Radu AN, Simionescu N. Endothelial cell plasma membrane obtained by chemically induced vesiculation. Exp Cell Res 1987;170:499–510.

43a. Nilsson M, Mölne J, Jörtsö E, Smeds S, Ericson LE. Plasma membrane shedding and colloid vacuoles in hyperactive human thyroid tissue. Virchows Archiv B Cell Pathol 1988;56:85–94.

44. Ostwald R. Cholesterol and membranes. In: Dupont J (ed). Cholesterol systems in insects and animals. Boca Raton: CRC Press, Inc., 1982, pp. 51–75.

45. Putney JW, Jr, Askari A. Modification of membrane function by drugs. In: Andreoli TE, Hoffman JF, Fanestil DD (eds). Physiology of membrane disorders. New York: Plenum Medical Book Company, 1978, pp. 417–445.

46. Rabbani GH. The search for a better oral rehydration solution for cholera. N Engl J Med 2000;342:345–347.

47. Rona G, Hüttner I, More RH. Fibrin as a natural tracer in cardiac muscle cell injury. Thromb Diath Haemm Suppl 1973;56:21–33.

47a. Rosai J, Carcangiu ML, DeLellis RA. Tumors of the thyroid gland. Atlas of tumors Pathology, 3rd Series, Fascicle 5. Washington, D.C.; MD: Armed Forces Institute of Pathology, 1992.

48. Rubenstein E. Diseases caused by impaired communication among cells. Sci Am 1980;242:102–116, 120–121.

49. Ryan US, Schultz DR, Ryan JW. Fc and C3b receptors on pulmonary endothelial cells: induction by injury. Science 1981;214:557–558.

50. Sage MD, Jennings RB. Cytoskeletal injury and subsarcolemmal bleb formation in dog heart during in vitro total ischemia. Am J Pathol 1988;133:327–337.

51. Schnaar RL. The membrane is the message. The Sciences 1986;May/June:34–40.

52. Schotland DL, Bonilla E, van Meter M. Duchenne dystrophy: alteration in muscle plasma membrane structure. Science 1977;196:1005–1007.

53. Schreiner GF, Unanue ER. Membrane and cytoplasmic changes in B lymphocytes induced by ligand-surface immunoglobulin interaction. Adv Immunol 1976;24:37–165.

54. Schwartz P, Piper HM, Spahr R, Spieckermann PG. Ultrastructure of cultured adult myocardial cells during anoxia and reoxygenation. Am J Pathol 1984;115:349–361.

55. Sebbagh M, Renvoizé C, Hamelin J, et al. Caspase-3-mediated cleavage of ROCK I induces MLC phosphorylation and apoptotic membrane blebbing. Nat Cell Biol 2001;3:346–352.

56. Seeman P. Transient holes in the erythrocyte membrane during hypotonic hemolysis and stable holes in the membrane after lysis by saponin and lysolecithin. J Cell Biol 1967;32:55–70.

57. Silver IA, Murrills RJ, Etherington DJ. Microelectrode studies on the acid microenvironment beneath adherent macrophages and osteoclasts. Exp Cell Res 1988;175:266–276.

58. Singer SJ, Nicolson GL. The fluid mosaic model of the structure of cell membranes. Science 1972;175:720–731.

59. Snyder LM, Fairbanks G, Trainor JP, et al. Properties and characterization of vesicles released by young and old human red cells. Br J Haematol 1985;59:513–522.

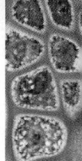

60. Stryer L. Biochemistry, 3rd ed. New York: WH Freeman and Company, 1988.

61. Tao M (ed). Membrane abnormalities and disease. Volumes I and II. Boca Raton, CRC Press, Inc., 1982.

62. Tao M, Conway RG. Biochemical aspects of normal and abnormal erythrocyte membranes. In: Tao M (ed). Membrane abnormalities and disease, volume I. Boca Raton, CRC Press, Inc., 1982, pp. 43–90.

63. Taraschi TF, Rubin E. Biology of disease: effects of ethanol on the chemical and structural properties of biologic membranes. Lab Invest 1985;52:120–131.

64. Teixeira JRM, Lapa AJ, Souccar C, Valle JR. Timbós. Ichthyotoxic plants used by Brazilian indians. J Ethnopharmacol 1984;10:311–318.

65. Trump BF, Laufer A, Jones RT (eds.) Cellular pathobiology of human disease. New York: Gustav Fischer, 1983.

66. Trump BF, Penttila A, Berezesky IK. Studies on cell surface conformation following injury. Virchows Arch. B Cell Pathol 1979;29:281–296.

67. Tu AT. Venoms: chemistry and molecular biology. New York: John Wiley & Sons, 1977.

68. Wagner R, Gabbert H, Höhn P. The mechanism of epithelial shedding after ischemic damage to the small intestinal mucosa. A light and electron microscopic investigation. Virchows Arch B Cell Pathol 1979;30:25–31.

69. Wagner R, Gabbert H, Höhn P. Ischemia and postischemic regeneration of the small intestinal mucosa. A light microscopic and autoradiographic study. Virchows Arch B Cell Pathol 1979;31:259–276.

70. Wallach DFH (ed). Plasma membranes and disease. London: Academic Press, 1979.

71. Weissmann G, Claiborne, R (eds). Cell membranes: biochemistry, cell biology & pathology. New York: HP Publishing Company, Inc., 1975.

72. Zubrzycka-Gaarn EE, Bulman DE, Karpati G, et al. The Duchenne muscular dystrophy gene product is localized in sarcolemma of human skeletal muscle. Nature 1988; 333:466–469.

Pathology of the Mitochondria

73. AFIP. The military uses mitochondrial DNA for human remains identification. AFIP Lett 1998;156:4–5.

74. Afzelius BA. Personal communication, 2001.

75. Andreu AL, Hanna MG, Reichmann H, et al. Exercise intolerance due to mutations in the cytochrome *b* gene of mitochondrial DNA. N Engl J Med 1999;341:1037–1044.

76. Bennett MJ, Rinaldo P, Strauss AW. Inborn errors of mitochondrial fatty acid oxidation. Crit Rev Clin Lab Sci 2000;37:1–44.

77. Berdanier CD, Everts HB. Mitochondrial DNA in aging and degenerative disease. Mutati Res 2001;475:169–184.

78. Carafoli E, Roman I. Mitochondria and disease. Mol Aspects Med 1980;3:295–429.

79. Johns DR. Mitochondrial DNA and disease. N Engl J Med 1995;333:638–644.

80. Joza N, Susin SA, Daugas E, et al. Essential role of the mitochondrial apoptosis-inducing factor in programmed cell death. Nature 2001;410:549–554.

81. Kirkinezos IG, Moraes CT. Reactive oxygen species and mitochondrial diseases. Cell Dev Biol 2001;12:449–457.

82. Kowald A. The mitochondrial theory of aging. Biol Signals Recept 2001;10:162–175.

83. Kroemer G, Reed JC. Mitochondrial control of cell death. Nat Med 2000;6:513–519.

84. Larsson N-G, Luft R. Revolution in mitochondrial medicine. FEBS Lett 1999;455:199–202.

85. Luft R, Ikkos D, Palmieri G, Ernster L, Afzelius B. A case of severe hypermetabolism of nonthyroid origin with a defect in the maintenance of mitochondrial respiratory control: a correlated clinical, biochemical, and morphological study. J Clin Invest 1962;41:1776–1804.

86. Luft R, Landau BR. Mitochondrial medicine. J Int Med 1995;238:405–421.

87. Margulis L. Origin of eukaryotic cells. Evidence and research implications for a theory of the origin and evolution of microbial, plant, and animal cells on the Precambrian earth. New Haven: Yale University Press, 1970.

88. Morgan-Hughes JA. Mitochondrial myopathies. In: Mastaglia FL, Walton J (eds). Skeletal muscle pathology. Edinburgh: Churchill Livingstone, 1982, pp. 309–339.

89. Ozawa T. Genetic and functional changes in mitochondria associated with aging. Physiol Rev 1997;77:425–464.

90. Pessayre D, Mansouri A, Fromenty B. Nonalcoholic steatosis and steatohepatitis v. mitochondrial dysfunction in steatohepatitis. Am J Physiol Gastrointest Liver Physiol 2002; 282:G193–G199.

91. Pfeifer U. Ultrastructural pathology of the human liver. In: Csomós G, Thaler H (eds). Clinical hepatology. Berlin: Springer-Verlag, 1983, pp. 159–194.

92. Robinson JM, Tanphaichitr N, Bellvé AR. Gossypol-induced damage to mitochondria of transformed Sertoli cells. Am J Pathol 1986;125:484–492.

93. Schwartz M, Vissing J. Paternal inheritance of mitochondrial DNA. N Engl J Med 2002;347:576–580.

94. Shanske AL, Shanske S, DiMauro S. The other human genome. Arch Pediatr Adolesc Med 2001;155:1210–1216.

95. Sjöstrand FS. Molecular pathology of Luft disease and structure and function of mitochondria. J Submicrosc Cytol Pathol 1999;31:41–50.

96. Sun CN, White HJ, Thompson BW. Oncocytoma (mitochondrioma) of the parotid gland. Arch Pathol 1975; 99:208–214.

97. Tandler B, Hutter RVP, Erlandson RA. Ultrastructure of oncocytoma of the parotid gland. Lab Invest 1970; 23:567–580.

98. Tandler B, Shipkey FH. Ultrastructure of Warthin's tumor. I. Mitochondria. J Ultrastruct Res 1964;11:292–305.

99. Wallace DC. Mitochondrial diseases in man and mouse. Science 1999;283:1482–1488.

Pathology of the Endoplasmic Reticulum and Golgi Apparatus

100. Bessis M. Cell death. Triangle 1970;9:191–199.

101. Bizzaro N, Pasini P, Ghirardello A, Finco B. High anti-Golgi autoantibody levels: an early sign of autoimmune disease? Clin Rheumatol 1999;18:346–348.

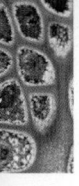

102. Bolmer S, Kleinerman J. Isolation and characterization of α_1-antitrypsin in PAS-positive hepatic granules from rats with experimental α_1-antitrypsin deficiency. Am J Pathol 1986;123:377–389.

103. Buckley IK. Phase contrast observations on the endoplasmic reticulum of living cells in culture. Protoplasma 1964; 59:569–588.

104. Callea F, Brisigotti M, Fabbretti G. Bonino F, Desmet VJ. Hepatic endoplasmic reticulum storage diseases. Liver 1992; 12:357–62.

105. Carlson JA, Rogers BB, Sifers RN, et al. Accumulation of PiZ α_1-antitrypsin causes liver damage in transgenic mice. J Clin Invest 1989;83:1183–1190.

106. Carlson JA, Rogers BB, Sifers RN, et al. Multiple tissues express alpha$_1$-antitrypsin in transgenic mice and man. J Clin Invest 1988;82:26–36.

107. Carrell RW, Lomas DA. Alpha$_1$-antitrypsin deficiency—a model for conformational diseases. N Engl J Med 2002; 346:45–53.

108. Castejon OJ. Ultrastructural pathology of Golgi apparatus of nerve cells in human brain edema associated to brain congenital malformations, tumours and trauma. J Submicrosc Cytol Pathol 1999;31:203–213.

109. Dawkins MJR. Carbon tetrachloride poisoning in the liver of the new-born rat. J Pathol Bacteriol 1963;85:189–196.

110. Durham SK, Boyd MR, Castleman WL. Pulmonary endothelial and bronchiolar epithelial lesions induced by 4-ipomeanol in mice. Am J Pathol 1985;118:66–75.

111. Eriksson S. Discovery of α_1-antitrypsin deficiency. Lung 1990;Suppl:523–529.

112. Eriksson S. Alpha$_1$-antitrypsin deficiency: lessons learned from the bedside to the gene and back again. Historic perspectives. Chest 1989;95:181–189.

113. Farber E, Liang H, Shinozuka H. Dissociation of effects on protein synthesis and ribosomes from membrane changes induced by carbon tetrachloride. Am J Pathol 1971; 64:601–617.

114. Farquhar MG, Bergeron JJM, Palade GE. Cytochemistry of Golgi fractions prepared from rat liver. J Cell Biol 1974; 60:8–25.

115. Ferreira ST, De Felice FG. Protein dynamic, folding and misfolding: from basic physical chemistry to human conformational diseases. FEBS Lett 2001;498:129–134.

116. Floersheim GL. Schutzwirkung hepatotoxischer Stoffe gegen letale Dosen eines Toxins aus Amanita phalloides (phalloidin). Biochem Pharmacol 1966;15:1589–1593.

117. Gonatas NK. Contributions to the physiology and pathology of the Golgi apparatus. Am J Pathol 1994;145:151–761.

118. Gonatas NK, Gonatas JO, Stieber A. The involvement of the Golgi apparatus in the pathogenesis of amyotrophic lateral sclerosis, Alzheimer's disease, and ricin intoxication. Histochem Biol 1998;109:591–600.

119. Gregersen N, Bross P, Jørgensen MM, Corydon TJ, Andresen BS. Defective folding and rapid degradation of mutant proteins is a proteins is a common disease mechanism in genetic disorders. J Inherit Metab Dis 2000;23:441–447.

120. Gregersen N, Bross P, Andresen BS, et al. The role of chaperone-assisted folding and quality control in inborn errors of metabolism: protein folding disorders. J Inherit Metab Dis 2001;24:189–212.

121. Jusko WJ. Smoking effects in pharmacokinetics. In: Benet LZ, Massoud N, Gambertoglio JG (eds). Pharmacokinetic basis for drug treatment. New York: Raven Press, 1984, pp. 311–320.

122. Kupfer D. Endogenous substrates of monooxygenases: fatty acids and prostaglandins. Pharmacol Ther 1980;11: 469–496.

123. Kuznetsov G, Nigam SK. Folding of secretory and membrane proteins. N Engl J Med 1998;339:1688–1695.

124. Langman J, Cardell L. Ultrastructural observations on FUdR-induced cell death and subsequent elimination of cell debris. Teratology 1978;17:229–270.

125. Lieberman J, Mittman C, Schneider AS. Screening for homozygous and heterozygous α_1-antitrypsin deficiency. Protein electrophoresis on cellulose acetate membranes. JAMA 1969;210:2055–2060.

126. Luczynska C, Wilson K. The clinical significance of the effects of cigarette smoking on drug disposition. Methods Find Exp Clin Pharmacol 1983;5:479–487.

127. Nelson DR, Kamataki T, Waxman DJ, et al. The P450 superfamily: update on new sequences, gene mapping, accession numbers, early trivial names of enzymes, and nomenclature. DNA Cell Biol 1993;12:1–51.

128. Ortiz de Montellano PR. Cytochrome P-450. New York: Plenum Press, 1986.

129. Pfeifer U, Ormanns W, Klinge O. Hepatocellular fibrinogen storage in familial hypofibrinogenemia. Virchows Arch Cell Pathol 1981;36:247–255.

130. Phillips MJ, Poucell S, Patterson J, Valencia P. The liver: an atlas and text of ultrastructural pathology. New York: Raven Press, 1987.

131. Porter KR. Electron microscopy of basophilic components of cytoplasm. J Histochem Cytochem 1954;2:346–373.

132. Porter KR, Claude A, Fullam EF. A study of tissue culture cells by electron microscopy. Methods and preliminary observations. J Exp Med 1945;81:233–246.

133. Recknagel RO, Ghoshal AK. Lipoperoxidation as a vector in carbon tetrachloride hepatotoxicity. Lab Invest 1966; 15:132–146.

134. Recknagel RO, Glende EA Jr, Hruszkewycz AM. Chemical mechanisms in carbon tetrachloride toxicity. In: Pryor WA (ed). Free radicals in biology. Vol. III. New York: Academic Press, 1977, pp. 97–132.

135. Roingeard P, Sureau C. Ultrastructural analysis of hepatitis B virus in HepG2-transfected cells with special emphasis on subviral filament morphogenesis. Hepatology 1998; 28: 1128–1133.

136. Rothman JE, Orci L. Budding vesicles in living cells. Sci Am 1996;274:70–75.

136a. Sifers RN, Finegold MJ, Woo SLC. Alpha-1-antitrypsin deficiency: accumulation or degradation of mutant variants within the hepatic endoplasmic reticulum. Am J Respir Cell Mol Biol 1989;1:341–345.

137. Singer HA, Saye JA, Peach MJ. Effects of cytochrome P-450 inhibitors on endothelium-dependent relaxation in rabbit aorta. Blood Vessels 1984;21:223–230.

138. Smuckler EA, Iseri OA, Benditt EP. An intracellular defect in protein synthesis induced by carbon tetrachloride. J Exp Med 1962;116:55–72.

139. Soto C. Protein misfolding and disease; protein refolding and therapy. FEBS Letters 2001;498:204–207.

140. Ugazio G, Danni O, Milillo P, Burdino E, Congiu AM. Mechanism of protection against carbon tetrachloride toxicity. I. Prevention of lethal effects by partial surgical hepatectomy. Drug Chem Toxicol 1982;5:115–124.

141. Ugazio G, Koch RR, Recknagel RO. Mechanism of protection against carbon tetrachloride by prior carbon tetrachloride administration. Exp Mol Pathol 1972;16:281–285.

142. Vesell ES. Pharmacogenetic perspectives: genes, drugs and disease. Hepatology 1984;4:959–965.

143. Waterman MR, John ME, Simpson ER. Regulation of synthesis and activity of cytochrome P-450 enzymes in physiological pathways. In: Ortiz de Montellano PR (ed). Cytochrome P-450. New York: Plenum Press, 1986, pp. 345–386.

Pathology of the Lysosomes and Peroxisomes

144. Allison AC, Morgan DML. Effects of silica, asbestos, and other particles on macrophage and neutrophil lysosomes. In: Dingle JT, Jacques PJ, Shaw IH (eds). Lysosomes in applied biology and therapeutics, vol. 6. Amsterdam: North-Holland Publishing Co., 1979, pp. 149–159.

145. Alroy J, Warren CD, Raghavan SS, Kolodny EH. Animal models for lysosomal storage diseases: their past and future contribution. Hum Pathol 1989;20:823–826.

146. Armstrong JA, D'Arcy Hart P. Response of cultured macrophages to Mycobacterium tuberculosis, with observations on fusion of lysosomes with phagosomes. J Exp Med 1971;134:713–740.

147. Aterman K. The development of the concept of lysosomes. A historical survey, with particular reference to the liver. Histochem J 1979;11:503–541.

148. Barranger JA, O'Rourke E. Lessons learned from the development of enzyme therapy for Gaucher disease. J Inherit Metab Dis 2001;24(suppl 2):89–96.

149. Baum H, Gergely J. Molecular aspects of medicine, vol. 2. Oxford: Pergamon Press, 1980.

150. Baumgart E, Stegmeier K, Schmidt, FH, Fahimi HD. Proliferation of peroxisomes in pericentral hepatocytes of rat liver after administration of a new hypocholesterolemic agent (BM 15766). Sex-dependent ultrastructural differences. Lab Invest 1987;56:554–564.

151. Beutler E. Gaucher's disease. N Engl J Med 1991;325:1354–1360.

152. Benson PF, Fensom AH. Genetic biochemical disorders. Oxford: Oxford University Press, 1985.

153. Brady RO, Barranger JA. Glucosylceramide lipidosis: Gaucher's disease. In: Stanbury JB, Wyngaarden JB, Frederickson DS, Goldstein JL, Brown MS (eds). The metabolic basis of inherited disease. 5th ed. New York: McGraw-Hill Book Company, 1983, pp. 842–856.

154. Cherian PV, Schumacher HR Jr. Immunochemical and ultrastructural characterization of serum proteins associated with monosodium urate crystals (MS) in synovial fluid cells from patients with gout. Ultrastruct Pathol 1986;10:209–219.

155. Cohn ZA, Hirsch JG. The isolation and properties of the specific cytoplasmic granules of rabbit polymorphonuclear leucocytes. J Exp Med 1960;112:983–1004.

156. Cox TM. Gaucher disease: understanding the molecular pathogenesis of sphingolipidoses. J Inherit Metab Dis 2001;24(suppl 2):106–121.

157. D'Alton ME, DeCherney AH. Prenatal diagnosis. N Engl J Med 1993;328:114–120.

158. de Duve C. The lysosome. Sci Am 1963;208:64–72.

159. de Duve C. A guided tour of the living cell. Vol I. New York: Scientific American Books, 1984.

160. DeGasperi R, Alroy J, Richard R, et al. Glycoprotein storage in Gaucher disease: lectin histochemistry and biochemical studies. Lab Invest 1990;63:385–393.

161. Dell'Angelica EC, Mullins C, Caplan S, Bonifacino JS. Lysosome-related organelles. FASEB J 2000;14:1265–1278.

162. Deretic V, Fratti RA. Mycobacterium tuberculosis phagosome. Mol Microbiol 1999;31:1603–1609.

163. Desnick RJ. Enzyme replacement and beyond. J Inherit Metab Dis 2001;24:251–265.

164. Dingle JT. Lysosomes in biology and pathology. Vol 3. New York: Elsevier-North Holland Publishing Co., 1973.

165. Dingle JT, Dean RT. Lysosomes in biology and pathology, vol. 5. Amsterdam: North-Holland Publishing Company, 1976.

166. Dzhekova-Stojkova S, Bogdanska J, Stojkova Z. Peroxisome proliferators: their biological and toxicological effects. Clin Chem Lab Med 2001;39:468–474.

167. Erikson A. Remaining problems in the management of patients with Gaucher disease. J Inherit Metab Dis 2001;24(suppl 2):122–126.

168. Fahimi HD, Kalmbach P, Stegmeier K, Stork H. Comparison between the effects of clofibrate and bezafibrate upon the ultrastructure of rat heart and liver. In: Greten H, Lang PD, Schettler G (eds). Lipoproteins and coronary heart disease. New York: Gerhard Witzstrock Publishing House, 1980, pp. 64–75.

169. Fujiki Y. Okumoto K, Otera H, Tamura S. Peroxisome biogenesis and molecular defects in peroxisome assembly disorders. Cell Biochem Biophys 2000;32:155–164.

170. Gagnon E, Duclos S, Rondeau C, et al. Endoplasmic reticulum-mediated phagocytosis is a mechanism of entry into macrophages. Cell 2002;110:119–131.

171. Gärtner J. Organelle disease: peroxisomal disorders. Eur J Pediatr 2000;159(suppl 3):S236–S239.

172. Gillooly DJ, Simonsen A, Stenmark H. Phosphoinositides and phagocytosis. J Cell Biol 2001;155:15–17.

173. Glew RH, Basu A, Prence EM, Remaley AT. Lysosomal storage disease. Lab Invest 1985;53:250–269.

174. Goren MB, Hart PD, Young MR, Armstrong JA. Prevention of phagosome-lysosome fusion in cultured macrophages by sulfatides of Mycobacterium tuberculosis. Proc Natl Acad Sci USA 1976;73:2510–2514.

175. Goren MB, Swendsen CL, Fiscus J, Miranti C. Fluorescent markers for studying phagosome-lysosome function. J Leukocyte Biol 1984;36:273–292.

176. Goren MB, Vatter AE, Fiscus J. Polyanionic agents do not inhibit phagosome-lysosome fusion in cultured macrophages. J Leukocyte Biol 1987;41:122–129.

177. Grabowski GA, Barton NW, Pastores G, et al. Enzyme therapy in type 1 Gaucher disease: comparative efficacy of mannose-terminated glucocerebrosidase from natural and recombinant sources. Ann Intern Med 1995;122:33–39.

178. Grabowski GG. Lysosomal storage diseases. In: Braunwald E, Fauci AS, Kasper DL, Hauser SL, Longo DL, Jameson JL (eds). Harrison's Principles of Internal Medicine, 15th ed. New York: McGraw-Hill, 2001, pp. 2276–2281.

179. Hannun UA, Bell RM. Lysosphingolipids inhibit protein kinase C: implications for the sphingolipidoses. Science 1987;235:670–674.

180. Harris L, McKenna WJ, Rowland E, Krikler DM. Side effects and possible contraindications of amiodarone use. Am Heart J 1983;106:916–923.

181. Holtzman E. Lysosomes: a survey. New York: Springer-Verlag, 1976.

182. Hortsmann G, Lüllmann-Rauch R. Mucopolysaccharidosis-like alterations in cardiac valves of rats treated with tilorone. Virchows Arch (Cell Pathol) 1985;48:33–45.

183. Hruban Z, Gotoh M, Slesers A, Chou S-F. Structure of hepatic microbodies in rats treated with acetylsalicylic acid, clofibrate, dimethrin. Lab Invest 1974;30:64–75.

184. Jackson LG. First-trimester diagnosis of fetal genetic disorders. Hosp Pract 1985;20:39–48.

185. Jägel M, Lüllmann-Rauch R. Lipidosis-like laterations in cultured macrophages exposed to local anesthetics. Arch Toxicol 1984;55:229–232.

186. Joiner KA, Fuhrman SA, Miettinen HM, Kasper LH, Mellman I. Toxoplasma gondii: fusion competence of parasitophorous vacuoles in Fc receptor-transfected fibroblasts. Science 1990;249:641–646.

187. Jones TC, Hirsch JG. The interaction between Toxoplasma gondii and mammalian cells. II. The absence of lysosomal fusion with phagocytic vacuoles containing living parasites. J Exp Med 1972;136:1173–1194.

188. Jones TC, Yeh S, Hirsch JG. The interaction between Toxoplasma gondii and mammalian cells. I. Mechanism of entry and intracellular fate of the parasite. J Exp Med 1972;136:1157–1172.

189. Kakkis ED, Muenzer J, Tiller GE, et al. Enzyme-replacement therapy in mucopolysaccharidosis I. N Engl J Med 2001;344:182–188.

190. Kane AB, Stanton RP, Raymond EG, et al. Dissociation of intracellular lysosomal rupture from the cell death caused by silica. J Cell Biol 1980;87:643–651.

191. Kaye EM, Alroy J, Raghavan SS, et al. Dysmyelinogenesis in animal model of GM₁ gangliosidosis. Pediatr Neurol 1992;8:255–261.

192. Kleijer WJ, Janse HC, Vosters RPL, Niermeijer MF, van de Kamp JJP. First-trimester diagnosis of mucopolysaccharidosis IIIA (Sanfilippo A disease). N Engl J Med 1986;314:185–186.

193. Kolodny EH, Cable WJL. Inborn errors of metabolism. Ann Neurol 1982;11:221–232.

194. Kornfeld S, Sly WS. Lysosomal storage defects. Hosp Pract 1985;20:71–82.

195. Krogstad DJ, Schlesinger PH, Gluzman IY. Antimalarials increase vesicle pH in Plasmodium falciparum. J Cell Biol 1985;101:2302–2309.

196. Kudo, RR. Protozozoology. Springfield: Charles C Thomas, 1966.

197. Lüllman-Rauch R, Reil GH. Chlorphentermine-induced ultrastructural changes in liver tissues of four animal species. Virchows Arch [B] 1975;13:307–320.

198. Lüllmann-Rauch R. Drug-induced lysosomal storage disorders. In: Dingle JT, Jacques PJ, Shaw IH (eds). Lysosomes in applied biology and therapeutics Vol 6. Amsterdam: North-Holland Publishing Company, 1979, pp. 49–130.

199. MacDonald RD, Engel AG. Experimental chloroquine myopathy. J Neuropathol Exp Neurol 1970;29:479–499.

200. Mankin HJ, Rosenthal DI, Xavier R. Gaucher disease: new approaches to an ancient disease. J Bone Joint Surg 2001;83-A(5):748–762.

201. McCarty DJ. Crystal deposition joint disease. Annu Rev Med 1974;25:279–288.

201a. McKinney JD, Gomez JE. Life on the inside for Mycobacterium tuberculosis. Nat Med 2003;9:1356–1357.

202. Moser HW, Goldfischer SL. The peroxisomal disorders. Hosp Pract 1985;20:61–70.

203. Neufeld EF, Cantz MJ. Corrective factors for inborn errors of mucopolysaccharide metabolism. Ann NY Acad Sci 1971;179:580–587.

204. Neufeld EF, Lim TW, Shapiro LJ. Inherited disorders of lysosomal metabolism. Annu Rev Biochem 1975;44:357–376.

205. Novikoff AB. Lysosomes: a personal account. In: Hers G, Van Hoof F (eds). Lysosomes and storage disease. New York: Academic Press, 1973, pp. 1–41.

206. Perkins DG, Haust MD. Ultrastructure of myocardium in the Hurler syndrome. Possible relation to cardiac function. Virchows Arch (Pathol Anat) 1982;394:195–205.

207. Peters SP, Lee RE, Glew RH. Gaucher's disease, a review. Medicine 1977;56:425–442.

208. Pfeifer U, Jeschke R. Cholesterylester-Speicherkrankheit. Virchows Arch B Cell Pathol 1980;33:17–34.

209. Ponder KP, Melniczek JR, Xu L, et al. Therapeutic neonatal hepatic gene therapy in mucopolysaccharidosis VII dogs. Proc Natl Acad Sci USA 2002;99:13102–13107.

210. Rao MS, Reddy JK. Peroxisome proliferation and hepatocarcinogenesis. Carcinogenesis 1987;8:631–636.

211. Reddy JK, Suga T, Mannaerts GP, Lazarow PB, Subramani S (eds). Peroxisomes. Biology and role in toxicology and disease. Ann NY Acad Sci 1996;804.

212. Riede UN, Fringes B, Moore GW. Peroxisomes in cellular injury and disease. In: Trump BF, Laufer A, Jones RT (eds). Cellular pathobiology of human disease. New York: Gustav Fischer, 1983, pp. 139–174.

213. Robinson JM, Karnovsky MJ. Ultrastructural localization of several phosphatases with Cerium. J Histochem Cytochem 1983;31:1197–1208.

214. Rusyn I, Rose ML, Bojes HK, Thurman RG. Novel role of oxidants in the molecular mechanism of action of peroxisome proliferators. Antiox Redox Signal 2000;2:607–621.

215. Sakuragawa N, Sakuragawa M, Kuwabara T, et al. Niemann-Pick disease experimental model: sphingomyelinase reduction induced by AY-9944. Science 1977;196:317–319.

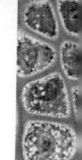

216. Schneider P, Korolenko TA, Busch U. A review of drug-induced lysosomal disorders of the liver in man and laboratory animals. Microsc Res Tech 1997;36:253–275.

217. Stanbury JD, Wyngaarden JB, Frederickson DS, Goldstein JL, Brown MS. The metabolic basis of inherited disease. 5th ed. New York: McGraw-Hill, 1983.

218. Starzl TE, Demetris AJ, Trucco M, et al. Chimerism after liver transplantation for type IV glycogen storage disease and type 1 Gaucher's disease. N Engl J Med 1993;328:745–749.

219. Wanders RJA. Peroxisomal disorders: clinical, biochemical, and molecular aspects. Neurochem Res 1999;24:565–580.

220. Weissmann G. The molecular basis of acute gout. In: Weissmann G, Claiborne R (eds). Cell membranes: biochemistry, cell biology and pathology. New York: HP Publishing, 1975, pp. 257–266.

Pathology of the Cytoskeleton

221. Afzelius BA. Disorders of ciliary motility. Hosp Pract 1986;21:73–80.

222. Afzelius BA. The immotile-cilia syndrome and other ciliary diseases. Int Rev Exp Pathol 1979;19:1–43.

223. Afzelius BA, Eliasson R, Johnsen O, Lindholmer C. Lack of dynein arms in immotile human spermatozoa. J Cell Biol 1975;66:225–232.

224. Allen RD. The microtubule as an intracellular engine. Sci Am 1987;256:42–49.

225. Bendall JR. Postmortem changes in muscle. In: Bourne GH (ed). The structure and function of muscle. 2nd ed. Vol II. New York: Academic Press, 1973, pp. 243–309.

226. Bloodgood RA. Resorption of organelles containing microtubules. Cytobios 1974;9:143–161.

227. Carter SB. Effects of cytochalasins on mammalian cells. Nature 1967;213:261–264.

228. Chan Y, Anton-Lamprecht I, Yu QC, et al. A human keratin 14 "knockout": the absence of K14 leads to severe epidermolysis bullosa simplex and a function for an intermediate filament protein. Genes Dev 1994;8:2574–2587.

229. Cooper JA. Effects of cytochalasin and phalloidin on actin. J Cell Biol 1987;105:1473–1478.

230. Copeman WSC. A short history of the gout and the rheumatic diseases. Berkeley: University of California Press, 1964.

231. Darnell J, Lodish H, Baltimore D. Molecular cell biology. New York: Scientific American Books, 1986.

232. Dustin P. Microtubules. 2nd ed. Berlin: Springer-Verlag, 1984.

232a. Eliasson R, Mossberg B, Camner P, Afzelius BA. The immotile-cilia syndrome. N Engl J Med 1977;297:1–6.

233. French SW. Present understanding of the development of Mallory's body. Arch Pathol Lab Med 1983;107:445–450.

234. Fuchs E. The cytoskeleton and disease: genetic disorders of intermediate filaments. Annu Rev Genet 1996;30:197–231.

235. Fuchs E, Weber K. Intermediate filaments: structure, dynamics, function, and disease. Annu Rev Biochem 1994; 63:345–382.

236. Fuchs E, Coulombe P, Cheng J, et al. Genetic bases of epidermolysis bullosa simplex and epidermolytic hyperkeratosis. J Invest Dermatol 1994;103(5 suppl):25S–30S.

237. Lillington GA. Dyskinetic cilia and Kartagener's syndrome. Clin Rev Allergy Immunol 2001;21:65–69.

238. Lowe JE, Jennings RB, Reimer KA. Cardiac rigor mortis in dogs. J Mol Cell Cardiol 1979;11:1017–1031.

239. McLean WHI, Lane EB. Intermediate filaments in disease. Curr Opin Cell Biol 1995;7:118–125.

240. Neumann PE, Horoupian DS, Goldman JE, Hess MA. Cytoplasmic filaments of Crooke's hyaline change belong to the cytokeratin class. Am J Pathol 1984;116:214–222.

241. Nonaka S, Tanaka Y, Okada Y, et al. Randomization of left-right asymmetry due to loss of nodal cilia generating leftward flow of extraembryonic fluid in mice lacking KIF3B motor protein. Cell 1998;95:829–837.

242. Pedersen H, Rebbe H. Absence of arms in the axoneme of immobile human spermatozoa. Biol Reprod 1975;12: 541–544.

243. Pernice B. Sulla cariocinesi delle cellule epiteliali e dell'endotelio dei vasi della mucosa dello stomaco e dell'intestino, nello studio della gastroenterite sperimentale (nell'avvelenamento per colchico). Sicilia Med 1889;1:265, 279.

244. Phillips MJ, Oda M, Funatsu K. Ece for microfilament involvement in norethandrolone-induced intrahepatic cholestasis. Am J Pathol 1978;93:729–744.

245. Phillips MJ, Poucell S, Oda M. Mechanisms of cholestasis. Lab Invest 1986;54:593–608.

246. Phillips MJ, Poucell S, Patterson J, Valencia P. Alcoholic liver disease and cirrhosis. In: Phillips MJ, Poucell S, Patterson J, Valencia P (eds). The liver. An atlas and text of ultrastructural pathology. New York: Raven Press, 1987, pp. 393–446.

246a. Plenck JG. Icones Plantarum Album, Centuria II/125, 1789.

247. Porter KR, Anderson KL. The structure of the cytoplasmic matrix preserved by freeze-drying and freeze-substitution. Eur J Cell Biol 1982;29:83–96.

248. Poste G, Lyon NC. Enucleation of cultured animal cells by cytochalasin B. In: Tanenbaum SW (ed). Cytochalasins—biochemical and cell biological aspects. Amsterdam: North-Holland Publishing Company, 1978, pp. 161–189.

249. Roberts WN, Liang MH, Stern SH. Colchicine in acute gout. JAMA 1987;257:1920–1922.

250. Schrek R, Stefani SS. Toxicity of microtubular drugs to leukemic lymphocytes. Exp Mol Pathol 1981;34:369–378.

251. Tanenbaum SW. Microbiological, preparative and analytical aspects of cytochalasin production. In: Tanenbaum SW (ed). Cytochalasins—biochemical and cell biological aspects. Amsterdam: North-Holland Publishing Company, 1978, pp. 1–14.

252. Vogel VJ. American indian medicine. Norman: University of Oklahoma Press, 1970.

253. Watanabe S, Phillips MJ. Acute phalloidin toxicity in living hepatocytes. Evidence for a possible disturbance in membrane flow and for multiple functions for actin in the liver cell. Am J Pathol 1986;122:101–111.

254. Weber K, Wehland J, Herzog W. Griseofulvin interacts with microtubules both in vivo and in vitro. J Mol Biol 1976; 102:817–829.

From Inclusion Bodies to Prions

255. Aronin N, Kim M, Laforet G, DiFiglia M. Are there multiple pathways in the pathogenesis of Huntington's disease? Philos Tans R Soc Lond B Biol Sci 1999;354:995–1003.

256. Brandner S, Klein MA, Frigg R, et al. Neuroinvasion of prions: insights from mouse models. Exp Physiol 2000; 85.6:705–712.

256a. Caughey B, Kocisko DA. A nucleic-acid accomplice? Nature 2003;425:673–674.

257. Chai Y, Shao J, Miller VM, Williams A, Paulson HL. Live-cell imaging reveals divergent intracellular dynamics of polyglutamine disease proteins and supports a sequestration model of pathogenesis. Proc Natl Acad Sci USA 2002;99:9310–9315.

258. Coles H. Nobel panel rewards prion theory after years of heated debate. Nature 1997;389:529.

258a. Couzin J. In a first, infected mice recover from prion disease. Science 2003;302:763–765.

259. Cummings CJ, Zoghbi HY. Fourteen and counting: unraveling trinucleotide repeat diseases. Hum Molec Genet 2000;9:909–916.

259a. Dawson TM, Dawson VL. Molecular pathways of neurodegeneration in Parkinson's disease. Science 2003;302: 819–822.

260. Denk H, Stumptner C, Zatloukal K. Mallory bodies revisited. J Hepat 2000;32:689–702.

261. French BA, van Leeuwen F, Riley NE, et al. Aggresome formation in liver cells in response to different toxic mechanisms: role of the ubiquitin-proteasome pathway and the frameshift mutant of ubiquitin. Exp Mol Pathol 2001; 71:241–246.

262. Fujiwara H, Hasegawa M, Dohmae N, et al. α-Synuclein is phosphorylated in synucleinopathy lesions. Nat Cell Biol 2002;4:160–164.

263. Gajdusek DC. Unconventional viruses and the origin and disappearance of kuru. Science 1977;197:943–960.

264. Goedert M. Filamentous nerve cell inclusions in neurodegenerative diseases: tauopathies and α-synucleinopathies. Phil Trans R Soc Lond 1999;354:1101–1118.

265. Goldberg MS, Lansbury PT. Is there a cause-and-effect relationship between α-synuclein fibrillization and Parkinson's disease? Nat Cell Biol 2000;2:E115–E119.

265a. He L, LU X-Y, Jolly AF, et al. Spongiform degeneration in *mahoganoid* mutant mice. Science 2003;299:710–712.

266. Heppner FL, Musahl C, Arrighi I, et al. Prevention of scrapie pathogenesis by transgenic expression of anti-prion protein antibodies. Science 2001;294:178–182.

267. Johnston JA, Ward CL, Kopito RR. Aggresomes: a cellular response to misfolded proteins. J Cell Biol 1998;143: 1883–1898.

268. Junn E, Mouradian MM. Human α-synuclein overexpression increases intracellular reactive oxygen species levels and susceptibility to dopamine. Neurosc Lett 2002; 320:146–150.

269. Kegel KB, Kim M, Sapp E, et al. Huntingtin expression stimulates endosomallysosomal activity, endosome tubulation, and autophagy. J Neurosci 2000;20:7268–7278.

270. Kopito RR, Sitia R. Aggresomes and Russell bodies. EMBO Rep 2000;1:225–231.

271. Kopito RR. Aggresomes, inclusion bodies and protein aggregation. Trends Cell Biol 2000;10:524–530.

272. Lam Y A, Pickart CM, Alban A, et al. Inhibition of the ubiquitin-proteasome system in Alzheimer's disease. Proc Natl Acad Sci USA 2000;97:9902–9906.

272a. Mallucci G, Dickinson A, Linehan J, et al. Depleting neuronal PrP in prion infection prevents disease and reverses spongiosis. Science 2003;302:871–874.

273. Okazawa H, Sudol M, Rich T. PQBP-1 (Np/PQ): a polyglutamine tract-binding and nuclear inclusion-forming protein. Brain Res Bull 2001;56:273–280.

274. Prusiner SB. Prions and neurodegenerative diseases. N Engl J Med 1987;317:1571–1581.

275. Prusiner SB. Neurodegenerative diseases and prions. N Engl J Med 2001;344:1516–1526.

276. Rifkind RA, Osserman EF, Hsu KC, Morgan C. The intracellular distribution of gamma globulin in a mouse plasma cell tumor (X5563) as revealed by fluorescence and electron microscopy. J Exp Med 1962;116:423–432.

277. Riley NE, Li J, Worrall S, et al. The Mallory body as an aggresome: *in vitro* studies. Exp Mol Pathol 2002;72:17–23.

277a. Ross CA, Poirier MA, Wanker EE, Amzel M. Polyglutamine fibrillogenesis: the pathway unfolds. Proc Natl Acad Sci USA 2003;100:1–3.

278. Russell W. An address on a characteristic organism of cancer. Br Med J 1890;2:1356–1360.

279. Schlossmacher MG, Frosch MP, Gai WP, et al. Parkin localizes to the Lewy bodies of Parkinson disease and dementia with Lewy bodies. Am J Pathol 2002;160: 1655–1667.

280. Shultz LD, Coman DR, Lyons BL, Sidman CL, Taylor S. Development of plasmacytoid cells with Russell bodies in autoimmune "viable motheaten" mice. Am J Pathol 1987; 127:38–50.

281. Sigurdsson B. Rida, a chronic encephalitis of sheep with general remarks of infections which develop slowly and some of their special characteristics. Br Vet J 1954; 110:341–354.

282. Sigurdsson B, Pálsson PA. Visna of sheep. A slow, demyelinating infection. Br J Exp Pathol 1958;39:519–528.

283. Smith MA, Drew KL, Nunomura A, et al. Amyloid-β, tau alterations and mitochondrial dysfunction in Alzheimer disease: the chickens or the eggs? Neurochem Intern 2002; 40:527–531.

284. Soto C, Saborío GP. Prions: disease propagation and disease therapy by conformational transmission. Trends Mol Med 2001;7:109–114.

285. Valetti C, Grossi CE, Milstein C, Sitia R. Russell bodies: a general response of secretory cells to synthesis of a mutant immunoglobulin which can neither exit from, nor be degraded in, the endoplasmic reticulum. J Cell Biol 1991; 115:983–994.

286. Weinstein T, Mittelman M, Djaldetti M. Electron microscopy study of Mott and Russell bodies in myeloma cells. J Submicrosc Cytol 1987;19:155–159.

287. Xu J, Kao S-Y, Lee FJS, et al. Dopamine-dependent neurotoxicity of α-synuclein: a mechanism for selective neurodegeneration in Parkinson disease. Nat Med 2002; 8:600–606.

288. Yuan QX, Marceau N, French BA, Fu P, French SW. Heat shock *in vivo* induces Mallory body formation in drug primed mouse liver. Exp Mol Pathol 1995;63:63–76.

289. Zatloukal K, Stumptner C, Lehner M, et al. Cytokeratin 8 protects from hepatotoxicity, and its ratio to cytokeratin 18

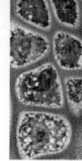

determines the ability of hepatocytes to form Mallory bodies. Am J Pathol 2000;156:1263–1274.

290. Zhou W, Hurlbert MS, Schaack J, Prasad KN, Freed CR. Overexpression of human α-synuclein causes dopamine neuron death in rat primary culture and immortalized mesencephalon-derived cells. Brain Res 2000;866:33–43.

Pathology of the Nucleus

291. Andersen JS, Lyon CE, Fox AH, et al. Directed proteomic analysis of the human nucleolus. Curr Biol 2002;12:1–11.

292. Avery OT, MacLeod CM, McCarty M. Studies on the chemical nature of the substance inducing transformation of pneumococcal types. Induction of transformation by a deoxyribonucleic acid fraction isolated from Pneumococcus Type III. J Exp Med 1944;79:137–158.

293. Bloom S, Cancilla PA. Conformational changes in myocardial nuclei of rats. Circ Res 1969;24:189–196.

294. Bohr VA, Evans MK, Fornace AJ Jr. DNA repair and its pathogenetic implications. Lab Invest 1989;61:143–161.

295. Brazma A, Hingamp P, Quackenbush J, et al. Minimum information about a microarray experiment (MIAME)—toward standards for microarray data. Nat Genet 2001; 29:365–371.

296. Farber E. Biochemical pathology. Annu Rev Pharmacol 1971;11:71–96.

297. Fenoglio-Preiser C (ed). Advances in pathology, vol 2. Chicago: Year Book Medical Publishers, Inc, 1989.

298. Fox JE. Molecular genetics—an overview for the clinician. Child Hosp Q 1989;1:43–47.

299. Gabrielson E, Berg K, Anbazhagan R. Functional genomics, gene arrays, and the future of pathology. Mod Pathol 2001;14:1294–1299.

300. Ghadially FN. Ultrastructural pathology of the cell and matrix. 2nd ed. London: Butterworths, 1982.

301. Goudie RB. DNA technology in histopathology. In: Anthony PP, MacSween RNM (eds). Recent advances in histopathology, No. 14. Edinburgh: Churchill Livingstone, 1989, pp. 1–21.

302. Goyer RA, Cherian MG. Tissue and cellular toxicology of metals. In: Brown SS (ed). Clinical chemistry and chemical toxicology of metals. Amsterdam: Elsevier Biomedical Press, 1977, pp. 89–103.

303. Griffith F. The significance of pneumococcal types. J Hyg 1928;27:113–159.

304. Grody WW, Gatti RA, Naeim F. Diagnostic molecular pathology. Mod Pathol 1989;2:553–568.

305. Guyer RL, Koshland DE Jr. The molecule of the year. Science 1989;246:1543–1546.

306. Jaenisch R. Transgenic animals. Science 1988;240: 1468–1474.

307. Kerkhoven P, Marti HR, Hug G. Electronmicroscopic and biochemical observations on erythroid cells in cogenital dyserythropoietic anemia type II. Virchows Arch A Pathol Anat Histol 1974;363:1–15.

308. Knight J, Abbott A. Full house. Nature 2002;417:785–786.

309. Korf B. Molecular medicine: Molecular diagnosis (Part one). N Engl J Med 1995;332:1218–1220.

310. Lako M, Hole N. (2000) Searching the unknown with gene trapping. Exp Rev Mol Med 6 July, http://www-ermm.cbcu.cam.ac.uk/00001824h.htm

311. Liotta LA, Kohn EC, Petricoin EF. Clinical proteomics. JAMA 2001;286:2211–2214.

312. Mak TW, Penninger JM, Ohashi PS. Knockout mice: a paradigm shift in modern immunology. Nat Rev Immunol 2001;1:11–19.

313. McLachlin JR, Goyer RA, Cherian MG. Formation of lead-induced inclusion bodies in primary rat kidney epithelial cell cultures: effect of actinomycin D and cycloheximide. Toxicol Appl Pharmacol 1980;56:418–431.

314. Pääbo S. Ancient DNA: extraction, characterization, molecular cloning, and enzymatic amplification. Proc Natl Acad Sci USA 1989;86:1939–1943.

315. Petters RM, Sommer JR. Transgenic animals as models for human disease. Transgenic Res 2000;9:347–351;discussion 345–346.

316. Portugal FH, Cohen JS. A century of DNA. Cambridge: The MIT Press, 1977.

317. Rubin EM, Tall A. Perspectives for vascular genomics. Nature 2000;407:265–269.

318. Scarpelli DG, Migaki G, Pletcher JM (eds). Transgenic animal models in biomedical research. Washington DC: Armed Forces Institute of Pathology, 1991.

319. Schoefl GI. The effect of actinomycin D on the fine structure of the nucleolus. J Ultrastruct Res 1964;10:224–243.

320. Schulze A, Downward J. Navigating gene expression using microarrays—a technology review. Nat Cell Biol 2001;3: E190–E195.

321. Skaar H, Ophus E, Gullvag BM. Lead accumulation within nuclei of moss leaf cells. Nature 1973;241:215–216.

322. van der Meer M (ed). Transgenesis and animal welfare: implications of transgenic procedures for the well-being of the laboratory mouse. Department of Laboratory Animal Science, Utrecht University; 2001.

323. Walton J, Buckley IK. The lead-poisoned cell: a fine structural study using cultured kidney cells. Exp Mol Pathol 1977; 27:167–182.

324. Westphal H. Transgenic mammals and biotechnology. FASEB J 1989;3:117–120.

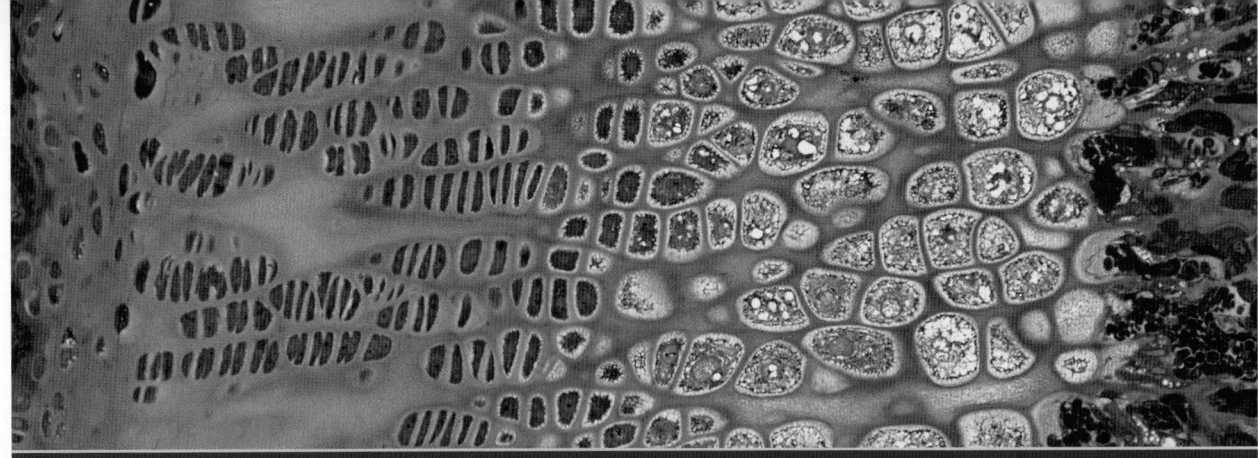

In Chapter 4 we dealt with the pathology of individual organelles; we will now consider the effects of injury on the cell as a whole.

As to the meaning of **injury,** dictionaries equate it with damage, which is good enough. The damage may be structural and/or functional. The main point is that the term injury does not include the response. Think of the term *wound,* which refers only to the damage; inflammation and repair are the responses.

Depending on the nature and intensity of the injury, cells may respond with an increased or decreased level of activity (Figure 5.1).

The Cellular Stress Response

Cells can be hurt by myriads of agents—physical, chemical, or biological. The catalog of responses is, of course, much shorter, because cells have a limited number of ways to react: one of these is a basic metabolic change, called the **stress** or **heat-shock response,** which takes place after any injury that may threaten the cell's life. The scientific community became aware of it late in the 1980s, but it was discovered in 1962. Stated in the simplest terms, this is the broadest known generalization regarding disease: *All the cells that have been tested—cells from animals, plants, and yeasts down to the simplest prokaryotes—when submitted to a stress such as a mild increase in temperature, temporarily turn down their usual protein synthesis and turn up the synthesis of certain selected proteins that have been called* **stress** *or* **heat-shock proteins** (HSPs) (341). The response develops within minutes (341) and lasts only a day or so. This time limit is probably a matter of survival: the cell cannot afford to turn off its regular protein synthesis indefinitely. In humans the stress response is triggered, for example, by ischemia, inflammation, fever, alcohol, and tissue damage in general (168, 219).

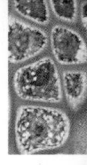

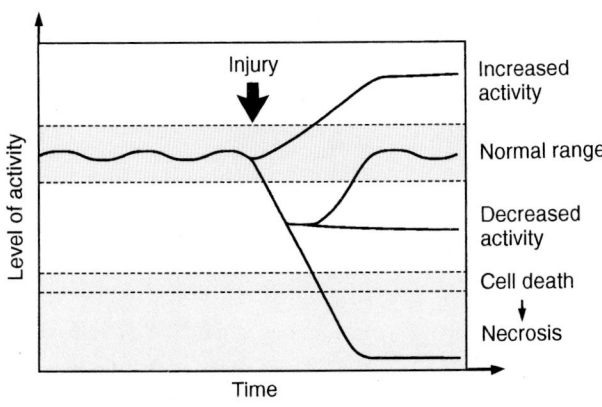

FIGURE 5.1 Responses of cells to injury. The activity of normal cells oscillates around a steady state, the physiologic range. After injury (**arrow**) cells may respond by increased activity (such as by the heat-shock response), by reversibly or irreversibly decreased activity, and eventually by cell death and necrosis. Enzymatic activity can persist for some time also in necrotic cells. (Adapted from [215].)

The seminal discovery was made in a genetics laboratory in Naples, in 1962, where Dr. Ferruccio Ritossa was working on the huge chromosomes of the salivary glands in fruit fly larvae. We have learned by the grapevine that the initial stimulus was accidental: someone knocked up the temperature of an incubator in which the larvae were kept, and Dr. Ritossa had the insight of using this accident as an experiment.

Eventually he found that after 30 minutes at 30°C (25°C being normal for the fruit flies), "puffs" appeared at certain sites—and always the same sites—on two chromosomes (Figure 5.2). The effect was reversible and could be elicited also with toxic chemicals (dinitrophenol, salicylate). It was known at that time that the puffs corresponded to sites of DNA uncoiling, a sign of enhanced transcription (RNA synthesis). In other words, the puffs represented activated genes. Twelve years later, in Geneva, A. Tissières and coworkers (318) showed by gel electrophoresis that protein synthesis was in fact enhanced: heat shock induced the appearance or increase of six proteins, accounting for about 30 percent of the total protein synthesis; the production of most other proteins was decreased. It seemed that the cell's protein-building machinery was being preempted for the manufacture of a small group of proteins. Within a few years similar results were obtained with all kinds of cells, from *E. coli* to slime molds and human tumors (279), and with all kinds of stressors.

The heat-shock response is about as ancient as it could be: the genes that code for its proteins have changed little in 3 billion years (345, 359). For example, if the amino acid sequences of equivalent heat-shock

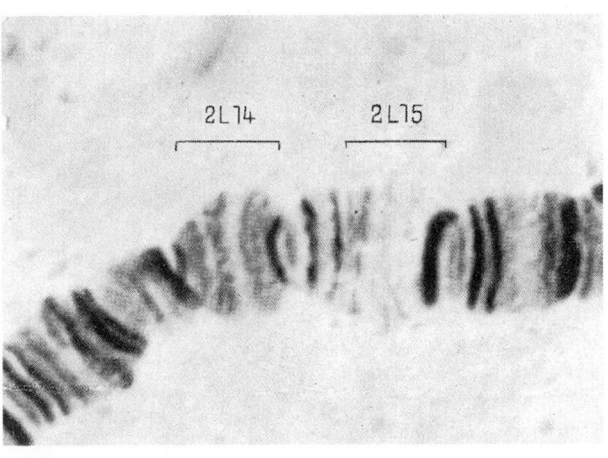

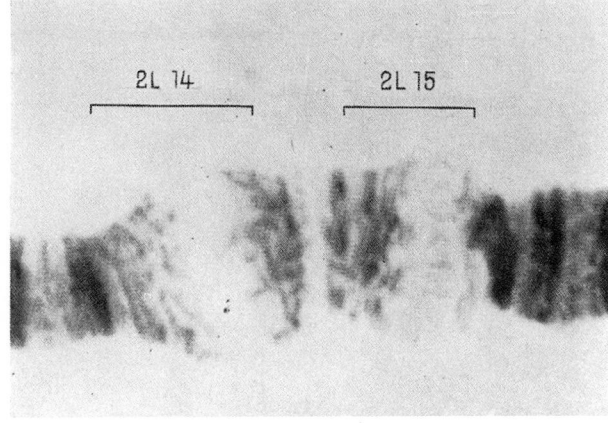

FIGURE 5.2 The original "puffing chromosomes" of Ritossa (1962), which led to the discovery of heat-shock proteins. *Top:* Brackets indicate two normal regions in salivary gland chromosomes of a larva of *Drosophila* reared at 25°C. *Bottom:* The same regions after receiving a thermal shock, administered by warming the larva for 30 minutes at 30°C. The key point is that the puffing occurred only in these regions, suggesting a specific phenomenon induced by heat. (Reproduced with permission from [266].)

proteins from prokaryotes and eukaryotes are compared, they are about 50 percent homologous, and many of the other residues are similar (359). Clearly the heat-shock response must play a key role for survival, and whatever that role may be, it must be intracellular because *the HSPs are not secreted.* The stressed cell keeps them for itself (a few exceptions will be mentioned further).

Other facts have emerged: *most of the HSPs are constitutive,* that is, they are always present in normal cells at low levels, as is well demonstrated by gel electrophoresis (Figure 5.3), and *all are key players in the normal cell's metabolism* (23).

The heat-shock proteins. As soon as the existence of the HSPs was recognized, it was easy enough to catalog

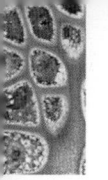

FIGURE 5.3 Gels of various mammalian cell lines showing heat-shock proteins after labeling with ^{35}S-methionine. **HeLa:** HeLa cells. **BHK:** Baby hamster kidney cells. **CHO:** Chinese hamster ovary cells. For each cell line, *lane 1* shows normal growth conditions, *lane 2* the effect of heat shock, and *lane 3* the effect of exposure to an amino acid analog of proline. **Arrowheads** point to heat-shock proteins. Note that the latter also exist in the normal control, but in lesser amounts. Figures at left indicate molecular mass in kilodaltons. (Reproduced with permission from [342].)

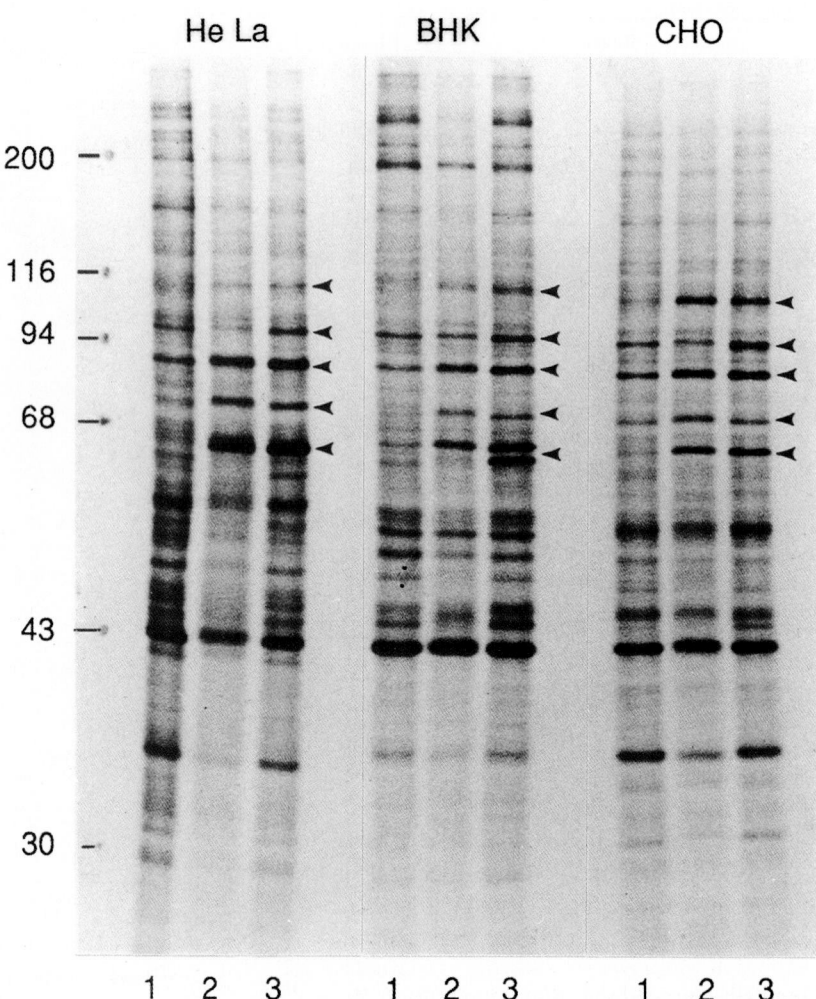

them—but their functions were largely unknown, so they were grouped by size and named HSP followed by the mass in kilodaltons. The 5 main families are HSPs 100, 90, 70, and 27 (26, 221); the last is a group of very small proteins, including **ubiquitin** (76 residues). This one was discovered accidentally during a search for thymic hormones and was found to be truly ubiquitous years before it was recognized as a HSP (36).

Eventually the tasks of the HSPs were worked out, and they were truly essential, in line with their great antiquity. They concerned **protein upkeep.** Proteins cannot function unless they are properly folded, a complex task even in a nonstressed cell, as we discussed in Chapter 4; stresses of many kinds (and especially heat) will tend to denature them, so it makes sense for the stressed cell to stop doing its daily chores and concentrate on straightening out its misfolded proteins, or getting rid of them. How the cell does it (more than 20 proteins are involved [76]) is best illustrated by a marvellous

bacterial HSP called GroEL (homologous to HSP60) extracted from *E. coli.* GroEL is shaped like a stack of four doughnuts, and oddly enough, it collaborates with a much smaller and entirely free protein, GroES, which acts like a lid or trap door for GroEL (Figure 5.4). First, the "lid" identifies a protein molecule that needs attention: the telltale sign of denaturation is that molecules of ubiquitin have become attached to it (i.e., it is *ubiquitinated*). The top "lid" somehow catches the protein and eases it into the central cavity of GroEL, where the corrective treatment is given (it has been visualized as a sort of massage). If the misfoding is corrected—which requires some energy, i.e., ATP—the captured protein is allowed to exit. If not, it is chopped up and the pieces are thrown out. The whole task is accomplished in about 13 seconds (285).

To the reader the story of GroEL-GroES may well sound like a *déjà vu:* indeed, by structure and behavior, this

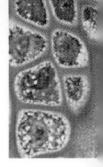

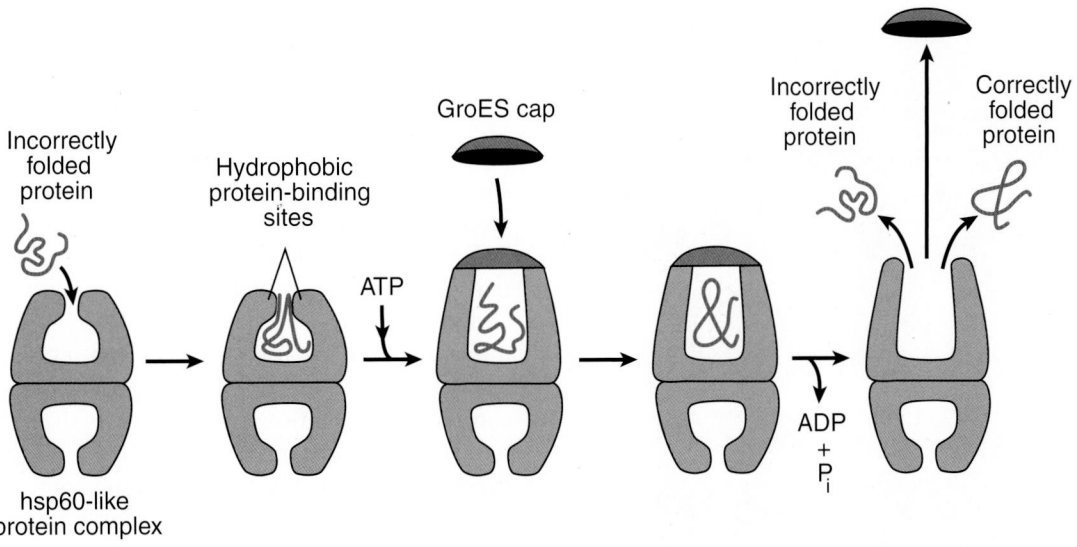

FIGURE 5.4   Structure and function of the bacterial GroEL proteins (homologous to the HSP60 family of chaperones). Initially, a misfolded protein is captured by hydrophobic interactions along a rim of the barrel and confined in the cavity of GroEL by the free-floating cap GroES. After about 15 seconds, ATP hydrolysis ejects the protein, whether folded or not, and the cycle is repeated. (Copyright 2002. From Molecular Biology of the Cell, 4th ed. Alberts B, Johnson A, Lewis J, et al. [eds]. Reproduced by permission of Routledge, Inc., part of The Taylor & Francis Group [2].)

tubular assembly is very similar to the proteasomes of eukaryotic cells. It so happens that, in the course of evolution, several proteases converged toward the same architecture, a non–membrane bound, extremely efficient protein-destroying machine (21).

Regarding assistance to protein molecules, some HSPs have another task that earned them the name *chaperonins:* they guide the newly born molecules to the right place (e.g., a mitochondrion), traversing, if necessary, an organelle membrane.

Thermotolerance and cell survival.   Here is more proof that the heat-shock response is important for the cell's survival: the phenomenon of thermotolerance.

Many experiments show that *cells challenged with mild heat become* **thermotolerant,** *that is, they can survive later exposure to a lethal temperature* (17, 349). Cultured fibroblasts grown at 37°C will survive a 30-minute thermal shock at 45°C, but if they are microinjected with an antibody against HSP 70, they die (Figure 5.5) (264). Various injurious agents bestow protection against other injurious agents (this is called **cross-protection**). For example, recovery from anoxia increases cellular thermotolerance as well as HSP synthesis; exposure to heat increases a cell's tolerance to adriamycin (57, 174). This works also *in vivo:* in rats maintained for 15 minutes at a body temperature of 41°C (reached by breathing air at 41–42°C), the retina is less sensitive to damage by bright light (17).

However, cross-protection between stresses is not always produced (139).

Morphology of the heat-shock response. Although the cell may perceive the heat-shock response as a major event, morphologically there is not much to see (besides the chromosome puffs noticed by Ritossa in 1962). Microscopic studies are usually carried out by immunochemistry, using antibodies against selected HSPs. Early in the heat-shock response, HSP 72 has been found to localize in the nucleolus; later, during recovery, it diffuses into the cytoplasm to areas rich in ribosomes (345). This distribution suggests that *HSP 72 may be involved in "rescuing" the complex molecular machinery involved in transcription and translation* (345).

The structural changes that occur during heat shock are mild and not necessarily related to the HSPs: condensation of the chromatin, appearance of bundles of filaments in the nucleus (247, 344), and breakup of the Golgi apparatus. The intermediate filament network tends to collect around the nucleus (341) as if it were providing it with a protective wrapping; however, HSPs tend to oppose this effect (343).

Functional changes during heat shock include a shift to anaerobic metabolism, with subtle changes in mitochondrial morphology. Also during the stress response, the cells abruptly stop growing (341), which fits with the survival plan: in an emergency, growth is a low priority.

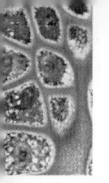

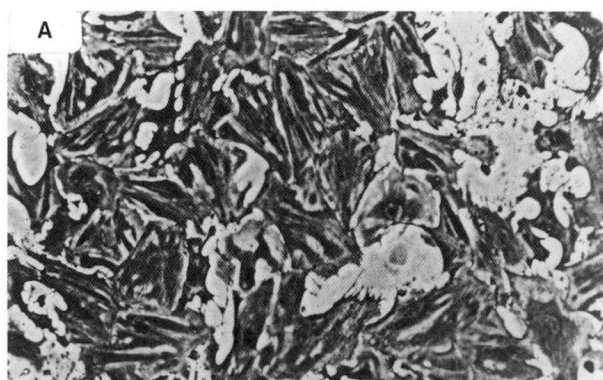

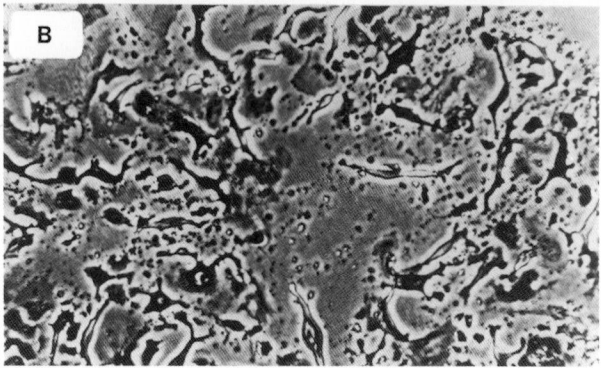

FIGURE 5.5   Cells individually microinjected with antibodies against heat-shock proteins are unable to survive a heat-shock challenge. The two panels show rat fibroblasts that have been submitted to heat shock at 43°C for 2 hours. *Top:* Cells microinjected with a "control" antibody have survived. *Bottom:* Cells microinjected with antibody against 72/73-kD stress proteins have not survived the heat shock. (Reprinted by permission from [264]. Copyright 1988 by the American Association for the Advancement for Science.)

How does the cell perceive the stress and transmit the information to the genes concerned? The task falls to a warning system that recalls the hypoxia-warning system (p. 699). The cytoplasm contains several heat-shock transcription factors (HTFs) which act on different cues; HSF-1, for example, is normally monomeric, but trimerizes under stress, shifts to the nucleus, and binds to the appropriate genes in seconds (72, 267). In mammalian cells the critical temperature for triggering the shock response is about 42°C; interestingly, the cells of the mouse testis—which are accustomed to live at 30°C—are triggered at 36–38°C (271).

By the way: **cold shock proteins** do exist in bacteria. They are different from HSPs; their tasks include freeze protection and mRNA chaperoning (351).

The heat shock proteins and disease. Important as it is in biology, the heat shock response is not (yet) a component of daily medical practice. The HSPs are largely intracellular, which means that they cannot be used as blood-borne markers of a given disease. However, a HSP has been found expressed on the surface of macrophages (336) and other cells (293). Also, when cells die, stress proteins can be released, and this may have important consequences that are just beginning to be appreciated: recent work shows that **stress proteins are powerful "adjuvants"** (5, 20, 236, 295, 296, 297). This means that they are able to increase the immune response to antigens: a polypeptide that is unable to induce an immune response by itself will become antigenic if attached to a HSP. Some HSPs have already been tested as components of anticancer vaccines, with encouraging results (5). We may expect significant developments in the near future in the field of immunology, regarding antitumor therapy and perhaps autoimmune disease. Other developments may occur regarding **infection.** Both the infectious agent and the host generate stress proteins; imagine the thermal shock it must be for a *Mycobacterium tuberculosis* to plunge from a wintery temperature into the 37°C oven of a human body. Since the stress proteins are highly conserved, they are necessarily similar in host and parasite; this means that the antibodies produced by the host against the bacterium may also behave—in part—as anti-host antibodies. So, which of the two will benefit most, host or parasite? There is no clear answer yet (152, 169, 173, 221, 303). Surprisingly, chlamydial and human HSP60 have been found *extracellularly* in human atherosclerosis, contributing to inflammation (161). Last but not least, HSPs, with their expertise in refolding the ill-folded, may help in the treatment of **conformational diseases.**

In closing, we should qualify our statement about the lack of "heat-shock therapy" in daily medical practice. The local application of heat is one of the most ancient forms of therapy; it is extensively discussed in the Hippocratic works as well as in the treatises of Ayurvedic medicine by Sushruta and Charaka (5, 192), and it probably helped, perhaps in part, by way of the heat-shock response. Nothing under the sun is entirely new.

An intriguing parallel: the liver has its own stress response. This discussion of the cellular stress response suggests another analogy between the cell—the elementary patient—and the body as a whole. *Severe, acute disease—such as trauma or infection—causes the liver to alter its pattern of protein synthesis,* a phenomenon known as the **acute phase response** (p. 504). It is not a heat-shock response: we are dealing with proteins that are secreted into the plasma rather than retained in the cell like HSPs; also, this reaction is slower and more prolonged than the heat-shock response. However, the purpose is the same: *survival of the cell* for the heat-shock proteins and *survival of the body* for the acute phase proteins.

Cell Wounds

Having examined the overall response of cells to stress, we will now see how they respond to the challenge of a wound.

Cells are sturdy; consider that we walk on them at every step. They can stand microsurgery with the laser, which can destroy minuscule targets such as one arm of a single chromosome (28). They have been seen to survive and even to divide (!) after surgical removal of the nucleus (182). Muscle fibers can be impaled many times with 0.5-μm microelectrodes and still maintain their resting potential (65), thus enabling electrophysiologists to make a living. And think of the enormous trauma endured by glial cells when they are isolated from a brain mash; yet they can be cultured (54).

Wounds in Individual Cells

Wounded cells can heal at an amazing speed; a few seconds for eggs of sea urchins. Happily so, because cell membranes are rather easily torn; even in the peaceful environment of cell culture, fibroblasts crawling around tend to tear their trailing edge (they heal in seconds [263]). *In vivo,* physical exercise can do some damage: in rats, after a night spent on spontaneous exercise in a rotating drum, the microscope will show that some fibers died by apoptosis (254), other fibers will have suffered surface tears, demonstrable by permeability markers (210).

In rats given a heart-stimulating drug for 1 hour, 60 percent of the myocardial cells will show surface "wounds"—but with no permanent damage (211).

Because the cell membrane consists mainly of lipids, it was thought at first that the mechanism of wound healing in cells could be studied on physical models, such as a lipid layer floating on water. Holes in such membranes do close (65, 238), but slowly, and the mechanism is very different from that seen in cells; for example, it is not calcium dependent, as it is in cells.

More suitable models are sea urchin or starfish eggs, which are huge by comparison with mammalian cells. In his pioneer experiments in the 1950s, the eminent physiologist L. V. Heilbrunn showed that starfish eggs punctured in sea water began to "bleed" cytoplasm, but the outflow stopped almost immediately as the cytoplasm appeared to clot. If calcium was removed from the sea water, the clotting did not occur, and the egg bled itself to death (Figure 5.6) (134). This suggested an analogy between starfish cytoplasm and mammalian blood: both are clotted by an excess of calcium. The facts were well

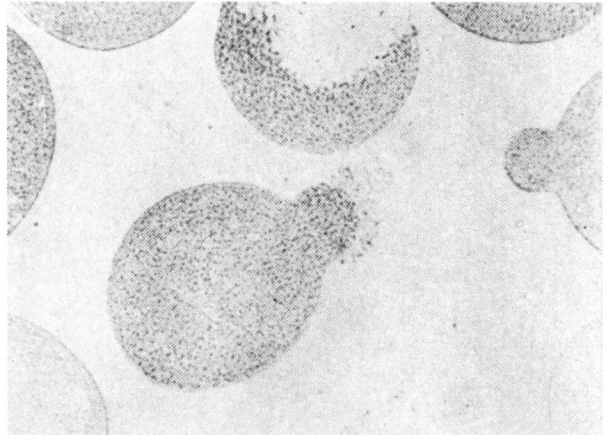
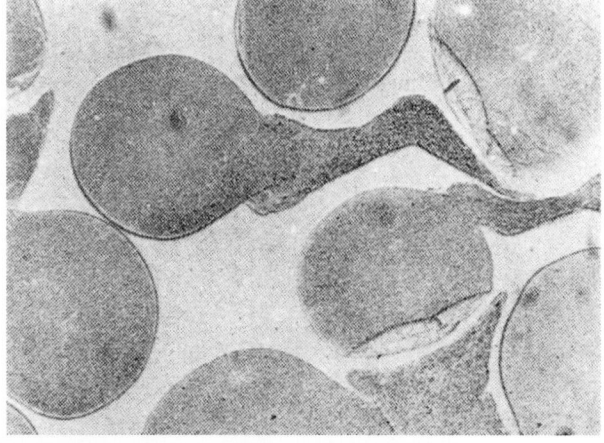

FIGURE 5.6   Effect of mechanical damage on starfish eggs. *Top:* Egg punctured in seawater. The small amount of escaping cytoplasm has seemingly "coagulated" and temporarily healed the injury. *Bottom:* In calcium-free seawater the cytoplasm fails to "coagulate" and bleeds out into the medium. (Reproduced with permission from [134].)

observed but the analogy proved wrong, as often occurs with reasoning by analogy.

Then came electron microscopy. Amoebae speared with the tip of a lady's eyelash appeared to heal, somehow, with new membrane (307, 308). But where did the membrane come from, and how could it heal so fast?

The data available at present indicate that *cell wounds heal by two mechanisms;* before reading further the reader might want to look at Figure 5.7 representing a wounded frog egg, in which the two mechanisms are shown or at least hinted.

First mechanism, best seen on frog or sea urchin eggs (25, 157): the wound quickly assumes a circular shape;

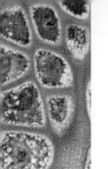

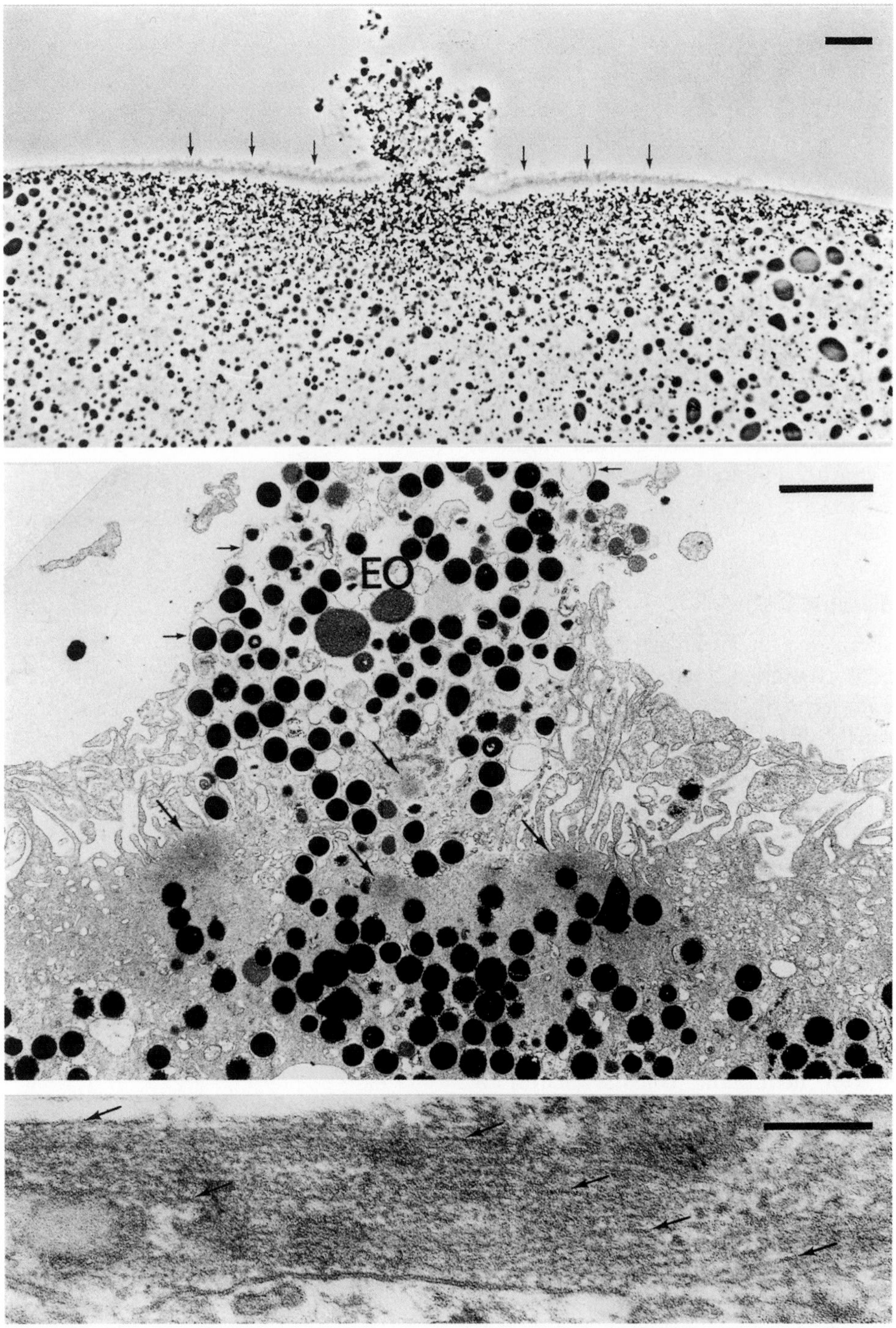

FIGURE 5.7　　*Top:* A punctured frog egg spills some of its yolk granules. **Bar** = 2 μm. *Center:* Detail of the punctured site. (**EO** = exovate.) **Bar** = 2 μm. *Bottom:* The puncture wound heals in purse-string fashion by the contraction of filaments (**arrows**) arranged in bundles. **Bar** = 0.2 μm. (Reproduced with permission from [34].)

then, within seconds, a ring of myosin and actin gathers around it, and contracts in purse-string fashion.

Second mechanism: this is not so intuitive; at first we were skeptical. What happens—with frog or sea urchin eggs—is that membrane-bound vesicles in the cytoplasm (mainly yolk granules) pile up at the level of the wound, fuse by a calcium-dependent mechanism (32), and create a sort of "instant dressing"

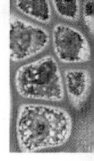

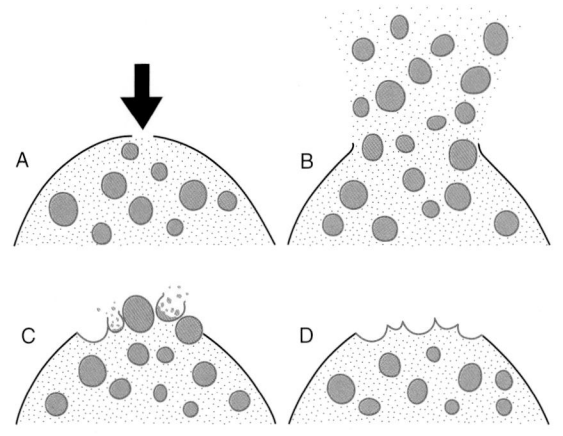

FIGURE 5.8 Wound healing in starfish oocytes (diameter, 180 μm) and sea urchin eggs (diameter, 100 μm): a new concept (314). Vesicular organelles, mainly yolk granules, pile up at the wound margin, fuse, and create a patch of new membrane. Time: A few seconds.

(Figure 5.8) (212, 263, 314). The investigators point out that this sequence could be interpreted as *endocytosis in reverse:* when a cell *takes in* a droplet of fluid, its surface loses the equivalent amount of plasma membrane; when it *expels* a droplet of fluid, a new patch of plasma membrane is added (212, 263). Similar findings were made with human fibroblasts, and here the vesicles were mainly lysosomes (263). An added bonus: as the lysosomes fuse with each other and with the cell membrane, they presumably secrete antibacterial agents into the surroundings.

Now we can understand why calcium is necessary for the instant healing of the cell's wound: the fusion of "vesicles" is calcium-dependent. Heilbrunn would have been pleased to learn it.

Wounds of Heart Cells: A Special Case

The heart is special for a number of reasons, but we might not have guessed that it is unique also regarding self-inflicted cellular wounds. In normal rats, *25 percent of the myocardial cells have surface injuries;* they can be recognized indirectly by injecting serum albumin intravenously: wherever the cell membrane is torn the albumin will seep into the cell (a variant of the dye exclusion test, p. 204) (51). The number of wounded cells increases if the heart is stimulated with isoproterenol; they *release acid and basic fibroblast growth factor,* perhaps helping recovery.

Joggers should know that their striated muscle are also subject to this kind of "work-related" injury. Strenuous exercise also increases HSP72 (86).

A special situation arises in the heart when a mass of cells is killed by sudden failure of blood flow (i.e., by infarction). When this happens, all around the infarct millions of dead cells are connected with surrounding live cells. This means that intracellular ions could leak out of the live, injured cells and initiate a lethal wave of depolarization. Fortunately, within 2–6 minutes a "healing-over" reaction occurs, indicating that a new ionic barrier is built up near the traumatized ends of the live cells and maintains the gradient of ionic concentration (63). Calcium is essential for this highly focal coagulation (66). Thanks to this ionic barrier a myocardial infarct can be sealed off and prevented from disrupting the function of the entire heart. The precise nature of the seal is not clear; it may be similar to the cytoplasmic coagulation discussed earlier.

Electrical effects of cell wounds are exploited in cardiology; recent myocardial infarcts, for example, affect the electrocardiogram because the live but injured part of the myocardium is negative with respect to the normal heart (126). Injury currents are mild and generally neglected in pathology; they were once thought to be involved in generating thrombi, but this was not confirmed. Biologists now believe that they can affect regeneration (p. 37) and be strong enough, in theory, to affect the orientation of surrounding cells (p. 370).

Cell Injury and Free Radical Pathology

The HSPs provided us with a sweeping generalization concerning the cellular *response* to injury; now we will examine another generalization concerning the *mechanisms* of cell injury: *many injurious agents, chemical, physical, and biological, cause damage by generating free radicals.* This is a relatively recent branch of chemistry: before the 1960s it would have been impossible to conceive that sunlight, many toxic agents, and reflow after ischemia cause damage by similar mechanisms, or that some liver poisons are innocuous molecules that the endoplasmic reticulum actively metabolizes into dangerous molecules. This discovery came in the 1960s

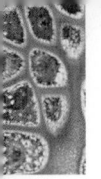

from the study of liver damage caused by carbon tetra-chloride, mentioned in Chapter 4 as causing cellular swelling and steatosis (pp. 142, 199). Later it turned out that *free radicals are involved in many pathologic and physiologic events,* far beyond the field of toxic agents; in fact they are turning up in all branches of pathology (12, 110, 128, 209, 311).

Free radicals had been waiting for a long time to be discovered (12, 128, 311). Two billion years ago, after the anaerobic blue-green algae had produced enough oxygen by photosynthesis, new types of cells evolved to exploit it for a life based on respiration. But these new cells were caught in a bind, as we are to this day: *oxygen is life-giving but toxic; no breathing animal can survive in pure oxygen.* Survival in our atmosphere is based on a precarious system of chemical mechanisms that mini-mize the production of oxygen-derived free radicals and inactivate (scavenge) those that are inevitable.

The reality of oxygen toxicity dawned on the med-ical profession quite late. Before 1967, when a critically ill patient was kept for many days on a respirator deliv-ering pure oxygen and then died of a peculiar lung disease, suspicions centered on a virus or on the ma-chine itself (227). Today, with the perfect clarity of hindsight (103), it is obvious that the toxicity of oxygen should have been predicted from its electronic struc-ture, because its reduction to water can proceed through a series of steps that generates highly reactive free radicals (96, 102). This is why this field is so closely linked with the metabolism of oxygen. However, let it be clear that *many free radicals have nothing to do with oxygen,* at least initially.

The existence of free radicals in the world of chem-istry was established by the turn of the century but remained shrouded in controversy, not all of which has disappeared. The food industry was the first to realize the importance of free-radical chemistry: by the 1940s it was clear that free radicals could explain the rancid-ity of foods. The great leap from cans of rancid peanuts to live people came about twenty years later, when it was realized that free radicals play a role in normal physiology, in disease, and even in aging (59) (are we slowly turning rancid?). The discovery, as mentioned earlier, was made not directly through the toxicity of oxygen but through studies of carbon tetrachloride poisoning (pp. 142, 199).

How Do Free Radicals Relate to Disease?

Let it be clear that we could not live without free radi-cals; however, they often cause damage. It should be helpful to begin with a bird's-eye view of the situations in which free-radical reactions are relevant to pathology. Here are a few.

- *Leukocytes use oxygen-derived free radicals for killing bacteria.* The price paid for this marvelous adaptation is that the same free radicals can turn against the leukocytes themselves or against any nearby tissue.
- *Because leukocytes produce free radicals also in the absence of bacterial stimulation,* many inflammatory diseases involve free-radical-induced damage, especially in the joints and lungs.
- *Injury spills blood, which releases iron;* iron catalyzes free-radical reactions that increase the damage, especially in the central nervous system.
- *Injury releases arachidonic acid from cell membranes;* the subsequent metabolism of arachidonic acid involves lipid peroxidation with release of free radicals (48).
- *Ischemia,* in theory, should be relieved by reperfu-sion; but when oxygen-rich blood is returned to the ischemic tissue, it raises havoc by a mechanism based in part on oxygen-derived free radicals (p. 714).
- *Organ preservation for transplants* is jeopardized by similar reperfusion problems.
- *Sunlight* damages the skin by singlet oxygen and free-radical mechanisms.
- *X-rays* kill tumors and cause tissue damage, in part by producing free radicals.
- *Tumors* are caused by many mechanisms; one is thought to be DNA damage by free radicals.
- *Many drugs, toxic agents, and pollutants* cause damage because they are metabolized in such a way as to produce injurious free radicals; the long list includes cigarette smoke, antibiotics, anticancer agents, and the ill-famed paraquat (315).
- *Atherosclerosis,* the great killer in Western cultures, involves the peroxidation of low-density lipoprotein (LDL), so much so that an antioxidant therapy was attempted.
- *Aging;* yes, there is also a free-radical theory of aging (59, 258).

We will spare you allergy, frostbite, and much more. This partial list should suffice to prove that the next 7 pages—perhaps rather dry for some tastes—is justified.

What Are Free Radicals?

Free radicals are atoms or molecules with an unpaired electron in the outermost orbital. As such they are un-stable and therefore highly reactive. Some last just milliseconds, and their existence can be established only indirectly: much of the controversy that still surrounds free radicals stems from this fact. They also tend to form chain reactions, which could be very destructive if the cells were not prepared to stop them by a number of defensive mechanisms. The brief existence of free radicals, reminiscent of a flare, has three phases: *initiation, propagation,* and *termination.* Because they are so reactive and easily trapped, free radicals can travel only very short distances within a cell, probably fractions of a micron. If this were not so, the DNA in the nucleus would be at the constant mercy of metabolic events in the endoplasmic reticulum and the mitochondria.

How, in a living tissue, can any atom or molecule find itself limited to a single electron in an outer orbit? This accident can occur in several ways.

- *Energy supplied by the environment can split the covalent bond between two atoms* in such a way that one electron remains attached to either side (homolytic fission). This is what happens when tissues are irradiated: water molecules are split into free radicals (**radiolysis**) which account for much of the tissue damage. The energy of sunlight does something similar to the skin (**photolysis**).
- Even without the application of external energy, *susceptible atoms can capture an electron;* for instance, an electron that strays off the electron transport chain in a mitochondrion. Normally, the electron-transfer reactions are carried out by enzymes that are firmly embedded and properly ordered in lipid membranes, so that the production of free radicals is minimized; but this order can be broken. Under normal conditions, about 1 percent of the electrons that pass along the transport chain stray away and react with molecular oxygen; fortunately, the resulting free radical is captured by defensive free-radical scavengers (to be discussed shortly) and damage is avoided (123). The rate of this electron escape is directly proportional to the partial pressure of oxygen. In a person breathing 100 percent O_2 the mitochondria of the pulmonary alveolar cells may produce five times the usual amount of free radicals, too much for the scavenger mechanisms to absorb.
- *Several oxidative enzymes can produce free radicals* (Figure 5.9) (102), in some cases because the substrate diffuses away from the enzyme surface before it is wholly oxidized or reduced to an even electron number (257).

The enzymes involved in redox reactions contain heavy metals such as Fe, Cu, and Zn (hence their color and their name: cytochromes). This is a key point: the so-called transitional metals, which can change valence, take part in electron transfers as acceptors or donors; when they are loose in the tissues they continue in these roles and generate free radicals in an uncontrolled fashion. Iron is the chief offender (11, 129, 218, 316).

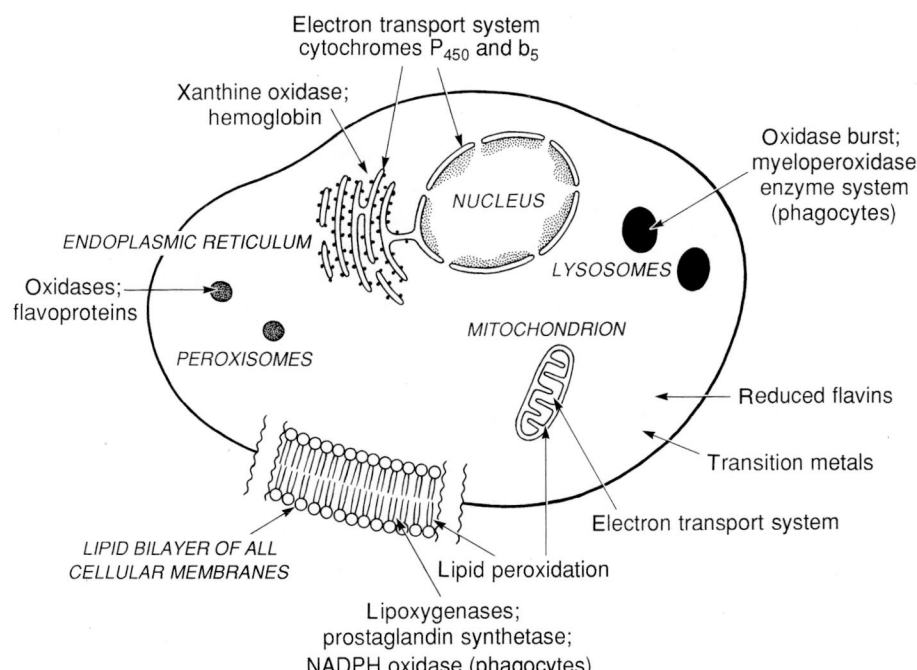

Electron transport system
cytochromes P_{450} and b_5

Xanthine oxidase;
hemoglobin

NUCLEUS

ENDOPLASMIC RETICULUM

Oxidases;
flavoproteins

PEROXISOMES

LYSOSOMES

MITOCHONDRION

Oxidase burst;
myeloperoxidase
enzyme system
(phagocytes)

Reduced flavins

Transition metals

Electron transport system

LIPID BILAYER OF ALL
CELLULAR MEMBRANES

Lipid peroxidation

Lipoxygenases;
prostaglandin synthetase;
NADPH oxidase (phagocytes)

FIGURE 5.9   Cellular sources of free radicals. (Adapted from [187].)

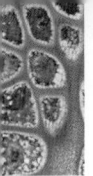

The ABCs of Free-Radical Reactions in Biological Systems

Let us begin by explaining the chain of events leading to the destruction of alveolar cells in the lungs of an animal exposed to 100 percent oxygen (pp. 194, 199). We know that cells derive most of their ATP from the stepwise reduction of oxygen to water by the mitochondrial transport system; each electron is conveyed along an orderly chain of enzyme molecules woven into the mitochondrial membrane. Although four electrons are needed for reducing each atom of oxygen, an oxygen atom can accept fewer than four; and in so doing it turns into one of several toxic free radicals, as summarized in Figure 5.10.

If oxygen accepts *one* electron, it becomes **superoxide anion radical:**

$$O_2 + 2e^- \rightarrow O_2^- \text{ (superoxide anion radical)}$$

Superoxide itself is not a very powerful oxidant; however, it can easily donate its electron to any nearby atom of Fe^{3+}, thereby reducing it to **divalent Fe:**

$$O_2^- + Fe^{3+} \rightarrow O_2 + Fe^{++}$$

If O_2 accepts *two* electrons, it produces the old-time antiseptic, **hydrogen peroxide:**

$$O_2 + 2e^- + 2H^+ \rightarrow H_2O_2 \text{ (hydrogen peroxide)}$$

Now, in the presence of divalent Fe, hydrogen peroxide produces OH·, the **hydroxyl radical,** which is the most reactive of all biological free radicals and the most potent biological oxidizing agent known:

$$H_2O_2 + Fe^{++} \rightarrow HO\cdot + OH^- + Fe^{3+}$$

Hydroxyl radical, HO· (also written OH·), is the real villain of most free-radical reactions in biology; it can react with almost any organic molecule. In fact, a classic method for hydroxylating organic molecules in Fenton's

reagent, a mixture of H_2O_2 and iron salts, which produces the reaction we have just outlined (123).

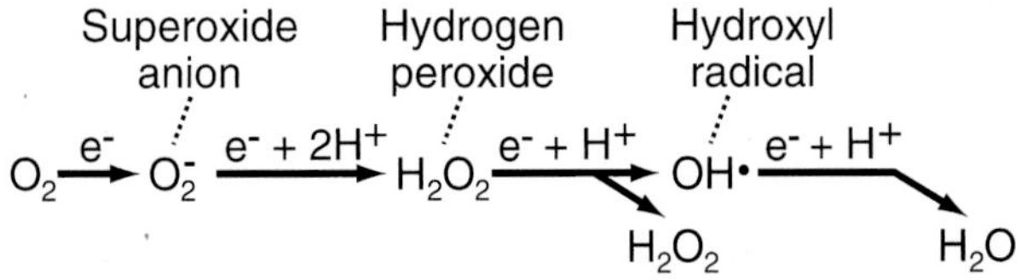

The last two reactions occur in the presence of iron, which acts as a catalyst; they can be summed up as follows, leaving out the Fe:

$$O_2^- + H_2O_2 \xrightarrow{\text{Fe}} OH\cdot + OH^- + O_2$$

This fundamental reaction has been called the iron-catalyzed Haber–Weiss reaction or the superoxide-driven Fenton reaction. Iron atoms for these reactions, inside and outside the cell, can be supplied by ferritin, transferrin, hemoglobin, and other heme-containing molecules. Here is an example: in blunt injuries to the central nervous system, blood escapes into the white or grey matter; part of the ensuing cellular damage is attributed not to trauma *per se* but to free radicals generated by the hemoglobin of spilled red blood cells (68) and by the iron transported by the plasma (p. 229) (346). We chose the central nervous system as an example, because this tissue is especially sensitive to free-radical damage on account of its high phospholipid content.

How Free Radicals Cause Damage

When a potent oxidizer such as OH· is set loose inside or near a cell, it can initiate a series of reactions that have irreparable effects on macromolecules. *Lipid, protein, carbohydrate, and even DNA molecules can be bent out of shape, broken, or cross-linked* (Figure 5.11). It is worth noting that commercial polymers such as Teflon, vinyl plastics, and even rubber are solidified (i.e., cross-linked) with the help of free radicals. Something similar happens normally *in vivo*: age pigment, lipofuscin, is made of cross-linked lipid (p. 102). On the other hand, in arthritis, the breakdown of hyaluronic acid, the essential macromolecular lubricant of all joints, is also attributed to free radicals.

Lipids are prime molecular targets for free radicals, which means that cell membranes are especially at risk. We will use them to illustrate the basic reactions.

Initiation. Consider the basic structure of the bimolecular leaflets, with the water-soluble, polar ends of the phospholipid molecules on the outer surfaces and the nonpolar ends pointing inward. Oxygen is 7 or 8 times more soluble in nonpolar solvents than in water, which means that it is more available in this midzone of the cell membrane. Here lie precisely those parts of the

$$O_2 \xrightarrow{e^-} O_2^- \xrightarrow{e^- + 2H^+} H_2O_2 \xrightarrow{e^- + H^+} OH\cdot \xrightarrow{e^- + H^+} H_2O$$

Superoxide anion   Hydrogen peroxide   Hydroxyl radical

FIGURE 5.10 The univalent pathway for the reduction of molecular oxygen to water. During this stepwise addition of electrons, toxic free-radical byproducts appear. This does not occur when oxygen is reduced quadrivalently by the mitochondrial cytochrome oxidase system. (Reproduced with permission from [64].)

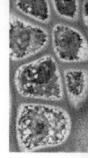

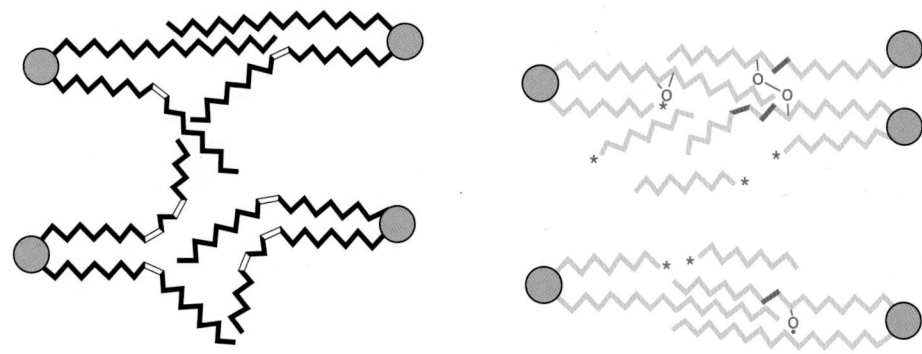

FIGURE 5.11 Types of damage that free radicals can produce in phospholipid molecules. *Left:* Four normal phospholipid molecules forming the skeleton of the plasma membrane. The circles are glycerophosphate head groups. In the fatty acid tails, unsaturated bonds create a bend with an angle of 123°. *Right:* As a result of free-radical attack, the fatty acid chains can be bent out of shape, broken, or cross-linked. ∗: Negative charge of carboxylic groups. —O—: Oxygen atoms. (Adapted from [67].)

phospholipid molecules—the polyunsaturated fatty acids—that are most susceptible to free-radical damage. Polyunsaturated fatty acids (PUFA) have an Achilles heal: the hydrogens on carbons between two double bonds are easily abstracted. A free radical comes along and abstracts the hydrogen, whereupon the double bonds rearrange themselves. This rearrangement causes the molecule to change shape because the normal *cis* form bends the chain to 123 degrees, whereas the *trans* form is straight (Figure 5.11).

Propagation. Now comes the phase of propagation. For instance,

$$PUFA\cdot + O_2 \rightarrow PUFA\text{--}OO\cdot$$
$$PUFA\text{--}OO\cdot + PUFA \rightarrow PUFA\text{--}OOH + PUFA\cdot$$

Another set of reactions causes the fatty-acid chains to break up and yield **malonaldehyde** (73). The smell of rancid foods is due to such aldehydes and to other lipid oxidation products (58, 97), but it has a useful counterpart: malonaldehyde can be used for quantitating free-radical reactions.

Termination. Eventually, before the whole cell and its neighbors are involved, *terminating reactions* set in. Note that in all the following examples, *the final result is that the fatty acids have been polymerized;* in other words, the net effect of the free-radical assault is a molecular lesion:

$$PUFA\cdot + PUFA\cdot \rightarrow PUFA\text{--}PUFA$$
$$PUFA\text{--}OO\cdot + PUFA\text{--}OO\cdot \rightarrow$$
$$O_2 + PUFA\text{--}OO\text{--}PUFA$$
$$PUFA\text{--}OO\cdot + PUFA \rightarrow PUFA\text{--}OO\text{--}PUFA$$

Other and more favorable terminating options occur when the roving free radical bumps into a scavenger

enzyme, or a scavenger phenolic compound such as vitamin E, embedded in the cell membrane. Such large molecules take part in free-radical reactions without propagating them: even though they acquire the change of a free radical, they can be considered "frozen," immobilized free radicals (95):

$$PUFA\cdot + (\text{vit. E})OH \rightarrow PUFA\text{--}H + (\text{vit. E})\cdot$$

The (vit. E)OH can then be regenerated by reacting with reduced glutathione (GSH) to yield GSSG, which in turn is reduced by glutathione reductase:

$$(\text{vit. E})O\cdot + GSH \rightarrow (\text{vit. E})OH + GS\cdot$$
$$GS\cdot + GS\cdot \rightarrow GSSG$$
$$GSSG + NADPH + H^+ \rightarrow 2GSH + NADP^+$$

Defenses against Free Radicals

Again, we must emphasize that free radicals are not to be thought of simply as enemies: we could not live, for example, without superoxide radical, our major ally as a bacterial killer (209). With this in mind, we can say that cells appear to have at least two neatly coordinated lines of defense: scavenger enzymes and antioxidants (Figure 5.12).

The first line of defense is a twin set of enzymes that eliminates the two principal reactants, superoxide radical (O_2^-) and hydrogen peroxide (H_2O_2), so that they cannot interact by the Haber–Weiss reaction and produce the dangerous hydroxyl radical OH·. Each of the two free radicals is counteracted by a specific type of enzyme:

Superoxide dismutase. This enzyme (called SOD) eliminates O_2^-:

$$O_2^- + O_2 + 2H \xrightarrow{\text{SOD}} H_2O_2 + O_2$$

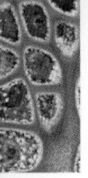

FIGURE 5.12 Cellular scavengers of free radicals. (Adapted
from [187].)

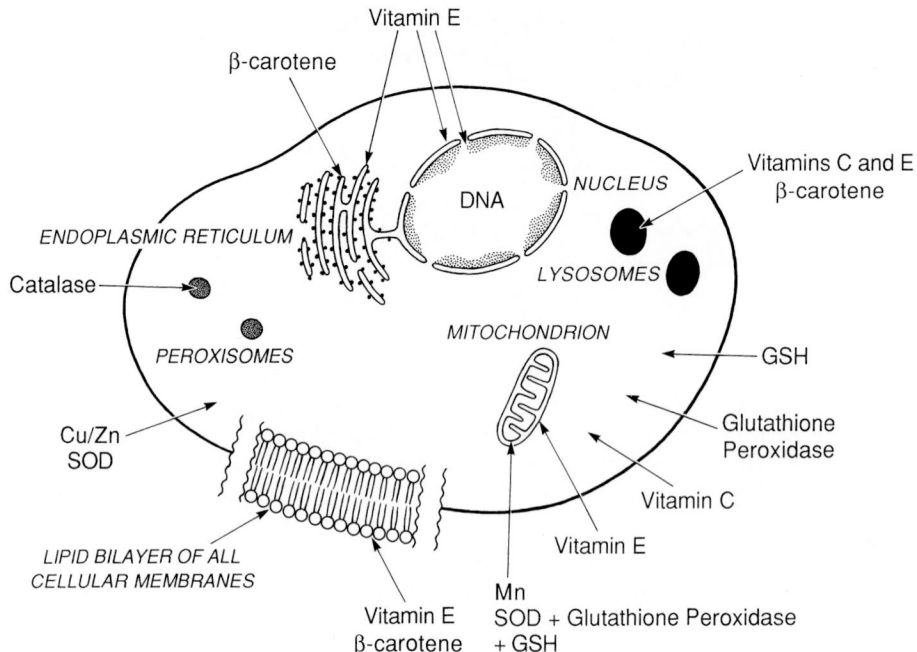

SOD, an inducible enzyme, is present in several isoen-
zyme forms: some are free in the cytosol, poised to
catch superoxide radicals wherever they may appear,
and some are in the mitochondria, where most of the
oxidative metabolism occurs. On the other hand, SOD
is present only in trace amounts in plasma and extracellular fluids, which means that free-radical reactions outside cells are not readily held in check (103). True to its
important function, SOD is very stable and one of the
most active enzymes known.

> SOD was discovered in 1938 in ox blood as a blue-green,
> copper-containing protein of unknown function and was
> called hemocuprein. Then cupreins were found in several
> tissues. In 1969 it was shown that they all represented
> SOD and contained zinc as well as copper (102). The
> metal atoms act as electron exchangers.
>
> An intellectually satisfying detail: aerobic bacteria also
> contain SOD, in which the copper is replaced by iron or
> manganese. Bacterial SOD belongs to a totally different
> evolutionary development, as shown by its amino acid se-
> quence. Guess which SOD is present in mitochondria?
> The bacterial type—one more bit of evidence that bacte-
> ria and mitochondria are close relatives (102).

Catalases and peroxidases. These enzymes eliminate
H_2O_2, the other potentially dangerous substrate; both
have hematin as a prosthetic group. Catalases act directly
on H_2O_2, whereas peroxidases require a cosubstrate
(reductant) other than H_2O_2 as electron donors (102).

$$H_2O_2 + H_2O_2 \rightarrow 2H_2O + O_2 \quad \text{(catalases)}$$
$$H_2O_2 + RH_2 \rightarrow 2H_2O + R \quad \text{(peroxidases)}$$

Antioxidants. The second line of defense is a group of
water- and lipid-soluble antioxidants. While SODs and
catalases/peroxidases hold to a minimum the two precursors of OH·, the small amount of OH· and other
radicals that may yet form are being neutralized by antioxidants strategically distributed in the membranes
and the cytosol:

Vitamin E
   (alpha-tocopherol)   ⎤
Beta-carotene   ⎥   *in the lipid phase*
   (precursor of
   vitamin A)   ⎦
Ascorbic acid   ⎤   *in the watery phase*
Glutathione   ⎦

In the extracellular spaces there is little or no superoxide dismutase; however, the plasma contains powerful scavengers, notably **ceruloplasmin.**

Enter Nitric Oxide

Nitric oxide, the "Molecule of the Year" for 1992 (348),
will be listed among the mediators of inflammation in
Chapter 9. However, its activities—both useful and
damaging—cover a wider range, including neurotrans-
mission, vasomotor tone, and modulation of immune
responses. Although nitric oxide is currently written as
NO, it is a free radical and should be written as NO·.
Alone it is relatively weak, but it can react with superoxide and generate the powerful oxidant peroxynitrite:

$$NO· + O_2^- \rightarrow ONOO^-$$

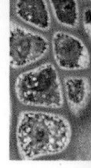

The chemical biology of NO is highly complex (13, 35, 92, 209, 347). In a nutshell, as a cell would see it, its reactions add **nitrosative stress** to **oxidative stress,** and the outcome may be good or bad depending on concentrations and circumstances (p. 369).

The **therapy** of diseases related to free radicals is not a topic for this book, but we should point out a key issue: *free radicals are produced mainly by inflammatory cells.* When the inflammation is due to infection, trying to stamp out the free radicals makes little sense, because they are the principal weapon of the leukocytes, our allies. When the inflammation is aseptic and unwanted, as in autoimmune diseases (such as rheumatoid arthritis), fighting inflammation in all its aspects becomes a top priority.

Examples of Free-Radical Disease

As we mentioned earlier, the trailblazer of this research was carbon tetrachloride poisoning—or rather Dr. R. O. Recknagel (p. 142). Only 2 hours after administration of the poison, electron microscopy of the liver already shows quite clearly that something is happening to the endoplasmic reticulum; the cisternae seen in profile become very thin and collapsed, as if they had lost their content (Figure 5.13) (82). Today

the molecular events are largely understood. The P-450 enzyme system, embedded in the membrane of the endoplasmic reticulum, adds an electron to the CCl_4 and splits it into a Cl^- ion and the highly reactive free radical $CCl_3^\cdot$, which attacks the membranes of the ER (Figure 5.14). This mechanism explains the toxic effects on the liver of many drugs (226), of environmental agents, and even of carcinogens (327).

Another classic example of free-radical injury (100, 199) is lung damage from exposure to pure oxygen. Adult rats breathing O_2 at one atmosphere die of pulmonary edema in less than 60 hours (96); histology shows destruction of the alveolar epithelium and of the underlying capillary endothelium (200). Chronic lung damage is caused by environmental pollutants, including ozone, NO, NO_2, and cigarette smoke, which initiate free-radical reactions.

Besides X-ray radiation, sunlight can be toxic (79, 93). Sunbathers protect themselves with sunscreen creams, and some aerobic bacteria protect themselves with SOD, but to strict anaerobes sunlight is lethal. The aerobe *Sarcina lutea* is yellow (lutea) because it contains the orange-yellow antioxidant beta-carotene in its membrane; the coating works like a suntan and makes the bacterium photoresistant. Indeed, the

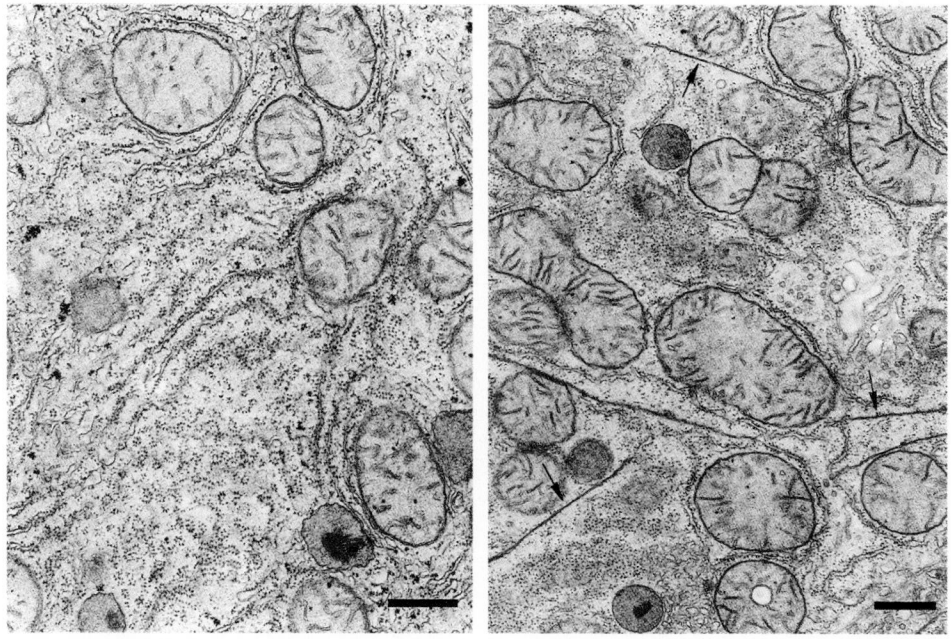

FIGURE 5.13   Effect of CCl_4 on rat liver. *Left:* Control (part of a liver cell). Note abundant endoplasmic reticulum and polyribosomes. *Right:* Two hours after intragastric administration of CCl_4. The rough ER cisternae have collapsed into thin, rigid plates; ribosomes have become detached; polyribosomes have broken up. **Bars** = 0.5 μm. (Reproduced with permission from [82], © American Society for Investigative Pathology.)

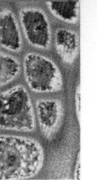

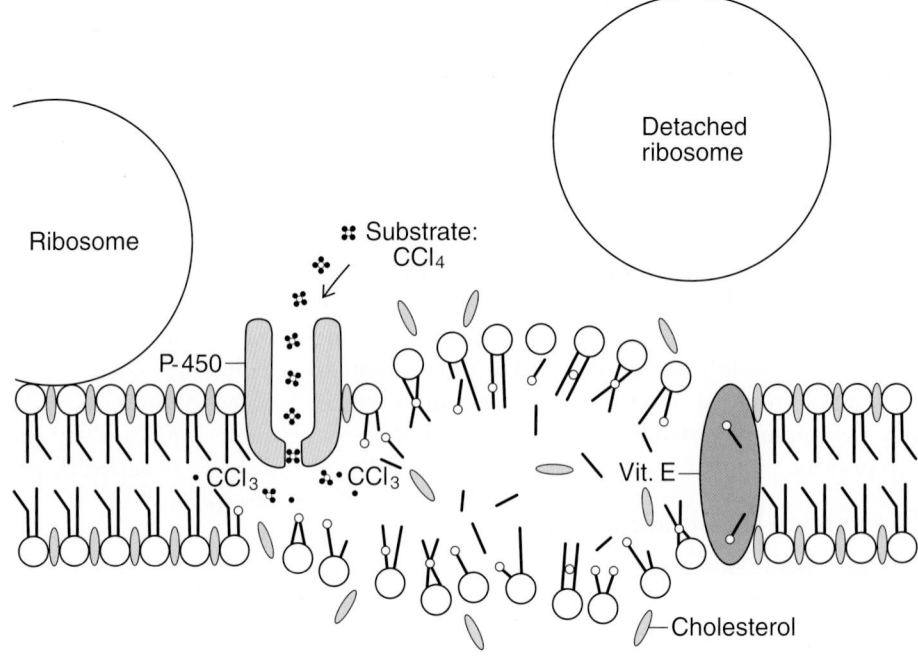

FIGURE 5.14 Artist's view of the catastrophic events in the membrane of the endoplasmic reticulum when the P-450 enzyme system metabolizes CCl_4. The CCl_4 breaks down into free radicals, which attack the surrounding phospholipid molecules (particularly their fatty acid tails), causing them to be deformed, cross-linked, or split; the chain reaction is then stopped by a molecule of vitamin E, which scavenges lipid peroxyl radicals. As a result of the membrane damage, the ribosomes become detached.

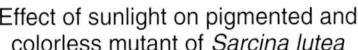

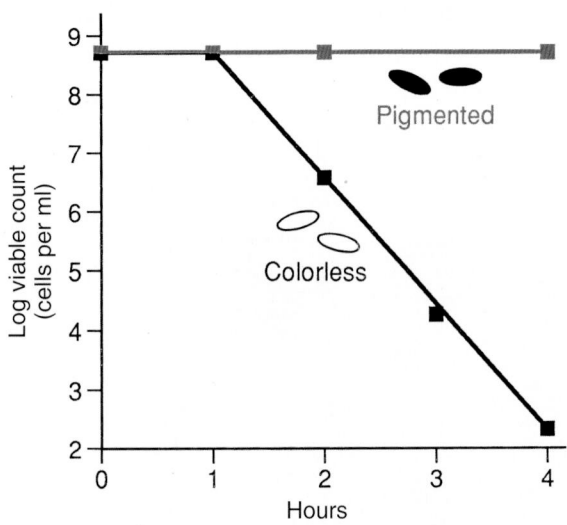

FIGURE 5.15 The bacterium *Sarcina lutea* is protected from the lethal effect of sunlight by its natural carotenoid pigment. (Adapted from [203].)

carotene-free mutant dies when exposed to light, becoming the victim of light-generated singlet oxygen and free radicals (Figure 5.15). This may sound like trivial information, but in 1970 it led Micheline Mathews-Roth and her collaborators to discover that previously incurable photosensitive patients could be treated with an antioxidant, β-carotene, a precursor of vitamin A. The inspiring thought: what is good for bacteria might also be good for people (202).

These photosensitive patients suffered from erythropoietic protoporphyria, a congenital anomaly in the metabolism of blood porphyrins (the ring-shaped, tetrapyrrolic, iron-free precursors of the heme in hemoglobin). Porphyrins have long been known as photosensitizers. Due to the lack of an enzyme, an excess of protoporphyrin accumulates in the blood and tissues. The precise chain of events is not clear, but it is believed that when protoporphyrin is struck by light, it generates free-radical reactions and singlet oxygen; therefore, exposing the skin to sunlight causes itching, burning, blisters, and even ulcerations and scarring. For some of these patients, condemned to lead a nocturnal life, treatment with beta-carotene makes it possible to reappear and work in broad daylight (Figure 5.16) (202).

How does one know that a disease is caused by free radicals? Ultimate proof is perhaps impossible. Many biochemical and biophysical methods are available for detecting and measuring free radicals (312). There are also some revealing experiments of nature: patients who lack glutathione peroxidase in their red blood cells suffer from hemolytic anemia because the red cell membranes are open to attack by H_2O_2. A similar defect is known for platelets in Glanzmann's thrombocytopenia (102). However, *the most compelling proof that a disease is caused by free radicals is the effect of prevention or*

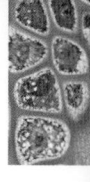

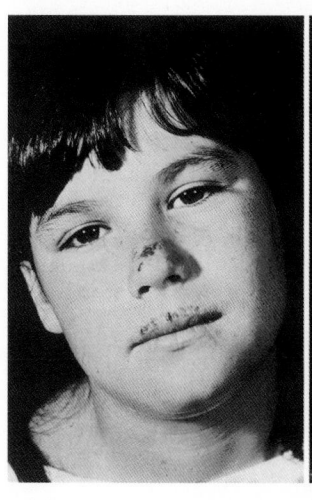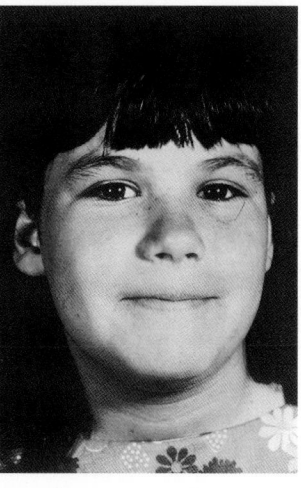

FIGURE 5.16 *Left:* Child with skin lesions typical of protoporphyria, an oversensitivity to light. *Right:* Same child after treatment with β-carotene, a precursor of vitamin A. (Courtesy of Dr. M. Mathews-Roth, Channing Laboratory, Harvard University, Boston, MA.)

treatment with antioxidants and/or with free-radical scavengers.

Experimentally, many reports indicate that treatment with superoxide dismutase (SOD), for instance, reduces X-ray damage or prolongs the life of rats exposed to pure oxygen (12, 311, 329). Cloned human SOD is now available and its clinical uses are being explored (12, 42); however, any therapy aimed at suppressing free radicals will not be without hazard because, after all, leukocytes need to retain their oxygen-radical generating mechanisms if they are to protect us from bacteria (22).

There are other problems. SOD injected intravenously is removed so fast by the littoral phagocytes (p. 316) that its half-life is of the order of minutes. The same is true for catalase. Furthermore, these enzymes are needed also, and perhaps, especially inside the cells where many free-radical reactions are initiated. Yet only a tiny fraction of the circulating enzyme is picked up by the endothelium, and even less is transcytosed into the tissues. Several tricks have been devised to evade the littoral phagocytes, with some success: packing the enzymes in liposomes (p. 225), in the hope that these will fuse with the endothelium of various organs and not just with phagocytes; and linking the enzyme with polyethylene glycol, which facilitates nonspecific cellular uptake and also makes the enzyme nonimmunogenic (22).

TO SUM UP: The study of free radicals has opened a window on some new mechanisms of disease, and therapeutic developments are bound to follow. A hot area of research is free-radical injury to the central nervous system. Myelin is made of cell membranes, which makes it a preferential target for free radicals; and injury spills red blood cells, which supply iron, a catalyst of free-radical reactions. Other major areas involve inflammation (free radicals are also among the chemical mediators of inflammation) and ischemia, a topic closely related to oxygen supply (p. 714). Free-radical research has come a long way since the cans of rancid peanuts.

Cell Death: Oncosis and Apoptosis

Cell death, once considered among the dullest topics in pathology, has moved to the cutting edge of biology research. This is due, in part, to the general trend of medical science, which is focussing more and more on the individual cell as the "elementary patient"; another factor has been the discovery of a fascinating modality of cell death, apoptosis, a topic that has permeated the entire field of biology. Whole books on cell death are now commonplace (40, 50, 62, 131, 149, 179, 214, 256, 306, 319, 320).

Cells can die in different ways; consider, for example, cell death by freezing, whereby ice crystals poke holes in the cell membrane; by toxic agents, which can target individual cell organelles; by fixatives, which are supposed to leave the cell structures intact; by acute ischemia, which makes the cells swell and burst; or by planned obsolescence, which usually involves apoptosis. In practice, however, we know a lot about only two forms of cell death: *cell death with shrinkage* (*apoptosis*), a physiologic event that balances mitosis in virtually all tissues, and *cell death with swelling,* a pathologic event typical of infarcts, which we restored to the old name of *oncosis.* Both forms of cell death are followed by secondary changes known as *necrosis* (Figure 5.17). Let us pause to clear up the wording.

The names of cell death. Before apoptosis appeared on the scene in the 1970s, as a single-cell, "physiologic"

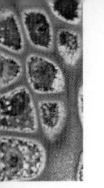

FIGURE 5.17   The two most common modes of cell death. *Top:* Normal cell. *Left:* **Death by oncosis.** Note: Swelling, blebbing, increased permeability (*double arrows*), incipient coagulation. During the stage of necrosis: coagulation, karyolysis, acute inflammation. *Right:* **Death by apoptosis.** Note: Shrinkage, increased density, pyknosis. During the stage of necrosis: budding, phagocytosis of apoptotic bodies. (Details in text.)

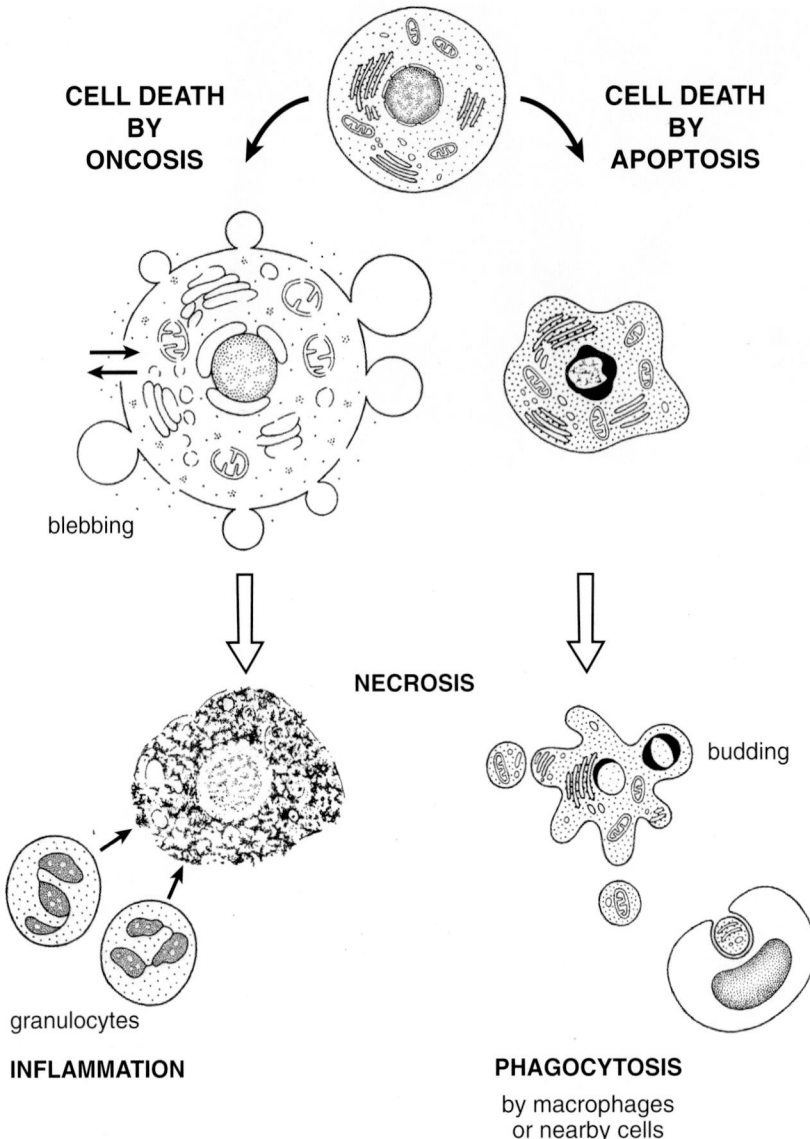

event, only one kind of cell death was recognized: namely the massive cellular breakdown as seen in infarcts. It had no particular name, except *cell death;* the term *necrosis* was applied to the secondary changes that appeared *after* cell death (193, 194). When apoptosis was so named in 1972 (156) it became necessary to find a name for "the other" form of cell death; the creators of the beautiful term apoptosis chose "necrosis." Not a fortunate choice in our view, because the term *necrosis* is long established in the nomenclature of pathology for any change that appears *after* cell death. In the sixth edition of the Robbins Pathology textbook (1999), we read that "*Necrosis refers to a spectrum of morphologic changes that **follow** cell death.* . . [emphasis ours]."

To solve this problem we proposed in 1995 to use **oncosis** for the massive "nonapoptotic" cell death (193). The choice is based on a neat symmetry between the two main forms of cell death: one is characterized by shrinking (it was called *shrinkage necrosis* at first [154]), the other by swelling (*ónkos* = Greek for "swelling"). The term *oncosis* was created in 1910 by a pupil of Virchow, F. von Recklinghausen, precisely to mean death with swelling (as he saw it in bone and cartilage). This terminology (329a) was recommended in 1999 by a committee of pathologists (171, 172). In the current literature, apoptosis has only one name, but the reader should be prepared to recognize half a dozen different terms for oncosis and postoncotic necrosis: **necrosis** (confusing, as explained above), **massive cell death** (acceptable), **accidental cell death, ischemic cell death** (partially correct, but accidental and ischemic injury can also cause apoptosis); and **nonapoptotic cell death** (acceptable, but there is more than one kind of nonapoptotic cell death).

The newcomer will probably be shocked to find that the nomenclature in this basic field is still so chaotic. This is what happens when a biological concept evolves over 2500 years; the career of "necrosis" is a perfect example. Furthermore, the field of cell death is complex and technically challenging. But there is hope, over time clarity tends to prevail.

Cell Death with Swelling: Oncosis

Oncosis is a form of cell death accompanied by acute cellular swelling. It is due mainly to deprivation of ATP and consequent failure of the Na/K ionic pumps.

This definition implies that experimental models of oncosis could be based on respiratory poisons (322, 324) or infarction (i.e., sudden deprivation of blood supply). To work out the basic steps of oncosis, we can use a simple experimental model that produces what we may call a "pseudoinfarct." All we need to do is to prepare (aseptically) cubes of fresh rat liver 1 cm on edge, weigh them, and introduce them into the peritoneal cavity of other rats (191, 194). Under these circumstances the liver cells will be dying as in an infarct; *immunologic phenomena are not involved,* at least up to 24 hours (but see p. 446). We will retrieve the implants at selected times, weigh them, and study them both microscopically and chemically. Figure 5.18 shows what the specimens look like to the naked eye, up to 9 days.

The basic changes are summarized in Figure 5.19.

- *Immediately the implants begin to swell,* as shown by an increase in weight
- Their internal pH drops precipitously
- The amount of extractable protein and of protein breakdown products rises, then falls
- In the meantime the implants become paler and paler to the naked eye

Translating these changes into cellular terms, we have:

- *The swelling (weight gain) of an implant means that the liver cells are starved of oxygen;* thus, the membrane ion pumps run down, and the cells swell as fluid is absorbed (in this setting) from the peritoneal cavity.

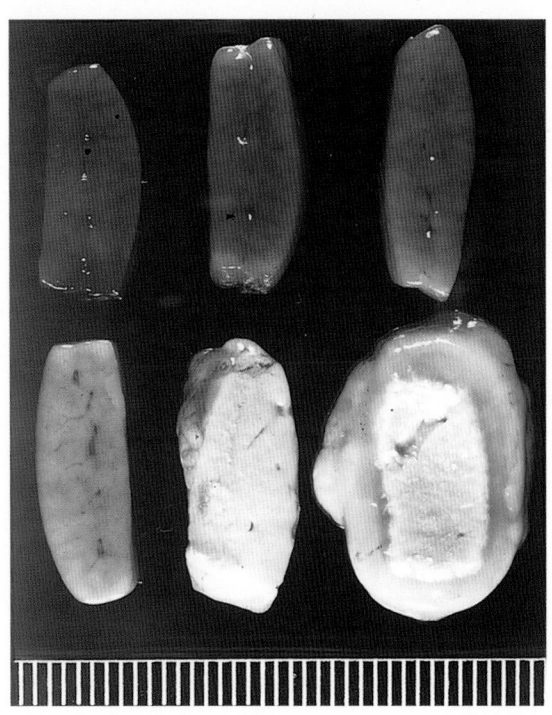

FIGURE 5.18   Gross aspect of rat liver, normal (*top left*) and after it was implanted in the peritoneal cavity for 2, 4, 12, and 24 hours, and for 9 days. Increasing whiteness is due to protein denaturation. After 9 days, the implant is wrapped in omentum. **Scale** in millimeters. (Reproduced with permission from [194].)

- *The drop in pH occurs because the cells must turn to their glycogen supplies* and limp along for some time by glycolysis, producing lactic acid, which cannot be removed because the dead or dying tissue has no circulation. In the meantime, some enzymes leak out of the lysosomes, and finding themselves in an acid pH (optimal for lysosomal hydrolases), they attack the cytoplasmic components. Eventually the pH returns to normal because the cell membranes are broken down, enabling the acids to diffuse away and be removed by the blood stream of the surrounding live tissues.

NOTE: *The drop in pH is actually protective, as can be shown in models of* **reversible ischemia.** *This is known as the "pH paradox." We shall return to this topic in relation to the pathophysiology of ischemia-reperfusion (p. 711).*

The microscopic changes, during the first few hours along this deadly path, are not impressive (Figure 5.20); even after 2 hours, when we know that most of the cells must

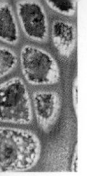

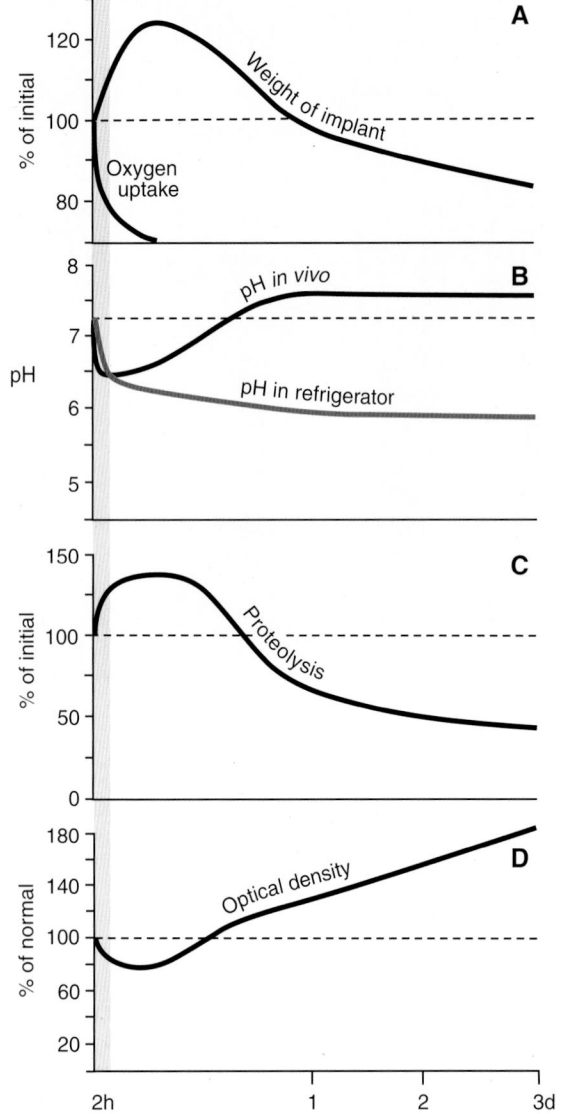

FIGURE 5.19   Changes occurring over 3 days in a mass of dying and dead liver tissue (peritoneal implants; oncosis → necrosis). The vertical pink band indicates the time during which the tissue is still alive. A: The implants swell, then shrink as the cells burst. The ability to take up oxygen (tested *in vitro*) reflects the condition of the mitochondria. B: Tissue pH drops precipitously *in vivo*, then rises as the acid diffuses away (which cannot happen in the refrigerator). C: The extractable protein rises (autolysis), then falls as coagulation prevails. D: Optical density reflects protein denaturation. During the first 12 hours, the effect is masked by cellular swelling. (Adapted from [194].)

be dead, no pathologist—however experienced—would make this diagnosis. Even the cellular swelling is hard to see: geometry tells us that *a doubling in volume would translate only as a 26 percent increase in diameter.* Overall, the cytoplasmic basophilia slowly disappears

because the ribosomes are partly denatured and partly digested by lysosomal ribonucleases; in the nucleus, the chromatin breaks up into small clumps that tend to stick to the nuclear membrane, but soon the nucleus loses its basophilia and fades away (*karyolysis*). By 24 hours or so the cell is reduced to an eosinophilic mass with little structural detail: this is **necrosis.**

Electron microscopy provides more detail. The progression from normal to oncosis and necrosis has been studied in several models by Trump and collaborators (322). The plasma membrane shows extensive blebbing; the actin filaments become detached from the plasma membrane and many disappear; the mitochondria show condensation, swelling of the inner compartment, eventually also calcification; the ER and Golgi apparatus swell and break up into vesicles. But when does the cell die? A necrotic cell without nucleus is surely dead—but it must have died long before.

The point of no return. At some critical time along the curves shown in Figure 5.19 the liver cells must become irreversibly damaged: this is the "point of no return," which we can identify with death. Morphology alone, as we have seen, does not give us the answer; but it can do so with this added trick.

> A mass of necrotic cells tends to become white to the naked eye (Figures 5.18, 5.21). We can exploit this phenomenon for determining the point of no return of liver tissue: in a rat, under anesthesia, and using an atraumatic forceps, we deprive a liver lobe of its blood supply. After a selected time interval we remove the clamp and allow the rat to survive 24 hours. If the liver lobe is normal in color, it survived that particular period of ischemia; if it is white, it did not.

This approach set the point of no return for rat liver at 2–2.5 hours (27, 99); 1–1.5 hours in our hands (of course, this figure varies enormously from one cell type to another). If we apply these figures with the data of our liver implant experiments, we learn three major lessons about cell death:

The swelling of oncosis continues after the death of the cell. In Figure 5.19 it peaks at ~6 hours; it is obviously a passive phenomenon that probably ends when the cell bursts (one review describes the event as "death by explosion" [8]). This fits with another well-established fact:

Cells that die by oncosis are permeable to dyes. Their membrane is riddled with holes and they are clearly unable to maintain their "milieu intérieur." This fact is used for identifying dead cells in a suspension (Figure 5.22): commercial kits are available for this "live/dead" test (**dye exclusion test**).

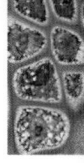

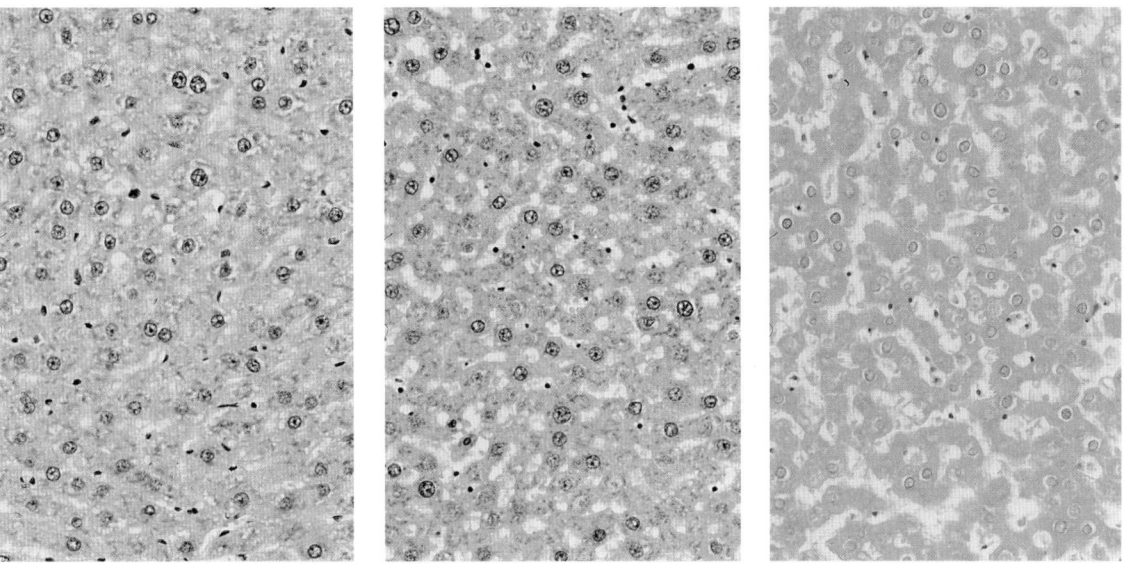

FIGURE 5.20   The difficulty of recognizing cell death by light microscopy. *Left:* Normal rat liver. *Center:* Section from a fragment of liver that has been implanted into the peritoneal cavity of another rat for 2 hours. Most of these cells are dead, but cannot be recognized as such on this routine microscopic section. *Right:* Section from a 24-hour liver implant. The cells are now clearly necrotic. The white halos around the nuclei are due to swelling of the perinuclear cisternae. (200x)

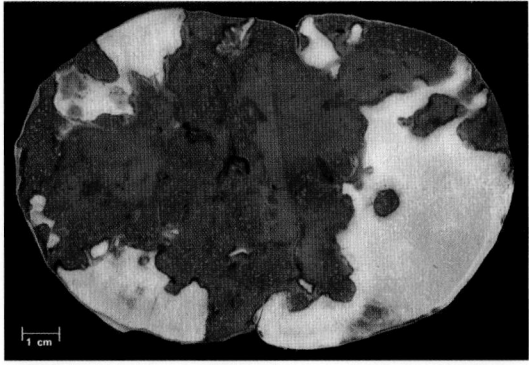

FIGURE 5.21   Multiple infarcts (white areas) in the enlarged spleen of a woman with a long history of heart disease.

Necrosis occurs long after cell death. Histologically at 2 hours the liver cells are far from being "necrotic" (Figure 5.20). In other words, **cell death and cell necrosis are two distinct phenomena.** By ignoring this fact many recent papers have simply raised the level of confusion.

Destruction of the Cellular Proteins: Two Pathways

Look at Figure 5.18: the 9-day specimen is striking. It is white, and would be quite firm to the touch. Why?

Common sense suggests protein denaturation, but proving it is not simple, because there is no histochemical method specific for denatured protein. In ordinary

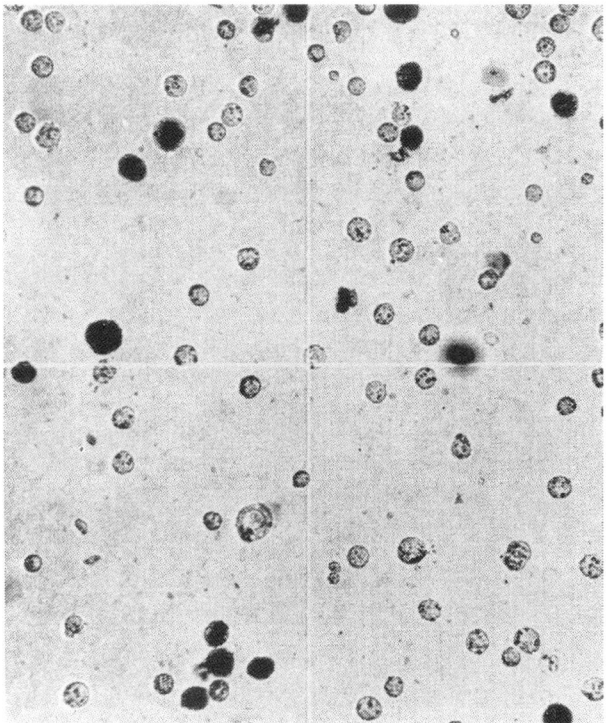

FIGURE 5.22   Dye exclusion test for identifying dead cells. Suspension of Ehrlich ascites carcinoma; the cells that have been permeated by the black dye (nigrosin) are dead. (Reproduced with permission from [147].)

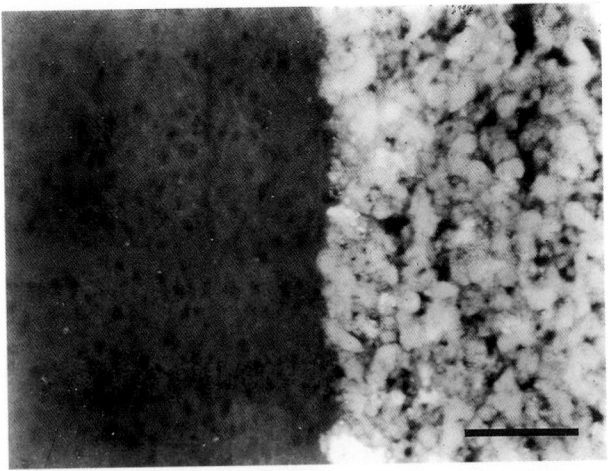

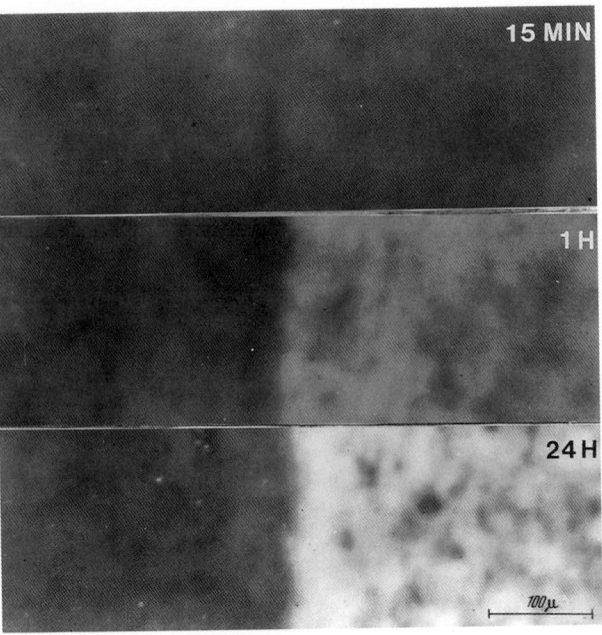

FIGURE 5.23   Precipitation of proteins in coagulation necrosis, as seen in fresh, unfixed sections of rat liver examined by dark field microscopy. *Left:* Normal liver. *Right:* Liver implant after 24 hours. The brightness is due to light diffraction by clumps of coagulated proteins. The earliest change is already visible, after only 30 minutes of anoxia. **Bar** = 100 μm. (Reproduced from [194] by permission from Springer-Verlag.)

FIGURE 5.24   Sections of unfixed rat liver (*left,* normal, *right,* implanted) viewed by ultraviolet light. The implants had been left in the peritoneal cavity for the time intervals indicated. Auto-fluorescence indicates protein denaturation. Note that protein denaturation begins while the cells are still alive, because it is already obvious at 1 hour, whereas it takes 2−2½ hours of ischemia to kill liver cells. (Reproduced from [194] by permission from Springer-Verlag.)

histologic sections *coagulated cells are eosinophilic* (which explains why neuropathologists sometimes speak of *red neurons* in injured brain tissue), but this is of course very nonspecific. The best way to demonstrate denatured proteins in a tissue is to examine thin slices of *fresh, unfixed* frozen sections using three types of illumination:

- By **transmitted light,** the implants become more and more opaque, as would be expected from the precipitation (coagulation) of denatured proteins.
- By **dark-field illumination,** the earliest signs of protein precipitation lie far beneath the limits of visibility by ordinary light microscopy, yet they can be beautifully visualized by means of the **Tyndall effect:** the optical phenomenon whereby, to an observer in a dark room, a ray of sunlight renders visible particles of dust that would be invisible in diffuse light. Each particle shines like a bright star. Under the microscope, this effect is obtained by illuminating the object from the side (dark-field microscopy) rather than from beneath. In this way one can visualize particles of ultramicroscopic size. Indeed, slices from a series of implants at different stages show a progressive increase in brightness (Figure 5.23).
- By **ultraviolet microscopy,** denatured proteins become autofluorescent, and slices of the implants show a progressive increase in autofluorescence (Figure 5.24). These results tell us, in essence, that

infarcts become white, opaque, and firm for the same reason that transparent egg white becomes white, opaque, and firm when boiled; the whiteness of snow, compared with the transparency of water, is based on the same Tyndall effect. As to the "dryness" of coagulated tissue, it is so only in appearance: a hard-boiled egg also appears dry but in fact contains the same amount of trapped water as a fresh egg (194).

A look at the time sequence of the various changes in dying tissue reveals an important fact: *protein lysis and coagulation are both occurring while the cell is still alive.*

Protein denaturation implies an uncoiling of the tertiary molecular structure (153); this exposes "buried" side chains, with several physicochemical results: denatured proteins become more reactive; they tend to aggregate; and some of the exposed radicals, if irradiated with ultraviolet light, emit visible light (i.e., become autofluorescent) (3, 37, 313).

Why is the sky blue? We are referring again to the Tyndall effect. Using gold colloids the smallest particles visible by dark-field microscopy are on the order of 50 Å (204). Theoretically, however, there is no limit to the size of an object that can be visualized by light diffraction as long as sufficient illumination is provided (197). After all, the sky is blue because of the light scattered by individual gas molecules in the atmosphere (291).

Although protein denaturation is one of the most prevalent pathologic cellular changes, until recently it was of interest (behold) only to the food industry (166). Yet it was recognized as early as 1886 by Weigert, one of Virchow's disciples, as *Koagulationsnekrose* (coagulation necrosis) (194). In one respect this term is ambiguous: it leaves open the question whether cell death is caused by or followed by coagulation. From what we have just said, however, the ambiguity is appropriate: *protein denaturation begins in the live cell, takes part in the killing, and then continues in the dead cell.* A major function of the heat-shock proteins is precisely to correct denaturation *in vivo*. We can venture to guess that a dying cell must be a busy place for ubiquitin, the monitor of denatured proteins (pp. 45, 187).

Protein denaturation has been observed also in plants (Figure 5.25) (125) and must be a general phenomenon. It has one striking clinical manifestation: the cataract (Figure 5.26). The progressive changes in a cataractous lens, although very slow (months and years), are in many ways parallel to those in the liver implants (194). As the cells of the crystalline lens die, water content and diffusible protein rise and then drop; the pH drops and then returns to normal; opacity and calcium content rise progressively.

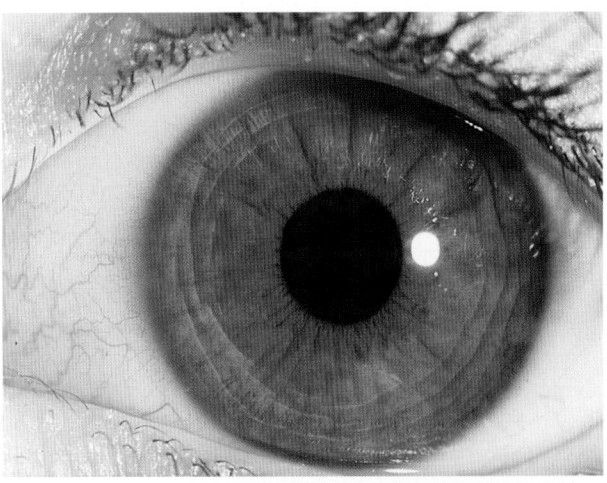

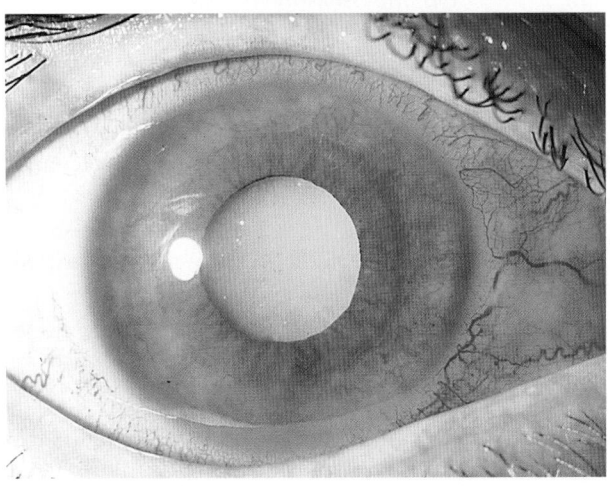

FIGURE 5.26 *Top:* Normal human eye. *Bottom:* Eye with a cataractous lens. The whiteness, due to protein denaturation, is common to most necrotic tissues. (Courtesy of Dr. J. Babel, Geneva, Switzerland.)

By electron microscopy the aggregates of denatured protein, if large enough, become recognizable as fluffy masses (322). During autolysis *in vitro,* within 1 hour the mitochondria swell and acquire small smudgy masses of osmiophilic material (144, 325). These masses are not lipid soluble, not rich in calcium, but digestible by proteases (142); they probably represent aggregates of denatured protein. All those who use fluorescence microscopy are familiar with the fact that dead cells are auto-fluorescent, but the phenomenon is known only as a nuisance. For obvious reasons, there are some studies on protein fluorescence in the crystalline lens (37).

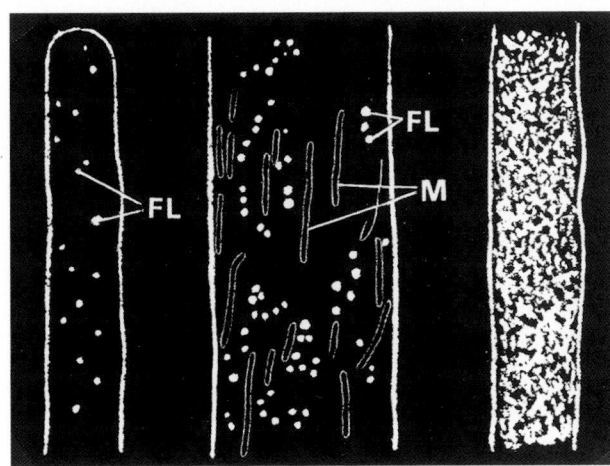

FIGURE 5.25 Denatured proteins in dead cells of plants. Three filaments of the fungus *Saprolegnia* seen by dark-field microscopy. *Left* and *center:* Two normal filaments. **FL:** Free lipid droplets. **M:** Mitochondria. *Right:* A dead filament; its cytoplasm is filled with precipitated proteins that diffract the light. (Slightly retouched from [125].)

As to the mechanism of protein denaturation in dying and dead cells: the drop in pH may be relevant initially, but the process continues even after the pH has returned to normal. Calcium may be involved (84, 85); indeed, denaturation occurs faster *in vivo* than in isolated tissues

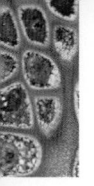

incubated at 37°C (194), suggesting that calcium supplies from the living tissues facilitate the process.

What is the biological significance of protein denaturation? We see it as a *protective device* on two counts. First, the dying cells are loaded with lysosomal proteolytic enzymes, ready to initiate self-digestion (autolysis). The products of protein digestion (peptides) are powerful irritants and set off an acute inflammatory reaction. *Denaturation puts a stop to autolysis (and to the acute inflammatory response) by inactivating the enzymes and removing their substrates.* Second, proteins released by dying cells can diffuse into the blood stream and become antigens, because intracellular proteins can be recognized by the immune system as nonself. *Denaturation interrupts this sequence by making the proteins insoluble and nonantigenic.*

Support for the latter suggestion comes from the cataract: if a crystalline lens is injured by trauma and not removed, its spilled proteins can give rise to antibodies that attack the lens in the other eye (**phacoanaphylactic ophthalmitis** [95]).

These concepts will be essential for understanding the evolution of an inflammatory reaction around infarcts (pp. 325, 446).

> Mild denaturation of soluble proteins is thought to increase their antigenicity, but in coagulation necrosis we are dealing with profound denaturation with loss of solubility; the aggregated proteins are no longer able to diffuse into the bloodstream, and histology shows that no response develops against an old coagulated protein mass.

> NOTE: cellular stress (such as heat or ischemia) induces denatured proteins, and conversely, denatured proteins induce the cellular stress response (87).

As a mechanism of cellular breakdown we emphasized protein denaturation, because it is rarely discussed in textbooks; but *the proteins of cells dying by the oncotic pathway are actually caught between two opposite destructive fates: denaturation, and digestion by cellular proteolytic enzymes* (autolysis). If denaturation prevails, both the enzymes and their substrates are made useless; if autolysis prevails, there will be no protein left to denature. Usually, denaturation wins the race, and the resulting amorphous mass is called **coagulation necrosis;** if autolysis wins, the process is called **liquefaction necrosis.**

> In the liver implants, coagulation wins: Figure 5.19 shows that extractable proteins (mainly polypeptides from autolysis) rise and fall, whereas denaturation progresses steadily for as long as 12 days.

It is important to remember that both processes, denaturation and proteolysis, begin while the cell is still alive. The very purpose of HSPs is to repair misfolded (including denatured) proteins.

> The two mechanisms are best observed in action in second-rate fish markets: fish fillets should be soft and semitransparent, but after they have been displayed for a day or two they look stiff, opaque, and whitish as if they had been partly cooked; this appearance—long known in pathology as *parboiled* (partially boiled)—is due to protein denaturation. On the other hand, outdated shellfish become flabby and seem to liquefy: this is autolysis.

What Is the Final Blow to the Oncotic Cell?

As the doomed cell slips from the stage of reversible to that of irreversible injury, there may well be a critical factor that can be held responsible for that transition; a cellular malfunction as obvious as "heart failure" or "respiratory failure" would be for the body as a whole. A great deal of effort has been spent in this search, because if we had the answer we might be able to improve the therapy of infarcts, and perhaps also the preservation of organs for transplants. There has been a tendency to blame single organelles; the **lysosome theory** of cell death was the first. Ischemic cells were supposedly killed from inside by the release of the lysosomal enzymes. This hypothesis was an outgrowth of the enthusiasm generated by the discovery of the lysosomes, which were often referred to by the rather sensational name of "suicide bags." Unfortunately, the theory did not fit the facts (83); cells do commit suicide, but not with their lysosomes (crystal-induced cell death may be the only exception, p. 147). The **mitochondria** are certainly involved in cell death by oncosis; progressive mitochondrial damage has been well demonstrated by electron microscopy (215) and a role for these organelles in ischemic cell death is all the more likely since it was found that cytochrome C is a powerful poison, and that mitochondria hold a key to cell death by apoptosis. Progressive **protein denaturation** surely plays a role (194) but it has not been studied as a mechanism of irreversibility. **Arrested protein synthesis** is unlikely to be the cause of acute cell death, since the hepatocytes can tolerate it for 24–48 hours in the course of ethionine poisoning (83). **Increased permeability of the plasma membrane with loss of K and inflow of Na ions** was long thought to be critical, but this theory remained dormant for a time, since it was shown—surprisingly—that cells could tolerate major fluxes of these ions (146). Eventually it was found that **calcium,** not Na or K, was responsible for the final blow; hence the theory, now prevalent, that

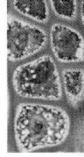

the mechanism of irreversible injury is **an increase in membrane permeability followed by influx of calcium** (49, 84, 85, 298, 321).

Calcium ions are biologically very active and liable to disrupt the myriad of interrelated metabolic reactions inside the cell. J. L. Farber proposed that a phospholipase, present in many cell membranes including the mitochondria, is activated by calcium, leading to membrane disruption. Some of the calcium may come from the ER and especially from the mitochondria: remember that the calcium content of the mitochondria is 1000 to 10,000 times greater than in the cytoplasm (10^{-3} vs. $10^{-6}-10^{-8}$ M). Whatever its source, the excess of free calcium can activate other enzymes besides phospholipases: *an ATPase* (49), which destroys what little ATP is generated; *proteases* (301), which may explain both the cytoskeletal damage (106, 300) and the surface blebbing; *endonucleases,* which may explain some of the nuclear changes.

The membrane damage caused by phospholipases is at least threefold: phospholipids are lost, and their breakdown products are membrane-toxic. By snipping a fatty acid from the phospholipid molecules, the phospholipase creates "one-legged" lysophospholipids. The wedge shape of these molecules causes them to break up the lipid bilayer into micelles (Figure 4.6); in the meantime the fatty acids, being fat soluble, also insert themselves into the membranes, contributing to the molecular disorder (Table 5.1) (55, 61).

Why should the cell membranes contain such dangerous enzymes as phospholipases? We are dealing with one of nature's many two-edged swords. Phospholipases have many essential functions, including phospholipid turnover and protein kinase activation (284). In the plasma membrane they are the key to eicosanoid metabolism. By cleaving arachidonic acid from phospholipid molecules, they initiate the cascade that leads to the production of prostaglandins and leukotrienes, important mediators of inflammation (p. 358).

So how can we summarize the drama of ischemic cell death? The drama varies from one tissue to another and with the type of injury, but for ischemic cell death of liver cells we can suggest the following, drawn from many sources. The reader should try to see it as a movie:

1. Mitochondrial ATP production stops.
2. The ATP-driven membrane ionic pumps run down.
3. Sodium and water seep into the cell.
4. The cell swells, and the plasma membrane is stretched.
5. Glycolysis enables the cell to limp on for a while.
6. The cell initiates a heat-shock (stress) response, which will probably not help if the ischemia persists.
7. The pH drops.
8. Calcium enters the cell.
9. Calcium activates phospholipases, causing the cell membranes to lose phospholipid and producing lysophosphatides and fatty acids, both of which cause more membrane damage, initiating a vicious circle.

   - Calcium activates proteases, damaging cytoskeletal structures; **blebbing** develops.
   - Calcium activates ATPase, causing more loss of ATP.
   - Calcium activates endonucleases, the nuclear chromatin forms clumps, some seeps out. Uric acid is released (p. 227).

10. Protein denaturation starts (calcium may be involved).
11. All cell membranes are damaged.
12. The ER and other organelles swell.
13. The final blow is probably related to the massive inflow of calcium.

Is Oncosis Reversible?

Oncosis is defined as death with swelling, and thus it cannot be reversible, but it is preceded by *acute cellular swelling* (p. 79) which is certainly reversible. Cells suffering from chronic ischemia can survive in a state of chronic swelling, and thus on the brink of death. This happens quite often in the heart, which is notoriously subject to ischemia (Figure 5.27).

The reversibility and prevention of ischemic damage are being studied intensively in models of ischemia/reperfusion (p. 714), a topic of great practical interest, which has joined the older field of *cytoprotection*. This term as now understood refers to protection against all relevant types of injury. The stomach, for example, is protected against mucosal injury by retinoids (223); in glomerulonephritis, nitric oxide synthase is protective (133), but when tested for *cardioprotection* nitric oxide can be both friend and foe (261). *Neuroprotection* against neuronal loss is being tried with nerve growth

Table 5.1 **Possible Mechanisms of Plasma Membrane Damage during Ischemic Cell Death (Oncosis)**

Stretching, secondary to cellular swelling
Loss of phospholipids*
Increased disorder due to insertion of fatty acids*
Increased disorder due to insertion of lysophospholipids*
Loss of connection with cytoskeleton, resulting in blebbing
Bursting of blebs

*Due to phospholipases; may affect internal membranes as well.

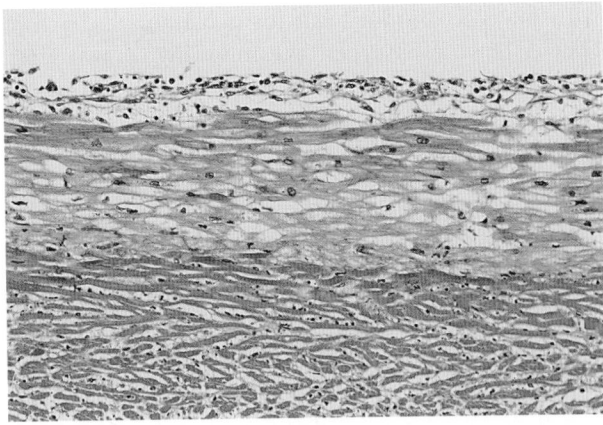

FIGURE 5.27   Human myocardium: left ventricle 1 day after infarction. Lumen of ventricle at top. *Bottom:* Typical coagulation necrosis of the myocardial fibers (the nuclei disappeared by cytolysis). *Center:* Layer of fibers, swollen (acute cellular swelling) but still alive, because of nourishment by the blood flowing in the ventricle. They have lost some of their fibrils and are certainly unable to contract. *Top:* Endocardium, with "too many cells" (some leukocytes have been attracted by the dead/dying tissue.)

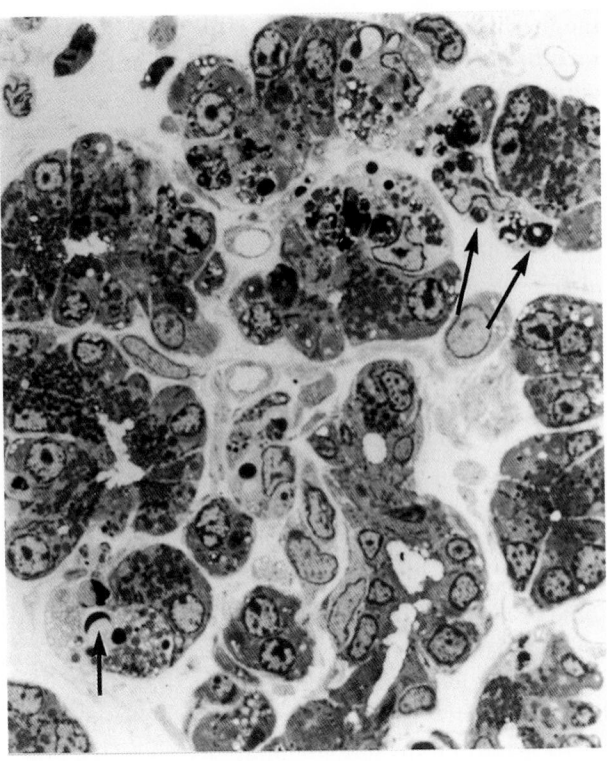

FIGURE 5.28   Parotid gland 24 hours after obstruction of the duct. Note the marginated, sharply defined, condensed chromatin in an apoptotic nucleus (**short arrow**) and apoptotic bodies within macrophages (**long arrows**). (Reproduced from [334]. Copyright © 1987 John Wiley & Sons. Reprinted by permission of John Wiley & Sons, Inc.)

factor (NGF) (292), erythropoietin (286), estrogen (70), and cytotoxin antagonists (231). Cytoprotection in the kidney has led to a fascinating development: an episode of acute renal failure protects against later ischemic or toxic damage (*acquired cytoresistance*); this effect was attributed to higher levels of cholesterol in the cell membranes (361). Similarly, cardioprotection against infarction was provided by "**ischemic preconditioning**" (p. 189) (272). Some of these effects may well reflect the healing touch of HSPs.

Cell Death with Shrinkage: Apoptosis

Apoptosis is a physiologic and genetically programmed type of cell death common to metazoans. It affects individual cells and acts as opposite to mitosis.

Until the mid-1980s, the only form of cell death described in textbooks was the massive cell death seen in infarcts. In 1971 J. F. R. Kerr, an Australian experimental pathologist, was studying the changes in rat liver induced by tying off branches of the portal vein. Depending on the branches tied, the liver did not show massive cell death; instead, in scattered individual cells, a distinctive form of death occurred: it was characterized by "condensation and compaction" of the chromatin, shrinkage and breakup of the cells, followed by phagocytosis of the debris by other parenchymal cells or by macrophages. Kerr called this phenomenon *shrinkage necrosis* (Figures 5.28, 5.29) (154). A year later, on

leave in Scotland, Kerr, with A. H. Currie and A. R. Wyllie, proposed for this form of death a more flamboyant name than shrinkage necrosis: **apoptosis,** a most felicitous choice by Prof. J. Cormack of the Department of Greek, University of Aberdeen. Apoptosis evokes the notion of "falling off": an allusion to the fact that cells did not die massively, but one by one, "much like individual leaves fall off a tree" (154, 156).

In a Hippocratic book on fractures and luxations, the word *apóptosis* was used precisely to describe *a falling off—* but of chunks of flesh and bones due to gangrene (141)— not quite the "leaves" and "petals" often mentioned in the apoptosis literature. The correct pronounciation calls for an accent on the first o (apóptosis). We found no reason for skipping the second p (apó'tosis) as suggested (156); we do not say "helico'ter." Beyond these details, we wish to congratulate the Scottish scholar who applied a Hippocratic term so aptly to a 20th century concept.

The new name drew some interest, but more bait was necessary to attract the attention of the scientific

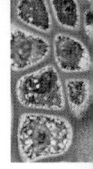

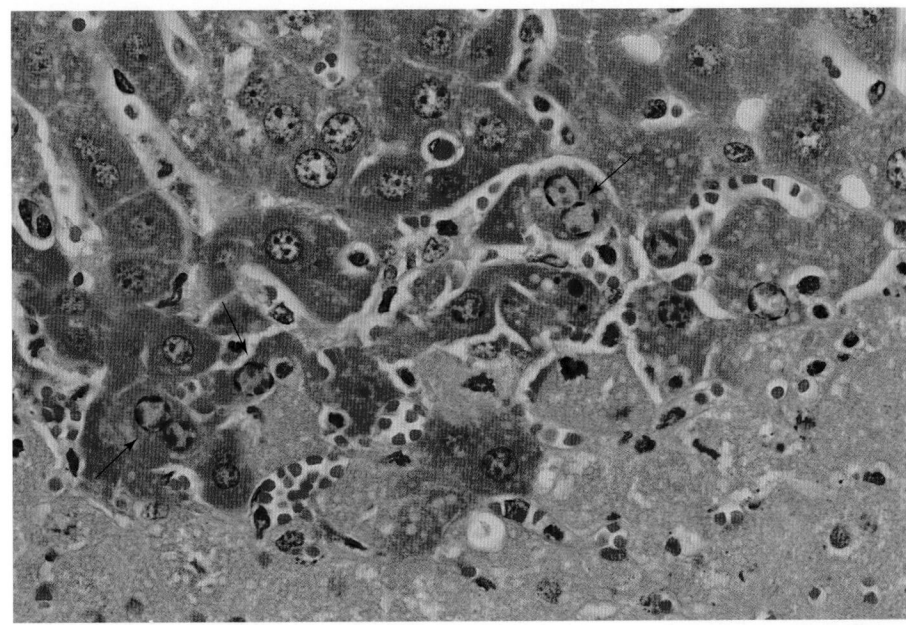

FIGURE 5.29 Two types of liver cell death caused by a single intravenous dose of a toxic agent (concanavalin A, a microtubular poison). *Bottom:* The pink cells show coagulation necrosis, indicating that they died by oncosis. Correspondingly, their nuclei are disappearing by karyolysis. At the margin between live and necrotic cells, several nuclei show the typical half-moons of apoptosis (**arrows**). (Preparation courtesy of Dr. G. Szabo, University of Massachusetts Medical School, Worcester, MA.)

community (154a). Wyllie et al. published some critical new facts in 1984 (356). The peculiar condensation of the chromatin seen microscopically could be defined in terms of biochemistry: the DNA was cleaved in internucleosomal fragments, presumably by an endonuclease, yielding a "ladder" pattern by electrophoresis, whereas ischemic cell death produced a continuous smear (Figure 5.30); also, apoptosis could be prevented by some protease inhibitors (198, 352, 356). What was the dying cell constructing? Tools to kill itself (180)? Whatever the answer might be, apoptosis ceased to be a purely microscopic event; it had become measurable and therefore accessible also to non-pathologists, and it skyrocketed. From 1991 to 1995 the number of papers on apoptosis was 283; from 1996 to 2000 it was 35,366. Today this topic ranks with the most intensely studied in virtually all fields of biological science (352–356). Paradoxically, the ladder pattern and the effect of protease inhibitors turned out to be less specific than hoped, so that morphology is still the basic criterion for defining apoptosis (153a).

Apoptosis continued to generate exciting news. First, the fact that it represented not only death but **cellular suicide.** In the meantime, immunologists discovered that cells can kill eachoter; **cell killing** became a closely related topic, even more closely when it turned out that cell killing is often accomplished by **enforced suicide.** In other words, a killer T cell can tell another cell "kill yourself"—and it will be obeyed, by apoptosis. It is no wonder that the terminology of apoptosis has become crudely human: *executioner* enzymes, removal of cell *corpses, cannibalization, eat me* signals.

Microscopic features of apoptosis. As usual, details vary, but the following description is representative; the whole performance lasts about an hour, sometimes less (220).

- *The cell shrinks, becomes denser (dark by electron microscopy), rounds up and detaches itself from its neighbors.* The loss of volume is the first change (190); it may be as high as 60 percent for eosinophils (207); it may have the purpose of reducing the labor of phagocytosis (362). Both shrinkage and density may reflect (a) *loss of fluid:* the smooth endoplasmic reticulum swells into vesicles that fuse with the cell membrane, dumping out fluid (7), while the Na/K-ATP pump extracts cations from the cell (207); and/or (b) *protein cross-linking by transglutaminases,* which may also explain the increased density (90).

- *The chromatin becomes very dense, and separates into deeply stained, homogeneous, often semilunar or sickle-shaped masses* plastered against the nuclear membrane (Figure 5.31). At least half a dozen factors are known to induce this chromatin condensation, including a factor called *acinus* and the caspases (see further) (362). If extracted and examined by electrophoresis, the DNA produces the pattern described above. We may wonder why the cell takes the trouble of shredding its DNA: the purpose may be to prevent it from being misused.

- *Budding:* Seen in a time-lapse movie the cell performs a striking "death dance": it sends out and pulls back short processes, which contain dense

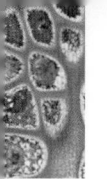

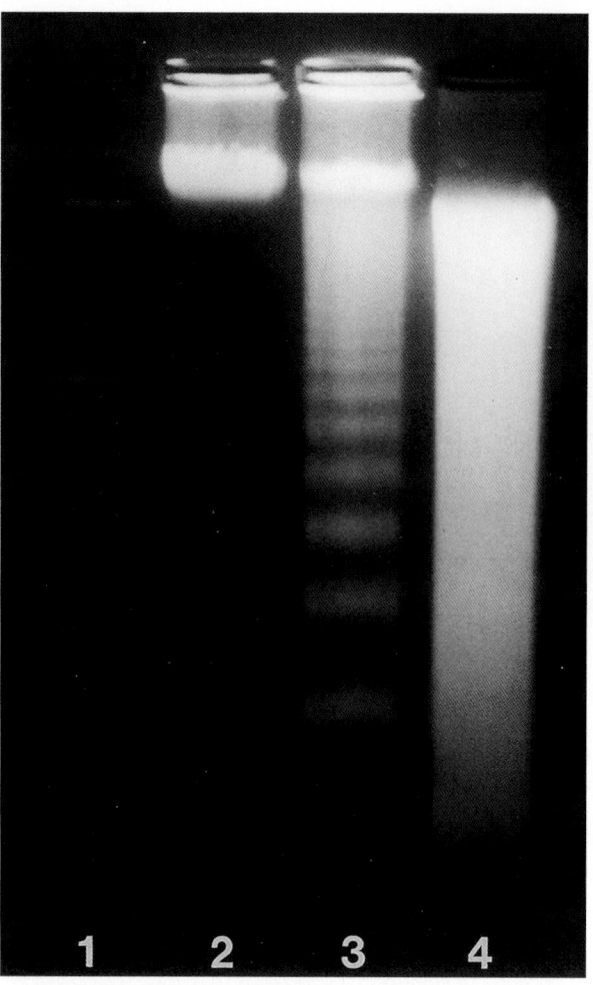

FIGURE 5.30   Comparing the DNA breakdown in apoptosis and massive cell death. Agarose gel electrophoresis of DNA extracted from cultures of mouse cells, stained with ethidium bromide and photographed under ultraviolet light. *Lane 1:* Molecular weight markers. *Lane 2:* Control culture. *Lane 3:* Culture heated for 30 minutes to 44°C, extracted 8 hours later, when it showed typical, extensive apoptosis. *Lane 4:* Culture submitted to repeated freezing and thawing, and extracted 72 hours later, when it showed massive necrosis. (Reproduced with permission from [155].)

cytoplasm and often a piece of the nucleus (29, 30).

- *Blebbing:* Small blebs may develop, but this is not typical of apoptosis, whereas it is constant and extensive in oncosis.

Blebs (p. 129), blister-like structures with a watery content (322), are biologically different phenomenon from budding. There has been some confusion between budding and blebbing, because scanning electron micrographs show balloon-like "protrusions" (354) that are difficult to interpret (53, 170). Another

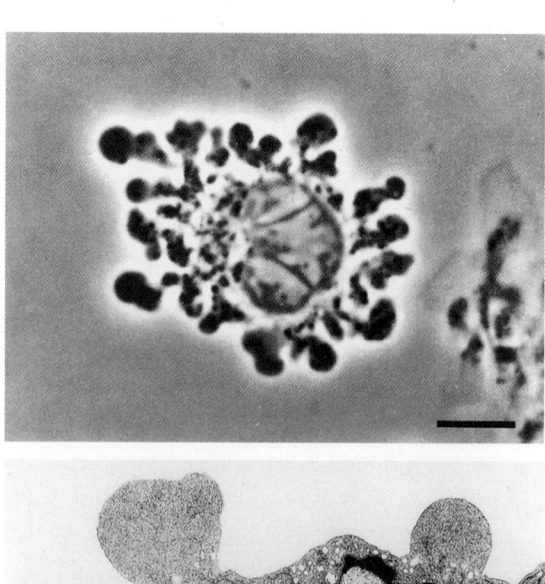

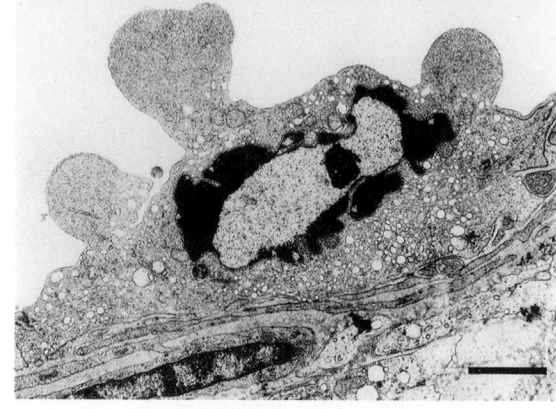

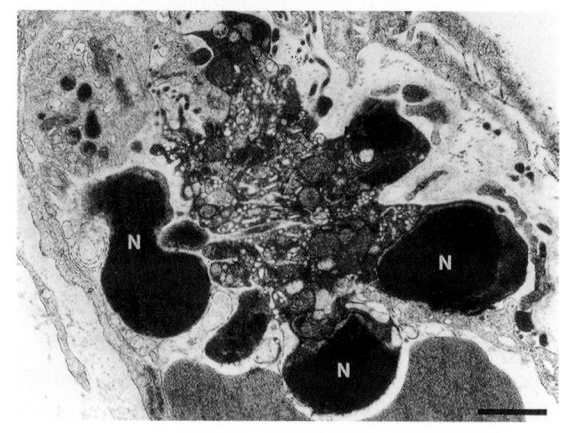

FIGURE 5.31   Three views of apoptosis. *Top:* The "death dance" of a leukocyte, recorded by a movie in the 1960s. This cell threw out and retracted "pseudopodia" and then broke up. Only a movie could do justice to this dramatic expression of cell suffering. **Bar** = 5 μm. (Reproduced from TRIANGLE, Sandoz J Med Science, 9(6):191–199, Copyright Sandoz Pharma Ltd, Basle, Switzerland [30].) *Center:* Apoptosis of endothelial cell in rat mammary gland 4 days after weaning. Note "pseudopodia" and peculiar clustering of chromatin. **Bar** = 2 μm. *Bottom:* Apoptosis in endothelial cell in mouse mammary gland 2 days after weaning. Note the *budding;* each bud contains a piece of the nucleus (**N**). **Bar** = 1 μm. (*Center and Bottom:* Reproduced from [333]. Copyright © 1989 John Wiley & Sons. Reprinted by permission of John Wiley & Sons, Inc.)

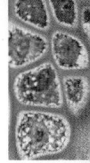

confusing factor is that intermediate forms may also occur.

- The "buds" break off, to become *apoptotic bodies.*
- What is left of the cell body is taken up by neighboring cells or extruded (in epithelia); or it is phagocytized by macrophages.

As seen *in vivo,* shrinkage and budding are over in minutes, and phagocytosis destroys the evidence very efficiently. In a tissue that is rapidly shrinking by apoptosis the cells may show only a peppering of nuclear remains, easily overlooked; which explains why apoptosis was escaped notice for so long.

By a stroke of good fortune, the entire sequence of apoptosis was captured cinematographically by a pioneering French hematologist, Marcel Bessis, 16 years before apoptosis was discovered (29): a leukocyte dying under the objective threw out bulky pseudopodia (the "budding" seen in fixed sections), then suddenly broke up into a cluster of separate bodies (Figure 5.32). The electron micrograph of an apoptotic cell shown in Figure 5.31 (*bottom*) illustrates this same, almost explosive breakup.

The corpses (130, 276) of apoptotic cells, if shed into a space such as a glandular lumen, may undergo what was called "secondary necrosis" (7). They can also be picked up by macrophages or by neighboring cells. These former neighbors are induced to cannibalize the remains because they express a number of "eat me signals" (69), perhaps as many as 10 (252); the most important are a vitronectin receptor, annexin 5, and molecules of phosphatidylserine, normally inserted into the inner leaflet of the cell membrane, but flipped out on the apoptotic cells (195). Remarkably absent around the corpses are the neutrophils. We will comment shortly on the meaning of their absence.

Molecular mechanisms of apoptosis. The stimuli to apoptosis can be positive, i.e., induced by specific ligands, chemicals, radiation; or negative, by withdrawal of growth factors; the latter has been called **death by neglect** (7). Recently, a new negative stimulus was discovered: cells that normally grow on a substrate die by apoptosis if they are removed from their customary substrate. This mechanism of death was named **anoikis,** Greek for *homelessness* (104). Its purpose may be to prevent loose cells from homing in the wrong places.

The molecular apparatus for self-killing is ready to be triggered and extremely powerful, but cellular suicide is a grave matter and must be tightly controlled, hence it is—in our eyes—extremely complicated. Basically, evolution has chosen that cellular suicide will

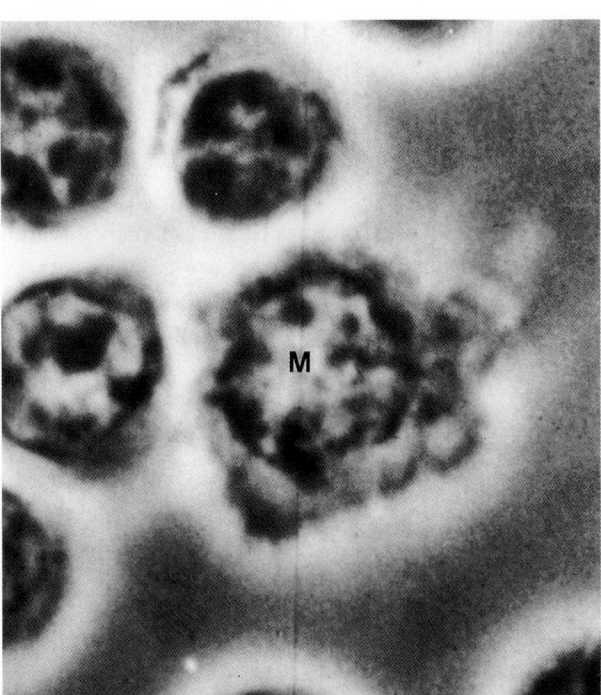

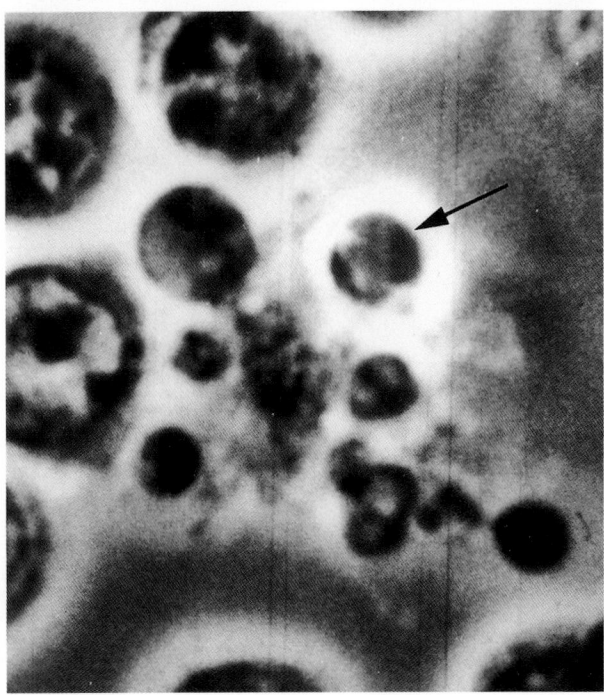

FIGURE 5.32 Apoptosis recorded on film before it had a name. Two frames of a movie taken by M. Bessis in 1955, showing the death of a white blood cell (**M**, probably a monocyte) in blood maintained *in vitro* at 37°C. *Top:* The cell just before it began to die; in later frames it began to throw out pseudopodia (the "budding" process) and at 33 minutes (*bottom*) it suddenly broke apart into what we now call apoptotic bodies. **Arrow:** this cell fragment contains half-moons of condensed chromatin typical of apoptosis.

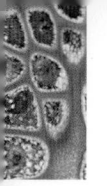

occur by a burst of intracellular proteolysis carried out by enzymes of at least 14 varieties called **caspases,** present in the cytosol as inactive pro-caspases. Once activated they have enough specificity to dismantle all the working parts of the cell; they are appropriately referred to as the "executioner enzymes." The search for mechanisms of apoptosis, therefore, becomes largely a search for mechanisms to activate the pro-caspases. As of 2003, at least four could be listed; they are identified by the cellular component that initiates the reaction: (A) *The surface receptor pathway (extrinsic pathway),* whereby the stimulation of specific surface receptors leads to intracellular pro-caspase activation, (B) *The mitochondrial pathway (intrinsic pathway),* whereby the mitochondria are induced to release cytochrome c, a pro-caspase activator; (C) *The endoplasmic reticulum pathway,* recently discovered (329a, 357a), whereby a pro-caspase residing in the ER is activated by "ER stress"; and (D) *The p53 pathway.* The superfamily of p53 transcription factors is a major device for the control of apoptosis, and as such also a cornerstone of tumor biology. Pathways (A) and (B) are shown in Figure 5.33, greatly simplified, because details are changing fast. Pathway (C) (via the ER) needs no further explanation at this time; pathway (D) (via p53) will be discussed in relation to tumors (pp. 216, 887).

The receptor pathway. The plasma membrane, rather surprisingly, is studded with receptors that function as molecular antennae ready to receive the order to commit suicide, and to forward it into the cytosol where the procaspases are waiting. Half a dozen of these receptors

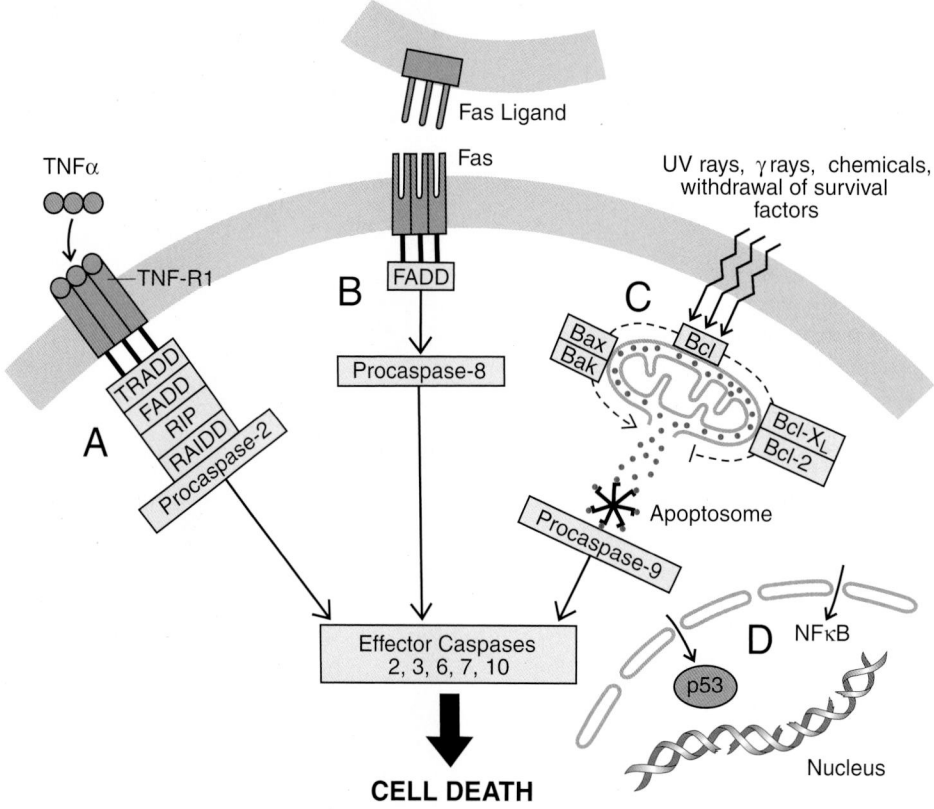

FIGURE 5.33   Mechanisms of apoptosis: a highly simplified diagram. *A:* **TNF (tumor necrosis factor) extrinsic pathway.** Soluble TNF binds to the specific receptor (TNF-R1) trimerized and thereby activated. Rectangular boxes represent proteins that assemble following activation (DD = death domain); activated procaspase-2 leads to the final, lethal activation of all the executor caspases. *B:* **Fas ligand extrinsic pathway:** Fas ligand, protruding from the membrane of a nearby (ill-intentioned) cell, binds to Fas and initiates another lethal cascade of activation through procaspase-8. *C:* **Intrinsic (mitochondrial) pathway:** physical and other causes lead to activation of Bcl, which activates both activators and inhibitors of cytochrome C release (red dots = cytochrome *c*). The escape of cytochrome *c* may occur through pores similar to those made by complement. Cytochrome *c* binds to Apaf-1 monomers, leading to the formation of the seven-spoked "wheel of death," the apoptosome. In turn, the apoptosome activates procaspase-9. *D:* Part of nucleus, indicating that p53 and NF-κB are also involved in apoptosis, another complex mechanism. (Adapted from many sources, including References 127a, 224, 228a, and 268a.)

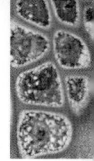

are known (224); the prototype of this pathway is a protein called **Fas,** similar, but not identical, to the TNF receptor. Fas can be triggered only by an extracellular signal, a molecule called **Fas ligand** (**FasL**), which can be either free-floating or bound to the surface of another cell. When FasL does bind to Fas, the deep end of Fas—which is protruding into the cytosol—recruits an "adaptor" molecule that connects the deep end of Fas with caspase 8 and activates it, whereby the entire caspase chain is called into action and dismantles the cell's machinery from inside.

Any cell expressing Fas is at the mercy of any cell expressing FasL; when the encounter occurs, the cell carrying only the ligand is safe, the Fas-carrying cell will die. This principle has some useful applications: since activated T cells express Fas, cells that want to be safe from the attack of T cells need only express Fas ligand. This is how the Sertoli cells and the epithelium of the anterior eye chamber maintain their immune-privileged status; and this is how some tumors have learned to fend off the attack of T cells (137). This is an important topic in immunology. Attempts have been made to protect allografts from immune attack by T cells along the Fas/FasL principle, but somehow it did not work; the result was more severe inflammation (234).

The mitochondrial pathway is activated by a variety of stimuli which stress the cell: environmental stimuli such as chemicals, radiation, and withdrawal of growth factors (205). In this emergency the mitochondria reveal that they are loaded with poison: namely cytochrome *c* (formerly known only as a life-giving enzyme) which is held in the narrow slit between the two mitochondrial membranes. Whether cytochrome *c* will or will not be spilled is decided by the balance of two sets of proteins (genes) of the Bcl-2 family.

Bcl-2 and Bcl-x_L oppose apoptosis, Bad and Bax favor it (56). By the way: how can a protein cause mitochondria to leak? in part, it seems, by inserting itself in the mitochondrial membrane, and/or by creating a pore (56). When cytochrome *c* does leak out, it becomes attached to a protein called APAF-1 (apoptotic protease activating factor), and the two self-assemble into an astounding, seven-spoke wheel (barely hinted in Figure 5.33) called **apoptosome** (268a). The apoptosome recruits procaspase-9, activates it and with it the whole caspase chain (119, 130, 158). Now it seems that Bcl-2 can also activate the caspases directly (196).

Death by Shrinkage, Death by Swelling: Who Decides?

In some situations the cell would appear to have no choice: apoptosis requires ATP; oncosis is caused by the *lack* of ATP; therefore, cells that are suddenly deprived of blood flow *should* die of oncosis. In fact, they can be induced to die by either apoptosis or oncosis by graded depletion of ATP (75, 175, 229, 328).

Using graded doses of antimycin A, a respiratory poison, it was possible to induce cultured fibroblasts to die of apoptosis, oncosis ("necrosis"), or by an intermediate mechanism that was named *aponecrosis* (94). Predictably, a single challenge can produce both types of cell death (244, 283, 309) These and similar experiments showed that virtually any cell can go down the path of oncosis or apoptosis, depending on (a) the type and intensity of the stimulus (Figure 5.34), (b) the available ATP, and (c) the degree of differentiation of the cell (232); furthermore, a cell may begin to die by apoptosis, but if its supply of ATP is suddenly cut off the apoptotic sequence may be aborted and turn into oncosis (143a, 237).

Knowing these facts, what should we expect to happen in an infarct? In experimental myocardial infarcts, studies by histology as well as histochemistry and DNA laddering, *a mixture of apoptosis and oncosis* ("necrosis") has been found (143a). This can mean one or both of the following: (a) the cells at the periphery of the infarct are not wholly anoxic/ischemic, and therefore have enough ATP to die by apoptosis (45, 78); and (b) there are intermediate forms of cell death.

Whether the two principal forms of cell death occur separately or together, understanding their diverse yet interconnected ways has a practical value: they may call for different therapy, especially for the heart. It is convenient to use the definitions proposed by Jaeschke and Lemasters (143a):

- Death by swelling is ATP-depletion dependent and caspase independent, and leads to oncotic necrosis;
- Death by shrinkage (apoptosis) is caspase-dependent and ATP-dependent, and may lead to apoptotic necrosis.

Apoptosis and Inflammation

Granulocytes are rarely seen around apoptotic cells. This in stark contrast with the response to ischemic necrosis: crowds of granulocytes and other inflammatory cells pour into the area. The "inflammatory silence" of apoptosis makes sense: if apoptosis is to carry out its discrete function of eliminating single unwanted cells, without damage to the tissue structure as a whole, the neutrophils must be kept out of the picture. When activated, these cells are known to secrete bactericidal molecules in such large amounts that collateral damage to bystander cells, as we will see in discussing Inflammation, is bound to occur. Actually, it is not quite

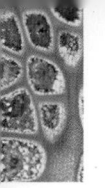

FIGURE 5.34 The two main ways of cell death (with shrinking, with swelling) illustrated by two cells of the same line (mastocytoma) shown at the same enlargement. *Left:* Shrunken, apoptotic cell 4 hours after a heat shock (30 minutes at 43°C). *Right:* Swollen cell that died by oncosis due to anoxia, after incubation for 30 hours in 95 percent N plus 5 percent CO. **Bar** = 0.2 μm. (Courtesy of Dr. B. V. Harmon, Medical School, Herston, Queensland, Australia.)

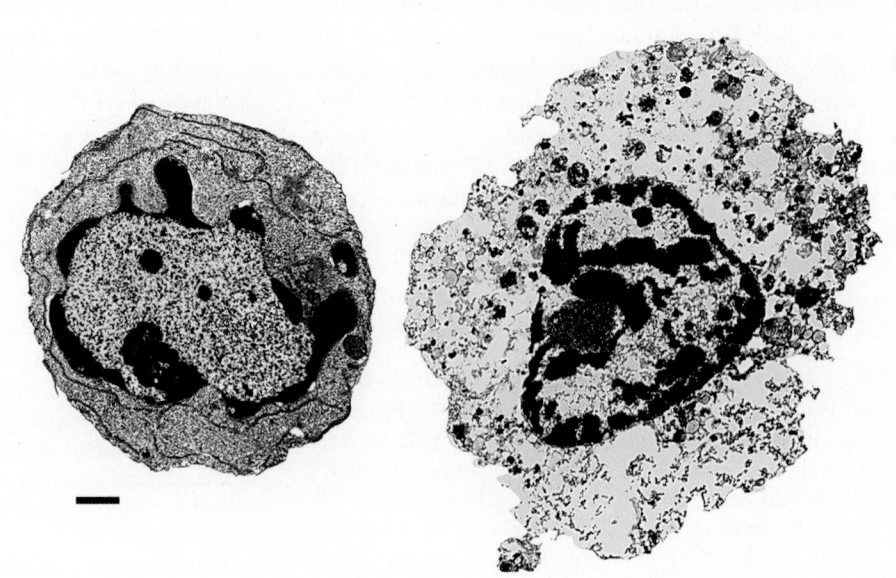

correct to say that apoptosis does not induce inflammation: macrophages do appear on the scene and phagocytize the apoptotic cells; and macrophages are almost the prototype of inflammatory cells.

It is a general rule of inflammation that when macrophages are activated, they secrete chemical messages to recruit other types of inflammatory cells; we rationalize this as a call for help. *But macrophages phagocytizing apoptotic cells do not call for help* (276). Quite to the contrary: *they secrete anti-inflammatory substances* (119) such as prostaglandin E_2 (80). It seems obvious that the overall plan for the apoptotic cells is to die *in incognito*.

> QUESTIONS: If the apoptotic cells are to die without leaving a trace, why do they induce autoimmune responses when injected intravenously (216)? And if the apoptotic cells release no chemical calls, how do the macrophages get to them? By random motion? By some secret call?

A single apoptotic cell in an epithelial sheet could still betray its presence by causing a leak in the sheet. Imagine what would happen to the intestinal mucosa if bacteria were to rush through every gap left by apoptotic cells that dropped off the epithelial lining. *In vitro,* apoptosis in a sheet of intestinal epithelium does cause a mild temporary leak (112, 189) but the trouble is minimized by two mechanisms: the dying cell and its neighbors develop tight junctions during the ejection, and the surrounding cells create a ring of actin-myosin that tightens around the critical area (268).

Apoptosis and the Immune Response

Apoptosis relates to the immune response in three entirely different ways, and each one may lead to autoimmune disease. First, *molecules from the apoptotic cell can behave as antigens.* Oddly enough, injected intravenously—in mice—they do (216). Second, *a genetic disruption of the apoptotic pathway* can cause failure to eliminate autoreactive lymphocytes (290, 305) (as mentioned above). Third, *given sets of cells may undergo premature, lymphocyte-independent apoptotic death.* Therefore, apoptosis is now an important mechanism to consider in the pathogenesis of autoimmune disease (77). Much of the evidence is indirect, but some is impressive: for example, in SLE (systemic lupus erythematosus, p. 590) the plasma contains antibodies against nucleosomes, a typical product of the apoptotic cell (77).

Apoptosis and the Heat-Shock Proteins

A basic function of the HSPs is to protect the cell from internal damage and to increase its chances of survival: not surprisingly, this task is accomplished in part by fending off apoptosis. To this end, several members of the HSP family interfere with apoptotic mechanisms: for example, HSP70 interferes with the assembly of the apoptosome (24, 269).

Apoptosis and Tumors

Since the size of all organs is maintained—somehow—by a perfect balance between cell gain by mitosis and

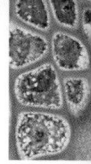

cell loss by apoptosis, it might seem logical to conclude that cancer could be a disease of too little apoptosis: but unfortunately the facts are much more complicated (355). To grasp the essentials, we can ask some basic questions;

1. *What would we find if we just counted mitotic and apoptotic cells in tissue sections?* The first to try this approach on a large scale found the task difficult and the results somewhat subjective (299). The two sets of counts can not be compared directly, because mitosis runs faster than apoptosis. Taking the number of apoptotic or mitotic cells per 100 tumor cells as the apoptotic or mitotic index, they found the apoptotic index low in benign tumors, but it was low also for melanoma. A high apoptotic index does not correlate with a high mitotic index, and does not predict or correlate with sensitivity to chemotherapy. Each tumor type appeared to have its own characteristic apoptotic index (299). Later studies found that contrary to expectations, high levels of apoptosis correlated with worse survival (246). So far, then, it seems that no nuggets were collected on this path.

2. *Supposing that a gene related to apoptosis developed a mutation: what would happen?* We have a fine example: children born with a mutation of Bcl-2, an antiapoptotic gene, develop chronic, non-malignant lymphocytic infiltrates and an autoimmune syndrome: the latter is explained by the persistence of autoreactive lymphocytes, which failed to be eliminated due to the apoptosis defect (150, 151, 183). This is the autoimmune lymphoproliferative syndrome (ALPS). This syndrome can also be produced by mutations of the all-important FAS gene, one of the doorways to apoptosis (330).

3. *Would it be possible to harness apoptosis against cancer?* Yes indeed, this is done all the time: chemotherapy and radiotherapy act by inducing apoptosis in tumor cells as well as in normal cells, mainly by the mitochondrial pathway (150, 151). It would be ideal to have a drug that induced apoptosis in tumor cells but not in normal cells. There is news from Holland that a protein of viral origin, named apoptin, does just that (250). Too good to be true?

Is Apoptosis Reversible?

At the present time the consensus appears to be that the death sentence may be reversible before the activation of the caspases. Prior to that point, along the mitochondrial pathway, the fate of the cell is in the hands of the large Bcl-2 family of proteins: with some 15 members, some for apoptosis, some against, the cell may still have a chance.

Apoptosis methodology. There are manuals on this topic (280, 364) and commercial catalogs of reagents for apoptosis, including antibodies to individual caspases. Histology remains the cornerstone: what used to be called karyorhexis is almost always apoptosis. Immunohistochemical methods designed to visualize single- or double-strand DNA breaks, still used, have been criticized because they sometimes fail to distinguish apoptotic from nonapoptotic cell death (116); the same criticism has been directed to the electrophoretic laddering effect (71, 241a). However, intermediate forms of cell death do exist, so the lack of specificity may also reflect a biological reality.

A surprising development: apoptosis can be made visible (experimentally) by *magnetic resonance imaging:* the principle is to inject intravenous radioactive annexin V, which binds very specifically to phosphatidylserine (363).

NOTE: How can one obtain a massive amount of apoptotic cells for analysis, since apoptosis is non-massive by definition? The current method is to expose a suspension of cells (e.g., thymocytes) to UV light; controls are prepared by repeated freezing and thawing of similar cells (216).

Cell Death: Loose Ends

- In plants, programmed cell death is "a way of life" (117). The bark and the spines are made of dead cells; vessels are formed by the planned sacrifice of long rows of cells (105) that line up and die. The so-called hypersensitive response around an area of infection (see Figure 16.4) consists of dead cells. As in animals, there are two modes of cell death; caspase-like enzymes have been described, but on the whole the differences with apoptosis are more impressive than the similarities (117, 163, 164). There also is a planned death for bacteria (357).

- Denatured proteins typical of postoncotic necrosis, as we have seen, are autofluorescent. Nobody to our knowledge has tried to find out whether apoptotic cells are also autofluorescent.

- Apoptotic cell death was seen, understood, and published in 1914 by a German anatomist, Ludwig Gräper ("A New Point of View Regarding the Elimination of Cells" ([193]). Gräper even pointed out that this form of cell death served to counterbalance mitosis. Times were not ripe (193).

"Programmed Cell Death" as "Cell Death on Schedule"

Beware of another hiccup of terminology (193). Today, *programmed cell death* is used as a synonym for apoptosis.

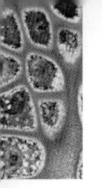

This is understandable, because all cells have at their disposal a genetically imprinted set of instructions—a program—for committing suicide. However, if you speak with an embryologist, you will discover another meaning of programmed cell death (193): this expression was actually coined by embryologists, to mean that some cells *die on schedule*. They die at a given time, suggesting that they have two kinds of genetic program: one to commit suicide (which may or may not be apoptosis) and the other to do so at a given time (41, 62, 177, 214, 319). This type of programmed cell death is an important mechanism for shaping the embryo (113): whole groups of cells die on schedule (113) as if they were deleted from the local development program (39). *Sometimes the deletion occurs because an organ has become obsolete;* such is the case of the pronephros. Cataclysmic examples of this kind occur during insect metamorphosis (178). *Nature also uses cell death to impart shape* (273, 274, 338), much as a sculptor hammers chips off a block of marble; this is how five digits are carved out of the rudimentary hand or foot, which initially looks like a solid paddle (14) (Figure 5.35). In the chick embryo, about the fourth day, a mass of cells dies in order to outline the rudimentary shape of the wing (Figure 5.36); if these cells are cut out and grafted to another part of the embryo, where their self-sacrifice

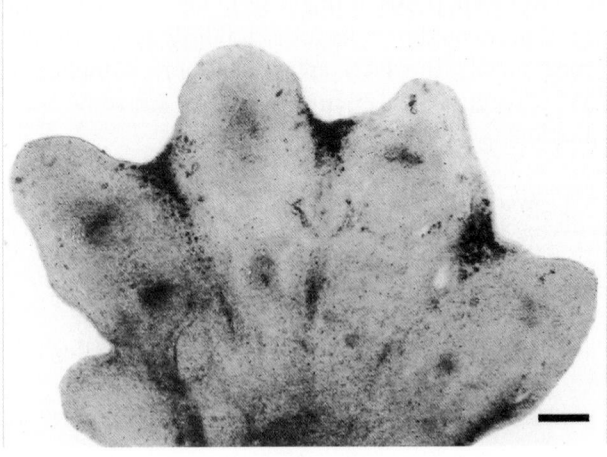

FIGURE 5.35　Section through the hind foot of a rat fetus at day 17, stained for acid phosphatase. The strong reaction in the interdigital tissues corresponds to areas where macrophages are busily removing the debris of dead tissue. The histochemical reaction is actually revealing the phagosomes of the macrophages. **Bar** = 200 μm. (Reproduced from [14] by permission from the Company of Biologists Ltd.)

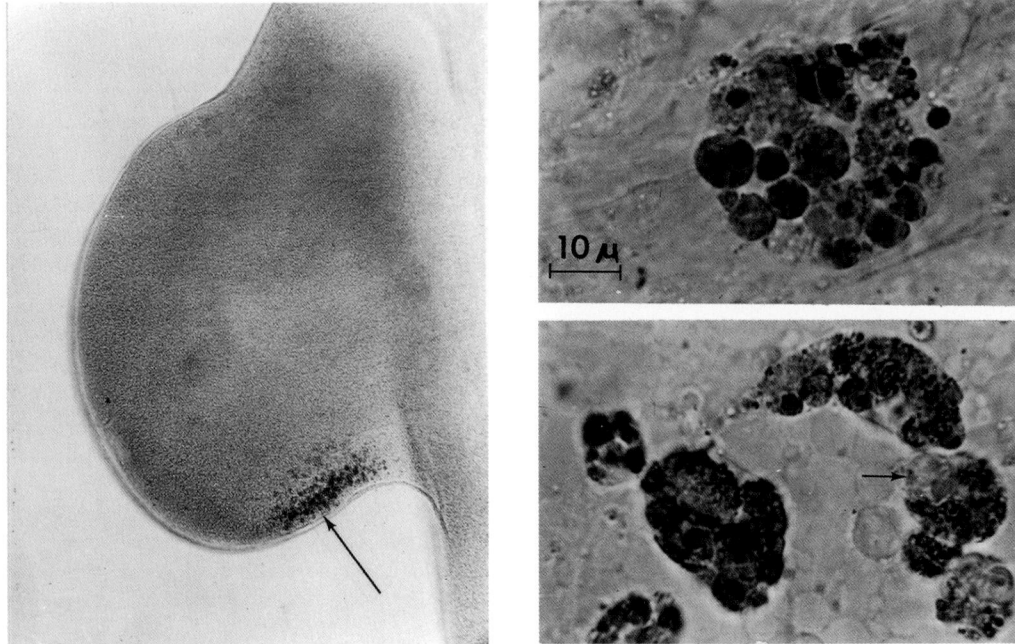

FIGURE 5.36　Typical "programmed cell death" in the original sense of *death on schedule*. *Left:* Wing bud of a 4-day chick embryo stained with neutral red and cleared (whole mount). **Arrow** points to a group of macrophages stained with neutral red and loaded with debris of dead cells. *Right:* Squash preparations to show the macrophages (**arrow**) filled with large phagosomes. (Reproduced by permission from [273]. Copyright 1966 by the American Association for the Advancement for Science.)

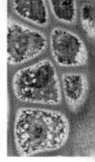

would not seem to be called for, they die anyway according to the original schedule (275).

Another fetal event dependent on cell death is the fusion of the two palatal shelves to produce a complete palate. For the two shelves to fuse, the covering epithelium must disappear, and it does so by apoptosis. There is some evidence that cortisone can prevent the fusion, suggesting a mechanism for certain malformations such as cleft palate (115).

Even tumors show programmed cell death (40). Those that arise from cells with an inborn deletion program, such as the epidermis, continue to express it: the malignant stem cells continue to multiply, producing cells that differentiate and progress to their death (p. 767) (39).

Cells programmed for deletion usually (but not always) die by apoptosis; therefore, programmed cell death in some models can be prevented by inhibitors of protein synthesis (81). Interestingly, in some forms of programmed cell death the ribosomes aggregate into crystals, a neat way to be put out of commission (Figure 5.37) (222, 235, 251).

Why Is Apoptosis Necessary?

The answers are spread throughout this book, but here are some points to keep in mind.

A perfectly healthy human being could live to 100 without experiencing massive cell death by the oncosis pathway (rare exceptions: e.g., bone cells can normally die by oncosis). Normally, billions of cells die every day by apoptosis. If they did not, disaster would follow. The embryo could not "chisel" itself into the proper shape;

the developing nervous system would be distorted by swarms of unwanted neurons; the maturing immune system would rapidly be overcome by autoimmune lymphocytes; the epidermis and other surface epithelia would become absurdly thick; and in the adult, the lack of a mechanism to counterbalance mitosis would lead to organ deformities incompatible with life.

Apoptosis is planned to perform as Nature's surgical knife: it acts swiftly (at least twice as fast as oncosis) and quietly (it does not trigger inflammation, as oncosis does).

Other Forms of Cell Death

The information available on apoptosis and oncosis could fill a large truck. There remains a small box of leftovers; the most challenging is the phenomenon of cell death in growth cartilage, illustrated in Figure 5.38 (145).

Long bones of young individuals grow in length because a transverse layer of cartilage at each end grows incessantly. Its cells form columns oriented along the axis of the bone; as they grow (in the direction *away* from the epiphysis) they swell progressively to many times their original volume (Figure 5.38) and eventually they die, leaving to capillaries, osteoblasts, and osteoclasts the job of turning cartilage trabeculae into bone trabeculae.

The expanding cells of the cartilage are traditionally known as hypertrophic ("zone of hypertrophic cartilage"), but in reality they are expanding until they burst and disappear. What is going on? The overall

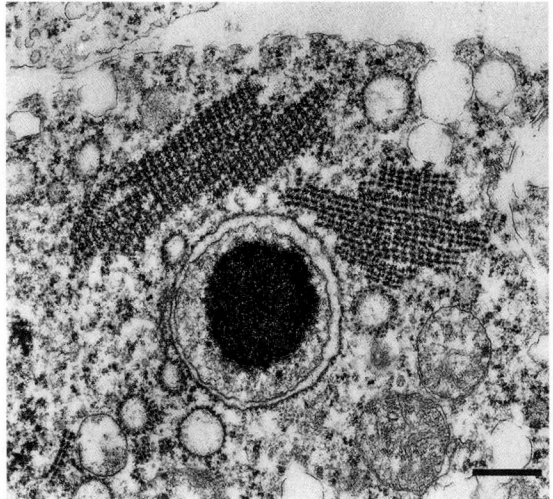
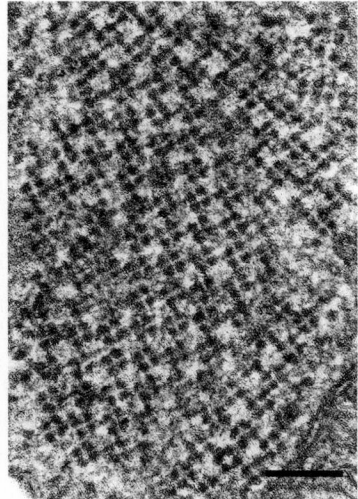

FIGURE 5.37 Crystallization of ribosomes during programmed cell death in a chick embryo. *Left:* In the limb bud ("posterior necrotic zone"). **Bar** = 0.5 μm. (Courtesy of N. Karle Mottet, M.D., Professor of Pathology, University of Washington School of Medicine, Seattle.) *Right:* In the spinal cord. **Bar** = 0.1 μm. (Reproduced from the **Journal of Cell Biology,** 1974;60:448–459, by copyright permission of The Rockefeller University Press [235].)

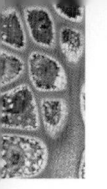

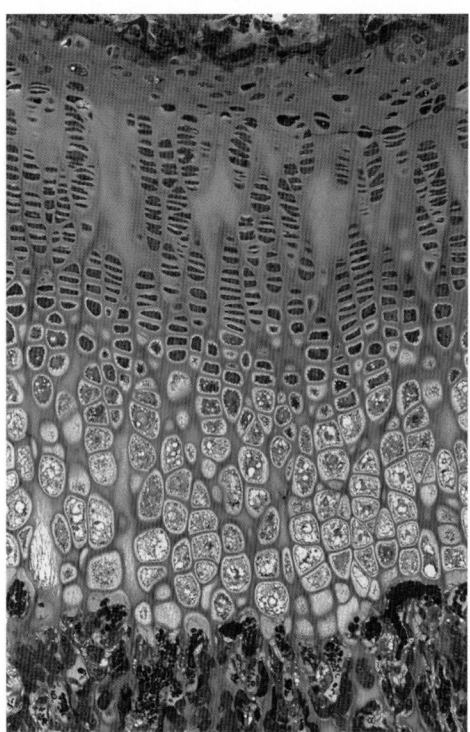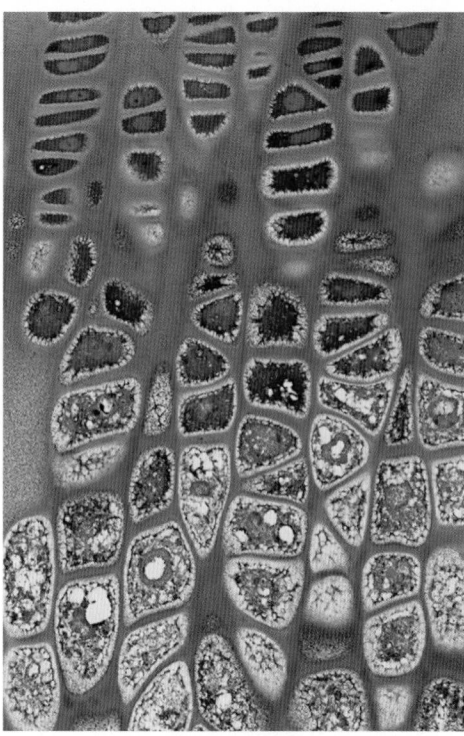

FIGURE 5.38   A common form of programmed cell death that fits no textbook category. Growth cartilage from the tibia of a newborn rat. *Left:* The cartilage cells (progressing from top to bottom) swell and eventually die, to be replaced by immature bone (far bottom). *Right:* Detail; the cells die by swelling and karyolysis, typical features of oncosis. (In other tissues, programmed cell death usually occurs by apoptosis; 1-μm section; toluidine blue stain.)

arrangement is a classic case of **programmed cell death:** these cells die on schedule. But instead of shrinking and performing apoptosis as most other cells programmed to die, they swell as is typical of oncosis.

To our knowledge, this type of cell death is unique; for the time being, we may call it **programmed cell death with oncosis.**

Another peculiar entity is **reproductive cell death.** Radiation can kill cells directly, but in low doses it only stops them from multiplying. The same effect is produced by many cytotoxic chemicals, also called radiomimetic for this very reason. The mechanism is damage to the DNA, best recognized microscopically as chromosomal abnormalities (p. 852). Some irradiated cells become gigantic (Figure 5.39). Many factors affect the extent of the damage: type and dosage of radiation, temperature, presence of protecting and sensitizing agents (especially oxygen), and stage of the mitotic cycle (135). Most affected are those tissues in which mature cells are produced by a relatively small number of rapidly dividing precursor cells, such as the bone marrow, the epidermis, the lining of the gut, and the testicular tubules. Cells thus deprived of their reproductive capacity may appear microscopically normal;

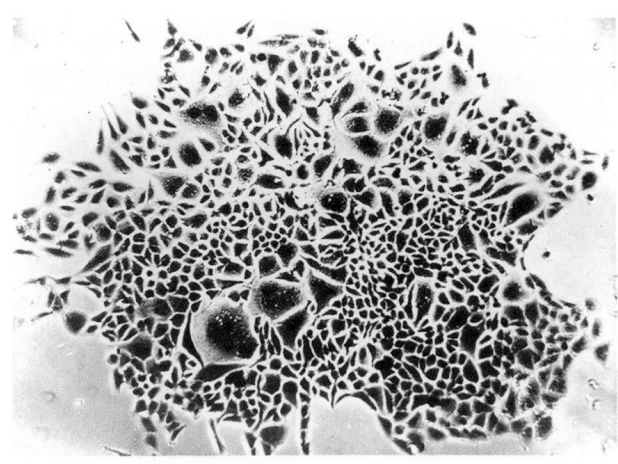

FIGURE 5.39   Changes induced by irradiation in a colony of cultured HeLa cancer cells. The large "monster" cells have lost their reproductive capacity but still carry on metabolic functions. (Reproduced with permission from [259].)

their defect can be brought to light experimentally by testing their ability to form colonies. This "hidden injury" is one of the long-term effects of radiation and cytotoxic therapy.

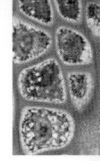

Other types of cell death have been described (262); we cannot review them here. Most are produced *in vitro* with toxic agents. Two themes recur: (a) there are intermediate forms between apoptosis and oncosis, and (b) different forms of cell death can be observed with different doses of the same toxic agent (339) or with a single agent at different times (167).

An example: Sanguinarine, an alkaloid of *Chelidonium majus* L., applied to a culture of erythroleukemic cells (12.5 μl/ml) induces "blister cell death," i.e., a single large "blister" (an intermediate between a bleb and an apoptotic "bud") without any blebbing. At 1.5 μl/ml it induces typical apoptosis (339).

Some bizarre manifestations of cell death, still unclassified, were made by Marcel Bessis in the cinematographic recordings mentioned earlier (29). The protagonists were leukocytes allowed to die in a thin layer of fluid between glass slide and coverslip. Here are two of their performances:

- In one neutrophil, the three lobes of the nucleus merged into one—perhaps a special case of pyknosis; this means that some of the mononuclear cells observed in inflammatory exudates could be obsolete neutrophils.

- Another granulocyte expelled the content of its nucleus, recalling the nuclear extrusion known to occur during the maturation of red blood cells and under the effect of cytochalasin (p. 158). This mechanism may be related to the process of self-amputation of cells recently reported as *autoschizis* (111). Nobody could ever guess that such events take place by looking at fixed cells, let alone homogenized cells in test tubes.

A final BEWARE: in the wake of apoptosis, new forms of cell death, or supposedly such, continue to be published. Some are real, some not. Among the latter is *autophagic cell death,* which can be traced to a misunderstanding: autophagocytosis and apoptosis can occur in the same cell, because both are induced by atrophy; but this does not mean that the cell is eating itself to death.

And a final teaser: there is no name for cell death by histologic fixatives, which—under ideal conditions—leave no visible trace. Cell death by protein crosslinking? By instant mummification?

After Cell Death: Necrosis

After the cells have died, they slowly proceed to lose all remnants of their normal structure; this is *necrosis,* a varied and interesting process despite its morbid name. Typically, it develops after oncotic cell death (*oncotic necrosis* [143a]) but when it is extensive, apoptosis too may undergo necrosis (apoptotic necrosis, "secondary necrosis" [7]).

Typically, massive necrosis develops after oncotic cell death (*oncotic necrosis* [143a]) but a large enough cluster of apoptotic cells can also become necrotic (*apoptotic necrosis*). In either case, necrosis will elicit an acute inflammatory response (p. 446). An *immune response* would seem to be against the interest of the individual: in fact protein denaturation in necrotic cells can be interpreted as a preventive measure against an immune response. However, an interesting picture is emerging: proteins from oncotic and apoptotic necrosis differ in their ability to activate dendritic cells (p. 227).

When necrosis is extensive enough it affects the body locally and generally, and within a few hours or days the necrotic mass itself undergoes three dynamic changes:

- *Calcium salts* accumulate.
- *Membrane cholesterol* becomes free and crystallizes.
- *Membrane phospholipids* form beautiful but pointless myelin figures.

Besides these relatively peaceful biochemical changes, a necrotic mass may be drastically modified by environmental effects (drying, infection) and turn into *gangrene:* an ancient and convenient clinical term that refers to necrosis modified either by exposure to air resulting in drying (dry gangrene), or by infection that turns it into a mixed bacterial culture (wet gangrene). Because both forms of gangrene are especially unsightly in animals, we will illustrate them in fruit (Figure 5.40).

The *drying up,* however ugly, is a favorable development relative to wet gangrene because bacteria cannot grow in dry tissue. An example of dry gangrene in mammals is the stump of the normal umbilical cord. The cord dies, dries up, and its connection with the live tissues is eventually severed; neutrophil enzymes do the actual surgery. Toes deprived of blood flow (e.g., by atherosclerotic arteries) share the same fate, and so do dead autumn leaves.

Wet gangrene is an ominous event. Bacteria swarming in the necrotic mass can easily diffuse into live tissue and into the bloodstream. *Gas gangrene* earns its name from anaerobic bacteria that produce visible and palpable bubbles of gas within the tissues. A typical setting: in a limb crushed in a motorcycle accident, the injured tissues

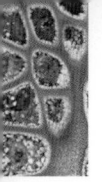

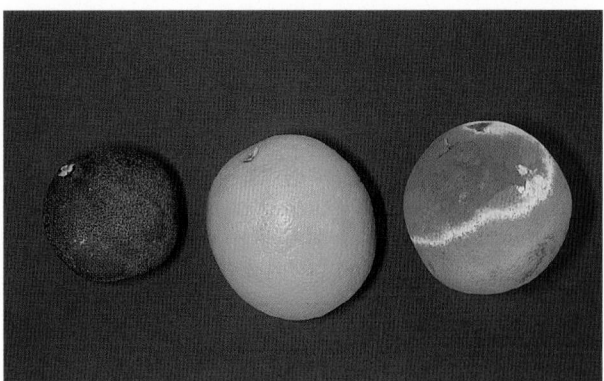

FIGURE 5.40 The notions of dry and moist gangrene illustrated with oranges. *Center:* Normal orange. *Left:* An orange that became dehydrated over several weeks at room temperature. It sustained no fungal or bacterial growth. This is essentially what happens to the umbilical cord after birth. *Right:* This orange became infected before it had the time to dry and is now overgrown by bacteria and molds, an equivalent of the fearful *moist gangrene* of animal tissues.

lose most or all of their blood supply and become a pasture for anaerobic bacteria picked up from the soil.

Calcium Deposition

Calcium begins to accumulate immediately, even before the cell dies (191). At first the deposits are not microscopically visible, but soon (hours, days) they appear as basophilic granules, usually smaller than nuclei. Occasionally the necrotic mass undergoes massive calcification. Because we are accustomed to think of cells as people, we visualize the macrophages nibbling at the necrotic mass as having a gritty meal. The complex process of calcification will be discussed later (Chapter 6). To underscore its importance, we will mention here only the most spectacular example, rarely seen in our days: the so-called **lithopedion,** or stone baby (Figure 5.41), in which the calcification actually makes the fetus stonelike.

> Today, the symptoms of tubal pregnancy call for immediate surgery. However, if a tubal pregnancy remains undiagnosed, it leads to rupture of the tube; thereby the embryo (or fetus) finds itself loose in the peritoneal cavity and dies. During past centuries, it was common for the "lost baby," incubated in the aseptic environment of the peritoneum, to undergo coagulative necrosis and then to calcify into a permanent lithopedion (365). This still happens occasionally (217).

There is a great deal of cholesterol in the plasma membranes: roughly half of the total lipid. When the cells die, the cholesterol slips out of the membranes, in which it

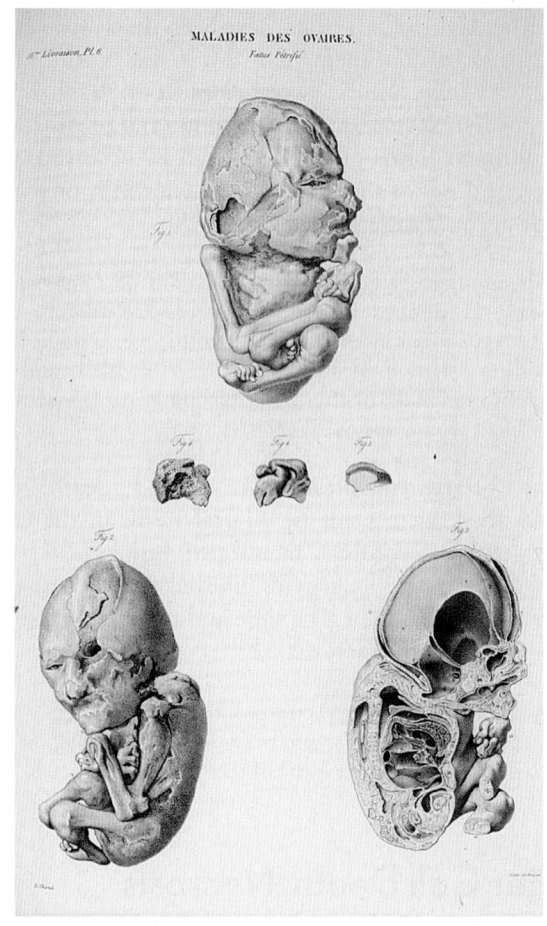

FIGURE 5.41 A "stone baby" (lithopedion) illustrated by Cruveilhier around 1842. A Parisian woman of 35, with one child, became pregnant. Toward the fourth or fifth month she suffered a prolonged episode of abdominal pain; then her abdomen shrank back to normal, the pain abated, and her periods reappeared. She had two more children, although she always felt that she had some kind of "foreign body" in her belly. In 1823, at age 77, she developed a strangulated hernia, was operated on, and died. At autopsy, this mummified, calcified fetus was discovered in the abdomen (60).

was floating almost freely, as you recall, not being held by covalent bonds. Because cholesterol is insoluble in water, it crystallizes into thin, flat rhomboid plates that have long attracted the curiosity of microscopists (Figure 5.42). In frozen sections they are birefringent; in paraffin sections they have been dissolved out, leaving the familiar cigar-shaped **cholesterol clefts,** which are cross sections of plates (Figure 5.43). The typical cigar shape, however, is an artefact due to tissue shrinkage; in tissues fixed for electron microscopy the clefts are always rectangular (Figure 5.44).

What happens next to the cholesterol crystals? Being insoluble in water they would persist indefinitely were

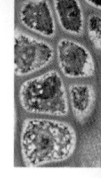

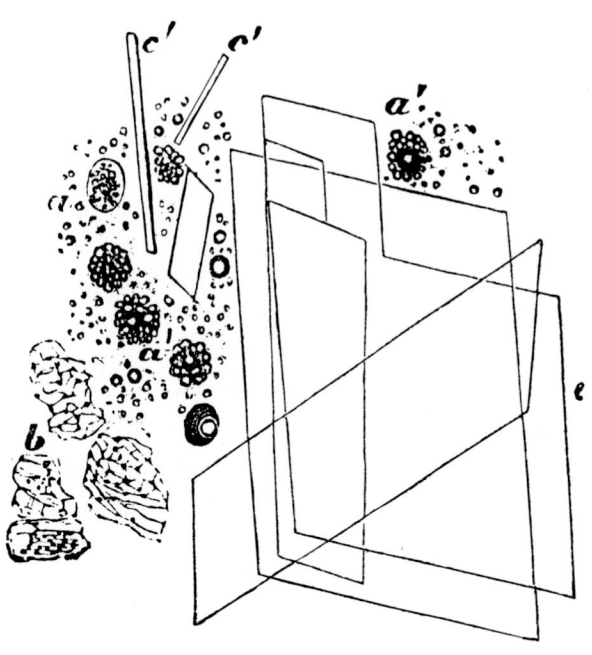

FIGURE 5.42   Microscopic crystals of cholesterol obtained from the necrotic center of an atheromatous plaque in an artery. Their typical shape is rhomboid, as shown in this drawing from 1873. (Reproduced with permission from [265].)

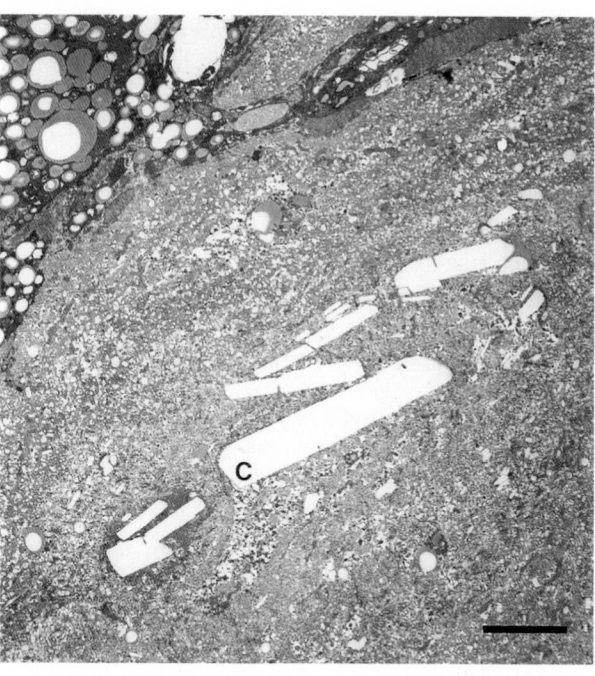

FIGURE 5.44   Crystals of cholesterol (**C**) in the necrotic core of a human atherosclerotic plaque as seen by electron microscopy. Part of a foam cell appears in the upper left corner. **Bar** = 5 μm.

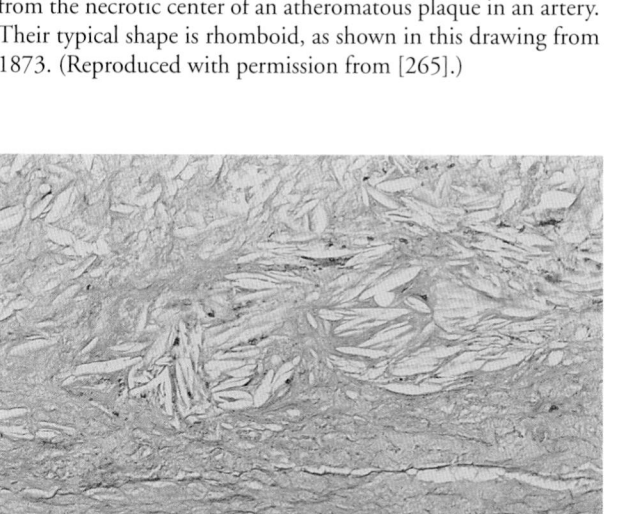

FIGURE 5.43   Empty, cigar-shaped clefts, about 50 μm in length, left by dissolved cholesterol crystals in the necrotic core of an atherosclerotic plaque. Such crystals are common in any necrotic mass; here they are especially prominent because the dead cells (foam cells) were loaded with cholesteryl esters.

it not for the macrophages, which are able to esterify cholesterol and then get rid of any excess via the HDL-lipoprotein pathway. From then on, there are only two ways for the body to rid itself of cholesterol: it can either excrete it through the bile (as the name

implies: *chole-sterol* means "bile sterol") or shed whole cells, cholesterol and all (p. 92).

Necrosis is a trap for calcium. Necrosis removes calcium from the plasma. So far we have emphasized the release of cell contents, but we should recall once again that necrosis absorbs calcium ions; if the necrosis is extensive, plasma calcium can drop low enough to cause tetany. This is, in our opinion, the mechanism of hypocalcemia in severe muscle necrosis (rhabdomyolysis) (159). We have already mentioned the special mechanism of hypocalcemia in fat necrosis: the formation of calcium soaps from triglycerides (302).

Necrosis elicits local and general reactions, namely inflammation, fever, and humoral changes.

We will deal with these events in the chapters on inflammation.

Myelin Figures

Myelin figures are stacks of phospholipid bilayers in the shape of spheres, cylinders, and spirals that develop wherever cells are destroyed. They are liquid crystals (288) and reflect the natural tendency of phospholipids to form bilayers. Because of their ordered molecular arrangement they can be birefringent, but in ordinary histologic sections they are usually invisible because they stain poorly. Presumably, when the cell dies, proteolysis

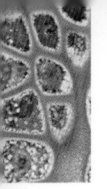

severs all links between cell membranes and cytoskeleton, and the phospholipids become free to follow the laws of physical chemistry. Phospholipids with a negative charge, such as phosphatidyl serine, swell the most (287).

Myelin figures grow like ghosts out of dead cells and are best seen if a fragment of tissue is allowed to die in water (Figure 5.45) (44). By electron microscopy, myelin figures can also be seen inside cells. In general, to the electron microscopist, *myelin figures (especially those free in tissue spaces) indicate that cell damage has occurred.*

The discovery of myelin figures by Virchow is a beautiful example of intuition and synthesis based on an extremely simple experiment. In his *Cellular Pathology* (1858) he

cells in which this substance quantity; still it is only in the

serve

Fɪɢ. 80.

substa

in all

contain

in the

only se

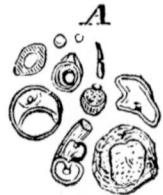 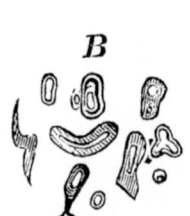

undergo a chemical change, or of chemical reagents. From

FIGURE 5.46   Myelin figures as drawn in 1858 by Virchow, who obtained them from nerves macerated in water.

explains that if bits of nerves are teased in water, their myelin sheaths expand into peculiar figures (Figure 5.46) (332). Anyone else would have dismissed these figures as unimpressive artefacts; but Virchow used them to argue, quite prophetically, that they represent a basic material present in all cells. What he really saw was phospholipid. In reading his lines, remember that he had described and named myelin but still knew nothing of phospholipids or cell membranes:

> Now it is very remarkable that this same substance [myelin] is one which most extensively prevails in the animal body. I had, curiously enough, in the first instance in the examination of lungs come across forms which presented very similar qualities to those we observe in the medulla of the nerves. Although this was very surprising, yet I did not really think there was an actual correspondence until I was gradually led [] to examine a number of tissues chemically. The result showed, that there scarcely exists a tissue rich in cells in which this substance does not occur in large quantity [] It is the same substance which forms the principal constituent of the yellow mass of yolk in the hen's egg [*perfectly true*], whence its taste and peculiarities, especially its peculiar tenacity and viscidity which are employed for the higher technical purposes of the kitchen, are familiar to everyone (332).

If we replace Virchow's *myelin* with *phospholipids*, we can readily understand why this key substance seemed to be present "in large quantities" in all cells. Virchow would have been delighted but not surprised to know that myelin and myelin figures, under the electron microscope, are very much alike (304).

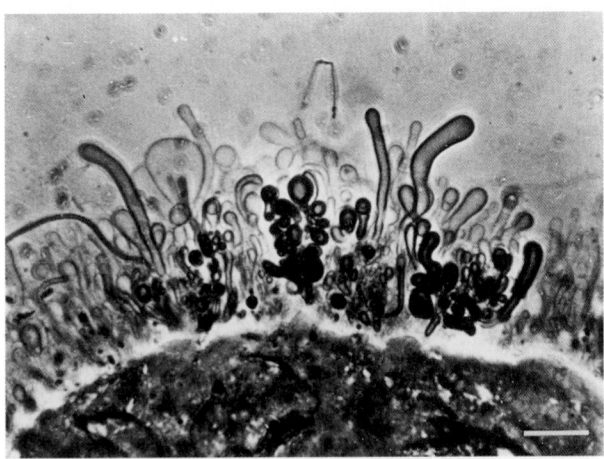

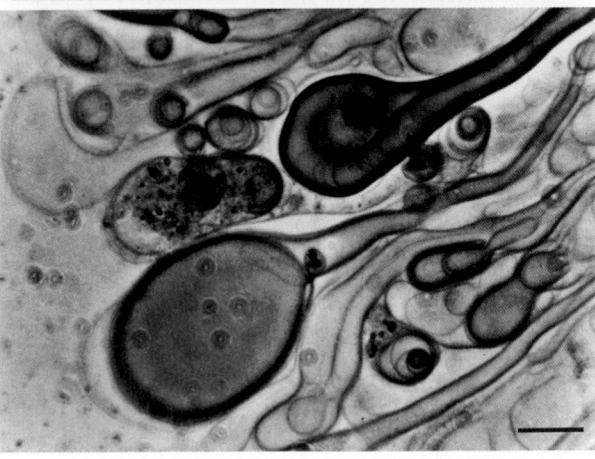

FIGURE 5.45   Myelin figures emerging from the edge of a piece of tissue (placenta) that was allowed to die in saline beneath a coverslip. *Top:* The phospholipid structures are enhanced by staining with Sudan black. *Bottom:* Multiple layers are visible in several of the myelin figures. Phase contrast microscopy. **Bars =** 10 μm. (Reproduced with permission from [44].)

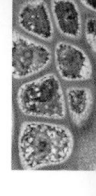

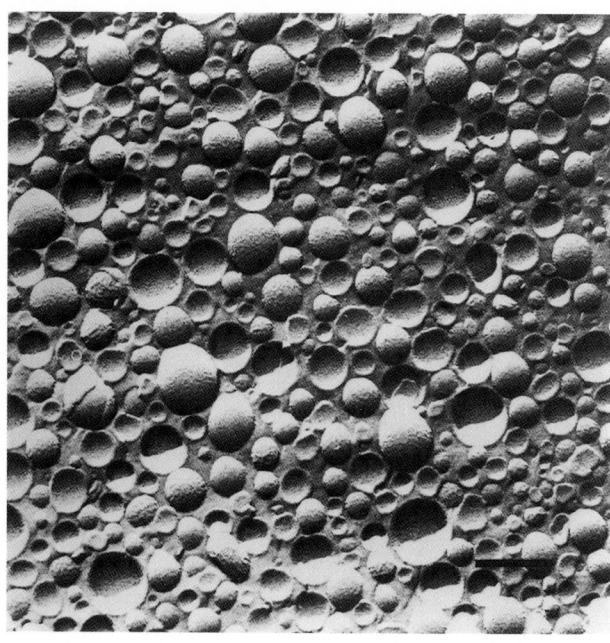

FIGURE 5.47 Liposomes, in a freeze-fracture electron micrograph of vesicles prepared from egg phospholipid. **Bar** = 0.2 μm. (Reproduced with permission from [206].)

Note also in passing that he found phospholipid in the lung; so he may well have discovered surfactant, the phospholipid that plays a key role in lung physiology, but it was not described until the 1950s (52, 188).

From myelin figures to liposomes. Once an interesting artefact, myelin figures have now leaped into prominence and even into commerce as **liposomes,** suspensions of standardized, spherical, microscopic myelin figures (Figure 5.47) (206, 240–242). They were born in the 1960s from studies of phospholipid emulsions (15). It had been clear for some time that phospholipid bilayers resembled cell membranes and could even be perforated by saponins just like them (16, 184); then Sessa and Weissmann (281, 282) proposed that spheres of such membranes, liposomes, could be made to represent actual models of cells by trapping in their cavity or incorporating into their membranes enzymes and a variety of water-soluble and lipid-soluble molecules. Because liposomes can be fused with real cells, they are used *in vitro* for transfection. Drug delivery by liposomes *in vivo* is another development (Figure 5.48) (43, 118, 213). The ultimate hope is that some day they may be injected intravenously and targeted to deliver their load in any selected organ, but at the present state of the art, when injected intravenously they are largely phagocytized by the sinusoidal phagocytes of the liver, spleen, and bone marrow (p. 314). This is a nuisance,

except for those cases in which the sinusoidal phagocytes happen to contain the target: a parasite.

Imagine this scenario. Certain fungal and parasitic agents hide and survive within phagosomes of the sinusoidal phagocytes. The phagocytic cells take up the parasites and cannot get rid of them. In essence, they nurture them. A classic case is Kala-azar (a tropical disease caused by the protozoan *Leishmania donovani*), which can be treated with antimonials, except that these compounds are very toxic if given intravenously (255). But if the antimonials are packaged in liposomes, they can be delivered into the blood quite safely; the liposomes are taken up by the sinusoidal phagocytes and then fused with the secondary phagosomes containing the parasites. It would be difficult to conceive a more advantageous delivery of the drug: the therapeutic index is multiplied by several hundred times (340).

Thus, myelin figures, that homely product of necrosis, are on the way to becoming a therapeutic weapon. Part of their fascination is that they bring biologists closer to an ancient dream: the artificial cell. The first cell, after all, must have been a globule about as simple as a liposome; and all living organisms, as George Palade once said, must represent a direct expansion of that original globule (243).

Molecules Released by Injured, Dying, and Dead Cells

Injured cells begin to spill their soluble contents even when the damage is reversible (1a); when they die they release what is left. The material leaching out of dying and dead tissue is relevant to pathology for several reasons:

- It is irritating to the surrounding normal tissues and sets up a local inflammatory response (p. 446).
- It may also have general effects, either toxic or injurious in some other way.
- It may attain blood levels high enough to be measured and thus become useful for diagnostic purposes.

The spilling is exploited *in vitro* and *in vivo* to measure the extent of cell damage and death; *in vivo,* the spilling raises the further issue of possible effects on surrounding tissues (inflammation) or even at a distance when the release is massive. Classic experimental and clinical settings in which this massive release can occur are infarction, especially of the heart (Figure 5.49), and the release of a tourniquet left too long in place.

The principal molecules released by dying and dead cells (besides excitotoxins, p. 228) are potassium, enzymes, uric acid, myoglobin, and other proteins.

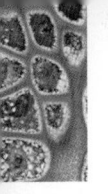

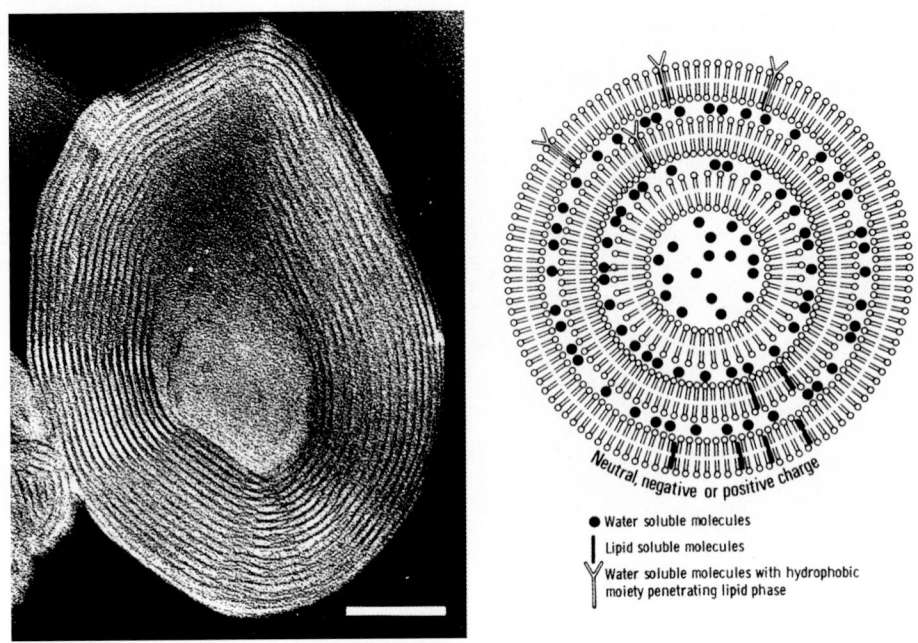

FIGURE 5.48 *Left:* A multilayered liposome as seen by electron microscopy in cross section. *Right:* Diagram of such a liposome, showing three bilayers of polar phospholipids alternating with aqueous compartments. Both water-soluble and lipid-soluble molecules can be inserted in such a structure, as indicated. **Bar** = 0.1 μm. (Reprinted, by permission of the New England Journal of Medicine 295:704–710,1976 [118].)

FIGURE 5.49 Time course of myocardial enzymes appearing in the blood after myocardial infarction. (Reproduced with permission from [350], copyright J. B. Lippincott Co. 1985.)

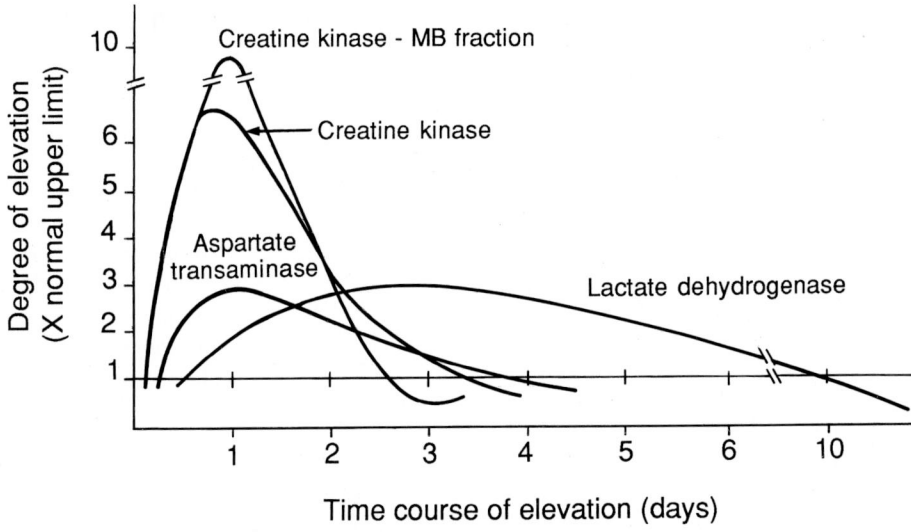

Potassium. Intracellular potassium is about 40 times the normal serum value (150–160 mEq/L versus 3.5–5.0 mEq/L); this means that *a dying cell is a small "potassium bomb."* The danger is greatest for the heart because it responds to high potassium concentrations quite simply by stopping (a solution of potassium at 25 mEq/L is used to hold the heart still during cardiac surgery). A life-threatening flood of potassium can reach the heart from two sources: a myocardial infarct or massive necrosis somewhere else in the body.

Electrocardiographic changes begin to occur at potassium plasma values of about 6 mEq/L and are severe at 8 mEq/L. To understand this potassium overload it helps to know that 100 gram of heart contain 250–293 mg of potassium (4); the adult body contains about 3600 mEq, about six times the lethal dose. About 300–600 mEq/L administered acutely can be lethal (148). During experimental ischemia, high potassium concentrations have actually been found in heart tissue spaces (140) and in coronary blood (132). An excess of extracellular potassium partially depolarizes the myocardial cells, first increasing and then decreasing ventricular conduction time (132). It has been postulated that the potassium gradient between normal and ischemic tissue creates an injury current that induces abnormal stimuli in the living, hyperexcitable tissue around infarcts (132), creating the risk of fatal arrythmia (91,132, 245).

A massive and lethal dose of potassium can be released from body tissues after **severe burns** and even under iatrogenic circumstances:

- In **tourniquet shock,** a life-threatening condition that develops when a tourniquet is maintained on a limb for several hours and then released, suddenly restoring blood flow (165, 225, 331);
- After **embolectomy:** when an embolus causing ischemia of a lower limb is removed surgically; blood flow is restored, and cardiac arrest can follow (127);
- In the **tumor lysis syndrome,** a paradoxical result of successful chemotherapy for leukemias and other highly proliferative malignancies that become acutely necrotic as a result of the treatment (47, 248, 337); this group of tumors includes Burkitt's lymphoma, a malignant tumor that is very sensitive to X-rays and chemotherapy (p. 830) (9).

Enzymes. As they leach out of dead cells *in vivo,* enzymes can find their way into the plasma, and when they do, they become invaluable clinically as signals that cellular injury and/or necrosis are occurring somewhere in the body (Figure 5.49). Oddly enough, the brain is an exception: dead brain tissue does not seem to release into the blood any significant amount of large molecules. Correspondingly, despite the frequency of cerebral infarcts (which occur in 80 percent of strokes), no test for brain enzymes is currently available (249). Presumably the blood–brain barrier interferes with the passage of enzymes across the endothelium. *The specific type of molecule, enzyme, or isozyme found in the plasma can indicate the organ involved (prostate, heart, etc.) and can even suggest the extent, timing, and evolution of the damage.* As might be expected, enzymes with smaller molecular weight are the first to escape.

Serious mistakes were made when it was not yet possible to distinguish similar enzymes originating from different tissues (isozymes). For example, the human heart and the human buttocks are very different, but both contain creatine kinase (CK). Years ago one of us was treated for myocardial infarction because of high plasma levels of this enzyme. It turned out later that the CK was coming from a poorly performed intramuscular injection.

The circulating enzymes rarely, if ever, cause any trouble. It may be relevant that 10 percent of plasma proteins are antiproteases. However, it is said that in severe acute pancreatitis, the heart, lungs, and kidneys may be affected (74, 185) and possibly also the brain (277).

Proteolytic enzymes in the blood can have general effects if their concentration is high enough. Pulmonary edema may develop as a result of myocardial ischemia, but the mechanism (not fully understood) seems to involve activated platelets (109). The effect of intravenous papain in the rabbit was studied by Lewis Thomas of literary (and pathologic) fame: the ears become droopy because the matrix of the cartilage is digested away (Figure 5.50) (208).

Myoglobin escapes from dead myocardium and striated muscle just as hemoglobin escapes from red blood cells (33). When large amounts of myoglobin are released by damaged striated muscles, the condition is called **rhabdomyolysis;** it can be initiated by severe trauma or burns, strenuous exercise, potassium depletion (e.g., by severe exercise in hot climates), alcohol and drug abuse, and many other factors (160, 201). The molecule of myoglobin (molecular weight about 16,000) escapes through the glomerular filter; if the urine is acid (360), the myoglobin precipitates in the tubules forming casts (solid plugs), which may lead to renal failure.

Troponin. Also escapes from injured myocardium, providing a very sensitive test for infarction (6).

Uric acid is normally present in cells and increases as a result of heat shock. When released in tissue spaces by damaged cells it stimulates the maturation of dendritic cells and acts locally as an immunologic adjuvant (p. 446). This means that it may play a role in initiating the immune response (282a). Uric acid becomes a problem in patients with malignancies that proliferate at a very high rate, especially leukemias (337), even in the absence of chemotherapy. Cellular purines are catabolized to xanthine and finally to uric acid; urate crystals precipitate in the renal tubules and can lead to acute renal failure. Hyperuricemia is actually a facet of the tumor lysis syndrome.

Other examples of bioactive materials released by necrotic tissue: renal infarcts release a short-acting vasopressor agent (124). Excitotoxins are released by neurons (p. 228). Toxic effects on the brain due to liver failure (hepatic encephalopathy) are due to several mechanisms, including the accumulation in the plasma of metabolic products that the liver failed to detoxify (98). Paradoxically, the slow destruction of the thyroid by an autoimmune process in

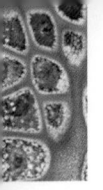

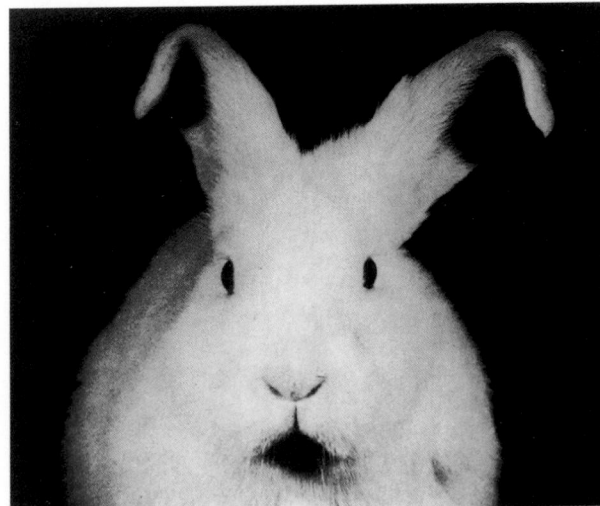

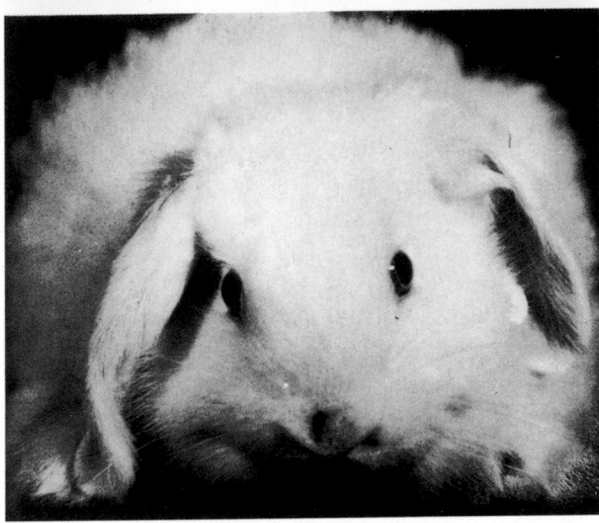

FIGURE 5.50 Illustrating the general effect of a proteolytic enzyme: two rabbits given 4 mg of papain intravenously, 4 hours (*top*) and 16 hours (*bottom*) before the photograph was taken. Enzymatic degradation of the cartilage matrix throughout the body caused the ears to collapse. (Reproduced from the **Journal of Experimental Medicine,** 1958;108:371–384, by copyright permission of The Rockefeller University Press [208].)

Hashimoto's disease can lead to hyperthyroidism, which is attributed to the reabsorption of colloid.

Some 30 years ago it was believed that liver necrosis releases products toxic to the kidney (162); the current belief is that those experiments, carried out on dogs, were misleading due to the presence of bacteria in normal dog livers.

Disposal of circulating cellular proteins. Enzymes and other cellular proteins that gain access to the plasma are eliminated via the kidney or slowly removed by the sinusoidal phagocytes of the liver, spleen, and bone marrow

(p. 315). Occasionally some intracellular material is recognized as foreign by the immune system and gives rise to autoantibodies.

Antibodies against heart tissue have been studied a great deal because of a mysterious syndrome that can appear 2–6 weeks after an infarct (pain, fever, leukocytosis, and a "pericardial rub" indicative of pericardial inflammation) (176). An autoimmune response was thought to be responsible, but the mechanism is still unknown. Antibodies against cardiolipin certainly do develop after myocardial infarction; in fact, high titers of these antibodies may be a marker for patients at increased risk for recurrent cardiovascular accidents (233). Cardiolipin is a phospholipid found only in mitochondria and bacteria (278).

Massive Bacterial Death

Treating a patient with an effective antibacterial drug, such as tetracycline for Lyme disease, can lead to a nasty surprise: within 1–2 hours a sudden chill is followed by fever, sweating, hyperventilation, hypertension, and then a drop in blood pressure (31). The mortality rate of about 5 percent (88). This is the **Jarisch-Herxheimer reaction,** first observed by these two men in 1895 and 1902 while treating syphilis with mercury. Herxheimer called it a *Quecksilberreaktion,* and incidentally, it *proves to us today that the ancient treatment with mercury did kill the spirochetes.* The pathogenesis is now believed to be similar to that of septic shock, namely: massive bacterial death → massive phagocytosis by macrophages → activation of the macrophages, which secrete TNF-alpha and other cytokines, which cause the symptoms (31, 88). An unpredictable price to pay for powerful antibiotics.

Cell Death and Necrosis in Special Tissues

The basic rules of cell death and necrosis do not change from tissue to tissue, but cells differ; thus, special problems arise with each type of tissue. The main examples follow.

Death of Central Nervous Tissue

Nervous tissue is special in many ways. Not surprisingly, the pathology of cell injury and cell death is also special (85). We will mention just three unusual features:

1. Excitotoxicity. This troublesome phenomenon (239) is specific to the brain, but it illustrates a general principle: stores of powerful chemical mediators are dangerous, rather like factories of fireworks (p. 315). The synapses in gray and white matter are loaded with excitatory neurotransmitters, which must be instantly available and are therefore preformed. The most prominent is **L-glutamate,** an essential and also very toxic molecule. Under normal conditions the extracellular portion of L-glutamate is highly controlled by five groups of glutamate transporters (310); but as a result of acute injuries, such as trauma, anoxia or ischemia, large amounts of L-glutamate are released from the cellular stores, resulting in overstimulation of the neurons' glutamate receptors, some of which control intracellular calcium. Toxic amounts of calcium seep into the neurons and may kill them; overstimulation of the neurons can also lead to further release of L-glutamate, initiating a vicious circle that is lethal to the neurons (10).

> Glutamate, of course (as monosodium glutamate) is one of the most common food additives. The so-called *Chinese restaurant syndrome* (headache, dizziness, nausea) is due to glutamate; in fact, "the neurotoxic effects of glutamate were discovered as a result of investigations into the use of MSG as a food additive" (10, 239).

2. Free radical damage. Almost any type of injury to the brain or cord will cause some red blood cells to spill into the tissue. In other organs these stray red blood cells would be quickly picked up by macrophages; in central nervous tissue this process is slower, and the iron of hemoglobin has the time to mediate free radical reactions, to which this tissue is especially sensitive.

3. Liquefaction. When a mass of brain tissue dies as a result of ischemia, many neuron cell bodies undergo coagulation necrosis (and turn into "red neurons" [107]) but the white matter and the tangle of cell processes in the grey matter (called "neuropil") break down into a milky fluid, a change that requires 5–10 days. Brain tissue does not contain more hydrolases than other organs, but the dead fibers and fibrils tend to break up into droplets, whereby the tissue disintegrates, producing the familiar "brain softening" (Figure 5.51). The resulting emulsion contains, besides myelin figures, large numbers of foam cells derived from blood monocytes and from the local population of macrophages (the **microglia**).

Death of Myocardial Tissue

Heart fibers are unique in that they beat. When they suddenly die, in an infarct, they cease to beat within one minute. We now have the situation of live, pulsating fibers rhythmically tugging at the ends of paralyzed but still live fibers. The result is that the paralyzed fibers are progressively drawn out and become long, thin, and wavy (38). Exactly how fast this occurs has not yet been determined, but the delay is certainly less than 3 hours and perhaps as short as 30 minutes. The wavy fibers,

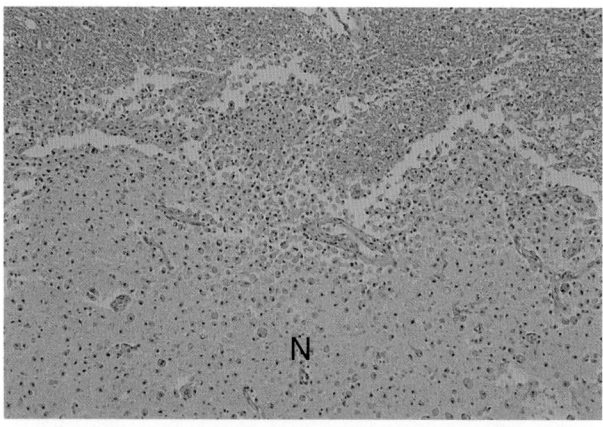

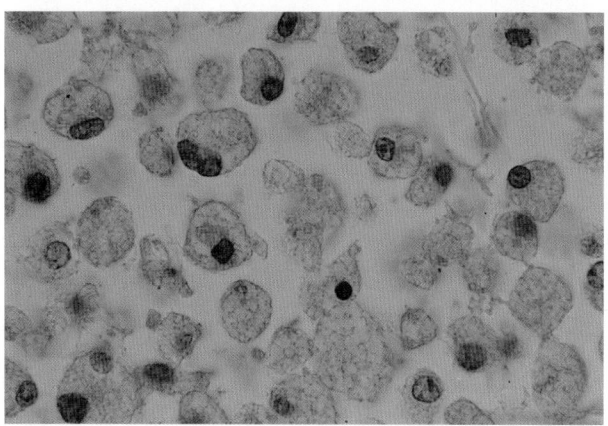

FIGURE 5.51 Cerebral infarction. *Top:* The necrotic brain tissue (**N**) liquefied and attracted swarms of macrophages (derived from blood monocytes and brain microglia) that are phagocytizing the debris. Note the sharp demarcation line between the necrotic tissue and the living tissue above it. This type of change can occur within 48 hours of infarction. *Bottom:* Detail showing macrophages loaded with myelin debris. (Courtesy of Dr. T. W. Smith, University of Massachusetts Medical School, Worcester, MA.)

initially, probably represent a reversible injury. *Thus, the heart offers a unique exception to the rule that cell death cannot be recognized before 6–8 hours* (p. 203).

Death of Adipose Tissue

Focal death of adipose tissue (also called fat necrosis or **steatonecrosis**) is not uncommon, especially after trauma or (in the abdomen) by spilling of pancreatic enzymes (Figure 5.52). *The distinctive biological feature of adipose tissue necrosis is that the fat released by the cells becomes an irritant.* First the macrophages feast on it and turn into foam cells or into multinucleated Touton cells (Figure 5.53). Then the fibroblasts take part in the action and lay down an abundance of

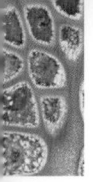

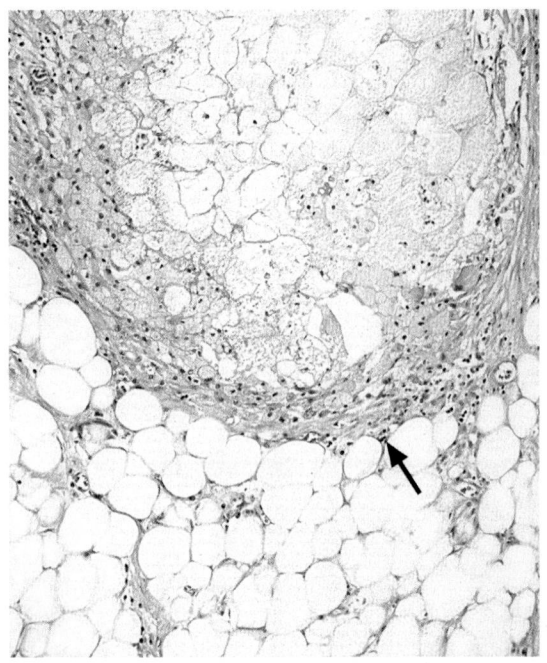

FIGURE 5.52   Necrosis of fat tissue (*top*) in a case of acute pancreatitis. Faint outlines of fat cells are still recognizable. *Bottom:* Normal fat tissue. **Arrow:** Fibrous layer indicating that the necrosis must be about 2–3 days old.

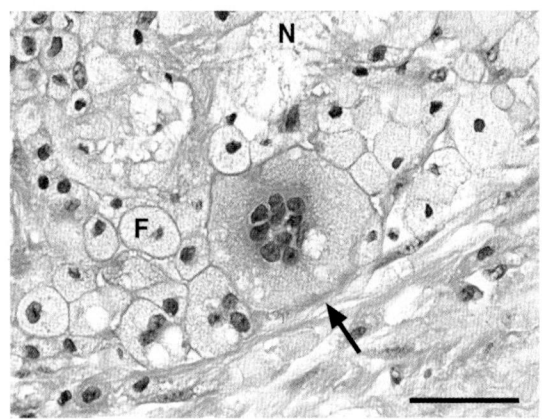

FIGURE 5.53   Cellular responses to necrotic fat cells (**N**). **F:** Foam cells (macrophages loaded with cholesteryl esters). The cholesteryl esters were dissolved in the triglycerides released by the necrotic fat cells. **Arrow:** Typical Touton cell, derived by fusion of foam cells. **Bar** = 50 μm.

collagen (Figure 5.54), which feels—if it can be palpated through the skin—like a firm mass. Now imagine a trauma to the female breast (e.g., by a car accident); a firm lump of fat necrosis leads to a difficult differential diagnosis with a tumor, benign or malignant.

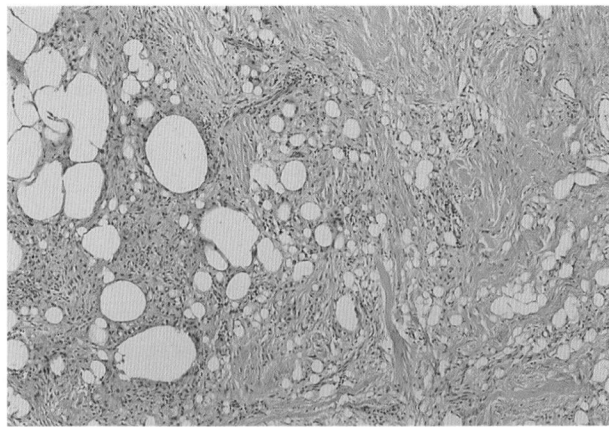

FIGURE 5.54   Long-term result of trauma on adipose tissue: intense fibrosis as a reaction to shattered fat cells. The clear spaces of irregular size and shape are droplets of free fat, which produced a macrophage response as well as a fibroblast response. When this sequence of events occurs in the female breast, the firm fibrotic lump may suggest the clinical diagnosis of tumor.

The lively tissue reaction occurs because the triglycerides break down giving rise to fatty acids, which are irritants. Some are probably inactivated by binding with the ever-present carrier, albumin. Another fraction of free fatty acids combines with calcium and becomes soap. Calcium soaps are recognizable in frozen sections as bundles of needles.

Fat necrosis in the abdominal cavity due to the spilling of pancreatic enzymes is a catastrophic event that occurs when the digestive enzymes are activated in the living pancreas. The cause of this explosive activation is not always clear; trauma, ischemia, infection, a huge meal, or alcoholic debauch are sometimes involved. Whatever the initial cause may be, masses of adipose tissue are damaged by the enzymes not only in the peritoneal cavity but even as far as the thoracic cavity or in the bone marrow. The lethal blow to the fat cells is probably given by pancreatic phospholipases that attack their membranes. Strangely enough, although the enzymes are spilled all over the peritoneal cavity, the resulting fat necrosis is typically focal; it presents as whitish, pea-sized, superficial spots on the omentum and wherever adipose tissue is present. These spots look very much like wax dropped from a candle (Figure 5.55), hence their very descriptive French name, *taches de bougie* (candle drops). Histologically these candle drops consist of necrotic fat cells surrounded by a halo of inflammation. *When fat necrosis is very extensive, the mass of dead cells and fatty acids can drain enough calcium from the plasma (forming calcium soaps) to induce hypocalcemic tetany.*

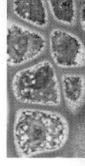

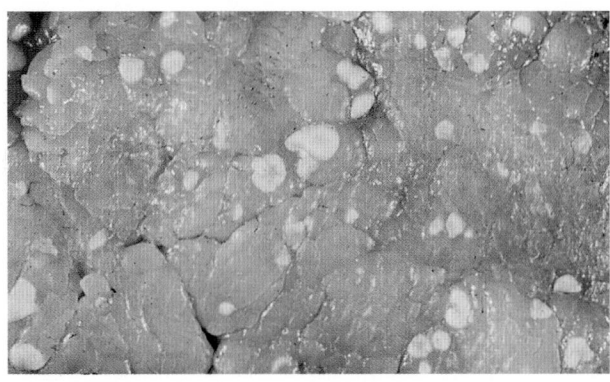

FIGURE 5.55   Small foci of fat necrosis ("candle drops") on retroperitoneal fat in a case of acute hemorrhagic pancreatitis. Natural size. (Courtesy of Dr. E. Soto, St. Vincent Hospital, Worcester, MA.)

Fat cells can sometimes be killed from inside by a crystallization of their own fat droplet. This can happen if the temperature drops beneath the melting point of the triglycerides, as in hypothermia, or because the triglycerides have an abnormally high melting point. This occurs physiologically in the newborn (101).

Death of Bone Tissue

Bone necrosis always occurs in fractures and sometimes after X-irradiation. The behavior of dead bone is unique in several respects. Bone is inhabited by *osteocytes,* cells imprisoned within the calcified matrix and communicating with each other and with bone surfaces by a network of microscopic canals. Whenever a group of osteocytes dies, the bone itself remains for a time outwardly and chemically unchanged; it does not become decalcified but simply loses its microscopic tenants (Figure 5.56). However, over days, weeks, and months, *the osteoblasts on the bone surfaces somehow receive the message that the bone tissue beneath them is dead; osteoclasts appear and slowly erode all the dead tissue while osteoblasts replace it with new bone.* After a fracture this process requires several months.

However, if the necrotic bone becomes infected, the sequence of events is entirely different. This can happen, for example, in an open fracture, or in the jaw after irradiation for a tumor in the mouth, which is a great source of bacteria. Once the necrotic bone is permeated with bacteria, the bone-resorbing cells no longer attack it; instead, they carve their way around it and isolate it. From this point on, the dead infected bone becomes an infected foreign body (a **sequestrum**), which can persist for years and continue to maintain the infection unless it is removed surgically. *Foreign bodies in general have the peculiar property of sustaining infection* (p. 494).

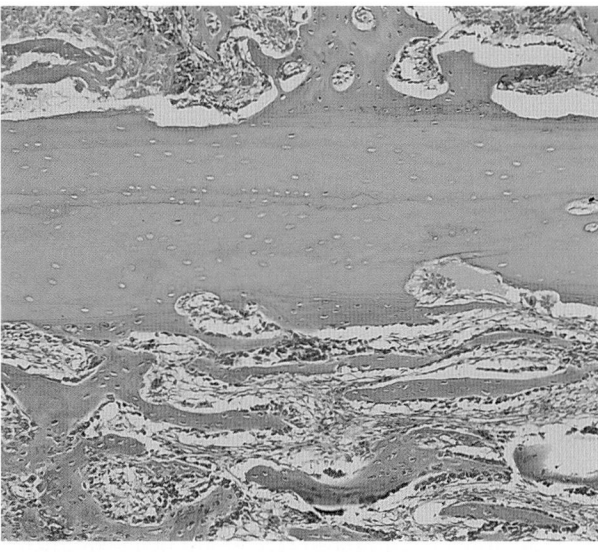

FIGURE 5.56   Rabbit tibia 21 days after an aseptic fracture. The original, compact tibial bone (*center*) is dead, as shown by the empty spaces (*lacunae*) left by the osteocytes. Note the two opposite repair processes at work: slow *reabsorption* of the dead bone (especially along the lower surface) and *outgrowth* of new, branching "osteophytes." Within weeks and months, the spaces between the branches of the osteophytes will be lined with layers of new bone.

Necrosis of Hollow Organs

So far we have discussed necrosis in solid organs, such as the brain or liver. Special problems arise when necrosis occurs in the wall of hollow organs such as the gut or the gall bladder. An example: if a segment of the intestine dies (e.g., by ischemia), the necrotic mucosa can no longer function as a barrier to the bacteria contained in the lumen; the muscular layer is paralyzed, peristaltic movements cease, and thus the necrotic segment of gut acts as an obstruction; the bacteria in the lumen produce gas, which stretches the weakened wall and may cause it to burst.

Epithelial cells that slough off from the mucosa of an injured hollow organ, such as an ischemic intestine, are generally thought to be dead; this may be too pessimistic. In renal ischemia, renal tubules shed many of their epithelial cells into the urine and eventually produce the histologic picture of "acute tubular necrosis." However, when cultured, 25–30 percent of the cells shed in the urine are found to be still alive. Shedding therefore precedes cell death (260).

Autolysis

The best way to study the capacity of tissues for "self-digestion" is to maintain them under sterile conditions

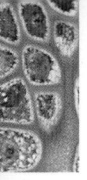

in a refrigerator. The cells slowly break up and release some of their lysosomal enzymes, which find the acid pH that they require. The digestive process is very slow, in part because protein denaturation is also taking place, although much more slowly than in an infarct: what takes hours *in vivo* will take months in a refrigerator (194).

In the context of an autopsy, of course, the process of autolysis is complicated by bacterial infection. Still, the breakdown is most severe in organs that are loaded with digestive enzymes, mainly the pancreas, which literally self-destructs in a few hours. For obscure reasons, the adrenal medulla also tends to liquefy: this is why early anatomists thought that the adrenals were empty bags (hence the name **adrenal capsules** in the older literature). Histologically, the destructive effects of lysis and denaturation vary from tissue to tissue; eventually the nuclei can no longer be stained (**karyolysis**). In the kidney, for instance, the glomeruli are relatively resistant, whereas the convoluted tubules autolyze very fast, perhaps because they contain more lysosomes. To the inexperienced eye, tubular autolysis can be mistaken for tubular necrosis due to circulatory failure or toxic agents (Figure 5.57). This "disappearance" of the nuclei may be only apparent; chemical analysis has shown that 50 percent of the DNA is still present in tissue autolyzing *in vitro* at 37°C when the nucleus in histologic sections appears only as a ghost (326).

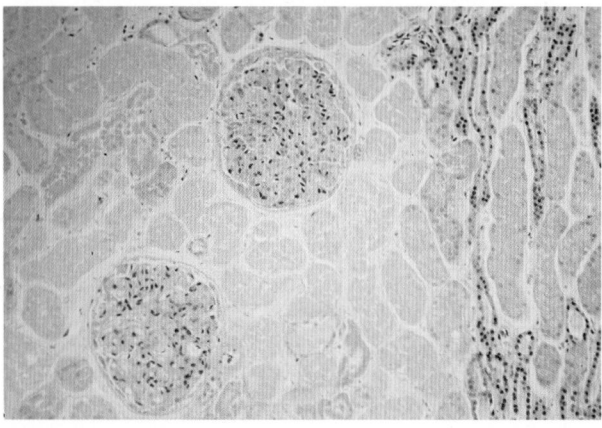

FIGURE 5.57 Postmortem autolysis in a human kidney, as often seen when the autopsy is performed as late as 18–24 hours after death. The nuclei in most of the tubules are no longer stainable. There is no doubt that this change occurred *post mortem* because necrosis of the tubules in a living kidney would have elicited a lively inflammatory reaction, and no such response is seen.

Obviously, it is best to perform autopsies as early as feasible. After 12 hours many structures are already marred by artefacts. Changes that occur within 3–5 hours can still be reversed if small samples are incubated in an oxygenated medium (18, 89, 294).

Does autolysis occur *in vivo?* It certainly does. As we mentioned earlier, whenever a cell dies, its proteins are caught between two fates: lysis, mainly by the cell's own enzymes, and denaturation, somehow favored by the surrounding live tissues, perhaps because they supply calcium. It follows that in the centers of very large infarcts autolysis prevails.

Autolysis raises an interesting question: when the whole body has been dead for 24 hours, why does it not appear like a massively coagulated infarct of the same age? The answer is that *postmortem autolysis and necrosis* in vivo *are very different phenomena.* Around a focus of necrosis, the circulation removes the breakdown products (thereby accelerating the breakdown reactions); it removes the acid, whereby the pH climbs back to slightly alkaline (Figure 5.19); it also removes pigments that are diffusing out, such as hemoglobin and its breakdown products, thus enhancing the whiteness of the necrosis; it supplies calcium (probably the main accelerator of denaturation) and other materials, including cells and enzymes that digest the tissues from outside (**heterolysis**). Therefore, paradoxically, the net effect of the surrounding blood flow is to accelerate the destruction. For example, a segment of kidney deprived of its blood supply dies, and after 2 or 3 days it will appear as a firm, white mass of necrotic tissue (white infarct); by contrast, if the kidneys are left in place after death, they will change aspect, but no matter how long we may wait, they will never look like a white infarct.

Some useful lessons have been learned from the study of tissue samples autolyzing *in vitro* (144, 194, 228, 325, 326), including contributions from food technology (166). (a) Refrigeration, of course, slows down the process. (b) Lysosomes in autolyzing tissues remain fairly well preserved (325, 326) and contain histochemically demonstrable acid phosphatase even after 4 hours of incubation at 37°C (114) (another blow to the suicide bag hypothesis). (c) Mitochondria lose their small dense granules (probably loaded with divalent cations) within 15 minutes; this can probably be taken as an index of ischemia *in vivo.*

On a more tasteful note, the sweetening that occurs as fruit ripens is partly an autolytic process; tasteless starch breaks down to tempting sucrose, glucose, and fructose. The chemical breakdown, however, occurs within the living cell (120, 121).

Autolysis in bacteria. In bacteria, autolysis is part of life. Enzymes called *autolysins* break down the bacterial wall, especially during cell division; antibiotics of the beta-lactam group (including penicillin) favor the action of autolysins in dividing bacteria, so that the wall becomes thinner, expands, and may eventually burst (317). If the wall contains endotoxins—as is the case for gram-negative bacteria—a dying bacterium that undergoes autolysis, releasing endotoxin and other irritating fragments of its wall, can be more irritating than a live bacterium (46).

How Cells Kill Each Other

When the rumor began to spread in the 1960s that cells could kill each other, it was greeted with skepticism. Could violence really extend to cells?

It certainly does. Without it we could not live: our immune system is based on killing the wrong kinds of lymphocytes and keeping the right ones. Much of the killing is directed against aggressors such as bacteria, viruses, and tumors. Killer (*cytotoxic*) cells in mammals are mainly the NK (natural killer) cells (Figure 5.58), cytotoxic T cells (including the T cell subset called NKT [186]), and sometimes B cells (230) and macrophages.

> Granulocytes are certainly professional killers, but highly specialized for killing bacteria by several means, including bactericidal *defensins* (p. 369). *Innocent bystander cells* can be killed by them accidentally, especially in acute inflammation when the tissue is soaked with enzymes from activated or dead granulocytes.

Killing by Lymphocytes

Killer lymphocytes can dispatch their victims in two ways: (a) by the rather brutal procedure of inserting cylindrical plugs into the victim's membrane and pouring proteolytic enzymes into them (the *perforin-granzyme* procedure) and (b) by instructing the victim (if it has the necessary molecular equipment) to kill itself by apoptosis. In either case the sequence, observed in live preparations of mixed killer and target cells, is impressive (136). The killer cells roam about until they make contact with a target cell; two or three killer cells may latch onto a single target cell (Figure 5.59). If the execution calls for apoptosis—it often does—the target cell undergoes violent budding (the "death dance," p. 211) and dies, sometimes in minutes;

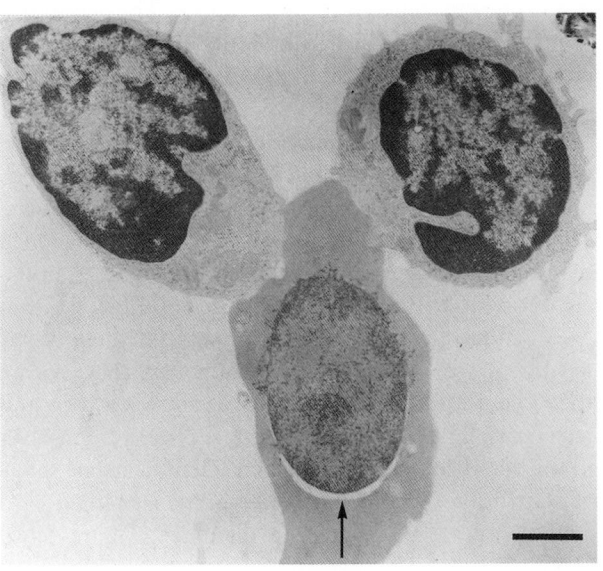

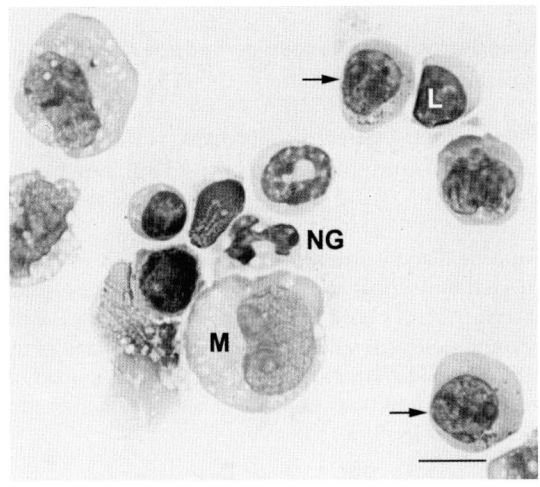

FIGURE 5.58   Cells obtained from mouse liver. **Arrows:** Natural killer cells, also called large granular leukocytes; **M** = monocyte/macrophage; **NG** = nucleus of granulocyte; **L** = lymphocyte. Stain: Wright-Giemsa. **Bar** = 10 μm. (Preparation courtesy of K.W. McIntyre, University of Massachusetts Medical School, Worcester, MA.)

FIGURE 5.59   Cell killing: Two B lymphocytes attacking an antibody-coated red blood cell of a chicken. The target cell shows signs of impending death: faintly staining chromatin, dilatation of the perinuclear cisterna (**arrow**). This task is normally reserved to T cells; very few B cells can perform it. Those here shown were obtained from tumor-bearing mice. **Bar** = 1 μm. (Reproduced with permission from [181].)

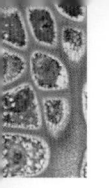

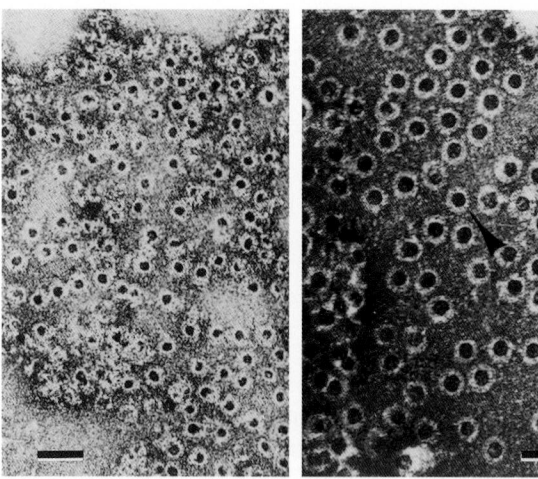

FIGURE 5.60 Comparing membrane lesions formed by complement and by cytotoxic lymphocytes. *Left:* Human complement lesions; internal diameter, 100 Å. *Right:* Lesions due to polymerized mouse perforin 1 (**arrowhead**), internal diameter, 160 Å. **Bars** = 0.05 μm. (Reproduced from Mechanisms of Host Resistance to Infectious Agents, Tumors, and Allografts 1986 by copyright permission of the Rockefeller University Press [253].)

in the meantime the killers wander off in search of new targets. Each killer lymphocyte can destroy up to a dozen target cells in a few hours. The apoptosis sequence in this setting runs faster than under other circumstances (136, 270, 358). A few submicroscopic details:

1) The Perforin-Granzyme Procedure is restricted to lymphocytes, including NK cells. The killer cell latches onto its target, tightly enough to form what was called an "immunological synapse" (19), and then rearranges its cytoplasm so that the toxic granules are brought to face the contact zone (122). Within 5–15 minutes the granules are extruded into the narrow space between the cells, where they release their chemical weapons, proteins called *perforin* and *granzymes*. The molecules of perforin insert themselves in the target cell's membrane and assemble in the shape of short tubes, whereby the membrane is riddled with gaping holes, 100–200 Å in diameter (Figure 5.60) (136).

A similar aggressive, perforating device is used by "complement," which we will describe with inflammation as *a machine for poking holes in cells, which normally circulates disassembled in about 20 pieces.* It sometimes happens that Nature uses similar molecular devices under different circumstances (recall the similarities between proteasomes and the HSP GroEL [p. 188]). In fact there is a 30 percent

homology between perforin and the corresponding molecule C9 of complement [136]).

At first the killing mechanism seemed obvious: the granzymes seep through the perforin holes, activate the caspases, and kill the target cell by apoptosis. Then the facts became much more complicated; there are 11 kinds of granzymes; they do not necessarily pass through pores; and sometimes the target cell dies not by apoptosis, but by *nonapoptotic death* (19). As to the inevitable question—how is the attacking lymphocyte protected against its own chemical weapons? we have a beginning of an answer: there is a protease inhibitor to granzyme B (19).

2) Death by the Fas/Fas Ligand Procedure does not require pore formation or enzyme secretion; the target cell, however, must express the Fas receptor on its surface. The killer comes along with Fas Ligand exposed, and the rest is predictable (p. 213). How the killer lymphocyte chooses to inflict one or the other type of death is not clear.

Killing by Macrophages

Macrophages can kill via three mechanisms:

1. Killing by TNF. Secreted TNF binds to TNF receptors on a target cell, and activates the target cell's apoptosis program (p. 213). (TNF was thought to be secreted only by macrophages, but NK cells and activated T cells can also secrete it, whereby another important cell-killing pathway is open [289]).

2. Killing by oxygen- or nitrogen-derived free radicals. This is how macrophages kill bacteria (p. 419).

3. Killing targets labeled by antibodies. This mechanism is part of an immune response (p. 539) but here is a summary.

Suppose that a worm settles in the tissues; it will soon be covered by a carpet of antibodies. Macrophages—sensing the tail ends [Fc] of the antibodies—will settle on them, become activated and discharge their arsenal of killer molecules. This situation is known in immunopathology as ADCC (antibody-dependent complement-mediated cytotoxicity [p. 539]).

In conclusion, it is obvious that the truly professional killers are the lymphocytes, mainly the NK cells. The macrophages are professional in almost everything they do (beginning with phagocytosis) but not in cell killing: they do not carry weapons especially designed for this purpose, such as the NK cells have as standard equipment.

TO SUM UP: Here ends our tale of cell injury and cell death. It is long, because it concerns virtually every disease. Each topic, from stress proteins to killer cells, recalls our basic theme, whereby the cell is the elementary patient; most pointedly the topic by the oxymoronic title "physiologic cell death." Indeed, for cells as well as for individuals, there can be no life without death.

Life and death, on this planet, are two faces of one reality. There is no better illustration of this concept than the famous puma cut out of stone by a pre-Columbian Aztec artist, and now exposed at the Anthropologic Museum of Mexico City: seen from the front, it is alive; seen from the back it is a skeleton (Figure 5.61).

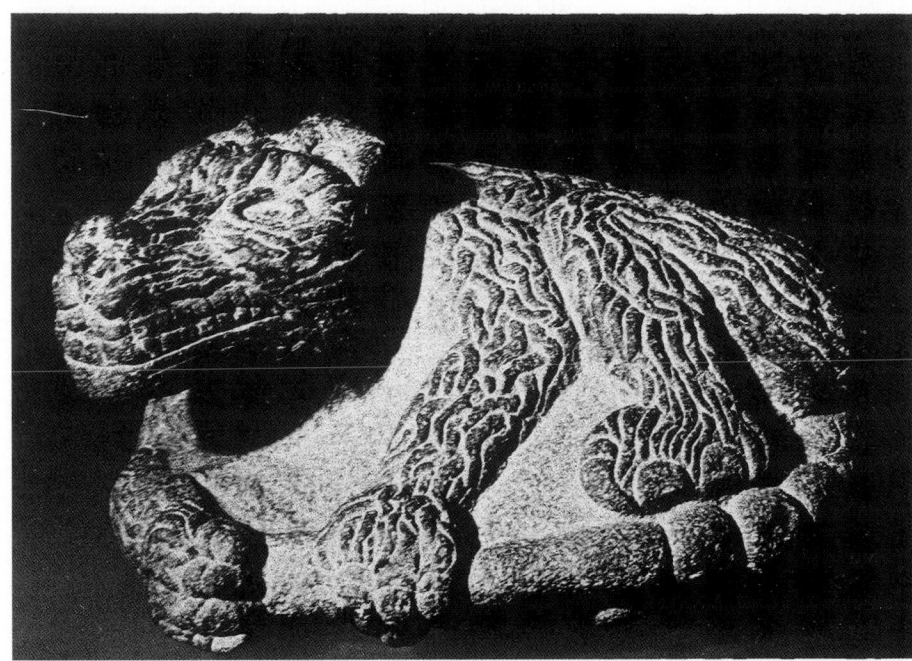

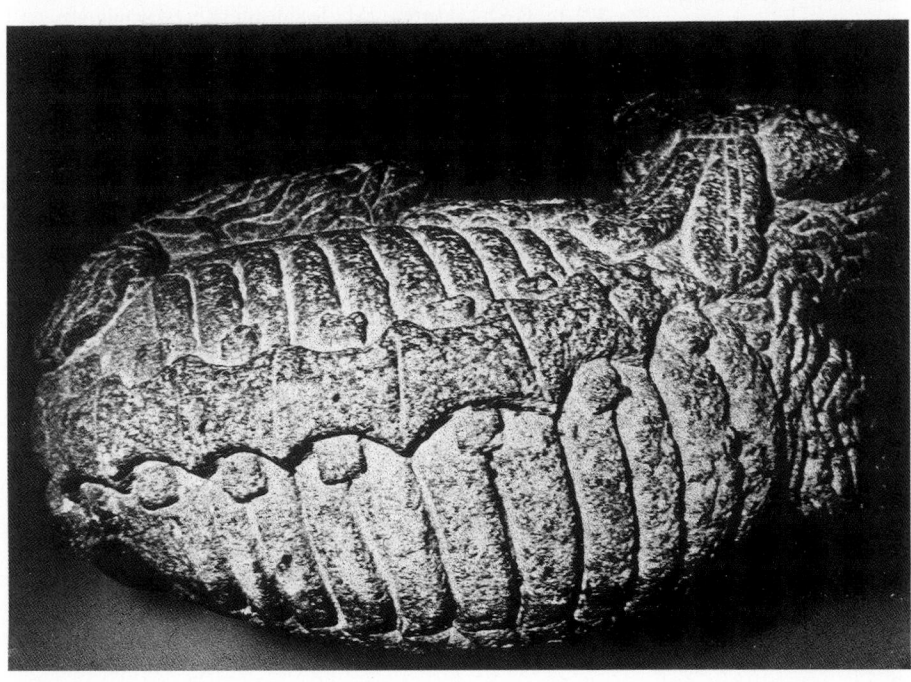

FIGURE 5.61 Life and death are inseparable. This concept is beautifully illustrated by this Aztec sculpture of a puma, from the Museum of Anthropology in Mexico City. *Top:* Viewed from the front, the puma is alive. *Bottom:* Viewed from the back, it is a skeleton. (Courtesy of the Museum of Anthropology, Mexico City, Mexico.)

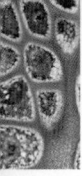
References

1. Acehan D, Jiang X, Morgan DG, et al. Three-dimensional structure of the apoptosome: implications for assembly, procaspase-9 binding, and activation. Mol Cell 2002;9:423–432.

1a. Acosta D, Puckett M, McMillin R. Ischemic myocardial injury in cultured heart cells: leakage of cytoplasmic enzymes from injured cells. In Vitro 1978;14:728–732.

2. Alberts B, Johnson A, Lewis J, et al (eds). Molecular biology of the cell. 4th ed. New York: Garland Science, 2002.

3. Altekar W, Paul P, Nadkarni GB. Changes in tryptophan microenvironment in horse heart myoglobin due to γ-irradiation. Biochim Biophys Acta 1977;495:203–211.

4. Altman PL, Dittmer DS (eds). Respiration and circulation. Bethesda: Federation of American Societies for Experimental Biology, 1971.

5. Anderson KM, Srivastava PK. Heat, heat shock, heat shock proteins and death: a central link in innate and adaptive immune responses. Immunol Lett 2000;74:35–39.

6. Antman EM. Decision making with cardiac troponin tests. N Engl J Med 2002;346:2079–2082.

7. Arends MJ, Wyllie AH. Apoptosis: mechanisms and roles in pathology. Int Rev Exp Pathol 1991;32:223–254.

8. Arrigo A-P. Small stress proteins: chaperones that act as regulators of intracellular redox state and programmed cell death. Biol Chem 1998;379:19–26.

9. Arsenau JC, Bagley CM, Anderson T, Canellos GP. Hyperkalaemia, a sequel to chemotherapy of Burkitt's lymphoma. Lancet 1973;1:10–14.

10. Ashcroft FM. Ion channels and disease. San Diego, CA: Academic Press, 2000.

11. Aust SD, Morehouse LA, Thomas CE. Role of metals in oxygen radical reactions. J Free Radic Biol Med 1985;1:3–25.

12. Autor AP (ed). Pathology of oxygen. New York: Academic Press, 1982.

13. Babior BM. Phagocytes and oxidative stress. Am J Med 2000;109:33–44.

14. Ballard KJ, Holt SJ. Cytological and cytochemical studies on cell death and digestion in the foetal rat foot: the role of macrophages and hydrolytic enzymes. J Cell Sci 1968; 3:245–262.

15. Bangham AD. Liposomes: realizing their promise. Hosp Pract 1992;27:51–62.

16. Bangham AD, Horne RW. Negative staining of phospholipids and their structural modification by surface-active agents as observed in the electron microscope. J Mol Biol 1964;8:660–668.

17. Barbe MF, Tytell M, Gower DJ, Welch WJ. Hyperthermia protects against light damage in the rat retina. Science 1988; 241:1817–1820.

18. Barrett LA, McDowell EM, Harris CC, Trump BF. Studies on the pathogenesis of ischemic cell injury. XV. Reversal of ischemic cell injury in hamster trachea and human bronchus by explant culture. Beitr Pathol 1977;161:109–121.

19. Barry M, Bleackley RC. Cytotoxic T lymphocytes: all roads lead to death. Nat Rev Immunol 2002;2:401–408.

20. Basu S, Binder RJ, Suto R, Anderson KM, Srivastava PK. Necrotic but not apoptotic cell death releases heat shock proteins, which deliver a partial maturation signal to dendritic cells and activate the NF-κB pathway. Int Immunol 2000;12: 1539–1546.

21. Baumeister W, Walz J, Zühl F, Seemüller E. The proteasome: paradigm of a self-compartmentalizing protease. Cell 1998; 92:367–380.

22. Beckman JS, Freeman BA. Antioxidant enzymes as mechanistic probes of oxygen-dependent toxicity. In: Taylor AE, Matalon S, Ward P (eds). Physiology of oxygen radicals. Bethesda: American Physiological Society, 1986, pp. 39–53.

23. Beckmann RP, Mizzen LA, Welch WJ. Interaction of Hsp 70 with newly synthesized proteins: implications for protein folding and assembly. Science 1990;248:850–854.

24. Beere HM. Stressed to death: regulation of apoptotic signaling pathways by heat shock proteins. Science's STKE (review as seen May 2002), http://www.stke.org/cgi/content/full/OC_sigtrans;2001/93/rel

25. Bement WM, Mandato CA, Kirsch MN. Wound-induced assembly and closure of an actomyosin purse string in *Xenopus* oocytes. Curr Biol 1999;9:579–587.

26. Benjamin IJ, McMillan DR. Stress (heat shock) proteins. Molecular chaperones in cardiovascular biology and disease. Circ Res 1998;83:117–132.

27. Bernelli-Zazzera A, Gaja G. Some aspects of glycogen metabolism following reversible or irreversible liver ischemia. Exp Mol Pathol 1964;3:351–368.

28. Berns MW, Aist J, Edwards J, et al. Laser microsurgery in cell and developmental biology. Science 1981;213:505–513.

29. Bessis M. Studies on cell agony and death: an attempt at classification. In: de Reuck AVS, Knight J (eds). Cellular injury. Ciba Foundation Symposium. London: J & A Churchill, Ltd, 1964, pp. 287–328.

30. Bessis M. La mort de la cellule. Triangle 1970;9:191–199.

31. Beutler B, Munford RS. Tumor necrosis factor and the Jarisch-Herxheimer reaction. N Engl J Med 1996;335:347–348.

32. Bi G-Q, Alderton JM, Steinhardt RA. Calcium-regulated exocytosis is required for cell membrane resealing. J Cell Biol 1995;131:1747–1758.

33. Block MI, Said JW, Siegel RJ, Fishbein MC. Myocardial myoglobin following coronary artery occlusion. An immunohistochemical study. Am J Pathol 1983;111:374–379.

34. Bluemink JG. Cortical wound healing in the amphibian egg: an electron microscopical study. J Ultrastruct Res 1972; 41:95–114.

35. Bogdan C, Röllinghoff M, Diefenbach A. Reactive oxygen and reactive nitrogen intermediates in innate and specific immunity. Curr Opin Immunol 2000;12:64–76.

36. Bond U, Schlesinger MJ. Ubiquitin is a heat shock protein in chicken embryo fibroblasts. Mol Cell Biol 1985;5:949–956.

37. Borkman RF, Lerman S. Fluorescence spectra of tryptophan residues in human and bovine lens proteins. Eye Res 1978; 26:705–713.

38. Bouchardy B, Majno G. Histopathology of early myocardial infarcts. A new approach. Am J Pathol 1974;74:301–330.

39. Bowen ID. Laboratory techniques for demonstrating cell death. In: Davies I, Sigee DC (eds). Cell ageing and cell death. Cambridge: Cambridge University Press, 1984, pp. 5–40.

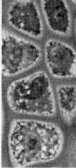

40. Bowen ID, Bowen SM. Programmed cell death in tumours and tissues. London: Chapman and Hall, 1990.

41. Bowen ID, Lockshin RA (eds). Cell death in biology and pathology. London: Chapman and Hall, 1981.

42. Bracken MB, Shepard MJ, Collins WF, et al. A randomized, controlled trial of methylprednisolone or naloxone in the treatment of acute spinal-cord injury. Results of the Second National Acute Spinal Cord Injury Study. N Engl J Med 1990;322:1405–1411.

43. Brandl M. Liposomes as drug carriers: a technological approach. Biotech Annu Rev 2001;7:59–85.

44. Buckley IK. Phosphatides in the morphology of injured tissue. QJ Exp Physiol 1961;46:229–237.

45. Buja LM, Entman, ML. Modes of myocardial cell injury and cell death in ischemic heart disease. Circulation 1998; 98:1355–1357.

46. Burroughs M, Cabellos C, Prasad S, Tuomanen E. Bacterial components and the pathophysiology of injury to the blood-brain barrier: does cell wall add to the effects of endotoxin in gram-negative meningitis? J Infect Dis 1992;165(suppl 1): S82–85.

47. Cech P, Block JB, Cone LA, Stone R. Tumor lysis syndrome after tamoxifen flare. N Engl J Med 1986;315:263–264.

48. Chan PH. The role of oxygen radicals in brain injury and edema. In: Chow CK (ed). Cellular antioxidant defense mechanisms, vol. III. Boca Raton: CRC Press, Inc., 1988, pp. 89–109.

49. Cheung JY, Bonventre JV, Malis CD, Leaf A. Calcium and ischemic injury. N Engl J Med 1986;314:1670–1676.

50. Chien KR, Abrams J, Pfau RG, Farber JL. Prevention by Chlorpromazine of ischemic liver cell death. Am J Pathol 1977;88:539–558.

51. Clarke MSF, Caldwell RW, Chiao H, Miyake K, McNeil PL. Contraction-induced cell wounding and release of fibroblast growth factor in heart. Circ Res 1995;76:927–934.

52. Clements JA, Tierney DF. Alveolar instability associated with altered surface tension. In: Fenn WO and Rahn H (eds). Handbook of physiology, Section 3: Respiration. Washington, DC: American Physiology Society, 1965, pp. 1565–1583.

53. Coleman ML, Sahai EA, Yeo M, et al. Membrane blebbing during apoptosis results from caspase-mediated activation of ROCK I. Nat Cell Biol 2001;3:339–345.

54. Collins VP. Cultured human glial and glioma cells. Int Rev Exp Pathol 1983;24:135–202.

55. Corr PB, Gross RW, Sobel BE. Amphipathic metabolites and membrane dysfunction in ischemic myocardium. Circ Res 1984;55:135–154.

56. Cory S, Adams JM. The BCL2 family: regulators of the cellular life-or-death switch. Nat Rev Cancer 2002;2:647–656.

57. Craig EA. The heat shock response. CRC Crit Rev Biochem 1985;18:239–280.

58. Cross HR, Leu R, Miller MF. Scope of warmed-over flavor and its importance to the meat industry. In: St Angelo AJ, Bailey ME (eds). Warmed-over flavor of meat. Orlando: Academic Press, Inc, 1987, pp. 1–18.

59. Cutler RG. Antioxidants, aging, and longevity. In: Pryor WA (ed). Free radicals in biology, vol. VI. Orlando: Academic Press, Inc., 1984, pp. 371–428.

60. Cruveilhier J. Anatomie pathologique du corps humain. Paris: J.B. Baillière, 1829–1842.

61. Das DK, Engelman RM, Rousou JA, et al. Role of membrane phospholipids in myocardial injury induced by ischemia and reperfusion. Am J Physiol 1986;251:H71–H79.

62. Davies I, Sigee DC (eds). Cell ageing and cell death. Cambridge: Cambridge University Press, 1984.

63. Délèze J. Calcium ions and the healing over of heart fibres. In: Taccardi B, Marchetti G (eds). International symposium on the electrophysiology of the heart. Oxford: Pergamon Press, 1965, pp. 147–148.

64. Del Maestro RF. An approach to free radicals in medicine and biology. Acta Physiol Scand [Suppl] 1980;492:153–168.

65. De Mello WC. Membrane sealing in frog skeletal-muscle fibers. Proc Natl Acad Sci USA 1973;70:982–984.

66. De Mello WC. Effect of intracellular injection of calcium and strontium on cell communication in heart. J Physiol 1975; 250:231–245.

67. Demopoulos HB, Flamm ES, Pietronigro DD, Seligman ML. The free radical pathology and the microcirculation in the major central nervous system disorders. Acta Physiol Scand [Suppl] 1980;492:91–118.

68. Demopoulos HB, Flamm E, Seligman M, Pietronigro DD. Oxygen free radicals in central nervous system ischemia and trauma. In: Autor AP (ed). Pathology of oxygen. New York: Academic Press, 1982, pp. 127–155.

69. Depraetere V. "Eat me" signals of apoptotic bodies. Nat Cell Biol 2000;2:E104.

70. Dluzen DE. Neuroprotective effects of estrogen upon the nigrostriatal dopaminergic system. J Neurocytol 2000; 29:387–399.

71. Dong Z, Saikumar P, Weinberg JM, Venkatachalam MA. Internucleosomal DNA cleavage triggered by plasma membrane damage during necrotic cell death. Involvement of serine but not cysteine proteases. Am J Pathol 1997;151:1205–1213.

72. Downes CP, Wolf CR, Lane DP (eds). Cellular responses to stress. Princeton, NJ: Princeton University Press, 1999.

73. Draper HH, Dhanakoti SN, Hadley M, Piché LA. Malondialdehyde in biological systems. In: Chow CK (ed). Cellular antioxidant defense mechanisms, vol. II. Boca Raton: CRC Press, Inc., 1988, pp. 97–109.

74. Dubick MA, Mayer AD, Majumdar APN, et al. Biochemical studies in peritoneal fluid from patients with acute pancreatitis. Relationship to etiology. Dig Dis Sci 1987;32:305–312.

75. Eguchi Y, Shimizu S, Tsujimoto Y. Intracellular ATP levels determine cell death fate by apoptosis or necrosis. Cancer Res 1997;57:1835–1840.

76. Eisenberg D. How chaperones protect virgin proteins. Science 1999;285:1021–1022.

77. Elkon KB. Apoptosis. In: Ruddy S, Harris ED, Sledge CB (eds). Kelley's textbook of rheumatology. 6th ed. Philadelphia, PA: WB Saunders Company. 2001, pp. 291–303.

78. Elsässer A, Suzuki K, Lorenz-Meyer S, Bode C, Schaper J. The role of apoptosis in myocardial ischemia: a critical appraisal. Basic Res Cardiol 2001;96:219–226.

79. Epstein JH. The pathological effects of light on the skin. In: Pryor WA (ed). Free radicals in biology, vol. III. New York: Academic Press, 1977, pp. 219–249.

80. Fadok VA, Bratton DL, Konowal A, et al. Macrophages that have ingested apoptotic cells in vitro inhibit proinflammatory cytokine production through autocrine/paracrine mechanisms involving TGF-β, PGE2, PAF. J Clin Invest 1998; 101:890–898.

81. Fahrbach SE, Truman JW. Mechanisms for programmed cell death in the nervous system of a moth. Ciba Found Symp 1987;126:65–81.

82. Farber E, Liang H, Shinozuka S. Dissociation of effects on protein synthesis and ribosomes from membrane changes induced by carbon tetrachloride. Am J Pathol 1971;64:601–622.

83. Farber JL. Reactions of the liver to injury. In: Farber E, Fisher MM (eds). Toxic injury of the liver, part A. New York: Marcel Dekker, Inc., 1979, pp. 215–241.

84. Farber JL. Calcium and the mechanisms of liver necrosis. Prog Liver Dis 1982;7:347–360.

85. Farber JL. Membrane injury and calcium homeostasis in the pathogenesis of coagulative necrosis. Lab Invest 1982; 47:114–123.

86. Febbraio MA, Koukoulas I. HSP72 gene expression progressively increases in human skeletal muscle during prolonged, exhaustive exercise. J Appl Physiol 2000;89:1055–1060.

87. Feder ME, Parsell DA, Lindquist SL. The stress response and stress proteins. In: Lemasters JJ, Oliver C (eds). Cell biology of trauma. Boca Raton, FL: CRC Press, 1995, pp. 177–191.

88. Fekade D, Knox K, Hussein K, et al. Prevention of Jarisch-Herxheimer reactions by treatment with antibodies against tumor necrosis factor α. N Engl J Med 1996;335:311–315.

89. Ferguson CC, Richardson JB. A simple technique for the utilization of postmortem tracheal and bronchial tissues for ultrastructural studies. Hum Pathol 1978;9:463–470.

90. Fesus L, Thomazy V, Falus A. Induction and activation of tissue transglutaminase during programmed cell death. FEBS Lett 1987;224:104–108.

91. Fisch C. Relation of electrolyte disturbances to cardiac arrhythmias. Circulation 1973;47:408–419.

92. Folkerts G, Kloek J, Muijsers RBR, Nijkamp FP. Reactive nitrogen and oxygen species in airway inflammation. Eur J Pharmacol 2001;429:251–262.

93. Foote CS. Light, oxygen, and toxicity. In: Autor AP (ed). Pathology of oxygen. New York: Academic Press, 1982, pp. 21–44.

94. Formigli L, Papucci L, Tani A, et al. Aponecrosis: morphological and biochemical exploration of a syncretic process of cell death sharing apoptosis and necrosis. J Cell Physiol 2000; 182:41–49.

95. Foulks GN (ed). Noninfectious inflammation of the anterior segment. International Ophthalmology Clinics, vol. 23. Boston: Little, Brown and Company, 1983.

96. Frank L. Oxygen toxicity in eucaryotes. In: Oberley LW (ed). Superoxide dismutase. Boca Raton: CRC Press, 1985, pp. 1–43.

97. Frankel EN. Volatile lipid oxidation products. Prog Lipid Res 1982;22:1–33.

98. Fraser CL, Arieff AI. Hepatic encephalopathy. N Engl J Med 1985;313:865–873.

99. Frederiks WM, Fronik GM, Hesseling JMG. A method for quantitative analysis of the extent of necrosis in ischemic rat liver. Exp Mol Pathol 1984;41:119–125.

100. Freeman BA, Crapo JD. Free radicals and tissue injury. Lab Invest 1982;47:412–426.

101. Fretzin DF, Arias AM. Sclerema neonatorum and subcutaneous fat necrosis of the newborn. Pediatr Dermatol 1987; 4:112–122.

102. Fridovich I. Oxygen radicals, hydrogen peroxide, and oxygen toxicity In: Pryor WA (ed). Free radicals in biology, vol. I. New York: Academic Press, 1976, pp. 239–277.

103. Fridovich I. Superoxide dismutase in biology and medicine. In: Autor AP (ed). Pathology of oxygen. New York: Academic Press, 1982, pp. 1–19.

104. Frisch SM, Ruoslahti E. Integrins and anoikis. Curr Opin Cell Biol 1997;9:701–706.

105. Gahan PB. Cell senescence and death in plants. In: Bowen ID, Lockshin RA (eds). Cell death in biology and pathology. London: Chapman and Hall, 1981, pp. 145–169.

106. Ganote CE, Vander Heide RS. Cytoskeletal lesions in anoxic myocardial injury. A conventional and high-voltage electron-microscopic and immunofluorescence study. Am J Pathol 1987;129:327–344.

107. Garcia JH, Conger KA, Lossinsky AS. The cellular pathology of ischemic stroke. In: Trump BF, Laufer A, Jones RT (eds). Cellular pathobiology of human disease. New York: Gustav Fischer, Inc., 1983, pp. 351–367.

108. Garcia JH, Yoshida Y, Chen H, et al. Progression from ischemic injury to infarct following middle cerebral artery occlusion in the rat. Am J Pathol 1993;142:623–635.

109. Gee MH, Flynn JT, Spath JA Jr. Pulmonary and coronary endothelial effects of acute myocardial ischemia in dogs. Am J Physiol 1982;242:H337–H348.

110. Gilbert DL, Colton CA. Reactive oxygen species in biological systems: an interdisciplinary approach. New York: Kluwer Academic/Plenum Publishers, 1999.

111. Gilloteaux J, Jamison JM, Arnold D, et al. Cancer cell necrosis by autoschizis: synergism of antitumor activity of vitamin C: vitamin K_3 on human bladder carcinoma T24 cells. Scanning 1998;20:564–575.

112. Gitter AH, Bendfeldt K, Schulzke J-D, Fromm M. Leaks in the epithelial barrier caused by spontaneous and TNF-α-induced single-cell apoptosis. FASEB J 2000;14: 1749–1753.

113. Glücksmann A. Cell deaths in normal vertebrate ontogeny. Biol Rev 1951;26:59–86.

114. Goldblatt PJ, Trump BF, Stowell RE. Studies on necrosis of mouse liver in vitro. Alterations in some histochemically demonstrable hepatocellular enzymes. Am J Pathol 1965; 47:183–208.

115. Goldman AS, Herold R, Piddington R. Inhibition of programmed cell death in the fetal palate by cortisol. Proc Soc Exp Biol Med 1981;166:418–424.

116. Grasl-Kraupp B, Ruttkay-Nedecky B, Koudelka H, et al. *In situ* detection of fragmented DNA (TUNEL assay) fails to discriminate among apoptosis, necrosis, and autolytic cell death: a cautionary note. Hepatol 1995;21:1465–1468.

117. Greenberg JT. Programmed cell death: a way of life for plants. Proc Natl Acad Sci USA 1996;93:12094–12097.

118. Gregoriadis G. The carrier potential of liposomes in biology and medicine. N Engl J Med 1976;295:704–710.

119. Gregory CD. CD14-dependent clearance of apoptotic cells: relevance to the immune system. Curr Opin Immunol 2000;12:27–34.

120. Grierson D. Nucleic acid and protein synthesis during fruit ripening and senescence. In: Davies I, Sigee DC (eds). Cell ageing and cell death. Cambridge: Cambridge University Press, 1984, pp. 189–202.

121. Grierson D, Maunders MJ, Slater A, et al. Gene expression during tomato ripening. Philos Trans R Soc Lond [Biol] 1986;314:399–410.

122. Griffiths GM. The cell biology of CTL killing. Curr Opin Immunol 1995;7:343–348.

123. Grisham MB, McCord JM. Chemistry and cytotoxicity of reactive oxygen metabolites. In: Taylor AE, Matalon S, Ward P (eds). Physiology of oxygen radicals. Bethesda: American Physiological Society, 1986, pp. 1–18.

124. Grollman A. Pressor activity of circulating blood after focal infarction of the kidney in the rat. Proc Soc Exp Biol Med 1970;134:1120–1122.

125. Guilliermond A. La structure des cellules végétales a l'ultramicroscope. Protoplasma (Berl) 1932;16:454–477.

126. Guyton AC. Textbook of medical physiology, 7th ed. Philadelphia: WB Saunders Company, 1986.

127. Haimovici H. Metabolic complications of acute arterial occlusions. J Cardiovasc Surg 1979;20:349–357.

127a. Hallenbeck JM. The many faces of tumor necrosis factor in stroke. Nat Med 2002;8:1363–1368.

128. Halliwell B. Oxidants and human disease: some new concepts. FASEB J 1987;1:358–364.

129. Halliwell B, Gutteridge JMC. Iron as a biological prooxidant. ISI Atlas of Science:Biochemistry 1988;1:48–52.

130. Hamon Y, Broccardo C, Chambenoit O, et al. ABC1 promotes engulfment of apoptotic cells and transbilayer redistribution of phosphatidylserine. Nat Cell Biol 2000;2:399–406.

131. Hannun YA, Boustany R-M (eds). Apoptosis in neurobiology. Boca Raton, FL: CRC Press, 1999.

132. Harris AS. Potassium and experimental coronary occlusion. Am Heart J 1966;71:797–802.

133. Heeringa P, Steenbergen E, van Goor, H. A protective role for endothelial nitric oxide synthase in glomerulonephritis. Kidney Int 2002;61:822–825.

134. Heilbrunn LV. The dynamics of living protoplasm. New York: Academic Press, Inc., 1956.

135. Hendry JH, Scott D. Loss of reproductive integrity of irradiated cells, and its importance in tissues. In: Potten CS (ed). Perspectives on mammalian cell death. Oxford: Oxford University Press, 1987, pp. 160–183.

136. Henkart PA. Cytotoxic T lymphocytes. In: Paul WE (ed). Fundamental immunology. 4th ed. Philadelphia, PA: Lippincott-Raven. 1999, pp. 1021–1049.

137. Hetts SW. To die or not to die. An overview of apoptosis and its role in disease. JAMA 1998;279:300–307.

138. Hickman ES, Moroni MC, Helin K. The role of p53 and pRB in apoptosis and cancer. Curr Opin Genet Dev 2002;12:60–66.

139. Hilden S. Stress proteins in renal ischemia. In: Lemasters JJ, Oliver C (eds). Cell biology of trauma. Boca Raton, FL: CRC Press, 1995, pp. 227–250.

140. Hill JL, Gettes LS. Ischemia induced changes in interstitial potassium in in situ myocardium. Circulation 1977; 56(suppl. III):III–108.

141. Hippocrates: Instruments of reduction. In: Hippocrates. With an English translation by Dr. E.T. Withington. Vol. III, pp. 398–449. Cambridge, MA: The Loeb Classical Library, Harvard University Press, 1959 (pp. 432–433).

142. Itkonen P, Collan Y. Mitochondrial flocculent densities in ischemia. Digestion experiments. Acta Pathol Microbiol Immunol Scand A 1983;91:463–468.

143. Itoh G, Tamura J, Suzuki M. DNA fragmentation of human infarcted myocardial cells demonstrated by the Nick End labeling method and DNA agarose gel electrophoresis. Am J Pathol 1995;146:1325–1331.

143a. Jaeschke H, Lemasters JJ. Apoptosis versus oncotic necrosis in hepatic ischemia/reperfusion injury. Gastroenterol 2003; 125:246–1257.

144. Jennings RB, Shen AC, Hill ML, Ganote CE, Herdson PB. Mitochondrial matrix densities in myocardial ischemia and autolysis. Exp Mol Pathol 1978;29:55–65.

145. Joris I, Underwood JM, Khan F, Majno G. Programmed cell death, oncosis and apoptosis: the case of growth cartilage. FASEB J 1998;12:A797.

146. Judah JD, Ahmed, K, Mclean AEM. Possible role of ion shifts in liver injury. In: deReuck AVS, Knight J (eds). Cellular injury. Ciba Foundation Symposium. Boston: Little, Brown, 1964, pp. 187–204.

147. Kaltenbach JP, Kaltenbach MH, Lyons WB. Nigrosin as a dye for differentiating live and dead ascites cells. Exp Cell Res 1958;15:112–117.

148. Kaplan M. Suicide by oral ingestion of a potassium preparation. Ann Intern Med 1969;71:363–364.

149. Kaufmann SH (ed). Apoptosis. Pharmacological implications and therapeutic opportunities. San Diego: Academic Press, 1997.

150. Kaufmann SH, Earnshaw WC. Induction of apoptosis by cancer chemotherapy. Exp Cell Res 2000;256:42–49.

151. Kaufmann SH, Gores GJ. Apoptosis in cancer: cause and cure. BioEssays 2000;22:1007–1017.

152. Kaufmann SHE. Heat shock proteins and the immune response. Immunol Today 1990;11:129–136.

153. Kauzmann W. Denaturation of proteins and enzymes. In: McElroy WD, Glass B (eds). A symposium on the mechanism of enzyme action. Baltimore: The Johns Hopkins Press, 1954, pp. 70–120.

154. Kerr JFR. Shrinkage necrosis: a distinct mode of cellular death. J Pathol 1971;105:13–20.

154a. Kerr JFR. History of the events leading to the formulation of the apoptosis concept. Toxicology 2002;181–182, 471–474.

155. Kerr JFR, Harmon BV. Definition and incidence of apoptosis: an historical perspective. In: Tomei LD, Cope FO (eds). Apoptosis: the molecular basis of cell death. Cold Spring Harbor: Cold Spring Harbor Laboratory Press, 1991, pp. 5–29.

156. Kerr JFR, Wyllie AH, Currie AR. Apoptosis: a basic biological phenomenon with wide-ranging implications in tissue kinetics. Br J Cancer 1972;26:239–257.

157. Kiehart DP. Wound healing: the power of the purse string. Curr Biol 1999;9:R602-R605.

158. Kluck RM, Bossy-Wetzel E, Green DR, Newmeyer DD. The release of cytochrome c from mitochondria: a primary site for Bcl-2 regulation of apoptosis. Science 1997;275:1132–1136.

159. Knochel JP. Serum calcium derangements in rhabdomyolysis. N Engl J Med 1981;305:161–163.

160. Knochel JP, Schlein EM. On the mechanism of rhabdomyolysis in potassium depletion. J Clin Invest 1972; 51:1750–1758.

161. Kol A, Bourcier T, Lichtman AH, Libby P. Chlamydial and human heat shock protein 60s activate human vascular endothelium, smooth muscle cells, and macrophages. J Clin Invest 1999;103:571–577.

162. Kraus GE, Costa G. Systemic effects of massive hepatic necrosis. I. Acute effects of hepatic infarction on the kidneys. Arch Surg 1963;87:957–962.

163. Lam E, del Pozo O. Caspase-like protease involvement in the control of plant cell death. Plant Mol Biol 2000;44:417–428.

164. Lam E, Kato N, Lawton M. Programmed cell death, mitochondria and the plant hypersensitive response. Nature 2001;411:848–853.

165. Larsson J, Bergström J. Electrolyte changes in muscle tissue and plasma in tourniquet-ischemia. Acta Chir Scand 1978;144:67–73.

166. Lawrie RA. Meat science, 3rd ed. Oxford: Pergamon Press, 1979.

167. Ledda-Columbano GM. Coni P, Curto M, et al. Induction of two different modes of cell death, apoptosis and necrosis, in rat liver after a single dose of thioacetamide. Am J Pathol 1991;139:1099–1109.

168. Lemasters JJ, Oliver C (eds). Cell biology of trauma. Boca Raton, FL: CRC Press, 1995.

169. Leppä S, Sistonen L. Heat shock response—pathophysiological implications. Ann Med 1997;29:73–78.

170. Leverrier Y, Ridley AJ. Apoptosis: caspases orchestrate the ROCK 'n' bleb. Nat Cell Biol 2001;3:E91–E94.

171. Levin S. Apoptosis, necrosis or oncosis: what is your diagnosis? A report from the Cell Death Nomenclature Committee of the Society of Toxicologic Pathologists. Toxicol Pathol 1999;27:484–490.

172. Levin S, Bucci TJ, Cohen SM, et al. The nomenclature of cell death: recommendations of an ad hoc committee of the Society of Toxicologic Pathologists. Toxicol Pathol 1999; 27:484–490.

173. Lewthwaite J, Skinner A, Henderson B. Are molecular chaperones microbial virulence factors? Trends Microbiol 1998; 6:426–428.

174. Li GC, Laszlo A. Thermotolerance in mammalian cells: a possible role for heat shock proteins. In: Atkinson BG, Walden DB (eds). Changes in eukaryotic gene expression in response to environmental stress. Orlando: Academic Press, 1985, pp. 227–254.

175. Lieberthal W, Menza SA, Levine JS. Graded ATP depletion can cause necrosis or apoptosis of cultured mouse proximal tubular cells. Am J Physiol 1998;274(Renal Physiol 43):F315–F327.

176. Liem KL, ten Veen JH, Lie KI, Feltkamp TEW, Durrer D. Incidence and significance of heartmuscle antibodies in patients with acute myocardial infarction and unstable angina. Acta Med Scand 1979;206:473–475.

177. Lockshin RA, Beaulaton J. Programmed cell death. Life Sci 1974;15:1549–1565.

178. Lockshin RA, Williams CM. Programmed cell death-IV. The influence of drugs on the breakdown of the intersegmental muscles of silkmoths. J Insect Physiol 1965;11:803–809.

179. Lockshin RA, Zakeri Z, Tilly JL (eds). When cells die. A comprehensive evaluation of apoptosis and programmed cell death. New York: Wiley-Liss, 1998.

180. Lockshin RA, Zakeri-Milovanovic Z. Nucleic acids in cell death. In: Davies I, Sigee DC (eds). Cell ageing and cell death. Cambridge: Cambridge University Press, 1984, pp. 243–268.

181. Lopez DM, Blomberg BB, Padmanabhan RR, Bourguignon LYW. Nuclear disintegration of target cells by killer B lymphocytes from tumor-bearing mice. FASEB J 1989;3:37–43.

182. Lorch IJ, Danielli JF, Hörstadius S. The effect of enucleation on the development of sea urchin eggs. Exp Cell Res 1952;4:253–274.

183. Lowe SW, Lin AW. Apoptosis in cancer. Carcinogenesis 2000;21:485–495.

184. Lucy JA, Glauert AM. Structure and assembly of macromolecular lipid complexes composed of globular micelles. J Mol Biol 1964;8:727–748.

185. Lungarella G, Gardi C, de Santi MM, Luzi P. Pulmonary vascular injury in pancreatitis: evidence for a major role played by pancreatic elastase. Exp Mol Pathol 1985;42:44–59.

186. MacDonald HR. Development and selection of NKT cells. Curr Opin Immunol 2002;14:250–254.

187. Machlin LJ, Bendich A. Free radical tissue damage: protective role of antioxidant nutrients. FASEB J 1987;1:441–445.

188. Macklin CC. The pulmonary alveolar mucoid film and the pneumonocytes. Lancet 1954;1:1099–1104.

189. Madara JL. Maintenance of the macromolecular barrier at cell extrusion sites in intestinal epithelium: physiological rearrangement of tight junctions. J Membrane Biol 1990; 116:177–184.

190. Maeno E, Ishizaki Y, Kanaseki T, Hazama A, Okada Y. Normotonic cell shrinkage because of disordered volume regulation is an early prerequisite to apoptosis. Proc Natl Acad Sci USA 2000;97:9487–9492.

191. Majno G. Death of liver tissue: a review of cell death, necrosis, and autolysis. In: Rouiller Ch. The liver, vol. 2. New York: Academic Press, 1964, pp. 267–313.

192. Majno G. The healing hand. Man and wound in the ancient world. Cambridge, MA: Harvard University Press, 1975.

193. Majno G, Joris I. Apoptosis, oncosis, and necrosis. An overview of cell death. Am J Pathol 1995;146:3–15.

194. Majno G, La Gattuta M, Thompson TE. Cellular death and necrosis: chemical, physical and morphologic changes in rat liver. Virchows Arch Path. Anat 1960;333:421–465.

195. Marguet D, Luciani M-F, Moynault A, Williamson P, Chimini G. Engulfment of apoptotic cells involves the redistribution of membrane phosphatidylserine on phagocyte and prey. Nat Cell Biol 1999;1:454–456.

196. Marsden VS, O'Connor L, O'Reilly LA, et al. Apoptosis initiated by Bcl-2-regulated caspase activation independently of the cytochrome c/Apaf-1/caspase-9 apoptosome. Nature 2002;419:634–637.

197. Martin LC, Johnson BK. Practical microscopy, 2nd ed. Brooklyn: Chemical Publishing Co, Inc., 1951.

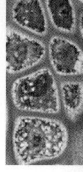

198. Martin DP, Schmidt RE, DiStefano PS, Lowry OH, Carter JG, Johnson EM Jr. Inhibitors of protein synthesis and RNA synthesis prevent neuronal death caused by nerve growth factor deprivation. J Cell Biol 1988;106: 829–844.

199. Marx JL. Oxygen free radicals linked to many diseases. Science 1987;235:529–531.

200. Matalon S, Nickerson PA. Alterations in mammalian blood-gas barrier exposed to hyperoxia. In: Taylor AE, Matalon S, Ward P (eds). Physiology of oxygen radicals. Bethesda: American Physiological Society, 1986, pp. 55–69.

201. Materson BJ, Preston RA. Myoglobinuria versus hemoglobinuria. Hosp Pract 1988;23:29–38.

202. Mathews-Roth MM. Carotenoid pigments and protection against photosensitization: how studies in bacteria suggested a treatment for a human disease. Perspect Biol Med 1984; 28:127–139.

203. Mathews-Roth MM, Pathak A, Fitzpatrick TB, Harber LC, Kass EH. Beta-carotene as a photoprotective agent in erythropoietic protoporphyria. Trans Assoc Am Physicians 1970; 83:176–184.

204. Mathieu JP. Optics, parts 1 and 2. Oxford: Pergamon Press, 1975.

205. Matsuyama S, Llopis J, Deveraux QL, Tsien RY, Reed JC. Changes in intramitochondrial and cytosolic pH: early events that modulate caspase activation during apoptosis. Nat Cell Biol 2000;2:318–325.

206. Mayer LD, Hope MJ, Cullis PR. Vesicles of variable sizes produced by a rapid extrusion procedure. Biochim Biophys Acta 1986;858:161–168.

207. McCarthy JV, Cotter TG. Cell shrinkage and apoptosis: a role for potassium and sodium ion efflux. Cell Death Differ 1997;4:756–770.

208. McCluskey RT, Thomas L. The removal of cartilage matrix, in vivo, by papain. Identification of crystalline papain protease as the cause of the phenomenon. J Exp Med 1958; 108:371–384.

209. McCord JM. The evolution of free radicals and oxidative stress. Am J Med 2000;108:652–659.

210. McNeil PL, Khakee R. Disruptions of muscle fiber plasma membranes. Role in exercise-induced damage. Am J Pathol 1992;140:1097–1109.

211. McNeil PL, Steinhardt RA. Loss, restoration, and maintenance of plasma membrane integrity. J Cell Biol 1997;137:1–4.

212. McNeil PL, Terasaki M. Coping with the inevitable: how cells repair a torn surface membrane. Nat Cell Biol 2001; 3:E124–E129.

213. Meers P. Enzyme-activated targeting of liposomes. Adv Drug Deliv Rev 2001;53:265–272.

214. Mergner WJ, Jones RT, Trump BF (eds). Cell death. Mechanisms of acute and lethal cell injury, vol. 1. New York: Field & Wood Medical Publishers, Inc., 1990.

215. Mergner WJ, Jones RT, Trump BF. Introduction. In: Mergner WJ, Jones RT, Trump BF (eds). Cell death. Mechanisms of acute and lethal cell injury, vol. 1. New York: Field & Wood Medical Publishers, Inc, 1990, pp. 1–11.

216. Mevorach D, Zhou JL, Song X, Elkon KB. Systemic exposure to irradiated apoptotic cells induces autoantibody production. J Exp Med 1998;188:387–392.

217. Miller DL, Dillon J. An unusual abdominal mass in an elderly woman. N Engl J Med 1989;321:1613–1614.

218. Minotti, G, Aust SD. The role of iron in the initiation of lipid peroxidation. Chem Phys Lipids 1987;44:191–208.

219. Morimoto RI, Tissières A, Georgopoulos C. The stress response, function of the proteins, and perspectives. In: Morimoto RI, Tissières A, Georgopoulos C (eds). Stress proteins in biology and medicine. Cold Spring Harbor: Cold Spring Harbor Laboratory Press, 1990, pp. 1–36.

220. Morris RG, Hargreaves AD, Duvall E, Wyllie AH. Hormone-induced cell death. 2. Surface changes in thymocytes undergoing apoptosis. Am J Pathol 1984; 115:426–436.

221. Moseley PL. Heat shock proteins. In: Mackowiak PA (ed). Fever: basic mechanisms and management, 2nd ed. Philadelphia: Lippincott-Raven Publishers, 1997, pp. 197–206.

222. Mottet NK, Hammar SP. Ribosome crystals in necrotizing cells from the posterior necrotic zone of the developing chick limb. J Cell Sci 1972;11:403–414.

223. Mózski G, Bódis B, Figler M, et al. Mechanisms of action of retinoids in gastrointestinal mucosal protection in animals, human healthy subjects and patients. Life Sci 2001; 69:3103–3112.

224. Müllauer L, Gruber P, Sebinger D, et al. Mutations in apoptosis genes: a pathogenetic factor for human disease. Mutat Res 2001;488:211–231.

225. Mullick S. The tourniquet in operations upon the extremities. Surg Gynecol Obstet 1978;146:821–826.

226. Myers CE, McGuire WP, Liss RH, et al. Adriamycin: the role of lipid peroxidation in cardiac toxicity and tumor response. Science 1977;197:165–167.

227. Nash G, Blennerhassett JB, Pontoppidan H. Pulmonary lesions associated with oxygen therapy and artificial ventilation. N Engl J Med 1967;276:368–374.

228. Nevalainen TJ, Anttinen J. Ultrastructural and functional changes in pancreatic acinar cells during autolysis. Virchows Arch B Cell Pathol 1977;24:197–207.

228a. Nicholson DW, Thornberry NA. Life and death decisions. Science 2003;299:214–215.

229. Nicotera P, Leist M. Energy supply and the shape of death in neurons and lymphoid cells. Cell Death Differ 1997; 4:435–442.

230. Nishioka WK, Welsh RM. B cells induce apoptosis via a novel mechanism in fibroblasts infected with mouse hepatitis virus. Natural Immun. 1993;12:113–127.

231. Nishizawa Y. Glutamate release and neuronal damage in ischemia. Life Sci 2001;69:369–381.

232. Nonaka T, Kuwae A, Sasakawa C, Imajoh-Ohmi S. *Shigella flexneri* YSH6000 induces two types of cell death, apoptosis and oncosis, in the differentiated human monoblastic cell line U937. FEMS Microbiol Lett 1999;174:89–95.

233. Norberg R, Ernerudh J, Hamsten A, Unander AM, Årfors L. Phospholipid antibodies in cardiovascular disease. Acta Med Scand Suppl 1987;715:93–98.

234. O'Connell J, Houston A, Bennett MW, O'Sullivan GC, Shanahan F. Immune privilege or inflammation? Insights into the Fas ligand enigma. Nat Med 2001;7:271–274.

235. O'Connor TM, Wyttenbach CR. Cell death in the embryonic chick spinal cord. J Cell Biol 1974;60:448–459.

236. Ohashi K, Burkart V, Flohé S, Kolb H. Cutting edge: heat shock protein 60 is a putative endogenous ligand of the toll-like receptor-4 complex. J Immunol 2000;164: 558–561.

237. Ohno M, Takemura G, Ohno A, et al. "Apoptotic" myocytes in infarct area in rabbit hearts may be oncotic myocytes with DNA fragmentation. Circulation 1998;98:1422–1430.

238. Oliveira-Castro GM, Loewenstein WR. Junctional membrane permeability. Effects of divalent cations. J Membrane Biol 1971;5:51–77.

239. Olney JW, Sharpe LG. Brain lesions in an infant rhesus monkey treated with monosodium glutamate. Science 1969; 166:386–388.

240. Ostro MJ (ed). Liposomes. New York: Marcel Dekker, Inc., 1983.

241. Ostro MJ (ed). Liposomes. From biophysics to therapeutics. New York: Marcel Dekker, Inc., 1987.

242. Ostro MJ. Liposomes. Sci Am 1987;256:102–111.

242a. Otsuki Y, Li Z, Shibata MA. Apoptotic detection methods—from morphology to gene. Prog Histochem Cytochem 2003; 38:275–339.

243. Palade GE. Membrane biogenesis: an overview. Methods Enzymol 1983;96:xxix-lv.

244. Park BS, Kim GC, Baek SJ, et al. Murine bone marrow-derived mast cells exhibit evidence of both apoptosis and oncosis after IL-3 deprivation. Immunol Invest 2000;29: 51–60.

245. Parker JO, Chiong MA, West RO, Case RB. The effect of ischemia and alterations of heart rate on myocardial potassium balance in man. Circulation 1970;42:205–217.

246. Parton M, Dowsett M, Smith I. Studies of apoptosis in breast cancer. Br Med J 2001;322:1528–1532.

247. Pekkala D, Heath IB, Silver JC. Changes in chromatin and the phosphorylation of nuclear proteins during heat shock of Achlya ambisexualis. Mol Cell Biol 1984;4:1198–1205.

248. Perry MC, Yarbro JW (eds). Toxicity of chemotherapy. Orlando: Grune & Stratton, 1984.

249. Pfeiffer FE, Homburger HA, Yanagihara T. Serum creatine kinase B concentrations in acute cerebrovascular diseases. Arch Neurol 1984;41:1175–1178.

250. Pietersen A, Noteborn MHM. Apoptin. Adv Exp Med Biol 2000;465:153–161.

251. Pilar G, Landmesser L. Ultrastructural differences during embryonic cell death in normal and peripherally deprived ciliary ganglia. J Cell Biol 1976;68:339–356.

252. Platt N, da Silva RP, Gordon S. Recognizing death: the phagocytosis of apoptotic cells. Trends Cell Biol 1998;8: 365–372.

253. Podack ER. Molecular assemblies in complement- and lymphocyte-mediated cytolysis. In: Steinman RM, North RJ, eds. Mechanisms of host resistance to infectious agents, tumors, and allografts. New York: Rockefeller University Press, 1986:217–230.

254. Podhorska-Okolow M, Sandri M, Zampieri S, et al. Apoptosis of myofibres and satellite cells: exercise-induced damage in skeletal muscle of the mouse. Neuropathol Appl Neurobiol 1998;24:518–531.

255. Popescu MC, Swenson CE, Ginsberg RS. Liposome-mediated treatment of viral, bacterial, and protozoal infections. In: Ostro MJ (ed). Liposomes. From biophysics to therapeutics. New York: Marcel Dekker, Inc., 1987, pp. 219–251.

256. Potten CS. Perspectives on mammalian cell death. Oxford: Oxford University Press, 1987.

257. Pryor WA (ed). Free radicals in biology, vol. I. New York: Academic Press, 1976.

258. Pryor WA. Free radical biology: xenobiotics, cancer, and aging. Ann NY Acad Sci 1982;393:1–23.

259. Puck TT. Radiation and the human cell. Sci Am 1960; 202:142–153.

260. Racusen LC. Alterations on human proximal tubule cell attachment in response to hypoxia: role of microfilaments. J Lab Clin Med 1994;123:357–364.

261. Rakhit RD, Marber MS. Nitric oxide: an emerging role in cardioprotection? Heart 2001;86:368–372.

262. Raloff J. Coming to terms with death. Accurate descriptions of a cell's demise may offer clues to diseases and treatments. Sci News 2001;159:378–380.

263. Reddy A, Caler EV, Andrews NW. Plasma membrane repair is mediated by Ca^{++}-regulated exocytosis of lysosomes. Cell 2001;106:157–169.

263a. Reed JC. Mechanisms of apoptosis. Am J Pathol 2000; 157:1415–1430.

264. Riabowol KT, Mizzen LA, Welch WJ. Heat shock is lethal to fibroblasts microinjected with antibodies against hsp 70. Science 1988;242:433–436.

265. Rindfleisch E. Traité d'histologie pathologique. Paris: Baillière et Fils, 1873.

266. Ritossa F. A new puffing pattern induced by temperature shock and DNP in Drosophila. Experentia 1962;18: 571–573.

267. Rokutan K, Hirakawa T, Teshima S, et al. Implications of heat shock/stress proteins for medicine and disease. J Med Invest 1998;44:137–147.

268. Rosenblatt J, Raff MC, Cramer LP. An epithelial cell destined for apoptosis signals its neighbors to extrude it by an actin- and myosin-dependent mechanism. Curr Biol 2001;11:1847–1857.

268a. Salvesen GY, Renatus M. Apoptosome: the seven-spoked death machine. Dev Cell 2002;2:256–257.

269. Samali A, Cotter TG. Heat shock proteins increase resistance to apoptosis. Exp Cell Res 1996;223:163–170.

270. Sanderson CJ. The mechanism of T cell mediated cytotoxicity. II. Morphological studies of cell death by time-lapse microcinematography. Proc R Soc Lond B 1976;192: 241–255.

271. Sarge KD, Bray, AE, Goodson ML. Altered Stress response in testis. Nature 1995;374:126.

272. Sato T, Marbán E. The role of mitochondrial K_{ATP} channels in cardioprotection. Basic Res Cardiol 2000;95:285–289.

273. Saunders JW. Death in embryonic systems. Science 1966;154:604–612.

274. Saunders JW, Fallon JF. Cell death in morphogenesis. In: Locke M (ed). Major problems in developmental biology. New York: Academic Press, 1966, pp. 289–314.

275. Saunders JW, Gasseling MT, Saunders LC. Cellular death in morphogenesis of the avian wing. Dev Biol 1962;5: 147–178.

276. Savill J, Fadok V. Corpse clearance defines the meaning of cell death. Nature 2000;407:784–788.

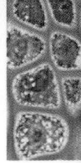

277. Schachenmayr W. Pankreatitis-assoziierte Gehirnbefunde: gibt es eine pankreatische encephalopathie? Pancreatitis-associated brain findings: does pancreatic encephalopathy exist? Verh Dtsch Ges Path 1987;71:280–283.

278. Schlame M, Rua D, Greenberg ML. The biosynthesis and functional role of cardiolipin. Prog Lipid Res 2000; 39:257–288.

279. Schlesinger MJ. Heat shock proteins: the search for functions. J Cell Biol 1986;103:321–325.

280. Schwartz LM, Osborne BA (eds). Cell death. In: Methods in cell biology, Vol 46. San Diego, CA: Academic Press, 1995.

281. Sessa G, Weissmann G. Phospholipid spherules (liposomes) as a model for biological membranes. J Lipid Res 1968;9: 310–318.

282. Sessa G, Weissmann G. Incorporation of lysozyme into liposomes. A model for structure-linked latency. J Biol Chem 1970;245:3295–3301.

282a. Shi Y, Evans JE, Rock KL. Molecular identification of a danger signal that alerts the immune system to dying cells. Nature 2003;425:516–521.

283. Shimizu S, Eguchi Y, Kamiike W, et al. Induction of apoptosis as well as necrosis by hypoxia and predominant prevention of apoptosis by Bcl-2 and Bcl-X$_L$. Cancer Res 1996;56:2161–2166.

284. Shirazi Y, Mergner WJ. Phospholipids, phospholipases, and cell injury. In: Mergner WJ, Jones RT, Trump BF (eds). Cell death. Mechanisms of acute and lethal cell injury, vol. 1. New York: Field & Wood Medical Publishers, Inc., 1990, pp. 201–220.

285. Shtilerman M, Lorimer GH, Englander SW. Chaperonin function: folding by forced unfolding. Science 1999;284: 822–825.

286. Sirén A-L, Ehrenreich H. Erythropoietin—a novel concept for neuroprotection. Eur Arch Psychiatry Clin Neurosci 2001;251:179–184.

287. Small DM. Phase equilibria and structure of dry and hydrated egg lecithin. J Lipid Res 1967;8:551–557.

288. Small DM. Liquid crystals in living and dying systems. J Colloid Interface Sci 1977;58:581–602.

289. Smyth MJ, Johnstone RW. Role of TNF in lymphocyte-mediated cytotoxicity. Microsc Res Tech 2000;50:196–208.

290. Sneller MC, Wang J, Dale JK, et al. Clinical, immunologic, and genetic features of an autoimmune lymphoproliferative syndrome associated with abnormal lymphocyte apoptosis. Blood 1997;4:1341–1348.

291. Sobel MI. Light. Chicago: The University of Chicago Press, 1987.

292. Sofroniew MV, Howe CL, Mobley WC. Nerve growth factor signaling, neuroprotection, and neural repair. Annu Rev Neurosci 2001;24:1217–1281.

293. Soltys BJ, Gupta RS. Cell surface localization of the 60 kDa heat shock chaperonin protein (hsp60) in mammalian cells. Cell Biol Int 1997;21:315–320.

294. Spacek J. Reoxygenation of anoxic human tissues. An application for electron microscopy and its limits. Virchows Arch [Cell Pathol] 1981;37:97–102.

295. Srivastava P. Roles of heat-shock proteins in innate and adaptive immunity. Nat Rev Immunol 2002;2:185–194.

296. Srivastava PK. Interaction of heat shock proteins with peptides and antigen presenting cells: chaperoning of the innate and adaptive immune responses. Annu Rev Immunol 2002; 20:395–425.

297. Srivastava PK, Amato RJ. Heat shock proteins: the 'Swiss Army Knife' vaccines against cancers and infectious agents. Vaccines 2001;19:2590–2597.

298. Starke PE, Hoek JB, Farber JL. Calcium-dependent and calcium-independent mechanisms of irreversible cell injury in cultured hepatocytes. J Biol Chem 1986;261:3006–3012.

299. Staunton MJ, Gaffney EF. Tumor type is a determinant of susceptibility to apoptosis. Am J Clin Pathol 1995; 103:300–307.

300. Steenbergen C, Hill ML, Jennings RB. Cytoskeletal damage during myocardial ischemia: changes in vinculin immunofluorescence staining during total in vitro ischemia in canine heart. Circ Res 1987;60:478–486.

301. Steenbergen C, Murphy E, Levy L, London RE. Elevation in cytosolic free calcium concentration early in myocardial ischemia in perfused rat heart. Circ Res 1987;60:700–707.

302. Stewart AF, Longo W, Kreutter D, Jacob R, Burtis WJ. Hypocalcemia associated with calcium-soap formation in a patient with a pancreatic fistula. N Engl J Med 1986;315: 496–498.

303. Stewart GR, Snewin VA, Walzl G, et al. Overexpression of heat-shock proteins reduces survival of *Mycobacterium tuberculosis* in the chronic phase of infection. Nat Med 2001;7:732–737.

304. Stoeckenius W. An electron microscope study of myelin figures. J Biophys Biochem Cytol 1959;5:491–500.

305. Strauss SE, moderator. An inherited disorder of lymphocyte apoptosis: the autoimmune lymphoproliferative syndrome. Ann Intern Med 1999;130:591–601.

306. Studzinski GP (ed). Cell growth and apoptosis. A practical approach. Oxford: IRL Press, 1995.

307. Szubinska B. "New membrane" formation in Amoeba proteus upon injury of individual cells. J Cell Biol 1971;49:747–772.

308. Szubinska B. Closure of the plasma membrane around microneedle in Amoeba proteus. An ultrastructural study. Exp Cell Res 1978;111:105–115.

309. Takeda M, Shirato I, Kobayashi M, Endou H. Hydrogen peroxide induces necrosis, apoptosis, oncosis and apoptotic oncosis of mouse terminal proximal straight tubule cells. Nephron 1999;81:234–238.

310. Tanaka K. Functions of glutamate transporters in the brain. Neurosci Res 2000;suppl 37:15–19.

311. Taylor AE, Matalon S, Ward P (eds). Physiology of oxygen radicals. Bethesda: American Physiological Society, 1986.

312. Taylor AE, Townsley MI. Assessment of oxygen radical tissue damage. In: Taylor AE, Matalon S, Ward P (eds). Physiology of oxygen radicals. Bethesda: American Physiological Society, 1986, pp. 19–38.

313. Teale FWJ, Weber G. Ultraviolet fluorescence of proteins. Biochem J 1959;72:15.

314. Terasaki M, Miyake K, McNeil PL. Large plasma membrane disruptions are rapidly resealed by Ca^{++}-dependent vesicle-vesicle fusion events. J Cell Biol 1997;139:63–74.

315. Thomas CE, Aust SD. Reductive release of iron from ferritin by cation free radicals of paraquat and other bipyridyls. J Biol Chem 1986;261:13064–13070.

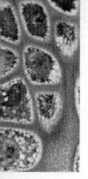

316. Thomas CE, Aust SD. Release of iron from ferritin by cardiotoxic anthracycline antibiotics. Arch Biochem Biophys 1986;248:684–689.

317. Tipper DJ. Mode of action of β-lactam antibodies. Pharmac Ther 1985;27:1–35.

318. Tissières A, Mitchell HK, Tracy UM. Protein synthesis in salivary glands of Drosophila melanogaster: relation to chromosome puffs. J Mol Biol 1974;84:389–398.

319. Tomei LD, Cope FO (eds). Apoptosis: the molecular basis of cell death. Cold Spring Harbor: Cold Spring Harbor Laboratory, 1991.

320. Tomei LD, Cope FO, (eds). Apoptosis II: the molecular basis of apoptosis in disease. New York: Cold Spring Harbor Laboratory Press, 1994.

321. Trump BF, Berezesky IK. Calcium-mediated cell injury and cell death. FASEB J 1995;9:219–228.

322. Trump BF, Berezesky IK. The reactions of cells to lethal injury: oncosis and necrosis—the role of calcium. In: Lockshin RA, Tilly JL, Zakeri Z (eds). Physiological cell death. New York: Wiley-Liss, 1998, pp. 57–96.

323. Trump BF, Berezesky IK. The reactions of cells to lethal injury: oncosis and necrosis—the role of calcium. In: Lockshin RA, Zakeri Z, Tilly JL (eds). When cells die. New York: Wiley-Liss, 1998.

324. Trump BF, Berezesky IK, Chang SH, Phelps PC. The pathways of cell death: oncosis, apoptosis, and necrosis. Toxicol Pathol 1997;25:82–88.

325. Trump BF, Goldblatt PJ, Stowell RE. Studies on necrosis of mouse liver in vitro. Ultrastructural alterations in the mitochondria of hepatic parenchymal cells. Lab Invest 1965;14:343–371.

326. Trump BF, Goldblatt PJ, Stowell RE. Studies of mouse liver necrosis in vitro. Ultrastructural and cytochemical alterations in hepatic parenchymal cell nuclei. Lab Invest 1965; 14:1969–1999.

327. Ts'o POP, Caspary WJ, Lorentzen RJ. The involvement of free radicals in chemical carcinogenesis. In: Pryor AW (ed). Free radicals in biology, vol. II. New York: Academic Press, 1977, pp. 251–303.

328. Tsujimoto Y. Apoptosis and necrosis: intracellular ATP level as a determinant for cell death modes. Cell Death Differ 1997;4:429–434.

329. Turrens JF, Crapo JD, Freeman BA. Protection against oxygen toxicity by intravenous injection of liposome-entrapped catalase and superoxide dismutase. J Clin Invest 1984;73:87–95.

329a. Van Cruchten S, Van den Broeck W. Morphological and biochemical aspects of apoptosis, oncosis and necrosis. Anat Histol Embryol 2002;31:214–223.

330. van den Berg A, Maggio E, Diepstra A, et al. Germline FAS gene mutation in a case of ALPS and NLP Hodgkin lymphoma. Blood 2002;99:1492–1494.

331. Van der Meer C, Valkenburg PW, Ariëns AT, van Benthem RMJ. Cause of death in tourniquet shock in rats. Am J Physiol 1966;210:513–525.

332. Virchow R. Cellular pathology as based upon physiological and pathological histology. 1859. (Translated from the Second German Edition by Frank Chance.) New York: Dover Publications, Inc., 1971, pp. 269–272.

333. Walker NI, Bennett RE, Kerr JFR. Cell death by apoptosis during involution of the lactating breast in mice and rats. Am J Anat 1989;185:19–32.

334. Walker NI, Gobé GC. Cell death and cell proliferation during atrophy of the rat parotid gland induced by duct obstruction. J Pathol 1987;153:333–344.

335. Wallevik K. Spontaneous in vivo isomerization of bovine serum albumin as a determinant of its normal catabolism. J Clin Invest 1976;57:398–407.

336. Wand-Württenberger A, Schoel, B, Ivanyi J, Kaufmann SHE. Surface expression by mononuclear phagocytes of an epitope shared with mycobacterial heat shock protein 60. Eur J Immunol 1999;21:1089–1092.

337. Warrell RP. Metabolic emergencies. In: DeVita VT Jr, Hellman S, Rosenberg SA (eds). Cancer Principles and practice of oncology, 6th ed. Philadelphia, PA: Lippincott, Williams & Wilkins. 2001, pp. 2633–2645.

338. Webster DA, Gross J. Studies on possible mechanisms of programmed cell death in the chick embryo. Dev Biol 1970;22:157–184.

339. Weerasinghe P, Hallock S, Tang S-C, Liepins A. Sanguinarine induces bimodal cell death in K562 but not in high Bcl-2-expressing JM 1 cells. Pathol Res Pract 2001;197:717–726.

340. Weinstein JN. Liposomes in the diagnosis and treatment of cancer. In: Ostro MJ (ed). Liposomes. From biophysics to therapeutics. New York: Marcel Dekker Inc., 1987, pp. 277–338.

341. Welch WJ. The mammalian stress response: cell physiology and biochemistry of stress proteins. In: Morimoto RI, Tissières A, Georgopoulos C (eds). Stress proteins in biology and medicine. Cold Spring Harbor: Cold Spring Harbor Laboratory Press, 1990, pp. 223–278.

342. Welch WJ, Garrels JI, Thomas GP, Lin JJ-C, Feramisco JR. Biochemical characterization of the mammalian stress proteins and identification of two stress proteins as glucose- and Ca^{++}-ionophore-regulated proteins. J Biol Chem 1983; 258:7102–7111.

343. Welch WJ, Mizzen LA. Characterization of the thermotolerant cell. II. Effects on the intracellular distribution of heat-shock protein 70, intermediate filaments, and small nuclear ribonucleoprotein complexes. J Cell Biol 1988; 106:1117–1130.

344. Welch WJ, Suhan JP. Morphological study of the mammalian stress response: characterization of changes in cytoplasmic organelles, cytoskeleton, and nucleoli, and appearance of intranuclear actin filaments in rat fibroblasts after heat-shock treatment. J Cell Biol 1985;101:1198–1211.

345. Welch WJ, Suhan JP. Cellular and biochemical events in mammalian cells during and after recovery from physiological stress. J Cell Biol 1986;103:2035–2052.

346. White BC, Aust SD, Arfors KE, Aronson LD. Brain injury by ischemic anoxia: hypothesis extension—a tale of two ions? Ann Emerg Med 1984;13:127–132.

347. Wink DA, Mitchell JB. Chemical biology of nitric oxide: insights into regulatory, cytotoxic, and cytoprotective mechanisms of nitric oxide. Free Radic Biol Med 1998;25: 434–456.

348. Wink DA, Feelisch M, Vodovotz Y, Fukuto J, Grisham MB. The chemical biology of nitric oxide. In: Gilbert DL, Colton CA. Reactive oxygen species in biological systems: an

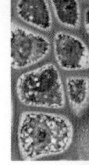

interdisciplinary approach. New York: Kluwer Academic/ Plenum Publishers, 1999, pp. 245–291.

349. Winrow VR, McLean L, Morris CJ, Blake DR. The heat shock protein response and its role in inflammatory disease. Ann Rheum Dis 1990;49:128–132.

350. Wise BL, Cockayne S. Enzymes. In: Bishop ML, Duben-Von Laufen JL, Fody EP (eds). Clinical chemistry. Philadelphia: JB Lippincott Company, 1985, pp. 205–239.

351. Wouters JA, Rombouts FM, Kuipers OP, de Vos WM, Abee T. The role of cold-shock proteins in low-temperature adaptation of food-related bacteria. System Appl Microbiol 2000;23:165–173.

352. Wyllie AH. Glucocorticoid-induced thymocyte apoptosis is associated with endogenous endonuclease activation. Nature 1980;284:555–556.

353. Wyllie AH. Cell death: the significance of apoptosis. Int Rev Cytol 1980;68:251–306.

354. Wyllie AH. Cell death: a new classification separating apoptosis from necrosis. In: Bowen ID, Lockshin RA (eds). Cell death in biology and pathology. London: Chapman and Hall. 1981, pp. 9–34.

355. Wyllie AH. Apoptosis: an overview. Br Med Bull 1997;53:451–465.

356. Wyllie AH, Morris RG, Smith AL, Dunlop D. Chromatin cleavage in apoptosis: association with condensed chromatin morphology and dependence on macromolecular synthesis. J Pathol 1984;142:67–77.

357. Yarmolinsky MB. Programmed cell death in bacterial populations. Science 1995;267:836–837.

357a. Yoneda T, Imaizumi K, Oono K, et al. Activation of caspase-12, an endoplastic reticulum (ER) resident caspase, through tumor necrosis factor-associated factor 2-dependent mechanism in response to the ER stress. J Biol Chem 2001;276: 13935–13940.

358. Young JD-E, Cohn ZA. How killer cells kill. Sci Am 1988; 258:38–44.

359. Young RA, Elliott TJ. Stress proteins, infection, and immune surveillance. Cell 1989;59:5–8.

360. Zager RA. Studies of mechanisms and protective maneuvers in myoglobinuric acute renal injury. Lab Invest 1989;60: 619–629.

361. Zager RA, Burkhart KM, Johnson ACM, Sacks BM. Increased proximal tubular cholesterol content: implications for cell injury and "acquired cytoresistance". Kidney Int 1999;56:1788–1797.

362. Zamzami N, Kroemer G. Condensed matter in cell death. Nature 1999;401:127–128.

363. Zhao M, Beauregard DA, Loizou L, Davletov B, Brindle KM. Non-invasive detection of apoptosis using magnetic resonance imaging and a targeted contrast agent. Nat Med 2001;7:1241–1244.

364. Zhu, L, Chun J (eds). Apoptosis detection and assay methods. BioTechniques® Books, Eaton Publishing, 1998.

365. Ziegler E. General pathology. New York: William Wood and Company, 1908.

366. Zivin JA, Choi DW. Stroke therapy. Sci Am 1991;265:56–63.

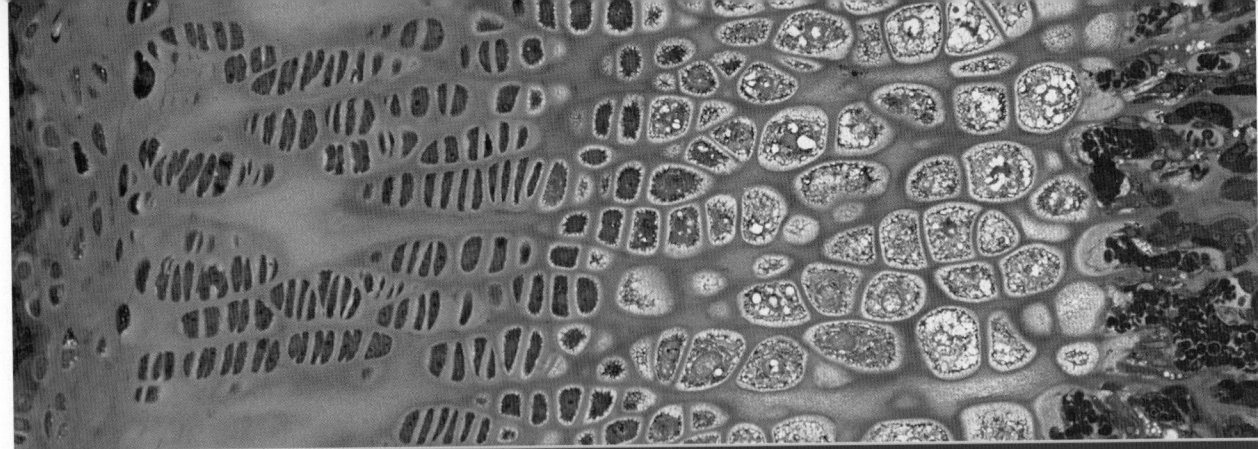

CHAPTER 6   PATHOLOGIC CALCIFICATION

Pathologic calcification is also known as *ectopic calcification,* meaning *calcification in the wrong place.* Overall, it is a fairly benign process, and fortunately so, because it is extremely common: to some degree it is found in every adult, be it in the arteries, in the kidney (66), or almost anywhere. Dead tissues are favorite targets for calcification, but even live cells and the extracellular matrix can calcify. The extent of calcification ranges from diffuse impregnations that only chemical analyses can detect, through granules that are visible microscopically as basophilic dots, to large stony masses that defy centuries and puzzle archaeologists (Figure 6.1). The topic is therefore broader than cellular pathology; we discuss it now because it is closely related to necrosis.

Why should calcium salts have the distinction of generating abnormal deposits? Why not sodium, potassium, or magnesium salts? If we include all forms of life, about 60 kinds of biominerals are known to exist (74). Noncalcific types of concretions do sometimes develop in humans, but calcification prevails because calcium homeostasis is always in precarious balance, easily upset to yield a precipitate of basic calcium phosphate, the mineral of bone. Pathologic calcification, in fact, is the price we pay for maintaining our skeleton, where more than 99 percent of body calcium is held (1), 99 percent of it as apatite (26).

For this very reason, the mineral of bone and of most pathologic calcifications is essentially the same, an analog of the naturally occurring mineral **hydroxyapatite,** $Ca_{10}(PO_4)_6(OH)_2$, which we will call **apatite** for short. *The main structural difference between bone and pathologic calcifications is in the calcified substrate:* in bone the substrate is **osteoid,** a particular organic matrix, and in pathologic calcifications it can be almost any tissue structure, dead or alive, intracellular or extracellular.

However, at the chemical level, there are also some similarities between the matrix of pathologic calcifications and bone: both contain specific proteins, including **osteopontin, osteonectin, osteocalcin,** and others (99a). The function of all these proteins is not clear, but osteopontin *prevents* the deposition of calcium (99a).

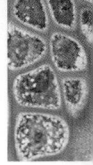

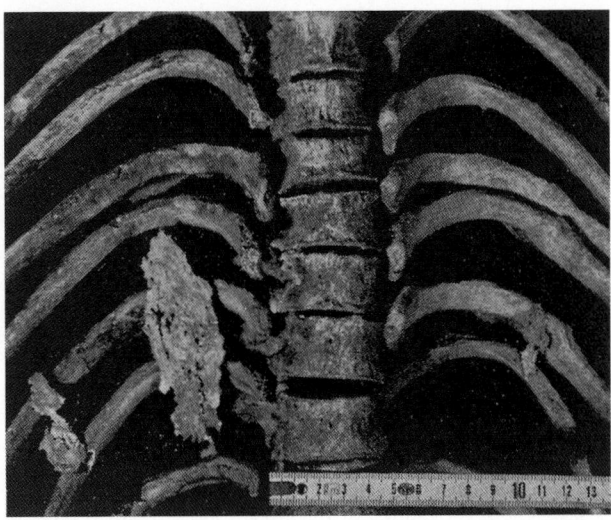

FIGURE 6.1 Plaques of pleural calcification in a medieval leprosy patient buried in Denmark between 1175 and 1500 A.D. The mineral of such pathologic calcifications is the same as that of bone and persists accordingly. (Reproduced from [82] by permission from the International Leprosy Association.)

From Plasma Calcium to Apatite: Some Basic Rules

To understand calcification we must first understand how serum calcium and phosphate relate to deposits of apatite.

What triggers the precipitation of calcium phosphate? Normally, total serum calcium is 10 ± 1 milligrams per deciliter (mg/dl), and total phosphate is 3.5 ± 0.5 mg/dl. Less than half of the serum calcium is ionized and physiologically active (Figure 6.2) (70), but it is generally agreed that the ionized fraction still represents a very high concentration of calcium. This is obvious to anyone who has tried to prepare a physiologic solution; when Ca^{++} is added, even the slightest shift to alkalinity is enough to give a cloudy precipitate of calcium phosphate. Which brings out a basic rule: *calcium phosphate precipitates in an alkaline medium and is dissolved by acid.* To prove the latter point, leave a chicken thigh bone in vinegar for 3 or 4 weeks: by that time you can tie it in a knot.

> Until the 1970s it was dogma that the normal serum concentration of ionized calcium is too low to allow the precipitation of calcium phosphate, but this concept has been challenged (101, 107). In the test tube, in the absence of proteins, even physiologic concentrations of calcium and phosphate may be sufficient to cause the precipitation of calcium phosphate. This precipitation does not generally occur *in vivo*, probably because calcification-inhibiting macromolecules are present.

Why do apatite crystals proliferate? The first detectable mineral deposited *in vivo* during calcification is a poorly crystallized apatite, which perfects with age (22). (Apatite may be preceded by some short-lived intermediates such as octacalcium phosphate (22), but we need not be concerned with them here.) *Once the first apatite crystals appear, they continue to grow—crystal after crystal—by extracting more calcium and phosphate from the solution.*

If the experiment is done *in vitro,* starting with the normal concentration of calcium, the tricky little crystals will go on proliferating until the concentration of calcium has dropped to one-third the normal level (63). In other words, the *serum concentration of calcium appears to be supersaturated with regard to growing crystals of apatite* (21, 63, 86).

How does a crystal begin? Apatite crystals grow out of other crystal surfaces by a phenomenon called **secondary nucleation** (86, 89), which means that the surface of an apatite crystal—when exposed to a supersaturated solution—acts as a growth site for another crystal. Apatite crystals can also grow on the surface of a different material—not necessarily a crystal—which acts as a primary nucleus; this phenomenon is called **epitaxy.** A crude example of epitaxy is provided by a high school experiment: if a cord is suspended in a saturated solution of sugar that is allowed slowly to evaporate, beautiful crystals of sugar grow on the cord (11). Epitaxy contributes a great deal to pathologic calcifications because it does not require that the seeding surface be that of another crystal. As the cord-and-sugar experiment shows, almost any surface works as long as

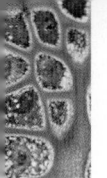

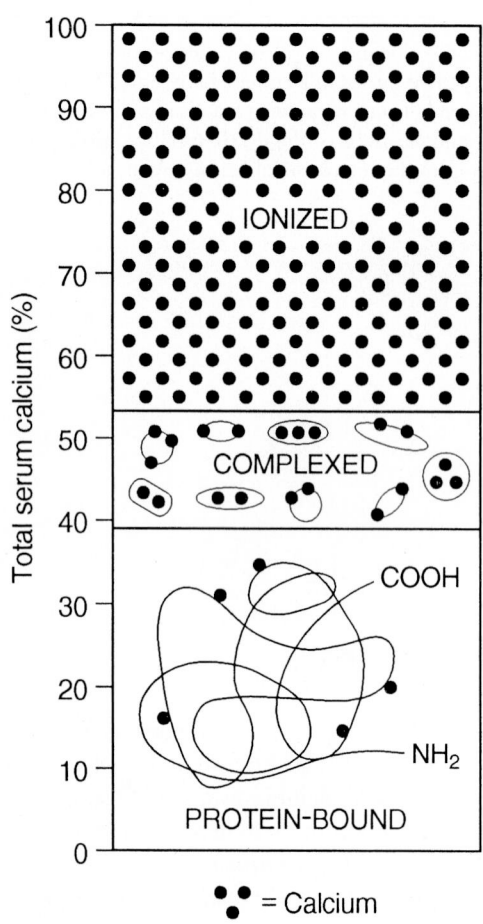

FIGURE 6.2　Total serum calcium consists of three fractions: ionized (the physiologically active fraction), protein-bound, and complexed (bound to several organic and inorganic anions). (Adapted from [70] with permission. Illustration by A. Miller.)

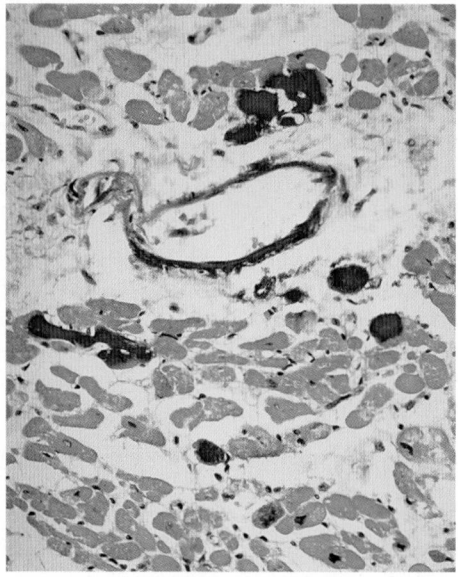

FIGURE 6.3　Calcification in the wall of an atherosclerotic artery. *Top right:* Lumen of the artery. *Top left:* Part of atherosclerotic plaque. *Center:* Calcified mass developing in the arterial media. Only the periphery of the mass is basophilic (hematoxylin and eosin stain).

its atomic lattice is sufficiently similar to that of the crystal. There are many examples of epitaxy (86); apatite crystals can be seeded even by organic surfaces, as we will explain shortly.

Microscopic Aspects of Calcification

It is fairly easy to recognize calcified structures in microscopic sections stained with hematoxylin and eosin: the basic rule is that *calcified structures are deeply basophilic or have at least a basophilic rim.* Therefore, they will be deep blue or have a deep blue rim.

FIGURE 6.4　*Left:* Myocardium with metastatic calcifications (basophilic). From a case of hypercalcemia due to a parathyroid adenoma. Calcification affects myocardial cells as well as vascular walls. *Right:* Dystrophic calcification of mitochondria in the same case.

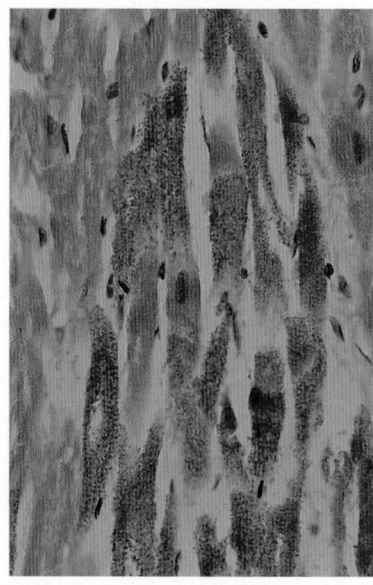

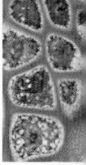

This basophilia is hard to explain. First of all, it is there whether the tissue sample has been decalcified or not. In other words, the basophilia is not a label for tissue calcium; it tells us that CALCIUM WAS HERE, BUT MAY NO LONGER BE HERE. Histochemically it means that the substrate has acquired negative charges, capable of binding calcium as well as the positively charged hematoxylin.

Another baffling fact is that a large calcified mass always has a basophilic rim; but as it expands, the central part tends to lose its basophilia and to stain pink with eosin (Figure 6.3). This means that the traditional rule whereby calcifications are always basophilic is not entirely correct. After all, bone—the prototype of calcified structures—is eosinophilic overall. The mechanism of the basophilic change needs to be worked out.

Dead, calcified cells, single or in groups, are often seen in histologic sections. This raises a question: *did the cells die because they were calcified, or did they calcify because they were dead*? Both events can occur. Calcifications in live cells usually start in mitochondria; this effect is common in injured cells (Figures 6.4, 6.5). It is easily produced, even *in vitro,* simply by prolonged incubation of mitochondria in physiologic solutions (65). These organelles are naturally predisposed to accumulate calcium.

Why are mitochondria prone to calcification? Remember that the cell membrane pumps calcium *out,* so the concentration of calcium in the cytoplasm is 1000–10,000 times lower than in the extracellular fluid. However, the mitochondrial membrane pumps calcium *into* the mitochondria, so these organelles have about ten times more free calcium than the extracellular fluid.

Whenever cytoplasmic calcium increases (e.g., because blood calcium is abnormally high or because the cell membrane is damaged), *the mitochondria come to the rescue as active calcium traps* (4, 7, 52): the calcium that they pump in is taken out of solution and appears as granules or amorphous masses, probably of calcium phosphate. Calcified mitochondria cease to function. When too many mitochondria are calcified, the cell dies.

Some technical problems arise when calcified tissues are to be examined histologically. If the calcifications are of microscopic size, the tissues can be embedded and cut as usual, although the calcifications may nick the knife; larger calcifications must be decalcified in acid after fixation, just like bone. Of course, if microscopic sections are being made for the very purpose of studying the mineral deposits, exposure to acids must be avoided.

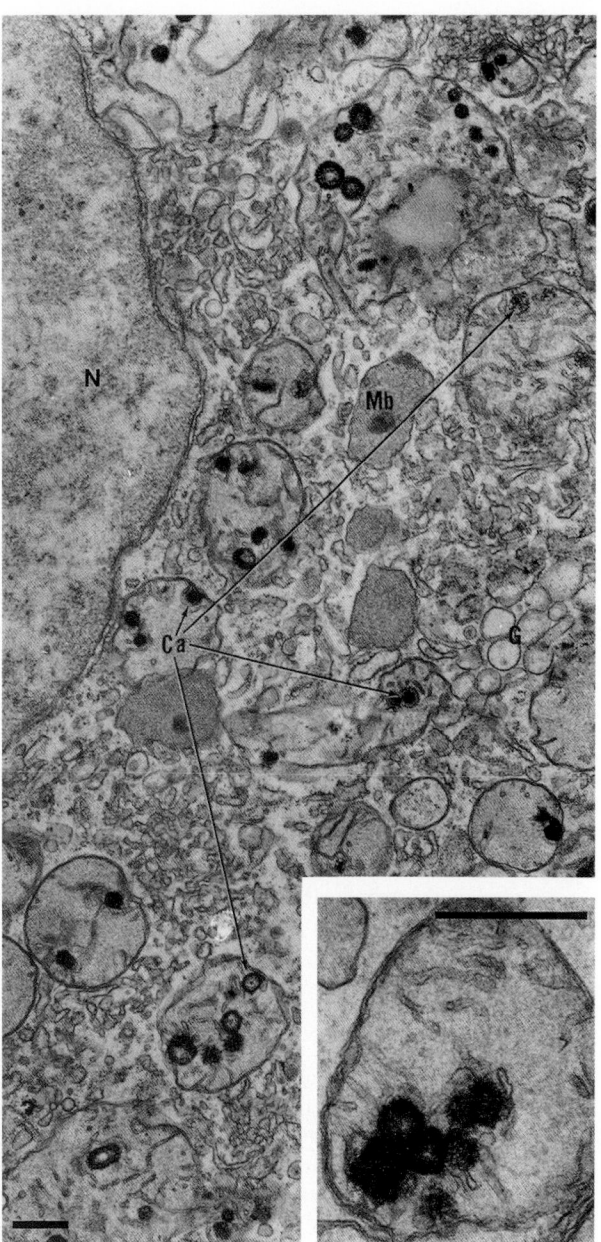

FIGURE 6.5 Part of a rat liver cell 16 hours after poisoning with carbon tetrachloride. **Ca:** Dark masses within mitochondria that represent calcification; some have a ringlike structure. **G:** Golgi apparatus. **Mb:** Microbody. **N:** Nucleus. **Bars** = 0.5 μm. (Reproduced from the **Journal of Cell Biology,** 1965; 25:53–75, by copyright permission of The Rockefeller University Press [92].)

Decalcification with a chelating agent (EDTA) at pH 7 is slow, but feasible. Histochemical methods are available to demonstrate either calcium or phosphate in the tissue sections.

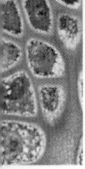

Two Roads to Pathologic Calcification

What should go through our mind when we encounter one or more ectopic calcifications, i.e., calcified cells or tissues that normally do not calcify? Experience has shown that such deposits may be caused by a **local** change, such as a focus of dead cells; or by a **body-wide** change, i.e., an excess of calcium or phosphate in the blood. Their names—**dystrophic** versus **metastatic** calcifications—are a bit awkward (they date from the 1800s) but the facts are rock-hard, and they are important, because the two types convey very different messages.

- In **dystrophic calcification,** by far the more common mechanism, *a local change or disturbance in the tissue favors the nucleation of apatite crystals. Serum calcium and phosphate concentrations are normal.* (The term *dystrophic* is supposed to remind us that there is a local disturbance, or "dystrophy.")
- In **metastatic calcification,** the disturbance is body-wide. It occurs *when the blood concentration of calcium (more rarely of phosphate) rises above a critical level,* whereby deposits of apatite crystals develop throughout the body. Because it is generalized, metastatic calcification can be lethal if the underlying metabolic defect is not removed.

Virchow saw the widespread calcifications as secondary deposits comparable to those of malignant tumors, and therefore called them calcium "metastases."

Dystrophic Calcification

Dystrophic calcification is always local, and blood levels of calcium and phosphate are normal.

Calcification of necrotic tissue. A classic example of dystrophic calcification is the calcification of necrosis. Even single dead endothelial cells can calcify, as was shown by injecting rats with tetracycline (54).

Tetracycline offers a simple and striking method for detecting ongoing calcification, normal (in bone and teeth) or pathologic. Whether it is injected or taken by mouth, it is somehow deposited in all structures that are becoming calcified. Although invisible *per se,* it has a beautiful gold autofluorescence in ultraviolet light.

Dead tissue, such as occurs in infarcts, is an excellent model for studying calcification. Enough calcium accumulates in liver (76) and myocardial infarcts to be visible histochemically (33) and sometimes grossly (Figure 6.6)

FIGURE 6.6   X-ray of a slice of heart, showing heavy calcification in an ancient infarct. Note also small calcifications in coronary arteries (**arrows**). (Courtesy of Dr. H. F. Cuénoud, University of Massachusetts Medical School, Worcester, MA.)

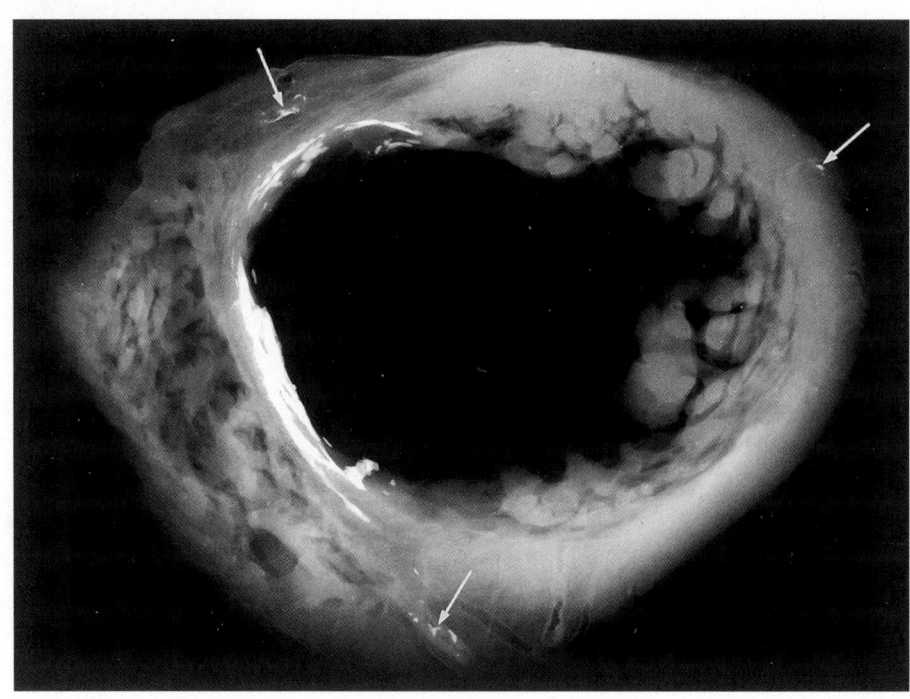

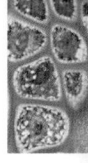

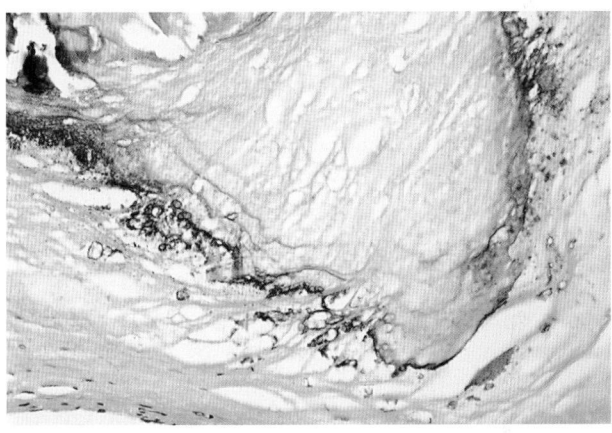

FIGURE 6.7 A calcified mass in the media of a human atherosclerotic artery. Calcospherites (basophilic granules) are peppered along the rim of the calcification. The multiple parallel lines are probably due to a Liesegang phenomenon (hematoxylin and eosin stain).

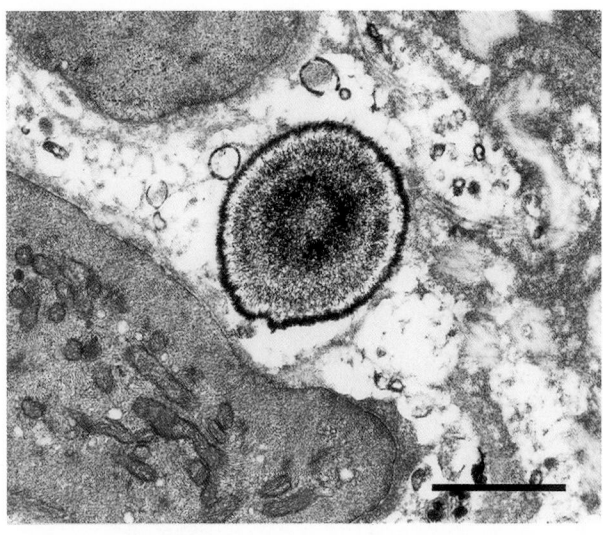

FIGURE 6.8 Typical target structure of a calcospherite in atherosclerosis (rat aorta). The target arrangement may be related to Liesegang rings (*see* Figure 6.9). Specimen not decalcified. **Bar** = 1 μm.

Because the calcium is supplied by the blood in the surrounding live tissues, calcification begins at the periphery of the infarct. Within a day or two, the process is announced by a powdering of tiny basophilic granules of uneven size, no larger than nuclei, and long known as **calcospherites** (117) (Figure 6.7). The largest granules have a targetlike structure, which was recognized as early as 1857 (117). Calcospherites tend to grow and to coalesce: the result is an expanding calcified area with a basophilic rim and a rather eosinophilic center. Electron microscopy shows that the target structure of the calcospherites is due to concentric rings of apatite crystals (Figure 6.8).

The growth of calcospherites by successive waves is best explained by analogy with the famous **Liesegang, rings,** known since the turn of the century (Figure 6.9) (44, 57, 105, 116). These systems of concentric rings can be produced by two reactants diffusing in a gel; they can be produced also with calcium and phosphate (24).

Calcification of the aortic valve. Another example of the dystrophic mechanism is the calcification of the aortic valve (Figure 6.10). Notice a striking feature of this condition: the valve cusps do not simply "turn to stone"; they are also *enlarged* by rough, bulky, wartlike masses. This tells us that calcification, under certain circumstances, increases the volume of the calcified tissue. Considering that calcospherites—at a microscopic level—do grow by concentric expansion, the progressive thickening of the aortic valves could be the effect of crystal growth over a long time.

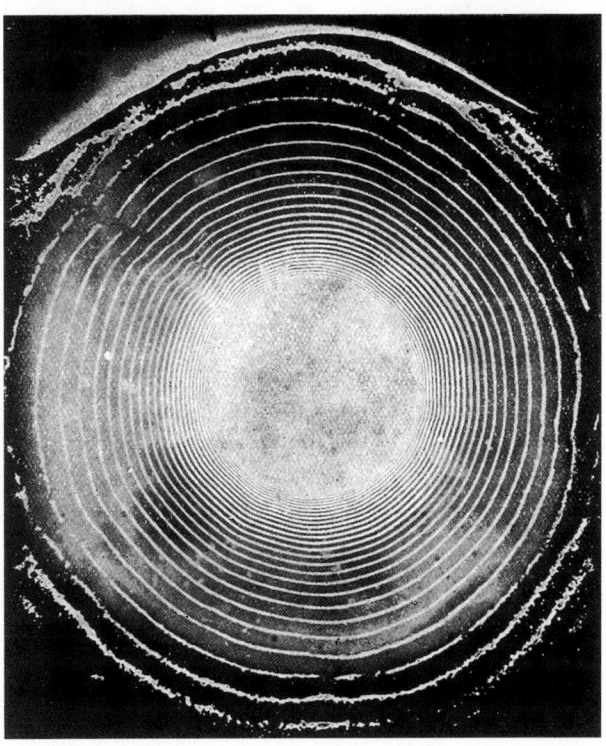

FIGURE 6.9 Example of a rhythmic chemical reaction: the Liesegang rings, as observed by Liesegang himself. A drop of 50 percent AgNo₃ is placed on a layer of gelatin containing 0.1 percent potassium bichromate. Precipitation occurs in concentric rings. (Reproduced from [44] by permission from Methuen & Co.)

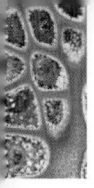

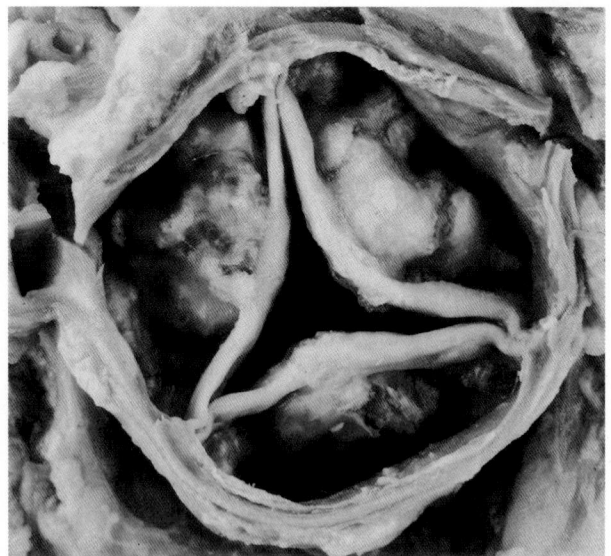

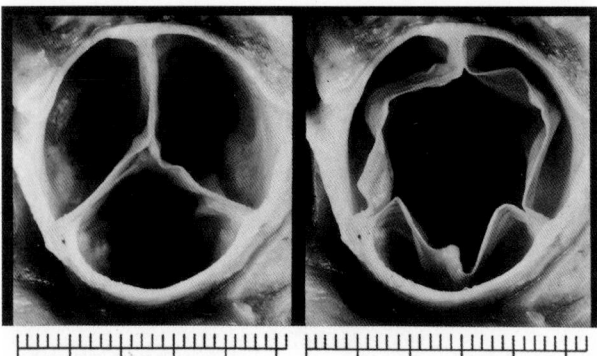

FIGURE 6.10 *Top:* Calcified aortic valve of an 80-year-old woman. Note that the tissue increases in volume as it calcifies. (Reproduced from [37] by permission of Mayo Foundation.) *Bottom:* Normal aortic valve viewed from above, in simulated closed (*left*) and open (*right*) positions. From a 33-year-old man. **Scale** in millimeters. (Reproduced with permission from [88].)

Histologically, the rock-hard aortic valves consist of calcium deposits in a mass of protein and lipid (66). What is this organic matrix? Is it some protein that seeped in from the plasma, and if so why? Did the lipid or the protein come first and the mineral later? Are we dealing with calcification triggered by proteolipids (90)? Does cholesterol nucleate apatite (95)? We have no answers.

Initiators of dystrophic calcification. To explain a localized calcification (which occurs despite normal values of blood calcium and phosphate), we need some local mechanism to set off the process by seeding apatite crystals. In theory, local calcification can be triggered in one of three ways (27): a local increase in the $Ca \times P$ product, exposure of nucleators (epitaxy), or removal of inhibitors. Examples of all three are known. However, *most crystal-seeding mechanisms assume that epitaxy is involved;* that is, an organic substrate has the property of binding calcium or phosphate in an orderly fashion, like a template, mimicking the crystalline surface of apatite and thereby triggering the birth of an apatite crystal. Perhaps each of the following mechanisms plays a role in initiating epitaxy in some circumstances.

- Phospholipids as initiators. *Phospholipids are amply proven to be nucleators* (23, 28), especially phosphatidyl serine, which is acidic and therefore able to bind calcium (Figure 6.11). This property of phospholipids would easily account for the prevalence of calcification in necrotic areas, where membrane phospholipids abound as myelin figures and **ultramicroscopic vesicles.** Such vesicles are especially common in atherosclerotic aortas (62, 101), from which source a proteolipid was extracted that actually caused nucleation of apatite *in vitro* (39) (**proteolipids** are integral membrane proteins that are soluble in organic solvents).

Here is the story of the **matrix vesicles.** Simple as they are, membrane-bound vesicles so common in necrotic

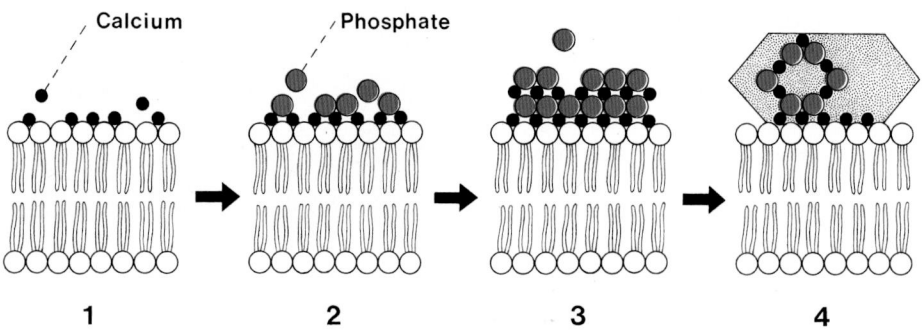

Calcium   Phosphate

1   2   3   4

FIGURE 6.11 Diagram of a possible model of membrane-facilitated calcification. *Stage 1:* Calcium ions bind to two adjacent polar heads of phospholipid molecules (water is displaced in the process). *Stage 2:* Phosphate groups bind to the layer of calcium. *Stage 3:* The cycle of calcium and phosphate binding is repeated. *Stage 4:* By an internal rearrangement of the calcium and phosphate ions, a microcrystal develops (paracrystalline apatite). (Adapted from [111].)

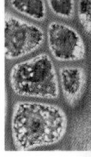

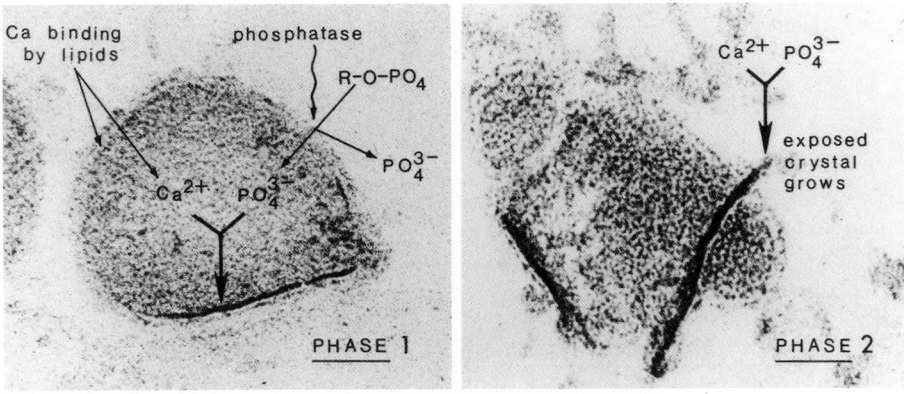

FIGURE 6.12 Scheme of the mineralization process operated by the matrix vesicles as it occurs in the growth plate cartilage of the rat. *Phase 1:* Intravesicular calcium concentration rises due to the affinity of calcium for the lipids of the inner membrane. Phosphatase in the membrane increases the local concentration of PO_4 in or near the vesicle. Thereby the $Ca \times PO_4$ product in the vesicle is raised, initiating a mineral deposit near the membrane. *Phase 2:* Apatite crystals grow because the medium is supersaturated with respect to apatite. The growing crystals perforate the membrane. (Reprinted from Metabol Bone Dis Relat Res *1*, Anderson HC. Introduction to the second conference on matrix vesicle calcification, pp. 83–87, Copyright 1978, with permission from Pergamon Press Ltd, Headington Hill Hall, Oxford OX3 OBW, UK [3].)

tissues raise an interesting question: are they related to the so-called extracellular "matrix vesicles" seen in normal enchondral ossification?

In the late 1960s, two research groups independently discovered 1000–2000 Å globules or vesicles in epiphyseal growth cartilage and proposed them as initiators of calcification in that system (2, 6, 16, 17). These matrix vesicles are thought to arise from local cells by a mechanism still under debate, perhaps by budding like viruses (6); the current concept is that calcium seeps into them and binds to the inner surfaces of their membranes by the phosphatidyl serine mechanism mentioned earlier; phosphatases in the membrane would then provide phosphate while also degrading pyrophosphate and ATP, which are "crystal poisons" (Figure 6.12). Vesicles of all sizes abound in necrotic tissues, including atherosclerotic arteries where many cells die leaving behind a magma of globules (62). Of course there is nothing specific about these "degenerative" vesicles; they are not necessarily the same as the "programmed" matrix vesicles of physiologically calcifying tissues. On the other hand, they might provide a protected environment in which the initial crystals form; they might also cause nucleation of apatite even without enzymatic intervention, by the surface mechanism shown in Figure 6.11 (6, 112).

Wherever the truth may lie, a feature of these nondescript vesicular remains is that they may offer a link between normal and dystrophic calcification (5). The link would become a very tight one if it is true that the normal matrix vesicles arise not only by budding but also by death and fragmentation of chondrocytes (17).

- Elastic fibers as initiators. Elastic fibers are susceptible to calcification; they may calcify while the

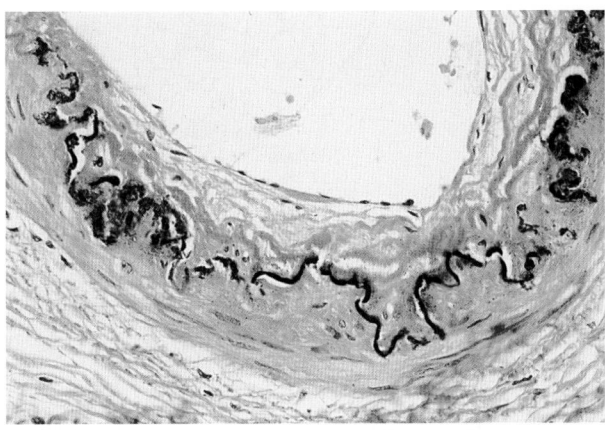

FIGURE 6.13 Selective calcification of the internal elastic lamina (basophilic wavy line) in a human artery. The intima is thickened.

tissues around them do not (Figure 6.13) (114). Several mechanisms have been proposed (63), including a progressive increase in carboxyl-bearing amino acids in the elastin molecule (69) and calcification of the microfibrils that surround the elastic fibers (56).

- Collagen fibrils as initiators. Collagen fibrils often calcify (96), for example, in poorly vascularized tissues such as tendons.
- Calcific deposits appear both around and within the fibrils; it has been proposed that there is a nucleation site within the fibril itself, where the quarter-staggered arrangement of the molecules leaves a space or "hole" (Figure 6.14) (11, 48).

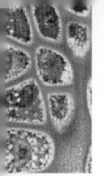

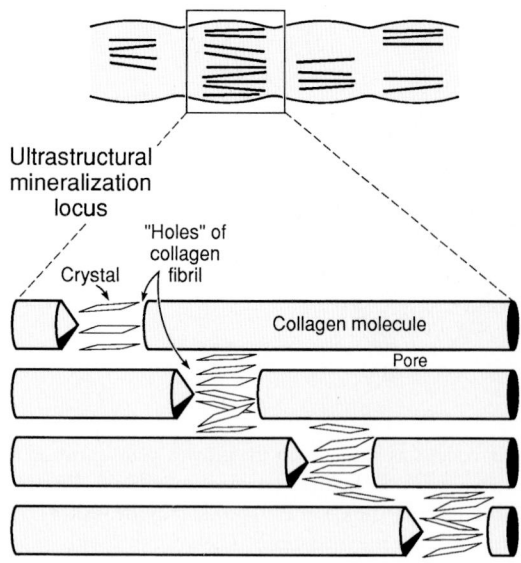

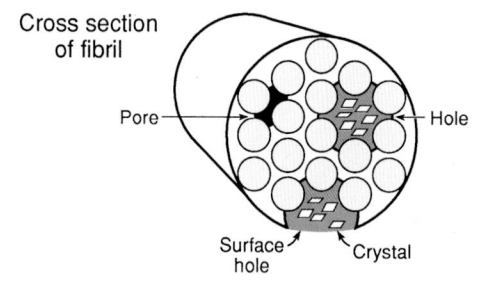

FIGURE 6.14   Pathologic calcification of the collagen fibrils is thought to begin in "holes" present in the fibrils, between the ends of the quarter-staggered molecules. (Adapted from [49].)

• Role of denatured proteins. Denatured proteins have not yet been studied as nucleators of calcium phosphates, but, in necrotic tissues, it is almost certain that denatured proteins bind calcium and/or phosphate (76).

• Role of GLA. GLA (gamma-carboxy-glutamic acid), a fairly recent addition to the family of amino acids, is formed from glutamic acid by carboxylation in the presence of vitamin K (47). Its two adjacent carboxyls make it suitable for tightly binding calcium, calcium phosphates, and (via the calcium) phospholipids. GLA is found in the blood, in mineralized tissues, and in pathologic calcifications; a GLA-rich protein in bone is abundant enough to qualify for the name **osteocalcin** (53). In atherosclerotic plaques, a related GLA protein was found and named **atherocalcin** (72); osteocalcin was also present (71). Whether these proteins have a primary or a secondary role—or no role at all—remains to be seen (115).

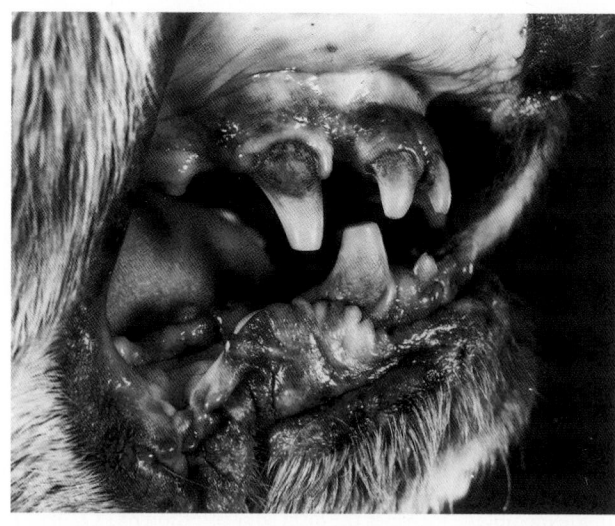

FIGURE 6.15   Bacterial calcification, as shown by dental calculus on the teeth of a 14-year-old dog. Similar calcified microbial plaques occur in humans. (Reproduced with permission from [34], © American Society for Investigative Pathology.)

Knockout mice lacking GLA protein provided a surprise: they developed to term but died within 2 months with diffuse arterial calcifications that led to arterial rupture. GLA proteins are normally produced by vascular smooth muscle cells, which do not normally calcify: this fact, and the findings on the GLA-deprived mice, suggests that calcification may need to be *actively inhibited* in soft tissues (75).

• Role of phosphoproteins. Phosphoproteins are thought to play a role in normal and pathologic calcifications (100).

• Role of fatty acids. Fatty acids certainly bind calcium to form soaps (p. 230), but their role in physiological calcification is not clear (13) and perhaps nil (117).

• Bacteria as initiators. Some bacteria can be very efficient nucleators. Because bacteria and mitochondria are related (p. 137) it is not too surprising that they should share also this bizarre property (110). It is the calcification of oral bacteria that produces **calculus,** that pernicious mineral periodically mined by dental hygienists (Figure 6.15). (We cannot resist mentioning the real meaning of *calculus:* it is Latin for "small stone." The Romans used pebbles for making simple "calculations.")

It was a member of the oral flora, *Bacterionema matruchotii* (Figure 6.16), that yielded the first phospholipid–protein complex capable of nucleating apatite *in vitro* (30, 39, 113). Actinomycetes are especially prone to calcify; they are thought to be responsible for calcified masses that sometimes form around intrauterine devices (IUDs) (6, 50).

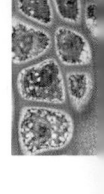

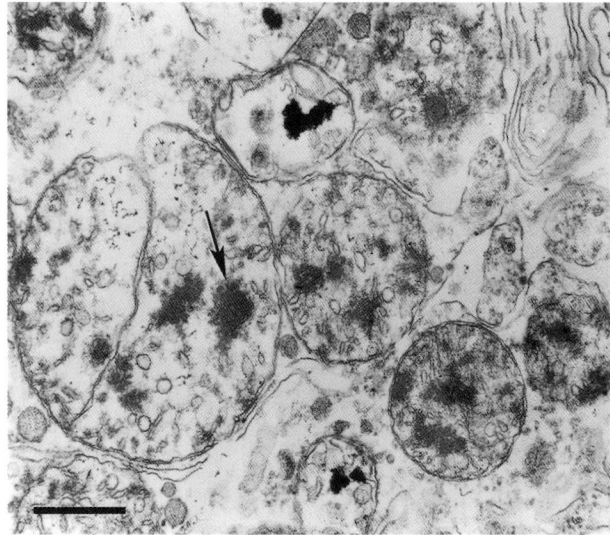

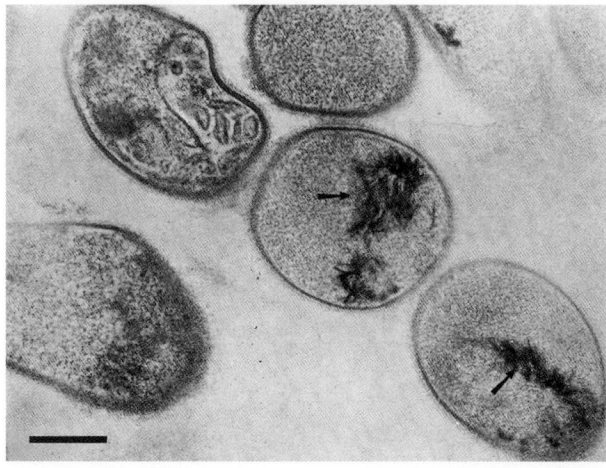

FIGURE 6.16   Calcification in mitochondria and bacteria. *Top:* Mitochondria incubated in physiologic concentrations of calcium and phosphate. **Arrow:** A type of density that contained calcium and phosphate when submitted to electron probe microanalysis. (Rat kidney cortex incubated in Earl's minimal essential medium plus Hanks' BSS.) **Bar** = 0.5 μm. (Reproduced with permission from [65].) *Bottom:* Crystals of apatite (**arrows**) forming inside *Bacterionema matruchotii,* a large filamentous microorganism from the oral flora. Ultimately such bacterial calcifications lead to the formation of dental calculus. **Bar** = 0.5 μm. (Reproduced from [113].)

Metastatic Calcification

The conditions that make metastatic calcification possible are **hypercalcemia** and, much more rarely, **hyperphosphatemia**. Hypercalcemia has many causes (Table 6.1). In hospitals it is seen most often in patients whose skeleton is rapidly destroyed by a malignant tumor, either metastatic or primary, such as multiple

Table 6.1 Hypercalcemia: The Principal Causes

Hypersecretion of parathyroid hormone (PTH) (→ increased bone resorption)

Primary (due to parathyroid hyperplasia or tumor)
Secondary to renal failure (which causes retention of phosphate)
Ectopic secretion of PTH by a malignant tumor (e.g., carcinoma of the lung)

Destruction of bone tissue

By a primary tumor of the bone marrow (e.g., multiple myeloma)
By diffuse skeletal metastases
By Paget's disease of bone (accelerated bone turnover)
By immobilization (immobility removes a stimulus to bone formation while resorption continues)

Other mechanisms

Poisoning with vitamin A or D (in food faddists)
Milk-alkali syndrome (from excess intake of both*)
Thiazide diuretics
Sarcoidosis (macrophages activate a vitamin D precursor)
Uremia and dialysis (mechanism unclear, probably multiple)

*Randall RE Jr, Strauss MB, McNeely WF. The milk-alkali syndrome. Arch Intern Med 1961;107:163–181.
Source: Adapted from Levine MM, Kleeman CR. Hypercalcemia: pathophysiology and treatment. Hosp Pract 1987;22:93–110.

myeloma. Another classic but less common cause is hyperparathyroidism, which is due to functional tumors of the parathyroid glands (about 50,000 cases per year in the United States). For calcium metastases to develop, the critical value of serum calcium is about 17 mg/dl (1); high phosphate can also lead to metastatic calcification (118). Phosphate usually rises as a result of chronic renal failure when the glomerular filtration rate drops to 25 percent or less.

A good rule of thumb is that the product of serum calcium and phosphate in adults is normally 35–40; above 60 or 70, metastatic calcification occurs (108). The main clinical sign of hypercalcemia is severe muscular weakness—the opposite of hypocalcemia, which induces tetany.

Preferred locations.   The so-called calcium metastases can appear almost anywhere as spotty deposits, but they have certain predilections. At first sight, a list of the tissues most afflicted by calcium metastases seems to make no sense at all:

- Mucosa of the stomach
- Kidneys and lungs
- Cornea
- Systemic arteries
- Pulmonary veins

It is quite a challenge to find a common feature among these disparate locations, but it does exist. The basic

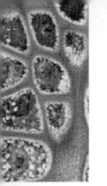

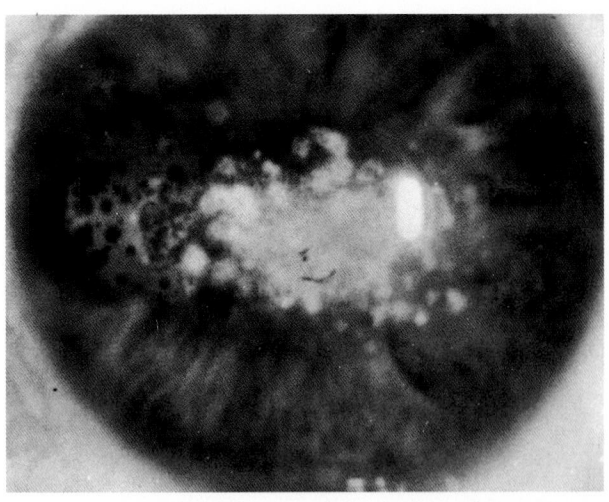

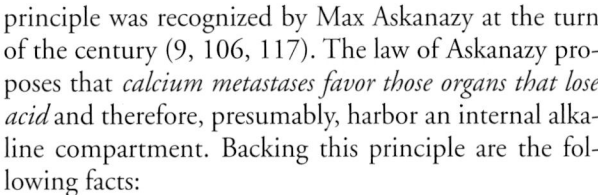

FIGURE 6.17　Calcification across the cornea in hypercalcemia (band keratopathy) attributed to local loss of CO_2. (Reproduced with permission from [58].)

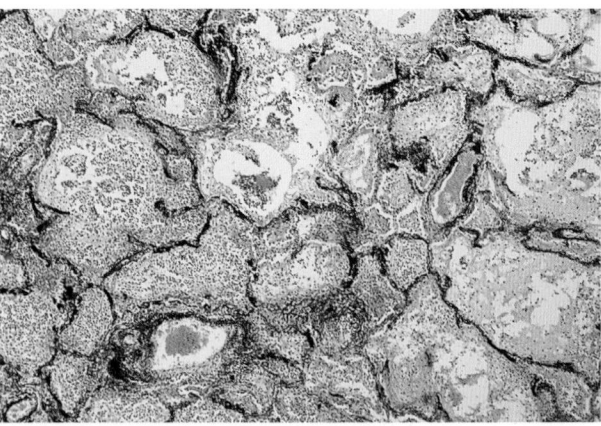

FIGURE 6.18　Lung tissue with diffuse calcification of the alveolar walls (basophilic network). The calcification was due to severe hypercalcemia caused by bone destruction secondary to multiple myeloma. (The alveoli are filled with cells; this is the pneumonia that eventually killed the patient.) (Hematoxylin and eosin stain.)

principle was recognized by Max Askanazy at the turn of the century (9, 106, 117). The law of Askanazy proposes that *calcium metastases favor those organs that lose acid* and therefore, presumably, harbor an internal alkaline compartment. Backing this principle are the following facts:

- The stomach secretes HCl, and the venous blood from the stomach does become more alkaline during the secretion of gastric juice (67).
- The renal tubules secrete acid urine.
- The lungs lose CO_2.
- The cornea loses CO_2 by diffusion (there is a carbonic anhydrase in the ciliary processes [77]), especially along the interpalpebral fissure where calcification is most common in association with renal failure (Figure 6.17).

Presumably, according to the same principle:

- The systemic veins are relatively spared because their blood is more acid (p. 259).
- The systemic arteries and pulmonary veins do calcify because they carry arterial blood in which carbonate is at its lowest (84, 117).
- There is also a tendency for heavier calcium deposition in the lining of the left side of the heart, where the blood is arterial (70, 84, 93).

Morphologic findings. The autopsy findings in cases of severe hypercalcemia are striking. Calcified tissues

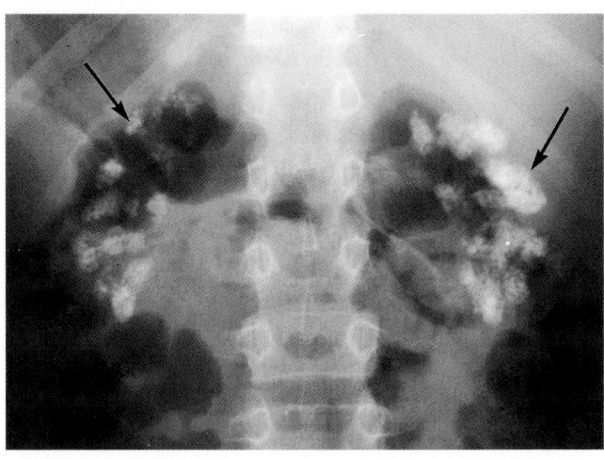

FIGURE 6.19　X-ray of a patient (boy aged 13) with bilateral renal calcifications. The opaque masses (**arrows**) represent the pattern of calcified pyramids. (Courtesy of Dr. A. Davidoff, University of Massachusetts Medical School, Worcester, MA.)

appear chalky. The gastric mucosa, for example, can appear strangely white: Virchow describes it as feeling like a rasp and grating under the knife, whereas the lung becomes "similar to a fine bathing sponge" (109), a very appropriate comparison because the alveolar walls become stiff with calcium deposits (Figure 6.18). Functionally the most damaging effect is **nephrocalcinosis,** calcification of the kidney (Figure 6.19), which causes retention of phosphate and secondary hyperparathyroidism, which in turn aggravates the

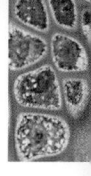

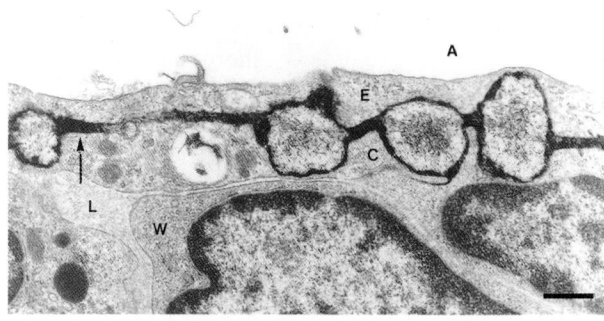

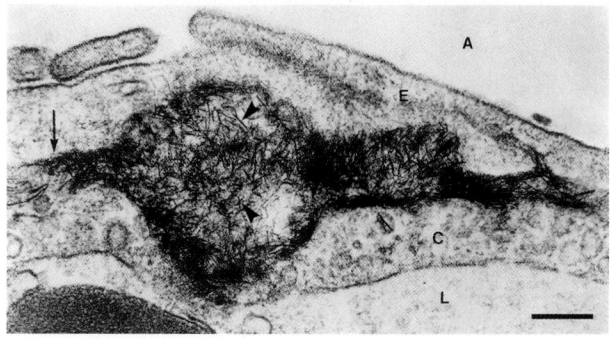

FIGURE 6.20 Calcification of the alveolar basement membrane in the lung of a rat, sacrificed 6 days after a single overdose of vitamin D by mouth. *Top:* The dystrophic calcification begins in the basement membrane and expands focally into a "rosary bead" pattern. **Bar** = 0.5 μm. *Bottom:* Detail showing the crystals of apatite (**arrowheads**). Although on electron micrographs these crystals appear as needles, they are in reality thin plates, 100–400 Å in length. **Bar** = 0.2 μm. **Arrows:** Basement membrane. **A:** Alveolar lumen. **E:** Alveolar epithelium. **C:** Capillary endothelium. **L:** Lumen of capillary. **W:** White blood cells. (Courtesy of Dr. Y. Kapanci, University of Geneva, Switzerland.)

hypercalcemia. In early stages it is reversible. Nephrocalcinosis should not be confused with nephrolithiasis (kidney stones).

Microscopically, mitochondria are the first cellular targets of hypercalcemia, especially in the heart and kidney. Deposits appear first as an amorphous mass and then as apatite needles (6, 79). Electron microscopy shows that calcified mitochondria appear at first in cells that are otherwise normal (18, 19); eventually the cells may die and become engulfed in mineral deposits.

In hypercalcemia due to hyperparathyroidism, the entry of calcium into the cell is favored by the parathyroid hormone itself (20). Primary mitochondrial calcification has been seen also in normocalcemic animals after various insults (e.g., in aortic smooth muscle after adrenaline administration) (32). In striated muscle, metastatic calcium deposits occur mainly along the fibrils and in the sarcoplasmic reticulum (18).

Basement membranes are another favorite site of metastatic calcification. Typical examples are seen in the lung (Figure 6.20) (38) and around the renal convoluted tubules (perhaps because this is where urine is being acidified) (31). The Ca^{++} ions probably bind to the negative charges of glycosaminoglycans or other basement membrane components (remember that basement membranes are also known to bind silver ions, Ag^+) (p. 278).

Growth and Fate of Calcifications

Once started, calcifications tend to grow (96). Of this there are many examples. At the electron microscopic level, the calcospherites grow by successive waves (Figure 6.21). The advancing rim seems to destroy all microscopic detail, as if the forest of growing crystals had the effect of grinding up all the structures they encounter. Most obviously, calcified aortic valves swell to several times their original thickness (see Figure 6.10).

Presumably, the growth of calcifications reflects the ability of apatite crystals to proliferate by secondary nucleation. But apatite crystals can continue to proliferate in a physiologic concentration of calcium, so why do calcifications ever stop growing? In the skeleton, where apatite crystals have a surface estimated at 500,000 m², their growing frenzy is probably restrained by the organic

matrix (25, 81); calcifications have no comparable barrier. Much evidence shows that **calcification inhibitors** come into play (41). Many have been described. Some are natural and have been found in the blood and urine (63, 94, 107). They include polyphosphates and macromolecules such as proteoglycans and heparin. Little is known of their behavior *in vivo,* but remember what happened to GLA-deficient mice (p. 254).

Macrophages derive from the same hematopoietic precursor as the osteoclasts (83), which means that nibbling at calcifications could well be included in their job description. In practice, they show little motivation to do so. Metastatic calcifications can regress, at least in part, if the cause of the hypercalcemia or hyperphosphatemia is removed (15, 98, 102, 104), but dystrophic

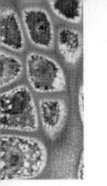
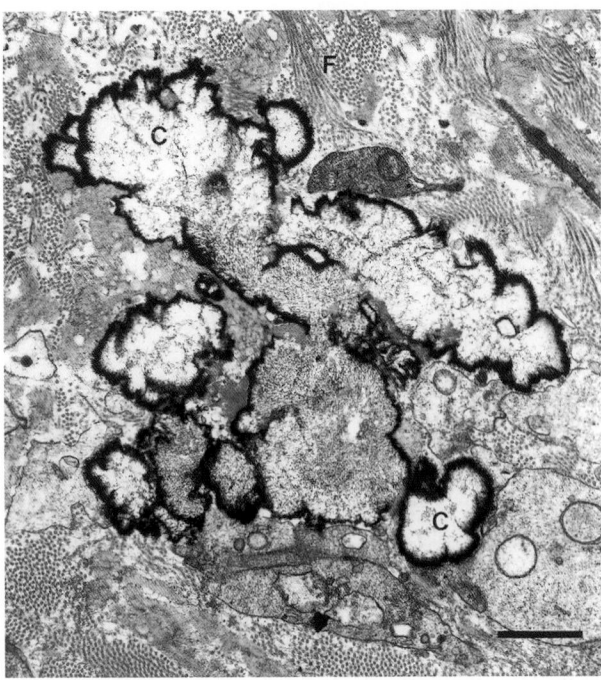

FIGURE 6.21   **C:** Foci of calcification (calcospherites) as seen by electron microscopy in a human atherosclerotic artery. **F:** Collagen fibers. The dark rims represent advancing fronts of apatite crystals. **Bar** = 1 μm.

FIGURE 6.22   Comparing the formulae of inorganic pyrophosphate and bisphosphonate.

calcifications such as a calcified lymph node of healed tuberculosis tend to persist for a lifetime.

Sometimes a layer of osteoid is laid down over a pathologic calcification; then a little patch of real bone tissue develops, and eventually hemopoietic bone marrow develops adjacent to the bone: a case of double differentiation not uncommon in human atherosclerotic arteries. The mechanism is not clear, but it may depend on local growth factors: osteocalcin, after collagen the protein most abundant in bone, may recruit osteoblasts (58a), and osteoblasts are a key component of the niches for hematopoietic cells (30a) (p. 18). These relationships may also help understand how bone became the home of bone marrow.

The calcifications caused by **chronic renal failure** (i.e., by hyperphosphatemia) have a natural history of their own (14, 51, 73, 104); some of the metastatic deposits (e.g., in the heart muscle) resemble those of hypercalcemia, but others are quite distinctive. They are aggravated by dialysis (60), a fact that is not well understood; one possibility is that dialysis removes an inhibitor. Serum calcium can be normal, but with a phosphate level of 9 the Ca × P product would rise well above the critical limit of 60 to 70 for metastatic calcification.

Massive, even tumorlike calcifications (104) develop especially over the hips, trunk, and joints; biopsies show calcification, necrosis, and intimal fibrosis (42) of small arteries and calcification of the subcutaneous fat and muscle with granulation tissue and giant cells, suggesting infarction secondary to arterial failure. Some unfortunate patients develop extensive, painful calcifications of the skin, which are usually—and incorrectly—diagnosed as *calciphylaxis* (see below). Yet another presentation is "pipe stem" calcification of the coronary arteries, in young patients after 5 years of dialysis (51); whether it relates to atherosclerosis is not known.

Prevention and treatment of calcifications can be attempted with bisphosphonates, which are related to pyrophosphates except that they have the structure P—C—P rather than P—O—P (Figure 6.22); remember that pyrophosphates are among the inhibitors of calcification. Bisphosphonates bind to the crystal surface and block its growth; by the same token they also prevent crystal dissolution. However, they also inhibit the osteoclasts and possibly shorten their life span (35). The P—C—P bond makes bisphosphonates resistant to all known enzymes. Their adoption for medical use was suggested by a curious analogy: they were used commercially to prevent scaling in water installations (43).

Calcification: Loose Ends

Some types of calcification are difficult to explain or downright mysterious. Listed below are a few that are especially intriguing.

Non-calcium phosphate deposits. Not all calcifications are apatite or other calcium phosphates. In the kidney (31) and in the lung (85), for example, they sometimes consist of **calcium carbonate.** (Eggshells, by the way, are also made of carbonate.) Using special electron microscopic techniques, it is possible to analyze the atomic composition of microscopic and ultramicroscopic granules. These methods were applied to specimens of human breast tissue that were surgically

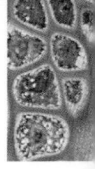

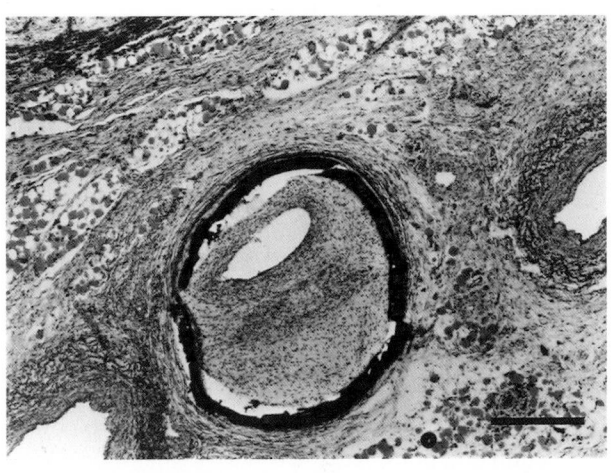

FIGURE 6.23 Calcified media (black circle) in a medium-sized artery from the thigh of a diabetic patient. The lumen is partially occluded by intimal thickening. **Bar** = 500 μm. (Reproduced from [12] with permission from Neurology.)

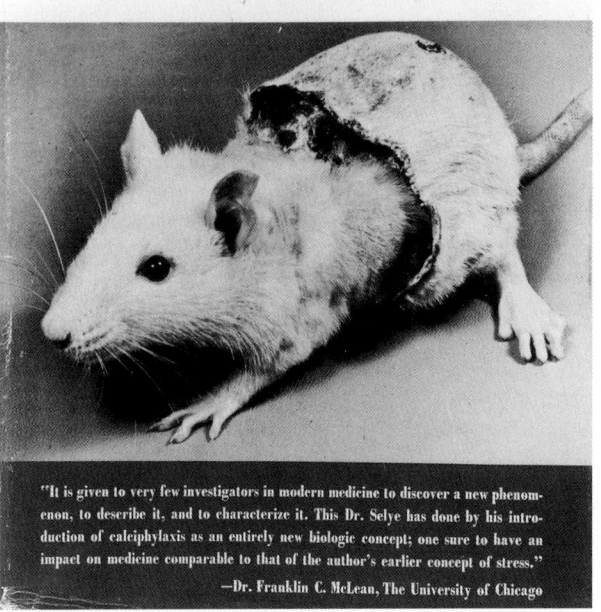

HANS SELYE

CALCIPHYLAXIS

"It is given to very few investigators in modern medicine to discover a new phenomenon, to describe it, and to characterize it. This Dr. Selye has done by his introduction of calciphylaxis as an entirely new biologic concept; one sure to have an impact on medicine comparable to that of the author's earlier concept of stress."
—Dr. Franklin C. McLean, The University of Chicago

FIGURE 6.24 The phenomenon of calciphylaxis, illustrated by calcification of the skin of a rat. (Reproduced with permission from [97].)

removed after mammography had shown them to contain "calcifications" associated with cancer. The radio-opaque nodules were then reported to contain calcium only, bound to some organic substrate, with little or no phosphate. Other concretions, more surprisingly, are noncalcifications containing Al, Fe, Mg, Si, Cu, Zn, Pb, Au, Ag, and other odd elements, alone or in combination (46); their significance is not known.

The case of small arteries. Arteries of a caliber in the range of 1–2 mm seem especially prone to calcify; about 9 percent of women who undergo mammography show segments of calcified arteries, clearly recognizable by the pattern of two fine parallel lines (61). This finding shows a correlation with diabetes (Figure 6.23) and hypertension; the mechanism is not clear.

Calcification and the heart valves. The valves of the pulmonary artery never calcify whereas the aortic valves do. Nobody knows why.

> We offer some speculations. The blood bathing the aortic valves is slightly more alkaline than that bathing the pulmonary valves: 7.45 versus 7.35 (99). This difference might be just enough to seed the first few apatite crystals, which would then continue to grow. This concept is an extension of the mechanism proposed to explain the different susceptibilities of arteries and veins to metastatic calcification (p. 256). Another major difference between right and left endocardium is that the transendothelial transport of lipid in early atherosclerosis is virtually limited to the valves on the left side; the subendocardial lipid deposit might be related to calcium deposition (36).

Calciphylaxis, a strange story. Calciphylaxis is a bizarre laboratory phenomenon described in the rat and so named by the late endocrinologist Hans Selye (45, 97). It refers to the precipitous calcification of certain organs or tissues in rats that are pretreated with a hypercalcemic agent (called a **sensitizer**) and then injected with one of many possible substances called **challengers.** For example, a large dose of the sensitizer (vitamin D or analog, parathyroid hormone) is given by mouth or parenterally, which induces (presumably) a mild hypercalcemia; but no calcifications develop. Then, after a critical period of 24–48 hours, the challenger is given either locally or systemically; this induces rapid calcifications, even though the challenger alone would have had no significant effect. Some examples:

- A rat is given by mouth 1 mg of dihydrotachysterol; the next day the skin is challenged subcutaneously with an innocuous substance such as egg albumin. Promptly the injected skin calcifies, and after 23 days it is shed, revealing, says Selye, a newly formed skin underneath (Figure 6.24).

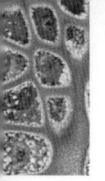

- After the use of the same sensitizer, an intravenous challenge with eggwhite produced an almost selective calcification of the pancreas, and egg yolk produced calcification of the whole spleen and of the Kupffer cells of the liver. The selectivity of the calcifications is astonishing.

- With the appropriate combination of sensitizer and challenger, Selye could calcify at will either the right auricular appendage of the heart, or the thymus, the salivary glands, the two vagus nerves, or even the carotid body. None of these localizations is explained. Though they were firmly established on some 60,000 rats (97), their relevance to human diseases is not clear. The lesions of certain human diseases show analogies with calciphylactic changes, but there is no hint that their mechanism could also be analogous (42, 78, 97).

The term calciphylaxis (defense by calcium) is probably a misnomer; there is no evidence that this strange phenomenon has any defensive value except under artificial (45) experimental conditions. However, the overall lesson one can draw from these experiments is that *the administration of two successive drugs, each one harmless, may have unpredictable effects.*

Arthritis due to crystals of apatite.

For reasons unknown, crystals of apatite can appear in joint spaces and cause inflammation (arthritis).

This peculiar phenomenon was discovered by investigating the joints of patients presumed to suffer from gout; it turned out that the crystals causing the damage were not sodium urate as expected, but calcium pyrophosphate dihydrate, a common product of intermediary metabolism (59). This disease, called *pseudo-gout* or **chondrocalcinosis,** is recognized as often asymptomatic and very common; it affects 5 percent of the adult population according to a study of autopsy cases (80). Later it was found that crystals of apatite are sometimes involved. Why should crystals inflame the joints? When phagocytized they can kill the phagocytic cell by perforating its lysosomes (p. 147). They may also adsorb and activate certain critical proteins specifically designed to trigger inflammation, such as those of the complement and kinin systems (to be discussed in Chapter 9). These properties are shared by several types of crystals, hence the unifying concept of *crystal-induced diseases.*

A post script on apatite: are stones our ancestors?

At the end of this chapter about live tissues turning to stone, it may be a shock to learn that stones may conceivably have something to do with the origins of life. We are referring to the fact that apatite crystals have a true enzymatic activity that cannot be destroyed by the heat; they function as an ATPase. The paper reporting this fact in 1962 (68) went curiously unnoticed, perhaps because of its forbidding technical title. Yet this is sensational news, not only because stones are not supposed to be enzymes but also because it is fascinating to speculate that some of the early enzymes in evolution may have been the stones that were lying around. The same idea was proposed by another group 11 years later ("In the Beginning There Was Apatite") (87). Could it be true? We will leave the rest to the imagination of the reader.

TO SUM UP: if pathologic calcification are the price we have to pay for our high levels of blood calcium and phosphate, necessary to maintain our skeleton, how high is the price? Overall not too high, but the answer will depend on who is asked. Small calcifications of the dystrophic type exist in virtually all people with normal blood calcium and phosphate; they are basically harmless, except for those that contribute to hardening the arteries and heart valves in atherosclerosis. In diabetics the arterial hardening is more severe. In individuals with high blood calcium or phosphate, metastatic calcifications can cause much damage—but then the underlying disease, such as bone cancer, may be the major problem. It is probably fair to say that *pathologic calcifications are never useful,* with the possible exception of those that develop in necrotic tuberculous lymph nodes: they might help to wall off the enemy.

References

1. Albright F, Reifenstein EC Jr. The parathyroid glands and metabolic bone disease. Baltimore: The Williams & Wilkins Company, 1948.

2. Anderson HC. Electron microscopic studies of induced cartilage development and calcification. J Cell Biol 1967; 35:81–101.

3. Anderson HC. Introduction to the second conference on matrix vesicle calcification. Metab Bone Dis Relat Res 1978; 1:83–87.

4. Anderson HC. Calcification processes. Pathol Annu 1980; 15:45–75.

5. Anderson HC. Calcific diseases. A concept. Arch Pathol Lab Med 1983;107:341–348.

6. Anderson HC. Matrix vesicle calcification: review and update. In: Peck WA (ed). Bone and mineral research/3: A yearly survey of developments in the field of bone and mineral metabolism. Amsterdam: Elsevier Science Publishers, 1985, pp. 109–149.

7. Anderson HC. Calcific diseases: the role of membranes in pathological calcification. In: Ali SY (ed). Cell mediated

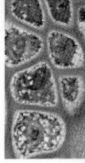

calcification and matrix vesicles. Amsterdam: Excerpta Medica, 1986, pp. 355–358.

8. Anderson HC. Mechanism of mineral formation in bone. Lab Invest 1989;60:320–330.

9. Askanazy M. Ueber Kalkmetastasen und progressive Knochenatrophie. In: Chemische und Medicinische Untersuchungen: Festschrift zur Feier des Sechzigsten Geburtstages von Max Jaffe. Braunschweig: Friedrich Vieweg und Sohn, 1901, pp. 188–240.

10. Atkinson J. Arterial calcification: mechanisms, consequences and animal models. Path Biol 1999;47:677–684.

11. Bachra BN. Nucleation in biological systems. In: Zipkin I (ed.) Biological mineralization. New York: John Wiley & Sons, 1973, pp. 845–881.

12. Banker BQ, Chester CS. Infarction of thigh muscle in the diabetic patient. Neurology 1973;23:667–677.

13. Berczi I. Fatty acids and soft tissue calcification. Exp Med Surg 1970;28:245–255.

14. Bleyer AJ, White WL, Choi MJ. Calcific small vessel ischemic disease (calciphylaxis) in dialysis patients. Int J Artif Organs 2000;23:351–355.

15. Boivin G, Walzer C, Baud CA. Ultrastructural study of the long-term development of two experimental cutaneous calcinoses (topical calciphylaxis and topical calcergy) in the rat. Cell Tissue Res 1987;247:525–532.

16. Bonucci E. Fine structure of early cartilage calcification. J Ultrastruct Res 1967;20:33–50.

17. Bonucci E. Fine structure and histochemistry of "calcifying globules" in epiphyseal cartilage. Z Zellforsch 1970;103:192–217.

18. Bonucci E, Sadun R. An electron microscope study on experimental calcification of skeletal muscle. Clin Orthop 1972;88:197–217.

19. Bonucci E, Sadun R. Experimental calcification of the myocardium. Ultrastructural and histochemical investigations. Am J Pathol 1973;71:167–184.

20. Borle AB. Control, modulation, and regulation of cell calcium. Rev Physiol Biochem Pharmacol 1981;90:13–153.

21. Boskey AL. Current concepts of the physiology and biochemistry of calcification. Clin Orthop 1981;157:225–257.

22. Boskey AL. Overview of cellular elements and macromolecules implicated in the initiation of mineralization. In: Butler WT (ed). The chemistry and biology of mineralized tissues. Birmingham: Ebsco Media Inc, 1985, pp. 335–343.

23. Boskey AL. Phospholipids and calcification: an overview. In: Ali SY (ed). Cell mediated calcification and matrix vesicles. Amsterdam: Excerpta Medica, 1986, pp. 175–179.

24. Boskey AL. Hydroxyapatite formation in a dynamic collagen gel system: effects of type I collagen, lipids, and proteoglycans. J Phys Chem 1989;93:1628–1633.

25. Boskey AL. Noncollagenous matrix proteins and their role in mineralization. Bone Miner 1989;6:111–123.

26. Boskey AL. Amorphous calcium phosphate: the contention of bone. J Dent Res 1997;76:1433–1436.

27. Boskey AL, Bullough PG. Cartilage calcification: normal and aberrant. Scan Electron Microsc 1984;II:943–952.

28. Boskey AL, Bullough PG, Posner AS. Calcium-acidic phospholipid-phosphate complexes in diseases and normal human bone. Metab Bone Dis Relat Res 1982;4:151–156.

29. Boyan BD, Swain LD, Boskey AL. Mechanisms of microbial calcification. In: ten Cate JM (ed). Recent advances in the study of dental calculus. Oxford: IRL Press, 1989, pp. 29–35.

30. Boyan-Salyers BD, Boskey AL. Relationship between proteolipids and calcium-phospholipid-phosphate complexes in Bacterionema matruchotii calcification. Calcif Tissue Int 1980;30:167–174.

30a. Calvi LM, Adams GB, Weilbrecht KW, et al. Osteoblastic cells regulate the haematopoeitic stem cell niche. Nature 2003;425:841–846.

31. Caulfield JB, Schrag PE. Electron microscopic study of renal calcification. Am J Pathol 1964;44:365–381.

32. Cavallero C, Spagnoli LG, Di Tondo U. Early mitochondrial calcifications in the rabbit aorta after adrenaline. Virch Arch A Pathol Anat Histol 1974;362:23–39.

33. Chatelain P, Kapanci Y. Histological diagnosis of myocardial infarction: the role of calcium. Appl Pathol 1984;2:233–239.

34. Coignoul F, Cheville N. Calcified microbial plaque. Dental calculus of dogs. Am J Pathol 1984;117:499–501.

35. Delmas PD. Bisphosphonates in the treatment of bone diseases. N Engl J Med 1996;335:1836–1837.

36. Eanes ED. Biophysical aspects of lipid interaction with mineral: liposome model studies. Anat Rec 1989;224:220–225.

37. Edwards WD. Applied anatomy of the heart. In: Brandenburg RO, Fuster V, Giulani ER, McGoon DC (eds). Cardiology: fundamentals and practice. Chicago: Year Book Medical Publishers, 1987, pp. 47–112.

38. Eggermann J, Kapanci Y. Experimental pulmonary calcinosis in the rat. Ultrastructural and morphometric studies. Lab Invest 1971;24:469–482.

39. Ennever J, Creamer H. Microbiologic calcification: bone mineral and bacteria. Calcif Tissue Res 1967;1:87–93.

40. Ennever J, Vogel JJ, Riggan LJ. Calcification by proteolipid from atherosclerotic aorta. Atherosclerosis 1980;35:209–213.

41. Ferrans VJ, Boyce SW, Billingham ME, et al. Calcific deposits in porcine bioprostheses: structure and pathogenesis. Am J Cardiol 1980;46:721–734.

42. Fischer AH, Morris DJ. Pathogenesis of calciphylaxis: study of three cases with literature review. Hum Pathol 1995;26:1055–1064.

43. Fleisch H. Diphosphonates: history and mechanisms of action. Metab Bone Dis Relat Res 1981;3:279–288.

44. Freundlich H, Hatfield HS. Colloid and capillary chemistry. London: Methuen & Co. Ltd, 1926.

45. Gabbiani G, Tuchweber B, Selye H. Experimental ectopic calcification (calciphylaxis and calcergy). In: Zipkin I (ed). Biological mineralization. New York: John Wiley & Sons, 1973, pp. 547–586.

46. Galkin BM, Frasca P, Feig SA, Holderness KE. Noncalcified breast particles. A possible new marker of breast cancer. Invest Radiol 1982;17:119–128.

47. Gallop PM, Lian JB, Hauschka PV. Carboxylated calcium-binding proteins and vitamin K. N Engl J Med 1980;302:1460–1466.

48. Glimcher MJ. A basic architectural principle in the organization of mineralized tissues. Clin Orthop 1968;61:16–36.

49. Glimcher MJ. On the form and function of bone: from molecules to organs. Wolff's Law revisited, 1981. In: Veis A (ed).

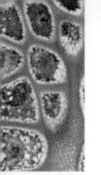
The chemistry and biology of mineralized connective tissue. Amsterdam: Elsevier North Holland, Inc, 1981, pp. 617–673.

50. Gonzalez ER. Calcium deposits on IUDs may play role in infections. JAMA 1981;245:1625–1626.

51. Goodman WG, Goldin J, Kuizon BD, et al. Coronary-artery calcification in young adults with end-stage renal disease who are undergoing dialysis. N Engl J Med 2000;342:1478–1483.

52. Greenawalt JW, Rossi CS, Lehninger AL. Effect of active accumulation of calcium and phosphate ions on the structure of rat liver mitochondria. J Cell Biol 1964;23:21–38.

53. Gundberg CM, Hauschka PV, Lian JB, Gallop PM. Osteocalcin: isolation, characterization, and detection. Methods Enzymol 1984;107:516–544.

54. Hansson GK, Schwartz SM. Evidence for cell death in the vascular endothelium in vivo and in vitro. Am J Pathol 1983;112:278–286.

55. Hasselbacher P. Crystal-protein interactions in crystal-induced arthritis. Adv Inflamm Res 1982;4:25–44.

56. Haust MD, Geer JC. Mechanism of calcification in spontaneous aortic arteriosclerotic lesions of the rabbit. Am J Pathol 1970;60:329–344.

57. Henisch HK. Crystals in gels and Liesegang rings. Cambridge: Cambridge University Press, 1988.

58. Hinzpeter EN, Naumann GOH. Cornea sclera. In: Naumann GOH, Apple DJ (eds). Pathology of the eye. New York: Springer-Verlag, 1986, pp. 317–412.

58a. Hoang QQ, Sicheri F, Howard AJ, Yang DSC. Bone recognition mechanism of porcine osteocalcin from crystal structure. Nature 2003;425:977–980.

59. Howell DS. Diseases due to the deposition of calcium pyrophosphate and hydroxyapatite. In: Kelley WN, Harris ED, Jr, Ruddy S, Sledge CB (eds). Textbook of rheumatology, vol 2, 2nd ed. Philadelphia: WB Saunders Company, 1985, pp. 1398–1416.

60. Ibels LS. The pathogenesis of metastatic calcification in uraemia. Prog Biochem Pharmacol 1980;17:242–250.

61. Kemmeren JM, van Noord PAH, Beijerinck D, et al. Arterial calcification found on breast cancer screening mammograms and cardiovascular mortality in women. The DOM Project. Am J Epidemiol 1998;147:333–341.

62. Kim KM. Calcification of matrix vesicles in human aortic valve and aortic media. Fed Proc 1976;35:156–162.

63. Kim KM. Pathological calcification. In: Trump BF, Arstila AU (eds). Pathobiology of cell membranes, vol III. New York: Academic Press, 1983, pp. 117–155.

64. Kim KM. Role of membranes in calcification. Surv Synth Pathol Res 1983;2:215–228.

65. Kim KM. Nephrocalcinosis in vitro. Scanning Electron Microsc 1983;III:1285–1292.

66. Kim KM. Huang S-N. Ultrastructural study of calcification of human aortic valve. Lab Invest 1971;25:357–366.

67. Kivilaakso E, Fromm D, Silen W. Effect of the acid secretory state on intramural pH of rabbit gastric mucosa. Gastroenterology 1978;75:641–648.

68. Krane SM, Glimcher MJ. Transphosphorylation from nucleoside di- and triphosphates by apatite crystals. J Biol Chem 1962;237:2991–2998.

69. Lansing AI, Alex M, Rosenthal TB. Calcium and elastin in human arteriosclerosis. J Gerontol 1950;5:112–119.

70. Levine MM, Kleeman CR. Hypercalcemia: pathophysiology and treatment. Hosp Pract 1987;22:93–109.

71. Levy RJ, Gundberg C, Scheinman R. The identification of the vitamin K-dependent bone protein osteocalcin as one of the t-carboxyglutamic acid containing proteins present in calcified atherosclerotic plaque and mineralized heart valves. Atherosclerosis 1983;46:49–56.

72. Levy RJ, Lian JB, Gallop P. Atherocalcin, a t-carboxyglutamic acid containing protein from atherosclerotic plaque. Biochem Biophys Res Commun 1979;91:41–49.

73. Llach F. Hyperphosphatemia in end-stage renal disease patients: pathophysiological consequences. Kidney Int 1999;56(Suppl 73):S31–S37.

74. Lowenstam HA, Weiner S. On biomineralization. New York: Oxford University Press, 1989.

75. Luo G, Ducy P, McKee MD, et al. Spontaneous calcification of arteries and cartilage in mice lacking matrix GLA protein. Nature 1997;386:78–81.

76. Majno G. Death and autolysis of liver tissue. In: Rouiller C (ed). The liver. Vol. II. New York: Academic Press, 1963, pp. 267–313.

77. Maren TH. Carbonic anhydrase: chemistry, physiology, and inhibition. Physiol Rev 1967;47:595–723.

78. Mastruserio DN, Nguyen EQ, Nielsen T, Hessel A, Pellegrini AE. Calciphylaxis associated with metastatic breast carcinoma. J Am Acad Dermatol 1999;41:295–298.

79. Matthews JL. Role of mitochondria in calcification. In: Ali SY (ed). Cell mediated calcification and matrix vesicles. Amsterdam: Excerpta Medica, 1986, pp. 115–118.

80. McCarty DJ. Crystal deposition joint disease. Annu Rev Med 1974;25:279–288.

81. Menanteau J, Neuman WF, Neuman MW. A study of bone proteins which can prevent hydroxyapatite formation. Metab Bone Dis Relat Res 1982;4:157–162.

82. Moller-Christensen V, Weiss DL. One of the oldest datable skeletons with leprous bone-changes from the Naeslved Leprosy Hospital Churchyard in Denmark. Int J Lepr 1971;39:172–182.

83. Mostov K, Werb Z. Journey across the osteoclast. Science 1997;276:219–220.

84. Mulligan RM, Stricker FL. Metastatic calcification produced in dogs by hypervitaminosis D and haliphagia. Am J Pathol 1948;24:451–473.

85. Neff M, Yalcin S, Gupta S, Berger H. Extensive metastatic calcification of the lung in an azotemic patient. Am J Med 1974;56:103–109.

86. Neuman WF, Neuman MW. The chemical dynamics of bone mineral. Chicago: The University of Chicago Press, 1958.

87. Neuman WF, Neuman MW. In the beginning there was apatite. In: Zipkin I (ed). Biological mineralization. New York: John Wiley and Sons, 1973, pp. 3–19.

88. Olson LH, Edwards WD, Tajik AJ. Aortic valve stenosis: etiology, pathophysiology, evaluation, and management. Curr Probl Cardiol 1987;12:459–508.

89. Posner AS, Betts F. Molecular control of tissue mineralization. In: Veis A (ed). The chemistry and biology of mineralized

connective tissue. Amsterdam: Elsevier North Holland, Inc, 1981, pp. 257–266.

90. Raggio CL, Boyan BD, Boskey AL. In vivo hydroxyapatite formation induced by lipids. J Bone Miner Res 1986;1: 409–415.

91. Randall RE Jr, Strauss MB, McNeely WF. The milk-alkali syndrome. Arch Intern Med 1961;107:163–181.

92. Reynolds ES. Liver parenchymal cell injury. III. The nature of calcium-associated electron-opaque masses in rat liver mitochondria following poisoning with carbon tetrachloride. J Cell Biol 1965;25:53–75.

93. Roberts WC, Waller BF. Effect of chronic hypercalcemia on the heart. An analysis of 18 necropsy patients. Am J Med 1981;71:371–384.

94. Russell RGG, Robertson WG, Fleisch H. Inhibitors of mineralization. In: Zipkin I (ed). Biological mineralization. New York: John Wiley & and Sons, 1973, pp. 807–825.

95. Sarig S, Weiss TA, Katz I, et al. Detection of cholesterol associated with calcium mineral using confocal fluorescence microscopy. Lab Invest 1994;71:782–787.

96. Schoen FJ, Levy RJ, Nelson AC, et al. Onset and progression of experimental bioprosthetic heart valve calcification. Lab Invest 1985;52:523–532.

97. Selye H. Calciphylaxis. Chicago: The University of Chicago Press, 1962.

98. Seymour HR, Cooke J, Given-Wilson RM. The significance of spontaneous resolution of breast calcification. Br J Radiol 1999;72:3–8.

99. Sherwood L. Human physiology. From cells to systems. St Paul: West Publishing Company, 1989.

99a. Steitz SA, Speer MY, McKee MD, et al. Osteopontin inhibits deposition and promotes regression of ectopic calcification. Am J Pathol 2002;161:2035–2046.

100. Strawich E, Glimcher MJ. Phosphoproteins of mineralized tissues: the chemistry and biosynthesis of the phosphoproteins of dental enamel. In: Akeson WH, Bornstein P, Glimcher MJ (eds). Symposium on heritable disorders of connective tissue. San Diego, CA, May, 1980. St Louis: The CV Mosby Company, 1982, pp. 173–191.

101. Tanimura A, McGregor DH, Anderson HC. Matrix vesicles in atherosclerotic calcification. Proc Soc Exp Biol Med 1983;172:173–177.

102. Taura S, Taura M, Imai H, Kummerow FA, Tokuyasu K, Cho-Simon BH. Ultrastructure of cardiovascular lesions induced by hypervitaminosis D and its withdrawal. Paroi artérielle 1978;4:245–259.

103. Termine JD, Eanes ED. Calcium phosphate deposition from balanced salt solutions. Calcif Tissue Res 1974;15:81–84.

104. Thakur A, Hines OJ, Thakur V, Gordon HE. Tumoral calcinosis regression after subtotal parathyroidectomy: a case presentation and review of the literature. Surgery 1999;126: 95–98.

105. Tuur SM, Nelson AM, Gibson DW, et al. Liesegang rings in tissue. How to distinguish Liesegang rings from the giant kidney worm, Dioctophyma renale. Am J Surg Pathol 1987; 11:598–605.

106. Urist MR. Biologic initiators of calcification. In: Zipkin I (ed). Biological mineralization. New York: John Wiley & Sons, 1973, pp. 757–805.

107. Urist MR. Biochemistry of calcification. In: Bourne GH (ed). The biochemistry and physiology of bone, 2nd ed., vol IV. New York: Academic Press, 1976, pp. 1–59.

108. Velentzas C, Meindok H, Oreopolous DG, et al. Visceral calcification and the Ca × P product. Adv Exp Mol Biol 1978;103:195–201.

109. Virchow R. Cellular pathology. Translated from the 2nd German Ed. by B Chance, 1859. Reproduced by Dover Publications, New York, 1971.

110. Vogel JJ. The microbial model in the study of calcification. In: Dickson GR (ed). Methods of calcified tissue preparation. Amsterdam: Elsevier Science Publishers BV, 1984, pp. 607–621.

111. Vogel JJ. The membrane interface in biologic calcification. In: Ali SY (ed). Cell mediated calcification and matrix vesicles. Amsterdam: Excerpta Medica, 1986, pp. 181–185.

112. Vogel JJ, Boyan-Salyers B, Campbell MM. Protein-phospholipid interactions in biologic calcification. Metab Bone Dis Relat Res 1978;1:149–153.

113. Vogel JJ, Ennever J. The role of a lipoprotein in the intracellular hydroxyapatite formation in Bacterionema Matruchotii. Clin Orthop 1971;78:218–222.

114. Vyavahare N, Ogle M, Schoen FJ, Levy RJ. Elastin calcification and its prevention with aluminum chloride pretreatment. Am J Pathol 1999;155:973–982.

115. Wallin R, Wajih N, Greenwood GT, Sane DC. Arterial calcification: a review of the mechanisms, animal models, and the prospects for therapy. Med Res Rev 2001;21:274–301.

116. Weiser HB. A textbook of colloid chemistry, 2nd ed. New York: John Wiley & Sons, Inc, 1949.

117. Wells HG. Chemical pathology, 5th ed. Philadelphia: WB Saunders Company, 1925.

118. Woodward SC. Mineralization of connective tissue surrounding implanted devices. Trans Am Soc Artif Intern Organs 1981;27:697–702.

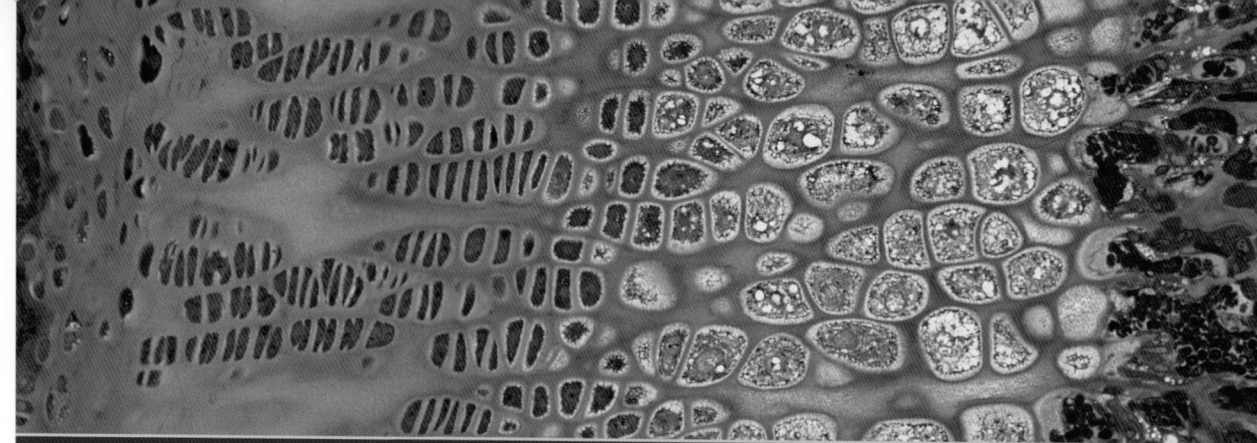

CHAPTER 7 EXTRACELLULAR PATHOLOGY

The Extracellular World

We have spoken of the cell as the elementary patient; now we turn to the patient's environment to see what we can learn there about disease.

Cells relate to their environment much more closely than humans do. They are physically attached to the extracellular matrix by a variety of receptors for collagen, laminin, fibronectin, fibrin, and many other molecules, so that signals may be transmitted from the matrix to the cell and vice versa (26).

It follows that the matrix can affect not only cell attachment but also cell function in general, including gene expression (2). Furthermore, the matrix is controlled by a family of more than 25 secreted and surface-borne enzymes, the **matrix metalloproteinases,** which can degrade or process virtually all the proteins of the extracellular world, including cell-to-cell adhesion proteins (45). Not surprisingly, a cell that has lost touch with its matrix may be obliged to commit suicide via apoptosis, on the grounds of **anoikis,** or "homelessness" (p. 213).

At the submicroscopic level the extracellular spaces are a jungle of molecules; the four major components, best seen in loose connective tissue, are

- Collagen fibers (non-branching)
- Elastic fibers (branching)
- Proteoglycans (a gel)
- Basement membranes (sheets)

Extracellular pathology includes changes in quantity and quality of these normal components, as well as the appearance of abnormal materials. The mechanism may be a congenital defect (about 150 are known) (38) but most of extracellular pathology is acquired. By light microscopy some pathologic conditions are easily identified

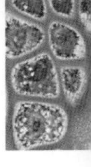

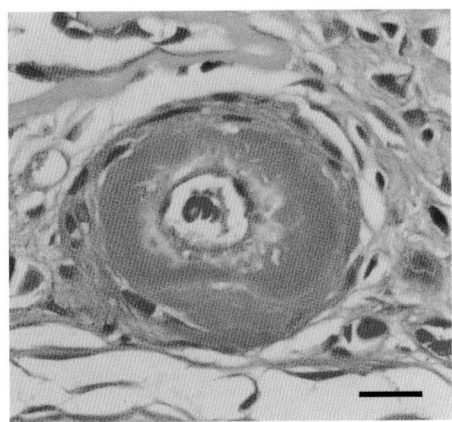 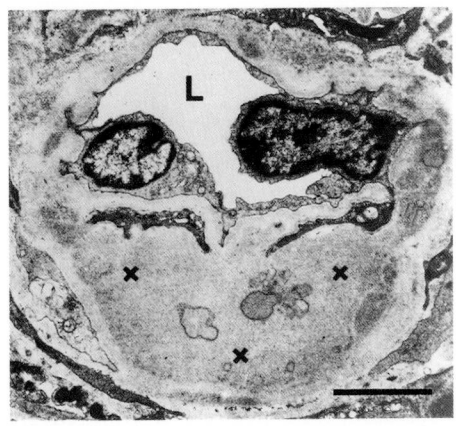

FIGURE 7.1   Hyalinized arterioles. *Left:* Glomerular afferent arteriole from a renal biopsy in long-standing diabetes. The media (smooth muscle layer) is largely replaced by a homogeneous hyalin mass. **Bar** = 10 μm. *Right:* Electron micrograph of a similar arteriole in a case of essential hypertension. The media is replaced by amorphous, basement-membranelike material (✕). **L:** Lumen. **Bar** = 2 μm. (Reproduced with permission from [12], © American Society for Investigative Pathology.)

(such as excess collagen in a cirrhotic liver), but quite often the picture is that of a nondescript extracellular material that cannot be identified without histochemical stains. To describe it in a noncommittal way, microscopists have come up with a handy bit of jargon: "hyalin," which means "glassy." In other words, *hyalin is not a substance; it is an adjective.*

A common example: with advancing age, many arterioles become hyalinized, especially in the spleen and kidney (Figure 7.1). What is that hyalin material made of? In the cases illustrated it consists mainly of hyaluronic acid bound to a plasma protein, the third component of complement (C3), which must have seeped out of the lumen (12). Why C3 should behave in this manner is not clear. In many arterioles, plasma-derived lipid is mixed into this hyalin, presumably because the endothelium has become leaky: this seems to be the usual condition of hyalinized arterioles.

In other situations, hyalin masses may consist of fibrin, packed collagen or basement membrane (Figure 7.2), mucopolysaccharides (glucosaminoglycans), or an abnormal material called amyloid. *It is important to identify the chemical nature of the hyalin because it may give a clue to a local or even a general*

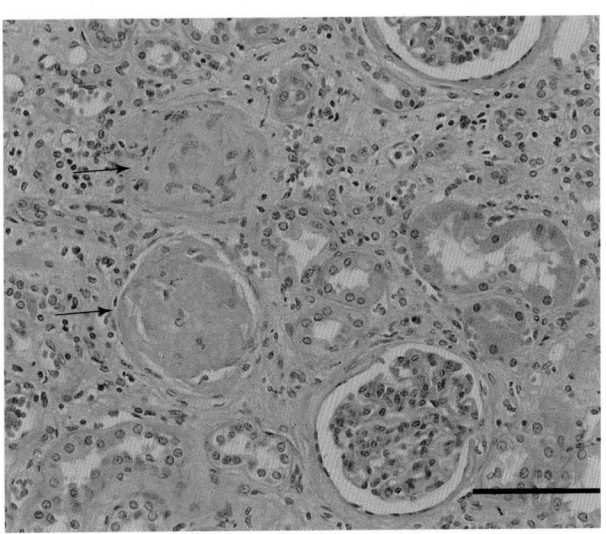

FIGURE 7.2   Two hyalinized glomeruli (**arrows**) next to a normal one. This hyalin represents an overproduction of capillary basement membrane.

disturbance, acute or chronic. Amyloid, for example, may indicate one of a whole gamut of problems, ranging from an incidental finding to a death sentence.

Pathology of Collagen

Considering that collagen is probably the most abundant protein in the animal world and that it accounts for almost one-third of the mammalian body's proteins, its contribution to the daily worries of physicians is relatively modest. This makes sense because collagen is a pillar of life; it is responsible for holding the body together, skeleton included, and for healing injuries. It is essential that such a vital protein be stable—and so it is.

FIGURE 7.3   Four common types of collagen. *Top:* Type 1, cut transversally and longitudinally (epineurium of a human nerve). *Center:* Type 2, from rat hyaline cartilage. The fibrils are thinner and do not have a clearly visible banding pattern. *Bottom:* Type 3 (human endoneurium), cut transversally, shows fibrils with a smaller diameter than Type 1. Parts of cells are included in this figure; they are covered with basement membrane (**arrow**) which contains collagen Type 4. **Bars** = 0.4 μm. (Reproduced by permission from [32a] and by courtesy of Dr. G. S. Montes, University of São Paulo Institute of Biomedical Sciences, Brazil.)

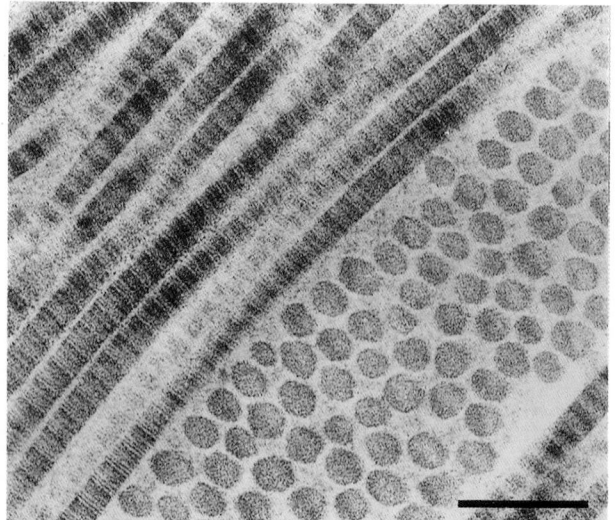

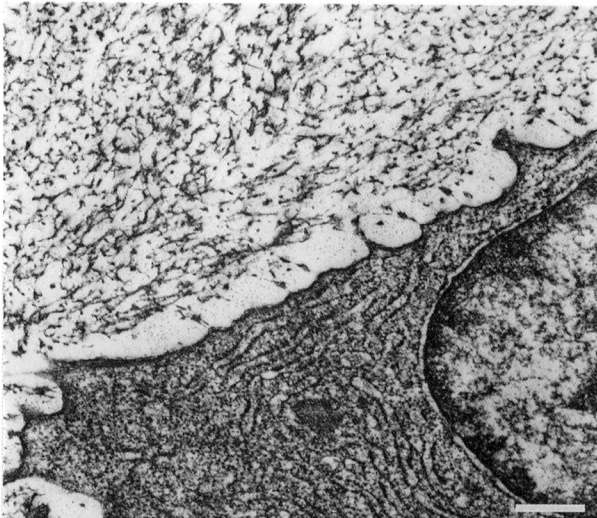

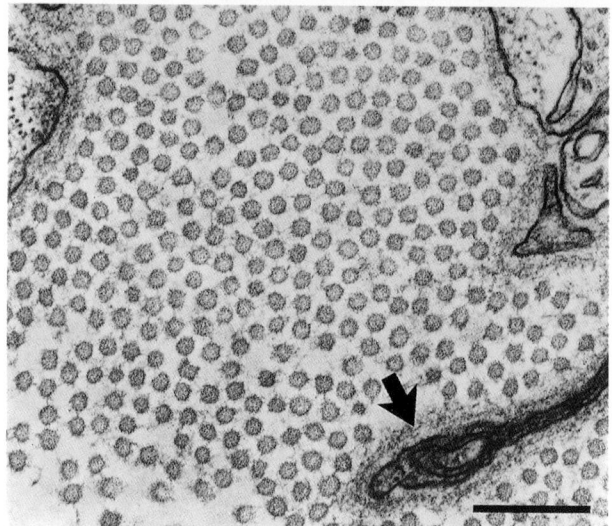

Full-blown, generalized abnormalities of collagen are rare: some are congenital, some are nutritional (e.g., scurvy), and others are toxic (e.g., osteolathyrism).

As usual, some of the metabolic diseases of collagen provided clues to its biology. Localized collagen-related problems are common and largely related to wound healing.

Warning: not all "collagen diseases" are diseases of collagen. One of the classic misnomers in clinical medicine is the term "**collagen diseases**" for a group of connective tissue diseases of autoimmune pathogenesis, such as systemic lupus erythematosus (SLE), rheumatoid arthritis, rheumatic fever, polyarteritis nodosa, dermatomyositis, and scleroderma (41). The misnaming dates from a time—not so long ago—when "collagen" could be used to mean "connective tissue." It was essentially an accident. In 1942, the eminent pathologist Paul Klemperer realized that these conditions had something in common; he could not yet recognize the autoimmune mechanism, but he correctly identified the common thread as an inflammatory condition in the connective tissue, and proposed the name collagen diseases (really meaning connective tissue diseases) (21). The name spread like wildfire, and when Klemperer attempted to change it in 1950, it was too late (20). Just remember that in these "collagen diseases" the collagen is normal. Better yet, avoid using that term.

Only one type of collagen was known before 1969; now we know of over 20, numbered in order of discovery. Each collagen molecule is made of three alpha-chains twisted in ropelike fashion; 38 different kinds of chains have been identified. A few details follow (Types 1 and 3 are listed consecutively because they are closely related).

- Type 1 is the principal fibrillar collagen, by far the most common. It provides tensile strength in tissues such as tendons and the cornea (Figure 7.3).
- Type 3 is made of thinner fibrils (Figure 7.3) and supports distensible organs such as blood vessels (when this collagen is defective, vessels tend to

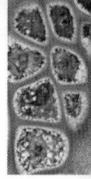

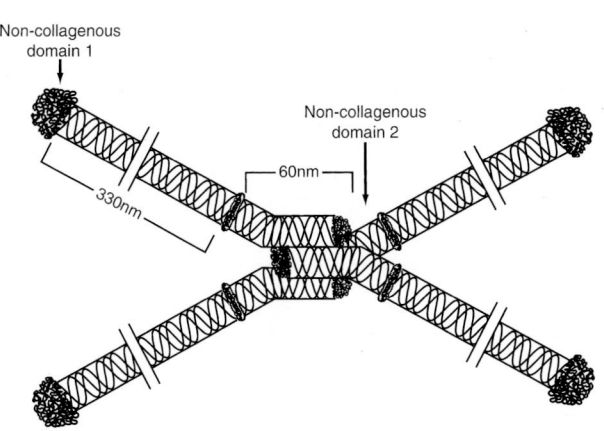

FIGURE 7.4   Model of collagen Type 4. Four molecules are assembled by stable interactions, producing an X-shaped structure that is the backbone of basement membranes. (Reproduced by permission from [46a], © Raven Press, 1982 and from [29], © by The US & Canadian Academy of Pathology, Inc.)

burst). *When new collagen is laid down, Type 3 tends to be deposited first, and is followed by Type 1.*

- Type 2 is also fibrillar but buried in cartilage, such as the hyaline cartilage of joints (Figure 7.3); correspondingly, when injected into susceptible rodents, it creates an immune response that affects the joints (46).

- Type 4 is nonfibrillar; its molecules tend to aggregate by fours into X-shaped units (Figure 7.4) that join up to make the skeleton of the basement membranes (Figure 7.3).

- Types 5, 6, 9, and 12 tend to coat other collagen fibrils.

Fibroblasts share the capacity to secrete collagen with many other mesenchymal cells, especially smooth-muscle cells, but also with epithelia, which synthesize their own basement membranes.

The rope-shaped, fibrillar varieties of collagen are mainly responsible for tissue strength. The genesis of these "ropes" (the collagen fibers as seen by light microscopy) must have presented an evolutionary production problem because their diameter is of the same order of magnitude as the cells themselves, and of course no cell is large enough to secrete such large objects. Nature solved the problem by having the cells secrete small precursors endowed with the power of self-assembly: a multistep process involving at least 13 enzymes and twice as many cofactors (Figure 7.5). The more complex a process is, the likelier it is to fail; thus, the pathology of collagen can fill a book, albeit a book of rare diseases. We will offer an overview,

emphasizing the basic principles. It will be apparent that some accidents beset the immature collagen molecule inside the cell; others concern the free fiber.

Follow the sequence in Figure 7.5. The messenger RNA coding for collagen emerges from the nucleus and is translated by ribosomes into two types of pro–alpha chains, tipped by terminal polypeptides that are critical for the manufacture of the molecule. Then the immature molecule, advancing in membranous structures (rough ER and Golgi apparatus), undergoes **hydroxylation** of its proline and lysine residues, as well as **glycation,** whereby glucose and other carbohydrates are added. The chains are now ready for self-twisting in groups of three into a helix, which is secreted, at long last, as **procollagen**—still bearing its terminal peptides. Outside of the cell, this newly born molecule cannot self-assemble unless its two bunches of terminal peptides are clipped off by extracellular peptidases, which finally release the true elementary collagen molecule: **tropocollagen.** The tropocollagen molecules then self-assemble into *microfibrils,* which are promptly cross-linked with the help of another extracellular enzyme, lysyl oxidase. This enzyme, in the presence of copper and ascorbic acid (two critical conditions), converts some of the hydroxyl terminals to aldehydes, which are essential for creating links within and between adjacent molecules. The microfibrils then continue to self-assemble into larger units, the *fibrils,* which are visible by electron microscopy and show a characteristic cross-banding; their diameter is about 50 nm. The collagen fibers seen by light microscopy are bundles of these banded units.

Now we will run through this scheme again and see how it can go awry. Keep this fact in mind: *collagen defects can be inborn or acquired.* Many errors are known or suspected for each of the steps in Figure 7.5; we will choose a few classic examples.

Genetic Defects of Collagen

Another glance at Figure 7.5 will show that in the elaborate sequence of collagen synthesis, which requires an hour or two (34), most of the modifications to the developing collagen molecule are posttranslational; this means that *congenital disease can arise from defects in two sets of genes: any of those that code for collagen, and any of those that code for the enzymes that are active in the posttranslational events.* In either case, the result is defective fibers. Dozens of congenital human and animal diseases arise through these mechanisms (38, 44). Symptoms arise from those organs whose mechanical functions depend most heavily on collagen: the bones (50 percent of their dry weight is collagen), the joints

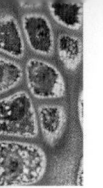

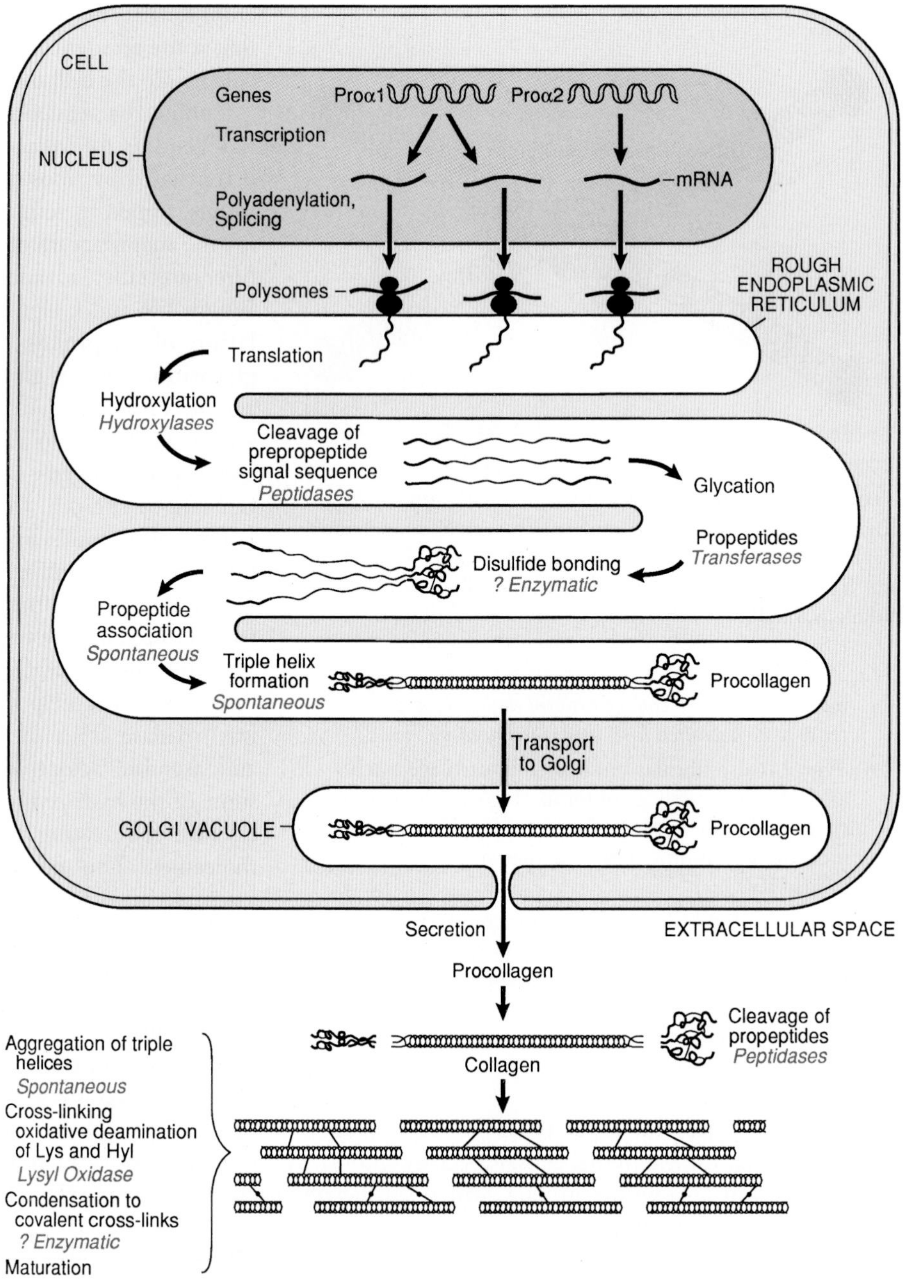

FIGURE 7.5 Biosynthesis of collagen Type 1. Note the complex posttranslational processing: at every step there is a chance for congenital or accidental disturbance. (Adapted with permission from [38]. Illustration by A. D. Iselin.)

CELL

NUCLEUS

Genes   Proα1   Proα2

Transcription

Polyadenylation, Splicing

—mRNA

Polysomes —

ROUGH ENDOPLASMIC RETICULUM

Translation

Hydroxylation
Hydroxylases

Cleavage of prepropeptide signal sequence
Peptidases

Glycation

Propeptides
Transferases

Disulfide bonding
? Enzymatic

Propeptide association
Spontaneous

Triple helix formation
Spontaneous

Procollagen

Transport to Golgi

GOLGI VACUOLE —

Procollagen

Secretion

EXTRACELLULAR SPACE

Procollagen

Cleavage of propeptides
Peptidases

Collagen

Aggregation of triple helices
Spontaneous

Cross-linking oxidative deamination of Lys and Hyl
Lysyl Oxidase

Condensation to covalent cross-links
? Enzymatic

Maturation

(held in place by fibrous ligaments), the skin (90 percent of its proteins are collagen), the large arteries (which have to withstand high internal pressure), the mitral valve (which is subjected to violent stresses at each heartbeat), and the eyes, especially the crystalline lens (which is held in place by a rim of collagen fibrils). Seen by electron microscopy, congenitally abnormal fibrils are somewhat disappointing: they can be a little too thick, a little too thin, or irregular, but they offer little help in differential diagnosis (48).

Several diseases of collagen have been known for centuries, because some of their manifestations are so striking that the patients were used for circus shows.

At the genetic level, as of 2001 more than 1,000 mutations had been identified in 22 collagen-related genes (33), but it is still too early to draw up a clinico-molecular classification of the collagen diseases. We sketch three typical clinical pictures to illustrate how a molecular defect can translate into a major human problem.

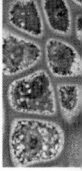

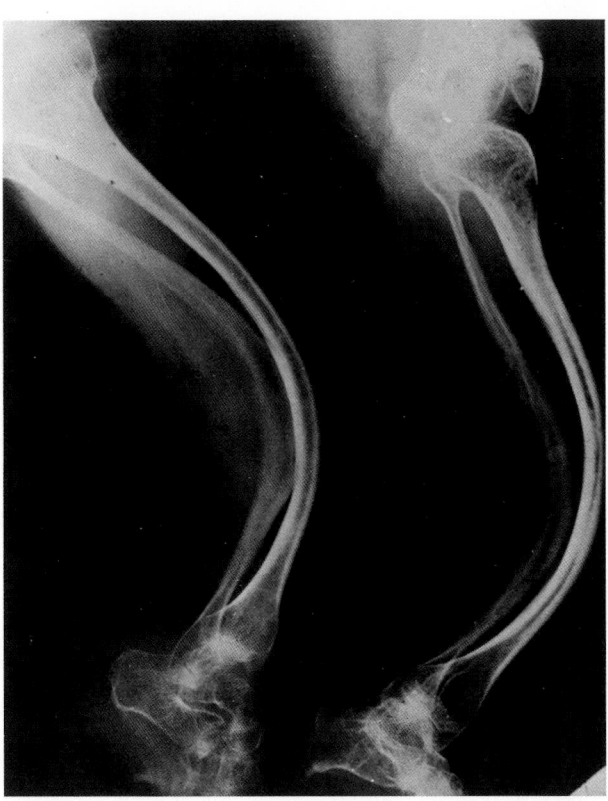

FIGURE 7.6   Osteogenesis imperfecta, a disease of the collagen molecule, as manifested in an adult. In this severe, progressive variant, the lower limbs are deformed. (Reproduced with permission from [22].)

Osteogenesis imperfecta. This disease is also called brittle bone disease or Lobstein's disease after the same Lobstein who coined the term arteriosclerosis in 1833. Its prevalence is about 1 in 25,000 people, and it has a surprisingly wide range of severity, depending on the mutation in one of the two procollagen genes (10). In some instances it is so severe that death occurs *in utero;* more fortunate individuals can lead normal lives by carefully avoiding mechanical stress (8); others are condemned to live with severe, progressive deformations of their long bones (Figure 7.6). Symptoms include "blue" (semitransparent) sclerae and opalescent teeth; both these tissues are rich in collagen Type 1.

The Ehler-Danlos syndrome. The 11 variants of this heterogeneous syndrome have two symptoms in common: *laxity of the joints,* which can be spectacular (Figure 7.7)—it produced the "rubber people" of circuses—and a *hyperextensible skin* (Figure 7.8). Although very thin, the skin folds can recoil because the elastic fibers are there; what is missing is the tethering effect of normal collagen fibers. The underlying defects

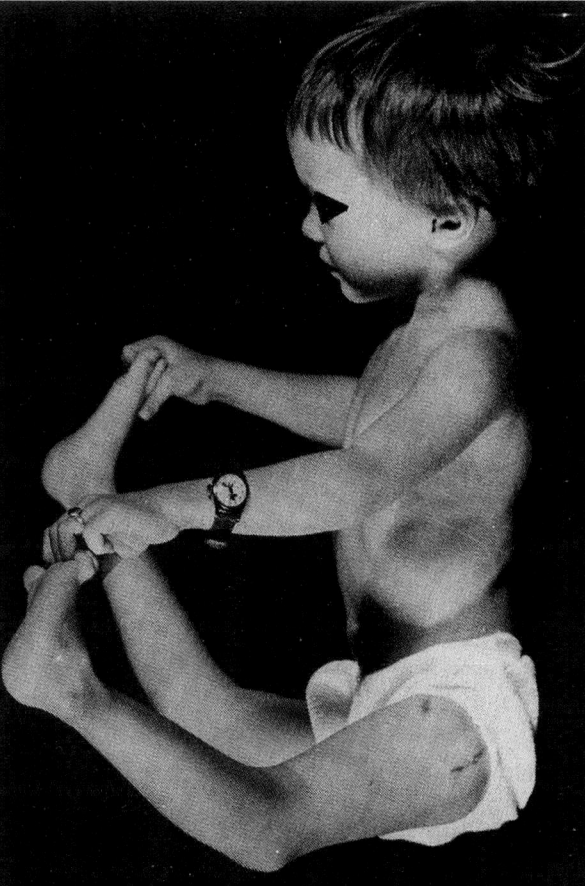

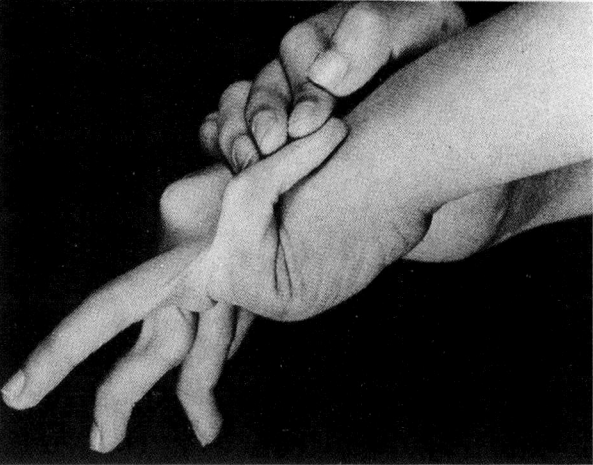

FIGURE 7.7   Joint laxity in a child affected by one type of Ehler-Danlos syndrome. Dislocated hips and hypermobile knee joints were noted at birth. (Reproduced with permission from [31].)

of the collagen molecule are varied and not all understood; the ultimate consequences include rupture of the aorta and other hollow organs such as the large bowel (13).

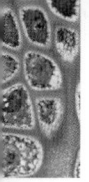

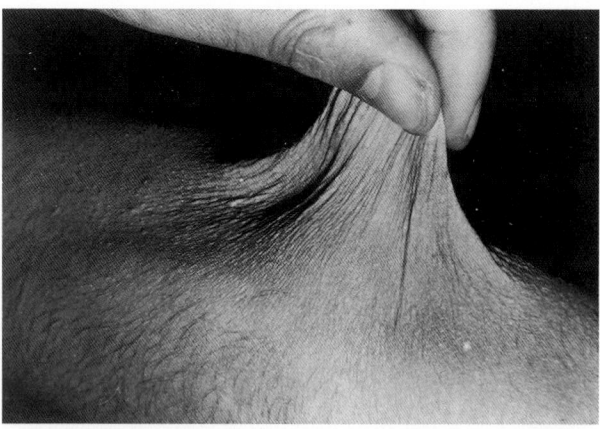

FIGURE 7.8   Abnormally stretchable skin from a case of Ehler-Danlos syndrome, probably Type 1. Elastic fibers are present, but the tethering effect of collagen fibers is missing. (Reproduced with permission from [22].)

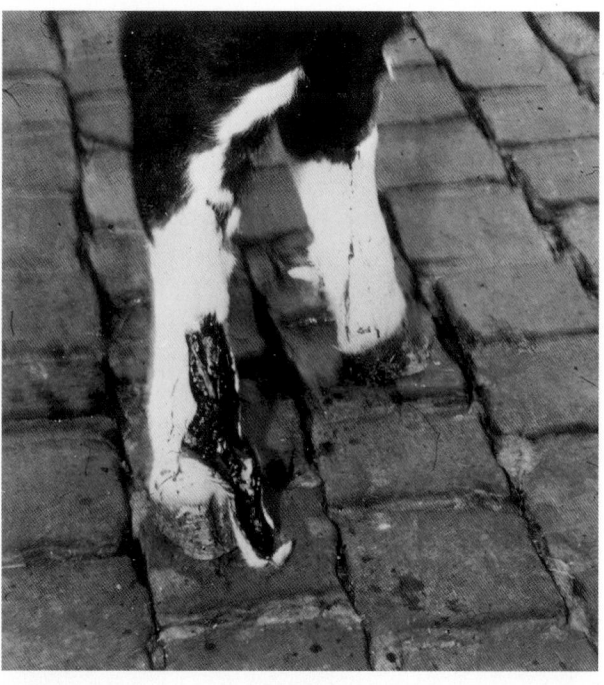

FIGURE 7.9   Dermatosparaxis (a disease of the collagen molecule). The skin of these calves has the consistency of wet blotting paper. The trauma of birth is sufficient to tear it and even to rip it off completely. (Reproduced with permission from [17].)

Dermatosparaxis: a failure of extracellular assembly. The collagen molecule is finally born when the procollagen molecule is assembled outside the cell (review this once again on Figure 7.5). But if the terminal peptides of procollagen are not removed, the nascent collagen molecules cannot assemble properly, and the mature collagen fibers are easily torn apart. This disturbance was the first proven collagen disease: it was discovered in calves by Belgian veterinarians (sheep are also affected) and named **dermatosparaxis,** from *derma,* "skin," and *sparássein,* "to tear" (Figure 7.9) (4, 17, 23). A few cases have been recognized in children; the principal sign is extreme fragility of the skin (49).

Originally, the gene of dermatosparaxis came to be selected because the heterozygous animals produce a more tender flesh (!) (36), which is not surprising if you take a look at the state of the collagen fibrils in dermatosparaxis (47) (Figure 7.10). Homozygous animals are doomed.

Acquired Defects of Collagen

If you had to design some way to produce weakened collagen fibers, your best bet would probably be to interfere with the cross-linking mechanisms within and between the fibrils. This is indeed what happens in real life, as a result of poor nutrition or toxic agents.

Deficient hydroxylation. We are now talking about **scurvy,** or vitamin C deficiency. Please refer once again to Figure 7.5: it will remind you that hydroxylation occurs *within* the fibroblast, as an early step in the genesis of the procollagen molecule. Historically, of course,

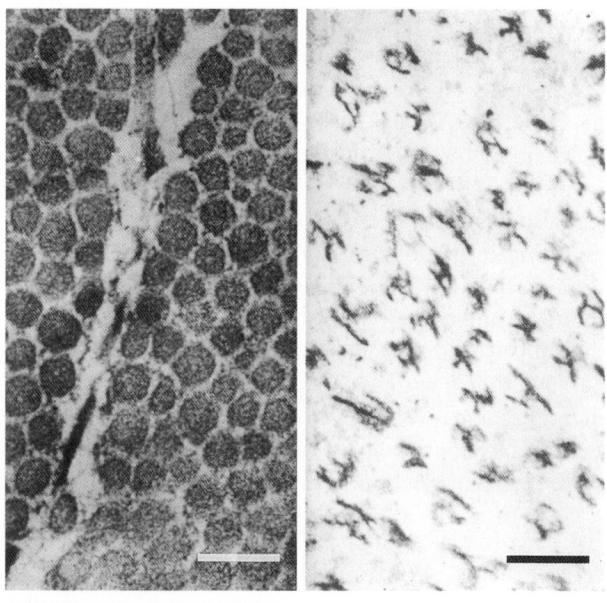

FIGURE 7.10   Dermatosparaxis. *Left:* Cross section of collagen fibers from the skin of a normal newborn lamb. *Right:* Collagen fibers from the skin of a dermatosparactic lamb. **Bar** = 0.2 μm. (Reproduced by permission from [47], © by Williams & Wilkins, 1976.)

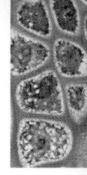

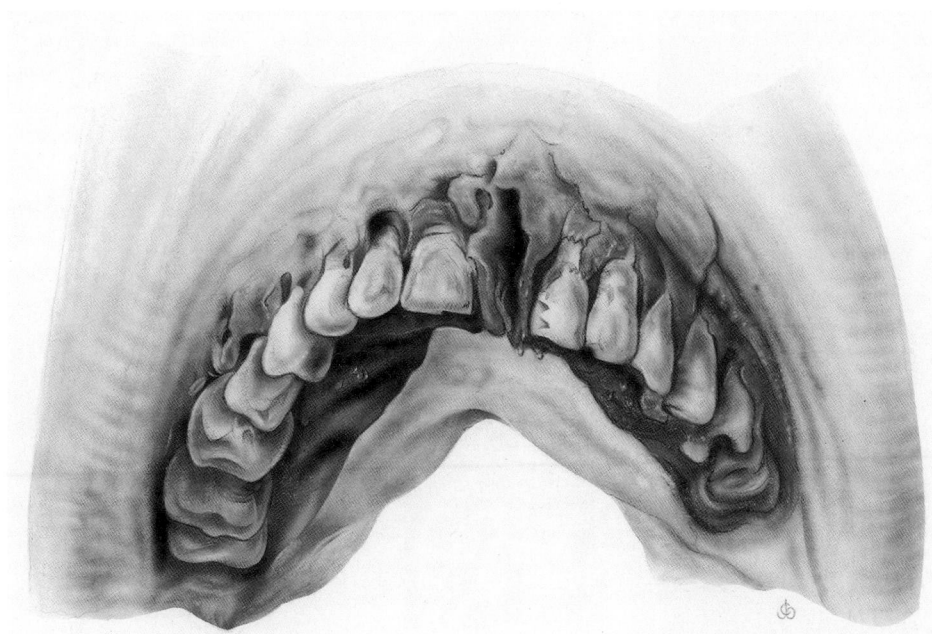

FIGURE 7.11 Effect of scurvy (avitaminosis C) on the gums and teeth. Lacking vitamin C, the fast-renewing collagen of the periodontal ligament is improperly hydroxylated, resulting in tooth mobility, tooth loss, bleeding, and periodontal infection. From the autopsy of a soldier who died of scurvy in 1919. (Redrawn with permission from [3].)

scurvy was the curse of long voyages at sea; it reappeared in malnourished armies during World War I. The unfortunate sailors and soldiers who lost their teeth (Figure 7.11) and saw their old scars break down to gape as fresh wounds could not have guessed that their problem was essentially one of inadequate hydroxylation. *Vitamin C, a redox agent and a cofactor in many hydroxylation reactions, is also required for the hydroxylation of the proline and lysine of collagen.* Low hydroxylation of lysine leads to reduced cross-linking and thus to defective collagen fibers. The sailors' teeth fall out because the collagen in the periodontal ligament that holds the teeth in place has a short half-life: 1 day (in the rat) compared with 15 days for skin collagen (43); therefore, the tough bundles of old but normal periodontal collagen are fast replaced by defective ones. The breakdown of old scars is explained by a similar mechanism; we will learn later that collagen turnover in scars remains elevated long after the healing process is clinically terminated (p. 482). The general bleeding tendency of scurvy may be due to a weakness of the microvascular basement membranes; the typical hemorrhages beneath the periosteum are probably due to tearing of weakened tendon insertions.

Defective cross-linking. Several nutritional and toxic mechanisms interfere with the cross-linking of collagen. For example, copper-deficient swine, sheep and chicks can die literally of broken hearts or aortas—because lysyl oxidase requires copper as a cofactor.

Among the toxic agents best known is a principle extracted from the sweet pea; in experimental animals it causes a most interesting condition, **osteolathyrism,** which taught us a great deal about collagen. During periods of starvation, people in India, Italy, and Spain once turned to a diet of chick peas (*Lathyrus sativus*), which caused neurologic problems (but no defect of collagen). While this form of poisoning—chick-pea lathyrism—was being worked out, it was accidentally discovered that the seeds of a related plant, the common sweet pea (*Lathyrus odoratus*), are also toxic but in a totally different way (24). The active principle of the sweet pea, BAPN (beta-aminopropionitrile), binds irreversibly to the enzyme lysyl oxidase, with the result that cross-linking is prevented, and correspondingly the mature collagen is extremely weak. Chicks and rats poisoned with BAPN have extremely soluble collagen and therefore brittle and misshapen bones (14) (Figure 7.12) and brittle skin. This "osteo-lathyrism" did not help us understand chick-pea lathyrism, but it became widely used experimentally as a model of defective collagen cross-linking.

As a matter of fact, there have been some attempts to harness the specific toxicity of BAPN for therapeutic purposes. Many distressing human diseases are characterized by fibrosis: too much fibrous tissue, which implies too much collagen. Understandably, this led to the idea that a therapeutically induced collagen defect might bring some benefit (37). The choice fell mainly on BAPN and penicillamine, the latter because it

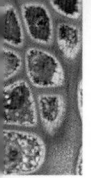

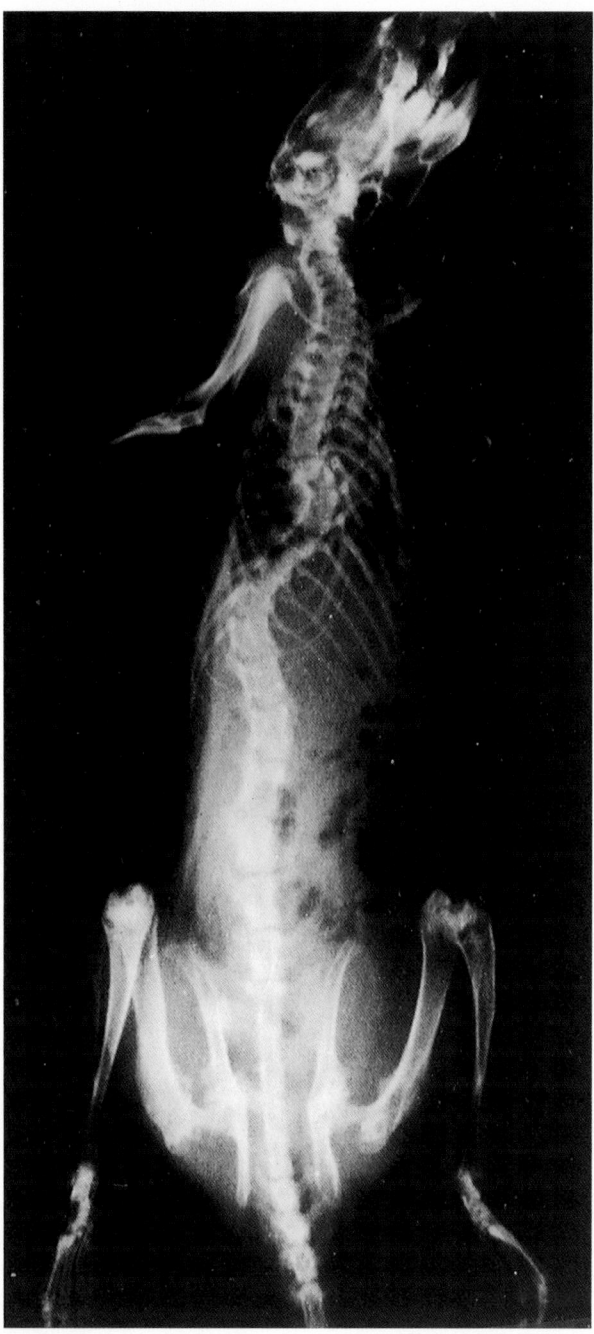

FIGURE 7.12   X-ray of a rat with experimental osteolathyrism: severe distortion of the spinal column, a result of inadequate cross-linking of collagen. (Reproduced from [14].)

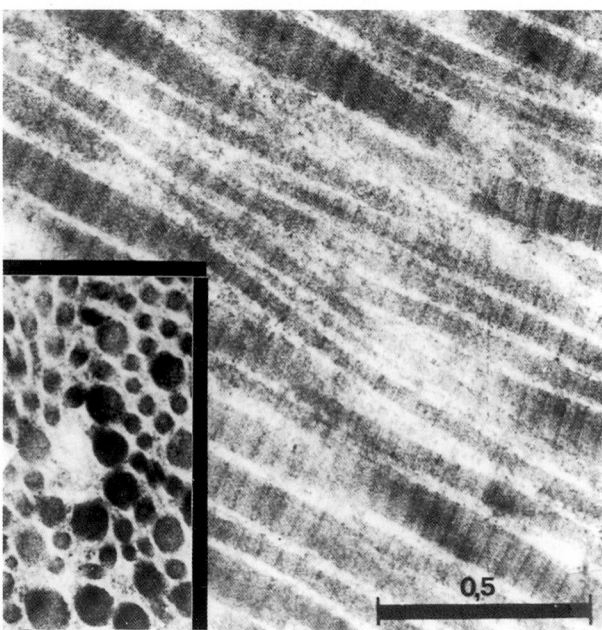

FIGURE 7.13   Collagen fibers of irregular thickness as seen by electron microscopy. *Inset:* Cross section. This was a side effect after 10 years of treatment for Wilson's disease with penicillamine. This drug, used clinically for chelating copper, is thought to interfere with cross-linking in both collagen and elastin. (Reproduced by permission from [40], © 1982 Munksgaard International Publishers Ltd., Copenhagen, Denmark.)

chelates copper and also competes for the aldehyde radicals required for cross-linking of collagen and elastin. Animal experiments gave some hope, but in human patients the results were disappointing. Penicillamine was also used in a totally different context. Because it

chelates copper, it can alleviate Wilson's disease, which is characterized by toxic cellular concentrations of free copper. The result: after several years, in some patients, the treatment produces faulty collagen (Figure 7.13) (40) and faulty elastin, clumps of which are then eliminated through the skin—a condition called **elastosis ulcerans serpiginosa** (5). Thus, the price for treating Wilson's disease was a subtype of lathyrism.

Interestingly, there is also a congenital metabolic disease that leads to a "toxic" defective cross-linking of collagen and elastin: ***homocystinuria.*** Due to the lack of an enzyme, homocysteine accumulates in the blood and tissues; it interacts with the aldehydes formed by lysyl oxidase, and thus blocks the development of stable cross-links (32). In other words, homocysteine functions here much like penicillamine; the two molecules are actually similar. The clinical picture includes a dislocation of the crystalline lens (which is held in place by a crown of collagen fibers) and was once confused with the Marfan syndrome (see further, *elastin*).

Excessive cross-linking. Excessive cross-linking is a typical effect of aging and diabetes (p. 284). If a joint is immobilized experimentally, the cross-linking of the capsular collagen increases as if it had prematurely aged (1). We suspect that this mechanism contributes to the stiffness that develops so rapidly in joints immobilized by plaster casts.

Digestion by enzymes. As we stated earlier, collagen is a very stable protein, especially when highly cross-linked. Its half-life ranges from hours to years. Native collagen is practically unaffected by trypsinlike proteolytic enzymes unless it is denatured; in fact the collagen in raw meat can be utilized as food only because the acid pH of the stomach denatures it, preparing it for digestion by pepsin. However, native collagen can be digested by one family of highly specific enzymes, the **collagenases.** This exposes the collagen fibers to a whole set of possible mishaps, such as bacterial attack. Until 1962, the only known collagenases were bacterial; animal collagenases remained a mystery. It was obvious that collagenous structures (such as bone) could be removed as part of normal tissue turnover, but nobody had ever succeeded in demonstrating collagenase activity in any tissue. It was rationalized, quite correctly, that collagenases in tissues would be potentially dangerous, because if let loose they could reduce the body to a pile of jelly. Indeed, today we know that tissue collagenases do exist, but they are kept in check by powerful inhibitors from the moment they are secreted (35); this is what makes these enzymes so difficult to find. Eventually they were discovered by an experiment *in vitro,* in which—by a fortunate technical accident—the inhibitors were left out (Figure 7.14) (15).

In pathology, the body's own collagenase is relevant mainly as an agent of collagen breakdown and turnover, such as occurs normally in wound healing, bone resorption, and receding gums. *Endogenous collagenase is thought to cause damage in at least three conditions: (a)* ***premature skin aging*** *induced by ultraviolet (UV) light; multiple exposures to UV light lead to sustained elevation of three matrix metalloproteinases, including collagenase (11); (b)* **osteoarthritis** *(so-called degenerative arthritis), in which part of the problem is a breakdown of the hyalin cartilage matrix (collagen included) by endogenous enzymes; and (c)* ***corneal diseases*** *of many kinds, in which the precious corneal stroma is destroyed by collagenases.* These enzymes can be produced by corneal fibroblasts, corneal epithelium, and inflammatory cells, as well as by bacteria; anticollagenase treatments have been devised (39).

Bacterial collagenase plays a major role in the pathogenesis of infection by the anaerobic, collagenase-producing *Clostridium histolyticum,* the agent of the

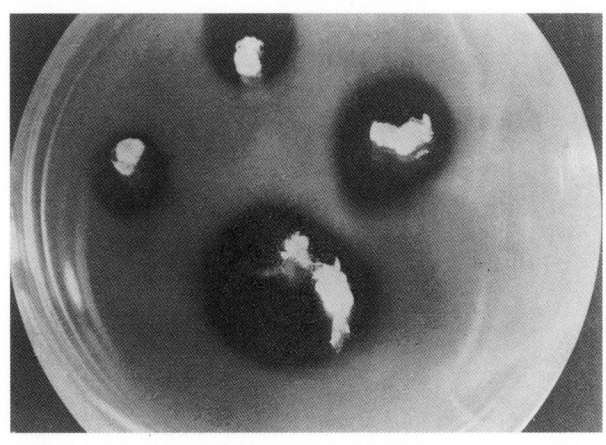

FIGURE 7.14 The discovery of collagenase. Fragments of tadpole tissue were placed on a layer of collagen gel (the opalescent area). The black regions around the explants show digestion of the gel by collagenase. By a stroke of good luck, the authors neglected to add serum or embryo extract to the culture medium, both of which contain a collagenase inhibitor that would have abolished the effect. (Reproduced with permission from [14].)

fast-spreading and life-threatening gas gangrene typical of wounds contaminated with soil. In these infections, collagenase favors the spread of the bacteria by clearing their path in the connective tissue (*histo-lyticum* means "tissue-dissolving"). The first inkling that a specific collagenase must exist came from the histologic study of gas gangrene (30). This is a fine example to show how morphology, well interpreted, can point the way to biochemistry.

Calcification. The price of aging includes a tendency of collagen to calcify (the same is true for elastin). Tendon collagen is especially at risk. The fibers become impregnated with apatite crystals—we might say fossilized—by a mechanism that was discussed earlier (p. 253).

Heat shrinkage of collagen: from Hippocrates to lasers. Heat shrinkage (thermal shrinkage) is a peculiar property of the collagen fibers. When heated to 65°C, they suddenly shrink to about one-third of their original length. Until recently, the only practical application—known to us—of this phenomenon was the shrinkage of deboned human heads as practiced in bygone days by Amazonian natives (28).

Collagen shrinkage explains the drastic shortening of bacon strips in the frying pan. The contracted fibers turn into a semitransparent mass, the common **gelatin** (34) (Figure 7.15). Gelatin today is best known as food, but it also has a significant tradition as **carpenter's glue:** a

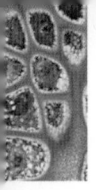

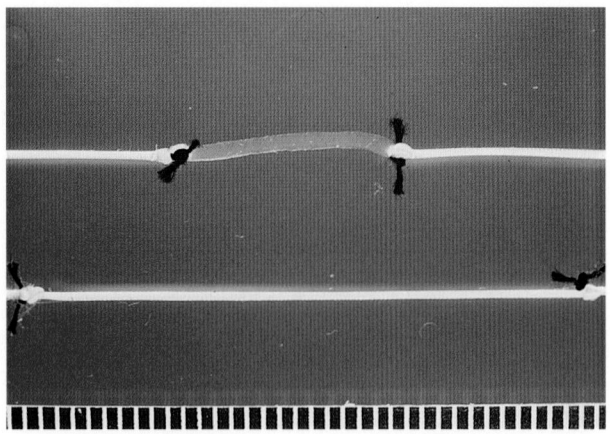

FIGURE 7.15　The phenomenon of thermal contraction of collagen. In these two rat-tail tendons, segments of equal length were marked with knots. In the upper tendon, the segment between the knots was briefly dipped in water at 80°C; it shrank to about one-third of its original size and became gelatinized in the process. The other tendon is a control. **Scale** in millimeters.

tradition that left its mark on the very word *colla-gen,* "generator of glue" (*colla* being Latin for "glue"). **Leather** is essentially dermal collagen made unshrinkable by tanning, a special variety of cross-linking (leather jackets should not shrink if boiled).

Pathologists learn to recognize the hyalin mass on the surface of skin biopsy samples as collagen gelatinized by the thermocautery (Figure 7.16); a similar change can be seen around the path of a bullet. Collagen shrinkage probably plays a role in the skin changes produced by *CO₂ skin laser resurfacing,* a procedure supposed to rejuvenate the skin (19, 42). Another application of collagen shrinkage has surfaced recently: orthopedic surgeons are using the heat of a laser to shrink parts of the shoulder joint capsule in "throwing athletes" who develop a tendency to dislocate the head of the humerus (9). A very similar operation was performed by the Hippocratic physicians on the same kind of athlete: they poked a red-hot iron through the skin of the armpit (27).

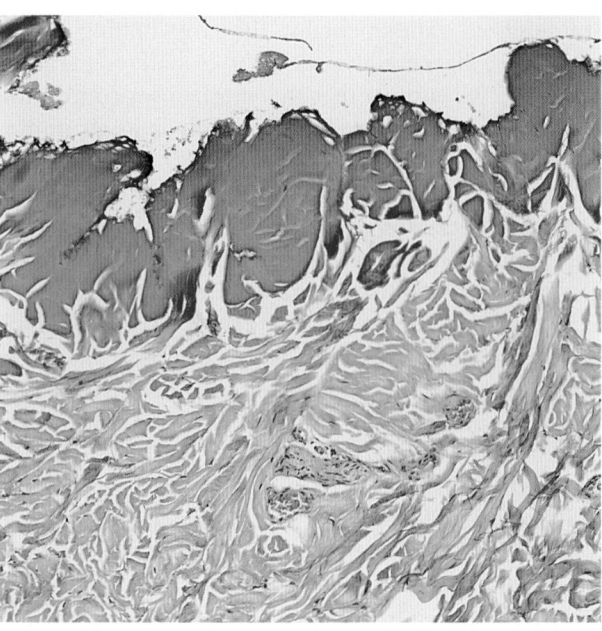

FIGURE 7.16　Thermal shrinkage of collagen along a cut made in human skin with an electrocautery. *Top:* Gelatinized fibers. *Bottom:* Normal collagen fibers.

The 400 B.C. rationale was to create a thick, contracting scar that would hold the head of the humerus in its socket; the 2002 rationale is to shrink the collagen and hope that the granulation tissue replacing it will maintain the shrinkage. We are not sure which one we prefer.

Alkaptonuria. This rare disease, also called **ochronosis,** can be interpreted as collagen tanning *in vivo.* The patients lack homogentisic acid oxidase, without which homogentisic acid (a normal metabolite of tyrosine and phenylalanine) accumulates in large amounts (13). The result is dark urine and a darkening or "staining" of articular cartilage, which dies and breaks down causing progressive joint disease. It has been suggested that homogentisic acid is a natural tanning agent that denatures the collagen (25). It may also inhibit lysyl hydroxylase, thus modifying the collagen by yet another mechanism (36).

Pathology of Elastin

The arteries need to be elastic, the skin needs to be elastic, and all soft tissues need some recoil. Elastin is the answer. Fibroblasts and smooth-muscle cells produce most of it.

Structurally, elastin is very different from collagen in that it is a complex polymer containing at least 19 proteins (72). It has received much attention because it changes (for the worse) with age. Its resistance to chemical agents is astonishing. Until recently, the standard method for extracting elastin from a piece of tissue was to autoclave the whole thing or to boil it in alkali, and the solid that was left was assumed to be

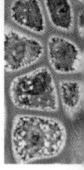

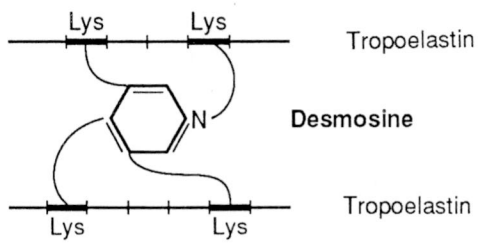

FIGURE 7.17 Desmosine, an amino acid unique to elastin. It develops from four lysine residues in two adjacent molecules of tropoelastin. (Adapted from [58].)

elastin. Elastin tends to persist in necrotic tissues after all other structures have disappeared.

Elastin shares with collagen the molecular feature of cross-linking as well as the cross-linking enzyme lysyl oxidase; for this reason it also shares some of collagen's pathology, namely the disturbances induced by cross-linking inhibitors such as those that occur in lathyrism, penicillamine treatment, and copper deficiency (p. 271).

> One type of cross-link is specific to elastin. Two lysine residues on one chain join two others of an adjacent chain, and the four together form a new amino acid: desmosine or its isomer isodesmosine (Figure 7.17) (58). This amino acid is not reused when elastin is broken down, so the amount of desmosine excreted in the urine can be used to measure elastin turnover (60), much as urinary proline can be used as a marker of collagen turnover.

Compared with rubber threads of the same size, isolated elastic fibers can stretch at least five times more (50), but in the context of tissues they cannot reach that limit because they are intertwined with collagen fibers, which are virtually inextensible. Elastin also differs from rubber in that water is required for its recoil. Its molecule contains hydrophobic regions, which may be related to its tendency to bind lipids (79). It also binds fatty acids, and once it is thus complexed, it is much more susceptible to digestion by elastase (76). These features may play a role in atherosclerotic plaques, where elastin and lipids abound.

Diseases of elastin can be congenital or acquired and can cause the elastic fibers to be increased, decreased, or abnormal (51).

Genetic Defects of the Elastic Fibers

These defects are many but rare, except for the Marfan syndrome. They may affect the fibrillin or elastin genes.

A Defect of Fibrillin: The Marfan Syndrome

One of the most common heritable disorders of connective tissue, Marfan syndrome affects about 1 in 10,000 people. It is typically represented by tall individuals with

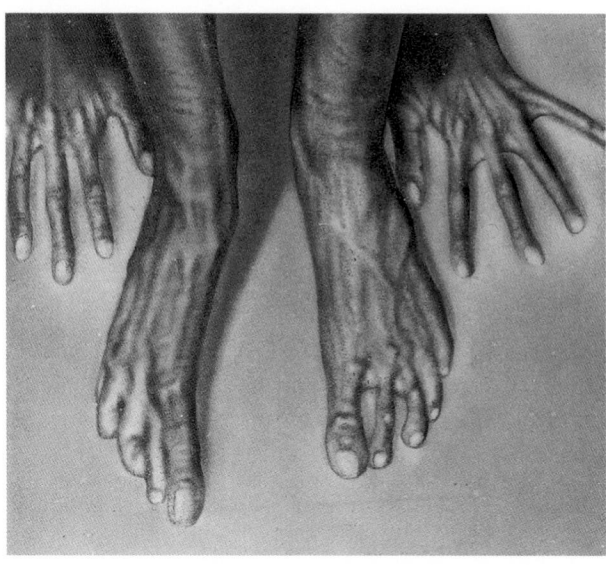

FIGURE 7.18 Arachnodactily (spider fingers) typical of Marfan syndrome, a congenital disease of fibrillin—a component of elastic fibers.(Reproduced from [74], © 1983 McGraw-Hill Book Co. with permission of The McGraw-Hill Companies.)

long, spidery fingers: "arachnodactily" (Figure 7.18). It has been suggested that President Lincoln and Paganini, two of history's tall men, were victims of the Marfan syndrome; regarding President Lincoln, permission to test his DNA was denied, but the diagnosis was ruled out on the basis of other available evidence (66).

The clinical picture includes loose joints, a deformed spine, floppy mitral valves (leading to regurgitation), and eye troubles such as dislocation of the lens. The main threat to life is a sudden rupture of the aorta; histology of the aortic wall shows a thickened wall with defective elastin (Figure 7.19) and pools of metachromatic material (Figure 7.20) (78). After a great deal of work, the molecular defect was linked to two fibrillin genes on chromosomes 5 and 15 (63, 69, 80). The glycoprotein **fibrillin,** identified only in 1986, is a component of the microfibrils associated with elastin, and it happens to be especially abundant in the aorta, the periosteum, and the ligament that holds the lens in place: the tissues most affected by Marfan syndrome (71). So, a century after it was described by a Paris pediatrician, Marfan syndrome is recognized as a disease of elastic fibers, which disturbs these fibers without affecting the elastin molecule itself. It includes a wide spectrum of clinical manifestations (55).

Congenital Defects of Elastin

Congenital supravalvular aortic stenosis. This rare human disease has been linked to a defect of the elastin gene. Children born with this problem have a special facies;

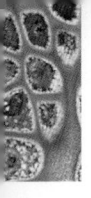

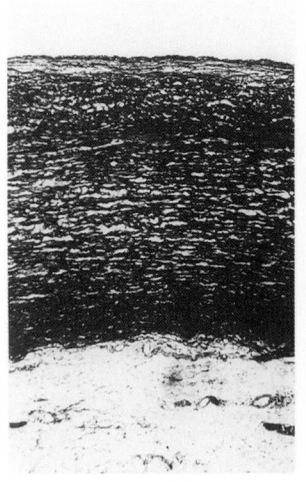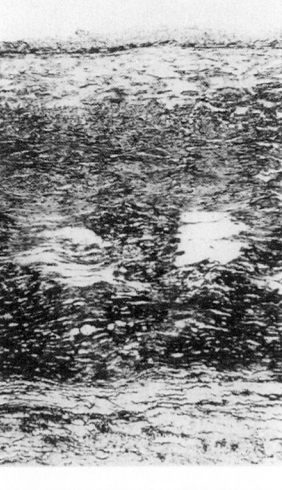

FIGURE 7.19   Example of elastin pathology: aortic wall in cystic medial necrosis (*right*) compared with the wall of a normal aorta (*left*). The pathogenesis of the elastin change in this condition is not understood. Verhoeff's elastic stain. (10x) (Reproduced with permission from [59].)

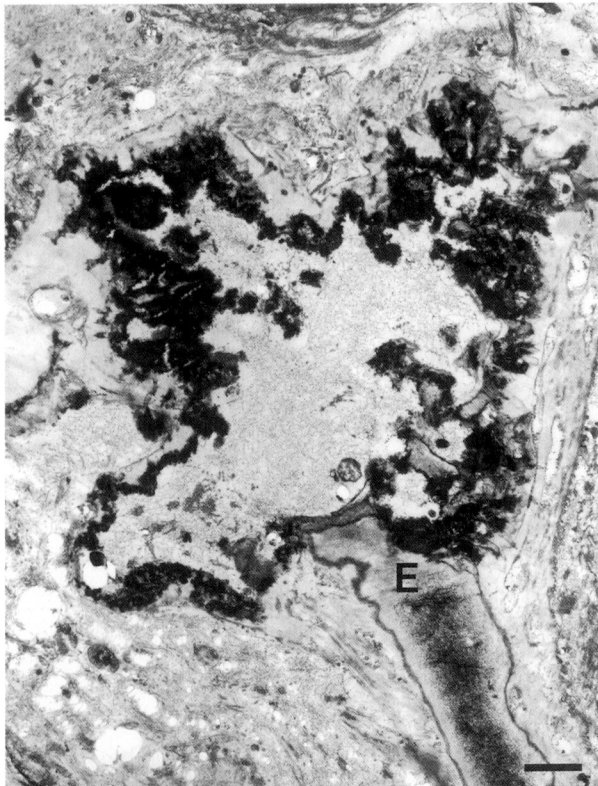

FIGURE 7.20   Faulty elastin in the wall of an artery in Marfan's syndrome. Electron micrograph. An elastic lamella (**L**) appears to break up into a disorganized mass. **Bar** = 2 μm. (Reproduced with permission from [78].)

the walls of their large arteries—lacking the elastic component—are greatly thickened by smooth muscle proliferation (77).

Knockout mice deprived of their elastin gene live only 4 days: the reason makes sense when explained—but it is quite surprising. The smooth muscle cells of the coronary arteries, not being restrained between sheets of elastin, multiply out of control and invade the lumen until the mouse dies (53).

Cutis laxa. This is a heterogenous group of congenital diseases that overlap in part with Ehler-Danlos syndrome but also have the distinctive feature that elastic fibers are too few. The skin lacks recoil and appears too large for the body; the face is typically droopy, recalling a bloodhound (Figure 7.21) (73), and the voice may be baritonal because the vocal cords lack tension. Our outward appearance depends a great deal on elastin.

Acquired Defects of the Elastic Fibers

Elastin is particularly sensitive to aging, as the cosmetic industry well knows, and elastogenesis in the skin is affected by sunlight, a problem shared—as we have seen—by collagen. The organs richest in elastin are the

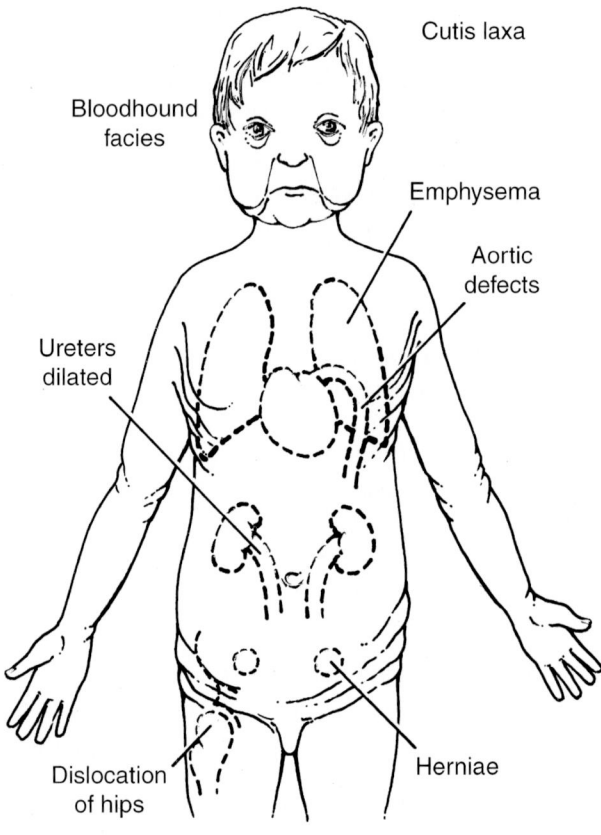

FIGURE 7.21   Multiple defects arising from the lack of normal elastin in *cutis laxa*. (Modified from [73].)

lungs, and the pathogenesis of emphysema is centered around the destruction of elastic fibers.

Aging. Cross-linking increases with age in elastin as it does in collagen, which means that the arteries become progressively stiffer. The amount of calcium bound to the elastic fibers also increases with age. This has been attributed to a progressive increase in acidic amino acids (aspartic and glutamic), which could bind calcium (64, 65); but it may also depend on an intrinsic property of the elastin molecule, which can nucleate apatite crystals (76). In some arteries the internal elastic lamina is specifically and strikingly calcified (Figure 6.13).

Solar elastosis. Among the acquired diseases of elastin, solar elastosis affects almost everybody's face after the age of 30. It is also called dermatoheliosis (54, 57) but should really be called sun-worshipers' disease. At first the skin becomes finely wrinkled and loses its elasticity; eventually it becomes lumpy, coarsely wrinkled, and even criss-crossed by deep furrows (Figure 7.22). A classic example is the "redneck," which you might never recognize under the pompous name of

cutis rhomboidalis nuchae. Microscopically, in all skin areas exposed to the sun, the dermis is thickened and contains seemingly amorphous pools of a basophilic hyalin (Figure 7.23). This material takes up dyes that normally stain elastic fibers, hence the name *elastosis;* in fact, by scanning electron microscopy, it corresponds to a dense matting of fine, abnormal elastic fibers (Figure 7.24) (81). It is believed that the dermal fibroblasts produce defective elastic fibers because they are damaged by the sun's rays. Note that the cells in the dermis do not live in total darkness: 50–75 percent of sunlight penetrates the epidermis. Experimentally, solar elastosis has been reproduced in hairless mice by exposure to UV light (75) or to X-rays (68).

Digestion by enzymes. Elastin is extremely resistant to enzymes, even more so than collagen. However, it can be digested by the elastases. These enzymes are not as specific as collagenases; they also digest many other proteins. Elastases are present in the pancreatic juice, in the granules of neutrophils (62), and on the surface of macrophages (67). Elastases are produced by many bacteria, such as *Pseudomonas;* they can play a role in the infectious process by "opening up" the connective tissue spaces and thus favoring bacterial spread. Many strains of *Clostridium histolyticum* produce elastase as well as collagenase (their name *histoLYTICUM* is well

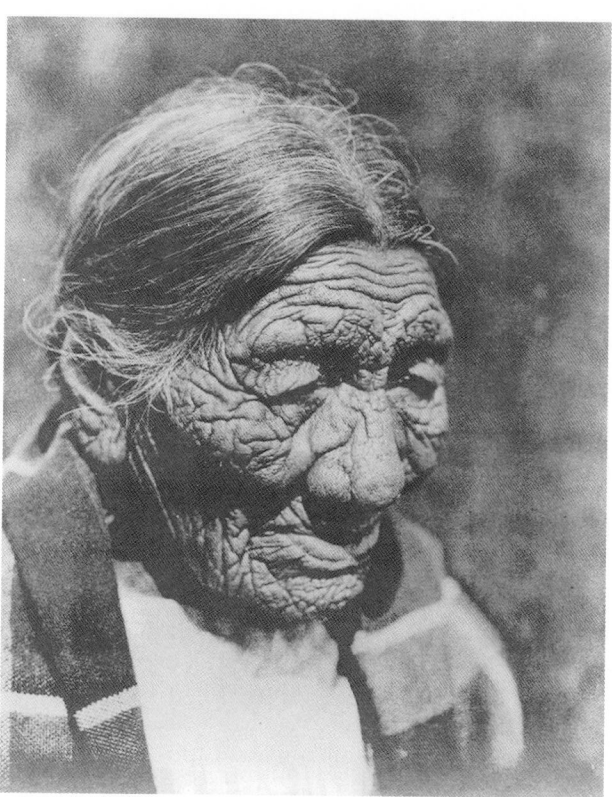

FIGURE 7.22 Portrait of Black Belly, a member of the Cheyenne tribe, taken by Edward S. Curtis at the turn of the century. The lumpy skin (solar elastosis) is a long-term effect of exposure to the sun. (Reproduced from [52].)

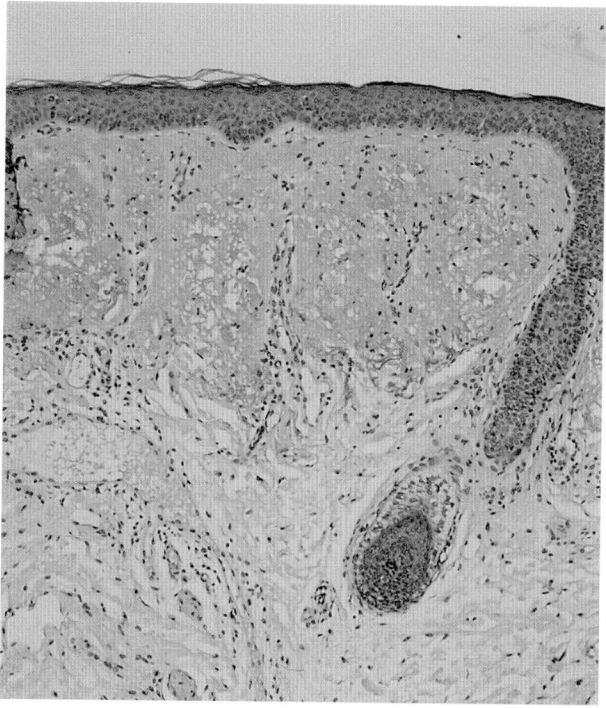

FIGURE 7.23 Solar elastosis (the hyalin, bluish layer beneath the epidermis) near a squamous cell carcinoma of the forehead in a 54-year-old man (hematoxylin and eosin stain).

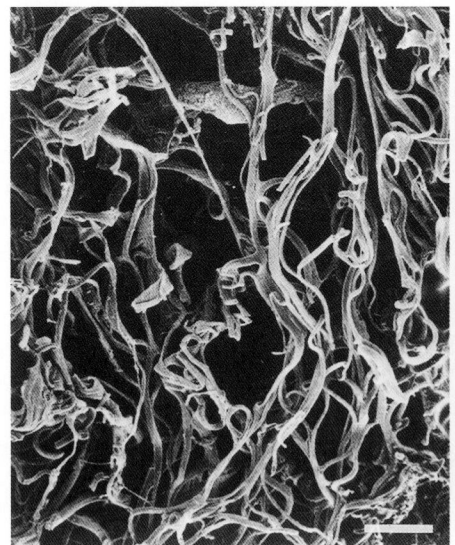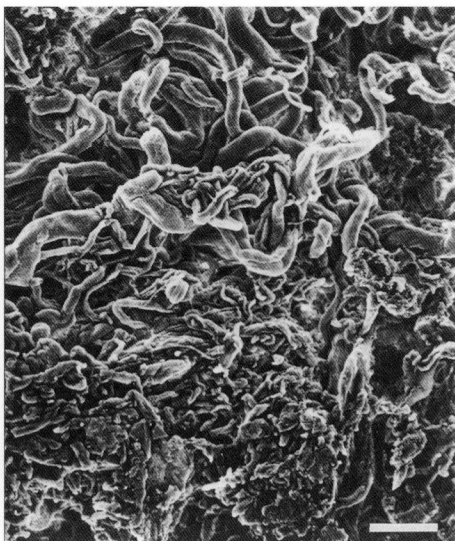

FIGURE 7.24 Elastin fibers obtained from samples of human dermis. (The collagen was destroyed by autoclaving.) *Left:* Normal skin. *Right:* Solar elastosis from the neck of a "redneck" (*cutis rhomboidalis nuchae*). Scanning electron micrographs. **Bars** = 25 μm. (Reproduced by permission from [81], © 1984 Munksgaard International Publishers Ltd., Copenhagen, Denmark.)

deserved). There is even a *Flavobacterium elastolyticum.* Some snake venoms, especially those of rattlesnakes and vipers, owe their local destructive properties to elastase. However, the elastase most relevant to human disease is endogenous: neutrophil elastase, the enzyme that leads to emphysema.

Emphysema. To understand emphysema, remember that the lung is subdivided into myriads of microscopic air spaces (the alveoli) that have the purpose of increasing the surface area available for gas exchanges. In emphysema the walls between the alveoli tend to break down, so that the air spaces become larger and larger, and the surface area available for gas exchanges is correspondingly reduced. The lung tissue is vanishing because it is being robbed of its critical elastin scaffolding, as a result of an *imbalance between elastase and antielastase (called alpha-1-antitrypsin)* combined with chronic inflammation (70). The correlation between emphysema and alpha-1-antitrypsin is complex (p. 140) (56, 61), but the essentials are as follows. Alpha-1-antitrypsin, despite its name, is important primarily as an anti*elastase* (it represents 90 percent of the antielastase activity of the blood). It is powerless against macrophage elastase but very effective against granulocyte elastase. In smokers, more granulocytes are attracted into the lungs, and there they release their enzymes, elastase included, either because they are activated or because they die. The enzymes cross the endothelial barrier (by transcytosis?), and the elastase attacks the functionally critical elastin framework of the alveoli. The elastase is, of course, more effective if the level of the plasma inhibitor is low (cigarette smoke itself renders the inhibitor ineffective). The final result is a breakdown of the alveolar walls: emphysema. The only enzyme that produces emphysema experimentally if instilled into the bronchi is elastase (62).

Pathology of Basement Membranes

Basement membranes are so thin that they remained ill-defined until the electron microscope came along (95, 96). They are thin indeed (less than 0.1 μm) but surprisingly tough. By electron microscopy, in damaged tissues, it is quite common to see that cells have been destroyed, whereas the basement membranes that supported them are still there. This ability to persist after the cells have disappeared has a definite survival value: it enables regenerating cells to grow back into the right places by creeping along a guiding surface (p. 34). The mechanical toughness of basement membranes is largely due to their skeleton of Type 4 collagen, which consists of molecules arranged in a network (Figure 7.25) (83). This collagenous structure is also their Achilles' heel: it makes them susceptible to destruction by collagenases, which are secreted by leukocytes, especially in the course of inflammation (pp. 335, 412).

Basement membranes as molecular traps. All basement membranes contain highly charged, "sticky" molecules such as heparan sulfate and fibronectin. This explains their affinity for calcium and silver ions; the latter

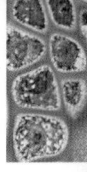

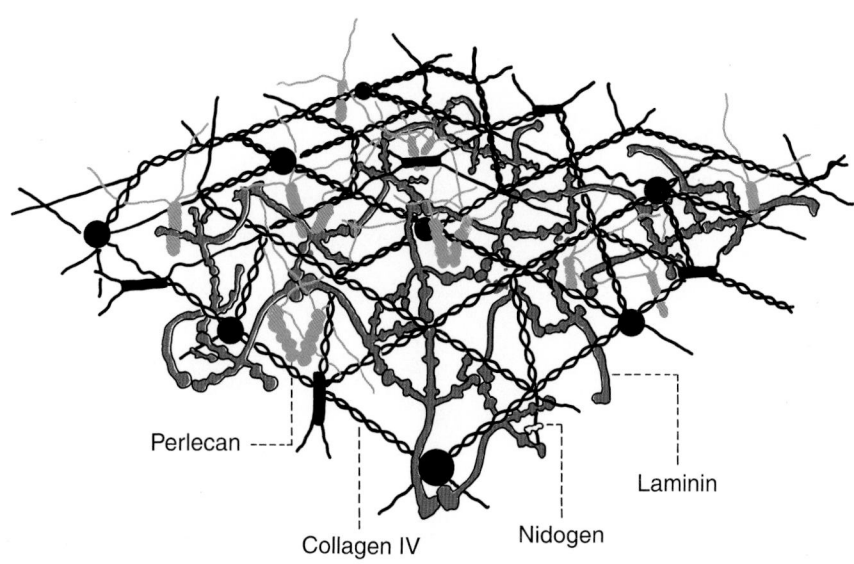

FIGURE 7.25 Molecular model of basement membrane showing the interactions between **collagen Type 4, perlecan** (proteoglycan), **laminin,** and **nidogen.** (Courtesy of Dr. P. D. Yurchenco, University of Medicine and Dentistry of New Jersey, Piscataway, NJ.)

Perlecan

Collagen IV   Nidogen   Laminin

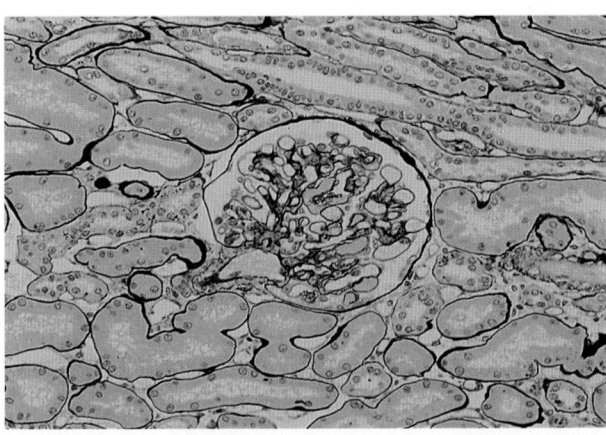

FIGURE 7.26 Basement membrane (thin black line) around kidney tubules and glomerular capillaries demonstrated by silver impregnation. (Courtesy of Geneviève Leyvraz, Department of Pathology, University of Geneva, Switzerland.)

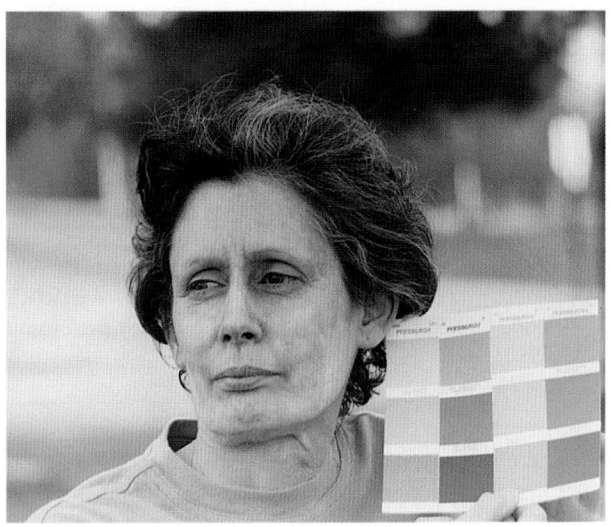

FIGURE 7.27 Argyria: the price to pay for an uncontrolled drug. At age 11, this 46-year-old lady was given unspecified drops for "allergies"; 3 years later, her skin turned gray. The facial pigmentation, initially diffuse, became patchy after dermabrasion. On one occasion, in the recovery room after unrelated surgery, the nurses became alarmed because they thought the patient was cyanotic. Silver nitrate solutions are still sold in some "health" food stores and pharmacies. (Photograph courtesy of Dr. B. A. Bouts, Blanchard Valley Medical Associates, Findlay, OH. Reproduced from [81a]. Copyright © 1999 Massachusetts Medical Society. All rights reserved.)

property is exploited to make them visible in histologic sections (Figure 7.26). The same property is displayed by basement membranes *in vivo.* So, imagine what might happen to individuals who continue to ingest preparations of colloidal silver, sold to this day as "dietary supplements" and therefore not submitted to any control. Recommended for almost any ailment and taken day after day, year after year, these "drugs" slowly impregnate with silver all of the basement membranes (and the pockets of the druggists); correspondingly, the skin acquires a grayish hue: a condition called **argyria** (Figure 7.27) (85, 87, 89). Industrial exposure can have the same effect; in any case argyria is unfortunately not reversible. It is easily reproduced in rats by adding silver nitrate to

the drinking water; this procedure has been useful for studying the growth of the thick basement membranes of the renal glomeruli (Figure 7.28) (91, 105), much as we use tree rings to study the growth of a tree (93).

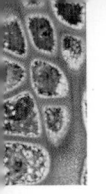

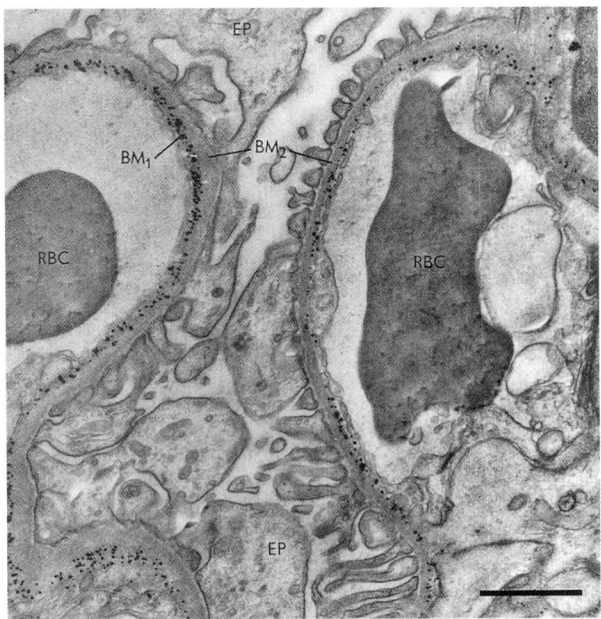

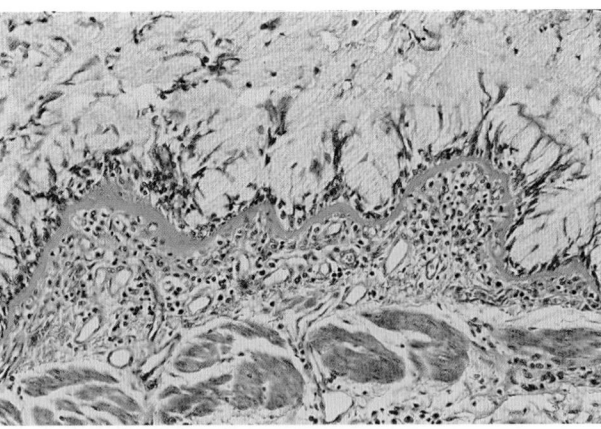

FIGURE 7.29   Thickening of the epithelial basement membrane in a bronchus from a case of asthma. *Top:* Lumen of the bronchus filled with mucus and desquamated epithelial cells. The thickened basement membrane is the pink wavy layer separating the epithelium from the inflamed mucosa.

FIGURE 7.28   Affinity of basement membranes for silver nitrate (argyrophilia). Glomerulus of a normal rat that was made argyric upon weaning and then allowed to live for another 5 months without silver in the drinking water. **BM₁:** Oldest layer of basement membrane synthesized during silver treatment; note the peppering of silver granules (black dots). The younger layer free of silver (**BM₂**) lies beneath the epithelial cells (**EP**), indicating that these are the cells that synthesized it. **RBC:** Red blood cell. **Bar** = 1 μm. (Reproduced with permission from [91].)

There is no saving grace to argyria, but it does reveal an important quality of the basement membranes: as we mentioned earlier, their strong negative charges allow them to trap growth factors and to release them locally when needed.

Pathologic thickening. Thickening of the basement membrane is fairly common, especially around capillaries and beneath epithelia. Perhaps it reflects a persistent, low-grade state of irritation of the cells that produce the basement membrane, be they epithelial or other. For example, in the bronchial mucosa of asthmatics, the subepithelial basement membrane can become thick enough to be visible by light microscopy, thus earning the name **lamina vitrea** (Figure 7.29); the bronchial epithelium of asthmatics is certainly in a chronic state of irritation (p. 537). The lamina vitrea seems to be harmless, but it is quite another matter when multiple thick layers of basement membrane are wrapped around capillaries; in such cases there must be some restriction of the lumen (94) although this effect has not been well

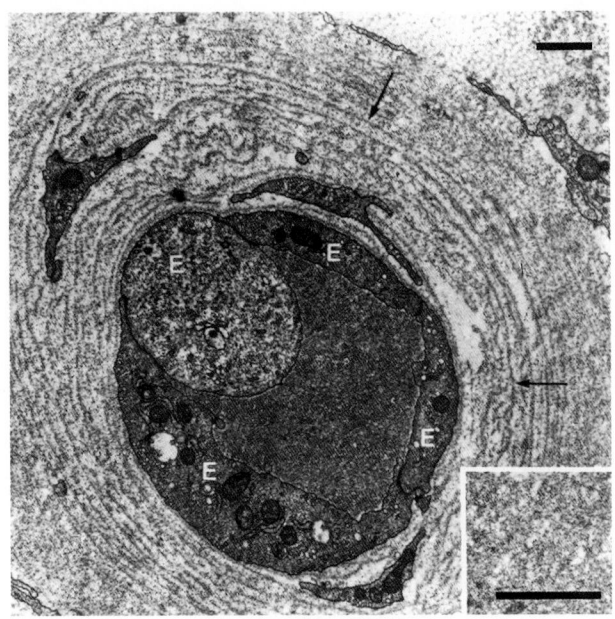

FIGURE 7.30   Multiple basement membranes (**arrows**) around a capillary of the dermis in a case of erythropoietic protoporphyria produced by long-wave UV light. **E:** Endothelial cells. *Inset:* detail. **Bars** = 1 μm. (Reproduced from [86] by permission from Blackwell Scientific Publications Ltd.)

studied. Just glance at two examples taken from tissues exposed to chronic, subtle injury, such as the skin of patients suffering from **porphyria,** a condition of abnormal sensitivity to sunlight (Figure 7.30), or the renal and

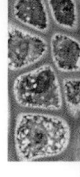

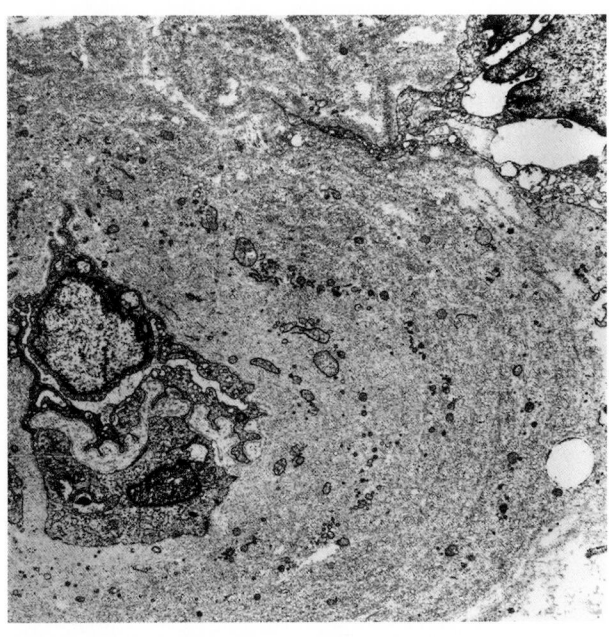

FIGURE 7.31 Thickening of the basement membrane in a ureteral capillary of a patient who abused the analgesic phenacetin. Severe restriction of the lumen. (Courtesy of M. J. Mihatsch, Institute for Pathology, Basel, Switzerland.)

perirenal tissues in individuals who abused the analgesic phenacetin (Figure 7.31) (86, 100).

The multilayered appearance of the pericapillary basement membrane was once explained by cycles of death and regeneration of pericytes, which are entirely wrapped in basement membrane. A more likely explanation is that endothelial cells are somehow turned on to form successive layers of basement membrane (96, 103, 104). What

irritant might turn them on remains unknown. Regarding the abuse of phenacetin, all we can say is that rats treated with analgesics can develop outright necrosis of the renal papilla (88). (Note: Multiple basement membranes around venules are a normal feature (107), but onion-skin arrangements such as illustrated in Figures 7.30 and 7.31 are clearly abnormal.)

A diffuse thickening of the pericapillary basement membranes is typical in diabetics (Figure 7.32) (106), which is puzzling in several respects. Why does it develop? Why does it select the capillary basement membranes? How does it affect the microcirculation? In diabetes the thickening around the glomerular capillaries can be extreme: irregular lumps of basement membrane material are large enough to be seen by light microscopy and to warrant a special name for this condition, **Kimmelstiel-Wilson glomerulosclerosis** (94). After pancreas transplantation, the basement membrane thickening is slowly reversible (5–10 years [84]).

The biochemical changes in the capillary basement membranes of diabetics are complex and not fully understood (101). In the glomerular basement membranes of diabetics the heparan sulfate component is reduced, which correlates well with the observed increase in glomerular permeability (95). Persistent hyperglycemia is harmful because it leads to cross-linking of proteins and thus to the formation of "advanced glycosylation end-products" (AGE, p. 284). The AGE in turn have a number of pernicious effects (Table 7.1). In rats the intravenous injection of glycosylated plasma proteins for 12 weeks caused glomerular changes similar to those of diabetes (99). Experimental diabetes induced in rats with streptozotocin (which selectively kills the pancreatic beta cells) also produces the typical glomerular changes. In humans this

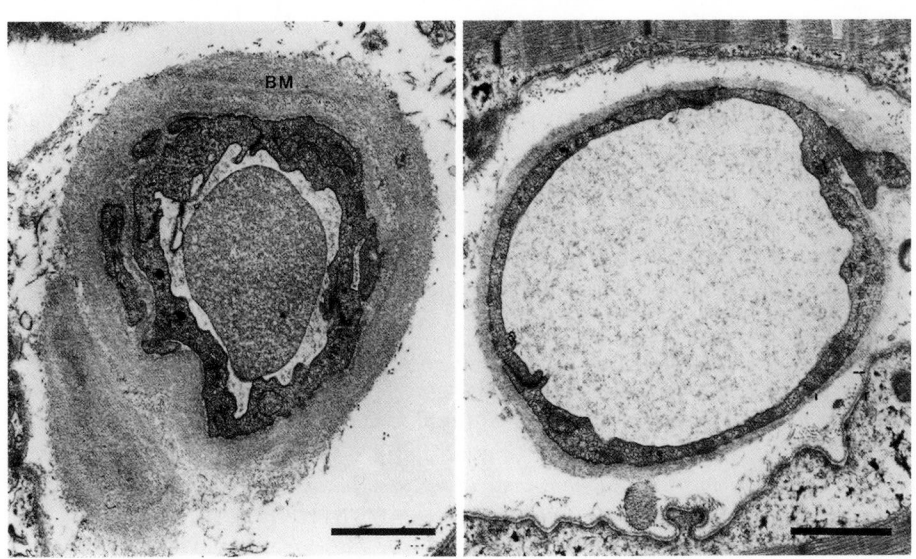

FIGURE 7.32 *Left:* Thickening of the pericapillary basement membrane (**BM**) in human diabetes. *Right:* Control. **Bars** = 1 μm. (Courtesy of Dr. J. R. Williamson, Washington University School of Medicine, St. Louis, MO.)

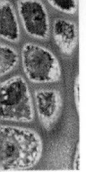
Table 7.1 Possible Effects of Hyperglycemia on Capillary Basement Membrane (BM)

AGE* develop on and between BM macromolecules; this
- Interferes with the self-assembly of BM
- Reduces the susceptibility of BM to enzymatic degradation
- Traps plasma proteins seeping into the BM
- Decreases BM affinity for growth-modulating heparan sulfate proteoglycans

AGE bind to macrophage receptors; the activated macrophages release cytokines (TNF, IL-1, etc.) with multiple effects:
- Stimulation of matrix synthesis
- Hypertrophy/hyperplasia of endothelial/smooth muscle cells
- Procoagulant changes of the endothelial surface

*Advanced glycosylation end-products.

(Adapted from [101] by permission from Blackwell Scientific Publications Ltd.)

lesion is at least partially reversible by control of the hyperglycemia (102). There is much evidence to show that diabetes affects the endothelium and the pericytes (pp. 496, 689).

Basement membranes are not all alike. Basement membranes look alike but differ chemically. The first evidence for this was provided in 1933 by a Japanese pathologist, M. Masugi, who injected rats with anti–rat-kidney antibodies prepared by injecting rat kidney into rabbits (98). The result was a glomerular disease now known as **Masugi nephrotoxic nephritis,** characterized by antibody deposition all along the glomerular basement membranes. What did *not* happen to Masugi's rats was very interesting: *the basement membranes in other organs remained intact (92, 97).* Therefore, they must be chemically different.

A similar lesson is taught by a human autoimmune disease, best known as the **Goodpasture syndrome.** This disease depends on an antigen present only in the basement membranes of the glomeruli and of the alveolar capillaries (pp. 542, 592).

Congenital diseases of the basement membrane. Best known but rare is the heterogenous **Alport syndrome (hereditary progressive glomerulopathy),** in which the glomerular basement membrane is thinned, allowing the escape of red blood cells (hematuria). Renal insufficiency may follow. Several mutations were found in genes for collagen Type 4 (90). A primary basement membrane defect may also be at the root of the nephrophtysis syndrome, a cause of renal failure in the young: cystic dilatations appear in the medullary tubules, and the cortex become atrophic (82).

Pathology of Proteoglycans

Proteoglycans are huge, feathery molecules shaped like test-tube brushes. The stem is a long molecule of hyaluronic acid (a **glycosaminoglycan,** formerly called mucopolysaccharide). Attached to this stem at regular intervals are **core proteins** bearing many chains of shorter glycosaminoglycans (e.g., chondroitin sulfate, keratan sulfate). Link proteins reinforce the attachment (Figure 7.33). Although typical of the connective tissue spaces, proteoglycans are also a component of basement membranes and of cell membranes, where their main functions relate to cell recognition, attachment, and growth control (116, 120).

When woven into the connective tissue matrix, *proteoglycans bind vast amounts of fluid and are therefore responsible for holding interstitial water in place;* without them, all the water would flow into our legs, as actually happens when their fluid-carrying capacity is exceeded (p. 621). *They also bind a variety of other molecules, such as growth factors* (111, 120).

Proteoglycans are involved in the pathology of joints. They form the bulk of the matrix in articular cartilage where they are synthesized by the chondrocytes under the stimulus of mechanical loading. They are essential for the protection of cartilage against overload; under pressure, some of the water squeezes out and mixes with the synovial fluid, helping lubrication. When joint cartilage is underloaded, as happens when a limb is immobilized in a plaster cast, there is a sharp decrease in proteoglycan synthesis within a few days (108, 118).

Extracellular "degeneration" of cartilage. The very common osteoarthritis (degenerative arthritis) begins with a reduction in the proteoglycan content of the articular cartilage (Figure 7.34). The mechanism is not clear (108, 112). Later the collagen fibers, which normally act as a scaffolding for the proteoglycans, are exposed and tend to separate like the hair of a brush, so that the normally shiny surface of the joint cartilage appears velvety (Figure 7.35). *This complex extracellular breakdown is one of the rare pathologic events that can properly be called "degenerative"* (p. 165).

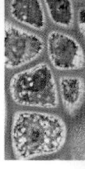

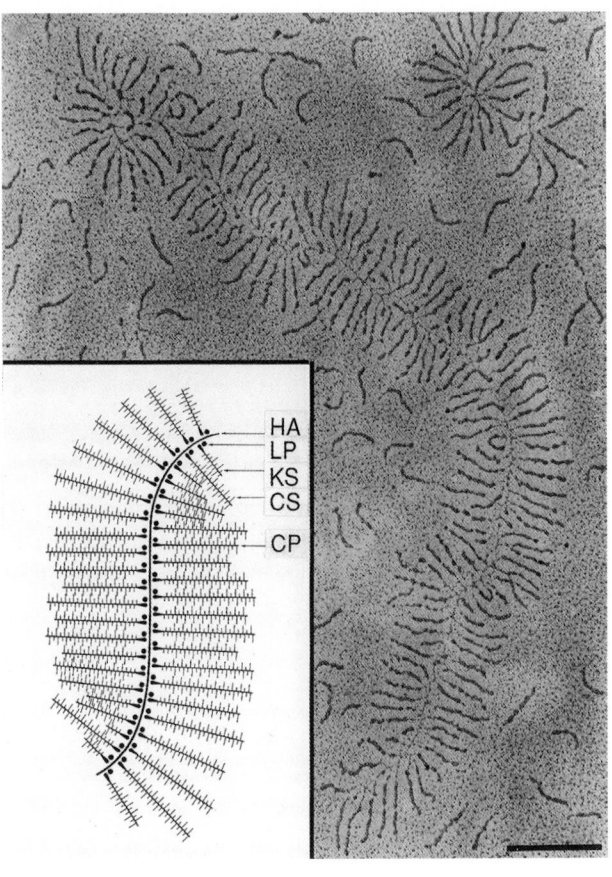

FIGURE 7.33 The feathery structure of a proteoglycan molecule seen with the electron microscope. (Reproduced with permission from [108a].) *Inset:* Diagram of the molecular architecture. **HA:** Backbone of hyaluronic acid. **LP:** Link protein. **KS:** Keratan sulfate. **CS:** Chondroitin sulfate. **CP:** Core protein. (Reproduced with permission from [119].)

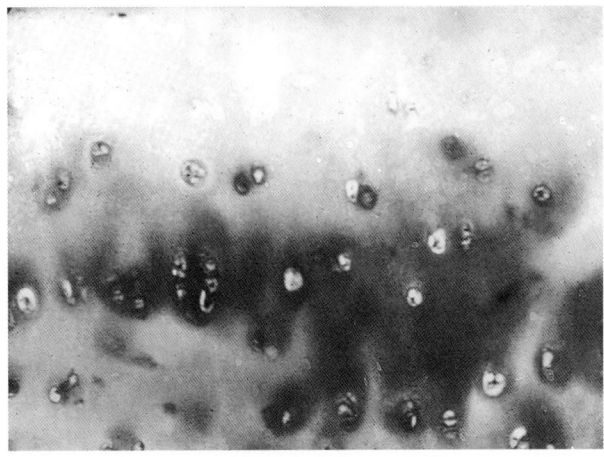

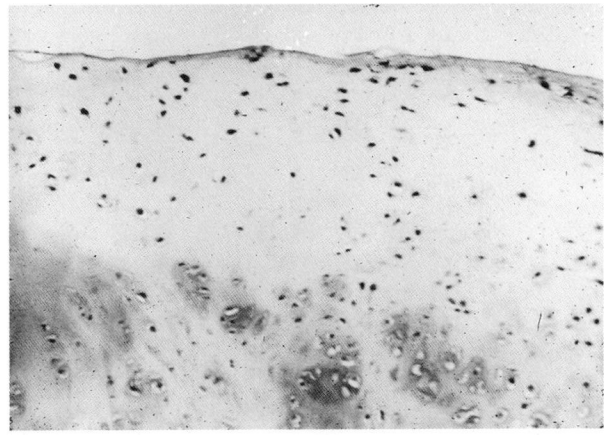

FIGURE 7.34 *Top:* Normal articular cartilage from the femoral head. The dark areas, red in the original, correspond to the dye Safranin-O and indicate a normal content of proteoglycans. *Bottom:* Similar cartilage in osteoarthrosis, showing extensive loss of proteoglycans. (Courtesy of the American Rheumatism Association, Atlanta, GA.)

Myxedema. Myxedema ("mucous edema") is the traditional name for a special variety of edema due to an excess of proteoglycans or their building blocks. It is nonpitting (p. 626) and limited to a few conditions, one of which is **advanced hypothyroidism,** now rarely seen (117). Hyaluronic acid accumulates in the tissue spaces (with some organ preferences) and causes symptoms accordingly: puffy face, thick cold skin, hoarse voice, swollen tongue, and stiff joints. The metabolic disturbance appears to be a reduction in hyaluronic acid degradation (110, 115). Paradoxically, Graves' disease, which leads to **hyperthyroidism,** also leads to an excessive deposition of glycosaminoglycans; even more strangely, this happens only in the pretibial area (pretibial myxedema) (Figure 7.36) (113). Because the thyroid in Graves' disease is overstimulated by an autoimmune mechanism (p. 588), it is possible that some fibroblasts may be stimulated by a similar mechanism (114). But why just the pretibial fibroblasts? Studies *in vitro* have shown that fibroblasts can be stimulated by a factor in the blood of these patients, whereas fibroblasts obtained from the shoulder area remain indifferent (109). This is a fine example of "homologous" cells from different parts of the body not being biologically identical.

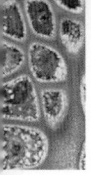

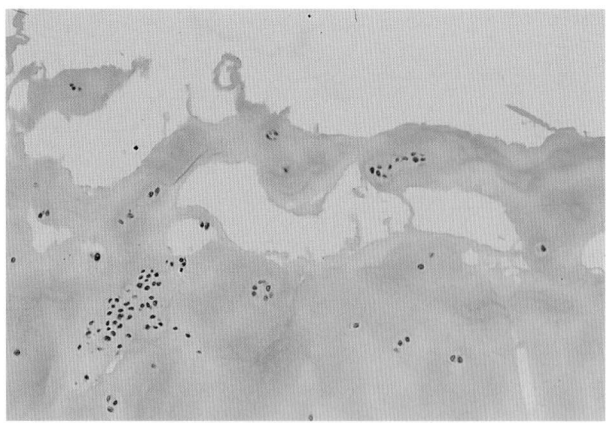

FIGURE 7.35   Breakdown of the extracellular matrix on the articular surface of a knee joint, in a case of "degenerative" arthritis. Bits of cartilage are flaking off; clusters of regenerating cells do develop (*center left*) but a coordinated replacement of the lost cartilage does not occur. (Biopsy specimen courtesy of Dr. Y. Kapanci, Department of Pathology, Geneva, Switzerland.)

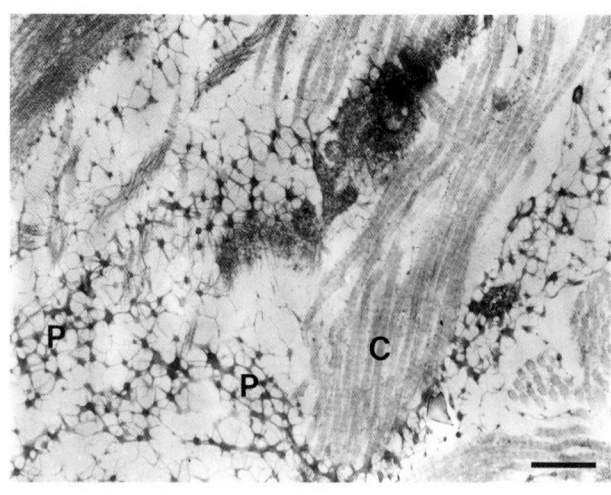

FIGURE 7.36   Electron microscopic view of myxedema: **P:** Proteoglycan. **C:** Collagen bundles. **Bar** = 0.5 μm. (Reproduced with permission from [113].)

Pathologic Changes due to Glucose

Our quest for mechanisms of disease leads us to discuss a danger that faces many of our macromolecules, be they extra- or intracellular. *Proteins that have very long lives, such as collagen and hemoglobin, are subject to chronic attack from an unlikely source: glucose.* The mechanism is **nonenzymatic glycation** (formerly called glycosylation).

Our story begins once again with the food industry, which has long been aware of the **browning reaction.** This reaction is essentially a nuisance: if milk is heated for a long time, sugar and proteins combine to form brown, bitter, burnt-tasting products called melanoidins (nothing to do with melanin, nor with the browning of

fruit, which is due to different compounds, p. 107). This reaction contributes to the brown color and toughness of cooked meat (128). Only recently did it dawn upon nonfood scientists that the same reaction is involved in aging (121) and especially in diabetes (124).

The reaction proceeds step by step without the help of enzymes, reversibly at first and then irreversibly. To begin, the aldehyde group of glucose reacts randomly with an amino group on a protein, giving rise to a ketoamine or Schiff base, which is unstable (Figure 7.37). This product quickly rearranges itself into a so-called Amadori product—still reversible. Now, if the protein persists in the body for months or years (or if food is

FIGURE 7.37   Mechanism of nonenzymatic glycation, showing how two molecules of protein become cross-linked by glucose. (Reproduced with permission from [124].)

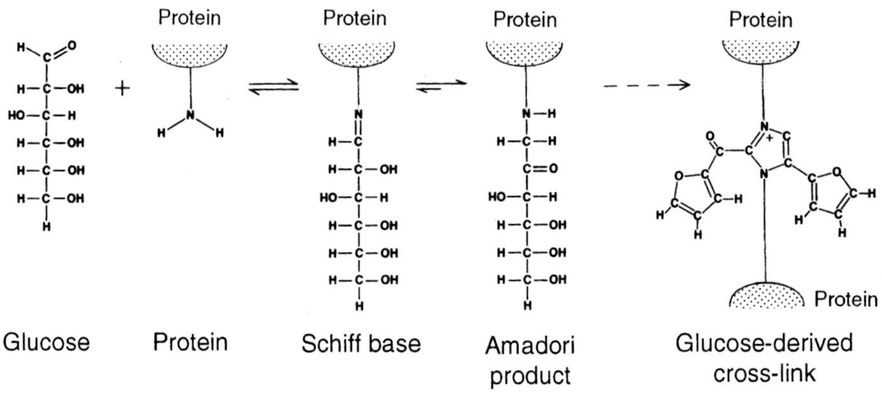

Glucose   Protein   Schiff base   Amadori product   Glucose-derived cross-link

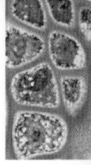

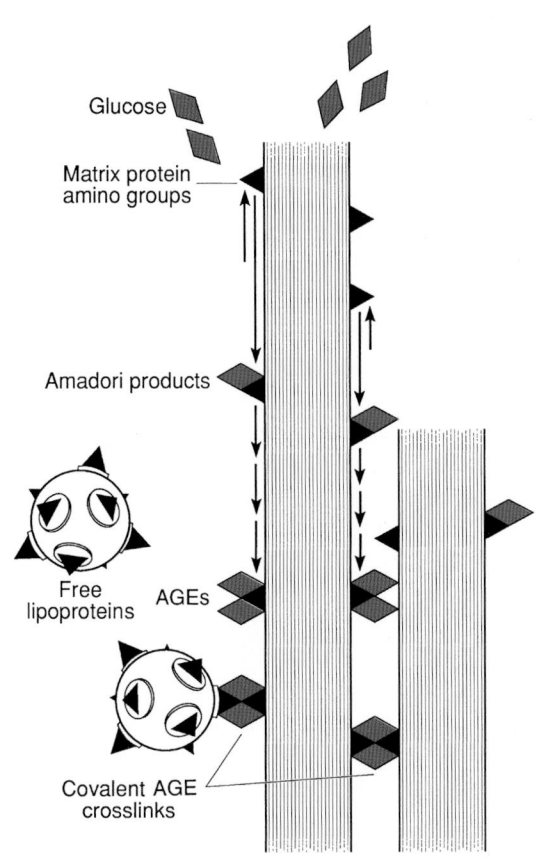

Glucose

Matrix protein
amino groups

Amadori products

Free
lipoproteins

AGEs

Covalent AGE
crosslinks

FIGURE 7.38   Formation of cross-links in matrix protein due to advanced glycosylation end-products (AGEs). The vertical columns represent collagen or other intersitial proteins. From the top downward, the figure shows the formation of irreversible AGE products. The lower part shows how lipoproteins can also become cross-linked with matrix proteins. The latter process may explain why atherosclerosis is accelerated in diabetics. (Reprinted, by permission of the New England Journal of Medicine, 318:1315–1321,1988 [122].)

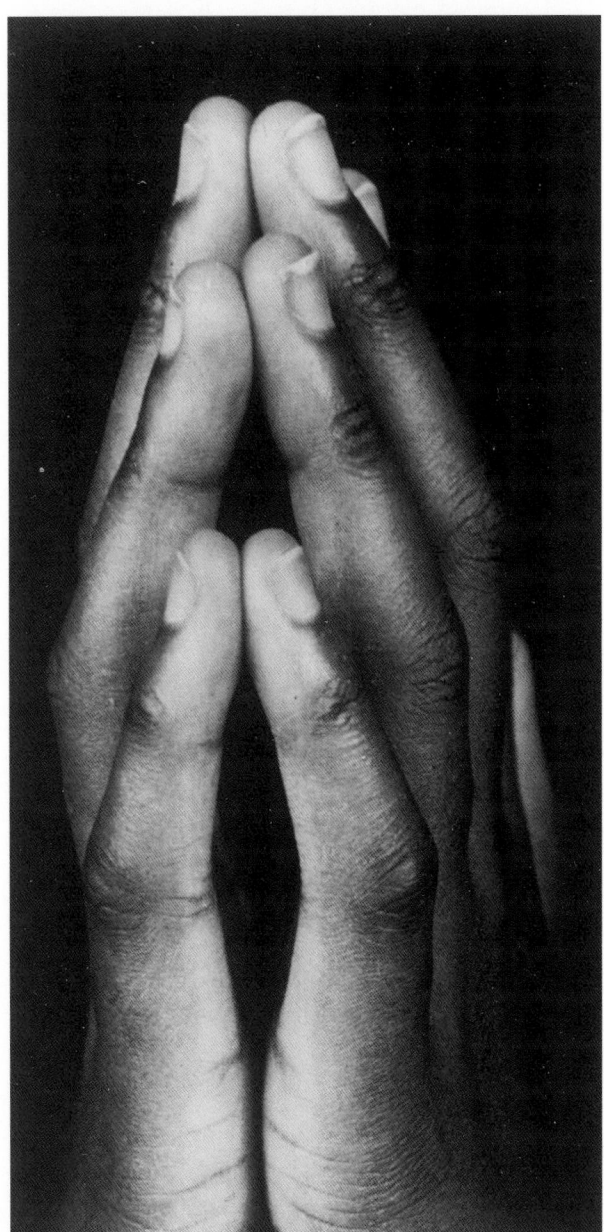

FIGURE 7.39   The "prayer sign" in diabetes. Pathologic cross-linking of collagen molecules results in stiff joints, including the inability to approximate the palmar surfaces. (Young woman of 17 with insulin-dependent diabetes for 14 years.) (Reprinted, by permission of the New England Journal of Medicine, 305:191–194,1981 [131].)

cooked longer), some of its Amadori products slowly dehydrate and rearrange themselves—again—into irreversible, brown, autofluorescent structures that Cerami and his group have called **advanced glycosylation end-products** or AGEs, a hint to their presumed role. Some of the AGEs can form cross-links between adjacent proteins, for instance, by condensation of two Amadori products (Figure 7.38) (122, 132).

This sequence has enormous implications, especially for diabetes. *If we list all the long-term complications of diabetes* (better known since insulin therapy was introduced in 1922), *a link with long-lived proteins now seems obvious for all:* accelerated arteriosclerosis (hardening of arteries), cataract, neuropathy, microangiopathy, and

stiffened joints (well illustrated in Figure 7.39 by the so-called prayer sign). In diabetes, collagen does indeed become more brown, more cross-linked, as if it were older (126, 127), and autofluorescent (129). The thickening of basement membranes could also be related to

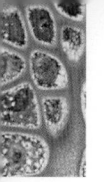

protein trapping and cross-linking (122, 125). In fact, the structural modification of proteins could have almost limitless consequences (125).

In this light, diabetes can be seen as a natural model of accelerated aging, a hypothesis that can be tested—to some extent—*in vitro:* Cerami et al. found that the long, thin tendons of young rat tails become tougher if incubated with glucose, and clear solutions of bovine lens proteins become cloudy if glucose is added, suggesting a "cataract in the test tube" (124). All these findings also mean that *blocking AGE formation could offer new hope against damage to proteins.*

In the meantime, at least one glycation product has found practical uses: hemoglobin (Hb), which is constantly exposed to blood glucose during its relatively long 4-month life; even normally about 5 percent of Hb is covalently linked to glucose and becomes chromatographically distinct as HbA_{1c}. *In diabetes, HbA_{1c} is increased 2- or 3-fold; thus the concentration HbA_{1c} is now used as a convenient measure of overall glucose control* (123, 127).

It is certainly a paradox that glucose, the principal cellular fuel, should also be an enemy of extracellular proteins. High glucose levels may even up-regulate the expression of Type 6 collagen genes (130). All this may explain nature's efforts to keep blood glucose below 200 mg/dl (127).

Currently, several drugs are being tested to prevent the formation of AGE and to disrupt already formed AGE-protein cross links (133).

Amyloid

The ways of disease are never-ending: one of them is to create deposits of a material called *amyloid.* This topic used to be quite bewildering (many facts, not much glue to hold them together), but the third millennium opened on a breakthrough: *amyloid is a classic case of protein misfolding.* So, this chapter should end on relief rather than on frustration. However, the path to this discovery was so challenging that we want the reader to share some of the excitement generated by the gradual closing in on the final truth (212). Two parts of the amyloid story (the Inclusion Body and the Prion connections) were told in Chapter 4 (128, 165).

We shall begin with a definition of amyloid such as was accepted around 1970; there is nothing wrong with it, even though it will have to be qualified in later pages: it just lacks the key.

*The term **amyloid** refers to a group of about 20 largely unrelated, pathologic, insoluble, extracellular, fibrous proteins that usually derive from precursors present in the blood, and have in common several properties:*

- *They are stained by the dye Congo red, and once so stained, they appear green in polarized light.*
- *They appear by electron microscopy as filaments 75–100 Å thick.*
- *By X-ray diffraction the polypeptide chains in the filaments do not run lengthwise but transversely back and forth, in the unusual beta or pleated-sheet pattern.*

Amyloidosis, the extracellular accumulation of amyloid, ranges from local microscopic deposits of no clinical significance to extensive, lethal infiltrations of vital organs (Figure 7.40). Because this massive form can arise as a side-effect of chronic inflammatory diseases, it was seen frequently in the past when tuberculosis and osteomyelitis were incurable. Massive amyloidosis of that kind (kilograms) is rare today in the Western world; the focus has shifted to microscopic deposits of amyloid that develop in the brain in old age and in Alzheimer's disease; hence, amyloidosis is in the news at least weekly.

Unveiling the Amyloid Mystery

When amyloid is present in kilogram amounts, it is hard to miss, at least at autopsy; anatomists in the

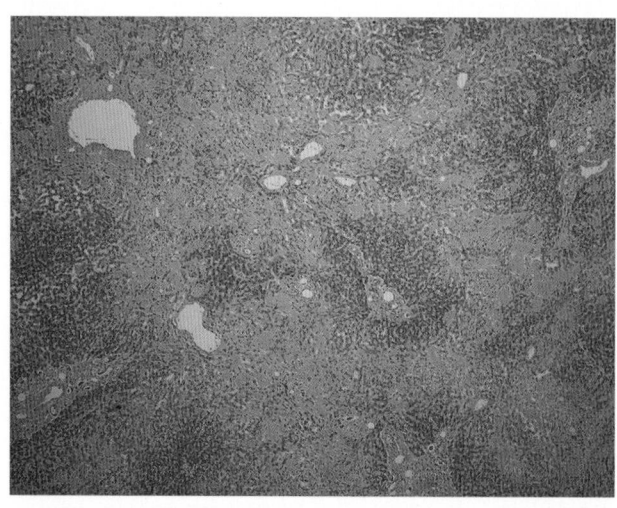

FIGURE 7.40   Amyloidosis (AL type) of the liver in a patient with multiple myeloma. The cords of liver cells are dissociated and atrophic due to compression by masses of amyloid (pink material), and possibly also to a toxic effect of the amyloid (hematoxylin and eosin stain.)

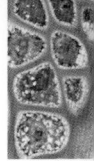

1700s knew very well that sometimes the liver, the spleen, and other organs appear strangely swollen and firm, as if they had been infiltrated by some abnormal stiff material. In the mid-1800s the Viennese school described such organs as "lardaceous" (baconlike); but this, Virchow objected, meant only that the Viennese understood little about bacon: waxy was more accurate (218). In any event, it was clear that some abnormal hyalin material was infiltrating the tissues, and in 1853 Virchow took the view that it was probably an "animal cellulose," a tempting synthesis of the plant and animal kingdoms (219). In his day it was known that cellulose treated with sulfuric acid was converted into a carbohydrate called amyloid (starchlike), which turned blue with iodine (205). Virchow convinced himself that fresh "waxy" organs gave this reaction and concluded that the mysterious material was indeed an animal cellulose. In retrospect, the color change produced on fresh organs was not always willing to appear, and the term amyloid was a misnomer. However, Virchow did confirm that the abnormal material was often found in the organs of patients who had died of some wasting disease and even hypothesized that a precursor material should exist in the blood. Promptly the chemists objected that amyloid was albuminous, that is, a protein, not a carbohydrate, and right they were.

From then onward progress was slow because all the proteins called amyloid (as we now know) seem to be planned to complicate the lives of chemists as well as histologists: *amyloids are almost insoluble, they are inert (poorly reactive), refractory to most stains, and poorly antigenic.*

However, in 1922, a step forward took place: the accidental discovery that the dye **Congo red** stained amyloid rather selectively. This staining method did not reveal anything about the nature of amyloid, but it made the microscopic diagnosis of amyloid much easier. It is used to this day.

The accidental discovery was made in a medical ward in Hamburg where Congo red was being used to study blood volume (140). In some patients the dye seemed to disappear faster, and a look at the records showed that all these patients suffered from amyloidosis. At the autopsy of one patient, the glomeruli on the cut surface of the kidney stood out as red dots, and the liver looked unusually red. The next step was obvious: try Congo red as a histologic stain for amyloid. This story also tells us that wasting diseases must have been very common in 1922.

The Congo red method came with a bonus. Although the stained amyloid on tissue sections looked rather pale, yellowish, and unimpressive, under polarized light it shone bright green (161). This means that stained amyloid is dichroic, i.e., that the absorption of light passing through it varies with the plane of polarization of the light (175). Today this apple-green effect is still the best method for the microscopic diagnosis of amyloid. Furthermore, unstained amyloid was reported to be birefringent, indicating that despite its smooth, glassy appearance it had to be, at the ultramicroscopic level, a fibrillar material (161). This turned out to be perfectly accurate.

By the 1950s it was apparent that amyloid infiltration of various organs developed under sets of conditions that had nothing in common. The best that one could do was to separate the cases of generalized amyloidosis into two categories: cases in which there seemed to be no underlying disease at all, called **primary amyloidosis,** and cases in which there was an associated wasting disease (as Virchow and others had noticed), called **secondary amyloidosis.** Furthermore, many cases—but not all—pointed to some association with the immune response; for instance, amyloidosis was common in the hyperimmunized horses used for the commercial production of antisera, yet the amyloid itself was different from antibody proteins (i.e., gamma globulins) and it certainly was no antigen–antibody precipitate. Amyloid was also discovered in certain tumors or in isolated lumps with no relation to tumors; it appeared even in the pancreatic islets of aging individuals. No unifying theory seemed possible. Amyloid was a depressing topic.

Enter the electron microscope. In 1959, Cohen and Calkins contributed some important new facts. Amyloid was indeed fibrillar (153) (Figure 7.41), and fibrils were nonbranching, 75–100 Å in diameter, and made of two filaments twisted around each other. Another component, a doughnut-shaped pentagonal molecule, was usually associated with them (Figure 7.42) (143). But this newly discovered unity was itself a puzzle. How could the same types of fibrils be formed under such diverse clinical conditions?

Eventually chemistry came through. Amyloid, which had been so stubbornly insoluble, yielded to more drastic extraction methods with denaturing solvents, and eventually it turned out—somewhat embarrassingly—that the best solvent was distilled water (204). Thanks to the availability of purified amyloid, the material from two cases of primary amyloidosis was sequenced in 1971 by Glenner and colleagues at the National Institutes of Health (NIH). Surprise: *that particular type of amyloid turned out to have the same amino acid sequence as the light chains of gamma globulin molecules* (Figure 7.43) (172). This was a great step: it echoed the prediction of an eminent immunologist, who used to say that someday amyloid would turn out

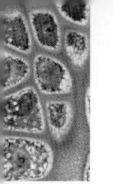
FIGURE 7.41   Experimental amyloidosis in the guinea pig. Renal peritubular deposit of typical amyloid fibrils: rigid, non-branching, diameter 70–100 Å, length indeterminate. **B:** Basement membrane. **Bar** = 0.5 μm. (Kindly provided by Dr. A. S. Cohen, Boston City Hospital, Boston, MA.)

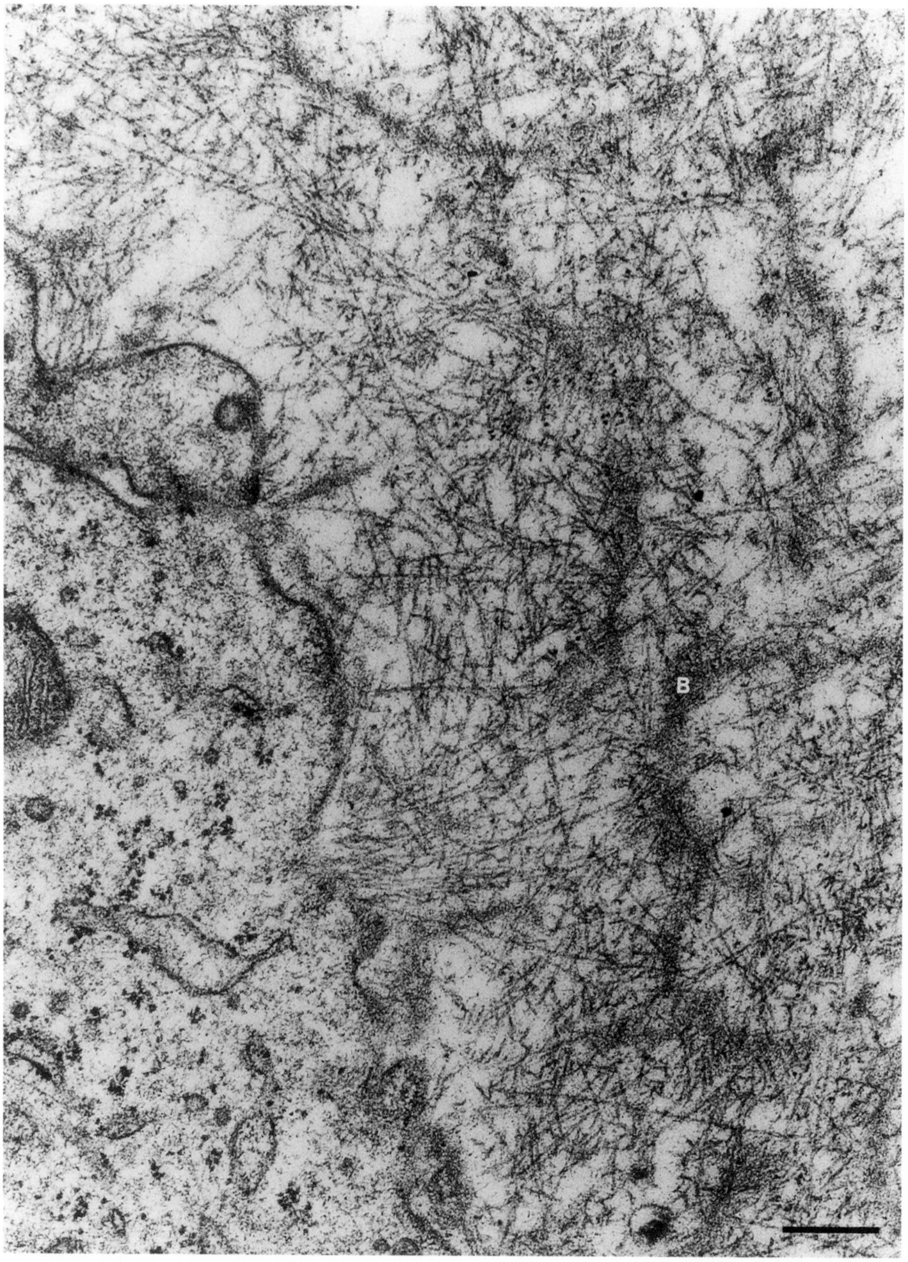

to be "gammyloid" (but not all amyloids are "gammyloids," as we will see).

However, every discovery raises new questions. If some amyloid fibrils were made of gamma globulin light chains, why did they aggregate into fibrils? One good place for studying the light chains of gamma globulins was the urine of patients with multiple myeloma, a tumor of the gamma globulin-secreting plasma cells. Apparently the malignant plasma cells produce not only gamma globulins but also an excess of one of their building blocks, the light chains. These are small

enough to pass into the urine, where they have long been known as **Bence-Jones protein.** This protein deserves the distinction of a personal name because it has an unusual property: it precipitates if the urine is heated to 40–50°C but then redissolves at the boiling point. The precipitate of Bence-Jones proteins was examined: it was not fibrillar. Why not? Here lay an obvious challenge.

The elegant answer came again from NIH: If the Bence-Jones protein is submitted to mild digestion with a proteolytic enzyme (trypsin), it promptly turns

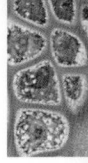

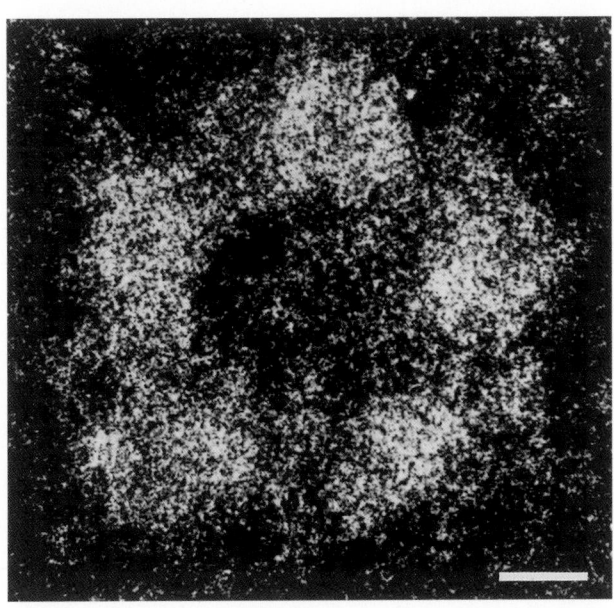

FIGURE 7.42 Ring-shaped component of human spleen amyloid, negatively stained with phosphotungstic acid. This enlargement clearly shows five globular subunits. **Bar** = 0.001 μm. (Reproduced with permission from [143].)

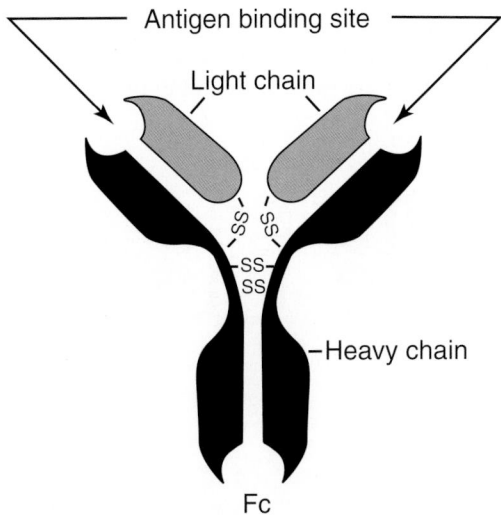

FIGURE 7.43 Diagram of an IgG molecule, emphasizing the light chains that are relevant to the genesis of amyloidosis. (Adapted from [178].)

into a cloudy precipitate made of fibrils that are stainable by Congo red and have the ultrastructure of amyloid (172).

This was an important hint. It suggested a new way of thinking about amyloid: *perhaps the secret bond between the disparate proteins called amyloid was not*

primarily in their sequence but rather in their shape—which could be altered by some environmental change such as mild proteolysis. It was not difficult to imagine how proteolysis could take place in the tissues: the cell most likely to carry out this task seemed to be the macrophage. A few macrophages do accompany the deposits of certain kinds of amyloid, but whether they are producing the amyloid or destroying it is not clear (183). Proteolysis, as we will see, is not the best answer, but it is close.

Enter X-ray diffraction (144, 155). This approach gave a precise verdict: the polypeptide chains of amyloid are arranged perpendicular to the axis of the fibril, in the *beta* or *pleated sheet* pattern (Figure 7.44). Because this

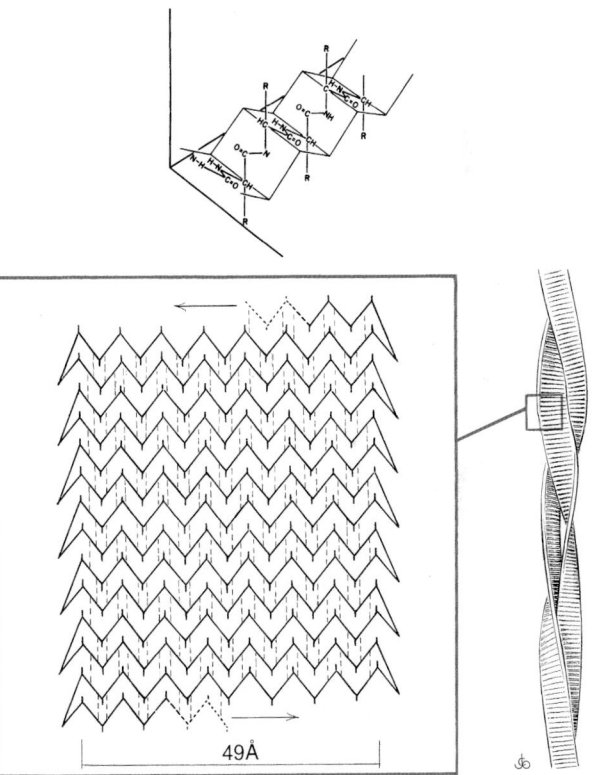

FIGURE 7.44 Molecular structure of amyloid fibrils. *Top:* Three-dimensional representation of a molecular chain in the beta conformation, showing the pleated sheet effect. (Reproduced by permission from [136a] © 1966 McGraw-Hill with permission of The McGraw-Hill Companies.) *Bottom Left:* Scheme of a "cross-beta" pleated sheet ribbon 49 Å in width. The long axis of the ribbon is from top to bottom. (Modified from [174], with permission from Blackwell Scientific Publications Ltd.) *Bottom right:* Entire fibril, made of two intertwined ribbons. (Reproduced by permission from [158], © The US & Canadian Academy of Pathology, Inc.)

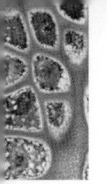
was recognized as the basic feature of amyloid, it was proposed that all diseases leading to amyloid deposition be grouped under the name of **beta fibrilloses** (170).

To visualize the pleating, it should be understood that the amyloid fibril is really a ribbon, as shown in Figure 7.44. Generally speaking, in filamentous proteins the polypeptide chains can assume two orderly arrangements, alpha and beta. The alpha pattern is a helix; the beta pattern is a flat sheet or ribbon in which the polypeptide chain runs back and forth transversely (the so-called antiparallel arrangement). The ribbon is finely corrugated, that is, pleated longitudinally (221). In amyloid, two such ribbons are twisted together. The beta pleated sheet structure of amyloid is consistent with its resistance to digestion *in vivo* and *in vitro,* with its optical properties, and also with the staining by Congo red (171). In one type of amyloid (AA) there seems to be an associated, longitudinal, non-beta component.

In other words, X-ray diffraction confirmed and aggravated the central paradox of amyloid already established by electron microscopy: *although biochemical methods define about 20 different amyloids, physical methods show unquestionably that amyloid fibrils are all the same.* Could it possibly be that all or most proteins, given the required conditions, can assume the conformation of beta-pleated sheets?

Problem solved: they can. *At long last, amyloid can be explained in the context of **protein misfolding.*** Without tracing all of the steps that led to this astonishing *finale,* here are the essentials (145, 148, 162, 212). Nascent proteins can fold into two orderly but very different states. The specific globular shape is probably reached by interaction of side chains; the hydrophobic peptide backbone remains hidden in the depths of the molecule. Under conditions of *mild denaturation,* such as incubation at pH 6 for several hours (162), a globular protein unfolds, exposing the main chain and making it available to interact with other main chains to form beta pleated sheets (Figure 7.45) (165a). With this treatment, even a typically globular protein such as myoglobin will yield fibrillar amyloid (148, 162, 168). Now we can understand why all of amyloid fibrils are alike: they reflect a basic feature of all proteins—the peptide bond backbone.

So we have learned enough about amyloid to prepare it in a test tube. How it forms *in vivo* is not quite as clear; many factors are probably involved. One is age.

Senile amyloidosis (see further) makes this point very clearly. Its precursor is a normal protein, **transthyretin,** so called because it **trans**ports **thy**roxin and **retin**ol, hence also amyloidosis TTR, or **ATTR.** Transthyretin does not change with age, yet it gives rise to amyloidosis only in old age.

Another factor is the amino acid sequence: certainly some sequences are more prone than others to generate

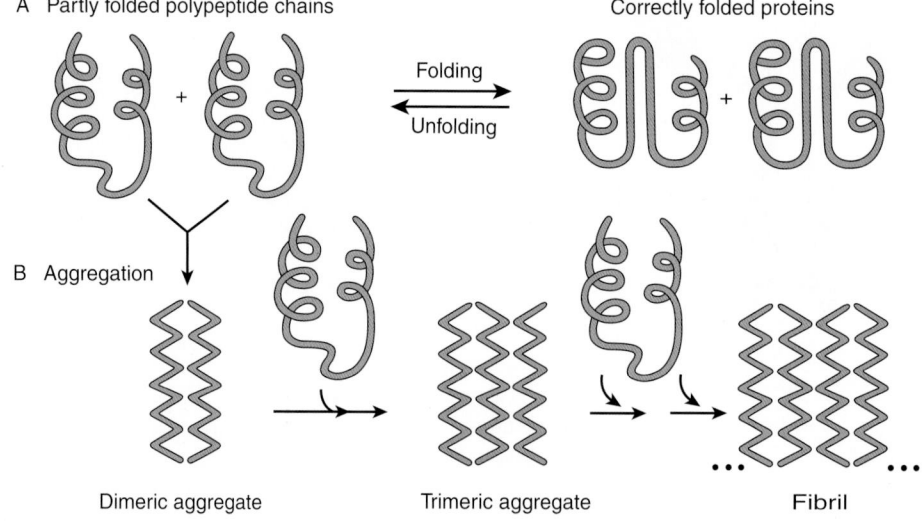

FIGURE 7.45 Diagram showing the generation of amyloid by partial unfolding, or by misfolding, of a normal protein. *Top right:* Correctly folded protein (in the alpha/helix conformation); the inner core contains hydrophobic domains. Partial denaturation (e.g., in acid) leads to partial unfolding (*top left*); the hydrophobic domains become exposed, stick together and force the protein to refold into a nonfunctional shape (*bottom left,* the beta/pleated sheet conformation). Further aggregation generates fibrils with the properties of amyloid to be visualized as growing along the horizontal plane. (Redrawn with permission from Nature. Danger—misfolding proteins, 2002;416:483–484. Copyright 2002 MacMillan Magazines Limited [165a].)

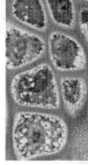

amyloid (162). Light chain amyloid (AL) produced by malignant myeloma cells contains mutation-induced amino acid substitutions that promote unfolding (212). There are some familial (hereditary) forms of amyloidosis in which the deposition of amyloid is again facilitated by a mutation in the amyloidogenic molecule; such is the case for the familial form of ATTR. Local conditions within the tissues surely play a role. We just mentioned *the prescription of physical chemists for transforming a globular protein into amyloid: incubation for several hours at an acid pH*. An acid pH does exist inside cells, in vacuoles such as phagosomes and endosomes. It seems most likely that nascent amyloid goes through an intracellular phase. The classic notion that amyloid is always extracellular does not hold any longer: immunostaining for amyloid shows that intracellular amyloid is common.

Is amyloid toxic? It is widely agreed that the solid form of amyloid causes little or no damage to cells, whereas the soluble amyloid monomers and polymers are toxic; it was shown experimentally that soluble amyloid peptides tend to penetrate into lipid layers and create pores permeable to ions, including calcium, the cell-killer (182, 199). Amyloid is beginning to make sense.

Gross and Microscopic Aspects of Amyloidosis

Mild deposits of amyloid escape the naked eye, but heavily infiltrated organs are pale, stiff, and waxy, just as Virchow insisted; after fixation the liver or spleen may be almost as hard as wood. Histologically, the connective tissue spaces are filled with an extraneous, insoluble, eosinophilic, hyaline material (149); the deposits have a strong tendency to infiltrate the vascular walls, especially the arterioles, recalling the fact that amyloid precursors come mostly from the blood (Figure 7.46). A small amount of highly sulfated glycosaminoglycans is incorporated in many and perhaps all amyloids (189, 196, 214, 215); perhaps it explains the occasional carbohydrate-like reaction dear to Virchow.

The bulk of amyloid is extracellular; however, bundles of fibrils can be found in plasma cells, macrophages, hepatocytes, neurons, and other cells, either free or in lysosomes (166, 209, 224). Amyloid sometimes develops in deep indentations of the surfaces of macrophages, much as collagen arises from deep infoldings of fibroblasts. *The tissues infiltrated with amyloid do not seem to react;* the macrophages do not perceive the fibrils as material to phagocytize. The parenchymal cells are crowded out, undergo atrophy, and fade away. This effect can be extreme in the spleen (Figure 7.47), and in the liver (see Figure 7.40); however, the functional

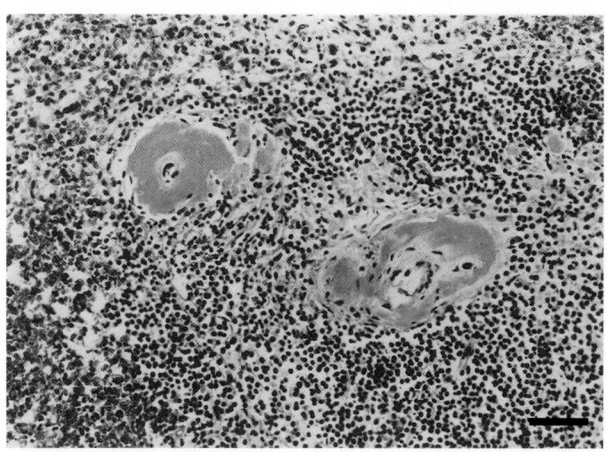

FIGURE 7.46 Amyloid deposition in two arterioles of the spleen. The media is hyalinized and destroyed. (Man aged 57 with AA amyloidosis.) **Bar** = 50 μm. (Reproduced by permission from [201], © The US & Canadian Academy of Pathology, Inc.)

reserve of the liver is such that liver failure in amyloidosis is rare. Amyloidosis of the heart is the main cause of death in generalized amyloidosis. Amyloid deposits in the wall of the glomerular capillaries cause them to become, rather paradoxically, *more permeable* to protein; renal insufficiency is the second major cause of death by amyloidosis (Figure 7.48).

Main Types of Amyloid and Their Genesis

Each type of amyloidosis is an interesting experiment of nature. We cannot discuss every type (151, 184), but we can summarize the current status (150, 152, 154, 170, 173, 174, 188, 192). There are *local and generalized forms,* all with different amyloid precursors. We will begin with the two best known generalized forms, which (like all amyloids) were saddled with rather skimpy names:

- **AL** (for **a**myloid/**l**ight chain, sometimes called *primary* or myeloma-related);
- **AA** (for amyloid A, so called because it was the first to be chemically characterized; also called *secondary*).

Amyloid AL. This is the light-chain variety and as such it includes the cases due to multiple myeloma (193). The reader may notice a contradiction: if this is also called primary amyloidosis, how can it be secondary to myeloma? The reason is that in earlier days some patients with this form of amyloidosis seemed to have no physical disease at all. Then plasma electrophoresis came

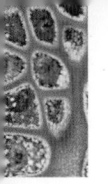

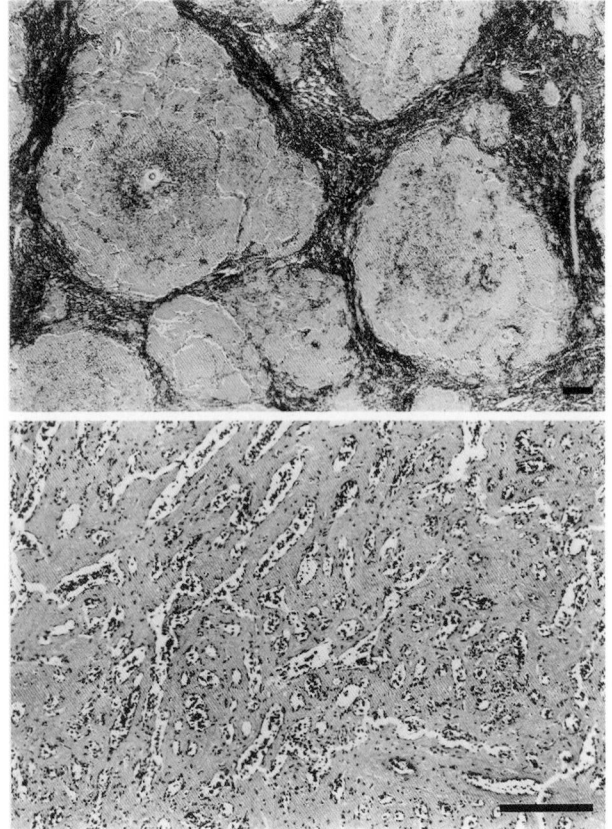

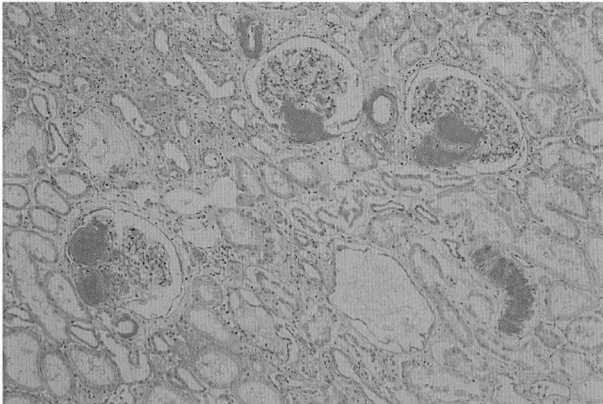

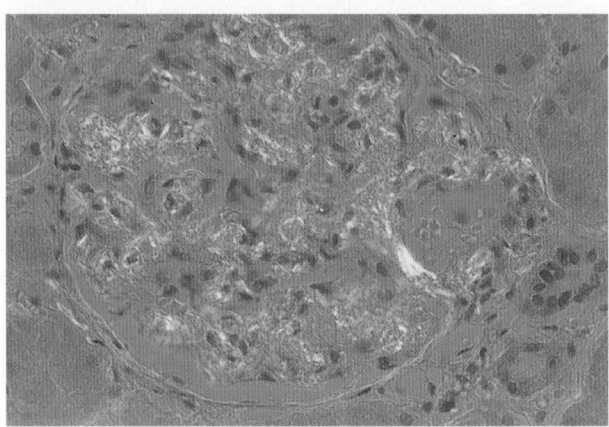

FIGURE 7.47 Two patterns of amyloid deposition in the human spleen. *Top:* "Sago spleen." Nodular deposition in the white pulp (AA amyloid). *Bottom:* "Lardaceous spleen." Diffuse deposition occurs in the red pulp (AL amyloid). The mechanisms leading to these patterns are not understood. **Bar** = 100 μm. (Reproduced by permission from [201], © The US & Canadian Academy of Pathology, Inc.)

FIGURE 7.48 Kidney of a 55-year-old man with a debilitating chronic disease and secondary amyloidosis. *Top:* Congo red stain shows massive amyloid deposits in the arterioles leading in and out of the glomeruli, as well as in other arterioles. (Specimen kindly provided by Dr. T. Watanabe, Saga Medical School, Nabeshima, Saga, Japan). *Bottom:* Same case: a glomerulus stained with Congo red and photographed by polarized light. "Apple green" fluorescence of the capillary basement membranes, thickened by amyloid deposits. (Color slide kindly provided by Dr. T. Watanabe.)

along and showed that these patients do indeed have an abnormality; the tracing shows a thick band of gamma globulins or of their light-chain fragment (Figure 7.49).

> These excess plasma proteins are immunoglobulins, and as such they can only be manufactured by B-cells (plasma cells); the electrophoretic pattern suggests that all the B-cells producing this protein belong to the same clone. Conclusion: somewhere in the bone marrow of these patients a clone of plasma cells is busily producing immunoglobulin, but without proliferating out of control (i.e., without behaving—yet—like a malignant tumor of the marrow). These clinical conditions are referred to as **B-cell dyscrasias** or benign monoclonal gammopathies. Actually about 10 percent go on to develop malignant B-cell tumors, that is, myelomas. This means that it is not very proper to call them benign (191). Regarding those patients who do have myelomas, 6–15 percent also develop amyloidosis.

Interestingly, bone marrow from a patient with myeloma, cultured *in vitro,* produced amyloid. The malignant plasma cells were closely apposed to macrophages (163).

AL amyloid is always plasma cell amyloid (be it from benign or malignant plasma cells). Because it represents—in essence—fragments of antibody, no two cases of AL amyloid can be exactly alike.

Regarding prognosis: if the underlying disease is a benign gammopathy, the patient is condemned to die in 14 months or so of the amyloidosis itself; if the underlying disease is multiple myeloma, the prognosis is even worse: death is inevitable because of the tumor.

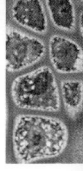

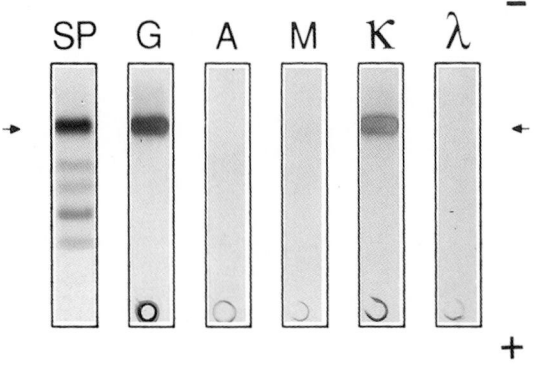

FIGURE 7.49   Electrophoresis of the serum from a 74-year-old woman with multiple myeloma. The small round well at the bottom of each strip is the point of application of the serum. All strips were overlaid with various antibodies, then the antigen-antibody complexes were stained with amido black. **SP:** Control strip overlaid with antibody against normal human serum. **G, A, M,** κ and λ: Strips overlaid with antibodies against IgG, IgA, IgM, and kappa or lambda light chains. The arrows indicate that the "myeloma protein" in this case is a monoclonal IgG with kappa light chains. No IgA or IgM is visible on the corresponding strips because the synthesis of these proteins is suppressed by the overproduced IgG. (Courtesy of Dr. R. B. Zurier, University of Massachusetts Medical School, Worcester, MA.)

Amyloid AA.   This form corresponds to secondary amyloidosis, also called reactive amyloidosis (171). Its precursor in the blood is serum amyloid A (SAA) (212).

Remember the term **reactive amyloidosis.** This form of amyloidosis is due to a general bodily reaction to chronic and wasting diseases, be they inflammatory or neoplastic—rheumatoid arthritis, chronic infections such as osteomyelitis and tuberculosis, and malignant tumors (especially renal cell carcinoma and Hodgkin's disease). Whatever the cause, the liver responds by changing its pattern of plasma protein synthesis (p. 504); the production of some proteins is reduced, and other proteins are secreted in vastly increased amounts. The latter go under the odd name of **acute-phase proteins.** The increased secretion of some of these can be explained; fibrinogen, for example, is necessary to make fibrin, and fibrin is necessary as a glue for injured vessels. For other proteins, however, the increase is baffling. Serum amyloid A, for example, has no known major function, and in the long run it may turn into deposits of amyloid A (it does not always do so). Medical students find this mechanism quite confusing, and they are not alone; what is the purpose of producing more SAA if it can lead to amyloidosis? We can only answer that the increase in SAA "must have" an overriding purpose that we do not yet comprehend.

Amyloid A was chemically defined by Benditt et al. in Seattle (138). Its circulating precursor (SAA) was discovered by searching for the target of antibodies against amyloid A. SAA is an apoprotein of high density lipoprotein (HDL) (139, 181)—another puzzle. Amyloid A can be produced experimentally in mice by the old and now classical method of injecting casein (200); obviously the mice produce amyloid A because they have a blood precursor homologous to human SAA.

Amyloid P (AP).   Amyloid P is the pentagonal molecule mentioned earlier (see Figure 7.42); *it does not occur alone but as a component* (5–10 percent) *of all other types of amyloid.* It is present under normal conditions in the basement membrane of glomerular capillaries, around small vessels of a few other sites (165), and in the microfibrils that surround elastic fibers (203). Like amyloid A, which has its circulating precursor (SAA) belonging to the acute-phase reactants, amyloid P has its serum amyloid P (SAP) precursor in a pentagonal protein identical to AP. SAP is similar to another pentagonal plasma protein, the C-reactive protein ([p. 505]) another acute-phase reactant, and also to the so-called hamster female protein. These proteins have been grouped into a family as **pentraxins** (from the Greek words for "five" and "berries").

Senile amyloid (AS).   Senile amyloid is much more prevalent than previously realized, especially in the heart and aorta (159). It is found in about one-third of all autopsies after the age of 70 and in 50 percent of all hearts after the age of 90. Its significance as a cause of death is not yet clear (159). In some cases its serum precursor is a protein confusingly called prealbumin although it has nothing to do with albumin. It transports thyroxin and retinol (vitamin A); hence its alternative name is **trans-thy-ret-in** (ATTR).

Endocrine amyloid (AE).   Five polypeptide hormones have a surprising tendency to self-aggregate into amyloid deposits: prolactin, calcitonin (produced by some medullary carcinomas of the thyroid), atrial natriuretic factor (ANF), and especially insulin and islet-associated polypeptide (IAPP) (222). The latter are responsibble for pancreatic islet amyloidosis, which is associated with adult-onset diabetes (Figure 7.50) and advanced age (197). The diabetes connection has produced new insights regarding both amyloid and diabetes (182, 185–187).

It has been known since 1900 that many pancreatic islets are hyalinized, especially in diabetics; now it turns out that the hyalin is a special type of amyloid derived from an islet-associated polypeptide (IAPP), synthesized

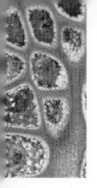

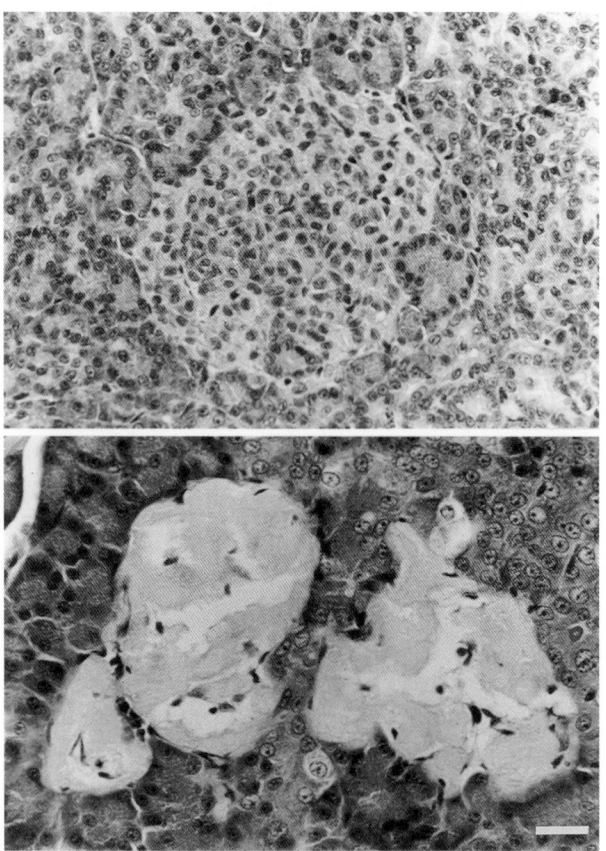

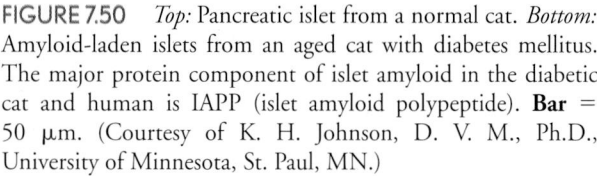

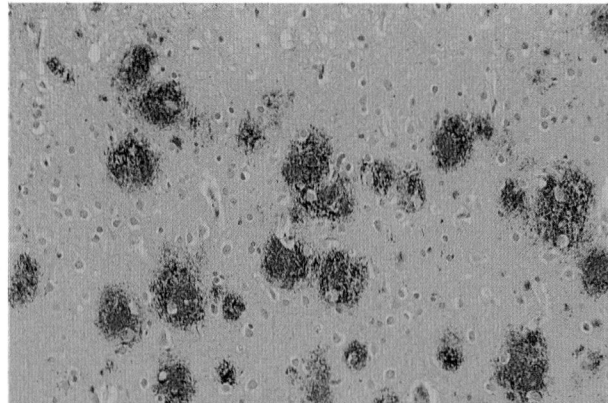

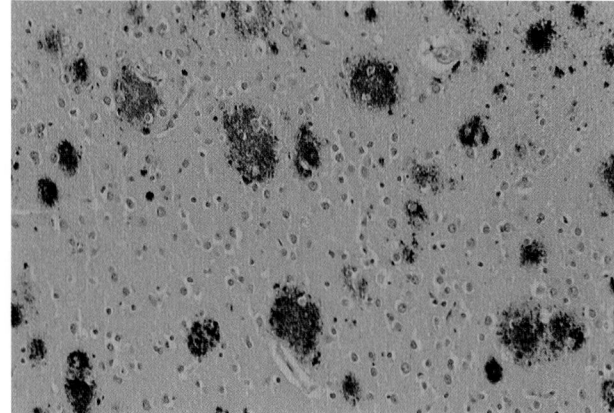

FIGURE 7.50 *Top:* Pancreatic islet from a normal cat. *Bottom:* Amyloid-laden islets from an aged cat with diabetes mellitus. The major protein component of islet amyloid in the diabetic cat and human is IAPP (islet amyloid polypeptide). **Bar** = 50 μm. (Courtesy of K. H. Johnson, D. V. M., Ph.D., University of Minnesota, St. Paul, MN.)

FIGURE 7.51 Senile plaques in Alzheimer's disease. *Top:* Bielschowsky's silver impregnation, which stains axons and dendrites black. *Bottom:* Immunoperoxidase stain for amyloid β: all plaques contain a core of amyloid. (Courtesy of Dr. T. W. Smith, University of Massachusetts Medical School, Worcester, MA.)

by normal beta cells and probably cosecreted with insulin. The story of IAPP is not yet completely worked out, but it appears that IAPP somehow opposes the action of insulin in peripheral tissues, thus explaining the pathogenesis of non–insulin-dependent diabetes. As time goes by, the deposition of amyloid in the islets may become a secondary cause of diabetes. The tendency of IAPP to polymerize spontaneously in the extracellular spaces is found only in a few species, such as human, cat, and raccoon (185, 187).

Alzheimer's disease: amyloid β. As mentioned in Chapter 4 (p. 166), three types of focal lesions (two of which contain amyloid) are found in the brain of patients with Alzheimer's disease *and in all aged brains:* senile plaques (Figure 7.51), blood vessels infiltrated with amyloid ("congophilic" or amyloid angiopathy) (Figure 7.52), and neurofibrillary tangles. The symptoms of the

disease are caused by the extensive destruction of gray matter wrought by these lesions (160, 208).

The plaques (Figure 7.51) consist of a core of amyloid with a wrapping of distorted neurofibrils, astrocytes and microglial cells (the brain equivalent of macrophages). The amyloid is of a special type, named amyloid beta (Aβ). Is amyloid the cause or the consequence of the disease? The evidence weighs heavily toward the causal hypothesis. Fortunately so, because it gives investigators a tangible lead (179). The genesis of Aβ is an intricate topic.

The precursor of Aβ is APP, a protein normally inserted in the membrane of most cell types, including brain cells, vascular smooth muscle cells, and platelets (190); its function is not clear (deletion of the *APP* gene in mice has no noticeable effect [208]), but we do know that APP is normally processed by two pathways: (a) on the cell surface, an enzyme, **α-secretase,** clips off the outer portion

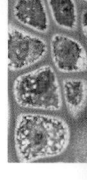

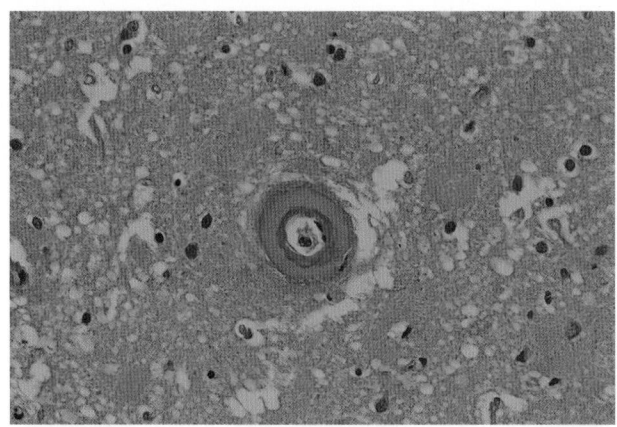

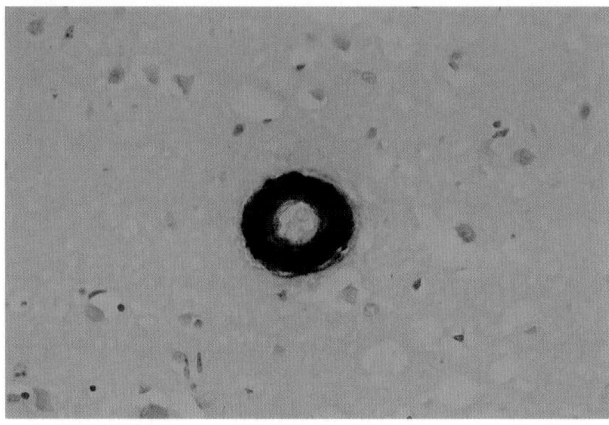

FIGURE 7.52 Amyloidosis of arterioles in the brain, the so-called congophilic angiopathy. *Top:* (Hematoxylin and eosin stain). *Bottom:* A similar arteriole demonstrated with an immunoperoxidase stain for beta amyloid. This type of amyloid deposition occurs spontaneously in old age, but it is exaggerated in Alzheimer's disease. (90x) (Courtesy of Dr. T. W. Smith, University of Massachusetts Medical School, Worcester, MA.)

of APP, yielding "soluble APP," which diffuses into the blood and other body fluids (207). However, this is NOT the precursor of the tissue amyloid. (b) The entire APP is internalized by cellular vesicles (endosomes, phagosomes) and processed by **β-** and **γ-secretases** into peptides 40–42 residues long. These are released to the extracellular space, where they tend to aggregate, generating amyloid β (199). **In the familial forms of Alzheimer's disease**—the most aggressive—mutations have been found in APP and in the enzymes that process it (198, 208); these mutations favor the aggregation of the amyloid peptides. An analogous correlation was mentioned earlier regarding the familial forms of ATTR. Two other proteins are involved in early-onset Alzheimer's disease: mutations in **presenilins 1 and 2** enhance the processing of APP to Aβ (179).

As for the damage caused by amyloid: when the "mature" form of Aβ—the insoluble, fibrillar form—was tested on living cells, it usually caused no harm (there were a few exceptions [145]), nor did the soluble monomers (179); however, *the soluble dimers and oligomers did cause functional and/or structural damage,* such as interference with synaptic function (142, 198, 220). When tested *in vivo* on the rat mesentery, Aβ caused inflammation: vascular leakage, diapedesis, and other damage, especially in the arterioles (206, 217).

All of these (179) and subsequent (187a) findings appear tantalizingly close to unveiling the secret of Alzheimer's disease. In the meantime they have suggested several new approaches to therapy. The secretases hinted to the possibility of using *enzyme inhibitors* (202). Because the peptide Aβ is the prime offender, *antibodies* against it were tried in transgenic mice and they helped: surprisingly, they were able to cross the blood-brain barrier (136). The injurious effect of Aβ peptides suggested the possibility of *vaccination* against them; in animals it seemed to work (211), but human trials had to be stopped because the procedure caused inflammation in the brain tissue. Because aggregation of Aβ depends in part on copper and zinc ions, *chelators* have reached the stage of clinical trials; so have *cholesterol-lowering diets,* because cholesterol—surprisingly—appears to favor Aβ deposition (179). This is merely a sample of current work, which shows the potential of a close collaboration between basic science and the practice of medicine.

Iatrogenic amyloidosis. A consequence of chronic hemodialysis, iatrogenic amyloidosis came to light because up to 50 percent of patients who had undergone hemodialysis for 20 years or longer developed the carpal tunnel syndrome (169) caused by a narrowing of the tunnel in the wrist where the medial nerve fits snugly along with nine tendons. Surgical release is required. The amyloid that develops in the tunnel belongs to a specific type whose precursor is beta-2-microglobulin (154, 176, 210). *The precursor protein is normally catabolized in the kidney—and these patients have no kidneys.* The resulting high concentration of precursor seems to be the critical factor; amyloid fibrils can be obtained from normal beta-2-microglobulin also *in vitro.*

Heredofamilial amyloidosis (AF). This amyloidosis is rare except in foci scattered around the world from Portugal to Brazil, Japan, England, and elsewhere—perhaps because a gene for it was spread by navigators (141). In most cases the amyloid consists of transthyretin (TTR) that is abnormal by a single amino acid; clinically the

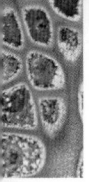

prevalent form of this disease is a polyneuropathy that appears around the age of 25–35 years (the delay is not well understood). Another rare hereditary form is familial Mediterranean fever, the only type of human amyloidosis that is treatable and preventable because the disease responds—for reasons unclear—to colchicine (146, 216, 223).

> New types of amyloidosis are still being found; the latest is **amyloidosis of the cornea** near an inflamed area (135). The precursor is lactoferrin, an antibacterial substance found in neutrophil leukocytes and in lacrimal glands. In all cases there was a mutation in the lactoferrin molecule; amyloid fibrils could be obtained *in vitro* from the mutated lactoferrin but not from the wild type. This novel amyloid behaved "just like in the books."

(Tumorlike) amyloidosis. Occasionally a small lump is surgically removed, especially from the upper respiratory mucosa, and found to be not a tumor but a mass of amyloid. These peculiar "amyloidomas" are thought to be the end-stage of a cluster of plasma cells and macrophages that produced a mass of amyloid and then burned out, leaving behind the amyloid and a few telltale plasma cells (170).

Amyloid bodies. Amyloid bodies have long been known to exist in the normal prostate and elsewhere. They do deserve their name (starchlike) because they resemble starch granules in size and concentric structure. They contain various materials including fibrils made of beta pleated sheets (177), perhaps arising from residues of epithelial cells that continue to slough off and die in the lumen (137). They are of little pathologic significance.

Diagnosis, Prognosis, and Therapy of Amyloidosis

Systemic amyloidosis can be discovered secondarily after the causal disease is recognized (e.g., myeloma). Clinical hints are a large liver or spleen, or proteinuria, especially in a patient suffering from chronic disease. An enlarged tongue carries the same message; **macroglossia** is caused by selective deposition of amyloid in the lingual muscles (Figure 7.53). Peculiar, but not uncommon, is the **carpal tunnel syndrome** already mentioned. *The final diagnosis of amyloid hinges on biopsy, staining with Congo red, and examination in polarized light.*

There is no blood test for amyloidosis. A group of imaginative British investigators proposed the following diagnostic method. Remember first that amyloid P (AP) occurs as a component of all amyloids; it also has a serum precursor called serum AP (SAP). Now, an

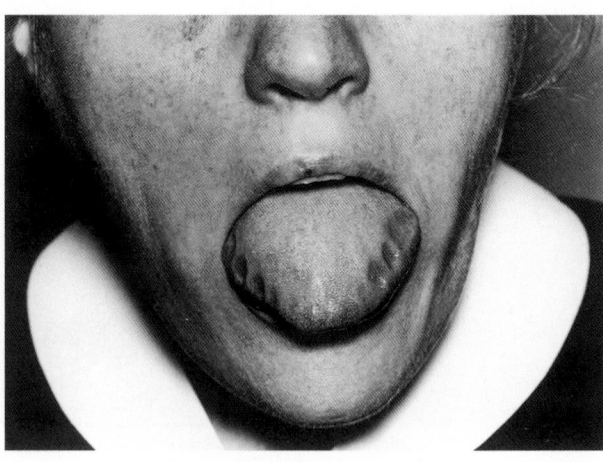

FIGURE 7.53   Macroglossia in a case of primary amyloidosis. Note the imprints of the teeth. (Reproduced with permission from [192].)

intravenous injection of radioactively labeled SAP should localize wherever there is a deposit of amyloid, and so it does (195). One of the difficulties is to procure SAP; the method is not current (180).

The rectal mucosa has long been the biopsy site of choice for diagnosing amyloid, the rationale being that the gastrointestinal tract is commonly affected; also, the rectal mucosa provides several varieties of tissues (sometimes even a lymphatic nodule) with practically no pain and surprisingly little risk of infection. Needle aspiration of abdominal fat is a less traumatic alternative (156, 164). Congo red staining of a tissue sample followed by study in polarized light is still the best method; staining with thioflavin followed by study under ultraviolet light gives a yellow fluorescence, but this technique is less specific. Other methods exist (156).

Regarding prognosis, when amyloid is deposited in association with a malignant tumor (such as myeloma or renal cell carcinoma), the outcome is of course bleak on account of the primary lesion. However, the relentless deposition of amyloid can be lethal in itself; survival in primary amyloidosis (AL) is on the order of 12–14 months; death is due mainly to cardiac and renal failure (194).

The prospects of reactive amyloidosis (AA) are not much better, but the underlying chronic disease may make life miserable (167). Moderately good news has been available only for the patients with the hereditary ATTR (transthyretin) amyloidosis: because transthyretin is made primarily in the liver, heart transplantation can be very helpful (167). It may even reduce the neuropathies typical of this form of amyloidosis. A great advance would be to find a drug that makes the amyloid deposits melt away; dimethylsulfoxide was tried, but it is not the answer.

NOTE: The pathology of amyloid includes the amazing story of **prions:** we have told it in Chapter 4 (p. 167), as a ramification of protein misfolding.

TO CLOSE: WHY SHOULD AMYLOIDOSIS EXIST? There is no use for amyloid in the life of a mammal. Amyloid is prevalent in the world of invertebrates; it is the backbone of silk (170) and even *Escherichia coli* knows how to make it (147). However, for mammals, medically speaking, amyloid is always bad news. So why should we have to put up with this invertebrate nuisance, which is hard to live with, hard to diagnose, and almost impossible to treat?

To be optimistic, there may be a reason: polymerized amyloid does not do much harm, but its soluble precursors are toxic. Perhaps we should accept amyloid as a quick way to inactivate its dangerous precursors (162).

References

Pathology of Collagen

1. Akeson WH, Amiel D, Mechanic GL, et al. Collagen cross-linking alterations in joint contractures: changes in the reducible cross-links in periarticular connective tissue collagen after nine weeks of immobilization. Connect Tissue Res 1977;5:15–19.
2. Alenghat FJ, Ingber DE. Mechanotransduction: all signals point to cytoskeleton, matrix and integrins. Sciences's STKE (Perspective). Available at: http://www.stke.org/cgi/content/full/OC_sigtrans;2002/119pe6. Accessed June 2002.
3. Aschoff L, Koch W. Skorbut. Eine pathologisch-anatomische Studie. Jena: Verlag Gustav Fischer, 1919.
4. Bailey AJ, Lapière CM. Effect of an additional peptide extension of the N-terminus of collagen from dermatosparactic calves on the cross-linking of the collagen fibers. Eur J Biochem 1973;34:91–96.
5. Bardach H, Gebhart W, Niebauer G. "Lumpy-bumpy" elastic fibers in the skin and lungs of a patient with a penicillamine-induced elastosis perforans serpiginosa. J Cutan Pathol 1979; 6:243–252.
6. Bauer EA. Collagenase in recessive dystrophic epidermolysis bullosa. Ann NY Acad Sci 1985;460:311–320.
7. Briggaman RA, Wheeler CE. Epidermolysis bullosa dystrophica-recessive: a possible role of anchoring fibrils in the pathogenesis. J Invest Dermatol 1975;65:203–211.
8. Byers PH, Barsh GS, Holbrook KA. Molecular pathology in inherited disorders of collagen metabolism. Hum Pathol 1982;13:89–95.
9. Carter TR, Bailie DS, Edinger S. Radiofrequency electrothermal shrinkage of the anterior cruciate ligament. Am J Sports Med 2002;30:221–226.
10. DePaepe A. Heritable collagen disorders: from phenotype to genotype. Verhandeligen-Koninklijke Academie voor Geneeskunde van Belgie. 1998;60:463–482; discussion 482–484.
11. Fisher GJ, Wang, ZQ, Datta SC, et al. Pathophysiology of premature skin aging induced by ultraviolet light. N Engl J Med 1997;337:1419–1428.
12. Gamble CN. The pathogenesis of hyaline arteriosclerosis. Am J Pathol 1986;122:410–420.
13. Gilbert-Barness E, Barness LA. Metabolic diseases: foundations of clinical management, genetics, and pathology. Natick, MA: Eaton Publishing, 2000.
14. Gross J. Collagen biology: structure, degradation, and disease. Harvey Lect 1974;68:351–432.
15. Gross J, Lapière CM. Collagenolytic activity in amphibian tissues: a tissue culture assay. Proc Natl Acad Sci USA 1962;48:1014–1022.
16. Hanna W, Silverman E, Boxall L, Krafchik BR. Ultrastructural features of epidermolysis bullosa. Ultrastruct Pathol 1983; 5:29–36.
17. Hanset R, Lapière CM. Inheritance of dermatosparaxis in the calf. J Heredit 1974;65:356–358.
18. Keene DR, Sakai LY, Lunstrum GP, Morris NP, Burgeson RE. Type VII collagen forms an extended network of anchoring fibrils. J Cell Biol 1987;104:611–621.
19. Kirsch KM, Zelickson BD, Zachary CB, Tope WD. Ultrastructure of collagen thermally denatured by microsecond domain pulsed carbon dioxide laser. Arch Dermatol 1998; 134:1255–1259.
20. Klemperer P. The concept of collagen diseases. Am J Pathol 1950;26:505–519.
21. Klemperer P, Pollack AD, Baehr G. Diffuse collagen disease. Acute disseminated lupus erythematosus and diffuse scleroderma. JAMA 1942;119:331–332.
22. Krane SM. Genetic and acquired disorders of collagen deposition. In: Piez KA, Reddi AH (eds). Extracellular matrix biochemistry. New York: Elsevier, 1984, pp. 413–463.
23. Lapière CM, Lenaers A, Kohn L. Procollagen peptidase: an enzyme excising the coordination peptides of procollagen. Proc Natl Acad Sci USA 1971;68:3054–3058.
24. Levene CI. Effect of lathyrogenic compounds on the cross-linking of collagen and elastin in vivo. In: Aldridge WN (ed). A symposium on mechanisms of toxicity. New York: St Martin's Press, 1971, pp. 67–81.
25. Levene CI. Diseases of the collagen molecule. J Clin Pathol 31 (Suppl Roy Coll Pathol) 1978;12:82–94.
26. Madri JA, Basson MD. Extracellular matrix-cell interactions: dynamic modulators of cells, tissue and organism structure and function. Lab Invest 1992;66:519–521.

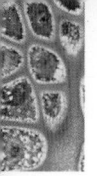

27. Majno G. The healing hand: man and wound in the ancient world. Cambridge, MA: Harvard University Press, 1975.

28. Majno G. The story of the myofibroblasts. Am J Surg Pathol 1979;3:535–542.

29. Martinez-Hernandez A, Amenta PS. The basement membrane in pathology. Lab Invest 1983;48:656–677.

30. Maschmann E. über Bakterienproteasen. IX. Mitteilung: Die Anaerobiase der Gasbranderreger. Biochem Z 1938; 297:284–296.

31. McKusick VA. Heritable disorders of connective tissue, 4th ed. St. Louis: The CV Mosby Company, 1972.

32. Minor RR. Collagen metabolism. A comparison of diseases of collagen and diseases affecting collagen. Am J Pathol 1980; 98:225–280.

32a. Montes GS, Junqueira LCU. Biology of collagen. Rev Can Biol Exp 1982;41:143–156.

33. Myllyharju J, Kivirikko KI. Collagens and collagen-related diseases. Ann Med 2001;33:7–21.

34. Nimni ME. Collagen: structure, function, and metabolism in normal and fibrotic tissues. Semin Arthritis Rheum 1983; 13:1–86.

35. Pérez Tamayo R. Pathology of collagen degradation. A review. Am J Pathol 1978;92:507–566.

36. Pinnell SR, Murad S. Disorders of collagen. In: Stanbury JB, Wyngaarden JB, Fredrickson DS, Goldstein JL, Brown MS (eds). The metabolic basis of inherited disease, 5th ed. New York: McGraw-Hill Book Company, 1983, pp. 1425–1449.

37. Prockop DJ, Kivirikko KI, Tuderman L, Guzman NA. The biosynthesis of collagen and its disorders. Parts I and II. N Engl J Med 1979;301:13–23 and 77–85.

38. Pyeritz RE. Heritable defects in connective tissue. Hosp Pract 1987;22:153–168.

39. Ralph RA. Chemical burns of the eye. In: Duane TD, Jaeger EA (eds). Clinical ophthalmology, vol 4. Philadelphia: Harper & Row, 1985, pp. 1–25.

40. Reymond JL, Stoebner P, Zambelli P, Beani JC, Amblard P. Penicillamine induced elastosis perforans serpiginosa: an ultrastructural study of two cases. J Cutan Pathol 1982;9: 352–357.

41. Reynolds MD. Origins of the concept of collagen-vascular diseases. Semin Arthrit Rheum 1985;15:127–131.

42. Ross EV, Yashar SS, Naseef GS, et al. A pilot study of in vivo immediate tissue contraction with CO_2 skin laser resurfacing in a live farm pig. Dermatol Surg 1999;25:851–856.

43. Sodek J. A comparison of the rates of synthesis and turnover of collagen and non-collagen proteins in adult rat periodontal tissues and skin using a microassay. Arch Oral Biol 1977; 22:655–665.

44. Stanbury JB, Wyngaarden JB, Fredrickson DS, Goldstein JL, Brown MS (eds). The metabolic basis of inherited disease, 5th ed. New York: McGraw-Hill Book Company, 1983.

45. Sternlicht MD, Werb Z. How matrix metalloproteinases regulate cell behavior. Annu Rev Cell Dev Biol 2001;17: 463–516.

46. Stuart JM, Townes AS, Kang AH. Type II collagen-induced arthritis. Ann NY Acad Sci 1985;460:355–362.

46a. Timpl R, Oberbäumer I, Furthmaayer H, Kuehn K. Macromolecular organization of type IV collagen. In: Kuehn K, Schoene H, Timpl R (eds). New trends in basement membrane research. New York: Raven Press, 1982, pp. 57–67.

47. Uitto J, Lichtenstein JR. Defects in the biochemistry of collagen in diseases of connective tissue. J Invest Dermatol 1976; 66:59–79.

48. Vogel A, Holbrook KA, Steinmann B, Gitzelmann R, Byers PH. Abnormal collagen fibril structure in the gravis form (type I) of Ehlers-Danlos syndrome. Lab Invest 1979; 40:201–206.

49. Watson RB, Holmes DF, Graham HK, Nusgens BV, Kadler KE. Surface located procollagen N-propeptides on dermatosparactic collagen fibrils are not cleaved by procollagen N-proteinase and do not inhibit binding of decorin to the fibril surface. J Molec Boil 1998;278:195–204.

Pathology of Elastin

50. Alberts B, Bray D, Lewis J, et al. Molecular biology of the cell. New York: Garland Publishing, Inc, 1989.

51. Bader, L. Disorders of elastic tissue: a review. Pathology 1973; 5:269–289.

52. Curtis ES. Portraits from North American Indian life. New York: Promontory Press, 1972.

53. Dietz HC, Mecham RP. Mouse models of genetic diseases resulting from mutations in elastic fiber proteins. Matrix Biol 2000;19:481–488.

54. Fitzpatrick TB, Eisen AZ, Wolff K, Freedberg IM, Austen KF. Update: dermatology in general medicine. New York: McGraw-Hill Book Company, 1983.

55. Francke U, Furthmayr H. Marfan's syndrome and other disorders of fibrillin. N Engl J Med 1994;330:1384–1385.

56. Gadek JE, Pacht ER. The protease-antiprotease balance within the human lung: implications for the pathogenesis of emphysema. Lung (Suppl) 1990;552–564.

57. Gilchrest BA. Skin and aging processes. Boca Raton: CRC Press, Inc, 1984.

58. Halme T. Elastin and collagen of human ascending aorta. Academic dissertation. Turku, Finland, 1987.

59. Halme T, Savunen T, Aho H, Vihersaari T, Penttinen R, Elastin and collagen in the aortic wall: changes in the Marfan syndrome and annuloaortic ectasia. Exp Mol Pathol 1985; 43:1–12.

60. Harel S, Janoff A, Yu SY, Hurewitz A, Bergofsky EH. Desmosine radioimmunoassay for measuring elastin degradation in vivo. Am Rev Respir Dis 1980;122:769–773.

61. Janoff A. Elastases and emphysema. Current assessment of the protease-antiprotease hypothesis. Am Rev Respir Dis 1985; 132:417–433.

62. Janoff A, Sloan B, Weinbaum G, et al. Experimental emphysema induced with purified human neutrophil elastase: tissue localization of the instilled protease: Am Rev Respir Dis 1977;115:461–478.

63. Kainulainen K, Pulkkinen L, Savolainen A, Kaitila I, Peltonen L. Location on chromosome 15 of the gene defect causing Marfan syndrome. N Engl J Med 1990;323:935–939.

64. Lansing AI, Alex M, Rosenthal TB. Calcium and elastin in human arteriosclerosis. J Gerontol 1950;5:112–119.

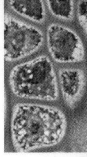

65. Lansing AI, Roberts E, Ramasarma GB, Rosenthal TB, Alex M. Changes with age in amino acid composition of arterial elastin. Proc Soc Exp Biol Med 1951;76:714–717.

66. Lattimer JK. Lincoln did not have the Marfan syndrome, documented evidence. NY State J Med 1981;81:1805–1813.

67. Lavie G, Zucker-Franklin D, Franklin EC. Elastase-type proteases on the surface of human blood monocytes: possible role in amyloid formation. J Immunol 1980;125:175–180.

68. Ledoux-Corbusier M, Achten G. Elastosis in chronic radiodermatitis. An ultrastructural study. Br J Dermatol 1974;91:287–295.

69. Lee B, Godfrey M, Vitale E, Hori H, et al. Linkage of Marfan syndrome and a phenotypically related disorder to two different fibrillin genes. Nature 1991;352:330–334.

70. Lucey EC, Keane J, Kuang PP, Snider GL, Goldstein RH. Severity of elastase-induced emphysema is decreased in tumor necrosis factor-α and interleukin-1β receptor-deficient mice. Lab Invest 2002;82:79–85.

71. McKusick VA. The defect in Marfan syndrome. Nature 1991;352:279–281.

72. Milewicz DM, Urban Z, Boyd C. Genetic disorders of the elastic fiber system. Matrix Biol 2000;19:471–480.

73. Newbold PCH. Inborn errors of skin. In: Holton JB, Ireland JT (eds). Inborn errors of skin, hair and connective tissue. Baltimore: University Park Press, 1975, pp. 3–14.

74. Pinnell SR, Murad S. Disorders of collagen. In: Stanbury JB, Wyngaarden JB, Frederickson DS, Goldstein JL, Brown MS (eds). The metabolic basis of inherited disease, 5th ed. New York: McGraw-Hill Book Company, 1983.

75. Poulsen JT, Staberg B, Wulf HC, Brodthagen H. Dermal elastosis in hairless mice after UV-B and UV-A applied simultaneously, separately or sequentially. Br J Dermatol 1984;110:531–538.

76. Rucker RB, Tinker D. Structure and metabolism of arterial elastin. Int Rev Exp Pathol 1977;17:1–47.

77. Stamm C, Friehs I, Ho SY, et al. Congenital supravalvar aortic stenosis: a simple lesion? Eur J Cardiothoracic Surg 2001;19:195–202.

78. Takebayashi S, Kubota I, Takagi T. Ultrastructural and histochemical studies of vascular lesions in Marfan's syndrome, with report of 4 autopsy cases. Acta Pathol Jpn 1973;23:847–866.

79. Tokita K, Kanno K, Ikeda K. Elastin sub-fraction as binding site for lipids. Atherosclerosis 1977;28:111–119.

80. Tsipouras P, Del Mastro R, Sarfarazi M, et al. Genetic linkage of the Marfan syndrome, ectopia lentis, and congenital contractural arachnodactyly to the fibrillin genes on chromosomes 15 and 5. N Engl J Med 1992;326:905–909.

81. Tsuji T. The surface structural alterations of elastic fibers and elastotic material in solar elastosis: a scanning electron microscopic study. J Cutan Pathol 1984;11:300–308.

Pathology of Basement Membranes

81a. Bouts BA. Images in clinical medicine. Argyria. N Engl J Med 1999;340:1554.

82. Cohen AH, Hoyer JR. Nephronophthisis. A primary tubular basement membrane defect. Lab Invest 1986;55:564–572.

83. Colognato H, Yurchenco PD. Form and function: the laminin family of heterotrimers. Dev Dyn 2000;218:213–234.

84. Fioretto P, Steffes MW, Sutherland DER, Goetz FC, Mauer M. Reversal of lesions of diabetic nephropathy after pancreas transplantation. N Engl J Med 1998;339:69–75.

85. Fung MC, Bowen DL. Silver products for medical indications: risk-benefit assessment. J Toxicol Clin Toxicol 1996;34:119–126.

86. Gschnait F, Wolff K, Konrad K. Erythropoietic protoporphyria—submicroscopic events during the acute photosensitivity flare. Br J Dermatol 1975;92:545–557.

87. Gulbranson SH, Hud JA, Hansen RC. Argyria following the use of dietary supplements containing colloidal silver protein. Cutis 2000;66:373–374.

88. Harper GS, Axelsen RA. Salicylate-induced renal papillary necrosis in the Gunn rat. The role of bilirubin. Lab Invest 1982;47:258–264.

89. Hill WR, Pillsbury DM. Argyria. The pharmacology of silver. Baltimore: Williams & Wilkins Company, 1939.

90. Kashtan CE. Alport syndrome. An inherited disorder of renal, ocular, and cochlear basement membranes. Medicine 1999;78:338–360.

91. Kurtz SM, Feldman JD. Experimental studies on the formation of the glomerular basement membrane. J Ultrastruct Res 1962;6:19–27.

92. Mackay IR, Burnet FM. Autoimmune diseases. Springfield, IL: Charles C Thomas, 1963.

93. Majno G. Ultrastructure of the vascular membrane. In: Hamilton WF, Dow P (eds). Handbook of physiology, sect 2, vol III. Washington, DC: American Physiological Society, 1965, pp. 2293–2375.

94. Makino H, Yamasaki Y, Haramoto T, et al. Ultrastructural changes of extracellular matrices in diabetic nephropathy revealed by high resolution scanning and immunoelectron microscopy. Lab Invest 1993; 68:45–55.

95. Martin GR, Rohrbach DH, Terranova VP, Liotta LA. Structure, function, and pathology of basement membranes. In: Wagner BM, Fleischmajer R, Kaufman N (eds). Connective tissue diseases. Baltimore: Williams & Wilkins, 1983, pp. 16–30.

96. Martinez-Hernandez A, Amenta PS. The basement membrane in pathology. Lab Invest 1983;48:656–677.

97. Masugi M. Über das Wesen der spezifischen Veränderungen der Niere und der Leber durch das Nephrotoxin bzw. das Hepatotoxin. Zugleich ein Beitrag zur Pathogenese der Glomerulonephritis und der eklamptischen Lebererkrankung. Beitr Pathol Anat 1933;91:82–112.

98. McCluskey RT, Vassalli P. Experimental glomerular diseases. In: Rouiller C, Muller AF (eds). The kidney: morphology, biochemistry, physiology, vol II. New York: Academic Press, 1969, pp. 83–198.

99. McVerry BA, Fisher C, Hopp A, Huehns ER. Production of pseudodiabetic renal glomerular changes in mice after repeated injections of glucosylated proteins. Lancet 1980;1:738–740.

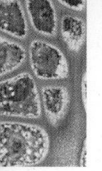

100. Mihatsch MJ, Torhorst J, Amsler B, Zollinger HU. Capillarosclerosis of the lower urinary tract in analgesic (phenacetin) abuse. An electron-microscopic study. Virchows Arch A Pathol Anat Histol 1978;381:41–47.

101. Mullarkey CJ, Brownlee M. Biochemical basis of microvascular disease. In: Pickup JC, Williams G (eds). Textbook of diabetes, vol 2. Oxford: Blackwell Scientific Publications, 1991, pp. 534–545.

102. Raskin P, Pietri AO, Unger R, Shannon WA. The effect of diabetic control on the width of skeletal-muscle capillary basement membrane in patients with type I diabetes mellitus. N Engl J Med 1983;309:1546–1550.

103. Vracko R. Basal lamina layering in diabetes mellitus. Evidence for accelerated rate of cell death and cell regeneration. Diabetes 1974;23:94–104.

104. Vracko R. Basal lamina scaffold—anatomy and significance for maintenance of orderly tissue structure. Am J Pathol 1974;77:314–346.

105. Walker F. Basement-membrane turnover in man. J Pathol 1972;107:123–125.

106. Williamson JR, Kilo C. Basement-membrane thickening and diabetic microangiopathy. Diabetes 1976;25(Suppl 2):925–927.

107. Yen A, Braverman IM. Ultrastructure of the human dermal microcirculation: the horizontal plexus of the papillary dermis. J Invest Dermatol 1976;66:131–142.

Pathology of Proteoglycans

108. Brandt KD, Radin E. The physiology of articular stress: osteoarthrosis. Hosp Pract 1987;22:103–126.

108a. Buckwalter JA, Rosenberg L. Structural changes during development in bovine fetal epiphyseal cartilage. Collagen Rel Res 1983;3:489–504.

109. Cheung HS, Nicoloff JT, Kamiel MB, Spolter L, Nimni ME. Stimulation of fibroblast biosynthetic activity by serum of patients with pretibial myxedema. J Invest Dermatol 1978;71:12–17.

110. DeMartino GN, Goldberg AL. A possible explanation of myxedema and hypercholesterolemia in hypothyroidism: control of lysosomal hyaluronidase and cholesterol esterase by thyroid hormones. Enzyme 1981;26:1–7.

111. Gordon MY, Riley GP, Watt SM, Greaves MF. Compartmentalization of a haematopoietic growth factor (GMCSF) by glycosaminoglycans in the bone marrow microenvironment. Nature 1987;326:403–405.

112. Hamerman D. The biology of osteoarthritis. N Engl J Med 1989;320:1322–1330.

113. Kobayasi T, Danielsen L, Asboe-Hansen G. Ultrastructure of localized myxedema. Acta Derm Venereol (Stockh) 1976;56:173–185.

114. Kohn LD. Connective tissue. In: Ingbar SH, Braverman LE (eds). Werner's the thyroid: a fundamental and clinical text, 5th ed. Philadelphia: JB Lippincott, 1986, pp. 816–839.

115. Kohn LD. Connective tissue. In: Ingbar SH, Braverman LE (eds). Werner's the thyroid: a fundamental and clinical text, 5th ed. Philadelphia: JB Lippincott, 1986, pp. 1128–1130.

116. Kresse H, Cantz M, von Figura K, Glössl J, Paschke E. The mucopolysaccharidoses: biochemistry and clinical symptoms. Klin Wochenschr 1981;59:867–876.

117. Niepomniszcze H, Amad RH. Skin disorders and thyroid diseases. J Endocrinol Invest 2001;24:628–638.

118. Palmoski M, Perricone E, Brandt KD. Development and reversal of a proteoglycan aggregation defect in normal canine knee cartilage after immobilization. Arthritis Rheum 1979;22:508–517.

119. Rosenberg L. Structure of cartilage proteoglycans. In: Burleigh PMC, Poole AR (eds). Dynamics of connective tissue macromolecules. Amsterdam: North-Holland Publishing Company, 1975, pp. 105–128.

120. Trelstad RL. Glycosaminoglycans: mortar, matrix, mentor. Lab Invest 1985;53:1–4.

Nonenzymatic Glycation

121. Baynes JW. The role of AGEs in aging: causation or correlation. Exp Gerontol 2001;36:1527–1537.

122. Brownlee M, Cerami A, Vlassara H. Advanced glycosylation end products in tissue and the biochemical basis of diabetic complications. N Engl J Med 1988;318:1315–1321.

123. Bunn HF, Gabbay KH, Gallop PM. The glycosylation of hemoglobin: relevance to diabetes mellitus. Science 1978;200:21–27.

124. Cerami A, Vlassara H, Brownlee M. Glucose and aging. Sci Am 1987;256:90–96.

125. Cohen MP. Nonenzymatic glycation: a central mechanism in diabetic microvasculopathy? J Diabetic Complications 1988;2:214–217.

126. Hamlin CR, Kohn RR, Luschin JH. Apparent accelerated aging of human collagen in diabetes mellitus. Diabetes 1975;24:902–904.

127. Kennedy L, Baynes JW. Non-enzymatic glycosylation and the chronic complications of diabetes: an overview. Diabetologia 1984;26:93–98.

128. Lawrie RA. Meat science, 3rd ed. Oxford: Pergamon Press, 1979.

129. Monnier VM, Kohn RR, Cerami A. Accelerated browning of collagen in diabetic humans. Diabetes 1982;31:28a.

130. Muona P, Jaakola S, Zhang R-Z, et al. Hyperglycemic glucose concentrations up-regulate the expression of type VI collagen in vitro. Am J Pathol 1993;142:1586–1597.

131. Rosenbloom AL, Silverstein JH, Lezotte DC, Richardson K, McCallum M. Limited joint mobility in childhood diabetes mellitus indicates increased risk for microvascular disease. N Engl J Med 1981;305:191–194.

132. Singh R, Barden A, Mori T, Beilin L. Advanced glycation end-products: a review. Diabetologia 2001;44:129–146.

133. Vasan S, Foiles PG, Founds HW. Therapeutic potential of AGE inhibitors and breakers of AGE protein cross-links. Expert Opin Investig Drugs 2001;10:1977–1987.

134. Vlassara H, Bucala R, Striker L. Pathogenic effects of advanced glycosylation: biochemical, biological, and clinical implications for diabetes and aging. Lab Invest 1994;70:138–151.

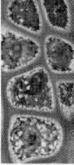

Amyloid

135. Ando Y, Nakamura M, Kai H, et al. A novel localized amyloidosis associated with lactoferrin in the cornea. Lab Invest 2002;82:757–765.

136. Bard F, Cannon C, Barbour R, et al. Peripherally administered antibodies against amyloid β-peptide enter the central nervous system and reduce pathology in a mouse model of Alzheimer disease. Nat Med 2000;6:916–919.

136a. Barrow GM. Physical chemistry. New York: McGraw-Hill, 1966.

137. Beems RB, Gruys E, Spit BJ. Amyloid in the corpora amylacea of the rat mammary gland. Vet Pathol 1978;15:347–352.

138. Benditt EP, Eriksen N. Chemical classes of amyloid substance. Am J Pathol 1971;65:231–252.

139. Benditt EP, Eriksen N. Amyloid protein SAA is associated with high density lipoprotein from human serum. Proc Natl Acad Sci USA 1977;74:4025–4028.

140. Bennhold H. Über die Ausscheidung intravenös einverleibter Farbstoffe bei Amyloidkranken. Verh Dtsch Ges Inn Med 1922;34:313–315.

141. Benson MD. Hereditary amyloidosis—disease entity and clinical model. Hosp Pract 1988;23:165–181.

142. Bhatia R, Lin H, Ratneshwar L. Fresh and globular amyloid β protein (1–42) induces rapid cellular degeneration: evidence for AβP channel-mediated cellular toxicity. FASEB J 2000;14:1233–1243.

143. Bladen HA, Nylen MU, Glenner GG. The ultrastructure of human amyloid as revealed by the negative staining technique. J Ultrastruct Res 1966;14:449–459.

144. Bonar L, Cohen AS, Skinner MM. Characterization of the amyloid fibril as a cross-beta protein. Proc Soc Exp Biol Med 1969;131:1373–1375.

145. Bucciantini M, Giannoni E, Chiti F, et al. Inherent toxicity of aggregates implies a common mechanism for protein misfolding diseases. Nature 2002;416:507–511.

146. Castaño EM, Frangione B. Human amyloidosis, Alzheimer disease and related disorders. Lab Invest 1988;58:122–132.

147. Chapman MR, Robinson LS, Pinkner JS, et al. Role of Escherichia coli curli operons in directing amyloid fiber formation. Science 2002;295:851–855.

148. Chiti F, Webster P, Taddei N, et al. Designing conditions for in vitro formation of amyloid protofilaments and fibrils. Proc Natl Acad Sci USA 1999;96:3590–3594.

149. Chopra S, Rubinow A, Koff RS, Cohen AS. Hepatic amyloidisis. A histopathologic analysis of primary (AL) and secondary (AA) forms. Am J Pathol 1984;115:186–193.

150. Cohen AS. An update of clinical, pathologic, and biochemical aspects of amyloidosis. Int J Dermatol 1981;20:515–530.

151. Cohen AS. Amyloidosis. Bull Rheum Dis 1991;40:1–12.

152. Cohen AS (ed). Amyloid. Int J Exp Clin Invest 2000;7:1–79.

153. Cohen AS, Calkins E. Electron microscopic observations on a fibrous component in amyloid of diverse origins. Nature 1959;183:1202–1203.

154. Cohen AS, Connors LH. The pathogenesis and biochemistry of amyloidosis. J Pathol 1987;151:1–10.

155. Cohen AS, Rubinow A, Kayne H, et al. The life span of patients with primary (AL) amyloidosis and the effect of colchicine treatment. In: Glenner GG, Osserman EF, Benditt EP, Calkins E, Cohen AS, Zucker-Franklin D (eds). Amyloidosis. New York: Plenum Press, 1986, pp. 559–565.

156. Cohen AS, Skinner M. The diagnosis of amyloidosis. In: Cohen AS (ed). Laboratory diagnostic procedures in the rheumatic diseases, 3rd ed. Orlando: Grune & Stratton, Inc, 1985, pp. 377–399.

157. Collinge J, Whittington MA, Sidle KCL, et al. Prion protein is necessary for normal synaptic function. Nature 1994;370:295–297.

158. Cooper JH. Selective amyloid staining as a function of amyloid composition and structure. Lab Invest 1974;31:232–238.

159. Cornwell GG III, Murdoch WL, Kyle RA, Westermark P, Pitkänen P. Frequency and distribution of senile cardiovascular amyloid. A clinicopathologic correlation. Am J Med 1983;75:618–623.

160. DeGirolami U, Anthony DC, Frosch MP. The central nervous system. In: Cotran RS, Kumar V, Collins T (eds). Robbins pathologic basis of disease. 6th ed. Philadelphia: WB Saunders Co., 1999.

161. Divry P, Florkin M. Sur les propriétés optiques de l'amyloïde. CR Soc Belg Biol 1927;97:1808–1810.

162. Dobson CM. Protein misfolding, evolution and disease. Trends Biol Sci 1999;24:329–332. Falk RH, Comenzo RL, Skinner M. The systemic amyloidoses. N Engl J Med 1997;337:898–909.

163. Durie BGM, Persky B, Soehnlen BJ, Grogan TM, Salmon SE. Amyloid production in human myeloma stem-cell culture, with morphologic evidence of amyloid secretion by associated macrophages. N Engl J Med 1982;307:1689–1692.

164. Duston MA, Skinner M, Shirahama T, Cohen AS. Diagnosis of amyloidosis by abdominal fat aspiration. Analysis of four years' experience. Am J Med 1987;82:412–414.

165. Dyck RF, Lockwood CM, Kershaw M, et al. Amyloid P-component is a constituent of normal human glomerular basement membrane. J Exp Med 1980;152:1162–1174.

165a. Ellis RJ, Pinheiro TJT. Danger—misfolding proteins. Nature 2002;416:483–484.

166. Eriksson L, Westermark P. Intracellular neurofibrillary tangle-like aggregations. A constantly present amyloid alteration in the aging choroid plexus. Am J Pathol 1986; 125:124–129.

167. Falk RH, Comenzo RL, Skinner M. The systemic amyloidoses. N Engl J Med 1997;337:898–909.

168. Fändrich M, Fletcher MA, Dobson CM. Amyloid fibrils from muscle myoglobin. Nature 2001;410:165–166.

169. Gejyo F. β2-Microglobulin amyloid. Amyloid. Int J Exp Clin Invest 2000;7:17–18.

170. Glenner GG. Amyloid deposits and amyloidosis. The beta-fibrilloses. Parts I and Part II. N Engl J Med 1980;302:1283–1292, 1333–1343.

171. Glenner GG, Eanes ED, Page DL. The relation of the properties of congo red-stained amyloid fibrils to the beta-conformation. J Histochem Cytochem 1972;20:821–826.

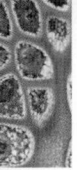
172. Glenner GG, Ein D, Eanes ED, et al. Creation of "amyloid" fibrils from Bence Jones proteins in vitro. Science 1971;174:712–714.

173. Glenner GG, Osserman EF, Benditt EP, et al. (eds). Amyloidosis. New York: Plenum Press, 1986.

174. Glenner GG, Page DL. Amyloid, amyloidosis, and amyloidogenesis. Int Rev Exp Pathol 1976;15:1–92.

175. Goldstein DJ. Detection of dichroism with the microscope. J Microsc 1969;89 (Pt. 1):19–36.

176. Gorevic PD, Casey TT, Stone WJ, et al. Beta-2 microglobulin is an amyloidogenic protein in man. J Clin Invest 1985;76:2425–2429.

177. Gueft B. The x-ray diffraction pattern of prostatic corpora amylacea. Acta Pathol Microbiol Scand 1972;Sect. A, 80 (Suppl. 233):132–134.

178. Halpern GM. L'immunoglobuline E, 20 ans après. Méd Hyg 1985;43:1074–1092.

179. Hardy J, Selkoe DJ. The amyloid hypothesis of Alzheimer's disease: progress and problems on the road to therapeutics. Science 2002;297:353–356.

180. Hawkins PN, Lavender JP, Pepys MB. Evaluation of systemic amyloidosis by scintigraphy with ^{123}I-labeled serum amyloid P component. N Engl J Med 1990;323:508–513.

181. Hoffman JS, Ericsson LM, Eriksen N, Walsh KA, Benditt EP. Murine tissue amyloid protein AA. NH_2-terminal sequence identity with only one of two serum amyloid protein (ApoSAA) gene products. J Exp Med 1984;159:641–646.

182. Höppener JWM, Ahrén B, Lips CTM. Islet amyloid and type 2 diabetes mellitus. N Engl J Med 2000;343:411–419.

183. Hou FF, Reddan DN, Seng WK, Owen WF. Jr. Pathogenesis of β_2-microglobulin amyloidosis: role of monocytes/macrophages. Semin Dialysis 2001;14:135–139.

184. Husby G, Araki S, Benditt EP, et al. The 1990 guidelines for nomenclature and classification of amyloid and amyloidosis. In: Natvig JB, Førre F, Husby G, et al. (eds). Amyloid and amyloidois 1990. Dordrecht: Kluwer Academic Publishers, 1991, pp. 7–11.

185. Johnson KH, O'Brien TD, Betsholtz C, Westermark P. Islet amyloid, islet-amyloid polypeptide, and diabetes mellitus. N Engl J Med 1989a;321:513–518.

186. Johnson KH, O'Brien TD, Hayden DW, et al. Immunolocalization of islet amyloid polypeptide (IAPP) in pancreatic beta cells by means of peroxidase-antiperoxidase (PAP) and protein A-gold techniques. Am J Pathol 1988;130:1–8.

187. Johnson KH, O'Brien TD, Jordan K, Westermark P. Impaired glucose tolerance is associated with increased islet amyloid polypeptide (IAPP) immunoreactivity in pancreatic beta cells. Am J Pathol 1989b;135:245–250.

187a. Kayed R, Head E, Thompson JL, et al. Common structure of soluble amyloid oligomers implies common mechanism of pathogenesis. Science 2003;300:486–489.

188. Kisilevsky R. Amyloidosis: a familiar problem in the light of current pathogenetic developments. Lab Invest 1983;49:381–390.

189. Kisilevsky R. Heparan sulfate proteoglycans in amyloidogenesis: an epiphenomenon, a unique factor, or the tip of a more fundamental process? Lab Invest 1990;63:589–591.

190. Kuo Y-M, Kokjohn TA, Watson MD, et al. Elevated Aβ42 in skeletal muscle of Alzheimer disease patients suggests peripheral alterations of AβPP metabolism. Am J Pathol 2000;156:797–805.

191. Kyle RA. "Benign" monoclonal gammopathy. A misnomer? JAMA 1984;251:1849–1854.

192. Kyle RA, Bayrd ED. Amyloidosis: review of 236 cases. Medicine 1975;54:271–299.

193. Kyle RA, Greipp PR. Amyloidosis (AL). Clinical and laboratory features in 229 cases. Mayo Clin Proc 1983;58:665–683.

194. Kyle RA, Greipp PR, Garton JP, Gertz MA. Primary systemic amyloidosis (AL): comparison of melphalan-prednisone vs. colchicine treatment in 101 cases. In: Glenner GG, Osserman EF, Benditt EP, Calkins E, Cohen AS, Zucker-Franklin D (eds). Amyloidosis. New York: Plenum Press, 1986, pp. 545–557.

195. Lachmann HJ, Booth DR, Booth SE, et al. Misdiagnosis of hereditary amyloidosis as AL (primary) amyloidosis. N Engl J Med 2002;346:1786–1791.

196. Linker A, Carney HC. Presence and role of glycosaminoglycans in amyloidosis. Lab Invest 1987;57:297–305.

197. Maloy AL, Longnecker DS, Greenberg ER. The relation of islet amyloid to the clinical type of diabetes. Hum Pathol 1981;12:917–922.

198. Matsuoka Y, Picciano M, Malester B, et al. Inflammatory responses to amyloidosis in a transgenic mouse model of Alzheimer's disease. Am J Pathol 2001;158:1345–1354.

199. McLaurin J, Yang D-S, Yip CM, Fraser PE. Review: modulating factors in amyloid-β fibril formation. J Struct Biol 2000;130:259–270.

200. Miura K, Takahashi Y, Shirasawa H. Immunohistochemical detection of serum amyloid A protein in the liver and the kidney after casein injection. Lab Invest 1985;53:453–463.

201. Ohyama T, Shimokama T, Yoshikawa Y, Watanabe T. Splenic amyloidosis: correlations between chemical types of amyloid protein and morphological features. Mod Pathol 1990;3:419–422.

202. Pennisi E. Enzymes point way to potential Alzheimer's therapies. Science 1999;286:650–651.

203. Pepys MB, Baltz ML, de Beer FC, et al. Biology of serum amyloid P component. Ann NY Acad Sci 1982;389:286–298.

204. Pras M, Schubert M, Zucker-Franklin D, Rimon A, Franklin EC. The characterization of soluble amyloid prepared in water. J Clin Invest 1968;47:924–933.

205. Puchtler H, Sweat F. A review of early concepts of amyloid in context with contemporary chemical literature from 1839 to 1859. J Histochem Cytochem 1966;14:123–134.

206. Rhodin JA, Thomas T. A vascular connection to Alzheimer's disease. Microcirculation 2001;8:207–220.

207. Selkoe DJ. Toward a comprehensive theory for Alzheimer's disease. Hypothesis: Alzheimer's disease is caused by the cerebral accumulation and cytotoxicity of amyloid β-protein. N Y Acad Sci 2000;924:17–25.

208. Selkoe DJ. Alzheimer's disease: genes, proteins, and therapy. Physiol Rev 2001;81:741–766.

209. Shirahama T, Cohen AS. Intralysosomal formation of amyloid fibrils. Am J Pathol 1975;81:101–116.

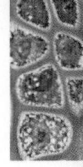
210. Shirahama T, Skinner M, Cohen AS, et al. Histochemical and immunohistochemical characterization of amyloid associated with chronic hemodialysis as beta-2-microglobulin. Lab Invest 1985;53:705–709.

211. Sigurdsson EM, Scholtzova H, Mehta PD, Frangione B, Wisniewski T. Immunization with a nontoxic/nonfibrillar amyloid-β homologous peptide reduces Alzheimer's disease-associated pathology in transgenic mice. Am J Pathol 2001;159:439–447.

212. Sipe JD. Serum amyloid A: from fibril to function. Current status. Amyloid. Int J Exp Clin Invest 2000;7:10–12.

213. Sipe JD, Cohen AS. Review: history of the amyloid fibril. J Struct Biol 2000;130:88–98.

214. Snow AD, Kisilevsky R, Stephens C, Anastassiades T. Characterization of tissue and plasma glycosaminoglycans during experimental AA amyloidosis and acute inflammation. Qualitative and quantitative analysis. Lab Invest 1987;56:665–675.

215. Snow AD, Willmer J, Kisilevsky R. Sulfated glycosaminoglycans: a common constituent of all amyloids? Lab Invest 1987;56:120–123.

216. Stone MJ. Amyloidosis: a final common pathway for protein deposition in tissues. Blood 1990;75:531–545.

217. Sutton ET, Thomas T, Bryant MW, et al. Amyloid-β peptide induced inflammatory reaction is mediated by the cytokines tumor necrosis factor and interleukin-1. J Submicrosc Cytol Pathol 1999;31:313–323.

218. Virchow R. Cellular pathology. Translated from the 2nd German ed. by B Chance, 1859. Reproduced by Dover Publications, New York, 1971.

219. Virchow R. Ueber eine im Gehirn und Rückenmark des Menschen aufgefundene Substanz mit der chemischen Reaction der Cellulose. Virchows Arch [Pathol Anat] 1854; 6:135–138.

220. Walsh DM, Klyubin I, Fadeeva JV, et al. Naturally secreted oligomers of amyloid β protein potently inhibit hippocampal long-term potentiation in vivo. Nature 2002;416:535–539.

221. Walton AG, Blackwell J. Biopolymers. New York: Academic Press, 1973.

222. Westermark P. The pathogenesis of amyloidosis. Am J Pathol 1998;152:1125–1127.

223. Zemer D, Pras M, Sohar E, et al. Colchicine in the prevention and treatment of the amyloidosis of familial Mediterranean fever. N Engl J Med 1986;314:1001–1005.

224. Zucker-Franklin D, Franklin EC. Intracellular localization of human amyloid by fluorescence and electron microscopy. Am J Pathol 1970;59:23–42.

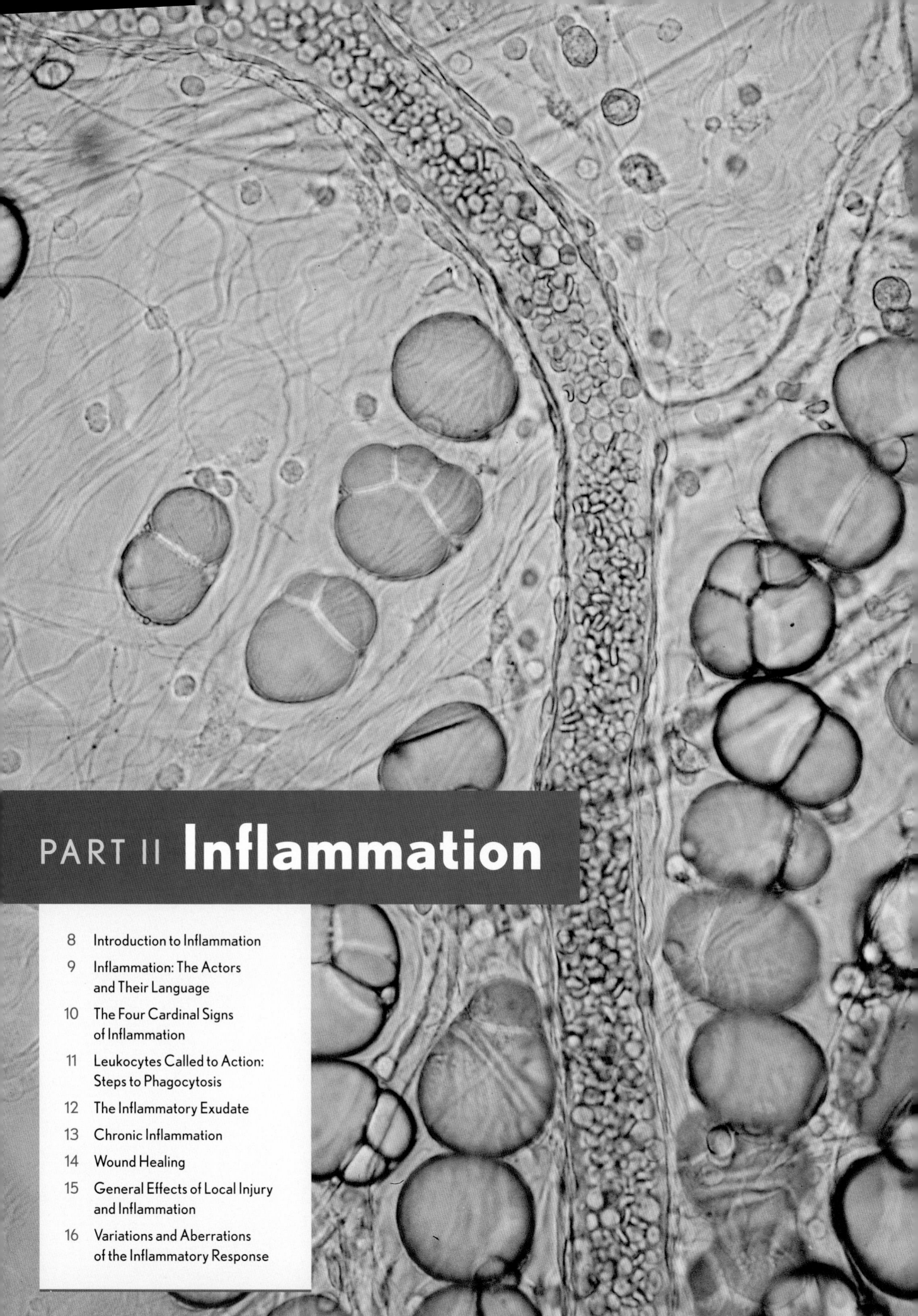

PART II Inflammation

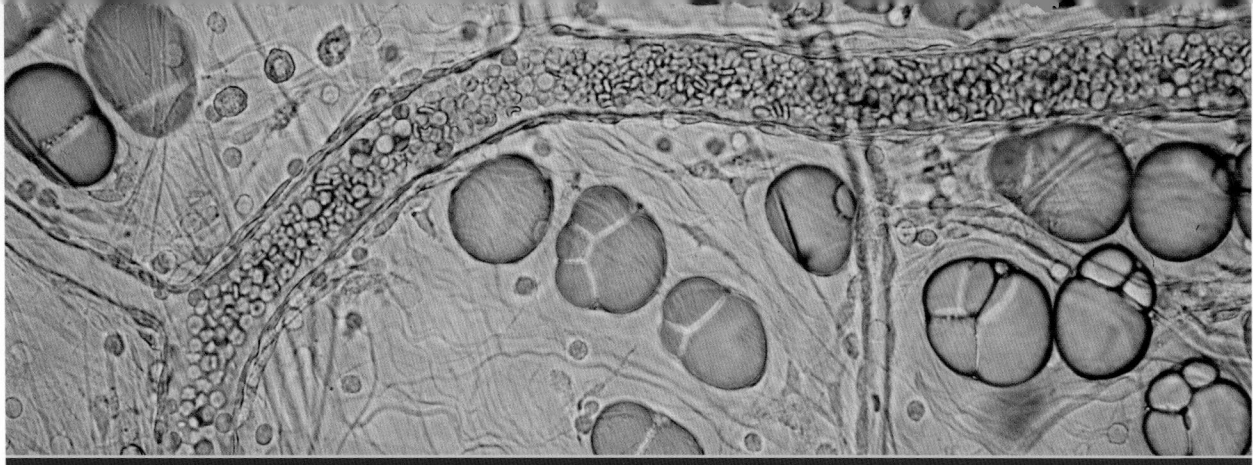

INTRODUCTION TO INFLAMMATION

With inflammation we step into a real-life drama, traditionally interpreted as the microscopic equivalent of warfare against true or perceived invaders, with its cellular heroes, villains, casualties, suicides, chemical weapons, and even victims of friendly fire. The setting is a battlefield in which real blood is shed, and the pace may be frantic or sluggish, but the action is always highly programmed, with messages flying in all directions. This makes cellular pathology sound rather tame in retrospect, but of course it was essential for understanding the performers on the battlefield.

A Working Definition

There are long and short definitions of inflammation; we will use the shortest, and build it up later:

Inflammation is a response to local injury in vascularized tissues. Its purpose is to deliver white blood cells and fluid (plasma) to a site of injury.

First of all, then, we must understand why we should need a special, local response to injury and why this response should be the delivery of blood components. Just examine the threats posed by a local injury such as a wound. The basic hazards are three (Figure 8.1): some vessels are severed, some tissue is destroyed, and the door is open to bacteria. The first problem, bleeding, is quite critical, but it is quickly, almost instantly, brought under control by the local mechanisms of hemostasis, which we will explain later. The second problem, loss of tissue, is less urgent; the loss will be compensated in due time (days, weeks) by regeneration while local scavenger cells clear up the debris. The third problem, infection, is critical, but for this task the local defenses are not adequate. The local antibacterial "national guard," spread out in the tissues, usually amounts to a few sleepy macrophages scattered among the fibroblasts. They are not enough to ward off a sudden bacterial

INJURY

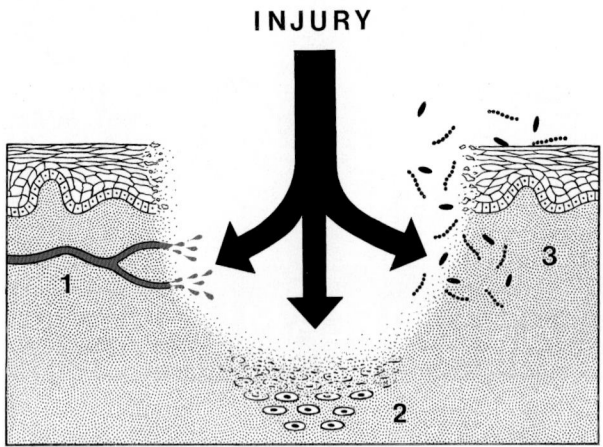

FIGURE 8.1   Injury to bacteria-laden surfaces creates three problems: **1.** Vessels bleed. **2.** Cells are destroyed. **3.** Microbial invaders penetrate.

attack. The reason for this inadequacy is that it would be extremely expensive, biologically speaking, and even dangerous to maintain fully alert defenses everywhere in the body. Nature has solved the problem by concentrating most of the defensive forces in the blood, where they circulate in inactive mode; then, wherever a problem arises, they are delivered—and activated. The delivery and the battle that ensues are the essence of inflammation.

The defensive materials supplied by the inflammatory response are of two kinds: (a) the *white blood cells,* which can handle different tasks related to tissue injury and infection; they respond to complex calls and actively crawl out of the microscopic vessels; and (b) *plasma,* which contains dozens of proteins able to perform defensive functions, such as killing bacteria. An immediate outpouring of plasma is easily supplied by the vessels, thanks to chemical messengers that induce the endothelium to become leaky. The red blood cells are not drafted, because their task is to provide general support in the guise of oxygen; this requires an active and intact microcirculation. Now imagine the complexity of the task for the microcirculation: make the vessels leaky enough to dispense some plasma but not enough to let out the red blood cells, while allowing the escape of the white blood cells, which are larger. The following chapters explain how this is done.

The mixture of cells and plasma that seeps out of the vessels is called *inflammatory exudate,* or simply *exudate;* it is generated in response to chemical messengers, better known as the *mediators* of inflammation. The first mediators to appear on the scene are products of cell injury. Notice the efficient feedback loop: the first steps of the defensive response are induced by chemicals released by the injured tissue (Figure 8.2).

Two Phases of the Inflammatory Response: Innate and Adaptive

Inflammation is not a permanent state but a dynamic process. Some cells die, some divide, others keep coming and going: not a simple matter to unravel. By the late 1900s paraffin embedding, microtome sections (31a) and histologic stains allowed pathologists to piece together a sketchy natural history of inflammation. One of the obvious findings was that *the inflammatory*

FIGURE 8.2   The basic feedback principle of inflammation. Injured tissue (**1**) releases chemical mediators (**2**) that diffuse to neighboring blood vessels and trigger an exudate of cells and fluid (**3**): the first step in the repair process.

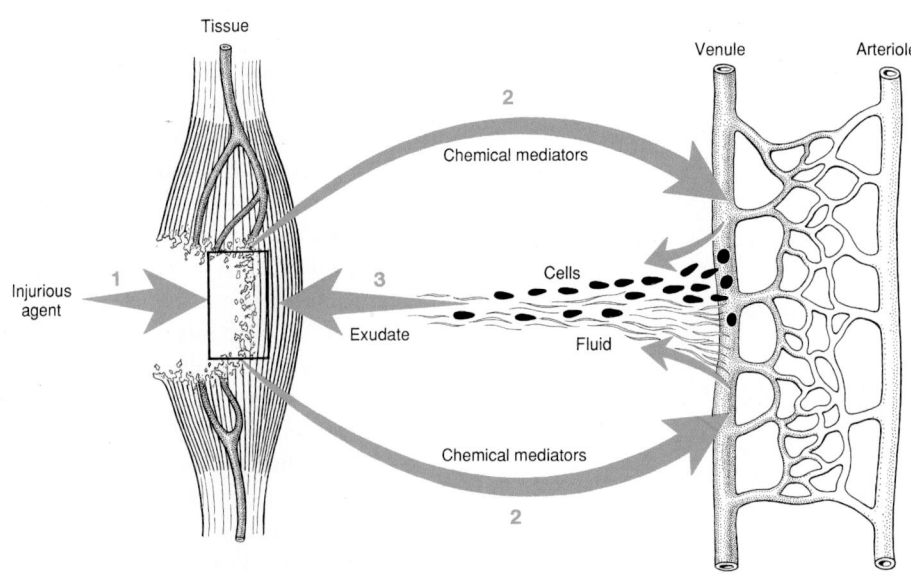

drama runs in two phases: at the very beginning (seconds, minutes, hours after injury), the events are quite standardized and almost immutable, regardless of the cause. This phase of the inflammatory response was called the **acute, stereotyped phase or nonspecific phase** of inflammation. The exudate consists mainly of edema and neutrophils.

About a week or two later, the inflammatory focus seemed to have adapted itself to the particular causal agent (a bacterium, a burn, a foreign body, etc.). New cell types appeared, in different proportions—lymphocytes, plasma cells, giant cells, eosinophils. This was called the **chronic, specific phase.** We now know that the immune response has taken place, specific indeed.

In recent years, immunologists made tremendous advances in unraveling the mysteries of inflammation. They also created new names for the two phases of inflammation. The first was called the *innate immune response.* We have no quarrel at all with the notion of "innate," but we firmly disagree with "immune": there is nothing immune about it, except that it was named by immunologists. The two key features of the immune response are memory and specificity; both are lacking in the innate response. We therefore call it, more simply and more accurately, the **innate inflammatory response** or just **innate response.** The second phase was called the *adaptive immune response.* It is certainly adaptive, in that the response is specific to the causal agent; but "immune adaptive" is redundant; every immune response is adaptive. We use, more simply, **immune response,** or adaptive response, which everybody understands. More about this when we discuss the evolution of inflammation (p. 430).

Apart from the terminology, the concept of dual response—innate versus immune—is important and led to some interesting discoveries, as we will see (p. 430).

Infection versus Inflammation

In the discussion above we may have given the impression that inflammation is primarily an antibacterial phenomenon, but we must hasten to add two important qualifications: (a) *inflammation operates against all invaders,* including viruses, worms, fungi, and other parasites. It just so happens that bacteria outnumber all other aggressors, so that evolution has patterned the defensive response especially against bacteria. (b) *Inflammation is also triggered aseptically by injured tissues,* a theme that will often recur in these pages.

Lay people, understandably, tend to confuse infection and inflammation. It is true that bacterial infection usually brings about inflammation, but the words infection and inflammation represent very different concepts. **Inflammation** is a reaction; **infection** simply means "contamination with microorganisms." There can be infection without inflammation, for example, in a severely immunosuppressed patient. There can also be inflammation without infection; remember that inflammation is triggered by products of tissue injury, thus any aseptic injury will trigger inflammation. A classic example is a myocardial infarct. The purpose of such programmed inflammation without infection is a semiphilosophical problem; we shall come to it on p. 430.

Terminology of Inflammation

The suffix *-itis* usually means inflammation of that organ or tissue (appendic-itis, mening-itis, pleur-itis). The terms **acute** and **chronic** are used loosely to mean events that evolve over *hours and days* versus *weeks, months, or years;* "acute" in a clinical setting means "coming sharply to a climax." **Injury** means damage: that is, the effect of an injurious agent. **Local injury** is damage inflicted to a limited part of the body. The term **exudate** always refers to the product of inflammation, namely the extravasated mixture of protein-rich fluid and cells; *it is opposed to* **transudate,** *the ultrafiltrate of plasma that arises from normal vessels* through hydrostatic mechanisms. If the diagnosis is not obvious, the noncommittal term **effusion** is handy. The term *inflammatory infiltrate* or simply **infiltrate** is often used for a swarm of inflammatory cells as seen under the microscope. The ancient terms *phlogistic* and *antiphlogistic* are still used to mean "inflammatory" and "antiinflammatory"; they come from the Greek *phlox* for "flame."

Understanding Inflammation: A Story of 5000 Years

Because local injury is part of everyday life, inflammation is probably the most common aspect of tissue pathology and has always been perceived as a central issue in the practice of medicine. It inspired theories that had enormous impact on medical treatment; some bad theories have killed many more people than the medical profession saved. It also inspired great discoveries; for example, the concept of bacterial infection,

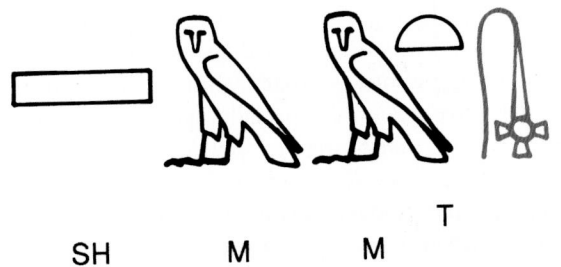

SH   M   M   T

FIGURE 8.3   One of the ancient Egyptian words for inflammation: SH-M-M-T, conventionally pronounced "shememet." The first four hieroglyphs stand for the consonants indicated. The last sign, called a "determinative," is not to be pronounced; it indicates the general meaning of the preceding word. This particular determinative represents a brazier filled with oil, with a flame arising from it and a trail of smoke curling downward. It therefore conveys the meaning "hot thing." (Reproduced with permission from [32].)

which was discovered in 1867 by the surgeon Joseph Lister, later Lord Lister, while studying inflamed wounds (31).

Inflammation Misunderstood as a Disease

A red eye, a hot and swollen finger, a wound that is surrounded by reddened skin and exuding pus are impressive sights: no healer of any era could fail to notice them. Accordingly, words for inflammation are found in the most ancient medical texts—Egyptian, Mesopotamian, Greek, and Chinese. The oldest known are the Egyptian papyri, which reach as far back as 2700 B.C. (Figure 8.3). The reader may wonder how any particular word of a dead language can be translated by our current term inflammation; but in fact, several of the ancient terms so translated refer most definitely to what we call inflammation because they relate to heat, to redness, or to an actual flame (32, 33).

Today we know that inflammation is a life-saving reaction, usually against infection. In ancient times, however, when the concept of bacterial infection did not exist, a swollen red finger was interpreted as meaning that the finger was "sick with inflammation." Inflammation was thought to be the disease—and was treated accordingly. How could one fight inflammation? Simple. The ancient Greeks argued, quite plausibly, that the redness is due to an excess of red blood. All excesses being bad, according to Greek culture, the obvious treatment was to draw blood. Such was the antiinflammatory therapy championed by the Hippocratic physicians and perpetuated by their heirs for some 2300 years. Bloodletting became the treatment of choice for any case of inflammation; eventually, blood was drawn even if no redness was visible, not only because this procedure seemed helpful as a form of drainage—removal of bad humors—but also because inflammation was thought to be at the root of most diseases (32). In Western medicine this aberrant therapy became extraordinarily popular because it seemed to make such good sense. The fashion continued well into the nineteenth century: Napoleon's wounded soldiers were bled of their last few ounces of blood on the battlefield to prevent inflammation of their wounds. Such is the power of theory.

The Romans went along with Greek theory, but they made one everlasting contribution. Cornelius Celsus, a writer of the first century, compiled a large encyclopedia; in the section on medicine (*De medicina*) he wrote: "*Notae vero inflammationis sunt quatuor: rubor et tumor cum calore et dolore,*" meaning "Truly the signs of inflammation are four, redness and swelling with heat and pain" (Figure 8.4). To this day, nobody has improved upon this definition of acute inflammation, which has been recited by medical students century after century and still appears on the National Board exams, though not in Latin.

Inflammation as a Useful Reaction

The thought that inflammation might be useful emerged as a speculation in the 1700s (41); it was spelled out unmistakably by John Hunter, a Scottish surgeon and naturalist endowed with tremendous insight and a genius for research. Hunter had tended hundreds of festering war wounds. His treatise *On the Blood, Inflammation and Gunshot Wounds,* published in 1794, contains this nugget: "Inflammation in itself is not to be considered as a disease, but as a salutary operation consequent either to some violence or some disease" (26). "Some violence" or "some disease" was his masterly intuition for "injured tissue" and "bacteria."

In the days of John Hunter, the microscope was used by few scientists. It had the reputation of being more a toy than a tool; its images were considered difficult to distinguish from artefacts and were therefore viewed with suspicion (34). Half a century later, Rudolf Virchow, the father of modern pathology and a firm believer in the microscope, published his revolutionary *Cellular Pathology* (1858). By his time it had become fashionable to study pus under the microscope, and it was well known that pus contained "pus corpuscles," which we now understand to be emigrated leukocytes.

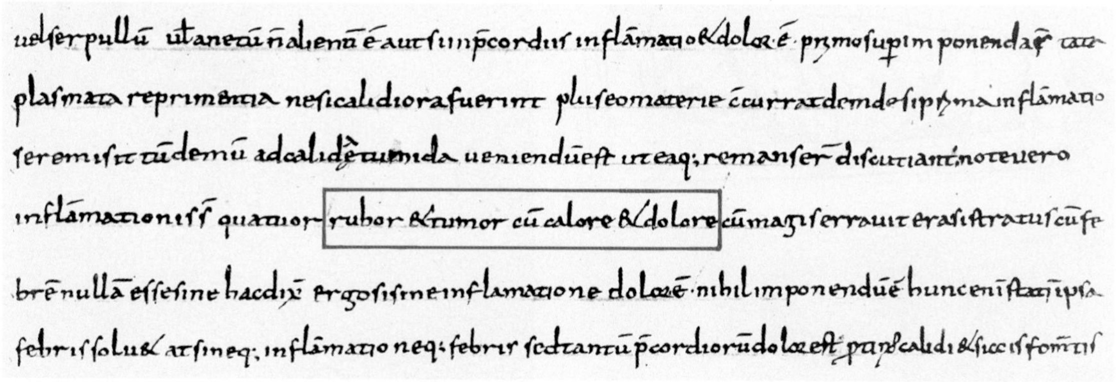

[Medieval manuscript text in handwritten Latin script]

FIGURE 8.4 The four cardinal signs of inflammation were codified by Celsus in the first century A.D. This is how they appeared much later in a codex of the tenth century. (Reproduced with permission from [32].)

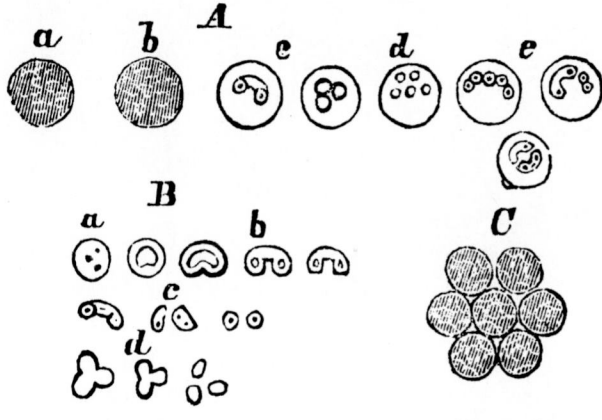

FIGURE 8.5 Pus corpuscles (leukocytes), as illustrated by Virchow in 1858. The darker ones (**Aab, C**) are fresh; all others have been treated with acetic acid, then a standard procedure for making tissues more transparent (stains were not yet used). The multilobed nucleus of the neutrophils is clearly shown in **Ac–e**, but Virchow was noncommittal as to the origin of the pus corpuscles, except for stating that "colorless blood-cells are so like pus corpuscles as easily to be mistaken for them." (Reproduced with permission from [47].)

Virchow portrayed them as he saw them (Figure 8.5) and noted their similarity to white blood cells, but he added that "it will probably still require a number of years" before anyone could decide whether they migrated from the blood into the pus or from the pus into the blood (47).

Actually, Virchow had not quite done his homework: the emigration of leukocytes from blood vessels had been clearly described by the Frenchman H. Dutrochet in 1824 (15), and the origin of the pus globules from "blood corpuscles perforating the capillaries" had been established in 1846 by an Englishman, Augustus Waller, who also described the "Wallerian degeneration" of resected nerves (16, 41, 48). Dutrochet and Waller having been forgotten, diapedesis had to be rediscovered in 1867 by one of Virchow's most famous pupils, Julius Cohnheim. At that time the thin histologic sections that we now take for granted did not exist. Like many of his contemporaries, including Waller, Cohnheim did his microscopic work on cumbersome but transparent living membranes such as the mesentery or the tongue of the frog (Figure 8.6): this limitation turned out to be a major advantage, because blood flow in living tissues offered the opportunity to observe dynamic events, such as the emigration of leukocytes (diapedesis). One day, as he was studying a preparation of frog mesentery, Cohnheim observed a sequence of events that gave inflammation a whole new meaning (11). He noticed that the arterioles in the irritated tissue became wider; flow at first was faster, then it slowed, and eventually white blood cells emigrated into the tissues while plasma also leaked out. Now the four cardinal signs stated by Celsus could be explained in scientific terms: the redness and heat were due to increased blood flow, the swelling to the exudation of cells and fluid, and the pain would follow. Cohnheim was understandably elated.

This was a big step forward, accomplished at the very limits of *in vivo* microscopy, in 1867 (Figure 8.7). Little does it matter that Cohnheim was not the first to see diapedesis (he acknowledges it in a footnote that reads very much like "oops": Professor Virchow, now partially updated, had just given him the reference to

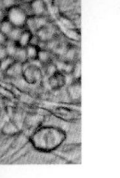

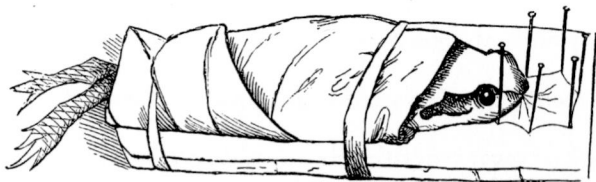

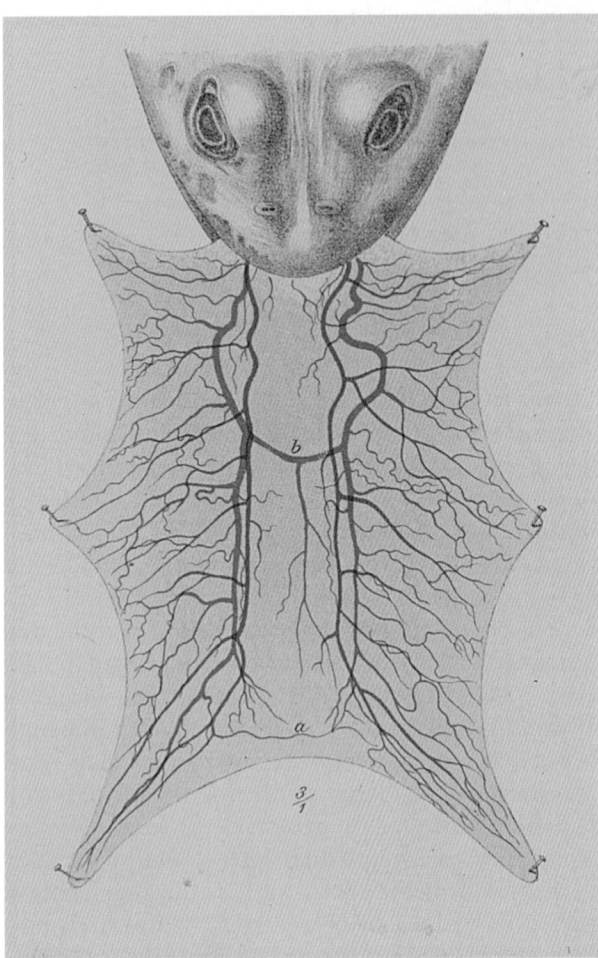

FIGURE 8.6   *Top:* A method for studying the circulation in the tongue of the living frog, as illustrated by Augustus Waller in 1846. (Reproduced from [48].) *Bottom:* Vessels in the tongue of the frog, as shown in Cohnheim's study of embolism. (Reproduced from [12].)

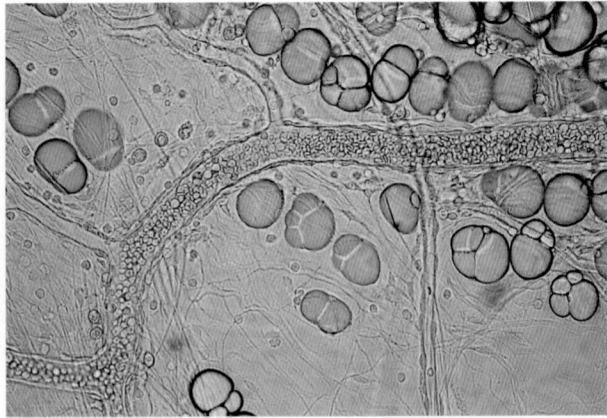

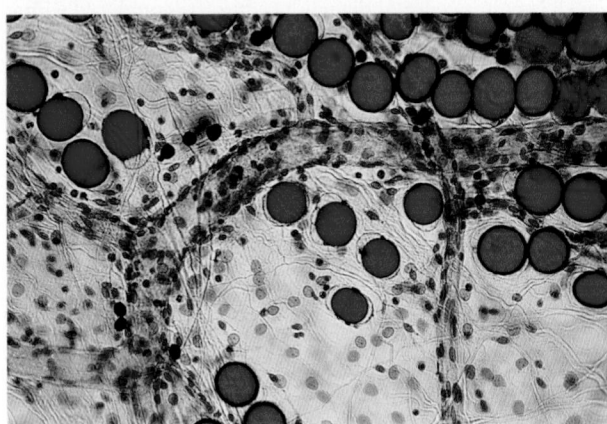

FIGURE 8.7   Acute inflammation as studied in 1867. Histologic sections did not exist; Julius Cohnheim used thin membranes such as rat omentum (shown here, 6 hours after mild irritation by laparotomy). *Top:* Even with a modern Zeiss microscope, it is virtually impossible to understand that leukocytes have escaped from the venules. *Bottom:* Same field stained with hematoxylin and scarlet red for fat (round red objects are fat cells). It is more obvious that there are "too many cells," but how did this happen? Cohnheim solved the problem by using living tissue membranes. (Reprinted from Majno G, Joris I. The microscope in the history of pathology. With a note on the pathology of fat cells. Virchows Arch Abt A Pathol Anat 1973;360:273–286. Copyright 1973, with permission from Springer-Verlag GmbH & Co. KG.)

Waller): Cohnheim's was the first scientific theory of inflammation.

Starfish and Phagocytes

Although Cohnheim did see the leukocytes emigrate, he had no idea what their functions could be out in the tissues. For that critical step we must skip to Messina, in Sicily, in 1882. The Russian zoologist Ilya Metchnikoff had just settled in Messina to escape turmoil in his native country. He had no job and worked at his home on the seaside, supported by his wealthy wife; the beach was a generous source of microscopic subjects for someone who knew where to look. In 1880 he discovered and named phagocytosis by studying the fate of carmine particles introduced into the mesoderm of transparent invertebrates. Then, in his words:

"One day when the whole family had gone to a circus to see some extraordinary performing apes, I remained alone with my microscope, observing the life in the mobile cells of transparent star-fish larvae, when a new thought suddenly flashed across my brain. It struck me that similar cells might serve in the defence of the organism against intruders. Feeling that there was in this something of surpassing interest, I felt so excited that I began striding up and down the room and even went to the seashore to collect my thoughts. I said to myself that, if my supposition was true, a splinter introduced into the body of a star-fish larva, devoid of blood vessels or of a nervous system, should soon be surrounded by mobile cells as is observed in a man who runs a splinter into his finger. This was no sooner said than done. There was a small garden in our dwelling, in which we had a few days previously organized a "Christmas tree" for the children on a little tangerine tree; I fetched from it a few rose thorns and introduced them at once under the skin of some beautiful star-fish larvae as transparent as water. I was too excited to sleep that night in the expectation of the result of my experiment, and very early the next morning I ascertained that it had fully succeeded. This experiment formed the basis of the phagocyte theory, to the development of which I devoted the next twenty-five years of my life. (37)"

Nobody could have done more with rose thorns and starfish larvae. This seminal experiment was soon confirmed by another masterly observation, this time on a tiny transparent crustacean, *Daphnia,* the water flea (Figure 8.8) (35, 36). The structure of this little creature is essentially that of an intestinal tube and a skin, separated by a space or coelom. Metchnikoff noticed that sometimes a rod-shaped microorganism, *Monospora,* escaped from the intestinal tube into the surrounding space, causing the animal to die. At other times the invading *Monospora* was attacked and engulfed by free-floating cells, and in these cases the animal survived. Once again, the phagocytes were proven to be defensive cells.

Metchnikoff had no medical training, but when he learned of Cohnheim's findings on inflammation and diapedesis he suddenly grasped the link: *the purpose of inflammation was to deliver phagocytes to a site of injury.* Fortunately he was not discouraged by a passing visitor, Professor Virchow, who politely advised him that the current theory of inflammation was quite the opposite: leukocytes were engaged in spreading bacteria (!) (37).

We tried to repeat some of Metchnikoff's "simple" experiments, but the sand fleas jumped out of the pail or

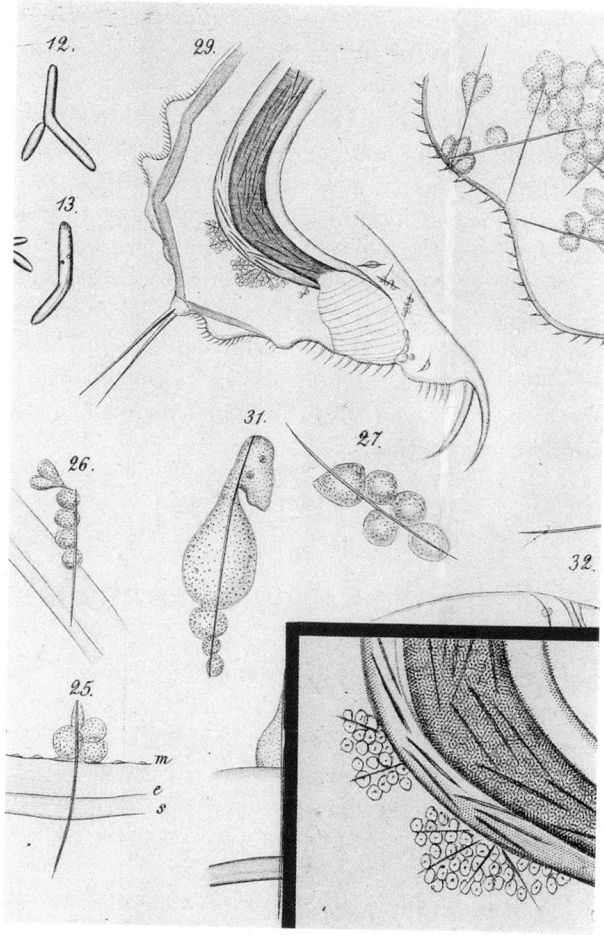

FIGURE 8.8   The defensive function of leukocytes as illustrated by Metchnikoff in 1884 from observations on the water flea, *Daphnia magna.* 29: Abdominal portion of a Daphnia. The intestinal lumen contains many rodlike spores of a primitive fungus that Metchnikoff called *Monospora bicuspidata. Inset:* Some of the spores have found their way into the wall of the intestine; others have emerged into the abdominal cavity where they are surrounded by leukocytes. 31, 27: Other spores surrounded by leukocytes. (Reproduced from [36].)

twirled around so fast that we could never get one under the microscope. Obviously Metchnikoff's "simple" is not everybody's "simple." He published the essence of his experiments in 1893 in a beautifully illustrated little book, *Lectures on the Comparative Pathology of Inflammation,* still unsurpassed. It was reprinted in 1968 (36).

Enter Antibodies

Then came another explosive novelty: in 1890 Behring and Kitasato discovered the life-saving effect of antibodies against diphtheria toxin. And so, a new (and German) theory of inflammation was launched: *the purpose of inflammation was to bring antibodies, not cells, to the site of infection.* This caused much bitterness to Metchnikoff, who was then working at the Pasteur Institute in Paris, and much energy was wasted by scientists of the two opposing sides, largely German versus French. The battle died away when it became obvious, as so often happens in the history of science, that both sides were right. The defensive power of inflammation hinges on phagocytes *and* on antibodies: cells and fluid, as stated in our definition. In 1908 Metchnikoff shared the Nobel prize with Paul Ehrlich, a member of the antibody faction (24).

Birth of the Reticuloendothelial System

A few years after Metchnikoff received the Nobel prize, his favorite cell, the macrophage, received the ultimate accolade. Metchnikoff had already used the expression "system of macrophages," but an eminent German pathologist, Ludwig Aschoff, seized upon it and proposed an even broader generalization: *all the phagocytic cells in the body can be considered as part of a "diffuse organ" with many functions, including defense.* He called this organ the reticuloendothelial system (RES) (2). We will now review it because it turned out to be even more important to survival than Aschoff had predicted: it plays a key role in orchestrating local and general defenses.

Exploring the Reticuloendothelial System

The reticuloendothelial system or RES (forgive this archaic name—we will discuss it shortly) was at first considered to be just a system of phagocytic cells. Now it is known to have many functions other than phagocytosis. Still, finding the sites where phagocytosis normally takes place is the simplest way to map the RES; so we will use phagocytosis as a guide.

To map the diffuse RES organ, Aschoff and his collaborators chose a number of colored materials (solutions of dyes and suspensions of particulate pigments), injected them either locally or intravenously, and found out which cells picked them up. They soon realized that almost any cell in the body will phagocytize if pushed to do so, and therefore decided to include only the most actively phagocytic cells in the RES. (Today the accepted term for these most active cells is **professional phagocytes.**) They also noticed that the most active "provinces" (their word) of the RES were **the liver, spleen, and bone marrow.**

The members of the RES family have changed somewhat since the time of Aschoff (17, 38a). The fibroblasts and endothelium have been thrown out as nonprofessional phagocytes, and other cells have been admitted (Figure 8.9). The members of the modern RES cells have a great deal in common, even their ancestry. It is now believed that a single cell type—the monocyte—is born in the bone marrow, is distributed throughout the body, and then differentiates, depending on where it lands, into cells as disparate as the microglia, the osteoclasts, the Kupffer cells of the liver, and the macrophages ("histiocytes") of all connective tissues. Phagocytosis is no longer the sole act of the RES. The monocyte/

macrophage has a mind-boggling series of functional properties: it is involved in the immune response, tumor cell control, hematopoiesis, angiogenesis, coagulation, and much else (30). Of course, the importance of the RES has skyrocketed, even though it remains an "invisible organ," hidden inside all other organs.

Before the versatility of the macrophages was recognized, in 1972 a committee of experts proposed that the name RES be changed to MPS (Mononuclear Phagocyte System), emphasizing phagocytosis. The new

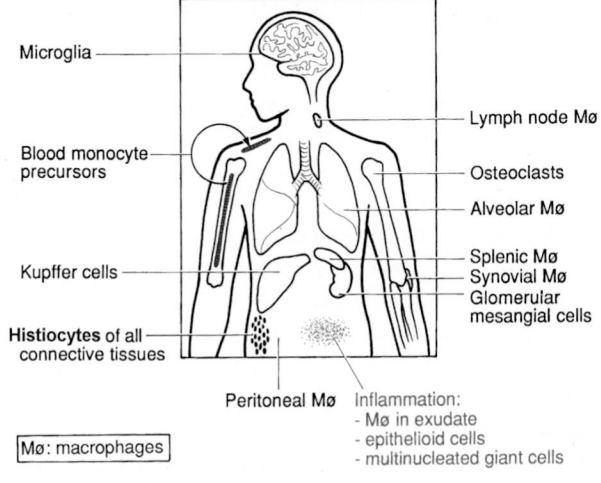

CELLS OF THE
MONONUCLEAR PHAGOCYTE SYSTEM

Microglia

Blood monocyte precursors

Kupffer cells

Histiocytes of all connective tissues

Lymph node Mø

Osteoclasts

Alveolar Mø

Splenic Mø
Synovial Mø
Glomerular mesangial cells

Peritoneal Mø   Inflammation:
- Mø in exudate
- epithelioid cells
- multinucleated giant cells

Mø: macrophages

FIGURE 8.9 Types of cells considered to belong to the reticuloendothelial system. (Adapted from [42] with permission of Blackwell Scientific Publications Ltd.)

name did not catch on; so we will retain the venerable, but generally accepted RES.

Membership in the RES club requires more than the capacity to phagocytize: the macrophages are distinguished as "big eaters," but also intervene in a number of cell and tissue functions, and carry a variety of marker antigens (38a). This is why the polymorphs, although unbeatable as phagocytes, will never be admitted to the club.

The provinces of the phagocytic system can be conveniently mapped, as Aschoff did, by injecting phagocytizable materials that are also colored; thus, each and every phagocyte will acquire its own label from one or another material. We now offer you a guided tour through these classic experiments; much is to be learned in the process. Just remember that no single material method can reveal all the phagocytes: one group or another will be excluded by each type of experiment. Predictably, the size of the labeling particles makes a difference: intravenously injected suspensions of colloidal pigments that cannot cross the endothelium will label only those phagocytes that line the bloodstream; solutions of dyes that can cross the endothelium will also label the phagocytes that lie outside the vessels, except in organs with endothelial "barriers." Therefore, several types of experiments are essential for understanding inflammation; they also illustrate what happens to foreign particles (including bacteria) in the blood or in the tissues.

Mapping the RES with an Intravenous Injection of Colloidal Particles

The beauty of this experiment is that it shows us the fate of foreign particles traveling in the bloodstream. Carbon black is the prototype of colloidal suspensions; its particles are 300 Å or more in diameter (the order of magnitude of lipoproteins) and cannot be transcytosed by the endothelium. Although they are much smaller than bacteria, they are picked up by the same cells that pick up bacteria.

Ordinary India ink is not recommended for these experiments because its shellac promotes clotting (20). A special "biological" suspension of carbon suspended in a gelatin solution should be used.

Three drops of carbon black suspension (0.3 ml) are enough to give the skin and mucosae of a 300-gram albino rat an ominous gray hue, but the discoloration fades away under the eyes of the experimenter, and in 5–10 minutes the normal pink color returns. Inspection of the internal organs after 15 minutes is absolutely striking. The novice will probably expect all

organs to be grey. Not at all: the **liver** and **spleen** are jet black, and all other organs are normal. If a long bone is opened, its **marrow** will also appear blackened, though not as intensely as the liver and spleen. The carbon black accumulates in the liver, spleen, and bone marrow because these organs have special, wide capillaries called **sinusoids** that are partially lined with flat macrophages (Figure 8.10). In ruminants also the capillaries of the lung are capable of performing some phagocytosis (8, 9, 49).

So we have learned that the RES has a special "province:" a set of phagocytes lining the finest blood

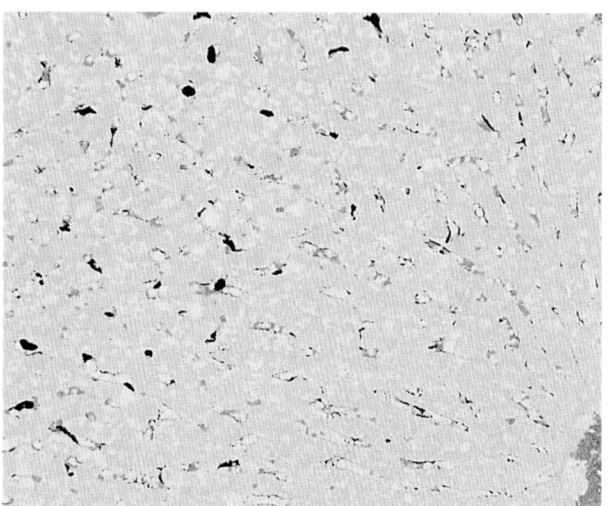

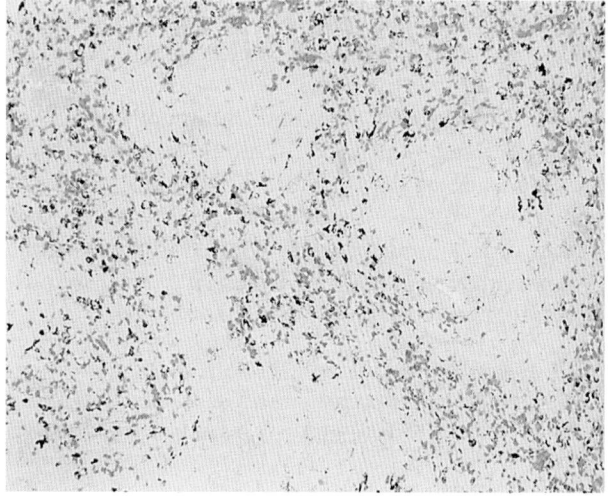

FIGURE 8.10 Littoral (or sinusoidal) phagocytes of the liver and spleen, in a rat injected 1 hour earlier with a colloidal suspension of carbon black. *Top:* Liver. The dots and streaks correspond to single Kupffer cells loaded with carbon. No carbon is picked up by the hepatocytes. *Bottom:* Spleen. The clear areas correspond to lymph follicles, because lymphocytes are not phagocytic. The dots represent phagocytes in the red pulp. Stain: Eosin only.

vessels in the liver, spleen, and bone marrow, and in ruminants also in the lung.

This particular province of phagocytes is called upon whenever some particulate foreign material is carried by the blood. There is no official name for it, which is regrettable, because we will often need to mention this sector of the RES. We will therefore adopt the rarely used but excellent name **littoral phagocytes;** littoral means "on the beach" (*litus* is Latin for "shore," here it refers to the "shores" of the bloodstream). *This system of littoral phagocytes includes about 90 percent of all mononuclear phagocytes (10) and is therefore the largest segment of the RES; it functions as the filter of the blood.*

> An alternative name for the littoral phagocytes is **sinusoidal phagocytes.** We find littoral more pictorial.

The littoral phagocytes of different organs do not have identical properties; for example, the spleen recognizes more easily those particles that are coated with immunoglobulin, of which it recognizes the "free end" (the so-called Fc portion) (p. 289). This may explain why the removal of the spleen can be followed by fulminating pneumococcal sepsis: the littoral phagocytes of the liver are not efficient in recognizing immunoglobulin-coated bacteria (22, 45).

Quantitative studies of the blood of rats injected intravenously with carbon show that, depending on the dose, most of the circulating carbon is removed in less than an hour (Figure 8.11) (4, 5). In general, the clearance of colloidal particles from the blood depends on their number (Figure 8.10), size, and nature. *Larger particles, including bacteria, are cleared faster than smaller particles* (10). Repeated intravenous injections lead to decreased uptake (5). This has been referred to as a **blockade of the RES** as if the diminished rate of clearance were due to overstuffing the phagocytes; in fact, it is more likely that repeated flooding of the plasma with foreign particles depletes it of phagocytosis-promoting proteins (opsonins) (43).

> The speed with which the RES clears the blood is amazing. In laboratory animals the liver alone clears about 80 percent of colloidal foreign material in a single passage; in fact, this rate can be used for measuring blood flow through the liver (6, 43).

We now discuss some lessons from these experiments with particles injected into the bloodstream.

Fate of Indigestible Material

Indigestible material stored in the littoral phagocytes is there for life. There is no way out of the RES—except

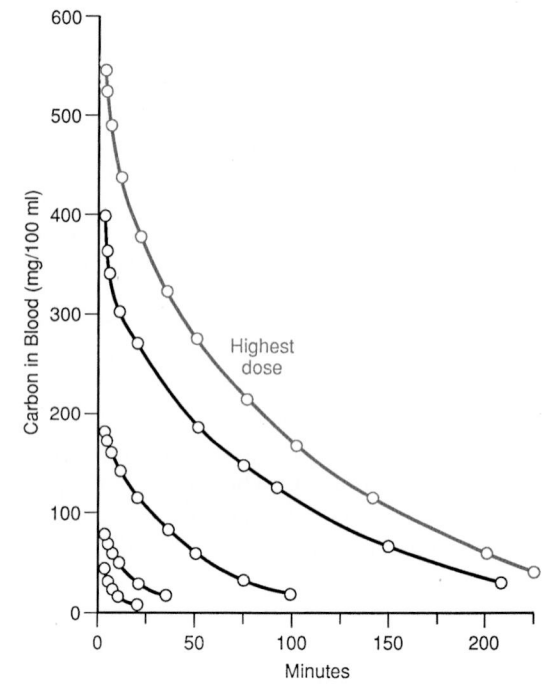

FIGURE 8.11   Rate of clearance of carbon black from the blood. Low doses are cleared faster. (Adapted from [5] with permission of Blackwell Scientific Publications Ltd.)

for some *inhaled* particles. When the littoral macrophages die, they may well spill their carbon into the bloodstream, but some other littoral macrophages will pick it up and repeat the cycle.

The only province of the RES that can dump some of its phagocytic cells—with or without carbon black—out of the body is represented by the alveolar macrophages, which are transported out by the ciliary conveyor belt (rats swallow about two million alveolar macrophages per hour) (8). Other monocytes/macrophages are probably lost into the gut, but neither group of cells can get rid of significant amounts of materials injected intravenously. Evolution has not prepared the RES for this housecleaning task.

> There was a time not long ago—in the early days of radiology—when thorotrast, a suspension of radioactive (!) thorium dioxide particles, was injected intraarterially to visualize arterial branches. It accumulated in the RES and damaged especially the liver (Figure 8.12). Its long-term effects included cancer.

Medical Uses for Littoral Phagocytes

Littoral phagocytes can be exploited for diagnosis or therapy. Colloidal sulfur technetium, a radioactive particle with a very short half-life, can be used to visualize the

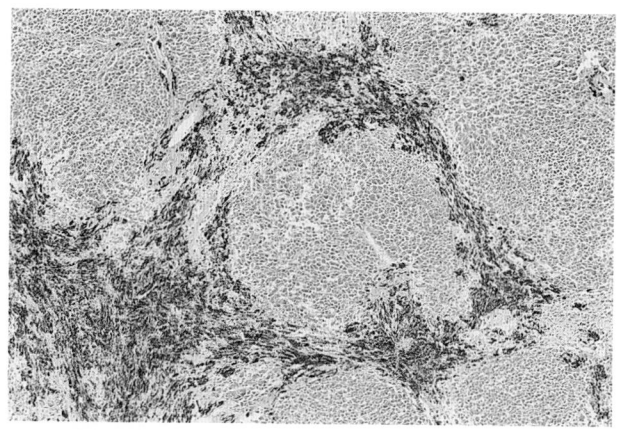

FIGURE 8.12   The scarred liver of a patient who died many years after an arteriography performed with an intra-arterial injection of thorotrast. The scars appear dark due to countless macrophages loaded with thorotrast. Autopsy was performed in 1940.

RES. Some parasites such as *Leishmania* have chosen the littoral phagocytes as a biological niche: they have found a way to survive inside them after being phagocytized. One imaginative way to sneak up on them is to inject a *colloidal* drug intravenously; the littoral phagocytes take it up, and with a little bit of luck—for the patient—parasite and drug will end up in the same phagosome (p. 225).

Relation of Lymph Nodes to the RES

Lymph nodes are certainly full of phagocytes, but remember that these are strategically placed to clear the *lymph*. The phagocytes in the lymph nodes line the lymphatics, not the blood vessels; therefore, in theory, an intravenous injection of carbon black should not label the lymph nodes at all. However, after an intravenous injection of carbon black some faint outlines of blackened vessels can be seen in the lymph nodes (Figure 8.13) (28) and in Peyer's patches of the intestine, another lymphatic organ (Figure 8.14) (38, 44, 50). Close study showed that *this does not represent phagocytosis*. The retention of particles is due to venular leakage of a special kind.

The blackened vessels are the famous high-endothelial venules, which are the doorway for lymphocyte recycling. The lymphocytes in the blood recognize this special endothelial surface, stick to it, crawl across the endothelium, and float away in the lymph, which will carry them back to the blood. As they perform their diapedesis across the endothelium of the high-endothelial venules, a few of the injected carbon particles can sneak across with them and then remain trapped against the basement membrane.

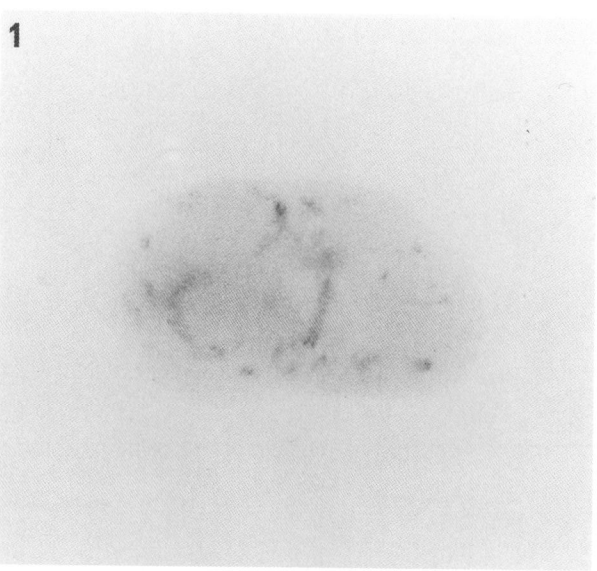

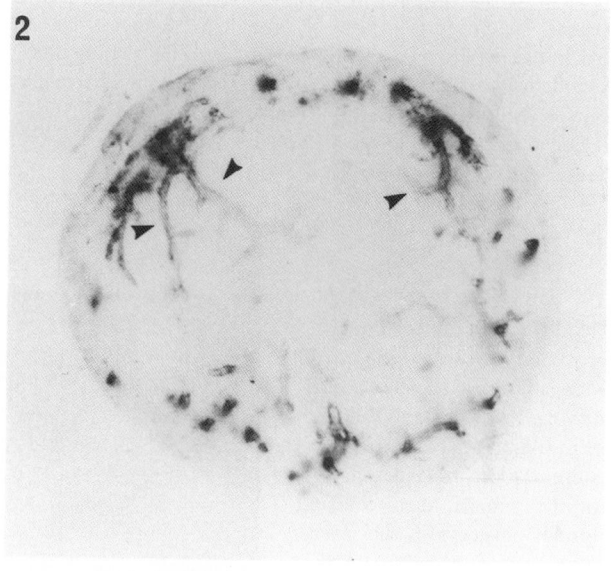

FIGURE 8.13   A special variety of vascular labeling in normal and acutely inflamed lymph nodes. *Top:* Normal mouse popliteal lymph node after a single intravenous injection of 0.1 ml of carbon black/100 gram body weight. There is some faint labeling of the venules, especially of the high-endothelial variety, due to leakage of carbon black accompanying lymphocyte diapedesis. *Bottom:* Mouse popliteal lymph node labeled with carbon black 12 hours after an injection of endotoxin in the footpad (which caused the lymph node to become acutely inflamed). Note the heavier labeling of the venules (**arrowheads**), representing an increased transendothelial traffic of lymphocytes. (Courtesy of Dr. M.C. Kowala [28].)

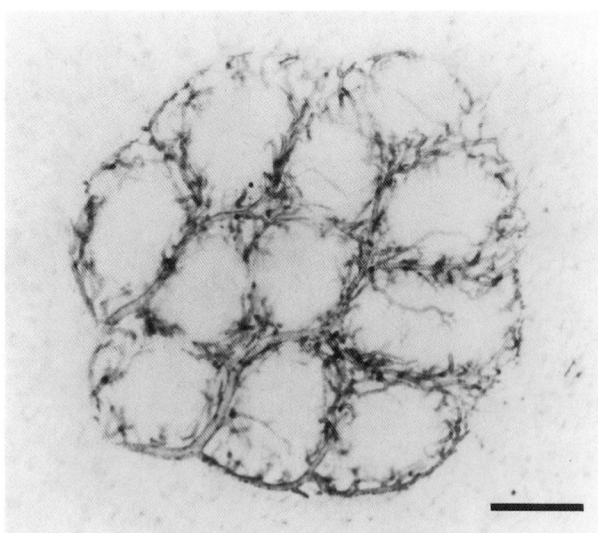

Bacteria in the Bloodstream

The littoral phagocytes probably save our lives on a daily basis. Any bacteria that find their way into the bloodstream—and this must happen all the time—are promptly removed, as can be shown experimentally (Figure 8.15). The simple act of chewing is said to cause bacteremia, bacteria being forced into the vessels of the pocket between tooth and gum. A door wide open to bacteria is created when a tooth is pulled (3). Using very sensitive culture methods, Fiore-Donno has grown as many as 32 varieties of oral bacteria from the bloodstream after tooth extractions (Fiore-Donno G, Faculty of Dental Medicine, Geneva, Switzerland; personal communication). Normally, this invasion is quickly overwhelmed by the littoral phagocytes.

FIGURE 8.14 Peyer's patch of a rat. The high-endothelial venules have been labeled in black by a hefty dose of carbon black injected intravenously 2 hours earlier. The labeling of the venules is due to carbon particles leaking out during the emigration of lymphocytes. **Bar** = 1 mm. (Courtesy of Dr. G. I. Schoefl, The John Curtin School of Medical Research, The Australian National University, Canberra.)

NOTE: The growth cartilage of young bones is normally eroded by leaky vessels, so that carbon black that is injected intravenously leaks out (Figure 8.16) (21). Bacteria can probably do the same: this area is a favored site for bone infections (osteomyelitis) in children.

FIGURE 8.15 Autoradiograph of sections of two mice injected with radioactive bacilli (*Bacillus cereus*) 15 minutes and 3 hours before sacrifice. Note the high concentration of radioactivity in the organs that contain littoral phagocytes: the liver, spleen, and bone marrow (vertebrae, **arrows**). (Reproduced with permission from [7].)

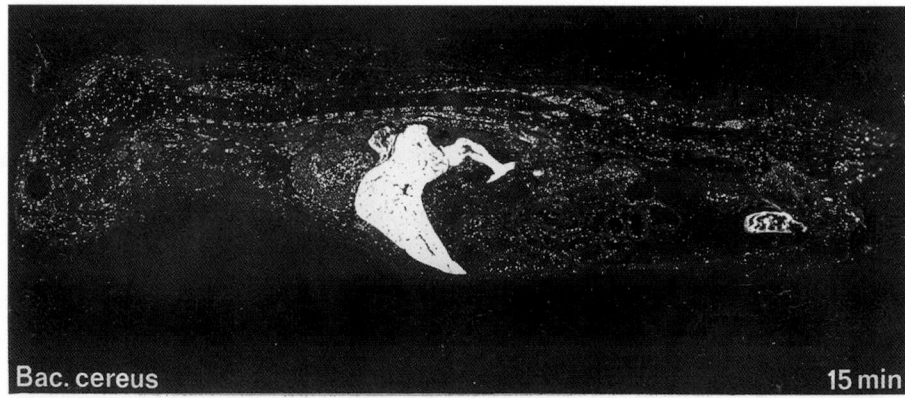

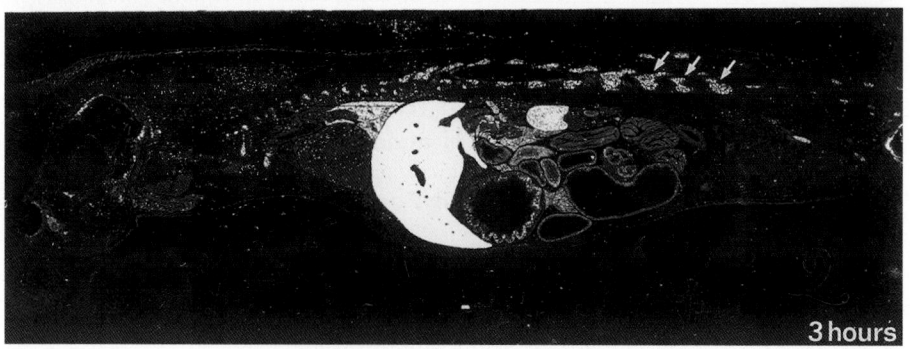

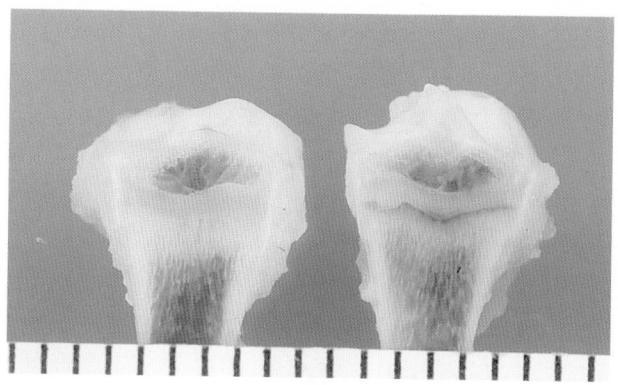

FIGURE 8.16   Upper end of the tibia of two newborn rats; cross section. *Left:* Control. *Right:* One hour after an intracardiac injection of carbon black. The deposition of carbon black along the growth cartilage indicates vascular leakage in this area, a normal condition. **Scale** in millimeters.

Mapping the RES with a Local Injection of Colloidal Particles

If a droplet of carbon black suspension is injected into the muscle or skin, most of it will remain in place, and the pigment will slowly be phagocytized by the macrophages of the connective tissue, with some reinforcements from the blood. This is, in essence, what tattoo artists do when they inject carbon black or other colloidal pigments into the skin. Blood monocytes attracted there by the trauma. These cells store the indigestible particles in their residual bodies until they die; at that time the debris will be taken up by other macrophages. A few particles will be swept into the lymphatics, especially during the trauma of tattooing, and will end their journey in the nearest filter: the regional lymph node. As a matter of fact, the filtering function of the lymph nodes was discovered by Virchow when performing the autopsy of a soldier who had a colored tattoo on the arm; the red cinnabar had persisted in the lymph node for nearly 50 years (47).

The lesson of this experiment is that *material injected into the tissues can find its way into the local lymphatic vessels and reach the regional lymph nodes.* This pathway is exploited in vaccination: the antigen is carried to the "antibody factory" in the lymph nodes.

Mapping the RES with Soluble Dyes Injected Intravenously

A favorite dye for this RES mapping experiment is Evans blue, which can also be used in humans to determine plasma volume. The dye binds to plasma albumin, so the result is much the same as that of injecting blue albumin. Water-soluble materials such as Evans blue, when injected intravenously, are taken up by all the macrophages in the body except those that lie beyond a blood-tissue barrier.

Trypan blue and Evans blue are traditionally used for this type of experiment simply because blue stands out well against the white skin of laboratory rodents. There is nothing magical about the blueness.

Do proteins cross the endothelium? Although the endothelium has the reputation of being a semipermeable barrier that is impermeable to protein, it is a fact that virtually all plasma proteins can be ferried across (however slowly) by transcytosis. This is true even for the large lipoprotein particles, which can be found in the tissue spaces. Furthermore, albumin is also taken up by specific receptors on the endothelial surface and then transcytosed (19, 40).

Over a few days a white rat or rabbit injected with Evans blue i.v. slowly turns blue because *all the phagocytes in the skin and connective tissues* pick up molecules of blue albumin emerging from the microcirculation. The circulating albumin–Evans blue complex is not recognized as extremely foreign by the littoral phagocytes, and its clearance is accordingly slower than that of carbon black (the clearance has not been studied in detail [25], but the dye probably remains in the circulation for more than 1 day). Of course, the littoral phagocytes are also blue; and once again, undigestible materials cannot escape from the RES: the animals will remain blue as long as they live.

It should be clear at this point that an intravenous injection of Evans blue demonstrates more macrophages than carbon black does. Besides the littoral phagocytes it demonstrates all the phagocytes in the connective tissue spaces *except those that lie behind blood-tissue barriers.* These are the blood-brain, blood-nerve, and blood-testis barriers and presumably also the blood-skin barrier (14) if its existence can be confirmed. At autopsy, the blue body of the rat or rabbit contrasts sharply with the bright white color of the brain and nerves (Figure 8.17).

The blood-skin barrier is intriguing. The evidence for such a barrier is the presence in the superficial capillaries of the dermis of the same marker that is present in brain capillaries (the P-glycoprotein or multidrug-resistance protein, p. 961). However, the skin does become blue in the Evans blue experiment; the role of this barrier is not yet clear.

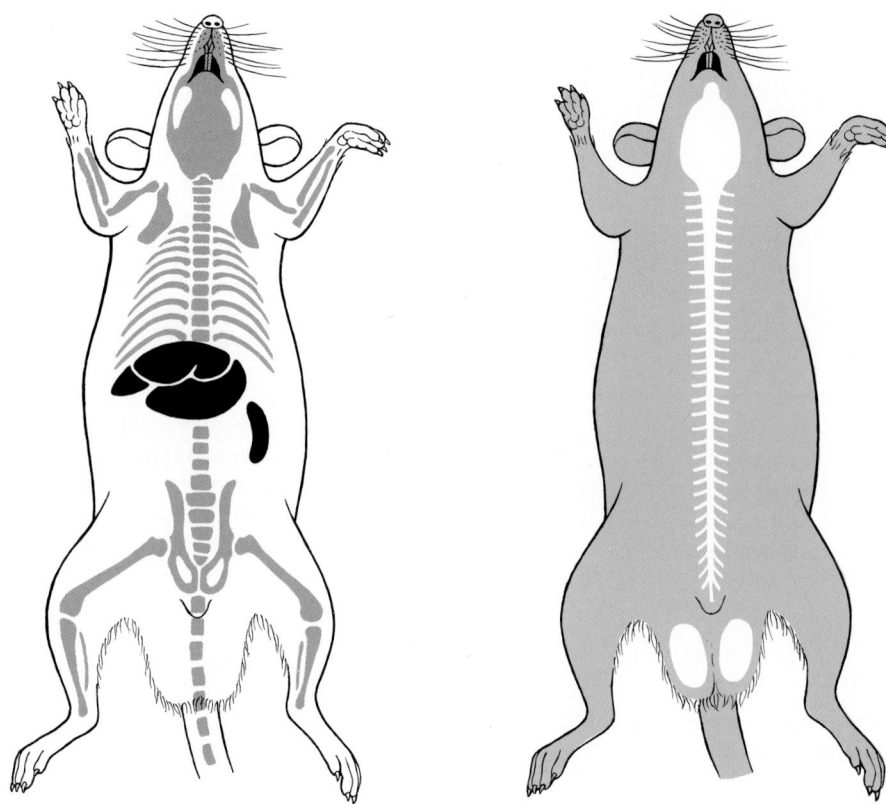

FIGURE 8.17   The fate of foreign materials carried by the bloodstream of a rat. *Left:* If the particles are too large to cross the normal endothelium (e.g., bacteria, or carbon black in the form of biological India ink), they are phagocytized by the littoral phagocytes in the liver, spleen, and bone marrow. In the lymph nodes (not shown), very little uptake occurs, and not by phagocytosis. *Right:* If the particles can be transported across normal endothelium (e.g., Evans blue dye, which binds to albumin), they will cross the endothelium throughout the body except where a blood–tissue barrier exists (in the brain, nerves, and testes). While in the bloodstream, these particles also are picked up by littoral phagocytes; once outside the vessels, they are picked up by interstitial macrophages.

In summary: to demonstrate the *littoral phagocytes* in the liver, spleen, and bone marrow, inject carbon black intravenously; to demonstrate the *phagocytes in the lymph nodes,* inject carbon black in the lymphatics (or in the tissues drained by those lymph nodes); to demonstrate *all phagocytes in the body* with one method is impossible, but Evans blue injected intravenously will eventually reach *all macrophages except those beyond the blood-tissue barriers.*

Some Highlights of RES Physiology

- *The role of blood flow.* It stands to reason that the littoral phagocytes can take up only what is delivered to them; therefore, in shock, when blood flow is poor, clearance is decreased (1).
- A few drugs and hormones such as small doses of steroids can increase phagocytosis (1).
- The system of littoral phagocytes can be a nuisance when it removes particles or molecules—such as

artificial red blood cells or enzymes for enzyme-deficient children—that the physician would like to circulate as long as possible. Recently it was discovered that the RES can be tricked: macromolecules such as enzymes are camouflaged with long, wavy molecules of polyethylene glycol. These "hairy" molecules become almost invisible to the RES because the so-called hairs, which are constantly in motion, tend to hide the surface sites that are usually recognized by the phagocytes (39).

The System of Phagocytes Comes of Age

Metchnikoff, who viewed his macrophages primarily as "big eaters" and named them accordingly, would be aghast to find out that phagocytosis is no longer seen as their main function. The insights of cell biology have proven macrophages to be secretory cells capable of manufacturing some 100 products, mainly cytokines, enough to compete with liver cells. Their local and general powers are mind-boggling: they can "present antigens" to lymphocytes and thereby initiate the immune response; they can stimulate the formation of new vessels and induce fibroblasts to produce collagen fibers; they can cause blood to clot and secrete cytokines that induce fever and sleep; in individuals with severe infections or malignant tumors they can even induce the miserable condition called *cachexia,* whereby the whole body withers away (they do so by secreting a factor called *cachexin* or *tumor necrosis factor*). And for a final bow, macrophages can pick up almost anything and become scavengers to clean up the place.

The Concept of Inflammation: Still Expanding

The 5000-year-old concept of inflammation sprouted several new branches; two are especially worthy of mention.

Neurogenic Inflammation

Obviously nerves take part in inflammation; witness the red flare that develops around a scratch on the skin (see the Triple Response, p. 385). Acetylcholine, the main parasympathetic neurotransmitter, inhibits inflammation; it even *deactivates activated macrophages;* stimulation of the vagus nerve also deactivates macrophages and inhibits the secretion of TNF by liver cells (44a). Oddly enough, pain and stress generate epinephrine and norepinephrine, which also inhibit macrophage activation, while increasing the secretion of interleukin 10, a powerful antiinflammatory cytokine: so here we have the sympathetic and parasympathetic systems working (unusually) in unison (44a).

But nerves can also *cause* inflammation. Nerve endings produce neuropeptides such as neurokinins and substance P ("P" stands for permeability), which degranulate mast cells (19a). Actually, this is the field of research now known as *neurogenic inflammation* (34a). It was founded in the 1960s by a pioneering Hungarian physician, N. Jancsó; it led to the discovery of capsaicin, the active principle of pepper (and paprika) and of substance P. A key observation is that if a sensory nerve of a rat is cut and the distal end is electrically stimulated (antidromically), plasma leakage from the venules and a mild leukocytic exudation occur in the corresponding field. In recent years, D. McDonald and collaborators produced beautiful light and electron microscopic studies showing venular leakage in the rat trachea after nerve stimulation (34b, 34c).

Whole Body Inflammation

This title may sound self-contradictory (how can a local process be generalized?), but it was successfully introduced in the 1960s by clinicians concerned with circulatory shock. The reason is straightforward: inflammation as a local phenomenon is driven by chemical mediators, and if these are poured into the bloodstream, serious trouble can develop, namely the life-threatening brand of shock called **s**ystemic **i**nflammatory **r**eaction **s**yndrome, or **SIRS** (p. 725).

> TO SUM UP: A recurring theme in this chapter is the elegance of simple experiments. The basic cellular events of inflammation—phagocytosis, diapedesis, and vascular leakage—were worked out with what we now call low-tech means: a monocular microscope, some starfish, sand flies, a rose thorn, the tongue of a live fog. Cohnheim did not illustrate his classic papers on diapedesis because—he wrote—the experiments are so simple that anybody can repeat them. Indeed, the main ingredient was thinking.

Inflammation: A Pictorial Overview

In the next 9 pages we will present a selection of microscopic views representing acute and chronic inflammation. We have two purposes in mind: (1) begin to familiarize the reader with one of the basic processes in general pathology; and (2) offer an opportunity to practice the fine art of interpreting a microscopic panorama. In the standard histologic sections stained with hematoxylin and eosin, there is no motion and no life: the reader must learn to fill in the motion. The task includes art and science. Each illustration will raise a number of questions, to be addressed in the next five chapters (Figures 8.18 to 8.31).

FIGURE 8.18 *Acute inflammation in the lung* produced experimentally by dripping a biological irritant (C5a desArg, a side product of complement activation) into a bronchus. *Top:* Normal rabbit lung with a few "resident" alveolar macrophages. *Middle:* 6 hours after irritation: the alveoli are filled with exudate, i.e., neutrophils in a protein-rich fluid (this condition of alveolar filling is known as *pneumonia* or *pneumonitis*). *Bottom:* Twenty-four to 48 hours later the neutrophils are replaced by macrophages, a sequence typical of acute inflammation. Once the irritant has disappeared, the exudate can be cleared out in a few days. In the lung, inflammatory exudate gathers at first within the thickness of the alveolar walls, but these are very tight spaces; soon the exudate spills out into the alveoli, as shown here. There is no visible damage to the lung tissue; this mild inflammatory response is entirely reversible. **Bar** = 50 μm. (Reproduced, with permission, from the Annual Review of Immunology, Vol. 1, © 1983 by Annual Reviews Inc. [29].)

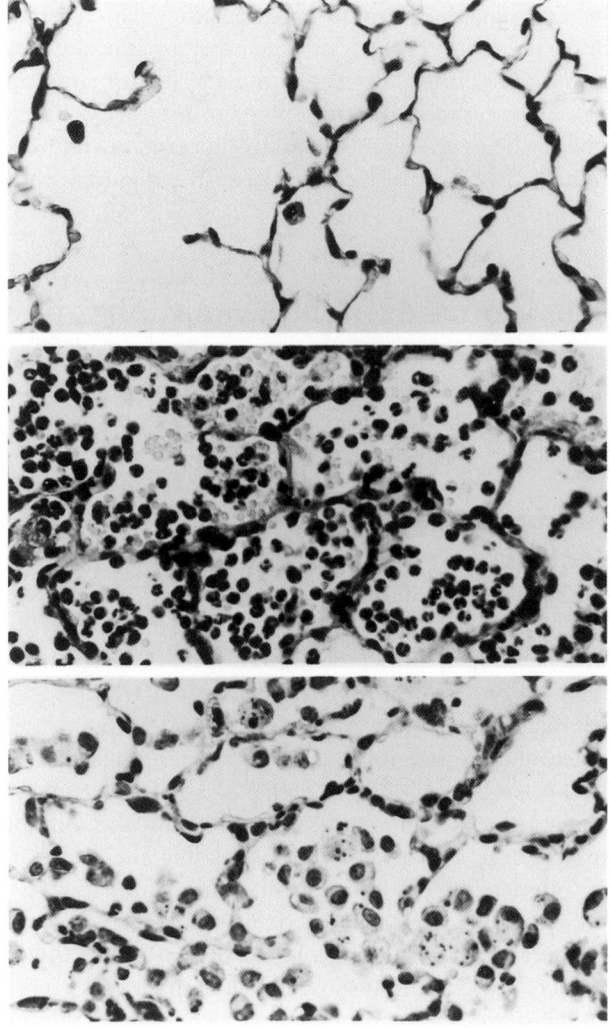

FIGURE 8.19 Biopsy of a pustule ("pimple"). Pustules are caused by bacteria on or in the epidermis. The bacteria attract a swarm of neutrophils, which emigrate from the venules in the dermis, crawl up into the epidermis, and form a droplet of pus beneath the horny layer. The detached horny layer appears here as a pencil line. The granular material beneath it is pus. (Preparation courtesy of Dr. A. B. Ackerman.)

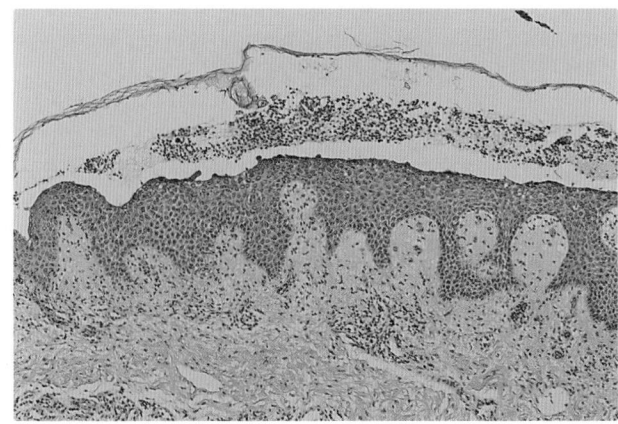

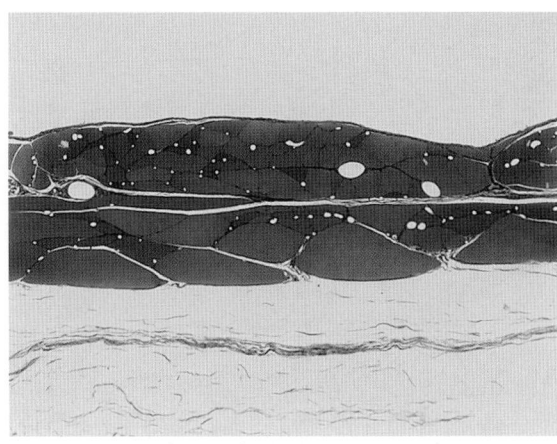
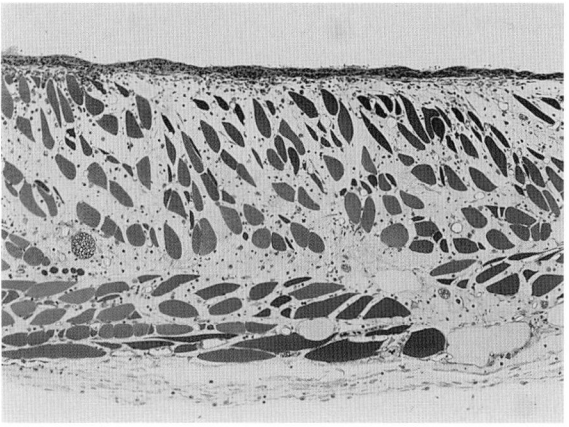

FIGURE 8.20 *Acute inflammation in a striated muscle. Left:* Control normal rat muscle. The muscle fibers, seen in cross section, are tightly packed (the vessels are open and empty because the tissue was fixed by perfusion). *Right:* Similar muscle after 2 days of exposure to an aseptic irritant (a piece of rat liver, not shown). The space between the muscle fibers represents edema; the cells free in this space indicate that this edema is inflammatory. The muscle fibers have shrunk (mechanism unclear). The number of fibroblasts seems normal, suggesting that the inflammation has not lasted long enough to stimulate their proliferation; they require 2–3 days to become visibly increased. (60x)

The main point: inflamed tissue becomes swollen with exudate, with some damage to the local parenchymal cells. If this inflammatory process were allowed to continue for another few days, the edema would be partly replaced by fibrous tissue.

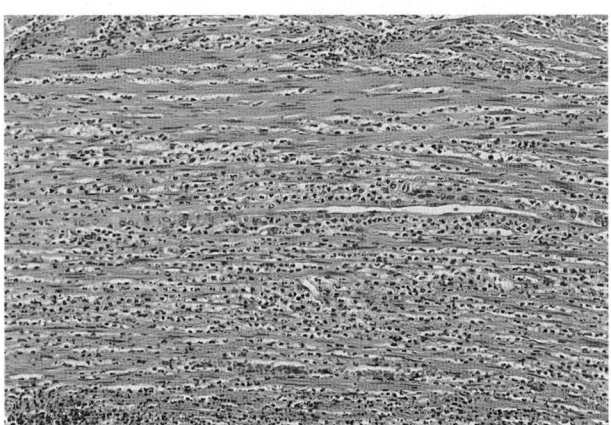
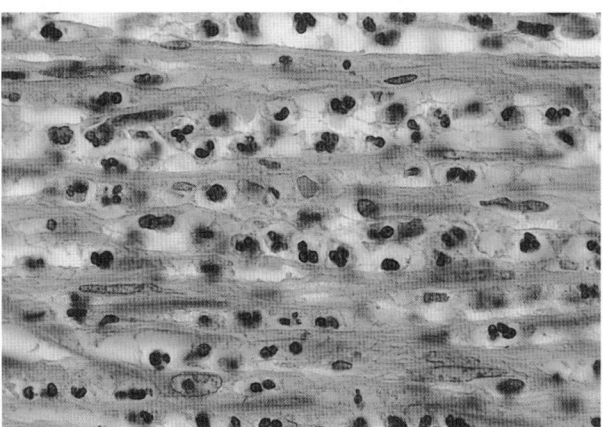

FIGURE 8.21 *Acute appendicitis.* The appendix becomes inflamed when bacteria contained in the lumen penetrate into the mucosa and spread centrifugally into the muscular and serosal layers. *Left:* The muscular wall of the appendix: a dramatic view of smooth muscle tissue overrun by an army of leukocytes chasing an invisible horde of bacteria. (120x) *Right:* A higher power shows that the cells packed between the muscle fibers are granulocytes (neutrophils), recognizable by their multilobed nucleus. (350x) In this and in most other bacterial infections the inflammatory response is obvious, but the bacteria are difficult to see unless special stains are used.

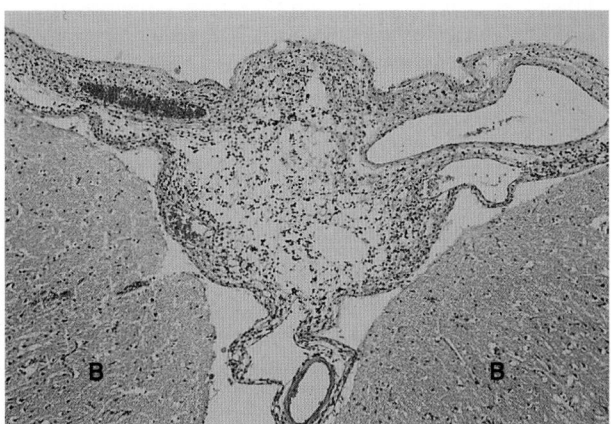

FIGURE 8.22 *Meningococcal meningitis.* Another example of bacteria attracting swarms of leukocytes. The branching structure at center and top is part of the meninges. Beneath it, the brain tissue (**B**) in this field is normal, but sometimes its outer layer does become inflamed. Bacteria are not visible at this enlargement.

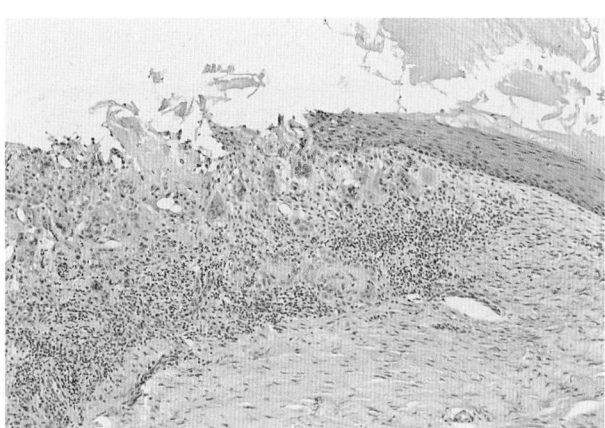

FIGURE 8.23 *Chronic aseptic inflammation in the skin* around an epidermal cyst that broke open. Epidermal cysts (wens) are common; they are spheres lined by epidermis with its horny layer inward, which explains why they are filled with desquamated cornified cells. Most of these cysts derive from hair follicles, a few arise by traumatic displacement of epidermal cells. When they break open, their aseptic content spills into the connective tissue and becomes a persistent irritant: it attracts a population of macrophages, some of which become multinucleated giant cells. All these cells contribute to phagocytize and eliminate the foreign material. The lumen of the cyst is at the top, with epithelial squames. To the right, the lining of the cyst is broken: the exposed content induced an intense, chronic inflammatory reaction (seen as a mass of basophilic cells). Among the macrophages, the large pink foreign body giant cells represent a response to the dead keratinized cells. The main points: chronic inflammatory exudates contain mostly mononuclear cells. Foreign bodies induce the formation of giant cells.

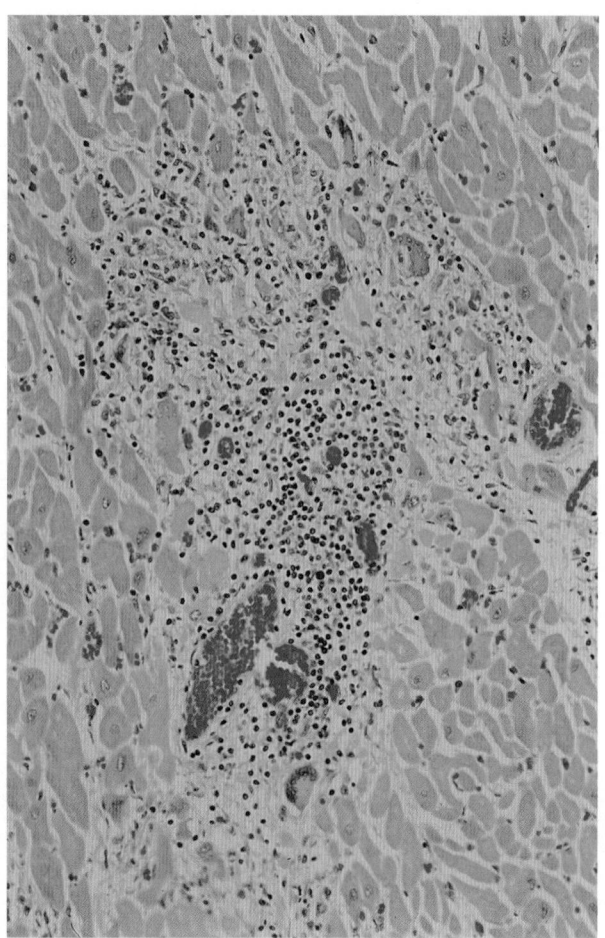

FIGURE 8.24 *Chronic, focal inflammation in the heart* (*myocarditis,* probably viral). *Lower center:* Two congested venules. Around and especially above them, a dense inflammatory infiltrate consisting mainly of lymphocytes. *Lower right:* Myocardium.

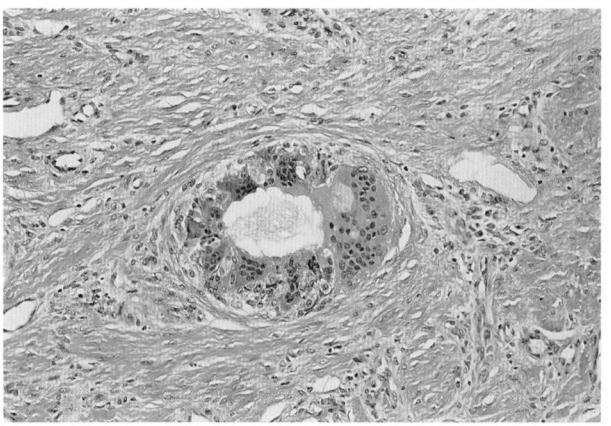

FIGURE 8.25 *Granulomatous inflammation* (*chronic*). When the irritant consists of tiny "quanta" dispersed in the tissues and difficult to eliminate, the inflammatory response consists mainly of clusters of macrophages called granulomas, gathered around each "quantum" of the irritant. Multinucleated cells are often present. This granuloma was caused by urate crystals in a case of gout.

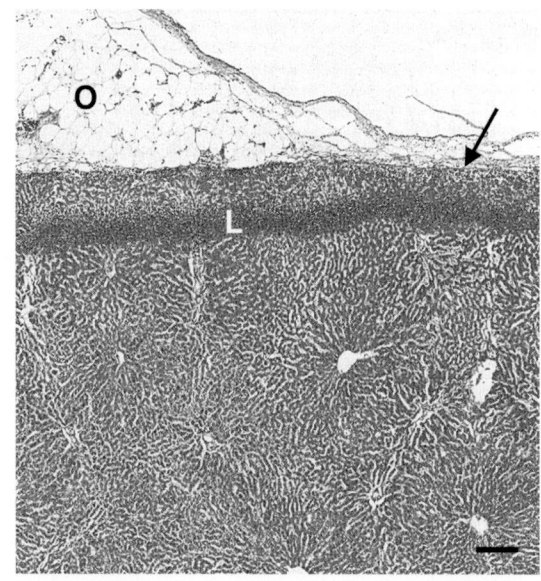

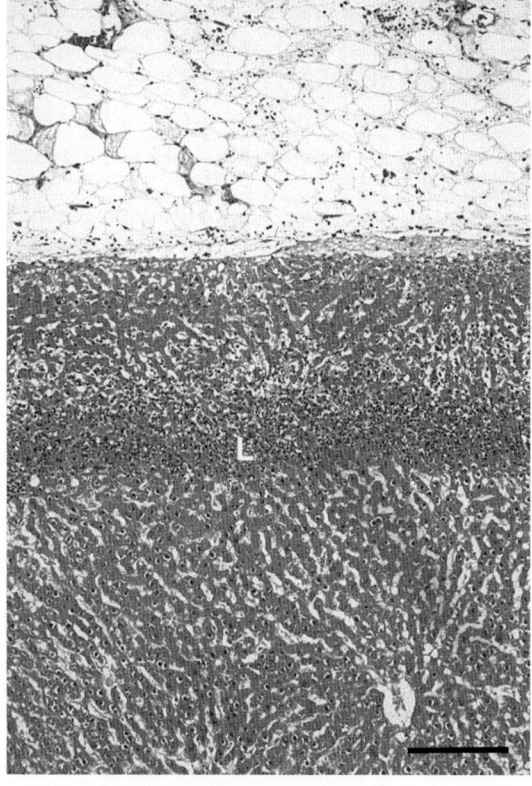

FIGURE 8.26   Stage: 1 day

DIAGRAM OF FIGURE 8.26 (top)   Stage: 1 day

FIGURE 8.26   *Top:* The liver implant, which by now is necrotic, is covered by the omentum (**O**) to which it is firmly glued by a layer of fibrin not visible at this enlargement. **Arrow:** Surface of the liver. The dark horizontal layer represents a cemetery of leukocytes: the blood vessels of the omentum, irritated by materials seeping from the dying tissue, have supplied swarms of leukocytes that penetrated into the liver implant. Note that all the leukocytes die very nearly at the same depth, probably where they run out of oxygen. *Bottom:* The leukocytes (**L**) appear as dots between the necrotic, coagulated liver cords.

FIGURES 8.26–8.31   *Inflammation around dead tissue.* This is a common setting of inflammation, because masses of tissue often die of inadequate blood flow (the process called *infarction*). Dying and dead tissue, even if aseptic, is an irritant and elicits acute, aseptic inflammation, which becomes chronic and ends with the removal of the mass and the formation of a scar; this removal process is called "organization." To illustrate this sequence we simulated an infarct by implanting a piece of sterile rat liver into the abdominal cavity of another rat. Under these conditions, the implant is promptly wrapped up by the omentum, a thin connective tissue membrane that hangs like an apron from the transverse colon. The omentum is highly vascularized and sets up an inflammatory response. Six stages are shown; *each stage is represented by a topographic view (top) and by a higher power (bottom).* **Bars** = 200 μm. Adjacent to each topographic view is a diagram showing its main features.

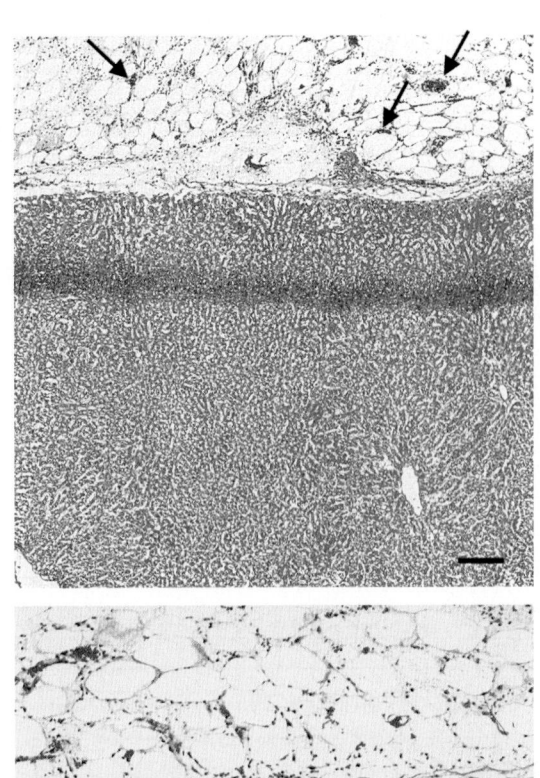

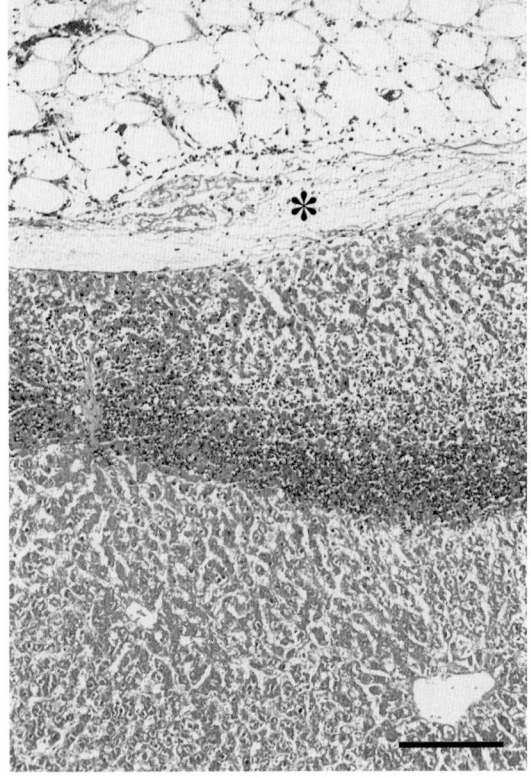

FIGURE 8.27   Stage: 2 days

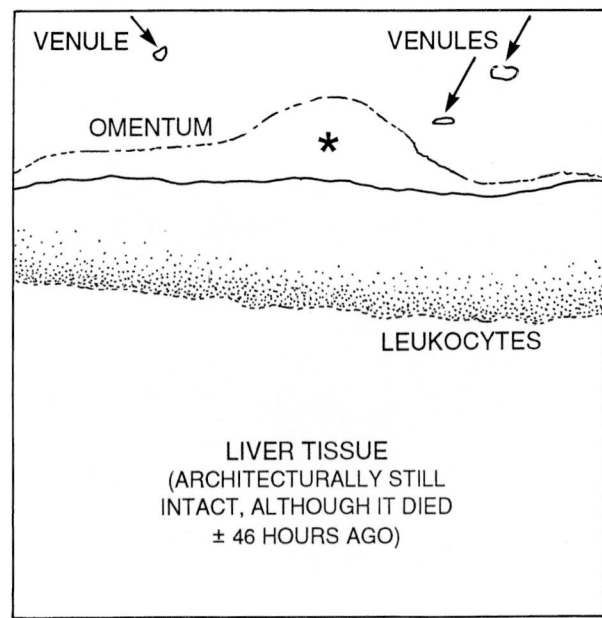

VENULE

VENULES

OMENTUM

*

LEUKOCYTES

LIVER TISSUE
(ARCHITECTURALLY STILL
INTACT, ALTHOUGH IT DIED
± 46 HOURS AGO)

DIAGRAM OF FIGURE 8.27 (top)   Stage: 2 days

FIGURE 8.27   *Top:* The omentum is visibly inflamed: it is peppered with inflammatory cells, and its venules are congested (**arrows**); they are the source of the emigrating leukocytes. *Bottom:* In the space between omentum and liver (**asterisk**) the thready material is fibrin, a polymer of a protein supplied by the blood as fibrinogen; it serves as a glue between the omentum and the dead tissue.

The main points: tissues that are dying or died recently attract leukocytes—which are doomed to die frustrated, because they find no bacteria to phagocytize. The omentum is rich in vessels, which are essential to its defensive function.

FIGURES 8.26–8.31   (*Continued*)

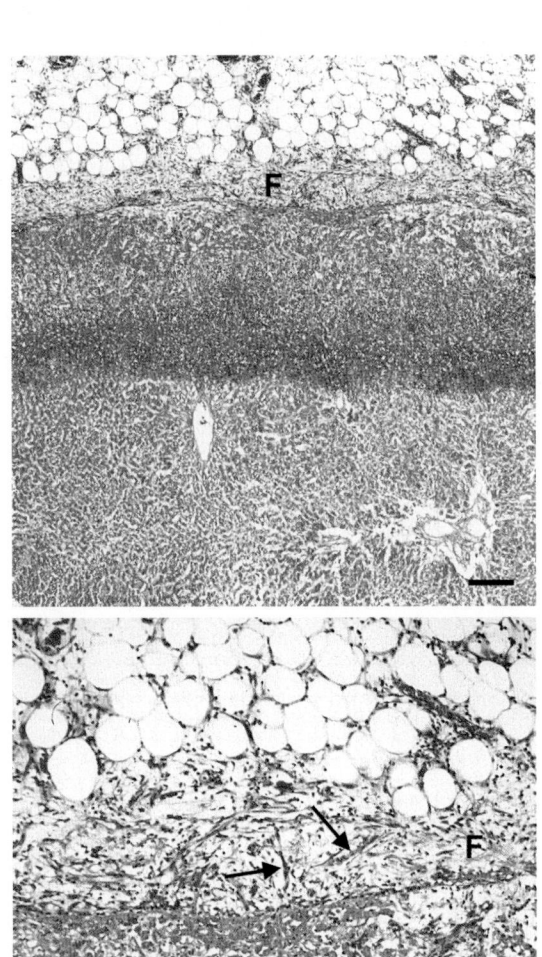

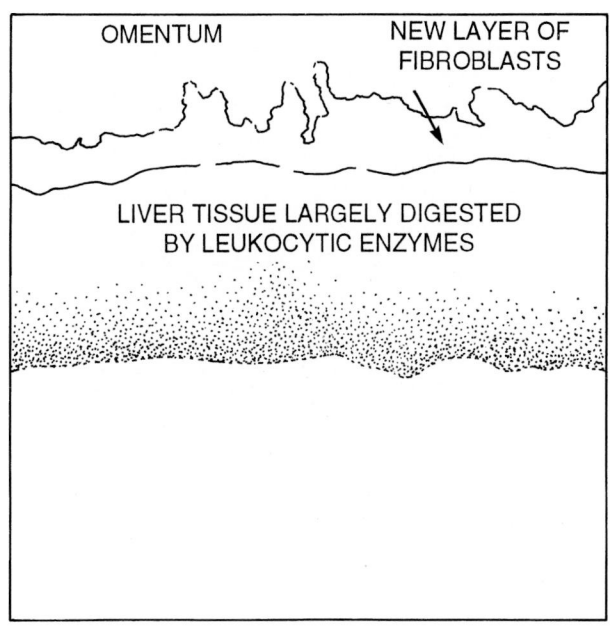

DIAGRAM OF FIGURE 8.28 (top)   Stage: 3 days

FIGURE 8.28   *Top: The salient novelty is the proliferation of fibroblasts* (**F**), which are now forming a new layer between the omentum and the dead tissue. This layer is the beginning of what will become "granulation tissue." The fibroblasts are supplied by the omentum as a component of the inflammatory response. The dark band of leukocytes is still there: new waves of leukocytes are probably still arriving. *Bottom:* The zone of fibroblast proliferation (**F**) contains streaks of nuclei (**arrows**), which represent capillary buds sprouting from the omentum.

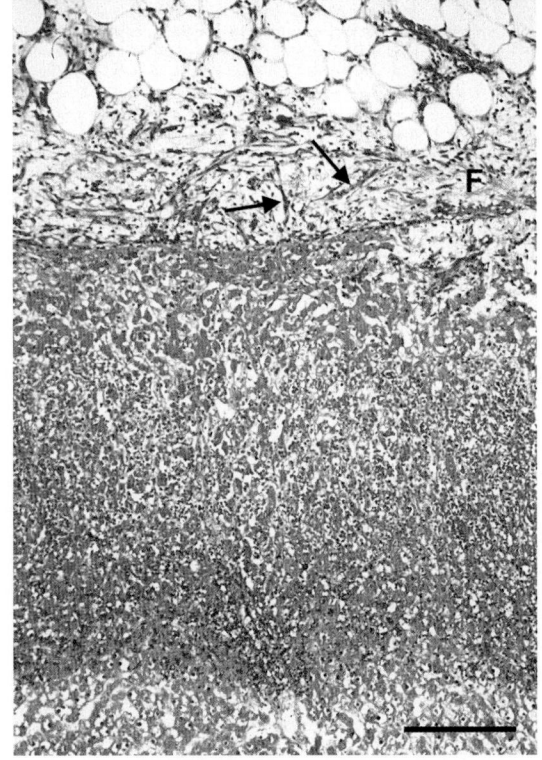

FIGURE 8.28   Stage: 3 days

FIGURES 8.26–8.31   (*Continued*)

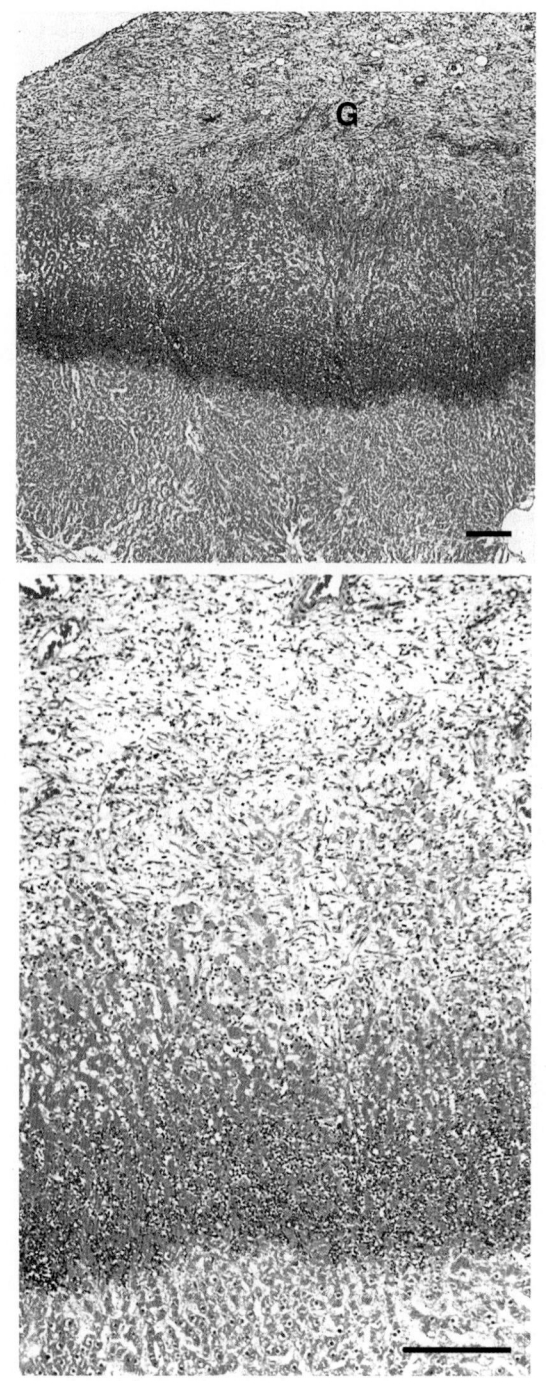

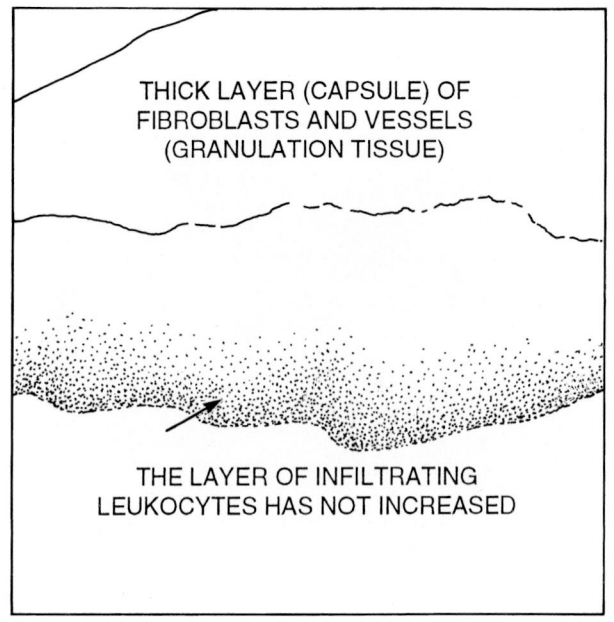

DIAGRAM OF FIGURE 8.29 (top)   Stage: 7 days

FIGURE 8.29   *Top:* The layer of fibroblasts has evolved into a thick layer of young connective tissue called *granulation tissue* (**G**) (young because it is rich in cells and sprouting vessels). This newly formed tissue behaves as a temporary organ, which (in this particular example) is responsible for removing the necrotic mass. *Bottom:* Detail showing how the granulation tissue begins to erode the surface of the necrotic mass (compare with the figure at left). This erosion is accomplished mainly by the phagocytic activity of macrophages, not well recognizable at this enlargement.

FIGURE 8.29   Stage: 7 days

FIGURES 8.26–8.31   *(Continued)*

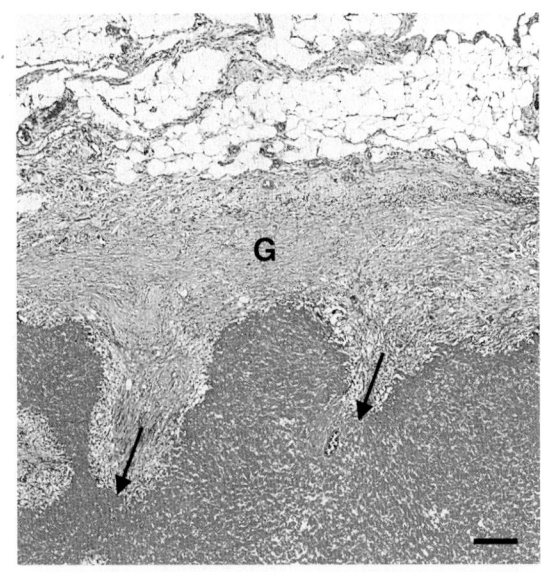

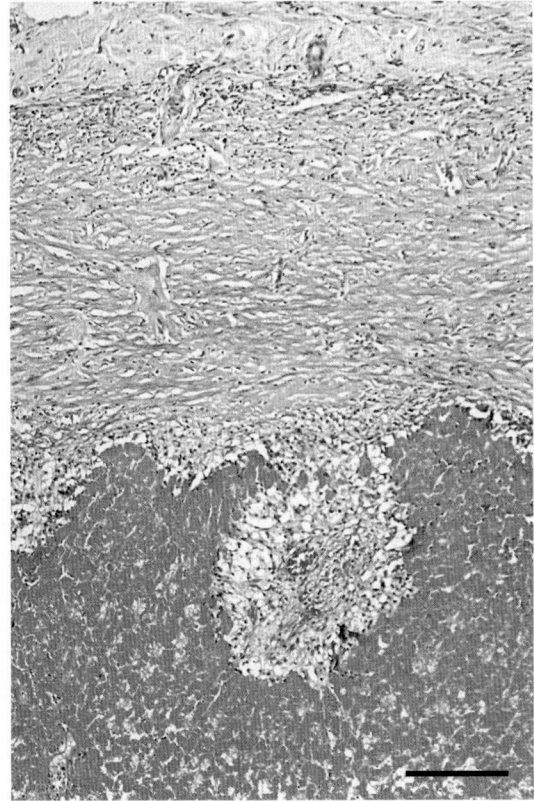

FIGURE 8.30   Stage: 1 month

OMENTUM

GRANULATION TISSUE
PENETRATING INTO
THE NECROTIC MASS

UNRECOGNIZABLE,
COAGULATED
LIVER TISSUE

DIAGRAM OF FIGURE 8.30 (top)   Stage: 1 month

FIGURE 8.30   *Top:* It is now obvious that the granulation tissue (**G**) is invading and reabsorbing (**arrows**) the necrotic mass. Note that this mass no longer contains a layer of leukocytes: it is fully coagulated (denatured) and has ceased to emit chemical messages that attract leukocytes. Its removal is entirely dependent on the granulation tissue. *Bottom:* Note the high number of cells in the granulation tissue in comparison with Figure 8.31.

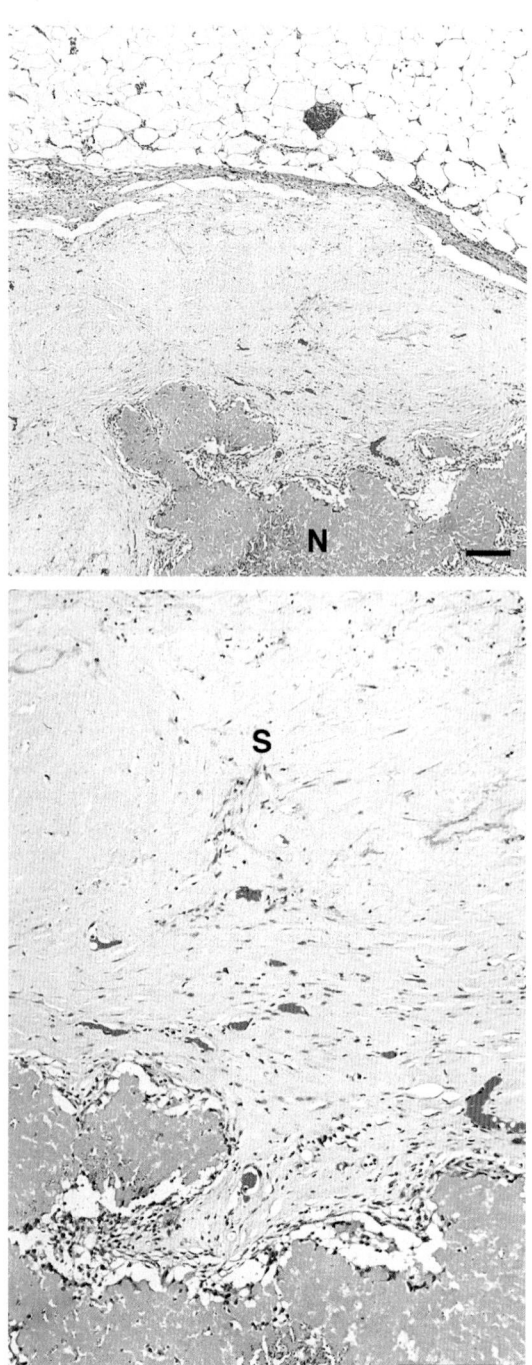

FIGURE 8.31   Stage: 13 months

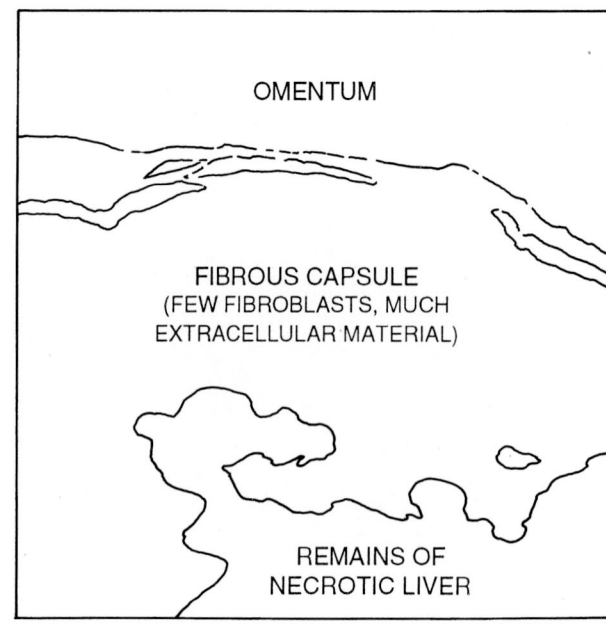

OMENTUM

FIBROUS CAPSULE
(FEW FIBROBLASTS, MUCH
EXTRACELLULAR MATERIAL)

REMAINS OF
NECROTIC LIVER

DIAGRAM OF FIGURE 8.31 (top)   Stage: 13 months

FIGURE 8.31   *Top:* The former granulation tissue appears clearer because it has lost most of its cells and capillaries and has acquired more collagen fibers. It has become a fibrous scar (**S**). The persistence of some necrotic material (**N**) at this late stage suggests that not much reabsorption is occurring, as might also be guessed from the structural change of the granulation tissue. Surprisingly, the outlines of liver tissue are still recognizable. Special stains would show that the necrotic mass is partly calcified. *Bottom:* The loss of cells in the former granulation tissue is obvious (compare with Figure 8.30).

The main point: granulation tissue—when its defensive (or reabsorptive) function is accomplished—matures into a fibrous scar. In this experiment, what was once one cubic centimeter of dead liver tissue has become a pinhead of mummified, calcified material wrapped in a fibrous capsule. A job well done.

References

1. Altura BM. Relationship of reticuloendothelial cell function to microcirculatory blood flow and low-flow states. In: Altura BM, Saba TM (eds). Pathophysiology of the reticuloendothelial system. New York: Raven Press, 1981, pp. 159–208.

2. Aschoff L. Lectures on pathology. New York: Paul B. Hoeber, Inc., 1924.

3. Baltch AL, Schaffer C, Hammer MC, et al. Bacteremia following dental cleaning in patients with and without penicillin prophylaxis. Am Heart J 1982;104:1335–1339.

4. Benacerraf B. Quantitative aspects of phagocytosis. In: Brauer RW (ed). Liver function. A symposium on approaches to the quantitative description of liver function. Washington: American Institute of Biological Sciences, 1958, pp. 205–234.

5. Biozzi G, Benacerraf B, Halpern BN. Quantitative study of the granulopectic activity of the reticulo-endothelial system. II. A study of the kinetics of the granulopectic activity of the R.E.S. in relation to the dose of carbon injected Relationship between the weight of the organs and their activity. Br J Exp Pathol 1953;34:441–457.

6. Biozzi G, Benacerraf B, Halpern BN, Stiffel C, Hillemand B. Exploration of the phagocytic function of the reticulo-endothelial system with heat denatured human serum albumin labeled with I^{131} and application to the measurement of liver blood flow, in normal man and in some pathologic conditions. J Lab Clin Med 1958;51:230–239.

7. Bonventre PF, Nordberg BK, Schmiterlöw CG. An autoradiographic study of radioactively labelled Bacillus cereus in the mouse. Acta Pathol Microbiol Scand 1961;51:157–163.

8. Brain JD. Physiology and pathophysiology of pulmonary macrophages. In: Reichard SM, Filkins JP (eds). The reticuloendothelial system. A comprehensive treatise, vol. 7B, Physiology. New York: Plenum Press, 1985, pp. 315–337.

9. Brain JD. Macrophages in the respiratory tract. In: Fishman AP, Fisher AB (eds). Handbook of physiology. Section 3: The respiratory system, vol. 1. Bethesda: American Physiological Society, 1985, pp. 447–471.

10. Buchanan JW, Wagner HN Jr. Regional phagocytosis in man. In: Reichard SM, Filkins JP. (eds). The reticulo-endothelial system. A comprehensive treatise, vol. 7B, Physiology. New York: Plenum Press, 1985, pp. 247–270.

11. Cohnheim J. Ueber Entzündung und Eiterung. Virchows Arch Pathol Anat Physiol Klin Med 1867;40:1–79.

12. Cohnheim J. Untersuchungen über die embolischen Processe. Berlin: Verlag von August Hirschwald, 1872.

13. Cohnheim J. Lectures in general pathology, 2nd ed, vol. 1 (translated from the second German edition). London: The New Sydenham Society, 1889.

14. Cordon-Cardo C, O'Brien JP, Casals D, et al. Multidrug-resistance gene (P-glycoprotein) is expressed by endothelial cells at blood-brain barrier sites. Proc Natl Acad Sci USA 1989;86:695–698.

15. Dutrochet MH. Recherches anatomiques et physiologiques sur la structure intime des animaux et des végétaux, et sur leur motilité. Paris: JB Baillière, 1824.

16. Florey HW. General pathology. Philadelphia: W.B. Saunders Co., 1970.

17. Friedman H, Escobar M, Reichard SM (series eds). The reticuloendothelial system: A comprehensive treatise. New York: Plenum Press, 1980–1988.

18. Gallin JI, Snyderman R (eds). Inflammation. Basic principles and clinical correlates, 3rd ed. Philadelphia: Lippincott Williams & Wilkins, 1999, pp. 865–881.

19. Ghinea N, Eskenasy M, Simionescu M, Simionescu N. Endothelial albumin binding proteins are membrane-associated components exposed on the cell surface. J Biol Chem 1989;264:4755–4758.

19a. Granstein RD. Neuropeptides in inflammation and immunity. In: Gallin JI, Snyderman R (eds). Inflammation. Basic principles and clinical correlates, 3rd ed. Philadelphia: Lippincott Williams & Wilkins. 1999, pp. 397–404.

20. Halpern BN, Benacerraf B, Biozzi G. Quantitative study of the granulopectic activity of the reticulo-endothelial system. I: The effect of the ingredients present in India ink and of substances affecting blood clotting in vivo on the fate of carbon particles administered intravenously in rats, mice and rabbits. Br J Exp Pathol 1953;34:426–440.

21. Ham KN, Hurley JV, Ryan GB, Storey E. Localization of particulate carbon in metaphyseal vessels of growing rats. Aust J Exp Biol Med Sci 1965;43:625–638.

22. Hamburger MI, Fields TR, Gerardi EN, Bennett RS. Assessment of reticuloendothelial system function in man using receptor specific probes. Adv Inflamm Res 1983;5:67–85.

23. Henson PM, Henson JE, Fittschen C, et al. Phagocytic cells: degranulation and secretion. In: Gallin JI, Goldstein IM, Snyderman R (eds). Inflammation: Basic principles and clinical correlates. New York: Raven Press, 1988, pp. 363–390.

24. Hirsch JG, Hirsch BI. Metchnikoff's life and scientific contributions in historical perspective. In: Karnovsky ML, Bolis L (eds). Phagocytosis—past and future. New York: Academic Press, 1982, pp. 1–12.

25. Hunsaker WG. Determination of Evans Blue in avian plasma by protein precipitation and extraction. Proc Soc Exp Biol Med 1965;120:747–749.

26. Hunter J. A treatise on the blood, inflammation, and gunshot wounds. London: John Richardson, 1794.

27. Joris I, Cuénoud HF, Doern GV, Underwood JM, Majno G. Capillary leakage in inflammation. A study by vascular labeling. Am J Pathol 1990;137:1353–1363.

28. Kowala MC. Acute inflammation of the lymph node. Ph.D. thesis, The Australian National University, 1982.

29. Larsen GL, Henson PM. Mediators of inflammation. Annu Rev Immunol 1983;1:335–359.

30. Lasser A. The mononuclear phagocytic system: a review. Hum Pathol 1983;14:108–126.

31. Lister J. On a new method of treating compound fracture, abscess, &c, with observations on the conditions of suppuration (Lancet, 1:326, 357, 387, 507; 2:95; 1867). In: The collected papers of Joseph, Baron Lister, 2 vols. Oxford: Clarendon Press, 1909, pp. 1–36.

31a. Long ER. A history of pathology. New York: Dover Publications, Inc., 1965, pp. 128–132.

32. Majno G. The healing hand. Man and wound in the ancient world. Cambridge: Harvard University Press, 1975.

33. Majno G. Inflammation and infection: historic highlights. In: Majno G, Cotran RS, Kaufman N (eds). Current topics in inflammation and infection. Baltimore: Williams & Wilkins, 1982, pp. 1–17.

34. Majno G, Joris I. The microscope in the history of pathology. Virchows Arch Abt A Pathol Anat 1973;360:273–286.

34a. McDonald DM. The concept of neurogenic inflammation in the respiratory tract. In: Kaliner MA, Barnes PJ, Kunkel GHH, Baraniuk JN (eds). Neuropeptides in respiratory medicine. New York: Marcel Dekker, Inc 1994, pp. 321–349.

34b. McDonald DM. Endothelial gaps and permeability of venules in rat tracheas exposed to inflammatory stimuli. Am J Physiol 1994(Lung Cell Mol Physiol 10);266:L61–L83.

34c. McDonald DM., Mitchell RA, Gabella G, Haskell A. Neurogenic inflammation in the rat trachea. II. Identity and distribution of nerves mediating the increase in vascular permeability. J Neurocytol 1988;17:605–628.

35. Metchnikoff E. Ueber eine Sprosspilzkrankheit der Daphnien. Beitrag zur Lehre über den Kampf der Phagocyten gegen Krankheitserreger. Virchows Arch Pathol Anat Physiol Klin Med 1884;96:177–195.

36. Metchnikoff E. Lectures on the comparative pathology of inflammation (translated from the French by FA Starling and EH Starling, MD), 1893. (Reproduced by Dover Publications, Inc., New York, 1968).

37. Metchnikoff O. Life of Elie Metchnikoff 1845–1916. Boston: Houghton Mifflin Company, 1921.

38. Nopajaroonsri C, Luk SC, Simon GT. The passage of intravenously injected colloidal carbon into lymph node parenchyma. Lab Invest 1974;30:533–538.

38a. Paul WE. Fundamental immunology. 4th ed. Philadelphia: Lippincott-Raven Publishers, 1999.

39. Pool R. PEG-treated enzymes are nearly invisible to the immune system. Science 1990;248:305.

40. Predescu D, Simionescu M, Simionescu N, Palade GE. Binding and transcytosis of glycoalbumin by the microvascular endothelium of the murine myocardium: evidence that glycoalbumin behaves as a bifunctional ligand. J Cell Biol 1988;107:1729–1738.

41. Rather LJ. Addison and the white corpuscles: An aspect of nineteenth-century biology. London: Wellcome Institute of the History of Medicine, 1972.

42. Roitt IM. Essential immunology, 6th ed. Oxford: Blackwell Scientific Publications, 1988.

43. Saba TM. Physiology and physiopathology of the reticuloendothelial system. Arch Intern Med 1970;126:1031–1052.

44. Schoefl GI. Structure and permeability of venules in lymphoid tissue. In: Société Française de Microscopie Electronique: Septième Congrès International de Microscopie Électronique, Grenoble, 1970, pp. 589–590.

44a. Tracey KJ. The inflammatory reflex. Nature 2002;420: 853–859.

45. Traub A, Giebink GS, Smith C, et al. Splenic reticuloendothelial function after splenectomy, spleen repair, and spleen autotransplantation. N Engl J Med 1987;317: 1559–1564.

46. van Furth R, Cohn ZA, Hirsch JG, et al. The mononuclear phagocyte system: a new classification of macrophages, monocytes, and their precursor cells. Bull WHO 1972;46:845–852.

47. Virchow R. Cellular pathology (translated from the second German edition by B. Chance), 1859. Reproduced by Dover Publications, New York: 1971, p. 182.

48. Waller A. Microscopic examination of some of the principal tissues of the animal frame, as observed in the tongue of the living frog, toad, &c. Lond Edinb Dublin Philo Magazine J Sci 1846;3:271–287.

49. Warner AE, Brain JD. Intravascular pulmonary macrophages: a novel cell removes particles from blood. Am J Physiol 1986;250:R728–R732.

50. Yamaguchi K, Schoefl GI. Blood vessels of the Peyer's patch in the mouse: II. In vivo observations. Anat Rec 1983;206: 403–417.

INFLAMMATION: THE ACTORS AND THEIR LANGUAGE

- The Actors of Inflammation
- Mediators: The Chemical Language of Inflammation

On a battle field we would expect to find three types of populations: the aggressors, the defenders, and the local people as innocent bystanders. In a focus of inflammation the setting is quite similar. The aggressor is not always apparent microscopically: it might be an invisible toxic chemical or a virus (even bacteria, as we saw in Chapter 8, are not always obvious). So the defending cells tend to dominate the field, at least visually; they belong to about 11 types (Table 9.1), and keep in touch by means of chemical messages, the mediators of inflammation, which include agents lethal for attacking cells. As for the local population of parenchymal cells, it is caught in the crossfire and suffers, sometimes more, sometimes less; but it does voice its involvement by producing chemical messages of its own.

The Actors of Inflammation

To pursue the military metaphor we should speak of the "soldiers" of inflammation: we prefer to adopt a more peaceful tone, and consider inflammation as a play with a cast of 11 main characters. Each type of inflammatory cell is specialized in some way, and therefore not all are called upon at every inflammatory occasion; plasma cells do not appear unless antibody formation is involved, eosinophils participate only in certain settings, and so on. *All 11 cell types are normally quiescent and become activated in the inflammatory focus; all have subtypes; and all 11 can produce inflammatory mediators.*

It is essential to know, at least in outline, what each cell type is programmed to do, so a short biography of each one follows. A large book is available for those who may want to know more (33).

Table 9.1 Inflammation: The Cellular Actors

Cell Type	Major Functions
Neutrophils	First line of defense against bacteria; not found in normal tissues; *end cells*
Eosinophils	Can kill worms; cause damage
Monocytes/macrophages (Mφ)	Key cells of *chronic, adaptive* inflammation; synthesize dozens of mediators; bactericidal; *long-lived*
Platelets	Upkeep of normal endothelium; key roles in blood clotting, hemostasis, thrombosis; source of preformed mediators
Mast cells/basophils	Related but not identical cells; loaded with histamine, can produce many cytokines. Triggers of acute inflammation.
T lymphocytes	T-cell immune responses; secrete cytokines; kill cells
B lymphocytes	B-cell immune responses; produce antibodies; become plasma cells
NK cells	Cell killing not dependent on the immune response
Dendritic cells	Antigen presentation
Endothelium	Mediates exchanges of fluid and cells between blood and tissues
Fibroblasts	Produce matrix; can modulate to myofibroblasts

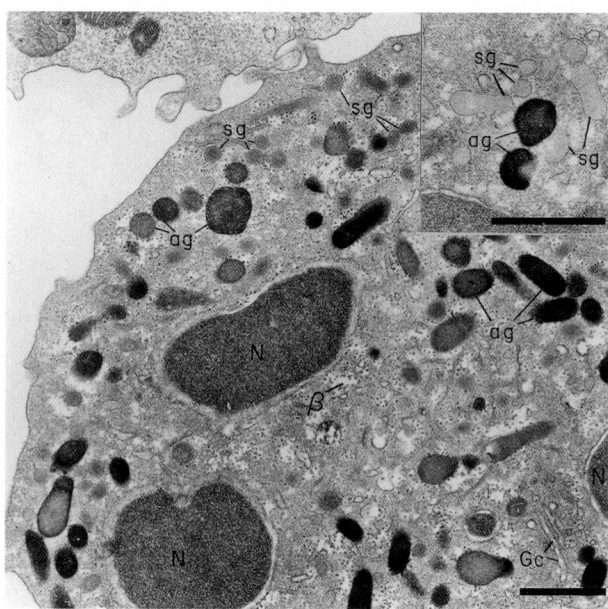

FIGURE 9.1 Part of a human neutrophil reacted for peroxidase. The cytoplasm is loaded with granules. The pale ones, negative for peroxidase, are the specific granules (**sg**). The darker, positive granules are the azurophilic granules (**ag**). Note the abundant supplies of beta particles of glycogen (**β**). **Gc:** Golgi cisternae. **N:** Lobes of the nucleus. **Bar** = 1 μm. **Inset bar** = 0.5 μm. (Reproduced with permission from [6].)

(1) Neutrophils: The Bactericidal Specialists

The neutrophil (Figure 9.1) seems to have been designed by Nature as a bacteria-killing machine. An important machine, as you may judge from these figures: the bone marrow weighs about 2600 gram; 55 to 60 percent of this mass is dedicated to making neutrophils (49). About 100 billion of them (100 cc) are poured every day into the blood, where they circulate for 12–20 hours (5) and then die. They cannot multiply; and they are not found in normal tissues, except in the mucosa of the gut, where they are probably responding to bacteria or bacterial products that found their way across the epithelial barrier. Although not all neutrophils can live to experience their moment of bactericidal glory, we must assume that many get to make their kill somewhere, even under normal conditions, because when the number of leukocytes in human blood drops below 1000–500/mm³ (**neutropenia**) from the normal 4000–11,000/mm³, bacterial infection becomes a threat.

When they float freely, neutrophils are spherical and a little larger than red blood cells, which means that every time a neutrophil is swept into a capillary (about twice a minute: once in the lung, once in a peripheral capillary), it must endure a squeeze. Like all other leukocytes, but unlike bacteria, neutrophils can only crawl, not swim. This is why they do a poor job against bacteria in waterlogged (edematous) tissue.

The vast chemical, enzymatic, and bactericidal equipment of the neutrophil is packed in some 2000 granules of four types (Table 9.2). The *azurophil granules,* also called *primary* because they are first to appear during maturation, contain large amounts of myeloperoxidase, which is involved in oxygen-derived bacterial killing (see further), and no less than *10 antimicrobial proteins* (110) including lysozyme, defensins, azurocidin, and BPI (bactericidal permeability-increasing protein, so named by its strategy in killing bacteria). The *specific granules* lack myeloperoxidase (by definition) but contain their own selection of antimicrobial proteins, including lactoferrin, which affects bacteria directly, as well as indirectly by removing iron (a growth requirement) from the medium. Some of the neutrophil antibiotic proteins are so effective that they are currently being tested in clinical trials (110).

The neutrophil granules also contain enzymes capable of hydrolyzing any component of the body, including collagen (*collagenase*) and the nearly indestructible

Table 9.2 Contents of Human Neutrophil Granules

Azurophil (Primary) Granules	Specific (Secondary) Granules	Gelatinase (Tertiary) Granules	Secretory Vesicles
Membrane	**Membrane**	**Membrane**	**Membrane**
CD63	CD15 antigens	Mac-1 (CD11b)	Alkaline phosphatase
CD66c	CD66a	fMLP receptor	Cytochrome b_{558}
CD68	CD66b	Diacylglycerol	Mac-1 (CD11b)
Matrix	Cytochrome b_{558}	deacylating enzyme	uPA receptor
Lysozyme	FMLP receptor	Cytochrome b_{558}	FMLP receptor
Defensins	Fibronectin receptor	Laminin receptor	CD10, CD13, CD45
Elastase	G-protein α-subunit	**Matrix**	CD16
Cathepsin G	Laminin receptor	Gelatinase	DAF (CD35)
Proteinase 3	MAC-1 (CD11b)	Acetyltransferase	CR1 (CD35)
Esterase N	NB 1 antigen	Lysozyme	**Matrix**
α$_1$-Antitrypsin	Rap 1, Rap 2		Plasma proteins (including
α-Mannosidase	Thrombospondin receptor		albumin)
Azurocidin	TNF receptor		pro-uPA/uPA
Bactericidal permeability-increasing protein (BPI)	Vitronectin receptor		
	uPA receptor		
β-Glycerophosphatase	**Matrix**		
β-Glucuronidase	Apolactoferrin		
β-Galactosidase	Lysozyme		
β-Glucosaminidase	β$_2$-Microglobulin		
α-Fucosidase	Collagenase		
Cathepsin B	Histaminase		
Cathepsin D	Heparinase		
Acid mucopolysaccharide	pro-u plasminogen activator		
Heparin binding protein	Vitamin B$_{12}$–binding protein		
N-Acetyl-β-glucosaminidase	Sialidase		
Sialidase	Protein kinase C inhibitor		
Ubiquitin	hCAP-18		
	SGP28		
	Neutrophil gelatinase-associated lipocalin		

Published with permission from Skubitz KM. Neutrophilic leukocytes. In Lee GR, Foerster J, Lukens J, et al. (eds). Wintrobe's Clinical Hematology, 10th ed. Baltimore, Lippincott, Williams & Wilkins, 1999, pp. 300–350.

elastin (*elastase*); this explains the "tenderizer" effect of pus—*especially on dead tissues*—which was known and even exploited in antiquity.

In Hippocratic times physicians noticed—quite correctly—that bruised wounds did not heal until the dead tissue had been "digested away" by the pus, so they tried to devise wound dressings that encouraged pus formation (57). An astute idea, but it probably did not work.

Besides their granules, the neutrophils are equipped with enough mitochondria to produce a massive "respiratory burst" (see further), some endoplasmic reticulum, and prominent glycogen reserves (Figure 9.2), from which they draw energy for their movements when they venture into poorly oxygenated areas of injury, as required by their job description.

Why their nuclei are subdivided into two to five lobes connected by a thread is not known, but the mul-

tilobed nuclei are excellent markers for recognizing neutrophils in tissue sections (Figure 9.3). When a neutrophil dies, the various lobes of its nucleus can flow into a single one, making it difficult to recognize the cell as a former granulocyte (p. 221).

Neutrophils are programmed to crawl out of the vessels and into the tissue spaces in response to many chemical calls, originating from bacteria, injured tissues, or other inflammatory cells. Because they are primarily bacteria killers they pour out by billions at sites of infection by certain bacteria; if they are concentrated enough the exudate becomes pus. Because of this high-profile performance at sites of injury or infection, the neutrophils have acquired a reputation of single-minded, kamikaze-type cells, programmed to chase bacteria, kill them, and die. To some extent this is true, although they would die young anyway, since their hours in the bloodstream are counted. However, we can

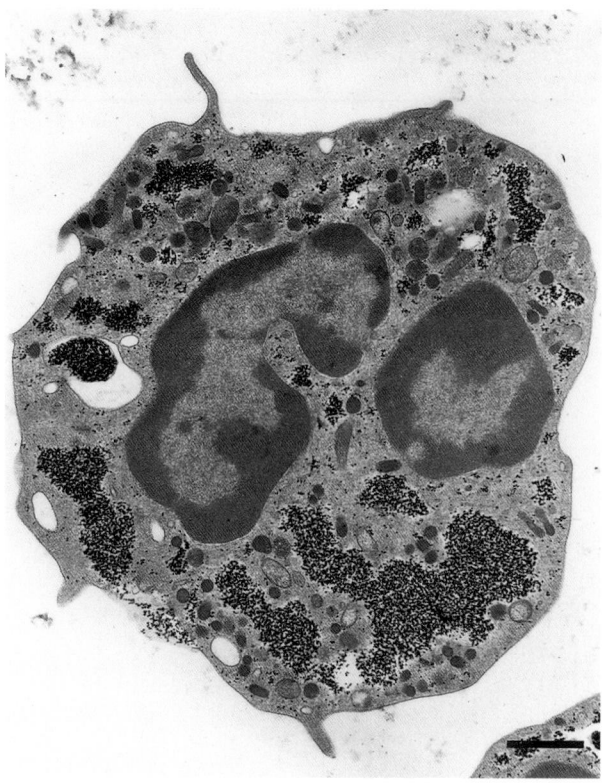

FIGURE 9.2   Human neutrophil stained with silver proteinate to demonstrate glycogen (the black, granular material). **Bar** = 1 μm.

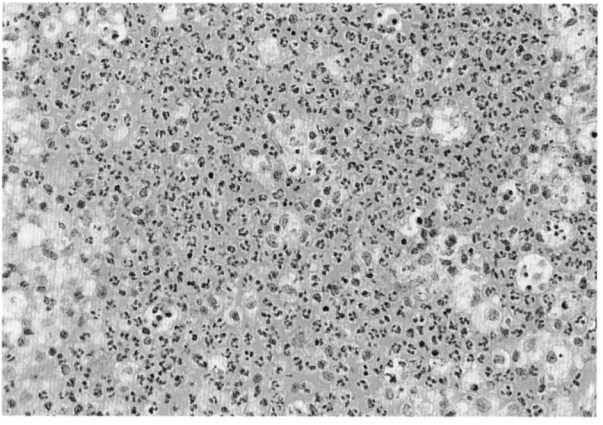

FIGURE 9.3   Pus, photographed in a dental abscess. The prevalent cell, the neutrophil, is clearly recognized by the multilobed structure of the nucleus. (230x)

also view them as powerful *secretory cells* (Figure 9.4), not only because they can release the content of their granules, but also because they have considerable synthetic possibilities: they respond to certain stimuli— such as endotoxin, TNF-α, TGF-β, certain bacteria

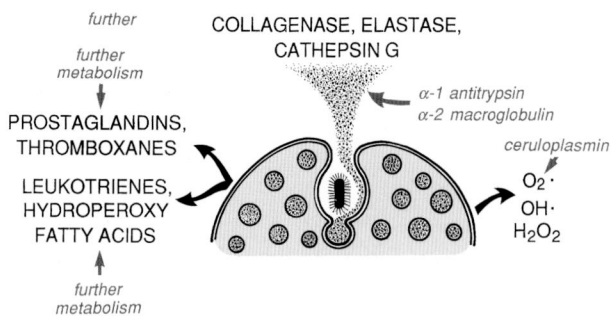

FIGURE 9.4   Principal mediators arising from an activated neutrophil and their principal inhibitors. (Reprinted by permission of the New England Journal of Medicine 303;27–34, 1980 [103].)

(110)—by producing cytokines, inflammatory and anti-inflammatory, including chemokines. They can also produce inflammatory mediators through the arachidonic acid cascade, and actively kill bacteria by generating a barrage of free radicals. The reverse of the coin is that the same activities that make the neutrophil a secretory cell also make it a *potentially harmful cell:* what kills a bacterium can also kill an innocent bystander cell. In fact, much of the injury that occurs during inflammation can be attributed to the neutrophils.

NOTE: Despite their tremendous appetite for bacteria, the neutrophils tend to shun other objects. They take to scavenging as a low priority; for this reason Metchnikoff called them *microphages* (62), a name that has not survived.

Surprisingly, it is not yet clear how and where the neutrophils normally end their lives. Many are thought to be taken up by the spleen or to break up in the capillaries of the lung; others are probably lost in the mouth and the gut. In inflammatory foci, spent or obsolete neutrophils are phagocytized by macrophages using a fascinating mechanism specifically designed for apoptotic cells (pp. 213, 216).

One might think that swallowing a neutrophil loaded with enzymes might be hazardous, but the macrophage is none the worse for its meal: the neutrophil's enzymes are probably denatured in the death process.

In essence: the neutrophil is a short-lived cell that can not multiply but can secrete or synthesize a vast array of bactericidal molecules, enzymes, and inflammatory mediators; its reputation of having "the hardware to kill but no software of its own" is certainly inaccurate

(110). Normally it is found only in the bone marrow, in the blood, and in mucosae exposed to bacterial trespassing. Its presence in other tissues signals two possible acute events: invasion by bacteria or some other parasite, and/or tissue injury.

(2) Eosinophils: The Worm Killers

The eosinophil seems to have evolved—like the neutrophil—in response to invaders, but to larger invaders, especially worms (Figure 9.5) (5, 20, 35, 36, 91, 105). *In vitro* it can kill, for example, a worm (*Schistosoma mansoni*) and a protozoan (*Trypanosoma cruzi*) responsible for two of the world's major tropical diseases. In relatively worm-free societies the eosinophil may be a frustrated cell. It is born in the bone marrow from precursor cells that differentiate under the influence of several cytokines, especially Interleukin 5 and 3 (blood levels of IL-5 are high in diseases with hypereosinophilia) (80). Although the eosinophil has some similarities to the neutrophil, the differences are great. It is much better equipped with mitochondria and endoplasmic reticulum and correspondingly has a much longer life span, perhaps 4 days in the blood, and weeks (for reasons unknown) in the tissues. It can phagocytize and kill bacteria, but much less efficiently than the neutrophil; on the other hand, when stimulated, the respiratory burst of the eosinophil lasts longer and produces twice the amount of superoxide anion (O_2^-) than that of the neutrophil (93).

In the blood, eosinophils represent only 1–3 percent of the leukocytes, but *in most tissues, where there are no neutrophils at all, eosinophils are scattered almost everywhere, especially where mast cells abound (104)*. To emigrate from the blood vessels the eosinophils can respond to a large number of mediators; the most specific are the recently discovered chemokines *eotaxin 1 and 2* (80, 82).

The granules of the eosinophils are larger and fewer (about 200, roughly one-tenth of the neutrophil's endowment) and are probably modified peroxisomes rather than lysosomes (5).

They contain several cationic (or positively charged) proteins (73), a fact that fits with their affinity for the acid stain eosin (*eosino*phils). Why should these proteins be cationic? It took a long time to find out that this property has a purpose; *it makes these proteins toxic by enabling them to bind with critical, negatively charged molecules on the surface of other cells,* a strategy presumably aimed at parasites. The so-called **major basic protein** (MBP) takes up more than half of each granule, in the form of a crystalloid mass (Figure 9.6); it can kill worms as well as normal mammalian cells (Figure 9.7) (27). Another cationic protein, **eosinophil cationic protein** (ECP), is said to create pores in cell membranes; it is harmless against bacteria but kills schistosoma larvae (73). At least three of the eosinophil cationic proteins can behave as neurotoxins; injected into the cerebral ventricles they cause selective death of the cerebellar Purkinje cells (Figure 9.8) (26).

When and where do the eosinophils accumulate in disease? This should tell us something about their functions (80, 82). In the blood, hypereosinophilia is a common effect of allergy and of parasitic infestation. In the tissues, a few eosinophils can be found in any acute inflammatory focus, along with the neutrophils, but they seem to be incidental. Large numbers are found in lesions due to parasites, in relation to some immune responses, in relation to angiogenesis, in healing wounds, and in some tumors (e.g., Hodgkin's disease). *Eosinophils have a special relationship with mast cells,* which secrete several eosinophil chemotactic factors, whereas major basic protein causes mast cells to release histamine.

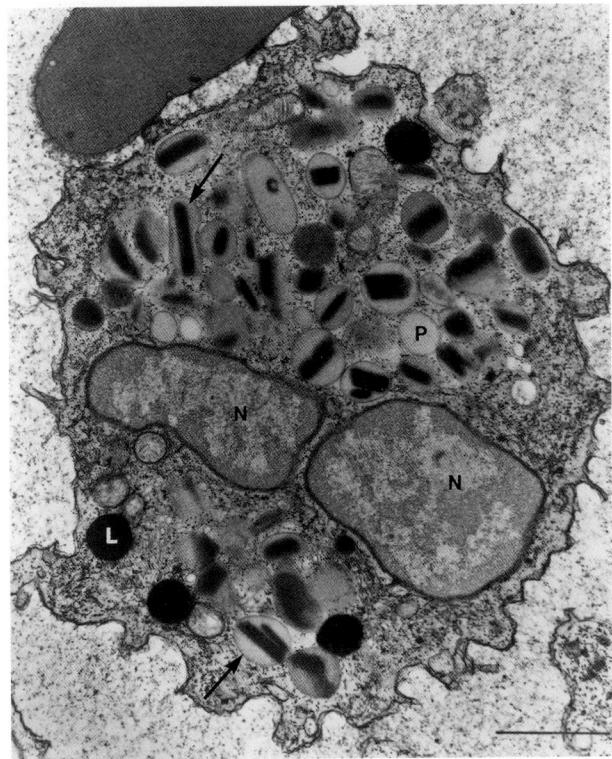

FIGURE 9.5   Human eosinophil. **N:** Typical bilobed nucleus. **Arrows:** Specific granules with dense central crystal. **P:** Primary granule, devoid of crystal. **L:** Lipid body. **Bar** = 1.4 μm. (Reproduced with permission from [20].)

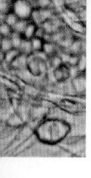

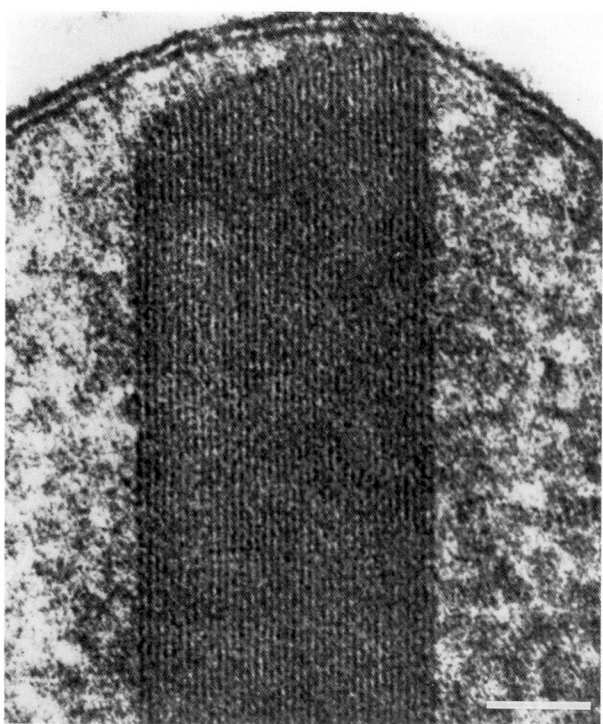

FIGURE 9.6   Part of a granule from a rat eosinophil, seen by electron microscopy; showing the typical central crystal of major basic protein. **Bar** = 0.05 μm. (Reproduced from the **Journal of Cell Biology,** 1966;31:349–362, by copyright permission of The Rockefeller University Press [63].)

It has been noticed that eosinophils contain enzymes that could be used for shutting off inflammation: histaminase, arylsulfatase (which inactivates leukotrienes), and a phospholipase that could inactivate the powerful platelet activating factor (36)—hence the suggestion that "the eosinophil can undo what the mast cell has done" (84). But before this can become a slogan, more data are needed (36).

It is clear that eosinophils can do a lot of damage.

- Asthma is always accompanied by an intense eosinophilic infiltration of the bronchi. MBP can paralyze the cilia of the bronchial epithelium (**ciliostasis,** 17), and cationic proteins have been demonstrated in damaged bronchial epithelium and in the sputum (90). Furthermore, the characteristic spasm of bronchial muscle can be correlated with the tendency of eosinophils to produce the spasmogenic leukotrienes LTC_4 and LTE_4 rather than the leukotactic LTB_4 produced by neutrophils (36, 90).

- The idiopathic *hypereosinophilic syndrome* is characterized by infiltration by eosinophils of many organs, including the heart; the result is a fibrosis that can be life-threatening, and eosinophil cationic

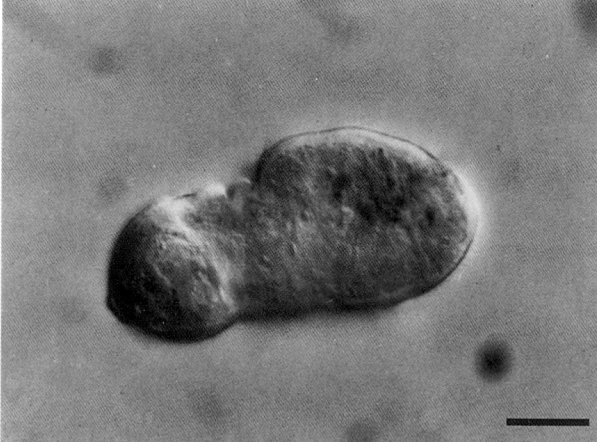

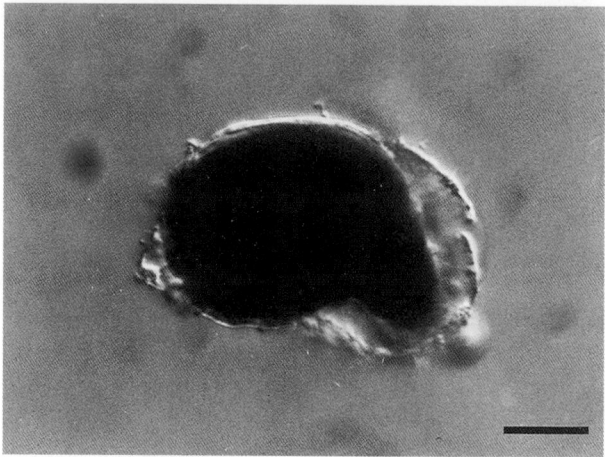

FIGURE 9.7   *Top:* Normal larva of *Schistosoma mansoni.* *Bottom:* After incubation with eosinophil major basic protein (MBP) the larva is damaged, as shown by the detached and ballooning membrane. **Bars** = 50 μm. (Reprinted from [36], Copyright 1986, with permission from Elsevier.)

proteins can be demonstrated in the tissue (36). Since 1989, a syndrome of hypereosinophilia and myalgia (muscle pain) has been described in individuals ingesting products that contain the "dietary supplement" L-tryptophan (19).

- Here is a teaser: the destructive major basic protein is contained in the placenta and in the plasma of pregnant women (98). It is tempting to speculate that this destructive protein may relate to the ability of fetal trophoblastic cells to invade the uterine wall (56).

- **Charcot-Leyden crystals** are microscopic, bipyramidal, hexagonal protein crystals (Figure 9.9) that have been known since the 1800s to be associated with eosinophils in the sputum of asthmatics. They can be obtained *in vitro* from eosinophils and also from basophils; they are made of lysophospholipase C from the cell membrane (20, 90).

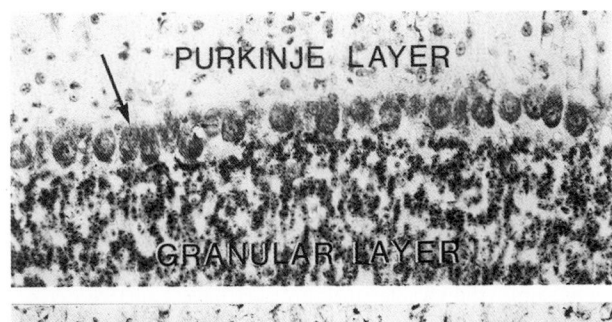

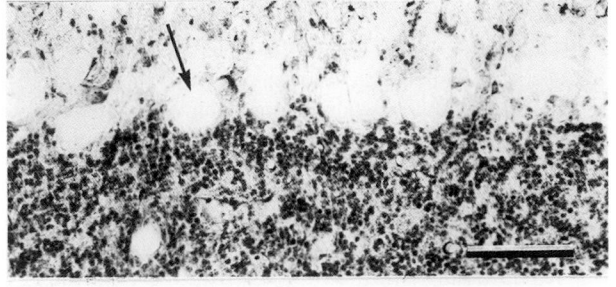

FIGURE 9.8 Destructive power of eosinophil cationic protein (ECP). *Top:* Cerebellum of a normal guinea pig; note the normal layer of Purkinje cells (**arrow**). *Bottom:* Seven days after an intraventricular injection of 0.3 micrograms of ECP; the Purkinje cells have disappeared, leaving empty spaces. **Bar** = 100 μm. (Reproduced with permission from [26].)

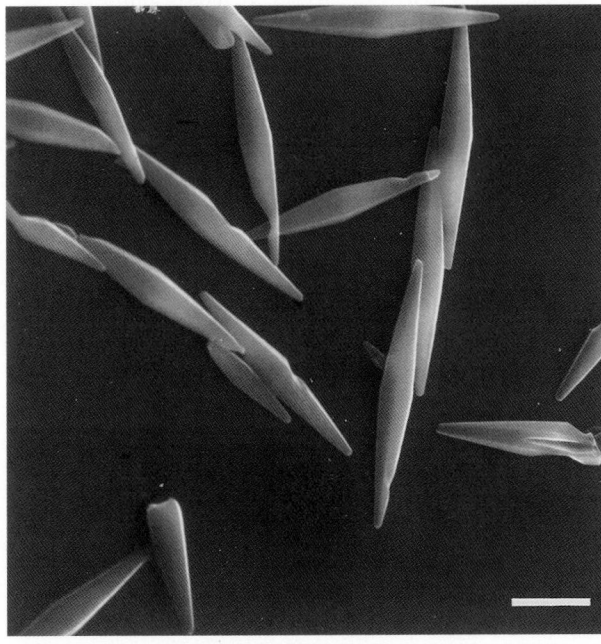

FIGURE 9.9 Charcot-Leyden crystals of lysophospholipase obtained from human eosinophils, seen by scanning electron microscopy. These protein crystals are commonly found in the sputum of asthmatics and are visible by light microscopy. **Bar** = 25 μm. (Reproduced with permission from [90].)

In essence: the eosinophil is loaded with powerful antiparasitic cytotoxins, which can also be misdirected and cause tissue damage, as happens in asthma. It has a mast cell connection, in that it can be summoned by several chemotaxins produced by mast cells: hence its presence in allergic lesions, in which mast cells are a key factor. This points to a primordial alliance between these two cells, originally intended to fight worms and other large parasites (p. 538). But worms apart, we still do not know why—or whether—we should be grateful for the existence of the eosinophil.

(3) Macrophages: The Master Minds

Monocytes and macrophages must be dealt with together because they represent two phases of the same cell—a circulating phase (49) and a tissue phase, respectively (Figure 9.10). Monocytes are born in the bone marrow; they circulate, in humans, for about 6 days (97), then migrate into the tissues and settle there as macrophages, quite turned off until they are activated by some local challenge (39, 71a). Macrophages found in tissues are also called *histiocytes*.

From the point of view of evolution, monocytes/macrophages derive from the ancestral invertebrate macrophage; this is the cell that Metchnikoff saw at work in his starfish larvae, and that evolved into the many phagocytic and multitalented cells of the vertebrate RES.

There is something stately and professional about the macrophages. In inflammation they make their appearance as a second wave, to finish what the neutrophils had started, and then they take over. On the whole, they can phagocytize the same bacteria as the

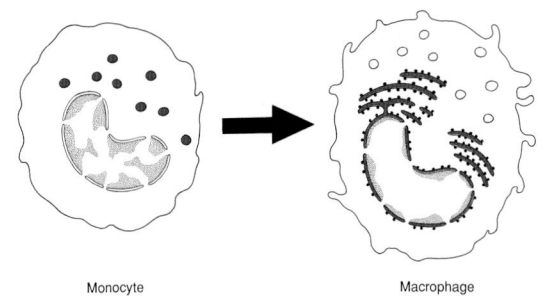

Monocyte   Macrophage

FIGURE 9.10 When a monocyte (*left*) migrates out of the vessels and becomes a resident macrophage (*right*), it becomes larger but downgrades its level of activity; peroxidase (*red*), present in the monocyte's granules, is restricted in the resident macrophage to the nuclear envelope and to the endoplasmic reticulum. (Adapted by permission from [96]. Copyright 1988 Raven Press Ltd.)

neutrophils, although not always as effectively; however, they are better equipped to handle hard-to-kill intracellular bacteria such as *Mycobacterium tuberculosis*. We have already alluded to the awesome capabilities of the macrophage besides phagocytosis: they include antigen presentation, which implies that it can be up to the macrophages to decide whether an immune response is required or not; they can turn on (or off) angiogenesis, unleash fibrosis or clotting; if enough of them are activated, they can affect the body as a whole by causing fever and even cachexia (p. 829). This wide range of activities implies the capability to produce a vast array of proteins and other molecules such as enzymes, cytokines, growth factors, and inflammatory mediators; the product list of the macrophage factory can compete with that of the liver cell (Table 9.3). The only major item we see missing in this list is the

production of antibodies. It is regrettable for the human observer, especially for a novice, that *the omnipotent macrophage has no morphologic marker* unless it has phagocytized something obvious. Fortunately, histochemical markers do exist.

The most specific methods for identifying macrophages are a histochemical stain for non-specific esterase and surface markers (antigens) (39) for subsets of macrophages. For example, the alveolar macrophages have a surface marker not present in resident peritoneal macrophages (96). Circulating monocytes are less heterogeneous but do have **subsets** (68) that vary in their response to chemotactic agents (24). The variations are probably due to microenvironmental effects and/or to maturation. Neutrophils are more uniform, but "fast" and "slow" sets have been described; there are also subsets of eosinophils (76).

Exactly how long macrophages live nobody knows, but it is probably months (33). Because they multiply, their individual life span matters little.

The "Angry" (Activated) Macrophage

Macrophages, like the endothelium, teach us that *activation is not an all-or-none process* (p. 60). The macrophages can be turned on in at least two ways: a quick, short-term and a slow, long-term activation.

- **Quick activation** (better called **stimulation**) is a burst of activity triggered in seconds or minutes, usually by phagocytosis. It causes exocytosis of lysosomal enzymes and the secretion of oxygen-derived free radicals. This is the equivalent of the respiratory burst of the neutrophils (p. 419) except that it is less dramatic: macrophages consume less than half the amount of oxygen and produce only 20 percent as much hydrogen peroxide as neutrophils (78).
- **Slow activation** is akin to hypertrophy; it implies changes in macrophages that occur over days. In the 1960s, G. B. Mackaness noticed that peritoneal macrophages of mice injected intravenously with *Listeria* (a facultative intracellular parasite) became more effective against other bacteria as well; they were larger, more ruffled, contained more granules, and had *in vitro* a much greater propensity to stick and spread over surfaces (Figure 9.11) (54). We now know that such macrophages, dubbed angry macrophages, also have a much more powerful respiratory burst and greater bactericidal and/or tumoricidal ability than resting macrophages. Histochemical studies have shown that the activation to angry macrophage is a multistep process, each step being defined by a particular set of surface markers and enzymatic content while given functions increase or decrease (2, 96).

The principal agents of this long-term activation are **cytokines,** especially interferon gamma produced by

Table 9.3 Products of Mononuclear Phagocytes: A Partial List

Enzymes	Reactive oxygen species
Acid hydrolases	Hydrogen peroxide
Angiotensin-converting enzyme	Hydroxyl radical
Arginase	Singlet oxygen
Catalase	Superoxide anion
Heme oxygenase	**Reactive nitric species**
Lipoprotein lipase	Nitric oxide
Lysozyme	Peroxynitrite
Neutral proteases	**Bioactive lipids**
Plasminogen activator	Arachidonate derivatives
Elastase	Hydroxyeicosatetranoic acids
Collagenase	Leukotrienes B_4, C_4, D_4, E_4
Nitric oxide synthases (type 2)	Prostacyclin
Nonspecific esterase	Prostaglandin E_2
Peroxidase	Prostaglandin F_{2a}
Phospholipase A_2	Thromboxane B_2
Superoxide dismutase	Lipoxins
Protease inhibitors	Platelet activating factor
α_2-Macroglobulin	**Chemotactic factors**
α_1-Antiprotease	Chemokines
Complement factors	**Cytokines/growth factors**
C1, C4, C2, C3, C5	Erythropoietin
Factors B, D, I, H	FGF
Properdin	TGF-α
Coagulation factors	IFN-α, -γ
XIII, X, IX, VII, V, II	IL-1, -3, -6, -8, -10, -12
Thrombomodulin	m-CSF
Thromboplastin	**Angiogenesis factors**
Plasminogen activator	**Angiogenesis inhibitors**
Binding proteins	
Transferrin	
Transcobalamin II	
Fibronectin	
Apolipoprotein E	

Published with permission from: Weinberg JB. Mononuclear phagocytes. In Lee GR, Foerster J, Lukens J, et al. (eds). Wintrobe's clinical hematology, 10th ed. Baltimore, Lippincott, Williams & Wilkins, 1999. pp. 377–414.

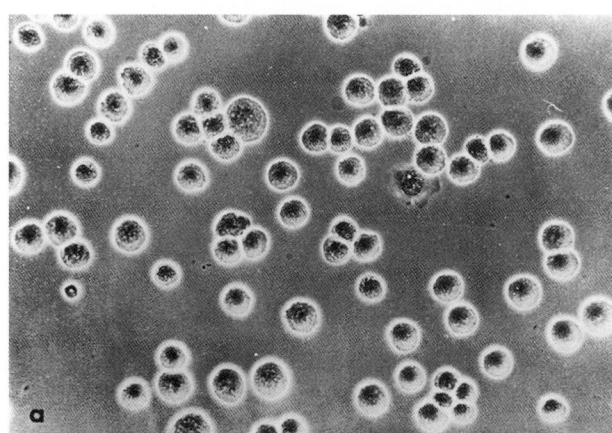

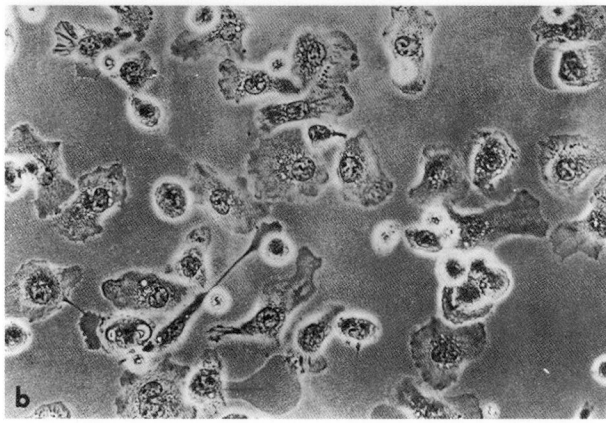

FIGURE 9.11 Structural and functional changes in activated macrophages. *Top:* Normal mouse macrophages obtained from the peritoneum; after 1 hour of incubation over a glass slide, they still retain their rounded shape, failing to attach and spread. *Bottom:* Activated peritoneal macrophages obtained by injecting a suspension of BCG bacteria into the peritoneum of a mouse vaccinated with BCG. After incubation for only 15 minutes, the macrophages have become attached and spread out. (Reproduced with permission from [55].)

lymphocytes (33), which means that this type of activation is to be expected mainly in infections and in immune responses. Macrophages can also stimulate themselves. When exposed to endotoxin, a powerful lipopolysaccharide produced by gram-negative bacteria, they produce tumor necrosis factor (TNF), which activates macrophages *in vitro* (33). Autostimulation should be an advantage because the macrophages can become "angry" immediately, without having to wait for several days—the time it would take for the immune response to develop and for lymphocytes to produce their interferon gamma.

Studies of macrophage activation have shown that a suspension of absolutely resting macrophages is not easily obtained. A classic way to obtain macrophages is to irritate the peritoneal cavity "slightly" with a mild substance such as glycogen. Today it is clear that macrophages answering this call, however gentle it may be, are partially activated, or **primed** (that is, ready to respond more intensely if stimulated) (46). Another established method for separating macrophages (for example, from the peritoneal fluid of a rat) is to place a drop of the peritoneal fluid on a glass or plastic surface: the macrophages adhere to it and spread (Figure 9.11), and the other cells can be washed away. However, adherence leads to partial activation (47). Alveolar macrophages can be obtained by bronchial lavage, a fairly uncomfortable procedure (18).

Besides activation, the macrophages can respond to external stimuli by undergoing either of two striking adaptations: they can become stuffed with lipid and become **foam cells,** the villains of atherosclerosis, or they can fuse with each other and become **giant cells,** the sometime heroes of chronic inflammation. Both changes deserve special treatment elsewhere (pp. 92 and 462).

There is also a dark side to the macrophages. Activated macrophages can be dangerous, just like neutrophils. In the lung, for example, they can attack the elastin scaffolding with their elastase (11, 107). One of their most powerful products, **tumor necrosis factor** (TNF), can destroy tumors under certain conditions (p. 365), but it also can be secreted in doses large enough to kill the host—hence TNF is also called **cachectin.** The syndrome of septic shock is caused by endotoxin, but that is largely because endotoxin stimulates macrophages and other cells to oversecrete cytokines, including TNF (p. 720). Macrophages can cause trouble also by becoming reservoirs for infectious agents, including the AIDS virus (33).

In essence: Unlike the single-minded, short-lived neutrophil, the macrophage is a highly versatile, long-lived cell with a multitude of biological properties that make it the mastermind of inflammation, especially in the chronic, adaptive stage (Figure 9.12). Like the neutrophil, it can become dangerous.

(4) Platelets

The platelets are stiff little discs, passively dragged around in the bloodstream (Figure 9.13). Their most obvious roles are intravascular: they maintain the integrity of the endothelium, probably by supplying it with a phospholipid, lysophosphatidic acid (169) (in the absence of platelets the endothelium falls apart [34]); they plug gaps in the endothelium; they are essential for stopping hemorrhage (p. 632); and they take part in blood clotting. However, *the platelets are also*

FIGURE 9.12 Basic functions of granulocytes and macrophages.

**MAIN FUNCTIONS OF
NEUTROPHILS AND MACROPHAGES**

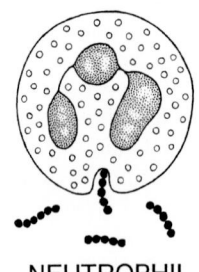

1. PHAGOCYTOSIS OF BACTERIA
   (especially pyogenic cocci)
2. RELEASE OF INFLAMMATORY MEDIATORS

NEUTROPHIL

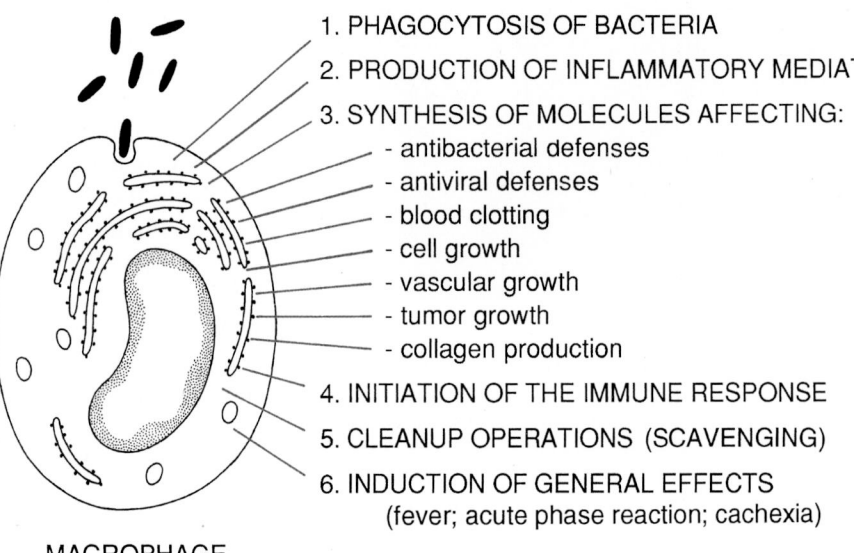

1. PHAGOCYTOSIS OF BACTERIA
2. PRODUCTION OF INFLAMMATORY MEDIATORS
3. SYNTHESIS OF MOLECULES AFFECTING:
   - antibacterial defenses
   - antiviral defenses
   - blood clotting
   - cell growth
   - vascular growth
   - tumor growth
   - collagen production
4. INITIATION OF THE IMMUNE RESPONSE
5. CLEANUP OPERATIONS (SCAVENGING)
6. INDUCTION OF GENERAL EFFECTS
   (fever; acute phase reaction; cachexia)

MACROPHAGE

loaded with at least 20 types of molecules that can play a number of useful roles in inflammation (65, 104, 108) (Figure 9.14). In fact, a subcutaneous injection of concentrated platelets produces a tremendous inflammatory response (12). But then, the platelets are unable to crawl out of the blood vessels, as the leukocytes do: so how can they reach the extracellular spaces where inflammation is raging, and use their arsenal of helpful molecules? The answer seems to be very simple: wherever injury occurs, millions of vessels are severed and bleed; the platelets rush those leaks, and within a matter of seconds or minutes they break up, releasing their load. In other words, despite the fact that they cannot actively emigrate from the blood vessels, they are the very first to supply mediators where they are urgently needed.

In essence: platelets, small as they are, are essential (a) for the daily upkeep of the blood vessels, (b) for blood clotting and hemostasis, and (c) for the instant delivery of inflammatory mediators and growth factors to injured tissues.

(5) Mast Cells and Basophils

Although mast cells live in tissues and basophils in the blood, these two types of cells must be mentioned together because they are very similar in structure and function; they both arise from bone marrow precursors (30, 48, 89) but—unlike the monocyte/macrophage tandem—the basophils are *not* precursors of the mast cells (79). Whenever we make general statements about mast cells, we should say "mast cells and basophils."

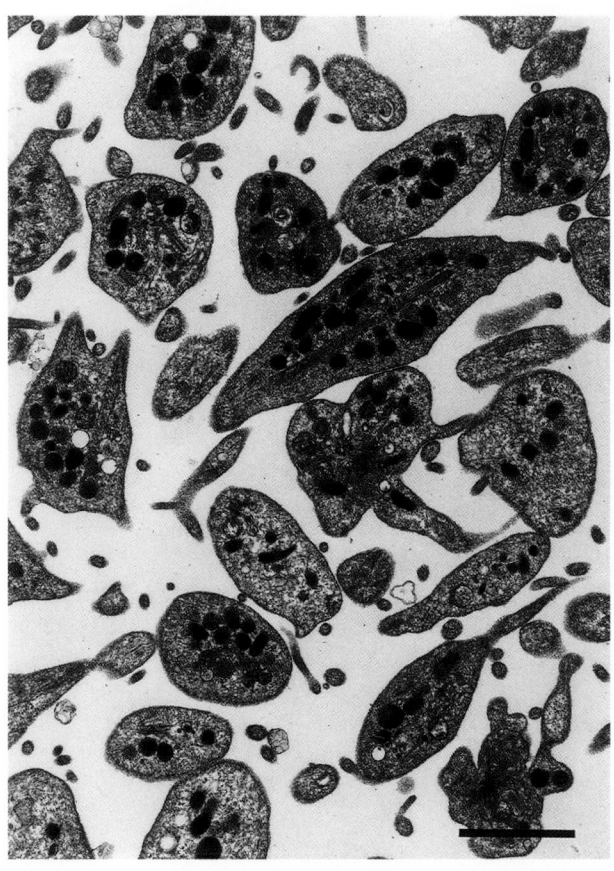

FIGURE 9.13   Normal rat platelets, isolated and spun down into a pellet. Note the abundant granular content. **Bar** = 0.2 μm. (Reproduced with permission from [12], © American Society for Investigative Pathology.)

There are, however, some clear-cut differences between the two cell types (33, 67): basophils are smaller, their nucleus is multilobed, they contain neither tryptase nor chymase (see further), they live only days compared with months (34, 103), and the responses to activators are different (33). In humans both types of cells can be grown from CD34 positive precursors, but using different growth factors (67).

By light and by electron microscopic standards, mast cells and basophils are spectacular; they are stuffed with large granules programmed to release histamine and other inflammatory mediators in such amounts that death can occur within minutes if the process is generalized, a catastrophe called anaphylactic shock (p. 532).

Mast cells were described around 1876 by a medical student who developed a passion for the newly available aniline dyes, which were being tested on tissues by his older cousin Carl Weigert, a famous pathologist. The young man soon noticed that some leukocytes stain with basic dyes, as do the mast cells (he called these *basophils*), others stain with acid dyes such as eosin (he called them *eosinophils*), and still others stain with neither (*neutrophils*). The medical student was Paul Ehrlich, who later originated the concept of receptors; it was he who shared the Nobel prize with Metchnikoff in 1908. After Ehrlich's work, interest in mast cells and basophils faded away for decades for the simple reason that their granules are almost invisible with the routine hematoxylin–eosin stain.

In the 1930s the granules of mast cells and basophils were found to contain the anticoagulant **heparin,** a

POSSIBLE ROLES OF PLATELET FACTORS IN INFLAMMATION

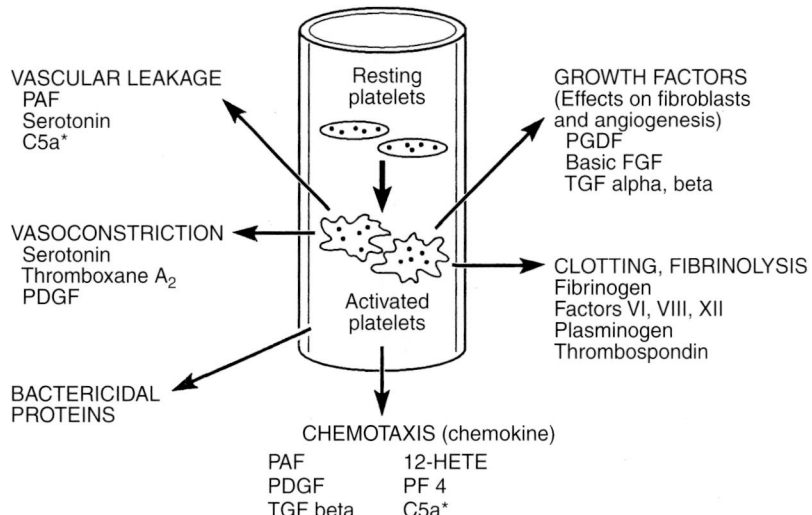

VASCULAR LEAKAGE
PAF
Serotonin
C5a*

Resting
platelets

GROWTH FACTORS
(Effects on fibroblasts
and angiogenesis)
PGDF
Basic FGF
TGF alpha, beta

VASOCONSTRICTION
Serotonin
Thromboxane A_2
PDGF

Activated
platelets

CLOTTING, FIBRINOLYSIS
Fibrinogen
Factors VI, VIII, XII
Plasminogen
Thrombospondin

BACTERICIDAL
PROTEINS

CHEMOTAXIS (chemokine)
PAF   12-HETE
PDGF   PF 4
TGF beta   C5a*

FIGURE 9.14   The platelets are loaded with molecules that are actual or potential inflammatory mediators. C5a* is generated secondarily by proteolytic cleavage of complement component C5.

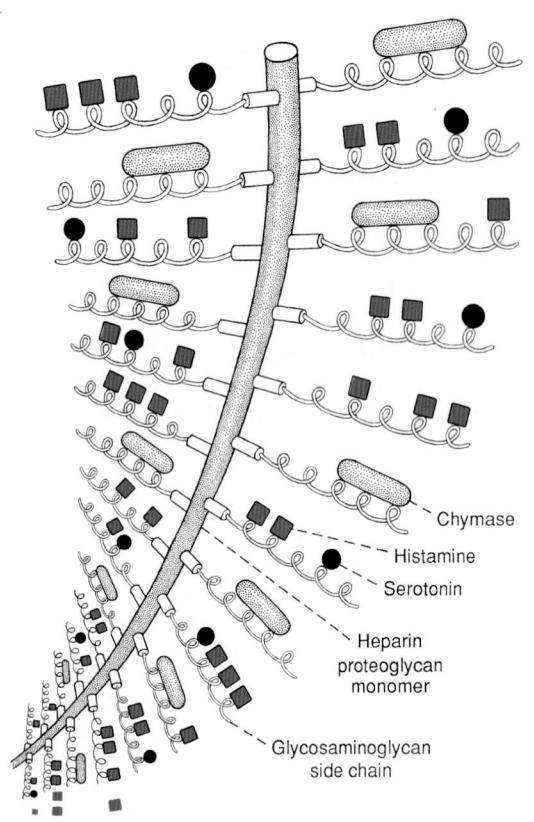

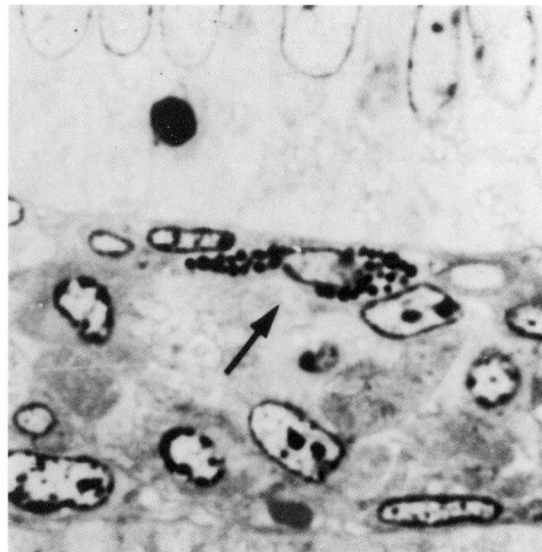

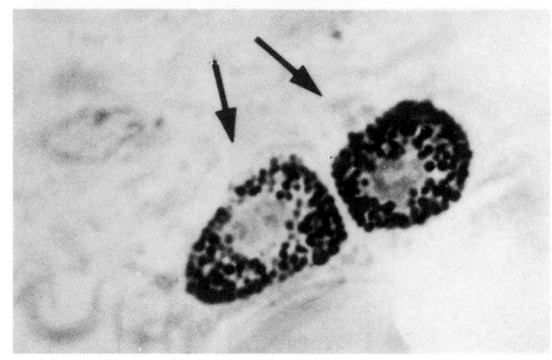

FIGURE 9.15 Artist's view of a feathery heparin molecule in a mast cell granule. The long axis is a protein, to which are attached glycosaminoglycan molecules. To the latter are bound (in noncovalent fashion) histamine, serotonin, and proteolytic enzymes (chymases of multiple types). (Adapted from [3, 61].)

FIGURE 9.16 Different aspects of mucosal mast cells (*top*) and connective tissue mast cells (*bottom*). Duodenal submucosa and tongue of the rat; toluidine blue stain. (Reproduced with permission from [23], © Raven Press 1986.)

highly acidic, sulfated glycosaminoglycan: its negative charge explains the basophilia of the granules, and some years later it was realized that **histamine** and (in rodents) **serotonin** are reversibly bound to the heparin (98). Today the macromolecular matrix of the mast cell and basophil granules can actually be conceived as a cation exchange resin to which positively charged molecules are reversibly attached (Figure 9.15) (70).

Mast cells are notoriously heterogeneous with respect to structure, mediator content, granule proteoglycan, and, most important, response to drugs (11, 31, 32, 33, 117). In rodents, two major types have been identified: the **connective tissue mast cells** and the **mucosal mast cells** (Figures 9.16, 9.17). These mucosal mast cells are smaller and more mobile, have fewer granules and less histamine, and have shorter life spans than those of the connective tissue (23).

In humans, again, two types can be distinguished histochemically, depending of their content of proteases: *positive for tryptase and chymase,* and *positive for tryptase only;* the two types correspond roughly to the connective tissue and mucosal mast cells of rodents.

Interestingly, there are differences in the pharmacologic responses of these subtypes: for example, in the rat, mast cells of the connective tissue type fail to respond to a powerful degranulating agent (a drug much used experimentally, called 48/80) and also to a powerful inhibitor of degranulation (disodium cromoglycate) (26). Such differences can be important in the treatment of allergies (p. 530).

The one great act of mast cells and basophils is degranulation and release of granule content (21).

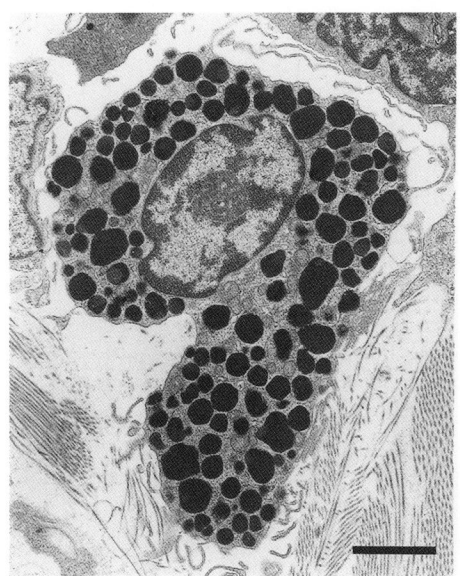 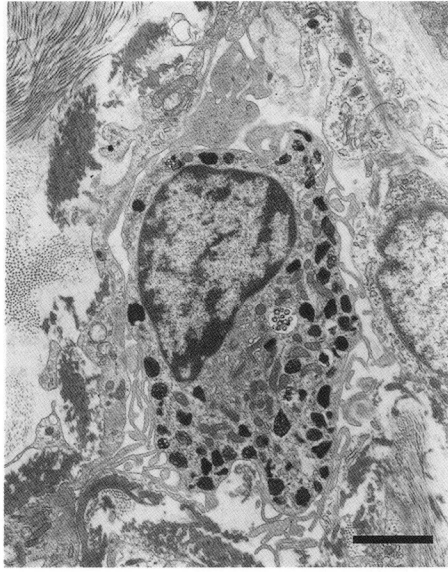

FIGURE 9.17 Two main types of human mast cells. *Left:* TC type (tryptase positive, chymase positive) found in the skin; it is analogous to the rodent "typical" or connective tissue type mast cells. *Right:* T-type (tryptase positive) mast cell from the lung, analogous to the rodent "atypical" or mucosal type. In the latter, the granules are fewer and smaller. **Bars** = 2 μm. (Reproduced by permission from [16], © by The US & Canadian Academy of Pathology, Inc.)

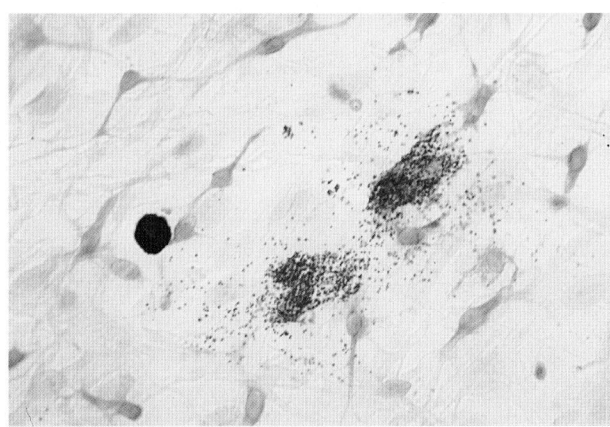

FIGURE 9.18 Mast cells in the rat mesentery. Two have degranulated, presumably during dissection; one (*left*) is in a resting state. Cresyl violet stain. (375x)

Because "exploded" mast cells are often seen in traumatized tissues, pathologists tend to see mast cells as fragile bags of granules ready to burst if prodded (Figure 9.18); in contrast, mast cell experts see degranulation as a biochemical response. Both views are probably right. One typical form of degranulation is mediated by an immunologic mechanism, which leads to anaphylaxis (p. 527). The details of degranulation vary, but the overall result is that the membranes surrounding the granules fuse to form tubes and the granules are extruded (21, 44). In rats the whole process takes about 2 minutes, in humans it spreads over 15 to 40 minutes. How long it takes for an individual mast cell to replace

its granules is not clear. Fawcett found (25) that all the mast cells in the peritoneum of a rat can be destroyed (not just degranulated) by an intraperitoneal injection of distilled water; this procedure appears drastic but is surprisingly well tolerated by the other peritoneal cells. Under these conditions, mast cells slowly reappear over 6 weeks (25); some may be newly supplied from the bone marrow, but degranulated mast cells can also produce a new set of granules (20a).

When they degranulate, the mast cells release a long list of mediators; some are preformed, namely histamine (plus serotonin in rodents) and TNFα (tumor necrosis factor α)—*the only cytokine known to be stored, ready for instant release* (33, 43). Other mediators follow within minutes: PAF (platelet activating factor), leukotrienes, chemokines (100a), and many cytokines (32, 37), including bFGF (basic fibroblast growth factor), reflecting a link between mast cells and fibrosis. Predictably, different types of mast cells, and mast cells of different species, secrete different mixes of mediators.

Mast cells can phagocytize colloidal particles as well as bacteria (*Escherichia coli, Salmonella*) (57a, 61), but they can also perform another and quite unusual type of uptake: they can absorb from the bloodstream and concentrate certain molecules such as metals, toxins, and enzymes (28, 85). Selye called this phenomenon "mastopexy", presumably without realizing that this is also the name of a surgical operation on the female breast, which may explain why his term never caught on.

Mast cells can multiply and even form tumors; in fact, mast cell tumors (*mastocytomas*) have been useful as sources of mast cells in bulk for chemical study.

There are conditions, called **mastocytoses**, that are excesses of mast cells, and can be localized, systemic (to the skin, as in *urticaria pigmentosa*), or generalized. Some of the symptoms of mastocytosis reflect an exaggerated release of histamine, such as skin eruptions, diarrhea, and flushes (71). Mast cells also appear in swarms in certain immune responses of the poison ivy type (p. 554), but their presence is not essential (31). Strains of mast-cell–deficient mice exist (30, 66).

But after all: what is the life purpose of the beautiful mast cells? They must have something better to do than producing allergies and anaphylactic shock, and it must be an important job, because they are everywhere (except behind the blood-brain barrier) and in vast numbers: 26,000 per mm^3 in the lung (67), for a total of at least 100 grams in humans (99). Another important clue is that they are heavily armed with mediators, more so than any other cell. The time has come to acknowledge that they are no longer mysterious: *they are the designated triggers of acute inflammation,* i.e., of the immediate, stereotyped, immutable, INNATE inflammatory response (31a, 100a, 107a). For this life-saving task, the mast cells are perfectly equipped. They can release instantly both histamine, to make vessels leak, and TNFα to attract leukocytes, and they can protect from infection, as has been shown in a model of peritonitis (22, 36a, 58). In mice that are genetically deficient in mast cells, the inflammatory response to local injury is seriously impaired (107a). Mast cells are beautiful *and* essential.

(6, 7) T and B Lymphocytes

T and B lymphocytes are agents of the immune system, and as such they have held the scientific and medical limelight for the past 30 years. An immunologist might have a fit at seeing that we deal with them here in only a few paragraphs. Our reason was stated in the preface: we assume that the reader has some background in immunology.

On the microscope stage, lymphocytes appear to be the least interesting of all cells. They are the smallest leukocytes, about as large as a red blood cell, and have so little cytoplasm that they look like plain nuclei in histologic sections. Their granules are tiny and rare; Ehrlich missed them altogether and branded the lymphocytes "physiologically inferior to the polymorphonuclear leukocytes" (43). Until the 1940s they were known only as "cells typical of chronic inflammation."

In human blood, lymphocytes make up 33 percent of the leukocytes; of these, 70–75 percent are T cells (95), 10–15 percent B cells, and 10 percent NK cells. Alas, none of these types can be distinguished from the others under the light microscope, so the only way to label them is to use immunochemical methods based on antibodies that recognize specific surface markers. Another difficulty in identifying lymphocytes is their ability to become much larger when undergoing the so-called blast transformation, which is a combination of hypertrophy and hyperplasia; the so-called *blasts* look distressingly similar to macrophages. The B cells, however, reveal their identity when they become elegant plasma cells, the antibody secretors (Figure 9.19).

Incidentally, rat blood swarms with lymphocytes (86 percent of their white blood cells). We have no explanation.

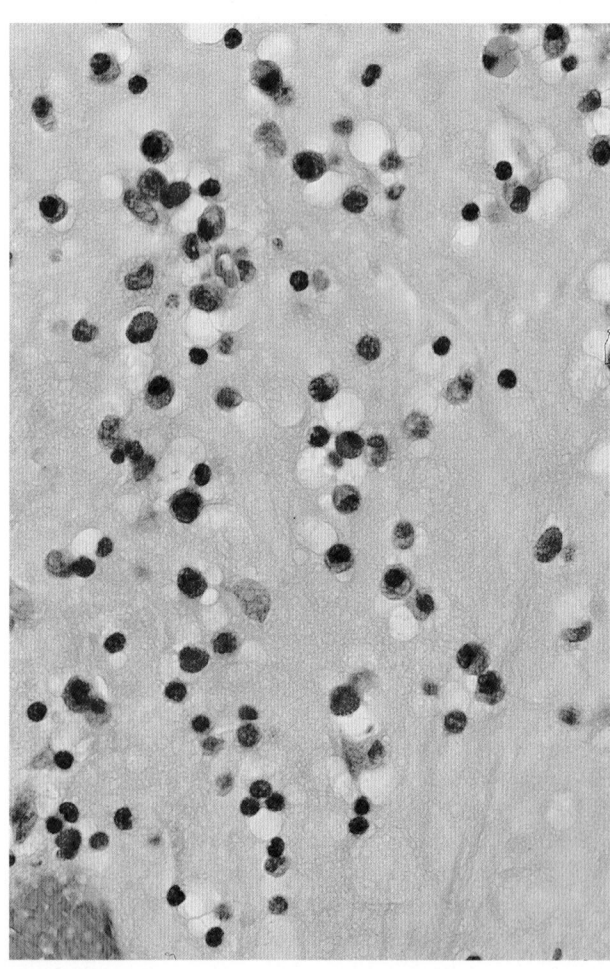

FIGURE 9.19 In this inflammatory exudate, plasma cells are easily identified by their eccentric nucleus and clear paranuclear halo. Note also the eosinophils (red), lymphocytes, and macrophages. The white circles are blebs, probably produced during fixation. (Edematous nasal mucosa of an allergic patient.) (530x)

The presence of lymphocytes in histologic sections of tissues normally devoid of these cells is suggestive of a local immune response (i.e., some antigenic material is or has been handled there). What a lymphocyte is actually doing in a given inflammatory focus can only by inferred from the enormous literature on lymphocyte functions: it might be

- Homing to an inflamed area
- Processing an antigen
- Secreting cytokines, and thereby
- Giving orders to surrounding cells
- Recruiting leukocytes from blood vessels
- Secreting antibody
- Killing a cell

Only the last two functions can be recognized under the microscope without immunostaining.

(8) Natural Killer Cells

Natural killer (NK) cells are also known as **large granular lymphocytes** (LGLs). They were identified as late as 1973 by their ability to kill tumor cells without prior sensitization (70). These amazing cells are programmed to kill selected enemies, namely tumors cells (unfortunately not all) and especially virus-infected cells. Therefore they accumulate in virus-infected organs (106). Normally they are found only in the blood, in the spleen, and in the liver, where they are called "pit cells" (109).

Compared with killer T-lymphocytes, NK cells choose their targets in a very distinctive way (94). Killer T-lymphocytes attack cells that are labeled as targets by the presence of antigen on their surface, combined with an "identity marker," a surface protein of the MHC family (p. 571). NK cells, in contrast, spare those cells that *do* wear the MHC class I label and *kill those that lack this passport.* This is the "missing self" hypothesis of cell killing (52). Their technique for dispatching target cells is discussed elsewhere (p. 233).

Because NK cells can eliminate virus-infected cells without the help of the immune response, they are vitally important as an early defense against virus infections (the immune system requires several days to mobilize its own counterattack). Overall NK cells seem to represent a primitive, nonspecific defense system that evolved after the macrophage but before the T-cell system (49). Recently, another small subset of killer lymphocytes was described, the NKT cells, which share receptors with both NK and T cells (53a).

The process of cell killing was discussed in Chapter 5 (p. 233).

(9) Dendritic Cells

These rather mysterious cells are the most powerful initiators of an immune response (7, 53, 77, 92). They are posted at the outer limits of the body, e.g., within the epidermis as Langerhans cells, seemingly as sentinels ready to pick up antigen; this being done, they float away to a lymph node with a gracious display of "veils" (lamellipodia), hence the nickname of *veiled cells,* and present their catch to the T cells. They arise from the bone marrow and are quite rare in the blood, *but with appropriate cytokine mixtures, they can be grown from circulating monocytes.* At this time, there is no single distinctive marker for the dendritic cells but rather a constellation of markers. It is said that dendritic cells are recruited rapidly at sites of inflammation, but the evidence (9, 10) is still meager.

(10) Endothelial Cells

Endothelial cells are critical to inflammation because they are the barrier that must be crossed by the two components of the inflammatory exudate, plasma and leukocytes. Rivers of ink continue to flow about these deceptively simple, flat cells, once thought to be as passive as a cellophane sheet (83, 86, 88, 278). The endothelial *renaissance* began when it became possible to study the endothelial cells by electron microscopy and to grow them *in vitro.* It turned out that they enjoy—among other distinctions—the rare privilege of a specific morphologic marker: the rod-shaped Weibel-Palade bodies, which are loaded with a specific protein (the von Willebrand factor) involved in clotting and other important functions.

We will discuss the endothelium in action when we analyze the various phases of inflammation; however, we must record here three endothelial concepts relevant to inflammation:

- *The endothelium is the largest endocrine organ,* weighing perhaps as much as one kilogram (86). Endothelial cells can secrete a great variety of molecules (87).
- *The endothelium can be activated:* if stimulated by cytokines or other agents, the endothelial cells respond instantly by producing prostaglandins, or in a few hours by secreting adhesion molecules and other proteins (74).
- *What is true for one set of endothelial cells may not be true for another.* The properties of endothelial cells vary a great deal along the vascular tree and from organ to organ.

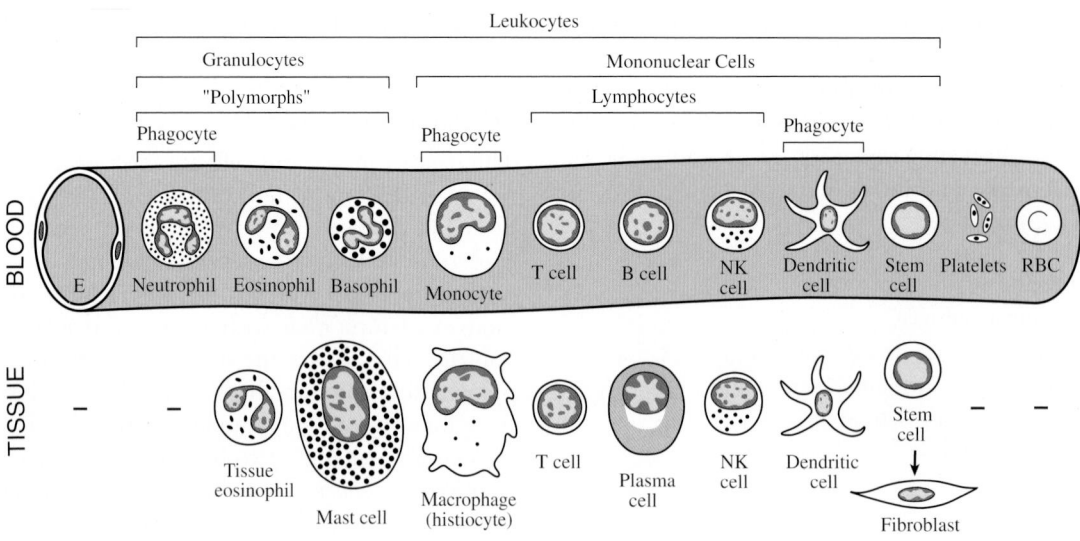

FIGURE 9.20 The family of inflammatory cells. Most are blood-borne but have a counterpart in the connective tissues; only the neutrophils and platelets do not. The fibroblast has a circulating relative among the stem cells. The role of the red cell in inflammation is mainly passive. **E** = Endothelial cell. *Top:* Alternate names often used for particular groups of inflammatory cells.

The permeability of the endothelium in the microcirculation is discussed on p. 387 and p. 614.

(11) Fibroblasts

Fibroblasts, once thought to be rather dull fibermakers, turn out to be quite dynamic; they can respond to chemotactic stimuli and move around (75); they are considered to be semiprofessional phagocytes; and they can also modulate into contractile cells the myofibroblasts (p. 485). On the other hand, they have lost their status as sole synthesizers of collagen, elastin, and glucoaminoglycans; it is now clear that these matrix molecules can also be produced also by smooth muscle cells and endothelium. They are broken down by a set of enzymes known as *metalloproteinases* generated by connective tissue and inflammatory cells (p. 815).

Another change in the status of the fibroblast: it has long been a typical tissue cell, with no counterpart in the blood, but recently it was shown that circulating, $CD34^+$ stem cells can be induced to produce collagen. We are living in a time of collapsing dogmas.

> TO SUM UP: At least 11 types of cells collaborate to repair injury and to preserve us against invaders. Figure 9.20 shows that most of these cells come from the blood but have a sister or a close relative living out in the tissue spaces. The fibroblasts, typical *tissue* cells, are finally understood to have an ancestor in the blood. Figure 9.20 should also help review the overlapping terms *leukocyte, polymorph, granulocyte, and phagocyte.* There are only two professional phagocytes: the monocytes/macrophages (omnivores) and the neutrophils (bacteria eaters). By comparison eosinophils, basophils, mast cells, and dendritic cells deserve to be called "microphages."

Mediators: The Chemical Language of Inflammation

An area of injury would turn into cellular chaos if all the cells concerned were unable to communicate. This disaster does not occur because the cells that are still alive immediately exchange messages in their language, the oldest on earth, using molecules for words. Surely a chemical language of this kind was spoken by the primal cells. Insects use it in their stings (a very effective means of communication), as does the nettle. Bacteria use messenger peptides that resemble our own (262). The language comes in many dialects (Table 9.4), Vertebrate

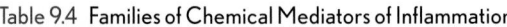

Table 9.4 Families of Chemical Mediators of Inflammation

Endogenous Mediators

1. Vasoactive amines (*histamine, serotonin*)
2. Vasoactive peptides (*bradykinin, substance P*)
3. Complement system by-products (*anaphylatoxins*)
4. Clotting and fibrinolytic system products (*fibrinopeptides, fibrin fragments*)
5. Phospholipid metabolites
   Eicosanoids
      Cyclooxygenase products (*prostaglandins, prostacyclin, thromboxanes*)
      5-Lipoxygenase products (*leukotrienes, HETEs, HPETEs*)
      15-Lipoxygenase products and cell-cell interaction products (*lipoxins, resolvins*)
   Platelet-activating factors (PAFs)
6. Cytokines (*interleukins, tumor necrosis factor*)
7. Chemotaxins (*chemokines*)
8. Free radicals (*nitric oxide, ozone*)
9. Lysosomal enzymes (*proteases*)
10. Nuclear factors (*NF-κB*)
11. Bactericidal peptides (*defensins, magainins*)
12. Cell components (*uric acid*)

Exogenous Mediators

1. Bacterial chemotaxins (*fMLP*)
2. Anti-leukocytic factors (*leukocidin*)
3. Macrophage activators (*endotoxin*)

cells seem to be fluent in all (plus the language of the aggressors), but no human can make that claim. People who speak "prostaglandin" have a strong accent when they speak free radicals, and those who speak "complement" are barely understandable to anyone else. We will do our best to steer you along a Berlitz-type path; for the faint of heart, the tables, the "bottom lines," and the summary figures may be enough.

We acknowledge one major difficulty: the size of the dictionary. In the blissful ignorance of the 1920s only one endogenous messenger was known, histamine, with only one target, blood vessels. Nobody dared think then that *all* aspects of inflammation were driven by chemical signals; Valy Menkin, a pathologist who proposed this concept in the 1930s (220, 221) was largely ignored.

What is a mediator of inflammation? In today's definition, *a mediator is any molecule that is generated in a focus of inflammation and modulates the inflammatory response in some way.* According to this definition, some of the molecules generated by aggressor parasites could also be considered as mediators; we will deal with them last as *exogenous mediators.*

The classic definition of **mediator** in physiologic processes is much more strict. According to an eminent

pharmacologist, an endogenous material can be accepted as a mediator in a physiopathologic phenomenon if (a) it is found in tissues in appropriate amounts, (b) it can be released by the stimulus that produces the phenomenon, (c) it has the same universality in various species as the phenomenon itself, (d) it is destroyed in the place of release, and (e) it can be blocked by inhibitors (259). Today we would add that a true mediator must bind to a specific receptor.

Autacoid has been proposed as an alternative term for inflammatory mediator. It comes from the Greek *autós + ákos,* meaning "self-drug," and may be more appropriate because many of the "inflammatory" mediators are just endogenous drugs that can be secreted under circumstances other than inflammation and that have noninflammatory effects (e.g., prostaglandin E_1 stimulates bone formation). By definition, autacoids are supposed to be pharmacologically active molecules that are secreted locally and are neither neurotransmitters nor hormones. We accept the basic concept, but the distinction is not sharp: prostaglandins should be typical autacoids, yet prostacyclin can circulate like a hormone. (The term autacoid, by the way, was proposed in 1916 as an improvement over the then new term "hormone" proposed by Starling. The latter term was considered inappropriate because it means "the exciting substance" whereas not all hormones excite [154, 172, 280]).

A peculiar development in the field of mediators is that they are currently referred to as **biological response modifiers** and discussed in a journal by that name (239). The reason: inflammatory mediators are potentially dangerous but also powerful molecules that can be tested for use as drugs; in fact many are already in clinical use.

Sources of Endogenous Inflammatory Mediators

Endogenous mediators are supplied by three sources: the plasma, the leukocytes, and the local tissues; that is, they are generated not only by the inflammatory cells but probably by all tissue cells. This is a recent discovery. When inflammation takes place in a parenchyma such as a gland or striated muscle, it certainly makes sense that the epithelial cells and the muscle fibers would have "their say." *Some parenchymal cells are known to speak out in terms of cytokines or prostaglandins;* to quote Sir John Vane, 1982 Nobel laureate for his work in this field, "mammalian cells seem to disgorge prostaglandins at the slightest provocation" (246).

The inflammatory mediators are chemically quite disparate. Some, like the cytokines, bind to specific receptors and thus behave like mediators in the strictest sense; free radicals can be considered mediators when they are produced to kill bacteria; lysosomal enzymes, once released, might be considered as injurious agents.

Here are some basic rules regarding inflammatory mediators:

- Any cellular function is a potential target: motion, secretion, multiplication are commonly affected.
- The cellular response may change depending on the concentration of the mediator; this is especially true for the cytokines.
- *For every mediator there are one or more inhibitors.* Without an inhibitor mechanism, the inflammatory exudate would become an enormous pool of messages that could seep into the bloodstream (via the lymphatics or by reabsorption into the microcirculation) and raise havoc everywhere. This is what actually happens, for example, in anaphylactic shock.
- *Mediators have short lives,* seconds or minutes, and their effects do not last much longer (minutes to an hour or so). Therefore, month-long and year-long chronic inflammation must be sustained by a well-orchestrated production and/or succession of mediators.
- *The effects of any mediator can vary from tissue to tissue and from species to species;* we must therefore be very cautious with generalizations. For example, histamine constricts large arteries and dilates small ones, but not uniformly in all species (132, 281). This variance justifies the use of the noncommittal term **vasoactive,** which implies that a given mediator may vasodilate, vasoconstrict, and/or increase vascular permeability.

We will now briefly describe the 12 known categories of mediators (Table 9.4) without implying any "pecking order" except that those in the first category are usually the first to appear during inflammation.

(1) Vasoactive Amines

The two amines histamine and serotonin (Figure 9.21) are especially important because—unlike most other mediators—*they are available from preformed supplies.* Histamine is stored in the granules of the mast cells and basophils, serotonin in granules of platelets (as well as in the mast cells of rodents). Correspondingly, *histamine and serotonin are the first mediators to be released* after injury. They seem to play little or no role in chronic inflammation.

The value of preformed mediators is easy to understand. If a defensive action is suddenly required, it is useful to have a store of mediators for immediate use. On the other hand, maintaining an arsenal has its dangers: this probably explains why most of the powerful mediators are manufactured when needed. Consider histamine. When mast cell degranulate suddenly throughout the body, they release most of their histamine—and the result is anaphylactic shock, one of the fastest way to die (p. 532). In adults, 0.33 milligrams of intravenous histamine will drop the pulse and blood pressure to dangerously low levels (299), and the skin alone contains about 100 times that critical dose (291). It seems that evolution has wisely equipped us with large supplies of very few readymade mediators; most are produced on short order, in even less than one minute.

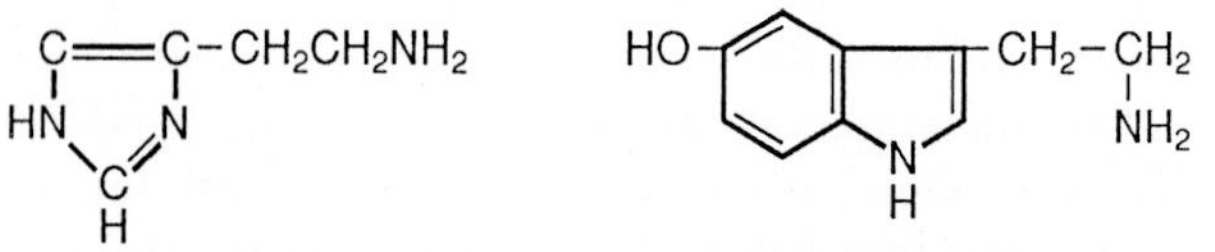

Histamine

Histamine as a mediator is stored primarily in mast cells and in platelets. It is also present in spinach and tomatoes, in wine, in the hairs of gypsy-moth caterpillars (276), and most prominently in the stingers of the nettle, where its function correlates with offense rather than defense (it discourages mammals that may have an appetite for nettles) (p. 537). It can be synthesized by many tissues, including granulation tissue, the new, young connective tissue that is produced in chronic inflammation; it is also found in the gastric mucosa and in the brain as a neurotransmitter (279).

In acute inflammation, histamine produces pain plus three major "vasoactive" effects, all related to cellular contraction:

- *Contraction of smooth muscle,*
- *Arteriolar dilatation, and*
- *Venular leakage (i.e., increased permeability) due to endothelial contraction.*

Therefore the overall effect of histamine injected into the skin is a wheal that looks very much like a mosquito bite.

Students are baffled by drugs that contract *and* dilate vessels. So are we. Whether the vessels respond by contracting or relaxing must depend on dosage, on the orientation of the smooth muscle cells, and on the physiology of the receptors, but the mechanism is incompletely understood (281, 283, 285). On the

FIGURE 9.21 Formulae of histamine and serotonin (5-hydroxytryptamine [5-HT]).

whole, *histamine tends to contract large arteries and to dilate small ones:* thus, the systemic effect of its release is either hypertension or hypotension, depending on the prevalent effect, which varies with the species. In humans there are two syndromes of acute histamine poisoning: anaphylactic shock (although histamine is not the only culprit; p. 532) and a bizarre culinary accident named scombroid poisoning (p. 539). The dramatic drop in blood pressure caused by histamine is due to arteriolar dilatation, aggravated by the loss of blood volume due to widespread venular leakage.

Histamine in low doses is said to attract eosinophils; it does not attract for neutrophils. However, histamine causes endothelial cells to expose, on their surface, the content of the Weibel-Palade bodies; this content includes the adhesion protein P-selectin, which induces leukocytes to stick (183). There are histamine receptors on all leukocytes, but their significance *in vivo* is not known (135). Three to four hours after a local injection of histamine, and probably of any permeability-increasing mediator, there will be a mild local infiltration of leukocytes (p. 433).

Serotonin

As a mediator, serotonin, or 5-hydroxytryptamine (163, 241), is distributed much like histamine: it is found mainly in the platelets (and in the mast cells of rodents) (Figure 9.15). It is also found in enterochromaffin cells, and in the central nervous system. On the whole *its basic vascular effects are similar to those of histamine: venular leakage (i.e., increased vascular permeability)—arterial contraction, and arteriolar dilatation, but with a greater tendency to induce contraction (vasospasm), as implied by its name* (serotonin means "serum substance that increases pressure").

Serotonin also has a property that histamine lacks: *it stimulates fibroblasts* (130). A good way to remember these disparate effects of serotonin is to picture the plight of individuals who carry a serotonin-secreting tumor of the gut. These tumors, called **carcinoids,** derive from chromaffin cells; they produce serotonin and other vasoactive substances, and because they are structured like endocrine glands their secretion is poured into the blood and carried away by the veins. The patients suffer from flushes of the skin, and at autopsy there is a **fibrosis of the endocardium on the right side of the heart** (Figure 9.22) but not on the left, because serotonin is inactivated by the pulmonary endothelium.

Serotonin is rapidly destroyed by monoamine oxidase, present in many cells including monocytes and the endothelium.

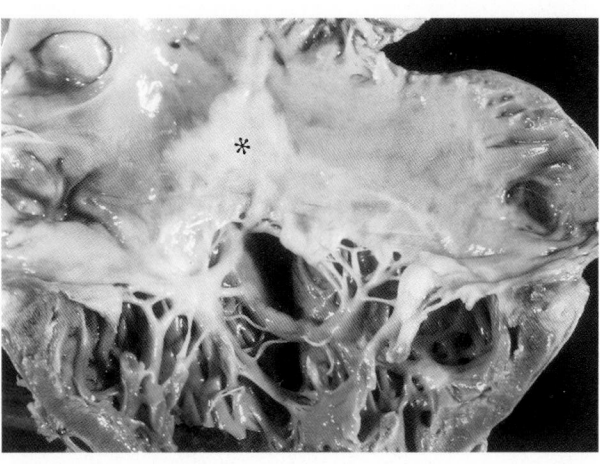

FIGURE 9.22   Plaque of fibrosis (*) in the right atrium of the heart in a case of carcinoid tumor with liver metastases. The fibrosis is an effect of serotonin and bradykinin secreted by the tumor and conveyed to the right side of the heart. The left side of the heart is rarely affected, because the causal agents are inactivated as they pass through the lungs. (Courtesy of Dr. F. J. Schoen, Harvard Medical School, Brigham and Women's Hospital, Boston, MA.)

(2) Vasoactive Peptides

Peptide mediators come from many sources, but they share one feature: they are bits of existing proteins, and have to be cleaved off by appropriate enzymes. Of course these enzymes are normally inactive; thus the genesis of these mediators begins with the activation of the corresponding enzymes.

The Kinin System

Kinins (the prototype is **bradykinin**) are extraordinarily potent vasoactive peptides that are normally carried in the blood in inactive form as parts of plasma molecules called **kininogens** (Figure 9.23). The kinins can be cleaved from the kininogens by specific proteases: the **kallikreins,** which are present in the blood and urine as well as in various body fluids and tissues (229). Obviously, the plasma kallikrein must circulate as an inactive precursor, prekallikrein. Plasma prekallikrein is activated in relation to blood clotting, namely when the plasma protein that initiates the clotting cascade—the Hageman factor—is activated by contact with collagen or with any other negatively charged surface. This means that *when blood clots, abundant kinins are produced,* mainly bradykinin (Figure 9.24).

We have just mentioned a pivotal factor carried by the blood, the ***Hageman factor.*** We recommend that the reader contemplate Figure 9.24, which conveys this

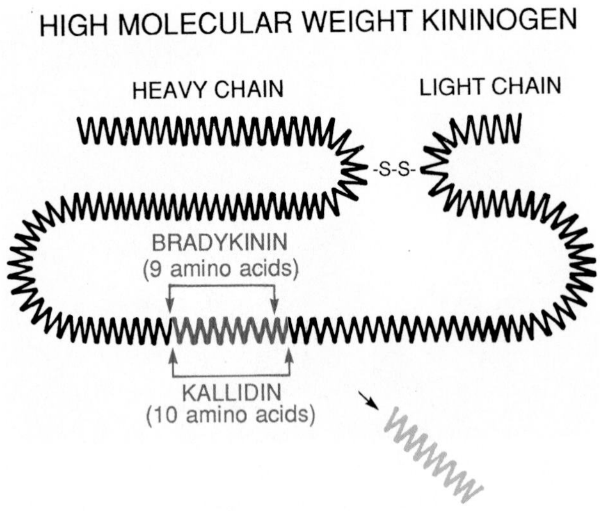

HIGH MOLECULAR WEIGHT KININOGEN

HEAVY CHAIN   **LIGHT CHAIN**

-S-S-

BRADYKININ
(9 amino acids)

KALLIDIN
(10 amino acids)

FIGURE 9.23   Showing how two vasoactive kinins (bradykinin and kallidin) are cleaved from the molecule of high molecular weight kininogen. (Adapted with permission from [204], © Raven Press 1988.)

important message: *nature has endowed the Hageman factor with the power of activating three enzyme cascades involved in the inflammatory response:*

- The **kinin system,** which produces kinins
- The **clotting system,** which produces fibrin
- The **fibrinolytic system,** which produces plasmin, which breaks down the fibrin.

Each cascade generates vasoactive molecules, as a main product or as a side-product.

The kallikreins have no monopoly on kinin release; kininogen can also be cleaved nonspecifically by neutrophil enzymes and by plasmin (151, 204). This reminds us of a general principle. *Plasmin and leukocyte proteases are often floating around in an inflammatory focus, and one of their effects is to generate bradykinin,* either directly or by cleaving the Hageman factor, which activates the clotting cascade (234).

The major component of the kinin family is the nonapeptide **bradykinin.** *Its effects are similar to those of histamine: increased vascular permeability, vasodilatation* or *vasoconstriction,* depending on the circumstances, *and burning pain.* As an **algogen** (pain inducer) bradykinin is even more powerful than histamine and serotonin; wasps and hornets use all three in their sting (155). All these effects are intense and immediate, quite out of line with the name bradykinin, which implies slow moving (the name was chosen when it was found that strips of gut, exposed to bradykinin *in vitro,* respond with a slow contraction). Instilled into the nose, *bradykinin reproduces the symptoms of a common cold with sore throat* (251).

Because the plasma carries substrate and proenzyme (kininogen and prekallikrein) in amounts large enough for a massive release of kinins, a powerful inactivating system is at hand: *the kininases cut the half-life of circulating active kinin to less than one minute* (155). Any remaining kinin is inactivated by a single passage through the lung, thanks to the **angiotensin-converting enzyme** (ACE, or kininase II), which is located on the endothelial surface. Paradoxically, this same enzyme (which inactivates the kinins) activates angiotensin I by cleaving it to angiotensin II, one of the most powerful vasoconstrictors known (267).

This homeostatic mechanism is disrupted in respiratory failure. Local acidosis increases the production of kinins,

FIGURE 9.24   Diagram illustrating the multiple roles of the Hageman factor, activated by contact with a negatively-charged surface. Thanks to the proximity of high molecular weight kininogen (H.M.W.K.) it can activate the kinin as well as the coagulation and the fibrinolytic cascades. Note the feedback activation from activated kallikrein.

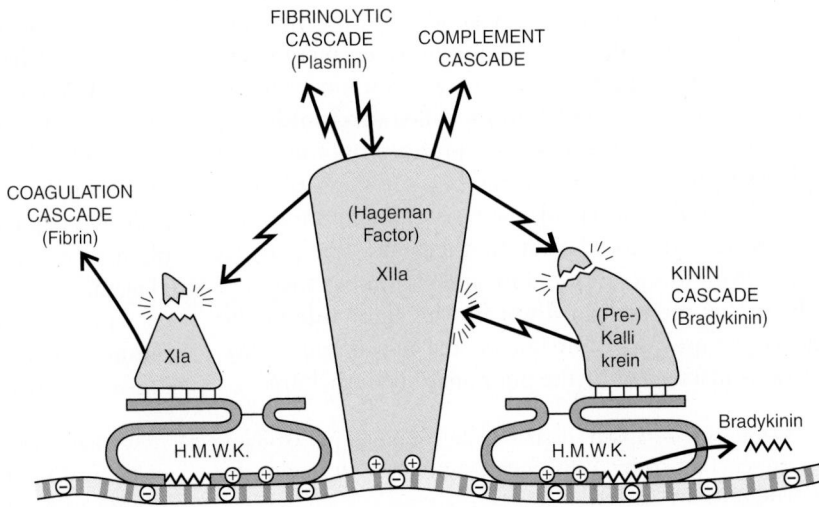

while hypoxia impairs the inactivation mechanism; the result is an excess of local bradykinin, with local and possibly also general effects (208, 236).

Bradykinin was discovered during a homely experiment: a few millileter of urine, injected intravenously into anesthetized dogs, lower blood pressure (154, 167) because it contains kallikrein. Later, various organ extracts were found to have a similar effect, especially those of pancreas (*kallikréas* in Greek, hence the name kallikrein). Tested *in vitro* these tissue kallikreins cleave the same substrate, kininogen, to form a decapeptide, kallidin.

> NOTE: **Histamine-type mediators** is a convenient term for referring to a group of mediators that dilate arterioles and cause venular leakage: histamine, serotonin, bradykinin and the anaphylatoxins, three products of activated complement (C3a, C4a, and C5a).

Other Peptides

Fibrinopeptides produced by digestion of fibrin increase vascular permeability and are also mild vasoconstrictors (120). Peptides of this kind should appear wherever fibrin appears, which includes most types of inflammation: fibrin formation and fibrin digestion are activated at the same time. We suspect that peptides produced by the self-digestion of dead cells (autolysis) have similar effects, but surprisingly they have not been tested.

> There are dozens of vasoactive peptides other than the kinins (269, 272), including *vasopressin,* the *angiotensins,* the *neurokinins, somatostatin,* the *endothelins*—powerful vasoconstrictors (117)—, *and* VIP—which happens to stand for *vasoactive intestinal peptide.* Some are related to hypertension or shock. **Substance P** is especially relevant to inflammation (242); it resembles bradykinin, is released by the endings of sensory C fibers, degranulates mast cells, and is involved in the pathogenesis of the so-called triple response (p. 385).

(3) Complement: A Simplified Version

Judged by power and by complexity, complement is the star of inflammatory mediators (33, 138, 151a, 228). Basically, *complement is a machine for perforating cells. It circulates in the blood stream disassembled into about 30 proteins; when it assembles itself, it also generates—as by-products—some powerful inflammatory mediators.*

This is enough to convey that complement is a very intricate topic (263). Eminent scientists have spent their lives on it. Presumably Nature made it so complicated for purposes of control. The basic concept, however, is simple (232). Many parasites, especially bacteria, can be killed if they are perforated (a very

human approach). However, just poking little holes in their surfaces would accomplish little because cell membranes heal very fast. A better plan is to perforate them with stiff little tubes or plugs that create persisting leaks: this is the ultimate purpose of complement (Figure 9.25). The little tubular plugs, called membrane attack complexes (MACs), are self-assembled mainly from 12 to 18 identical molecules that circulate in the plasma under the name of C9.

There is a bonus in this complicated assembly mechanism. Remember that complement is typically needed for killing invaders, which must also be fought off with inflammation. Well, as the proteins of complement are activated by enzymatic action, some of them release

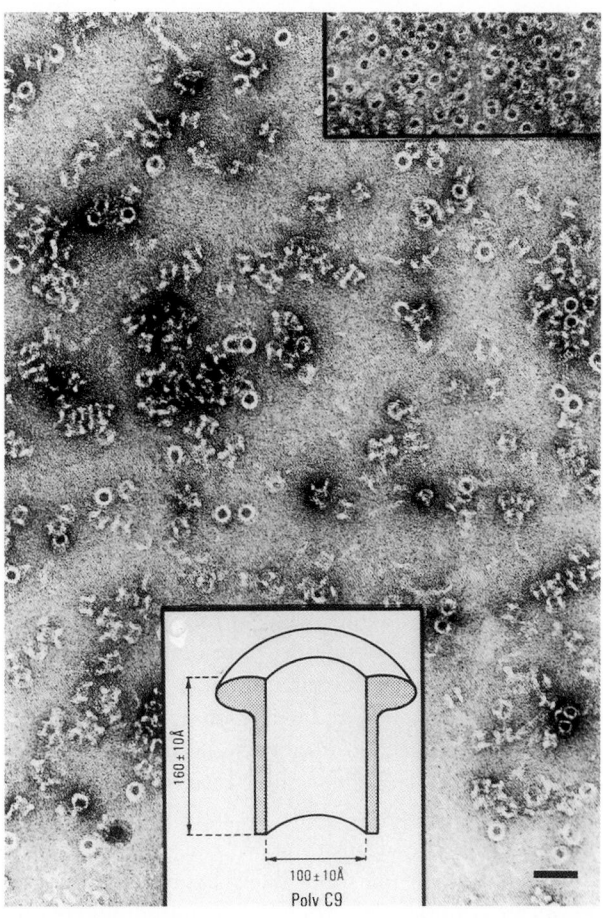

FIGURE 9.25 Electron microscopic image of free "membrane attack complexes" formed by C9 polymerized *in vitro.* Viewed from the top they appear as rings with a 100 Å internal diameter; viewed from the side they are rectangular. **Bar** = 0.05 μm. *Upper inset:* Complement lesions on rabbit erythrocytes (internal diameter about 100 Å). *Lower inset:* Schematic drawing of "poly C9." (Reproduced with permission from [247].)

small fragments that fly off and trigger or enhance the main functions of inflammation, such as summoning leukocytes, causing exudation of plasma, and assisting phagocytosis.

It follows, of course, that complement is extremely useful, but also extremely dangerous. If it were activated in the wrong circumstance, it would perforate and kill any cell. *Evolution has taken care of this problem by creating a machine that circulates disassembled in many pieces* that can be fitted together only under highly controlled circumstances with inhibitors at every step. The system is so complex than only the experts have memorized it all, and we will outline only the essentials, enough to appreciate this marvel of Nature.

Vocabulary of complement—and some helpful hints. Consider that the plug-shaped MAC is not thrust into the target cell like an arrowhead, but created within the membrane, at a site selected by the first component of complement (C1). The nine basic pieces required for triggering the assembly of the MAC are numbered in the order in which they settle on the target membrane (C1 to C9) with the exception of C4, which was named before it was understood. *So the order, alas, really is 1 → 423 → 56789* (followed by more C9 to make up the ring). We clustered these numbers to point out that the nine components actually form three little heaps: 1 by itself, 423 nearby, and 56789 near 423. Those components that are activated by proteolysis are split into a large piece (b), which takes part in further reactions, and a small piece (a), which flies off as a mediator. (Beware: *a* does not mean "activated" as it does in the clotting cascade. This is not our fault.)

The Encounter Complement-Bacterium

A typical scenario could begin as follows: a colony of *E. coli* sets up an inflammatory reaction in the skin (coli endotoxin is a powerful inflammatory agent). Plasma seeps out of the vessels and with it come all the complement components, so the bacteria find themselves exposed to the still-disassembled complement. *Now there are two possibilities:* the plasma may or may not contain antibodies against the bacteria.

Let us assume the more likely hypothesis. Because *E. coli* are common infecting agents, antibodies are present in the plasma, and so complement activation follows the so-called **classical pathway.** The antibodies promptly coat the bacteria, and thereby label them as targets for killer cells; contrary to traditional thought, antibodies can also participate in bacterial killing by producing ozone (292a). How do circulating antibodies reach the bacteria? Remember that we are on a

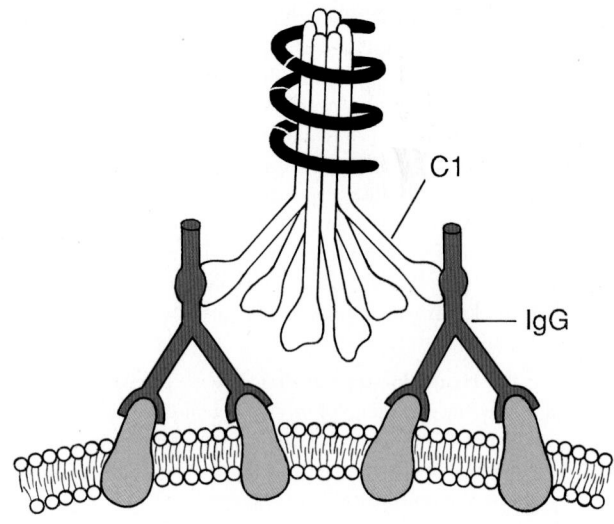

FIGURE 9.26   How C1, the first component of complement, is activated by contact with the Fc portion of two precisely spaced IgG molecules. (Adapted from [111a].)

battlefield: the bacteria have set up an inflammatory response, whereby the vessels are leaking, and the tissue spaces are soaked with plasma. At this point, then, visualize the bacterial surfaces bristling with antibody molecules, say of the immunoglobin (IgG) type: these molecules are shaped like Ys, and they are attached by their two branches, with the stems (called Fc segments) sticking out (see Figure 7.43).

Now, suspended in the plasma is also C1, a marvelous molecule shaped like a flower (its six petals resemble collagen). If a molecule of C1, hovering above the bacterial surface, binds to two Fc segments that are spaced just right, it becomes activated (Figure 9.26); then the next three components are activated as a chain reaction (C2, C3, C4) and settle onto the bacterial surface nearby (the actual order, remember, is C423). These three molecules are caught up in the action simply because they are present in the mixture of plasma proteins. Activated C3 and C4 give off the fragments C3a and C4a, which are mediators of inflammation (anaphylatoxins). At this stage *we can visualize the first assembly (C1 + antibody molecules) sitting on the bacterial surface, surrounded by little piles of C234* (more precisely C2 + C3b + C4b) (Figure 9.27).

Note: some additional C3b fragments settle on the bacterial membrane on their own, as shown in Figure 9.28. Their function is to make the bacterium more appetizing for the phagocytes. Details follow.

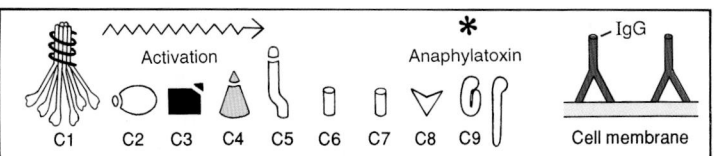

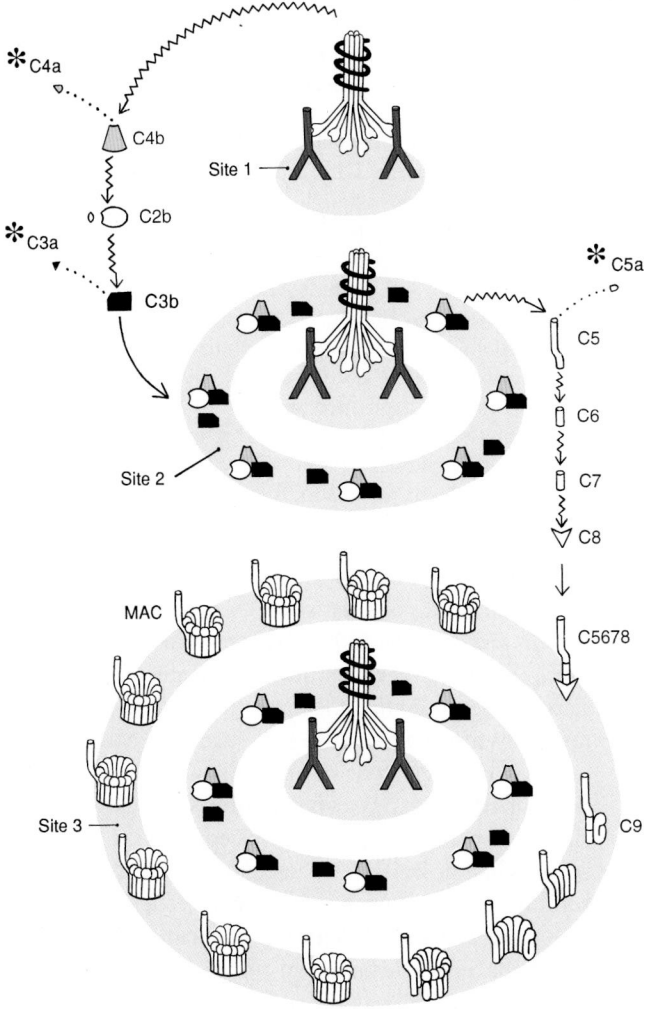

FIGURE 9.27 Geography of complement activation on the surface of a cell to be destroyed. The diagram emphasizes that three sites are involved. *Site 1* is chosen by C1 when it meets two appropriately spaced immunoglobulin molecules; C1 then activates C4, C2, and C3, which form an enzyme complex that settles nearby on the cell membrane (*Site 2*). Note that some molecules of C3b also settle singly on the cell membrane, where they perform as opsonins. The enzyme complex C234 now acts on other complement molecules floating around, and modifies them in such a way that they assemble into membrane attack complexes (*Site 3*). At sites 2 and 3, anaphylatoxins are released (C3a, C4a, C5a), whereby inflammation is induced.

Each little pile of C234 acts as an enzyme and splits any C5 that may be floating by. The smaller fragment (C5a) flies off to become the most powerful of the three anaphylatoxins. The larger fragment (C5b) settles onto the nearby bacterial surface and performs an amazing feat: it develops into a stiff rod by lining up with C6, C7, and C8 (which also happen to be floating by). The rod has a hydrophobic head that is thrust into the bacterial membrane: *perforation has begun*. The rod formed by C5b678 *acts like a shoehorn for* C9, the last arrival, which can be visualized as an egg-shaped molecule (248). When C9 hits the shoehorn it becomes acti-vated and straightens out into a rigid stick that enlarges the hole. More C9 molecules (as many as 19) bump into the settled C9, straighten out and begin to form a circular palisade. In the end the completed MAC looks like a short tube with a handle made up of C5b678 (Figure 9.28). The entire MAC can therefore be summed up as C5b678+999999999999. Milliseconds from the start, the mission is accomplished. The whole sequence—as visualized on a perforated cell membrane—has involved three types of complement sites, which we can imagine as set in three concentric areas (Figure 9.27): the C1 site in the center,

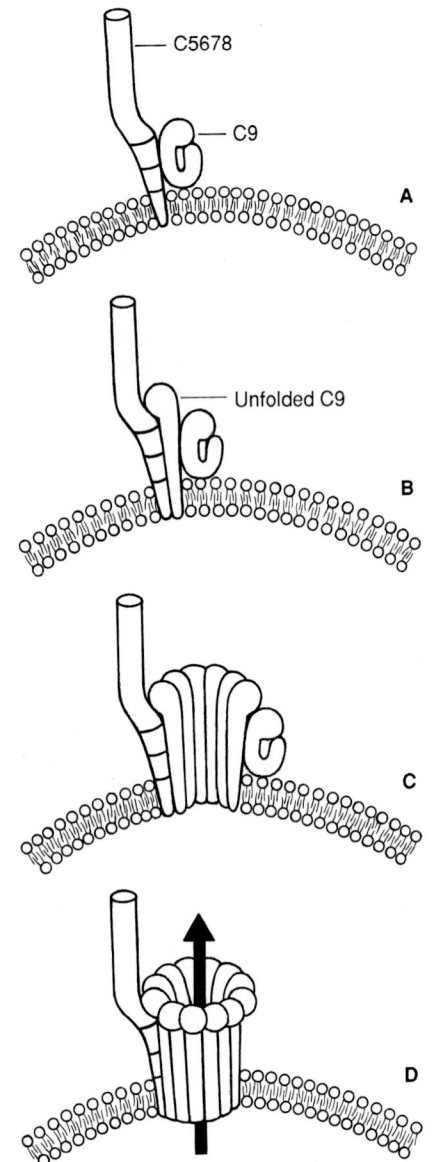

FIGURE 9.28   Development of the complement-derived membrane attack complex (MAC). **A:** a rod-shaped structure formed by four complement components (5b, 6, 7, and 8 [C5678 on the figure]). The hydrophobic end of this complex stabs the cell membrane, and then comes in contact with a folded molecule of C9. **B:** The molecule of C9 is induced to unfold and to penetrate into the cell membrane; the long C5b678 complex appears to act as a "shoehorn." Now another molecule of ~~un~~folded C9 comes in contact with the previous one, and it is also induced to unfold, as shown in **C.** The process is repeated until a complete tubular structure is formed (**D**). (Adapted with permission from [249], © 1984 Pergamon Press Ltd.)

surrounded by a ring of C234 sites and by an outer ring of C5b6789 sites (many more than C234 sites). The perforations can be demonstrated by electron microscopy (Figure 9.25, upper inset). Some cells, including blood cells and the endothelium, carry a membrane glycoprotein called *protectin* or CD59 that acts as a partial shield against the thrust of the MACs (222, 228).

The principle of perforating membranes by means of a plug is not unique to complement; several killer cells of the immune system perforate their targets by a similar mechanism. However, leukocytes can kill without assembling MAC-like pores; one such agent is tumor necrosis factor (see below).

A few details: the dagger-shaped, four-molecule assembly C5b678 (without C9) causes some leakage from the bacterium but not enough to kill it. The size of the MACs varies somewhat depending on the number of C9 molecules that participate. Regarding the "dosage" of MACs required for a kill, a single MAC hit is said to be lethal to red blood cells, but nucleated cells perforated by MACs have defenses that they can mobilize; in one experiment the cells somehow got rid of the MACs in about 2 minutes (254). If a purified solution of C9 is incubated, it polymerizes into typical tubular assemblies (Figure 9.25) (248); this takes 3 days at 37°C, but just 10 minutes in the presence of the C5b678 complex, which acts, as expected, as an accelerator of C9 polymerization (282).

Let us now return to the mechanism of complement activation, and consider the other possibility: *the coli bacilli attack a host that has no anti-coli antibodies.* Clearly, complement cannot be activated as we just described, because that mechanism required a carpet of antibody molecules coating the bacteria. Still, complement is not defeated: it can still be activated by two other pathways: (a) The **mannose pathway** (very similar to the classic pathway, except that C1 is replaced by another flower-like molecular complex, capable of binding to mannose residues on the bacterium) (138, 228) and (b) the **alternative** or **properdin pathway** (173). Bacterial surfaces can themselves attract C3b (a small amount is always present in the plasma); this C3b then activates C3 in a special manner that causes it to interact with five proteins (B, D, P [properdin], H, and I), which also circulate in plasma. The final result is the activation of the typical cascade, amputated of its early components C1, C4, and C2. Note the most important feature of these alternative pathways for survival: *complement attacks bacteria even when they are "seen" for the first time, without the benefit of antibodies.*

The discovery of the alternative pathway took place in sad circumstances. In the early 1950s, Dr. Louis Pillemer—a "tormented genius" (256)—was sure that he had discovered an important new type of anti-bacterial defense, independent of antibody and therefore nonspecific; it involved a protein that activated complement "in midstream" without using up the early components C1, C4, and C2 (but C3 was essential) (244). He called it *properdin,* suggesting an enzyme that intervened before (*pro*) the loss (*perdo,* "I lose [from the solution, by consumption]") C3 (256). Pillemer met with a storm of opposition and ridicule; when he suddenly died of a barbiturate overdose, at the height of the controversy, the properdin story was certainly involved (209, 256). Shortly thereafter his views were vindicated: the discovery of complement activation in guinea pigs that genetically lacked C4 proved that there was, indeed, an alternative pathway.

The inflammatory effects of complement derive from two sources.

(a) The small fragments C3a, C4a, and C5a. They have similar effects and are called **anaphylatoxins** because they cause mast cell degranulation, which—if extensive—leads to anaphylactic shock. The anaphylatoxins also attract and activate leukocytes and stimulate other cells to produce mediators; for example, C5a causes leukocytes to release prostaglandins (189). There is evidence that anaphylatoxins can also increase vascular permeability directly (i.e., not via the mast cells) (296).

> The biological potency of the three anaphylatoxins is C5a > C3a > C4a, dropping by a factor of roughly 100 from one peptide to the next (this is why C5a is often mentioned alone) (129).

(b) Another important proinflammatory effect is due to C3b, which settles on cell membranes and prepares them for phagocytosis by the leukocytes, which have C3b receptors (C3b gets swallowed in the process). This prophagocytic effect is called **opsonization** (p. 415).

The bacterium, as planned, loses its *milieu intérieur* through the many MAC perforations, dies, and is eventually scavenged. Bacteria that are resistant to complement attack, such as Gram-positive bacteria and some strains of Gram-negative bacteria, seem to be protected by a coat of filamentous molecules that keep the MACs at a distance from the cell membrane (Figure 9.29) (197). Viruses can also be killed by MACs if they are duly coated with antibody (Figure 9.30) (292).

> In certain conditions complement can also become activated in the plasma, that is, in a fluid phase. This could be a disaster for any cell exposed to free-floating MACs, but these are promptly deactivated by a providential plasma inhibitor known as protein S (128, 232).

Pathology of Complement

As may be expected, the complement sequence is sometimes activated inappropriately. For example, in autoimmune diseases based on the antibody mechanism, the problem is that antibodies label a "friendly" structure; and complement, their blind accomplice,

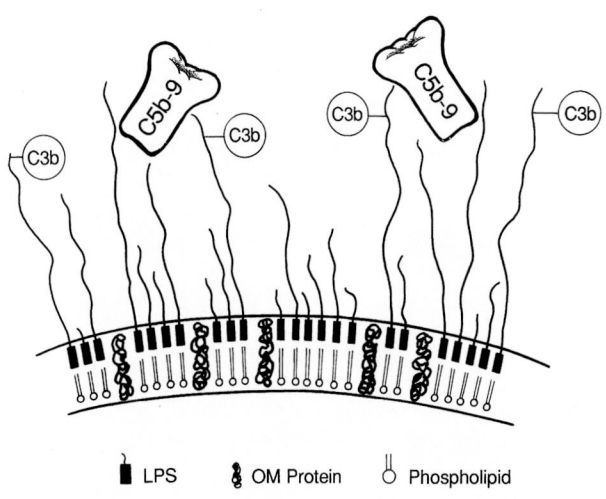

FIGURE 9.29   Why certain bacteria are not harmed by the MAC of complement. Complement is activated when C3b becomes attached to the side chains of endotoxin molecules (LPS for lipopolysaccharide). Steric hindrance by the long endotoxin molecules prevents the MAC from reaching the bacterial wall; the MAC is eventually shed. (Adapted from [197], with permission from Springer-Verlag.)

destroys it. This is what happens to the neuromuscular plaques in myasthenia gravis (p. 593) (268). In immunologic diseases based on the formation of antigen–antibody complexes (e.g., in the wall of arteries; p. 549), the complexes themselves do no harm. Arteritis develops because the complexes activate complement. Traumatized and necrotic tissues activate complement even if no bacteria are involved; whether this is good or bad is not clear (pp. 434, 447). The plastic membranes used for hemodialysis and those of cardiopulmonary bypass pumps can activate complement too and therefore lead to hemolysis; they can also activate leukocytes that will be trapped in the lung and cause damage (Adult Respiratory Distress Syndrome or ARDS) (136, 179, 270).

> Congenital deficiencies of a complement component are rare and can be troublesome, but they are not usually lethal because the bodily defenses against microorganisms are so redundant. C3 deficiency causes increased susceptibility to pyogenic infections, in keeping with the loss of the C3b opsonin, but it is something of a shock to find that the lack of C9 is usually asymptomatic (260). The most important congenital deficiency is the lack of the inhibitor to C1 (C1 esterase inhibitor): as a result of physical or even emotional trauma these patients suffer acute episodes of edema of the skin and mucosae, which can be fatal if it affects the airways (***angioneurotic edema*** or better ***angioedema***) (152, 240). The kinin and clotting systems also appear to be involved in the pathogenesis of angioedema.

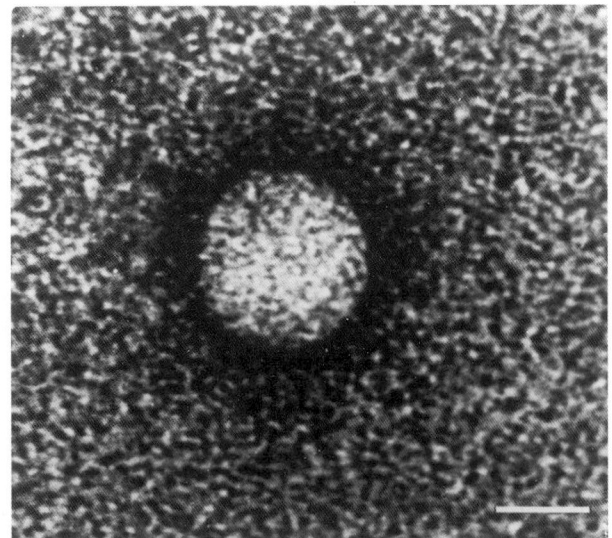

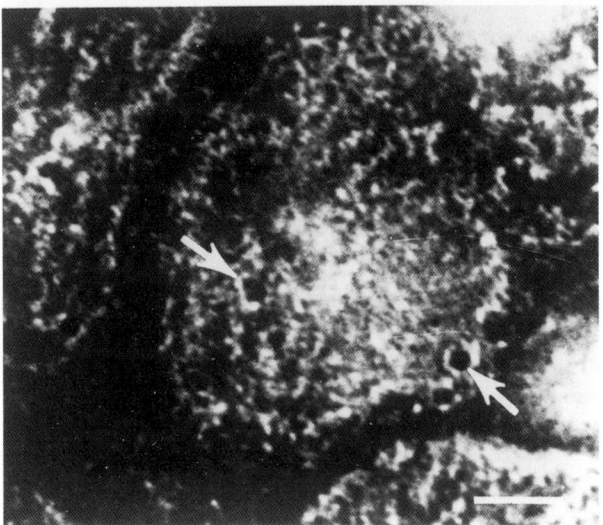

FIGURE 9.30   Scanning electron microscopic view of a virus exploded by complement. *Top:* Normal particle of murine leukemia virus. *Bottom:* The arrows point to one of several holes produced by complement. **Bars** = 500 Å. (Reproduced with permission from [141].)

Has the reader wondered how complement earned its peculiar name? In 1896 Bordet found that specific antisera against vibrios, if heated, could not destroy their targets (the vibrios were coated with antibody, but heating had destroyed complement); however, lysis took place if a little "complement" of nonspecific fresh serum was added (166, 212).

(4) The Clotting and Fibrinolytic Cascades

Blood becomes a solid clot when the soluble protein fibrinogen turns into a network of fibrin filaments (Figure 9.31). Opposing processes in nature are often linked: for example, the dissolution of clots (**fibrinolysis**) is linked with clot formation. The two processes combined generate inflammatory mediators by several mechanisms.

- To aggregate into fibrin, the fibrinogen molecule must lose two couples of peptides, fibrinopeptides A and B (Figure 9.32), which are chemotactic and increase vascular permeability (265).
- Destruction of the polymer occurs at the same time. As fibrinogen aggregates, the opposite (fibrinolytic) system is also activated, and **plasmin,** a proteolytic enzyme, breaks down the fibrin filaments. The resulting *fibrin degradation products* increase vascular permeability by releasing histamine from mast cells (162).
- Plasmin, as a protease, can release inflammatory peptides from substrates other than fibrin, such as kininogen (to release kinins) and C3 (to release the anaphylatoxin C3a) (271).

Plasmin also has a feedback loop (Figure 9.24): it activates a critical molecule, the Hageman factor, which reactivates the whole clotting cascade, plus the fibrinolytic and kinin cascades.

(5) Mediators Derived from Phospholipids

By the late 1960s, the medicoscientific commumity had come to think of inflammatory mediators largely as amines or small peptides. Then everything changed: the arrival of new, *lipid* mediators was announced. The largest family consisted of *eicosanoids,* from the Greek word *éikosi* for "twenty," because they derived from the 20-carbon arachidonic acid. There also was a bunch of new (lipid) *platelet-activating factors* (PAFs), and it took a while to understand why they *had* to be there as well.

The Eicosanoids

However complicated their pharmacology (170, 171, 178) the eicosanoids have to be admired for their architecture. They are built into the structure of the cell membranes, including the endoplasmic reticulum and the plasma membrane; one of the two fatty acid legs of the phospholipid molecules being arachidonic acid, that leg can be chopped out, processed and sent on its way in a hurry: an ideal arrangement for molecules that have to be "spoken into the outer spaces" by the cell. The original arachidonic acid molecule can be processed along three pathways: the **cyclooxygenase pathway,** first to be discovered, which leads to the prostaglandins and thromboxanes; the **lipoxygenase**

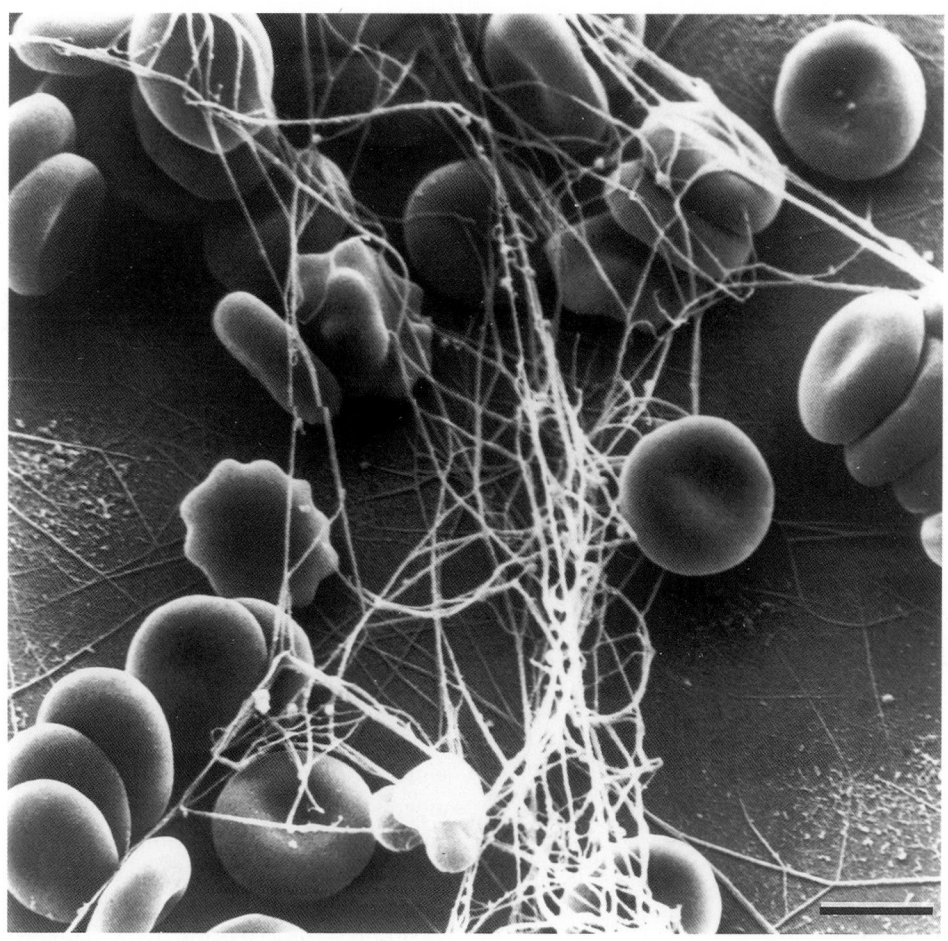

FIGURE 9.31 Scanning electron micrograph of a developing blood clot: red blood cells enmeshed in a network of fibrin filaments. **Bar** = 5 μm. (Courtesy of Dr. M. J. Karnovsky, Harvard Medical School, Boston, MA.)

pathway, which produces the leukotrienes; and the **lipoxin cell-cell interaction pathway,** which produces the **lipoxins** (Figure 9.33). The expression "cell-cell interaction" refers to an interesting mechanism: when two cells are in contact, they can generate in the virtual slit between them metabolic products that neither cell alone could produce (275a). *Each type of cell—if appropriately stimulated—generates its own particular choice of eicosanoids.* For example, endothelium responds to stimulation by producing prostacyclin, whereas platelets go the way of thromboxanes. The stimulus may be injury or another mediator: for example, inter-leukin-1 prods endothelial and smooth muscle cells to secrete prostacyclin (PGI$_2$) (261).

Prostaglandins. The prostaglandins owe their name to a misunderstanding.

In 1930 two gynecologists at Columbia University noticed that during artificial insemination the uterus sometimes contracted violently, sometimes relaxed (122). Later research proved the existence of a contracting agent thought to come from the prostate; it actually comes from the seminal vesicles. To this day the prostaglandins have retained important gynecologic connections, for instance, the initiation of labor by uterine contraction and the control of bleeding (122).

It is now clear that *all mammalian cells, from brain to fat, from skin to stomach, produce prostaglandins if duly stimulated* (227).

A simplified scheme of prostaglandins and other arachidonic acid derivatives is shown in Figure 9.33. Leaving details to specialized treatises, we will only summarize the effects of prostaglandins that are relevant to inflammation. The most important

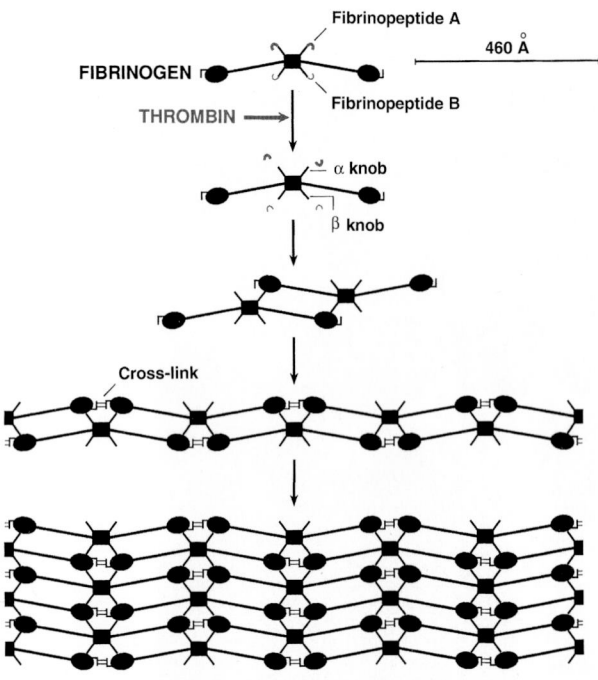

FIGURE 9.32   Polymerization of fibrinogen to fibrin. The first step is accomplished by the enzyme thrombin. The fibrinopeptides A and B are clipped off and join the pool of inflammatory mediators; the fibrinogen molecule is then converted to fibrin monomer, which self-assembles into filaments of fibrin. (Adapted from [153]. © George V. Klein.)

prostaglandins in this respect are two: PGE_2 (produced, e.g., by stimulated macrophages) (131) and $PG1_2$, also called prostacyclin (produced, e.g., by vascular tissues).

> **Prostacyclin** is just another prostaglandin, but it deserved a special name because it is extremely potent and because it is the only prostaglandin to escape immediate inactivation as it passes through the lung. It therefore qualifies as a hormone, as opposed to an autacoid (225).

The principal effect of PGE_2 and PGI_2 is vasodilatation; they can therefore increase the exudation of fluid and the supply of leukocytes (193) by increasing flow through vessels that are already leaky but without increasing permeability or causing diapedesis (p. 388) (187).

Prostaglandins of the PGE series are intensely *hyperalgesic:* that is, they make the skin hypersensitive to painful stimuli. Yet, no prostaglandins cause pain directly. PGE_2 is also one of the most potent agents for producing *fever* (187).

Prostaglandins are not chemotactic, in fact they tend to oppose leukocyte activities.

In essence, the prostaglandins contribute to all four cardinal signs of inflammation listed by Cornelius Celsus, *rubor et tumor cum calore et dolore:* by increasing

blood flow they favor *rubor* and *calor;* they increase the *dolor* if some other agent causes pain and the *tumor* if some other agent causes vascular leakage. Besides increasing pain, their main effects are vascular. Overall, *the main role of prostaglandins in inflammation could be that of guaranteeing an ample supply of blood* (i.e., cells and fluid for the exudate) despite local controlling factors (165).

But then, to remind us that nothing is absolutely clear-cut, *PGE_1 is a typical antiinflammatory agent:* it counteracts histamine, serotonin, and other mediators (164, 252).

We might add that prostaglandins are metabolized in minutes, but "the effects of PGE_2 greatly outlast its presence" (297), perhaps by an hour or two. Drugs that inhibit prostaglandin synthesis are the best proof that prostaglandins are involved in inflammation. The drugs include aspirin, corticoids, and nonsteroidal inhibitors such as indomethacin (Figure 9.33).

Thromboxanes. These mediators have received much attention thanks largely to the platelets because thromboxane A_2 (produced by platelets) is a potent platelet aggregator and vasoconstrictor, two properties that suggest an important role in bleeding vessels. Also, there is a classic opposition between platelets, which metabolize arachidonic acid in the direction of thromboxanes, and endothelium, which metabolize it to produce prostacyclin, with diametrically opposite effects.

Leukotrienes. Just like their relatives the prostaglandins, the leukotrienes were first identified through their effect on smooth muscle.

> Perfused lungs, challenged with snake venom, release into the perfusing medium a substance that, when applied to strips of smooth muscle, caused a slow, persistent contraction. It was named slow-reacting substance (SRS). Later it was found that anaphylactic challenge of the lungs yielded a similar material, SRS-A (SRS of Anaphylaxis). In 1979 the agent was identified as a metabolite of arachidonic acid and the name leukotriene was adopted for this class of compounds (180).

This brief history points out three characteristics of the leukotrienes: they play a special role in lung pathology, they can be generated by an allergic mechanism, and they can cause smooth muscle spasm.

The leukotrienes (Figure 9.33) are generated from arachidonic acid by an enzyme, 5-lipoxygenase, which is present in only a few cells (210, 211). Hence *the leukotrienes, unlike the prostaglandins, are produced by few cell types:* all the leukocytes (as the name implies), including some subsets of lymphocytes; mast cells; and

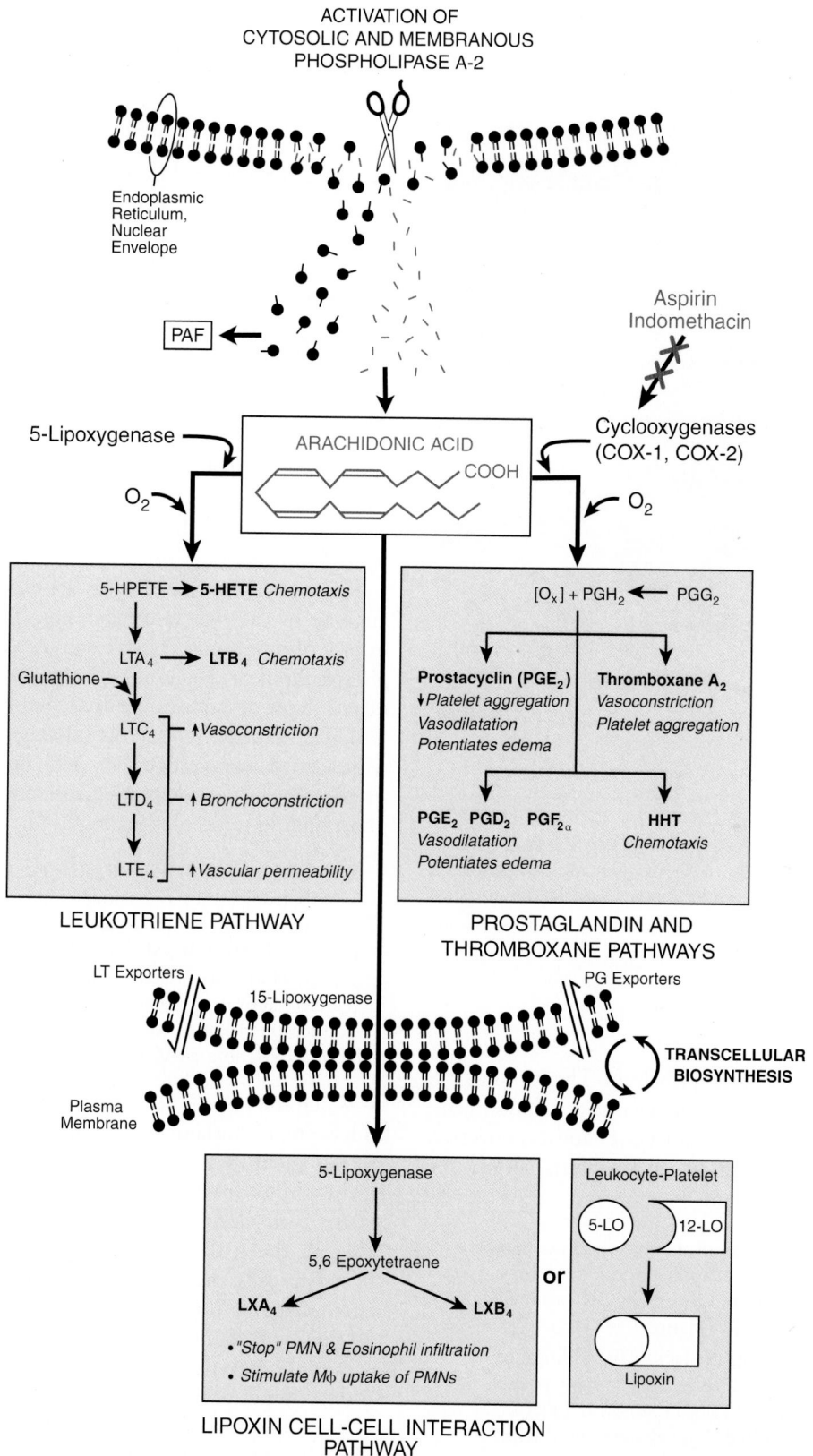

FIGURE 9.33   Arachidonic acid and its metabolites relevant to inflammation. The first step is the activation of phospholipase A₂; the location of this enzyme (cytosol, membranes) is uncertain. Notice that the splitting of each phospholipid molecule generates two sets of mediators: the larger part of the molecule becomes platelet activating factor (PAF). Arachidonic acid can follow three paths, leading to leukotrienes, prostaglandins/thromboxanes, and lipoxins (LO). The latter can be produced via cell-cell interaction. (Adapted from [142], copyright 1989 with permission from Elsevier and updated courtesy of Dr. C. N. Serhan, Brigham and Women's Hospital, Boston, MA.)

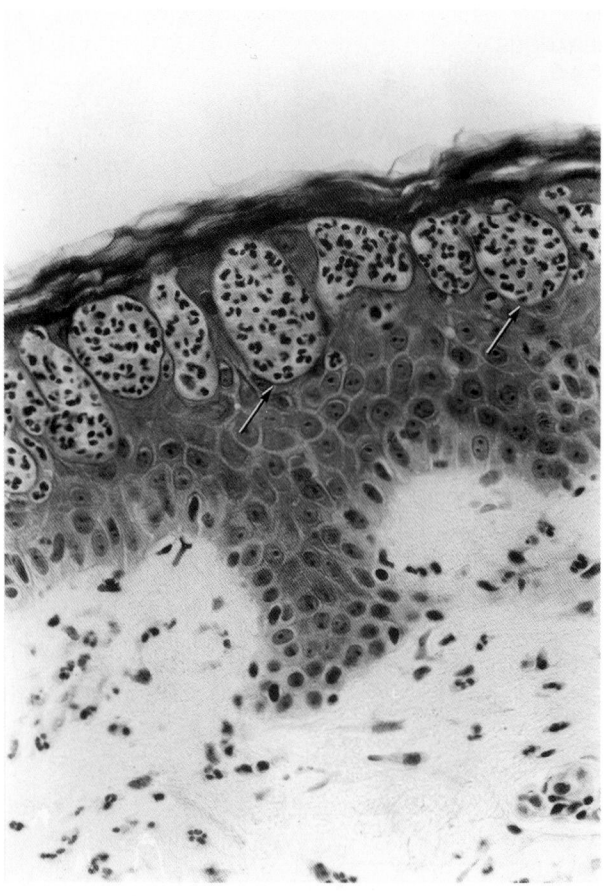

FIGURE 9.34   Chemotactic effect of leukotriene B$_4$. Photomicrograph from a skin biopsy, 24 hours after topical application of 100 ng of LTB$_4$. The granulocytes attracted by the mediator have collected in intraepidermal microabcesses (**arrows**). (Courtesy of Dr. R. D. R. Camp, Guy's and St. Thomas's Hospitals, University of London, London, United Kingdom.)

perhaps human bronchial epithelium. The stimulus can be allergic, as in the antigenic challenge of mast cells, but endotoxin and certain hormones are also effective.

Regarding inflammation, a few facts about the leukotrienes are important.

- Leukotriene B$_4$ is one of the most potent chemotactic substances known; applied to human skin it draws neutrophils into the epidermis, producing microscopic abscesses (Figure 9.34) (133).
- Other lipid chemotactic factors (in addition to LTB$_4$) are produced by the lipoxygenase pathway: they are called HPETEs and HETEs (for hydroperoxy- or hydroxyeicosatetraenoic acid derivatives) (Figure 9.33).
- Leukotrienes C$_4$, D$_4$, and E$_4$ cause leakage from the venules (180, 198).

- The same leukotrienes C$_4$, D$_4$, and E$_4$ cause a combination of vasospasm and vasodilatation, but the tendency to spasm prevails, hence their role in the bronchospasm of asthma and possibly of the coronary arteries (186).

Lipoxins and resolvins. Lipoxins are another family of eicosanoid mediators, which are attracting special attention because of their anti-inflammatory properties (275b), hence the name **resolvins** recently proposed for a subgroup (di- and tri-hydroxydocosanoids) (275c).

Platelet Activating Factors

Platelet activating factors (PAFs) are unforgettable, because, as mediators, they can do almost everything: just glance at Figure 9.35. Their direct effects include everything needed to induce inflammation with the possible exception of vasodilatation. The PAFs also illustrate the extraordinary economy of Nature: *they are made from leftovers of eicosanoid production.*

Remember that eicosanoids are made by chopping out one of the two fatty acid legs (arachidonic acid) from a phospholipid. This leaves us with a one-legged phospholipid, a dangerous leftover, because its asymmetric shape destablizes the lipid membrane (see Figure 4.6). The remedy: replace the missing arachidonic acid with a small, two-carbon fatty acid, and now you have a typical PAF. Two potent mediators for the price of one phospholipid molecule (Figure 9.36).

> The first inkling of PAF was found around 1970. Basophils from a rabbit sensitized against an antigen were exposed *in vitro* to the same antigen, in the presence of platelets. It was noticed that the platelets around the basophils clumped—a sign of activation, hence the name platelet activating factor. An alternative but unpronounceable name for PAF is acetyl-glyceryl-ether-phosphorylcholine (AGEPC) (190).

When the PAF molecule was identified it turned out to have many variants, depending on slight changes in the fatty acid chains; this is why we now speak of PAFs in the plural. It was confirmed that PAFs are released primarily in allergic reactions from a limited number of cells: all the leukocytes (basophils and their cousins the mast cells, neutrophils, eosinophils, monocytes/macrophages, NK cells), endothelium, platelets, mesangial cells, and some epithelial cells (245, 301).

Because they are not water-soluble, PAFs are carried to their target organ bound to albumin. They do dissolve in lipoproteins, in which they are found in surprisingly large amounts (121).

When PAFs are injected into the skin, they cause immediate blanching followed by vascular leakage

FIGURE 9.35 Versatility of Platelet Activating Factor as an inflammatory mediator. (Adapted with permission from [245], © Raven Press 1988.)

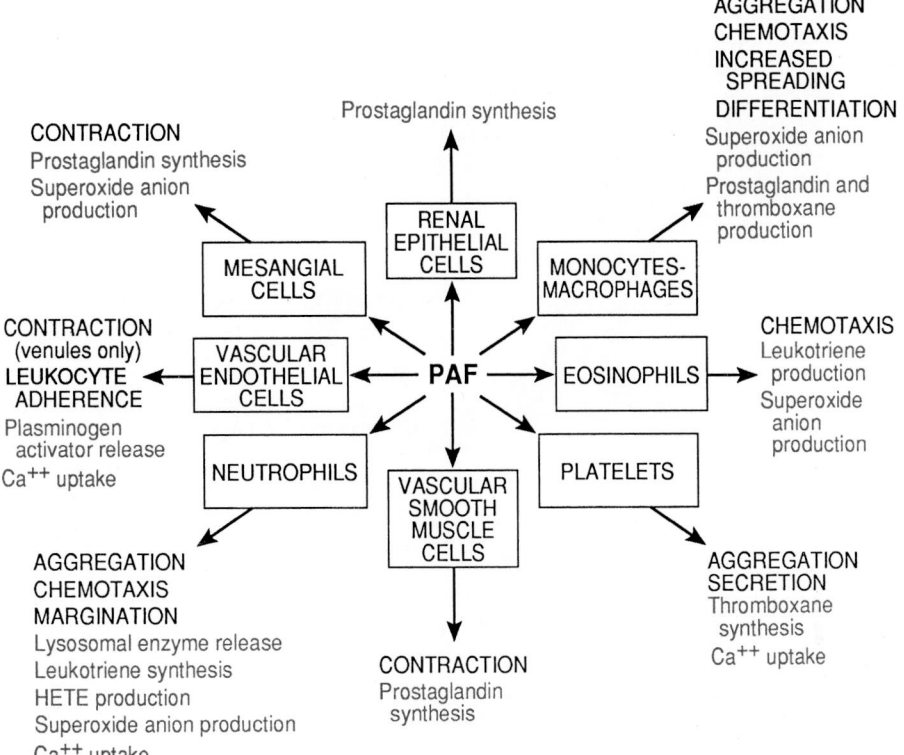

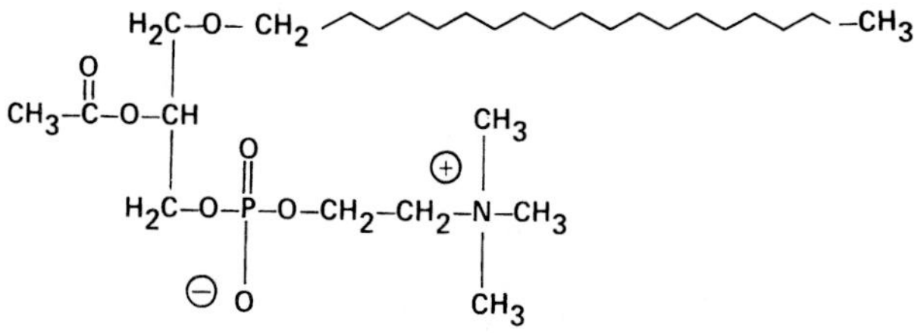

FIGURE 9.36 Structural formula of PAF. A typical phospholipid molecule, characterized by two fatty acids attached to a glycerol backbone, the third carbon being occupied by a phosphate group bound to choline. Critical features are the long-chain fatty acid in position A and the very short chain in position B (acetyl).

(at molar concentrations 100–10,000 times lower than any other autacoid, including histamine), accumulation of leukocytes and burning pain, and eventually a red flare, perhaps due to histamine release. When injected intravenously, they cause, as their name promises, instant aggregation of platelets and leukocytes, which embolize the lungs (Figure 9.37) while the number of circulating leukocytes and platelets, understandably, drops (218).

After all this buildup, it is somewhat sobering to conclude that the role of PAFs as presently understood is limited to acute allergic reactions. Their effects help explain the air hunger (bronchial constriction) and the immediate drop in circulating leukocytes typical of anaphylactic shock. Yet there is no indication that the PAFs, despite their amazing versatility, are put to use in ordinary, nonallergic inflammation. Time will tell.

(6) Cytokines

This large and varied group of chemical messages includes many "prima donna" type of molecules; its scope exceeds inflammation and covers much of biology (235, 240a, 257). Cytokines are small, stable regulatory proteins secreted by virtually all cells (not just inflammatory cells); they control the survival, growth, differentiation and function of other cells, usually over a short distance (235). Each one can be secreted by several types of cells, sometimes without apparent stimulus. All cytokines bind to specific receptors, whereupon they are endocytosed and destroyed. Some bind also to the extracellular matrix near the responder cells, and thus provide them with an immediate local supply of the message. *In essence, the cytokines provide a system of communication and information between cells;* they also provide biologists with "cytokine soups" for tissue culture, whereby cells can be instructed to behave almost at will. Some found applications in the therapy

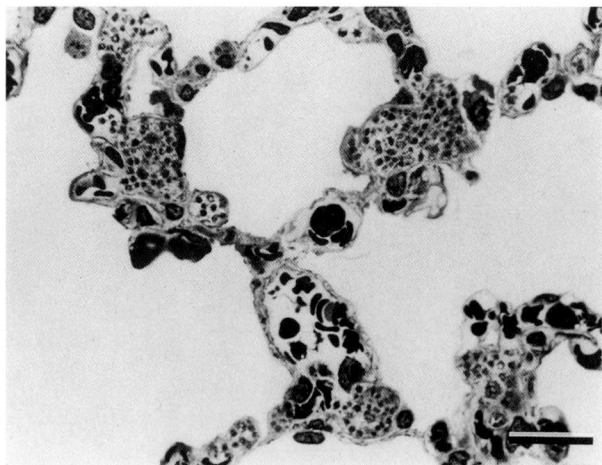

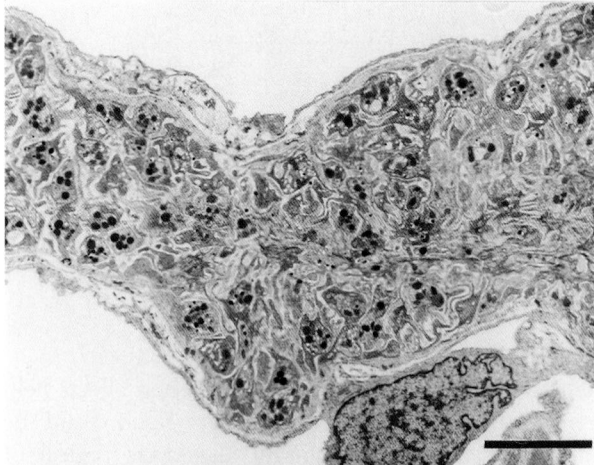

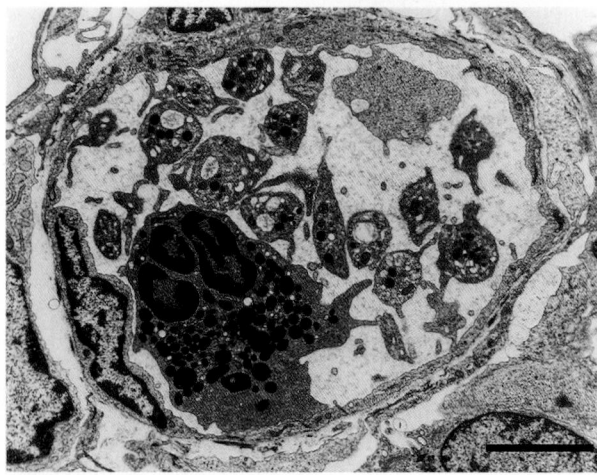

FIGURE 9.37   Platelet-aggregating effect of PAF in a rabbit lung fixed 30 seconds after an intravenous infusion of PAF. *Top:* Alveolar capillaries are stretched by large platelet aggregates. **Bar** = 25 μm. *Center:* Alveolar capillary filled with aggregated platelets. **Bar** = 5 μm. *Bottom:* Leukocytes participate in the platelet aggregates produced by PAF. **Bar** = 5 μm. (Reproduced from [219].)

of inflammation, tumors, and even HIV infection (235, 257).

Cytokines number in the hundreds. They are difficult to classify, because they are multifunctional, with tremendous redundancy in their effects. Paradoxically, gene deletion experiments have shown that *most cytokines are not essential for life,* not because they are unimportant but because their effects are so important that they must be backed up by other cytokines. Another complicating factor: the effects of one cytokine can be altered by the presence of another; e.g., interleukin 2 induces interleukin 1 (203). Their nomenclature is utterly confusing, because—starting in the 1960s—the same molecules were discovered several times in different fields, misinterpreted at first as very specific, named and renamed accordingly, and assigned to overlapping groups, including *growth factors, colony stimulating factors, lymphokines, monokines, transforming growth factors, interferons, interleukins,* and, finally, *chemokines.* Interleukin 1 held 11 separate names until it became IL-1 (235).

> Perhaps there is some hope in a future classification based on the receptors, which fall into four distinct groups (235). By international agreement in 1986, any new cytokine discovered and sequenced receives the name "interleukin" followed by a number.

Under these circumstances, for all but those who are doing research in this field, it is clearly impossible—and actually unnecessary—to memorize the facts about every cytokine. All we can do is to develop some familiarity with a handful of the most common; two are summarized below, others will be introduced later or can be found elsewhere in books (170, 184, 235, 257). The basic concept to retain is that, given a certain cell behavior, it can probably be explained by a cytokine or, more likely, by a group of cytokines.

Interleukin-1

Interleukin-1 (17–20 kD) comes in six forms: three agonists, two antagonists, and one inert (147, 148, 149, 170, 235). It is produced by monocytes/macrophages and an assortment of other cells including NK cells, smooth muscle, and some epithelia. Injected locally, IL-1 increases vascular permeability and causes leukocyte emigration (143, 145). Its general effects, listed in Figure 9.38, seem to reach every corner of the body. Notice the familiar clinical symptoms that accompany "dis-ease": fever, sleepiness, and loss of appetite. Muscle aches may also be due to IL-1-mediated muscle breakdown (115), but this was not confirmed with

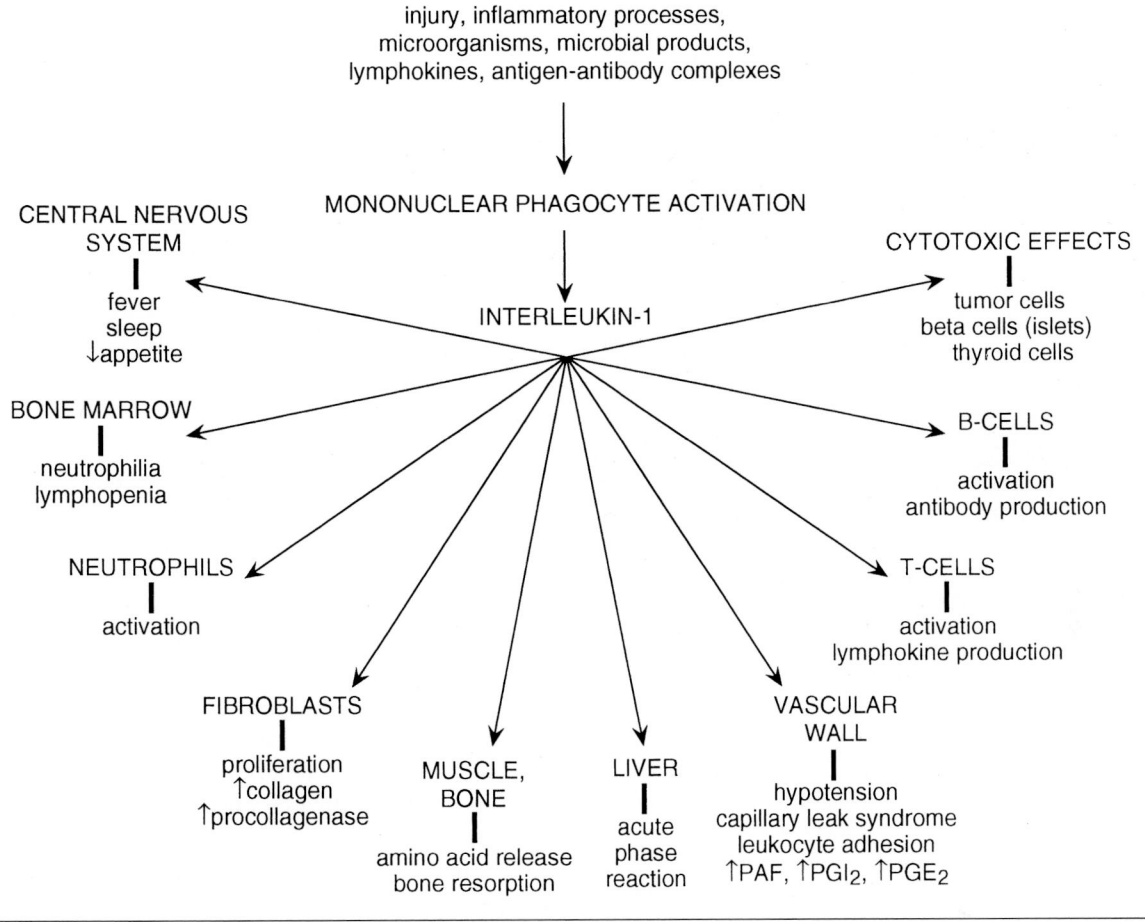

injury, inflammatory processes,
microorganisms, microbial products,
lymphokines, antigen-antibody complexes

MONONUCLEAR PHAGOCYTE ACTIVATION

CENTRAL NERVOUS
SYSTEM

fever
sleep
↓appetite

INTERLEUKIN-1

CYTOTOXIC EFFECTS

tumor cells
beta cells (islets)
thyroid cells

BONE MARROW

neutrophilia
lymphopenia

B-CELLS

activation
antibody production

NEUTROPHILS

activation

T-CELLS

activation
lymphokine production

FIBROBLASTS

proliferation
↑collagen
↑procollagenase

MUSCLE,
BONE

amino acid release
bone resorption

LIVER

acute
phase
reaction

VASCULAR
WALL

hypotension
capillary leak syndrome
leukocyte adhesion
↑PAF, ↑PGI₂, ↑PGE₂

FIGURE 9.38   Main biological effects of Interleukin-1. (Adapted from information appearing in The New England Journal of Medicine [147].)

recombinant IL-1; the effect may have been due to a contaminant, perhaps tumor necrosis factor (148).

Some of the general effects are clearly beneficial (e.g., leukocytosis), and others are puzzling. For example, the ability to induce PGE_2 and collagenase secretion by macrophages in the joints looks like a mechanism that is certain to cause arthritis; the production of IL-1 by gingival epithelium can activate the adjacent osteoclasts, causing bone loss and receding gums. More problems of this nature are raised by tumor necrosis factor.

Tumor Necrosis Factor Alpha

This powerful and dangerous agent, often called just TNF, is produced mainly by macrophages in response to bacterial infection and many other stimuli, in amounts that can be large enough to induce cachexia, hence the alternative name *cachexin*. Its biological effects are indistinguishable from those of TNF beta or lymphotoxin, produced by activated T lymphocytes. TNF (alpha) is so

powerful that it came to the attention of the medical world in the late 1800s (125, 237, 238).

At that time it was observed that occasional cancers regressed when the patient suffered a concurrent bacterial infection. A few courageous physicians attempted to induce infections in their cancer patients. Some regressions were obtained, but the risk was great, so a New York surgeon, William B. Coley, turned to killed bacteria. The name *Coley's toxin was applied to a mixture of killed Streptococcus pyogenes and Serratia marcescens,* which were reported to induce some complete regressions (Figure 9.39) (140). As late as 1934 there was no other medical treatment for cancer. Then came radio- and chemotherapy, and Coley's toxins were relegated to the controversial; they might have been forgotten entirely if Coley's daughter had not collected his and other similar records (233). But experimental work continued: tumor-bearing mice were challenged with bacteria or culture filtrates. Eventually, endotoxin was found to produce hemorrhagic necrosis in certain mouse tumors, especially

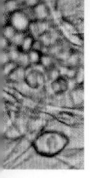

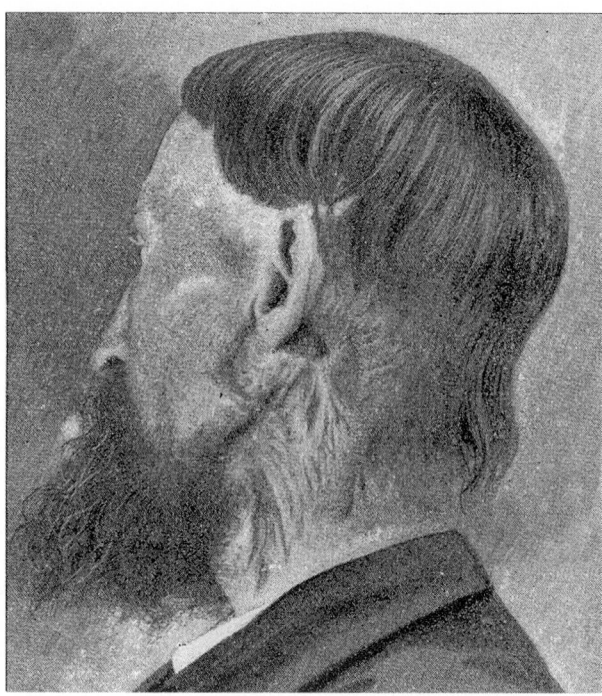

FIGURE 9.39 An infection (note the scar below the ear) reportedly cured this patient of a malignant tumor. This was one of the cases that inspired William B. Coley (1893) to try infection as a cure for malignancy. This patient was operated on five times in 3 years for a "round-celled sarcoma of the neck" at age 31. "At the last operation it was found impossible to remove all of the tumor, and the case was considered hopeless. Two weeks after the operation a severe (*spontaneous*) attack of erysipelas occurred, followed by a second attack shortly after the first had subsided. . . . The sarcoma entirely disappeared, the wound rapidly healed, and the patient was seen . . . by myself seven years afterward, at which time this photograph was taken." (Reproduced with permission from [140].)

if the mice had been "primed" with an infection by *bacillus Calmette-Guérin* (BCG), an attenuated *Mycobacterium tuberculosis* used for vaccinating humans against tuberculosis (134, 223). It was in the serum of these mice that TNF was first discovered; further work showed that the hemorrhagic necrosis in the tumors was not produced by the endotoxin but by the TNF that the macrophages secreted under the stimulus of endotoxin (Figure 9.40).

> **NOTE:** TNF was discovered again in relation to sleeping sickness, another fascinating story (p. 829).

When they were first discovered, the properties of TNF raised high hopes for tumor therapy. When 39 types of tumor cells were exposed to TNF *in vitro*, about 30 percent were killed, but the choice of targets seemed capricious: some were sarcomas, some were carcinomas. Normal cells were spared. TNF injected intravenously killed the same tumors that were affected *in vitro* (124).

> As to the mechanism of TNF killing, the cells exposed to TNF become much more sensitive to its toxic effect if they are previously treated with an inhibitor of protein synthesis—and the reader may recall what this suggests: cells that commit suicide and die by apoptosis seem to require a burst of protein synthesis before they die (p. 211). The cells killed by TNF undergo the structural and biochemical changes of apoptosis (Figure 9.41) (207). Normal cells exposed to TNF *in vitro* are stimulated in a variety of ways (126, 206), but mysteriously, they are not killed at the doses that kill tumor cells.

When TNF is injected intravenously to tumor-bearing animals, the typical effect—hemorrhagic necrosis—is spectacular. The mechanism may be related—in part—to the fact that TNF induces apoptosis in cultured endothelial cells; furthermore, TNF has microvascular effects (such as fibrin thrombi), which preclude its therapeutic use (194). After all, TNF is a major link in the pathogenesis of septic shock.

When TNF is injected into the skin, it induces acute inflammation (143). When infused subcutaneously, it induces acute and then chronic inflammation; in high doses massive necrosis develops, suggesting a direct toxic effect (243). A single intravenous injection in mice produces a "vascular leak syndrome" and necrosis of the villi in the small bowel (258). In human pathology TNF is currently turning up as a link in the pathogenesis of various diseases such as cerebral malaria (176) and graft-versus-host disease (p. 579). Alas, TNF is not a magic bullet that hits tumors only. Clinical trials have been disappointing (125).

(7) Chemotactic Agents (Chemotaxins)

Chemotaxis refers to the movement of a cell along a chemical gradient. It plays a major role in inflammation (displacement of the troops!) especially, but not only, for leukocytes.

If we had to guess the sources of leukotactic stimuli, knowing that leukocytes must be summoned into infected lesions, we would probably suggest three possibilities: bacterial products, injured cells, and spilled blood with its enzyme cascades (pp. 372, 373). All guesses would be correct, except that today we have to include almost all cell types, from epithelial to cartilage and neurons. Most chemotaxins are peptides.

Bacterial chemotaxins. The chemotactic effect of pyogenic bacteria is easily seen *in vitro*. It is of course suicidal for bacteria to attract leukocytes, but they do it anyway

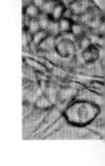

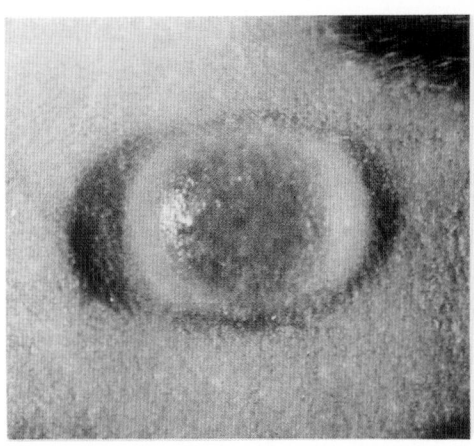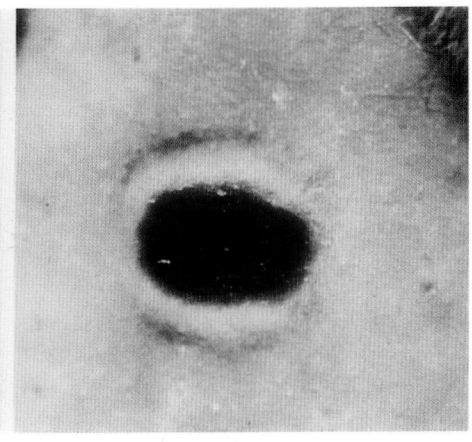

FIGURE 9.40   Sometimes, some tumors can be killed by injecting a dangerous bacterial product, endotoxin. *Left:* A tumor growing freely in the subcutaneous tissue of a rat. *Right:* A similar tumor 6 hours after an intravenous injection of endotoxin: the vessels *of the tumor only* are damaged and bleed, and the tumor dies. This effect is now interpreted as indirect: endotoxin induces macrophages to secrete a potent cytokine, tumor necrosis factor (TNF). For the mechanism of cell killing by TNF, see Figure 5.33. (Reproduced with permission from Dr. L. J. Old [238].)

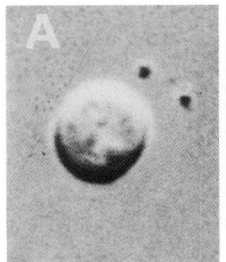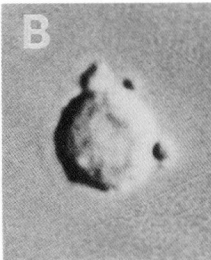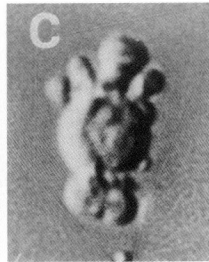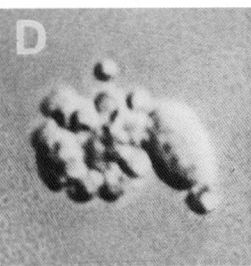

FIGURE 9.41   Stages of apoptosis induced by TNF in cells of a monocyte-like line (U937). The target cells emit buds and eventually appear to burst. The process requires 1 or 2 hours from stage A (normal cell binding TNF) to stage D. (~1,300x) (Adapted with permission from [207].)

(p. 403). *Pyogenic* means "pus-producing": because pus is a suspension of leukocytes, chemotactic bacteria are (by clinical definition) pyogenic.

A great deal was learned from *Escherichia coli*. Like all gram-negative bacteria, *E. coli* contains in its wall a complex lipopolysaccharide also known as LPS or endotoxin, which is responsible for a great deal of human disease. An intracutaneous injection of endotoxin causes an influx of neutrophils with a peak at 2 hours, a little later than after an injection of TNF or IL-1, presumably because the endotoxin effect requires two steps: stimulation of macrophages and secretion of TNF and IL-1.

Studies of bacterial chemotaxins have been very fruitful and have led to the discovery of the prototype chemoattractant fMLP (formyl-methionyl-leucyl-phenylalanine).

It was noticed at first that cultures of *E. coli* are highly chemotactic. Following this lead, it has been possible to pinpoint the chemical structure of these peptides that is critical for chemotaxis, and thus to synthesize dozens of chemotactic di-, tri-, and tetrapeptides. Today the most widely used chemotactic peptide is the potent fMLP active even in dilutions of 10^{-11} (17). Hundreds of similar peptides are commercially available for experimental purposes.

The biological (and pathological) significance of fMLP is clear: prokaryotic cells initiate protein synthesis with formyl-methionyl tRNA, in contrast to the methionyl-tRNA of eukaryotic cells. Thus the polypeptides produced by the growing *E. coli* can be interpreted by eukaryotic cells as evidence of protein synthesis by an expanding bacterial population (163). Obviously the leukocytes have evolved the ability to recognize this ancestral call: the smell of a growing, aggressive bacterial colony.

The potencies of several chemotaxins are compared in Figure 9.42.

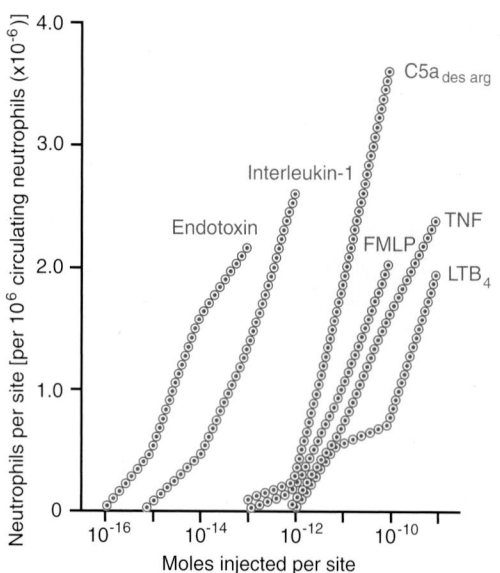

FIGURE 9.42 Effectiveness of six inflammatory agents in causing neutrophil emigration into rabbit skin. Endotoxin is considerably more powerful than leukotriene B_4 or the complement-derived chemotaxin C5a des Arg. (Adapted from [230], with permission from S. Karger AG, Basel.)

Chemotaxins released by dead or dying cells. This apparently simple situation was difficult to work out. *In vivo* it was obvious that leukocytes rush toward dead tissue and crawl into it as far as they can (Figures 8.26 and 8.27). The confusion began when the chemotactic effect was sought *in vitro*. We will present the reader with the puzzle as it originated in 1953.

An eminent scientist (75) published a paper showing that dead tissue was not chemotactic *in vitro*. His test objects were liver and muscle autolyzed aseptically for 3–24 hours. He concluded that chemotaxis could not play much of a role in disease, and so interest in chemotaxis sagged for a while (203). Then a French hematologist, Marcel Bessis, showed very dramatically that when a single leukocyte was killed under the microscope by a laser beam, other leukocytes converged on it "like sharks . . . upon one of their number which has blood escaping from a wound" (21, 215). Bessis actually coined the term *necrotaxis*. How can these opposite findings be reconciled?

The answer: *WHILE cells are dying,* they release or produce chemotaxins; but when this terminal outburst is over, no more messages are sent and so the necrotic lump ceases to attract the "sharks" (p. 453) (124). Today nobody doubts that dying and recently dead cells release a soup of chemotactic molecules, although their chemical nature has not been studied.

Chemotaxins released from spilled blood. Clotting blood generates four proteolytic cascades, as we have seen, and

you can expect that Nature would take advantage of this automatic event to generate chemotaxins. Indeed, the *clotting cascade* leads to thrombin, which is chemotactic for monocytes; as thrombin acts on fibrinogen it releases a chemotactic polypeptide. When fibrin is attacked by the *fibrinolytic cascade,* the breakdown products are again chemotactic. *Activated complement* supplies anaphylatoxins, i.e., C3a, C4a, and C5a (p. 357), which are also chemotactic. Not enough? In injured tissues, inactive complement proteins will be floating around, including C3, C4, and C5. If any of these runs into a proteolytic enzyme—there can be many in injured tissues—it will be split, releasing anaphylatoxin.

Sundry chemotaxins (214). Several families of inflammatory mediators include chemotactic effects: some lipid mediators of the arachidonic acid group (leukotrienes, HETEs), PAF, PDGF, exogenous cyclic AMP (205), and beta-endorphin (156).

So we have plenty of chemotaxins from plenty of sources, but they are rather disappointing: overall, they tend to attract the whole motley crowd of leukocytes, whereas we know that in some diseases very specific subgroups of leukocytes are drafted. The really "professional" chemotaxins were discovered belatedly (around 1990) among the cytokines.

Chemokines. In 1987 it was noticed that three known chemotactic cytokines, including interleukin 8, shared a molecular structure, pointing to a whole new class of chemotaxins. They had four conserved cysteines (C), of which the first two could be separated by an amino acid (X), producing a C-X-C structure: these were called *alpha chemokines* (Figure 9.43). In the *beta chemokines,* the first two cysteine residues are adjacent (CC) (Figure 9.43). There are other types (C, CXXXC), but the main point is that we have here a class of more than 40 chemotactic molecules with more specificity for leukocytes than any previously known chemotaxin family: e.g., lymphotactin for resting T cells, IL-8 for neutrophils, IP-10 and MCP-1 for monocytes, eotaxin for eosinophils (113, 114, 216).

A sample of the nomenclature: **IP-10** = interferon-inducible protein 10; **MCP** = monocyte chemoattractant protein; **RANTES** is supposed to mean **r**egulated upon **a**ctivation **n**ormal **T** cell **e**xpressed and **s**ecreted, but a rumor reached us whereby the name was actually due to a joke.

Chemokines: the HIV connection. Some bacteria and viruses use receptors for gaining entry into cells: e.g., the Epstein-Barr virus uses complement receptor 3(CR3). Similarly, HIV-1 binds to several chemokine receptors; individuals with a defective receptor cannot be infected by

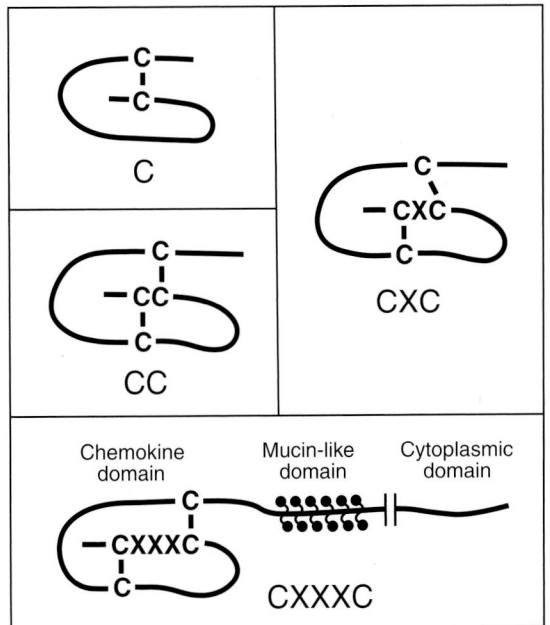

FIGURE 9.43   Basic structure of the four principal families of chemokines: C, CC, CXC, CXXC. C = Cysteine residue. See text. (Adapted with permission from New Engl. J. Med. "Chemokines—Chemotactic Cytokines that Mediate Inflammation" Luster AD. 338:436–445, 1998. Copyright © 1998 Massachusetts Medical Society. All rights reserved.)

this virus, and their cells cannot be infected even *in vitro* (216).

Inhibitors of chemotaxis. Plasma and serum usually contain several factors that deactivate either the leukocytes or the chemotaxins (195). For example, chemotactic factor inactivator (CFI) (93) and cell-directed inhibitor (CDI), present in normal serum, increased in 70 percent of patients with malignant tumors, resulting in a leukotactic defect (205). Another endogenous inhibitor is prostaglandin A_1 (154).

(8) Free Radicals

Many of the oxygen- and nitrogen-derived free radicals were discussed earlier (p. 196). The latest addition is **ozone** (p. 539). The smallest of all mediators, and the latest to procure the Nobel prize (1998) is nitric oxide: NO (short for NO·), produced by the enzyme NO synthase (NOS) acting on L-arginine (213, 224, 300). As a free radical it is not very reactive: this allows it to diffuse several microns before running into an inactivating collision. It scavenges free radicals. In the endothelium, diffusing from its vantage point in the endothelial caveolae (where NOS is located), it dilates vessels, opposes platelet aggregation, and inhibits leukocyte-platelet adhesion.

(9) Lysosomal Enzymes

Lysosomal enzymes can find their way into an area of injury when cells break up or neutrophils spill the content of their granules. Enzymes are not true mediators, in the sense that they do not bind to receptors; however, we list them here because the small molecules resulting from enzymatic digestion can have important biological effects. This is especially true for proteases: they can cleave kininogen to produce bradykinin; they also cleave C3 and C5 to yield chemotactic fragments, or fibrin to yield active "split products." *Wherever proteases are on the loose, inflammatory mediators appear.* Proteases can also stimulate mitosis and differentiation; there is even a human leukemia line that can be stimulated by trypsin to mature *in vitro* (273).

> A practical example of proteases as a nuisance: some individuals who wear **contact lenses** complain of irritation of the cornea (keratitis). In some cases this is due to infection by bacteria that secrete a protease; this protease, besides its direct effect on the cornea, activates the omnipotent Hageman factor and releases kinins, which are powerful inflammatory mediators (200).

Inhibitors of free proteases are mainly alpha-1-antitrypsin and alpha-2-macroglobulin.

(10) Nuclear Factors

It is high time to include these powerful molecules among the mediators of inflammation. They operate as intermediates between the primary mediator and the gene or group of genes that the primary mediator normally activates. Take the best known, NF-κB: normally it is sequestered in the cytoplasm, being held in an inactive state by the inhibitor I-κB. When the cell receives the required signal, i.e., TNF has bound its membrane receptor, NF-κB is released, migrates into the nucleus, and activates *a group of about 60 genes* related to inflammation. Obviously NF-κB holds the key to vital functions: but if it overstimulates its dependent genes, it generates an excessive inflammatory response—which opens the gates to some of our worst enemies, such as shock and multiple organ failure, as we will see in due time (211a, 279a). Just as interesting is the story of **chromatin protein HMGB1,** an inflammatory nuclear factor released from necrotic (but not apoptotic) cells (272a).

(11) Bactericidal Peptides

This category, long ignored, is rapidly expanding. Some of the families are the *magainins* (from a Hebrew word for "shield"), *defensins,* and *cathelicidins.* Bactericidal peptides were found in macrophages and granulocytes (the azurophil granules alone contain 10 types, representing 30 percent of the cell's total proteins), and in covering epithelia, e.g., in the granules of the Paneth cells. They are especially concentrated in regenerating epithelia. They show a high degree of specificity; overall they are positively charged, which allows them to come close to their target cell, and amphipathic; their mode of action is direct disruption of the cell membrane (this distinguishes them from complement and antibodies, which act indirectly) (112).

(12) Cellular Components

This new category was just born with the discovery of **uric acid** as a mediator (p. 227).

Exogenous Mediators of Inflammation

Bacteria produce toxins; this we can rationalize as part of their calling. But they also produce real inflammatory mediators, such as chemotaxins (288). Why should bacteria, or any other parasite, encourage inflammation? It is obviously against their interest.

> There may be an evolutionary explanation for the apparent indifference of bacteria to being eaten by leukocytes. Bacteria are about 3.6 billion years old; multicellular creatures appeared only 700 million years ago (174). By then the metabolic pathways of bacteria were probably set, and the vertebrate tissues had ample time to learn how to sniff them out.

A fine example of exogenous mediator is the typical bacterial tetrapeptide **fMLP** produced by *E. coli* (217). Mammalian tissues respond to it with a wave of leukocytes (p. 404). Another example: *Streptococcus faecalis* cannot mate in peace in the tissues because leukocytes are attracted by its sex pheromones (159).

The most formidable bacterial mediator is **endotoxin,** a product of gram-negative bacteria (p. 720).

Actually, bacterial toxins are best considered as injurious agents rather than inflammatory mediators. They can generate an inflammatory response indirectly, by killing or damaging cells (192, 214) or by triggering immunologic mechanisms (293).

We also know of a few bacterial *antiinflammatory* mediators, such as the leukocyte-killing **leukocidin** produced by staphylococci (298). Bacteria have also evolved several antioxidant defenses against the oxygen-derived offensive weapons of the leukocytes (182).

One of the marvels of evolution is the pharmacologic cunning of stinging insects: bees, wasps, and hornets borrow pain-producing *mammalian* inflammatory mediators for their stings. The painful cocktail includes histamine, serotonin, and bradykinin, plus the histamine liberator acetylcholine. A similar combination is found in some snake poisons (177). We will learn later the fascinating technique used by the nettle (p. 537) (160). What we are witnessing in all these cases is the exogenous use of endogenous mediators.

Mediators: Some Afterthoughts

- *Are all the inflammatory messages necessarily soluble, extracellular, or even chemical?* Probably not.
(a) ***Electrical stimuli*** were once thought to play a role in chemotaxis and thrombosis, but the topic has disappeared from the literature (175). However, it is still thought that the arrangement of fibroblasts in wounds may have something to do with injury potentials. Figure 9.44 shows that fibroblasts do respond to electrical fields of a magnitude that can be expected from injury potentials *in vivo* (161, 290). Electrical stimuli are currently used to assist bone repair (116). (b) ***Heat*** may play a role in directing the motion of leukocytes (*thermotaxis*) (p. 407). (c) ***Intracellular messages*** are exchanged

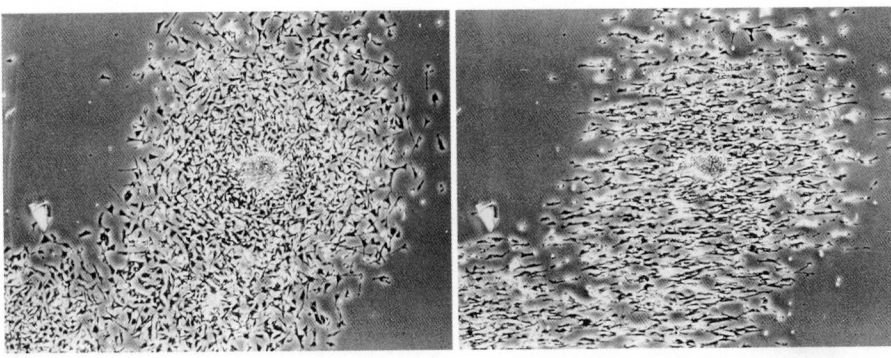

FIGURE 9.44   Cultured fibroblasts before and after 90 minutes of exposure to an electric field of 400 mV/mm. This field strength is only about three times higher than the field strength measured in guinea pig wounds. (30x) (Reproduced from the **Journal of Cell Biology,** 1984;98,296–307 by copyright permission of The Rockefeller University Press [161].)

across junctions or by direct contact; in this manner, the news of a wound travels some distance within the epidermis, and there is evidence that this actually happens. Knowledge in this area is just beginning to develop.

- The mediators as a whole are easily generated, but surely not all are called upon for every inflammatory focus.
- In humans, histamine and TNF from mast cells, serotonin from platelets, and neuropeptides from nerve endings are probably the first mediators to be released locally.

If the pleura of the rat is irritated with 1 percent kaolin, at 20 minutes the exudation is mediated mainly by kinins, histamine, and serotonin; at 3 hours mainly by prostaglandins and possibly kinins (188). There are other such examples (195).

- Aseptic wound healing is largely driven by growth factors; it has very little to do with histamine, with prostaglandins (215), with complement, or with the immune response.
- Chronic inflammation is driven mainly by cytokines.
- Infection requires complement for destroying bacteria.
- In bronchi (asthma) there is a tendency to produce leukotrienes; in the joints (arthritis), prostaglandins and IL-1.
- Remember the dictum of Sir John Vane: *"Virtually all cells, when irritated by injury or even by inflammation are ready to disgorge prostaglandins."*

TO SUM UP: Yes, we do have many mediators to learn about, far too many to remember in detail. At one time we wondered how the cells could cope with such a cacophony of messages (Figure 9.45), but it is obvious that they have no problem at all: they know their job far better than we do. The frustration is entirely our own.

Entirely missing from this chapter is a histochemical attempt to localize mediators by microscopy. Antibodies against cytokines are easily prepared, but virtually all mediators are water-soluble and are washed away during fixation (we understand that new histochemical methods are in the works). There are hundreds of mediators floating in and around the cells and there is no way to see them. This is why we reluctantly compared the experience of "reading a slide" to watching a **silent movie**. Imagine watching an opera without sound.

An overview of the inflammatory mediators is provided in Figures 9.46 and 9.47, and Table 9.5 groups the principal mediators according to their effects. Beyond these capsule summaries, we will refer to the principle spelled out in the Preface: *Faced with too much to learn, each one of us must choose his or her own maximum admissible level of ignorance.* However, if we suffered from an inflammatory disease, we would choose a physician well conversant with these basic facts.

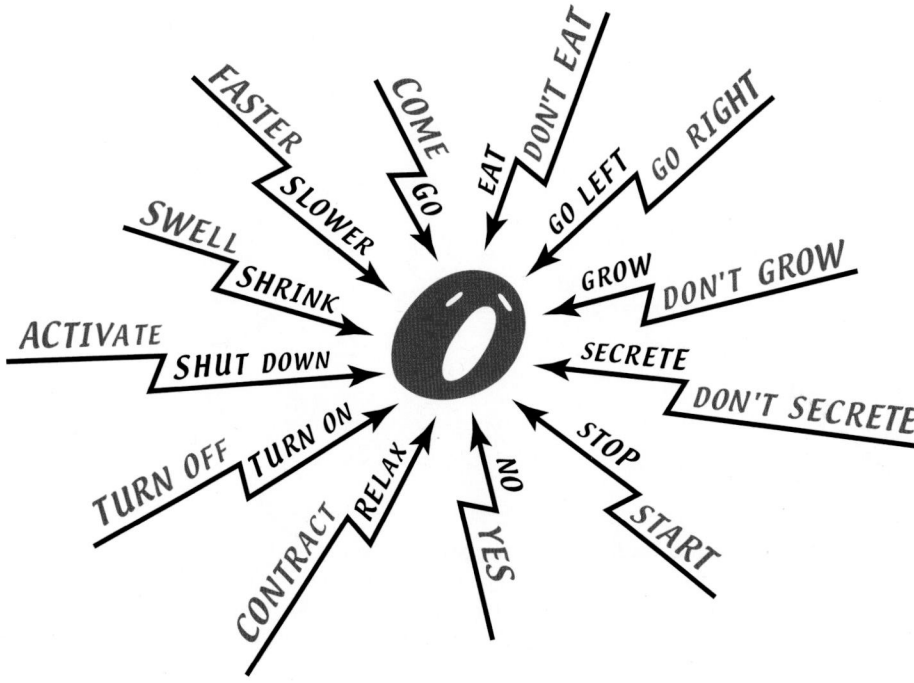

FIGURE 9.45 In inflamed tissues, each cell is submitted to a myriad of contradictory messages. The cell can handle them—a mind-boggling feat from the human perspective.

PLASMA-DERIVED MEDIATORS

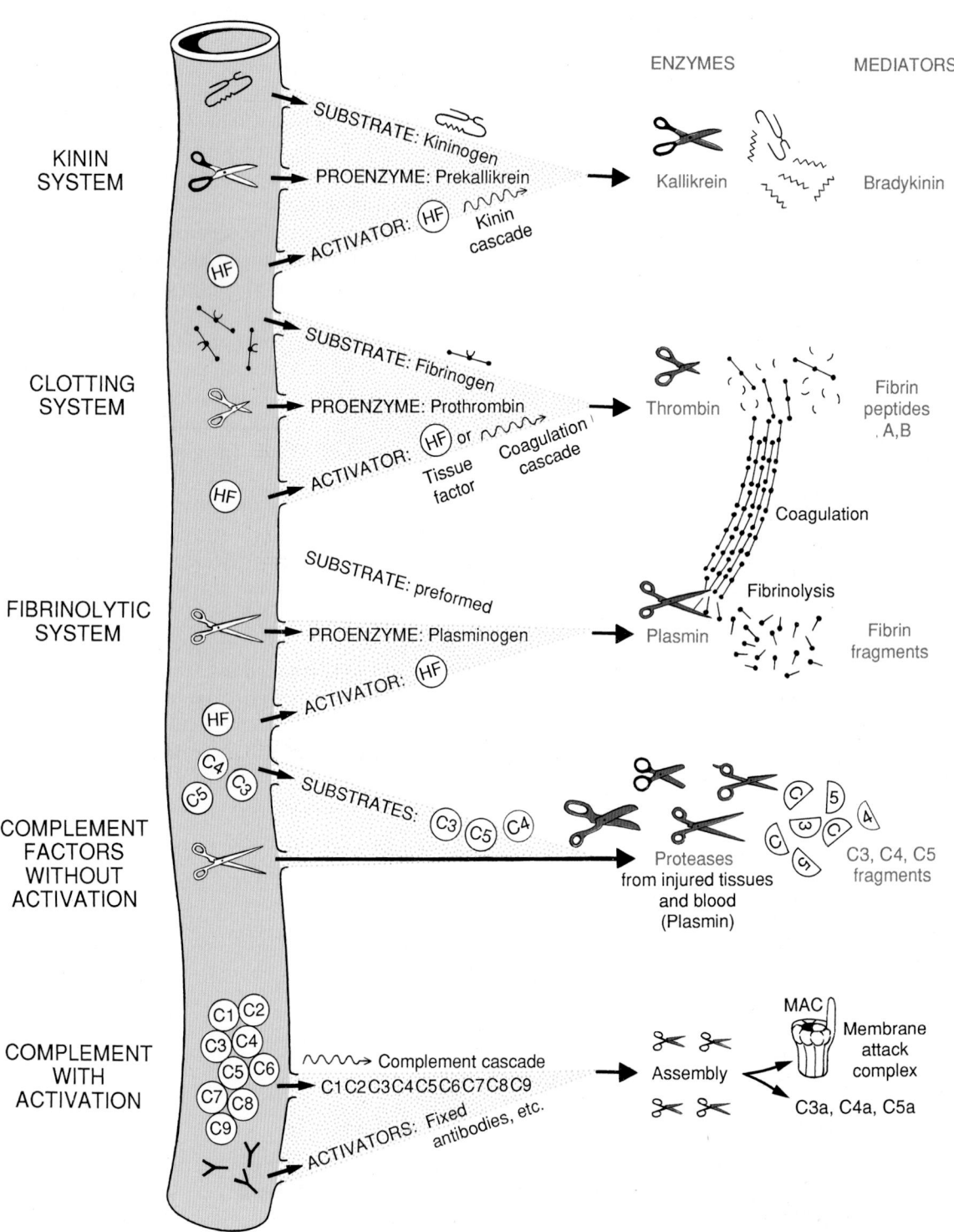

FIGURE 9.46   Overview of the plasma-derived inflammatory mediators. A damaged blood vessel (which could be of any kind) is shown as containing the inactive precursors of five mediators. The vessel allows plasma to escape through five leaks, and for each one of these, the activation of an inflammatory mediator is illustrated. The various types of scissors represent proteolytic enzymes; note that enzymes are always involved in generating the mediators. **HF** = Hageman factor.

PRINCIPAL SOURCES OF CELL-DERIVED MEDIATORS

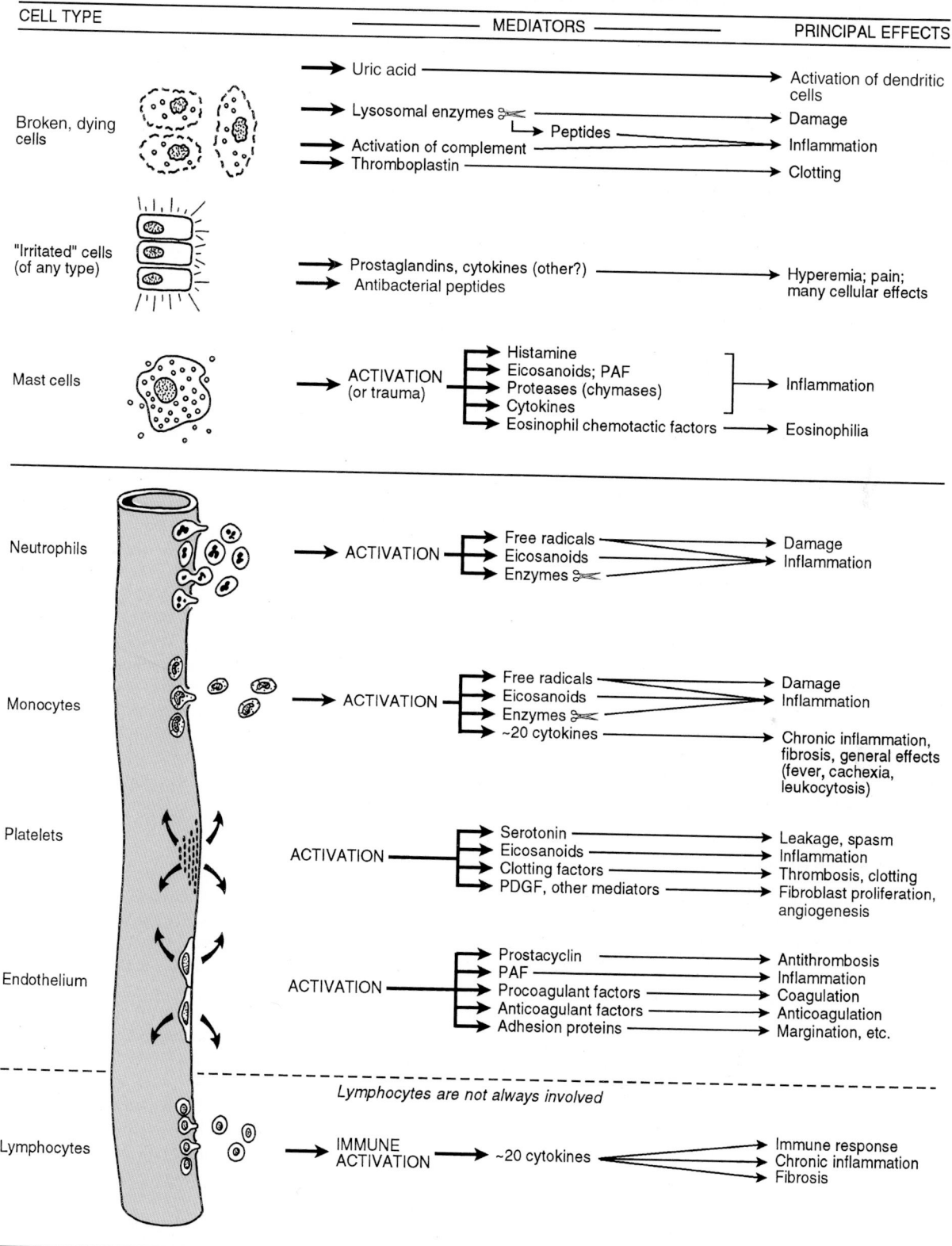

FIGURE 9.47   Overview of the cell-derived inflammatory mediators and their major effects. The cells capable of supplying mediators are mainly leukocytes and platelets, but many and perhaps all tissue cells can be induced to participate.

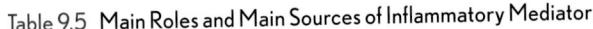

Table 9.5 Main Roles and Main Sources of Inflammatory Mediators

Vasodilatation

Histamine, serotonin	Mast cells, platelets
Prostaglandins	Probably all cells

Immediate vascular leakage

Histamine, serotonin	Mast cells, platelets
Bradykinin	Plasma
Leukotrienes C_4, D_4, E_4	Leukocytes, mast cells
PAF	Membrane phospholipids
C5a, C3a, C4a	Plasma

Chemotaxis

Chemokines	Macrophages, neutrophils, other cell types
Leukotriene B_4, HETEs	Leukocytes, mast cells
PAF	Membrane phospholipids of some cell types
C5a, C3a, C4a	Plasma

Pain

Bradykinin	Plasma
[Prostaglandins, by lowering pain threshold]	Probably all cells

Opsonins

C3b, IgG	Plasma

Tissue damage

Bacterial products	Bacteria
Free radicals	Activated leukocytes
Leukocytic enzymes	Leukocyte regurgitation
Lysosomal enzymes	Damaged cells
Uric acid	Dying/dead cells
	Broken/dying cells

References

Inflammation: The Actors

NOTE: For this and other chapters on Inflammation, extensive bibliography can be found in Gallin JI, Snyderman R (eds). Inflammation: Basic principles and clinical correlates. 3rd ed. Philadelphia: Lippincott Williams & Wilkins, 1999.

1. Adams DO, Hamilton TA. The cell biology of macrophage activation. Annu Rev Immunol 1984;2:283–318.
2. Adams DO, Hamilton TA. Phagocytic cells: cytotoxic activities of macrophages. In: Gallin JI, Goldstein IM, Snyderman R (eds). Inflammation. Basic principles and clinical correlates. New York: Raven Press 1988, pp. 471–492.
3. Austen KF. Biologic implications of the structural and functional characteristics of the chemical mediators of immediate-type hypersensitivity. Harvey Lect 1979;73:93–161.
4. Austen KF. The heterogeneity of mast cell populations and products. Hosp Pract 1984;19:135–146.
5. Bainton DF. Phagocytic cells: developmental biology of neutrophils and eosinophils. In: Gallin JI, Goldstein IM, Snyderman R (eds). Inflammation. Basic principles and clinical correlates. New York: Raven Press 1988, pp. 265–280.
6. Bainton DF, Friedlander LM, Shohet SB. Abnormalities in granule formation in acute myelogenous leukemia. Blood 1977;49:693–704.
7. Bancereau J, Steinman RM. Dendritic cells and the control of immunity. Nature 1998;392:245–252.
8. Befus AD, Bienenstock J, Denburg JA (eds). Mast cell differentiation and heterogeneity. New York: Raven Press, 1986.
9. Bobryshev YV, Konovalov HV, Lord RSA. Ultrastructural recognition of dendritic cells in the intimal lesions of aortas of chickens affected with Marek's disease. J Submicrosc Cytol Pathol 1999;31:179–185.
10. Bobryshev YV, Lord RSA. Mapping of vascular dendritic cells in atherosclerotic arteries suggests their involvement in local immune-inflammatory reactions. Cardiovasc Res 1998;37:799–810.
11. Brain JD. Toxicological aspects of alterations of pulmonary macrophage function. Annu Rev Pharmacol Toxicol 1986;26:547–565.
12. Braunstein PW Jr, Cuénoud HF, Joris I, Majno G. Platelets, fibroblasts, and inflammation. Tissue reactions to platelets injected subcutaneously. Am J Pathol 1980;99:53–66.
13. Bucala R, Spiegel LA, Chesney J, Hogan M, Cerami A. Circulating fibrocytes define a new leukocyte subpopulation that mediates tissue repair. Molec Med 1994;1:71–81.
14. Buchanan JW, Wagner HN Jr. Regional phagocytosis in man. In: Reichard SM, Filkins JP (eds). The reticulo-endothelial system. A comprehensive treatise. Vol. 7B Physiology. New York: Plenum Press, 1985, pp. 247–270.
15. Capron M, Capron A, Joseph M, Verwaerde C. IgE receptors on phagocytic cells and immune response to schistosome infection. Monogr Allergy 1983;18:33–44.
16. Craig SS, Schechter NM, Schwartz LB. Ultrastructural analysis of human T and TC mast cells identified by immunoelectron microscopy. Lab Invest 1988;58:682–691.
17. Dahl R, Venge P, Fredens K. Eosinophils. In: Barnes PJ, Rodger IW, Thomson NC (eds). Asthma: Basic mechanisms and clinical management. London: Academic Press 1988, pp. 115–129.
18. Daniele RP, Dauber JH. Collection and enrichment of human alveolar macrophages. In: Herscowitz HB, Holden HT, Bellanti JA, Ghaffar A (eds). Manual of Macrophage Methodology. New York: Marcel Dekker, Inc., 1981, pp. 23–30.
19. Duffy J. The lessons of eosinophilia-myalgia syndrome. Hosp Pract 1992;27:65–88.
20. Dvorak AM, Ackerman SJ, Weller PF. Subcellular morphology and biochemistry of eosinophils. In: Harris JR (ed). Blood cell biochemistry, vol. 2. New York: Plenum Publishing Company, 1991, pp. 237–344.
20a. Dvorak AM, Schleimer RP, Lichtenstein LM. Human mast cells synthesize new granules during recovery from degranulation. In vitro studies with mast cells purified from human lungs. Blood 1988;71:76–85.
21. Dvorak AM, Schulman ES, Peters SP, et al. Immunoglobulin E-mediated degranulation of isolated human lung mast cells. Lab Invest 1985;53:45–56.
22. Echtencher B, Männel DN, Hültner L. Critical protective role of mast cells in a model of acute septic peritonitis. Nature 1996;381:75–77.

23. Enerback L. Mast cell heterogeneity: the evolution of the concept of a specific mucosal mast cell. In: Befus AD, Bienenstock J, Denburg JA (eds). Mast cell differentiation and heterogeneity. New York: Raven Press, 1986, pp. 1–26.

24. Falk W, Leonard EJ. Human monocyte chemotaxis: migrating cells are a subpopulation with multiple chemotaxin specificities on each cell. Infect Immun 1980;29: 953–959.

25. Fawcett DW. An experimental study of mast cell degranulation and regeneration. Anat Rec 1955;121:29–51.

26. Fredens K, Dahl R, Venge P. The Gordon phenomenon induced by the eosinophil cationic protein and eosinophil protein X. J Allergy Clin Immunol 1982;70:361–366.

27. Frigas E, Loegering DA, Gleich GJ. Cytotoxic effects of the guinea pig eosinophil major basic protein on tracheal epithelium. Lab Invest 1980;42:35–43.

28. Galli SJ. New approaches for the analysis of mast cell maturation, heterogeneity, and function. Fed Proc 1987; 46:1906–1914.

29. Galli SJ. New insights into "the riddle of the mast cells": microenvironmental regulation of mast cell development and phenotypic heterogeneity. Lab Invest 1990;62:5–33.

30. Galli SJ. New concepts about the mast cell. N Engl J Med 1993;328:257–265.

31. Galli SJ, Dvorak AM, Dvorak HF. Basophils and mast cells: morphologic insights into their biology, secretory patterns, and function. Prog Allergy 1984;34:1–141.

31a. Galli SJ, Maurer M, Lantz CS. Mast cells as sentinels of innate immunity. Curr Opin Immunol 1999;11:53–59.

32. Galli SJ, Wershil BK, Gordon JR, Martin TR. Mast cells: immunologically specific effectors and potential sources of multiple cytokines during IgE-dependent responses. Ciba Found Symp 1989;147:53–73.

33. Gallin JI, Snyderman R. Inflammation: Basic Principles and Clinical Correlates, 3rd ed. Philadelphia: Lippincott Williams & Wilkins, 1999.

34. Gimbrone MA, Aster RH, Cotran RS, et al. Preservation of vascular integrity in organs perfused in vitro with a platelet-rich medium. Nature 1969;222:33–36.

35. Gleich GJ. Current understanding of eosinophil function. Hosp Pract 1988;23:137–160.

36. Gleich GJ, Adolphson CR. The eosinophilic leukocyte: structure and function. Adv Immunol 1986;39:177–253.

36a. Gommerman JL, Oh DY, Zhou X, et al. A role for CD21/CD35 and CD19 in responses to acute septic peritonitis: a potential mechanism for mast cell activation. J Immunol 2000;165:6915–6921.

37. Gordon JR, Burd PR, Galli SJ. Mast cells as a source of multifunctional cytokines. Immunol Today 1990;11:458–464.

38. Gordon JR, Galli SJ. Mast cells as a source of both preformed and immunologically inducible TNF-a/cachectin. Nature 1990;346:274–276.

39. Gordon S. Development and Distribution of Mononuclear Phagocytes: Relevance to Inflammation. In: Gallin JI, Snyderman R. (eds). Inflammation: Basic principles and clinical correlates. 3rd ed. Philadelphia: Lippincott Williams & Wilkins, 1999, pp. 35–48.

40. Grützkau A, Krüger-Krasagakes S, Baumeister H, et al. Synthesis, storage, and release of vascular endothelial growth factor/vascular permeability factor (VEGF/VPF) by human mast cells: implications for the biological significance of $VEGF_{206}$. Mol Biol Cell 1998;9:875–884.

41. Gurish MF, Austen KF. Different mast cell mediators produced by different mast cell phenotypes. Ciba Found Symp 1989;147:36–52.

42. Herscowitz HB, Holden HT, Bellanti JA, Ghaffar A (eds). Manual of macrophage methodology. New York: Marcel Dekker, Inc., 1981.

43. Hirsch JG, Hirsch BI. Paul Ehrlich and the discovery of the eosinophil. In: Mahmooud AAF, Austen KF, Simon AS (eds). The eosinophil in health and disease. New York: Grune & Stratton, 1980, pp. 3–23.

44. Ishizaka K (ed). Mast cell activation and mediator release. Basel S. Karger, 1984.

45. Janeway CA. A primitive immune system. Nature 1989; 341:108.

46. Johnston RB Jr, Kitagawa S. Molecular basis for the enhanced respiratory burst of activated macrophages. Fed Proc 1985; 44:2927–2932.

47. Kelley JL, Rozek MM, Suenram CA, Schwartz CJ. Activation of human blood monocytes by adherence to tissue culture plastic surfaces. Exp Mol Pathol 1987;46:266–278.

48. Kirshenbaum AS, Kessler SW, Goff JP, Metcalfe DD. Demonstration of the origin of human mast cells from CD34+ bone marrow progenitor cells. J Immunol 1991;146:1410–1415.

49. Lee GR, Foerster J, Lukens J et al. (eds). Wintrobe's clinical hematology, 10th ed. Baltimore: Williams & Wilkins, 1999.

50. LeRoith D, Roth J. Evolutionary origins of messenger peptides: materials in microbes that resemble vertebrate hormones In: Falkmer S, Hakanson R, Sundler F (eds). evolution and tumour pathology of the neuroendocrine system. New York: Elsevier Science Publishers, 1984, pp. 147–164.

51. Levitt D, Mertelsmann R. (eds.) Hematopoietic Stem Cells. New York, Marcel Dekker, Inc. 1995.

52. Ljunggren H-G, Kärre K. In search of the "missing self": MHC molecules and NK cell recognition. Immunol Today 1990;11:237–244.

53. Lotze MT, Thomson AW (eds). Dendritic Cells. London: Academic Press, 1999.

53a. MacDonald HR. T before NK. Science 2002;296:481–482.

54. Mackaness GB. The mechanism of macrophage activation. In: Mudd S (ed). Infectious agents and host reactions. Philadelphia: W.B. Saunders Company, 1970, pp. 61–75.

55. Mackaness GB. The monocyte in cellular immunity. Semin Hematol 1970;7:172–184.

56. Maddox DE, Kephart GM, Coulam CB, et al. Localization of a molecule immunochemically similar to eosiniphil major basic protein in human placenta. J Exp Med 1984;160: 29–41.

57. Majno G. The healing hand. Man and wound in the ancient world. Cambridge: Harvard University Press, 1975.

57a. Malaviya R, Abraham SN. Mast cell modulation of immune response to bacteria. Immunol Rev 2001;179:16–24.

58. Malaviya R, Ikeda T, Ross E, Abraham SN. Mast cell modulation of neutrophil influx and bacterial clearance at sites. Nature 1996;381:77–80.

59. Malech HL. Phagocytic cells: egress from marrow and diapedesis. In: Gallin JI, Goldstein IM, Snyderman R (eds).

Inflammation. Basic principles and clinical correlates. New York: Raven Press, 1988, pp. 297–308.

60. McIntyre KW, Welsh RM. Accumulation of natural killer and cytotoxic T large granular lymphocytes in the liver during virus infection. J Exp Med 1986;164:1667–1681.

61. Metcalfe DD, Kaliner M, Donlon MA. The mast cell. CRC Crit Rev Immunol 1981;3:23–74.

62. Metchnikoff E. Sur la lutte des cellules de l'organisme contre l'invasion des microbes. Ann Instit Pasteur 1887;1:321–336.

63. Miller F, DeHarven E, Palade GE. The structure of eosinophil leukocyte granules in rodents and in man. J Cell Biol 1966;31:349–362.

64. Nabel G, Galli SJ, Dvorak AM, Dvorak HF, Cantor H. Inducer T lymphocytes synthesize a factor that stimulates proliferation of cloned mast cells. Nature 1981;291:332–334.

65. Nachman RL, Weksler BB. The platelet as an inflammatory cell. In: Weissmann G (ed). The cell biology of inflammation. Amsterdam: Elsevier/North-Holland Biomedical Press, 1980, pp. 145–162.

66. Nakano T, Kanakuba Y, Nakahata T, Matsuda H, Kitamura Y. Genetically mast cell-deficient W/Wᵛ mice as a tool for studies of differentiation and function of mast cells. Fed Proc 1987;46:1920–1923.

67. Nilsson G, Costa JJ, Metcalfe DD. Mast Cells and Basophils. In: Gallin JI, Snyderman R. (eds). Inflammation: Basic principles and clinical correlates. 3rd ed. Philadelphia: Lippincott Williams & Wilkins, 1999, pp. 97–117.

68. Noga SJ, Normann SJ, Weiner RS. Isolation of guinea pig monocytes and Kurloff cells: characterization of monocyte subsets by morphology, cytochemistry, and adherence. Lab Invest 1984;51:244–252.

69. Old LJ. Tumor necrosis factor. Sci Am 1988;258:59–75.

70. Oldham RK. Natural killer cells: artifact to reality: an odyssey in biology. Cancer Metastasis Rev 1983;2:323–336.

71. Parwaresch MR., Horny H-P, Lennert K. Tissue mast cells in health and disease. Pathol Res Pract 1985;179:439–461.

71a. Paul WE. Fundamental immunology, 4th ed. Philadelphia: Lippincott-Raven, 1998.

72. Pennington DG, Streatfield K, Roxburgh AE. Megakaryocytes and the heterogeneity of circulating platelets. Br J Haematol 1976;34:639–653.

73. Peters MS, Rodriguez M, Gleich GJ. Localization of human eosinophil granule major basic protein, eosinophil cationic protein, and eosinophil-derived neurotoxin by immuno-electron microscopy. Lab Invest 1986;54:656–662.

74. Pober JS, Cotran RS. The role of endothelial cells inflammation. Transplantation 1990;50:537–544.

75. Postlethwaite AE, Kang AH. Fibroblasts. In: Gallin JI, Goldstein IM, Snyderman R (eds). Inflammation. Basic principles and clinical correlates. New York: Raven Press, 1988, pp. 577–597.

76. Prin L, Charon J, Capron M, et al. Heterogeneity of human eosinophils. II. Variability of respiratory burst activity related to cell density. Clin Exp Immunol 1984;57:735–742.

77. Randolph GJ, Beaulieu S, Lebecque S, Steinman RM, Muller WA. Differentiation of monocytes into dendritic cells in a model of transendothelial trafficking. Science 1998;282:480–483.

78. Reiss M, Roos D. Differences in oxygen metabolism of phagocytosing monocytes and neutrophils. J Clin Invest 1978;61:480–488.

79. Rodewald H-R, Dessing M, Dvorak AM, Galli SJ. Identification of a committed precursor for the mast cell lineage. Science 1996;271:818–822.

80. Rosenberg HF. Eosinophils. In: Gallin JI, Snyderman R. (eds). Inflammation: Basic principles and clinical correlates. 3rd ed. Philadelphia: Lippincott Williams & Wilkins, 1999, pp. 61–76.

81. Rosmalen JGM, Martin T, Dobbs C, et al. Subsets of macrophages and dendritic cells in nonobese diabetic mouse pancreatic inflammatory infiltrates: correlation with the development of diabetes. Lab Invest 2000;80:23–30.

82. Rothenberg ME. Eosinophilia. N Engl J Med 1998;338:1592–1600.

83. Ryan US. Endothelial Cells, Vols I, II, III. Boca Raton: CRC Press, Inc., 1988.

84. Samter M. Eosinophils—nominated but not elected. N Engl J Med 1980;303:1175–1176.

85. Selye H. The mast cells. Washington: Butterworths, 1965.

86. Simionescu M. Receptor-mediated transcytosis of plasma molecules by vascular endothelium. In: Simionescu N, Simionescu M (eds). Endothelial cell biology in health and disease. New York: Plenum Press, 1988, pp. 69–104.

87. Simionescu N, Simionescu M (eds). Endothelial cell biology in health and disease. New York: Plenum Press, 1988.

88. Simionescu N, Simionescu M (eds). Endothelial cell dysfunction. New York: Plenum Press, 1992.

89. Siraganian RP. Mast cells and basophils. In: Gallin JI, Goldstein IM, Snyderman R (eds). Inflammation. Basic principles and clinical correlates. New York: Raven Press, 1988, pp. 513–542.

90. Slifman NR, Adolphson CR, Gleich GJ. Eosinophils: biochemical and cellular aspects. In: Middleton E Jr, Reed CE, Ellis EF, Adkinson NF Jr, Yunginger JW (eds). Allergy Principles and Practice, 3rd ed. St. Louis: The C.V. Mosby Company, 1988, pp. 179–205.

91. Spry CJF. Eosinophils. Oxford: Oxford University Press, 1988.

92. Steinman RM, Bhardwaj N. Dendritic Cells. In: Gallin JI, Snyderman R. (eds). Inflammation: Basic principles and clinical correlates. 3rd ed. Philadelphia: Lippincott Williams & Wilkins, 1999, pp. 49–59.

93. Tauber AI, Goetzl EJ, Babior BM. Unique characteristics of superoxide production by human eosinophils in eosinophilic states. Inflammation 1979;3:261–272.

94. Timonen T. Natural killer cells: endothelial interactions, migration, and target cell recognition. J Leukoc Biol 1997;62:693–701.

95. von Andrian UH, Mackay CR. T-cell function and migration. N Engl J Med 2000;343:1020–1034.

96. van Furth R. Phagocytic cells: development and distribution of mononuclear phagocytes in normal steady state and inflammation. In: Gallin JI, Goldstein IM, Snyderman R (eds). Inflammation. Basic principles and clinical correlates. New York: Raven Press, 1988, pp. 281–295.

97. van Furth R, Raeburn JA, van Zwet TL. Characteristics of human mononuclear phagocytes. Blood 1979;54:485–500.

98. Wasmoen TL, McKean DJ, Benirschke K, Coulam CB, Gleich GJ. Evidence of eosinophil granule major basic protein in human placenta. J Exp Med 1989;170: 2051–2063.

99. Wasserman SI. The mast cell and the inflammatory response. In: Pepys J, Edwards AM (eds). The mast cell. Bath: The Pitman Press, 1979, pp. 9–20.

100. Watzl C, Long EO. Exposing tumor cells to killer cell attack. Nature Med 2000;6:867–868.

100a. Wedemeyer J, Tsai M, Galli SJ. Roles of mast cells and basophils in innate and acquired immunity. Curr Opin Immunol 2000;12:624–631.

101. Weidner N, Austen KF. Evidence for morphologic diversity of human mast cells. An ultrastructural study of mast cells from multiple body sites. Lab Invest 1990;63:63–72.

102. Weissmann G, Korchak HM, Perez HD, et al. Leukocytes as secretory organs of inflammation. In: Weissmann G, Samuelsson B, Paoletti R (eds). Advances in inflammation research, vol. 1. New York: Raven Press, 1979, pp. 95–112.

103. Weissmann G, Smolen JE, Korchak HM. Release of inflammatory mediators from stimulated neutrophils. N Engl J Med 303:27–34,1980.

104. Weksler BB. Platelets. In: Gallin JI, Goldstein IM, Snyderman R (eds). Inflammation. Basic principles and clinical correlates. New York: Raven Press, 1988, pp. 543–557.

105. Weller PF. The immunobiology of eosinophils. N Engl J Med 1991;324:1110–1118.

106. Welsh RM, Vargas-Cortes M. Natural killer cells in viral infection. In: Lewis CE, McGee JO'D (eds). The Natural Killer Cell. Oxford: IRL Press, 1992, pp. 107–150.

107. Werb Z, Gordon S. Elastase secretion by stimulated macrophages. Characterization and regulation. J Exp Med 1975;142:361–377.

107a. Wershil BK, Murakami T, Galli SJ. Mast cell-dependent amplification of an immunologically nonspecific inflammatory response. Mast cells are required for the full expression of cutaneous acute inflammation induced by phorbol 12-myristate 13-acetate. J Immunol 1988;140:2356–2360.

108. White JG. Platelet secretory granules and associated proteins. Lab Invest 1993;68:497–498.

109. Wisse E, Braet F, Luo D, et al. Sinusoidal Liver Cells. In: Bircher J, Benhamou JP, McIntyre N, Rizzetto M, Rodés J. Oxford textbook of medical hepatology. 2nd ed., Vol 1. Oxford: Oxford University Press, 1999, pp. 33–49.

110. Witko-Sarsat V, Riew P, Descamps-Latscha B, Lesavre P, Halbwachs-Mecarelli L. Neutrophils: molecules, functions and pathophysiological aspects. Lab Invest 2000;80: 617–653.

111. Wright DG. The neutrophil as a secretory organ of host defense. In: Gallin JI, Fauci AS (eds). Advances in host defense mechanisms. vol. 1, Phagocytic cells. New York: Raven Press, 1982, pp. 75–110.

Inflammation: The Chemical Language

111a. Alberts B, Bray D, Lewis J, et al. Molecular biology of the cell. 3rd ed. New York: Garland Publishing, Inc., 1994.

112. Anderson M, Zasloff M. Antimicrobial peptides: complementing classical inflammatory mechanisms of defense. In: Gallin JI, Snyderman R. (eds). Inflammation. Basic principles and clinical correlates. 3rd ed. Philadelphia: Lippincott Williams & Wilkins, 1999, pp. 1279–1292.

113. Baggiolini M. Chemokines and leukocyte traffic. Nature 1998;392:565–568.

114. Baggiolini M, Dewald B, Moser B. Human chemokines: an update. Annu Rev Immunol 1997;15:675–705.

115. Baracos V, Rodemann HP, Dinarello CA, Goldberg AL. Stimulation of muscle protein degradation and prostagnaldin E2 release by leukocytic pyrogen (interleukin-1). N Engl J Med 1983;308:553–558.

116. Bassett CAL, Jackson SF. A critique of medical uses of weak pulsing electromagnetic fields. In: Chiabrera A, Nicolini C, Schwan HP (eds). Interactions between electromagnetic fields and cells. New York: Plenum Press, 1985, pp. 569–579.

117. Battistini B, D'Orleans-Juste P, Sirois P Biology of disease endothelins: circulating plasma levels and presence in other biologic fluids. Lab Invest 1993;68:600–628.

118. Becker EL. The formylpeptide receptor of the neutrophil. A search and conserve operation. Am J Pathol 1987;129:16–24.

119. Beer DJ, Matloff SM, Rocklin RE. The influence of histamine on immune and inflammatory responses. Adv Immunol 1984; 35:209–268.

120. Belew M, Gerdin B, Porath J, Saldeen T. Isolation of vasoactive peptides from human fibrin and fibrinogen degraded by plasmin. Thromb Res 1978;13:983–994.

121. Benveniste J, Nunez D, Duriez P, et al. Preformed PAF-acether and lyso PAF-acether are bound to blood lipoproteins. FEBS Lett 1998;226:371–376.

122. Bergström S. The prostaglandins: from the laboratory to the clinic. In: Les Prix Nobel en 1982. The Nobel Foundation, 1983;127–148.

123. Bessis M. Studies on cell agony and death: an attempt at classification. In: deReuck, AVS, Knight, J, eds. Ciba Foundation Symposium on Cellular Injury. London: J & A Churchill, 1964, pp. 287–328.

124. Beutler B. The tumor necrosis factors: cachectin and lymphotoxin. Hosp Pract 1990;25:45–56.

125. Beutler B. Tumor Necrosis Factors: The molecules & their emerging role in medicine. New York: Raven Press, 1992.

126. Beutler B, Cerami A. Cachectin and tumour necrosis factor as two sides of the same biological coin. Nature 1986;320: 584–588.

127. Beutler B, Cerami A. The biology of cachectin/TNF—a primary mediator of the host response. Annu Rev Immunol 1989;7:625–655.

128. Bhakdi S, Roth M. Fluid-phase SC5b-8 complex of human complement: generation and isolation from serum. J Immunol 1981;127:576–580.

129. Bitter-Suermann D. The anaphylatoxins. In: Rother K, Till GO (eds). The complement system. Berlin: Springer-Verlag, 1988, pp. 367–395.

130. Boucek RJ, Speropoulos AJ, Noble NL. Serotonin and ribonucleic acid and collagen metabolism of fibroblasts in vitro. Proc Soc Exp Biol Med 1972;140:599–603.

131. Brune K, Kälin H, Schmidt R, Hecker E. Regulation of prostaglandin release from macrophages. In: Weissmann G,

Samuelsson B, Paoletti R (eds). Advances in inflammation research, Vol. 1. New York: Raven Press, 1979, pp. 467–475.

132. Burn JH, Dale HH. The vaso-dilator action of histamine, and its physiological significance. J Physiol (Lond) 1926; 61:185–214.

133. Camp R, Jones RR, Brain S, Woollard P, Greaves M. Production of intraepidermal microabscesses by topical application of leukotriene B_4. J Invest Dermatol 1984;82:202–204.

134. Carswell EA, Old LJ, Kassel RL, et al. An endotoxin-induced serum factor that causes necrosis of tumors. Proc Natl Acad Sci USA 1975;72:3666–3670.

135. Casale TB, Wescott S, Rodbard D, Kaliner M. Characterization of histamine H-1 receptors on human mononuclear cells. Int J Immunopharmacol 1985;7:639–645.

136. Chenoweth DE, Cooper SW, Hugli TE, et al. Complement activation during cardiopulmonary bypass. Evidence for generation of C3a and C5a anaphylatoxins. N Engl J Med 1981;304:497–503.

137. Colditz IG, Movat HZ. Kinetics of neutrophil accumulation in acute inflammatory lesions induced by chemotaxins and chemotaxinigens. J Immunol 1984;133:2169–2173.

138. Collard CD, Väkevä A, Morrissey MA, et al. Complement activation after oxidative stress. Role of the lectin complement pathway. Am J Pathol 2000;156:1549–1556.

139. Clemens MJ. Cytokines. Oxford: BIOS Scientific Publishers Ltd., 1991.

140. Coley WB. The treatment of malignant tumors by repeated inoculations of erysipelas: with a report of ten original cases. Am J Med Sci 1983;105:487–511.

141. Cooper NR, Welsh RM Jr. Antibody and complement-dependent viral neutralization. Springer Semin Immunopathol 1979;2:285–310.

142. Cotran RS, Kumar V, Robbins SL. Robbins pathologic basis of disease, 4th ed. Philadelphia: W.B. Saunders Company, 1989, pp. 56.

143. Cybulsky MI, Chan MKW, Movat HZ. Acute inflammation and microthrombosis induced by endotoxin, interleukin-1, and tumor necrosis factor and their implication in gram-negative infection. Lab Invest 1988;58:365–378.

144. Cybulsky MI, McComb DJ, Movat HZ. Neutrophil leukocyte emigration induced by endotoxin. Mediator roles of interleukin 1 and tumor necrosis factor a. J Immunol 1988; 140:3144–3149.

145. Cybulsky MI, Movat HZ, Dinarello CA. Role of interleukin-1 and tumour necrosis factor$_x$ in acute inflammation. Ann Inst Pasteur Immunol 1987;138:505–512.

146. Dale HH, Richards AN. The vasodilator action of histamine and of some other substances. J Physiol 1918;52: 110–165.

147. Dinarello CA. Interleukin-1 and the pathogenesis of the acute-phase response. N Engl J Med 1984;311:1413–1418.

148. Dinarello CA. Biology of interleukin 1. FASEB J 1988;2: 108–115.

149. Dinarello CA. Interleukin-1: a proinflammatory cytokine. In: Gallin JI, Snyderman R. (eds). Inflammation: Basic principles and clinical correlates. 3rd ed. Philadelphia: Lippincott Williams & Wilkins, 1999, pp. 443–461.

150. Dinarello CA, Cannon JG, Wolff SM, et al. Tumor necrosis factor (cachectin) is an endogenous pyrogen and induces production of interleukin 1. J Exp Med 1986;163: 1433–1450.

151. Dittman B, Wimmer R, Mindermann R, Ohlsson K. The effect of human granulocyte proteinases on kininogens. Adv Exp Med Biol 1979;120B:297–304.

151a. Dodds AW, Sim RB. Complement. Oxford: IRL Press at Oxford University Press, 1997.

152. Donaldson VH. The challenge of hereditary angioneurotic edema. N Engl J Med 1983;308:1094–1095.

153. Doolittle RF. Fibrinogen and fibrin. Sci Am 1981; 245:126–135.

154. Douglas WW. Autacoids. Introduction. In: Goodman LS, Gilman A (eds). The Pharmacological basis of therapeutics, 4th ed. London: Collier-MacMillan Limited, 1970, pp. 620–621.

155. Douglas WW. Polypeptides—angiotensin, plasma kinins, and other vasoactive agents; prostaglandins. In: Goodman LS, Gilman A (eds). The pharmacological basis of therapeutics, 4th ed. London: Collier-MacMillan Limited, 1970, pp. 663–676.

156. Dunn CJ. Cytokines as mediators of chronic inflammatory disease. In: Kimball ES (ed). Cytokines and inflammation. Boca Raton: CRC Press, 1991, pp. 1–33.

157. Dvorak AN, Schulman ES, Peters SP, et al. Immunoglobulin E-mediated degranulation of isolated human lung mast cells. Lab Invest 1985;53:45–56.

158. Eichler O, Farah A (eds). Handbook of experimental pharmacology. vol. 18, Pt. 1. Histamine and anti-histaminics. New York: Springer-Verlag, 1966.

159. Ember JA, Hugli TE. Characterization of the human neutrophil response to sex pheromones from Streptococcus faecalis. Am J Pathol 1989;134:797–805.

160. Emmelin N, Feldberg W. The mechanism of the sting of the common nettle (Urtica Urens). J Physiol 1947; 106:440–455.

161. Erickson CA, Nuccitelli R. Embryonic fibroblast motility and orientation can be influenced by physiological electric fields. J Cell Biol 1984;98:296–307.

162. Eriksson M, Saldeen K, Saldeen T, Strandberg K, Wallin R. Fibrin-derived vasoactive peptides release histamine. Int J Microcirc: Clin Exp 1983;2:337–345.

163. Erspamer V. Half a century of comparative research on biogenic amines and active peptides in amphibian skin and molluscan tissues. Comp Biochem Physiol 1984;79C:1–7.

164. Fantone JC, Kunkel SL, Ward PA, Zurier RB. Suppression by prostaglandin E_1 of vascular permeability induced by vasoactive inflammatory mediators. J Immunol 1980;125: 2591–2596.

165. Forrest MJ, Jose PJ, Williams TJ. The role of the complement-derived polypeptide C5a in inflammatory reactions. In: Higgs GA, Williams TJ (eds). Inflammatory mediators. London: MacMillan, 1985, pp. 99–115.

166. Frank MM. The complement system in host defense and inflammation. Rev Infect Dis 1979;1:483–501.

167. Frey EK, Kraut H, Werle E. Das Kallikrein-Kinin-System und Seine Inhibitoren. Stuttgart: F Enke Verlag, 1968.

168. Furie MB, Randolph GH. Chemokines and tissue injury. Am J Pathol 1995;146:1287–1301.

169. Gainor JP, Morton CA, Bell DR, Vincent PA, Minnear FL. Platelet phospholipids decrease vascular endothelial permeability via a novel signaling pathway independent of cAMP/protein kinase A. In: Goetzl EJ, Lynch KR. (eds). Lysophospholipids and Eicosanoids in Biology and Pathophysiology. New York: Annals of the New York Academy of Sciences. Vol. 905, 2000.

170. Gallin JI, Snyderman R. Inflammation: Basic principles and clinical correlates, 3rd ed. Philadelphia: Lippincott Williams & Wilkins, 1999.

171. Goetzl EJ, Lynch KR. (eds). Lysophospholipids and Eicosanoids in Biology and Pathophysiology. New York: Annals of the New York Academy of Sciences. Vol. 905, 2000.

172. Goodman LS, Gilman A (eds). The pharmacological basis of therapeutics, 3rd ed. New York: MacMillan, 1965.

173. Gordon DL, Hostetter MK. Complement and host defence against microorganisms. Pathology 1986;18:365–375.

174. Gould SJ. Wonderful life: The burgess shale and the nature of history. New York: WW Norton, 1989.

175. Grant L. The sticking and emigration of white blood cells in inflammation. In: Zweifach BW, Grant L, McCluskey RT (eds). The inflammatory process, 2nd ed., vol. 2. New York: Academic Press, 1973, pp. 205–249.

176. Grau GE, Fajardo LF, Piguet P-F, et al. Tumor necrosis factor (cachectin) as an essential mediator in murine cerebral malaria. Science 1987;237:1210–1212.

177. Habermann E. Chemistry, pharmacology, and toxicology of bee, wasp, and hornet venoms. In: Bücherl W, Buckley EE (eds). Venomous animals and their venoms. Vol. III, Venomous invertebrates. New York: Academic Press, 1971, pp. 61–93.

178. Haeggström JZ, Serhan CN. Update on Arachidonic Acid Cascade. In: Serhan CN, Ward PA (eds). Molecular and cellular basis of inflammation. Totowa, NJ: Humana Press, 1999, pp. 51–92.

179. Hakim RM, Breillatt J, Lazarus JM, Port FK. Complement activation and hypersensitivity reactions to dialysis membranes. N Engl J Med 1984;311:878–882.

180. Hammarström S. The leukotrienes. In: Litwak G (ed). Biochemical actions of hormones, vol. XI. New York: Academic Press, 1984, pp. 1–23.

181. Harris H. Chemotaxis of monocytes. Br J Exp Pathol 1953;34:276–279.

182. Hassett DJ, Cohen MS. Bacterial adaptation to oxidative stress: implications for pathogenesis and interaction with phagocytic cells. FASEB J 1989;3:2574–2582.

183. Hattori R, Hamilton KK, Fugate RD, McEver RP, Sims PJ. Stimulated secretion of endothelial von Willebrand factor is accompanied by rapid redistribution to the cell surface of the intracellular granule membrane protein GMP-140. J Biol Chem 1989;264:7768–7771.

184. Hébert CA. (ed). Chemokines in disease. Totowa, NJ: Humana Press, 1999.

185. Hendrzak JA, Brunda MJ. Biology of Disease, Interleukin-12. Biologic activity, therapeutic utility and, role in disease. Lab Invest 1995;72:619–637.

186. Higgs GA, Moncada S. Leukotrienes in disease. Implications for drug development. Drugs 1985;30:1–5.

187. Higgs GA, Moncada S, Vane JR. Eicosanoids in inflammation. Ann Clin Res 1984;16:287–299.

188. Hori Y, Jyoyama H, Yamada K, et al. Time course analyses of kinins and other mediators in plasma exudation of rat kaolin-induced pleurisy. Eur J Pharmacol 1988;152:235–245.

189. Hugli TE. Structure and function of the anaphylatoxins. Springer Semin Immunopathol 1984;7:193–219.

190. Humphrey DM, McManus LM, Satouchi K, Hanahan DJ, Pinckard RN. Vasoactive properties of acetyl glyceryl ether phosphorylcholine and analogues. Lab Invest 1982;46:422–427.

191. Hunt JD, Ward PA. Chemotactic factor inactivator release from rat leukocytes. Inflammation 1979;3:203–214.

192. Issekutz AC, Megyeri P, Issekutz TB. Role for macrophage products in endotoxin-induced polymorpho-nuclear leukocyte accumulation during inflammation. Lab Invest 1987;56:49–59.

193. Issekutz AC, Movat HZ. The effect of vasodilator prostaglandins on polymorphonuclear leukocyte infiltration and vascular injury. Am J Pathol 1982;107:300–309.

194. Jäättelä M. Biologic activities and mechanisms of action of tumor necrosis factor-a/cachectin. Lab Invest 1991;64:724–742.

195. Johnston MG, Hay JB, Movat HZ. The role of prostaglandins in inflammation. Curr Top Pathol 1979;68:259–287.

196. Johnston RB Jr. Monocytes and macrophages. N Engl J Med 1988;318:747–752.

197. Joiner KA, Frank MM. Mechanisms of bacterial resistance to complement-mediated killing. In: Jackson GG, Thomas H (eds). The pathogenesis of bacterial infections. Berlin: Springer-Verlag, 1985, pp. 122–136.

198. Joris I, Majno G, Corey EJ, Lewis RA. The mechanism of vascular leakage induced by leukotriene E_4. Endothelial contraction. Am J Pathol 1987;126:19–24.

199. Kaliner M, Wasserman SI, Austen, KF. Immunologic release of chemical mediators from human nasal polyps. N Engl J Med 1973;289:277–281.

200. Kamata R, Yamamoto T, Matsumoto K, Maeda H. A serratial protease causes vascular permeability reaction by activation of the Hageman factor-dependent pathway in Guinea pigs. Infect Immun 1985;48:747–753.

201. Kimball ES. Involvement of cytokines in neurogenic inflammation. In: Kimball ES (ed). Cytokines and inflammation. Boca Raton: CRC Press, 1991, pp. 169–189.

202. Kimball ES (ed). Cytokines and inflammation. Boca Raton: CRC Press, 1991.

203. Kovacs EJ. Control of IL-1 and TNFa production at the level of second messenger pathways. In: Kimball ES (ed). Cytokines and inflammation. Boca Raton: CRC Press, 1991, pp. 89–107.

204. Kozin F, Cochrane CG. The contact activation system of plasma: biochemistry and pathophysiology. In: Gallin JI, Goldstein IM, Snyderman R (eds). Inflammation: Basic principles and clinical correlates. New York: Raven Press, 1988, pp. 101–120.

205. Kuhlman M, Joiner K, Ezekowitz RAB. The human mannose-binding protein functions as an opsonin. J Exp Med 1989;169:1733–1745.

206. Kunkel SL, Remick DG, Strieter RM, Larrick JW. Mechanisms that regulate the production and effects of tumor necrosis factor-a. CRC Crit Rev Immunol 1989; 9:93–117.

207. Larrick JW, Wright SC. Cytotoxic mechanism of tumor necrosis factor-a. FASEB J 1990;4:3215–3223.

208. Larsen GL, Henson PM. Mediators of inflammation. Annu Rev Immunol 1983;1:335–359.

209. Lepow IH. Louis Pillemer, properdin, and scientific controversy. J Immunol 1980;125:471–478.

210. Lewis RA, Austen KF. Leukotrienes. In: Gallin JI, Goldstein IM, Snyderman R (eds). Inflammation: Basic principles and clinical correlates. New York: Raven Press, 1988, pp. 121–128.

211. Lewis RA, Austen KF, Soberman RJ. Leukotrienes and other products of the 5-lipoxygenase pathway. Biochemistry and relation to pathobiology in human diseases. N Engl J Med 1990;323:645–655.

211a. Li Q, Verma IM. NF-κB regulation in the immune system. Nat Rev Immunol 2002;2:725–734.

212. Loos M. Bacteria and complement—A historical review. Curr Topics Microbiol Immunol 1985;121:1–5.

213. Loscalzo J, Vita JA (eds). Nitric oxide and the cardiovascular system. Totowa, NJ: Humana Press, 2000.

214. Lubran MM. Bacterial toxins. Ann Clin Lab Sci 1988; 18:58–71.

215. Lundberg C, Gerdin B. The inflammatory reaction in an experimental model of open wounds in the rat. The effect of arachidonic acid metabolites. Eur J Pharmacol 1984;97: 229–238.

216. Luster AD. Chemokines—chemotactic cytokines that mediate inflammation. N Eng J Med 1998;338:436–445.

217. Marasco WA, Phan SH, Krutzsch H, et al. Purification and identification of formyl-methionyl-leucyl-phenylalanine as the major peptide neutrophil chemotactic factor produced by Escherichia coli. J Biol Chem 1984;259:5430–5439.

218. McManus LM, Pinckard RN. Kinetics of acetyl glyceryl ether phosphorylcholine (AGEPC)-induced acute lung alterations in the rabbit. Am J Pathol 1985;121:55–68.

219. McManus LM, Pincard RN, Hanahan DJ. Acetyl glyceryl ether phosphorylcholine (AGEPC) in allergy and inflammation. In: Theoretical and clinical aspects of allergic diseases symposium Oct. 12–14. Stockholm: Skandia Group, 1982, pp. 165–182.

220. Menkin V. Newer Concepts of Inflammation. Springfield: Charles C. Thomas, 1950.

221. Menkin V. Modern views on inflammation. Int Arch Allergy Appl Immunol 1953;4:131–168.

222. Meri S, Waldmann H, Lachmann PJ. Distribution of protectin (CD59), a complement membrane attack inhibitor, in normal human tissues. Lab Invest 1991;65:532–537.

223. Michie HR, Manogue KR, Spriggs DR, et al. Detection of circulating tumor necrosis factor after endotoxin administration. N Engl J Med 1988;318:1481–1486.

224. Moncada S. Nitric oxide: discovery and impact on clinical medicine. J R Soc Med 1999;92:164–169.

225. Moncada S, Korbut R, Bunting S, Vane JR. Prostacyclin is a circulating hormone. Nature 1978;273:767–768.

226. Moncad S, Higgs EA. Endogenous nitric oxide: physiology, pathology and clinical relevance. Eur J Clin Invest 1991; 21:361–374.

227. Moncada S, Radomski MW. The problems and the promise of prostaglandin influences in atherogenesis. Ann NY Acad Sci 1985;454:121–130.

228. Morley BJ, Walport MJ. The complement facts book. London: Academic Press Inc., 2000.

229. Movat HZ. The kinin system and its relations to other systems. Curr Top Pathol 1979;68:111–134.

230. Movat HZ, Cybulsky MI. Neutrophil emigration and microvascular injury. Role of chemotaxins, endotoxin, interleukin-1 and tumor necrosis factor alpha. Pathol Immunopathol Res 1987:6:153–176.

231. Müller-Eberhard HJ. The significance of complement activity in shock. In: Proceedings of a symposium on recent research developments and current clinical practice in shock: The cell in shock. A scope publication. Upjohn, 1975, pp. 35–38.

232. Müller-Eberhard HJ. The membrane attack complex. Springer Semin Immunopathol 1984;7:93–141.

233. Nauts HC. The Beneficial Effects of Bacterial Infections on Host Resistance to Cancer. End Results in 449 Cases. Monograph No. 8, 2nd ed. New York: Cancer Research Institute, Inc., 1980.

234. Newball HH, Revak SD, Cochrane CG, Griffin JH, Lichtenstein LM. Activation of human Hageman factor by a leukocytic protease. Adv Exp Med Biol 1979;120B:139–151.

235. Nicola NA (ed). Guidebook to cytokines and their receptors. Oxford: Oxford University Press, 1994.

236. O'Brodovich HM, Stalcup SA, Pang LM, Lipset JS, Mellins RB. Bradykinin production and increased pulmonary endothelial permeability during acute respiratory failure in unanesthetized sheep. J Clin Invest 1981;67:514–522.

237. Old LJ. Tumor necrosis factor (TNF). Science 1985;230: 630–632.

238. Old LJ. Tumor necrosis factor. Sci Am 1988;258:59–75.

239. Oldham RK. Journal of biological response modifiers: why another journal? J Biol Resp Modif 1982;1:1–2.

240. Oltvai ZM, Wong ECC, Atkinson JP, Tung KSK. C1 inhibitor deficiency: molecular and immunologic basis of hereditary and acquired angioedema. Lab Invest 1991;65: 381–388.

240a. Oppenheim JJ. Cytokines: past, present, and future. Int J Hematol 2001;74:3–8.

241. Page IH. The discovery of serotonin. Perspect Biol Med 1976;20:1–8.

242. Pernow B. Substance P. Pharmacol Rev 1983;35:85–141.

243. Piguet PF, Collart MA, Grau GE, Sappino A-P, Vassalli P. Requirement of tumour necrosis factor for development of silica-induced pulmonary fibrosis. Nature 1990;344: 245–247.

244. Pillemer L, Blum L, Lepow IH, et al. The properdin system and immunity: I. Demonstration and isolation of a new

serum protein, properdin, and its role in immune phenomena. Science 1954;120:279–285.

245. Pinckard RN, Ludwig JC, McManus LM. Platelet-activating factors. In: Gallin JI, Goldstein IM, Snyderman R (eds). Inflammation: Basic principles and clinical correlates. New York: Raven Press, 1988, pp. 139–167.

246. Piper P, Vane J. The release of prostaglandins from lung and other tissues. Ann NY Acad Sci 1971;180:363–385.

247. Podack ER. Assembly of transmembrane tubules (poly perforins) on target membranes by cloned NK and TK cells: comparison to poly C9 of complement. In: Hoshino T, Koren HS, Uchida A (eds). Natural killer activity and its regulation. Amsterdam: Excerpta Medica, 1984, pp. 101–106.

248. Podack ER, Tschopp J. Circular polymerization of the ninth component of complement. J Biol Chem 1982; 257:15204–15212.

249. Podack ER, Tschopp J. Membrane attack by complement. Mol Immunol 1984;21:589–603.

250. Proud D, Reynolds CJ, Lacapra S, et al. Nasal provocation with bradykinin induces symptoms of rhinitis and a sore throat. Am Rev Respir Dis 1988;137:613–616.

251. Proud D, Togias, A, Naclerio RM, et al. Kinins are generated in vivo following nasal airway challenge of allergic individuals with allergen. J Clin Invest 1983;72:1678–1685.

252. Pullman-Mooar S, Laposata M, Lem D, et al. Alteration of the cellular fatty acid profile and the production of eicosanoids in human monocytes by gamma-linolenic acid. Arthritis Rheum 1990;33:1526–1533.

253. Rabson AR, Anderson R, Glover A, Lomnitzer R. Inhibitory effect of prostaglandin A$_1$ on neutrophil motility. Br J Exp Pathol 1978;59:298–304.

254. Ramm LE, Whitlow MB, Koski CL, Shin ML, Mayer MM. Elimination of complement channels from the plasma membranes of U937, a nucleated mammalian cell line: temperature dependence of the elimination rate. J Immunol 1983; 131:1411–1415.

255. Rampart M, Van Damme J, Zonnekeyn L, Herman AG. Granulocyte chemotactic protein/interlueukin-8 induces plasma leakage and neutrophil accumulation in rabbit skin. Am L Pathol 1989;135:21–25.

256. Ratnoff WD. A war with the molecules: Louis Pillemer and the history of properdin. Perspect Biol Med 1980; 23:638–657.

257. Remick DG, Friedland JS (eds). Cytokines in health and disease. New York: Marcel Dekker, Inc., 1997.

258. Remick DG, Kunkel RG, Larrick JW, Kunkel SL. Acute in vivo effects of human recombinant tumor necrosis factor. Lab Invest 1987;56:583–590.

259. Rocha e Silva M. A brief history of inflammation. In: Vane JR, Ferreira SH (eds). Inflammation. Handbook of experimental pharmacology, vol. 50/I. Berlin: Springer-Verlag, 1978, pp. 6–25.

260. Rosen FS, Alper CA. Genetic deficiencies of the complement system. Clin Immunol Allergy 1985;5:371–377.

261. Rossi V, Breviario F, Ghezzi P, Dejana E, Mantovani A. Prostacyclin synthesis induced in vascular cells by interleukin-1. Science 1985;229:174–176.

262. Roth J, Leroith D, Collier ES, Watkinson A, Lesniak MA. The evolutionary origins of intercellular communication and the Maginot lines of the mind. Ann NY Acad Sci 1986;463:1–11.

263. Rother K, Till GO (eds). The complement system. Berlin: Springer-Verlag, 1988.

264. Ruff MR, Pert CB, Weber RJ, et al. Benzodiazepine receptor-mediated chemotaxis of human monocytes. Science 1985; 229:1281–1283.

265. Ryan GB. Inflammation. Mediators of inflammation. Beitr Pathol 1974;152:272–291.

266. Ryan GB, Majno G. Inflammation (A Scope Publication). Kalamazoo, MI: The Upjohn Company, 1977.

267. Ryan JW, Ryan US. Biochemical and morphological aspects of the actions and metabolism of kinins. In: Pisano JJ, Austen KF (eds). Chemistry and biology of the Kallikrein-Kinin system in health and disease, Fogarty Int Center Proc, No. 27. Washington, DC: US Government Printing Office, 1976, pp. 315–333.

268. Sahashi K, Engel AG, Lambert EH, Howard FM Jr. Ultrastructural localization of the terminal lytic ninth complement component (C9) at the motor end-plate in myasthesia gravis. J Neuropathol Exp Neurol 1980;39:160–172.

269. Said SI. Vasoactive peptides. State-of-the-art review. Hypertension 1983;5 (Suppl I):I-17–I-26.

270. Salama A, Hugo F, Heinrich D, et al. Deposition of terminal C5b-9 complement complexes on erythrocytes and leukocytes during cardiopulmonary bypass. N Engl J Med 1988; 318:408–414.

271. Saldeen T. The fibrinolytic system in inflammation. In: Higgs GA, Williams TJ (eds). Inflammatory Mediators. London: MacMillan 1985, pp. 87–97.

272. Saria A, Lundberg JM. Neurogenic inflammation. In: Higgs GA, Williams TJ (eds). Inflammatory mediators. London: MacMillan 1985, pp. 73–85.

272a. Scaffidi P, Misteli T, Bianchi ME. Release of chromatin protein HMGB1 by necrotic cells triggers inflammation. Nature 2002;418:191–195.

273. Scher W. The role of extracellular proteases in cell proliferation and differentiation. Lab Invest 1987;57:607–633.

274. Schiffmann E, Gallin JI. Biochemistry of phagocyte chemotaxis. Curr Top Cell Regulation 1979;15:203–261.

275. Selvan RS, Butterfield JH, Krangel MS. Expression of multiple chemokine genes by a human mast cell leukemia. J Biol Chem 1994;269:13893–13898.

275a. Serhan CN. Lipoxins and aspirin-triggered 15-epi-lipoxins. In: Gallin JI, Snyderman R (eds). Inflammation. Basic principles and clinical correlates. 3rd ed. Philadelphia: Lippincott Williams & Wilkins, 1999, pp. 373–385.

275b. Serhan CN, Oliw E. Unorthodox routes to prostanoid formation: new twists in cyclooxygenase-initiated pathways. J Clin Invest 2001;107:1481–1489.

275c. Serhan CN, Hong S, Gronert K, et al. Resolvins: a family of bioactive products of omega-3 fatty acid transformation circuits initiated by aspirin treatment that counter proinflammation signals. J Exp Med 2002;196:1025–1037.

276. Shama SK, Etkind PH, Odell TM, et al. Gypsy-moth-caterpillar dermatitis. N Engl J Med 1982;306:1300–1301.

277. Siemion IZ, Kluczyk A. Tuftsin: on the 30-year anniversary of Victor Najjar's discovery. Peptides 1999;20:645–674.

278. Silverstein RL. The Vascular endothelium. In: Gallin JI, Snyderman R (eds). Inflammation: Basic principles and clinical correlates. 3rd ed. Philadelphia: Lippincott Williams & Wilkins, 1999, pp. 207–225.

279. Steinbusch HWM, Mulder AH. Localization and projections of histamine-immunocreactive neurons in the central nervous system of the rat. In: Ganellin CR, Schwartz J-C (eds). Frontiers in Histamine Research. Oxford: Pergamon Press, 1985, pp. 119–130.

279a. Tak PP, Firestein GS. NF-κB: a key role in inflammatory diseases. J Clin Invest 2001;107:7–11.

280. Thorgeirsson G. Endothelial autacoids. Acta Med Scand 1985;217:453–456.

281. Toda N. Heterogeneous responses to histamine in blood vessels. In: Vanhoutte PM (ed). Vasodilatation. New York: Raven Press, 1988, pp. 531–535.

282. Tschopp J, Podack ER, Müller-Eberhard HJ. The membrane attack complex of complement: C5b-8 complex as accelerator of C9 polymerization. J Immunol 1985;134:495–499.

283. Tsuru H. Heterogeneity of the vascular effects of bradykinin. In: Vanhoutte PM (ed). Vasodilatation. New York: Raven Press, 1988, pp. 479–482.

284. Van Epps DE, Williams RC. Serum inhibitors of leukocyte chemotaxis and their relationship to skin test energy. In: Gallin JI, Quie, PG (eds). Leukocyte chemotaxis: methods, physiology, and clinical implications. New York: Raven Press, 1978, pp. 237–253.

285. Vanhoutte PM, Cohen RA, Van Nueten JM. Serotonin and arterial vessels. J Cardiovasc Pharmacol 1984;6 (suppl 2):S421–S428.

286. Ward PA. Overview. In: Gallin JI, Quie PG (eds). Leukocyte chemotaxis: Methods, physiology, and clinical implications. New York: Raven Press, 1978, pp. 405–411.

287. Ward PA, Becker EL. Biology of leukotaxis. Rev. Physiol Biochem Pharmacol 1977;77:125–148.

288. Ward PA, Lepow IH, Newman LJ. Bacterial factors chemotactic for polymorphonuclear leukocytes. Am J Pathol 1968; 52:725–736.

289. Warren JS, Ward PA, Johnson KJ. Tumor necrosis factor: a plurifunctional mediator of acute inflammation. Mod Pathol 1988;1:242–247.

290. Weaver JC, Astumian RD. The response of living cells to very weak electric fields: the thermal noise limit. Science 1990;247:459–462.

291. Weissmann G. Mediators of inflammation. New York: Plenum Press, 1974.

292. Welsh RM Jr, Lampert PW, Burner PA, Oldstone MBA. Antibody-complement interactions with purified lymphocytic choriomeningitis virus. Virology 1976;73:59–71.

292a. Wentworth P Jr, Wentworth AD, Zhu X, et al. Evidence for the production of trioxygen species during antibody-catalyzed chemical modification of antigens. PNAS 2003; 100:1490–1493; published online before print as 10.1073/pnas.0437831100.

293. Wilder RL. Proinflammatory microbial products as etiologic agents of inflammatory arthritis. Rheum Dis Clin North Am 1987;13:293–306.

294. Wilkinson PC. Chemotaxis and inflammation, 2nd ed. Edinburgh: Churchill Livingstone, 1982.

295. Wilkinson PC, Lackie JM. The adhesion, migration and chemotaxis of leucocytes in inflammation. Curr Top Pathol 1979;68:47–88.

296. Williams T, Jose PJ. Mediation of increased vascular permeability after complement activation. J Exp Med 1981; 153:136–153.

297. Willis AL. The eicosanoids: an introduction and an overview. In: Willis AL (ed). CRC Handbook of Eicosanoids: Prostaglandins and Related Lipids vol. 1. Boca Raton: CEC Press Inc., 1987, pp. 3–46.

298. Woodin AM, Wieneke AA. Leukocidin, tetraethylammonium ions, and the membrane acyl phosphatases in relation to the leukocyte potassium pump. J Gen Physiol, 1970;56: 16–32.

299. Yurt RW. Role of the mast cell in trauma. In: Dineen P, Hildick-Smith G (eds). The Surgical Wound. Philadelphia: Lea & Febiger, 1981, pp. 37–62.

300. Zamora R, Vodovotz Y, Billiar TR. Inducible nitric oxide synthase and inflammatory diseases. Mol Med 2000;6: 347–373.

301. Zhou W, Chao W, Levine BA, Olson MS Evidence for platelet-activating factor as a late-phase mediator of chronic pancreatitis in the rat. Am J Pathol 1990;137:1501–1508.

302. Zurier RB. Prostaglandin E_1: is it useful? J Rheumatol 1990; 17:1439–1441.

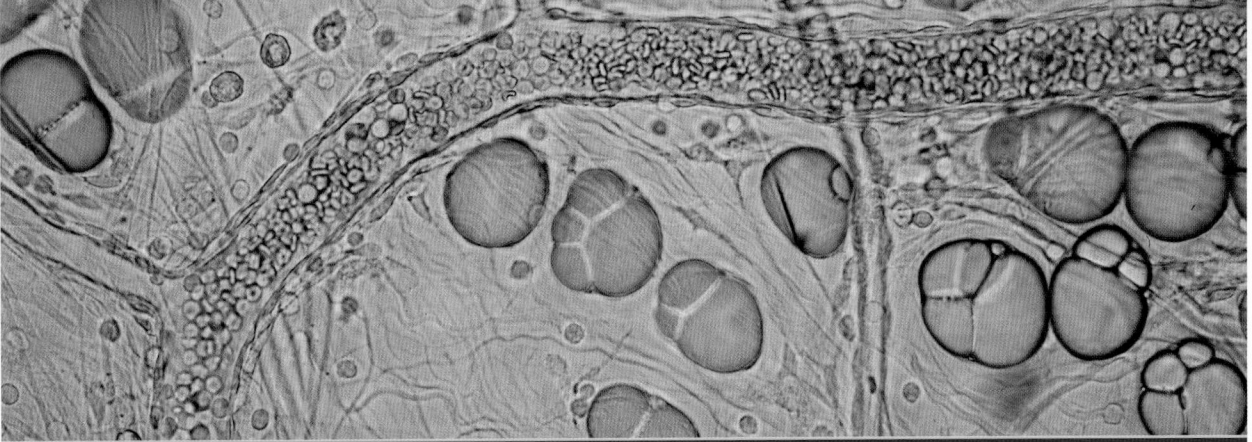

CHAPTER 10

THE FOUR CARDINAL SIGNS OF INFLAMMATION

- Mechanisms of Redness, Heat and Pain
- Inflammatory Swelling: Mechanisms of Vascular Leakage

Having introduced the actors of inflammation and their language, we can now view the play: "redness and swelling with heat and pain" (*rubor et tumor cum calore et dolore*).

Mechanisms of Redness, Heat, and Pain

The Greeks, who believed that inflamed organs contained "too much blood," had observed correctly. To this day, a clinician who has to describe a blood-shot eye or a flaming red larynx (Figure 10.1) will use the Greek term for "much blood," *hyperemia.* Its mechanism began to be understood when it became possible to witness the vascular events of inflammation in live tissues under the microscope. Cohnheim marveled over them in 1867, in the mesentery of the living frog (6). Note that he did not need to injure the mesentery; it became inflamed on its own due to the trauma of exposure. Here is what he saw:

> The first thing you notice in the exposed vessels is a dilation which occurs chiefly in the arteries, then in the veins, and least of all in the capillaries. With the dilatation which is gradually developed, but which during the space of fifteen to twenty minutes has usually attained considerable proportions (often exceeding twice the original diameter) there immediately sets in the mesentery an acceleration of the bloodstream, most striking again in the arteries. . . . Yet this acceleration never lasts long; after half an hour or an hour . . . it invariably gives place to a decided retardation, the velocity of the stream falling more or less below the normal (8).

The dilatation of the arterioles (small arteries) is the cumulative effect of vasoactive mediators (histamine and many others) and probably also of nervous impulses.

What happens when arterioles dilate? Physiology teaches us that the arterioles are the resistance vessels of the arterial tree.

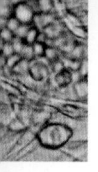

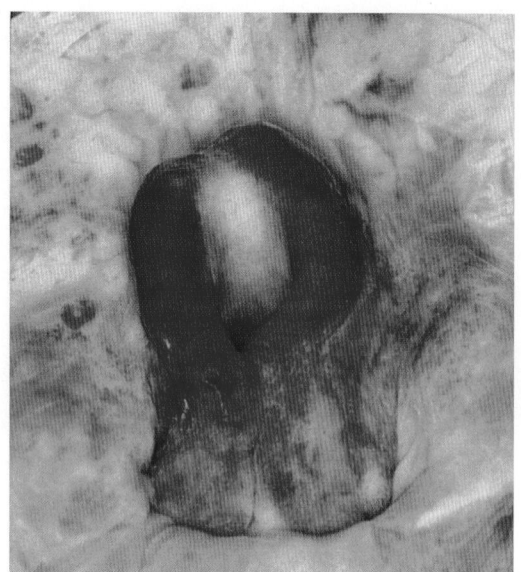

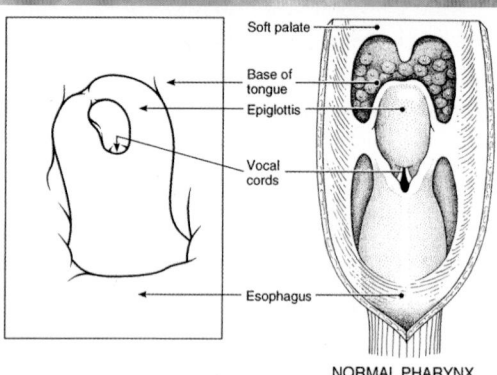

Soft palate

Base of tongue

Epiglottis

Vocal cords

Esophagus

NORMAL PHARYNX

FIGURE 10.1 Inflammatory RUBOR: the acutely inflamed epiglottis of a 7-year-old child who died of asphyxia. Such infections are usually caused by *Haemophilus influenzae,* the epiglottis swells and becomes cherry red. Stridor (harsh sound during respiration) is a warning and should be treated as an emergency. (Magnification approximately × 2.) *Bottom:* Diagram of top figure and scheme of the pharynx as seen from behind the soft palate, looking forward. (Courtesy of Dr. F. J. Krolikowski, Medical Examiner, Commonwealth of Massachusetts.)

Under normal conditions they bring about the largest drop in blood pressure (from ~85 to 30 mm Hg), which means that normally their upstream effect is to provide the heart pump with a resistance, while their downstream effect is that of floodgates: they protect the capillaries from the high arterial pressure. *If all the arterioles throughout the body were to dilate at the same time, the arterial blood pressure would drop precipitously* (this is what happens in anaphylactic shock). In inflammation they dilate only in a limited area, so that systemic arterial pressure is not affected. However, *downstream from*

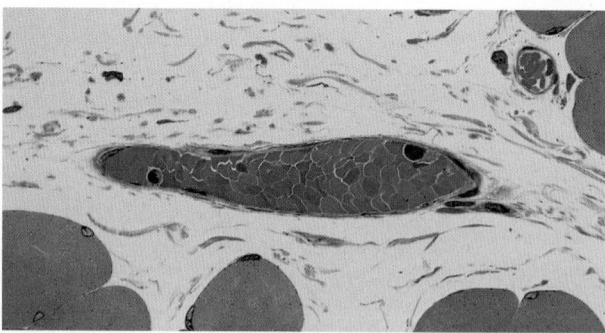

FIGURE 10.2 Congested venule in an acutely inflamed muscle. The vessel is filled with compacted red blood cells; under normal circumstances about half of the space in the lumen should be occupied by plasma. The tissue surrounding the venule is edematous, presumably from plasma lost by this and other leaky venules. (~350x)

the dilated arterioles, flow accelerates and capillary pressure rises: the floodgates are open, and capillaries that are normally empty are filled by the incoming tide, enough to give the gross impression of a blush. This is what happens when people blush. Blood flow can increase as much as tenfold (26).

Capillary dilatation is minimal, but the venules become distended. The cause can be guessed from Figure 10.2, which portrays a typical venule in an inflamed area. This venule contains only blood cells, no plasma. Normally, blood cells make up about 44 percent of the total blood volume. Thus, 56 percent should be plasma, yet little or no plasma is left in "inflamed" venules. Where did it go? Light microscopy cannot clearly show it, but the walls of these venules have become leaky: plasma has escaped through tiny, temporary gaps between endothelial cells. The semisolid cylinder of red blood cells that now fills the lumen opposes a much greater resistance to flow (Figure 10.3). The increased resistance raises the pressure upstream, and the lumen expands. Now flow becomes slower, as Cohnheim observed. All this happens within a few minutes. The leakiness of venules will be explained later.

Notice how these venular changes fit the overall plan: the increased flow from the arterioles, combined with an obstacle in the leaky venules, leads to greater exudation of fluid—which is one of the two basic purposes of inflammation: to deliver fluid and cells to the site of injury.

To better understand the "redness," we will resort to a simple experiment on human skin: the so-called *triple response.*

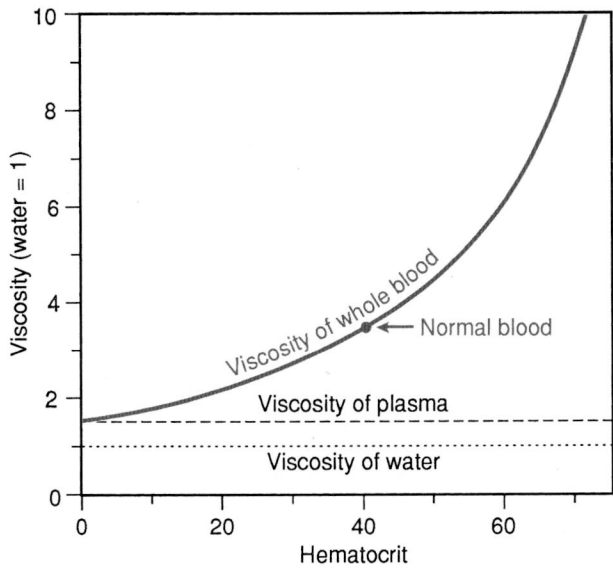

FIGURE 10.3   The viscosity of the blood rises sharply as the hematocrit increases. This explains the slow flow in leaky venules of inflammatory foci: the plasma has leaked out, and the hematocrit inside the venule approaches 100 percent. (Reproduced with permission from [21].)

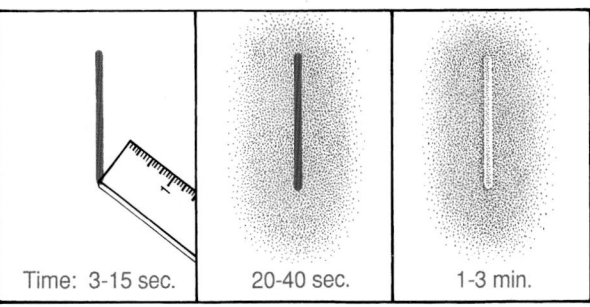

FIGURE 10.4   The "triple response" of Lewis, produced by firmly stroking the skin with a blunt object. First a red line appears; then a red flare develops along the red line; eventually the red line turns into a wheal.

The Triple Response of the Skin

The mechanisms of arterial dilatation were worked out in the skin as early as the 1920s by the pioneer studies of a British clinician, Sir Thomas Lewis (44). His experiments, though extremely simple, were a landmark because they led to discover the first inflammatory mediator, histamine, cautiously referred to in those days as "substance H". You can try his basic experiment as you read these lines. Take a ruler, and pull one of its corners rather firmly along the skin of your forearm (Figure 10.4). A three-step reaction will follow:

1. A red line appears within seconds (vasodilatation).
2. A red flare appears after 15–30 seconds, spreading all around the line to a distance of several centimeters (again vasodilatation).
3. The red line becomes a wheal (a transient swelling of the skin, such as is produced by the sting of a nettle). This takes a little longer, 1–3 minutes, because it is due to vascular leakage, which requires time. At first the wheal is red; as it swells further it pales.

The triple response is explained as follows. The trauma caused by the ruler breaks up or somehow degranulates the mast cells in the dermis; the mast cells spill their histamine, which causes local vasodilatation (red line) followed by vascular leakage (wheal). As to

the flare, it is not conceivable that histamine could diffuse several centimeters in a matter of seconds. Sir Thomas found that it is due to an axon reflex, as explained in Figure 10.5 (5, 75). He tried the triple response experiment in accident victims in whom the sensory nerve leading to the test area had been severed; for the first 5 days after the nerve was cut, the flare did develop; then it disappeared, coincidentally with the slow breakdown of the severed axons.

The triple response helps us understand the redness of the skin around an injury (look for the flare around your next mosquito bite). As to the meaning of the response itself: it increases local blood flow and may therefore have a protective effect (44).

> The triple response is reduced in diabetics, presumably because of the diabetic neuropathy (31). Whether it occurs also in internal organs is not clear (26); however, it has been proposed that the bronchial spasm of asthma is due to an axon reflex, which in this case would be obnoxious. The bronchial epithelium, damaged by the eosinophils exposes C fibers, which generate an axon reflex leading to bronchial spasm and hypersecretion of mucus (2).

Heat and Pain

The heat of inflamed skin is due to the increased perfusion of the tissues with blood, and so the temperature can never be higher than that of blood. It follows that *calor* can develop only in the skin, which is normally cool. Inflamed inner organs cannot become hotter because they are already as hot as they can be. Does the increased temperature of the skin have any significance? It has been shown that leukocytes maintained in a thermal gradient *in vitro* move toward warmer temperatures (**thermotaxis**) (38); but whether this is actually helpful *in vivo* is not known. However, in discussing fever, we will mention several potentially beneficial effects of

FIGURE 10.5 Mechanism of the triple response shown in Figure 10.4. The stimulation of a sensory fiber and the mast cell degranulation initiate an impulse; by an antidromic pathway the impulse reaches an arteriole, where the nerve endings release substance P and/or ATP. This causes mast cells to degranulate, producing further sensory and vasomotor effects. (Adapted with permission from [75], Raven Press, 1988.)

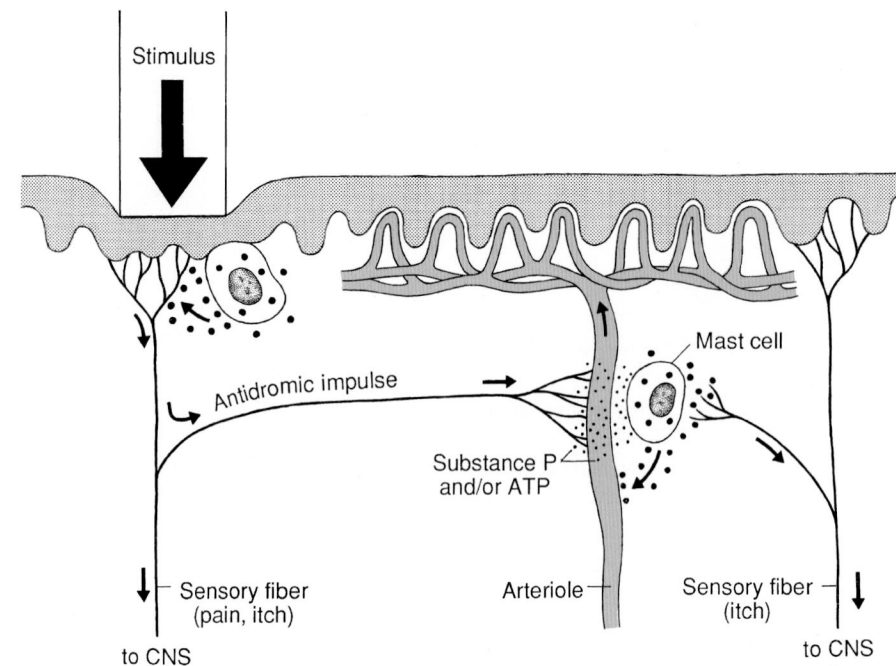

higher temperatures; for example, leukocytes move faster. It is therefore possible that the *calor* of inflamed skin may have a survival value.

The pain occurs when specialized nerve-fiber endings are stimulated by mediators, especially bradykinin (remember that many insects use bradykinin to make their stings painful).

A standard test for pain mediators (**algogens**) in humans is to raise a blister on the forearm with the ancient blistering agent cantharidin (prepared from the dried, crushed bodies of a special kind of beetle), cut off the roof of the blister, and drip the substance to be tested on the denuded dermis. This test shows that bradykinin is about 50 times more potent than histamine or serotonin in eliciting pain (18).

It is possible that tissue pressure may enhance the pain, but there is no good evidence of correlation between tissue swelling and pain; *noninflammatory edema is painless*. Prostaglandins sensitize the nerve endings to the effects of bradykinin and other algogens (56). Once again, *aspirin reduces the pain of inflammation by cutting off the supply of prostaglandins*. This explains why aspirin is of no help in many types of noninflammatory pain (56).

Itching is probably not the same modality as pain, but little is known about it. Histamine is certainly involved: a small intradermal dose of histamine causes itching, a larger dose pain. Proteases are also involved (3, 16). How itching powder works (cowhage, the spicules of a tropical fruit) is still not clear (3, 16).

Can There Be Acute Inflammation without Redness?

Not really, except for one special case: on a slice of lung, seen at autopsy, a focus of acute inflammation (bronchopneumonia) appears whitish instead of red, because the color that prevails (at least at autopsy) is the color of fibrin and leukocytes that fill the alveoli (Figure 10.6). In chronic inflammation, however, redness is often lacking.

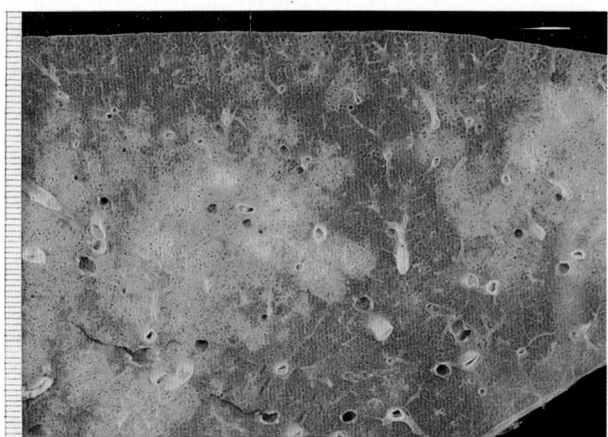

FIGURE 10.6 Slice of human lung showing foci of bronchopneumonia: an inflammatory condition in which the air spaces are replaced by white blood cells and fibrin. A combination of these produces the whitish discoloration of the lung's cut surface. **Scale** in millimeters.

Can There Be Acute Inflammation without Pain?

Certainly. In internal organs, such as the lung, inflammation is painless unless it reaches the pleura, as proven by the phenomenon of "walking pneumonia": you can have a focus of acute inflammation in a lung and walk around feeling sick but without realizing that your problem is pneumonia. Many dermatologic inflammatory conditions cause redness with little or no pain. In our experience, the purple-red erythema of Lyme disease is painless to the point of escaping notice. Perhaps a special mixture of mediators is involved.

> **TO SUM UP: Rubor** represents good news, more blood supplies for the defenses; **dolor** is incidental, although it may help by pointing to an area of trouble; **calor** is limited to inflammation in the skin, where it may have a protective value. We now turn to the **tumor**.

Inflammatory Swelling: Mechanisms of Vascular Leakage

The basic mechanism of the inflammatory swelling was proposed by Cohnheim in 1873 when he ventured a guess beyond the resolving power of his microscope: *plasma escapes from the blood vessels, which have somehow become leaky* (7). Correct but unproven, this explanation held for about 80 years, pending the arrival of more powerful microscopes.

> Electron microscopes existed in the 1930s, but it was "common knowledge" that they could not be used in biology, because no known blade could cut tissue slices thin enough for the electrons to go through them (about 500 Å, roughly the wavelength of light). A young American pathologist, H. Latta, changed all that by discovering that a piece of broken glass was the long-sought "perfect" blade (47); after 1955 anybody with patience, including the authors of this book, could cut ultrathin sections.

Looking into an electron microscope in the 1950s was a dream come true. A pathologist could see the cell slowly come to life as the "elementary patient," with new organelles discovered every year. At Rockefeller University, Dr. George E. Palade discovered the ribosomes (Nobel prize in 1974) and chose the endothelium as another tissue that called for urgent definition, as the barrier between blood and tissues. Until then, the endothelium had been the private hunting ground of physiologists; in 1951 a distinguished group of them published a physicomathematical study of endothelial permeability based largely on perfusion of isolated dog limbs, and concluded that the endothelium behaved as an inert plastic sheet, equipped with two sets of pores of given sizes. To this date, they have not quite forgiven Dr. Palade for not confirming their calculations.

Electron microscopy revealed no pores of the required size, and worse yet, it found something quite different, which did not fit with the plastic sheet concept and would escape the mathematics: the endothelial cells contained a set of vesicles that appeared to actively transport droplets of plasma across the cell, probably in both directions (60).

All of this is pertinent to our story, because inflammatory leakage is understood as a disturbance of Starling's law—and Starling's law is based on the endothelium behaving as a passive, semipermeable membrane—which it is not. For readers who would like a reminder of the forces supposed to be involved in the Starling equilibrium, Tables 10.1 and 10.2 will do, but we must be sure to understand that these figures are based, with all due respect, on a theoretical nonexisting kind of endothelium. As of 2003, there is no agreement between physiologists (54) and electron microscopists (60)

Table 10.1 Forces Involved in Filtration and Reabsorption Along the Capillary and Venule

At the Arterial End of the Capillary		At the Venular End of the Capillary	
Forces tending to move fluid outward:		**Force tending to move fluid inward:**	
Capillary pressure	30.0	Plasma colloid osmotic pressure	28.0
Negative interstitial free fluid pressure	5.3	Total inward force	28.0
Interstitial fluid colloid osmotic pressure	6.0	**Forces tending to move fluid outward:**	
Total outward force	41.3	Capillary pressure	10.0
Forces tending to move fluid inward:		Negative interstitial free fluid pressure	5.3
Plasma colloid osmotic pressure	28.0	Interstitial fluid colloid osmotic pressure	6.0
Total inward force	28.0	Total outward force	21.3
Summation of forces:		**Summation of forces:**	
Outward	41.3	Inward	28.0
Inward	28.0	Outward	21.3
Net outward force	13.3	Net inward force	6.7

(Reprinted from [21], Copyright 1986, with permission from Elsevier.) Values given in millimeter Hg.

Table 10.2 Concentration and Osmotic Pressure
of Plasma Proteins

Protein	Concentration (G %)	Osmotic Pressure (mm Hg)
Albumin	4.5	21.8
Globulins	2.5	6.0
Fibrinogen	0.3	0.2
Total	7.3	28.0

(Reprinted from [21], Copyright 1986, with permission from Elsevier.)

regarding the physiologic pathways across the endothelial barrier.

The Dynamics of Fluid Exudation

With these limitations in mind, we can safely state that acute inflammation throws off the equilibrium of fluid exchanges governed by the hydrostatic and osmotic forces acting on both sides of the endothelium (Tables 10.1 and 10.2).

Normally the main force driving fluid OUT of the vessels is the hydrostatic pressure of the blood; the main force driving fluid BACK INTO THE BLOOD is the colloidal osmotic pressure of the plasma proteins. (Table 10.1 also conveys the notion that the extravascular hydrostatic pressure is negative: we will return to this astonishing fact elsewhere [p. 615]).

In acute inflammation all elements of this equilibrium are perturbed. The semipermeable membrane is riddled with leaks. Furthermore, the main force driving fluid out of the vessels is increased because the arterioles are dilated, which increases downstream pressure; the main force driving fluid back into the blood is decreased, because some plasma proteins are escaping into the tissue spaces, and create there an osmotic pressure that competes with that of the plasma remaining in the vessel (Figure 10.7). Inflammatory mediators that dilate arterioles—but do not increase vascular permeability—will still increase the loss of fluid (30). This effect can be measured (Figure 10.8).

There is, in principle, no limit to the amount of exudate that can seep out of an inflamed *body surface*, such as a burn; but when exudation occurs in the tissue spaces, the tissues are distended, and the corresponding increase in tissue pressure opposes further exudation. In a dog's knee that is experimentally inflamed by injected urate crystals (a sort of artificial gout), the joint pressure rises to a level approaching diastolic pressure (Figure 10.9).

The turnover of extractable (i.e., unbound) exudate proteins was measured in rabbit skin after burns produced with the ill-famed vesicant war gas nitrogen mustard. In one-day lesions the total renewal of the extractable proteins required about 8 hours; in three- and five-day lesions, about 35 hours (14).

The next step is to find out the meaning of "leaky endothelium" at the level of ultrastructure. This was the task for one of us who joined Dr. Palade's team in the 1950s. Fortunately, pathologic leaks were somewhat easier to find than the pathways of normal endothelial permeability (by the way: the term *leaky*, strangely enough, does not exist in Latin languages).

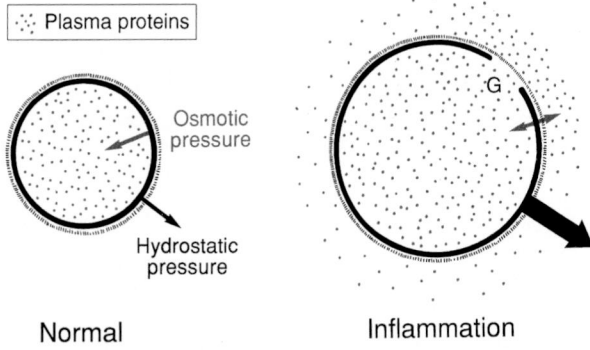

FIGURE 10.7 Schematic cross section of two capillaries or venules, represented as membranes impermeable to plasma protein molecules (**dots**). *Left:* The normal condition. The two main opposing forces causing filtration and reabsorption (**arrows**) are balanced. *Right:* In inflammation, the membrane is interrupted by gaps (**G**); proteins escape, so that intra- and extravascular osmotic pressures tend to cancel each other; intravascular hydrostatic pressure is greatly increased (*heavy arrow*). Result: inflammatory edema.

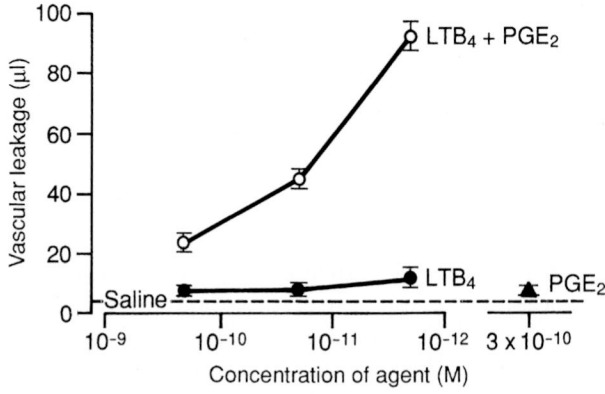

FIGURE 10.8 Demonstrating that vasodilators increase vascular leakage. Leukotriene B_4—injected alone into the skin of a rabbit—causes very little vascular leakage; if it is injected together with a powerful vasodilator (prostaglandin E_2) the loss of fluid is greatly increased. (Adapted with permission from [77a].)

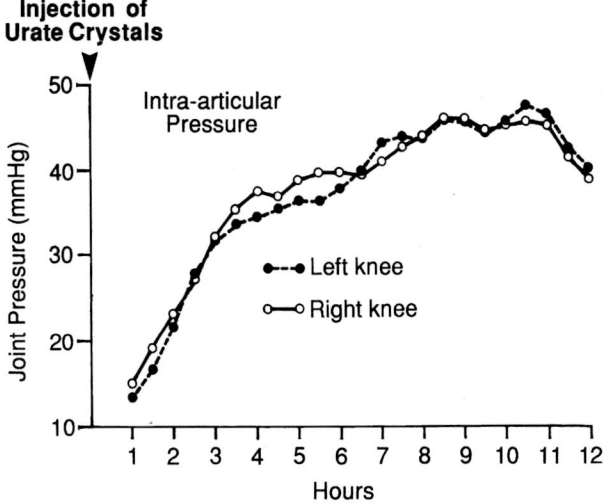

Injection of Urate Crystals

Intra-articular Pressure

Joint Pressure (mmHg)

●—● Left knee
○—○ Right knee

Hours

FIGURE 10.9 Experiment illustrating tissue pressure in acute inflammation. Intraarticular pressure of two joints (dog knees) inflamed by injection of urate crystals. The curves rise to a level approaching diastolic blood pressure. The joint space can be taken to represent an "enlarged interstitial space." (Reproduced from [50a] with permission from Springer-Verlag.)

We began by working out the structure of the vessels involved. The capillaries and venules, the vessels most susceptible to leakage, are made of a single layer of endothelial cells, hugged on the outside by long, spidery cells called pericytes, beautifully described in 1923 by Zimmermann (Figure 10.10) (79). Their function is not

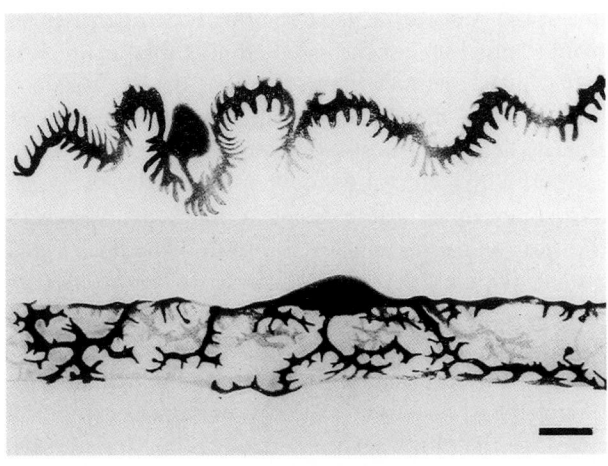

FIGURE 10.10 Pericytes, impregnated (blackened) with silver as illustrated by K. W. Zimmermann in 1923. *Top:* Pericyte stretched along capillaries of the human tongue (actual length about 0.15 mm). *Bottom:* Pericytes on a postcapillary venule in cat heart. **Bar** = 5 μm. (Reproduced from [79] with permission from Springer-Verlag.)

known, but they can phagocytize, and when grown in cultures they appear to "give orders" to the endothelial cells (59). *The permeability barrier* in all vessels is the endothelium; each vessel is surrounded by a clearly identifiable **basement membrane,** which provides mechanical support. What happens if these layers are damaged?

- *If the endothelial layer alone is interrupted,* the permeability barrier is lost and plasma leaks out, but the basement membrane remains and holds the vessel together; it acts temporarily as a coarse filter (and a guide to regenerating cells) until the endothelium is repaired.

- *If the basement membrane alone is destroyed* (by enzymes), the vessel tends to break apart: for example, if collagenase is injected into the skin of a rat, it produces extensive hemorrhage. This shows the mechanical role of the basement membrane.

- *If both layers are destroyed,* the result is not leakage but hemorrhage.

Methods for Demonstrating Vascular Leakage

The diagram in Figure 10.7 has a practical application: if leaky vessels lose enough fluid, it should be possible to detect the leakage with the naked eye by injecting colored material into the blood stream. The basic principle would be the same that civil engineers use when they look for a leak in a septic tank: they pour fluorescein into the tank and see where the fluorescence turns up. In fact, intravenous fluorescein is used by ophthalmologists for demonstrating leaky vessels in the retina.

However, the study of leaky vessels includes a refinement not available for testing septic tanks. In experimental animals, two kinds of colored materials can be used, with different but complementary results: *a soluble dye* such as Evans blue and *colloidal particles* such as India ink. These are the same two sets of colored materials that we used for mapping the RES (p. 314); in that context, of course, we used them for testing phagocytosis, whereas here we are testing permeability. The critical difference between the two materials is the size of the colored particles (Figure 10.11).

Testing permeability with soluble dyes. This classic method is often referred to as **bluing,** notwithstanding the fact that red dyes can also be used (43, 51). As seen on the shaved skin of a white rabbit, the result is striking. If 3 ml of a 1 percent solution of trypan blue or Evans blue are injected intravenously, the rabbit shows little change, except that within hours and days it slowly acquires a blue-gray tinge. However, if the skin is slightly irritated in one area, that area will turn bright blue in 2–3 minutes (Figure 10.12).

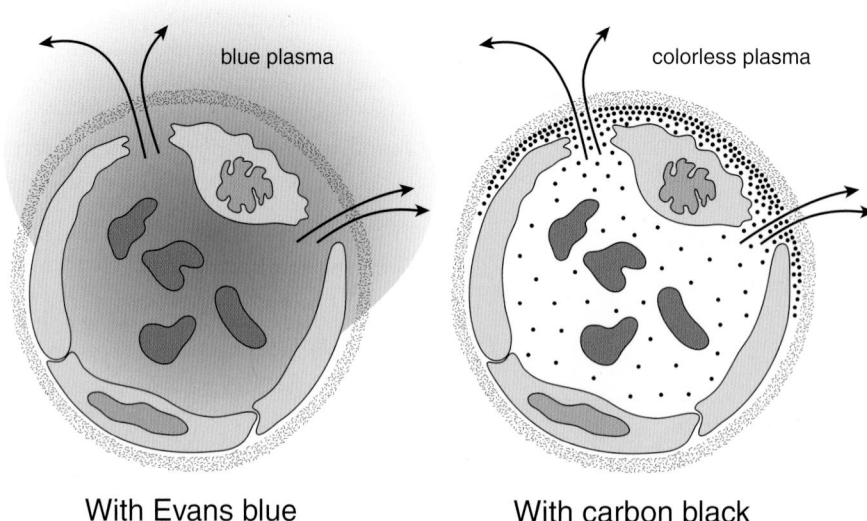

With Evans blue   **With carbon black**

FIGURE 10.11 Explaining two methods for studying vascular leakage. It is assumed that the permeability barrier (the endothelium) is broken, e.g., by trauma, leaving the basement membrane intact. *Left: By injecting a blue dye intravenously;* the plasma proteins, stained by the dye, seep across the basement membrane and diffuse into the extracellular spaces. *Right: By injecting a colloidal suspension of a pigment* (e.g., carbon black): being too large to seep across the basement membrane, the particles of pigment are retained, and cause the leaky vessel to remain "labeled." Details in text.

This test is very sensitive because albumin, which carries the blue dye (p. 85), is among the smallest plasma proteins: just what is needed for detecting fine leaks.

In the skin, the severity of the leakage is roughly proportional to the diameter of the blue spot, which is better seen by dissecting off the skin and examining its underside (Figure 10.13) (57). It is also possible to extract and quantitate the amount of extravasated dye (37). The bluing test is currently used experimentally not only for measuring the ability of given compounds to increase vascular permeability but also for testing the effectiveness of antiinflammatory drugs. The leakage of protein can also be quantitated using intravenous injections of ^{125}I-labeled albumin (58).

The bluing test is easy and sensitive, and it does demonstrate the general area in which vessels are leaking, but it does not indicate precisely which vessels are leaking (Figure 10.14). To do this we must inject into the blood some colored material that can be trapped in the wall of the leaking vessels.

Testing permeability with colloidal suspensions (vascular labeling). We choose this method when we want to pinpoint individual leaky vessels, that is, vessels that have a *leaky endothelium and an intact basement membrane.* Knowing that histamine produces leaky vessels, we pre-

pare a rat with a subcutaneous injection of histamine. Experience has shown that the basement membrane retains particles larger than 200–300 Å (the exact figure probably varies from site to site), so we will inject intravenously a colloidal suspension such as carbon black (biological India ink), which consists of particles about 300 Å in diameter. As the carbon-loaded plasma rushes out of the endothelial gaps, the suspended particles remain trapped against the basement membrane, much as coffee piles up on a filter (Figure 10.11). Within a minute or so the deposit can be dense enough to be seen by light microscopy or even by the naked eye. In contrast with the diffuse blue spot obtained with trypan blue, one can see a fine design of blackened vessels in the skin and especially in the more vascular striated muscle (Figure 10.14). *The advantage over the bluing method is that each leaky vessel remains permanently marked,* so it is easy to determine precisely where the leakage has occurred. This is important; the type of leaking vessel (arteriole, capillary, or venule) can give a clue as to the causal agent.

Tissues with labeled vessels can be studied in ordinary histologic sections; however, imagine how frustrating it would be to work out the damage in the wires of a telephone exchange by studying cross sections of the whole system. It would make more sense to leave the damaged wires intact and to examine them in their

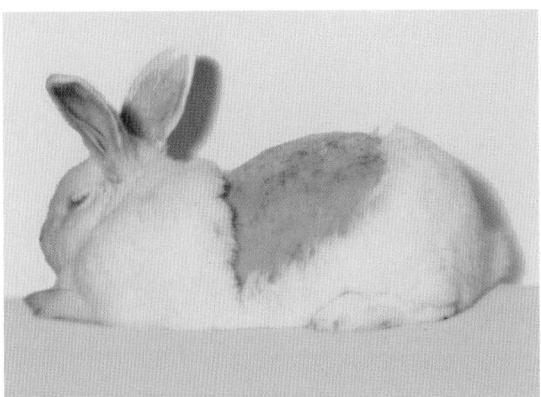

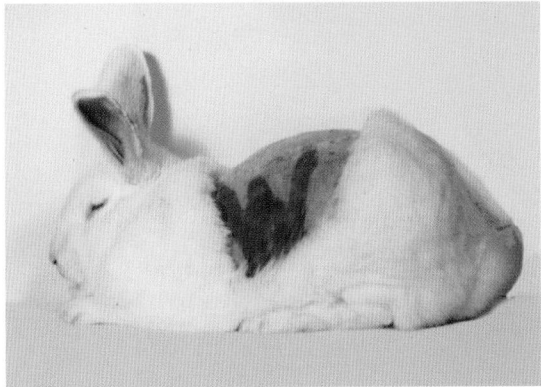

FIGURE 10.12   Experiment demonstrating the speed of the permeability-increasing response. *Top:* a white rabbit with back and flanks shaved, 1 minute after an intravenous injection of trypan blue, and after a "W" (for Worcester) was painted on the skin with xylene, a very mild irritant. Comparison with the photograph below will show that the outline of the W is just beginning to appear. *Bottom:* The same rabbit 5 minutes later. Trypan blue leaked out of the vessels only where the skin had been irritated.

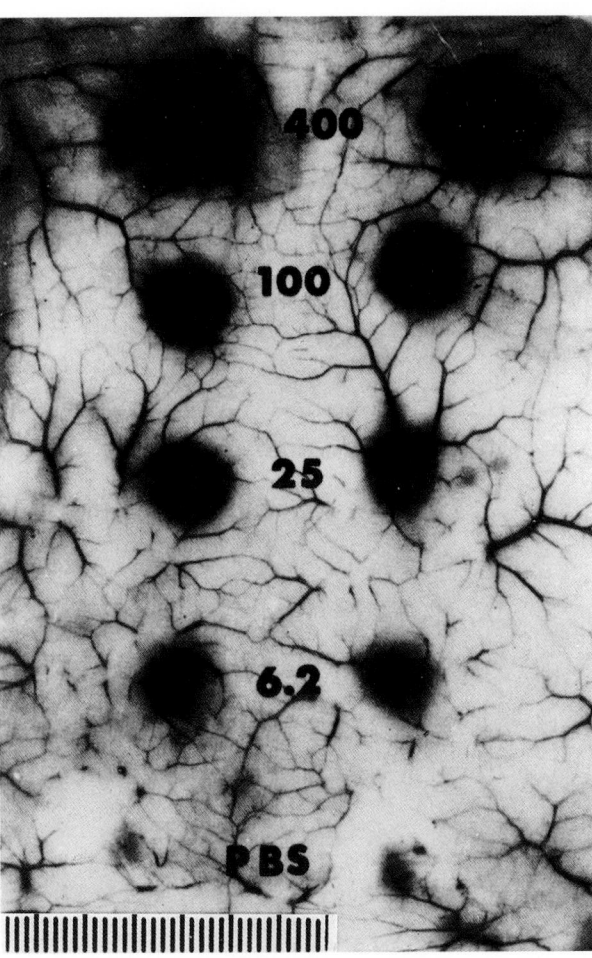

FIGURE 10.13   Bluing method for measuring increased vascular permeability. The undersurface of guinea pig skin after an intravenous injection of Evans blue and intradermal injections of brady-kinin (doses expressed in nanograms). **PBS:** Phosphate-buffered saline. **Scale** in millimeters. (Reproduced from [57] with permission from Springer-Verlag.)

proper context. The same is true for the circulatory network: damaged (and especially labeled) vessels are best studied either in living, transparent tissues, or in fixed tissues examined as a whole after they have been made transparent by glycerin. Several of our illustrations were obtained by photographing a thin striated muscle, the cremaster of the rat, cleared in glycerin; in this manner arterioles, capillaries and venules are easily identified.

The rat cremaster preparation. In the rat, each testicle is contained in a thin bag of striated muscle, the cremaster, which is continuous with the abdominal internal oblique muscle. An inflammatory mediator injected into the skin of the scrotum diffuses into the cremaster; carbon black (biological India ink) is then injected intravenously, and leaky vessels in the cremaster become labeled. Because the carbon black is cleared very quickly from the blood stream (thanks to the littoral phagocytes, p. 316) vascular labeling can occur only within the first 1–2 minutes after the intravenous injection. The cremaster is then excised, fixed, cleared in glycerin, and examined by transillumination (49).

Types of Vascular Leakage

A wide array of agents—chemical, physical, biological—can cause the vessels of the microcirculation to leak, and each agent may affect arterioles, capillaries, and venules in different combinations. The labeling method

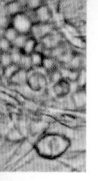

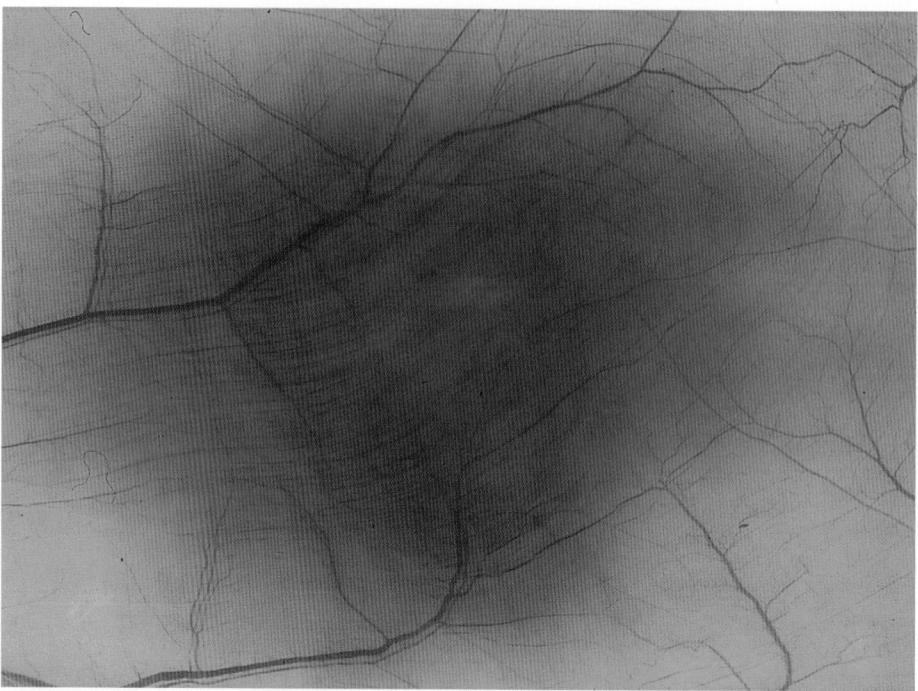

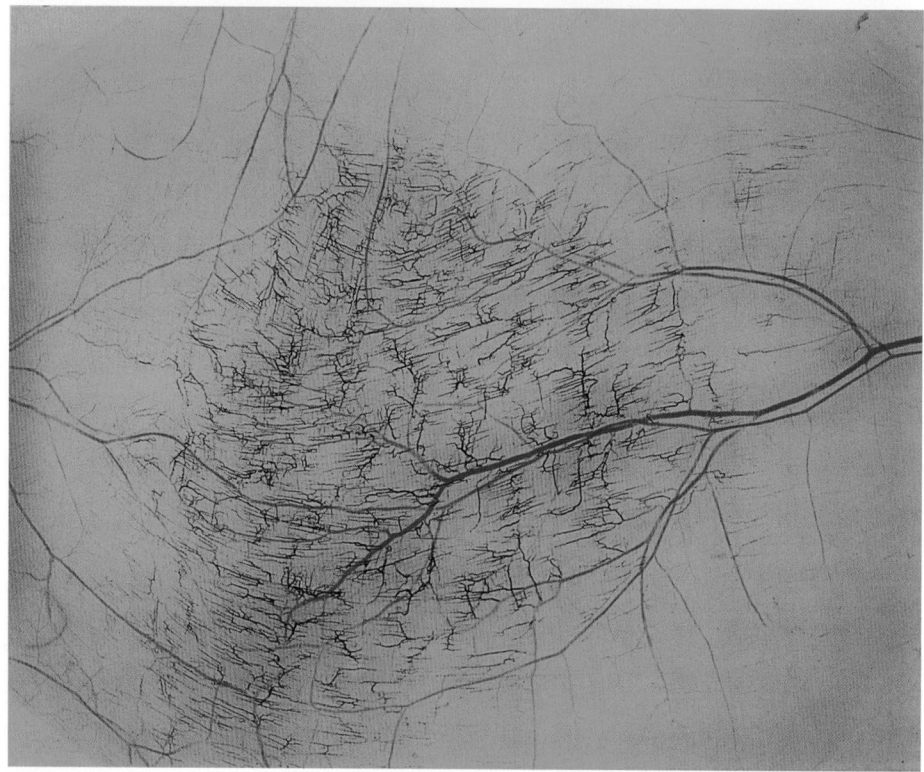

FIGURE 10.14   Contrasting two methods for demonstrating vascular leakage. Cremaster muscle *30 minutes* after a local injection of histamine and intravenous injection of *either* trypan blue or carbon black. Cremasters are mounted in glycerine jelly and transillumi- nated. *Top:* If blue is injected, the local escape of dye is impressive, but no dye is retained in the walls of the leaking vessels. (Repro- duced from [65].) *Bottom:* If colloidal carbon black is injected intravenously instead of trypan blue, some particles of carbon are retained within the wall of the leaky vessels and produce "vascular labeling." (Reproduced from **The Journal of Biophysical and Biochemical Cytology, 1961;11:607–626** by copyright permission of the Rockefeller University Press.)

has been instrumental in working out this topic. At this time we can identify three clearcut patterns of microvascular leakage, induced by (a) direct injury, (b) histamine-type mediators, and (c) angiogenesis, plus a fourth category of "sundry mechanisms."

(1) Leakage by Direct Injury of Vessels

This is self-explanatory, but we must distinguish between severe injury (severe enough to kill tissues, which causes immediate leakage), and mild injury, which causes delayed leakage.

Direct injury, severe. A crude physical or toxic insult damages the vascular walls *in all types of vessels* (9, 45). *Leakage begins immediately and continues* until the vessels are repaired or plugged. For example, after a severe experimental burn of the skin, all of the vessels in the subcutaneous tissue show labeling (Figure 10.15). Over the next day or two, these vessels will be lined by new endothelial cells gliding along the basement membrane; failing this, they will be plugged by platelets and "condemned."

Direct injury, mild. The prototype is the sunburn: as everyone knows, exposure to the sun in the morning is followed by a sunburn at night, with swelling and inflammation that can last several days. The leakage is therefore *delayed* and *prolonged*. A similar response can be produced experimentally with UV light, X-rays, mild heat (9, 11, 66), toxins (10, 28), infection, and a variety of chemicals (12). This delayed-prolonged type of leakage often occurs as the second bump of a biphasic curve (Figure 10.16): the early spike portrays immediate leakage, due mainly to histamine-type mediators released by degranulated mast cells. The late phase usually begins after 2–3 hours or longer and lasts a few hours. Even a triphasic curve has been described (77).

A late phase of leakage is common in certain allergic reactions and is thought to represent secretion of cytokines by the mast cells (p. 529). It is not abolished by antihistamines. The few electron microscopic studies of delayed-prolonged leakage found some endothelial damage (8, 9), especially in capillaries, but this may simply reflect the fact that the injurious agent was applied directly over capillary networks, e.g., in the dermis.

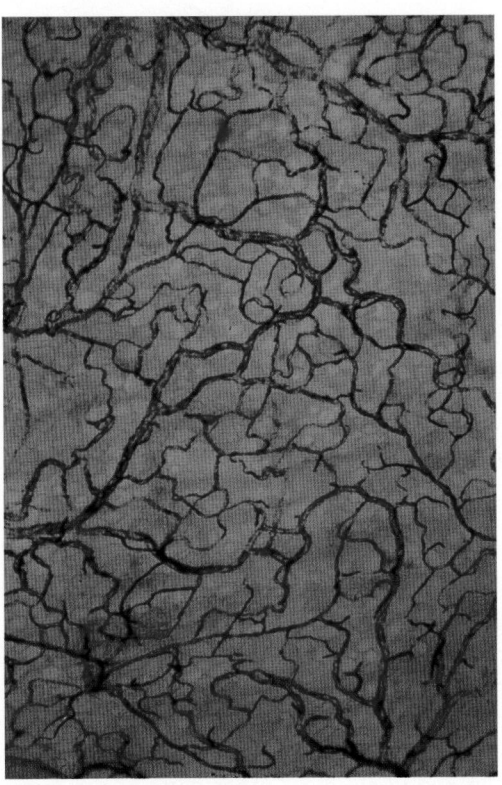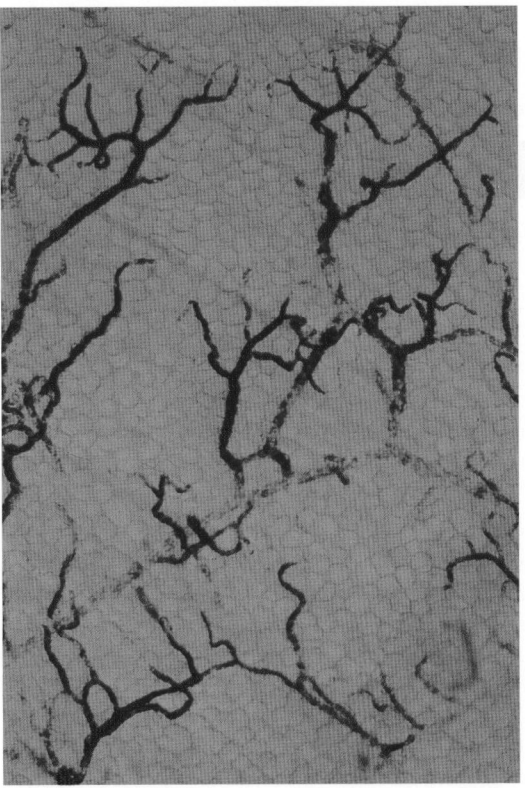

FIGURE 10.15   Comparing vascular labeling by direct injury (*left*, mild skin burn) and by histamine injection (*right*). In the burn, vessels of all types are labeled. (Subcutaneous adipose tissue of a rabbit.)

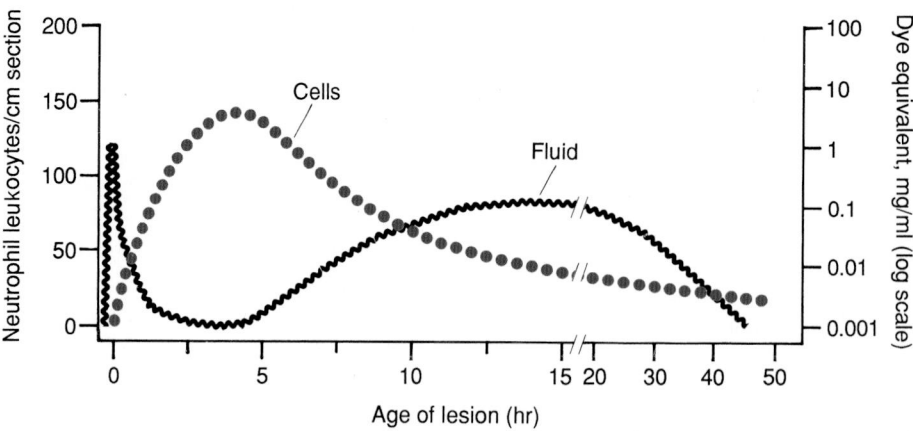

FIGURE 10.16 Example of biphasic fluid exudation (**wavy line**) obtained by painting xylene on guinea pig skin; chloroform, benzene, and many other irritants have a similar effect. The mechanism of delayed leakage in this model has not been worked out (delayed direct injury as by UV?). Note that the neutrophil response (**dotted line**) follows a different curve. (Adapted with permission from [69].)

(2) Leakage by Histamine-Type Mediators

This type of leakage is induced by a disparate group of fast-acting inflammatory mediators that are either preformed (such as histamine in mast cells) or produced within a minute or so after injury (such as bradykinin, platelet activating factor [PAF], leukotrienes). Injected into the skin of a rat, these mediators produce a patch of vascular leakage that is

- immediate
- limited to the venules, and
- Lasts only 20–30 minutes

It is convenient to call this *histamine-type vascular leakage (49)*. Its specificity for the venules is remarkable (Figure 10.17); it demolished a physiologic dogma going back to the 1920s, whereby histamine was supposed to increase *capillary* permeability (68). Physiologists, with notable exceptions (24), have been slow in accepting this singular behavior of the venules. Many continue to speak of the "capillary effect" of histamine, even though the astonishing fact is that *capillaries are specifically spared* not only by histamine but also by the other mediators mentioned above. To this day, the single *physiological* agent known to us that causes a mild degree of capillary leakage (beyond the predominant venular leakage) is a cytokine, vascular endothelial growth factor (VEGF) (64).

Why are the capillaries spared? We can only answer that nature must have some good reasons for protecting the capillary from histamine-type mediators, but we do not know them. We did once speculate that leaky capillaries would soon become clogged with blood cells; however, this line of reasoning collapsed when we realized that

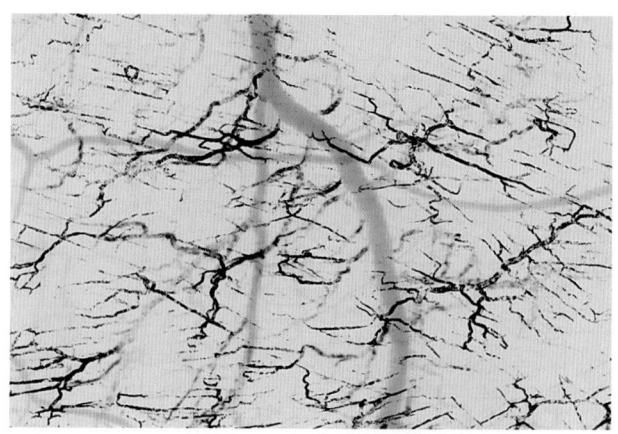

FIGURE 10.17 Typical example of "histamine-type" vascular leakage. Cremaster muscle seen by transillumination, 1 hour after a local injection of histamine immediately followed by an intravenous injection of carbon black. Leaky vessels are black; from their branching pattern it is obvious that they are venules. To compare with an example of capillary labeling, see Figure 10.21. (10x)

Nature had in store a planned variety of capillary leakage (see next section). The reverse question, "how are the venules selected?" is easier to answer: using histamine complexed with ferritin (which is visible by electron microscopy), Heltianu et al. (23) showed that venular endothelium has more histamine receptors than endothelium in other parts of the microvascular tree. But then, again—why so?

Mechanism of venular leakage. Within a minute or so after the local injection of a mediator, transmission

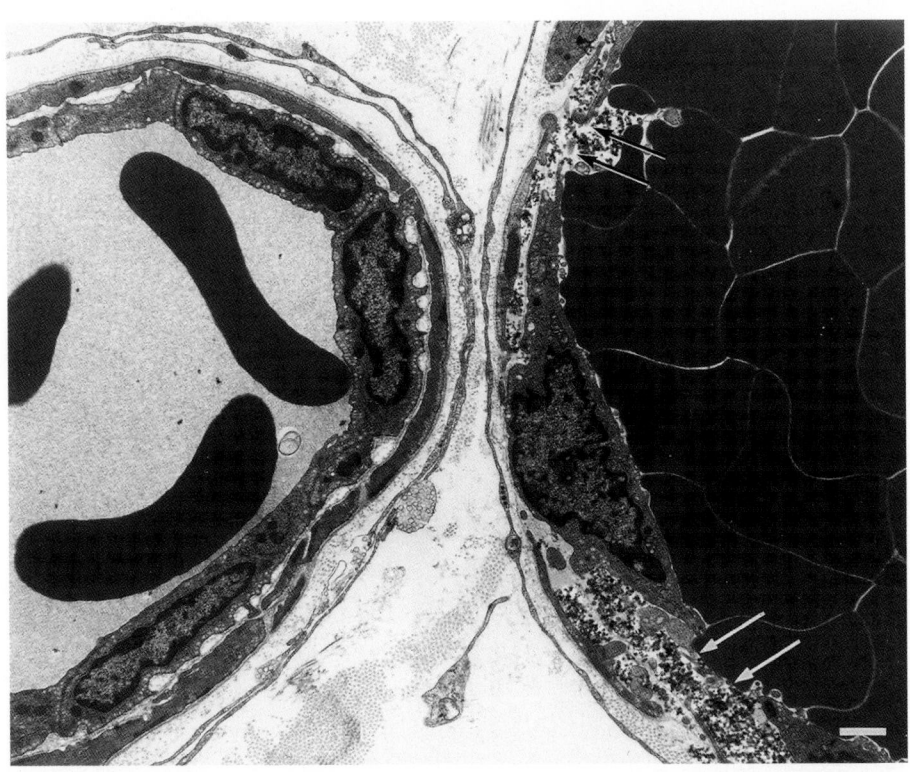

FIGURE 10.18 Arteriole (left) and venule (right) of a guinea pig 12 minutes after a local injection of histamine and an intravenous injection of carbon black. In the venule, two endothelial gaps have developed (**arrows**); escaping carbon particles are trapped in the venular wall. Because plasma has leaked out, the red blood cells are compacted ("stasis"). Note the contrast with the arteriole, whose endothelium did not become leaky: the arteriolar lumen contains a normal amount of plasma. **Bar** = 1 μm.

electron microscopy shows small gaps here and there between endothelial cells of the venules; the gaps are only ~1 μm in diameter, as if two endothelial cells had pulled apart and become disconnected at one limited spot (Figures 10.18, 10.19) (35, 48). Occasionally a gap is plugged by a platelet, or by a red blood cell that has been sucked in by the escaping plasma. In so doing, the red blood cells demonstrate their extraordinary plasticity: whereas in blood smears they look deceptively like stiff little coins, in reality they behave much more like "plastic bags filled with syrup" (we owe this analogy to the late Dr. Eugene M. Landis, the first physiologist to measure capillary pressure). It is not unusual to see a single red blood cell sucked into two adjacent gaps, presumably about to be torn apart.

How do the gaps develop? Electron microscopy shows that the cells on either side of a gap bulge into the lumen, and their nucleus shows unusual, tight infoldings (Figure 10.19). This is strong evidence of cellular contraction. Whenever a contractile cell shortens (be it striated muscle, myocardium, or other), its nucleus is thrown into folds rather like an accordion (35, 50). We can therefore propose that *venular gaps develop because adjacent endothelial cells contract and pull apart* at a limited point.

This pathogenesis of the venular gaps, suggested by studies *in vivo*, has been confirmed *in vitro: endothelial cultures* exposed of histamine or thrombin (which has histamine-like effects) have shown increased permeability, formation of intercellular gaps, a large increase in actin stress fibers (1), and contraction of the endothelial cells; the latter event is sometimes described as "retraction," to mean that it occurs along a limited part of the cell margin (4, 39, 42; reviewed in 63). The recent proposal that the gaps are artefacts created by the carbon black or other injected material and that the leakage occurs *through* the endothelial cells (17) goes against a mountain of evidence and is based, in our opinion, on artefacts).

Important new bits of information have been added to the "endothelial gap" story. Thrombin, for example, which causes blood to clot, also increases vascular permeability in a histamine-type fashion; it does so by disassembling the intercellular junctions of the *adhaerens* type (63), which are built like a zipper (15). Scanning electron microscopy has overwhelmingly confirmed that the gaps develop *between* cells. It has also shown that the gaps are complex structures, bridged by long, thread-like cellular projections that may help to close the gap (Figure 10.20) (52).

(3) Leakage by Angiogenesis

Angiogenesis can occur in two patterns: *by sprouting,* whereby new vessels grow out of existing ones, and *by remodeling,* when preexisting vessels enlarge.

Leakage from capillary sprouts. This modality is self-explanatory, and typical of wound healing. When new

FIGURE 10.19 *Top:* Venule in the abdominal muscle of a guinea pig, 11 minutes after an intradermal injection of LTE$_4$ and an intravenous injection of carbon black. Endothelial contraction has caused the cells to become thicker and the nuclear membranes to fold. Between the endothelial cells is a gap filled with carbon particles. **Arrow:** Basement membrane. Note the packed red blood cells in the lumen, a consequence of plasma loss. *Bottom:* Wall of a normal venule in the abdominal muscle of a guinea pig. **Bars** = 1 μm. (Reproduced with permission from [35], © American Society for Investigative Pathology.)

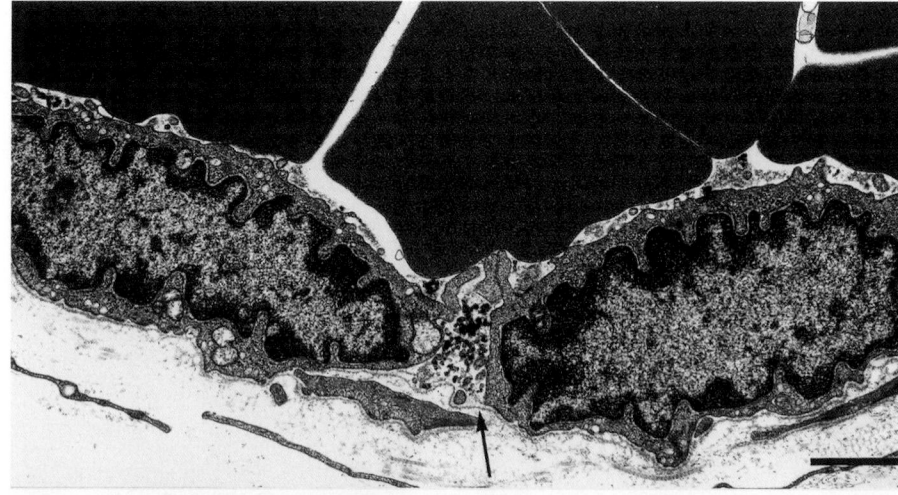

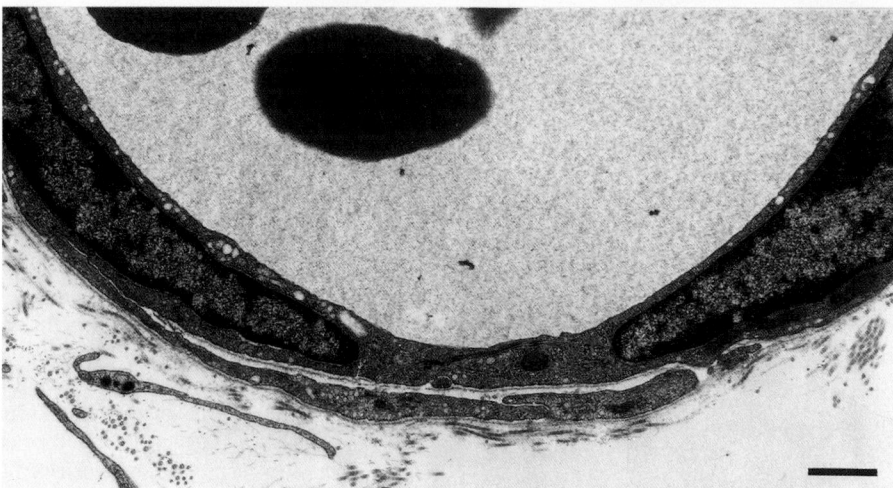

capillaries sprout from existing vessels (usually venules), at first their wall is loosely built, and they leak: fluid and even some red blood cells seep out (see Figure 13.7).

Capillary leakage by vascular remodeling. We stumbled upon this interesting phenomenon by reasoning as follows. Virtually all experiments on permeability-increasing mediators had focussed on the immediate effect of a single mediator, as pure as possible, injected into the skin—an experimentally clean but quite unnatural situation. What type of leakage would occur in a "dirty" but natural situation, e.g., when a mass of tissue dies, as in an infarct? The surrounding normal tissue is exposed to a highly impure mixture of mediators and breakdown products that has never even been analyzed. So we devised an experimental "pseudo-infarct": we slipped a piece of rat liver into a cremasteric pouch of another rat and watched what happened in the overlying cremaster muscle. When we injected carbon black intravenously after 3 hours, we found

what we expected: some venular labeling. But after 18–48 hours, the labeling was largely capillary (Figure 10.21): the tight pattern of parallel vessels (running along the muscle fibers) contrasted sharply with the tree-shaped venules that we had been accustomed to see with histamine-type mediators. After that time the labeling ceased abruptly.

This capillary leakage was mystifying, because no known mediator was capable of producing so specific a pattern. On electron micrographs the capillary endothelium looked plump and "activated," with no evidence of contraction; many junctions appeared to be loose and leaky; mitoses were common. Overall, these features recalled the capillaries of granulation tissue.

Our interpretation: in this inflamed muscle the microcirculation is undergoing a rearrangement; *the capillaries are enlarging to venules* due to the persisting inflammatory hyperemia (33), and in the process, for 1 or 2 days, they are leaky. A similar shift of capillaries to venules in an inflamed mucosa was described

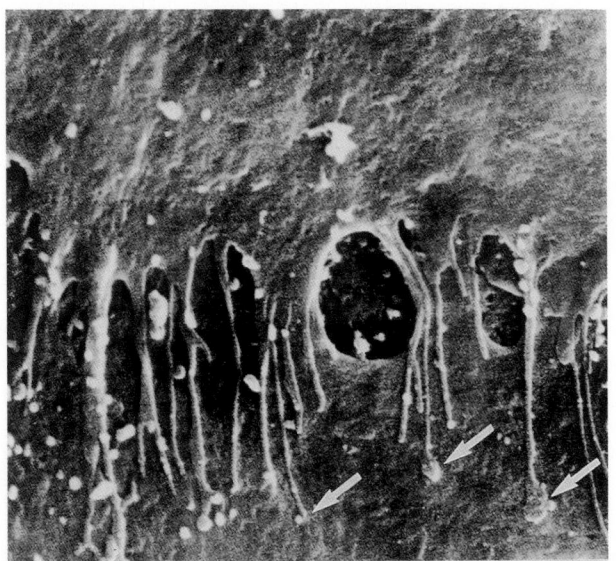

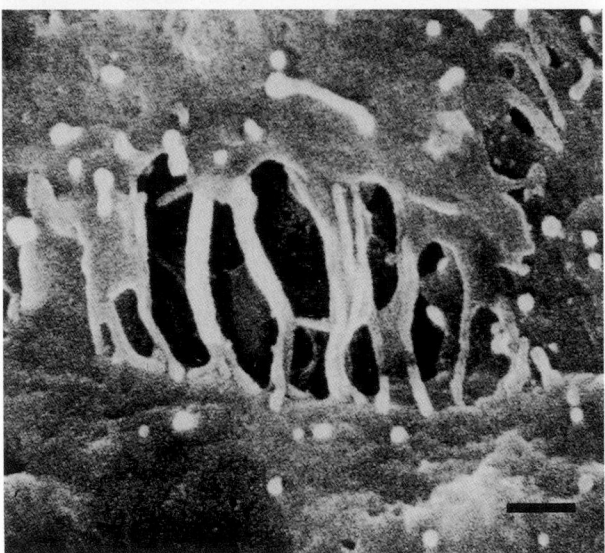

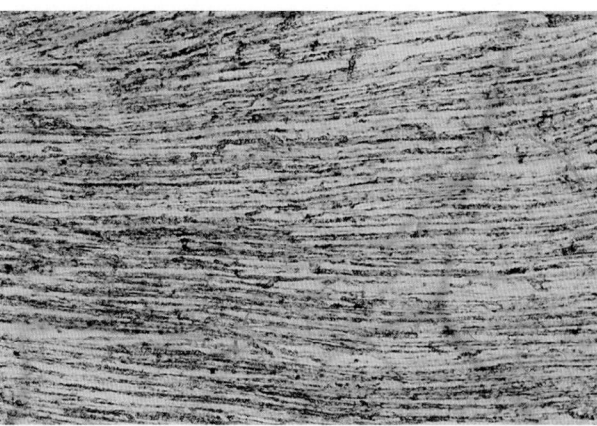

FIGURE 10.21 Capillary leakage in aseptic inflammation: cremaster muscle of a rat, 48-hour stage. The leaky vessels, labeled with carbon black, form a pattern of parallel lines: in striated muscles the capillaries run primarily along the muscle fibers, hence this parallel pattern indicates capillary leakage. (10x)

they go in and out of the brain without a significant disruption of the blood-brain barrier (67).

LEUKOCYTES can also damage the endothelium, in another manner, namely by means of their secretions, when ischemic tissues are reperfused (p. 711, ischemia-reperfusion syndrome).

Many CYTOKINES affect the endothelium (13, 14, 61, 62, 64, 70) but not in the straightforward manner of the histamine-type mediators: cytokines, as the reader may recall, are multifunctional, they tend to generate "cascades" of other cytokines, they may reverse their effects at different concentrations, they can act in an autocrine or endocrine manner, and their effects are so redundant that they are difficult to inhibit. As regards vascular leakage, their most notorious misdeed is the *capillary leak syndrome* due to the intravenous administration of interleukin 2 for immunotherapy (p. 916).

Questions Raised by Vascular Leakage

Many years of teaching tell us that the following topics need to be addressed.

(1) In Ordinary Histologic Sections, without the Help of Vascular Labeling, How Can Vascular Leakage Be Recognized?

When we look for leaky vessels in a microscopic section of acutely inflamed tissue, we are not much better off than Cohnheim because the endothelial gaps are usually very small, of the order of one micrometer. However, anyone can diagnose increased permeability

FIGURE 10.20 Venule of a rat trachea 1 minute after an intravenous injection of substance P (a histamine-type vasoactive mediator). Scanning electron microscopy. Intercellular endothelial gaps have formed (mean diameter, 0.36–0.47 μm). Two gaps are shown; finger-like cell processes (**white arrows**) partition each opening. **Bar** = 1 μm. (Reproduced with permission from [52].)

by Thurston et al. (72). In essence, this is a form of "adaptive angiogenesis."

(4) Sundry Mechanisms of Vascular Leakage

DIAPEDESIS tops this list but only marginally: although in some experimental models emigrating leukocytes cause a modest amount of leakage (41), the overall message is rather in the opposite direction: the leukocytes manage to sneak across the endothelium without turning it into a sieve (p. 410). Even normally

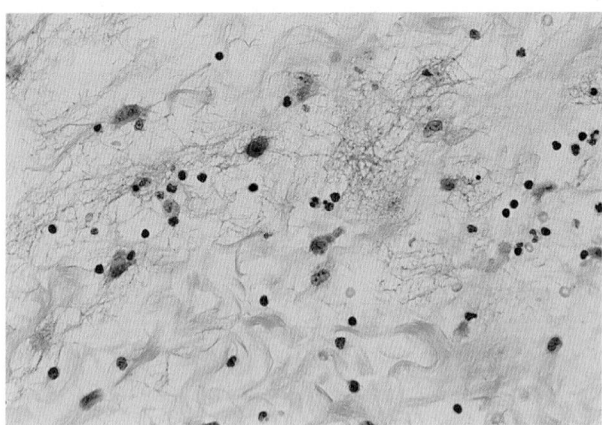

FIGURE 10.22 Deposition of fibrin in acutely inflamed, edematous tissue. There are many ways to distinguish fibrin from collagen, but in a section stained with hematoxylin and eosin it can be difficult. The pattern helps: collagen fibers are wavy and do not branch (*bottom right*). A typical cluster of fibrin is shown at right of center.

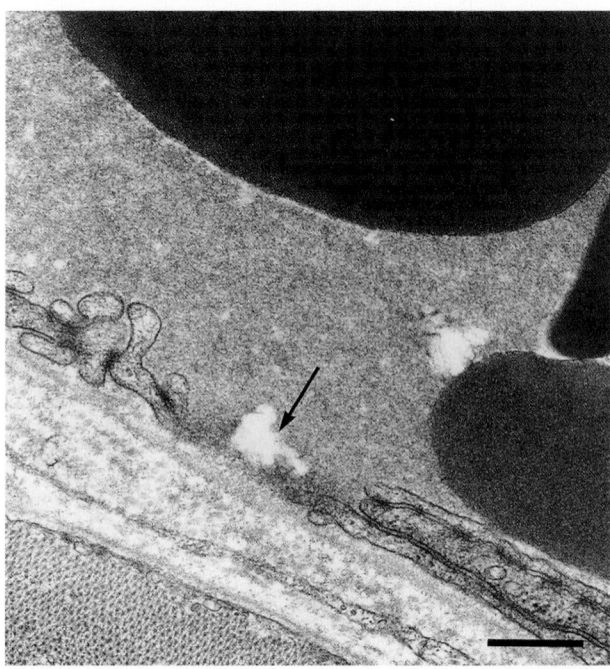

FIGURE 10.23 "Natural" vascular labeling in a hyperlipidemic man. Part of a venule from a biopsy of striated muscle. **Arrow:** a chylomicron, which lies against the basement membrane in a gap between two endothelial cells. **Bar** = 0.5 μm.

indirectly, on purely morphologic grounds. One good lead is **edema,** the presence of excess fluid in the tissue spaces: edema is not always inflammatory, but *if it is accompanied by inflammatory cells* it is likely to reflect inflammatory vascular leakage. Another hint is the presence of **fibrin** filaments in the extracellular spaces (Figure 10.22). Fibrin is a polymer of fibrinogen, a rod-shaped molecule about 460 Å long that cannot escape in bulk unless the endothelium is leaky. In other words, the presence of fibrin means that the building block, fibrinogen, must have escaped from leaky blood vessels. And so, if enough fibrin has formed, the diagnosis of leaky vessels can be made indirectly with the naked eye.

(2) Does Normal Plasma Contain Particles that Can Be Retained by the Vascular Basement Membrane?

Vessels develop leaks all the time, in bruises and insect bites, and are labeled in a natural way by natural "marker particles" that exist in the bloodstream—namely, chylomicrons and the larger lipoproteins. Wherever there is an endothelial gap, the basement membrane retains these particles and the blood vessel remains labeled with lipid (45). We once had the opportunity to demonstrate that a cup of heavy cream (with chocolate) produces in an adult human, after 4 hours, enough chylomicrons to label leaky vessels (Figure 10.23). Platelets, of course, tend to plug any leak (p. 632).

> This mechanism does not explain the accumulation of lipid in arteries in atherosclerosis. In this disease lipoproteins

are actively picked up by the endothelium and transferred into the wall of the artery; gaps do not seem to play an important role (p. 674).

We should recall here that *circulating bacteria tend to localize in inflamed tissues.* This is an old observation (20, 53); the mechanism is probably the same as that of vascular labeling: bacteria become trapped in the wall of leaky vessels. This principle can be extended to explain the development of bone infection (osteomyelitis) in the metaphyses of growing children: an electron microscopic study of the metaphyses in growing rats has shown that the capillaries in this zone are riddled with large gaps, through which even red blood cells can escape; carbon black injected intravenously produces a grossly visible black band of labeling in this area (22). We will see later that injured tissues tend to retain also circulating cancer cells (p. 822).

(3) What Happens to Labeled Vessels?

If the label is indigestible (like carbon black), the vessel is essentially tattooed and will remain so for life (9). The particles piled up against the basement membrane are slowly taken up by the endothelium and pericytes; a few seep out and are caught by the tissue macrophages.

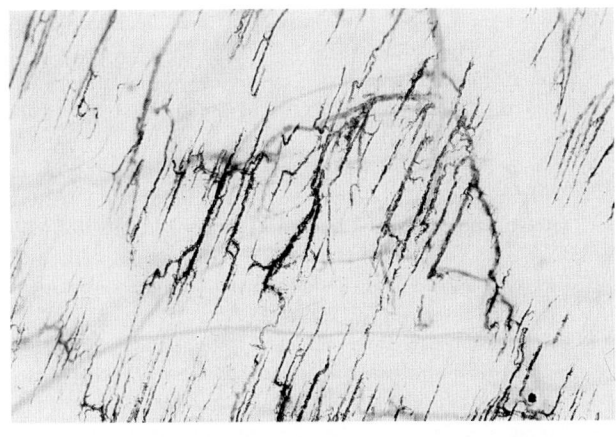

FIGURE 10.24 "Double labeling" with black and blue, to demonstrate that challenging the same site with histamine, 24 hours apart, causes the same venules to leak. Cremaster muscle; after the first injection of histamine, carbon black was injected intravenously; after the second, Monastral blue was injected intravenously. (~20x)

(4) Are There Any Colored Labeling Particles?

There is a lovely *Monastral blue* (34). It can be used, e.g., for comparing the same lesion at two different times, once with carbon and once with the blue (Figure 10.24). Regretfully this suspension is no longer available.

(5) Is It Possible that Labeling Particles Create Gaps?

Certainly not, because the gaps are identical with or without labeling particles.

This finding has been confirmed many times. A study from one laboratory (17) concluded that colloidal pigments create gaps in tissues injected with histamine. We have no doubt that this conclusion is based on some sort of misunderstanding.

(6) In a Typical Inflamed Lesion—Say, an Infected Wound—How Is Vascular Leakage Maintained?

Over time, leakage is caused or maintained by several mechanisms (Figure 10.25). Physicians must know about them, because they can be opposed by different drugs. To the naked eye—in rats as well as in people—vascular leakage in a given lesion appears to be a continuum; there is no evidence of successive phases. However, to visualize the mechanisms that might be operative at any given time, the following facts should be kept in mind:

- ***Direct injury*** causes leakage that starts immediately and continues until the damaged vessels are repaired or closed. In some infections, a steady release of bacterial products may continue to damage the vessels until the infection is overcome.

- ***Histamine-type mediators*** are released immediately: mast cell histamine at time zero, platelet serotonin shortly thereafter, while PAF and leukotrienes are secreted mainly from leukocyte membranes.

- ***Cytokines*** are discharged at a site of injury almost immediately by platelets, but as regards vascular leakage the most important has to be synthesized locally: it is VEGF, initially called vascular permeability factor (VPF), which has two microvascular functions. It increases the permeability of existing vessels and creates new ones (which are leaky until they are mature). VEGF can be expected to appear on the scene of injury in a matter of hours.

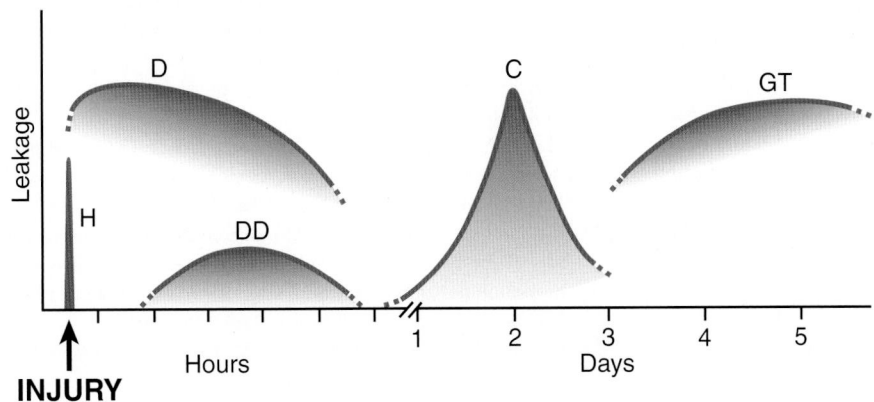

D = Direct injury/immediate
H = Histamine-type (venular)
DD = Direct injury/delayed
C = Capillary leakage
GT = Granulation tissue

FIGURE 10.25 Five mechanisms of vascular leakage, within 5 days of injury. **H** = A burst of histamine-type leakage, occurring immediately after most types of injury. **D** = Direct injury, severe. **DD** = Direct injury, mild, with a delayed effect (typical of the sunburn). **C** = Capillary leakage (e.g., around infarcts) due to capillary remodeling and possibly to cytokines. **GT** = Leakage from granulation tissue (due to regenerating capillary sprouts, and probably to VEGF and other cytokines.)

- **_Vasodilatation by prostaglandins_** increases blood flow and therefore tends to exaggerate vascular leakage due to any mechanism.
- **_Leaky regenerating vessels_** contribute their share of leakage in chronic inflammation.

(7) Is Any Factor Involved in Modulating Vascular Leakage, Besides Tissue Pressure?

An important limiting factor is BLOOD FLOW. The perfusion of tissues with blood can drop to very low levels in the state of **shock** (which is actually defined as a state of "generalized hypoperfusion"). Under such conditions, vascular leakage—and inflammation altogether—are greatly reduced. _In the skin of a rat in shock, the phenomenon of vascular labeling cannot be demonstrated._ Correspondingly, in a patient in shock, infection is more likely to occur because inflammation cannot run its natural course.

> **TO SUM UP:** This chapter is centered on problems of vascular permeability, a classic meeting ground for morphology, physiology, pharmacology, and cell biology. The basic contributions, we believe, were made by the electron microscope, because _it can translate physiologic problems into tangible morphology._ Cell bioogy of endothelial cultures has also been invaluable, by giving us a relatively pure model of the blood-tissue barrier—the ancestral barrier between the body and the sea.

References

NOTE: For this and other chapters on inflammation, an extensive bibliography can be found in Gallin JI, Snyderman R. Inflammation: Basic principles and clinical correlates, 3rd ed. Philadelphia: Lippincott Williams & Wilkins. 1999.

1. Andriopoulou P, Navarro P, Zanetti A, Lampugnani MG, Dejana E. Histamine induces tyrosine phosphorylation of endothelial cell-to-cell adherens junctions. Arterioscler Thromb Vasc Biol 1999;19:2286–2297.
2. Barnes PJ. Asthma as an axon reflex. Lancet 1986;1:242–245.
3. Berhard, JD (ed.), Itch: Mechanisms and management of pruritus. McGraw-Hill, Inc. 1994.
4. Boswell CA, Joris I, Majno G. The concept of cellular tone: reflections on the endothelium, fibroblasts and smooth muscle cells. Perspect Biol Med 1992.
5. Burnstock G. Autonomic neuroeffector junctions—reflex vasodilatation of the skin. J Invest Dermatol 1977;69:47–57.
6. Cohnheim J. Über Éntuzündung und Eiterung. Virchows Arch Pathol Ana Physiol Klin Med 1867;40:1–79.
7. Cohnheim J. Neue Úntersuchungen über die Entzündung. Berlin: A. Hirschwald, 1873.
8. Cohnheim J. Lectures on general pathology, vol. 1 (translated from the 2nd German edition). London: New Sydenham Society, 1889, pp. 248.
9. Cotran RS. The delayed and prolonged vascular leakage in inflammation. II. An electron microscopic study of the vascular response after thermal injury. Am J Pathol 1965;46:589–620.
10. Cotran RS. Studies on inflammation. Ultrastructure of the prolonged vascular response induced by Clostridium oedematiens toxin. Lab Invest 1967a;17:39–60.
11. Cotran RS. Delayed and prolonged vascular leakage in inflammation. III. Immediate and delayed vascular reactions in skeletal muscle. Exp Mol Pathol 1967b;6:143–155.
12. Cotran RS, Majno G. The delayed and prolonged vascular leakage in inflammation. I. Topography of the leaking vessels after thermal injury. Am J Pathol 1964;45:261–281.
13. Cotran RS, Pober JS. Effects of cytokines on vascular endothelium: their role in vascular and immune injury. Kidney Int 1989;35:969–975.
14. Cotran RS, Pober JS, Gimbrone MA Jr, et al. Endothelial activation during interleukin 2 immunotherapy: a possible mechanism for the vascular leak syndrome. J Immunol 1987;139:1883–1888.
15. Dejana E, DelMaschio A. Molecular organization and functional regulation of cell to cell junctions in the endothelium. Thromb Haemost 1995;74:309–312.
16. Denman T. A review of pruritis. J Am Acad Dermatol 1986 14:375–392.
17. Feng BD, Nagy JA, Hipp J, Dvorak HF, Dvorak AM. Vesiculovacuolar organelles and the regulation of venule permeability to macromolecules by vascular permeability factor, histamine, and serotonin. J Exp Med 1996;183:1981–1986.
18. Garcia Leme J. Bradykinin-system. In: Vane JR, Ferreira SH, eds. Inflammation. Berlin: Springer-Verlag, 1978, pp. 464–522.
19. Gawlowski DM, Ritter AB, Duran WN. Reproducibility of microvascular permeability responses to successive topical applications of bradykinin in the hamster cheek pouch. Microvasc Res 1982;24:354–363.
20. Ginsburg I, Gallis HA, Cole R.M, Green I. Group A streptococci: localization in rabbits and Guinea pigs following tissue injury. Science 1969;166:1161–1163.
21. Guyton AC. Textbook of medical physiology. 7th edition. Philadelphia: WB Saunders, 1986, pp. 358.
22. Ham KN, Hurley JV, Ryan GB, Storey E. Localization of particulate carbon in metaphyseal vessels of growing rats. Aust J Exp Biol Med Sci 1965;43:625–638.
23. Heltianu C, Simionescu M, Simionescu N. Histamine receptors of the microvascular endothelium revealed in situ with a histamine-ferritin conjugate: characteristic high-affinity binding sites in venules. J Cell Biol 1982;93:357–364.
24. Horan KL, Adamski SW, Ayele W, Langone JJ, Grega GJ. Evidence that prolonged histamine suffusions produce transient increases in vascular permeability subsequent to the formation of venular macromolecular leakage sites. Proof of the Majno-Palade hypothesis. Am J Pathol 1986;123:570–576.

25. Humphrey DM, McManus LM, Satouchi K, Hanahan DJ, Pinckard RN. Vasoactive properties of acetyl glyceryl ether phosphorylcholine and analogues. Lab Invest 1982;46:422–427.

26. Hurley JV. The sequence of early events. In: Vane JR and Ferreira SH, eds. Inflammation. Berlin: Springer-Verlag, 1978, pp. 26–67.

27. Hurley JV, Ham N, Ryan G.B. The mechanism of the delayed prolonged phase of increased vascular permeability in mild thermal injury in the rat. J Pathol Bacteriol 1967;94:1–12.

28. Hurley JV, Jago MV. Delayed and prolonged vascular leakage in inflammation: the effects of dehydromonocrotaline on blood vessels in the rat cremaster. Pathology 1976;8:7–20.

29. Hurley JV, Ryan GB. A delayed prolonged increase in venular permeability following intrapleural injections in the rat. J Pathol Bacteriol 1967;93:87–99.

30. Hurley JV, Spector WG. Delayed leucocytic emigration after intradermal injections and thermal injury. J Pathol Bacteriol 1961;82:421–429.

31. Hutchison KJ, Johnson BW, Williams HTG, Brown GD. The histamine flare response in diabetes mellitus. Surg Gynecol Obstet 1974;139:566–568.

32. Joris I, Cuénoud HF, Doern G.V, Underwood JM, Majno G. Capillary leakage in inflammation. A study by vascular labeling. Am J Pathol 1990;137:1353–1363.

33. Joris I, Cuénoud HF, Underwood JM, Majno G. Capillary remodeling in acute inflammation: a form of angiogenesis. FASEB J 1994;6:A938.

34. Joris I, DeGirolami U, Wortham K, Majno G. Vascular labelling with Monastral blue B. Stain Technol 1982;57:177–183.

35. Joris I, Majno G, Corey EJ, Lewis RA. The mechanism of vascular leakage induced by leukotriene E_4. Endothelial contraction. Am J Pathol 1987;126:19–24.

36. Joris I, Majno G, Ryan GB. Endothelial contraction *in vivo:* a study of the rat mesentery. Virchows Arch Abt B Zellpath 1972;12:73–83.

37. Judah JD, Willoughby DA. A quantitative method for the study of capillary permeability: extraction and determination of Trypan blue in tissues. J Pathol Bacteriol 1962;83:567–572.

38. Kessler JO, Jarvik LF, Fu TK, Matsuyama SS. Thermotaxis, chemotaxis and age. Age 1979;2:5–11.

39. Killackey JJF, Johnston MG, Movat HZ. Increased permeability of microcarrier-cultured endothelial monolayers in response to histamine and thrombin. Am J Pathol 1986;122:50–61.

40. Kopaniak MM, Hay JB, Movat HZ. The effect of hyperemia on vascular permeability. Microvasc Res 1978;15:77–82.

41. Kubes P, Grisham MB, Barrowman JA, Gaginella T, Granger DN. Leukocyte-induced vascular protein leakage in cat mesentery. Am J Physiol 1991;261:H1872–H1879.

42. Laposata M, Dovnarsky DK, Shin HS. Thrombin-induced gap formation in confluent endothelial cell monolayers *in vitro.* Blood 1983;62:549–556.

43. Lewis PA. The distribution of Trypan-red to the tissues and vessels of the eye as influenced by congestion and early inflammation. J Exp Med 1916;23:669–676.

44. Lewis T. The blood vessels of the human skin and their responses. London: Shaw & Sons, 1927.

45. Majno G. Mechanisms of abnormal vascular permeability in acute inflammation. In: Thomas L, Uhr JW, Grant L, eds. Injury, inflammation and immunity. Baltimore: Williams & Wilkins, 1964, pp. 58–93.

46. Majno G. The healing hand. Man and wound in the ancient world. Cambridge: Harvard University Press, 1975.

47. Majno G. Historical events in Pathology: the glass knife. Am J Pathol 1978;92:226.

48. Majno G, Palade GE. Studies on inflammation. I. The effect of histamine and serotonin on vascular permeability: an electron microscopic study. J Biophys Biochem Cytol 1961;11:571–605.

49. Majno G, Palade GE, Schoefl GI. Studies on inflammation. II. The site of action of histamine and serotonin along the vascular tree: a topographic study. J Biophys. Biochem Cytol 1961;11:607–626.

50. Majno G, Shea SM, Leventhal M. Endothelial contraction induced by histamine-type mediators. An electron microscopic study. J Cell Biol 1969;42:647–672.

50a. McCarty DJ. Short-term drug control of crystal-induced inflammation. In: Vane JR, Ferreira SH, eds. Anti-inflammatory drugs, Handbook of Experimental Pharmacology, vol. 50/II. Berlin: Springer-Verlag, 1979, pp. 92–107.

51. McClellan RH, Goodpasture EW. A method of demonstrating experimental gross lesions of the central nervous system. J Med Res 1923;44:201–206.

52. McDonald DM, Thurston G, Baluk P. Endothelial gaps as sites for plasma leakage in inflammation. Microcirculation 1999;6:7–22.

53. Menkin V. Studies on inflammation. VII. Fixation of bacteria and of particulate matter at the site of inflammation. J Exp Med 1931;53:647–660.

54. Michel CC, Curry FE. Microvascular permeability. Physiol Rev 1999;79:703–16.

55. Miller FN, Sims DE. Contractile elements in the regulation of macromolecular permeability. Fed Proc 1986;45:84–88.

56. Moncada S, Ferreira SH, Vane JR. Pain and inflammatory mediators. In: Vane JR, Ferreira SH, eds. Inflammation. Berlin: Springer-Verlag, 1978, pp. 588–616.

57. Movat H.Z. The kinin system and its relation to other systems. Curr Top Pathol 1979;68:111–134.

58. Movat HZ, Cybulsky MI, Colditz IG, William Chan MK, Minarello CA. Acute inflammation in Gram-negative infection: endotoxin interleukin 1, tumor necrosis factor, and neutrophils. FASEB 1987;46:97–104.

59. Orlidge A, D'Amore PA. Inhibition of capillary endothelial cell growth by pericytes and smooth muscle cells. J Cell Biol 1987;105:1455–1462.

60. Palade GE, Predescu D, Predescu S, Stan RV. Malpighi's heritage three centuries later. In: Motta PM (ed). Recent advances in microscopy of cells, tissues and organs. Rome: Antonio Delfino Editore, 1997, pp. 9–19.

61. Pober JS, Cotran RS. Cytokines and endothelial cell biology. Physiol Rev 1990;70:427–451.

62. Pober JS, Cotran RS. The role of endothelial cells in inflammation. Transplantation 1990;50:537–544.

63. Rabiet M-J, Plantier J-L, Rival Y, et al. Thrombin-induced increase in endothelial permeability is associated with changes in cell-to-cell junction organization. Arterioscler Thromb Vasc Biol 1996;16:488–496.

64. Roberts WG, Palade GE. Increased microvascular permeability and endothelial fenestration induced by vascular endothelial growth factor. J Cell Sci 1995;108:2369–2379.

65. Ryan GB, Majno G. Inflammation. A SCOPE monograph. Kalamazoo, Mich.: Upjohn, 1977.

66. Sevitt S. Early and delayed oedema and increase in capillary permeability after burns of the skin. J Pathol Bacteriol 1958; 75:27–37.

67. Silverstein RL. The vascular endothelium. In: Gallin JI, Snyderman R (eds). Inflammation: Basic principles and clinical correlates, 3rd ed. Philadelphia: Lippincott Williams & Wilkins, 1999, pp. 207–225.

68. Spector WG. Substances which affect capillary permeability. Pharmacol Rev 1958;10:475–505.

69. Steele RH, Wilhelm DL. The inflammatory reaction in chemical injury. III. Leucocytosis and other histological changes induced by superficial injury. Br J Exp Pathol 1970;51: 265–279.

70. Stolpen AH, Guinan EC, Fiers W, Pober JS. Recombinant tumor necrosis factor and immune interferon act singly and in combination to reorganize human vascular endothelial cell monolayers. Am J Pathol 1986;123:16–24.

71. Sundy JS, Patel DD, Haynes BF. Cytokines in normal and pathogenic inflammatory responses. In: Gallin JI, Snyderman R (eds). Inflammation: Basic principles and clinical correlates, 3rd ed. Philadelphia: Lippincott Williams & Wilkins, 1999, pp. 433–441.

72. Thurston G, Murphy TJ, Baluk P, Lindsey JR, McDonald DM. Angiogenesis in mice with chronic airway. Strain-dependent Differences. Am J Pathol 1998;153:1099–1112.

73. Wasi S, Movat HZ. Phlogistic substances in neutrophil leukocyte lyosomes: their possible role *in vivo* and their *in vitro* properties. Curr Top Pathol 1979;68:213–237.

74. Wells F.R, Miles A.A. Site of the vascular response to thermal injury. Nature, 200:1015–1016, 1963.

75. Westerman RA, Magerl FW, Szolcsanyi J, et al. Vasodilator axon reflexes. In: Vanhoutte, PM, ed. Vasodilatation. New York: Raven Press, 1988:107–112.

76. Wilhelm DL. Chemical mediators. In: Zweifach BW, Grant L, McCluskey RT, eds. The inflammatory process, vol. II, 2nd ed. New York: Academic Press, 1973a:251–301.

77. Wilhelm D.L. Mechanisms responsible for increased vascular permeability in acute inflammation. Agents Action 1973b; 3:297–306.

77a. Williams TJ. Factors that affect vessel reactivity and leukocyte emigration. In: Clark, RAF., Henson PM., eds. The molecular and cellular biology of wound repair. New York: Plenum Press, 1988:115–147.

78. Yi Eunhee S, Ulich Thomas R. Endotoxin, interleukin-1, and tumor necrosis factor cause neutrophildependent microvascular leakage in postcapillary venules. Am J Pathol 1992;140: 659–663.

79. Zimmerman KW. Der feinere Bau der Blutcapillaren. Z Anat Entwicklungsgeschichte 1923;69:29–109.

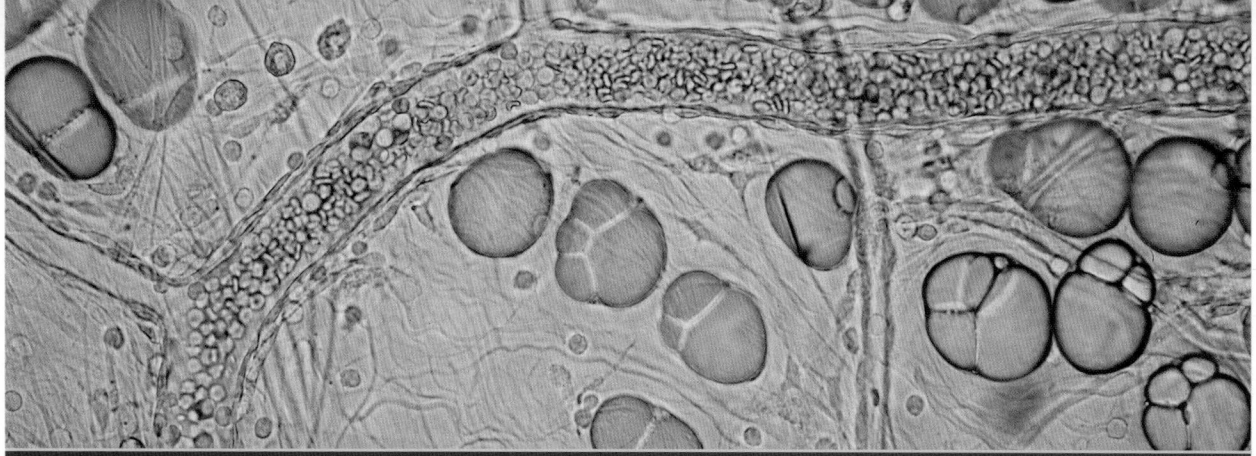

CHAPTER 11

LEUKOCYTES CALLED TO ACTION: STEPS TO PHAGOCYTOSIS

The purpose of inflammation, as we defined it, is to convey fluid and cells to a site of injury. Fluid is delivered first, in a matter of seconds; cells take a little longer (minutes) because they cannot just pour out of the vascular system. Indeed, before a circulating leukocyte can kill a bacterium seeded in a wound, a complex string of events must take place. This sequence, which aims first of all at recruiting leukocytes out of the blood stream, was worked out by some of the most elegant and "simple" experiments in modern biology. The steps—indicated by the subtitles—are not arbitrary: each one can be blocked by inhibitors (82, 83). In real life the whole sequence takes several minutes.

Chemotaxis

We will begin with chemotaxis: its role in diapedesis is crucial.

Biology of Chemotaxis

All free cells, from bacteria (Figure 11.1) and amoebae to spermatozoa and fibroblasts, have the privilege of moving toward a chemical attractant, to pursue food, to escape danger, or even to meet their sexual counterparts; in fact, chemotaxis was discovered by studying the fertilization of ferns. This is but one of many basic discoveries that cell biology owes to botanists; earlier discoveries include the nucleus and the very notion of cell.

It was 1884 when Wilhelm Pfeffer showed that the antherozoids of the male fern, trapped in a fine glass tube, would migrate toward higher concentrations of malic acid (92, 127). Four years later a German ophthamologist, Theodor Leber, followed the lead and began implanting capillary tubes into the corneas or anterior chambers of rabbit eyes. In those days the cornea was a favorite tool for

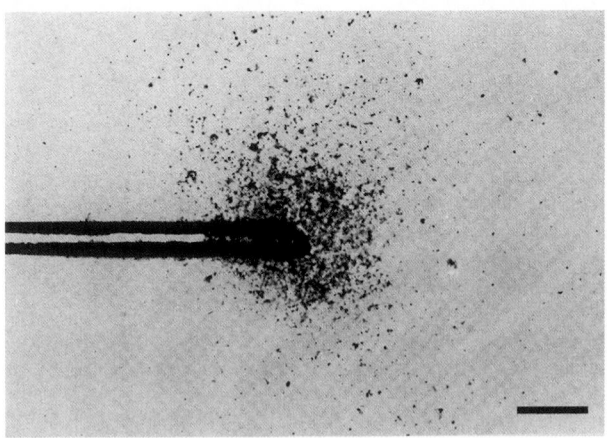

FIGURE 11.1 Photomicrograph showing that *Escherichia coli* are attracted by chemical stimuli. The capillary tube contained aspartate ($2 \leq 10^{-3}$ M). **Bar** = 50 μm. (Reprinted with permission from [95]. Copyright 1969 by the American Association for the Advancement of Science.)

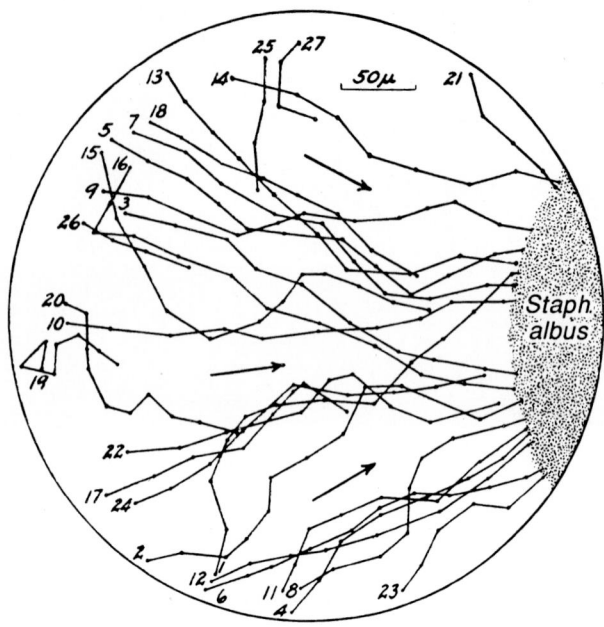

FIGURE 11.2 Microscopic field showing that leukocytes are attracted by a mass of staphylococci. The starting points of 27 leukocytes are indicated by numbers. Most of the cells head directly toward the staphylococci; after 30 minutes 17 had made contact. (Reproduced by permission from [77]. Copyright 1934, American Medical Association.)

experimental pathology: as a transparent tissue, easily excised and studied directly under the microscope, it offered better visibility than the thick tissue slices of the time. Leber found that capillary tubes loaded with bacteria or extracts of putrefying tissues attracted leukocytes, and concluded that chemotaxis was the force drawing leukocytes into an inflammatory focus. Metchnikoff, who had just discovered phagocytosis, promptly incorporated this new phenomenon into his own theory of inflammation (80).

In the 1930s it was clearly shown that some bacteria attract leukocytes (Figure 11.2). Later studies added some numbers: neutrophils moving up a chemotactic gradient crawl at a speed of about 30 μm per minute, almost 2 mm per hour (131) and in a reasonably straight line; monocytes are a little slower (45, 91).

The next major advance came in 1962, when it became possible to study chemotaxis quantitatively thanks to a simple, ingenious Australian device: the **Boyden chamber** (Figure 11.3) (15). This is essentially a small vertical plastic cylinder subdivided into an upper and a lower compartment by a filter; the upper chamber is filled with a suspension of leukocytes, the lower with the chemotactic solution to be tested. After 30 minutes at 37°C the filter is removed and examined microscopically: the number of leukocytes that can be counted, either in the thickness of the filter as seen in cross sections or on the lower surface, gives a measure of the chemotactic response (Figure 11.4).

To use the Boyden chamber properly it is essential to distinguish between chemotaxis and **chemokinesis.** The latter is simply accelerated motion of cells, without any directional preference in response to a chemical stimulus. It can mimic chemotaxis. Suppose that some chemical accelerated the random leukocyte motion in the neighborhood of a leukocyte "trap" such as a porous surface. More leukocytes would end up being trapped simply because they moved around faster, even though the porous surface exerted no attraction. The accepted control for this possible artefact when using the Boyden chamber is to mix the chemotaxin with the leukocytes in the upper chamber and count how many cells become trapped in the filter by accelerated random motion. This procedure shows that many chemotaxins are also chemokinetic; after all, chemokinesis could also be beneficial in a focus of inflammation.

In Chapter 9 we listed the many sources of chemotaxins, which are responsible for bringing leukocytes and invaders face to face. Now try to imagine a duel between a neutrophil and a flagellated bacterium (the two, of course, cannot see, but they do smell each other). The bacterium has several advantages: it can swim, and in so doing it can also choose to swim

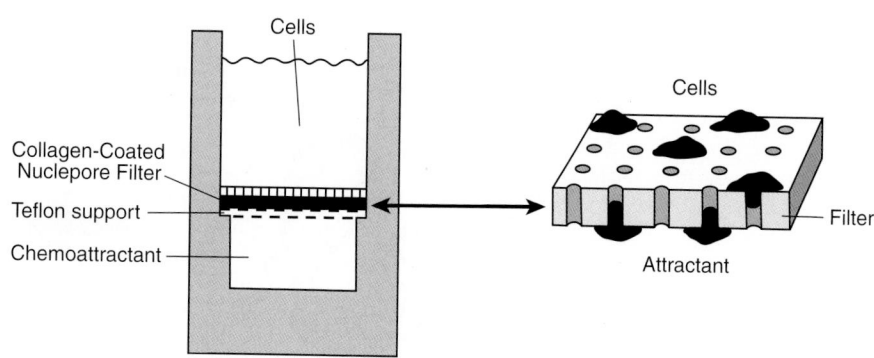

FIGURE 11.3 Diagram of the Boyden chamber (*left*) showing two compartments separated by a porous filter (*right*). Migrating cells cross the filter and appear on the underside; they can be quantitated by several methods. (Reproduced from [42] by permission of S. Karger AG, Basel.)

toward a good thing, such as sugar or amino acids (3, 79), or *away* from the threat of a disinfectant, like phenol (1, 63, 120) or from the breath of a panting, activated leukocyte (117). This is **negative chemotaxis.**

Oddly enough, very little is known about negative chemotaxis in the world of cells (other that bacterial). We did mention in Chapter 2 that the growth cones of nerves are guided by semaphorins by positive and negative

chemotaxis; leukocytes were not known to run away from anything, but subsets of human T cells are repelled by high concentrations of a chemokine (94a).

How do cells respond to directional clues? Overall, there are three options. A highly motile cell might be able to compare concentrations at two points in time, in quick succession, which would require some sort of memory (*temporal mechanism*). Flagellated bacteria, for example, swim in a zigzag fashion: short runs interrupted by "tumbles," at which point they change direction randomly (the tumble is brought about by changing the beat of the flagellum to clockwise (Figure 11.5) [61]). When submitted to a chemical

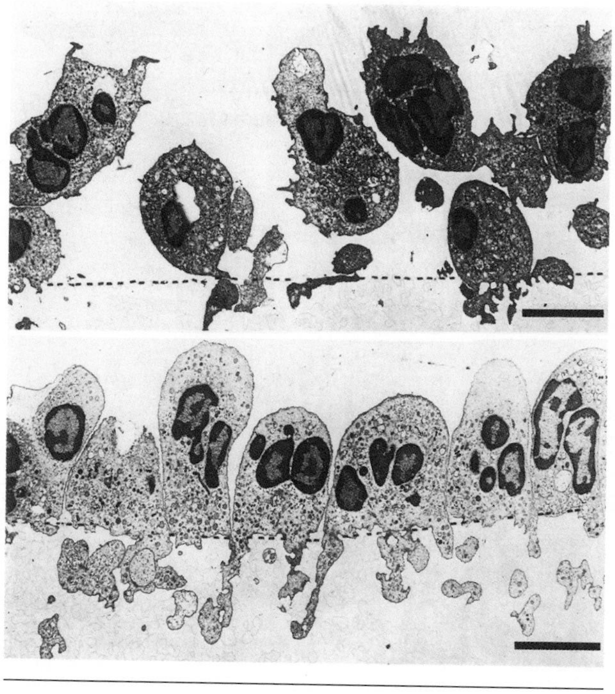

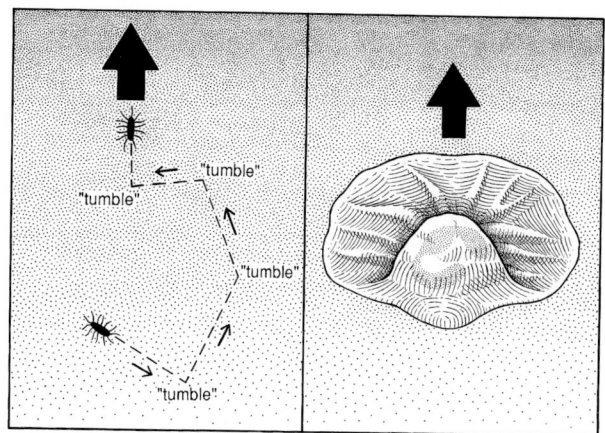

FIGURE 11.4   Behavior of neutrophils on a 0.45 μm pore filter in the Boyden chamber. The surface of the filter is indicated by a dotted line. *Top:* Condition of "activated random migration." A chemotactic agent is present on both sides of the filter in equal concentrations. *Bottom:* The chemotactic agent is present only below the filter. **Bars** = 5 μm. (Reproduced from the **Journal of Cell Biology,** 1977;75:666–693, by copyright permission of The Rockefeller University Press [71].)

FIGURE 11.5   Mechanisms of chemotaxis. *Left:* Motile bacteria move about by short, seemingly random "darts" interrupted by "tumbles". They advance along a gradient by prolonging the darts in the favorable direction, as if they had a memory of the concentration from which they have last moved. *Right:* Leukocytes can obey a chemotactic call only when attached to a surface. This leukocyte can be visualized either as crawling up a concentration gradient sensed in a solute along its length, or as crawling by haptotaxis toward an area of greater stickiness.

FIGURE 11.6 Illustrating how receptors, stored on the inner surface of leukocytes granules, can be transferred to the surface of the cell and increase its responsiveness to a chemotactic stimulus such as the bacterial peptide fMLP. (Reproduced by permission from [37a]. Copyright 1988 by Raven Press Ltd.)

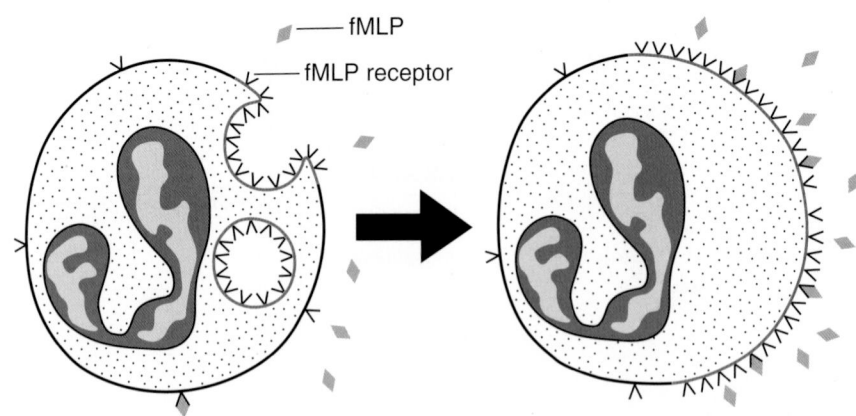

FIGURE 11.7 Under normal and near-normal conditions, leukocytes emerging from capillaries are pushed toward the walls of the venules. Here are three of the four known mechanisms. *Top:* In the smallest venules the red blood cells flow faster than the leukocytes, overtake them, and in so doing push them toward the wall. *Center:* Leukocytes reaching a venule from a tributary capillary are swept along the wall of the venule by laminar flow. *Bottom:* In conditions of low flow, red blood cells tend to aggregate into rouleaux, and these larger structures tend to occupy the center, displacing the leukocytes toward the periphery.

THREE MECHANISMS CAUSING LEUKOCYTES TO MARGINATE IN THE VENULES

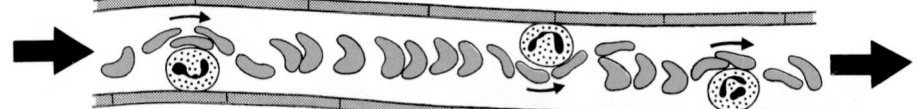

RBCs flow faster than leukocytes, overtake them, push them toward wall

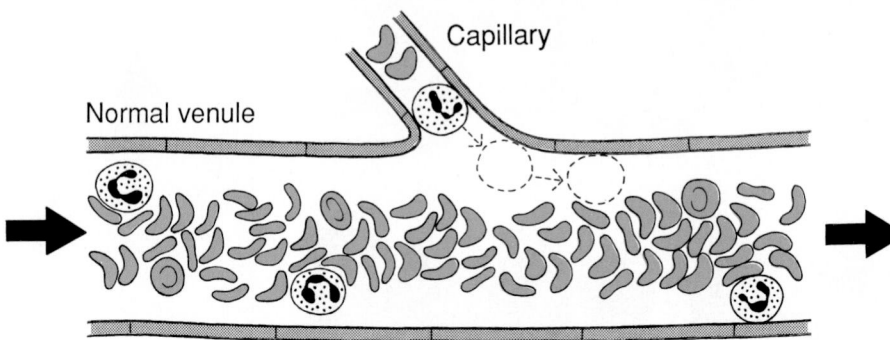

Laminar flow maintains leukocytes against venular wall

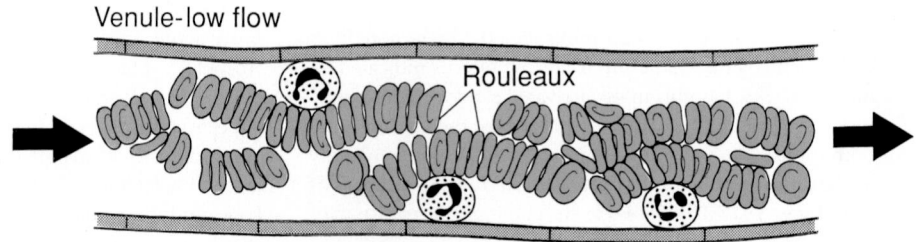

Rouleaux displace leukocytes from axial flow

gradient, creating a choice between a "favorable" and "unfavorable" direction, they continue to swim and tumble in random fashion—but they prolong the straight runs in the favorable direction. The net effect is movement in the favorable direction (63, 69, 120).

As to the leukocytes, it is possible that they use a *spatial mechanism* and compare concentrations along their own body (Figure 11.5) (25, 26), but they are so slow that one wonders how they could keep up with the changes in concentration gradients in the swirling body fluids (124). And so, it has been suggested that *solid gradients* might be the answer: if the molecules of chemotaxins were somehow bound to a substrate, and made it sticky, the roaming leukocyte could feel them and move in the direction of greater stickiness: this is **haptotaxis** (9, 101). The evidence compelling. Many chemokines are positively charged; they could become attached to the negative charges of the proteoglycan molecules both in the connective tissue spaces and on the endothelium (9, 128). In this way the leukocyte would find a solid trail, marked by a carpet of molecules (9).

> Rethinking about the Boyden chamber (p. 404) in this light: if some of the chemotaxins bind to the filter, the result of the test will be a sum of chemotaxis and haptotaxis. In fact, control experiments are needed to separate the two (101).

> There is a **thermotaxis chamber** for studying cell responses to heat gradients: spermatozoa do navigate toward a warmer climate (10a) and leukemic leukocytes lose some of their thermotaxis (130a) but more work is needed.

Chemotaxis and Inflammation

Now, returning to the battlefield of inflammation: how can chemotaxis help in recruiting leukocytes out of the vessels? Even without experiments, we can guess that a chemotactic call reaching a venule (the favorite vessel for diapedesis) would do little to entice a leukocyte directly. By the time a few molecules of chemotaxin reached it, the leukocyte has been washed away. We need a better strategy: rather than trying to call the evasive leukocyte, it would make more sense to work on the endothelium, which cannot run away, and *trap the leukocyte* by activating (i.e., instructing) the endothelium to become sticky. This is what actually happens. Many mediators can activate the endothelium, and after this is done, chemotaxins help by activating also the leukocytes (Figure 11.6). A wonderful stratagem, and even more wonderful if we consider that there are theoretical reasons to anticipate that it should be bound to failure: the laws of blood flow in the microcirculation tell us that the leukocytes—being the largest objects

carried by the blood—should travel in the axis of the bloodstream, where they would be out of reach of the sticky trap (29, 86). But fortunately Nature, who makes the rules, also knows how to break them: in the microcirculation there are at least four arrangements that force some of the leukocytes to travel at the periphery of the stream (Figure 11.7):

- *In the smallest venules, where cells have just emerged from capillaries, special flow conditions prevail.* There the large, spherical leukocytes tend to advance more slowly than the smaller, disc-shaped red blood cells; as the red blood cells overtake and pass by the leukocytes, they tend to push them to the sides (108).

- *Whenever a capillary feeds into the side of a venule,* like a tributary into a river, *the cells in the capillary blood are swept by laminar flow along the wall of the venule.*

- *In low-flow conditions, red blood cells tend to aggregate and form rouleaux.* Now rouleaux become the largest elements of the blood, so they occupy the center of the stream and push the leukocytes to the side (Figures 11.7, 11.8) (86). If inflammation persists long enough to trigger an increased erythrocyte sedimentation rate (p. 506), the tendency to form rouleaux is much increased.

- *As wall shear stress decreases* (as should happen in the venules), models show that *the leukocytes tend to move away from the center and toward the periphery* (86).

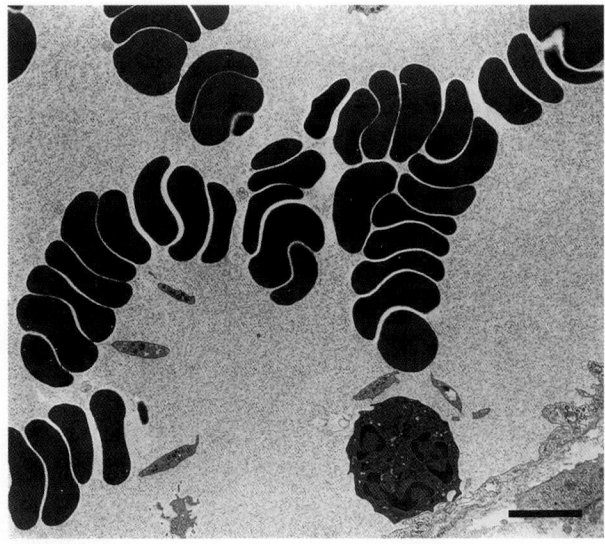

FIGURE 11.8 Typical rouleaux of red blood cells in a venule of an acutely inflamed omentum. Note marginating neutrophil. **Bar** = 0.5 μm.

Endothelial Activation, Leukocyte Rolling

In his 1867 study of inflammation in living tissues (p. 311), Cohnheim described what he called *margination:* in the venules, many leukocytes rolled along the endothelium, while others remained stuck to it. A surprise finding of the past 10 years is that these two aspects of margination, now called leukocyte *rolling* and *sticking,* are separate phenomena governed by different adhesion molecules. This was proved *in vitro* by experiments of almost artistic beauty: imagine a suspension of leukocytes being washed, at known shear rates, over a lipid bilayer in which known adhesion molecules are incorporated (65). In this system the role of a given protein can be verified by inactivating it with a specific antibody.

Thanks to this and many other models we can safely state that ROLLING is due to an endothelial change, with no active contribution of the leukocytes. The endothelial cell covers itself with a gentle glue that will bind to the leukocyte just enough to make it roll, not enough to stop it. There must be many variants to this mechanism (depending on species, tissue, cause of inflammation, stage, etc.) but the following sequence is

well proven (59, 82, 83, 89, 128). Since we are dealing with inflammation, i.e., a response to injury, there must be injured tissues nearby, and they must be releasing a whole soup of mediators, including *histamine* from crushed mast cells and *thrombin* from clotted blood, *anaphylatoxins* from complement components, *kinins* from plasma, and many more. All these molecules reach the venules and make them leak, as we described in the previous chapter, but at least two of these mediators (histamine and thrombin) also activate the endothelium. In this context, endothelial activation means that the Weibel-Palade bodies in the endothelial cells make contact with the luminal cell membrane and spread over it the adhesive molecules that they hoard (*P-selectin,* a glycoprotein). As soon as a leukocyte comes along—neutrophil, monocyte, or other—ligands ("sticky sugars") on the surface of the leukocyte bind to the P-selectin spread on the endothelium, and the leukocyte, partially stuck, will begin to roll along the endothelial surface (Figure 11.9) (82, 83, 128). This is the first phase of margination; it may last seconds or minutes.

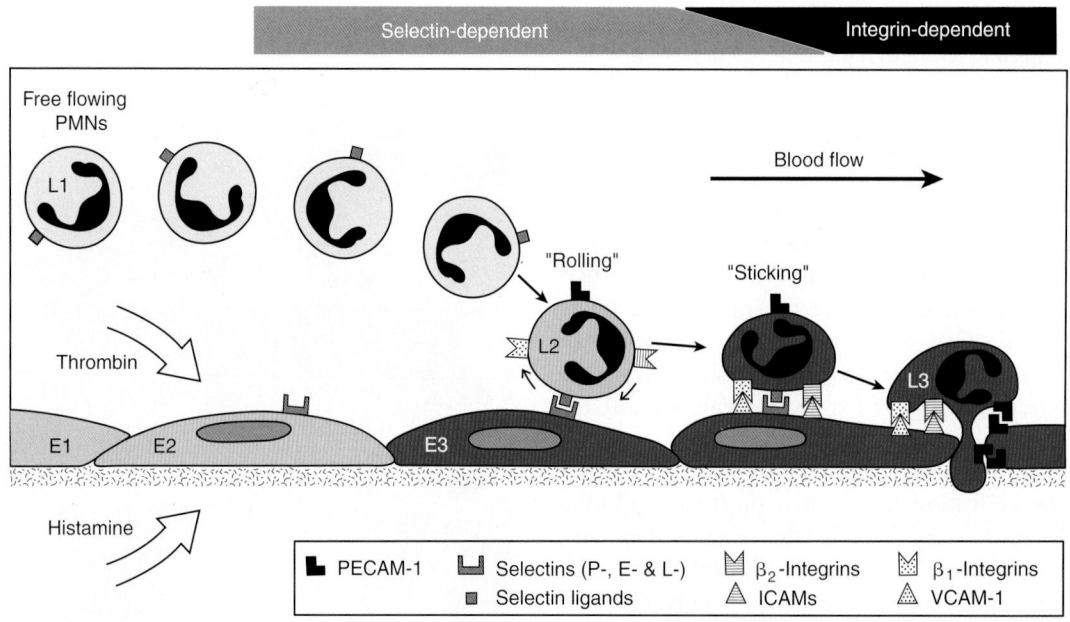

FIGURE 11.9　Mechanisms of leukocyte sticking and diapedesis in a venule. E1 = non-activated endothelial cell. E2, E3 = cells partially/fully activated by intraluminal thrombin and/or by extravascular histamine. L1 = Leukocyte about to be swept toward the wall by flow. L2 = Leukocyte trapped by P-selectin begins to roll. L3 = beginning of diapedesis. NOTE: endothelial gaps induced by histamine/thrombin are not shown. (Adapted with permission from [89].)

Leukocyte Activation and Sticking

Now the leukocyte, partially (and passively) tethered, actively puts on the brakes to come to a full stop. To this end it uses special surface proteins, heterodimers of the *integrin* family (Figure 11.10) (102, 122); they undergo a small change in configuration, which makes them more avid for their endothelial ligand, a protein called ICAM-1 (intercellular adhesion molecule 1, of the *immunoglobulin* family). As soon as the integrins and ICAMS are linked, the leukocyte is firmly anchored—often, and conveniently, just above a junction (82, 83). It appears that fibrinogen may contribute to this phase of margination, by coating the endothelium as well as the leukocytes (114a).

A curious feature of marginating leukocytes is that they also appear to be sticky to eachother, as manifested by their tendency to aggregate and pile up (Figure 11.11) (49). This property may help recruit more leukocytes at a site of diapedesis; it also explains why *agents that activate leukocytes also cause neutropenia when injected intravenously* (44): clumps of leukocytes are retained in the lungs. Activated platelets also aggregate, more understandably, because one of their callings is to build up hemostatic plugs (p. 632). We are reminded of an intriguing phenomenon observed in starfish: clumping of this creature's amoebocytes is a standard reaction to injury (Figure 11.12).

Note the economy and speed of the "sticking" episode: no new proteins need to be synthesized; ligand and counter-ligand are both in place; all that is needed is a small change in shape of the leukocyte ligand. This is what we would expect of an emergency response.

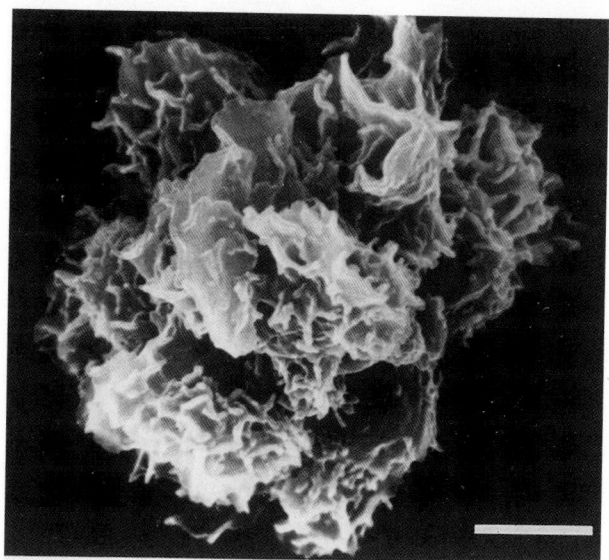

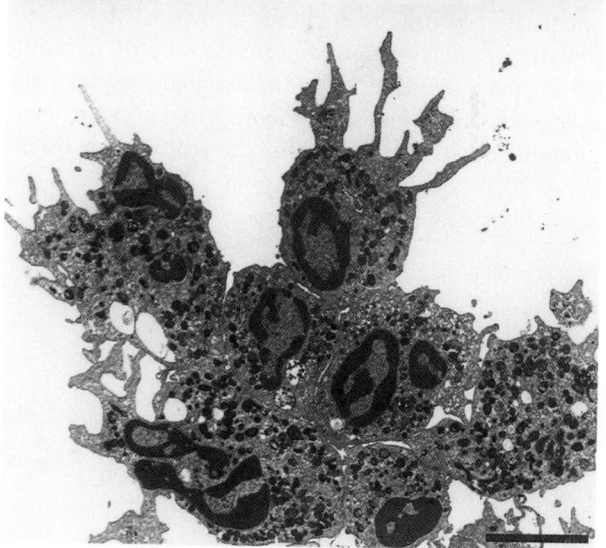

FIGURE 11.11   Activated leukocytes tend to aggregate. These human neutrophils were stimulated with a chemotactic factor (fMLP) and stirred; 1 minute later they were fixed. *Top:* Scanning electron micrograph shows a cluster of aggregated neutrophils with ruffles, evidence of activation. *Bottom:* Transmission electron micrograph of a similar cluster. The ruffles are obvious on the free surfaces. **Bars** = 5 μm. (Reproduced from the **Journal of Cell Biology,** 1982;95:234–241, by copyright permission of The Rockefeller University Press [49].)

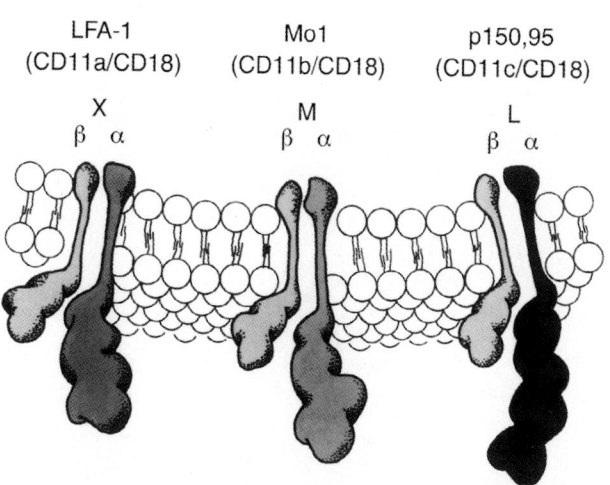

FIGURE 11.10   Schematic representation of the leukocyte adhesion molecules of the CD11/CD18 (integrin) family. Each transmembrane glycoprotein is a heterodimer consisting of a distinctive higher molecular weight α subunit, noncovalently associated with an identical lower molecular weight β subunit. (Adapted from [118] with permission from Springer-Verlag.)

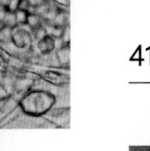

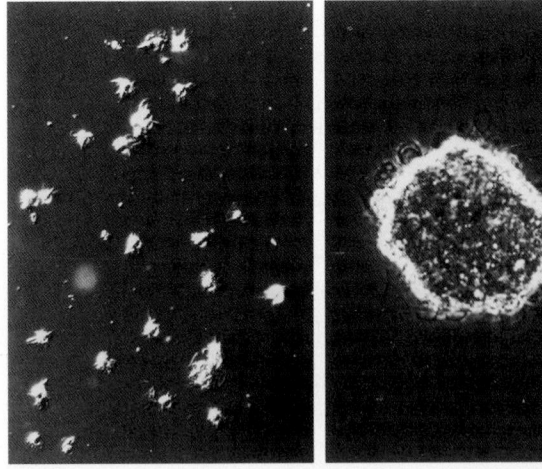

FIGURE 11.12 Cell aggregation as it occurs with amoebocytes from a starfish. *Left:* Dispersed amoebocytes. *Right:* Mass of amoebocytes that have aggregated upon contact with the glass. The phenomenon requires 15–20 minutes. Nomarski optics. (Reproduced with permission from [11].)

How does the leukocyte become activated? As soon as it starts rolling it is brought in closer contact with the endothelial surface, where some very active (and activating) molecules are appearing, especially chemotaxins (*chemotaxis and activation are linked*): interleukin-8 (IL-8), the prototype chemokine, is stored in the Weibel-Palade bodies together with P-selectin and released with it (121); if an additional dose of IL-8 is being supplied from tissue sources, it is transcytosed across the venule and offered to the endothelium (81); the powerful platelet activating factor (PAF) is also being produced at the endothelial surface (62, 133, 134). These mediators activate the rolling leukocyte in such a way that its latent surface "glue," the integrin dimer, is turned on, and locks to its endothelial counterpart. Now the leukocyte, firmly tethered to the endothelial surface, is ready for the critical step.

Diapedesis

No photograph taken through the light microscope can adequately portray diapedesis: a white blood cell, drawn by an ancestral call, sneaks out of a venule through an invisible hole. In histologic sections the event can only be guessed: some leukocytes are marginating, others are lying within the venular wall, others yet are free outside (Figure 11.13). It is no wonder that diapedesis was discovered in living tissues. Electron microscopy, however, succeeds in bringing the event to life: marginating leukocytes are held onto the endothelium by an invisible glue; many are astride a junction and pushing a pseudopod into it (Figure 11.14). The

FIGURE 11.13 A venule in the wall of an acutely inflamed colon. Granulocytes (mainly neutrophils) are recognizable by the 2–3 lobes of the nucleus. Careful study, better with a lens, will show leukocytes in all phases of diapedesis. Leukocytes "free" in the lumen are in reality attached either to other activated and sticky leukocytes, or to filaments of fibrin waving in the current.

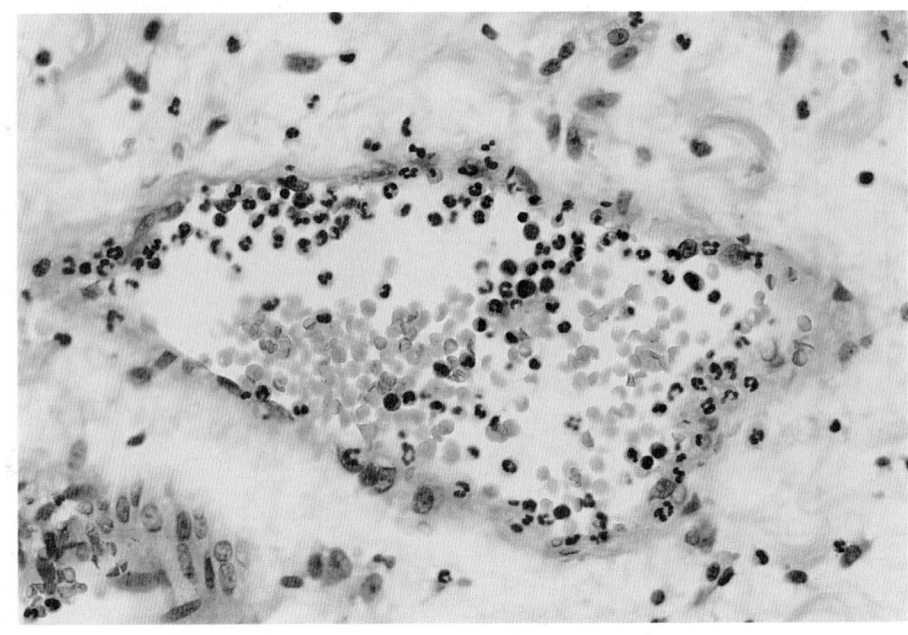

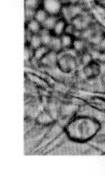

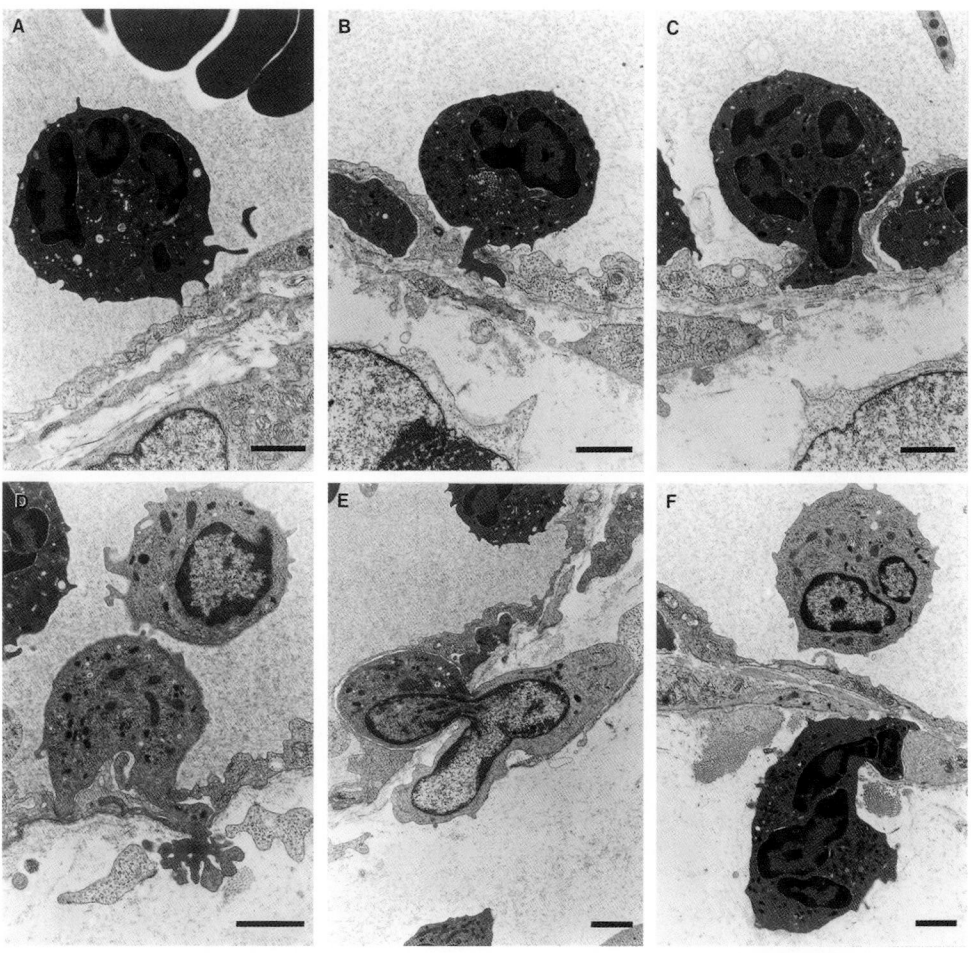

FIGURE 11.14 Margination of a neutrophil (**A**) followed by 5 stages of diapedesis (**B–F**). In **B** and **C** the emigrating neutrophil is temporarily held up by the basement membrane. In **D** and **E** the emigrating cells are monocytes. In **F** the neutrophil has reached the extravascular space. The reason for the high electron density of the neutrophils is not known. From the inflamed omentum of a rat. **Bars** = 2 μm.

first electron micrographs of diapedesis were provided in 1960 by Vincent T. Marchesi, an American medical student working in Oxford with Lord Florey (73, 74). They showed that the leukocyte fits tightly in its narrow passage, so that very little fluid escapes around it, as shown by loading the plasma with visible colloidal particles. Interestingly, the leukocyte appears to be burrowing its own way out, rather than using intercellular gaps previously induced by permeability-increasing mediators. This can be rationalized; these gaps are created for a purpose, i.e., to deliver the fluid portion of the exudate. If they were immediately plugged by leukocytes, this purpose would be defeated.

More recent work has provided further proof that the leukocytes do indeed exit through endothelial junctions (Figure 11.15), and especially at corners where

three cells meet and the junction is discontinuous (18, 19). Furthermore, the endothelial intercellular adhesion protein PECAM-1 (**p**latelet-**e**ndothelial **c**ell **a**dhesion **m**olecule-1) is (almost) essential for diapedesis: antibodies against it reduce diapedesis by 75 percent (82, 83). Few phenomena in biology obey the rules by 100 percent: antibodies against another intercellular protein (JAM [junctional adhesion molecule]) reduce diapedesis only by 50 percent (76). Neutrophils create some disarray in the junctional proteins just by adhering to the endothelium (24). Claims that leukocytes choose to punch their way *through* the endothelial cells (30) conflict with many facts.

Having negotiated the endothelial barrier the leukocyte runs into another obstacle: the basement membrane. Here it usually pauses for a while (30 minutes in

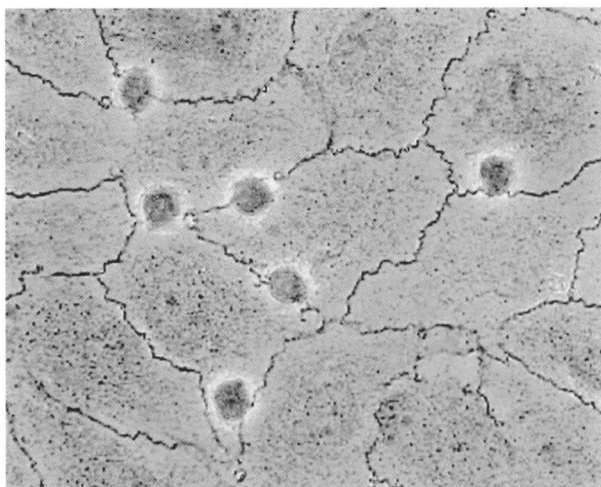

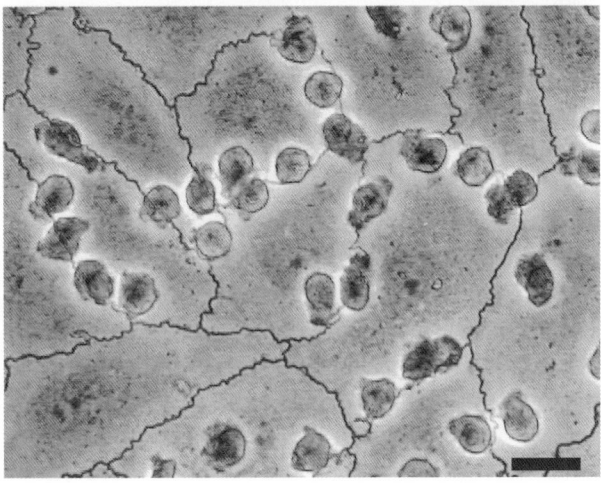

FIGURE 11.15   The tendency of leukocytes to seek interendothelial junctions. Human endothelium and leukocytes, costimulated for 4 minutes with histamine under conditions of flow; poststained with silver nitrate to emphasize the junctions. Over 75 percent of the leukocytes are over a junction (they may be seeking a tricellular corner, where the tight junction is discontinuous). **Bar** = 10 μm. (Reprinted with permission from "P-selectin mediates neutrophil adhesion to endodthelial cell borders," by Burns AR, et al., J. Leukoc. Biol. 65: 299–306,1999)

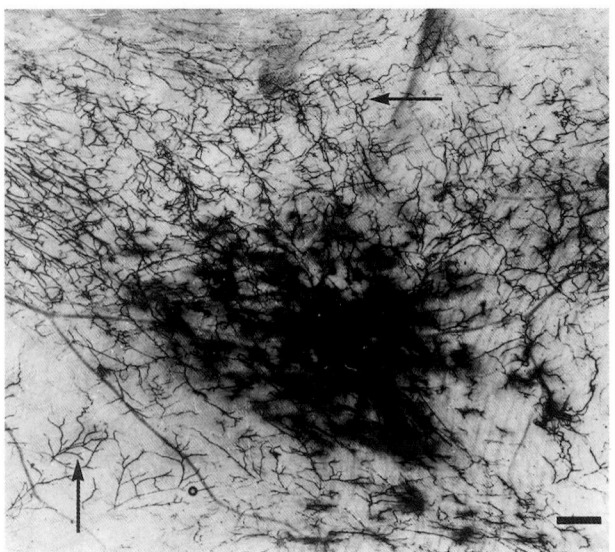

FIGURE 11.16   Demonstrating how the basement membranes are torn by diapedesis. Rat cremaster muscle. One hour before this tissue was fixed, histamine was injected locally, and carbon black was injected intravenously. Typical venular labeling developed as expected (**arrows**) except in the central zone: here, diapedesis had been induced 5 hours previously with an injection of serum. The black mass is carbon that spilled out of the basement membranes. **Bar** = 1 mm. (Reproduced with permission from [51].)

one model [87]) as if waiting for something to happen (110). Eventually it breaks through; does it succeed by sheer violence, or does it nibble at the basement membrane with some enzyme? It probably uses both means. Monocytes produce a surface elastase (64) and neutrophil elastase can attack basement membranes (7).

Anyway, an episode of diapedesis leaves the basement membrane in shambles. This was shown by an ingenious experiment (52) based on the principle of vascular labeling. In a normal rat, if the venules are labeled in black by a local injection of histamine followed by an intravenous injection of carbon black, the outlines of the blackened venules are sharp (see Figure 10.17). If the experiment is repeated 4 hours after a local injection of serum, which causes a burst of diapedesis, the torn-up basement membranes are unable to hold back the carbon, which spills out as a cloud of black fuzz (Figure 11.16). It is not known how long it takes for the basement membrane to be repaired.

Free at long last in the tissue spaces, the leukocyte has to find its way to the target. This process has been called "navigation," but it has nothing marine about it: the leukocyte has to painstakingly haul itself along in a semisolid jungle of fibers (72), while keeping track of the overall direction. Amazingly, it is able to integrate and prioritize multiple chemotactic calls (31, 59, 128); and just as amazingly it has a built-in device to avoid wasting ammunition: *there is a 15- to 45-minute delay between the initial activation and free radical respiratory burst,* so the leukocyte can pounce on its pray with maximum efficiency (34, 128). While on the way, if it happens to fall into a fluid-filled cavity such as the peritoneum or a joint, it will be condemned to float aimlessly until a random collision brings it in contact with its bacterial prey. In any event, it must hurry, because—remember—it has only hours to live.

The Second Wave of Margination and Diapedesis

The sequence described above shows that endothelium and leukocytes can collaborate to produce an *immediate* episode of margination (within seconds) and diapedesis (within minutes). This speed is possible because neither type of cell needs to synthesize new materials.

> *In vitro* the integrin-activating effect of the chemoattractants is very fast: by pretreating leukocytes or endothelial cells with fMLP, C5a, LTB$_4$ and PAF, it was shown that stickiness peaked at 2 minutes (119). Cytokines such as TNF and IL-1 are also effective (122).

There is also a *delayed and prolonged* response (Figure 11.17), much as we described for vascular leakage. In this modality the endothelium is exposed to inflammatory cytokines or toxins, and allowed the time necessary to synthesize new adhesion proteins and to express them on its surface (89, 93).

This was first shown in 1985 by M. Bevilacqua and colleagues (13). The plan was to expose an endothelial culture to a cytokine, then flood it with a suspension of leukocytes for a few minutes, wash it, and count how many leukocytes remained stuck to the endothelium.

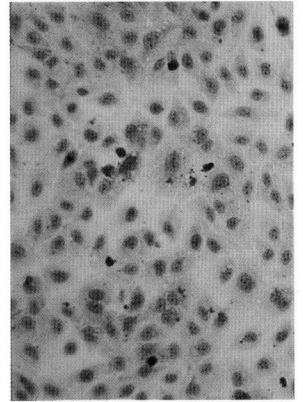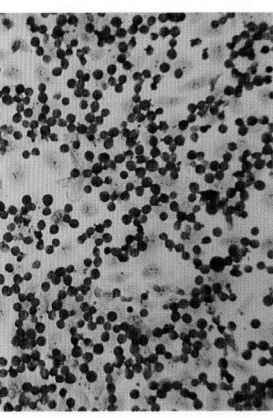

FIGURE 11.18   Monolayers of human endothelium incubated with a suspension of human promyelocytes (HL-60 cell line) for 10 minutes, then washed. *Left:* Control experiment with untreated endothelium. After washing, only scattered promyelocytes have remained attached. *Right:* This endothelium was pretreated with interleukin-1 for 4 hours. The cytokine has greatly increased the adhesiveness of the endothelial cells for the promyelocytes. A similar result is obtained with polymorphonuclear cells. (Courtesy of Dr. M. P. Bevilacqua, Brigham and Women's Hospital, Boston, MA.)

The result was impressive (Figure 11.18). The effect peaked at 4–6 hours, was reversible, and prevented by inhibitors of protein synthesis. Similar effects were obtained with tumor necrosis factor and endotoxin (21, 107). In this manner the first **e**ndothelial-**l**eukocyte **a**dhesion **m**olecule was identified and labeled ELAM-1 (Table 11.1).

Why does diapedesis occur from the venules? A moment's thought suggests that the use of capillaries for diapedesis would be disastrous (70). Monocytes and granulocytes are about twice as large as the lumen of most capillaries and experience a tight squeeze every time they pass through them (p. 713). Because the process takes 3–9 minutes, every single leukocyte that emigrated from a capillary would cause a 3–9 minute traffic jam; blood flow in that capillary would stop, defeating the very purpose of inflammation. By contrast, the leukocytes can marginate in the venules at their leisure while blood continues to flow past—however slowly—and to supply more leukocytes for margination.

There is one exception to venular diapedesis: *in the lung, the leukocytes emigrate from the alveolar capillaries* (67). However, the layout of these capillaries is unique. The alveolar capillaries are extremely short, averaging 8 μm (50), and form a very tight gridlike network, beautifully shown by plastic casts (Figure 11.19) (20). This layout means that many leukocytes can stick here

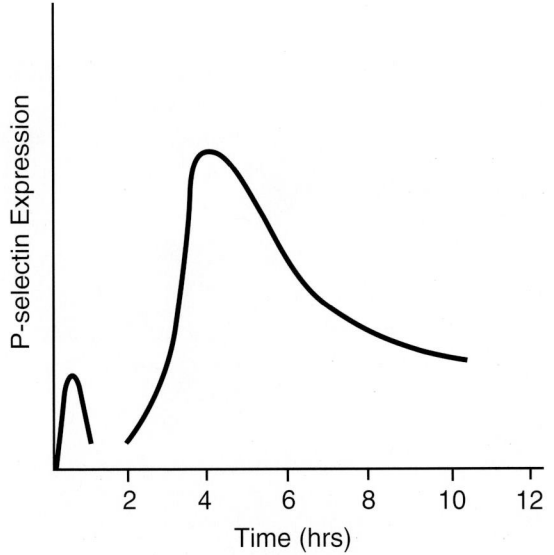

FIGURE 11.17   Expression of an endothelial cell adhesion molecule, P-selectin, by mouse intestine challenged with histamine (*left*) or with endotoxin (*right*). (Adapted from [89]; copyright 1998 American Gastroenterological Association, with permission from Elsevier.)

Table 11.1 Adhesion Glycoproteins Involved in Leukocyte-Endothelial Cell Adhesive Interactions

Adhesion molecule	Alternative designation	Localization	Ligand	Function
Selectin family				
L-selectin	LAM-1, LECAM-1 MEL-14 Ag, CD62L	All leukocytes	P-selectin, E-selectin. GlyCAM CD14, MAdCAM	Rolling
P-selectin	PADGEM, GMP-140, CD62P	Endothelial cells platelets	L-selectin, PSGL-1, 120-kD PSL	Rolling
E-selectin	ELAM-1, CD62E	Endothelial cells	L-selectin, CLA, SSEA-1, 250-kD ESL	Rolling
Integrin family				
CD11a/CD18	LFA-1, $\alpha_L\beta_2$	All leukocytes	ICAM-1, ICAM-2	Adherence/emigration
CD11b/CD18	Mac-1, MO1, CR3, $\alpha_M\beta_2$	Granulocytes monocytes	ICAM-1, iC3b; Fb	Adherence/emigration
CD11c/CD18	p150.95, $\alpha_x\beta_2$	Granulocytes monocytes	Fb; iC3b?	?
CD49d/CD29	VLA-4, $\alpha_4\beta_1$	Lymphocytes monocytes eosinophils, basophils	VCAM-1, extracellular matrix molecules	Adherence
CD49d/β_7	$\alpha_4\beta_7$	Lymphocytes	MadCAM-1, VCAM-1, fibronectin	Adherence
Ig supergene family				
ICAM-1	CD54a	Endothelium, Monocytes	LFA-1, Mac-1 CD43	Adherence/emigration
ICAM-2	CD102	Endothelium	LFA-1	Adherence/emigration
VCAM-1	CD106	Endothelium	VLA-4	Adherence
PECAM-1	CD31	Endothelium, leukocytes, platelets	PECAM-1 (homophilic)	Adherence/emigration
MAdCAM-1		Endothelium (intestine)	L-selectin, CD49d/β_7	Adherence/emigration

CLA, cutaneous lymphocyte antigen; ELAM, endothelial leukocyte adhesion molecule; ESL, E-selectin ligand; GMP, granule membrane protein; LAM, leukocyte adhesion molecule; LECAM, lymphocyte-endothelial cell adhesion molecule; LFA, lymphocyte function-associated antigen; PADGEM, platelet activation-dependent granule external membrane protein; PSL, P-selectin ligand; SSEA, sialyl stage-specific embryonic antigen.

Source: Adapted with permission from (89).

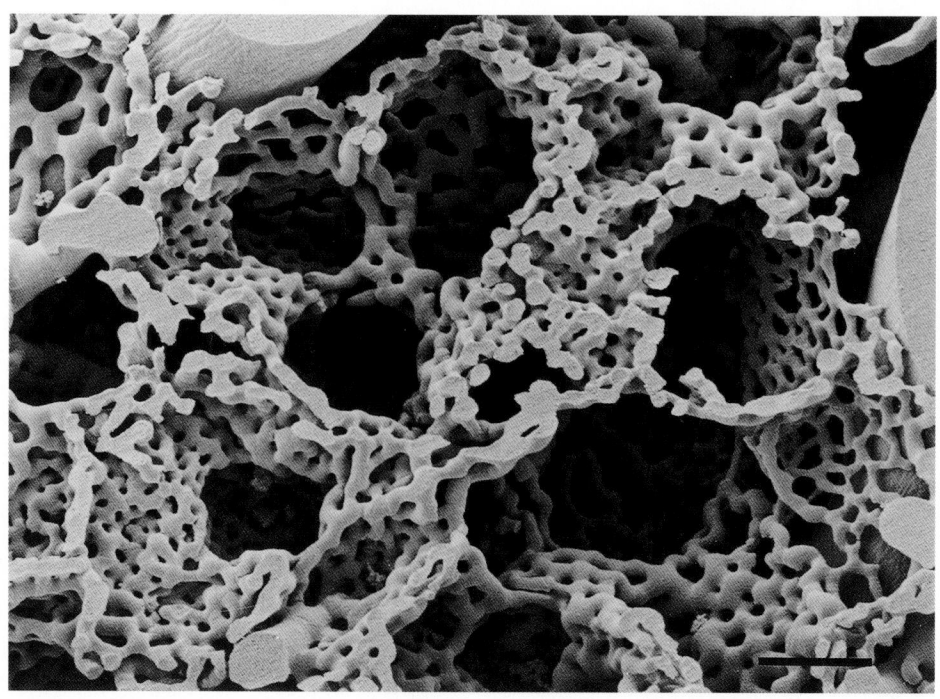

FIGURE 11.19 Demonstrating why leukocytes do not cause traffic jams in alveolar capillaries of the lungs. The capillary network is so richly branched that many capillaries are as long as they are wide (about 8 μm). Muscle capillaries are about 100 times longer. (Rat lung capillaries injected with plastic; the tissue has been removed.) **Bar** = 25 μm. (Courtesy of Drs. L. Fisher and P. H. Burri, University of Berne, Switzerland.)

and there in the grid without stopping the red-cell traffic. It is calculated that even if half of all the leukocytes in the blood were trapped in the human lung, only 10 percent of the alveolar capillary segments would be blocked (50).

Reverse Diapedesis

Reverse diapedesis (outside-in) has not been observed in living vessels. However, read this surprising story.

To reproduce *in vitro* the conditions of an early atherosclerotic plaque (where diapedesis of monocytes from the lumen into the wall of the artery is known to occur), G. J. Randolph *et al.* seeded blood monocytes on a culture of endothelial cells growing on a collagen base. Within an hour all the monocytes climbed out into the collagen, but after a few hours they began to climb back, and within a week 75 percent had returned, *but*—with the phenotype of dendritic cells! Whatever the message, the puzzle is tantalizing (83, 96).

Recognition and Attachment

After the leukocyte has been lured into the extravascular world, it must identify what to attack, and then stick to the target (116). How it does so is not entirely clear to us, but it is certainly clear to the leukocyte, which moves about in crowded quarters and knows enough to push aside a normal red blood cell, for example, but to seize an aged one. The clues to recognition must be subtle cell-surface differences, such as charge, hydrophilic properties, and molecular structure; some have been worked out regarding apoptotic cells (p. 213).

Opsonization. If the surface of the target is prepared (*opsonized*) by plasma proteins, phagocytosis is made easier, though some targets can be taken up without this coating (Figure 11.20).

> Opsonization (116, 125, 126) was discovered in 1903. Two Englishmen, Wright and Douglas, noticed that serum contains factors that coat bacteria and make them more palatable for the leukocytes; they called them opsonins (ópson is Greek for "prepared food").

There are three types of opsonins:

- *IgG antibody.* This is the most important opsonin, which means that whenever a bacterium is encountered for the *first* time, this important defense mechanism will be lacking. However, life exposes us to so many subclinical infections that some antibody-opsonin is usually available. IgG antibody works like a ligand: the Fab part of the globulin (see Figure 7.44) binds to the surface of the microorganism while the Fc portion sticks out and fits into the membrane receptors of the phagocyte.
- *C3b fragment of complement.* Being a fragment of C3, C3b is set free when complement is activated. Like IgG, C3b has a tail end that fits into a receptor on the surfaces of phagocytic cells.
- *Nonspecific opsonins.* Several proteins have opsonic properties (125), for example, Hageman factor, fibronectin (somewhat debated), Serum amyloid A (SAA, p. 505) and C-reactive protein.

Phagocytosis without opsonization. In some situations, however, opsonization is not needed. Consider an alveolar macrophage: the dust that it is supposed to clean up must be phagocytized in the absence of serum—and so it is, quite avidly (90). In this regard, the macrophage lives up to the prowess of its distant ancestor, the ameba, which takes all of its meals, presumably, without the benefit of having them labeled as dinner. Neutrophils do the same but with less enthusiasm. The molecular mechanism is not clear (126). Better understood is the uptake of nonopsonized bacteria, another feat of the macrophage: certain sugars on the

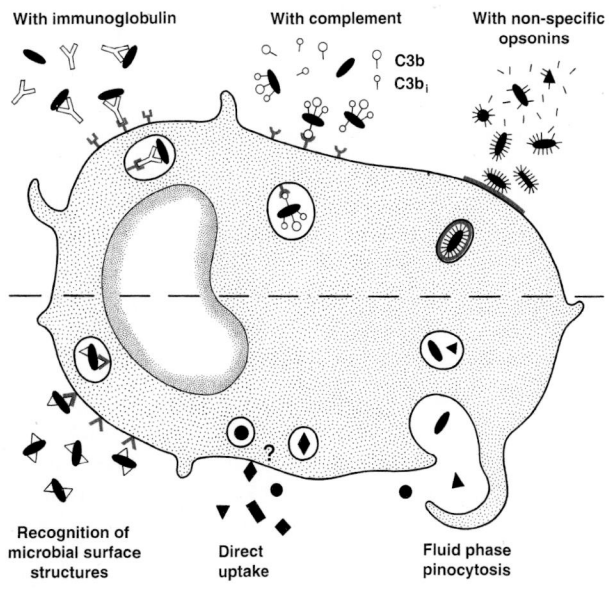

WITH OPSONIZATION

FIGURE 11.20   A macrophage can phagocytize by at least six pathways: three require opsonization, three do not. The small oval objects represent bacteria. (Adapted with permission from [2]. Copyright Raven Press 1988.)

surface of the phagocyte are recognized by a receptor on the bacterial surface, or vice versa (39). Also, of course, very small particles, of the order of magnitude of proteins, can be taken in accidentally by the macrophage in the course of pinocytosis. This has been called piggy-back phagocytosis.

Reverse opsonization. Reverse opsonization modifies the surface of the phagocyte, which amounts to whetting the appetite rather than spicing the meal. Because phagocytosis is facilitated by conditioning the surface of the target, it would be strange if there were no way to condition the surface of the phagocyte. Such is the function of the tetrapeptide **tuftsin,** which is incorporated in IgG1 molecules (33) and is cleaved off in two steps, in the spleen and on the surface of phagocytic cells (39, 84, 85, 109). Tuftsin stimulates phagocytosis, motility, cytotoxicity, and other leukocytic functions.

Phagocytosis

After a target has been recognized and seized by a phagocyte it must be ingested to be eliminated. Transmission electron microscopy gives the impression that two pseudopods emerge from the surface of the phagocyte and surround the target like a pair of arms (Figure 11.21), but in three dimensions the event looks different. Usually, a circular ridge rises around the attached particle, grows to form a cup, and develops into a crater (Figure 11.22) (88). Eventually the crater closes up, the apposed plasma membranes fuse, and the particle finds itself in an intracellular vacuole (phagosome).

Then the digestion process begins. As seen in phagocytes that have been fixed and stained, this event appears utterly bland; somehow the phagocyte looses its granules (it is said to become "degranulated"), and the phagocytized bacteria may or may not die. In reality, what happens in living cells is truly dramatic. It has been recorded in a movie that every biologist should see (47).

How granulocytes loose their granules. In the early 1960s James Hirsch and Gordon Archer recorded on film the behavior of granulocytes phagocytizing various types of particles (6, 47). In each sequence, a cell creeps toward its immobile target until it engulfs it in a pocket of cytoplasm. Eventually the pocket closes up and becomes a phagosome. In the meantime, in a matter of seconds, the cell's granules move to the pocket, fuse with it, and eject their enzymes into it. This is literally an explosive event: the granules pop one by one like ammunition, until the phagocyte is degranulated. Two representative frames are shown in Figure 11.23. The specific granules are the first to be expended (130), perhaps because of their high content of antibacterial molecules.

> Movies of phagocytosis had been taken before, but by the more "hi-tech" time-lapse method, whereby the popping event, which lasts only one-tenth of a second, was regularly missed. Hirsch and Archer took the movie by the ordinary and cheaper method, which produced a slow but complete recording.

An important detail: *the popping of granules begins to occur even before the particule is completely engulfed.* This can be seen also on electron micrographs (Figure 11.24). The result is that some of the extruded

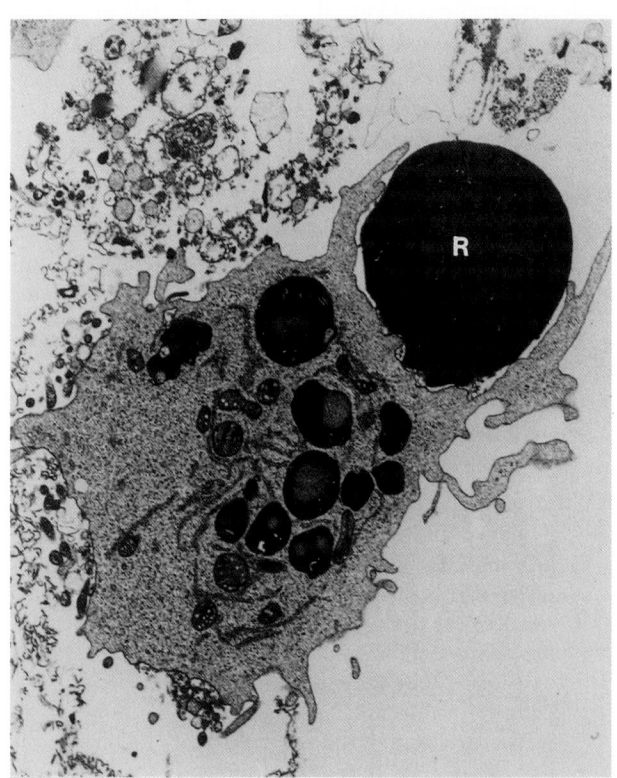

FIGURE 11.21   Phagocytosis of a red blood cell (**R**): The phagocyte here shown is a cloned NK cell engulfing a red blood cell coated with antibody. Note that the granules have moved toward the contact site. In this two-dimensional view the phagocyte appears to "throw two arms" around its prey, but compare it with the three-dimensional crater seen by scanning electron microscopy (Fig. 11.22). (Reproduced from **Mechanisms of Host Resistance to Infectious Agents, Tumors, and Allografts,** 1986, pp. 217–230, by copyright permission of The Rockefeller University Press [94].)

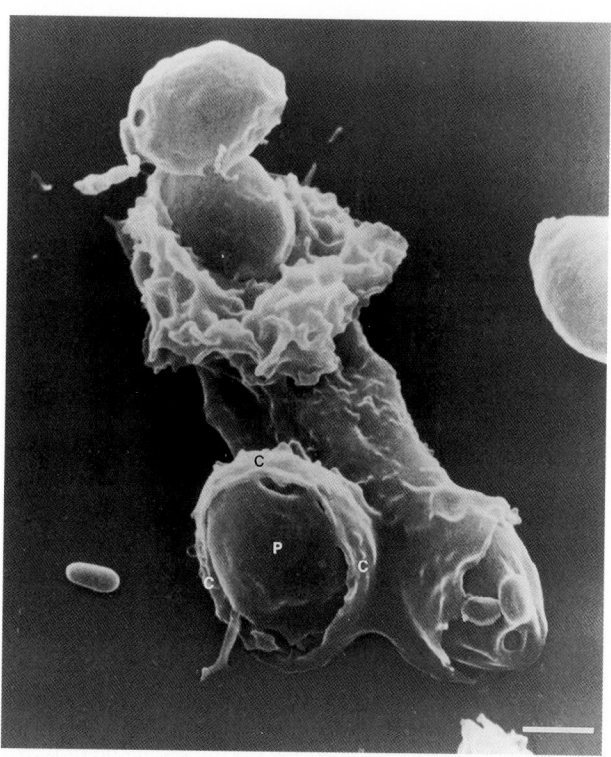

FIGURE 11.22 Human neutrophil phagocytizing foreign particles: a three dimensional view. Note how the membrane rises to form a cup (**C**) surrounding the particle (**P**). **Bar** = 2 μm. (Courtesy of Dr. M. J. Karnovsky, Harvard Medical School, Boston MA.)

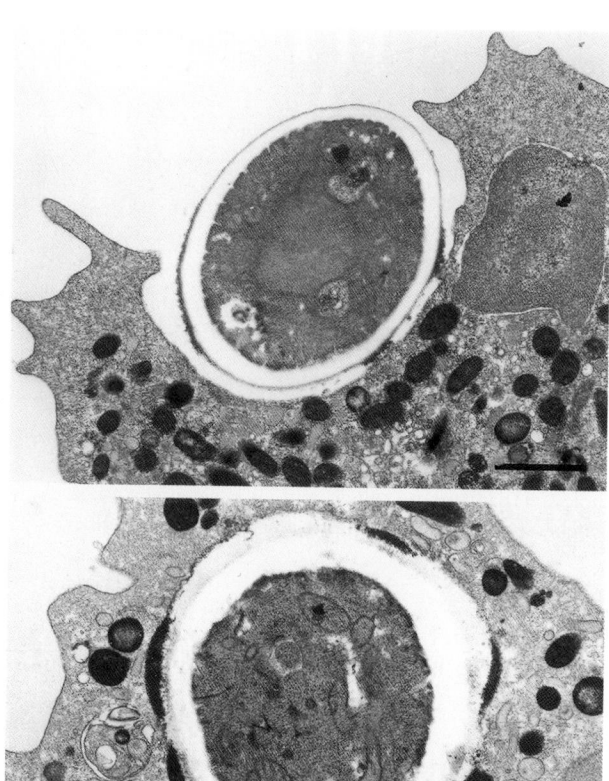

FIGURE 11.24 Human neutrophils phagocytizing opsonized yeast. Section reacted for peroxidase: the peroxidase-positive, electron-dense azurophil granules stand out against the peroxidase-negative specific granules. *Top:* The neutrophil has recognized the yeast cell and is about to engulf it. Already at this early stage, enzymes of the azurophil granules are present at the surface of the yeast cell. *Bottom:* Detail of a yeast cell fully enclosed in a phagocytic vacuole. Note the massive release of granule contents. **Bars** = 1 μm. (Reproduced from [10] with permission from Elsevier Science Publishers.)

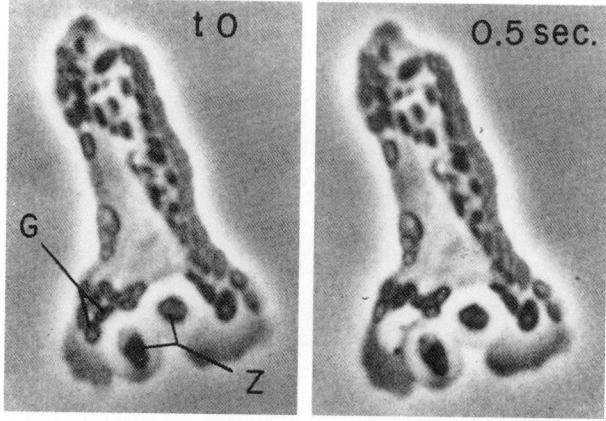

FIGURE 11.23 Two frames from a movie showing that the leukocyte's granules (**G**) burst into the phagosomes during phagocytosis. Chicken leukocytes phagocytizing a particle of zymosan (**Z**). At *time 0*: Two granules are intact. At *0.5 second*: they have burst, leaving a clear space. (Reproduced from the **Journal of Experimental Medicine,** 1962;116:827–834, by copyright permission of The Rockefeller University Press [47].)

enzymes leak out into the tissue spaces, a messy event known as **regurgitation while feeding** (which helps us understand why the inflammatory exudate is rich in hydrolytic enzymes).

Frustrated phagocytosis. This colorful term fits the following situation: when a phagocyte runs into a large, flat surface that it recognizes as foreign, it "attempts" to phagocytize it by lying on it; it pops its granules against it but of course is never be able to take it in (46). The frustration, however, may be only in the mind of the beholder; the phagocyte can cause plenty of damage to

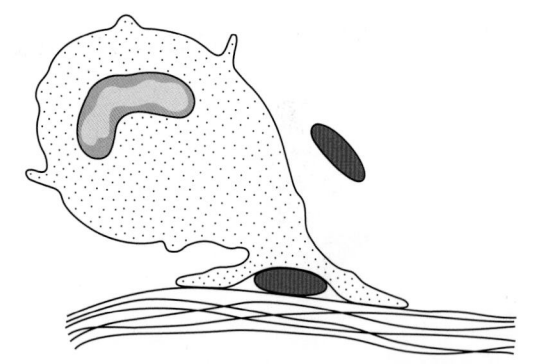

FIGURE 11.25 *Surface phagocytosis*. A macrophage in the connective tissue spaces cannot catch a free-floating bacterium—unless it happens to collide with it accidentally—but easily catches another one by trapping it against a collagen fiber.

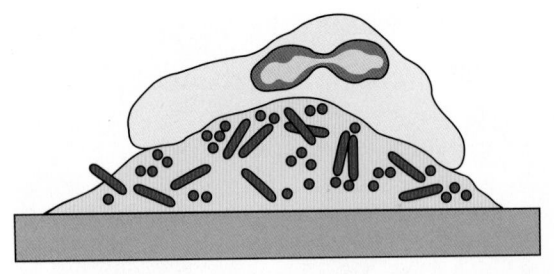

FIGURE 11.26 Bacteria attached to a surface may evade the attack of leukocytes by burying themselves in a mucous "biofilm" (slime). (Adapted with permission from [41]. Copyright 1985 by the American Association for the Advancement of Science.)

this type of prey without swallowing it. This is the very principle of a killing mechanism known in immunology as ADCC (p. 539).

Surface phagocytosis. Surface phagocytosis is a mechanism for relieving frustrated phagocytes (111, 129). Imagine a phagocyte hopelessly chasing around a slippery particle without being able to grab it (recalling the popular game of trying to bite an apple floating on water). The chase can end only if the particle is backed against a resistant surface; collagen fibers or filaments of fibrin may perform this function in inflammatory foci (Figure 11.25).

> Surface phagocytosis can be demonstrated by an elegant experiment: phagocytes are incubated with encapsulated pneumococci (notoriously slippery) in a rotating tube; after 30 minutes, few of the phagocytes contain bacteria because it was hard for them to phagocytize while floating. If a piece of filter paper or strands of fibrin are added to the mixture, after 30 minutes many more bacteria have been ingested (111).

Phagocytosis frustrated by slime. Phagocytes sometimes encounter a third type of surface problem. Some bacteria are able to attach themselves to a surface, such as a catheter, and then coat themselves with a layer of slime In so doing they create what is now known as a *bacterial biofilm* (Figure 11.26). This makes them almost inaccessible to phagocytes. Perhaps we should call this **frustrated surface phagocytosis.** This phenomenon explains why physicians are reluctant to insert catheters, and why surgeons are always worried about foreign bodies. We shall return to biofilms in dealing with foreign bodies (p. 494).

Coiling phagocytosis. This variant of phagocytosis can be identified only by electron microscopy (97, 98). Imagine a bacterium stuck on a phagocyte; instead of drawing the bacterium into a phagosome, the phagocyte produces a lamellipodium that wraps itself several times around the bacterium. In cross section the result is a spiral with the microorganism in its center. Then the whole structure sinks into the cell and is somehow dissolved, bacterium and all, without forming a phagosome and without the help of lysosomes. Biologically the interesting point is that the bacterial antigens become free in the cytosol, and available to be processed immunologically like cytosolic viral antigens (97). A microorganism that is taken up preferentially in this manner is the spirochete *Borrelia burgdorferi,* the agent of Lyme disease; but coiling phagocytosis is not specific to any bacterium or phagocyte. Time will tell whether it is a mere curiosity or a significant phenomenon.

Phagokinesis is a curious *in vitro* phenomenon. Cells are seeded on a surface coated with colloidal gold particles. As the cells move about, they phagocytize the gold, leaving a clear area (Figure 11.27) (4).

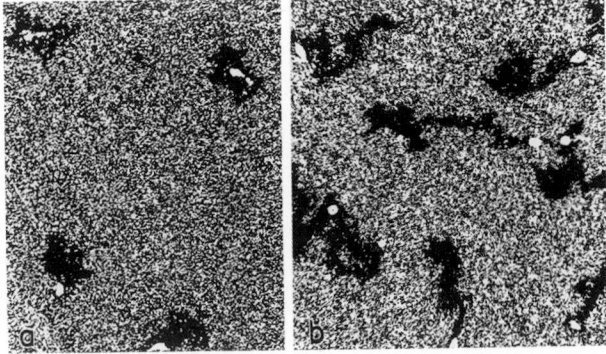

FIGURE 11.27 Two scenes of phagokinesis. *Left:* Cultured capillary endothelial cells deposited on a surface covered with gold particles. *Right:* Similar setting except that the cells have been stimulated with the supernatant from a culture of tumor cells. As the cells move about, they pick up gold particles. (Courtesy of Dr. B. R. Zetter, Harvard Medical School, Boston, MA.)

Bacterial Killing: Metabolic Aspects of Phagocytosis

Phagocytosis of bacteria is a prelude to bacterial killing. Bacteria engulfed by neutrophils or macrophages can be destroyed by two mechanisms: oxygen-dependent (thanks to oxygen-derived free radicals) and oxygen-independent (14). The latter mechanism reminds us that leukocytes are often called upon to kill bacteria in injured tissues, in which the oxygen supply is low. The two mechanisms are almost equally powerful, but the oxygen dependent mechanism has a slight edge (123).

Oxygen-Dependent Antibacterial Mechanisms

Phagocytosis (38) was once considered a purely physical phenomenon based on surface tensions, and there may be some truth in this concept (125). Yet in 1933 it was shown that oxygen uptake increases during phagocytosis (55). The topic attracted little interest for 26 years until Anthony Sbarra and Manfred Karnovsky returned to it during a study of host–parasite relations (57, 105). They discovered some startling facts: granulocytes incubated with polystyrene particles phagocytized them equally well under aerobic or anaerobic conditions. The phagocytizing cells did show an increased oxygen uptake (Figure 11.28); but they continued to phagocytize if they were poisoned with cyanide, which uncouples oxidative phosphorylation. In other words, the extra oxygen uptake did not represent mitochondrial respiration. The energy for phagocytosis seemed to derive from glycolysis because poisoning with

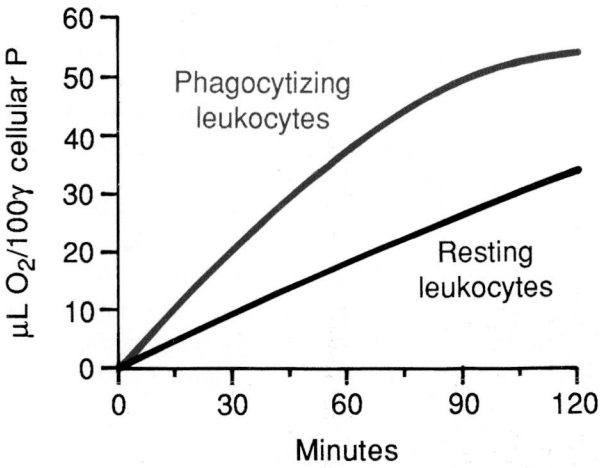

FIGURE 11.28   The respiratory burst induced by phagocytosis: respiration of guinea pig peritoneal cells (80 percent neutrophils) at rest and during phagocytosis. The particles to be phagocytized were introduced at zero time. (Adapted with permission from [105].)

iodoacetate or fluoride did inhibit the uptake of particles. This last finding made good sense, at least for the leukocytes. Because these cells are often called on to perform in traumatized areas where the circulation is impaired, it is certainly convenient that they should be able to engulf bacteria in the absence of oxygen by drawing energy from their built-in supply of glycogen. But then why would phagocytizing leukocytes need more oxygen? The increased uptake can be huge, over 50 times the normal (8).

The answer came two years later. Stimulated (activated) phagocytes release H_2O_2 (hydrogen peroxide) and *superoxide anion* (O_2^-), and these molecules are further metabolized into highly toxic oxidants, so *the purpose of the respiratory burst is not to provide energy, but to produce lethal oxidants as antibacterial agents* (8, 35, 56).

The enzyme responsible for the increased oxygen uptake (NADPH oxidase) is built into the cell membrane; its NADPH binding site projects into the cytosol. But its products are released outside of the cell, and therefore into phagosomes, as required for killing bacteria (a phagosome is lined with internalized cell membrane). In a resting cell the enzyme remains dormant, but when activated it catalyzes the one-electron reductions of oxygen at the expense of NADPH:

$$O_2 + NADPH \rightarrow O_2^- + NADP^+ + H^+$$

It is no mean feat of histochemistry that superoxide, which lasts only milliseconds, can be demonstrated on electron micrographs (Figure 11.29) (17), but we find it even more astonishing that the generation of oxygen-derived free radicals is accompanied by the emission of *light* (photons), so that a standard method for measuring the activation of leukocytes is to monitor their chemoluminescence. Most of the O_2^- promptly reacts with itself, producing oxygen and hydrogen peroxide:

$$2O_2^- + 2H^+ \rightarrow H_2O_2 + O_2$$

At the same time, glucose is metabolized via the hexose monophosphate (HMP) shunt in order to regenerate the NADPH (this explains why Sbarra and Karnovsky found that during phagocytosis the catabolism of glucose via the HMP shunt is greatly accelerated). Today, the expression *respiratory burst* refers to the four events: increased oxygen uptake, increased catabolism of glucose via the HMP shunt, release of H_2O_2, and release of O_2^-.

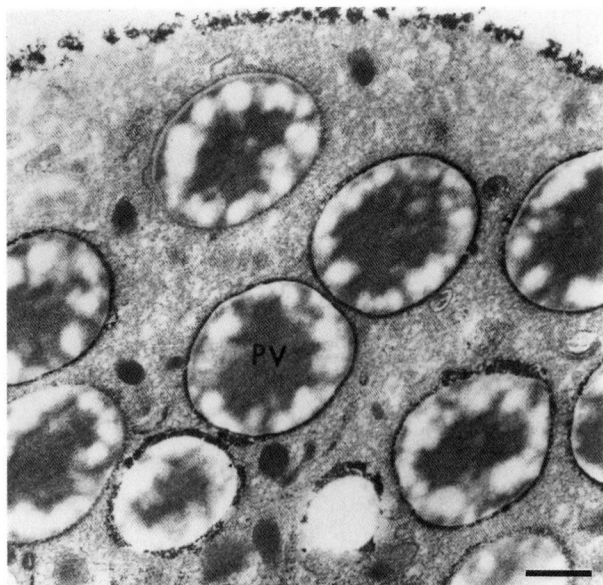

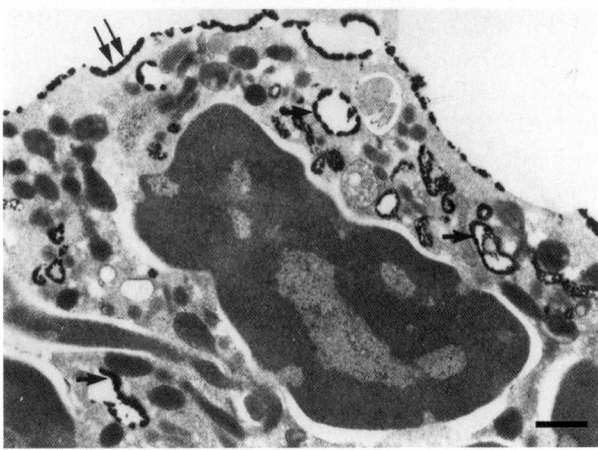

FIGURE 11.29 Electron micrographs of activated neutrophils treated by a histochemical method to show the sites of H_2O_2 generation. The black precipitate represents the reaction product. *Top:* Neutrophil activated by phagocytosis of polystyrene spheres. Reaction product on the cell surface and on the membranes of phagocytic vacuoles (**PV**). (Reproduced from the **Journal of Cell Biology,** 1975;67:566–586, by copyright permission of The Rockefeller University Press [16].) *Bottom:* Neutrophil stimulated with phorbol myristate acetate. **Arrows:** Reaction product on surface and on surface-derived membranes. (Courtesy of Dr. M. J. Karnovsky, Harvard Medical School, Boston, MA.) **Bars** = 0.5 μm.

Up to this point we have H_2O_2 and superoxide radical, neither of which is very effective at killing bacteria, but they are used as starting materials for producing the really effective antiseptics, which belong to two categories: *oxidizing radicals* and *oxidized halogens.*

The best-known oxidizing radical is the hydroxyl radical (OH·), which is produced by a metal-catalyzed

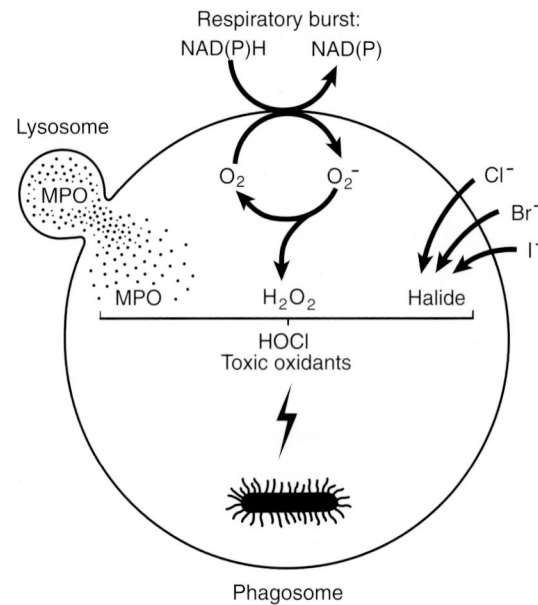

FIGURE 11.30 The Klebanoff system, an oxygen dependent antibacterial weapon of phagocytes, has three components: myeloperoxidase (MPO) supplied by lysosomes; H_2O_2 supplied by the respiratory burst (some H_2O_2 may be supplied by the bacterium itself), and a halide. The interaction of these three components supplies toxic oxidants.

reaction, the Haber-Weiss reaction (p. 196):

$$O_2^- + H_2O_2 \xrightarrow{Fe^{++} or Cu^{++}} OH\cdot + OH^- + O_2$$

Hydroxyl radical is formed and released not only in the phagocytic vacuole but also around the activated phagocyte, because all the reagents are available there.

The prototype of the oxidized halogens is hypochlorite (**HOCl**), which can only be generated with the collaboration of myeloperoxidase (MPO), an enzyme present in the azurophil (primary) granules. Thus, the antiseptic power of the hypochlorite can only be exploited in the phagocytic vacuole, in which MPO conspires with two other reactants to produce a variety of toxic agents, including hypochlorite (60). This three-pronged myeloperoxidase—H_2O_2—halide system, more simply known as the *Klebanoff system,* works inside the phagosome as follows (Figure 11.30):

- Myeloperoxidase is supplied by fusion of the phagosome with a primary granule.
- H_2O_2 is supplied mostly by the oxygen burst occurring in the phagosome membrane (which really represents activated cell membrane) by means of the NADPH-oxidase; some H_2O_2 can also be contributed by the bacterium in the phagosome.
- Halide is supplied by the cell; it can be Cl^-, I^-, or Br^-.

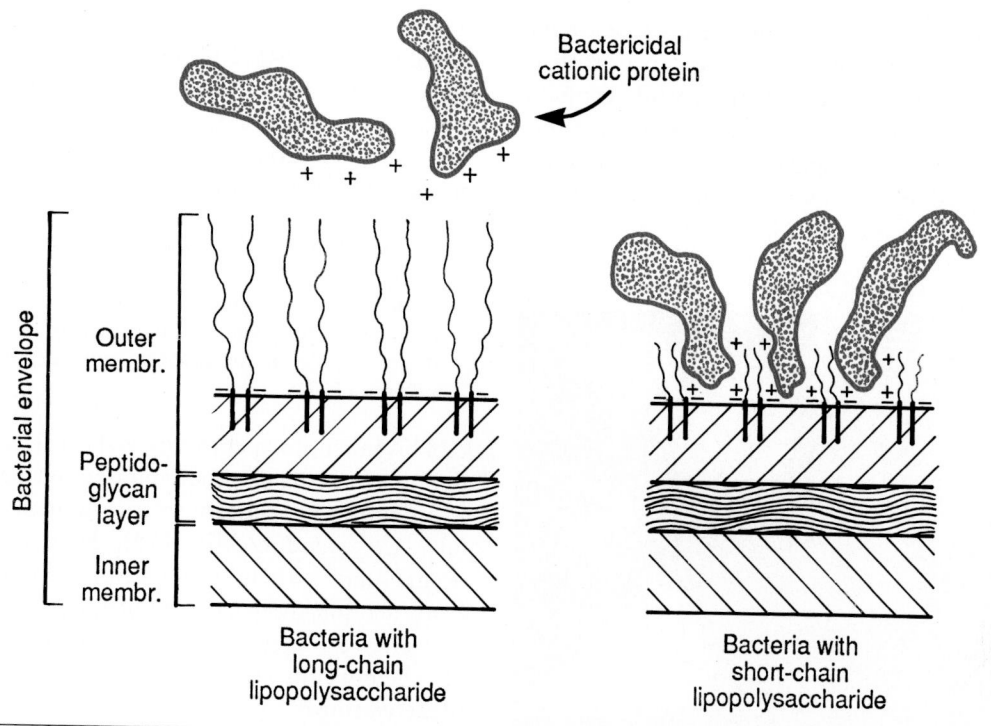

FIGURE 11.31 Bactericidal cationic proteins are among the oxygen-independent bactericidal systems of neutrophils (they are also called Bacterial Permeability-Increasing Proteins, or BPI proteins). This scheme shows how these proteins are thought to interact with negative charges on the surface of gram-negative bacteria; the interaction is more effective when the polysaccharide chains of the lipopolysaccharide are short. (Adapted from [27].)

The basic reaction is the following:

$$H^+ + Cl^- + H_2O_2 \xrightarrow{\text{myeloperoxidase}} HOCl + H_2O$$

All this being said, we find that the choice of antiseptics used by the phagocytic cells is absolutely fascinating. We invite our readers to give it a moment's thought (think simply) and we will give our own perspective at the very end of this chapter.

Oxygen-Independent Antibacterial Mechanisms

Leukocytes are well equipped to kill bacteria by a variety of mechanisms unrelated to oxygen metabolism (28, 113). Ground up, leukocytes that are congenitally unable to produce a respiratory burst can still kill some bacteria. Each type of phagocyte has its own mix of antibacterial molecules (28). These are in part enzymatic: proteases, phospholipases, nucleases, and lysozyme, which is powerful against a few gram-positive bacteria. Many other antibacterial mechanisms such as the cationic proteins are nonenzymatic. Especially effective against gram-negative bacteria is a cationic protein that kills bacteria by increasing their permeability (BPI

for bacterial permeability-increasing protein). Its possible mechanism of action is shown in Figure 11.31. *Defensins* (66) are small cytotoxic proteins. Other cytotoxic proteins are contained in eosinophils; one of them, the eosinophil cationic protein (ECP), is a pore-forming molecule (p. 337). *Lactoferrin* acts mainly as an iron-binding protein, depriving bacteria of iron as a growth factor; persons congenitally lacking in neutrophil lactoferrin may be prone to infections.

Triggers of Phagocyte Activation

The respiratory burst can be induced by phagocytosis (60, 106) as well as by the stimulation of surface receptors, especially those for chemotaxins. Experimentally the prototype activator is phorbol myristate acetate (TPA, p. 61), the active principle of croton oil; the use of this pharmacologic agent is of course highly artificial, but it is also extremely effective and has been invaluable for working out the details of leukocyte activation. It is possible experimentally to trigger each one of the various leukocyte functions separately (chemotaxis, phagocytosis, respiratory burst, etc.); a typical, full-blown sequence induced by chemotaxins could run as follows. Within less than 5 seconds after the chemotaxins have bound to the cell's surface receptors, Ca^{++} and Na^+ rush in and the concentration of cAMP rises, while cytosolic pH drops; the cell swells, reorganizes its cytoskeleton, assuming a roughly triangular shape, and becomes polarized in the direction of the stimulus (Figure 11.32).

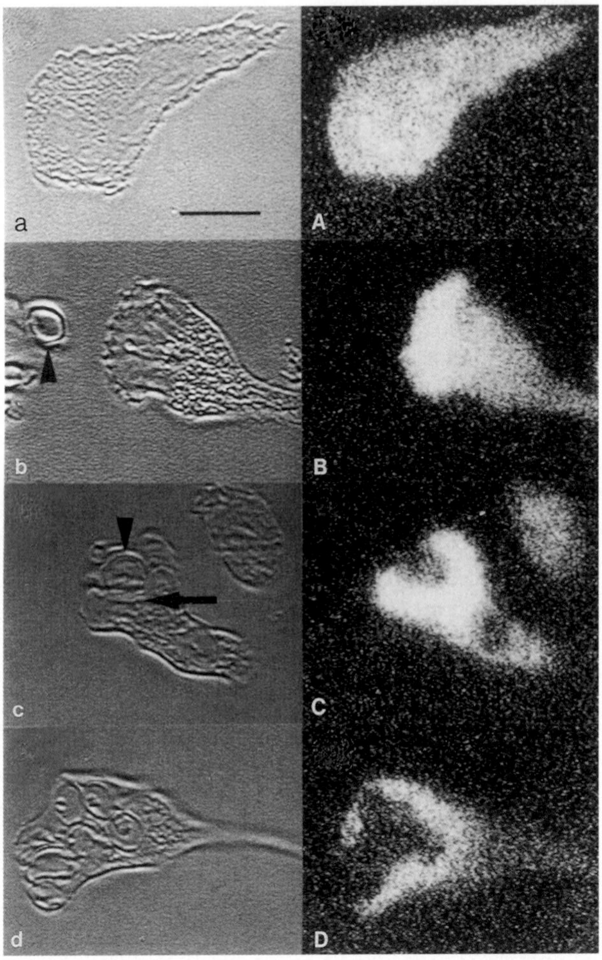

In 5–10 seconds it begins to send out pseudopodia or a lamellipodium (Figure 11.33) in which Ca^{++} reaches its highest concentration (104), and the chemotactic receptors begin to cluster at the front end (37). Superoxide is also generated from the cell's outer membrane while arachidonic acid is released.

The biochemical mechanism of leukocyte activation is partly worked out. When the receptor for the chemotaxin is occupied, phospholipase C is activated by a G protein to produce IP_3 and diacylglycerol; PIP_2 hydrolysis leads to increased membrane permeability to calcium (112).

This burst of hyperactivity is short-lived: degranulation and superoxide production do not persist beyond 2–5 minutes and the same is true for increased intracellular Ca^{++} and cAMP (112). How this shutdown occurs is not entirely clear. Chemotaxins, like all mediators, are quickly inactivated; it is also well established that after prolonged exposure to high concentrations of chemotaxins the leukocytes cease to respond (**deactivation**) (131).

Reversibility of activation. Granulocytes stimulated by phagocytosis cannot be stopped in their tracks: in this respect they quite justify their kamikaze reputation. However, if they are chemically stimulated *in vitro* (e.g., by fluoride) the respiratory burst can be reversed by washing away the fluoride (22).

FIGURE 11.32 Displacements of intracellular free calcium in a human neutrophil during chemotaxis and phagocytosis. **a:** Unstimulated neutrophil that is already polarized (it has a head and a tail). **A:** Calcium distribution in the same neutrophil: white areas represent the highest concentration. **b:** Neutrophil migrating toward an opsonized zymosan particle (**arrowhead**). **B:** Calcium distribution in the same cell. Calcium is migrating to the lamellipodium. **c:** Neutrophil engulfing a zymosan particle. **C:** Calcium distribution. **d, D:** Neutrophil that has ingested several zymosan particles. High regional calcium appears to be important for oxidative metabolism, chemotaxis, phagocytosis, and degranulation. **Bar** = 10 μm. (Reprinted with permission from [104]. Copyright 1985 by the American Association for the Advancement of Science.)

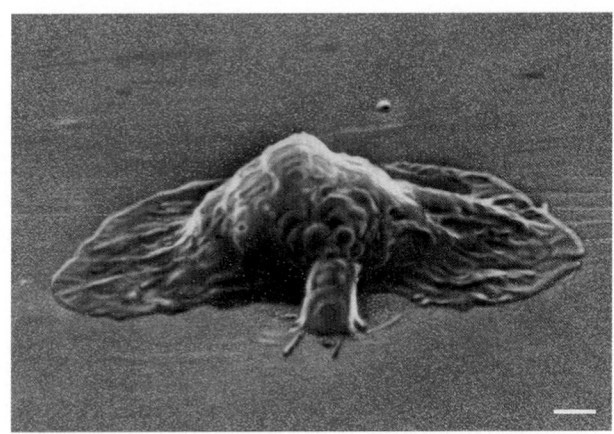

FIGURE 11.33 Scanning electron micrograph of a granulocyte moving away from the observer on a glass surface. Notice the tail end (uropod) and the extremely thin, advancing lamellipodium. **Bar** = 1 μm. (Reproduced from [12] with permission from Springer-Verlag.)

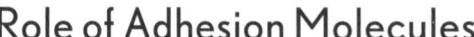

Role of Adhesion Molecules

The cellular adhesion proteins surfaced in the mid-1980s (102) and soon revealed that they play major roles in health and disease (32, 40). The inflammatory "rolling and sticking" phenomenon turned out to be a variant of the normal "homing" phenomenon, whereby lymphocytes circulating in the blood stream are captured by adhesion molecules on the endothelium of the *high endothelial venules* in lymphoid organs (115).

The endothelial adhesion proteins belong to four main groups: *the integrins; the immunoglobulin family* (no relation to immunology); *cadherins* and *selectins*. The *integrins,* as we have seen, consist of two subunits, alpha and beta, which are normally inactive and can be activated. They are heterophilic, that is, they bind to ligand molecules of a different structure. Members of the *immunoglobulin group* can be heterophilic or homophilic: the latter work like zippers, which have a clearly symmetric (homophilic) structure. The same is true for the *cadherins,* which take part in forming junctions of the *adhaerens* type. The *selectins* are unique in that they bind to carbohydrate molecules.

Adhesion molecules contribute to pathology in many ways; perhaps the worst is the following.

Leukocyte adhesion deficiency (LAD). The molecular defect varies; in *type I* (about 100 patients world wide, plus a few dogs and cows) it concerns the beta 2 integrin subunit on the leukocytes (58); this results in the paradox of *leukocytosis accompanied by the incapacity to produce an effective inflammatory response,* especially against bacteria (as opposed to viruses). The latter feature suggests that the lymphocytes are less affected than the neutrophils and monocytes. Depending on the severity of the defect some of the patients can survive to adulthood, despite dreadful-looking, necrotizing infections especially of the skin, and dental problems (Figure 11.34). The earliest detectable sign is *delayed separation of the umbilical cord.* Normally the dried-up stump of the umbilical cord attracts leukocytes and falls off in 7–10 days, severed by the leukocytic enzymes (Figure 11.35). In LAD patients, the leukocytes in the umbilical circulation are condemned to circulate perpetually without stopping for a chemotactic call, the

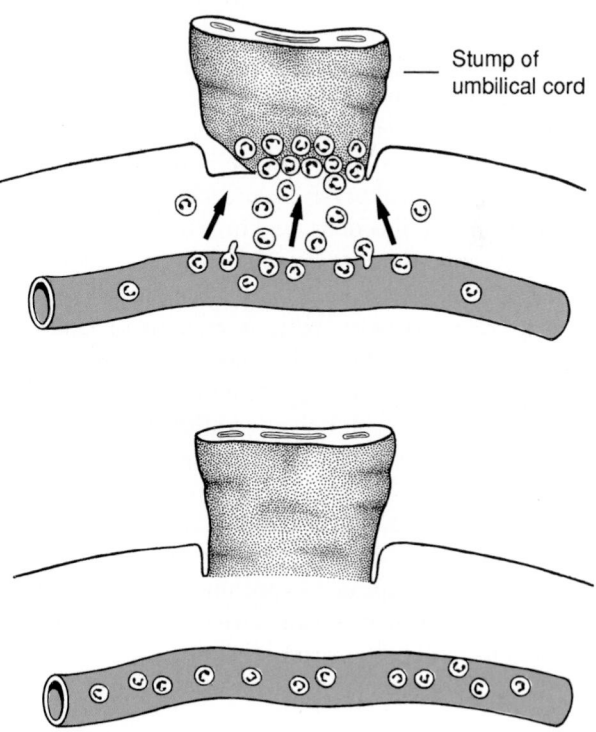

Stump of umbilical cord

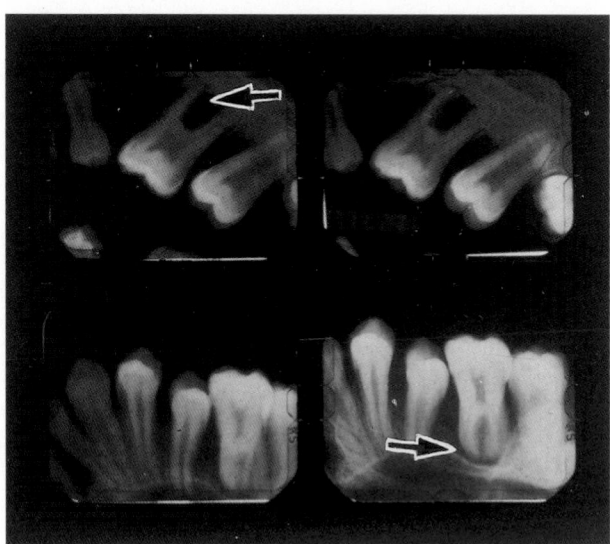

FIGURE 11.34   X-rays of the jaws in a 12-year-old child affected by leukocyte adhesion deficiency. **Arrows** point to severe bone loss due to infection. The gums were inflamed and deep periodontal pockets had formed. (Reproduced from [5] by permission of The University of Chicago Press. © 1985 by The University of Chicago. All rights reserved.)

FIGURE 11.35   The "umbilical cord phenomenon" in leukocyte adhesion deficiency. *Top:* Normal situation: within 7–10 days the necrotic stump of the umbilical cord, acting as an irritant, attracts leukocytes and is cut off by their enzymes. *Bottom:* In leukocyte adhesion deficiency the leukocytes cannot emigrate, and the umbilical stump is retained.

essential prelude to diapedesis and to the enzymatic surgery of the umbilical stump.

LAD type 2 is due to impaired synthesis of fucosylated carbohydrates, which include the ligands of the selectins (32).

Adhesion molecules play a role, directly or indirectly, in almost all diseases. Some **tumor cells** circulating in the blood express adhesion molecules which cause them to be retained in given organs (p. 823). One of the very first steps of **arteriosclerosis** is the sticking and emigration of monocytes and lymphocytes into the arterial intima (53, 54, 100) (p. 674). **Pathogenic bacteria** carry negative surface charges, and so do tissue cells; to overcome the resulting charge repulsion bacteria depend on powerful protein **adhesins** (108a). These and other examples have suggested that the course of many diseases—not typically "inflammatory"—might be slowed down or stopped by antiinflammatory therapy, *targeted against adhesion proteins;* but this approach is always a two-edged sword. Inflammation is a defensive response; suppressing it may come with a price.

> **TO SUM UP:** The performance of the leukocytes in inflammation is awesome, and it has been dissected and worked out in masterly fashion. Even a bland and apparently nonspecific phenomenon such as "leukocyte rolling" now has its molecular explanation. We are especially impressed by the ability of the leukocytes to integrate calls coming from various directions, and to save their ammunition while they are doing so. We have enough detail to say that if bacteria had eyes, they would perceive a terrifying sight: as millions of leukocytes are hauling themselves along the connective tissue fibers and closing in, following their sniff, they are swelling, huffing and puffing (their respiration is greatly increased), reaching out with long pseudopodia, drooling acid juices, and emitting sparks (real photons). And when they reach their arch-enemies, the bacteria, they douse them with hydrogen peroxide and hypochlorite—two of our household antiseptics. Leukocytes have been using them for millions of years.

References

1. Aaronson S. Chemical communication at the microbial level, vol. 1. Boca Raton: CRC Press, 1981.
2. Adams DO, Hamilton TA. Phagocytic cells: cytotoxic activities of macrophages. In: Gallin, JI., Goldstein IM, Snyderman R, eds. Inflammation: basic principles and clinical correlates. New York: Raven Press, 1988, pp. 471–492.
3. Adler J. Chemoreceptors in bacteria. Science 1969;166: 1588–1597.
4. Albrecht-Buehler G. The phagokinetic tracks of 3T3 cells. Cell 1977;11:395–404.
5. Anderson DC, Schmalsteig FC, Finegold MJ, et al. The severe and moderate phenotypes of heritable Mac-1, LFA-1 deficiency: their quantitative definition and relation to leukocyte dysfunction and clinical features. J Infect Dis 1985;152: 668–689.
6. Archer GT, Hirsch JG. Motion picture studies on degranulation of horse eosinophils during phagocytosis. J Exp Med 1963; 118:287–294. (Available from Rockefeller University Press, Film Service, 222 East 70th Street, New York, NY 10021.)
7. Arsenis C, Kuettner KE, Schwartz DE Degradation of intact basement membranes by human neutrophil elastase. A model for enzyme degradation of intact collagenous matrices. In: Sen A, Thornhill T, eds. development and diseases of cartilage and bone matrix. New York: Alan R. Liss, 1987, pp. 45–54.
8. Babior BM. The respiratory burst of phagocytes. J Clin Invest 1984;73:599–601.
9. Bacon KB, Schall TJ. Chemokines as mediators of allergic inflammation. Int Arch Allergy Immunol 1996;109:97–109.
10. Baggiolini M. Phagocyte activation and its modulation by drugs. In: Glynn LE, Houck JC, Weissmann, G Handbook of inflammation, vol. 5. Amsterdam: Elsevier, 1985, pp. 117–121.
10a. Bahat A, Tur-Kaspa I, Gakamsky A, et al. Thermotaxis of mammalian sperm cells: a potential navigation system in the female genital tract. Nature Med 2003;9:149–150.
11. Bang FB. Disease processes in seastars: a Metchnikovian challenge. Biol Bull 1982;162:135–148.
12. Bessis M, Boisfleury AD. Les mouvements des leucocytes étudiés au microscope électronique à balayage. Nouv Rev Fr Hématol 1971;11:377–400.
13. Bevilacqua MP, Pober JS, Wheeler ME, Cotran RS, Gimbrone MA Jr. Interleukin-1 activation of vascular endothelium. Effects on procoagulant activity and leukocyte adhesion. Am J Pathol 1985;121:394–403.
14. Boxer GJ, Curnutte JT, Boxer LA. Polymorphonuclear leukocyte function. Hosp Pract 1985;20:69–90.
15. Boyden S. The chemotactic effect of mixtures of antibody and antigen on polymorphonuclear leucocytes. J Exp Med 1962; 115:453–466.
16. Briggs RT, Drath DB, Karnovsky ML, Karnovsky MJ. Localization of NADH oxidase on the surface of human polymorphonuclear leukocytes by a new cytochemical method. J Cell Biol 1975;67:566–586.
17. Briggs RT, Robinson JM, Karnovsky ML, Karnovsky MJ. Superoxide production by polymorphonuclear leukocytes. A cytochemical approach. Histochemistry 1986;84:371–378.
18. Burns AR, Bowden RA, Abe Y, et al. P-selectin mediates neutrophil adhesion to endothelial cell borders. J Leukoc Biol 1999;65:299–306.
19. Burns AR, Bowden RA, MacDonell SD, et al. Analysis of tight junctions during neutrophil transendothelial migration. J Cell Sci 2000;113:45–57.

20. Caduff JH, Fischer LC, Burri PH Scanning electron microscope study of the developing microvasculature in the postnatal rat lung. Anat Rec 1986;216:154–164.

21. Cotran RS, Pober JS. Cytokine-endothelial interactions in inflammation, immunity, and vascular injury. J Am Soc Nephrol 1990;1:225–235.

22. Curnutte JT, Babior BM, Karnovsky ML. Fluoride-mediated activation of the respiratory burst in human neutrophils. A reversible process. J Clin Invest 1979;63:637–647.

23. Dejana E, Corada M, Lampugnani MG. Endothelial cell-to-cell junctions. FASEB J 1995;9:910–918.

24. Del Maschio A, Zanetti A, Corada M, et al. Polymorphonuclear leukocyte adhesion triggers the disorganization of endothelial cell-to-cell adherens junctions. J Cell Biol 1996;135:497–510.

25. Devreotes PN, Zigmond SH. Chemotaxis in eukaryotic cells: a focus on leukocytes and Dictyostelium. Annu Rev Cell Biol 1988;4:649–686.

26. Eckert R. Bioelectric control of ciliary activity. Locomotion in the ciliated protozoa is regulated by membrane-limited calcium fluxes. Science 1972;176:473–481.

27. Elsbach P, Weiss J. Oxygen-independent bactericidal systems of polymorphonuclear leukocytes. Adv Inflam Res 1981;2:95–113.

28. Elsbach P, Weiss J. Phagocytic cells: oxygen-independent antimicrobial systems. In: Gallin JI, Goldstein IM, Snyderman R, eds. Inflammation: Basic principles and clinical correlates. New York: Raven Press, 1988:445–470.

29. Fåhraeus R. The suspension stability of the blood. Physiol Rev 1929;9:241–274.

30. Feng D, Nagy JA, Pyne K, Dvorak HF, Dvorak AM. Neutrophils emigrate from venules by a transendothelial cell pathway in response to FMLP. J Exp Med 1998;187:903–915.

31. Foxman EF, Kunkel EJ, Butcher EC. Integrating conflicting chemotactic signals: the role of memory in leukocyte navigation. J Cell Biol 1999;147:577–587.

32. Frenette PS, Wagner DD. Adhesion molecules—Part I. N Engl J Med 1996;334:1526–1529.

33. Fridkin M, Najjar VA. Tuftsin: its chemistry, biology, and clinical potential. Crit Rev Biochem Mol Biol 1989;24:1–40.

34. Fuortes M, Jin W-w, Nathan C. Ceramide selectively inhibits early events in the response of human neutrophils to tumor necrosis factor. J Leukoc Biol 1996;59:451–460.

35. Gabig TG, Babior BM. Oxygen-dependent microbial killing by neutrophils. In: Oberley, LW, ed. Superoxide Dismutase, vol. 2. Boca Raton: CRC Press, 1982, pp. 1–13.

36. Gallin JI, Quie PG. Leukocyte Chemotaxis: methods, physiology, and clinical implications. New York: Raven Press, 1978.

37. Gallin JI, Seligmann BE Mobilization and adaptation of human neutrophil chemoattractant fMet-Leu-Phe receptors. Fed Proc 1984;43:2732–2736.

37a. Gallin JI. Phagocytic cells: disorders of functions. In: Gallin JI, Goldstein IM, Snyderman R, eds. Inflammation: basic principles and clinical correlates. New York: Raven Press, 1988:493–511.

38. Gallin JI, Snyderman R. (eds). Inflammation: basic principles and clinical correlates. 3rd ed. Philadelphia: Lippincott Williams & Wilkins, 1999.

39. Goldman R, Bar-Shavit Z. Phagocytosis—modes of particle recognition and stimulation by natural peptides. In: Karnovsky ML, and Bolis L, eds. Phagocytosis—past and future. New York: Academic Press, 1982, pp. 259–285.

40. Granger DN, Schmid-Schönbein GW. (eds). Physiology and pathophysiology of leukocyte adhesion. New York: Oxford University Press, Inc., 1995.

41. Gristina AG, Oga M, Webb LK, Hobgood CD. Adherent bacterial colonization in the pathogenesis of osteomyelitis. Science 1985;228:990–993.

42. Grotendorst GR, Martin GR. Cell movements in wound-healing and fibrosis. Rheumatology 1986;10:385–403.

43. Harlan JM, Liu DY, eds. Adhesion: its role in inflammatory disease. New York: WH Freeman, 1992.

44. Harlan JM. Leukocyte-endothelial interactions. Blood 1985;65:513–525.

45. Harris H. Chemotaxis of monocytes. Br J Exp Pathol 1953;34:276–279.

46. Henson PM, Henson JE, Fittschen C, et al. Phagocytic cells: degranulation and secretion. In: Gallin JI, Goldstein, IM, Snyderman R, eds. Inflammation: basic principles and clinical correlates. New York: Raven Press, 1988, pp. 363.

47. Hirsch JG. Cinemicrophotographic observations on granule lysis in polymorphonuclear leucocytes during phagocytosis. J Exp Med 1962;116:827–834.

48. Hirsch JG. Phagocytosis and degranulation. A 16mm silent movie. (Available from the Film Service Department, The Rockefeller University, York Avenue and E 66th Street, New York City, NY 10021.)

49. Hoffstein ST, Friedman RS, Weissmann G. Degranulation, membrane addition, and shape change during chemotactic factor-induced aggregation of human neutrophils. J Cell Biol 1982;95:234–241.

50. Hogg JC. Neutrophil kinetics and lung injury. Physiol Rev 1987;67:1249–1295.

51. Hurley JV. Acute inflammation: the effect of concurrent leucocytic emigration and increased permeability on particle retention by the vascular wall. Br J Exp Pathol 1964;45:627–633.

52. Hurley JV. Acute inflammation. Baltimore: Williams and Wilkins, 1972.

53. Joris I, Majno G. Atherosclerosis and inflammation. In: Chandler EB, Eurenius K, McMillan GC, Nelson CB, Schwartz CJ, Wessler S (eds). The thrombotic process in atherogenesis. Adv Exp Med Biol vol. 104. New York: Plenum Publishing Corp, 1978.

54. Joris I, Zand T, Nunnari JJ, Krolikowski FJ, Majno G. Studies on the pathogenesis of atherosclerosis. I. Adhesion and emigration of mononuclear cells in the aorta of hypercholesterolemic rats. Am J Pathol 1983;113:341–358.

55. Karnovsky ML. Metabolic basis of phagocytic activity. Physiol Rev 1962;42:143–168.

56. Karnovsky MJ, Robinson JM, Briggs RT, Karnovsky ML. Oxidative cytochemistry in phagocytosis: the interface between structure and function. Histochem J 1981;13:1–22.

57. Karnovsky ML, Sbarra AJ. Metabolic changes accompanying the ingestion of particulate matter by cells. Am J Clin Nutr 1960;8:147–155.

58. Kishimoto TK, Baldwin ET, Anderson DC. The role of β_2 integrins in inflammation. In: Gallin JI, Snyderman R (eds). Inflammation: basic principles and clinical correlates. 3rd ed. Philadelphia: Lippincott Williams & Wilkins, 1999, pp. 537–569.

59. Kitayama J, Carr MW, Roth SJ, Buccola J, Springer TA. Contrasting responses to multiple chemotactic stimuli in transendothelial migration. J Immunol 1997;158:2340–2349.

60. Klebanoff SJ. Oxygen Metabolites from Phagocytes. In: Gallin JI, Snyderman R (eds). Inflammation: basic principles and clinical correlates. 3rd ed. Philadelphia: Lippincott Williams & Wilkins, 1999, pp. 721–768.

61. Larsen SH, Reader RW, Kort EN, Tso W-W, Adler J. Change in direction of flagellar rotation is the basis of the chemotactic response in Escherichia coli. Nature 1974;249:74–77.

62. Lorant DE, Topham MK, Whatley RE, et al. Inflammatory roles of P-selectin. J Clin Invest 1993;92:559–570.

63. Lauffenburger DA, Rivero M, Kelly F, Ford R, DiRienzo J. Bacterial chemotaxis. Cell flux model, parameter measurement, population dynamics, and genetic manipulation. Ann NY Acad Sci 1987b;506:281–295.

64. Lavie G, Zucker-Franklin D, Franklin EC. Elastase-type proteases on the surface of human blood monocytes: possible role in amyloid formation. J Immunol 1980;125:175–180.

65. Lawrence MB, Springer TA. Leukocytes roll on a selectin at physiologic flow rates: distinction from and prerequisite for adhesion through integrins. Cell 1991;65:859–873.

66. Lehrer RI, Ganz T, Selsted ME. Defensins: endogenous antibiotic peptides of animal cells. Cell 1991;64:229–230.

67. Lien DC, Henson PM, Capen RL, et al. Neutrophil kinetics in the pulmonary microcirculation during acute inflammation. Lab Invest 1991;65:145–159.

68. MacGregor RR, Macarak EJ, Kefalides NA. Comparative adherence of granulocytes to endothelial monolayers and nylon fiber. J Clin Invest 1978;61:697–702.

69. Macnab RM, Koshland DE Jr. The gradient-sensing mechanism in bacterial chemotaxis. Proc Natl Acad Sci USA 1972;69:2509–2512.

70. Majno G. The capillary then and now: an overview of capillary pathology. Mod Pathol 1992;5:9–22.

71. Malech HL, Root RK, Gallin JI. Structural analysis of human neutrophil migration. J Cell Biol 1977;75:666–693.

72. Mandeville JTH, Lawson MA, Maxfield FR. Dynamic imaging of neutrophil migration in three dimensions: mechanical interactions between cells and matrix. J Leukoc Biol 1997;61:188–200.

73. Marchesi VT. The site of leucocyte emigration during inflammation. Q J Exp Physiol 1961;46:115–118.

74. Marchesi VT, Florey HW. Electron micrographic observations on the emigration of leucocytes. Q J Exp Physiol 1960;45:343–348.

75. Marlin SD, Springer TA. Purified intercellular adhesion molecule-1 (ICAM-1) is a ligand for lymphocyte function-associated antigen 1 (LFA-1). Cell 1987;51:813–819.

76. Martin-Padura I, Lostaglio S, Schneemann M, et al. Junctional adhesion molecule, a novel member of the immunoglobulin superfamily that distributes at intercellular junctions and modulates monocyte transmigration. J Cell Biol 1998;142:117–127.

77. McCutcheon M, Wartman WB, Dixon HM. Chemotropism of leukocytes in vitro. Arch Pathol 1934;17:607–614.

78. McEver RP. Leukocyte interactions mediated by selectins. Thromb. Haemost 1991;66:80–87.

79. Mesibov R, Adler J. Chemotaxis toward amino acids in Escherichia coli. J Bacteriol 1972;112:315–326.

80. Metchnikoff E. Lectures on the comparative pathology of inflammation. Translated from the French by FA Starling, EH Starling, 1892. New York: Dover Publications, 1968.

81. Middleton J, Neil S, Wintle J, et al. Transcytosis and surface presentation of IL-8 by venular edothelial cells. Cell 1997;91:385–395.

82. Muller WA. Leukocyte-endothelial cell adhesion molecules in transendothelial migration. In: Gallin JI, Snyderman R (eds). Inflammation: Basic Principles and Clinical Correlates. 3rd ed. Philadelphia:Lippincott Williams & Wilkins, 1999, pp. 585–592.

83. Muller WA, Randolph GJ. Migration of leukocytes across endothelium and beyond: molecules involved in the transmigration and fate of monocytes. J Leukoc Biol 1999;66:698–704.

84. Najjar VA, Nishioka K. "Tuftsin": a natural phagocytosis stimulating peptide. Nature 1970;228:672–673.

85. Najjar VA. Tuftsin, a natural activator of phagocyte cells: an overview. In: Najjar VA, Fridkin M. (eds). Antineoplastic, immunogenic and other effects of the tetrapeptide tuftsin: a natural macrophage activator. New York: The New York Academy of Sciences, 1983, pp. 1–11.

86. Nobis U, Pries AR, Cokelet GR, Gaehtgens P. Radial distribution of white cells during blood flow in small tubes. Microvasc Res 1985;29:295–304.

87. Oda T, Katori M, Hatanaka K, Yamashina S. Five steps in leukocyte extravasation in the microcirculation by chemoattractants. Mediators of inflammation 1992;1:403–409.

88. Orenstein JM, Shelton E. Membrane phenomena accompanying erythrophagocytosis. A scanning electron microscope study. Lab Invest 1977;36:363–374.

89. Panés J, Granger DN. Leukocyte-endothelial cell interactions: molecular mechanisms and implications in gastrointestinal disease. Gastroenterol 1998;114:1066–1090.

90. Parod RJ, Brain JD. Immune opsonin-independent phagocytosis by pulmonary macrophages. J Immunol 1986;136:2041–2047.

91. Payling Wright G. Introduction to pathology. Boston: Little, Brown, 1958.

92. Pfeffer W. Locomotorische Rchtungs-bewegungen durch chemische Reize. Ber Dtsch Bot Ges 1883;1:524–533.

93. Pober JS. Cotran RS. Cytokines and endothelial cell biology. Physiol Rev 1990;70:427–451.

94. Podack ER. Molecular assemblies in complement—and lymphocyte-mediated cytolysis. In: Steinman RM, and North RJ, eds. Mechanisms of host resistance to infectious agents, tumors and allografts. New York: The Rockefeller Press, 1986, pp. 217–230.

94a. Poznansky MC, Olszak IT, Foxall R, et al. Active movement of T cells away from a chemokine. Nature Med 2000; 6:543–548.

95. Ramsey SW, Adler J. Chemoreceptors in bacteria. Science 1969;166:1588–1597.

96. Randolph GJ, Furie MB. Mononuclear phagocytes egress from an in vitro model of the vascular wall by migrating across endothelium in the basal to apical direction: role of intercellular adhesion molecule 1 and the CD11/CD18 integrins. J Exp Med 1995;183:451–462.

97. Rittig MG, Häupl T, Burmester GR. Coiling phagocytosis: a way for MHC Class I presentation of bacterial antigens? Int Arch Allergy Immunol 1994;103:4–10.

98. Rittig MG, Kuhn K-H, Dechant CA, et al. Phagocytes from both vertebrate and invertebrate species use "coiling" phagocytosis. Dev & Comp Immunol 1996; 20:393–406.

99. Ross R. Atherogenesis. In: Gallin JI, Snyderman R (eds). Inflammation: Basic Principles and Clinical Correlates. 3rd ed. Philadelphia:Lippincott Williams & Wilkins, 1999, pp. 1083–1095.

100. Ross R. Atherosclerosis—an inflammatory disease. N Engl J Med 1999;340:115–126.

101. Rot A. Neutrophil attractant/activation protein-1 (interleukin-8) induces in vitro neutrophil migration by haptotactic mechanism. Eur J Immunol 1993;23:303–306.

102. Ruoslahti E, Pierschbacher MD. New perspectives in cell adhesion: RGD and integrins. Science 1987;238:491–497.

103. Savage DC, Fletcher M. Bacterial Adhesion: Mechanisms and Physiological Significance. New York: Plenum Press, 1985.

104. Sawyer DW, Sullivan JA, Mandell GL. Intracellular free calcium localization in neutrophils during phagocytosis. Science 1985;230:663–666.

105. Sbarra AJ, Karnovsky ML. The biochemical basis of phagocytosis. I. Metabolic changes during the ingestion of particles by polymorphonuclear leukocytes. J Biol Chem 1959;234:1355–1362.

106. Sbarra AJ, Selvaraj RJ, Paul BB, et al. Biochemical aspects of phagocytic cells: relationship between metabolic activities and physiological function. In: Altura BM, Saba TM, eds. Pathophysiology of the reticuloendothelial system. New York: Raven Press, 1981, pp. 19819–19829.

107. Schleimer RP, Rutledge BK. Cultured human vascular endothelial cells acquire adhesiveness for neutrophils after stimulation with interleukin 1, endotoxin, and tumor-promoting phorbol diesters. J Immunol 1986;136:649–654.

108. Schmid-Schönbein GW, Usami S, Skalak R, Chien S. The interaction of leukocytes and erythrocytes in capillary and postcapillary vessels. Microvasc Res 1980;19:45–70.

108a. Shulman ST, Phair JP, Peterson LR, Warren JR (eds). The biologic and clinical basis of infectious diseases. 5th ed. Philadelphia: WB Saunders Company, 1997.

109. Siemion IZ, Kluczyk A. Tuftsin: on the 30-year anniversary of Victor Najjar's discovery. Peptides 1999;20:645–674.

110. Smith CW. Transendothelial migration. In: Harlan JM, Liu DY, eds. Adhesion: its role in inflammatory disease. New York: WH Freeman, 1992, pp. 83–115.

111. Smith MR, Wood WB Jr. Surface phagocytosis. Further evidence of its destructive action upon fully encapsulated pneumococci in the absence of type-specific antibody. J Exp Med 1958;107:1–12.

112. Snyderman R, Uhing RJ. Phagocytic cells: stimulus-response coupling mechanisms. In: Gallin JI, Goldstein IM, Snyderman R, eds. Inflammation: basic principles and clinical correlates. New York: Raven Press, 1988, pp. 309–323.

113. Spitznagel JK. Antibiotic proteins of human neutrophils. J Clin Invest 1990;86:1381–1386.

114. Springer TA, Lasky LA. Sticky sugars for selectins. Nature 1991;349:196–197.

114a. Sriramarao P, Languino LR, Altieri DC. Fibrinogen mediates leukocyte-endothelium bridging in vivo at low shear forces. Blood 1996;9:3416–3423.

115. Steeber DA, Tedder TF. Molecular basis of lymphocyte migration. In: Gallin JI, Snyderman R (eds). Inflammation: Basic Principles and Clinical Correlates. 3rd ed. Philadelphia:Lippincott Williams & Wilkins, 1999, pp. 593–605.

116. Stossel TP. Phagocytosis. New Eng J Med 1974;290: 717–723, 774–780, and 833–839.

117. Styrt B, Sugerman B, Mummaw N, White JC. Chemorepulsion of trichomonads by products of neutrophil oxidative metabolism. J Inf Dis 1991;163:176–179.

118. Todd RF, Simpson PJ, Lucchesi BR. Anti–inflammatory properties of monoclonal anti-Mol (CD11b/CD18) antibodies in vitro and in vivo. In: Springer TA, Anderson DC, Rosenthal AS, Rothlein R, eds. Leukocyte adhesion molecules. New York: Springer-Verlag, 1988, pp. 125–137.

119. Tonnesen MG. Neutrophil-endothelial cell interactions: mechanisms of neutrophil adherence to vascular endothelium. J Invest Dermatol, 1989;93 (suppl. 2): 53S–58S.

120. Tsang N, Macnab R, Koshland DE Common mechanism for repellents and attractants in bacterial chemotaxis. Science 1973;181:60–63.

121. Utgaard JO, Jahnsen FL, Bakka A, Brandtzaeg P, Haraldsen G. Rapid secretion of prestored interleukin 8 from Weibel-Palade bodies of microvascular endothelial cells. J Exp Med 1998;188:1751–1756.

122. Vadas MA, Gamble JR, Smith WB. Regulation of myeloid blood cell-endothelial interaction by cytokines. In: Harlan, JM, Liu, DY, eds. Adhesion: its role in inflammatory disease. New York: WH Freeman, 1992, pp. 65–81.

123. Vel WAC, Namavar F, Verweij AMJJ, Pubben ANB, MacLaren DM. Killing capacity of human polymorphonuclear leukocytes in aerobic and anaerobic conditions. J Med Microbiol 1984;18:173–180.

124. Vicker MG, Lackie JM, Schill W. Neutrophil leucocyte chemotaxis is not induced by a spatial gradient of chemoattractant. J Cell Sci 1986;84:263–280.

125. von Oss C.J Phagocytosis as a surface phenomenon. Annu Rev Microbiol 1978;32:19–39.

126. Walters MN-I, Papadimitriou JM. Phagocytosis: a review. CRC Crit Rev Toxicol 1978;5:377–421.

127. Wilkinson PC. Chemotaxis and inflammation, 2nd ed. Edinburgh: Churchill Livingstone, 1982.

128. Witko-Sarsat V, Rieu P, Descamps-Latscha B, Lesavre P, Halbwachs-Mecarelli L. Neutrophils: molecules, functions and pathophysiological aspects. Lab Invest 2000;80: 617–653.

129. Wood WB Jr. White blood cells v. bacteria. Sci Am 1951;184:48–52.

130. Wright DG, Gallin JI. Secretory responses of human neutrophils: exocytosis of specific (secondary) granules by human neutrophils during adherence *in vitro* and during exudation *in vivo*. J Immunol 1979;123:285–294.

130a. Wysocki H, Wierusz-Wysocka B, Siekierka H, et al. Polymorphonuclear neutrophils function in untreated patients with chronic myeloid leukemia. 1988; Oncology 45:79–83.

131. Zigmond SH. Ability of polymorphonuclear leukocytes to orient in gradients of chemotactic factors. J Cell Biol 1977;75: 606–616.

132. Zigmond SH. Chemotaxis by polymorphonuclear leukocytes. J Cell Biol 1978;77:269–287.

133. Zimmerman GA, McIntyre TM, Mehra M, Prescott SM. Endothelial cell-associated platelet-activating factor: a novel mechanism for signaling intercellular adhesion. J Cell Biol 1990;110:529–540.

134. Zimmerman GA, Prescott SM, McIntyre TM. Endothelial cell interactions with granulocytes: tethering and signaling molecules. Immunol Today 1992;13:93–100.

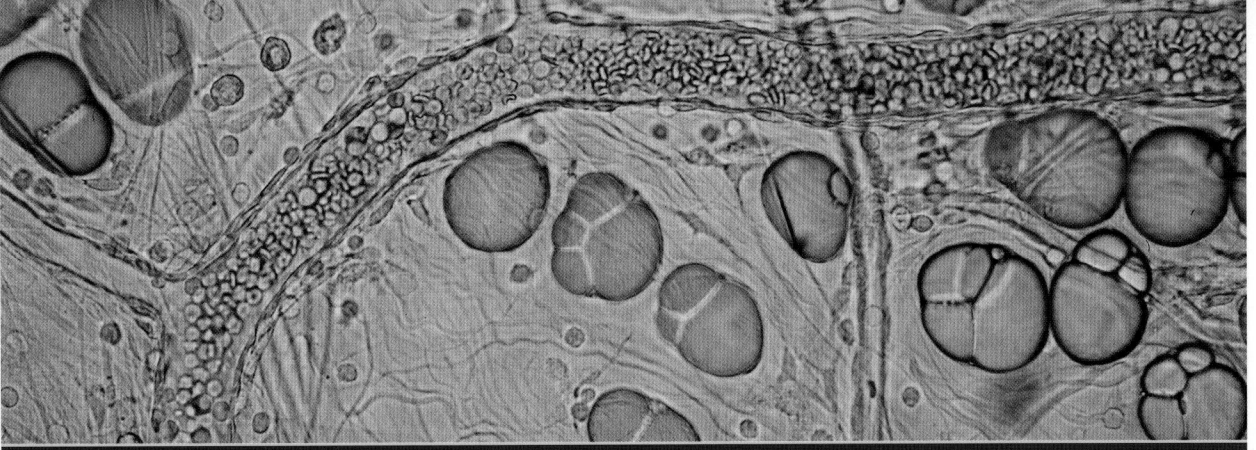

THE INFLAMMATORY EXUDATE

*E*xudate is the distinctive product of an inflammatory focus. It is a varied mixture of cells and fluid. Up to this point we have explained how these two components are conveyed to the area in distress; now we will see what we can learn from the exudate itself, which mirrors the events developing in the inflammatory focus.

The Cellular Sequence and Its Roots in Evolution

A basic feature of the exudate is that *the first cells to emigrate from the microcirculation are the neutrophils, followed by the monocytes and lymphocytes.* This sequence can be demonstrated by many simple experiments, such as the so-called *skin window:* a glass coverslip is taped over a few fine scratches on the skin of a volunteer; white blood cells climb out and stick to the coverslip, which is removed at a selected time, stained, and examined microscopically (Figure 12.1). Another model: inject into the peritoneum of a rat or mouse a very mild irritant, such as glycogen in saline, and then look at smears of the exudate every few hours (Figures 12.2, 12.3). The result is qualitatively always the same: the neutrophils respond first, the mononuclear cells follow a few hours later.

How is this sequence engineered? It used to be said that the neutrophils recruit the mononuclear cells; which is not entirely wrong, but it cannot be the basic explanation, because if the granulocytes are experimentally eliminated from the circulating blood, the mononuclear cells emigrate on schedule (29). The current view is that the endothelium is programmed to express the adhesion molecules that trap the required leukocytes (see Table 11.1). So be it, *but is this an innate, stereotyped inflammatory response, an immune response, or both? And more generally, how does the innate inflammatory response relate to the immune response?* These are

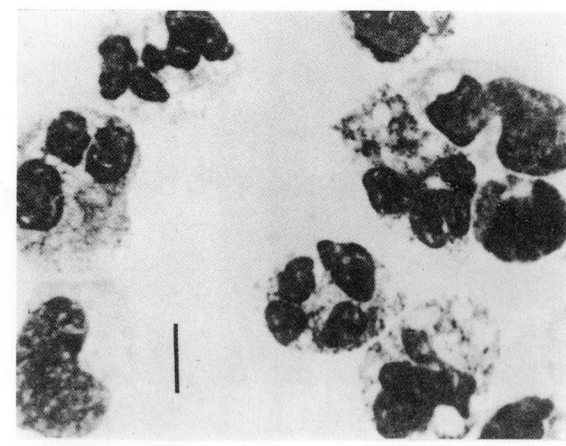

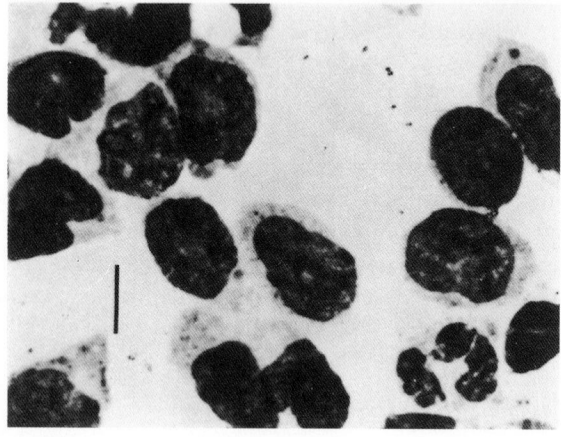

FIGURE 12.1 The sequence neutrophils–monocytes illustrated by the method of the "skin window." An area of skin 3 mm wide is scarified, and a coverslip is taped over it. *Top:* After 3 hours the predominant cell type on the coverslip is the neutrophil. *Bottom:* After 12 hours, the monocyte is predominant. **Bars** = 10 μm. (Reproduced with permission from [40].)

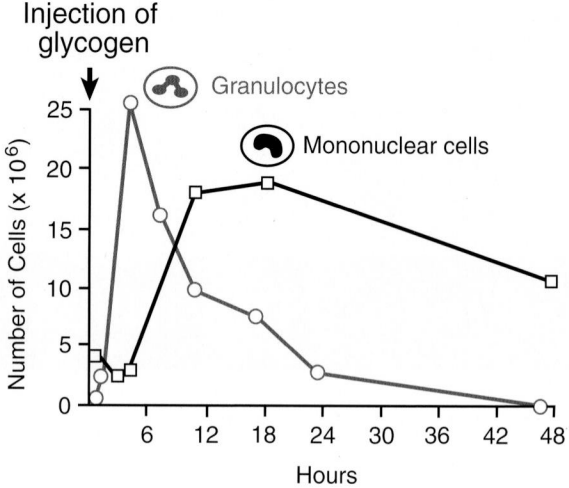

FIGURE 12.2 The cellular sequence of a typical acute inflammatory response, illustrated by injecting a mild irritant (glycogen) into the rat peritoneum. An early neutrophil response is followed by a more protracted mononuclear response. (Adapted with permission from [23].)

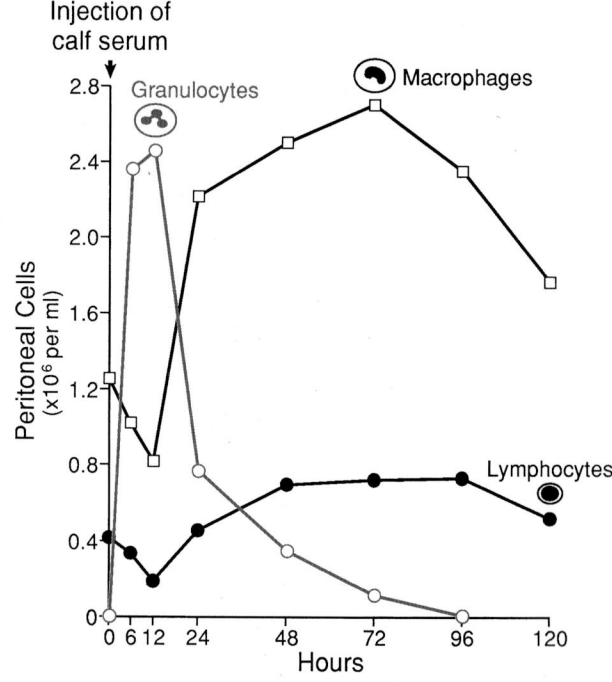

FIGURE 12.3 Changing numbers of granulocytes, macrophages, and lymphocytes in the mouse peritoneal cavity, which has been irritated by an injection of calf serum. (Reproduced from [45] with permission from Springer-Verlag.)

fundamental questions; to answer them we shall turn to evolution. We have no fossil lymphocytes, but we can climb down the evolutionary tree on which we now live, and find out—very succinctly—how our distant ancestors reacted to local injury (a complete story, not available, should include the evolution of wound healing, inflammation, infection, regeneration, and graft rejection).

Evolution and Inflammation

The inflammatory response to local injury (inflammation) developed in two phases (Figure 12.4) (7), which correspond by and large to invertebrates and vertebrates.

Phase 1. There was a time, about 1.4 billion years ago (50), when eukaryotes existed only as single cells; they crawled around, and ate—and so they invented

phagocytosis as a feeding device. They probably acted rather like Metchnikoff's starfish macrophages, and dealt with bacterial aggressors by eating them; we know for sure that they did phagocytize bacteria,

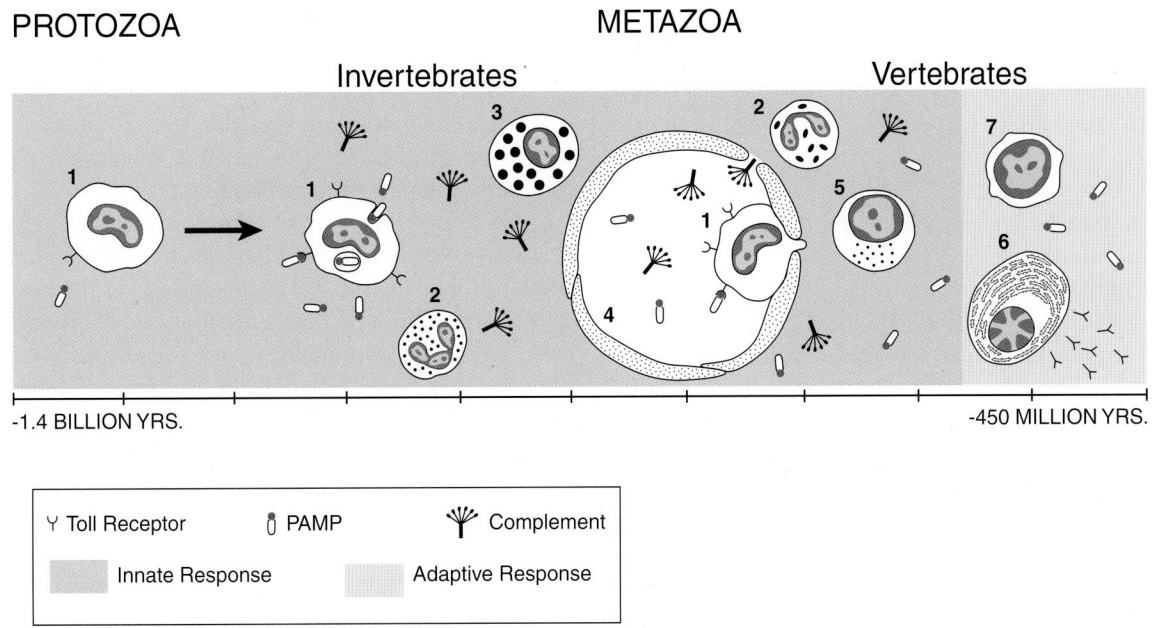

FIGURE 12.4   Evolution of the inflammatory response, innate and adaptive. A tentative scheme. (**Time scale:** 100 million years). 1 = primal macrophages; 2 = granulocytes (neutrophil and eosinophil); 3 = mast cell; 4 = endothelium; 5 = natural killer cell; 6 = plasma cell secreting antibody; 7 = T lymphocyte.

because some of the bacterial meals were not digested and became permanent intracellular guests as mitochondria. When multicellular creatures appeared they had internal fluid-filled spaces; some of the primal macrophages lived in them as defensive cells, mainly as antibacterial guardians. And when a circulatory system developed, a set of macrophages took to the bloodstream as monocytes, ready to be delivered where injury and/or infection called. In the blood they were joined by *granulocytes,* equipped with more efficient bactericidal molecules. In the meantime a noncellular device for killing bacteria appeared in the blood (34): that was *complement,* a mixture of proteins that could self-assemble into a bacteria-perforating machine. To pour out a large supply of complement in a hurry, in areas of injury, mechanisms of *controlled vascular leakage* developed; this included developing a large, redundant group of leakage-producing mediators, as well as sentinel cells ready to pour some out in an instant, the *mast cells,* which can trigger the whole innate inflammatory cascade. Rather late, small cells called *natural killer cells* appeared, specialized in killing virus-infected and tumor cells. A large number of antibiotic molecules also developed in many cell types, especially in the surface epithelia (antibiotic = antibacterial, antiviral, antifungal).

All these defenses could be summoned within minutes or faster: an important consideration in a world in which some pathogenic bacteria have a doubling time of 20 minutes. However, these defenses had two flaws: as antibiotic devices they lacked *specificity,* and they lacked *memory,* i.e., the ability to become more effective after repeated exposure to the same agent.

Phase 2. Both flaws were addressed about 450 million years ago by adding a new set of fighting cells endowed with both specificity and memory (19): *the T and B lymphocytes.* When instructed by activated dendritic cells (a type of cell related to the macrophage), the T cells could be trained to kill other cells with great specificity, while the B cells produced antibodies that could latch onto specific proteins (antigens) thereby adding a new dimension to the defense system.

Overall, then, Phase 1 defenses correspond to the innate, nonspecific, non-adaptive, stereotyped inflammatory response (typical of Invertebrates); Phase 2 defenses correspond to the immune, specific, adaptive, modulated inflammatory response (typical of Vertebrates).

At this point, take another look at the diagram of Figure 12.4. The innate defensive system is endowed with the largest arsenal; the immune system includes only two types of cells, the T and B lymphocytes. *In practice, the immune system, when called on, "borrows" the extensive resources of the innate system,* so it does not need to reinvent the blood vessels, the mechanisms of margination and diapedesis, the granulocytes, and so on. The two systems are constantly collaborating.

And now, as a bonus, we will share with you a nugget that emerged from the study of the innate defensive system.

Novel twist to the innate response: The TLR story.
The trail blazers on this new frontier have been the late Dr. Charles Janeway and collaborators at the Yale Medical School. Beginning in the 1990s, this group began publishing papers on the innate inflammatory response—but on an experimental animal that had little or no appeal to us: the fruit fly, *Drosophila* (31, 32). How could one learn the rules of mammalian inflammation in a tiny fly that has no closed vascular system and no adaptive immune response?

It turned out that the fruit fly had indeed little to teach us concerning "our" classic mammalian types of inflammation, but the fly faces bacteria, viruses, and fungi with a wholly different strategy. Over millions of years, evolution has taught *Drosophila* cells to "look" at (or better, scan) the surface of microscopic invaders, and to recognize on it some essential, repetitive molecular patterns (Parasite-Associated Molecular Patterns, **PAMP**s) which are vital to the aggressor and therefore unlikely to change with time; for example, lipopolysaccharide (LPS) for gram-negative bacteria. Each PAMP elicits the formation of specific receptors, called **Toll receptors;** when these receptors bind to the corresponding PAMP, the cell responds by showering the parasite with the appropriate antiparasitic peptides. These molecules are not as subtle as antibiotics, but they are very effective: *they poke holes in the cell membrane* (12). About 500 such peptides are known (including *Metchnikowin*); a prototype, **defensin,** is

so ancient that the molecule is similar in mammals, insects, and plants (19). In essence, *the fruit flies have learned to kill their parasites by hitting their most sensitive molecular targets.* Note that the Toll receptors are encoded in the *Drosophila* genes and immutable, so they are very different from antibodies.

The important part of this story is that it is not a purely invertebrate affair: humans have Toll-like receptors (TLRs), in fact, 10 at this time (31). Microbiologists have estimated that with about 20 TLRs most of the important pathogens would be covered (bacteria, viruses, and fungi) (3). To sum up, Janeway *et al.* discovered a new mechanism of defense against microscopic invaders. It is certainly innate, since it is recorded in the genes. It also has the two main features of the adaptive immune response—specificity and memory—but can one speak of immunologic memory if the specific encounter occurred 500 million years ago, rather than during the lifetime of an insect? We may need a new classification of innate defenses.

After this excursion into fruit-fly territory, we can return to the more familiar topic of mammalian exudates.

Correlation between escaping fluid and cells.
It is fairly easy to measure the time course of local accumulation of fluid and cells—for example, in the skin of a rabbit after a standard injection of live *E. coli* (Figure 12.5). As the figure shows, the curves are almost parallel. Fluid begins to pour out of the vessels immediately after injury; the leukocytes appear after a slight delay because they need some time to crawl out of the vessels (11, 18, 33). Some red blood cells, too, tend to escape across the leaky endothelium.

Why should an injection of *E. coli* increase vascular permeability? Because the endotoxin on the surface of these

FIGURE 12.5 Time course of inflammatory events in the skin of a rabbit after intradermal injection of live *E. coli* (2×10^7). Vascular permeability increases immediately and is promptly followed by microhemorrhage and extravasation of neutrophils. (Adapted from [33] with permission from S. Karger AG, Basel.)

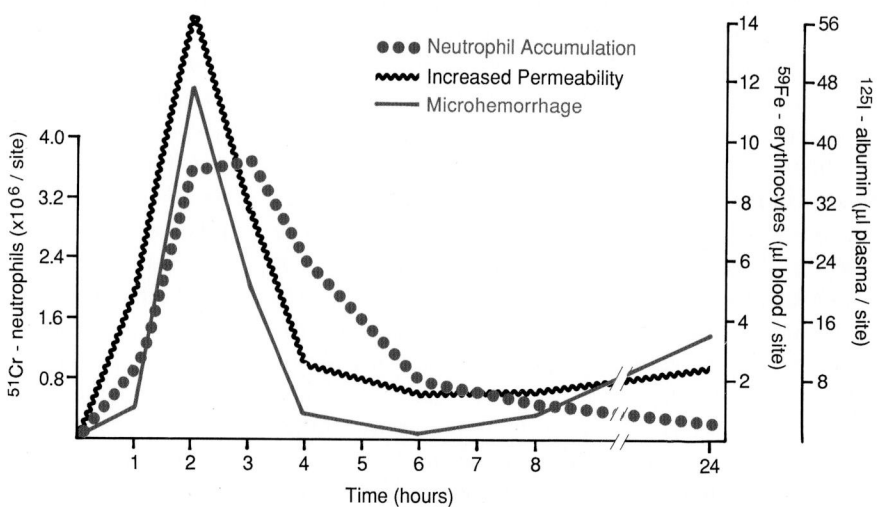

gram-negative bacteria activates complement; and when this happens, permeability-increasing molecules are released (p. 720).

Does the microcirculation become leaky as a result of diapedesis? We have mentioned that the passage of leukocytes tears up the basement membrane; it would not be surprising if persistent diapedesis also wore down the interendothelial junctions. Results vary, depending on the model, but on the whole it seems that diapedesis causes little or no leakage (6, 28).

> A bizarre development: it has been reported that rabbits made leukopenic with nitrogen mustard do not respond to the permeability-increasing mediator C5a desArg, a breakdown product of C5a (24, 47). Perhaps the nitrogen mustard makes the venules insensitive to permeability agents? Not so, because they still respond to histamine and bradykinin. We must conclude, rather surprisingly, that under certain conditions, "no leukocytes, no leakage."

Vascular leakage of any kind seems to be followed by a mild delayed episode of leukocyte emigration (Figure 12.6) (22), as if a plasma factor had become activated out in the tissues.

> The mechanism is not clear, but here is a possibility: exudate includes the plasma protein Hageman factor, which is activated by collagen fibers. Activated Hageman factor triggers three enzyme cascades, all of which produce chemotactic factors (p. 351).

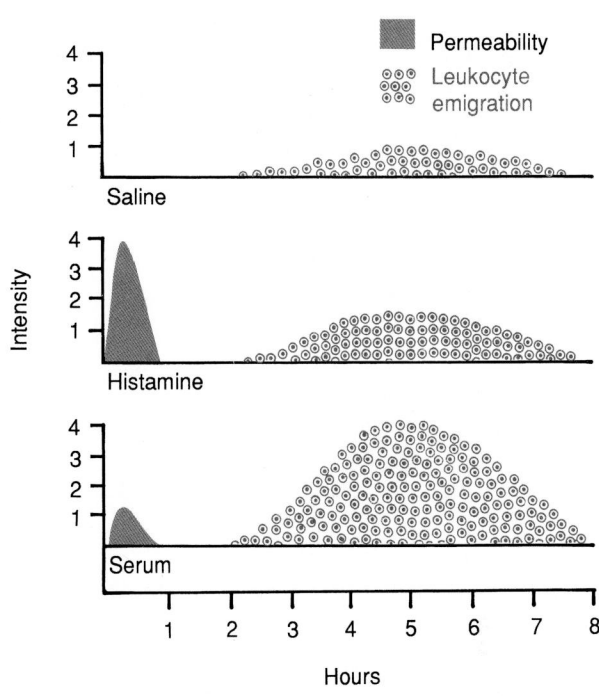

FIGURE 12.6 Examples of delayed leukocyte emigration, mainly of neutrophils, in rat skin after a local injection of vascular permeability-increasing agents such as normal saline, histamine, and serum. (Adapted with permission from [21].)

Functions of the Inflammatory Exudate

Assuming that the exudate was designed by evolution as an anti-parasitic and especially anti-bacterial fluid, we can rationalize a defensive function for its components. The mere bulk of fluid may be beneficial by diluting bacterial toxins (but we could also argue that the associated swelling should tend to diminish tissue oxygenation by increasing the distance between capillaries). The leukocytes phagocytize bacteria and debris, while delivering chemical commands to other cells; if an immune response is required, the dendritic cells and the macrophages initiate it, while the macrophages are also orchestrating general effects such as fever. The proteins of the exudate assist in the antibacterial fight by providing opsonins, antibodies, and the killing devices of complement; as to the fibrin network, even though there is no proof that it acts as a bacterial trap as tradition maintains, it probably does hamper bacteria in a different way: by providing leukocytes with a surface against which they can better trap their prey (*surface phagocytosis,* p. 418).

But then, what is the purpose of the exudate when there are no parasites to eliminate? Why, for example, should a myocardial infarct—a typically aseptic lesion—trigger acute inflammation?

The answer, we believe, lies once again in the evolutionary significance of inflammation as a primarily antibacterial response. It is a matter of urgency. The doubling time of common pathogenic bacteria is of the order of 20 minutes. The number of bacteria required to produce clinical infection is about 10^5 per gram of tissue (much less for beta-hemolytic streptococcus [14]); a single bacterium could reach that number in just 6 hours. Therefore, it is essential to destroy the colony as soon as possible. This is true also for antibiotic treatment (5) (Figure 12.7). Once bacteria have penetrated a tissue, there is a grace period of

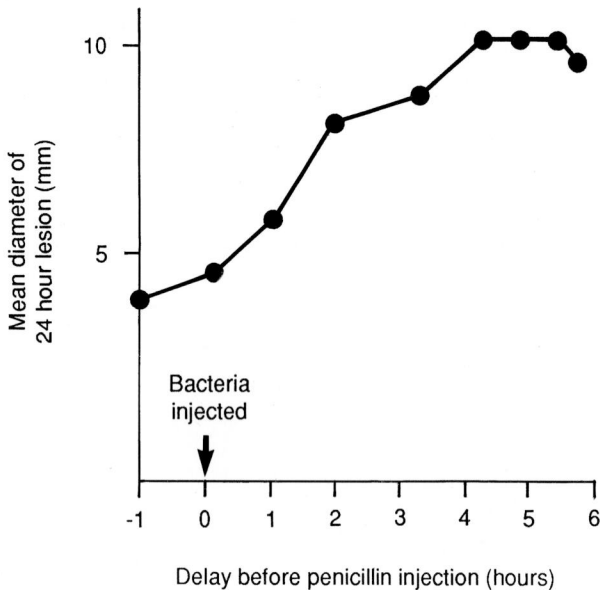

FIGURE 12.7 Effect of delaying antibiotic therapy after injection. Staphylococci were injected in the skin, and the size of the resulting lesion was measured 24 hours later. Penicillin was injected at various times during the 24 hours. As can be seen, the later the penicillin injection, the larger the lesion. (Adapted with permission from [5].)

2–4 hours during which the course of the infection can be influenced most successfully; after 6 hours the beachhead is well-entrenched and treatment is more difficult.

Therefore, *an efficient antibacterial defense program requires that the acute inflammatory response be triggered BEFORE the bacteria reveal their presence.* The price to pay is that any kind of tissue damage, infected or not, will induce an immediate acute inflammatory response. So the activated bactericidal neutrophils invading an infarct find "nothing to do"; they just rush in because they follow a program, dictated by chemical messages. In infarcts of the heart's left ventricle the neutrophils probably make matters worse: their enzymes tenderize the dead tissue and make it more prone to burst under the pressure from within the ventricle.

However, it would be presumptuous to conclude that the inflammatory response to an infarct is totally useless. All infarcts must be reabsorbed (organized) anyway, and inflammation is needed for that purpose. The first wave of inflammatory cells may be wasted, but the second, healing phase will perform a helpful function.

Transudates and Exudates

Recall: an **effusion** is any collection of fluid in a body cavity; a **transudate** is an effusion caused by a hydrostatic imbalance, an **exudate** is caused by inflammation. It is important to distinguish these two types of effusion, because they call for very different treatment.

Transudate. Described as "serous" (i.e., slightly yellowish but clear), transudates contain few cells, hence the comparison with *serum* (p. 638). A typical example is a bilateral pleural effusion in congestive heart failure. Being produced by ultrafiltration of plasma across a normal endothelium (no gaps!), transudates contain less protein than exudates. Exudates have the opposite properties: they are milky, due to large number of suspended leukocytes; and their protein content is closer to that of plasma (5 mg/100 ml), because the fluid component of exudates is made of plasma escaping from leaky venules (p. 388).

> Strictly speaking, all exudates should contain a portion of transudate, because the increased blood pressure in the inflamed microcirculation should force some fluid (a) out of endothelial gaps, but also (b) out of normal endothelial junctions, where ultrafiltration occurs. Picky readers will also remember that some filtration occurs also at the level of the gaps: the basement membrane retains some lipoproteins (p. 398). However, the basic point remains: transudates contain less protein than exudates.

The dividing line between transudates and exudates has long been set at ~3 grams protein/100 ml for pleural fluid, and 2.00–2.5 grams protein/100 ml for peritoneal fluid (2, 16, 39). Currently a more precise method is to compare the albumin level in blood and in the effusion: if the albumin level in the effusion is 12 grams/liter lower than in serum, the diagnosis is transudate (29a). Another useful test is the comparison of the levels of lactate dehydrogenase (LDH) between the blood and the effusion. LDH is a cytoplasmic enzyme present in almost all cells; its extracellular level therefore reflects cell destruction. In effusions it parallels the number of dead/dying cells (29a).

Inflammation and hydrostatic disturbances do not explain all effusions. A fluid tinged with blood—a **hemorrhagic** effusion—suggests either trauma, malignant tumor, or infarction (e.g., pulmonary infarct). Milky, so-called **chylous effusions** in the pleural space are due to the rupture of the thoracic duct. Rare **pseudochylous (cholesterol) effusions** with a greenish-golden iridescence contain visible cholesterol crystals and suggest chronic inflammation, e.g., tuberculosis (2).

Seroma, a pocket filled with clear, sterile fluid, is a postoperative complication; the term appears almost exclusively in the surgical literature (36, 42). Seromas develop in several surgical settings, and correspondingly the fluid may not always be quite the same. For example, a seroma can develop in the free tissue space created when surgery (e.g., mastectomy) requires the undermining of a large skin flap; in this case the fluid is mainly lymph. Seromas can also develop around a tubular Dacron graft inserted along an artery; suggested causes include "weeping" of fluid across the Dacron, a serous inflammatory reaction, and a collection of lymph escaping from severed lymphatics. In any event, seromas should be removed by needle aspiration because they are a good culture medium for bacteria.

Pus. A purulent exudate, or more simply pus, is an exudate rich in cells; its high cell content gives it a creamy look (a greenish hue is due to the high content of myeloperoxidase in the neutrophils [27]). Pus is typical of infections by strongly chemotactic bacteria such as staphylococci (Figure 12.8). It follows that the formation of pus (**suppuration**) denotes a healthy and vigorous

Table 12.1 Chemistry of Human Pus

Assay	Units	Value	Range	Normal plasma values
pH	pH	**6.17**	5.5–6.8	7.35–7.45
Osmolality	mOsm/kg H$_2$O	402	207–535	280–296
Sodium	mEq/L	119	92–134	135–145
Potassium	mEq/L	**18.5**	10–33.5	3.5–5.0
Chloride	mEq/L	87.9	60–109	100–108
Calcium	mg/dl	6.2	2.8–9.3	8.5–10.5
Phosphate	mg/dl	**14.5**	6.2[†]–28.2	3.0–4.5
Protein[a]	g/L	29.9	±12.6	60–84

(Adapted from [4], copyright 1987, with permission from Elsevier.)
[a]From [46].
[†]6.2 originally published as 62, which we take to be an error.

leukocytic response. This fact was recognized in antiquity, however dimly: "creamy pus" was considered good news and was known as *pus bonum et laudabile,* good and laudable pus, in contrast to relatively thin, bloody pus of rapidly progressing infections.

Pus is acidic, which discourages the bacteria as well as the leukocytes. Compared with plasma (Table 12.1) it has higher concentrations of two intracellular ions, potassium and phosphate, presumably from dead cells. The levels of potassium correlate with hemolysis and are high enough to activate neutrophils (50), perhaps a useful feature. Proteolytic activity is high, which may account for the low immunoglobulin and complement levels (46). The "digestive" activity of pus was mentioned earlier (p. 335) (30). The cell count in pleural pus has given figures on the order of 10^8 cells/ml (95 percent neutrophils, 60–90 percent alive) (46). Pus provides roughly *one neutrophil per bacterium:* a generous but not a wasteful supply. The percentage of live leukocytes varies a great deal (Figure 12.8); overall the phagocytic prowess of the leukocytes has been rather disappointing. Excuses for the leukocytes may be a low oxygen content and lack of an appropriate firm surface for practicing surface phagocytosis (p. 418) (3a); or more simply, that life is too short.

Fibrinous exudates. Solid masses or sheets of fibrin are often seen on an inflamed surface (e.g., peritoneum, pleura, an infected wound). They indicate that plasma has been oozing from that surface and fibrin was polymerized from it. With the microscope, some fibrin is found in all acutely inflamed tissues, but an exudate is called fibrinous when fibrin deposition is the dominant feature. Fibrin is essentially a blood clot without blood cells, thus it appears to the naked eye as a whitish material that might be compared to wet paper: a bland but

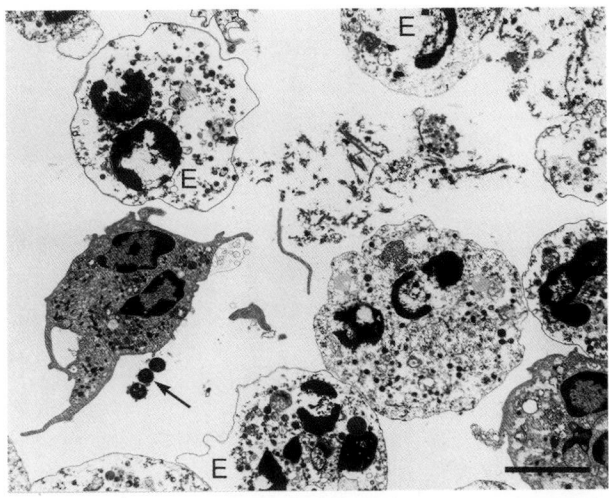

FIGURE 12.8   Electron microscopic aspect of pus from a subcutaneous infection of a guinea pig with *Staphylococcus aureus*. Most of the leukocytes are dead or dying as shown by cellular edema (**E**), nuclear changes, and cell debris. One live neutrophil has three bacteria (**arrow**) attached to it. **Bar** = 5 μm.

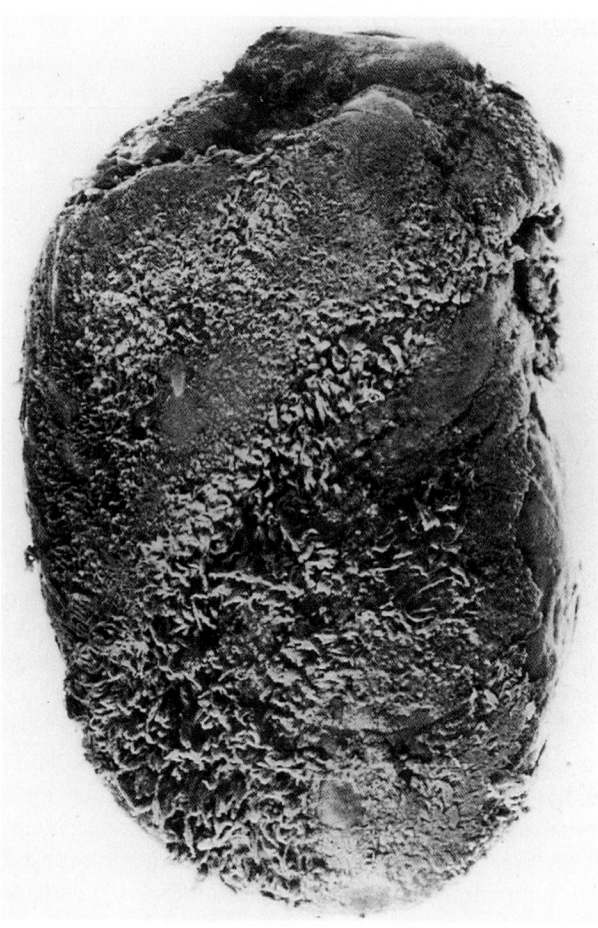

FIGURE 12.9   A human heart covered by a layer of fibrin. This is *fibrinous pericarditis,* once known as *cor villosum* ("hairy heart"), typical of uremia. The shaggy aspect of the fibrin deposit is thought to be due to the beating action of the heart. (Reproduced with permission from [10].)

unmistakable sight. When a thick fibrinous deposit coats the heart (*pericarditis*) it becomes furry, presumably because the heartbeat rubs it into threads (Figure 12.9); on the acutely inflamed peritoneum it looks rather like wet cotton wool (Figure 12.10). The presence of a fibrin coat on the heart or lung can be inferred clinically by a rubbing sound, due to the fact that the serosal surfaces are no longer smooth and slippery. The rub of an inflamed pleura was noticed even by the Hippocratic physicians, by placing an ear to the chest (30). Histologically, a thick fibrin deposit appears as an eosinophilic mass (Figure 12.11); it cannot persist indefinitely, because macrophages recognize it as abnormal and destroy it.

The mechanism of fibrin formation seems clear. Any plasma that seeps out of the vessels into tissue spaces contains the monomer fibrinogen as well as the protein Hageman factor, which is capable of triggering the clotting system. The Hageman factor is activated by contact with collagen, which is plentiful in the tissue spaces (p. 637). Activated macrophages may help clotting by producing procoagulant factors (15).

It is important to recognize fibrin because it signals trouble, as injury, inflammation, or both. Its monomer, fibrinogen, is normally retained by the endothelial barrier; the small amount that normally seeps into the tissues has presumably crossed the endothelium by pinocytosis. Therefore, fibrin in the tissue spaces means that plasma proteins have escaped from leaky blood vessels.

FIGURE 12.10   *Left:* Fibrin on the peritoneal surface. Compare this ragged coating with the smooth surface of the normal peritoneum (*right*). From a case of acute peritonitis. Photograph taken under fluid. **Scale** in millimeters.

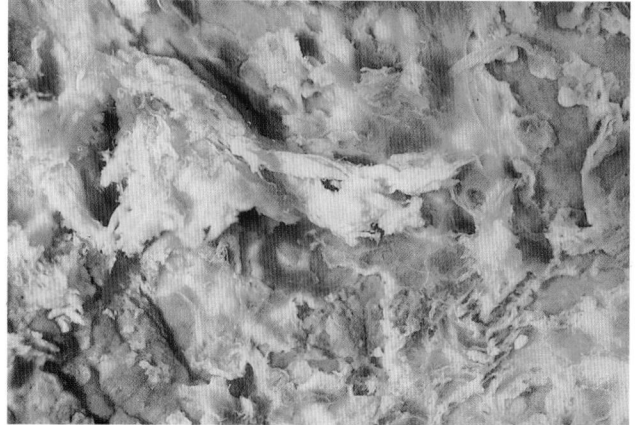 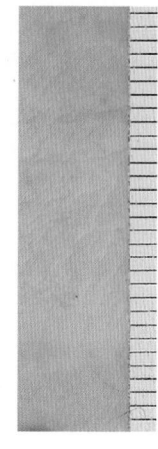

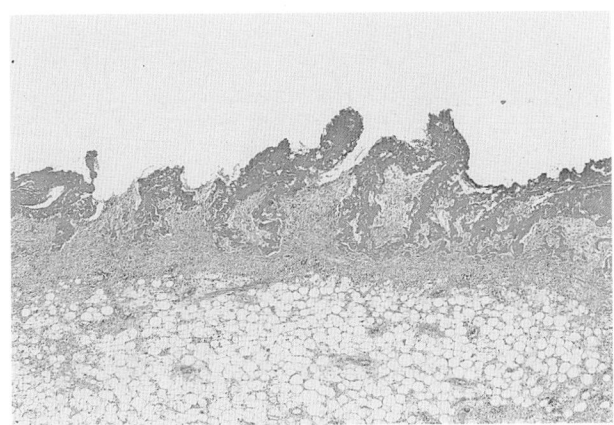

FIGURE 12.11 Histology of fibrinous pericarditis. The adipose tissue (lower half) corresponds to the epicardium. Above it is a layer of granulation tissue exuding lumps of fibrin (red material). The nature of the irritant in this condition is not known.

The Lymphatics in Inflammation

Much less is known about the lymphatics than about their distinguished relatives the blood vessels, in part because they are difficult to see by light microscopy. Imagine the smallest, "initial" lymphatics (41) as branching, open-ended tubes a little wider than blood capillaries, lined with thin, loosely overlapping endothelial cells architectured to function as one-way valves. Normally they reabsorb about 10 percent of the transudate oozing out of the blood capillaries, the remainder being reabsorbed by the venules. The initial lymphatics drain into collecting lymphatics, which have smooth muscle cells in their wall.

In acutely inflamed tissues the lymphatics have two functions: one hydraulic and one biological. *The hydraulic function* is to drain away the inflammatory edema, which is under high pressure (normally in most tissue spaces the pressure is negative, p. 615). We might guess that the thin-walled lymphatics, caught in the high pressure of the inflamed connective tissue, would be squeezed flat. Not so: they open up. Their outer walls are anchored to connective tissue fibers; when the tissue swells, the fibers are placed under tension, and the lymphatic is pulled open (Figure 12.12) (37). There is a limit to this mechanism: if the swelling is too great, the lymphatic is pulled apart and becomes nonfunctional.

The rising tissue pressure is transmitted to the lymph; values as high as 120 cm of water have been measured in the lymphatics of the ankle, after scalding the foot of anesthetized dogs (control values were close to zero) (9, 49).

Of course, the fluid drained off under such circumstances is not normal lymph: it is exudate, with a fibrinogen content approaching that of plasma, and it can clot. This is a rare event; Figure 12.13 shows an example, taken from a severe infection.

The biological function of the lymphatic vessels is to convey to the nearest lymph node, for processing, cells, bacteria and other antigenic and/or particulate foreign material. In this regard, the lymph nodes are placed along the lymphatic vessels like filtering stations;

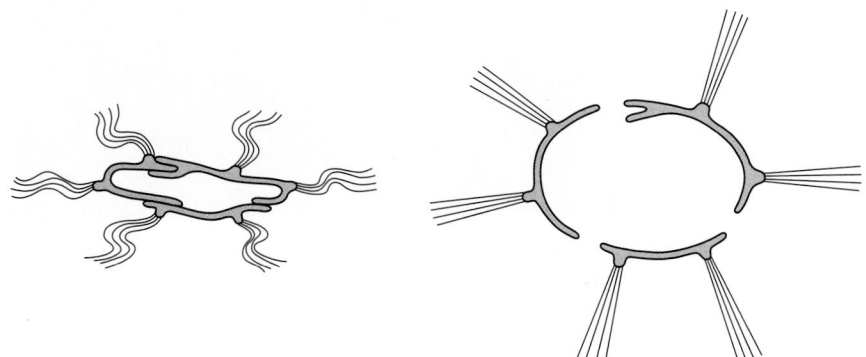

FIGURE 12.12 Behavior of lymphatic capillaries in edema: a diagram. *Left:* Normal condition: the lumen is narrow, the collagen fibers attached to the outer surface (anchoring fibrils) are relaxed. *Right:* In edematous tissue the anchoring fibrils are stretched; the lumen is dilated, and gaps develop in the wall of the capillary.

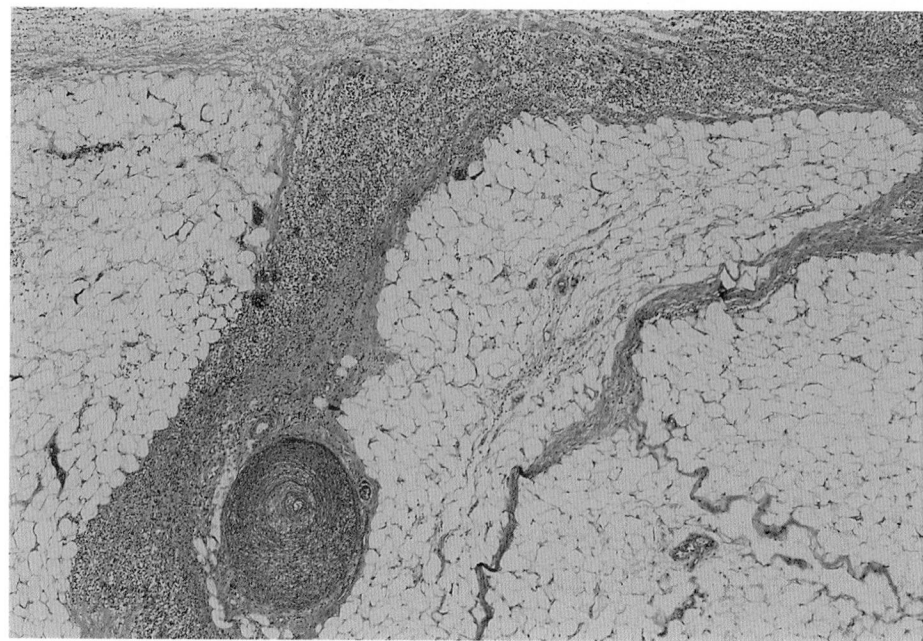

FIGURE 12.13 Subcutaneous tissue of the abdomen in a case of fulminant infection (*necrotizing fasciitis*). The greatly dilated lymphatic (lower left) carried so much exudate and cell debris that the fibrinogen clotted and the lumen became obstructed by layers of fibrin. (35x)

the incoming lymph (not the blood!) trickles through a three-dimensional maze of macrophages, which explains the efficiency of the system.

The filtering capacity of the lymph node can be tested with colloidal materials such as carbon black (remember the tattoo pigments) or with live bacteria. In one classic experiment, the popliteal lymph node of a dog was perfused (through an afferent lymphatic) with 5 ml of a culture medium containing 600 million bacteria per ml. After 80 minutes, cultures of the lymph draining out of the node showed that filtration had been 99 percent complete: "An efficiency so great as to make it fairly certain that in a part kept at rest [to minimize lymph flow] early in an infection, practically no microorganisms would escape the nodes in the line of drainage" (8). And if any did escape into the efferent lymph, and therefrom into the blood stream, they would run into another extremely efficient filter—the littoral phagocytes (p. 316).

Lympho-venous Anastomoses. There is evidence that some lymph—under high pressure—may find its way into small veins through lympho-venous anastomoses. Peripheral connections between blood and lymph are probably not open normally, but they seem to exist as "safety valves" that open during emergencies, certainly after the ligature of large lymphatic ducts, and perhaps during exercise (43). Under normal conditions, connections between blood and lymph have been demonstrated (functionally) in the lymph nodes (49). A recent study appears to fit with these data (38a), which leaves us somewhat skeptical.

If the challenge to the lymph node is mild (e.g., antigens only, no live bacteria) the node may simply enlarge, by a process that we can define as *hypertrophy;* in such cases it can become clinically palpable but remains painless. If it is overloaded by an infectious agent, the response will include *inflammation (lymphadenitis)*, and the swollen node is usually painful.

The lymphatic vessels conveying exudate to a lymph node are exposed to a "job-related" disease known clinically as the *lymphangitic streak;* we mention it here because it is generally misunderstood.

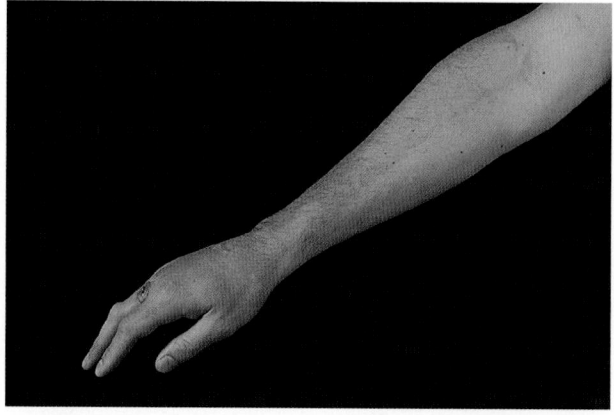

FIGURE 12.14 Example of noninfectious lymphangitic streak. Arm of a 32-year-old man, 36 hours after uprooting, without gloves, a stem of poison ivy. Note the faint red streak running from the wrist to the elbow crease. The hand is swollen and a blister has appeared. (Courtesy of Mr. R. J. Madison.)

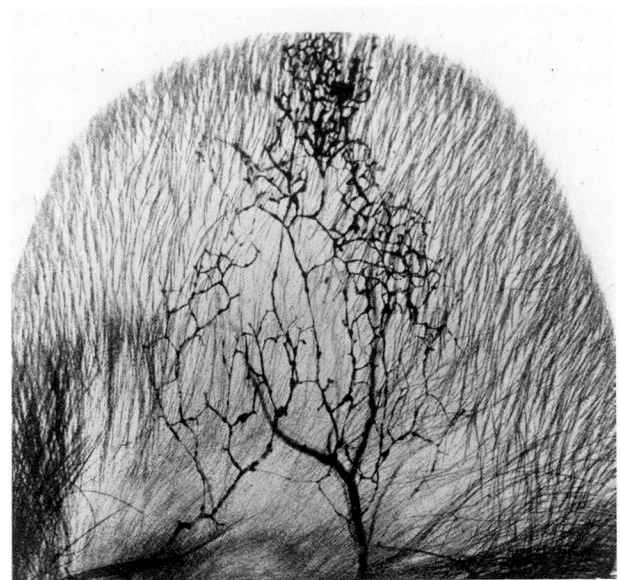

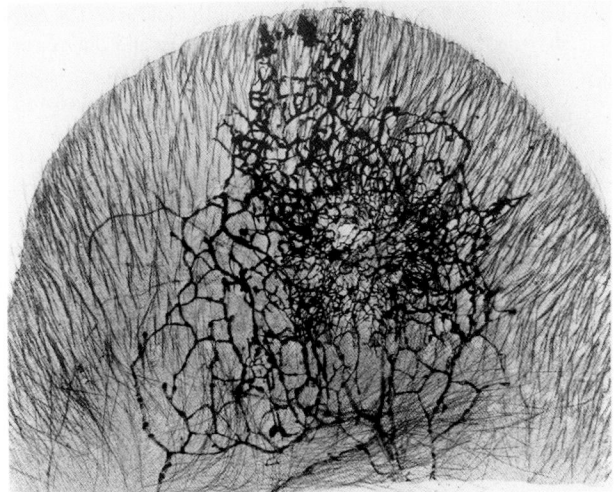

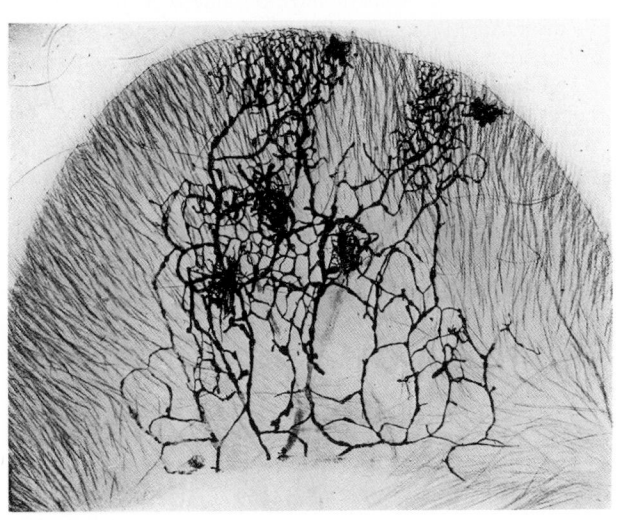

FIGURE 12.15 Proliferation of lymphatics in chronically inflamed skin (mouse ear). A black colloidal suspension of graphite was injected in the margin of the ear. *Top:* Lymphatics of a normal mouse ear. *Center:* Lymphatics, 21 days after induction, with a drop of turpentine, of a small abscess that perforated the ear. *Bottom:* Proliferation of lymphatics at three points where amorphous silica had been injected subcutaneously 3 months previously. (Reproduced with permission from [38].)

The lymphangitic streak. This rather frightening red streak is observed only in human skin (Figure 12.14), and as far as we know it has not been studied since John Hunter described it in 1794 (20). The usual setting: there is a severe infection of a hand or foot; suddenly one or two red streaks appear on the skin, running from the infected part to the elbow or knee. It is clear that they indicate inflammation along the large collecting lymphatic vessels (*lymphangitis*). Current thinking is that bacteria are escaping from the focus of infection, swarming in the lymphatics, and threatening to reach, ultimately, the bloodstream.

Nobody has seen the histology of a red streak; we assume that it would show inflammation around a lymphatic, but would it be *bacterial* inflammation? Not necessarily. We have seen typical red streaks developing in the arm after a severe, noninfected inflammation of the hand due to poison ivy (Figure 12.14) and from the red patch of a strongly positive tuberculin test. Both settings correspond to delayed hypersensitivity. This means that **a lymphangitic streak can also be generated by a focus of ASEPTIC inflammation.** The lymph draining a focus of acute inflammation is loaded with mediators (25) which a lymph node can easily handle (13). So, in some cases, the lymphangitic streak is just telling us that the lymph contains a high concentration of cytokines, which are oozing out of a lymphatic trunk and inflaming the skin: not a life-threatening situation. The clinical reflex of running to the antibiotics, in our opinion, needs rethinking.

Lymphangiogenesis. This term is new (it appeared in the wake of *angiogenesis*) but the phenomenon had been observed in England as far back as 1937: striking photographs of mouse ears showed dense networks of new lymphatics at sites of irritation (Figure 12.15). Little is known about lymphangiogenesis, except that it occurs in granulation tissue, with some delay after angiogenesis (49). So there is no doubt that new lymphatics can grow in inflamed tissues; they are just hard to see.

Injury to the cornea produces lymphatic vessel growth in the limbus (17, 26); and when a limb is experimentally amputated, lymph flow reappears after 3–6 days, indicating that the lymphatics have reconnected (1). We shall return to lymphangiogenesis in Chapter 26 (p. 778).

TO SUM UP: Nobody would doubt that inflammatory exudation is a marvellously orchestrated life-saving phenomenon. But then, we should not forget that parenchymal cells—in the tissues where inflammation rages—must take a dim view of the inflammatory exudate. To them it must be an acid, corrosive, hypertonic, asphyxiating medium, thick with proteolytic enzymes only partially controlled by plasma antiproteases (48). The trigger-happy activated neutrophils, spewing enzymes and free radicals, must be especially dangerous neighbors. These side effects of the exudate come to the foreground when inflammation involves tissues very sensitive to hydrolysis, such as articular cartilage, or to anoxia, such as the nervous system. In essence, a war—even if defensive—comes at a price.

References

1. Anthony JP, Foster RD, Price DC, Mahdavian M, Inoue Y. Lymphatic regeneration following microvascular limb replantation: a qualitative and quantitative animal study. J Reconstr Microsurg 1997;13:327–330.

2. Beers MH, Berkow R (eds). The Merck manual of diagnosis and therapy. Whitehouse Station, NJ: Merck Research Laboratories, 1999.

3. Brown P. Cinderella goes to the ball. Nature 2001:410: 1018–1020.

3a. Bryant RE. Effect of the suppurative environment on antibiotic activity. In: Root RK, Sande MA (eds). New dimensions in antimicrobial therapy. New York: Churchill Livingstone, 1984, pp. 313–337.

4. Bryant RE. Pus: friend or foe? In: Root RK, Trunkey DD, Sande, MA, eds. New surgical and medical approaches in infectious diseases. New York: Churchill Livingstone, 1987, pp. 31–48.

5. Burke JF. The effective period of preventive antibiotic action in experimental incisions and dermal lesions. Surgery 1961; 50:161–168.

6. Burns AR, Bowden RA, MacDonell SD, et al. Analysis of tight junctions during neutrophil transendothelial migration. J Cell Sci 2000;113:45–57.

7. Delves PJ, Roitt IM. The immune system. N Engl J Med 2000;343:37–49.

8. Drinker CK, Field ME, Ward HK. The filtering capacity of lymph nodes. J Exp Med 1934;59:393–407.

9. Field ME, Drinker CK, White JC. Lymph pressures in sterile inflammation. J Exp Med 1932;56:363–370.

10. Florey HW. General pathology, 4th ed. London: Lloyd-Luke (Medical Books), 1970, p. 29.

11. Forrest MJ, Jose PJ, Williams TJ. The role of the complement-derived polypeptide C5a in inflammatory reactions. In: Higgs GA, Williams TJ (eds). Inflammatory mediators. New York: MacMillan, 1985, pp. 99–115.

12. Gura T. Innate immunity: ancient system gets new respect. Science 2001;291:2068–2071.

13. Hall JG, Sinnett HD. The endolymphatic perfusion of lymph nodes with toxic materials. Br J Exp Pathol 1989;70: 283–292.

14. Heggers JP Variations on a theme. In Heggers JP, and Robsonn MC *Quantitative Bacteriology: Its Role in the Armamentarium of the Surgeon.* Boca Raton: CRC Press, 1991, pp. 15–23.

15. Helin H. Macrophage procoagulant factors—mediators of inflammatory and neoplastic tissue lesions. Med Biol 1986; 64:167–176.

16. Henry JB. Clinical diagnosis and management by laboratory methods. Philadelphia: W.B. Saunders Company, 1984.

17. Henson PM, Henson JE, Fittschen C, et al. Phagocytic cells: degranulation and secretion. In: Gallin JI, Goldstein, IM, Snyderman R, eds. Inflammation: basic principles and clinical correlates. New York: Raven Press, 1988, pp. 363–390.

18. Higgs GA, Williams TJ, eds. Inflammatory mediators. New York: MacMillan, 1985, pp. 99–115.

19. Hoffmann JA, Kafatos FC, Janeway CA, Ezekowitz RAB. Phylogenetic perspectives in innate immunity. Science 1999; 284:1313–1318.

20. Hunter J. A treatise on the blood, inflammation and gun-shot wounds. London: J. Richardson, 1794.

21. Hurley JV. Substances promoting leukocyte emigration. Ann NY Acad Sci 1964;116:918–935.

22. Hurley JV. Acute inflammation. Baltimore: Williams and Wilkins, 1972.

23. Hurley JV, Ryan GB, Friedman A. The mononuclear response to intrapleural injection in the rat. J Pathol Bacteriol 1966; 91:575–587.

24. Issekutz TB, Issekutz AC, Movat HZ. The *in vivo* quantitation and kinetics of monocyte migration into acute inflammatory tissue. Am J Pathol 1981;103:47–55.

25. Johnston MG, Hay JB, Movat HZ. Kinetics of prostaglandin production in various inflammatory lesions, measured in draining lymph. Am J Pathol 1979;95:225–238.

26. Junghans BM, Collin HB. Limbal lymphangiogenesis after corneal injury: an autoradiographic study. Curr Eye Res 1989; 8:91–100.

27. Klebanoff SJ. Oxygen Metabolites from Phagocytes. In: Gallin JI, Snyderman R (eds). Inflammation: basic principles and clinical correlates. 3rd ed. Philadelphia: Lippincott Williams & Wilkins, 1999, pp. 721–768.

28. Kubes P, Grisham MB, Barrowman JA, Gaginella T, Granger DN. Leukocyte-induced vascular protein leakage in cat mesentery. Am J Physiol 1991;261:H1872–H1879.

29. Leibovich SJ, Ross R. The role of the macrophage in wound repair. A study with hydrocortisone and antimacrophage serum. Am J Pathol 1975;78:71–100.

29a. Light RW. Pleural Effusion. New Engl J Med 2002;346: 1971–1977.

30. Majno G. The healing hand: man and wound in the ancient world. Cambridge: Harvard University Press, 1975.

31. Medzhitov R. Toll-like receptors and innate immunity. Nat Rev Immunol 2001;1:135–145.

32. Medzhitov R, Janeway C. Innate immunity. N Engl J Med 2000;343:338–344.

33. Movat HZ, Cybulsky MI. Neutrophil emigration and microvascular injury. Role of chemotaxins, endotoxin, interleukin-1 and tumor necrosis factor alpha. Pathol Immunopathol Res 1987;6:153–176.

34. Nonaka M. Evolution of the complement system. Curr Opin Immunol 2001;13:69–73.

35. Paavonen K, Puolakkainen P, Jussila L, Jahkola T, Alitalo K. Vascular endothelial growth factor receptor-3 in lymphangio-genesis in wound healing. Am J Pathol 2000;156:1499–1504.

36. Pricolo VE, Potenti F, Soderberg CH. Effect of perigraft seroma fluid on fibroblast proliferation *in vitro*. Ann Vas Surg 1991;5:462–466.

37. Pullinger BD, Florey HW. Some observations on the structure and functions of lymphatics: their behaviour in local oedema. Br J Exp Pathol 1935;16:49–61.

38. Pullinger BD, Florey HW. Proliferation of lymphatics in inflammation. J Pathol Bacteriol 1937;45:157–170.

38a. Rafii S, Skobe M. Splitting vessels: keeping lymph apart from the blood. Nat Med 2003;9:166–168.

39. Ravel R. Clinical Laboratory Medicine. St. Louis: Mosby, 1995.

40. Rebuck JW. Inflammatory cell dynamics in man. In: Reichard SM, Filkins JP (eds). The reticuloendothelial system. New York: Plenum Press, 1985, pp. 271–288.

41. Schmid-Schönbein. Mechanisms causing initial lymphatics to expand and compress to promote lymph flow. Arch Histol Cytol 1993;53 Suppl.:107–114.

42. Shaw JHF, Rumball EM. Complications and local recurrence following lymphadenectomy. Br J Surg 1990;77:760–764.

43. Threefoot SA. Lymphovenous anastomoses. In: Földi M, Casley-Smith, JR (eds). Lymphangiology. Stuttgart: FK Schattauer, 1983, pp. 177–184.

44. Tortora GJ, Funke BR, Case CL. Microbiology. An introduction. San Francisco: Benjamin Cummings, 2001, p. 278.

45. van Furth R. Mononuclear phagocytes in inflammation. In: Vane JR, Ferreira SH (eds). Inflammation. Berlin: Springer-Verlag, 1978, pp. 68–108.

46. Waldvogel FA. Pathophysiological mechanisms in pyogenic infections: two examples—pleural empyema and acute bacterial meningitis. In: Majno G, Cotran, RS, Kaufman N (eds). Current topics in inflammation and infection. Baltimore: Williams & Wilkins, 1982, pp. 115–122.

47. Wedmore CV, Williams TJ. Control of vascular permeability by polymorphonuclear leukocytes in inflammation. Nature 1981;289:646–650.

48. Woessner JF Jr, Dannenberg AM Jr, Pula PJ, et al. Extracellular collagenase, proteoglycanase and products of their activity, released in organ culture by intact dermal inflammatory lesions produced by sulfur mustard. J Invest Dermatol 1990;95:717–726.

49. Yoffey JM, Courtice FC. Lymphatics, lymph and the lymphomyeloid complex. London: Academic Press, 1970.

50. Zimmerli W, Gallin JI Pus potassium. Inflammation 1988; 12:37–43.

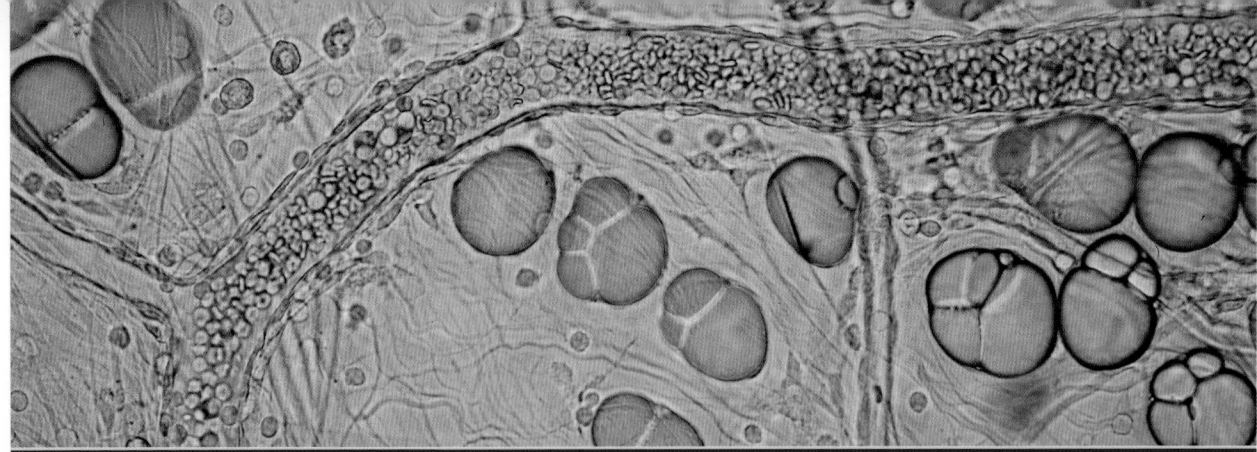

CHAPTER 13

CHRONIC INFLAMMATION

Chronic Inflammation: Defense at a Price

Chronic inflammation is good news and bad news. Good, because it means that the body's defenses are able to keep up a good fight; bad, because neither side is winning, and the collateral damage keeps rising.

> Remember that all organs are made up of two components: **parenchyma** (the functional part, i.e., glands, ducts, muscle) and **stroma** (the "bed" in which the parenchyma lies: connective tissue, vessels, and nerves). Inflammation takes place in the connective tissue.

To visualize the situation, look at Figure 13.1: it shows a section from a kidney suffering from chronic pyelonephritis, a bacterial infection. How can a beautiful kidney cortex come to look like this? Three major changes must have taken place:

1) Massive infiltration of mononuclear cells. The macrophages and lymphocytes in the tissue include cells recruited from the blood and their local offspring. Mechanism: the endothelium of the venules in chronically inflamed tissue modulates into a "high endothelium" phenotype (Figure 13.2), which expresses the adhesion molecules necessary for recruiting mononuclear cells (2, 7, 12–14, 24, 37, 64); the recruitment mechanism is similar to that for recruiting normal lymphocytes in the lymph nodes (Figure 13.3), but not identical (24, 40). Histochemically the activation (as manifested by the expression of adhesion molecules) is limited to the endothelium (Figure 13.4) (1a, 4a) (p. 408).

2) Massive loss of renal parenchyma (i.e., of epithelial structures). This is due in part to the bacteria, in part to the inflammatory cells; the large number of cells in Figure 13.1 suggests a rather severe infection, but the bacteria are not visible without special stains.

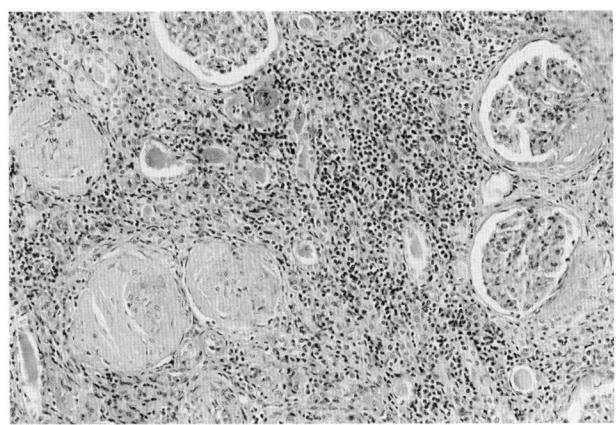

FIGURE 13.1 Typical example of chronic inflammation: pyelonephritis (bacterial infection of the kidney). The renal epithelial structures have been largely destroyed. Some glomeruli are hyalinized (*bottom left*), others show little change but they are not connected to a system of tubules. The latter have been destroyed; the space they occupied is taken over by connective tissue (granulation tissue) with a heavy infiltrate of mononuclear cells and remnants of tubules (rounded or oval masses without nuclei). (120x)

Research in this important field—we referred to it above as **collateral damage** of inflammation—is surprisingly rare. Anyway, we can assume that normal cells do not thrive in a bath of inflammatory cytokines.

3) Development of new and special connective tissue. This is somewhat hidden among the inflammatory cells, but

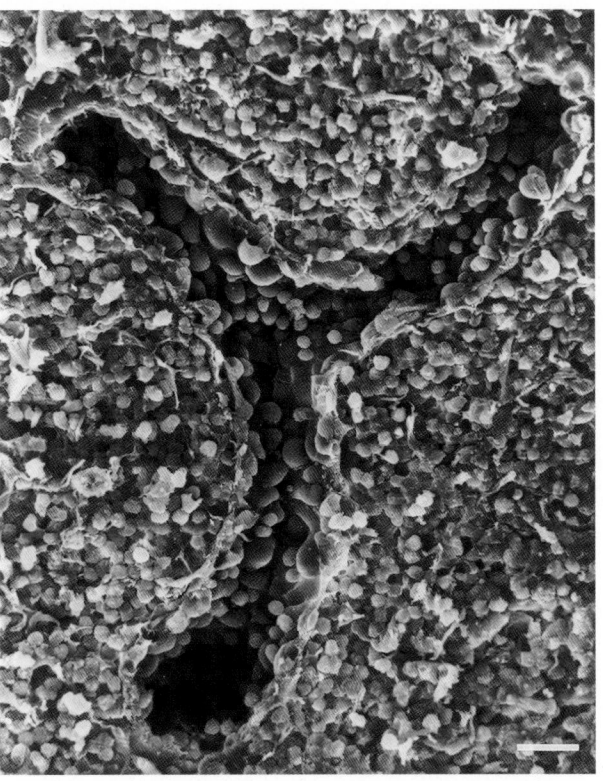

FIGURE 13.3 A high-endothelial venule: scanning electron micrograph showing the cut surface of a mouse lymph node. Note many lymphocytes attached to the plump endothelial cells; nonadherent blood elements were removed by perfusion before fixation. **Bar** = 50 μm. (Reprinted from [187], Copyright 1980, with permission from Elsevier.)

FIGURE 13.2 Large postcapillary venule in the synovium from a case of rheumatoid arthritis. Note the thickened ("activated") endothelium and two emigrating lymphocytes (**arrowheads**). Both features recall the high-endothelial venules of normal lymph nodes. **Bar** = 5 μm. (Reproduced with permission from the Journal of Clinical Investigation [23]. Copyright 1986 by the American Society for Clinical Investigation via the Copyright Clearance Center.)

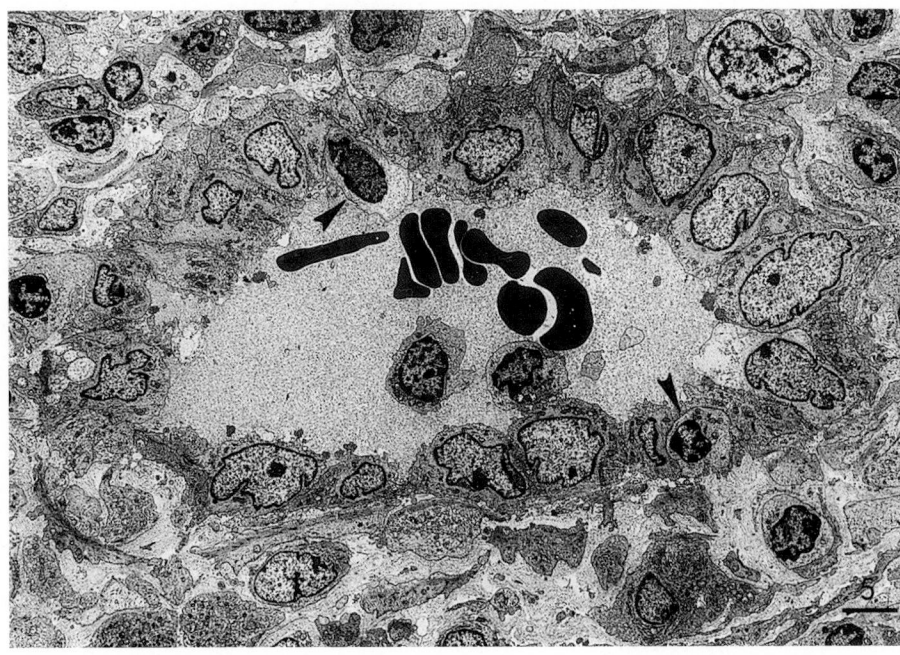

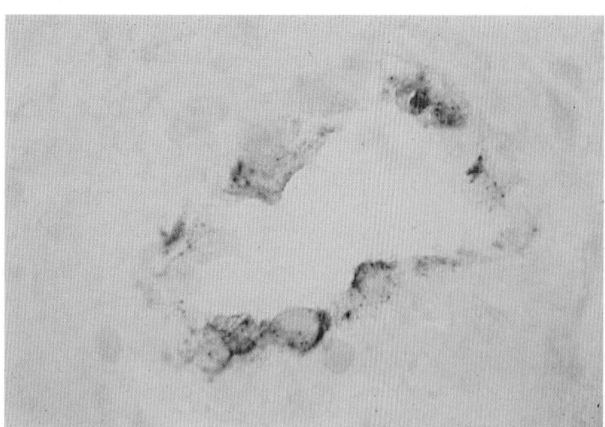

FIGURE 13.4 Typical activated, thickened endothelium 23 hours after local injection of streptococcal antigens. Immunoperoxidase demonstration of an adhesion molecule, the first so identified: ELAM-1 (endothelium-leukocyte adhesion molecule 1). The staining is limited to the endothelial cells; from a human volunteer. (Reproduced from Cotran RS, Gimbrone MA Jr, Bevilacqua MP, et al. Induction and detection of a human activation antigen *in vivo*. J Exp Med 1986;164:661–666 by copyright permission of the Rockefeller University Press [5].)

it is there: it is known as *granulation tissue,* a key component of chronic inflammation. *The concept of granulation tissue* was explained in the panoramic overview of inflammation (Figures 8.26–8.31). In essence: after a day or two of acute inflammation, the connective tissue—in which the inflammatory reaction is unfolding—begins to react, producing more fibroblasts, more capillaries, more cells—more tissue. In other words, granulation tissue arises from normal connective tissue by a process akin to regeneration, but it cannot be mistaken for normal connective tissue, because its fibroblasts are plump and activated, it contains many budding capillaries, and a sprinkling of inflammatory cells, including plasma cells if there is infection (Figures 13.5, 13.6). The sprouting capillaries are typical (Figure 13.7); being incompletely formed they are leaky and contribute to the inflammatory exudate.

This basic structure varies depending on the stimulus, which may be septic or aseptic. *Granulation tissue often acts as a barrier, e.g., forming a sheet between normal and dead tissue,* or between normal and infected tissue, or lining the bottom of a wound; in such cases it has an inner "active" face and an outer, more fibrous face (Figure 13.8). With time, its function accomplished, granulation tissue loses most of its cells, the collagen component increases, and the terminal picture blends with that of a scar.

Granulation tissue is an old surgical term related to wound healing: originally it applied to the little lumps or "granules" of young connective tissue that glisten on the raw surface of a healing wound. Later it was adopted in the terminology of chronic inflammation. In either case we are dealing with new, growing, richly vascularized and inflamed connective tissue.

FIGURE 13.5 *Typical young granulation tissue.* It surrounds a hematoma produced by injecting 3 ml of blood into the perirenal fat pad of a rat. After 5 days the blood had clotted; between the clot and the fat there was no sharp limit. *Top left:* part of the clot. Empty circles at right: adipocytes of the fat pad. Swarms of fibroblasts infiltrate the fat and connect it to the clot. This is an early step in the process of *organization.* For cellular details see Figure 13.6. (90x)

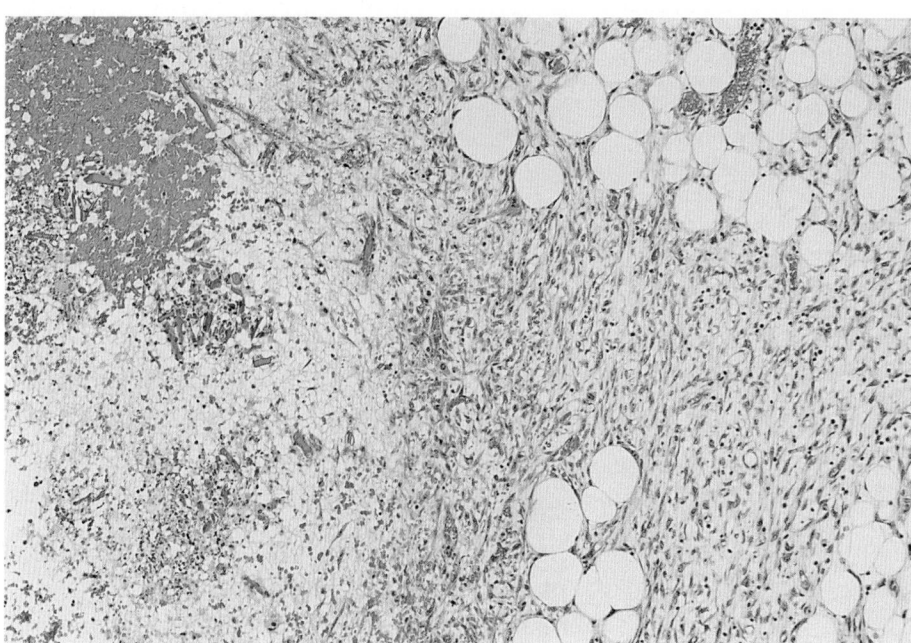

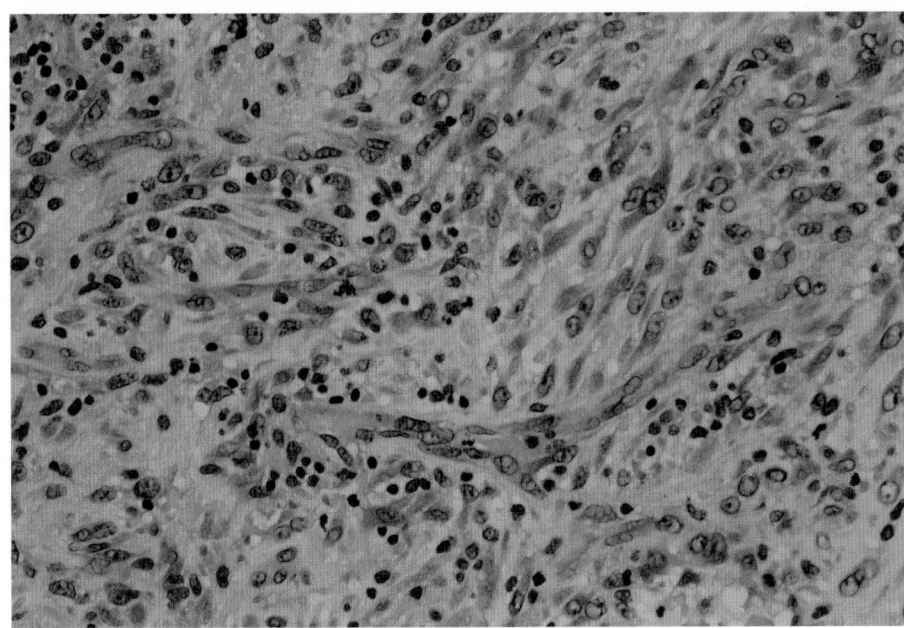

FIGURE 13.6 Typical granulation tissue (human epicardium, 7 days after open heart surgery). The tissue consists mainly of oblong cells (fibroblasts), macrophages, and capillary sprouts (streaks of elongated cells). Red blood cells (pink) help identify capillaries and capillary sprouts. There also is a sprinkling of lymphocytes (dark nuclei). The overall bluish tinge is due to the basophilia of the cells, which are actively synthesizing protein.

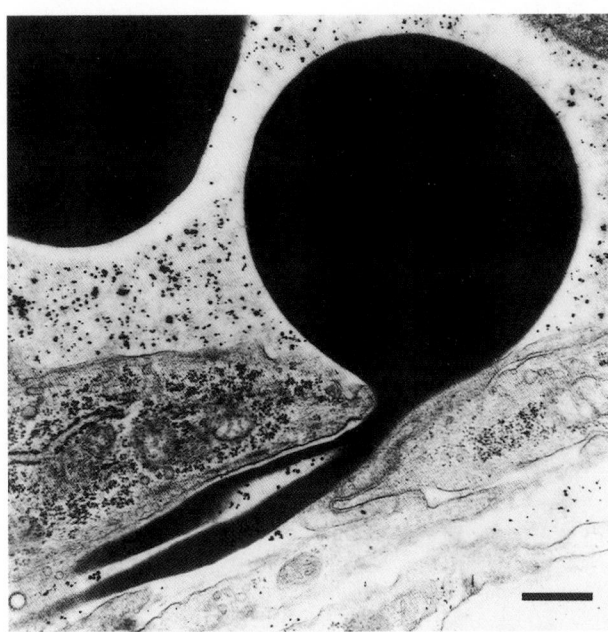

FIGURE 13.7 Red blood cell squeezing out of a regenerating capillary through a junction between two endothelial cells. This electron micrograph illustrates the excessive permeability of newly formed capillaries in granulation tissue, as well as the great plasticity of the red blood cells. **Bar** = 0.5 μm. (Reproduced by permission from [48]. Copyright Springer-Verlag GmbH & Co. KG.)

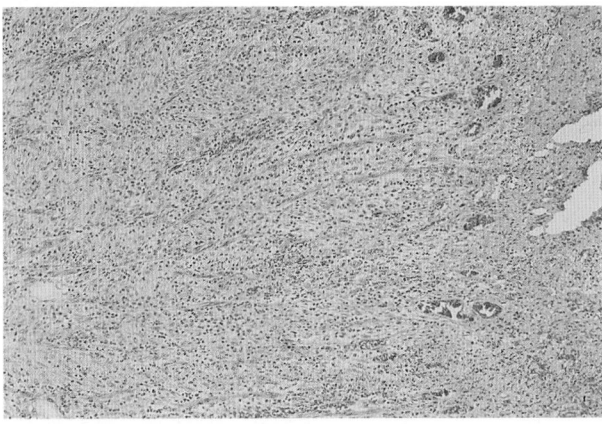

FIGURE 13.8 Granulation tissue from a case of empyema of the pleura in a 30-year-old man. The pleura had been infected 3 weeks earlier, and the inner surface of the chest wall had become lined with a layer of granulation tissue about 8 mm thick. The surface of the layer facing the pleural cavity and exuding pus is seen here at the right. The cellular population consists mainly of fibroblasts, macrophages (not distinguishable at this enlargement) and many newly formed capillaries, recognizable as long, thin streaks of nuclei. (60x)

The Many Faces of Chronic Inflammation

Chronic inflammation takes on a variety of aspects depending mainly on the setting (to maintain the military metaphor, we would say the geography of the battlefield) and on the agent, infectious or aseptic. The typical settings are five: "organization", i.e., aseptic reabsorption; the abscess; ulcers; adhesions; and granulomatus inflammation.

"Organization": Aseptic Reabsorption

*Organization is the process whereby a layer of granulation tissue removes **aseptic,** absorbable material* such as dead tissue, fibrin, or a surgical sponge. In essence, this is a large-scale scavenging operation, and correspondingly the cells that do most of the work are macrophages. A classic example is the reabsorption of an infarct, presumed to be aseptic (the septic counterpart of this process is the *abscess*). The reabsorption of an aseptic infarct can be demonstrated experimentally by placing a fragment of sterile rat liver in the peritoneal cavity of another rat: after a brief episode of acute inflammation, the omentum surrounds the dead tissue and its organization is under way (see Figures 8.26–8.31). Notice, in

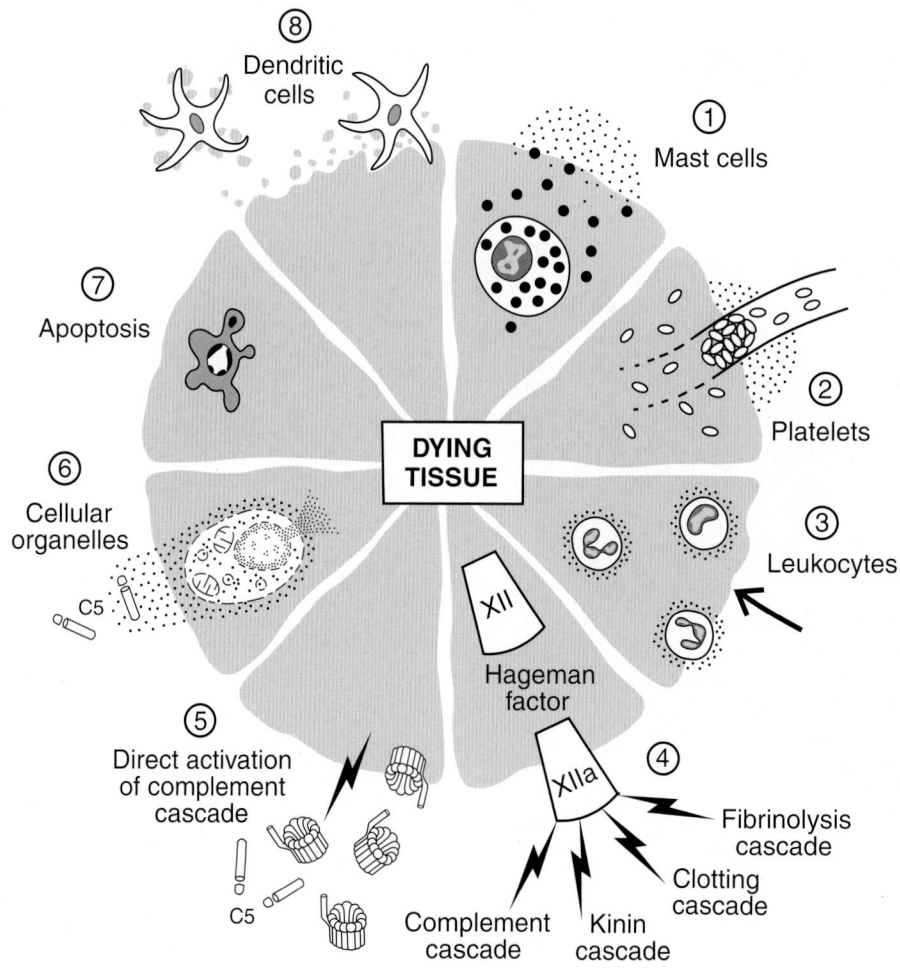

FIGURE 13.9 **Why is inflammation induced by dying tissue?** Some of the basic mechanisms. (1) Degranulating mast cells release preformed mediators (histamine, TNF). (2) Platelets release at least 20 preformed mediators. (3) Leukocytes attracted to dying cells release enzymes which generate secondary mediators. (4) Hageman factor (in plasma) is activated; it activates four enzyme cascades, each one generating inflammatory molecules. (5) Direct activation of complement by cell breakdown products. (6) Cells that die by swelling release irritant materials from the nucleus, from mitochondria, from lysosomes and from the cytoplasm. (7) Apoptotic cells release minimal amounts of irritants. (8) Dendritic cells acquire antigens from the dying cells and initiate an immune response.

these figures, the natural history of the granulation tissue, which starts out as highly cellular and slowly becomes more fibrous.

The term *organization,* although very handy, sounds like a rather peculiar choice, and indeed it derives from an obsolete concept of the 1800s: *"Where there was dead tissue there is now granulation tissue; so, the dead tissue must have been revitalized or "organized" into live tissue."*

How Does Dead Tissue Trigger Inflammation?

Cells in the throes of death release hundreds of molecular species, hereafter referred to as **irritants;** this oozing stops only after 12–24 hours, when the cell has become a mass of inert denatured proteins (p. 205). The main sources or groups of irritants are listed below (Figure 13.9).

1. **Mast cells** release histamine, preformed TNF, derivatives of arachidonic acid, and much else.

2. **Platelets** clog the capillaries where they penetrate into dying tissue; they burst and release at least 20 mediators (p. 341).

3. **Leukocytes** attracted to the dying tissue release dozens of enzymes, bactericidal peptides, etc. (p. 334).

4. **Hageman Factor (Clotting Factor XII),** a component of plasma, is activated when exposed to collagen fibers, and in turn activates four enzyme cascades, each one leading to inflammatory products (p. 351).

5. **Complement** is activated directly by necrotic tissue (Figure 13.10) (8, 47, 57) and by components of injured cells (38, 44, 50, 53). Complement activation means, of course, release of inflammatory anaphylatoxins C3a, C4a, and C5a (19, 23, 36, 39, 60) (p. 354).

   Does this mean that precious complement is being wasted on killing dead cells? Perhaps it does give some dying cells the *coup de grâce* (39). Experiments on myocardial ischemia showed that **anticomplement treatment** reduced the size of the infarct (35, 61); it also reduced the influx of leukocytes (27).

6. **Cells that die by swelling (oncosis)** release a variety of materials from their swollen organelles: from the *nucleus,* chromatin proteins (46b); from the *mitochondria,* N-formylmethionyl peptides, typical of prokaryotes (1b), not surprisingly, because the mitochondria are the descendants of bacteria; from the *lysosomes,* proteases that can cleave complement components and generate anaphylatoxins as in (5) and from the cytoplasm (uric acid, p. 227).

7. **Apoptotic** cells were thought to die *in incognito* (p. 210), but it was recently shown that they do emit soluble signals, conveying messages such as

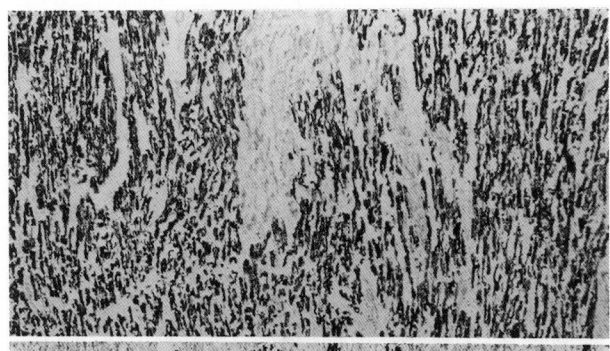
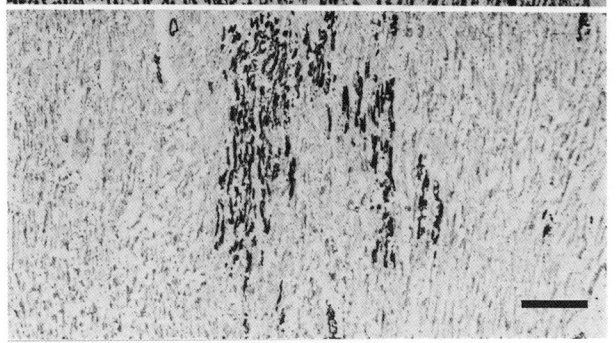

FIGURE 13.10 Presence of complement membrane-attack complex (MAC) in necrotic tissue. *Top:* Myocardium stained for succinic dehydrogenase: the central area devoid of enzyme represents a 6–7 day old infarct. *Bottom:* A consecutive section stained for the C5b-9 complex shows the reverse staining pattern: the complex is present only in the infarct. **Bar** = 250 μm. (Reproduced by permission from [47], © by Williams & Wilkins, 1986.)

"come hither, scavengers", "eat me" and possibly also "eat me or die." Scavengers carry a receptor that recognizes phosphatidylserine on the apoptotic cell (46a).

8. **Dendritic cells** take up cellular proteins, migrate to the draining lymph node and stimulate cytotoxic T-cell responses (51a).

The Abscess

An abscess is a collection of pus in a newly formed cavity (*abscess* is from the Latin *abscessum,* "cut off", in the sense of "material set aside", first used by Celsus; a literal translation of the Greek *apóstema*). Collections of pus can also develop in preexisting spaces, but they are given special names that have been consecrated by the centuries, such as *empyema* for the pleural cavity and *pyosalpinx* for the fallopian tube (remember that the Greek *py-* is the root for *pus*).

An abscess begins as a microscopic battle between a parasite—usually a pyogenic bacterium, sometimes amoebae (56)—and an army of neutrophils. The bacteria, which may have arrived by the blood stream or by

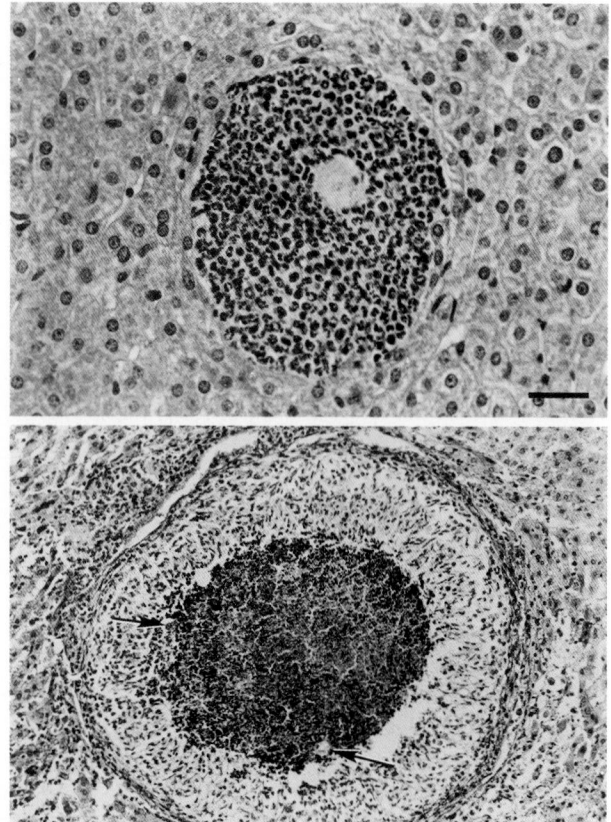

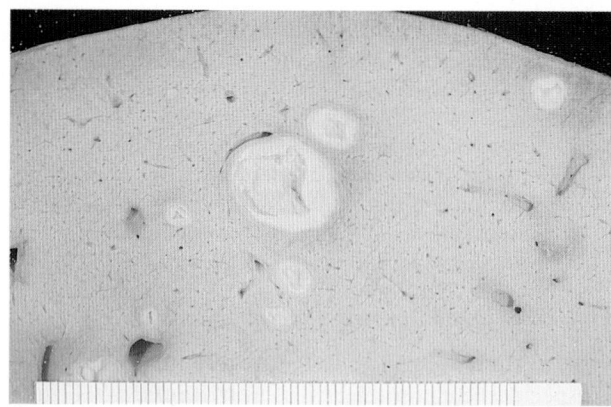

FIGURE 13.12   Multiple abscesses in the liver (pale round structures). From the liver of a 59-year-old man with acute leukemia, who died of sepsis with abscesses in many organs. (Because the liver was fixed before being cut, the pus did not flow out of the abscesses.) **Scale** in millimeters.

FIGURE 13.11   Microscopic abscesses induced in the liver of hamsters by injecting amoebae (*Entamoeba histolytica*) into the portal vein. *Top:* 6 hours after the inoculation: an amoeba is visible in the upper center of the abscess. **Bar** = 50 μm. *Bottom:* 4-day stage: **arrows** point to amoebae, and the necrotic mass is surrounded by a rim of macrophages and fibroblasts. **Bar** = 100 μm. (Reproduced with permission from [56], © American Society for Investigative Pathology.)

any other route, produce toxins that kill the local cells; the neutrophils, as they attack the bacteria, secrete enzymes that digest the dead cells, and perhaps some live ones as well. Within a few hours the result is a microscopic cavity filled with cell debris and neutrophils: a *microabscess* (Figure 13.11). Within 2–3 days a thin layer of granulation tissue begins to develop all around the microabscess (Figure 13.11, bottom); it continues to pour into the cavity leukocytes, mainly neutrophils, while fibroblasts build layers of a collagen-rich tissue on the outside. This lifesaving wall of granulation tissue is known as "*pyogenic*" *membrane* because its inner surface (in contact with the offending agent) "produces pus"; overall it performs as a highly effective barrier to the spread of infection. What happens next depends on the

balance of forces (including the effect of antibiotics [1a']):

- *All the bacteria (or amoebae) are killed, the pus becomes sterile, and healing occurs* by reabsorption of the sterilized pus. The influx of leukocytes stops because the chemotactic stimulus has disappeared; the content of the abscess becomes essentially a mass of denatured proteins, which macrophages slowly erode. Eventually the pyogenic membrane shrinks concentrically into a scar; its shrinkage is probably helped by an outer layer of fibroblasts that have modulated into contractile cells, *myofibroblasts* (p. 485).

- *The battle continues, and the abscess expands* (Figure 13.12). Presumably the imprisoned bacteria attack and destroy the inner surface of the pyogenic membrane while new layers are added to its outer surface. Pressure within the cavity, both hydrostatic and osmotic, could help enlarge the abscess (pus is hypertonic).

- *The abscess empties its contents through a **fistula**. A fistula (Latin for tube) is any pathologic channel from a body cavity to another internal cavity or to the body surface.* A lung abscess can erode its way into a bronchus; an abscess that develops at the tip of the root of a carious tooth can work its way out into the mouth or toward the skin. Fistulae can be congenital, traumatic, or inflammatory. In the case of a ruptured abscess, the wall of the fistula gradually becomes lined with granulation tissue: this is an *inflammatory fistula.* Drainage of pus through the fistula continues as long as the infection persists.

NOTE: An abscess can be sterile from the beginning if it is induced by sterile chemotactic materials.

An established experimental method for producing sterile subcutaneous abscesses in mice is to inject the autoclaved content of mouse cecum (25). In the nineteenth century, a rather barbaric method for treating septicemic patients was to create sterile intramuscular "fixation abscesses" by injecting turpentine. It was hoped that the circulating bacteria would somehow become localized in the abscesses. Some probably did, but we would not recommend the procedure.

The dental abscess is an odd case. An infected root canal is a routine event, but it leads to a biologically unique situation: granulation tissue mixed with epithelium. Here is what happens. Cavities in teeth are caused by bacteria that may work their way down the dentin canals (Figure 13.13) and eventually reach the pulp, spread along the root, emerge at the tip, and cause a small abscess (Figure 9.3): a collection of pus surrounded by granulation tissue (Figure 13.14). Here is the unique feature: this granulation tissue is often covered by or mixed with layer of squamous stratified epithelium. The mechanism: embryologically the tooth develops inside a cup of epithelium (the *enamel organ*) that determines its shape. The epithelial cup then disappears but leaves behind, on the surface of the tooth's root, little clusters of residual epithelial cells called *rests of Malassez* (52). When granulation tissue develops at the tip of a root, some of these rests wake up—

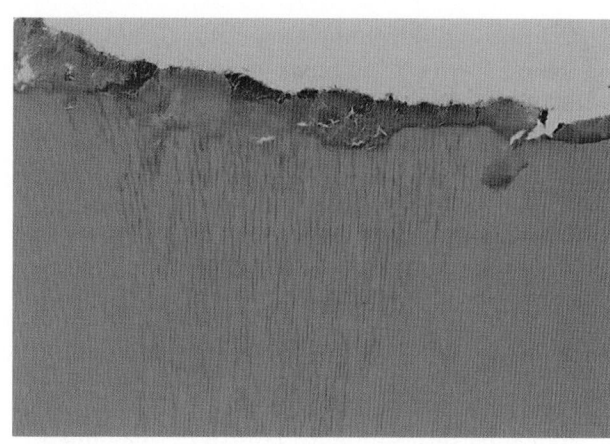

FIGURE 13.13   Human tooth; section at the level of a cavity (*top*). The basophilic material lining the cavity is a mixture of bacteria and dentin (the major "bony" component of the tooth) decalcified by the bacteria. The pale blue streaks descending from the cavity are the dentin canals stuffed with bacteria (hence the basophilia) which are creeping toward the dental pulp, not visible here. All this catastrophe begins with a bacterial biofilm (*plaque*) on the tooth surface. (40x) (Tooth provided courtesy of Dr. P. J. Alizzeo, Shrewsbury, MA.)

presumably under the influence of inflammatory growth factors—and grow with the granulation tissue. As far as we know, they never reach the stage of cancerous growth.

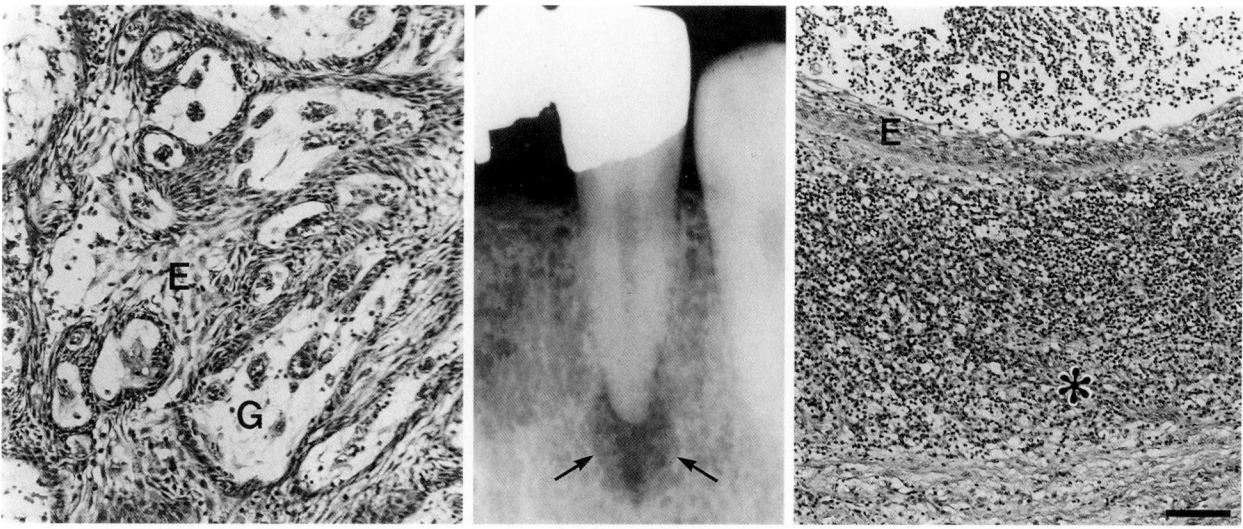

FIGURE 13.14   A mix of granulation tissue and epithelium as observed in dental pathology. *Center:* X-ray of a tooth that has undergone repair for caries (note the metal crown). Some bacteria survived, emerged from the tip of the root, and set up an inflammatory process that caused the bone to be reabsorbed (lucent space between **arrows**). The bone loss could be due to a granuloma, a cyst, or an abscess. Embryologic remains of epithelium (**E**) stimulated by the inflammatory process often proliferate and either mix with the granulation tissue (**G**) (*left, dental granuloma*), or line the surface of a pus-filled cavity (*right*). **P** = pus; **E** = epithelium; **asterisk** = granulation tissue overloaded with inflammatory cells. **Bar** = 100 μm. (Left and center reproduced from [42]. *Right:* Specimen courtesy of Dr. D. J. Krutchkoff, University of Connecticut, Farmington, CT.)

Cellulitis or **phlegmon** is essentially the opposite of an abscess: it refers to an acute, overwhelming infection without clear borders that spreads along the skin and subcutaneous connective tissue before local defenses have a chance to wall it off. Malaise, chills, and fever are usually present; common causes are group A streptococci and *staphylococcus aureus* (31).

> NOTE: *The medical term* **cellulitis** *has nothing to do with cells as we now understand them.* Until the late 1800s *cellular tissue* was an alternate term for connective tissue. The reason: a technique for separating the skin, much favored by anatomists as well as by butchers, was to blow air beneath it. If you try this, you will find that bubbles of air remain trapped between thin, transparent connective tissue membranes, presumably made of collagen. These bubbles were called "cells"; in this context, a phlegmon that spread along the connective tissue spaces—like air—was appropriately called cellulitis.

In a totally different context: In the non-medical world, the term **cellulitis** is applied to a puckered aspect of the skin over fat thighs. Whatever this may be, it is not a recognized pathologic entity.

Ulcers

An ulcer is a gap in the skin or in a mucosa, **with no tendency to heal.** The latter property is the key difference between a wound and an ulcer. Ulcers in vascularized tissues, such as the mucosa of the gut, are lined by granulation tissue (Figure 13.15); in skin ulcers the "granules" of granulation tissue can be very obvious (Figure 13.16). Wherever an ulcer may be, two questions need to be answered: what was the initial injury, and why did it not heal? Answers are surprisingly varied.

In ancient times virtually all wounds became infected and turned into ulcers, which explains why the Greek word for *wound* and *ulcer* was the same, *hélkos* (34). The painful gnawing of **gastric ulcers** has long been attributed to the corrosive action of digestive juices; another theory blames the lack of fibroblast growth factor (FGF), said to be degraded by hydrochloric acid (11, 54, 55). And so, the medical world was aghast in the mid-1980s when an Australian pathologist found that many gastric ulcers are caused by *Helicobacter pylori* and can be treated with antibiotics (59). **Acute stress ulcers of the stomach** (Figure 13.17) are attributed to low flow and vasoconstriction (10). **Ulcers about the ankles** in patients with varicose veins and poor circulation show fibrin cuffs around capillary loops, suggesting the possibility of an

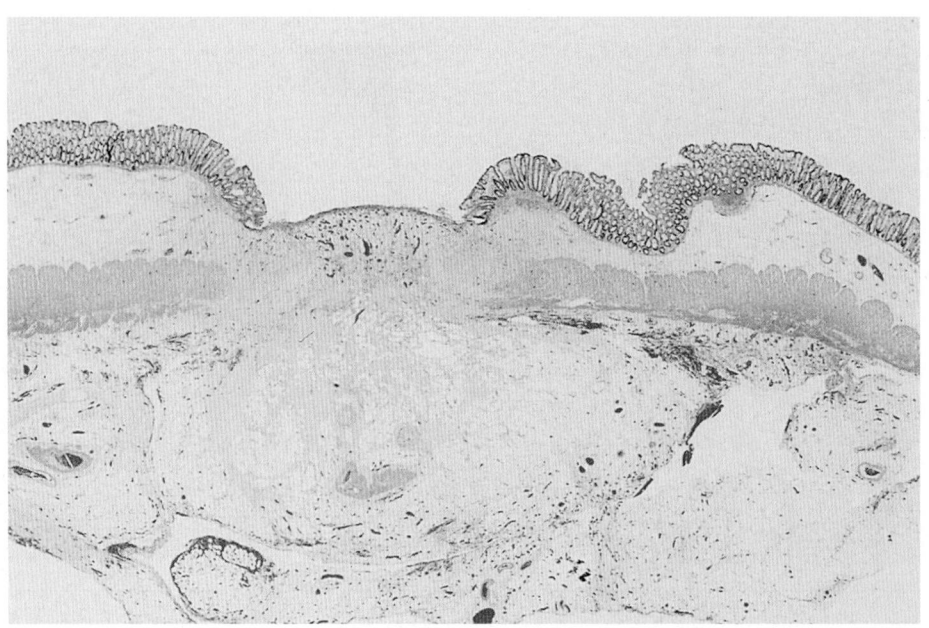

FIGURE 13.15   A small ulcer of the colon (area without mucosa, left of center) where a polyp had been excised 12 days earlier. The exposed submucosa has become a wall of granulation tissue, containing many dilated venules. This inflammatory response has probably destroyed the underlying smooth muscle layer and is spreading into the adipose tissue around the colon (how much of the damage is done by the bacterial infection, as opposed to the inflammatory response, can not be decided on this slide alone).

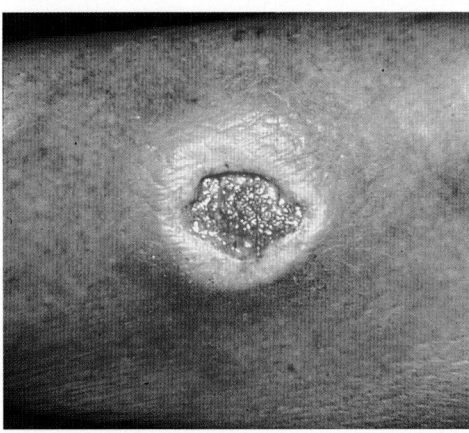

FIGURE 13.16 Example of granulation tissue: "granulating ulcer" after trauma of the leg in a dark-skinned patient. The highlights represent granulations. The pale rim represents regenerating epidermis; the melanocytes regenerate poorly and unpredictably. Actual size. (Courtesy of Dr. R. L. Walton, Chicago Medical School, Chicago, IL.)

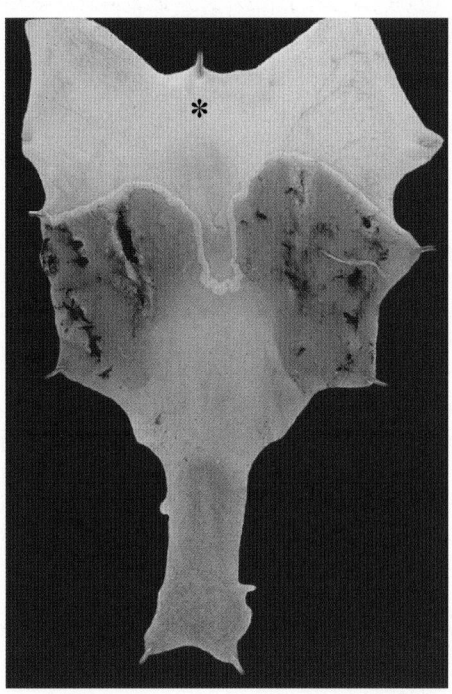

FIGURE 13.17 Stress ulcers in the stomach of a rat, euthanized in the winter of 1952. It had escaped and was found semistarved in a cellar. Note the typical stress ulcers (black areas). (*) Top part of the stomach: in the rat it contains no glands, and is lined by an epithelium similar to that of the esophagus. Slightly enlarged.

oxygen diffusion barrier, inadequate fibrinolysis, and/or trapping of growth factors (1, 9, 29), hence therapeutic attempts with oxygen and growth factors. The causes of **ulcers of the foot** in diabetics must be sought in diabetic neuropathy (loss of sensation) and in the many problems of the microcirculation in diabetes. **Pressure ulcers** ("bedsores") are probably maintained by the large amount of necrotic fat tissue that surrounds them; shearing forces are thought to play a major role (62). They are best treated by removing the pressure. **Buruli ulcer** is a scourge of several African countries; it is caused by *Mycobacterium ulcerans,* which produces a toxin that kills fat cells and impairs the immune system. Children are mainly affected. The ulcer can be healed by warming it to fever temperature (40°C) because the mycobacterium dies at 35°C, but electricity for a controlled heater is rarely available in rural settings (17). **Neurotrophic ulcers** of the cornea—the most innervated tissue of the body—develop as a result of local loss of sensation; they used to be hopeless but were recently healed with nerve growth factor, perhaps the greatest therapeutic success of a growth factor (28).

Adhesions: Inflammation of Serosal Surfaces

A serosal space, such as the pleura or the peritoneum, creates special conditions for inflammation because it offers a large cavity in which the exudate can accumulate, rather than infiltrating the tight spaces of connective tissue. Accordingly, inflamed serosal spaces can become filled with serous exudate (e.g., *serous pleuritis*)

or pus (e.g., *pleural empyema*); or the apposed serosal surfaces may become coated with fibrin (e.g., *fibrinous pericarditis, fibrinous peritonitis*) (see Figures 12.9, 12.10, 12.11). Whenever a fibrin coat is present, the serosal lining (mesothelium is destroyed and replaced by a layer of granulation tissue, which is exuding the fibrin (Figure 13.18). Healing often occurs via fusion of the apposed surfaces: a permanent complication called *adhesion.*

Adhesions. Normal serosal surfaces are kept apart by the lubricating effect of their mesothelial lining, which is coated with surfactant (20). When they are irritated by bacteria or some other agent, their mesothelial lining is locally destroyed; the two surfaces become inflamed and are glued together, at first, by fibrin. This is a *fibrinous adhesion,* which can be separated by gentle pulling.

The next step is critical: if the fibrin is digested away by macrophages or by the fibrinolytic activity of the serosal fluid, the mesothelium regenerates and healing is complete (46). But if the fibrin is replaced (organized) by granulation tissue, the result is a permanent *fibrous adhesion.* A fibrous adhesion of the entire pleura, pericardium or peritoneum is called a *symphysis.*

For the function of the lung, a focal adhesion is not critical, but a symphysis is life-threatening. Pericardial symphysis increases the cardiac workload and causes myocardial hypertrophy.

Overall, adhesions are of concern especially for the peritoneum, where a single adhesion can cause trouble by creating a noose through which an intestinal loop can slip and become strangulated. Peritoneal adhesions occur after 70–90 percent of abdominal operations and cause significant trouble (43). A key factor is serosal fibrinolytic activity, which is decreased after surgery (21).

Peritoneal fibrosis with diffuse adhesions is also a common complication of chronic **peritoneal dialysis.** Recent work has shown that in about 20 percent of the cases the mesothelial cells shift from an epithelial to a mesenchymal phenotype (188). This is one of the best-documented examples of metaplasia from epithelium (admittedly of a special kind) to fibroblast (see p. 59).

> Until the 1940s, an inordinate number of patients who had undergone abdominal surgery developed peritoneal adhesions that contained mysterious microscopic foreign bodies. Finally, it was realized that the talcum powder used to lubricate surgical gloves induced a chronic inflammatory reaction: *talcum granulomas* (51). The problem was not completely solved by replacing talcum with starch (22).

The omentum: an organ planned for adhesions. The omentum is a peculiar organ (30). Hanging as it does in front of the intestines, it looks like an afterthought, or maybe a leftover from some embryologic maneuver (which it is, as a large fold of excess peritoneal lining). In fact, the omentum is poised there waiting for trouble. It is programmed to prevent the spread of infection, as signaled by inflammation. If it happens to float over an infected and inflamed appendix, for example, it too becomes infected and inflamed; it generates fibrin, which mixes with the fibrin oozing from the appendix and becomes trapped over the inflamed appendix, creating a barrier against the further spread of the bacteria. In essence, it performs as an easily inflammable organ for producing life-saving adhesions. We believe that in this function the omentum is helped by its structure: it is a vascularized membrane perforated by countless holes, making it look like a net (Figure 13.19). In fact, its name in German is *Netz* (45). Because of these meshes, it is more easily trapped in a network of inflammatory fibrin (45). Its medical nickname of "policeman of the abdominal cavity" is well earned.

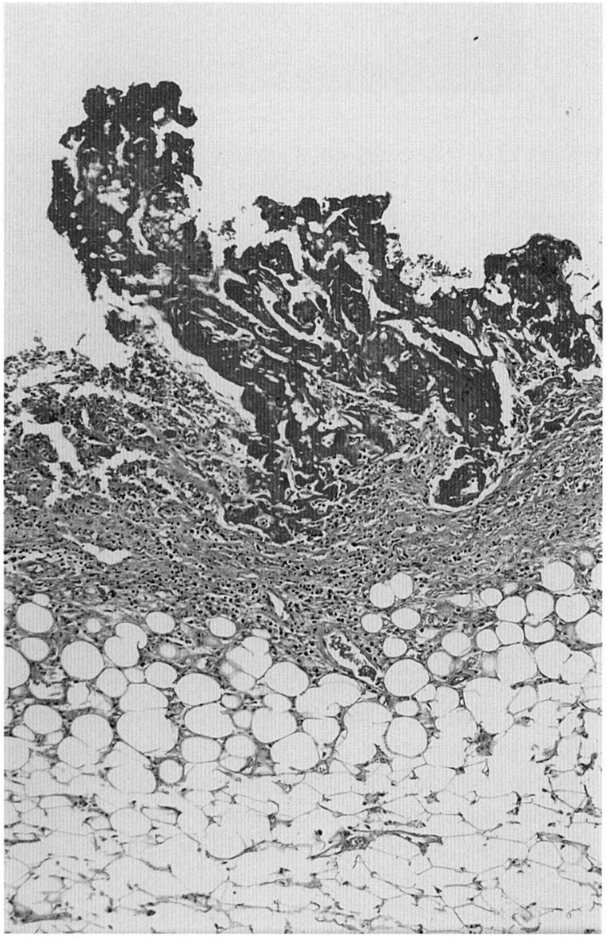

FIGURE 13.18 Inflamed epicardium in uremia: *fibrinous pericarditis* (see Figure 12.9 for gross aspect). Epicardial surface at top. Dense material = fibrin. Between the fibrin and the adipose tissue is a layer of granulation tissue; plasma oozing out of its vessels generates the fibrin. (90x)

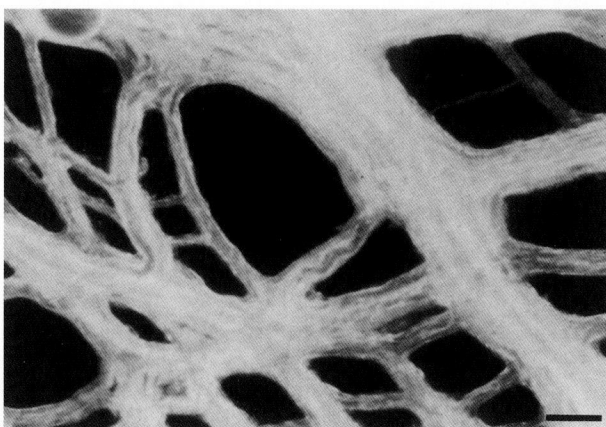

FIGURE 13.19 Human omentum, seen by dark field microscopy to emphasize the net-like structure. (Omentum mounted on a glass slide, unstained). **Bar** = 100 μm. (Courtesy of Dr. G. B. Ryan, University of Melbourne, Parkville, Australia.)

Banjo-string adhesions. The type of adhesions described so far are sometimes called *flat adhesions,* to distinguish them from string-shaped ("banjo-string") adhesions that have a different pathogenesis. These arise in the peritoneum as follows. Imagine that some blood is spilled in the abdominal cavity, that it clots, and that the clot becomes attached to the peritoneal surface at two points 10–15 cm apart. Two organs are thus connected by a soft, rubbery clot. No harm is done, but the end result depends on what happens next. If the clot is dissolved by fibrinolysis or by macrophages, no trouble will develop. But if the clot is colonized by fibroblasts (organized), it will turn into a taut string ready to choke an intestinal loop that may wind around it Figure 13.20 (45). Needless to say, banjo-string adhesions are always a nuisance.

At this point the reader should find it interesting to attempt a two-part quiz, combining cell death and inflammation (note: immunology is not involved):

Questions:

(a) If we open the abdomen of a rat 48 hours after implanting a piece of *fresh* liver, what are we likely to see?
(b) If we open the abdomen of a rat 48 hours after implanting a piece of *boiled* liver, what are we likely to see?

Answers:

(a) The fresh liver will be wrapped in inflamed omentum; the two will be glued together by fibrinous adhesions. Mechanism: the dying liver cells released a variety of peptides, eicosanoids, and other inflammatory mediators that inflamed the omentum, causing it to become attached to the implant. This acute inflammation will slowly merge into chronic inflammation, and eventually the implant will be organized.
(b) The boiled liver can release no mediators: it is essentially an inert mass of denatured protein from which no inflammatory messages arise. It will therefore be ignored by the omentum and will remain free in the abdominal cavity. In other words, it will not be organized. Eventually its surface will be colonized by peritoneal cells, probably macrophages, which will very slowly nibble at it while it slowly calcifies.

> NOTE: After two or three days, an implant of *fresh* liver has released most of its chemical inflammatory messages and has turned into a mass of coagulated protein; therefore, it should no longer be an irritant. Indeed, if it is surgically removed and transplanted into another rat, it will remain free, like the boiled liver (33). *This explains why infarcts are removed very slowly:* after a fiery burst of acute inflammation they no longer attract leukocytes and are only nibbled at by the macrophages that happen to be in contact with their surface; sometimes they calcify.

These concepts are illustrated in Figures 13.21 and 13.22.

Granulomatous Inflammation

In an organ that is *chronically* inflamed, the cellular infiltrate tends to follow one of two patterns: it can spread more or less evenly throughout the tissue—this is the more common arrangement—or it can gather

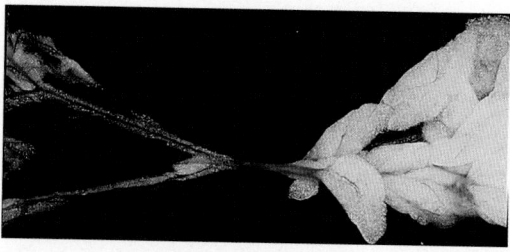

FIGURE 13.20   Genesis of a banjo-string adhesion in a rat. Two milliliters of rat blood were injected 7 days earlier into the peritoneum, as the blood clotted it became attached to the omentum (*left*) and to a mass of adipose tissue (*right*). Fibrinolysis failed to remove the clot; fibroblast-like cells settled on it (perhaps from free, undifferentiated peritoneal cells) and made it permanent. The brown color at the point of junction is due to remains of blood. Magnification approximately × 2. (Reproduced with permission from [45], © American Society for Investigative Pathology.)

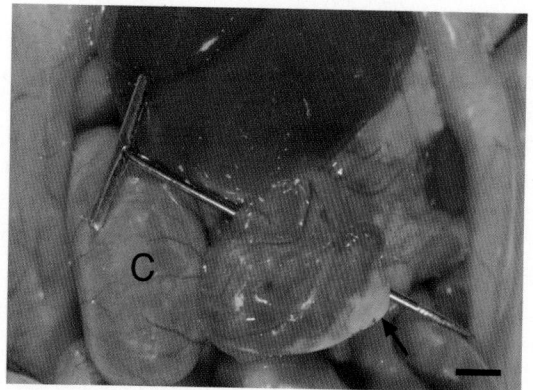

FIGURE 13.21   Abdominal cavity of a rat 2 days after implantation of a fragment of sterile, fresh liver. The implant has inflamed the omentum, which has wrapped it up. A small area of white, necrotic liver is still visible at lower right (**arrow**). **C:** cecum. **Bar** = 5 mm.

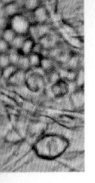

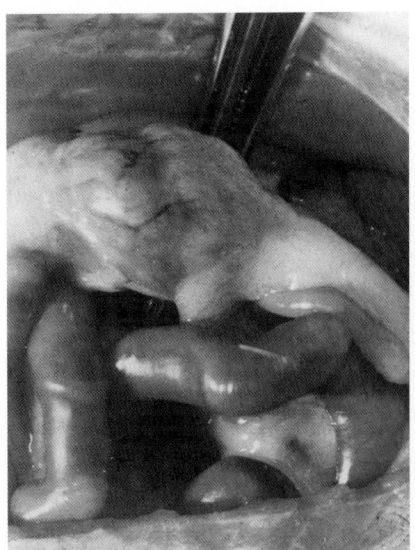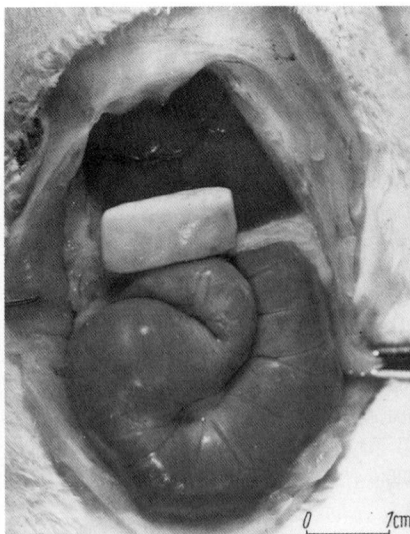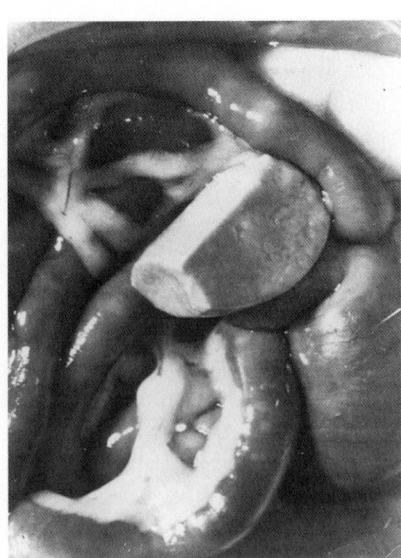

FIGURE 13.22 Long-standing necrotic tissue has lost its ability to trigger acute inflammation. The three panels show the fate of various kinds of liver fragments 1 week after introduction into the peritoneal cavity. *Left:* Fresh liver. Note complete wrapping by the omentum. *Center:* Sterile liver implant that has been transferred daily for 5 days to new recipient animals. It has failed to irritate the peritoneum and is ignored by the omentum. *Right:* A boiled implant has been similarly ignored. (Reproduced from [33] with permission from Springer-Verlag.)

into tiny, separate, rounded clusters of macrophages with a sprinkling of other cell types. These intriguing clusters, roughly of the size of a pinhead, are called *granulomas* (*granulomata* by purists). What do they mean?

The granuloma is Nature's device for isolating and destroying materials that are difficult to eliminate because they are poorly soluble and/or poorly degradable (127). The offending agent may be antigenic or non-antigenic, alive or inert; it is often distributed in minuscule amounts, which macrophages tend to imprison in granulomas. In any case, it must be understood that **granulomas are not a disease:** they are part of our defenses—especially for killing hardy bacteria—and as such they can also cause collateral damage. A typical granuloma is shown in Figure 13.23; it was elicited by *Mycobacterium tuberculosis.* We now know that this type of granuloma is meant to kill mycobacteria; and in so doing, it destroys some lung tissue.

A peculiar feature of granulomas—which we tend to conceive as a "hyperactive" form of connective tissue—is that **they have no blood vessels** (exceptions are rare). Their small diameter, on the order of 1 mm, apparently allows them to survive by diffusion of oxygen and nutrients from the surrounding fluid. It would be interesting to compare isolated granulomas regarding the secretion of angiogenic (98a) and anti-angiogenic factors.

The study of granulomas is helped by the fact that they are fairly easy to produce experimentally. Sterile granulomas can be produced by injecting microscopic plastic beads, bland or loaded with cytokines and other agents to be tested. Suspensions of various materials can be injected into the peripheral veins to produce granulomas in the lungs, or into the portal vein to produce granulomas in the liver. Schistosoma eggs are often used, mainly for injection into the portal vein. An advantage of liver

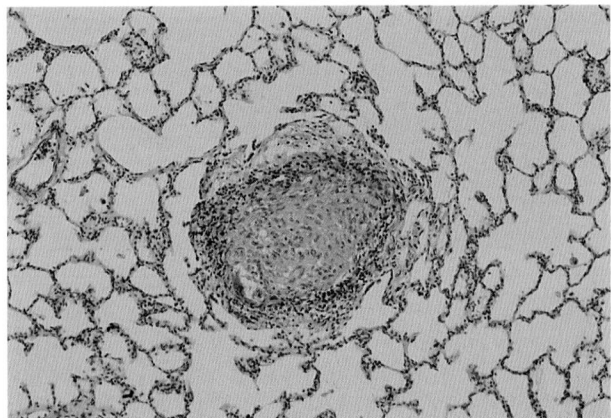

FIGURE 13.23 Tuberculous granuloma ("tubercle") in a case of mycobacterial dissemination by the blood stream ("miliary" tuberculosis). The granuloma consists of epithelioid cells surrounded by a layer of lymphocytes. (80x)

granulomas is that they can be isolated: a suspension of schistosoma eggs is injected into the portal vein of a mouse; a week or two later the liver is "gently homogenized" in a blender, and the granulomas can be spun down as tiny grains (Figure 13.24) (104). These can

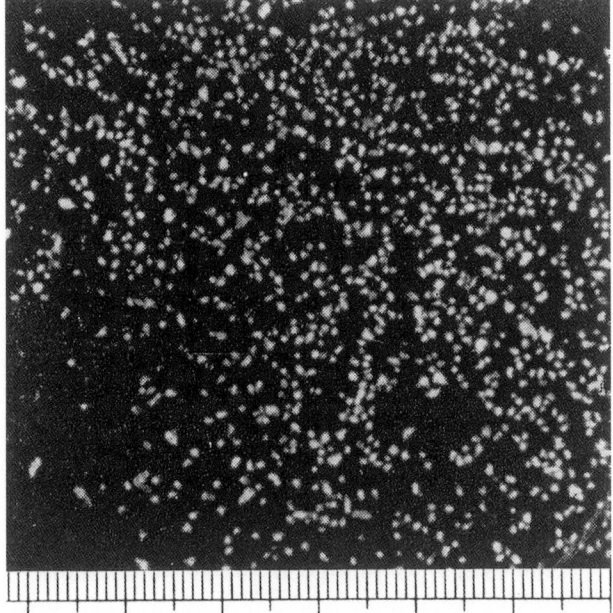

FIGURE 13.24   Suspension of *Schistosoma* granulomas isolated from mouse liver 8 weeks after infection. Granulomas prepared in this manner can be used for metabolic studies *in vitro*. **Scale** in millimeters. (Reproduced with permission from [104].)

be incubated for metabolic studies, analyzed chemically, or dissociated into individual cell types.

Incubated granulomas secrete a host of inflammatory mediators, including cytokines, free radicals, prostaglandins, collagenase (108) and other enzymes (77, 80, 84, 97, 114). In essence, they behave like **miniature endocrine organs**: a fact to keep in mind in dealing with granulomatous diseases (see below). Artificial granulomas have also been tried (Figure 13.25).

Types of granulomas

Currently two types of granulomas are recognized (Figure 13.26). If the material that induced the granuloma is an irritant only in a mechanical sense, we are dealing with a **foreign-body type granuloma** (typical agents are surgical sutures, glass splinters, crystals, small thorns); if the material is antigenic, the response will be an **immune granuloma** (sometimes called **hypersensitivity granuloma**). Mixed types are obviously possible (p. 557). This distinction is biologically relevant because the two types represent the innate and the immune response, respectively (69a, 72, 73, 91, 122).

Foreign-body granulomas tend to be smaller and contain fewer cells than their immune counterparts; the foreign body is usually visible in the center of the granuloma, and its visibility is often enhanced by polarized light (Figure 13.27). A layer or two of activated macrophages lie on its surface; although activated, they look quite bland. They are much more numerous in the

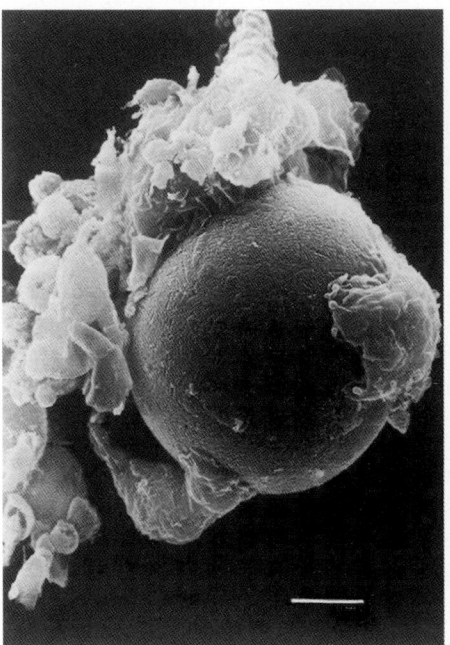
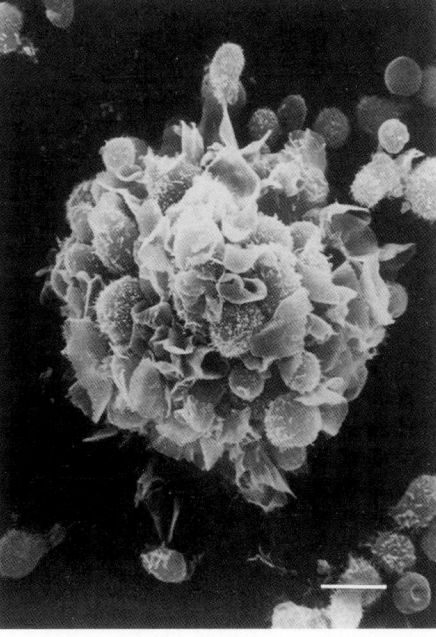

FIGURE 13.25 "Granuloma" formation *in vitro*. Latex beads were incubated with mouse spleen cells (over 95 percent macrophages). After incubation for 1 day (**A**) and 3 days (**B**) the beads became progressively covered with macrophages. The effect was enhanced by incubation in the presence of interleukin-1 and tumor necrosis factor α but not in the presence of interleukin-2 or interferon-γ. **Bars** = 5 μm.   (Reproduced with permission from [110], © American Society for Investigative Pathology.)

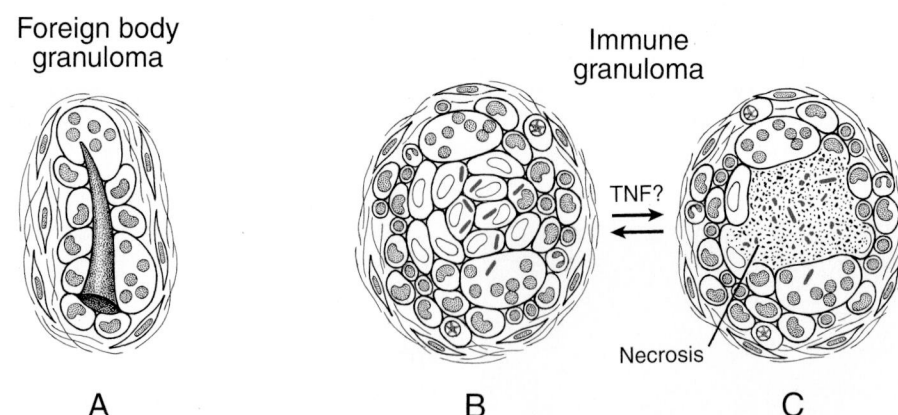

Foreign body
granuloma

Immune
granuloma

TNF?

Necrosis

A   B   C

FIGURE 13.26   *Two types of granulomas.* **A:** *Foreign body granuloma,* as caused by a thorn. The granuloma contains macrophages, giant cells, and fibroblasts, *but no lymphocytes.* **B, C:** *Immune granulomas,* as caused by *Mycobaterium tuberculosis.* The core is made of epithelioid cells (some with bacilli) surrounded by lymphocytes, macrophages, plasma cells, giant cells and perhaps dendritic cells. Necrosis may develop in the center (**C**).

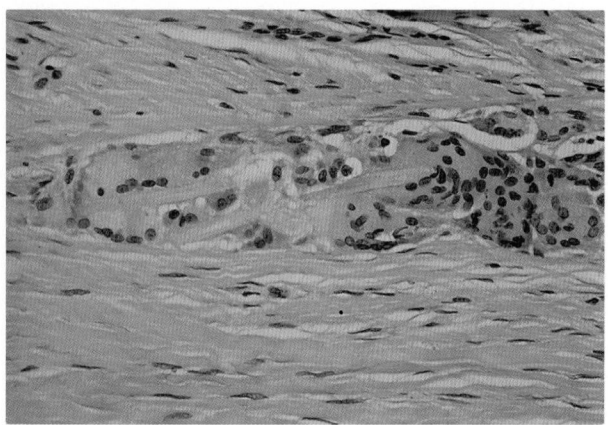

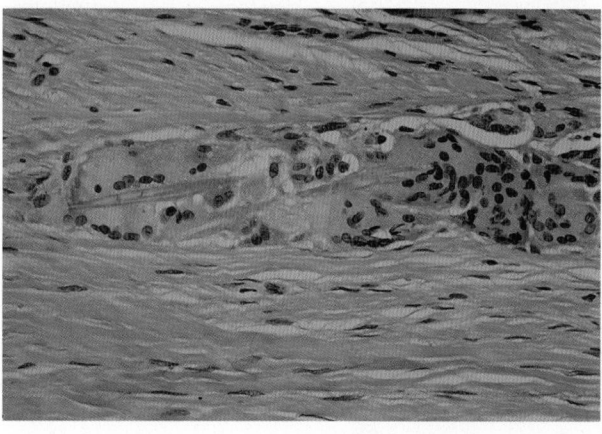

FIGURE 13.27   *Top:* In an old surgical scar, a foreign body granuloma presumably containing the remains of a suture thread. The granuloma consists mainly of giant cells and macrophages. *Bottom:* Using partially polarized light the foreign object is more clearly visible.

core of immune granulomas, where they are called **epithelioid cells**. If animals bearing granulomas are made hyperlipidemic, the epithelioid cells pick up the lipid and turn into foam cells (109).

Giant cells are a prominent feature of all granulomas, both foreign-body type and immune. These huge cells arise primarily by fusion of macrophages, although some degree of internal mitosis is possible (83, 107). If a foreign body is small enough, it can be entirely engulfed by a giant cell, producing what might be called a single-cell granuloma. We shall give giant cells a closer look at the end of this section.

Fibroblasts form a loose coat around the foreign-body granuloma. As time passes—months, even years—the macrophage component tends to disappear, and the foreign body remains surrounded by a thin fibrous layer, sometimes so thin that the extraneous body appears to lie free in the tissue.

How does a foreign body granuloma get started, if the foreign body itself does not attract macrophages? Studies with plastic beads injected intravenously suggested that the surface of a foreign body activates the Hageman factor, an important source of inflammatory mediators. Pigeons are deficient in Hageman factor, and they do not develop granulomas in response to intravenous beads (93, 123).

Immune granulomas. The cellular population of immune granulomas is more rich and varied, as expected, because it reflects the many aspects of the immune response. Typically, an immune granuloma has a concentric arrangement. The core is a small lump of tightly packed *epithelioid cells,* similar to those of foreign body

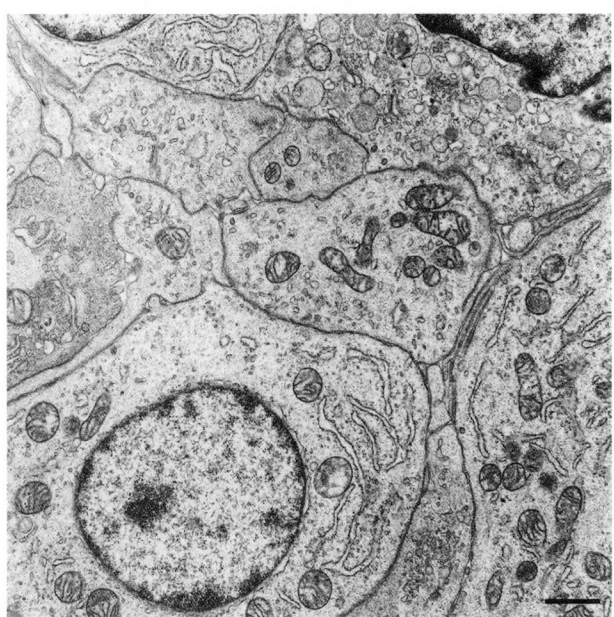

FIGURE 13.28 Electron microscopic aspect of epithelioid cells from a human beryllium granuloma, induced in the skin of a volunteer (chronic berylliosis is caused by industrial exposure to beryllium dust, which induces an immune response). Note the densely packed and interdigitating processes of macrophages. **Bar** = 1 μm. (Courtesy of Dr. W. L. Epstein, University of California, San Francisco, CA.)

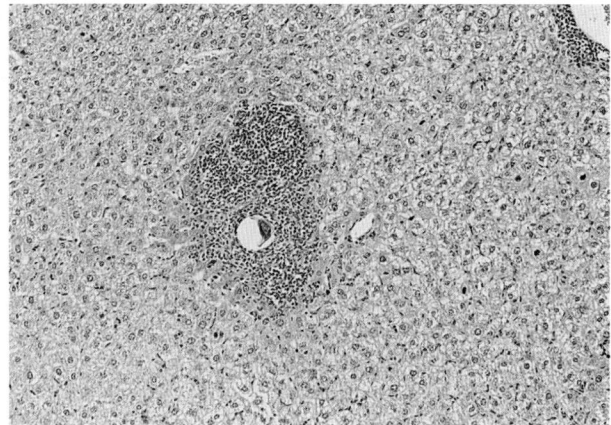

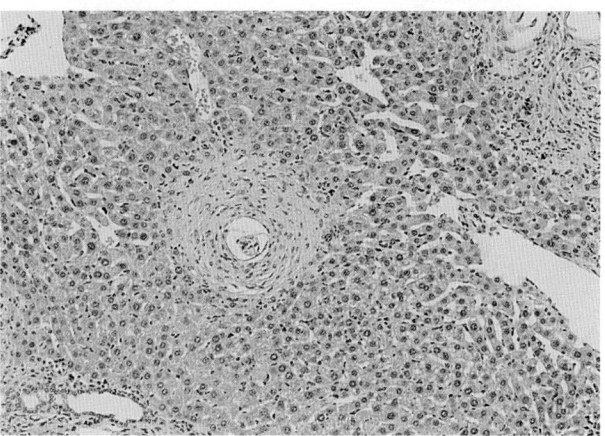

FIGURE 13.29 Variability of tissue responses of mouse liver to eggs of *Schistosoma. Top:* A live egg has attracted a dense population of leukocytes, mainly neutrophils and eosinophils. This response is therefore a microabscess (80x) (see Figure 13.11). *Bottom:* A dead Schistosoma egg is surrounded by a dense layer of fibroblasts, macrophages and collagen. This can be considered a scar (80x). The different cellular responses are due—in part—to the age of the lesion. (Specimens kindly provided by Dr. M. J. Stadecker, Tufts University School of Medicine, Boston, MA.)

granulomas but more numerous; by electron microscopy they appear tightly apposed and interdigitated (Figure 13.28), perhaps an adaptation for retaining an offensive agent (71). Surrounding the core is a layer of *lymphocytes* with or without plasma cells, and a thin outer rim of *fibroblasts* (Figures 13.23, 13.26) (91, 102); the latter, in *Schistosoma* granulomas, produce macrophage chemoattractants, thereby recruiting cells for the granuloma (99): a logical arrangement, but we should not visualize granulomas as standardized, predictable structures. They vary a great deal because they adapt their cell population to the agent. The initial response may even be a microabscess (Figure 13.29; see also Figure 13.11). When the battle is over a granuloma may turn into a scar (Figure 13.29).

As to the immune response, it is mainly (but not only) of the *cellular* type; if plasma cells are present, we know that antibody formation (i.e., the *humoral* response) is involved.

To demonstrate the role of the immune response in the pathogenesis of these granulomas, a standard experiment is to instill into the bronchi of mice a suspension of microscopic plastic beads, with or without an added antigen (76). In a normal animal both kinds of beads will induce a mild foreign body reaction; in an animal immunized against the specific antigen immune granulomas will develop (115). The same type of experiment can be used to demonstrate the role of different cytokines in generating an immune granuloma (Figure 13.30).

Experimental models also taught us that *granulomas represent a favorable outcome.* For example: two strains of mice were compared regarding infection with *Mycobacterium tuberculosis.* In one strain all the mice died in less than 14 days with diffuse, necrotizing

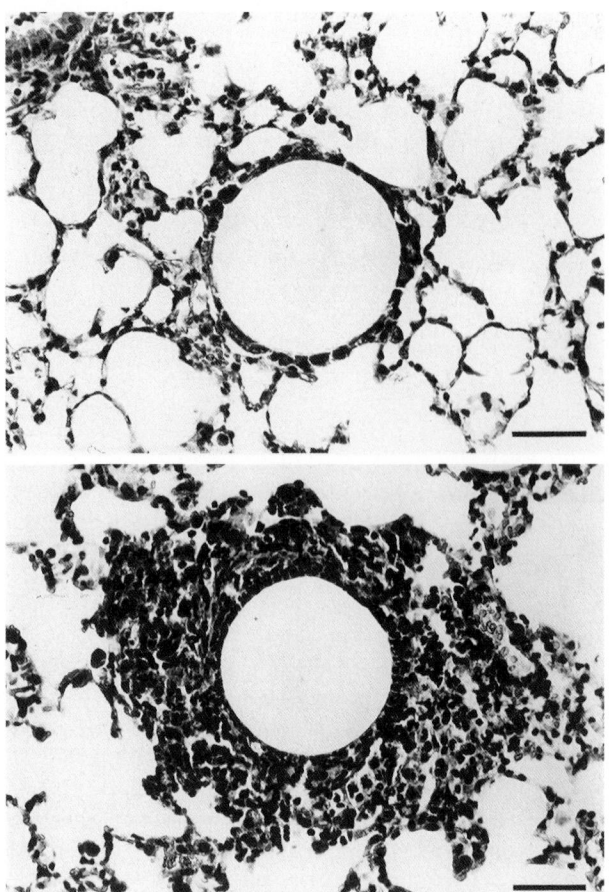

FIGURE 13.30   Role of interleukin-1 in the pathogenesis of granulomas. *Top:* The central white disk represents the cross section of a plain Sepharose (control) bead injected through the trachea into the lung of a mouse. After 3 days it has caused a very mild inflammatory reaction, represented by a single layer of macrophages. *Bottom:* Effect of a bead coupled with interleukin-1. After 3 days it has produced a large granuloma consisting mainly of macrophages. **Bars** = 100 μm. (Reproduced with permission from [92], © American Society for Investigative Pathology.)

lesions in the lungs and widely disseminated bacilli; in the other the mice lived twice as long, and the bacilli were mainly contained within granulomas (65). Immune granulomas develop very poorly in nude rats, which are incapable of mounting a cell-mediated immune response (72–74, 76, 119,121).

So be it: but the immune system has two sets of weapons (effector arms): killer cells and antibodies. Who decides which one has to be mobilized? The short answer lies in the T-helper cells, or more precisely in the T_H1-T_H2 paradigm. We will discuss this later (p. 530), but the reader may be interested to know how it came about.

In the 1980s, Mosmann et al. tested different clones of T-helper cells with regard to their output of cytokines, and found that they fell into two groups, which were labeled T_H1 and T_H2 (100a). Then it turned out that these two groups made sense also with regard to function: T_H1 cytokines provided help toward setting up cellular responses (*which include granulomas*), and T_H2 cytokines did the same for humoral (i.e., antibody) responses. Dendritic cells are critical to the process.

The choice between the T_H1 and T_H2 pathways is dictated by the cytokine environment that prevails during and after antigen presentation. If it is IL-12, T_H1 cells will develop (leading to a cell-mediated response); if it is IL-4, T_H2 cells will guide B cells to produce antibody. Rather surprisingly, the choice of the pathway depends in part on the organ (65).

Necrosis in immune granulomas. Necrosis is NOT the rule in immune granulomas; it is seen, typically, in those of tuberculosis, syphilis, and rheumatoid arthritis. The necrosis is always of the "coagulation" type (p. 558) and develops in the centers of the granulomas. When adjacent granulomas fuse, the result can be a large mass of necrosis surrounded by a rim of "granuloma" tissue (Figure 13.31); we can call it "tuberculous granulation tissue" because it is richly vascularized (81) (in contrast

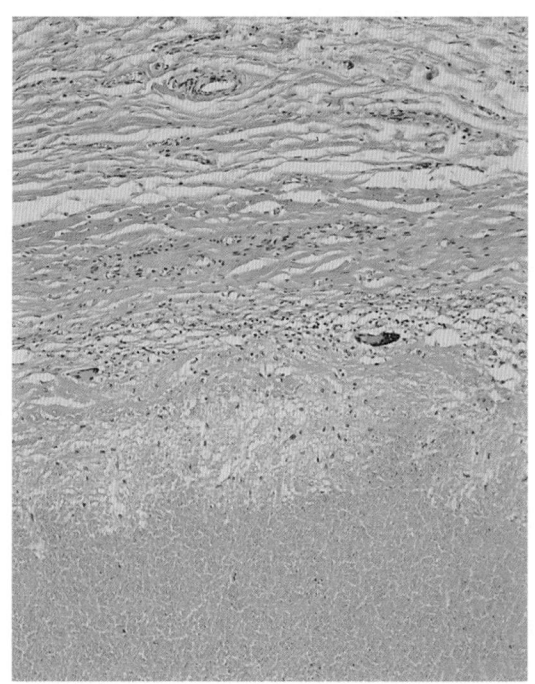

FIGURE 13.31   Caseous necrosis: mode of progression as seen in a tuberculous lymph node. *Bottom:* caseous necrosis. *Top:* fibrous, vascularized capsule of the node. *In between:* thin layer of granulation tissue: note lymphocytes and one giant cell. (80x)

FIGURE 13.32 Regression of schistosomal granulomas in mice treated with a single dose of hycanthone and oxamniquine. *Top:* Granuloma in an untreated mouse. *Center:* After 2 months of treatment the granuloma is sharply defined and contains fewer cells. In the center are an empty and shrunken egg shell. *Bottom:* After 4.5 months, remnants of a Schistosoma egg are surrounded by pigment-laden phagocytic cells and some collagen fibers. Spontaneous healing can occur also without drugs, as part of the life cycle of immune granulomas. **Bars** = 50 μm. (Reproduced with permission from [68], © American Society for Investigative Pathology.)

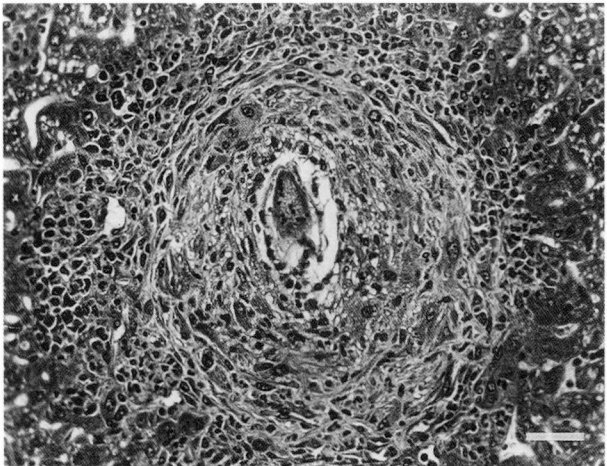

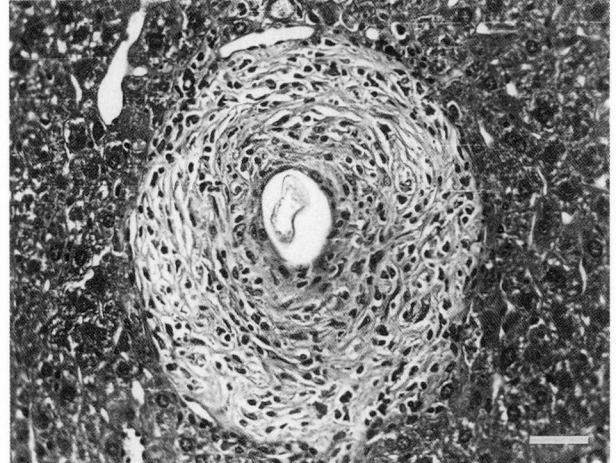

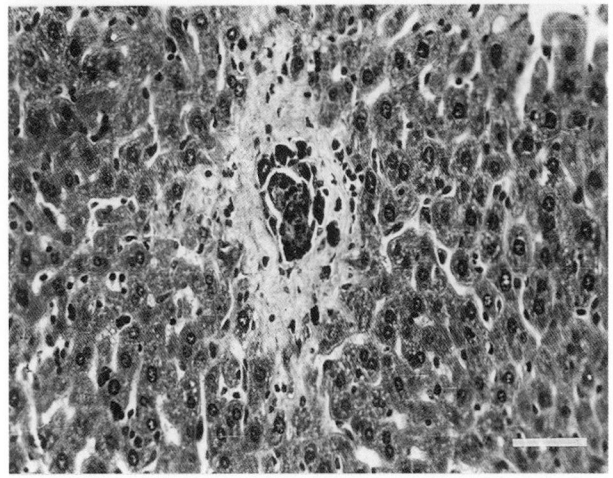

with tiny individual granulomas, which may contain no capillaries). The resulting mass can reach several centimeters in diameter, resembling a tumor, hence the names *tuberculoma* for such lumps that develop in tuberculosis, *gumma* in syphilis and *rheumatoid nodule* in rheumatoid arthritis. The syphilitic gumma is so-called because the necrosis gives it a rubbery consistency. In tuberculosis the necrosis is rather dry and cheesy, hence the name *caseous necrosis.*

Why does necrosis develop in some immune granulomas? It is natural to blame the bacilli and spirochetes for the granulomas of tuberculosis and syphilis, but a very similar necrosis develops in the sterile granulomas of rheumatoid arthritis, which is a nonbacterial, autoimmune disease (p. 591). So, there must be a nonbacterial explanation for the necrosis of immune granulomas. Nobody knows for sure (82), but it is generally felt that the necrosis in granulomas has something to do with the immunologic phenomenon called hypersensitivity. Prime suspects as chemical indicators are macrophage-derived cytokines such as tumor necrosis factor. We will discuss caseous necrosis in the chapter on hypersensitivity (p. 558).

Natural history of granulomas. Immune granulomas change with time in both structure and function (79, 122). It has been suggested that during the life of a granuloma there is a constant flux of macrophages from the periphery to the center (112), but how those in the center disappear is not understood. The growth of the granuloma appears to be autostimulated by TNF secreted by macrophages: antibodies against TNF inhibit the formation of granulomas induced by the attenuated tubercle bacillus BCG (94). The outer fibrous wrapping, which can be striking, is probably accounted for by fibroblast-stimulating factors from macrophages or lymphocytes (119, 121, 126) but especially from transforming growth factor beta (TGFβ): studies with mice overexpressing and underexpressing the *TGFβ* gene

show corresponding modulations of the fibrosis (120). Eventually, *if a granuloma succeeds in eliminating the irritant, it shrinks and disappears,* sometimes leaving a small scar; the same happens if the causal agent is killed by treatment (Figure 13.32). On the other hand, *adjacent granulomas may expand and fuse;* this is

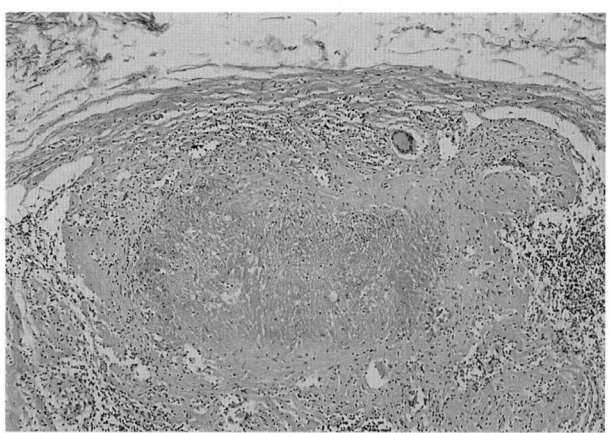

FIGURE 13.33 Tuberculous infection in a human lymph node, from the hilus of a tuberculous lung. At this advanced stage the lymph node is replaced by caseous necrosis (the eosinophilic area in the center). Individual tubercles have coalesced and are not identifiable. The necrotic mass reaches the capsule (*top*) of the lymph node. Note one large giant cell. (60x)

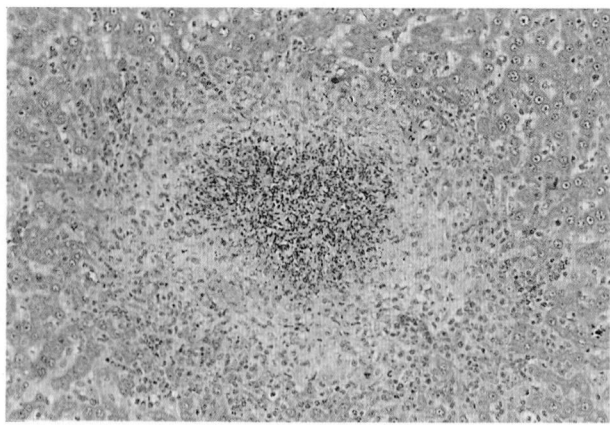

FIGURE 13.34 A sterile "granuloma" produced in the rat by injecting intravenously a preparation of streptococcal cell walls. These so-called granulomas consist of a central mass of neutrophils surrounded by a crown of macrophages: they are hybrid lesions, intermediate between granulomas and abscesses. (120x) (From a slide kindly provided by Dr. J. D. Geratz of the University of North Carolina, Chapel Hill, NC.)

especially true of bacterial granulomas such as those of tuberculosis and leprosy (Figure 13.33).

What is special about granulomas? Clearly the basic purpose of granulomas is to participate in defense, especially against bacteria; but what is their particular strength? the inflammatory mediators that they produce can be found also in chronic inflammation without granulomas. Their power does not seem to lie in a single bactericidal "magic bullet," but rather in the timing, sequence and concentration of mediators produced (mainly cytokines). *We like to think of the granuloma as a specialized device for focusing and concentrating the cellular counterattack.* It performs its task, then regresses and disappears. In this respect it behaves as a **temporary organ** made of connective tissue. The only other temporary organ known to us is granulation tissue (p. 443).

Granulomas and abscesses: how do they relate? Both are inflammatory responses to irritating agents. The typical abscess is a large (~10 cm) hollow structure filled with dead and dying neutrophils; the typical granuloma is a solid, near-microscopic structure (1 mm) built mainly of live macrophages. There are some interesting intermediate forms in which the two responses overlap: (1) *Preparations of streptococcal wall,* when injected, have been reported to produce focal "granulomas" rich in capillaries and infiltrated with neutrophils (Figure 13.34) (85, 119, 121). There is no name for these

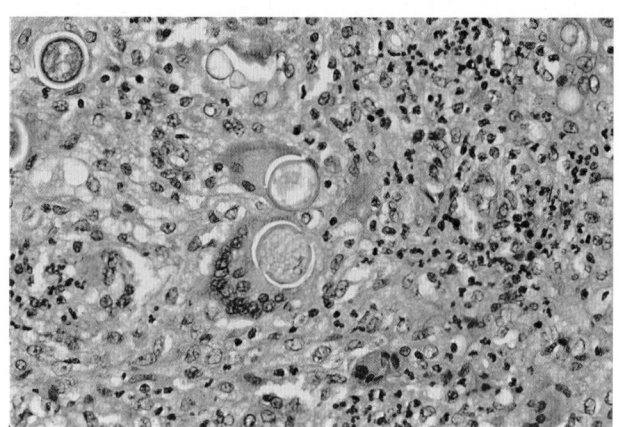

FIGURE 13.35 Focus of infection by a fungus, *Coccidioides immitis,* in a lymph node (not recognizable as such). Spherules of the fungus are partly surrounded by giant cells. When the spherules break open, they induce an acute inflammatory response, as indicated by the neutrophils seen on the left. This fungus therefore induces both a specific (granulomatous) and a nonspecific (neutrophilic) response. Coccidiomycosis is endemic in the American Southwest. (230x)

small granuloma-abscesses, but privately we refer to them as *granulabscesses.* This mixture of acute and chronic response reminds us of coccidiomycosis, a fungal infection endemic in the American Southwest (84a) in which *the fungus secretes materials that induce a diffuse, mixed response of both macrophages and neutrophils* (Figure 13.35). (2) *A microscopic abscess can be the first stage of a granuloma,* as seen when Schistosoma eggs are embolized into the liver (Figures 13.29). We can explain this sequence by assuming that the pattern of cytokines induced by the foreign eggs changes over time. Predictably, *a microscopic abscess can also be the first stage of a larger abscess,* as shown in Figure 13.11. The larger cavity is truly an abscess, because it is lined by a pus-producing "pyogenic membrane" (p. 484) made of granulation tissue.

A Note on Vocabulary: Granulocyte, Granuloma, Granulation Tissue. In our teaching experience, these "granular" words can suggest nonexisting links. **Granulocytes** are cells with microscopic granules within them—nothing to do with granulation tissue or granulomas. The **"granules"** of granulation tissue can be seen with the naked eye on the raw, "granulating" surface of wounds and ulcers (p. 444; see Figure 13.16). Some pathologists tend to think that **granulomas** are lumps of granulation tissue—but they are not: granulation tissue is made largely of capillaries; granulomas have no vessels. However, it is true that together they create a category of **temporary organs of connective tissue.**

Pros and Cons of the Granulomatous Response

Foreign-body granulomas are probably useful; after all, they tend to free the tissues of extraneous material. Immune granulomas have, basically, great survival value. Excellent proof of their value is found in leprosy, which comes in two forms: *tuberculoid,* in which patients produce a hefty granulomatous response, and *lepromatous,* in which the granulomatous response is impaired (Figure 13.36). Prognosis for the latter form is relatively poor.

On the other hand, immune granulomas can be harmful. They occupy space, much of which is not added but is removed from an organ. A tubercle in the lung, for example, is formed at the expense of a small portion of the lung. It is as if macrophages prepared the site for the expanding granuloma by removing local structures. For this reason, granulomas in the retina cause irreversible damage. Furthermore, granulomas recruit cells by secreting cytokines. These cytokines are presumably washed into the blood and lymph, but any excess might produce unwanted local reactions such as fibrosis, or even general effects ranging from fever to immunosuppression.

Granulomatous diseases number in the hundreds and affect all organs (74, 78, 90). They can be limited to one organ, especially the lung (from inhaled particles) or generalized. The agents can be infectious (syphilis, tuberculosis, leprosy, cat-scratch disease), fungal (cryptococcosis), parasitic (schistosomiasis), autoimmune

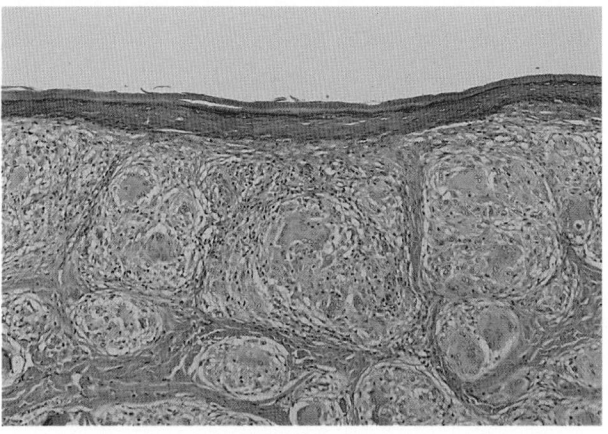

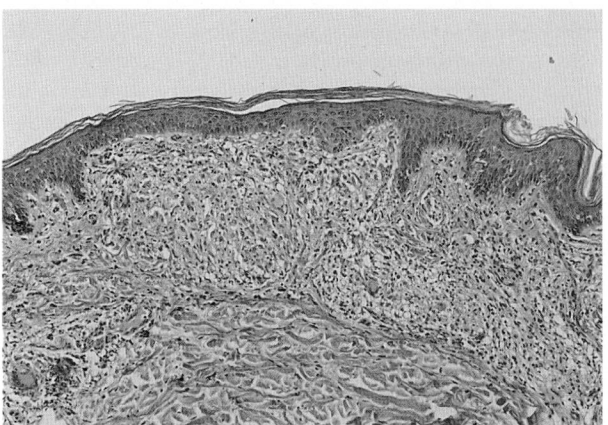

FIGURE 13.36 Two forms of leprosy. *Top:* Tuberculoid leprosy of the skin. The dermis is packed with granulomas; almost every one contains one or more giant cells. This pattern corresponds to a vigorous response of the immune system. *Bottom:* Lepromatous leprosy. There is a diffuse, although not very obvious, inflammatory infiltrate of the dermis, with no tendency to form granulomas. This is the pattern of an immunocompromised patient. (80x)

(rheumatic fever), or inorganic (inhaled beryllium compounds); often the cause remains unknown.

Most frustrating of all granulomatous diseases is **sarcoidosis,** in which classic, immune-type, giant-cell, noncaseating granulomas are scattered bodywide, yet no agent can be seen within them or grown out of them (Figure 13.37). Because the granulomas appear almost anywhere, symptoms are extremely variable and may even be lacking. About two thirds of the cases recover, either completely or with lung or eye impairment. Tuberculosis remains the prime suspect: mycobacterial DNA was found in more than half of biopsies (88), but there may be several causal agents (103). Another frustrating feature is that in the absence of a known cause the diagnosis has to be made by exclusion.

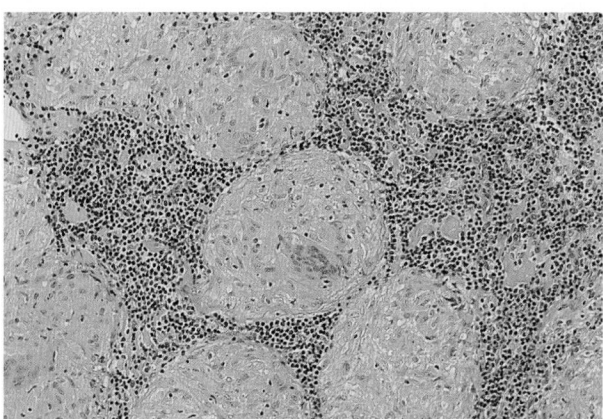

FIGURE 13.37 Granulomas of sarcoidosis in a lymph node. They consist mainly of packed macrophages (*epithelioid cells*) with a few lymphocytes. Note the presence of a giant cell in the central granuloma and the absence of central necrosis. Capillaries are also absent, as in all granulomas. (120x)

> **TO SUM UP:** In the big picture of chronic inflammation, granulomas behave like specialized, temporary subcommittees designed to handle tough local problems. They may or may not use the mechanisms of the immune response, but they always depend on the omnipotent macrophage.

The Giant Cell Story

Once regarded as a pathologist's curiosity, giant cells—short for multinucleated giant cells—turned out to be the ticket to a Nobel prize and then to a commercial boom. They derive from macrophages and are therefore close relatives of the osteoclasts (multinucleated cells associated with bone resorption). The story of the giant cells should be recorded here as a perfect example of how a little seed, in the proper hands, can grow into a forest.

Giant cells were first described by Johannes Müller, Virchow's teacher, in 1838. For a long time they were thought to be pregnant "mother cells" (Mutterzellen); that is, a type of cell that contains many baby cells, perhaps by analogy with the sporocysts of protozoa. Then it was realized that macrophages can give rise to giant cells, either by cell fusion or by nuclear division that is not followed by cell division (142, 151).

Structurally, the giant cells of chronic inflammation are essentially macrophages with many nuclei. It is traditional to mention that the nuclei can be arranged in two patterns: either randomly (as often seen in foreign-body granulomas) or around the cell periphery

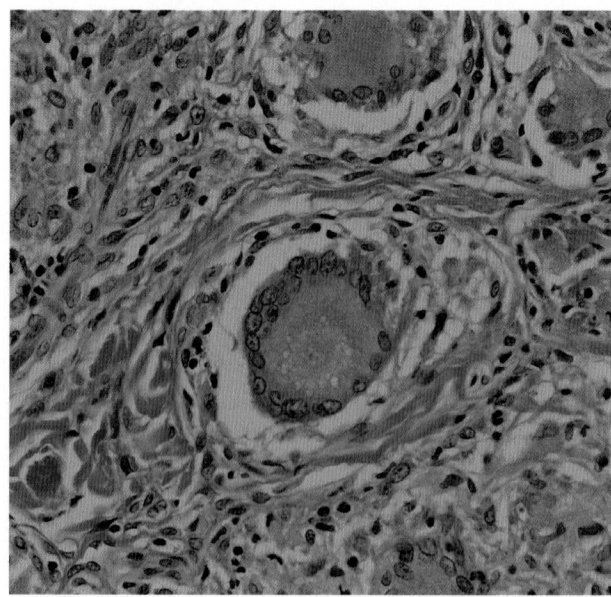

FIGURE 13.38 Typical multi-nucleated giant cell in a case of leprosy of the skin. It occupies much of the granuloma; the surrounding clear halo is an artefact.

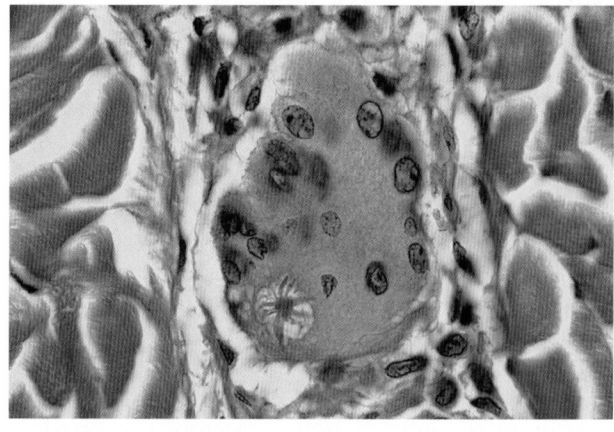

FIGURE 13.39 Giant cell containing a typical asteroid body, in a case of leprosy of the skin. (600x)

(*Langhans-type* giant cells, often seen in tuberculosis) (Figure 13.38). The peripheral arrangement is caused by a giant centrosphere in the middle of the cell (147). However, the distinction between the two arrangements has no known significance. Sometimes, especially in sarcoidosis, the giant cells contain beautiful **asteroid bodies** composed of cytoskeletal material (including tubulin) and phospholipid (Figure 13.39)(133). They may also contain rounded calcified structures called Schaumann bodies. What these inclusions mean is not known (139).

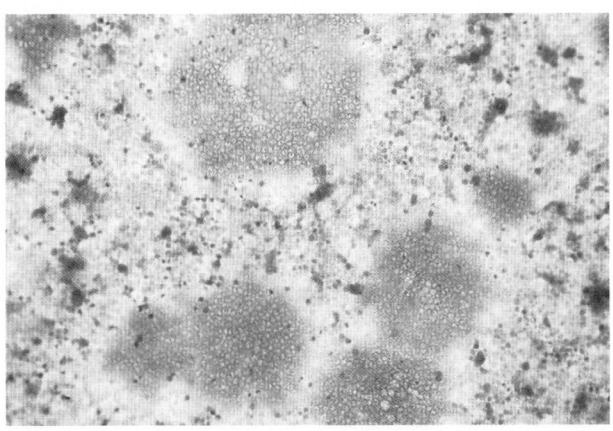

FIGURE 13.40   An example of cell fusion by a virus. Culture of human malignant epithelial cells (Hep-2) 24 hours after infection with a herpes virus. Many cells have been induced to fuse, producing large syncytia (toluidine blue stain).

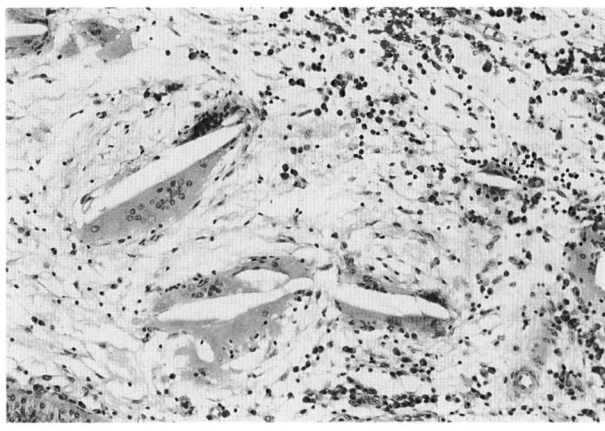

FIGURE 13.41   Multinucleated giant cells around crystals of cholesterol.

Spontaneous cell fusion. Cell fusion can be a normal process and does not necessarily produce giant cells: think of fertilization. As a pathologic process, it occurs in at least four settings:

(a) *In tissues infected by certain bacteria or viruses* (e.g., tubercle bacillus, papilloma viruses). These giant cells develop from macrophages as well as from epithelia (Figure 13.40). Adjacent cells are being zipped together by a physicochemical effect of lipids or proteins of the infectious particles (130). Cytokines can also accomplish the fusion (141, 148) including Interferon gamma (130).

(b) *By contact of macrophages with sterile foreign bodies* (Figure 13.41). The microscopic picture suggests that the cells are becoming larger and larger so as to take in a particle larger than themselves. Figure 13.42 shows that the zipping up recalls phagocytosis.

(c) Tumors of all sorts contain giant cells, neoplastic (as in "giant cell tumors of bone") or incidental.

(d) *Most unexpectedly, bone-marrow derived stem cells injected in vivo fuse with Purkinje neurons* (140a, 149a), *heart cells and liver cells* (p. 19) (127a). The documents are truly exciting. Will this be a new path to therapy?

How do macrophages fuse over a foreign body? Direct studies are lacking, but we can speculate. It is known that the converging edges of two extremely flattened cells creeping over a surface can meet and fuse where they touch, the reason being that the two tightly folded cell membranes no longer repel each other (Figure 13.42) (128). By this mechanism two macrophages could fuse while attempting to engulf the same particle (131).

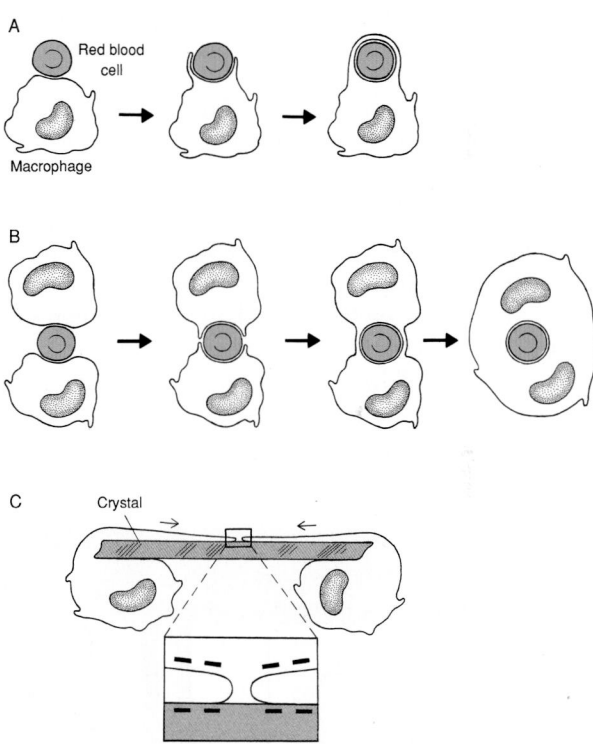

FIGURE 13.42   Showing how phagocytosis may lead to the fusion of macrophages. **A:** Phagocytosis of a red blood cell by a macrophage. The red blood cell is engulfed by a "crater" arising from the cell membrane; the rim of the crater then fuses with itself and closes over the red blood cell. **B:** Two macrophages attempting to engulf the same red blood cell. The two apposed craters may fuse along their rims. **C:** Fusion of two macrophages over the surface of a crystal. The two thin lamellipodia may fuse because the radius of curvature of the cell membranes at their advancing edge (*inset*) is so small that the negative charges are spread apart, whereby the apposed folds do not repel each other. (Adapted with permission from [131].)

Mechanisms of cell fusion. Giant cells have played a major historical role by reviving interest in cell fusion. Cells can fuse spontaneously; they can also be induced to do so. Both phenomena were well known early in the 1900s by botanists, who even used cell fusion to produce hybrids (132). But somehow the news did not reach the "animal people." Then came, in 1965, Drs. H. Harris and J. F. Watkins of the Sir William Dunn School of Pathology in Oxford (167). Taking the hint from virus-induced giant cells, Harris and Watkins reasoned that if viruses can zip together cells of the same kind, they might also join cells of different species. Sure enough, human cells and mouse cells, in the presence of Sendai virus (convenient because it is not pathogenic for humans), merged into beautiful giant cells; and most important, the giant cells survived (136, 137). These cells were called *heterokarya.* The virus worked even if it was inactivated by UV light, proving that the effect was chemical or physicochemical, unrelated to the infective process.

> Just 48 hours after this study appeared in *Nature,* a cartoon in the *London Daily Mirror* (Figure 13.43) (135) showed that the press was quick to grasp some implications of the experiment.

Not all experimental fusions are successful, although some mind-boggling combinations have survived for a time, such as between human and carrot, or human and tobacco leaf (138). A typical result of such disparate fusions is the following: the two nuclei of the heterokaryon enter mitosis together; then a single spindle is formed, and the two mononuclear daughter cells

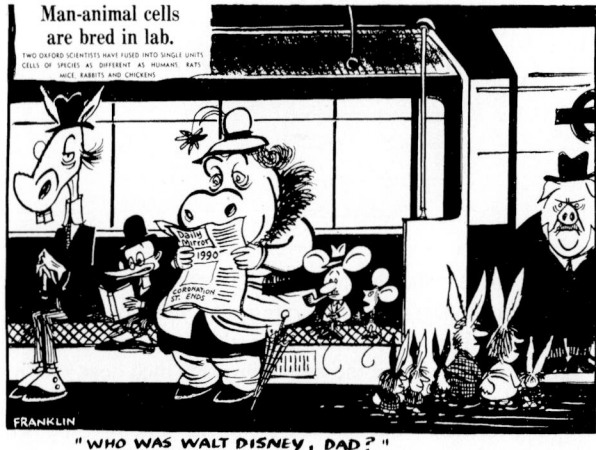

Man-animal cells are bred in lab.
TWO OXFORD SCIENTISTS HAVE FUSED INTO SINGLE UNITS CELLS OF SPECIES AS DIFFERENT AS HUMANS, RATS, MICE, RABBITS AND CHICKENS

FRANKLIN

"WHO WAS WALT DISNEY, DAD?"

FIGURE 13.43 Cartoon from *The London Daily Mirror* of February 15, 1965. Response to the news that cells "from man and mouse" had been fused into viable hybrids. (Reproduced from [135] by permission of Oxford University Press.)

contain, *in a single nucleus,* the chromosomes of both parent cells (135). In successive mitoses, some chromosomes can be eliminated, a fact that can be used for mapping single human chromosomes. This approach has opened up a new branch of genetics.

Of course, *fusions between normal and tumor cells* came early in the experimental agenda. At first they seemed to show that malignancy (as a pessimist might have guessed) tends to be dominant, but more work reversed this conclusion (p. 929). This is where the commercial boom occurred: two imaginative scientists (140) had the idea of fusing a malignant, and therefore immortal, plasma cell with a normal, mortal cell that secretes a certain protein: *this fusion produces a protein-secreting cell that is also immortal.* From this single fused cell one can then grow an artificial tumor or *hybridoma* that will continue to secrete that protein *in vitro* in potentially unlimited amounts: at long last a contribution to human welfare by tumors. This was the key to monoclonal antibodies. Cell fusion can now be induced by a host of reagents such as polyethylene glycol, even with electricity (129, 149). In 1984 the Nobel prize committee chose to reward the application of cell fusion to the production monoclonal antibodies rather than to the original idea.

> One hope raised by the heterokarya did not materialize: the possibility of alleviating world famine by creating a new generation of plant hybrids. The advent of genetic engineering in 1977 provided a more effective method (134).

Biological significance of giant cells. Apart from the inspiration that they provided to researchers, to this day we know of no specific function of giant cells, beyond the status of glorified macrophages. For some time they were maligned: it was said that they were less phagocytic (144) and slower moving (143) than their parent cells, and even that they represented a way to get rid of obsolete macrophages. Their half-life, estimated from transplantation experiments, was said to be only a few days (145), a figure that we find unlikely. More recent work finds the giant cells to be metabolically at least as active as a regular macrophage (146); one study found their respiratory burst to be 20–30 times greater (141).

It has been suggested that giant cells may have a survival value for viruses, by allowing them to jump from one cell to the next without being exposed to the intercellular fluid, which might contain dangerous antibodies. They are certainly useful to the pathologist: they provide a diagnostic hint that something abnormal is lurking in the tissue, perhaps a foreign body, perhaps an infectious agent.

Fibrosis

Fibrosis means an excess of fibrous connective tissue. It implies an excess of collagen fibers, with a varying admixture of other matrix components. It can be a *local* phenomenon, as an end result of chronic inflammation and of wound healing, and overlaps with the concept of scar. It can also be a *bodywide* phenomenon, in the autoimmune disease **scleroderma.**

> **Elastosis** applies to two very different conditions: (a) a localized excess of elastic fibers, seen microscopically (e.g., in some breast cancers), and (b) a pathologic change of elastic fibers in the skin (see *dermatoheliosis*, p. 277).

When fibrosis develops in the course of inflammation it may contribute to the healing process; such is the fibrosis that surrounds an abscess. By contrast, an excessive or inappropriate stimulus can produce severe fibrosis throughout an organ, and impair its function; typical examples are liver cirrhosis and idiopathic pulmonary fibrosis.

> *Cirrhosis* is now applied rather loosely to mean a severe, progressive fibrosis of the liver (Figure 13.44) and occasionally of the pancreas, although the term was originally coined to mean *yellowness* (p. 83).

Fibrotic tissue is whitish to the naked eye because of its high collagen content (Figure 13.45). For the same reason it is also firm, or even hard: hence the terms *sclerosis* and *sclerotic* (from the Greek *sklerós* for "hard"). It consists of cells and fibers, with few vessels; and it tends to contract very slowly, over weeks and months or longer.

The collagen of fibrotic tissues consists of the ordinary types I and III (156), and its chemical composition is normal. But there is evidence, at least in the lung, for a "fibrotic" collagen characterized by an *excess of hydroxylation and cross-linking* (178). Another exception occurs in the fibrosis of diabetes, in which glycation is thought to make the fibers more resistant to enzymatic attack (p. 284). As fibrotic lesions age, collagen becomes more and more cross-linked and reabsorption becomes more difficult (178). Furthermore, there are two special cases, special because the type of fibrotic tissue produced is clearly different from ordinary scar tissue: *inhaled silica particles* produce, in the lungs, deposits of thick, "hyalin" collagen fibers that contain few cells and are quite distinctive (Figure 13.46); the mechanism of this response in the early phase is clearly inflammatory, and related in part to the generation of oxygen- or nitrogen-derived free radicals (184); *inhaled asbestos particles* (Figure 13.47) produce on the pleura thick plaques of collagen that are almost as hard as wood (Figure 13.48) (152, 154, 161, 169, 179).

The cells of fibrous tissue, seen by light microscopy, seem to include only fibroblasts, sometimes admixed with inflammatory cells of the "chronic" type: macrophages and lymphocytes. Before 1971, none of these features explained the slow contraction typical of fibrous tissue; in fact it was the pursuit of this tantalizing phenomenon—the contraction of a supposedly noncontractile tissue—that led us to discover the

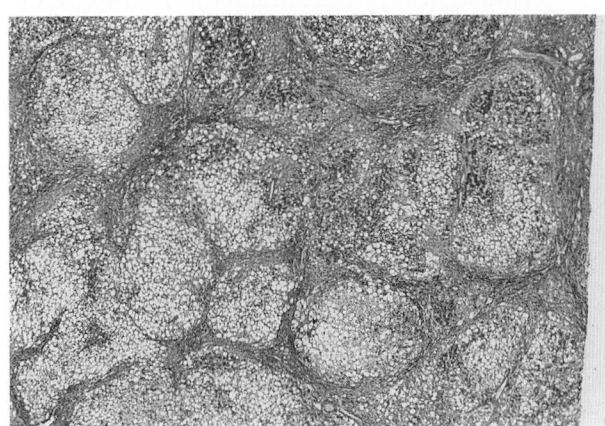

FIGURE 13.44 Example of scarring: cirrhosis of the liver in an alcoholic. The liver tissue is criss-crossed by bands of fibrous tissues. Many hepatocytes contain droplets of fat. (Masson trichrome, a special blue stain for collagen; 15x.)

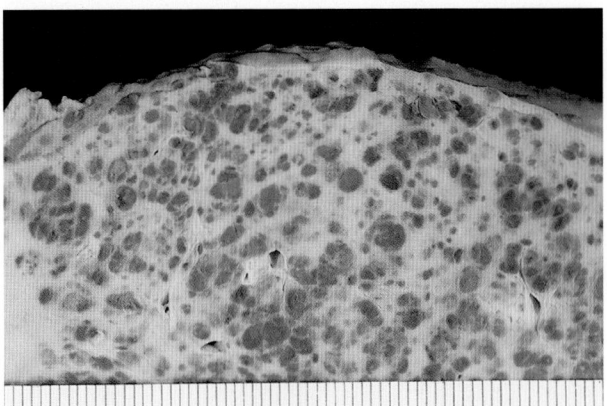

FIGURE 13.45 Example of fibrosis: cut surface of a cirrhotic liver from a chronic alcoholic. The green nodules represent regenerating liver tissue; the whitish background is the newly formed fibrous tissue typical of cirrhosis. **Scale** in millimeters.

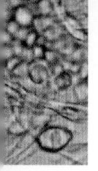

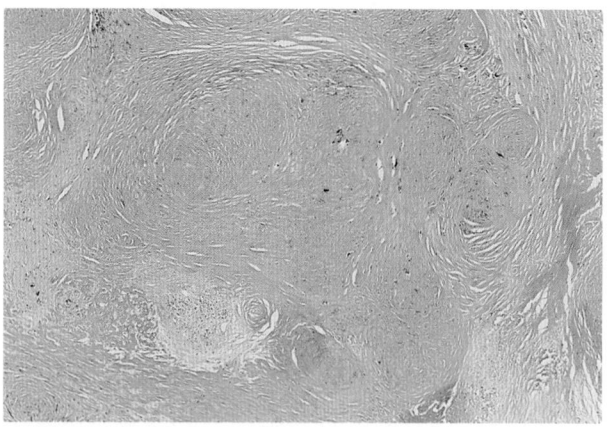

FIGURE 13.46   Silicotic nodules in the hilar node of a miner's lung: dense whorls of collagen fibers with few cells. A view of this field in polarized light would show scattered grains of silica. (25x)

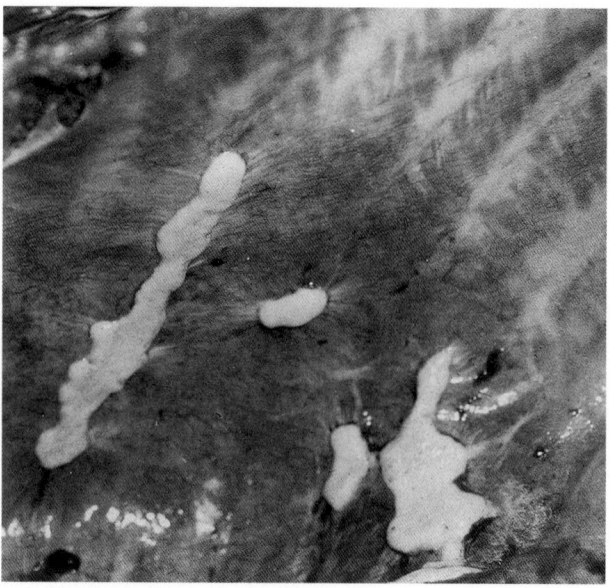

FIGURE 13.48   Thick, whitish fibrous plaques typical of exposure to asbestos. Photograph taken at autopsy, showing the inner surface of the chest; natural size.

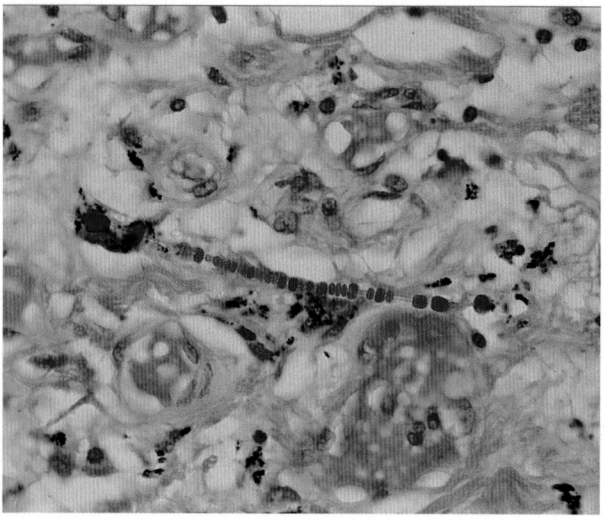

FIGURE 13.47   Asbestos body in the lung of a patient who had been chronically exposed to asbestos and developed fibrosis of the lung (asbestosis). Note typical beaded structure, and rusty color due to hemosiderin.

myofibroblasts, as we will see in the next chapter. Myofibroblasts have been found in most types of fibrosis and in all types of pathologically contracted organs or connective tissues; but the modulation of fibroblast to myofibroblast is too subtle to be recognized by the routine stains of light microscopy.

Why Does Fibrosis Develop?

In most cases the beginning clearly involves chronic inflammation; for example, *idiopathic* (i.e., unexplained) *pulmonary fibrosis,* a very distressing disease,

begins as a mild form of inflammation, followed by a wholly "unnecessary" scarring, i.e., fibrosis (Figure 13.49). Whether there is a truly primary fibrosis, not preceded by inflammation, we are not sure; even silicosis begins with activated macrophages. If fibrosis is largely secondary to inflammation, its genesis must be related to cytokines; this topic has produced a mountain of literature, because fibrosis includes many incurable diseases, and there is hope in anti-cytokine therapies.

Proof that a given cytokine is truly involved in fibrosis can be sought: (a) by infusing the cytokine into the tissues; (b) by testing the effect of anti-cytokine antibodies; (c) by proving by immunohistochemistry that local cells are synthesizing a given cytokine (Figure 13.50) (177); and (d) by creating genetically altered strains of mice. Cytokines, furthermore, may cause fibroblasts to divide, to move, and to secrete matrix of various kinds and/or matrix-destroying enzymes (metalloproteinases); the same functions may also be inhibited.

The long list of cytokines involved in fibrosis includes platelet-derived growth factor (PDGF) (163), insulin-like growth factor (IGF-1), the fibroblast growth factors (FGF), acid and basic, and also fibronectin, which can act as a growth factor; most of the responsibility is given to (TGFβ), which seems to be the driving force behind inflammation, wound healing, and most connective tissue activities (Figure 13.51) (4, 58, 181).

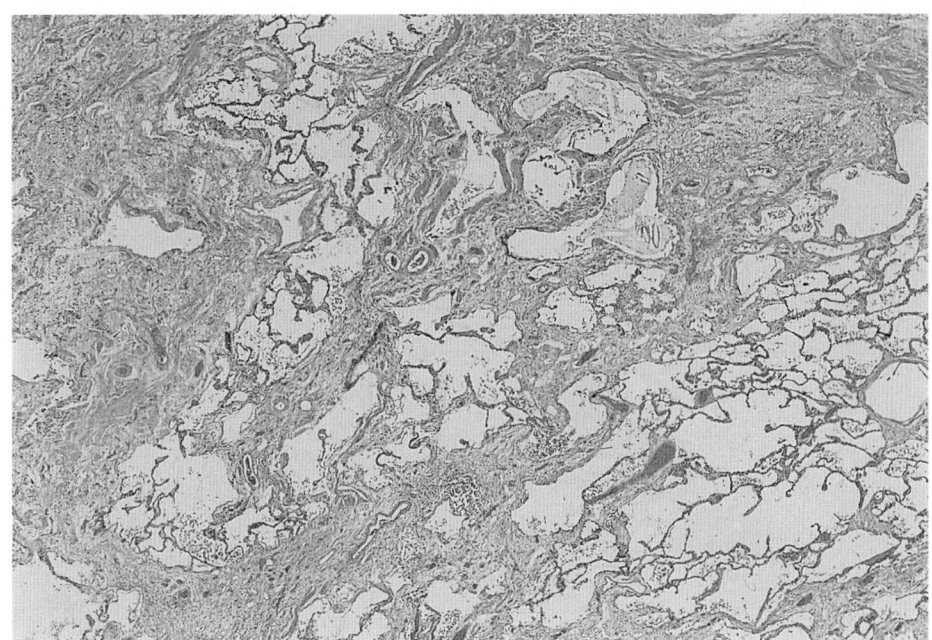

FIGURE 13.49 Idiopathic fibrosis of the lung. Strands of fibrous tissue infiltrate the parenchyma: very small patches of lung tissue are still recognizable. The paucity of inflammatory cells indicates that this is a long-standing lesion. (20x)

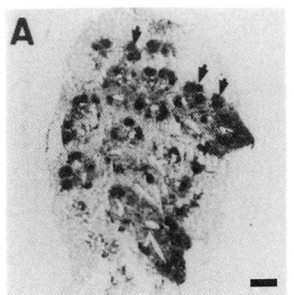 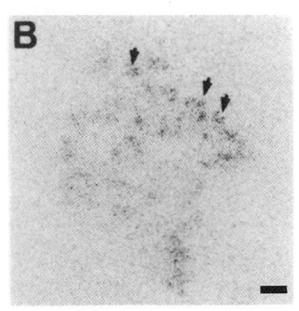

FIGURE 13.50 Tumor necrosis factor is involved in fibrosis. **A:** Histologic section of mouse lung. Instilled silica particles produced densely fibrous silicotic nodules (**arrowheads**). **B:** Autoradiograph of the same section after it was hybridized with a probe for TNF messenger RNA. The silver grains of the autoradiograph are deposited over the silicotic nodules (**arrows**) but not over the rest of the lung. **Bars** = 1000 μm. (Reprinted by permission from [177]. Copyright 1990 Macmillan Magazines Limited.)

Causes of Fibrosis

Besides inflammation, wound healing, and the inhalation of silica or asbestos, fibrosis can be induced by the following:

Ischemia. That ischemia is well-established as a cause of fibrosis may strike the reader as peculiar because lack of blood supply should tend to inhibit all cellular activities, including collagen synthesis. Yet hypoxia favors collagen synthesis *in vitro* (172), possibly because lactate, a product of anaerobic metabolism, favors collagen synthesis (164, 182).

In **retrolental fibroplasia** (or retinopathy of prematurity) the mechanism is thought to be spasm of the immature retinal arterioles in response to oxygen therapy, followed by retinal damage and a proliferative fibrovascular response.

Note also a special case: in experimental ischemia of the kidney, some of the fibrosis is perpetrated by the *epithelium* of the tubules (185), a finding that we believe but will cause much debate.

Alcohol abuse. It causes fibrosis (cirrhosis) of the liver (Figure 13.44), but the mechanism that stimulates collagen synthesis by the lipocytes (Ito cells) appears to be indirect, via acetaldehyde (162); in the cirrhotic liver it is possible that the lipocytes are further activated by growth factors provided by surrounding cells (157). Alcoholics are especially prone to develop a bizarre condition, *Dupuytren's disease:* a fibrosis and contraction of the palmar fascia, which deforms the hand.

Radiation. Fibrosis is usually an unwanted effect of gamma rays; in irradiated tissues, TGFβ can be demonstrated within 6 hours of the treatment (173).

Drugs. Several forms of sclerosis are iatrogenic: a disturbing development, because some of the drugs are invaluable. Bleomycin, a standard drug for producing

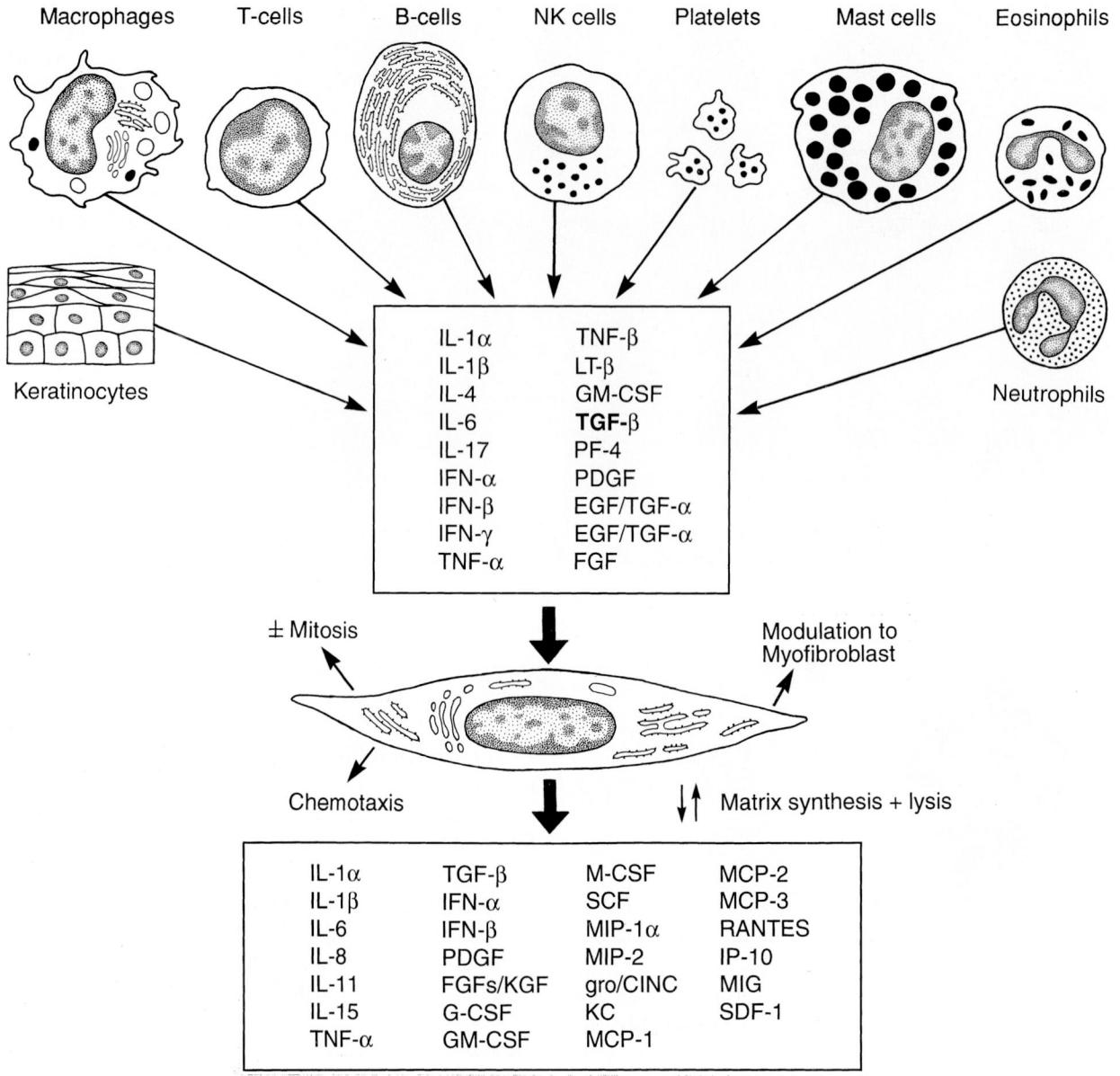

FIGURE 13.51 Many types of cells can stimulate the fibroblasts, by means of the chemical messengers shown in the box. The stimulated fibroblasts may respond by chemotaxis, by proliferation, by secretion of collagen and other macromolecules, and by modulation to myofibroblasts.

experimental pulmonary fibrosis, is currently used for cancer therapy.

A few patients treated for migraine develop ureteral constriction caused by retroperitoneal fibrosis (170), whereby a tough, glistening, wood-hard mass of fibrous tissue 2–6 cm thick (170, 175) encases the ureters, the large vessels, and other retroperitoneal structures. The main drug involved is methysergide, a vasoconstricting ergot derivative. Several other drug families have been incriminated, including beta blockers. Beta blockers include in their list

of possible side effect: Peyronies's disease, a slow retraction of the penile shaft.

Another peculiar disease in this category is ***idiopathic retractile mesenteritis,*** in which the mesentery becomes fibrous and contracts into a palpable mass, sometimes leading to intestinal obstruction (166).

The last example points out that some of the localizations of idiopathic fibrosis are surprisingly selective. A full explanation is not available, but it is well to remember that fibroblasts in different locations are at least functionally different (165, 174). They may have different life spans (171), different surface markers or patterns of synthesis (186), or varying propensities to modulate into myofibroblasts (159); even two cells arising from the same mitosis may grow at very different rates (171).

Fibrosis has a reputation of being irreversible, but it is more accurate to say that we do not yet have a magic wand to make fibrous tissue disappear, Yet, liver fibrosis (due to biliary obstruction) tends to reverse spontaneously if the obstruction is removed (153, 160). Renal fibrosis, the end result of chronic renal disease, was decreased—in rats—by subtle manipulations of the mesangial matrix (164a). Interferon gamma-1b is a strong antifibrotic (189). *There is nothing intrinsically irreversible even in the toughest fibrotic plaques.* We tend to think of collagen fibers as dead ropes, but they are organic structures with a metabolism. Recall the lesson of scurvy in the old days: the sailors' scars broke down, *because collagen has a turnover* (see Chapter 7). Fibroblasts produce collagen as well as collagenase. Dozens of cytokines are involved in the metabolism of the matrix. A dynamic construct is more easily affected than an inert one: there is definite hope for the treatment of fibrosis.

The End of the Show

Inflammation burns out if its cause is eliminated; the local effort turns to regeneration and healing. In the tissues, exudation stops; excess fluid is drained away; if fibrin had formed, the macrophages recognize it as something that should not be there and clean it out. If neutrophils are present, the macrophages remove them as well. This is a dangerous task, because the neutrophils are loaded with powerful enzymes that must not be spilled (Figure 13.52). So the macrophages wait until the neutrophils die by apoptosis; at that point they sweep up the corpses so fast—in minutes—that the experimenters must hurry to catch them in the act (Figure 13.53). This is admirable, but there is more to it. During phagocytosis the macrophages usually "drool," spilling some of their own enzymes, which could produce exactly the kind of environmental catastrophe that the macrophages have come to prevent. And so these well-trained scavengers, just as they take in that apoptotic morsel, refrain from drooling—although they will do so if swallowing anything else (18).

What happens to the other inflammatory cells is not well known. A few macrophages, fibroblasts, and perhaps lymphocytes may remain as permanent residents; all others will disappear, the myofibroblasts by apoptosis (16). The parenchyma of the inflamed organ will regenerate if it can; otherwise, a fibrous patch will mark the site. The few studies of parenchymal damage by inflammation have focused on increased permeability of the gut induced by diapedesis (32) or by free radicals (6) and on damage by hypersensitivity in tuberculosis (p. 558).

We have barely sketched the events of resolution, but how do all the cells know what to do? What causes the rise(s) and fall(s) of the inflammatory episode? We are just beginning to understand. The show depends on the interplay of *cells and matrix, mediators and receptors.* All cells are guided by GO and STOP signals (see Figure 9.45) (174a). The STOP signals are essential, to prevent a destructive and lethal cascade release of all the ammunition. In most tissues the first GO signal comes from the sentinels: their preformed

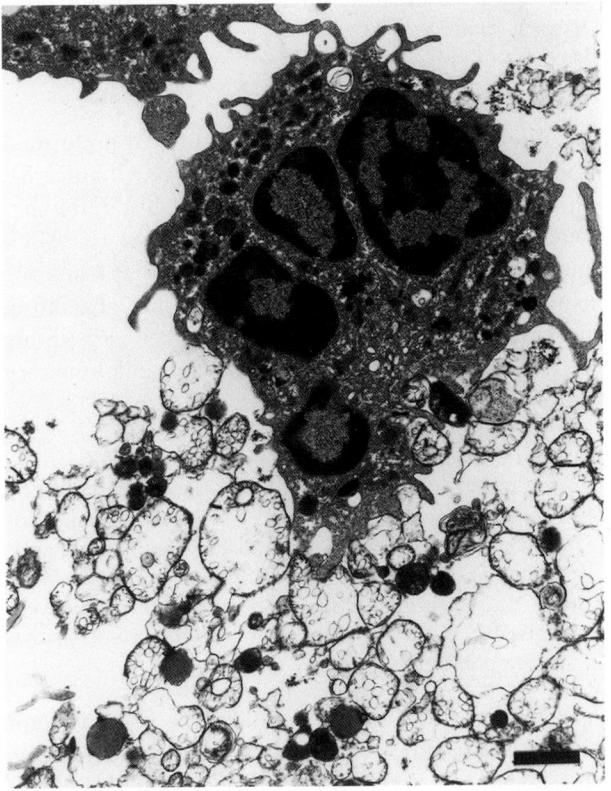

FIGURE 13.52   The destructive power of activated neutrophils. This human neutrophil sits over the debris of endothelial cells it has destroyed. It had been stimulated by a combination of endotoxin and chemotactic factors and then placed over a monolayer of cultured human endothelium. **Bar** = 1 μm. (Reproduced by permission from [160a]. Copyright 1988 Raven Press Ltd.)

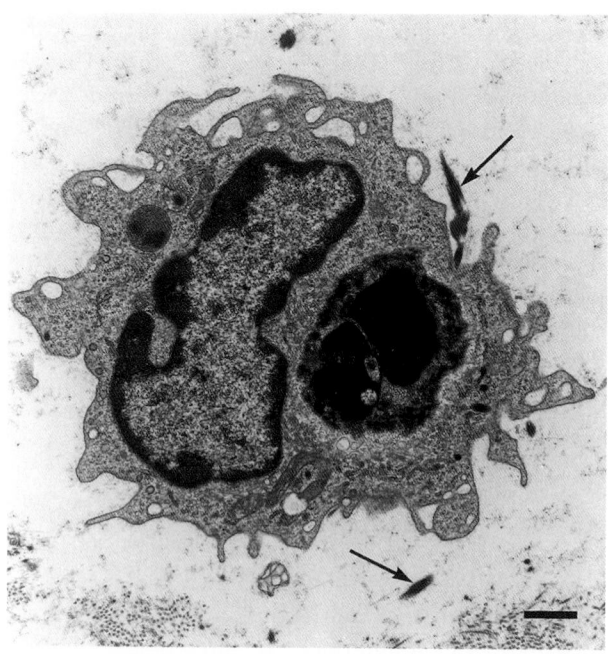

FIGURE 13.53 Macrophage that just engulfed a polymorph; the nuclear lobes are still recognizable. Note the wisps of fibrin (**arrows**). From a focus of acute inflammation in rat skin. **Bar** = 1 μm.

histamine triggers vascular leakage, and their preformed TNF triggers leukocyte recruitment (see Chapter 8). This episode is self-limiting, because histamine becomes ineffective after about 20 minutes (p. 371). Among its successors are derivatives of arachidonic acid; neutrophils supply arachidonate for generating the inflammatory leukotriene B_4, but they also supply arachidonate to cells that produce the anti-inflammatory lipoxins and *resolvins* (168a, 172a, 182a).

> Another example of the GO-STOP sequence (58). In the early phase of inflammation, TGFβ—secreted in part by macrophages—is inflammatory: it helps recruit and activate cells. On reaching a higher dose, it shifts to an anti-inflammatory role, downregulating macrophage activation and favoring fibrosis. The mechanism: the cells targeted by TGFβ modify their receptor profile so that they respond in the opposite fashion.

As a regulator of cytokine synthesis, the nuclear factor NK-κB may also play a role; it is presently being considered as a target for therapy (168b). Inhibitors of NF-κB include glucocorticoids and the anti-inflammatory cytokine IL-10 (69).

Sometimes There Is No End to the Show

This can happen, first, when an infectious agent cannot be destroyed; the classic example is tuberculosis.

In such cases the problem of local infection becomes a whole body problem (p. 717). Another setting is autoimmune disease: again, the causal agent cannot be eliminated because it is a normal component of the body. Under these circumstances, **inflammation becomes the disease,** and therefore the legitimate target of therapy.

> TO SUM UP: In discussing inflammation, we recognized the terminology introduced by immunologists, but in practice we used the traditional terms, better adapted to common language. Whatever the terms, it must be clear that there are two phases to the inflammatory response—innate/nonspecific ("acute") and modulated/specific ("chronic")—and that, despite the different level of sophistication, they have much in common. Both are planned to convey fluid and cells to the war front, and both do it largely (although not exclusively) by using the venules, which control the escape of fluid through the junctions, and the trapping and escape of leukocytes by means of adhesion molecules. In the meantime, the capillaries maintain the life-giving blood flow. A fine division of labor, made possible by a marvelous temporary organ, granulation tissue, with special arrangements for special situations—abscesses, adhesions, and granulomas.

References

Chronic Inflammation

1. Bello YM, Phillips TJ. Chronic leg ulcers: types and treatment. Hosp Pract 2000; February 15:101–107.
1a. Bevilacqua MP, Pober JS, Mendrick DL, Cotran RS, Gimbrone MA Jr. Identification of an inducible endothelial-leukocyte adhesion molecule. Proc Natl Acad Sci USA 1987;84:9238–9242.
1a′. Bryant RE. Effect of the suppurative environment on antibiotic activity. In: Root RK, Sande MA (eds). New dimensions in antimicrobial therapy. New York: Churchill Livingstone, 1984, pp. 313–337.
1b. Carp H. Mitochondrial N-formylmethionyl proteins as chemoattractants for neutrophils. J Exp Med 1982;155:264–275.
2. Cavender DE. Lymphocyte adhesion to endothelial cells in vitro: models for the study of normal lymphocyte recirculation and lymphocyte emigration into chronic inflammatory lesions. J Invest Dermatol 1989;93(suppl.):88S–95S.
3. Clark RAF (ed). The molecular and cellular biology of wound repair. New York: Plenum Press, 1996.

4. Clark RAF. Wound repair. Overview and general considerations. In: Clark RAF (ed). The molecular and cellular biology of wound repair. New York: Plenum Press, 1996, pp. 3–50.

5. Cotran RS, Gimbrone MA Jr, Bevilacqua MP, Mendrick DL, Pober JS. Induction and detection of a human activation antigen in vivo. J Exp Med 1986;164:661–666.

6. Cuzzocrea S, Mazzon E, De Sarro A, Caputi AP. Role of free radicals and poly (ADP-ribose) synthetase in intestinal tight junction permeability. Mol Med 2000;6:766–788.

7. Duijvestijn AM, Horst E, Pals ST, et al. High endothelial differentiation in human lymphoid and inflammatory tissues defined by monoclonal antibody HECA-452. Am J Pathol 1988;130:147–155.

8. Engel AG, Biesecker G. Complement activation in muscle fiber necrosis: demonstration of the membrane attack complex of complement in necrotic fibers. Ann Neurol 1982;12:289–296.

9. Falanga V, Eaglstein WH. The "trap" hypothesis of venous ulceration. Lancet 1993;341:1006–1008.

10. Fiddian-Green RG. Stress ulceration: a focal manifestation of mucosal ischemia. In: Marson A, Bulkley GB, Fiddian RG, Haglund UH (eds). Splanchnic ischemia and multiple organ failure. St. Louis: The C. V. Mosby Co., 1989, pp. 253–259.

11. Folkman J, Szabo S, Stovroff M, et al. Duodenal ulcer. Ann Surg 1991;214:414–427.

12. Freemont AJ, Ford WL. Functional and morphological changes in post-capillary venules in relation to lymphocytic infiltration into BCG-induced granulomata in rat skin. J Pathol 1985;147:1–12.

13. Freemont AJ, Jones CJP. Endothelial specialization of salivary gland vessels for accelerated lymphocyte transfer in Sjögren's syndrome. J Rheumatol 1983;10:801–804.

14. Freemont AJ, Jones CJP, Bromley M, Andrews P. Changes in vascular endothelium related to lymphocyte collections in diseased synovia. Arthritis Rheum 1983;26:1427–1433.

15. Goldstein IM, Weissmann G. Generation of C5-derived lysosomal enzyme-releasing activity (C5a) by lysates of leukocyte lysosomes. J Immunol 1974;113:1583–1588.

16. Greenhalgh DG. The role of apoptosis in wound healing. Int J Biochem Cell Biol 1998;30:1019–1030.

17. Ham A. AFIP mycobacteriology chief continues to attack Buruli ulcer in Third World countries. AFIP Lett 2000;158:4,5,14.

18. Haslett C, Henson P. Resolution of inflammation. In: Clark RAF (ed). The molecular and cellular biology of wound repair. New York: Plenum Press, 1996, pp. 143–168.

19. Hill JH, Ward PA. The phlogistic role of C3 leukotactic fragments in myocardial infarcts of rats. J Exp Med 1971; 133:885–900.

20. Hills BA, Burke JR, Thomas K. Surfactant barrier lining peritoneal mesothelium: lubricant and release agent. Periton Dialy Int 1998;18:157–165.

21. Holmdahl L, Ivarsson ML. The role of cytokines, coagulation, and fibrinolysis in peritoneal tissue repair. Eur J Surg 1999;165:1012–1019.

22. Holmdahl L, Risberg B. Beck DE, et al. Adhesions: pathogenesis and prevention-panel discussion and summary. Eur J Surg Suppl 1997;577:56–62.

23. Iguchi T, Ziff M. Electron microscopic study of rheumatoid synovial vasculature. J Clin Invest 1986;77:355–361.

24. Jalkanen S, Steere AC, Fox RI, Butcher EC. A distinct endothelial cell recognition system that controls lymphocyte traffic into inflamed synovium. Science 1986;233:556–558.

25. Joiner KA, Onderdonk AB, Gelfand JA, Bartlett JG, Gorbach SL. A quantitative model for subcutaneous abscess formation in mice. Br J Exp Pathol 1980;61:97–107.

26. Junghans BM, Collin HB. Limbal lymphangiogenesis after corneal injury: an autoradiographic study. Curr Eye Res 1989; 8:91–100.

27. Katori M, Kanayama T, Sasaki K, et al. Biphasic accumulation of leukocytes in rat cardiac infarct tissue caused by leukotriene B4 and complement. Jpn J Pharmacol 1989;50:234–238.

28. Lambiase A, Rama P, Bonini S, Caprioglio G, Aloe L. Topical treatment with nerve growth factor for corneal neurotrophic ulcers. N Engl J Med 1998;338:1174–1180.

29. Leu HJ. Morphology of chronic venous insufficiency—light and electron microscopic examinations. VASA 1991;20:330–342.

30. Liebermann-Meffert D, White H. The greater omentum. Berlin: Springer-Verlag, 1983.

31. Lindbeck G, Powers R. Cellulitis. Hosp Pract 1993;28 (suppl. 2):10–14.

32. Madara JL. Pathobiology of neutrophil interactions with polarized columnar epithelia. In: Serhan CN, Ward PA (eds). Molecular and cellular basis of inflammation. Totowa, NJ: Humana Press Inc., 1999.

33. Majno G, LaGattuta M, Thompson TE. Cellular death and necrosis: chemical, physical and morphologic changes in rat liver. Virchows Arch Pathol Anat 1960;333:421–465.

34. Majno G. The healing hand: man and wound in the ancient world. Cambridge, MA: Harvard University Press, 1975.

35. Maroko PR, Carpenter CB, Chiariello M, et al. Reduction by cobra venom factor of myocardial necrosis after coronary artery occlusion. J Clin Invest 1978;61:661–670.

36. McManus LM, Kolb WP, Crawford MH, et al. Complement localization in ischemic baboon myocardium. Lab Invest 1983;48:436–447.

37. Oppenheimer-Marks N, Ziff M. Binding of normal human mononuclear cells to blood vessels in rheumatoid arthritis synovial membrane. Arthritis Rheum 1986;29:789–792.

38. Pinckard RN, Olson MS, Giclas PC, et al. Consumption of classical complement components by heart subcellular membranes in vitro and in patients after acute myocardial infarction. J Clin Invest 1975;56:740–750.

39. Pinckard RN, O'Rourke RA, Crawford MH, et al. Complement localization and mediation of ischemic injury in baboon myocardium. J Clin Invest 1980;66:1050–1056.

40. Pitzalis C, Kingsley G, Haskard D, Panayi G. The preferential accumulation of helper-induced T lymphocytes in inflammatory lesions: evidence for regulation by selective endothelial and homotypic adhesion. Eur J Immunol 1988;18:1397–1404.

41. Pullinger BD, Florey HW. Proliferation of lymphatics in inflammation. J Pathol Bacteriol 1937;45:157–170.

42. Regezi JA, Sciubba JJ. Oral pathology. Clinical-pathologic correlations. Philadelphia, PA: WB Saunders, 1989.

43. Risberg B. Adhesions: preventive strategies. Eur J Surg Suppl 1997;577:32–39.

44. Rossen RD, Swain JL, Michael LH, et al. Selective accumulation of the first component of complement and leukocytes in ischemic canine heart muscle. A possible initiator of an extra

myocardial mechanism of ischemic injury. Circ Res 1985;57: 119–130.

45. Ryan GB, Grobéty J, Majno G. Postoperative peritoneal adhesions. A study of the mechanisms. Am J Pathol 1971; 65:117–148.

46. Ryan GB, Grobéty J, Majno G. Mesothelial injury and recovery. Am J Pathol 1973;71:93–112.

46a. Savill J, Gregory C, Haslett C. Eat me or die. Science 2003; 302:1516–1517.

46b. Scaffidi P, Misteli T, Bianchi ME. Release of chromatin protein HGMGB1 by necrotic cells triggers inflammation. Nature 2002;418;191–195.

47. Schäfer H, Mathey D, Hugo F, Bhakdi, S. Deposition of the terminal C5b-9 complement complex in infarcted areas of human myocardium. J Immunol 1986;137:1945–1949.

48. Schoefl GI. Studies on inflammation. III. Growing capillaries: their structure and permeability. Virchows Arch Pathol Anat 1963;337:97–141.

49. Schoefl GI, Majno G. Regeneration of blood vessels in wound healing. Adv Biol Skin 1964;5:173–193.

50. Seifert PS, Catalfamo JL, Dodds WJ. Complement C5a (desArg) generation in serum exposed to damaged aortic endothelium. Exp Mol Pathol 1988;48:216–225.

51. Sheikh KMA, Duggal K, Relfson M, Gignac S, Rowden G. An experimental histopathologic study of surgical glove powders. Arch Surg 1984;119:215–219.

51a. Shi, Y, Rock KL. Cell death releases endogenous adjuvants that selectively enhance immune surveillance of particulate antigens. Eur J Immunol 2002;32:155–162.

52. Spouge JD. A new look at the rests of Malassez. A review of their embryological origin, anatomy, and possible role in periodontal health and disease. J Periodontol 1980;51: 437–444.

53. Storrs SB, Kolb WP, Pinckard RN, Olson MS. Characterization of the binding of purified human C1q to heart mitochondrial membranes. J Biol Chem 1981;256:10924–10929.

54. Szabo S, Folkman J, Vattay P, Morales RE, Kato K. Duodenal ulcerogens: effect of FGF on cysteamine-induced duodenal ulcer. In: Halter F, Garner A, Tytgat GNJ, eds. Mechanisms of peptic ulcer healing. (Falk Symposium 59). Dordrecht: Kluwer Academic Publishers, 1990:139–150.

55. Szabo S, Vattay P, Scarbrough E, Folkman J. Role of vascular factors, including angiogenesis, in the mechanisms of action of sucralfate. Am J Med 1991;91(suppl 2A):158S–160S.

56. Tsutsumi V, Mena-Lopez R, Anaya-Velazquez F, Martinez-Palomo A. Cellular bases of experimental amebic liver abscess formation. Am J Pathol 1984;117:81–91.

57. Väkevä A, Laurila P, Meri S. Regulation of complement membrane attack complex formation in myocardial infarction. Am J Pathol 1993;143:65–75.

58. Wahl SM. Transforming growth factor-β (TGF-β) in the resolution and repair of inflammation. In: Gallin JI, Snyderman R. (eds). Inflammation: Basic principles and clinical correlates. 3rd ed. Philadelphia: Lippincott Williams & Wilkins, 1999, pp. 883–892.

59. Walsh JH, Peterson WL. The treatment of *Helicobacter pylori* infection in the management of peptic ulcer disease. N Engl J Med 1995;333:984–999.

60. Ward PA, Hill JH. C5 chemotactic fragments produced by an enzyme in lysosomal granules of neutrophils. J Immunol 1970;104:535–543.

61. Weisman HF, Bartow T, Leppo MK, et al. Soluble human complement receptor type 1: in vivo inhibitor of complement suppressing post-ischemic myocardial inflammation and necrosis. Science 1990;249:146–151.

61a. Weissman IL, Butcher EC, Rouse RV, Scollay RG. Cell-cell interactions in the establishment and maintenance of lymphoid tissue architecture. In: Sercarz E, Cunningham AJ, eds. Strategies of immune regulation. New York: Academic Press, 1980:77–94.

62. Yarkony GM. Pressure ulcers: a review. Arch Phys Med Rehabil 1994;75:908–917.

63. Yoffey JM, Courtice FC. Lympathics, lymph and the lymphomyeloid complex. London: Academic Press, 1970.

64. Ziff M, Cavender D, Haskard D. Pathogenetic factors in rheumatoid synovitis. Br J Rheumatol 1988;27(suppl II): 153–156.

Granulomatous Inflammation

65. Actor JK, Olsen M, Jagannath C, Hunter RL. Relationship of survival, organism containment, and granuloma formation in acute murine tuberculosis. J Interfer Cytokine Res 1999; 19:1183–1193.

66. Adams DO. The biology of the granuloma. In: Ioachim HL, ed. Pathology of granulomas. New York: Raven Press, 1983, pp. 1–20.

67. Allred DC, Kobayashi K, Yoshida T. Anergy-like immunosuppression in mice bearing pulmonary foreign-body granulomatous inflammation. Am J Pathol 1985;121:466–473.

68. Andrade ZA, Grimaud J-A. Morphology of chronic collagen resorption. A study on the late stages of schistosomal granuloma involution. Am J Pathol 1988;132:389–399.

69. Barnes PF, Lu S, Abrams JS, et al. Cytokine production at the site of disease in human tuberculosis. Inf Immunol 1993;61: 3482–3489.

69a. Boros, DL, ed. Granulomatous Infections and Inflammation. Cellular and molecular mechanisms. Washington, DC: ASM Press, 2003.

70. Boros DL. The granulomatous inflammatory response: an overview. In: Boros DL, Yoshida T, eds. Basic and clinical aspects of granulomatous diseases. New York: Elsevier-North Holland, 1980, pp. 1–14.

71. Boros DL. Experimental granulomatous disease. In: Fanburg BL, ed. Sarcoidosis and other granulomatous diseases of the lung. New York: Marcel Dekker, 1983, pp. 403–449.

72. Boros DL. Experimental granulomatosis. Clin Dermatol 1986;4:10–21.

73. Boros DL. Immunoregulation of granuloma formation in murine *Schistosomiasis mansoni*. Ann NY Acad Sci 1986; 465:313–323.

74. Boros DL. Hypersensitivity granulomas. In: Middleton E Jr, Reed CE, Ellis EF, Adkinson NF Jr, Yunginger JW, eds. Allergy: principles and practice, 3rd ed, vol 1. St. Louis: CV Mosby, 1988, pp. 275–294.

75. Boros DL, Warren KS. Delayed hypersensitivity-type granuloma formation and dermal reaction induced and elicited by a

soluble factor isolated from *Schistosoma mansoni* eggs. J Exp Med 1970;132:488–507.

76. Boros DL, Warren KS. Specific granulomatous hypersensitivity elicited by bentonite particles coated with soluble antigens from schistosome eggs and tubercle bacilli. Nature 1971; 229:200–201.

77. Boros DL, Warren KS, Pelley RP. The secretion of migration inhibitory factor by intact schistosome egg granulomas maintained in vitro. Nature 1973;246:224–226.

78. Boris DL, Yoshida T, eds. Basic and clinical aspects of granulomatous diseases. New York: Elsevier-North Holland, 1980.

79. Chensue SW, Boros DL. Modulation of granulomatous hypersensitivity. I. Characterization of T lymphocytes involved in the adoptive suppression of granuloma formation in *Schistosoma mansoni*-infected mice. J Immunol 1979;123: 1409–1414.

80. Chensue SW, Kunkel SL, Higashi GI, Ward PA, Boros DL. Production of superoxide anion, prostaglandins, and hydroxyeicosatetraenoic acids by macrophages from hypersensitivity-type (*Schistosoma mansoni* egg) and foreign body-type granulomas. Infect Immun 1983;42:1116–1125.

81. Courtade ET, Tsuda T, Thomas CR, Dannenberg AM Jr. Capillary density in developing and healing tuberculous lesions produced by BCG in rabbits. Am J Pathol 1975; 78:243–260.

82. Dannenberg AM Jr, Tomashefski JF Jr. Pathogenesis of pulmonary tuberculosis. In: Fishman AP, ed. Pulmonary diseases and disorders, 2nd ed, vol 3. New York: McGraw-Hill, 1988, pp. 1821–1842.

83. Dreher R, Keller HU, Hess MW, Roos B, Cottier H. Early appearance and mitotic activity of multinucleated giant cells in mice after combined injection of talc and prednisolone acetate. A model for studying rapid histiocytic polykarion formation in vivo. Lab Invest 1978;38:149–156.

84. Elliott DE, Righthand VF, Boros DL. Characterization of regulatory (interferon-α/β) and accessory (LAF/IL 1) monokine activities from liver granuloma macrophages of *Schistosoma mansoni*-infected mice. J Immunol 1987;138: 2653–2662.

84a. Galgiani JN. Coccidiomycosis: a regional disease of national importance. I. Approaches for control. Ann Intern Med 1999;130(4 Pt 1):293–300.

85. Geratz JD, Tidwell RR, Schwab JH, Anderle SK, Pryzwansky KB. Sequential events in the pathogenesis of streptococcal cell wall-induced arthritis and their modulation by bis(5-amidino-2-benzimidazolyl)methane (BABIM). Am J Pathol 1990;136:909–921.

86. Ginsburg CH, McCluskey RT, Nepom JT, et al. Antigen- and receptor-driven regulatory mechanisms. X. The induction and suppression of hapten-specific granulomas. Am J Pathol 1982;106:421–431.

87. Greenaway TM, Caterson ID. Hypercalcemia and lipoid pneumonia. Aust N Z J Med 1989;19:713–715.

88. Grosser M, Luther T, Müller J, et al. Detection of *M. tuberculosis* DNA in sarcoidosis: correlation with T-cell response. Lab Invest 1999;79:775–784.

89. Hoffman KF, Cheever AW, Wynn TA. IL-10 and the dangers of immune polarization: excessive type 1 and type 2 cytokine responses induce distinct forms of lethal immunopathology in murine schistosomiasis. J Immunol 2000;164:6406–6416.

90. Ioachim HL, ed. Pathology of granulomas. New York: Raven Press, 1983.

91. James DG, Zumla A (eds). The granulomatous disorders. Cambridge: Cambridge University Press, 1999.

92. Kasahara K, Kobayashi K, Shikama Y, et al. Direct evidence for granuloma-inducing activity of interleukin-1. Am J Pathol 1988;130:629–638.

93. Kellermeyer RW, Warren KS. The role of chemical mediators in the inflammatory response induced by foreign bodies: comparison with the schistosome egg granuloma. J Exp Med 1970;131:21–39.

94. Kindler V, Sappino A-P, Grau GE, Piguet P-F, Vassalli P. The inducing role of tumor necrosis factor in the development of bactericidal granulomas during BCG infection. Cell 1989;56:731–740.

95. Kobayashi K, Allred C, Castriotta R, Yoshida, T. Strain variation of bacillus Calmette-Guerin-induced pulmonary granuloma formation is correlated with anergy and the local production of migration inhibition factor and interleukin 1. Am J Pathol 1985;119:223–235.

96. Kozeny GA, Barbato AL, Bansal VK, Vertuno LL, Hano JE. Hypercalcemia associated with silicone-induced granulomas. N Engl J Med 1984;311:1103–1105.

97. Krulewitz AH, Stadecker MJ, Wright JA, Fanburg BL. Angiotensin-1-converting enzyme activity of murine macrophages isolated from granulomas elicited by eggs of *Schistosoma mansoni*. Infect Immun 1983;41:39–43.

98. Lemann J Jr, Gray RW. Calcitriol, calcium, and granulomatous disease. N Engl J Med 1984;311:1115–1117.

98a. Loeffler DA, Lundy SK, Singh KP, et al. Soluble egg antigens from Schistosoma mansoni induce angiogenesis-related abscesses by upregulating vascular endothelial growth factor in human endothelial cells. J Infect Dis 2002;185: 1650–1656.

99. Lukacs NW, Chensue SW, Smith RE, et al. Production of monocyte chemoattractant protein-1 and macrophage inflammatory protein-1α by inflammatory granuloma fibroblasts. Am J Pathol 1994;144:711–718.

100. Lurie MB. Resistance to tuberculosis: experimental studies in native and acquired defensive mechanisms. Cambridge, MA: Harvard University Press, 1964.

100a. Mosmann TR, Sad S. The expanding universe of T-cell subsets: Th1, Th2 and more. Immunol Today 1996;17:138–146.

101. Murray HW. Granulomatous inflammation: Host antimicrobial defense in the tissues in visceral leishmaniasis. In: Gallin JI, Snyderman R (eds). Inflammation: Basic principles and clinical correlates. 3rd ed. Philadelphia: Lippincott Williams & Wilkins, 1999, pp. 977–994.

102. Narayanan RB, Badenoch-Jones P, Turk JL. Experimental mycobacterial granulomas in guinea pig lymph nodes: ultrastructural observations. J Pathol 1981;134:253–265.

103. Newman LS, Rose CS, Maier LA. Sarcoidosis. N Engl J Med 1997;336:1224–1234.

104. Pellegrino J, Brener Z. Method for isolating schistosome granulomas from mouse liver. J Parasitol 1956;42:564.

105. Perrotto JL, Warren KS. Inhibition of granuloma formation around *Schistosoma mansoni* eggs. IV. X-irradiation. Am J Pathol 1969;56:279–291.

106. Rook GAW, Taverne J, Leveton C, Steele J. The role of gamma-interferon, vitamin D$_3$ metabolites and tumour necrosis factor in the pathogenesis of tuberculosis. Immunology 1987;62:229–234.

106a. Rutitzky LI, Hernandez HJ, Stadecker MJ. Th1-polarizing immunization with egg antigens correlates with severe exacerbation of immunopathology and death in schistosome infection. Proc Natl Acad Sci USA 2002;98:13243–12348.

107. Ryan GB, Majno G. Inflammation. Kalamazoo, MI: The Upjohn Company, 1977.

108. Salthouse TN, Matlaga BF. Collagenase associated with macrophage and giant cell activity. Experientia 1972;28:326.

109. Schwartz CJ, Ghidoni JJ, Kelley JL, et al. Evolution of foam cells in subcutaneous rabbit carrageenan granulomas. I. Light-microscopic and ultrastructural study. Am J Pathol 1985;118:134–150.

110. Shikama Y, Kobayashi K, Kasahara K, et al. Granuloma formation by artificial microparticles in vitro. Am J Pathol 1989;134:1189–1199.

111. Stadecker MJ. The regulatory role of the antigen-presenting cell in the development of hepatic immunopathology during infection with Schistosoma mansoni. Pathobiology 1999;67:269–272.

111a. Stadecker MJ. Personal communication, December 2002.

112. Stadecker MJ, Wright JA. Distribution and kinetics of mononuclear phagocytes in granulomas elicited by eggs of *Schistosoma mansoni*. Am J Pathol 1984;116:245–252.

113. Tanaka A, Emori K, Nagao S, et al. Epitheloid granuloma formation requiring no T-cell function. Am J Pathol 1982;106:165–170.

114. Truden JL, Boros DL. Collagenase, elastase, and nonspecific protease production by vigorous or immunomodulated liver granulomas and granuloma macrophages/eosinophils of *S. mansoni*-infected mice. Am J Pathol 1985;121:166–175.

115. Unanue ER, Benacerraf B. Immunologic events in experimental hypersensitivity granulomas. Am J Pathol 1973;71:349–364.

116. van der Rhee HJ, van der Burgh-de Winter CPM, Daems WT. The differentiation of monocytes into macrophages, epitheloid cells, and multinucleated giant cells in subcutaneous granulomas. I. Fine structure. Cell Tissue Res 1979;197:355–378.

117. von Lichtenberg F. Studies on granuloma formation. III. Antigen sequestration and destruction in the schistosome pseudotubercle. Am J Pathol 1964;45:75–93.

118. Wahl SM. Fibrosis: bacterial-cell-wall-induced hepatic granulomas. In: Gallin JI, Goldstein IM, Snyderman R, eds. Inflammation. Basic principles and clinical correlates. New York: Raven Press, 1988, pp. 841–860.

119. Wahl SM, Allen JB, Dougherty S, et al. T lymphocyte-dependent evolution of bacterial cell wall-induced hepatic granulomas. J Immunol 1986;137:2199–2209.

120. Wahl SM, Frazier-Jessen M, Jin WW, et al. Cytokine regulation of schistosome-induced granuloma and fibrosis. Kidney Int 1997;51:1370–1375.

121. Wahl SM, Hunt DA, Allen JB, Wilder RL, Paglia L, Hand AR. Bacterial cell wall-incuded hepatic granulomas. An in vivo model of T cell-dependent fibrosis. J Exp Med 1986;163:884–902.

122. Warren KS. A functional classification of granulomatous inflammation. Ann NY Acad Sci 1976;278:7–18.

123. Warren KS. The cell biology of granulomas (aggregates of inflammatory cells) with a note on giant cells. In: Weissmann G, ed. The cell biology of inflammation. Amsterdam: Elsevier-North Holland Biomedical Press, 1980, pp. 543–557.

124. Warren KS, Domingo EO, Cowan RBT. Granuloma formation around schistosome eggs as a manifestation of delayed hypersensitivity. Am J Pathol 1967;51:735–756.

125. Weinstock JV, Boros DL. Organ-dependent differences in composition and function observed in hepatic and intestinal granulomas isolated from mice with schistosomiasis mansoni. J Immunol 1983;130:418–422.

126. Wyler DJ, Stadecker MJ, Dinarello CA, O'Dea JF. Fibroblast stimulation in schistosomiasis. V. Egg granuloma macrophages spontaneously secrete a fibroblast-stimulating factor. J Immunol 1984;132:3142–3148.

127. Zumla A, Mwaba P, Rook G, Lucas S. Tuberculosis. In: The granulomatous disorders. Cambridge: Cambridge University Press, 1999, pp. 132–160.

The Giant Cell Story

127a. Alvarez-Dolado M, Pardal R, Garcia-Verdugo JM, et al. Fusion of bone-marrow derived cells with Purkinje neurons, cardiomyocytes and hepatocytes. Nature 2003;425:968–973.

128. Bangham AD. The adhesiveness of leukocytes with special reference to zeta potential. Ann NY Acad Sci 1964;116:945–949.

129. Beers RF Jr, Bassett EG, eds. Cell fusion: gene transfer and transformation (Miles International Symposium Series, No. 14). New York: Raven Press, 1984.

130. Blobel CP, Wolfsberg TG, Turck CW, et al. A potential fusion peptide and an integrin ligand domain in a protein active in spermegg fusion. Nature 1992;356:248–252.

131. Chambers TJ. Fusion of macrophages following simultaneous attempted phagocytosis of glutaraldehyde-fixed red cells. J Pathol 1977;122:71–80.

132. Constabel F, Cutler AJ. Protoplast fusion. In: Fowke LC, Constabel F, eds. Plant protoplasts. Boca Raton, FL: CRC Press, 1985, pp. 53–65.

133. Gadde PS, Moscovic EA. Asteroid bodies: products of unusual microtubule dynamics in monocyte-derived giant cells. An immunohistochemical study. Histol Histopathol 1994;9:633–642.

134. Gasser CS, Fraley RT. Genetically engineering plants for crop improvement. Science 1989;244:1293–1299.

135. Harris H. Cell fusion. The Dunham Lectures. Oxford: Clarendon Press, 1970.

136. Harris H, Watkins JF. Hybrid cells derived from mouse and man: artificial heterokaryons of mammalian cells from different species. Nature 1965;205:640–646.

137. Harris H, Watkins JF, Ford CE, Schoefl GI. Artificial heterokaryons of animal cells from different species. J Cell Sci 1966;1:1–30.

138. Jones CW, Mastrangelo IA, Smith HH, Liu HZ, Meck RA. Interkingdom fusion between human (HeLa) cells and tobacco hybrid (GGLL) protoplasts. Science 1976;193:401–403.

139. Kirkpatrick CJ, Curry A, Bisset DL. Light- and electron-microscopic studies on multinucleated giant cells in sarcoid granuloma: new aspects of asteroid and Schaumann bodies. Ultrastruct Pathol 1988;12:581–597.

140. Köhler G, Milstein C. Continuous cultures of fused cells secreting antibody of predefined specificity. Nature 1975; 256:495–497.

140a. Kozorovitskiy Y, Gould E. Stem cell fusion in the brain. Nat Cell Biol 2003;5:952–954.

141. Kreipe H, Radzun HJ, Rudolph P, et al. Multinucleated giant cells generated in vitro. Terminally differentiated macrophages with down-regulated c-fms expression. Am J Pathol 1988;130:232–243.

142. Mariano M, Spector WG. The formation and properties of macrophage polykaryons (inflammatory giant cells). J Pathol 1974;113:1–19.

143. Papadimitriou JM, Kingston KJ. The locomotory behaviour of the multinucleate giant cells of foreign body reactions. J Pathol 1976;121:27–36.

144. Papadimitriou JM, Robertson TA, Walters MN-I. An analysis of the phagocytic potential of multinucleate foreign body giant cells. Am J Pathol 1975;78:343–358.

145. Papadimitriou JM, Sforsina D, Papaelias L. Kinetics of multinucleate giant cell formation and their modification by various agents in foreign body reactions. Am J Pathol 1973;73:349–364.

146. Papadimitriou JM, Van Bruggen I. Evidence that multinucleate giant cells are examples of mononuclear phagocytic differentiation. J Pathol 1986;148:149–157.

147. Sapp JP. An ultrastructural study of nuclear and centriolar configurations in multinucleated giant cells. Lab Invest 1976;34:109–114.

148. Sone S. Functions of multinucleated giant cells formed by fusing rat alveolar macrophages with lymphokines containing macrophage fusion factor. Lymphokine Res 1984;3:163–173.

149. Sowers AE, ed. Cell fusion. New York: Plenum Press, 1987.

149a. Weimann JM, Johnasson CB, Trejo A, Blau HM. Stable reprogrammed heterokaryons form spontaneously in Purkinje neurons after bone marrow transplant. Nat Cell Biol 2003; 11:959–966.

150. Weinberg JB, Hobbs MM, Misukonis MA. Phenotypic characterization of gamma interferon-induced human monocyte polykaryons. Blood 1985;66:1241–1246.

151. Weiss LP, Fawcett DW. Cytochemical observations on chicken monocytes macrophages and giant cells in tissue culture. J Histochem Cytochem 1953;1:47–65.

Fibrosis

152. Aalto M, Potila M, Kulonen E. The effect of silica-treated macrophages on the synthesis of collagen and other proteins in vitro. Exp Cell Res 1976;97:193–202.

153. Abdel-Aziz G, Lebeau G, Rescan P-Y, et al. Reversibility of hepatic fibrosis in experimentally induced cholestasis in rat. Am J Pathol 1990;137:1333–1342.

154. Craighead JE, Mossman BT. The pathogenesis of asbestos-associated diseases. N Engl J Med 1982;306:1446–1455.

155. Davis GS. Pathogenesis of silicosis: current concepts and hypotheses. Lung 1986;164:139–154.

156. De Crombrugghe B, Liau G, Setoyama C, et al. Structural and functional studies on the interstitial collagen genes. Ciba Found Symp 1985;114:20–33.

157. Friedman SL, Bissell DM. Hepatic fibrosis: new insights into pathogenesis. Hosp Pract 1990;25:43–50.

158. Friedman SL, Roll FJ, Boyles J, Bissell DM. Hepatic lipocytes: the principal collagen-producing cells of normal rat liver. Proc Natl Acad Sci USA 1985;82:8681–8685.

159. Gabbiani G, Hirschel BJ, Ryan GB, Statkov PR, Majno G. Granulation tissue as a contractile organ. A study of structure and function. J Exp Med 1972;135:719–734.

160. Hammel P, Couvelard A, O'Toole D, et al. Regression of liver fibrosis after biliary drainage in patients with chronic pancreatitis and stenosis of the common bile duct. N Engl J Med 2001;344:418–423.

160a. Henson PM, Henson JE, Fittschen C, et al. Phagocytic cells: degranulation and secretion. In: Gallin JI, Goldstein, IM, Snyderman R, eds. Inflammation: basic principles and clinical correlates. New York: Raven Press, 1988:363–390.

161. Heppleston AG. Cellular reactions with silica. In: Bendz G, Lindqvist I, eds. Biochemistry of silicon and related problems. New York: Plenum Press, 1977, pp. 357–379.

162. Holt K, Bennett M, Chojkier M. Acetaldehyde stimulates collagen and noncollagen protein production by human myofibroblasts. Hepatology 1984;4:843–848.

163. Hoyle GW, Li J, Finkelstein JB, et al. Emphysematous lesions, inflammation, and fibrosis in the lungs of transgenic mice overexpressing platelet-derived growth factor. Am J Pathol 1999;154:1763–1775.

164. Hunt TK, Conolly WB, Aronson SB, Goldstein P. Anaerobic metabolism and wound healing: an hypothesis for the initiation and cessation of collagen synthesis in wounds. Am J Surg 1978;135:328–332.

164a. Ingelfinger JR. Forestalling fibrosis. New Engl J Med 2003; 348:2265–2266.

165. Jelaska A, Strehlow D, Korn JH. Fibroblast heterogeneity in physiological conditions and fibrotic disease. Springer Semin Immunopathol 2000;21:385–395.

166. Kelly JK, Hwang W-S. Idiopathic retractile (sclerosing) mesenteritis and its differential diagnosis. Am J Surg Pathol 1989;13:513–521.

167. Kovacs EJ. Fibrogenic cytokines: the role of immune mediators in the development of scar tissue. Immunol Today 1991;12:17–23.

168. Kuhn C, McDonald JA. The roles of the myofibroblast in idiopathic pulmonary fibrosis. Ultrastructural and immunohistochemical features of sites of active extracellular matrix synthesis. Am J Pathol 1991;138:1257–1265.

168a. Lawrence T, Willoughby DA, Gilroy DW. Anti-inflammatory lipid mediators and insights into the resolution of inflammation. Nat Rev Immunol 2002;2:787–795.

168b. Lawrence T, Gilroy DW, Colville-Nash PR, Willoughby DA. Possible new role for NF-κB in the resolution of inflammation. Nat Med 2001;7:1291–1297.

169. Lemaire I, Beaudoin H, Massé S, Grondin, C. Alveolar macrophage stimulation of lung fibroblast growth in asbestos-induced pulmonary fibrosis. Am J Pathol 1986; 122:205–211.

170. Lepor H, Walsh PC. Idiopathic retroperitoneal fibrosis. J Urol 1979;122:1–6.

171. Leroy EC. Collagen deposition in autoimmune diseases: the expanding role of the fibroblast in human fibrotic disease. Ciba Found Symp 1985;114:196–207.

172. Levene CI, Bates CJ. The effect of hypoxia on collagen synthesis in cultured 3T6 fibroblasts and its relationship to the mode of action of ascorbate. Biochim Biophys Acta 1976;444:446–452.

172a. Levy BD, Clish CB, Schmidt B, Gronert K, Serhan CN. Lipid mediator class switching during acute inflammation: signals in resolution. Nat Immunol 2001;7:612–619.

173. Martin M, Lefaix J-L, Delanian S. TGF-β1 and radiation fibrosis: a master switch and a specific therapeutic target? Int J Radiat Oncol Biol Phys 2000;47:277–290.

174. Müller GA, Strutz FM. Renal fibroblast heterogeneity. Kidney Int 1995;48(Suppl. 50):S33–S36.

174a. Nathan C. Points of control in inflammation. Nature 2002;420:846–852.

175. Ormond JK. Idiopathic retroperitoneal fibrosis: a discussion of the etiology. J Urol 1965;94:385–390.

176. Pérez Tamayo R. Cirrhosis of the liver: a reversible disease? Pathol Annu 1979;14:183–213.

177. Piguet PF, Collart MA, Grau GE, Sappino A-P, Vassalli P. Requirement of tumour necrosis factor for development of silica-induced pulmonary fibrosis. Nature 1990;344: 245–247.

178. Reiser KM, Last JA. A molecular marker for fibrotic collagen in lungs of infants with respiratory distress syndrome. Biochem Med Metab Biol 1987;37:16–21.

179. Roberts WC, Ferrans VJ. Pure collagen plaques on the diaphragm and pleura. Gross, histologic and electron microscopic observations. Chest 1972;61:357–360.

180. Roberts WC, Sjoerdsma A. The cardiac disease associated with the carcinoid syndrome (carcinoid heart disease). Am J Med 1964;36:5–34.

181. Roberts AB, Sporn MB. Transforming growth factor-β. In: Clark RAF (ed). The molecular and cellular biology of wound repair. New York: Plenum Press, 1996, pp. 275–308.

182. Savolainen E-R, Leo MA, Timpl R, Lieber CS. Acetaldehyde and lactate stimulate collagen synthesis of cultured baboon liver myofibroblasts. Gastroenterology 1984;87:777–787.

182a. Serhan CN, Hong S, Gronert K, et al. Resolvins: a family of bioactive products of omega-3 fatty acid transformation circuits initiated by aspirin treatment that counter pro-inflammation signals. J. Exp Med 2002;196:1025–1037.

183. Seuwen K, Magnaldo I, Pouysségur J. Serotonin stimulates DNA synthesis in fibroblasts acting through 5-HT$_{1B}$ receptors coupled to a G$_i$-protein. Nature 1988;35:254–256.

184. Spech RW, Wisniowski P, Kachel DL, Wright JR, Martin WJ II. Surfactant protein A prevents silica-mediated toxicity to rat alveolar macrophages. Am J Physiol Lung Cell Mol Physiol 2000;278:L713–L718.

185. Suzuki T, Kimura M, Ansano M, Fujigaki Y, Hishida A. Role of atrophic tubules in development of interstitial fibrosis in microembolism-induced renal failure in rat. Am J Pathol 2001;158:75–85.

186. Trelstad RL, Birk DE. The fibroblast in morphogenesis and fibrosis: cell topography and surface-related functions. Ciba Found Symp 1985;114:4–19.

187. Weissmann IL, Butcher EC, Rouse RV, Scollay RG. Cell-cell interactions in the establishment and maintenance of lymphoid tissue architecture. In: Sercarz E, Cunningham AJ (eds). Strategies of immune regulation. New York: Academic Press, 1980, pp. 77–84.

188. Yañez-Mó M, Lara-Pezzi E, Selgas R et al. Peritoneal dialysis and epithelial-to-mesenchymal transition of mesothelial cells. N Engl J Med 2003;348:403–413.

189. Ziesche R, Block L-H. Mechanisms of antifibrotic action of interferon gamma-1b in pulmonary fibrosis. Wien Klin Wochenschr 2000;112:785–790.

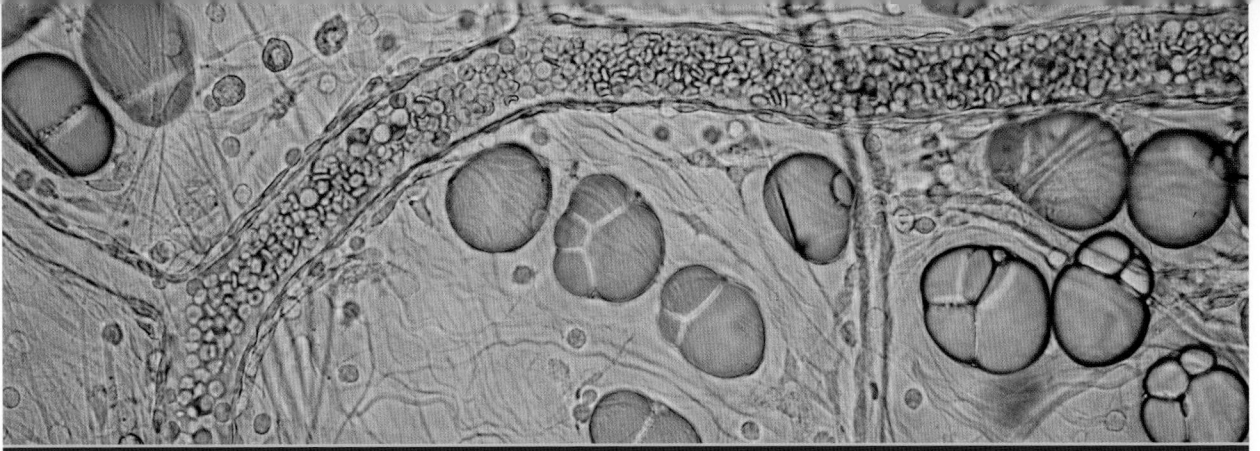

CHAPTER 14   WOUND HEALING

The grand scenario of wound healing is the sum of three responses: *hemostasis,* because vessels bleed; *inflammation,* because there has been injury, with or without infection; and *regeneration,* because structures have been severed or destroyed (see Figure 8.1). These three healing processes are orchestrated according to the type of injury; the final result, barring complications, is to close the gap with a fibrous seal called a *scar.*

The clinical path from wound to scar runs most smoothly if the margins are apposed, naturally or by a suture, and are neither infected nor bruised. The prototype of this *closed wound* is a sutured aseptic surgical incision; healing can start immediately, because there is no gap to close, no infection to overcome, and no dead tissue to eliminate or to reabsorb. The traditional surgical term for this optimal clinical course is *healing by first intention* (Figure 14.1).

By contrast, if the margins are separated (*open wound*), and/or infected, and/or bruised, the wound must correct these three situations before it can close; this is called *healing by second intention* (Figure 14.1).

> There is something rather quaint about this ancient notion of "intention." For one thing, *who is supposed to have the intention, the wound or the surgeon?* Almost 1000 years ago, in the *Canon* of Avicenna—one of the pillars of Arabic medicine—it was clearly the surgeon who displayed therapeutic "intentions" appropriate to the type of injury (4). In the surgical writings of the later Middle Ages, e.g. by Guy de Chauliac (1300–1368), healing intentions are sometimes attributed to the surgeon, sometimes to the wound or to Nature (37). In today's medical jargon it is assumed that the intention is expressed by the wound itself.

Healing by First Intention: Closed Aseptic Wounds

We will now describe the healing of a noninfected, sutured wound. Technically all wounds are infected to some degree, but in aseptic surgery the number of bacteria is so small that healing is

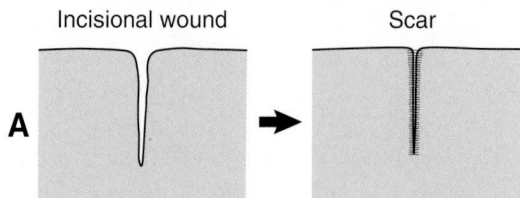

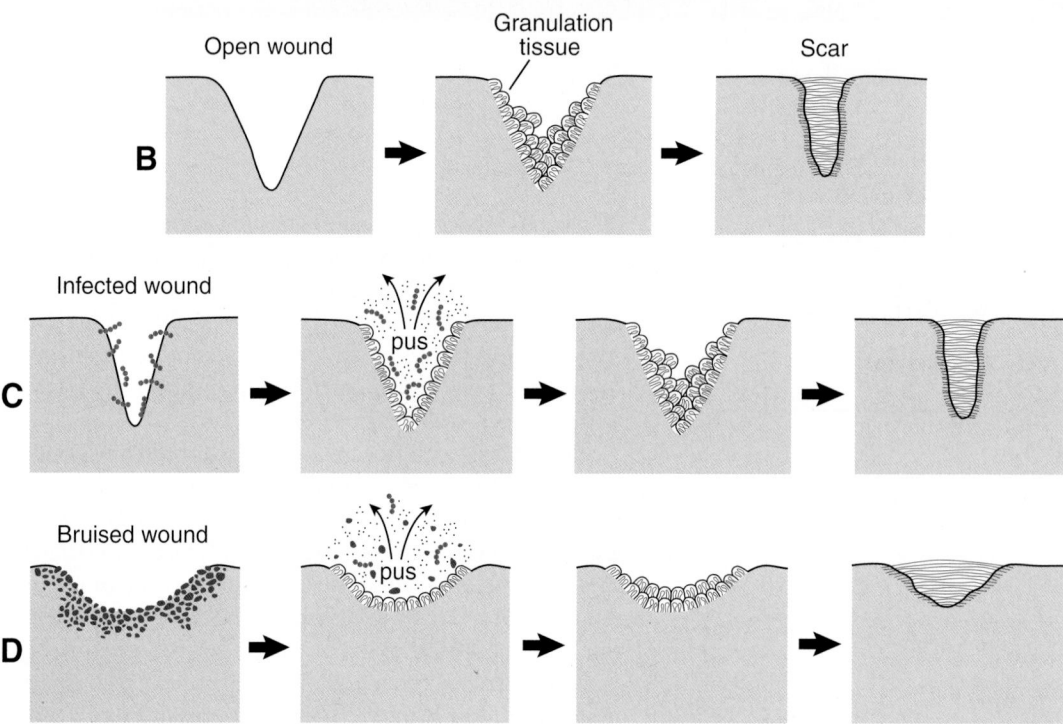

FIGURE 14.1 Wound healing by first and second intention. **A:** *Healing by first intention* in a closed, noninfected wound, such as a surgical incision. The margins are apposed; healing occurs directly, with a minimum of granulation tissue. **B:** *Healing by second intention* in an open, aseptic wound. The wound space fills with granulation tissue, which contracts and closes the wound. **C:** *Healing by second intention* in an infected wound (red dots represent bacteria). The wound becomes lined with granulation tissue, which produces pus until the bacteria are eliminated, then contracts. **D:** *Healing by second intention* in a bruised (and infected) wound: process similar to **C,** except that the granulation tissue must eliminate the necrotic tissue as well as the bacteria.

not disturbed. The sequence of events (Figure 14.2) is fairly constant, but the timing indicated below is merely indicative: depending on the conditions it may be cut by half or doubled.

Hemostasis: Within Seconds to Minutes

The first priority is to stop the bleeding (hemostasis); and as usual the programming is admirable. The severed arterioles contract and the spilled blood clots. Generally speaking, blood can be induced to clot by either one

of two mechanisms, (a) by coming in contact with collagen, and (b) by mixing with a "tissue factor" released by injured cells. Both mechanisms are triggered in a wound, and so the spilled blood clots without delay. This helps to stop the bleeding. In the meantime, platelets pile up on the mouths of the bleeding vessels and create plugs called *thrombi,* another essential mechanism of hemostasis. The details will be discussed later (p. 631).

The clotted blood also forms a tenuous network (not quite a glue) that connects the two faces of the wound in

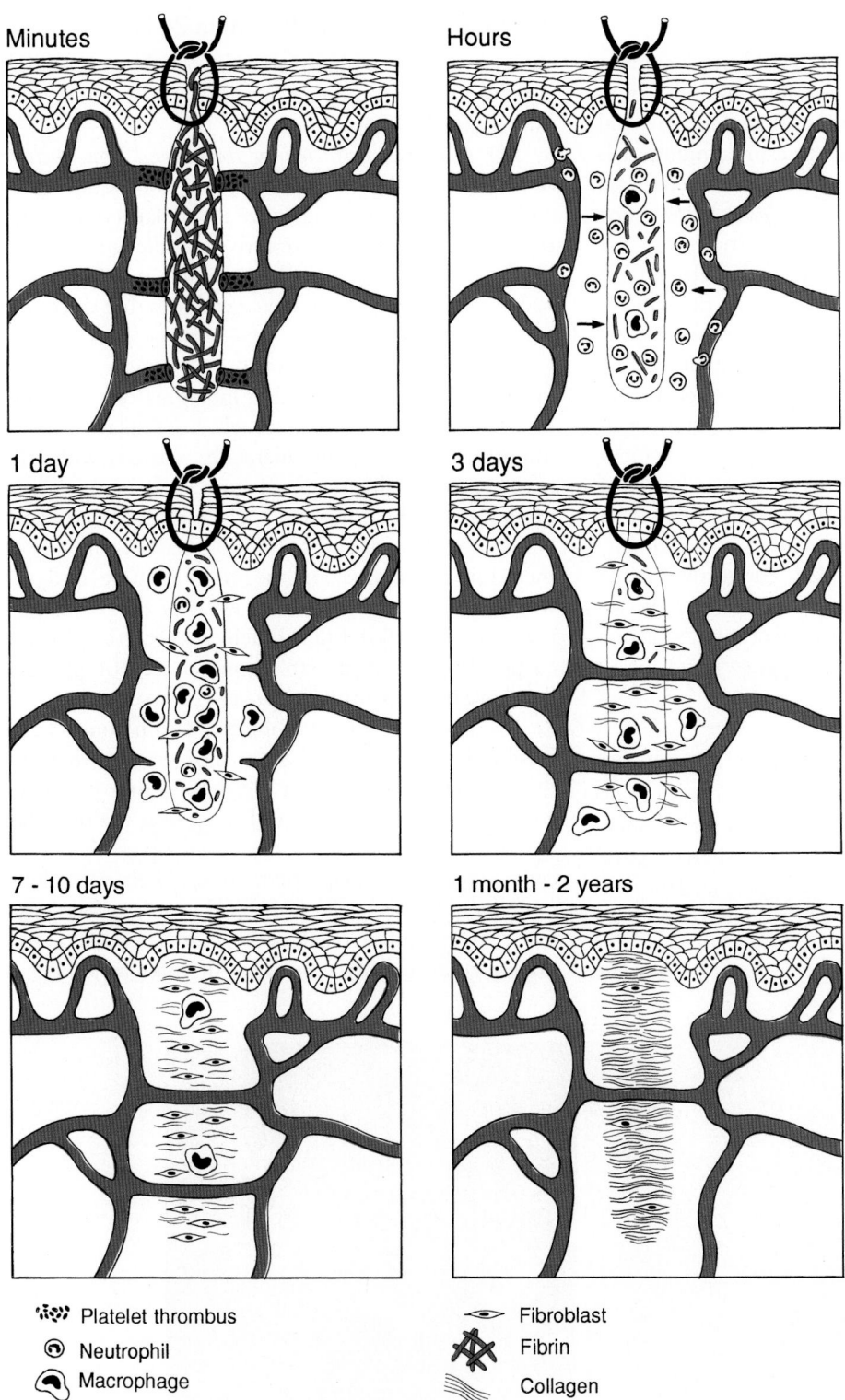

Minutes

Hours

1 day

3 days

7 - 10 days

1 month - 2 years

Platelet thrombus

Neutrophil

Macrophage

Fibroblast

Fibrin

Collagen

FIGURE 14.2 Wound healing by first intention: diagram of the principal steps.

the so-called "wound space". Here is another example of Nature's economy: products of the clotting mechanism also help initiate the healing processes. Thrombin, the enzyme that generates fibrin, attracts macrophages and causes fibroblasts to replicate; and platelet-derived growth-factor (PDGF), released by degranulating platelets, is also a mitogen and a chemotaxin for fibroblasts (29).

Inflammation: Within Minutes to Hours

The next priority is to ward off bacteria. Here is another example of prudent design. The wound has no way to "know" whether it is infected or not; therefore, to avoid a potentially dangerous loss of time, inflammation is triggered automatically without waiting for the bacteria to do it. In other words, *the wound prepares for the worst case scenario,* and fires all the ammunition ready at hand: the trauma itself causes mast cells to release their stores, and platelets from injured vessels do the same—but die in the process. Arterioles dilate to increase the supply, and leukocytes crawl around looking for prey. (If they find any, the battle is on, and more leukocytes are called in.) However, in a sterile wound the number of leukocytes in the exudate is never large enough to qualify as pus. Scavenging of debris, including the remains of spent neutrophils, begins immediately. The tissues next to the wound swell up a little because of the inflammatory edema. In the expanded connective tissue spaces, the exudate clots and forms a fine network of fibrin; this offers the leukocytes an extra surface against which they can trap bacteria (*surface phagocytosis*).

Scab Formation

Exudate seeps out of the sutured wound; it clots, and eventually dries up. This process continues and builds up a scab, which has two important functions: in open wounds, it shrinks by dehydration and thereby contributes to wound contraction (see Figure 14.10); and it seals off the wound from the environment, preventing bacteria from penetrating. *The scab is a natural dressing* (57).

Migration of Fixed Cells: Within 24 Hours

By 24 hours even some stationary cells begin to move: the fibroblasts, the epidermal cells and even the endothelium (70).

The leukocytes attracted to the wound now include more monocytes (158), which settle in the wound space and around it; they phagocytize the remains of the neutrophils, which continue to arrive and die within hours of their arrival. As the macrophages scavenge, they become activated; they secrete cytokines that direct the activities of all other cells.

The network of fibrin continues to grow from the fibrinogen supplied by the inflammatory exudate. Mechanically it is not very tough, but it plays another important role: fibrin filaments coated with the plasma protein **fibronectin** (Figure 14.3) are suitable as footholds for the epidermal cells and migrating fibroblasts (65). By 24 hours, the fibroblasts come out of their torpor, enlarge and begin to migrate into the wound space, hauling themselves along the coated filaments of fibrin (66). One of their chemotactic calls may be platelet-derived growth factor released by platelets that have been spent in the process of hemostasis.

The epidermal cells are mobilized within hours (128). Basal cells on the edge of the cut, triggered perhaps by the sudden absence of a neighbor—the "free-edge effect" (116)—flatten out and creep over the denuded area; the cells at the leading edge are temporarily phagocytic, which may help them to eat their way along *under the forming scab* (116). This migration is an apparent exception to the rule that basement membranes guide epithelia because, in this case, there is

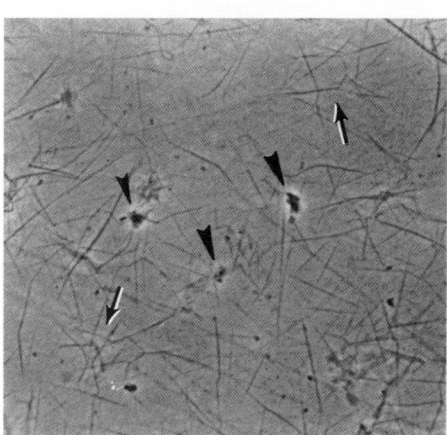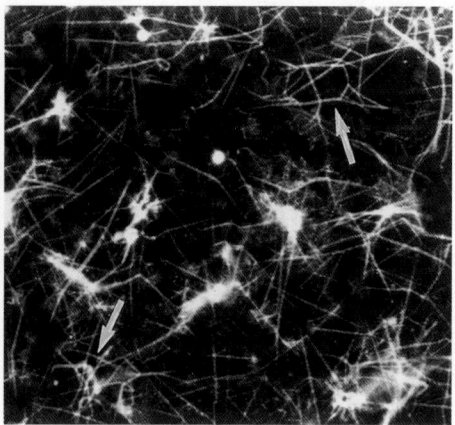

FIGURE 14.3 Clot of human blood. *Left:* Phase contrast photograph shows fibrin strands (**arrows**) and platelets (**arrowheads**). *Right:* Photograph in ultraviolet light after immunofluorescent staining of fibronectin with specific antibody, showing that fibronectin is present in the fibrin strands (**arrow**). (From [58], Copyright © 1984 Alan R. Liss, Inc. Reprinted by permission of Wiley-Liss, a division of John Wiley & Sons, Inc.)

no basement membrane. Histochemical studies have shown that the substrate over which the epithelial cells accept to glide is a mixture of fibrin and fibronectin (61,166); the latter is supplied by plasma and by the activated fibroblasts (22). Normal basal cells of the epidermis have no receptors for fibronectin, but regenerating ones do (59,67). The gliding cells advance at a rate of 2–3 cell diameters per hour or roughly 0.5 mm/day; the speed record is held by amphibian epidermis, which migrates 10 times faster (176).

It may seem strange that the epithelium should advance faster in a cold-blooded animal, but we can theorize as follows. Imagine an open wound in the skin of a frog that is out in the air; the surface will be covered by a clot, which becomes a dry scab. Now, if the frog goes swimming, the scab becomes soggy and will allow precious electrolytes to be lost to the hypotonic water of the pond. Therefore it is urgent to cover the wound with a watertight layer: the fastest way is for the regenerating epithelium to creep *over* the scab (140) instead of having to burrow beneath it.

Capillary sprouts are not easy to see at 24 hours by light microscopy (the earliest are simply endothelial pseudopodia reaching out through the basement membrane [151a]) but they are already developing in both faces of the wound in response to angiogenic factors, and grow toward the wound space. Anoxia is a major factor in stimulating vascular ingrowth. In the wound space, oxygen tension is close to zero; if it is artificially raised, angiogenesis stops (91). This phase of angiogenesis is another feat of the macrophages. Those that have migrated into the wound space become anoxic, and *anoxia causes them to secrete a factor that stimulates capillary outgrowth* (90), probably TNF alpha (99). High concentrations of lactate, such as occur in wounds, have the same effect (83). Again, two admirable feedback mechanisms.

Regeneration: 3 Days

As regards inflammatory cells, by 2–3 days the monocytes begin to outnumber the neutrophils (158). Regeneration, which had started by day one, now dominates the picture. The advancing epidermal cells undermine the scab, which eventually falls off; the timing depends a great deal on the size of the scab. Where the epidermis is perforated by a suture thread, a strange thing may happen: epidermal cells grow down into the suture track like a tube surrounding the thread (Figure 14.4). After all, this should be expected because epithelia tend to grow over raw tissue surfaces. (This is the principle exploited when earlobes are perforated and a wire is left in place until healing occurs.)

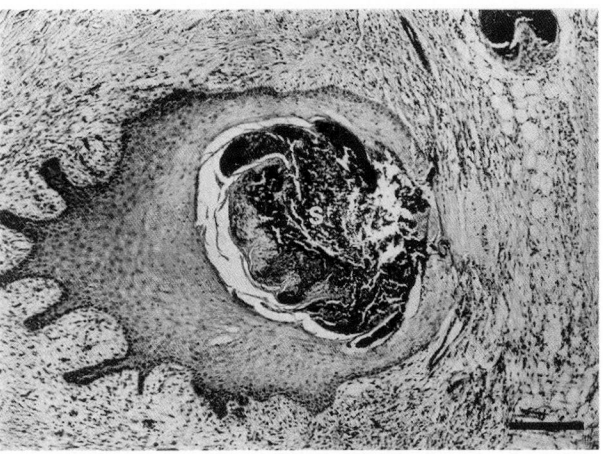

FIGURE 14.4 Cross section of a suture thread (**S**) in the depth of a wound in the skin of a pig. The thread is almost completely surrounded by epidermis. The mechanism: on the surface of the skin, where the suture thread penetrates into the tissue, the regenerating epidermis tends to plunge into the tunnel created by the suture. **Bar** = 200 μm. (Reproduced with permission from Arch. Surg. [128]. Copyright 1966 American Medical Association.)

The activated fibroblasts are in full swing. Responding to growth factors they multiply and produce collagen fibrils (Type 3 as a start [117]) and other matrix components—but for reasons unknown few elastic fibers.

Angiogenesis (the regeneration of blood vessels) (p. 774) has progressed enough after 2–3 days for some sprouts to join up tip to tip (80). This critical encounter is called *inosculation* (*osculare* is Latin for kissing) (36, 146). The crowd of new fibroblasts mingles with the new capillaries to form the beginning of granulation tissue.

Early Scarring: 7–10 Days

Within a week the wound space has had the time to fill with granulation tissue: very little is needed, because the two faces of the wound are apposed. A network of capillaries has bridged the wound space. The lymphatics begin to regenerate with some delay after the blood capillaries; their advancing tips never seem to link up with tips of blood vessels (176), presumably because they carry different recognition molecules. Slowly the granulation tissue acquires more and more collagen fibers and begins to look more and more like the fibrous mass called a scar.

Throughout the wound, scavenging by the macrophages continues and eventually the fibrin is also removed. Collagen Type 1 begins to appear (24, 50, 117).

Although the epidermis has regenerated, skin appendages such as hair and sweat glands do not develop; this lack is an everyday observation in surgical wards. (The rabbit stands out as a rare exception [11].) Human scars are not only hairless but usually also pale, especially on black skin, because melanocytes regenerate poorly (p. 20). Yet hyperpigmented scars do occur, in white as well as in black skin; the reason is not understood.

Scar Maturation: 1 Month–2 Years

Ultimately, the scar will be a mass of fibrous tissue with many collagen fibers, few cells and few vessels (Figure 14.5), but the process of maturation is slow. As time

passes, most cells vanish; apoptosis has been observed in fibroblasts and endothelial cells (33). Eosinophils maintain a low profile in healing wounds, but they are there, and contribute their share of TGF-alpha and beta-1 (177). The collagen becomes more and more cross-linked; elastic fibers remain few, so that scars have little recoil, and eventually tend to stretch. Many capillaries disappear so that old scars appear white (3).

However, it takes many months, even a year or two, for a surgical scar to change from pink to white. The local turnover of collagen remains high for years; this is why, in the days of scurvy, old scars would break down during a long trip at sea (p. 271).

Even a mature scar is never as strong as normal skin. The tensile strength remains below normal (Figure 14.6) (100, 131). Boxers are aware of this problem: scars break open more easily than normal skin.

The term *scar* is applied also to the end result of injuries other than wounds. An infarct, for example, is said to heal with a scar (Figure 14.7).

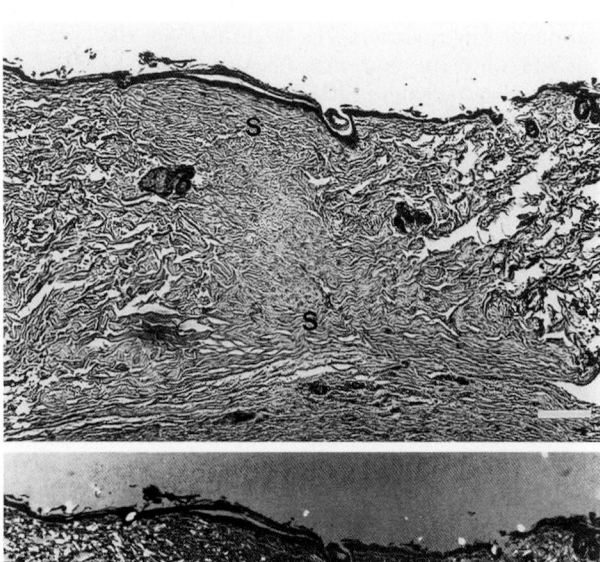

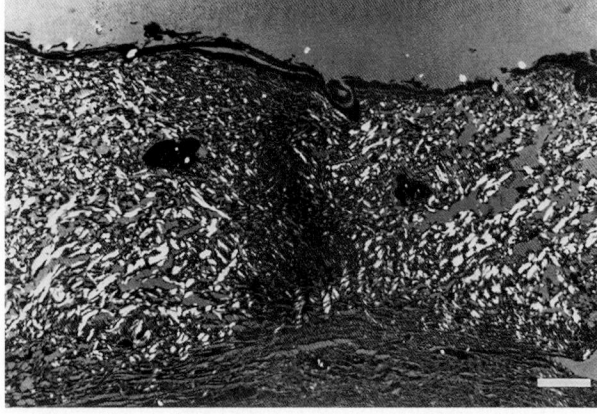

FIGURE 14.5   The arrangement of scar collagen is not "normal." Dermal scar from a 100-day-old (tape-closed) skin wound in the rat. *Top:* Viewed in ordinary light. The scar (**S-S**) can be recognized because it is made of collagen bundles thinner than those of the surrounding dermis. *Bottom:* Viewed in polarized light, normal collagen appears bright (birefringent) because it consists of thick bundles of parallel fibrils; scar collagen is dark (not birefringent) because it is made of thin fibrils arranged in a disorderly fashion. **Bars** = 250 μm. (Reproduced by permission from [45] © 1969 with permission of The McGraw-Hill Companies.)

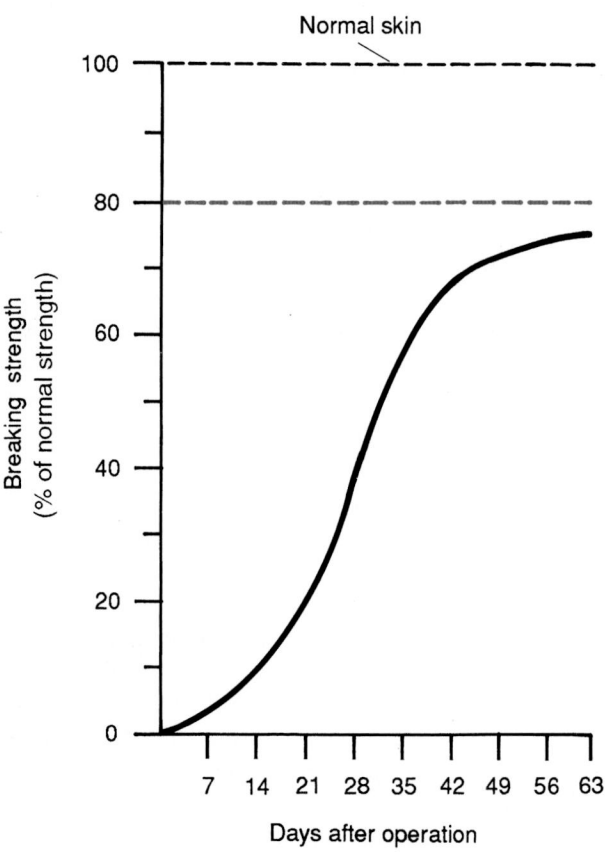

FIGURE 14.6   Breaking strength of a healing wound in rat skin. The strength of the final scar is about 80 percent of that of normal skin. (Reproduced with permission from [100].)

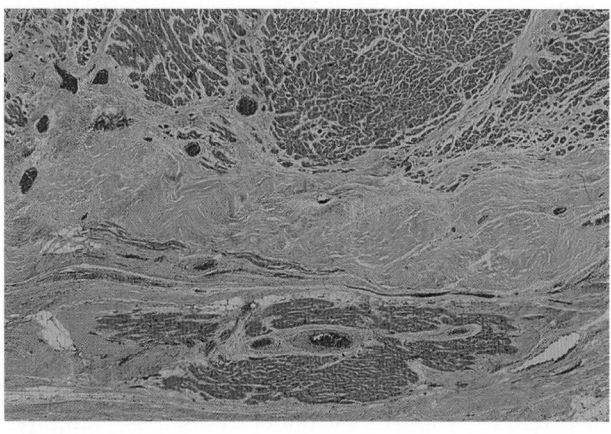

FIGURE 14.7 Typical scars (lightly stained) between bundles of myocardial fibers: the signature of a healed infarct. The scar tissue consists mainly of collagen fibers with few cells. (25x)

The Cells and Mediators of Wound Healing

In an inflamed wound, the cells and the mediators involved are very much the same as discussed in previous chapters. Key concepts to retain:

- Wounds *will heal by first or second intention* depending mainly on the loss of tissue, the presence of infection and of necrotic tissue (Figure 14.1).
- *Healing is somewhat different in different organs:* a topic not sufficiently explored.

- It is convenient to think of *two stages:* (a) an early, "acute," non-specific response of the tissues—an innate response supplying fluid and granulocytes, dominated by "histamine-type" mediators. This stage is followed by (b) a "chronic" phase, dominated by a different set of mediators—and a population of cells pertaining to the immune (i.e., adaptive) response (pp. 308, 430).
- We like to think that a dominant cell initiates each phase: as the macrophage is the non-contested master for the immune response, *we see the mast cell as the queen for the acute response.* The mast cells are the first to ring the alarm after injury: otherwise, why would they carry such a huge dose of dangerous histamine? The platelets behave much the same as the mast cells, the main difference being that mast cells do not die as they degranulate, whereas platelets do; and platelets contain more types of mediators.

This early phase leaves the matrix edematous and infiltrated with filaments of **fibrin,** which prepare the way for the inward migration of macrophages and fibroblasts. Thereafter the chemical guidance for the reconstruction (including angiogenesis) belongs to cytokines and growth factors; Table 14.1 offers a glimpse of this complex molecular soup. The principal suppliers are the macrophages and the fibroblasts (144); even the keratinocytes contribute: they supply VEGF (vascular endothelial growth factor) for angiogenesis (13), as well as TGF-beta and PDGF to instruct the fibroblasts,

Table 14.1 Cytokines that Affect Wound Healing

Cytokine	Major Source	Target Cells and Major Effects
Epidermal growth factor family		Epidermal and mesenchymal regeneration
Epidermal growth factor	Platelets	Pleiotropic-cell motility and proliferation
Transforming growth factor α	Macrophages, epidermal cells	Pleiotropic-cell motility and proliferation
Heparin-binding epidermal growth factor	Macrophages	Pleiotropic-cell motility and proliferation
Fibroblast growth factor family		Wound vascularization
Basic fibroblast growth factor	Macrophages, endothelial cells	Angiogenesis and fibroblast proliferation
Acidic fibroblast growth factor	Macrophages, endothelial cells	Angiogenesis and fibroblast proliferation
Keratinocyte growth factor	Fibroblasts	Epidermal-cell motility and proliferation
Transforming growth factor β family		Fibrosis and increased tensile strength
Transforming growth factors β1 and β2	Platelets, macrophages	Epidermal-cell motility, chemotaxis of macrophages and fibroblasts, extracellular-matrix synthesis and remodeling
Transforming growth factor β3	Macrophages	Antiscarring effects
Other		
Platelet-derived growth factor	Platelets, macrophages, epidermal cells	Fibroblast proliferation and chemoattraction, macrophage chemoattraction and activation
Vascular endothelial growth factor	Epidermal cells, macrophages	Angiogenesis and increased vascular permeability
Tumor necrosis factor α	Neutrophils	Pleiotropic expression of growth factors
Interleukin-1	Neutrophils	Pleiotropic expression of growth factors
Insulin-like growth factor I	Fibroblasts, epidermal cells	Reepithelialization and granulation-tissue formation
Colony-stimulating factor 1	Multiple cells	Macrophage activation and granulation-tissue formation

(Reproduced with permission from: New Engl. J. Med. "Cutaneous Wound Healing," Singer A. J, Clark, R. A. F., 341:738–746, 1999. Copyright © 1999 Massachusetts Medical Society. All rights reserved.)

which reciprocate with KGF, keratinocyte growth factor (159).

A good way to find out "who does what" is of course to eliminate the various players one at a time. For example: if the neutrophils are depleted, wound healing proceeds on schedule—at least in rats (158). By contrast, in the absence of monocytes and macrophages the wound becomes filled with fibrin and all manner of debris, including dead neutrophils; fibroblasts do not appear until day 5, and fibrosis is significantly reduced, so that by 10 days the wound appears "extremely immature" (98):

Clearly the macrophages are playing the leading role, as they do in chronic inflammation. As for eliminating mediators, here are some samples. In transgenic mice lacking *plasminogen,* and therefore unable to generate plasmin, the keratinocytes could not dissect their way under the scab and reepithelialize the wound (141).

Mice deprived of P- and E-selectin showed impaired recruitment of inflammatory cells, as expected (122). An amazing generalized inflammatory disease develops in TGF-beta-1 knockout mice: intense macrophage and lymphocyte infiltrates develop all over the body, especially in the heart and lung, and the mice die (94). This would suggests that TGF-beta-1 is a potent immunosuppressor, but, as mentioned earlier, its role with regard to inflammation is ambivalent.

Overall, the mediators at work in the various phases of wound healing overlap with those of acute and chronic inflammation and fibrosis. As regards the anti-inflammatory eicosanoids found in the resolving phase of inflammation, lipoxins, and *resolvins* (153a, 153b), they have not yet been studied in wounds, but it would be surprising if they did not take part in the noble enterprise of wound healing.

Healing by Second Intention: The Contraction of Wounds

Wound healing is delayed if the margins are not ready to become attached to eachother; they may be *too far removed,* due to loss of tissue; they may also be *infected* and/or *devitalized,* i.e., bruised or necrotic (Figure 14.1). If any one or more of these conditions prevail the wound is left open. Why so?

The Healing of Infected Wounds

Imagine a wound of the leg by a motorcycle accident on a dusty country road. The wound surface will be heavily seeded with bacteria and particles of dirt (the latter are of great help to the bacteria, as we will see later). Chemotaxis begins to operate within minutes; swarms of neutrophils will crawl to the surface of the wound; within a day or so they will be numerous enough to be called "pus." Polymorphs are great as bacterial fighters, which is what we want them to be, but they are not equipped to build new tissue. As long as they are around, little healing can take place. However, a millimeter or two beneath the surface, angiogenesis sets in, fibroblasts and macrophages are stimulated, and within a week or so the wound is covered with granulation tissue, virtually identical to the **pyogenic membrane** of an abscess. Pus is loaded with proteolytic enzymes; again, this is excellent for removing dead tissue (which is a fine culture medium for bacteria) but it can also destroy the new capillary sprouts. Still, the granulation tissue will continue to pour out leukocytes, until most of the bacteria are dead and the "devitalized" tissue is removed. The latter operation is called biological

débridement; the surgeon in charge of the wound will also perform some surgical *débridement,* but in a fresh wound it is difficult to decide which tissue is dead or bound to die. As the battle continues, at some point most of the bacteria are eliminated, and healing can get under way: the open wound, lined with granulation tissue, is ready to heal *by second intention.* Try to imagine how this could happen.

In theory, there are two options. The simplest would be to have tissue grow in from all around the wound, and cover the gap. This is the solution that trees have adopted (Figure 14.8). We vertebrates can also provide some ingrowth of tissue (as granulation tissue) but we also have another and faster way. Consider the large open wound shown in Figure 14.9. After a lag period of a few days the margins move toward eachother as if pulled by an invisible force (131). This is *wound contraction,* obvious but not easy to explain: in fact it has been and still is a central puzzle in the biology of wound healing.

The Contraction of Open Wounds

That contraction occurs is easily demonstrated; the problem is to identify the pulling force—or forces. *In a wounded tissue at least three kinds of pulling forces are available—at least in theory.* Let us briefly examine them.

(1) The Contraction of Fibrin

We have encountered fibrin in Chapter 9 as a product of inflammation; however, the specific task of fibrin is to

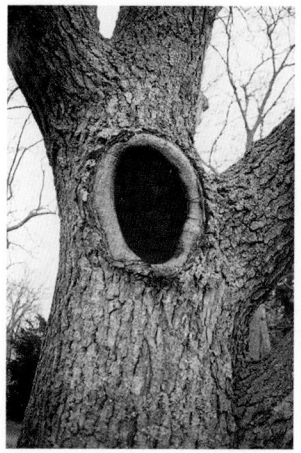 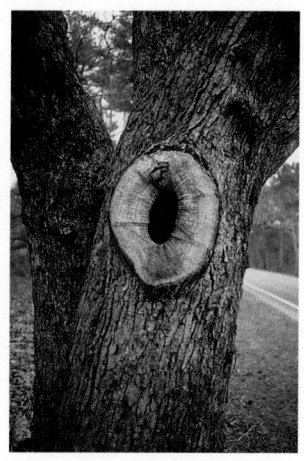 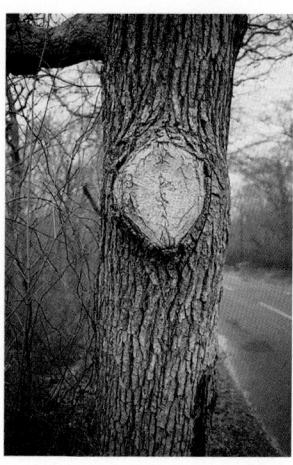

FIGURE 14.8   Open wounds in trees heal by ingrowth from the margins. The process takes years; tarring (*left* and *center*) reduces the risk of infection.

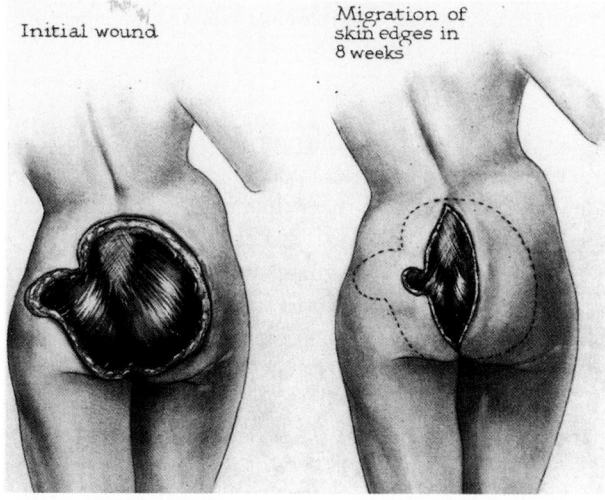

Initial wound   Migration of skin edges in 8 weeks

FIGURE 14.9   Contraction of an open wound. *Left:* Patient who lost nearly all the skin of both buttocks when run over by a bus. *Right:* Three weeks later, the wound area is reduced by contraction to 50 percent. (Reproduced from [41].)

stop hemorrhage. In small bleeding vessels, fibrin creates a three-dimensional network of ultramicroscopic fibrils that entrap the red blood cells. Then, by a process that is not fully understood (p. 638) (26), platelets in the clot emit pseudopods that tug at the fibrin network and squeeze the fluid out of the clot. Most relevant is a study *in vitro* showing that platelets can be replaced by fibroblasts in causing the clotted fibrin to retract (124).

Actually there may be a fourth "pulling force" in open wounds: the **drying and contraction of the scab.** This concept used to be part of traditional, rather than scientific surgical teaching; it makes sense, but lacks research support, hence we will not list it as a separate

contractile force. Furthermore, the scab is made largely of fibrin, hence the mechanism of scab contraction may overlap with the contraction of fibrin. The best model to show the scab effect is an excisional wound. In an anesthetized rat or rabbit, a 10 × 10 mm square of skin is cut out, and the wounded area is NOT covered with a dressing. After a few hours the wound begins to dry by evaporation; a thin scab develops; as it dries it shrinks, and being firmly anchored to the tissues beneath, it can significantly reduce the wound surface within one day (Figure 14.10).

(2) The Myofibroblasts

Biologists have known since the 1940s that some fibroblasts can be induced to contract (110, 169), but this fact was largely forgotten. Eventually it was the good fortune of our laboratory to show that *open wounds* acquire a special set of modulated, contractile fibroblasts. They are nestled in the granulation tissue and resemble smooth muscle.

The adventurous quest for the myofibroblasts has been told elsewhere (110). It led us as far as investigating the method used for head-shrinking, Amazonian style. Eventually we became convinced that the secret was in the fibroblasts, and after moving to Geneva we joined forces with G. Gabbiani and G. B. Ryan. Using the electron microscope, we looked at several kinds of granulation tissue (including that of open wounds) and found that many fibroblasts contained more fibrils than usual. But did these fibrils have anything to do with contraction? In a previous study on endothelial cells, Majno and Leventhal (112) had used the "accordeon" deformation of the nucleus as an indicator of cellular contraction, and we found to our delight that many of the fibroblast nuclei did show the typical accordeon folds (48). However, when these findings were reported at an international meeting, the reception was cool: morphologic evidence could only

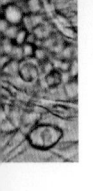

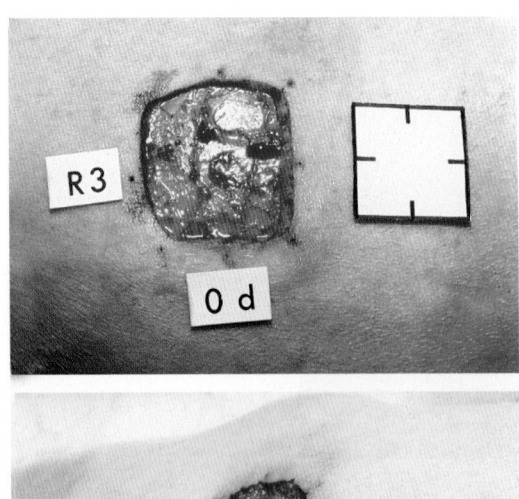

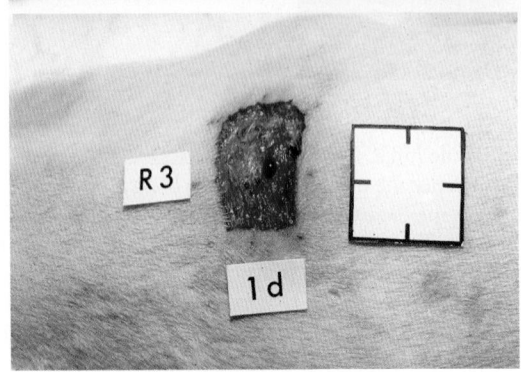

FIGURE 14.10   Early contraction of a 2 × 2 cm excisional wound on the flank of a rabbit (at time 0 and 1 day). Immediately after surgery the wound enlarges slightly; after 24 hours it is reduced by about 40 percent, through dehydration of the scab. (Courtesy of Dr. G. B. Ryan, University of Melbourne, Parkville, Australia.)

suggest contraction, it could not prove it. We had submitted a hypothesis, not a fact. The challenge, at this point, was to provide *functional* evidence that wound fibroblasts contract.

We offer this challenge, year after year, to the students in our Pathology course, adding that the solution has to be simple and inexpensive. The answer that we reward goes to the student who proposes to take a strip of granulation tissue, suspend it in a bath as physiologists do with smooth muscle, stimulate it with a smooth muscle contractant such as bradykinin, and record the response. This was the method that we actually used (111), and it worked (Figure 14.11). To behold that strip of supposedly inert connective tissue shorten under our eyes was a rare experience. The first granulation tissue that we tested we obtained from a "rat granuloma pouch" (p. 490); it responded to contractants and relaxants much like smooth muscle, only not as intensely. It was fortunate that we began with that preparation: our first experiment with wound tissue (from a 10-day open wound of a rat) was negative. The wound had already contracted *in vivo* and

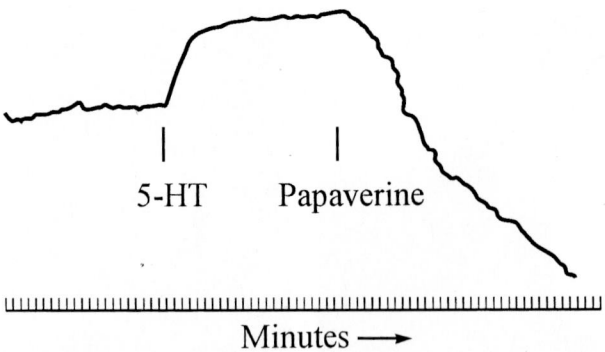

5-HT   Papaverine

Minutes ⟶

FIGURE 14.11   Proof that granulation tissue is a contractile organ. Responses of a strip of granulation tissue obtained from a 25-day-old granuloma pouch. The strip was connected to a recording needle and then stimulated with a contractant (5-hydroxytryptamine = serotonin), followed by a relaxant, papaverin. (Adapted from [148].)

understandably the granulation tissue refused to contract any further. Minutes later we realized our conceptual error and dowsed the strip with a smooth muscle relaxant: it relaxed—and so did we.

We concluded from these and other experiments that under certain conditions, such as in open wounds, fibroblasts modulate into a contractile phenotype (48, 49) for which one of us (GM) proposed the name **myofibroblast** (111). The reason for introducing a new name was largely the notion, well known to anthropologists, that in the human world things truly exist only when they have a name. The successful career of the myofibroblast confirmed this notion. In essence, we had shown that *the granulation tissue that fills an open wound is a temporary contractile organ.*

Biology of the myofibroblasts. Most myofibroblasts arise from fibroblasts; possibly a few derive from pericytes and other cells including leukocytes, but such discussions have lost much of their relevance in today's biological climate, since we have seen in Chapter 2 that "brain can turn into blood." It is more important to define the myofibroblast. At the level of light microscopy, the transient expression of *alpha-smooth muscle actin* is the most valid criterion (38); this is not a specific criterion, but then we must remember that as of 2003 we still have no cytologic marker for fibroblasts. Seen by electron microscopy, fully developed myofibroblasts show distinctive features (Figure 14.12): (a) an overall shape of branching cells containing bundles of fibrils with dense bodies (*stress fibers*), (b) extensive gap junctions between such cells, and (c) *microtendons* (a name more descriptive than *fibronexus*): bundles of fibrils emerge from a cell, continuing the direction of a stress fiber. These

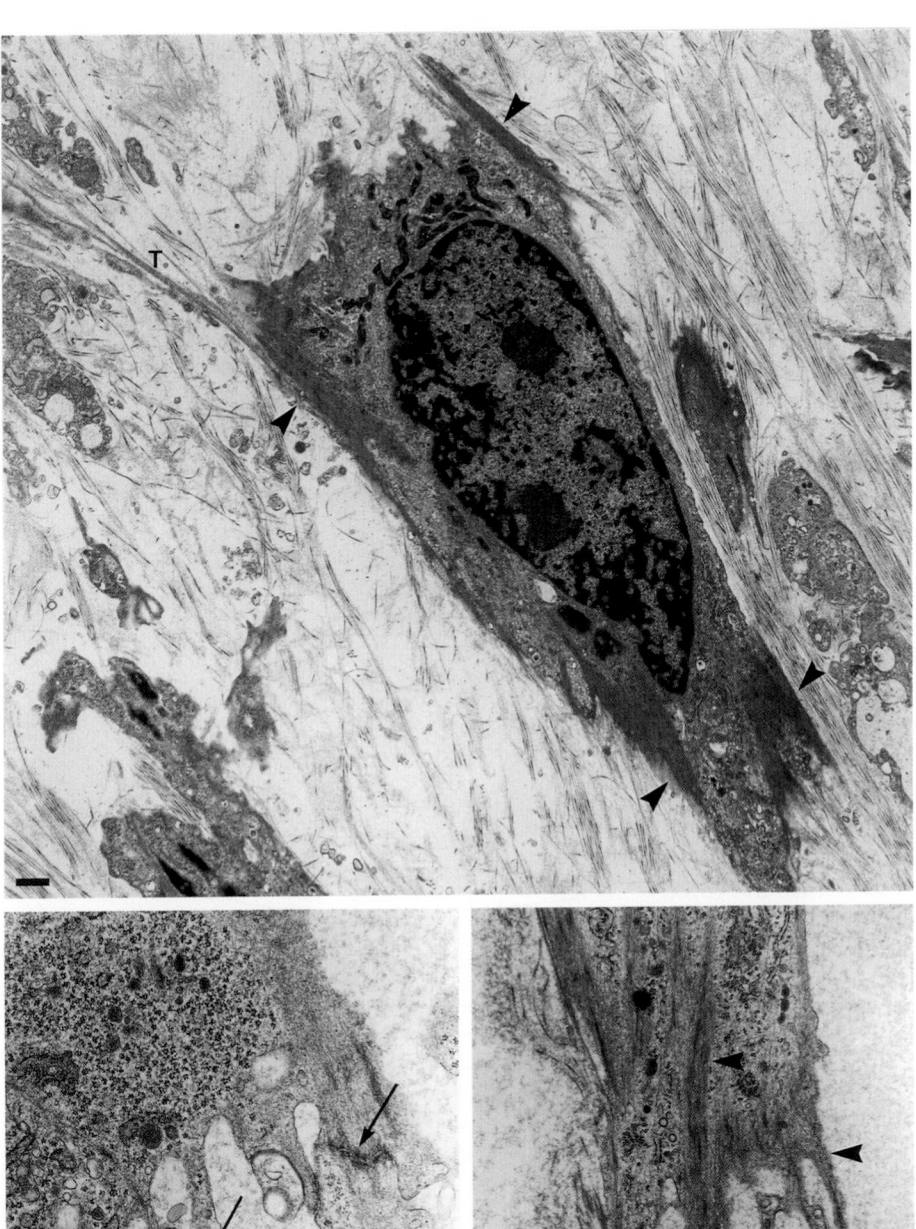

FIGURE 14.12 Myofibro-blasts. *Top:* Overall view. Bundles of intracellular fibrils (**arrowheads**), some of which are continuous with extracellular "microtendons" (**T**). (From a human stenotic mitral valve). *Bottom left:* Junctions (**arrows**) between adjacent myofibroblasts. *Bottom right:* Bundles of fibrils (**arrowheads**) extending into cell processes. (From an 11-day open wound in a rat). **Bars** = 1 μm.

features are quite unlike those of a typical fibroblast, which uses contact inhibition to avoid touching its neighbors. The extensive junctions between cells are obviously related to the contractile function: a chain of myofibroblasts pulling while connected in series is more effective than cells contracting in isolation.

What makes a fibroblast modulate into a myofibroblast? Several cytokines, especially transforming growth factor beta (TGFb) (47, 169), but also mechanical factors. Stretching the skin of a mouse with a spring-loaded device for 4–6 days generates myofibroblasts (164). A tantalizing fact is that myofibroblasts do not develop in closed wounds, where they are not needed, whereas they do develop in open wounds, where they are needed.

> In fact this is why the myofibroblasts were not discovered earlier: a leading group of experimenters who had studied wound healing extensively before us by electron microscopy never saw a myofibroblast, because they had chosen to work only with incisional wounds.

So much for the myofibroblasts, which have become very popular cells. But there is yet another and more mysterious "contractile" force to deal with.

(3) Fibroblasts and the Collagen Lattice

Do normal fibroblasts contract, as some biologists have been saying for half a century (109, 169)? It depends in part on what we call a fibroblast and what we mean by contraction. In some normal organs there are fibroblasts that certainly do contract, e.g., in the lung and liver, but morphologically they are *myo*fibroblasts. In cell cultures, all fibroblasts tend to develop myofibroblast features (169)—which makes sense, because the fibroblasts presumably "feel" as if they were in an open wound, and modulate accordingly. The latter statement, incidentally, is also troublesome, because it implies that we may never have a culture of entirely "normal," nonactivated fibroblasts.

But then, in 1972, the same year that the myofibroblasts appeared on the scene, a new experimental model revealed a highly puzzling trait of the fibroblasts: they are able to exert a pull without becoming shorter. The method, described by a British group, was based on preparing thin buttons a collagen gel seeded with cultured fibroblasts (43). These "collagen lattices," as they are now called, were originally intended as engineered tissue substitutes for plastic surgery, but they became interesting also scientifically (62, 63, 64, 66). The name "lattice" is more accurate than "gel," because under the electron microscope the gel is not amorphous: it is a three-dimensional network of fibrils, to which the cells become attached.

> The lattice can be set up for isometric contraction (by leaving it attached to the dish) or for isotonic contraction (by detaching it, as indicated in Figure 14.13). If prepared without cells and maintained in medium, the lattice just sits there; nothing happens. If fibroblasts are added, over the next few days the lattice contracts to a small, dense object about 1/10 of the original volume (62, 63). The shortening is so great that it cannot be due to shortening or shrinking of the cells. Microscopic study shows that the fibroblasts are not connected. Myofibroblastic morphology develops only under isometric conditions, i.e., when the cells are kept under tension. If the tension is released, the fibroblasts die by apoptosis (62, 63, 66).

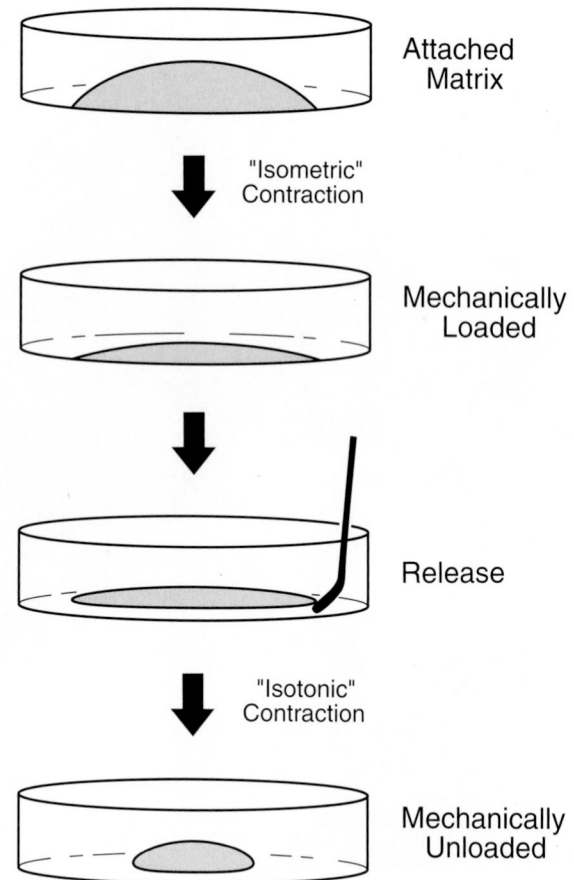

FIGURE 14.13 Use of a collagen matrix seeded with fibroblasts for the study of wound contraction. The gel settles in about 30 minutes, and remains anchored to the dish. Thereafter the cells begin to pull, under *isometric* conditions, and develop stress fibers. At this point, if the gel is artificially detached from the dish, it shrinks as the cells pull under *isotonic* conditions; after 3–6 hours a wave of apoptosis occurs, recalling the death of myofibroblasts in a healed wound. (Reprinted from Exp Cell Res Grinnell F, Zhu M, Carlson MA, Abrams JM. Release of mechanical tension triggers apoptosis of human fibroblasts in a model of regressing granulation tissue, 608–619, Copyright 1999, with permission from Elsevier Science.)

How can we explain the contraction of the lattice without shortening of the cells enclosed within it? Comparing the fibroblasts with muscle is probably misleading. An alternative: the fibroblasts, as they crawl around, could become transiently attached to the collagen fibrils and gather them up; a corresponding rearrangement of the collagen fibers around the cells can be seen microscopically. Yet another mechanism is best explained by comparing each cell with a lobsterman who hauls in the trap by pulling it in *hand over hand* (and does not become shorter in the process).

Fibroblasts in collagen gels do emit and retract pseudopodia (62, 63, 66).

And now, returning to the whole-wound level, *how does an open wound contract?* Few would disagree that myofibroblasts are on the scene after about a week, ready to perform in the style of smooth muscle cells, by shortening of the cell body. *During* the first week, fibroblasts (or better, activated fibroblasts) must be pulling by some other mechanism that does not require cell shortening. The "hand-over-hand" pulling described above is an obvious candidate; but there is yet another one, quite forgotten and not included in the collagen gels, the **fibrin network,** which is probably involved in the early stages of wound healing; it is high time to study it, especially since *there is a striking analogy between the shrinkage of the collagen lattice and the "syneresis" (retraction) of a fibrin-platelet thrombus.*

Current reviews of wound contraction tend to fall into two camps: the fibroblast camp versus the myofibroblast camp. Such polarizations are common in medical history; the final verdict of time is almost unfailingly that both sides were right, or almost right.

Pathology of contraction. The contraction of open wounds is not always wanted. Burns are the best example: a burn encircling an arm is an open wound; accordingly, myofibroblasts appear and produce enough traction to lock the elbow into a permanent flexed position or even to hamper the circulation. By the same mechanism, burns of the face or neck can produce disfiguring scars. Besides wounds, myofibroblasts have been found in cirrhosis of the liver, in the so-called *contracted kidney,* and in many diseases in which fibrosis and contraction of connective tissue are central features (152).

To this day the only method for preventing the contraction of an open wound in humans is to cover it with a graft. Drugs have been tried but without much success.

Shapes of Open Wounds and Shapes of Scars

An open wound contracts as if its margins were being drawn toward the center; this means that the final shape of the scar depends on the original shape of the wound. For example, as is well known to plastic surgeons, a square wound will lead to a star-shaped scar and a triangular wound to a Y-shaped scar (Figure 14.14). One way to understand these geometric results is to imagine 40 turtles standing in a square and facing inward at right angles to the sides of the square; if they all walk straight forward, they must come to a halt in the formation of a star (Figure 14.15) (109). Using the same example, we

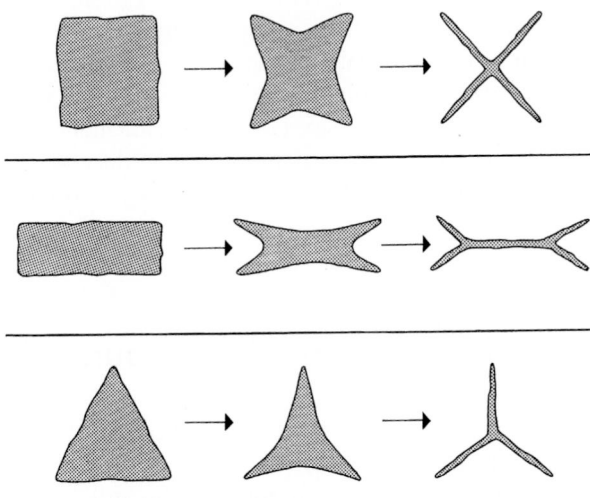

FIGURE 14.14 Open wounds of the three shapes shown (*left*) will contract and produce scars of predictable geometric patterns (*right*). (Reproduced with permission from [109].)

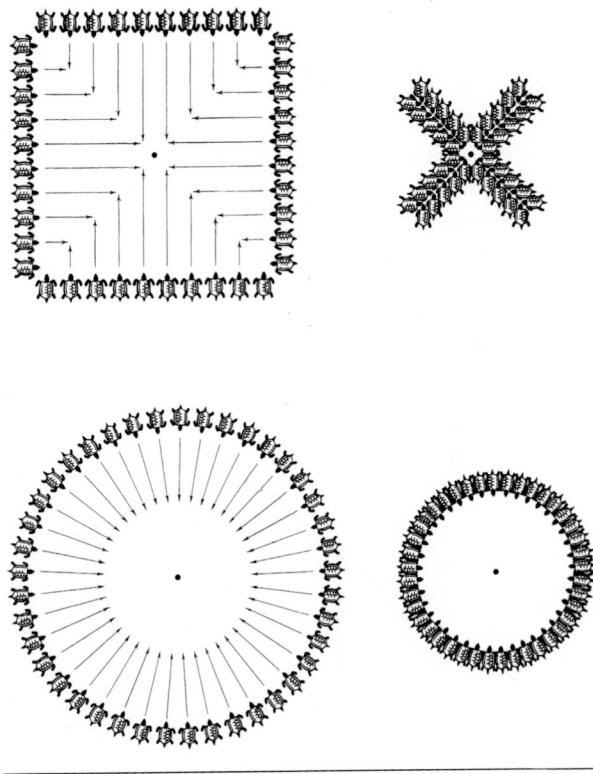

FIGURE 14.15 The "turtle experiment" illustrating how open wounds heal. The rows of turtles represent the margins of skin wounds. *Top:* In a square wound, an inward motion of the margins leads to a star-shaped scar. *Bottom:* If the wound is perfectly circular, it cannot heal solely by contraction because its margins cannot condense into a point. Large circular wounds heal by becoming oblong; later they close with a linear scar. (Reproduced with permission from [109].)

can predict that there must be a problem in the healing of round wounds; as matter of fact, it was known in Hippocratic times that a round wound heals more quickly if it is cut into a different shape (109). Experimental round wounds in rabbits do heal more slowly than square wounds of the same surface area: eventually they do heal because the circular shape slowly turns into an oval, then the oval becomes narrower, and finally it heals like a linear wound. This is intuitive. If a round wound were to heal by contraction, its margins would have to condense to a point, which is patently impossible.

Experimental Models of Wound Healing

Because wounds are such a basic medical problem, a great deal of effort has gone into developing experimental models (28): not a simple task, because laboratory animals naturally tend to "work" on their wounds and interfere with the experiment.

The Rabbit Ear Chamber

A classic device is the rabbit ear chamber (Figure 14.16): in essence, a small hole is punched in a rabbit ear, which is then sandwiched between two coverslips; the hole fills up with blood, and over the next few weeks one can observe, under the microscope, the ingrowth of blood vessels that organize the clot, i.e., replace it with living tissue (Figure 14.17). Careful drawings made by Sandison and by the Clarks in the 1920s and 1930s show very nicely how the vascular network develops (Figure 14.18) (20, 149). A recent improvement to the ear chamber has been the introduction of oxygen electrodes, which have confirmed that oxygen pressure in the center of the wound, where the macrophages are at work, is close to zero (Figure 14.19) (77).

Sponges and Cylinders

To examine the chemistry of granulation tissue, one can implant a small absorbable sponge, let it be infiltrated by granulation tissue, and then recover it for study at various times (74). To analyze the nature and properties of "wound fluid," one can slip a hollow object such as a cylinder of wire mesh under the skin of an experimental animal (77, 181); after a few days the space is filled with wound fluid, which is similar to the inflammatory exudate.

Eye Injuries

Studies on eye injuries have illustrated many points, such as the angiogenic power of macrophages (Figure 14.20); they have also provided spectacular three-dimensional views of angiogenesis (Figure 14.21).

The Air Pouch (Selye Pouch)

Besides open wounds, a highly standardized method for producing sheets of granulation tissue is the "granuloma pouch" or "Selye pouch" (Figure 14.22) (49). On the back of a rat, using a syringe, 20 ml of air are injected subcutaneously, followed by 1 ml of 1 percent croton oil, a powerful irritant. Within a few days the wall of the air pouch is filled with exudate and lined by granulation tissue. It can be excised as an egg-shaped organ, and the granulation tissue (which, unlike that of an open wound, is aseptic) can be studied microscopically or measured in various ways. If left alone, the pouch shrinks—it is loaded with myofibroblasts (49)—and disappears in about 3 months.

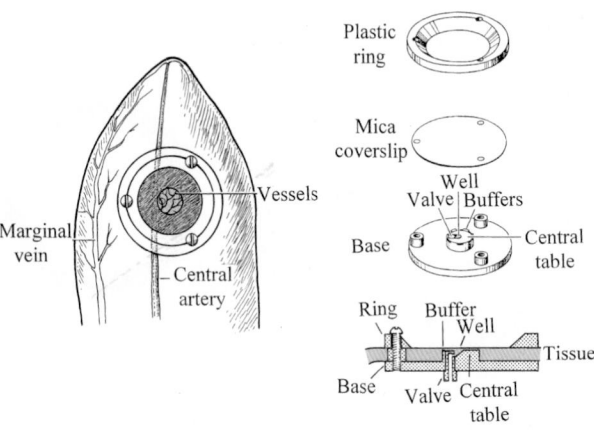

FIGURE 14.16 Rabbit ear chamber, a tool for the study of wound healing *in vivo. Left:* The chamber as installed in the ear. *Right:* Exploded view of the chamber and cross section of the chamber installed *in vivo.* (Adapted from the **Journal of Experimental Medicine,** 1964; 120:57–82, by copyright permission of The Rockefeller University Press [121].)

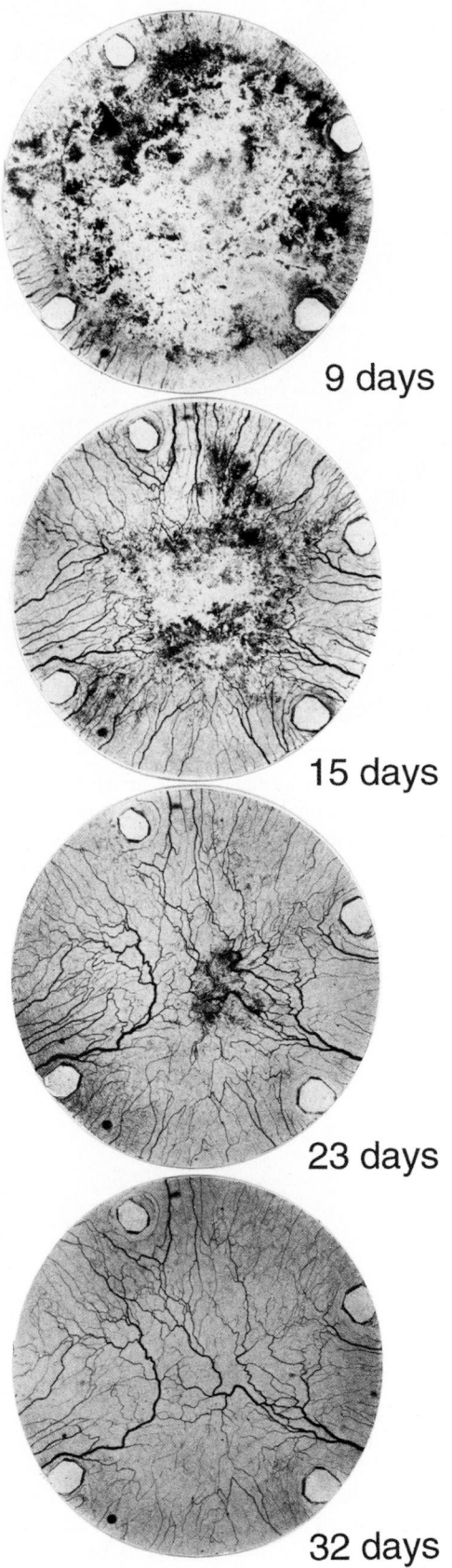

9 days

15 days

23 days

32 days

FIGURE 14.17   Serial photographs through a rabbit ear chamber, showing the progressive ingrowth of blood vessels and the organization of the central blood clot at various times after chamber was installed. (Reprinted from [21], copyright 1931, by permission of Wiley-Liss, a division of John Wiley & Sons, Inc.)

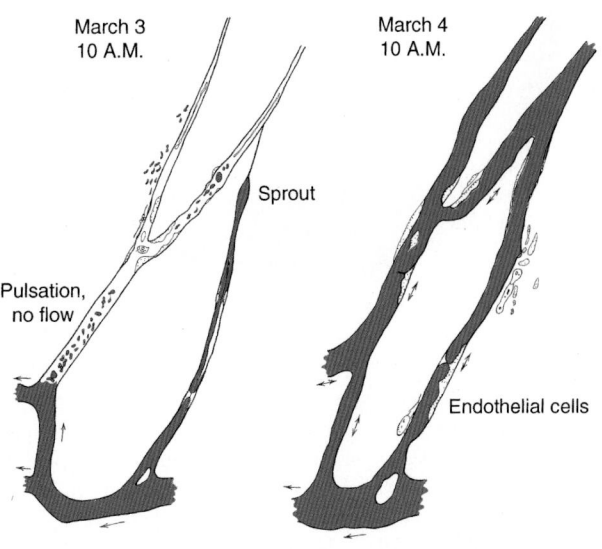

FIGURE 14.18   Advancing edge of a capillary network as seen in the rabbit ear chamber. The two drawings are of the same field and were made 24 hours apart. (Reprinted from [149], copyright 1928, by permission of Wiley-Liss, a division of John Wiley & Sons, Inc.)

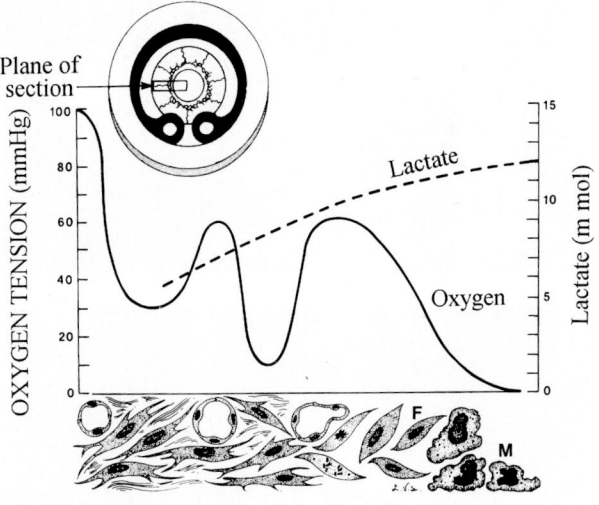

FIGURE 14.19   Oxygen and lactate levels in the rabbit ear chamber. Tissue sample oriented as shown in the inset at top. The peaks of oxygen concentration correspond to vessels. The cells at the advancing front, shown at bottom, are macrophages (M) and fibroblasts (F); they live in a low-oxygen, high-lactate environment. (Reproduced with permission from [76].)

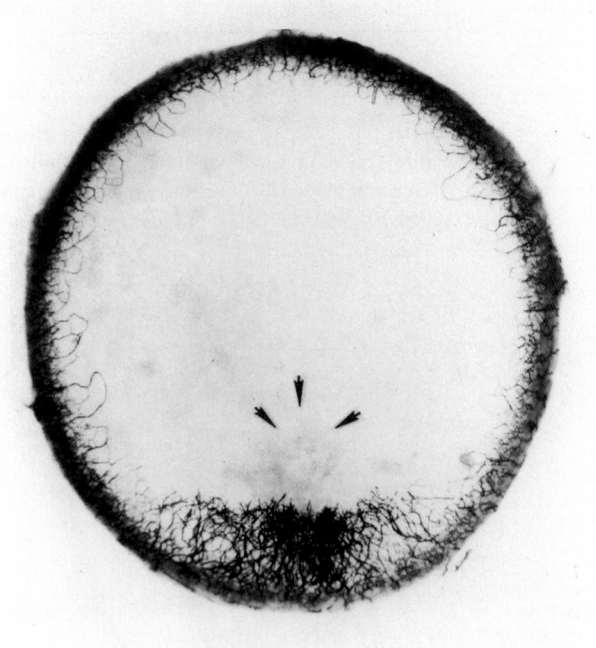

FIGURE 14.20 Dense growth of vascular sprouts in guinea pig cornea. To illustrate the angiogenic property of macrophages, the cornea was injected with activated peritoneal macrophages, and 7 days later all vessels were perfused with carbon black. **Arrowheads:** Injection site. (Reprinted by permission from [136]; Copyright © 1977 Macmillan Magazines Limited.)

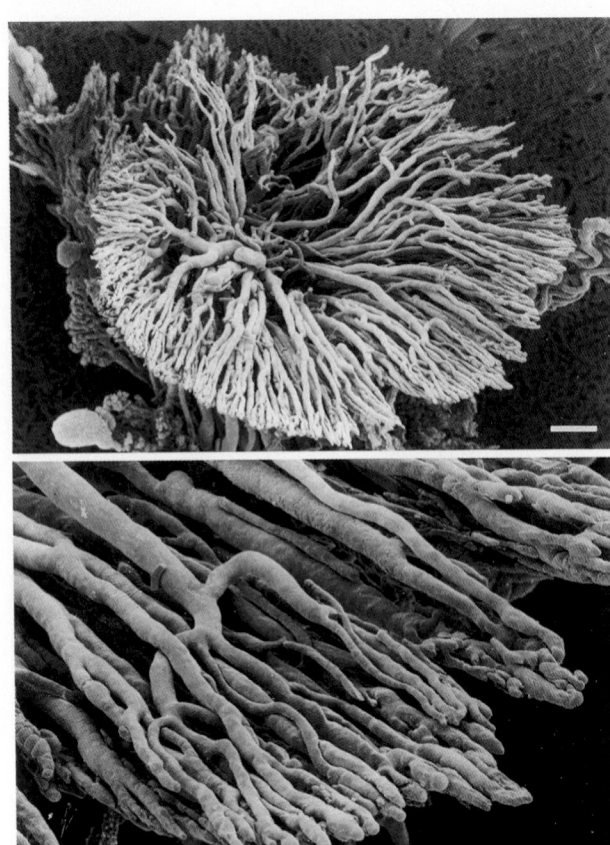

FIGURE 14.21 Burst of angiogenesis in the eye of a rabbit. These vessels grew into the vitreous body (normally avascular) in response to an injection of cultured skin fibroblasts 3 months earlier. The vessels were then injected with plastic, and all tissues were removed by corrosion. *Top:* Normal view of the vascular fan. **Bar** = 200 μm. *Bottom:* Higher power showing advancing vascular loops. **Bar** = 100 μm. (Reprinted from [168], copyright 1981, with permission from Elsevier.)

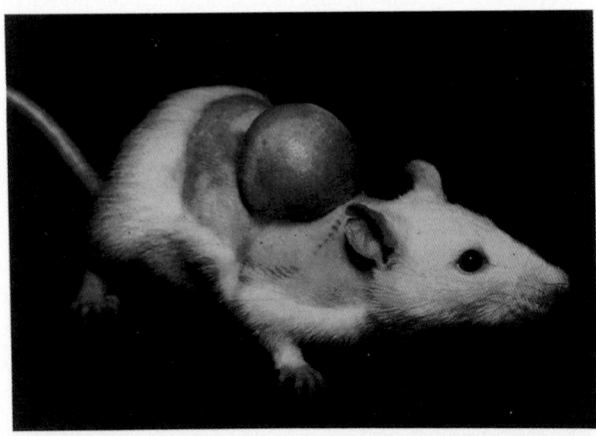

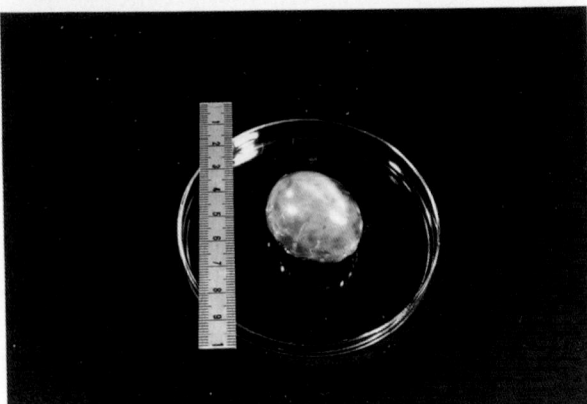

FIGURE 14.22 *Top:* The "granuloma pouch" method for the study of inflammation. Air (20 ml) is injected under the rat's skin, followed by a small volume of irritant in oil; the skin remains intact. *Bottom:* 2–3 weeks later a pouch of granulation tissue can be excised and studied. It contains air and exudate. **Scale** in centimeters. (Courtesy of Dr. G. B. Ryan, University of Melbourne, Melbourne, Australia.)

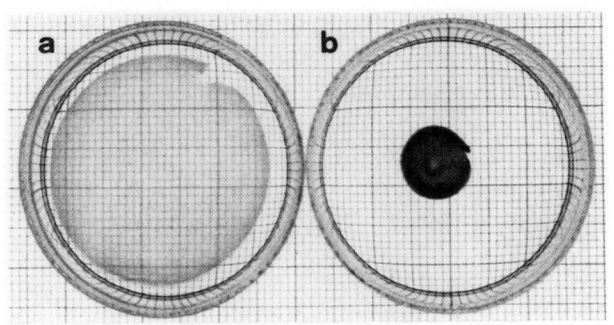

FIGURE 14.23 Stimulation of "cultured fibroblasts" to contract their substrate. Two dishes were coated with a layer of collagen, seeded with 1 million fibroblasts, and stained after 5 days. **a:** Control. **b:** Stimulation with transforming growth factor beta (TGF-β). **Scale** in millimeters. (Reproduced with permission from [120].)

Collagen Lattice

This model was described above. It opened a window on a new mechanism of fibroblast contraction. It is excellent for testing the effect of cytokines and other agents on contraction (Figure 14.23). It also has a flaw: the cells with which the lattice is seeded are cultured fibroblasts, and therefore partially activated.

The Pace of Wound Healing

Mankind has been trying for millennia to accelerate wound healing, be it with spider webs, manure, or more orthodox drugs (139). However, by the early twentieth century, pessimism began to prevail: the view was widely adopted that *wounds heal at maximal rate,* meaning that no drug could possibly speed up the process. This dogma is now collapsing as growth factors are tested on wounds; some growth factors do stimulate wound healing in experimental models (Figure 14.24)

(55, 102) and in humans, for whom the need is great, especially for treating "recalcitrant" diabetic ulcers (86, 118).

> Mammals lick their wounds. Mouse salivary glands secrete large amounts of nerve growth factor and epidermal growth factor. In mice deprived of sublingual and submaxillary glands, open wounds contract more slowly (76) and corneal ulcers heal poorly (170). Even in humans, wounds in the mouth heal quickly and without infectious

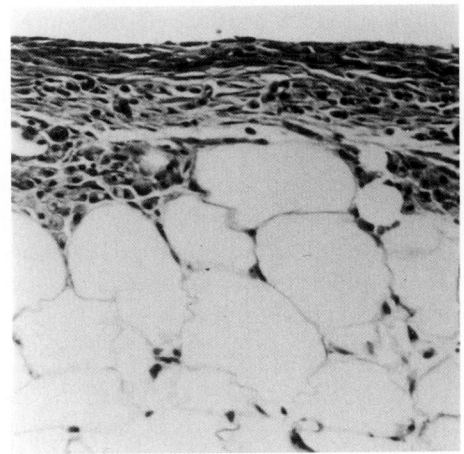
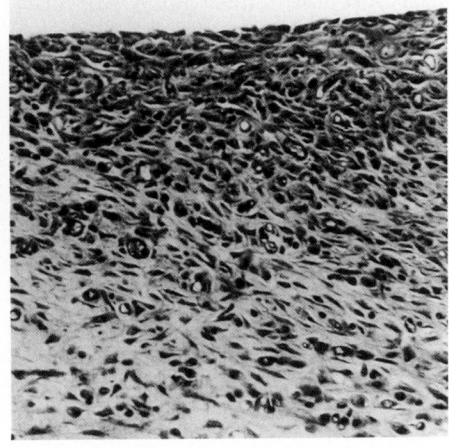

FIGURE 14.24 Stimulation of wound healing with recombinant PDGF in square open wounds on the backs of genetically diabetic mice. *Left:* Control wound in a diabetic mouse treated with control solution for 5 days shows minimal cellular invasion and granulation tissue formation. *Right:* 5-day diabetic wound treated with recombinant PDGF shows marked increase in the thickness, cellularity, and vascularity of the granulation tissue. (25x) (Reproduced with permission from [55], © American Society for Investigative Pathology.)

complications, despite a teeming bacterial flora. The mechanism is not clear.

Mucosal wounds in general heal faster than skin wounds (153). When a *muscularis mucosae* exists, it contracts and reduces the area of the wound. This is why mucosal biopsies can be taken routinely, even from the rectum.

Age is a factor in the rate of healing. Although armies are not known for basic research, an exception should be made for the wound healing laboratory of the French army during World War I: Alexis Carrel and his group discovered that open wounds in older persons close more slowly (52). Wound healing in the fetus will be discussed shortly.

Disorders of Wound Healing

The process of healing is powerfully programmed and very difficult to obstruct, but it has its enemies. Some are iatrogenic: glucocorticoids, given during the first 3 days after injury, retard wound healing. Delays are caused also by the cachexia induced by malignant tumors, X-ray therapy, and many antineoplastic agents; this can create a problem when surgery is needed during the treatment of tumors (15, 157). Diabetics have a fivefold greater risk than nondiabetics of wound infection (15); not only is their inflammatory response defective (p. 519) but also there are subtle defects of the microcirculation, of phagocytosis and of the granulation tissue (53, 175). Malnutrition, including lack of vitamin C (scurvy), can also impair wound healing.

The two main complications of wound healing are infection, the most common (75), and keloids.

Wound Infection

No skin wound can be totally free from bacterial contamination, but there is a critical number of bacteria beyond which clinical infection results: this is currently set at 10^5 bacteria per gram of tissue or per milliliter of biologic fluid. This figure varies surprisingly little with different organisms (73).

Infection and oxygen. It is an axiom of surgery that *the resistance of wounds to infection is proportional to their blood supply* (78). As we have seen, blood protects against infection in many ways. A key factor is the oxygen supply. Leukocytes can move about and phagocytize anaerobically, but they depend on oxygen for killing some bacteria; for example, *Staphylococcus aureus* and *E. coli* are killed at rates proportional to oxygen tension, whereas pneumococci are killed independently of oxygen tension. In essence, *leukocytes deprived of oxygen behave like leukocytes in chronic granulomatous disease: the respiratory burst is impaired* (78).

If wounded rabbits are kept in various concentrations of oxygen, and *Pseudomonas aeruginosa* are injected into the wounds, the bacteria are cleared much faster from the rabbits breathing the highest oxygen concentrations (78, 79). In this context, it has been said that oxygen acts as an antibiotic (88). By the year 2000, a study of 500 patients submitted to colorectal surgery showed that breathing 30–80 percent oxygen during and 2 hours after surgery reduced the number of postoperative wound infections (56).

Infection and foreign bodies: the role of biofilms. Foreign bodies such as dirt or splinters can create serious complications even if they are chemically inert because they have the odd property of favoring infection. This is why surgeons submit accidental wounds to careful cleaning and do not immediately suture dirty wounds. Foreign bodies favor infection in three ways:

- They can be a source of bacteria.
- They lower the infectious dose of bacteria.
- They make the infection harder to treat.

The first way is self-evident. The second has been more difficult to understand, but the facts are impressive: in experiments on courageous volunteers in the 1950s, virulent staphylococci were introduced into the skin, with or without a surgical suture. The suture lowered the infectious dose of bacteria to 100 staphylococci, enhancing their virulence at least 10,000 times (42, 125). Something has tipped the balance in favor of bacteria. It has been shown experimentally that the foreign body acts as a decoy and distracts the phagocytes, which waste their precious granules in attempts to phagocytize it. In other words, frustrated phagocytosis becomes distracting phagocytosis.

> If a small, sterile plastic cage is implanted under the skin of a guinea pig, as few as 100 *Staph aureus* suffice to infect, whereas even 10^8 bacteria fail to produce an abscess in normal guinea-pig skin (181). If the neutrophils in the cage are tested later, they are found to have developed a phagocytic defect (180): loss of ammunition.

The third problem created by foreign bodies (infections are harder to treat) is due to the fact that many bacteria can switch to the **biofilm** mode of life: they settle on a surface, switch on the appropriate genes, and cover themselves

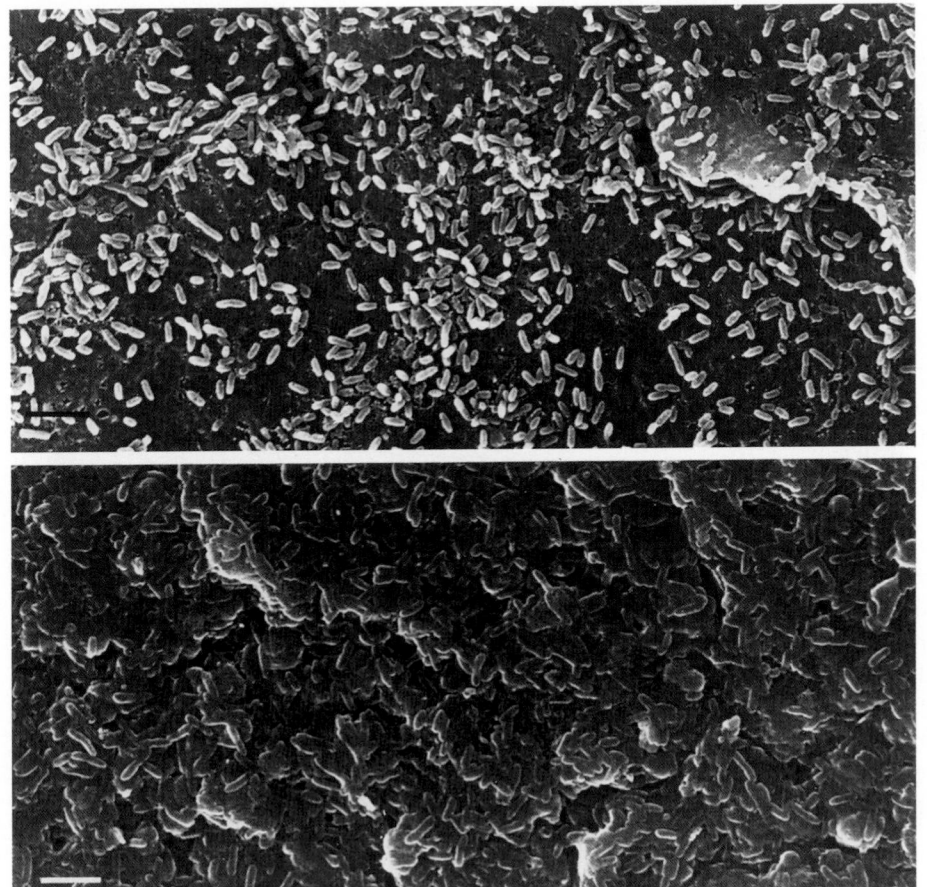

FIGURE 14.25 Behavior of *Pseudomonas aeruginosa* on the surface of a piece of catheter that is bathed in artificial urine. *Top:* Colonization of the surface after 2 hours of exposure to the bacteria-laden medium. *Bottom:* The same after 8 hours; the surface is now covered by a thick film in which the bacterial cells are buried. **Bars** = 5 μm. (Reprinted from [35], copyright 1987, with permission from Elsevier.)

with a thick layer of mucus (more elegantly called *biopolymer*) (Figure 14.25). This gel protects the bacteria at least partially from phagocytes (84, 171), from lymphocytes (132) as well as from antibodies, and even from antibiotics (31, 151). In ordinary bacterial cultures on a solid medium, biofilms do not develop because the prime requirement—a watery habitat—is lacking.

> Awareness of biofilms, today a booming science (34, 93) dates back only to the 1970s and 1980s. It is now realized that biofilms constitute a major part of the bacterial biomass. For every planktonic bacterium there are 10^3–10^4 held in the slime layer of submerged surfaces: a complex habitat, with a special physiology, pH, flow of water and food, metabolism, antibiotic resistance (108a), and the response to noxious agents (Figure 14.26).

Medically, biofilms are relevant because they develop not only on catheters and on foreign bodies, but also on bone surfaces, heart valves, and almost any conduits, especially the bronchi of patents suffering from *cystic fibrosis* (34, 137, 138). Urinary catheters can become coated with slimy layers of bacteria, dozens of cells and hundreds of micrometers thick (32). In essence, *staphylococci growing on a urinary catheter are simply doing*

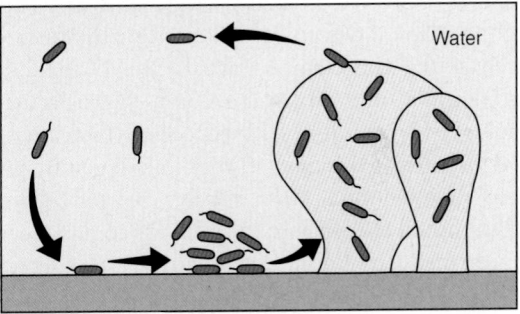

FIGURE 14.26 Genesis of a biofilm on a submerged surface. Free, "planktonic" bacteria secrete molecules that function as "quorum sensors" (not shown); when so instructed, the bacteria secrete *adhesins* that make them stick to a surface and secrete a mucous matrix. (Reprinted with permission from Science "One for All and All for One," Kolter R, Losick R. 226:226–227, 1998. Copyright 1998 American Association for the Advancement of Science.)

what they would do in their natural environment (18). Dentists have been aware of these facts for a long time because the crevices around a tooth, where dental plaque flourishes, is one of these natural ecosystems

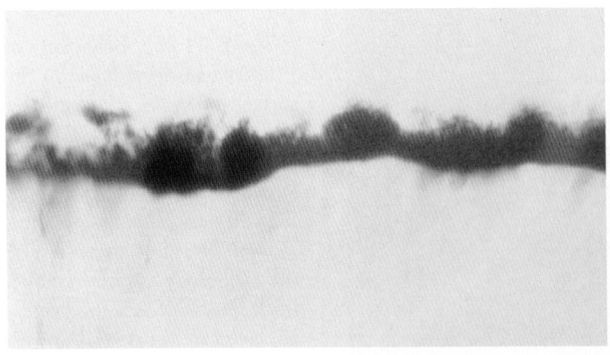

FIGURE 14.27   Dental plaque is a biofilm. Here it is empha-sized by a red stain, on the teeth of a patient who did not believe in brushing. Acid produced by some of these bacteria cause decay. (Courtesy of Dr. G. Cimasoni, Geneva, Switzerland.)

(Figure 14.27) (167). To reduce the risk of infection by surgical sutures, the Centers for Disease Control now recommends monofilament threads (44).

But not all is necessarily bad about bacteria. A 1968 paper reported normal healing of incisional wounds in germ-free mice (6), but a more recent study found *impaired* healing in the *germ-free* state, and concluded that bacterial products from the gut may be beneficial to wound healing (127).

Diabetes and wound healing. Diabetes increases the risk of wound infection, but in diabetics the course of wound healing is defective in many ways, due to a mind-boggling series of defects, which frustrate the researcher as well as the clinician. A partial list: (1) inadequate blood supply due to macro- and microcirculatory pathology; (2) rigidity of blood cells, which increases blood viscosity; (3) higher affinity for oxygen by glyco-sylated hemoglobin: this impairs oxygen delivery; (4) diminished chemotaxis; (5) diminished phagocytosis and intracellular killing of bacteria; (6) decreased fibroblast proliferation and collagen synthesis; (7) inad-equate formation of granulation tissue (53a, 101, 133, 165); diabetic neuropathy. Currently several of these defects have been reinterpreted as different aspects of one basic disorder, **endothelial cell dysfunction,** in which prominent features are the scavenging of nitric oxide by glucose and the excessive generation of AGE products (51, 53a, 133). The latter concept has led to treat diabetic mice with soluble receptors for AGE products. In the mice it worked…

Hypertrophic Scars and Keloids

Aberrations of scar formation are the nightmare of plas-tic surgeons and of their patients. In some individuals the smallest wound, even that left by piercing an ear,

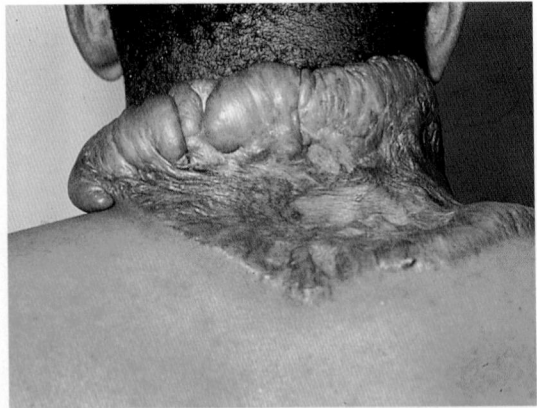

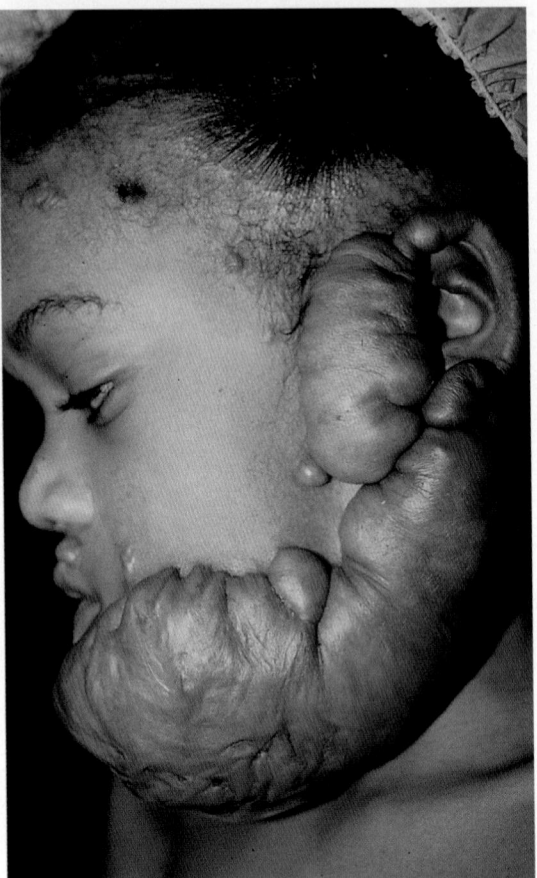

FIGURE 14.28   *Top:* Keloid of the neck, following an infection. *Bottom:* Extensive keloid of the face, following a burn of the ear and two grafting operations. (*Top:* Reprinted from [130], copy-right 1984, with permission from Elsevier. *Bottom:* Reprinted from [129].)

can lead to an overgrowth of the scar. If the scar develops into a raised, firm ridge, it is called a *hy-pertrophic scar* (103, 108) which can regress. If the overgrowth exceeds the borders of the scar, it is called a *keloid,* which does not regress. Keloid is Greek for claw-like, and therefore cancer-like. This cancer connection

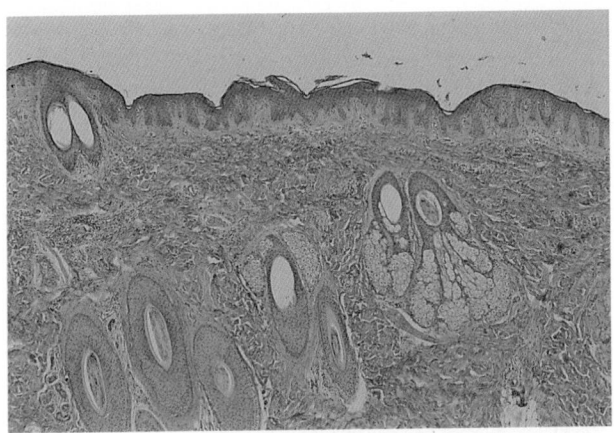

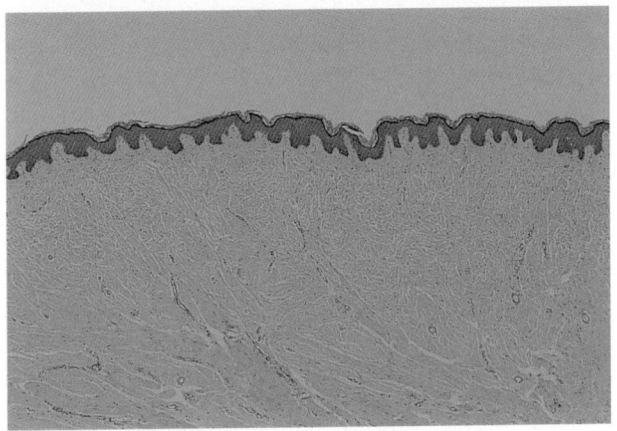

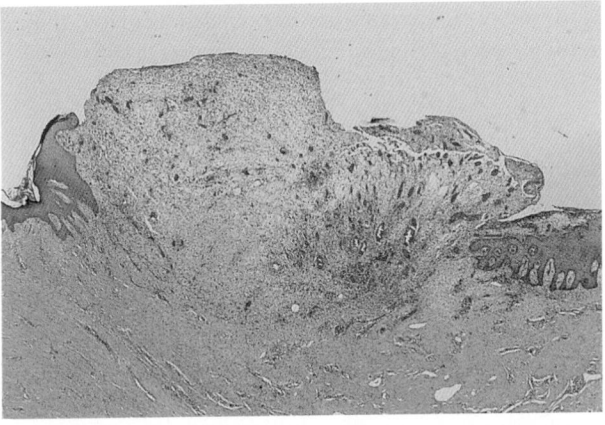

FIGURE 14.30   Excessive granulation tissue ("proud flesh") in an ulcer of the skin. The mass of granulation tissue (*center*) rises higher than the epidermis, visible on either side. Cauterization with silver nitrate controls the overgrowth, but its genesis is not understood. (10x)

FIGURE 14.29   Comparison of normal skin and keloid tissue. *Top:* Control skin. *Bottom:* Keloid. The dermis is replaced by a meshwork of thick collagen fibers without many cells. Note lack of glands and hair. (25x)

has yet to be proven, although some keloids truly suggest tumor growth (Figure 14.28). Histologically, all one sees is a tremendous overproduction of collagen (Figure 14.29); biochemically, collagen metabolism is abnormally high in keloids even after 10 years (5). Excision of a keloid simply creates another one. However, keloids are capricious: a wound in one part of the body may produce a keloid, but in another it may not. Blacks (whose skin is privileged in other ways—such as the rarity of melanoma) are especially prone to keloid development. Theories abound (27), but there is no explanation for this distressing condition.

"Proud flesh." Hypertrophy of granulation tissue sometimes occurs during wound healing. An overenthusiastic granulation tissue grows above the surface of the surrounding skin (Figure 14.30), but it can be brought under control by cauterization with silver nitrate. This condition was once known by the antique name of *proud flesh* (a similar expression is still current in

carpentry: in covering a wall with plaster the surface above a hole must be slightly "prouded"). In children, an overgrowth of granulation tissue can obstruct the opening of a long-term tracheostomy tube (143); occasionally an overgrowth occurs at the naval after shedding of the umbilical cord ("umbilical granuloma").

Fetal wounds. These wounds attracted much attention because early work showed that they could heal without a scar, and therefore might teach some important lesson to plastic surgeons (115). Fetal wounds heal in the milieu of amniotic fluid, but this can not be their secret, because wounds in the fetus of a marsupial heal just as well. Experimentally, incisional wounds in the fetus can heal perfectly; open wounds may heal by contraction, but in some species they do not heal at all (104, 105, 163). Fetal wounds in general heal with minimal inflammation, and their cytokine profile is different from that of the adult wound.

> Here is an imaginative use of the rabbit fetal model, in which excisional wonds heal without contraction: local treatment of such wounds with TGF-beta induced healing by contraction, thereby confirming that (a) TGF-beta induces the modulation of fibroblasts to myofibroblasts, and (b) myofibroblasts are responsible for the contraction of open wounds (96).

Current thought regarding the scarless healing of fetal wounds is not the fetal environment, but the age of the fetus: this is what decides whether the wound will or will not heal with a scar (115). We tend to think of embryonic and fetal tissues as omnipotent, but we should also remember that the fetus is neutropenic, lacks an immune response, and has less oxygen available than a mountaineer at the top of Mount Everest (105).

> **TO SUM UP:** We consider wound healing as one of the marvels of Nature, considering its ability to succeed despite the repulsive materials that humanity has used to help it (Galen's favorite was dove droppings [109]). This amazing resistance may be due to the fact that the process of wound healing evolved in a world saturated with bacteria.
>
> We have begun to understand the process of wound contraction, and we have at hand a variety of growth factors that experimentally can help wound healing, but so far none is effective enough for large scale use in humans. There are still many challenges, including the following:
>
> - What is the basic connection, if any (72, 113, 150), between wound healing and the immune response?
> - Do the circulating "fibrocytes" contribute significantly to wound healing (16, 178)?
> - What can we do to stop the myofibroblasts—and the activated fibroblasts—from pulling when it causes damage?
> - Why do spleen wounds heal without a scar (87)?

References

1. Allen TD, Schor SL. The contraction of collagen matrices by dermal fibroblasts. J Ultrastruct Res 1983;83:205–219.
2. Arora PD, Narani N, McCulloch CAG. The compliance of collaen gels regulates transforming growth factor-β induction of α-smooth muscle actin in fibroblasts. Am J Pathol 1999;154:871–882.
3. Ausprunk DH, Falterman K, Folkman J. The sequence of events in the regression of corneal capillaries. Lab Invest 1978;38:284–294.
4. Avicenna. *Liber Canonis.* Translated from Arabic to Latin by Gerard of Cremona. Printed in Venice, 1507; photographically reproduced by G. Olms Verlag, Hildesheim, 1964; pp. 79/r col.2, 446 r/col.2.
5. Bailey AJ, Bazin S, Sims TJ, et al. Characterization of the collagen of human hypertrophic and normal scars. Biochim Biophys Acta 1975;405:412–421.
6. Bauer H. Cellular defence mechanisms. In: Coates ME, Gordon HA, Wostmann BS, eds. The germ-free animal in research. London and New York: Academic Press, 1968, pp. 210–226.
7. Bell E, Ivarsson B, Merrill C. Production of a tissue-like structure by contraction of collagen lattices by human fibroblasts of different proliferative potential in vitro. Proc Natl Acad Sci USA 1979;76:1274–1278.
8. Bhawan J, Bacchetta C, Joris I, Majno G. A myofibroblastic tumor: Infantile digital fibrome (recurrent digital fibrous tumor of childhood). Am J Pathol 1979;94:19–36.
9. Bhawan J, Majno G. The myofibroblast. Possible derivation from macrophages in xanthogranuloma. Am J Dermatopathol 1989;11:255–258.
10. Blobe GC, Schiemann WP, Lodish HF. Role of transforming growth factor β in human disease. N Eng J Med 2000;342:1350–1358.
11. Breedis C. Regeneration of hair follicles and sebaceous glands from the epithelium of scars in the rabbit. Cancer Res 1954;14:575–579.
12. Brown GL, Nanney LB, Griffen J, et al. Enhancement of wound healing by topical treatment with epidermal growth factor. N Engl J Med 1989;321:76–79.
13. Brown LF, Yeo K-T, Berse B, et al. Expression of vascular permeability factor (vascular endothelial growth factor) by epidermal keratinocytes during wound healing. J Exp Med 1992;176:1375–1379.
14. Campbell GR, Ryan GB. Origin of myofibroblasts in the avascular capsule around free-floating intraperitoneal blood clots. Pathology 1983;15:253–264.
15. Carrico TJ, Mehrhof AI Jr, Cohen IK. Biology of wound healing. Surg Clin North Am 1984;64:721–733.
16. Chesney J, Bucala R. Peripheral blood fibrocytes: mesenchymal precursor cells and the pathogenesis of fibrosis. Curr Rheumatol Reports 2000;2:501–505.
17. Chettibi S, Ferguson MWJ. Wound repair: an overview. In: Gallin JI, Snyderman R. (eds). Inflammation. Basic Principles and Clinical Correlates. 3rd ed. Philadelphia: Lippincott Williams & Wilkins, 1999.
18. Christensen GD, Baddour LM, Hasty DL, Lowrance JH, Simpson WA. Microbial and foreign body factors in the pathogenesis of medical device infections. In: Bisno AL, Waldvogel FA, eds. Infections associated with indwelling medical devices. Washington, DC: American Society for Microbiology, 1989, pp. 27–59.
19. Chvapil M, Koopmann CF Jr. Scar formation: physiology and pathological states. Otolaryngol Clin North Am 1984;17:265–272.
20. Clark ER, Clark EL. Observations on living preformed blood vessels as seen in a transparent chamber inserted into the rabbit's ear. Am J Anat 1931;49:441–477.
21. Clark ER, Hitschler WJ, Kirby-Smith HT, Rex RO, Smith JH. General observations on the ingrowth of new blood vessels into standardized chambers in the rabbit's ear, and the subsequent changes in the newly grown vessels over a period of months. Anat Rec 1931;50:129–160.
22. Clark RAF, Winn HJ, Dvorak HF, Colvin RB. Fibronectin beneath reepithelializing epidermis in vivo: sources and significance. J Invest Dermatol 1983;80:026s–030s.
23. Clark RAF. Overview and general considerations of wound repair. In: Clark RAF, Henson PM, eds. The molecular and cellular biology of wound repair. New York: Plenum Press, 1988, pp. 3–33.
24. Clark RAF, Henson PM, eds. The molecular and cellular biology of wound repair. New York: Plenum Press, 1988.
25. Clark RAF (ed). The Molecular and Cellular Biology of Wound Repair. New York: Plenum Press. 1996.

26. Cohen I. The contractile system of blood platelets and its function. Methods Achiev Exp Pathol 1979;9:40–86.

27. Cohen IK, McCoy BJ. Keloid: biology and treatment. In: Dineen P, Hildick-Smith G, eds. The surgical wound. Philadelphia: Lea & Febiger, 1981, pp. 123–131.

28. Cohen K, Mast BA. Models of wound healing. J Trauma 1990;30(12 Suppl):S149–S155.

29. Colvin RB. Wound healing processes in hemostasis and thrombosis. In: Gimbrone MA Jr, ed. Vascular endothelium in hemostasis and thrombosis. Edinburgh: Churchill Livingstone, 1986, pp. 220–241.

30. Converse JM, Smahel J, Ballantyne DL Jr, Harper AD. Inosculation of vessels of skin graft and host bed: a fortuitous encounter. Br J Plast Surg 1975;28:274–282.

31. Costerton JW. Effects of antibiotics on adherent bacteria. In: Sabath LD, ed. Action of antibiotics in patients. Bern: Hans Huber Publishers, 1982, pp. 160–176.

32. Costerton JW. The etiology and persistence of cryptic bacterial infections: a hypothesis. Rev Infect Dis 1984; 6(suppl 3): S608–S616.

33. Costerton JW, Geesey GG, Chen, K-J. How bacteria stick. Sci Am 1978;238:86–95.

34. Costerton JW, Stewart PS, Greenberg EP. Bacterial biofilms: a common cause of persistent infection. Science 1999;284: 1318–1322.

35. Costerton JW, Watkins L. Adherence of bacteria to foreign bodies: the role of the biofilm. In: Root RK, Trunkey DD, Sande MA. New surgical and medical approaches in infectious diseases. New York: Churchill Livingstone, 1987, pp. 17–30.

36. Darby I, Skalli O, Gabbiani G. α-Smooth muscle actin is transiently expressed by myofibroblasts during experimental wound healing. Lab Invest 1990;63:21–29.

37. de Chauliac G. On wounds and fractures. (Translated by WA Brennan). Chicago: Translator, 1923.

38. Desmoulière A, Gabbiani G. Myofibroblast differentiation during fibrosis. Exp Nephrol 1995;3:134–139.

39. Desmoulière A, Rubbia-Brandt L, Crau G, Gabbiani G. Heparin induces α-smooth muscle actin expression in cultured fibroblasts and in granulation tissue myofibroblasts. Lab Invest 1992;67:716–726.

40. de Vries HJC, Middelkeep E, van Heemstra-Hoen M, Wildevuur CHR, Westerhof W. Stromal cells from subcutaneous adipose tissue seeded in a native collagen/elastin dermal substitute reduce wound contraction in full thickness skin defects. Lab Invest 1995;73:532–540.

41. Dunphy JE. Practical accomplishments and future prospects. In: Dunphy JE, Van Winkle W Jr, eds. Repair and regeneration. New York: McGraw-Hill, 1969, pp. 349–358.

42. Elek SD, Conen PE. The virulence of Staphylococcus pyogenes for man. A study of the problems of wound infection. Br J Exp Pathol 1957;38:573–586.

43. Elsdale T, Bard J. Collagen substrata for studies on cell behavior. J Cell Biol 1972;54:626–637.

44. Fishman M. Microbial adherence and infection—clinical relevance. Infect Control 1986;7:181–184.

45. Forrester JC, Zederfeldt BH, Hayes TL, Hunt TK. Mechanical, biochemical and architectural features of repair. In: Dunphy JE, Van Winkle W Jr, eds. Repair and regeneration. New York: McGraw-Hill, 1969, pp. 71–85.

46. Gabbiani G. The cellular derivation and the life span of the myofibroblast. Path Res Pract 1996;192:708–711.

47. Gabbiani G. Evolution and clinical implications of the myofibroblast concept. Cadiovasc Res 1998;38:545–548.

48. Gabbiani G, Ryan GB, Majno G. Presence of modified fibroblasts in granulation tissue and their possible role in wound contraction. Experientia 1971;27:449–550.

49. Gabbiani G, Hirschel BJ, Ryan GB, Statkov PR, Majno G. Granulation tissue as a contractile organ. A study of structure and function. J Exp Med 1972;135:719–734.

50. Gay S, Viljanto J, Raekallio J, Pentinnen R. Collagen types in early phases of wound healing in children. Acta Chir Scand 1978;144:205–211.

51. Goligorsky MS, Chen J, Brodsky S. Endothelial dysfunction leading to diabetic nephropathy. Focus on nitric oxide. Hypertension 2001;37:744–748.

52. Goodson WH III, Hunt TK. Wound healing and aging. J Invest Dermatol 1979;73:88–91.

53. Goodson WH III, Radolf J, Hunt TK. Wound healing and diabetes. In: Hunt TK, ed. Wound healing and wound infection. New York: Appleton-Century-Crofts, 1980, pp. 106–117.

53a. Goova MT, Li J, Kislinger T, et al. Blockade of receptor for advanced glycation end-products restores effective wound healing in diabetic mice. Am J Pathol 2001;159:513–525.

54. Gown AM. The mysteries of the myofibroblast (partially) unmasked. Lab Invest 1990;63:1–3.

55. Greenhalgh DG, Sprugel KH, Murray MJ, Ross R. PDGF and FGF stimulate wound healing in the genetically diabetic mouse. Am J Pathol 1990;136:1235–1246.

56. Greif R, Akça O, Horn E-P, Kurz A, Sessler DI. Supplemental perioperative oxygen to reduce the incidence of surgical-wound infection. N Engl J Med 2000;342:161–167.

57. Grillo HC. Research in wound healing. In: Ballinger F, ed. Research methods in surgery. The National Cancer Institute, 1964, pp. 235–254.

58. Grinnell F. Fibronectin and wound healing. J Cell Biochem 1984;26:107–116.

59. Grinnell F. The activated keratinocyte: up regulation of cell adhesion and migration during wound healing. J Trauma 1990;30(suppl 12):S144–S149.

60. Grinnell F. Fibroblast reorganization of three-dimensional collagen gels and regulation of cell biosynthetic function. In: Okamura S, Tsuruta S, Imanishi Y, Sunamoto J, eds. Fundamental investigations on the creation of biofunctional materials. Kyoto, Japan: Kagaku-Dojin, 1991, pp. 33–43.

61. Grinnell F. Wound repair, keratinocyte activation and integrin modulation. J Cell Sci 1992;101:1–5.

62. Grinnell F. Fibroblasts, myofibroblasts, and wound contraction. J Cell Biol 1994;124:401–404.

63. Grinnell F. Fibroblast-collagen-matrix contraction: growth–factor signalling and mechanical loading. Trends Cell Biol 2000; 10:362–365.

64. Grinnell F, Ho C-H. Transforming growth factor β stimulates fibroblast-collagen matrix contraction by different mechanisms in mechanically loaded and unloaded matrices. Exp Cell Res 2002;273:248–255.

65. Grinnell F, Billingham RE, Burgess L. Distribution of fibronectin during wound healing in vivo. J Invest Dermatol 1981;76:181–189.

66. Grinnell F, Ho CH, Tamariz E, Lee DJ, Skuta G. Dendritic fibroblasts in three-dimensional collagen matrices. Mol Biol Cell. 2003;14:384–395.

67. Grinnell F, Toda, K-I, Takashima A. Activation of keratinocyte fibronectin receptor function during cutaneous wound healing. J Cell Sci Suppl 1987;8:199–209.

68. Grinnell F, Zhu M, Carlson MA, Abrams JM. Release of mechanical tension triggers apoptosis of human fibroblasts in a model of regressing granulation tissue. Exp Cell Res 1999; 248:608–619.

69. Gristina AG, Oga M, Webb LK, Hobgood CD. Adherent bacterial colonization in the pathogenesis of osteomyelitis. Science 1985;228:990–993.

70. Grotendorst GR, Martin GR. Cell movements in wound-healing and fibrosis. Rheumatology 1986;10:385–403.

71. Harris AK, Wild P, Stopak D. Silicone rubber substrata: a new wrinkle in the study of cell locomotion. Science 1980; 208:177–179.

72. Havran WL. A role for epithelial $\gamma\delta$ T cells in tissue repair. Immunol Res 2000;21/2–3:63–69.

73. Heggers JP. Variations on a theme. In: Heggers JP, Robson MC, eds. Quantitative bacteriology: its role in the armamentarium of the surgeon. Boca Raton, FL: CRC Press, 1991, pp. 15–23.

74. Holund B, Junker P, Garbarsch C, Christoffersen P, Lorenzen I. Formation of granulation tissue in subcutaneously implanted sponses in rats. Acta Pathol Microbiol Scand Sect A 1979; 87:367–374.

75. Hunt TK, ed. Wound healing and wound infection. New York: Appleton-Century-Crofts, 1980.

76. Hunt TK. Prospective: a retrospective perspective on the nature of wounds. Prog Clin Biol Res 1988;266:xiii–xx.

77. Hunt TK, Andrews WS, Halliday B, et al. Coagulation and macrophage stimulation of angiogenesis and wound healing. In: Dineen P, Hildick-Smith G, eds. The surgical wound. Philadelphia: Lea & Febiger, 1981, pp. 1–18.

78. Hunt TK, Knighton DR, Price DC, et al. Oxygen in the prevention and treatment of infection. In: Root RK, Trunkey DD, Sande MA, eds. New surgical and medical approaches in infectious diseases. New York: Churchill Livingstone, 1987, pp. 1–16.

79. Hunt TK, Linsey M, Grislis G, Sonne M, Jawetz E. The effect of differing ambient oxygen tensions on wound infection. Ann Surg 1975;181:35–39.

80. Hunt TK, Van Winkle W Jr. Normal repair. In: Hunt TK, Dunphy JE, eds. Fundamentals of wound management. New York: Appleton-Century-Crofts, 1979, pp. 2–67.

81. Hutson JM, Niall M, Evans D, Fowler R. Effect of salivary glands on wound contraction in mice. Nature 1979; 279:793–795.

82. James DW. Wound contraction—-a synthesis. Adv Biol Skin 1964;5:216–230.

83. Jensen JA, Hunt TK, Scheuenstuhl H, Banda MJ. Effect of lactate, pyruvate, and pH on secretion of angiogenesis and mitogenesis factors by macrophages. Lab Invest 1986;54: 574–578.

84. Johnson GM, Lee DA, Regelmann WE, et al. Interference with granulocyte function by Staphylococcus epidermis slime. Infect Immun 1986;54:13–20.

85. Kapanci Y, Burgan S, Pietra GG, Conne B, Gabbiani G. Modulation of actin isoform expression in alveolar myofibroblasts (contractile interstitial cells) during pulmonary hypertension. Am J Pathol 1990;136:881–889.

86. Karukonda SRK, Flyn TC, Boh EE, et al. The effects of drugs on wound healing: part 1. Int J Dermatol 2000;39: 250–257.

87. Kluger Y, Rabau M, Rub R, et al. Comparative study of splenic wound healing in young and adult rats. J Trauma Injury Inf & Crit Care 1999;47:261–264.

88. Knighton DR, Halliday B, Hunt TK. Oxygen as an antibiotic. A comparison of the effects of inspired oxygen concentration and antibiotic administration on in vivo bacterial clearance. Arch Surg 1986;121:191–195.

89. Knighton DR, Fiegel VD. The macrophages: effector cell wound repair. Prog Clin Biol Res 1989;299:217–226.

90. Knighton DR, Hunt TK, Scheuenstuhl H, et al. Oxygen tension regulates the expression of angiogenesis factor by macrophages. Science 1983;221:1283–1285.

91. Knighton DR, Silver IA, Hunt TK. Regulation of wound-healing angiogenesis——effect of oxygen gradients and inspired oxygen concentration. Surgery 1981;90:262–270.

92. Knox P, Crooks S, Rimmer CS. Role of fibronectin in the migration of fibroblasts into plasma clots. J Cell Biol 1986; 102:2318–2323.

93. Kolter R, Losick R. One for all and all for one. Science 1998;280:226–227.

94. Kulkarni AB, Karlsson S. Transforming growth factor-β_1 knockout mice. Am J Pathol 1993;143:3–9.

95. Kuwabara T, Perkins DG, Cogan DG. Sliding of the epithelium in experimental corneal wounds. Invest Ophthalmol 1976;15:4–14.

96. Lanning DA, Diegelmann RF, Yager DR, et al. Myofibroblast induction with transforming growth factors-β_1 and -β_3 in cutaneous fetal excisional wounds. J Pediatr Surg 2000;35: 183–188.

97. Lawrence WT. Physiology of the acute wound. Clin Plast Surg 1998;25:321–340.

98. Leibovich SJ, Ross R. The role of the macrophage in wound repair. A study with hydrocortisone and anti-macrophage serum. Am J Pathol 1975;78:71–100.

99. Leibovich SJ, Wiseman DM. Macrophages, wound repair and angiogenesis. Prog Clin Biol Res 1988;266:131–145.

100. Levenson SM, Geever EF, Crowley LV, et al. The healing of rat skin wounds. Ann Surg 1965;161:293–308.

101. Levenson SM, Demetriou AA. Metabolic factors. In: Cohen IK, Diegelmann RF, Lindblad WJ, eds. Wound healing: biochemical and clinical aspects. Philadelphia: WB Saunders, 1992, pp. 248–273.

102. Li AKC, Koroly MJ, Schattenkerk ME, Malt RA, Young M. Nerve growth factor: acceleration of the rate of wound healing in mice. Proc Natl Acad Sci USA 1980;77:4379–4381.

103. Linares HA, Larson DL, Willis-Galstaun BA. Historical notes on the use of pressure in the treatment of hypertrophic scars or keloids. Burns 1993;19:17–21.

104. Longaker MT, Whitby DJ, Adzick NS, et al. Studies in fetal wound healing. VI. Second and early third trimester fetal wounds demonstrate rapid collagen deposition without scar formation. J Pediatr Surg 1990;25:63–69.

105. Longaker MT, Adzick NS. The biology of fetal wound healing: a review. Plast Reconstr Surg 1991;87:788–798.

106. Lusthaus S, Shoshan S, Benmeir P, et al. Effect of denervation on incision wound scars in rabbits. J Geriat Dermatol 1993;1:11–14.

107. Vardy D. Effect of denervation on incision wound scars in rabbits. J Geriat Dermatol 1993;1:11–14.

108. Machesney M, Tidman N, Waseem A, Kirby L, Leigh I. Activated keratinocytes in the epidermis of hypertrophic scars. Am J Pathol 1998;152:1133–1141.

108a. Mah T-F, Pitts B, Pellock B, et al. A genetic basis for *Pseudomonas aeruginosa* biofilm antibiotic resistance. Nature 2003;426:306–310.

109. Majno G. The Healing Hand. Man and Wound in the Ancient World. Cambridge, MA: Harvard University Press, 1975.

110. Majno G. The story of the myofibroblasts. Am J Surg Pathol 1979;3:535–542.

111. Majno G, Gabbiani G, Hirschel BJ, Ryan GB, Statkov PR. Contraction of granulation tissue in vitro: similarity to smooth muscle. Science 1971;173:548–550.

112. Majno G, Leventhal M. Pathogenesis of histamine-type vascular leakage. Lancet 1967;2:99–100.

113. Martin CW, Muir IFK. The role of lymphocytes in wound healing. Br J Plastic Surg 1990;43:655–662.

114. Martin P. Wound healing—aiming for perfect skin regeneration. Science 1997;276:75–81.

115. McCallion RL, Ferguson WJ. Fetal wound healing and the development of antiscarring therapies for adult wound healing. In: Clark RAF (ed). The Molecular and Cellular Biology of Wound Repair. New York: Plenum Press, 1996, pp. 561–600.

116. McCarthy JB, Sas DF, Furcht LT. Mechanisms of parenchymal cell migration into wounds. In: Clark RAF, Henson PM, eds. The molecular and cellular biology of wound repair. New York: Plenum Press, 1988, pp. 281–319.

117. McPherson JM, Piez KA. Collagen in dermal wound repair. In: Clark RAF, Henson PM, eds. The molecular and cellular biology of wound repair. New York: Plenum Press, 1988, pp. 471–496.

118. Millington JT, Norris TW. Effective treatment strategies for diabetic foot wounds. J Fam Pract 2000;49(suppl):S40–S48.

119. Mochitate K, Pawelek P, Grinnell F. Stress relaxation of contracted collagen gels: disruption of actin filament bundles, release of cell surface fibronectin, and down-regulation of DNA and protein synthesis. Exp Cell Res 1991;193:198–207.

120. Montesano R, Orci L. Transforming growth factor β stimulates collagen-matrix contraction by fibroblasts: implications for wound healing. Proc Natl Acad Sci USA 1988;85: 4894–4897.

121. Moses JM, Ebert RH, Graham RC, Brine KL. Pathogenesis of inflammation. I. The production of an inflammatory substance from rabbit granulocytes in vitro and its relationship to leucocyte pyrogen. J Exp Med 1964;120:57–82.

122. Nagaoka T, Kaburagi Y, Hamaguchi Y, et al. Delayed wound healing in the absence of intercellular adhesion molecule-1 of L-selectin expression. Am J Pathol 2000;157:237–247.

123. Nedelec B, Ghahary A, Scott PG, Tredget EE. Control of wound contraction. Hand Clinics 2000;2:289–302.

124. Niewiarowski S, Goldstein S. Interaction of cultured human fibroblasts with fibrin: modification by drugs and aging in vitro. J Lab Clin Med 1973;82:605–610.

125. Noble WC. The production of subcutaneous staphylococcal skin lesions in mice. Br J Exp Pathol 1965;46:254–262.

126. Oh S-J, Kurz H, Christ B, Wilting J. Platelet-derived growth factor-B induces transformation of fibrocytes into spindle-shaped myofibroblasts in vivo. Histochem Cell Biol 1998; 109:349–357.

127. Okada M. The influence of intestinal flora on wound healing in mice. Surgery Today Jpn J Surg 1994;24:347–355.

128. Ordman LJ, Gillman T. Studies in the healing of cutaneous wounds. I. The healing of incisions through the skin of pigs. Arch Surg 1966;93:857–882.

129. Peacock EE Jr. Pharmacologic control of surface scarring in human beings. Ann Surg 1981;193:592–597.

130. Peacock EE Jr. The wound repair. Philadelphia: WB Saunders, 1984.

131. Peacock EE Jr, Van Winkle W Jr. Surgery and biology of wound repair. Philadelphia: WB Saunders, 1970.

132. Peters G, Gray ED, Johnson GM. Immunomodulating properties of extracellular slime substance. In: Bisno AL, Waldvogel FA, eds. Infections associated with indwelling medical devices. Washington, DC: American Society for Microbiology, 1989, pp. 61–74.

133. Pierce GF. Inflammation in nonhealing diabetic wounds. The space-time continuum does matter. Am J Pathol 2001; 159:399–403.

134. Pierce GF, Tarpley JE, Yanagihara D, et al. Platelet-derived growth factor (BB Homodimer), transforming growth factor-β1, and basic fibroblast growth factor in dermal wound healing. Am J Pathol 1992;140:1375–1388.

135. Pierce GF, Vande Berg J, Rudolph R, Tarpley J, Mustoe TA. Platelet-derived growth factor-BB and transforming growth factor beta-1 selectively modulate glycosaminoglycans, collagen, and myofibroblasts in excisional wounds. Am J Pathol 1991;138:629–646.

136. Polverini PJ, Cotran RS, Gimbrone MA Jr, Unanue ER. Activated macrophages induce vascular proliferation. Nature 1977;269:804–806.

137. Potera C. Forging a link between biofilms and disease. Science 1999;283:1837–1839.

138. Prince AS. Biofilms, antimicrobial resistance, and airway infection. New Engl J Med 2002;347:1110–1111.

139. Prudden JF, Wolarsky ER, Balassa L. The acceleration of healing. Surg Gynecol Obstet 1969;128:1321–1326.

140. Repesh LA, Oberpiller JC. Ultrastructural studies on migrating epidermal cells during the wound healing stage of regeneration in the adult newt, *Notophthalmus viridescens*. Am J Anat 1980;159:187–208.

141. Romer J, Bugge TH, Pyke C, et al. Impaired wound healing in mice with a disrupted plasminogen gene. Nature Med 1996;2:287–292.

142. Root RK, Trunkey DD, Sande MA. New surgical and medical approaches in infectious diseases. Contemporary issues in infectious diseases, vol 6. New York: Churchill Livingstone, 1987.

143. Rosenfeld RM, Stool SE. Should granulomas be excised in children with long-term tracheotomy? Arch Otolaryngol Head Neck Surg 1992;118:1323–1327.

144. Rowlatt U. Intrauterine wound healing in a 20 week human fetus. Virchows Arch A Path Anat Histol 1979;381:353–361.

145. Rudolph R. Inhibition of myofibroblasts by skin grafts. Plast Reconstr Surg 1979;63:473–480.

146. Rudolph R, Ballantyne DL Jr. Skin grafts. In: McCarthy JG, May JW Jr, Littler JW. Plastic surgery, vol 1. Philadelphia: WB Saunders, 1990.

147. Ryan GB, Cliff WJ, Gabbiani G, et al. Myofibroblasts in human granulation tissue. Hum Pathol 1974;5:55–67.

148. Ryan GB, Majno G. Inflammation. (A Scope Publication.) Kalamazoo, MI: The Upjohn Company, 1977.

149. Sandison JC. Observations on the growth of blood vessels as seen in the transparent chamber introduced into the rabbit's ear. Am J Anat 1928;41:475–496.

150. Schäffer M, Barbul A. Lymphocyte function in wound healing and following injury. Br J Surg 1998;85:444–460.

151. Schembri MA, Givskov M, Klemm P. An attractive surface: Gram-negative bacterial biofilms. Science's STKE 2002, www.stke.org/cgi/content/full/OC_sigtrans;2001/132/re6

151a. Schoefl GI. Studies on inflammation. III. Growing capillaries: their structure and permeability. Virchows Arch Pathol Anat 1963;337:97–141.

152. Schürch W, Seemayer TA, Gabbiani G. Myofibroblast. In: Sternberg SS, ed. Histology for pathologists. New York: Raven Press, 1992.

153. Sciubba JJ, Waterhouse JP, Meyer J. A fine structural comparison of the healing of incisional wounds of mucosa and skin. J Oral Pathol 1978;7:214–227.

153a. Serhan CN. Lipoxins and aspirin-triggered 15-epi-lipoxins. In: Gallin JI, Snyderman R. (eds). Inflammation. Basic Principles and Clinical Correlates. 3rd ed. Philadelphia: Lippincott Williams & Wilkins, 1999, pp. 373–385.

153b. Serhan CN, Hong S, Gronert K, et al. Resolvins: a family of bioactive products of omega-3 fatty acid transformation circuits initiated by aspirin treatment that counter pro-inflammation signals. J. Exp Med 2002;196:1025–1037.

154. Serini G, Gabbiani G. Mechanisms of myofibroblast activity and phenotypic modulation. Exp Cell Res 1999;250:273–283.

155. Serini G, Bochaton-Piallat M-L, Ropraz P, et al. The fibronectin domain ED-A is crucial for myofibroblastic phenotype induction by transforming growth factor-β1. J Cell Biol 1998;142:873–881.

156. Shah M, Foreman DM, Ferguson MWJ. Neutralisation of TGF-β_1 and TGF-β_2 or exogenous addition of TGF-β_3 to cutaneous rat wounds reduces scarring. J Cell Sci 1995;108:985–1002.

157. Shamberger R. Effect of chemotherapy and radiotherapy on wound healing: experimental studies. Recent Results Cancer Res 1985;98:17–34.

158. Simpson DM, Ross R. The neutrophilic leukocyte in wound repair. A study with antineutrophil serum. J Clin Invest 1972;51:2009–2023.

159. Singer AJ, Clark RAF. Cutaneous Wound Healing. N Eng J Med 1999;341:738–746.

160. Skalli O, Schürch W, Seemayer T, et al. Myofibroblasts from diverse pathologic settings are heterogeneous in their content of actin isoforms and intermediate filament proteins. Lab Invest 1989;60:275–285.

161. Smith RS, Smith TJ, Blieden TM, Phipps RP. Fibroblasts as sentinel cells. Synthesis of chemokines and regulation of inflammation. Am J Pathol 1997;151:317–322.

162. Somasundaram K, Prathap K. Intra-uterine healing of skin wounds in rabbit foetuses. J Pathol 1970;100:81–86.

163. Somasundaram K, Prathap K. The effect of exclusion of amniotic fluid on intra-uterine healing of skin wounds in rabbit foetuses. J Pathol 1972;107:127–130.

164. Squier CA. The effect of stretching on formation of myofibroblasts in mouse skin. Cell Tissue Res 1981;220:325–335.

165. Stadelmann WK, Digenis AG, Tobin GR. Impediments to wound healing. Am J Surg 1998;176(Suppl 2A):39S–47S.

166. Stenn KS, DePalma L. Re-epithelialization. In: Clark RAF, Henson PM, eds. The molecular and cellular biology of wound repair. New York: Plenum Press, 1988, pp. 321–335.

167. Taichman NS, Tsai C-C, Shenker BJ, Boehringer H. Neutrophil interactions with oral bacteria as a pathogenic mechanism in periodontal diseases. Adv Inflam Res 1984;8:113–142.

168. Tano Y, Chandler DB, Machemer R. Vascular casts of experimental retinal neovascularization. Am J Ophthalmol 1981;92:110–120.

169. Tomasek JJ, Gabbiani G, Hinz B, Chaponnier C, Brown RA. Myofibroblasts and mechano-regulation of connective tissue remodelling. Nature Rev Molec Cell Biol 2002;3:349–363.

170. Tsutsumi O, Tsutsumi A, Oka T. Epidermal growth factor-like, corneal wound healing substance in mouse tears. J Clin Invest 1988;81:1067–1071.

171. Vaudaux PE, Zulian G, Huggler E, Waldvogel FA. Attachment of *Staphylococcus aureus* to polymethyl-methacrylate increases its resistance to phagocytosis in foreign body infection. Infect Immun 1985;50:472–477.

172. Vaughan MB, Howard EW, Tomasek JJ. Transforming growth factor-β1 promotes the morphological and functional differentiation of the myofibroblast. Exp Cell Res 2000;257:180–189.

173. Wahl SM, Arend WP, Ross R. The effect of complement depletion on wound healing. Am J Pathol 1974;74:73–90.

174. Williams TJ. Factors that affect vessel reactivity and leukocyte emigration. In: Clark RAF, Henson PM, eds. The molecular and cellular biology of wound repair. New York: Plenum Press, 1988, pp. 115–147.

175. Williamson JR, Chang K, Rowold E, et al. Diabetes-induced increases in vascular permeability and changes in granulation tissue levels of sorbitol, *myo*-inositol, *chiro*-inositol, and *scyllo*-inositol are prevented by sorbinil. Metabolism 1986;35(suppl 1):41–45.

176. Winter GD. Movement of epidermal cells over the wound surface. Adv Biol Skin 1964;5:113–127.

177. Wong DTW, Donoff RB, Yang J, et al. Sequential expression of transforming growth factors α and β₁ by eosinophils during cutaneous wound healing in the hamster. Am J Pathol 1993;143:130–142.

178. Yang L, Scott PG, Giuffre J et al. Peripheral blood fibrocytes from burn patients: identification and quantification of fibrocytes in adherent cells cultured from peripheral blood mononuclear cells. Lab Invest 2002;82:1183–1192.

179. Yoffey JM, Courtice FC. Lymphatics, lymph and the lymphomyeloid complex. London: Academic Press, 1970.

180. Zimmerli W, Lew PD, Waldvogel FA. Pathogenesis of foreign body infection. Evidence for a local granulocyte defect. J Clin Invest 1984;73:1191–1200.

181. Zimmerli W, Waldvogel FA, Vaudaux P, Nydegger UE. Pathogenesis of foreign body infection: description and characteristics of an animal model. J Infect Dis 1982;146:487–497.

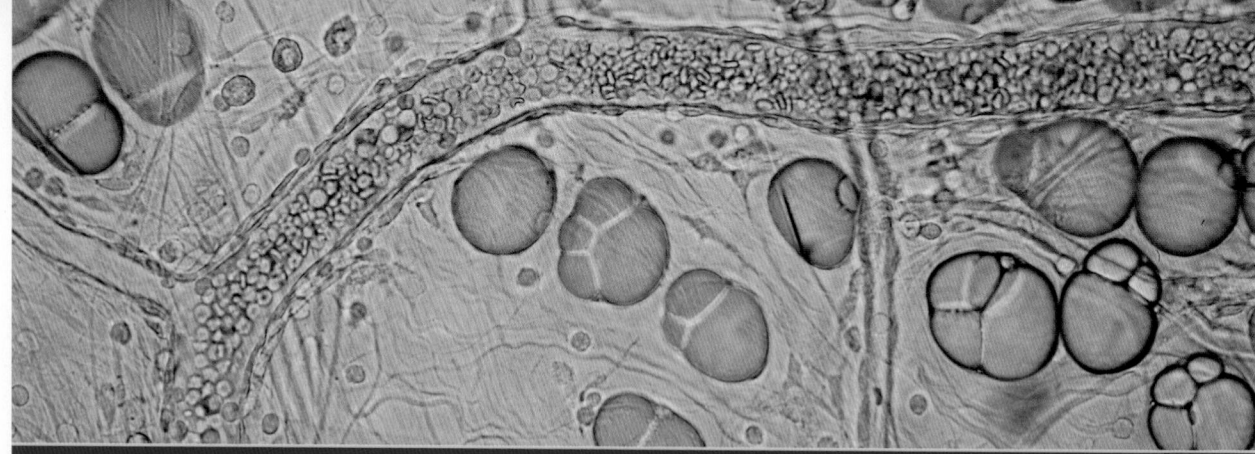

CHAPTER 15

GENERAL EFFECTS OF LOCAL INJURY AND INFLAMMATION

- Acute Phase Proteins
- Increased Erythrocyte Sedimentation Rate
- Fever
- Leukocytosis
- Other General Effects of Local Injury

The inflammatory response is by definition a local event, a response to local injury. It is based on the local production of hundreds of chemical mediators, which instruct the local cells as to "what to do next." The mediators, as a group, are powerful molecules, to be destroyed on the spot after their task is accomplished; however, some cytokines find their way in to the bloodstream, and induce a variety of general effects. These have been grouped, for historical reasons, under the peculiar name of *acute phase response* (20, 21, 35), although they may be associated with utterly chronic inflammatory conditions. They are of two kinds:

1. *Changes in the concentration of certain plasma proteins,* which thereby acquire the right to be called *acute phase proteins;* these changes are reflected—strange as this may seem—on the speed of sedimentation of the red blood cells (*erythrocyte sedimentation rate* [ESR]).
2. *An assortment of functional changes* (biochemical, physiologic, nutritional, behavioral) such as fever, anorexia, somnolence, negative nitrogen balance, muscular atrophy, osteoporosis, lysis of adipose tissue, leukocytosis and thrombocytosis (21).

All these effects can be reproduced experimentally by injecting the appropriate cytokines, mainly interleukin-6 (IL-6), interleukin-1 beta (IL-1β), tumor necrosis factor alpha (TNF-α), transforming growth factor beta (TGF-β), or interferon gamma (IFN-γ) (21). Hormones are also involved. In real life the cytokines are produced by fibroblasts and other cells, but mainly by macrophages. Apart from the scientific interest, these changes are important because they can be used to measure the severity or the evolution of a given inflammatory focus.

Acute Phase Proteins

This is essentially a liver story. Within hours of injury (such as trauma or surgery), the pattern of protein synthesis by the liver is altered, as can be seen by following the composition of the plasma: for some proteins, such as albumin, liver synthesis is decreased (these have been called "negative" acute phase proteins); for others, such as fibrinogen, it is increased (these are the "positive" acute phase proteins). To be recognized in either category, a plasma protein must vary its concentration by at least 25 percent.

To adjust its level of protein synthesis, the liver is responding mainly to IL-6, and in a roughly quantitative manner: maximal responses are induced by trauma, burns, infections, infarcts, advanced cancer; moderate responses by childbirth, heat stroke, strenuous exercise; and minimal responses by psychological stress (20).

Complement components can rise by a modest 50 percent, but C-reactive protein (CRP) and serum amyloid A (SAA) (discussed in Chapter 7) can rise in a spectacular way, up to 1000-fold (Figure 15.1). Not all the changes are understood; we tend to believe that they must have some protective value, but this is not always necessarily the case. For example:

• *Decrease in plasma iron* (hypoferremia or hyposideremia): this can be understood as an

antibacterial measure, because iron is a growth factor for many bacteria (9, 57).

This change has a complicated 3-step mechanism: activated neutrophils release lactoferrin, an iron-binding protein; lactoferrin snatches away the iron from serum transferrin, another iron-binding protein; and finally, the iron-laden lactoferrin is phagocytized by the monocyte-macrophage system and stored away as ferritin (56). A hyposideremia after infection was found even in lizards (24).

• *Increase in C3:* this molecule is a key component of complement; as such it is an essential antibacterial weapon.

• *Increase in ceruloplasmin:* this blue, copper-containing protein, can act as a scavenger of free radicals, clearly a defensive function (23).

• *Increase in CRP:* CRP appears to be part of a beautiful system: IL-1 stimulates the secretion of CRP; CRP binds to damaged tissue components, and makes them better suited for phagocytosis (i.e., it is an opsonin); the macrophages take up the complex, and become activated, thereby secreting more IL-1 (60).

• *Increase in alpha-1-antitrypsin:* this protein inactivates dangerous proteases that might be released by damaged cells.

• *Increase in fibrinogen:* this molecule is essential for coagulation, which is be needed for stopping hemorrhages resulting from injury.

• *Increase in SAA.* The plasma concentration of SAA can rise 1000-fold, suggesting that this molecule has some important task, but all we knew until recently was that it could cause a deadly disease, amyloidosis (p. 293). Now it appears that SAA does indeed deserve to be called on in emergencies: it is a potent activator of neutrophils, making them more effective against bacteria (4).

The molecular structure of SAA recalls a cluster of five berries, hence the name **pentraxins** for this class of proteins (which includes CRP). CRP has an interesting history (42, 48).

The C-reactive protein was discovered in 1930 at the Hospital of the Rockefeller Institute in the days when pneumococcal pneumonia was deadly. The study of type-specific antibodies against pneumococci was a top priority because they were the only known way to treat the disease. Something very strange turned up in the serum of febrile patients admitted with pneumonia: it invariably contained a protein that reacted specifically with a crude pneumococcal antigen named "fraction C"; however, it was not likely to be an antibody because it appeared too soon. In fact, it behaved in a way that was opposite to that of antibodies: it began to drop while type-specific agglutinating antibodies rose. Even more baffling was the

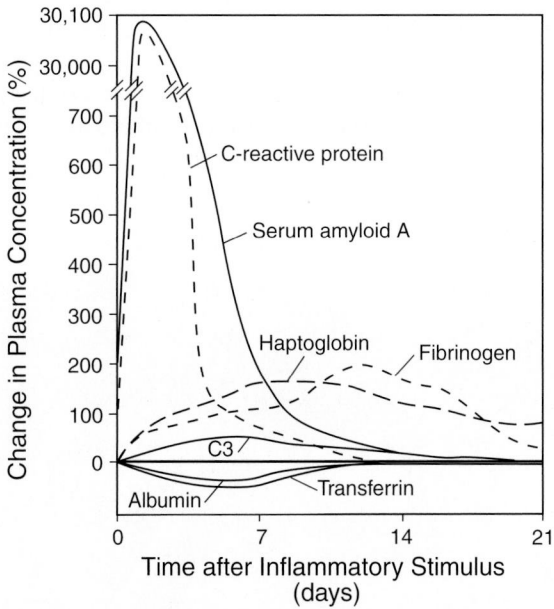

FIGURE 15.1   Typical pattern of changes in plasma concentration of some acute-phase proteins ("positive" or "negative" with respect to baseline) after a moderate inflammatory stimulus. (Reproduced with permission from: Gabay C, Kushner I., New Engl J Med "Acute-Phase Proteins and Other Systemic Responses to Inflammation" 340:448–454, 1999. Copyright © 1999 Massachusetts Medical Society. All rights reserved.)

subsequent finding that this C-reactive protein also appeared in the serum of patients with other acute diseases (42). The logical conclusion was that CRP could not be a specific effect of pneumonia; it was somehow related to the acute phase of disease in general. Soon, other proteins were found to behave in a similar fashion. Thus were born two rather unwieldy names, the C-reactive protein and the acute phase response.

Intensive studies of CRP (21, 60) suggest that it can bind to a number of surfaces and influence several functions of the blood (e.g., platelet aggregation).

CRP responds so fast to acute disease that it has been proposed as a clinical barometer to assess the severity of a patient's condition (21). In practice, few hospitals use this test (55); it is much simpler to measure the erythrocyte sedimentation rate, which reflects the rise of another acute phase protein, fibrinogen. However, the CRP test may be about to gain popularity thanks to a typically chronic disease. Atherosclerosis is now recognized to be at least in part an inflammatory condition, and the CRP test was found to be more predictive of cardiovascular complications than the LDL cholesterol test (48a).

Increased Erythrocyte Sedimentation Rate

Although some authors (29) consider it quaint, the simple test of measuring the ESR continues to be a reliable screening test for the medical practitioner (8a). In about 1 hour it can answer two basic questions: *Is there tissue damage somewhere in this patient? If so, how severe is the damage?* For this reason, this test was widely used for the prognosis of tuberculosis and syphilis before the advent of antibiotics and to this day it remains the most demanded laboratory test in many hospitals, including our own. The principle was discovered in 1894 and forgotten (34), and then rediscovered in a classic paper by Fårhaeus in 1929 (16).

In essence: normally, the blood forms a stable suspension because the density of the red blood cells (1.09) is close to that of the plasma (1.03). Therefore, if blood (2 ml) is anticoagulated and poured into a vertical tube, the red blood cells settle very slowly; after 1 hour, they have settled only 0–10 mm in men and 1–15 mm in women as measured by the commonly used Westergren method.

The driving force that causes the red blood cells to fall is their weight (generally speaking, the weight of spherical particles increases by the cube of the radius). This driving force is opposed by the resistance offered by the plasma, which increases only with the radius of the falling particles (17). This means that the larger the particles, the faster they fall: stones sink faster than sand. Now, the red blood cells in blood taken during an acute phase reaction tend to aggregate into **rouleaux** (rolls) resembling piles of coins (Figure 15.2). The rouleaux are the equivalent of stones: they sink faster.

What produces rouleaux? Under normal conditions the red blood cells repel each other by their similar charges; but if the plasma contains a large number of elongated molecules such as fibrinogen, these molecules tend to become attracted by the surfaces of the red blood cells, and this coating reduces the repelling effect of the surface charges (21). Because fibrinogen is one of the positive acute phase proteins, the ESR reflects the acute phase response (Figure 15.3). Rouleaux can also be seen on blood smears (Figure 15.4), but this fact is not used as a test.

It must be understood that the ESR test is very nonspecific; after all, it reflects the nonspecific acute phase response. It should be used only as a quick way to find out if "something is really wrong" while remembering that a normal value may not exclude diseases that are unrelated to tissue damage, including many malignancies. It can even reflect pregnancy. As a matter of fact, it was discovered in the course of a study of blood changes in pregnancy.

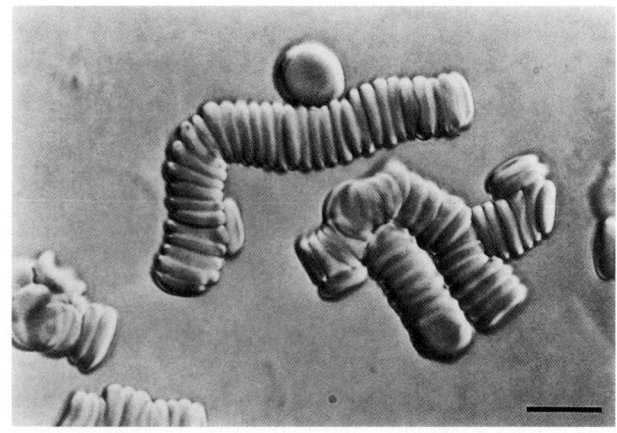

FIGURE 15.2   Red blood cells forming typical rouleaux, by interference microscopy. **Bar** = 10 μm. (Reproduced from [8] by permission from Springer-Verlag.)

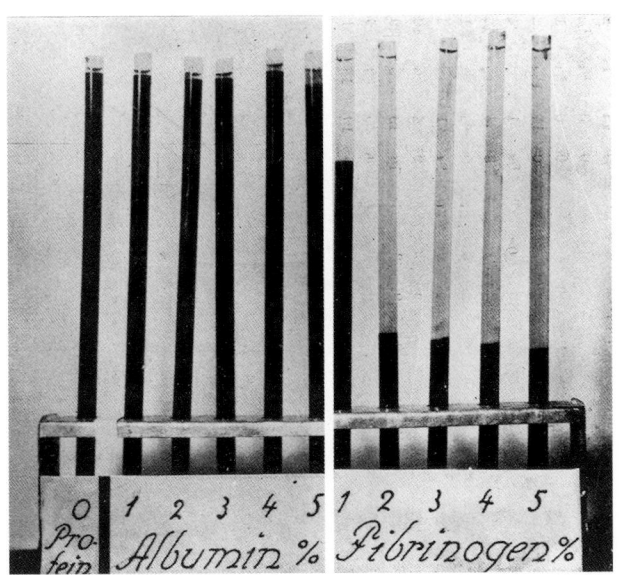

FIGURE 15.3 Mechanism of accelerated sedimentation rate, demonstrated by suspending red blood cells in solutions of plasma proteins. Albumin solutions of increasing concentrations (1.3–6.3 percent) do not increase the sedimentation rate of red blood cells after 3 hours. Fibrinogen solutions of 1–5 percent do increase the sedimentation rate (normal concentration of fibrinogen in plasma: 0.15–0.35 g/100 ml). (Reproduced with permission form [15].)

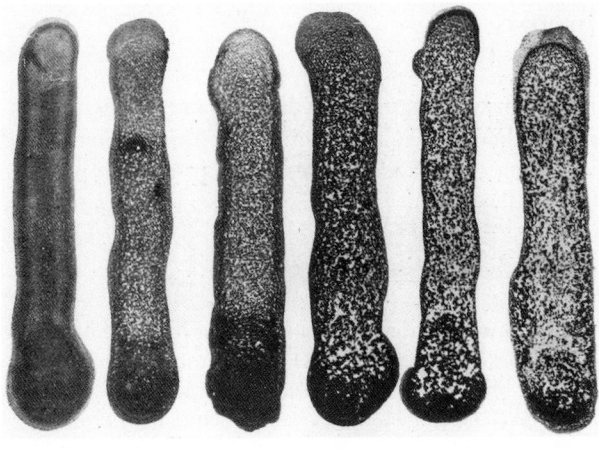

FIGURE 15.4 Blood smears prepared from six drops of blood with sedimentation rates of 2, 7, 28, 40, 68, and 102 mm/h (from left to right). The subjects were, respectively, a healthy man, a healthy woman, a pregnant woman, a man with appendicitis, a man with pneumonia, and a man with sepsis. The increasingly granular aspect of the smears is due to the formation of rouleaux. (Reproduced with permission from [15].)

The phenomenon of increased sedimentation rate was observed in antiquity and had an enormous impact on medical practice well into the 1800s. It was customary in bloodletting, from the time of Hippocrates and for 2200 years afterward, to collect the blood in a basin, where it eventually clotted. If a patient's ESR was high, the red blood cells might be able to settle a few millimeters before clotting; then, when clotting did occur, the blood would be divided into two layers as in Figure 15.5: a bottom red layer and a superficial whitish jelly (actually a fibrin clot) called the buffy coat. To ancient observers this meant that the blood of that patient contained an abnormal whitish material, supposedly the pernicious "phlegm"; such blood was referred to as "sizy" and the fibrin layer became known as the phlogistic crust (*crusta phlogistica*). The logical therapy was to draw more blood so as to remove more of that pernicious phlegm. As more and more blood was drawn, the patient became anemic; and because anemia accelerates the sedimentation rate, the cycle was self-perpetuating (16). Worse yet, pregnant women were systematically bled well into the past century, because, as we mentioned, their ESR is always accelerated (16). Nobody knows how many patients died of this therapy. Such is the power of theory.

Up to this point, in discussing the general effects of local injury, we have considered the acute phase

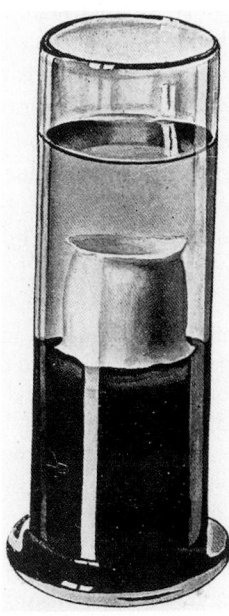

FIGURE 15.5 Buffy coat produced by blood with a high sedimentation rate: a phenomenon that had a tremendous impact on the history of medicine. (Reproduced with permission from [15].)

proteins and a related effect, the accelerated erythrocyte sedimentation rate. Other repercussions of local injury on the body as a whole (21) were listed above. We will now briefly consider fever and leukocytosis.

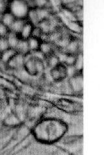

Fever

Fever can be recognized by doctors, and mothers, without the benefit of a thermometer. It is often mentioned in the oldest Akkadian tablets and in the Hippocratic books (2, 3, 40). The Romans, perhaps because they were harassed by malaria, saw fit to give it a heavenly patron, the goddess *Febris*.

> The first thermometer for measuring body temperature was designed around 1611 by Santorio Santorio, who probably borrowed the basic idea from his colleague in Padua, Galileo. However, the principle of thermometry was not adopted in routine medical practice until the mid-1800s (30).

The Genesis of Fever

Body temperature is regulated by a nucleus in the anterior hypothalamus, which functions as a thermostat, controlling the balance between heat production and heat loss. Stated in the simplest terms: fever develops when the thermostat is switched to a higher setting. For the body to reach a higher temperature, heat loss by the skin must be reduced by vasoconstriction, so for a short time during a rising fever the skin, paradoxically, becomes cool. The moment of switching is clinically apparent as a chill, which means that the environmental temperature is suddenly perceived as too cool.

What resets the thermostat? The hunt for a chemical cause goes back to the 1800s.

> In 1866 a German medical student, inspired by Billroth, the eminent surgeon–musician friend of Brahms, injected filtered autogenous pus into a cat and found that it produced fever (3, 59). The cat escaped, but the experiment proved that pus contained "pyrogens." However, it remained to be decided whether these pyrogens were bacterial, leukocytic, or both. After nearly a century, in 1953, in a series of experiments that were hailed as classic, Bennett and Beeson proved that a preparation of "granulocytes" produced fever (7, 59); many years later it turned out that the effect of Bennett's and Beeson's preparation was due primarily to a small fraction of contaminating monocytes (26).

Even after these early experiments suggested that leukocytes were the source of endogenous pyrogens, the next step was difficult to accomplish because fresh leukocytes contain no fever-inducing material. Monocytes *produce* endogenous pyrogenic cytokines (including TNF, IL-1, IL-6, and MPI-1) (12) only when they are exposed to certain phagocytizable exogenous (bacterial) pyrogens, especially endotoxin. These cytokine pyrogens affect the anterior hypothalamus by increasing the local synthesis of prostaglandin E_2 (PGE_2). *Aspirin opposes fever precisely by inhibiting cyclooxygenase in the hypothalamus.* TNF can also stimulate the hypothalamic center directly (36). With these facts at hand, it was easy to understand why endogenous pyrogens, injected intravenously, act almost immediately, whereas exogenous (bacterial) pyrogens act only after a delay of at least 30 minutes.

> Exogenous pyrogens are many. The prototype is endotoxin, a lipopolysaccharide from the wall of gram-negative bacteria. Endotoxin lurks almost everywhere and causes much trouble to manufacturers of medical supplies, whose products must be pyrogen-free. Other exogenous pyrogens are found in gram-positive bacteria. Overall the pathogenesis of fever is well understood, but some pieces of the puzzle still need to be fit (22, 49).

Is Fever Useful?

Sir William Osler, the "modern Hippocrates," once wrote that "Humanity has but three great enemies: fever, famine and war. Of these by far the greatest, by far the most terrible, is fever" (47). A century later it appears that Osler was equating fever with infection, and infections are indeed a great scourge. And they cause fever. But blaming fever for the misdeeds of infection is assuming guilt by association. In 1927, just eight years after the death of Osler, the Nobel prize for medicine was given to Wagner-Jauregg for his method of treating neurosyphilis with fever by actually giving malaria to the patients (30); the basic idea was to cook the spirochetes, which are known to die at temperatures above 41°C (30). There are strains of pneumococci that die at temperatures as low as 40°C, easily within reach of fever in rabbits; pneumococcal virulence in this animal can actually be correlated with the ability of the cocci to survive at 41°C (30). These facts and many others (30, 32, 39) argue for a useful effect of fever in infections. (It is certainly useful indirectly, for diagnosing infections, but some tumors, especially leukemias and lymphomas, can also secrete fever-producing cytokines [21].)

In mammals, however, it has been difficult to prove beyond doubt that fever has a general survival value. The experimental procedure is to compare the survival

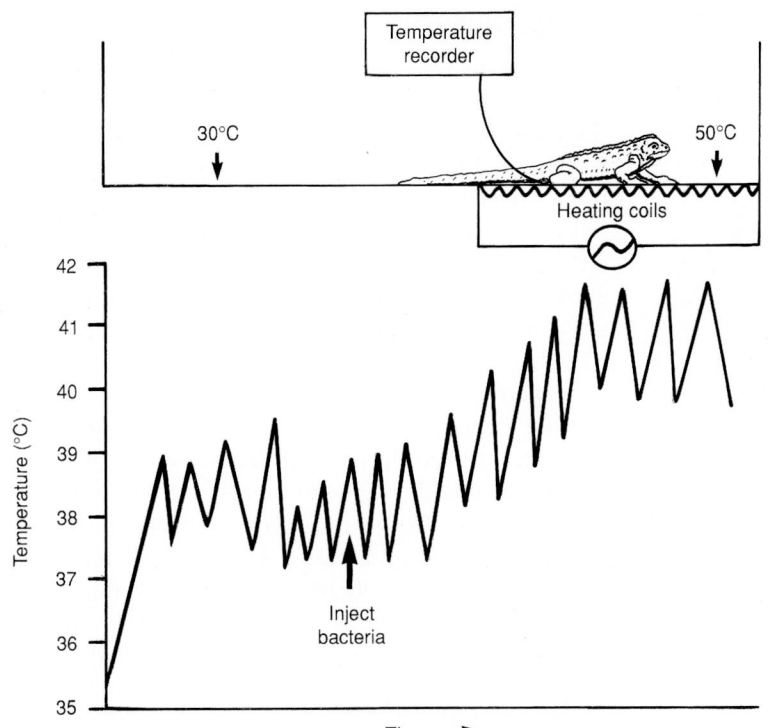

FIGURE 15.6 *Top:* Self-regulation of body temperature in the lizard *Dipsosaurus dorsalis,* kept in a sand box. Left side of sand box is set at 30°C. The lizard moves back and forth between the two sides, thereby selecting its appropriate body temperature, 38°C (measured by a thermocouple inserted into the cloaca and taped to the tail). *Bottom:* Self-induced fever in a lizard injected with pathogenic bacteria. Before the injection: The lizard migrates back and forth, maintaining an average temperature of about 38°C.) A few hours after being inoculated with pathogenic bacteria (**arrow**), the lizard begins to adjust its body to higher temperatures, eventually reaching 43°C. (From [30], Copyright © 1979 by Princeton University Press. Reproduced by permission of Princeton University Press.)

of two feverish groups, one treated and one not treated with antipyretics; thus one can always argue that antipyretics might have effects other than decreasing body temperature. The problem was solved ingeniously by a physiologist who chose to study animals in which body temperature can be raised or lowered without drugs: lizards (Figure 15.6) (30).

Like snakes and other poikilotherms, lizards set their own temperature either by exposing part of their body to the sun, just enough to produce the desired overall temperature, or by moving back and forth between sun and shade. Kluger placed his small iguanas in a sand box, part of which was warmed by heat lamps; the lizards were free to shuttle back and forth between the warm and the cool parts, and thereby to choose their own temperature anywhere between that of the room and 50°C. They chose about 38°C; but if they had been injected with appropriate gram-negative bacteria (reptilian pathogens) they gave themselves fever by choosing 42°C. If they were prevented from doing so and kept at 38°C, within 24 hours half of them were dead. A similar experiment can be done with fish swimming in communicating tanks at different temperatures (30).

Kluger's experiments prove beyond doubt that fever *can* have survival value. In retrospect, this is logical. The capacity to react to infection with fever has been found in all vertebrates that have been tested (30). If evolution has preserved this energy-consuming reaction for so long, it is not likely to be worthless. An exception should be made for high fevers, beyond the 40–41°C range, which are generally considered dangerous. The truth therefore seems to be in the camp of Thomas Sydenham, the "English Hippocrates" (1624–1689), who wrote some 300 years ago that "fever is Nature's engine which she brings into the field to remove her enemy" (30).

How can fever be useful? The iguana experiment provides one answer: fever increases the bactericidal effect (in the iguana, against iguana bacteria), and it is comforting to know that leukocytes move faster at higher temperatures (Figure 15.7). However, a review of the published experiments on the effects of higher temperatures on bodily defenses (27a) shows that in the plethora of results it is easy to choose a model that will prove almost any point, including a *decreased* ability of human leukocytes to ingest *Escherichia coli* at 42°C compared with 39°C. In another review [38], 13 experimental models showed that fever helped against infection, and 3 showed that it made matters worse.

To conclude, we can understand—regretfully—why the wonderful iguana experiment has not yet abolished

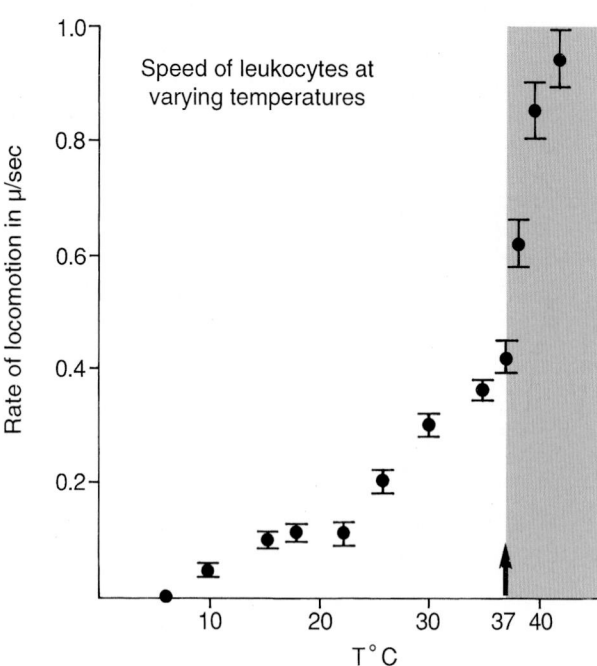

Speed of leukocytes at varying temperatures

FIGURE 15.7   Rate of locomotion of human neutrophils as a function of temperature. **Red bar:** Range of fever. (Adapted with permission from [45], © 1971 by the Society for Experimental Biology and Medicine.)

Comparison with Hyperthermia

Hyperthermia refers to an increase in body temperature *above* the thermostat setting which remains normal; it is therefore improper to use this term interchangeably with fever (53, 54, 45a). The body becomes hyperthemic *when heat dissipation cannot keep up with the amount of heat produced or absorbed.* Classic examples are heat stroke, a hazard of hot environments, and exertion heat stroke, typically seen in untrained joggers; in this latter case rectal temperatures can exceed 41.5°C (27).

Hyperthermia has attracted some interest since it became a therapeutic modality in cancer. Using focal hyperthermia produced with radio waves, minimal necrosis of muscle begins to occur after 30 minutes at 40–43°C (43). Cell membranes are irreversibly damaged at temperatures between 41 and 45°C; both proteins and lipids are probably affected (37). It is no wonder that body temperatures exceeding 41°C (106°F) should be regarded as medical emergencies (14).

Malignant hyperthermia syndrome (fulminant hyperthermia) is a genetic disease of humans, swine, cats, dogs, and horses; it is a sudden hypermetabolic state of striated muscle that is unleashed accidentally in 1 in 10,000–15,000 general anesthesias. The cause appears to be an excessive release of calcium by the sarcoplasmic reticulum in response to neuronal stimulation (45a, 50). The syndrome can be triggered in swine and horses by sudden stress (46). In the 1950s, 30 members of one family died of anesthesia before the disease was recognized (25). The temperature can rise at the rate of 1°C every 5 minutes, reaching 44.4°C in humans and 48.2°C in a strain of predisposed swine. Aspirin is quite useless in such cases because the target of aspirin is the thermostat, which is not involved.

the reflex habit of "curing fevers" with antipyretics (30, 31). Besides the uncertainties of the literature, antipyretics are also analgesics and make the patients feel more comfortable; the only reason for withdrawing aspirin from children is the fear of a toxic effect, the Reye syndrome, which is now rare but carries a mortality risk of about 30 percent (p. 91).

Leukocytosis

Human blood contains 4000–10,000 leukocytes per mm³; numbers above and below these limits denote *leukocytosis* and *leukopenia*. The predominant leukocyte in human blood is the neutrophil; in rats and mice, the predominant cell is the lymphocyte (Table 15.1).

Neutrophilia (neutrophil leukocytosis) is a common effect of injury and especially of infections with pyogenic (pus-generating) bacteria (Table 15.2). It has survival value by helping to recruit more leukocytes to the battlefield. Normally more than half of all neutrophils are not circulating but are held in a "loosely marginating" pool (1); *loosely* means that wherever these neutrophils may be, margination is not followed by diapedesis. These neutrophils are immediately available and *can be released by stress and exercise, and artifically by an injection of epinephrine.*

Leukocytosis induced by trauma or infection is sustained by the colony-stimulating factors (CSFs) (44), small glycoproteins that promote bone-marrow hyperplasia; in and around injured tissues they can be produced by many cell types, including monocytes and endothelial cells (52). After trauma, greatly increased

Table 15.1 White Blood Cells: Normal Counts

	Human Adults	Rats
Total (per μl)	4000–11,000	6000–18,000
Neutrophils	60%	15–20%
Eosinophils	3%	1–4%
Basophils	0.6%	Rare
Monocytes	4%	6%
Lymphocytes	33%	86%

Table 15.2 Neutrophil Leukocytosis: Major Causes

Physiologic	Exercise
	Stress
	Epinephrine
	Steriod therapy
Infections	Bacterial, especially pyogenic bacteria; some fungal, parasitic, and viral diseases
Inflammation	Burns
	Necrosis (e.g., myocardial and pulmonary infarction, trauma)
	Autoimmune diseases: myositis, vasculitis
Metabolic disorders	Ketoacidosis
	Uremia
	Eclampsia
	Gout
Other:	Tumors of many types
	Acute hemorrhage or hemolysis
	Idiopathic

Adapted from (11).

levels of CSFs appear in the serum and in the urine, where they were first detected (58).

Few drugs cause leukocytosis, in contrast with the many that cause leukopenia. Corticosteroids lead to leukocytosis by several mechanisms: they impair the diapedesis of leukocytes, prolong their life span, and enhance their release from the bone marrow.

Other General Effects of Local Injury

The *sleepiness* and *lack of appetite* (anorexia) that appear after serious injury are best considered as part of the acute phase response, and therefore as cytokine-induced (35). The same is true for the typical anemia of chronic inflammation, due in part to *depressed production of erythropoietin. The mechanism of muscular pain* (myalgia) so common in fever is not well understood; however, it is a fact that striated muscle during the acute phase response shows accelerated proteolysis; the effect can be duplicated by IL-1, and it is reversed by aspirin, which suggests that it is mediated by prostaglandins (6).

Severe injury also elicits what is known to the public as *stress,* scientifically the *hypothalamic-pituitary-adrenal stress response.* This is a complex, non-specific endocrine response that has been the topic of many volumes (51). It may occur also after psychological challenges, in the absence of physical damage (20, 41). Among its many effects we will cite two: it depresses some cellular inflammatory functions (28) and increases the susceptibility to the common cold in humans (10).

This endocrine stress response intersects with the acute phase response in that it can be initiated by IL-1 and IL-6 (35); indeed, corticosteroids can be considered as cofactors of the acute phase response (35). It is no wonder that the metabolic consequences of injury are so complex.

Last but not least, *a generalized protective effect of inflammation* has been described at the Pasteur Institute in Paris (18), using an experimental model based on granulomas in mice, and on the notion that granulomas can be construed as organs of internal secretion (p. 455). Talcum-induced granulomas generate a protein that protects mice against an otherwise lethal infection (19) and exerts a cytostatic effect against a highly malignant mouse tumor (18). This amounts to a general increase in resistance, which is a sort of bonus in addition to the local protective effect of inflammation.

TO SUM UP: Strictly speaking, there is no such thing as a purely local injury. The news of local damage spreads quickly throughout the body, even in the absence of infection. In Chapters 8–12 we learned that the tissues surrounding an injury respond within seconds or minutes with inflammation, and that all cells adapt to noxious stimuli in a matter of hours by generating intracellular stress (heat-shock) proteins; within the same time span, the liver brings the blood to readiness by readjusting the levels of the plasma proteins. One may wonder why this frenzy of preparedness takes place even if the damage is aseptic (as in a fracture)—but the defense systems have no way to decide whether infection is present or not, and respond, as we have already noticed (p. 480), according to the worst case scenario.

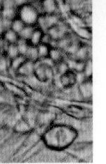

References

1. Athens JW, Haab OP, Raab SO, et al. Leukokinetic studies. IV. The total blood, circulating and marginal granulocyte pools and the granulocyte turnover rate in normal subjects. J Clin Invest 1961;40:989–995.

2. Atkins E. Fever: its history, cause, and function. Yale J Biol Med 1982;55:283–289.

3. Atkins E. Fever: the old and the new. J Infect Dis 1984;149:339–348.

4. Badolato R, Wang JM, Stornello S-L, et al. Serum amyloid A is an activator of PMN antimicrobial functions: induction of degranulation, phagocytosis, and enhancement of anti-Candida activity. J Leukoc Biol 2000;67:381–386.

5. Baltz ML, de Beer FC, Feinstein A, et al. Phylogenetic aspects of C-reactive protein and related proteins. Ann NY Acad Sci 1982;389:49–75.

6. Baracos V, Rodemann HP, Dinarello CA, Goldberg AL. Stimulation of muscle protein degradation and prostaglandin E$_2$ release by leukocytic pyrogen (interleukin-1). N Engl J Med 1983;308:553–558.

7. Bennett IL Jr, Beeson PB. Studies on the pathogenesis of fever. I. The effect of injection of extracts and suspensions of uninfected rabbit tissues upon the body temperature of normal rabbits. J Exp Med 1953;98:477–492.

8. Bessis M. Living blood cells and their ultrastructure. New York: Springer-Verlag, 1973.

8a. Brigden M. The erythrocyte sedimentation rate. Postgrad Med 1998;103:257–274.

9. Bullen JJ. The significance of iron in infection. Rev Infect Dis 1981;3:1127–1138.

10. Cohen S, Tyrrell DAJ, Smith AP. Psychological stress and susceptibility to the common cold. N Engl J Med 1991;325:606–612.

11. Dale DC. Leukocytosis, leukopenia, and eosinophilia. In: Wilson JD, Braunwald E, Isselbacher KJ, et al., eds. Harrison's principles of internal medicine, 12th ed. New York: McGraw-Hill, 1991.

12. Davatelis G, Wolpe SD, Sherry B, et al. Macrophage inflammatory protein-1: a prostaglandin-independent endogenous pyrogen. Science 1989;243:1066–1068.

13. Dinarello CA, Bunn PA. Fever. Semin Oncol 1997;24:288–298.

14. Donaldson JF. Therapy of acute fever: a comparative approach. Hosp Pract 1981;16:125–138.

15. Fåhraeus R. The suspension-stability of the blood. Acta Med Scand 1921;55:1–228.

16. Fåhraeus R. The suspension stability of the blood. Physiol Rev 1929;9:241–274.

17. Florey HW. General pathology, 4th ed. Philadelphia: WB Saunders, 1970.

18. Fontan E, Fauve RM. Inflammation and anti-tumor resistance. IV. Induction of cytostatic activity of murine peritoneal cells by a mouse granuloma protein. Int J Cancer 1988;42:267–272.

19. Fontan E, Fauve RM, Hevin B, Jusforgues H. Immuno-stimulatory mouse granuloma protein. Proc Natl Acad Sci USA 1983;80:6395–6398.

20. Ganong WF. The stress response—a dynamic overview. Hosp Pract 1988;23:155–171.

21. Gabay C, Kushner I. Acute-phase proteins and other systemic responses to inflammation. N Engl J Med 1999;340:448–454, correction, N Engl J Med 1999;340:1376.

22. Goldbach J-M, Roth J, Zeisberger E. Fever suppression by subdiaphragmatic vagotomy in guinea pigs depends on the route of pyrogen administration. Am J Physiol 1997;272:R675–R681.

23. Goldstein IM, Kaplan HB, Edelson HS, Weissmann G. Ceruloplasmin. A scavenger of superoxide anion radicals. J Biol Chem 1979;254:4040–4045.

24. Grieger TA, Kluger MJ. Fever and survival: the role of serum iron. J Physiol 1978;279:187–196.

25. Gronert GA. Malignant hyperthermia. Anesthesiology 1980;53:395–423.

26. Hanson DF, Murphy PA, Windle BE. Failure of rabbit neutrophils to secrete endogenous pyrogen when stimulated with staphylococci. J Exp Med 1980;151:1360–1371.

27. Hanson PG, Zimmerman SW. Heatstroke in road races. N Engl J Med 1979;300:96–97.

27a. Hasday JD. The influence of temperature on host defenses. In: Mackowiak PA (ed). Fever: Basic mechanisms and management. 2nd ed. Philadelphia: Lippincott-Raven Publishers, 1997, pp. 177–196.

28. Henricks PAJ, Binkhorst GJ, Nijkamp FP. Stress diminishes infiltration and oxygen metabolism of phagocytic cells in calves. Inflammation 1987;11:427–437.

29. Jandl JH. Blood. Boston: Little, Brown, 1987.

30. Kluger MJ. Fever. Its biology, evolution, and function. Princeton, NJ: Princeton University Press, 1979.

31. Kluger MJ. Phylogeny of fever. Fed Proc 1979;38:30–34.

32. Kluger MT, Bartfai T, Dinarello C (eds). Molecular mechanisms of fever. New York: Annals of the New York Academy of Sciences, Vol 856, 1998.

33. Konijn AM, Hershko C. Ferritin synthesis in inflammation. I. Pathogenesis of impaired iron release. Br J Haematol 1977;37:7–16.

34. Kucharz E. 80th anniversary of the discovery of erythrocyte sedimentation rate. Mater Med Pol 1975;7:344–346.

35. Kushner I, Rzewnicki O. Acute Phase Response. In: Gallin JI, Snyderman R. (eds). Inflammation: Basic principles and clinical correlates. 3rd ed. Philadelphia: Lippincott William & Wilkins, 1999, pp. 317–329.

36. Le J, Vilcek J. Tumor necrosis factor and interleukin 1: cytokines with multiple overlapping biological activities. Lab Invest 19872;56:234–248.

37. Lepock JR. Involvement of membranes in cellular responses to hyperthermia. Radiat Res 1982;92:433–438.

38. Mackowiak P. Fever: modern insights into an ancient clinical sign. Contemp Intern Med 1992;4:17–28.

39. Mackowiak PA (ed). Fever: Basic mechanisms and management. 2nd ed. Philadelphia: Lippincott-Raven Publishers, 1997.

40. Majno G. The healing hand: man and wound in the ancient world. Cambridge, MA: Harvard University Press, 1975.

41. Makara GB. Mechanisms by which stressful stimuli activate the pituitary-adrenal system. Fed Proc 1985;44:149–153.

42. McCarty M. Historical perspective on C-reactive protein. Ann NY Acad Sci 1982;389:1–10.

43. Meshorer A, Prionas SD, Fajardo LF, et al. The effects of hyperthermia on normal mesenchymal tissues. Arch Pathol Lab Med 1983;107:328–334.

44. Metcalf D. The molecular control of normal and leukaemic granulocytes and macrophages. Proc R Soc Lond [Biol] 1987; 230:389–423.

45. Nahas GG, Tannieres ML, Lennon JF. Direct measurement of leukocyte motility: effects of pH and temperature. Proc Soc Exp Biol Med 1971;138:350–352.

45a. Ohnishi ST, Ohnishi T (eds). Malignant hyperthermia: A genetic membrane disease. Boca Raton: CRC Press Inc., 1994.

46. Olgin J, Argov Z, Rosenberg H, Tuchler M, Chance B. Noninvasive evaluation of malignant hyperthermia susceptibility with phosphorus nuclear magnetic resonance spectroscopy. Anesthesiology 1988;68:507–513.

47. Osler W. The study of the fevers of the South. JAMA 1896; 26:999–1004.

48. Pepys MB, Baltz ML. Acute phase proteins with special reference to C-reactive protein and related proteins (pentaxins) and serum amyloid A protein. Adv Immunol 1983;34:141–212.

48a. Ridker PM, Rifai N, Rose L, Buring JE, Cook NR. Comparison of C-reactive protein and low-density lipoprotein cholesterol levels in the prediction of first cardiovascular events. N Engl J Med 2002;347:1557–1565.

49. Riedel W, Maulik G. Fever: an integrated response of the central nervous system to oxidative stress. Mol Cell Biochem 1999;196:125–132.

50. Rubenstein E. Malignant hyperthermia. In: Rubenstein E, Federman DD (eds). *Scientific American Medicine.* New York: Scientific American, Inc., 1993;Sect. 8V, pp. 1–2.

51. Selye H. Stress without distress. Philadelphia: JB Lippincott, 1974.

52. Sieff CA, Tsai S, Faller DV. Interleukin 1 induces cultured human endothelial cell production of granulocyte-macrophage colony-stimulating factor. J Clin Invest 1987;79:48–51.

53. Simon HB. Hyperthemia. In: Desforges JF, ed. Current concepts. N Engl J Med 1993;329:483–488.

54. Stitt JT. Fever versus hyperthermia. Fed Proc 1979;38:39–43.

55. Van Lente F. The diagnostic utility of C-reactive protein. Hum Pathol 1982;13:1061–1063.

56. Van Snick JL, Masson PL, Heremans JF. The involvement of lactoferrin in the hyposideremia of acute inflammation. J Exp Med 1974;140:1068–1084.

57. Ward CG, Hammond JS, Bullen JJ. Effect of iron compounds on antibacterial function of human polymorphs and plasma. Infect Immun 1986;51:723–730.

58. Weiner HL, Robinson WA. Leukopoietic activity in human urine following operative procedures. Proc Soc Exp Biol Med 1971;136:29–33.

59. Wood WB Jr. Studies on the cause of fever. N Engl J Med 1958;258:1023–1031.

60. Yamada Y, Kimball K, Okusawa S, et al. Cytokines, acute phase proteins, and tissue injury. Ann NY Acad Sci 1990;587: 351–361.

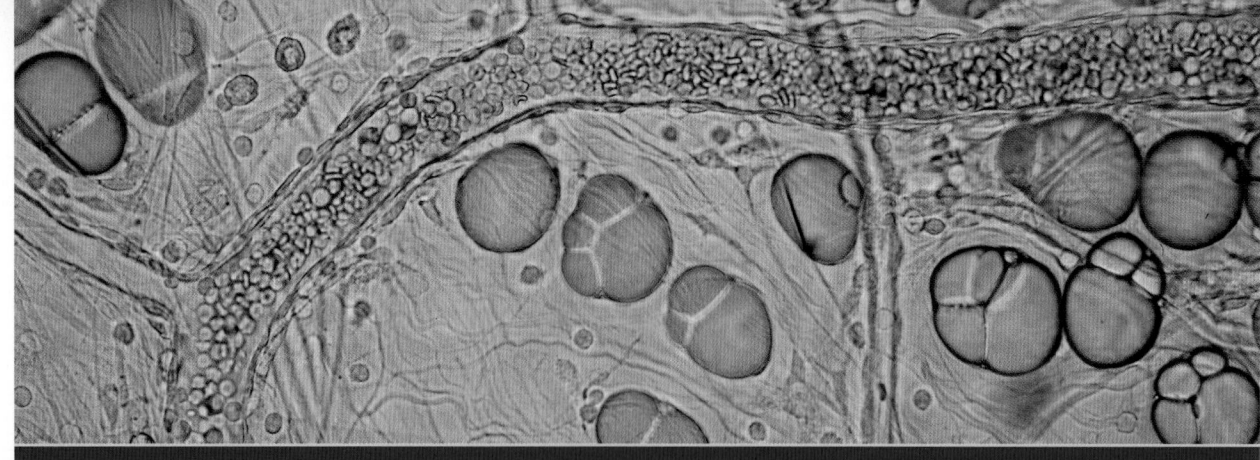

VARIATIONS AND ABERRATIONS OF THE INFLAMMATORY RESPONSE

The inflammatory response always obeys its own basic rule—to create an exudate—but the intensity of the process, its side effects and the final result vary a great deal according to the tissue, the age and state of health of the subject, as well as many other factors. The inflammatory response can also be defective for congenital or acquired reasons.

Inflammation in Tissues Devoid of Blood Vessels

By definition, inflammation is a response to injury of *vascularized* tissues. What happens if no vessels are present? The damaged cells will simply regenerate if they can, and their debris may incite an inflammatory reaction in the nearest vascularized tissue.

The Case of the Cornea

The cornea has no vessels. If it is scratched, surprisingly, some neutrophils appear in the scratch, but they do not crawl in from the rim (the *limbus*)—they "jump over" from the covering eyelid (51). Historically these leukocytes caused much trouble: because they were not seen wandering in from the rim, they were taken as proof that corneal fibroblasts could turn into leukocytes. The scratch itself will heal by epithelial regeneration, without becoming truly inflamed, unless bacteria take over. If the injury is severe or persistent, blood vessels grow toward it from the limbus; they advance within the thickness of the cornea like a whitish, opaque sheet called **pannus** (Latin for sheet). The pannus reaches its target, becomes granulation tissue, and the cornea then can develop inflammation as any other vascularized tissue. Eventually the pannus may regress.

Articular Cartilage

In arthritis the inflammatory process takes place in the synovial membrane; the cartilage itself is involved only passively, being bathed in the inflammatory exudate. This kind of bath is not a treat, because leukocytes can damage the cartilage matrix. In the long run the entire layer of cartilage may be destroyed and replaced by a vascular *pannus* arising from the rim of the articular surface.

Inflammation in Different Organs

This topic has not been studied in detail, except for the following two organs.

Inflammation in the Central Nervous System

Inflammation in the central nervous system is quite predictably a special case. By definition, inflammation takes place in the extracellular spaces, and there are virtually no such spaces in the brain and spinal cord. Inflamed tissues swell, but both brain and spinal cord are contained in a box of bone that cannot expand. In other organs excess fluid is drained away by the lymphatic vessels, but there are none of these in the central nervous system. Accordingly, an episode of acute inflammation—e.g., after a local trauma—will raise the tissue pressure within the nervous tissue, whereby the traumatic injury will be complicated by ischemic injury, and possibly also by the damage caused by reflow after ischemia (p. 713) (10, 19).

Then there are problems related to inflammatory mediators. *Some inflammatory cytokines can modulate neural function, and conversely, neurotransmitters released locally can modulate the inflammatory response* (57a) (remember glutamate, the neurotransmitter and "excitotoxin," p. 228). *Free radicals* released during an acute inflammatory episode tend to target the nerve fibers, because they are rich in lipid (p. 196); and any red blood cells spilled out by injury will favor the production of free radicals by releasing hemoglobin and iron (p. 196), which catalyzes the production of iron-dependent free radicals (44). Other features that complicate inflammation in the central nervous tissue are the (apparent?) lack of significant regeneration and the presence of the blood-brain barrier. Inflammation *caused* by stimulating nerve fibers experimentally (**neurogenic inflammation**) was mentioned earlier (p. 321) (57b).

Pathophysiology of the blood-brain barrier. Progress in this area is slow. We will limit our remarks to a few established facts. (a) Why the barrier should exist at all is not well understood. (b) In the short run (hours), breaking the barrier is not critical; in fact it is a routine procedure for increasing the local delivery of drugs, such as chemotherapy for tumors. The standard method is to inject a hypertonic solution into the carotid artery (Figure 16.1); the effect lasts about 10 minutes (40a). (c) We would expect inflammation to break the barrier, and in fact this what happens around a brain abscess

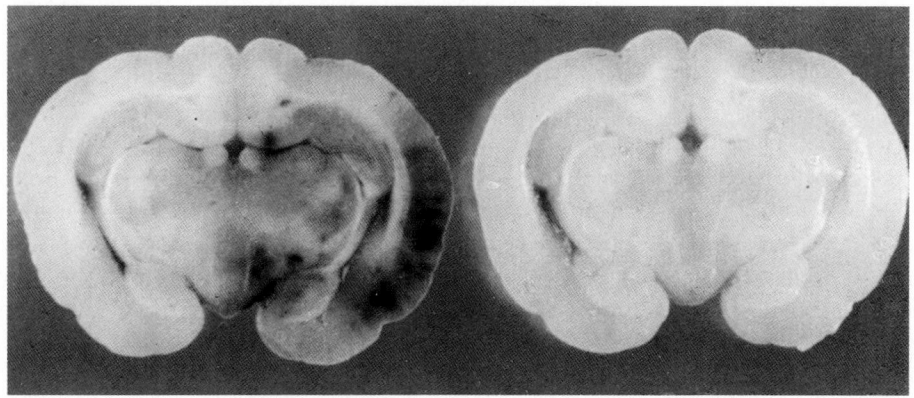

FIGURE 16.1   Coronal sections of two rabbit brains. In both rabbits the blood–brain barrier was broken with a hypertonic solution of urea (2 Osm) injected into the right carotid artery. Evans blue was injected intravenously before the dose of urea in the first animal (*left*) and 30 minutes after the dose of urea in the second animal (*right*). A broken barrier is indicated by the dark staining; the damage is repaired within 30 minutes. (Reproduced with permission from [41].)

(37). However, macrophages enter the brain during development and in several diseases without a demonstrable breach of permeability (37a). Injection of a cytokine into the brain will summon neutrophils, and they do break the barrier; so do activated T cells (37a).

Some cytokines traverse the barrier by active transport (62). Overall, the term "barrier" may be too strong a word for the physiologic phenomenon involved.

> **NOTE:** *The effects of injury and inflammation are stronger in the spinal cord than in the brain,* including the breakdown of the blood-brain barrier (44a).

Inflammation in the Newborn

The inflammatory response in the newborn is defective in almost all respects, and the immune response is also defective. In fact, *the human neonate can be considered an immunocompromised host* (Table 16.1). (12, 55). The diminished responsiveness of the newborn extends to the blood vessels (30), as has been demonstrated quite dramatically in rodents (26). Correspondingly, and disappointingly, neonatal sepsis is still a major problem in the United States; its incidence is still 1–10 cases for every 1000 live births, accounting for 30 percent of all neonatal deaths (59). It is clear that newborns are not well prepared to fight infections.

Inflammation in the Kidney

As few as 10 *Escherichia coli* or staphylococci injected into the renal medulla of some experimental animals can start an infection, whereas over 10,000 are needed to infect the cortex (25). The inflammatory response in the medulla is thought to be poor for several reasons, including a lower blood supply and a hypertonic extracellular fluid that depresses phagocytosis by the polymorphs.

Table 16.1 Defects of Inflammation in the Newborn

Increased neutrophil rigidity
Reduced neutrophil and monocyte chemotaxis
Reduced neutrophil and monocyte locomotion
Reduced neutrophil and monocyte adherence
Reduced neutrophil anaerobic glycolysis
Reduced neutrophil bactericidal ability
Reduced serum opsonic ability
Reduced complement components (one-third to one-half)
Reduced antibody response
Reduced cell-mediated immune response

Adapted from (42).

Inflammation in Invertebrates

The classic studies of Metchnikoff on starfish eggs and sand fleas (Chapter 8) still make for the best reading (32). Since then, much has been learned about inflammation in mollusks and especially oysters, presumably because they make good food and beautiful pearls. Foreign bodies that penetrate into the body of mollusks are submitted to *encapsulation* (13): they are surrounded by all-purpose blood cells called *hemocytes,* which form a sort of granuloma, with an outer fibrous layer as one might also expect in vertebrates. Any parasite or foreign body that is trapped between the body of an oyster and its shell will irritate the covering epithelium of the body, called *mantle;* eventually it will be coated—on the mantle side—with the normal secretion of the mantle, which is *nacre* or mother-of-pearl. This accident, called *nacrezation,* produces half a pearl; the trick of producing a whole pearl is accomplished by grafting into the body of an oyster a piece of mantle, next to a spherical

object; the epithelium of the mantle then will grow over the sphere and continue to produce mother-of-pearl. In 2–3 years the coat will be thick enough to produce the effect of a natural pearl (Figure 16.2).

There are analogous processes in human pathology. In certain malignant tumors of the epidermis (squamous cell carcinomas), pegs of epidermis invade the dermis. The basal cells are on the outside, and they tend to differentiate into mature squamous cells toward the core of the peg. Under these conditions the center of the peg, seen in cross section, appears to contain a lump of shed keratinocytes, actually called a "pearl" (see Figure 26.41). The same process occurs on a larger scale when a sphere of epidermal cells grows beneath the skin, as an *epidermoid cyst* filled with shed cells. Such cysts are sometimes formed by traumatic displacement of epidermis into the subcutaneous tissue; more often they develop from hair follicles (Figure 16.3).

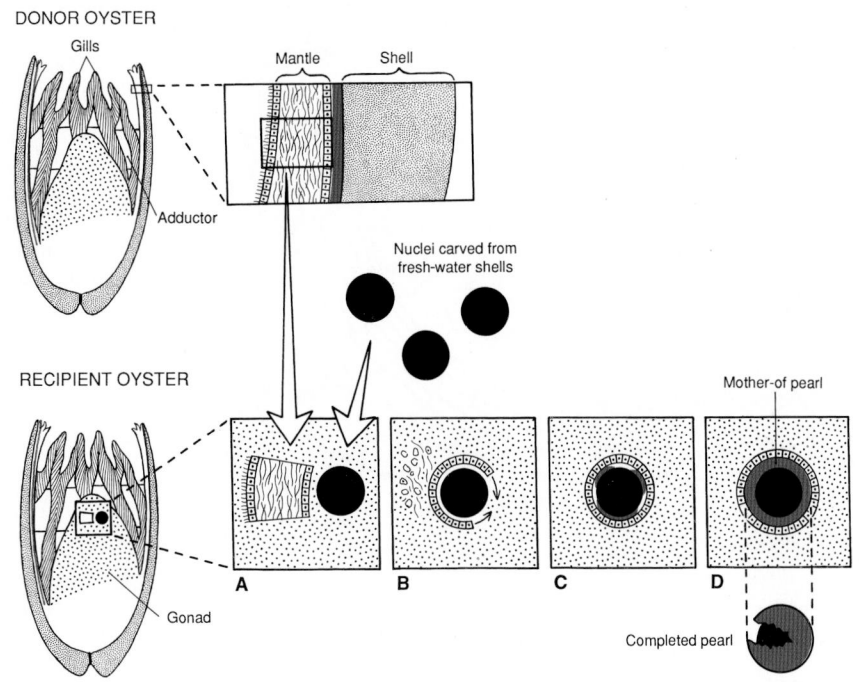

FIGURE 16.2 The method used in Japan for producing cultured pearl exploits mechanisms of normal wound healing. *Top:* A square piece of mantle is obtained from an oyster (the deep epithelium of the mantle normally secretes the mother-of-pearl). *Center:* Spheres carved out of fresh water shells are obtained, as nuclei for the pearls; the size of the nucleus determines the size of the future pearl. *Bottom:* **A:** The two objects are implanted side by side in the gonad of another oyster; the epithelium in charge of making the mother-of-pearl must face the nucleus. **B:** The epithelium begins to cover the nucleus. **C:** The epithelium begins to secrete mother-of-pearl. **D:** After 2 years the pearl is ready. (Drawn with the aid of Prof. Koji Wada, Faculty of Bioresources, Mie University, Japan.)

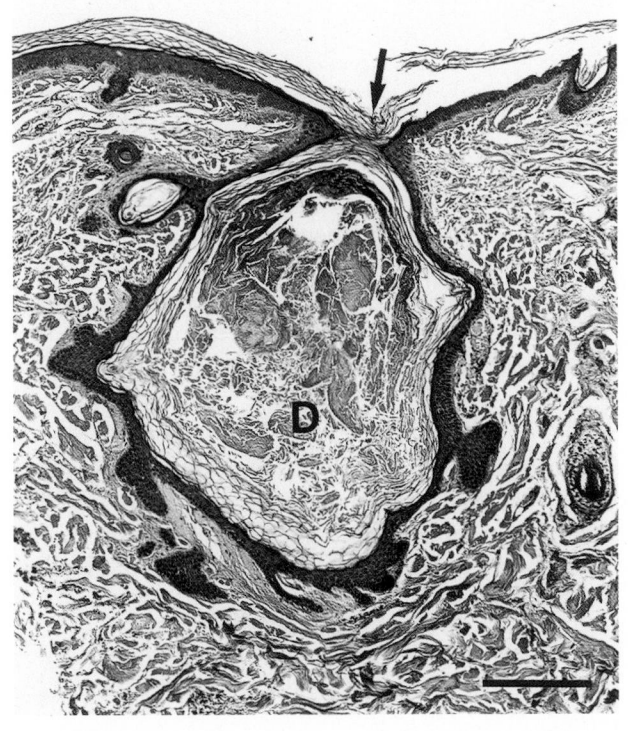

FIGURE 16.3 Epidermoid cyst filled with desquamated cells (**D**). In this case a connection with the epidermis is present (**arrow**). **Bar** = 250 μm. (Specimen kindly provided by Dr. A. B. Ackerman, Thomas Jefferson University Medical Center Philadelphia, PA.)

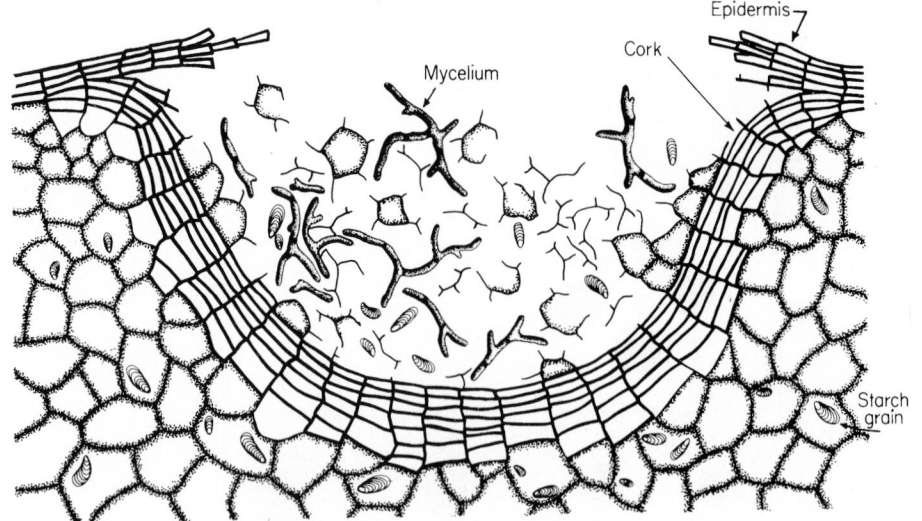

FIGURE 16.4 Surface of a potato invaded by a fungus. The potato responds by forming a dense layer of cork cells beyond the point of infection; this inhibits further invasion, blocks the spread of toxic substances, and deprives the pathogen of nourishment. (Adapted from [40].)

Life Without Inflammation: The Case of Plants

Plants have no migrating cells and no phagocytes; to defend themselves against invading organisms, plant tissues depend on a variety of mechanisms. One is to *sacrifice the injured part* by walling it off so that it will die, and with it dies the pathogen (Figure 16.4) (1). In animal tissues a similar process is called **sequestration:** a piece of infected tissue is isolated in a cavity (i.e., in an abscess) and contained there for long periods; bone sequestra in osteomyelitis can be retained for years. Plants also respond with general adaptations such as the production of protease inhibitors, which happen to be toxic to pathogens and pests (4). It certainly is amazing that phagocytosis plays no role in defense. However, chemotaxis does exist in plants; it was actually discovered in fern gametes (p. 403).

Last, plants rely heavily on **antibiotics,** including bactericidal agents. A powerful member of this group are the **defensins,** molecules so ancient that three types can also be found in human neutrophils (pp. 369, 432).

Failures of the Inflammatory Response

As all mechanisms in biology, inflammation can fail, by excess and by default, and for reasons inherited or acquired.

The theme of failure by excess has run through all the preceding chapters. Prolonged inflammation can destroy an organ; we have defined this as "collateral damage." An extreme case of malfunction by excess occurs when inflammation is unleashed—by the immune system—against a normal tissue (Chapter 18). A unique mechanism of inflammatory damage is represented by the so-called **crystal diseases,** which cause much pain despite the beautiful name.

The "crystal diseases." Several diseases are based on the deposition of microscopic endogenous crystals in the tissues, especially in the joints (pp. 147, 260). The crystals themselves are not greatly irritating to the tissues; but when they are deposited in a joint, an acute inflammatory response ensues. Why? One theory is that the crystal surface binds IgG and thereby activates complement (20). The resulting influx of activated leukocytes is deleterious to the articular cartilage.

Acquired Defects of Inflammation

Leukocytes fail because they cannot be properly delivered to an injury site by the microcirculation, because they are too few, or because they are defective; plasma components can be insufficient or exhausted. Here are some examples of leukocyte failure:

- *Inadequate delivery of blood.* Every surgeon knows that poor blood supply is a major cause of

Table 16.2 Neutropenia: Major Causes

By Decreased Production

- X-rays
- A large variety of drugs (antineoplastic agents, some antihistamines, antibiotics, analgesics, tranquilizers, antiinflammatory agents, many others)
- Some infections (tuberculosis, malaria, hepatitis, typhoid, overwhelming sepsis)
- Starvation, anorexia nervosa
- Folate deficiency, especially in alcoholics
- Vitamin B12 deficiency

By Peripheral Trapping or Destruction

- Diseases with splenomegaly (e.g., congestive splenomegaly, Gaucher disease, sarcoidosis)
- Anaphylaxis, cardiopulmonary bypass (due to clumping followed by trapping)
- Some autoimmune disorders (e.g., systemic lupus erythematosus)
- Autoimmune neutropenia (antineutrophil antibodies)
- Some drugs (e.g., mercurial diuretics)

Adapted from (7).

inadequate inflammation and therefore of infection, especially in skin flaps. Remember that hypoxic leukocytes are ineffective against many bacteria. It follows that hypoxic tissues are much more susceptible to infection than normal tissues, as can be shown most dramatically with experimental skin flaps (22). Hypoxia and ischemia are multiplied in *circulatory shock*, which is generalized inadequate flow: in shock, bacteria can multiply out of control almost anywhere, but especially in the gut. In essence, ischemia frustrates inflammation: it allows bacteria to multiply, unhindered by leukocytes, by complement, and by antibiotics injected intravenously.

- *Inadequate numbers of leukocytes.* Neutropenia can be due to a variety of conditions (Table 16.2). In general, the risk of infection becomes critical as the number of neutrophils per cubic millimeter drops below 1000–500. Monocytopenia appears to be less dangerous than neutropenia; it is seen after stress or glucocorticosteroid therapy and during many acute infections.

- *Lack of spleen.* Splenectomy exposes a patient to the risk of sepsis, especially by pneumococci. There is a heightened risk of infection immediately after splenectomy (48) as well as a long range risk due to several factors. One is, obviously, the loss of macrophages (those of the spleen are especially able to phagocytize bacteria that are not well opsonized, hence they play a critical role in the nonimmune host [3]). Add to this a loss of antibody production; a defect in monocyte chemotaxis; and an impairment of phagocytosis due to reduced production of two opsonins, tuftsin and properdin (49, 50, 56).

- *Overworked littoral macrophages.* Whenever the RES system (p. 314) is flooded with excess material to phagocytize, a so-called blockade develops. This

event has been measured: in rats, if the system is challenged twice in a sequence with intravenous injections of carbon black, the second time it will respond less effectively (p. 316) (2). Clinical settings of blockade can be induced by intravascular hemolysis, which amounts to blockade by hemoglobin and red cell ghosts (27). Circulating antigen–antibody complexes have a similar effect.

- *Impairment of leukocytes by severe burns.* Extensive burns imply a greatly increased risk of infection, due at least in part to leukocyte "exhaustion": thermal injury generates large amounts of chemotaxins, especially C5a, resulting in generalized activation of neutrophils. The neutrophils respond by secreting their specific granules and become ineffective (8, 34). When the leukocyte population has lost most of its granules (5–15 days), septic complications reach their peak (9).

- *Impairment of leukocytes by alcoholic intoxication.* Alcohol abuse carries a risk of infection, especially of the lungs (23). In the preantibiotic era, lobar pneumonia of drunkards was an everyday occurrence in city hospitals. In alcohol intoxication, leukocytes adhere abnormally and migrate poorly. This was shown by adherence tests *in vitro* using nylon wool and by skin-window tests on volunteers (18).

- *Drugs.* Many drugs depress leukocyte function or production. Leukocyte adherence *in vitro* is decreased by steroids, salicylates, colchicine, and local anesthetics; and because adherence is the first step to leukocyte emigration, these same drugs decrease chemotaxis *in vivo* (43). Other drugs with antiinflammatory side-effects are tetracycline, chloroquine, chloramphenicol, and halothane (43, 58). Anti-inflammatory drugs are the basis of treatment for autoimmune diseases, and of course they are a two-edged sword (45).

- *Diabetes.* A variety of defects in inflammation and wound healing accompany diabetes (38): impaired chemotaxis and phagocytosis (14, 35), delayed wound closure and contraction, defective granulation tissue (61), inhibition of collagen synthesis (54), and microcirculatory disturbances, including increased vascular permeability (60). (See also pp. 281, 496, 689.)

- *Cancer.* Defects of leukocyte function are often associated with cancer, and at least two types of chemotaxis inhibitors have been found in the serum of cancer patients (28). However, the principal mechanism of inflammatory failure in cancer is chemotherapy, which affects the bone marrow as well as the cancer.

Interestingly, the same French laboratory that described an antiinflammatory effect of cancer cells (11) later found an antitumor effect of inflammatory cells (21).

- *Viral and bacterial infections.* Certain infectious agents interfere with leukocyte function. The dangerous *Entamoeba histolytica* evades the only cell that can engulf it, the monocyte/macrophage, by means of a specific chemotaxis inhibitor; neutrophils are not affected by it (17).
- *Malnutrition.* Though it is known that malnutrition impairs the leukocytes (46, 47), this topic has been poorly explored (36).

Congenital Defects of Inflammation

The most common congenital defect of inflammation in humans is just being a newborn, as mentioned above. In addition, there are about 20 congenital diseases of the inflammatory response. Although generally rare, as experiments of nature they have been very useful for deciphering normal mechanisms of inflammation (16).

Congenital defects of leukocytes. When a malfunction of leukocytes is suspected, a battery of tests is available (31, 58). Defects include anomalies of leukocyte adherence, chemotaxis, phagocytosis, and bacterial killing— alone or combined. The lack of one function may affect several others; for instance, the lack of adhesion also affects motility over a substrate (14, 39, 58). Leukocyte adhesion deficiency (LAD) has already been mentioned (p. 423) (Figure 16.5); a few other examples are listed:

- *Chronic granulomatous disease (CGD).* In this miserable condition, neutrophils, macrophages and eosinophils are unable to produce a respiratory burst in response to stimulation (Figure 16.5). Chronic infections usually develop during the first year of life; inflammation, both suppurative and granulomatous, is excessive but ineffective. This syndrome can be produced by several molecular defects; although rare, it has attracted great interest for studying the leukocytes' respiratory burst (16).
- *Myeloperoxidase (MPO) deficiency.* This deficiency is quite common: the use of peroxidase stain for routine leukocyte differential counts has revealed it in one of every 1,200 individuals. It affects neutrophils and monocytes but not eosinophils. Oddly enough, few of these patients have problems with bacterial infections, probably because the defective cells show increased activity of the NADPH-oxidase system producing superoxide anion. MPO deficiency can also be acquired: for instance, in pregnancy, anemia, and leukemia.
- *Congenital lack of specific granules.* Discovered in children with recurrent infections, this lack was "useful" in showing that these granules are a source not only of the anti-bacterial lactoferrin but also of receptors for chemotaxins. As the granules fuse with

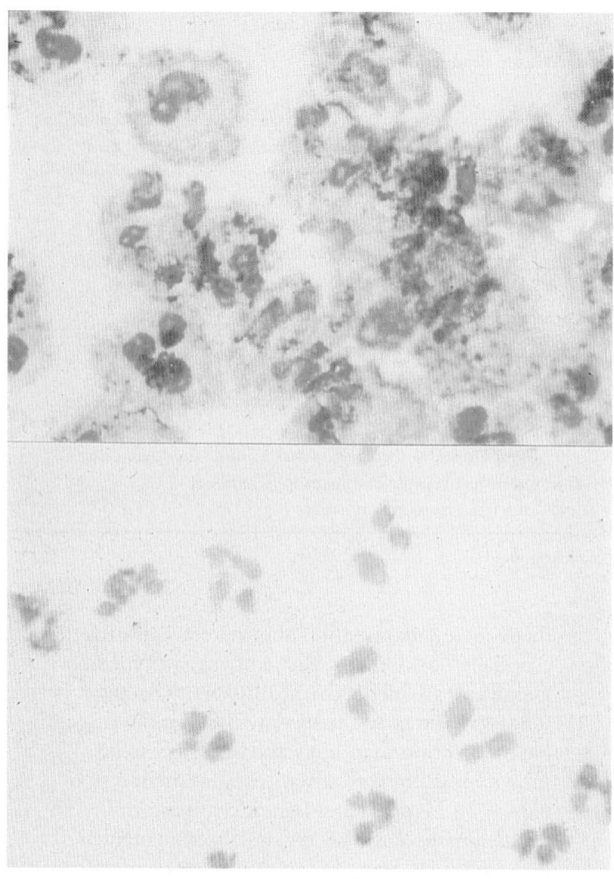

FIGURE 16.5 Oxidative defect of neutrophils, from a child with chronic granulomatous disease. *Top:* Normal human neutrophils stimulated for 40 minutes with phorbol myristate acetate and tested for their ability to reduce the dye nitroblue tetrazolium (NBT). Note the abundance of dark granules, blue in the original specimen. *Bottom:* Defective leukocytes can be demonstrated by a nuclear stain; they contain no reaction product. (Courtesy of Ms. Julia Metcalf and Dr. John I. Gallin, National Institute of Allergy and Infectious Diseases.)

the plasma membrane, the receptors on the inner surfaces of the granules are transferred to the outer surface of the plasma membrane (Figure 11.6) (15).

- *Job's syndrome.* This skin disease was named, somewhat inaccurately, from the Bible: *So went Satan forth from the presence of the Lord, and smote Job with sore boils from the sole of his foot unto his crown* (Job 2:7). The biblical Job was an adult, whereas most of Job's syndrome patients begin to suffer from infections during the first weeks of life (multiple, torpid, skin abscesses) (39). These patients turn out to have very high IgE levels (hyper-IgE syndrome). How this syndrome relates to the disease is not clear. Chemotaxis is depressed, especially for monocytes, but not always.

- *Other congenital defects of inflammation are attributed to dysfunction of the microtubules,* which are important for locomotion as well as for phagocytosis. Instances are the *Chediak–Higashi syndrome,* characterized by multiple phagocytosis defects and large granules in all granulocytes; and the *Primary Ciliary Dyskinesia,* which mainly concerns a dysfunction of the ciliary microtubules (p. 161).
- *Congenital defects of the complement system* are discussed on p. 357.

TO SUM UP: We take inflammation for granted because (speaking for all vertebrates) it rarely lets us down; but when it does, we realize how essential it is for survival. It works even behind the scenes, in everyday life, even in the absence of overt disease. Individuals with leukocyte adhesion deficiency develop overwhelming gum infections: this tells us that anonymous leukocytes are constantly fighting duels around our teeth, keeping the bacteria under control. Among the congenital failures of inflammation, it is interesting to see that the most common is represented by the neonatal state. Among the acquired failures, many are iatrogenic and accompany immunosuppression, the ultimate failure of our defense systems (p. 604). We should not complain that the mechanisms of inflammation are so redundant.

References

1. Agrios GN. Plant Pathology. San Diego: Academic Press, 1988.
2. Biozzi G, Benacerraf B, Halpern BN. Quantitative study of the granulopectic activity of the reticuloendothelial system. II. A study of the kinetics of the granulopectic activity of the R.E.S. in relation to the dose of carbon injected. Relationship between the weight of the organs and their activity. Br J Exp Pathol 1953;34:441–457.
3. Bohnsack JF, Brown EJ. The role of the spleen in resistance to infection. Annu Rev Med 1986;37:49–59.
4. Bowles D. Signals in the wounded plant. Nature 1990; 343:314–315.
5. Bryant RE. Pus: friend or foe? In: Root RK, Trunkey DD, Sande MA, eds. New surgical and medical approaches in infectious diseases. Contemporary issues in infectious diseases, vol 6. New York: Churchill Living-stone, 1987, pp. 31–48.
6. Cohen N, Sigel MM, eds. The reticuloendothelial system. A comprehensive treatise, vol 3, phylogeny and ontogeny. New York: Plenum Press, 1982.
7. Dale DC. Leukocytosis, leukopenia, and eosinophilia. In: Wilson JD, Braunwald E, Isselbacher KJ, et al., eds. Harrison's principles of internal medicine, 12th ed. New York: McGraw-HIll, 1991.

8. Davis JM, Dineen P, Gallin JI. Neutrophil degranulation and abnormal chemotaxis after thermal injury. J Immunol 1980; 124:1467–1471.
9. Duque RE, Phan SH, Hudson JL, Till GO, Ward PA. Functional defects in phagocytic cells following thermal injury. Am J Pathol 1985;118:116–127.
10. Faden AI. Pharmacotherapy in spinal cord injury: a critical review of recent developments. Clin Neuropharmacol 1987; 10:193–204.
11. Fauve RM, Hevin B, Jacob H, Gaillard JA, Jacob F. Anti-inflammatory effects of murine malignant cells. Proc Natl Acad Sci USA 1974;71:4052–4056.
12. Fleer A, Gerards LJ, Verhoef J. Host defence to bacterial infection in the neonate. J Hosp Infect 1988;11(suppl A):320–327.
13. Fletcher TC, Cooper-Willis CA. Cellular defense systems of the mollusca. In: Cohen N, Sigel MM, eds. The reticuloendothelial system. A comprehensive treatise, vol 3, phylogeny and ontogeny. New York: Plenum Press, 1982, pp. 141–166.
14. Forehand JR, Johnston RB. Phagocytic defects. Clin Immunol Allergy 1985;5:351–369.
15. Gallin JI, Fletcher MP, Seligmann BE, et al. Human neutrophil-specific granule deficiency: a model to assess the role of neutrophil-specific granules in the evolution of the inflammatory response. Blood 1982;59:1317–1329.
16. Gallin JI, Snyderman R (eds). Inflammation: Basic principles and clinical correlates. 3rd ed. Philadelphia: Lippincott Williams and Wilkins, 1999.
17. Giménez-Scherer JA, Pacheco-Cano MG, de Lavín EC, et al. Ultrastructural changes associated with the inhibition of monocyte chemotaxis caused by products of axenically grown *Entamoeba histolytica.* Lab Invest 1987;57:45–51.
18. Gluckman SJ, MacGregor RR. Effect of acute alcohol intoxication on granulocyte mobilization and kinetics. Blood 1978; 52:551–559.
19. Hall ED. Free radicals and CNS injury. Crit Care Clin 1989; 5:793–805.
20. Hasselbacher P. Crystal-protein interactions in crystal-induced arthritis. In: Weissmann G, ed. Advances in inflammation research. New York: Raven Press, 1982, pp. 25–44.
21. Hevin M-B, Friguet B, Fauve RM. Inflammation and anti-tumor resistance. V. Production of a cytostatic factor following cooperation of elicited polymorphonuclear leukocytes and macrophages. Int J Cancer 1990;46:533–538.
22. Hunt TK, Knighton DR, Price DC, et al. Oxygen in the prevention and treatment of infection. In: Root RK, Trunkey DD, Sande MA, eds. New surgical and medical approaches in infectious diseases. New York: Churchill Livingstone, 1987, pp. 1–16.
23. Kass EH. Changing ecology of bacterial infections. Arch Environ Health 1963;6:19–25.
24. Kucharz E. 80th anniversary of the discovery of erythrocyte sedimentation rate. Mater Med Pol 1975;7:344–346.
25. Leaf A, Cotran RS. Renal pathophysiology. New York: Oxford University Press, 1976.
26. Little RA. Changes in the reactivity of the skin blood vessels of the rabbit with age. J Pathol 1969;99:131–138.
27. Loegering DJ, Grover GJ, Schneidkraut MJ. Effect of red blood cells and red blood cell ghosts on reticulo-endothelial system function. Exp Mol Pathol 1984;41:67–73.

28. Maderazo EG, Anton TF, Ward PA. Serum-associated inhibition of leukotaxis in humans with cancer. Clin Immunol Immunopathol 1978;9:166–176.

29. Malech HL, Gallin JI. Neutrophils in human diseases. N Engl J Med 1987;317:687–694.

30. Matheson A, Nierenberg M, Greengard J. Reactivity of the skin of the newborn infant. Pediatrics 1962;10:181–197.

31. Metcalf JA, Gallin JI, Nauseef WM, Root RK. Laboratory manual of neutrophil function. New York: Raven Press, 1986.

32. Metchnikoff E. Lectures on the comparative pathology of inflammation, 1892. (Translated from the French by Starling FA, Starling EH). New York: Dover Publications, 1968.

33. Mims CA. The pathogenesis of infectious disease. London: Academic Press, 1976.

34. Moore FD Jr, Davis C, Rodrick M, Mannick JA, Fearon DT. Neutrophil activation in thermal injury as assessed by increased expression of complement receptors. N Engl J Med 1986;314:948–953.

35. Naghibi M, Smith RP, Baltch AL, et al. The effect of diabetes mellitus on chemotactic and bactericidal activity of human polymorphonuclear leukocytes. Diabetes Res Clin Pract 1987; 4:27–35.

36. Neumann CG. Nonspecific host factors and infection in malnutrition—a review. In: Suskind RM, ed. Kroc Foundation series vol 7. Malnutrition and the immune response. New York: Raven Press, 1977, pp. 355–374.

37. Neuwelt EA, ed. Implications of the blood-brain barrier and its manipulation, vol 2. New York: Plenum Medical Book Company, 1989.

37a. Perry VH, Anthony DC, Bolton SJ, Brown HC. The blood-brain barrier and the inflammatory response. Mol Med Today 1997;3:335–341.

38. Pickup JD, Williams G. Textbook of diabetes, vol 2. Oxford: Blackwell Scientific Publications, 1991.

39. Quie PG. Phagocytic cell dysfunction. J Allergy Clin Immunol 1986;77:387–398.

40. Ramsey GB. A form of potato disease produced by Rhizoctonia. J Agric Res 1917;9:421–426.

40a. Rapoport SI: Osmotic opening of the blood-brain barrier: principles, mechanisms, and therapeutic applications. Cell Mol Neurobiol 2000;20:217–320.

41. Rapoport SI, Hori M, Klatzo I. Testing of a hypothesis for osmotic opening of the blood-brain barrier. Am J Physiol 1972;223:323–327.

42. Regelmann WE, Mills EL, Quie PG. Immunology of the newborn. In: Feigin RD, Cherry JD, eds. Textbook of pediatric infectious diseases, vol 1, 2nd ed. Philadelphia: WB Saunders, 1987, pp. 921–939.

43. Roberts R, Gallin JI. The phagocytic cell and its disorders. Ann Allergy 1983;50:330–343.

44. Sadrzadeh SMH, Anderson DK, Panter SS, Hallaway PE, Eaton JW. Hemoglobin potentiates central nervous system damage. J Clin Invest 1987;79:662–664.

44a. Schnell L, Fearn S, Klassen, et al. Acute inflammatory responses to mechanical lesions in the CNS: differences between brain and spinal cord. Eur J Neurosc 1999;11:3648–3658.

45. Seldin MF, Steinberg AD. Immunoregulatory agents. In: Gallin JI, Goldstein IM, Snyderman R, eds. Inflammation: basic principles and clinical correlates. New York: Raven Press, 1988, pp. 911–934.

46. Selvaraj RJ, Bhat KS. Phagocytosis and leucocyte enzymes in protein-calorie malnutrition. Biochem J 1972;127:255–259.

47. Seth V, Chandra RK. Opsonic activity, phagocytosis, and bactericidal capacity of polymorphs in undernutrition. Arch Dis Child 1972;47:282–284.

48. Shatney ClH. Complications of splenectomy. Acta Anaesth Belg 1987;38:333–339.

49. Shaw JHF, Print CG. Postsplenectomy sepsis. Br J Surg 1989; 76:1074–1081.

50. Simon M Jr, Djawari D, Hohenberger W. Impairment of polymorphonuclear leukocyte and macrophage functions in splenectomized patients. N Engl J Med 1985;313:1092.

51. Sloop G, Moreau JM, Conerly LL, Dajcs JJ, O'Callaghan RJ. Acute inflammation of the eyelid and cornea in *Staphylococcus* keratitis in the rabbit. Invest Ophthalmol Vis Sci 1999;40: 385–391.

52. Smedley LA, Tonnesen MG, Sandhaus RA, et al. Neutrophil-mediated injury to endothelial cells. Enhancement by endotoxin and essential role of neutrophil elastase. J Clin Invest 1986;77:1233–1243.

53. Smith RM, Curnutte JT. Molecular basis of chronic granulomatous disease. Blood 1991;77:673–686.

54. Spanheimer RG. Direct inhibition of collagen production in vitro by diabetic rat serum. Metabolism 1988;37:479–485.

55. Stiehm ER. The human neonate as an immunocompromised host. In: Verhoef J, Peterson PK, Quie PG, eds. Infections in the immunocompromised host—pathogenesis, prevention and therapy. Amsterdam: Elsevier-North Holland Biomedical Press, 1980, pp. 77–94.

56. Styrt B. Infection associated with asplenia: risks, mechanisms, and prevention. Am J Med 1990;88(suppl 5N):33N–42N.

57. Suckling AJ, Rumsby MG, Bradbury MWB, eds. The blood-brain barrier in health and disease. Chichester, England: Ellis Horwood Ltd., 1986.

57a. Szelényi J. Cytokines and the central nervous system. Brain Res Bull 2001;54:329–338.

57b. Tracey KJ. The inflammatory reflex. Nature 2002;420: 853–859.

58. van der Valk P, Herman CJ. Leukocyte functions. Lab Invest 1987;57:127–137.

59. Wasserman RL. Neonatal sepsis: the potential of granulocyte transfusion. Hosp Pract 1982;17:95–104.

60. Williamson JR, Chang K, Tilton RG, et al. Increased vascular permeability in spontaneously diabetic BB/W rats and in rats with mild versus severe streptozocininduced diabetes. Diabetes 1987;36:813–821.

61. Yue DK, Swanson B, McLennan S, et al. Abnormalities of granulation tissue and collagen formation in experimental diabetes, uraemia and malnutrition. Diab Med 1986;3: 221–225.

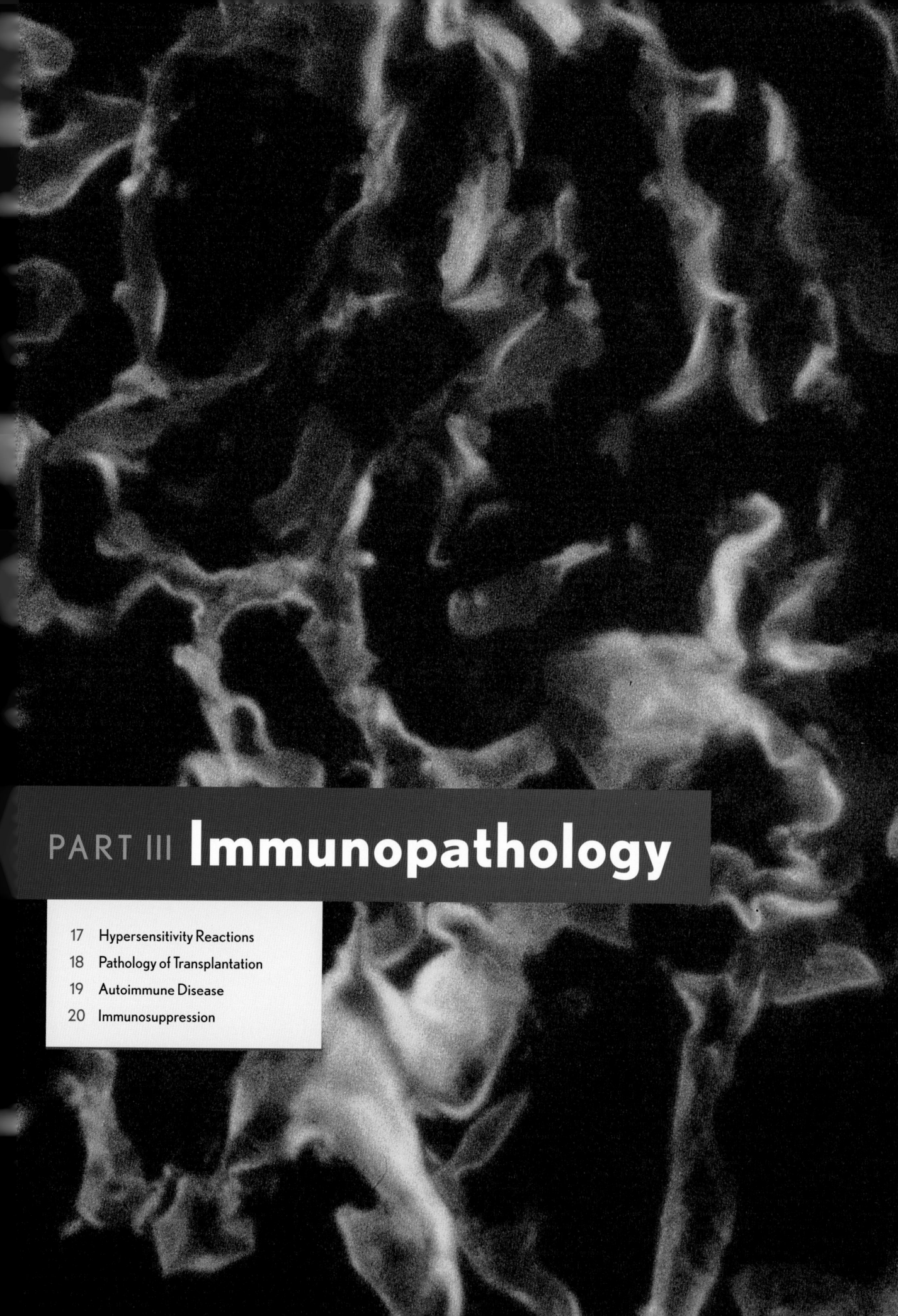

PART III **Immunopathology**

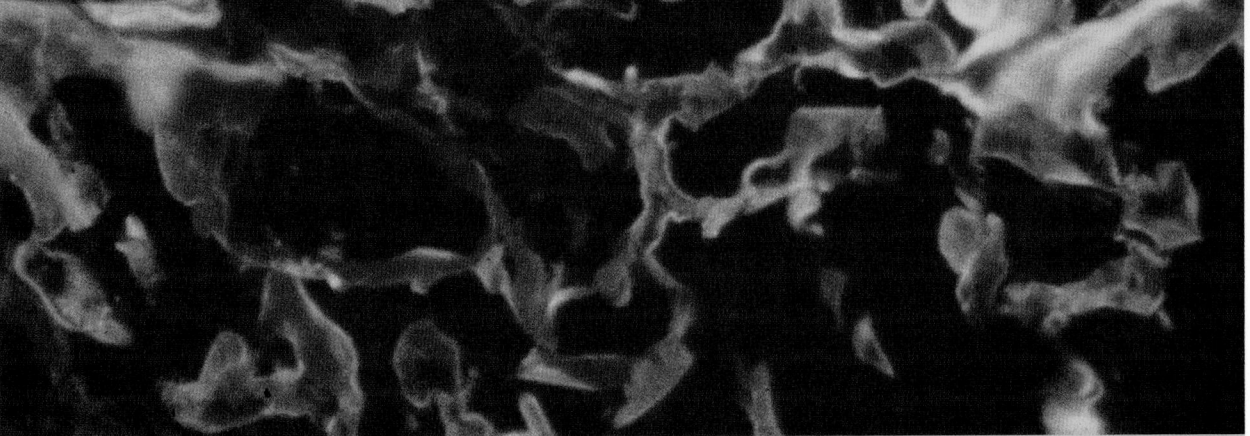

HYPERSENSITIVITY REACTIONS

We are now stepping into the field of immunopathology. This and the next three chapters will describe how the immune response can fail: it can do too much (*hypersensitivity*) or too little (*immunodeficiency*) or it can attack the "wrong" target (*autoimmunity*).

We assume that the reader is familiar with the basic concepts of immunology. However, classroom experience tells us that it would be wise to clarify the ambivalent use of the word **immune.**

In common language, to be *immune* from a disease, or from anything else, is a good thing. It was certainly a good thing to be *immunis* in Roman times, because it meant to be **tax exempt** (from *in-*, "not," and *munus,* "money"). In the late 1800s the new science of immunology focused on *immunizing* humans and other animals against a disease, and the two basic characteristics of the immune response were established: **specificity** and **memory** (example: to be immune to smallpox you need *previous* exposure to a *specific* vaccine). Then in 1901 a conceptual disaster struck: a dog injected twice with the same toxin died instead of being "immunized," and unwittingly contributed to the birth of allergy. *From then on the word "immune" came to have a double meaning: an "immune" phenomenon may have a good or bad result, as long as it is defined by specificity and memory.* Multiple sclerosis destroys the nervous tissue of the patient, yet it is called an *immune* disease.

Hypersensitivity Reactions

This group of diseases afflicts a large part of humankind. The problem here is that *the immune system reacts against an antigen that in itself is harmless.* The classic example is hay fever: pollen is certainly a collection of antigens, but by themselves these antigens cause no harm, and to battle them *creates a problem where there was none.* Pollen is exogenous, but the antigens responsible

Table 17.1 The Four Principal Types of Hypersensitivity

Type 1: Anaphylactic

Key is the mast cell

Antibody (IgE) is bound to mast cells "by the tail" (Fc segment: *cytophilic binding*)

Degranulation occurs when antigen hits the mast cell

No cells die

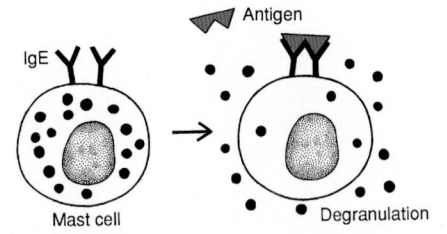

Type 2: Cytotoxic

Antibody (non-IgE) binds to an antigenic surface, cell or basement membrane, by the Fab segments (*cytotoxic binding*)

The carpet of fixed antibody fixes leukocytes and activates complement, thereby attracting more leukocytes

Damage to the antigenic surface is done by complement and by leukocytes

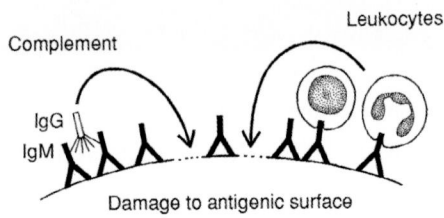

Type 3: Complex-Mediated

Complexes are formed by antigen + antibody

Complexes fix leukocytes and activate complement, thereby attracting more leukocytes

Damage to any tissue nearby is done mainly by neutrophils

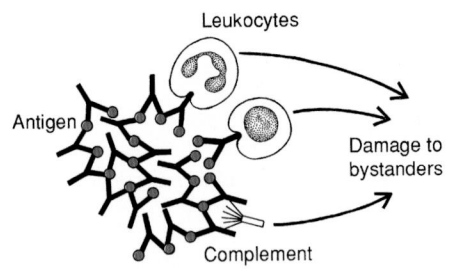

Type 4: Cell-Mediated

No antibody is involved

Only cells participate

Target antigenic cells are killed by killer cells and lymphokines

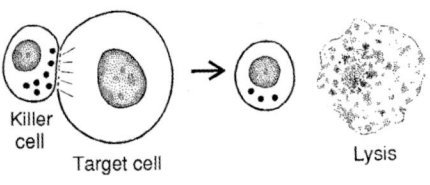

(left margin: Immediate — applied to Types 1–3; Delayed — applied to Type 4)

for hypersensitivity reactions can also be endogenous, and they can produce damage by one or the other effector arm of the immune response, namely *antibodies* or *effector T cells*. Accordingly, it is helpful to adopt the classification suggested by Coombs and Gell in 1975 (12). Follow Table 17.1: just as there are two ways to deal with antigens (by the B cell and the T cell pathway) there are two main categories of hypersensitivity responses. *One category is called* **antibody mediated** *because it depends on antibody production,* and includes Types 1, 2 and 3. Type 1 involves the rather unusual IgE antibodies; Types 2 and 3 involve IgG, IgM, and IgA antibodies. *The other category (***cell mediated***) depends on effector T cells.* Because we are dealing with immune responses, the general rule is that both types of hypersensitivity reactions do not occur on first contact with the antigen: there must be a period of sensitization followed by elicitation. Another basic rule: reactions mediated by antibodies tend to occur rapidly—in seconds or minutes—because the reagents are in solution; therefore the top three types listed in Table 17.1 are called **immediate hypersensitivity reactions.** The fourth type depends on mobilizing cells, which, however activated, move slowly and require 12–18 hours to gather in sufficient numbers: hence the name **delayed-type hypersensitivity (DTH).**

The key feature of Table 17.1 is the right-hand column: note the various arrangements of the antibody molecules. Once these are understood, the three antibody-mediated types of hypersensitivity are not difficult to remember. Besides, Type 1 is unforgettable.

Hypersensitivity Type 1: Anaphylactic

Many of us have heard of an outdoor party that turned to tragedy when someone was stung by a bee, collapsed, and died. An episode of this kind happens at least 40 times a year in the United States (68).

This is **anaphylactic shock,** due to massive degranulation of the mast cells. The chain of events that led to explain its mechanism began with a cruise on a royal yacht, as we will see shortly. Decades later it turned out that anaphylactic shock was just the tip of an iceberg: today we can produce a list of reactions due to the same mechanism (but not as life-threatening), such as asthma and food allergies. An acute degranulation of mast cells occurs when individuals whose mast cells are coated with antibody to a given antigen are again exposed to that antigen. In essence, we are dealing with endogenous overdoses of mast-cell products (70). The villains, to be precise, are not only the mast cells but also their circulating relatives, the basophils (other cells play lesser roles).

When it was realized that mast cells are programmed to coat themselves with antibody and to act in that uniform as agents of the immune reaction, something like a mast-cell cult developed. And rightly so: no other group of cells is equipped to kill the whole body in a few minutes.

But let us begin from the beginning, aboard the royal yacht (Figure 17.1).

In 1901 Prince Albert of Monaco, who was interested in marine biology, set to sea on the *Princess Alice II* to work out the mechanism of poisoning by the Portuguese man-of-war, a stinging jellyfish that can be a nuisance on Mediterranean beaches (Figure 17.2). The ship was equipped with labs for animal experiments; Paul Portier was the resident scientist. To supervise the experiments, Prince Albert invited a senior scholar, Charles Richet (1850–1935), who was also a writer and an eminent physiologist; it was he who found that dog panting is a cooling device (24). As the ship cruised along, a number of dogs, ducks, pigeons, and frogs were injected with toxic jellyfish extracts; the only finding worthy of note was that the animals tended to "fall asleep," perhaps by a neurotoxic effect. After the voyage, Richet continued the experiments on dogs using sea anemones, which cost less. Would their poison have the same "narcotic" effect as that of the

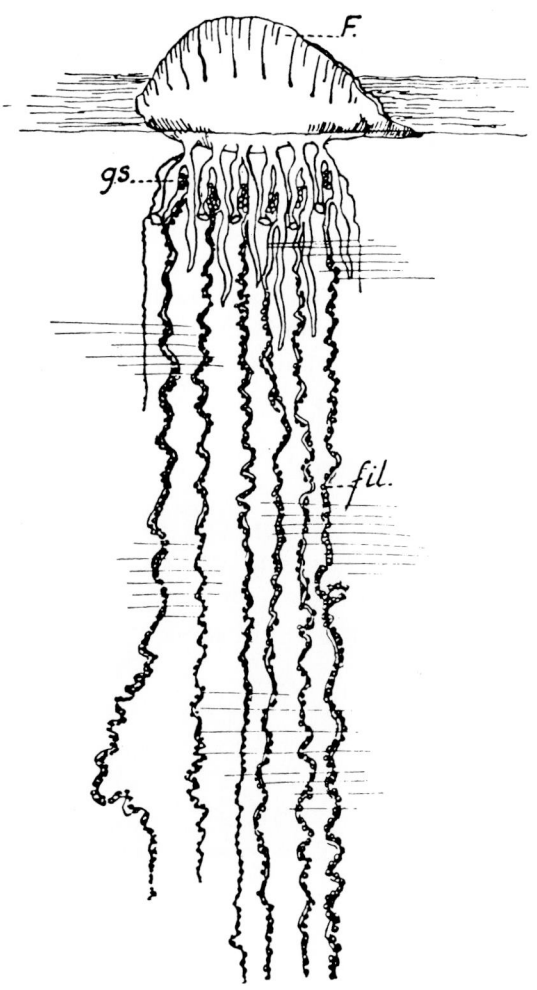

FIGURE 17.2 Portuguese man-of-war floating in the sea. The dangerous sting of this mollusk inspired the Prince of Monaco to initiate research that led to the discovery of anaphylaxis. (Reproduced with permission from [54].)

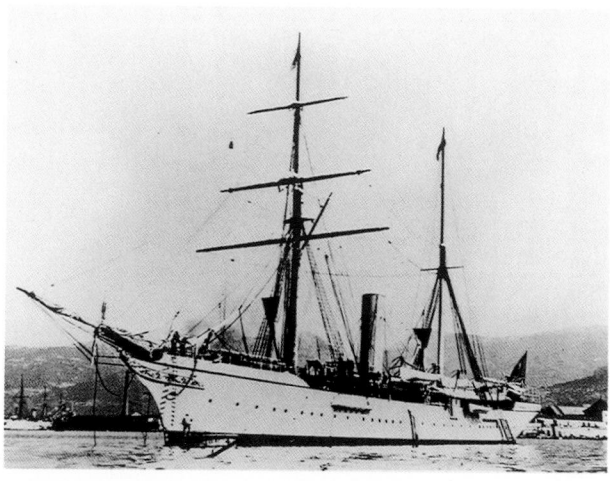

FIGURE 17.1 The *Princesse Alice II,* the yacht used by Prince Albert 1st of Monaco for the oceanographic cruise that led to the discovery of anaphylaxis. (By courtesy of, and with the authorization of, The Oceanographic Museum of Monaco.)

Portuguese man-of-war? Richet tried several doses, and, again for economic reasons, he used the same dog for more than one injection. So, Dog Neptune, for example, received three *nonlethal* doses on days 1, 3, and 27 (61); the first two had no apparent harmful effect, but after the third one, the unfortunate Neptune suddenly keeled over, convulsed, vomited, and died within 25 minutes (55). Portier and Richet were utterly amazed, having anticipated, if anything, an immunizing (prophylactic) effect of repeated doses. Dog Neptune—and others after him—seemed to show the reverse effect. Groping for a Greek word to mean "reversed protection" they settled on *anaphylaxis*, supposedly the opposite of prophylaxis (54, 67). As Greek goes it was a poor choice, but 12 years later Richet was awarded the Nobel prize for having opened a new field of immunology. Actually, anaphylaxis had been seen by others before him, but nobody had generalized from it. Neither Richet nor Portier lived long enough to learn its basic mechanism.

Mechanisms of Anaphylactic Hypersensitivity

We are now able to explain in some detail what happened to those unfortunate dogs. Portier and Richet had come upon the phenomenon of *generalized* anaphylactic hypersensitivity: massive, allergic mast-cell degranulation (Figure 17.3). For an anaphylactic response to occur—whether it be local (as in hay fever) or generalized—the antigenic material must have the property of inducing antibodies of the IgE class. In most mammals, IgE antibodies bind to the surface of mast cells, basophils and activated eosinophils; but note this key fact: if we liken the shapes of immunoglobulin molecules to lobsters, an IgE molecule binds to a mast cell by its "tail" (i.e., by the Fc portion), and the "claws" float free, ready to bind antigen (see Figure 17.18). This type of binding is called *cytophilic* (cell-friendly), and in fact, the mast cell is not at all troubled by its antigenic coat: it has receptors for the very purpose of acquiring it as part of its normal life (we will see why). When the specific antigen to these antibodies comes along and binds to their outstretched claws, it triggers degranulation; to do so it must be at least divalent so that it can bind two adjacent molecules of IgE (Figure 17.4).

But beware: *mast cells can be induced to degranulate by hundreds of molecules that are wholly unrelated to IgE and to anaphylactic hypersensitivity*, the so-called **histamine liberators** (p. 538). Mast cells also degranulate in response to two purely experimental tricks: one is to use antibodies against the bound IgE antibody, the other is to use antibodies against the surface IgE receptor.

Degranulation: Two Waves of Mast-Cell Products

We have mentioned earlier (p. 342) that the mast cells carry a heavy load of chemical weapons, the heaviest among all cells. When the mast cells become troublemakers, their awesome arsenal comes to light. The response is immediate; its effects become clinically apparent in two waves (29, 30).

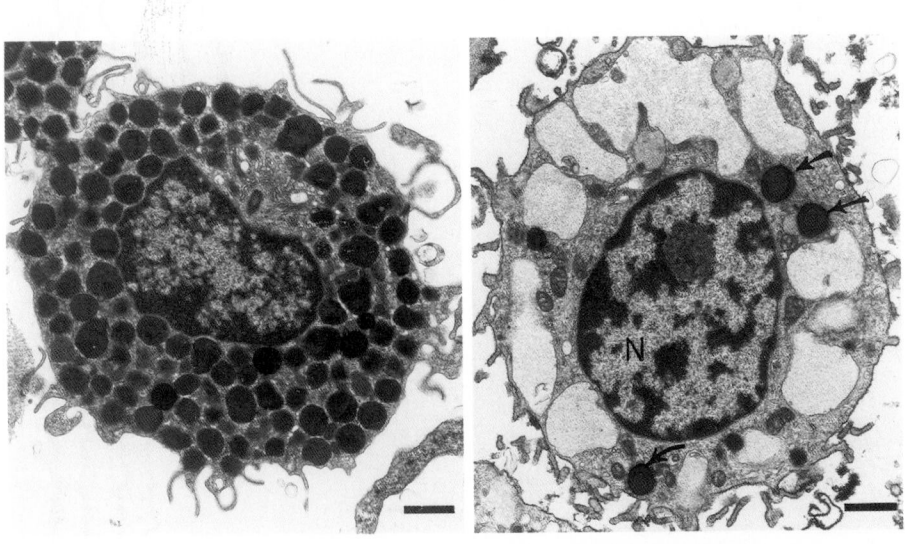

FIGURE 17.3   Mast cells isolated from the human lung. *Left:* Normal cell. *Right:* Degranulating cell, fixed 10 minutes after the degranulation stimulus (challenge with anti-IgE); clear spaces represent swollen granules; there are few residual granules. **Arrows:** Lipid bodies. **N:** Nucleus. **Bars** = 1 μm. (*Left:* From : Dvorak AM, Schleimer RP, Lichtenstein LM. Human mast cells synthesize new granules during recovery from degranulation. *In vitro* studies with mast cells purified from human lungs. *Blood* 1988;71:76–85. Copyright American Society of Hematology, used with permission. *Right:* Reproduced by permission from [17], © by The US & Canadian Academy of Pathology, Inc.)

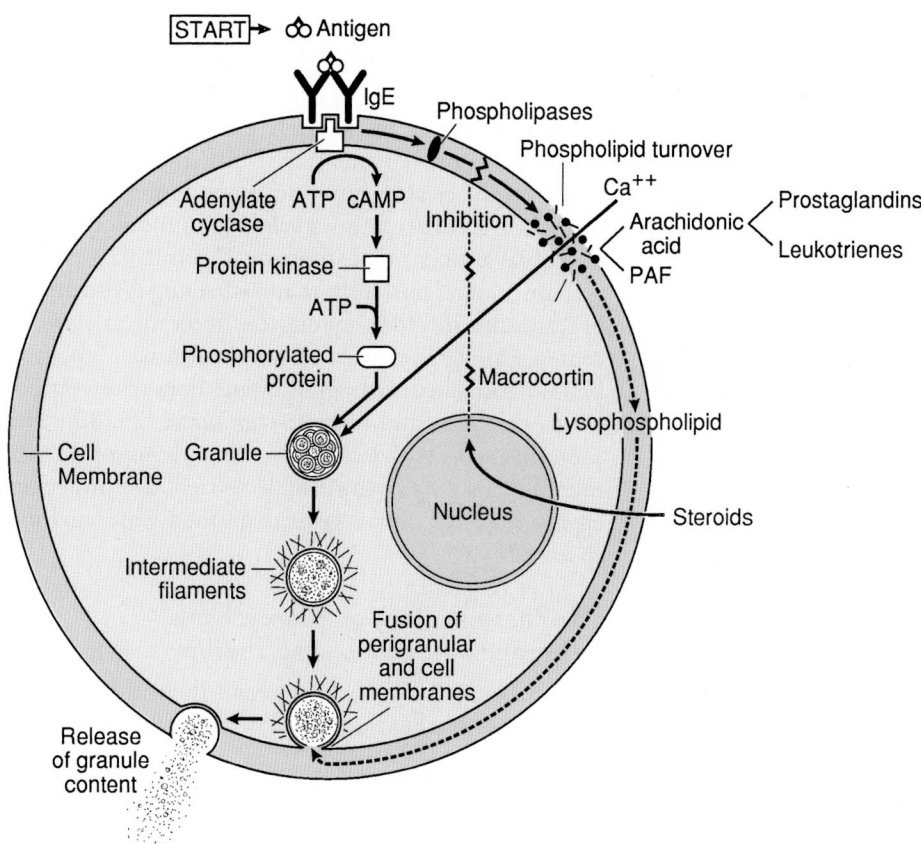

FIGURE 17.4 Proposed sequence of metabolic events in a mast cell activated by antigen bridging a pair of IgE molecules. Transduction of the stimulus leads to degranulation as well as to perturbation of cell-membrane phospholipids; this leads to the production of arachidonic acid metabolites and of platelet activating factor. Note the inhibitory pathway mediated by macrocortin. (Adapted and reproduced with permission from [4]. Illustration by B. Tagawa.)

The immediate response. Within seconds after the stimulus to degranulate, histamine is released from storage in the granules; *in rats, serotonin comes with it.* The result is vascular leakage, which causes local swelling in many places, including the skin and (more ominously) the larynx. Circulating histamine contributes to a drop in blood pressure, to constriction of the bronchi, and to other smooth muscle effects. At the same time the mast cell releases preformed TNF. It also puts the phospholipids in its membranes to work, producing four sets of mediators (pp. 345, 358): leukotrienes, prostaglandins, lipoxins, and platelet activating factors (PAF) (64–66, 89). Prostaglandin D2 and leukotriene C4 are powerful bronchoconstrictors, and the latter makes the spasm worse by stimulating the secretion of mucus: thus the victim has plenty of reasons for suffering from air hunger, although the greatest threat of suffocation (in anaphylaxis) comes from edema of the larynx. Other factors released during this phase are chemotactic for neutrophils and eosinophils, but it takes some time (hours) for these cells to respond in significant numbers.

At this point the mast cells have fired their first, double-barreled shot, but there is more to come.

The late-phase reaction. After 2–4 hours the late-phase reaction begins; it peaks at 6–12 hours and can last 1–2 days or longer. It has been observed not only in the skin but also in the nose (in hay fever) and in the bronchi (35). *Biopsies have shown an inflammatory exudate* (whereas during the early reaction there is almost pure edema) with eosinophils, basophils, neutrophils, and some macrophages; many granules are spilled around, from degranulated mast cells, basophils, and eosinophils (Figure 17.5). One hypothesis is that the granules spilled from the mast cells slowly release their bound proteases (tryptase and chymase, p. 344), which act on plasma proteins of the edema to produce inflammatory mediators; the eosinophils participate with their own toxic products (10, 34). In other words, at this stage the initiating antigen is not necessarily involved (32). *Intradermal injections of mast-cell granules produce late-phase reactions* (27). It has also been suggested that late-phase reactions involve activated eosinophils, which secrete their cytolytic *major basic protein* (66).

Why Do Some Antigens Induce an IgE Response?

The crucial feature that makes some antigens capable of inducing anaphylactic reactions is their ability to induce the formation of IgE antibodies. This effect,

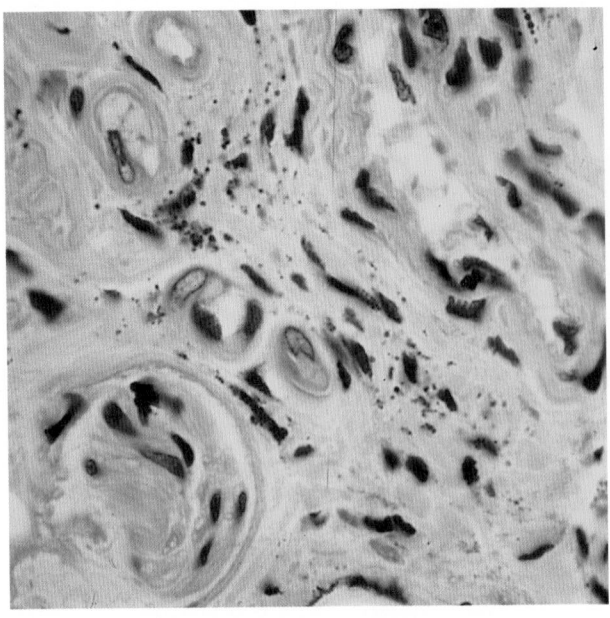

FIGURE 17.5   Pathogenesis of the late-phase allergic reaction. Biopsy of the skin 5 hours after the intradermal injection of antigen in a sensitized patient. Note the degranulating mast cells and the free mast-cell granules which are thought to be responsible for the late-phase reaction. (Reproduced with permission from [27].)

however, is the combined result of many factors; in our perspective it is a bizarre collaboration, because the choice to produce IgE leads to trouble, whereas IgG or IgM would lead to no harm and possibly to protection. The road to IgE depends on the following: (a) *the type of antigen:* typically a small protein, easily soluble, resistant to drying, often an enzyme; and (b) *processing by antigen-presenting cells,* which depends on the local cytokine environment (Figure 17.6). If it is IL-4, T_H2 helper cells will develop, and they will steer B cells to producing IgE; but if it is IL-12, T_H1 helper cells will develop, and they will steer the response in the direction of delayed-type hypersensitivity (the cell-mediated response). We must assume that the cells in the lymphoid organs, in their collective wisdom, know what cytokines are called for (13, 25). (c) *The route of administration and dosage:* The antigen is usually applied to a mucosal surface, and in a very small dose. (d) *Genetic factors:* Allergies run in families. In children, the cumulative risk of developing some allergic condition is 10 percent if neither parent has a history of allergy; if one or both parents are allergic, it is about 25 and 50 percent, respectively (Figure 17.7) (75). (e) *Environmental factors:* Many allergens are clearly environmental, such as pollen, dandruff from pet animals, feces of house mites, and house dust. Furthermore,

epidemiologic studies have connected allergies with a "Western" lifestyle. After the unification of Germany in October 1989, it was expected that allergies would be more prevalent in the more polluted Eastern cities; the opposite proved true (76, 77). Perhaps in Western countries the cleaner environment and more liberal use of antibiotics deprive the developing immune system of microbial antigens that stimulate T_H1 cells (29).

Protection against asthma and wheezing is also offered by exposure to older children at home or at day-care centers (5). Lower levels of **atopic disease** ("allergies" p. 534) correlated with an intestinal flora of lactobacilli versus coliforms and *Stapylococcus aureus* (29, 30). This protective effect of lactobacilli reminds us of Metchnikoff's passion for yogurt and lactobacilli as a protection against the onset of old age: perhaps there was something to his theory.

The Pharmacology of Allergy: Links between Pathogenesis and Therapy

Pharmacology helps us understand the mechanisms of allergic lesions (Figure 17.8). For example (52):

- *Inhibitors of degranulation* prevent but do not treat anaphylactic manifestations; it is useless to give cromolyn sodium, the best known inhibitor of degranulation, to someone who has already degranulated.

- *Epinephrine and other adrenergic agonists* can be lifesaving. They act by stimulating adrenergic alpha and beta receptors, which raise the cell's level of cAMP and stop degranulation. Epinephrine also dilates the bronchi and constricts arteries; hence it has long been the drug of choice in anaphylactic shock and other allergies. Even the Romans knew that a decoction of *ephedra* is helpful for asthma (40).

- *Antihistamines* are effective in many conditions (such as urticaria), but not in others (such as asthma), because *histamine is only one of the mediators released by mast cells.* It is also well to remember that mast cells differ from one body site to another (p. 344).

- *Antiinflammatory agents:* aspirin is generally avoided in treating asthma because it makes things worse. The mechanism is thought to be the following: aspirin inhibits the cyclo-oxygenase pathway of arachidonic acid metabolism, which releases prostaglandins; this inhibition makes more substrate available for the lipoxygenase pathway, which produces leukotrienes, some of which are bronchoconstrictors, and make asthma worse. Corticoids take effect only after several hours, so they are useful for preventing and treating late reactions.

- Desensitization therapy by injecting the offending antigen might sound contradictory and dangerous to the novice, but there is of course a theory behind

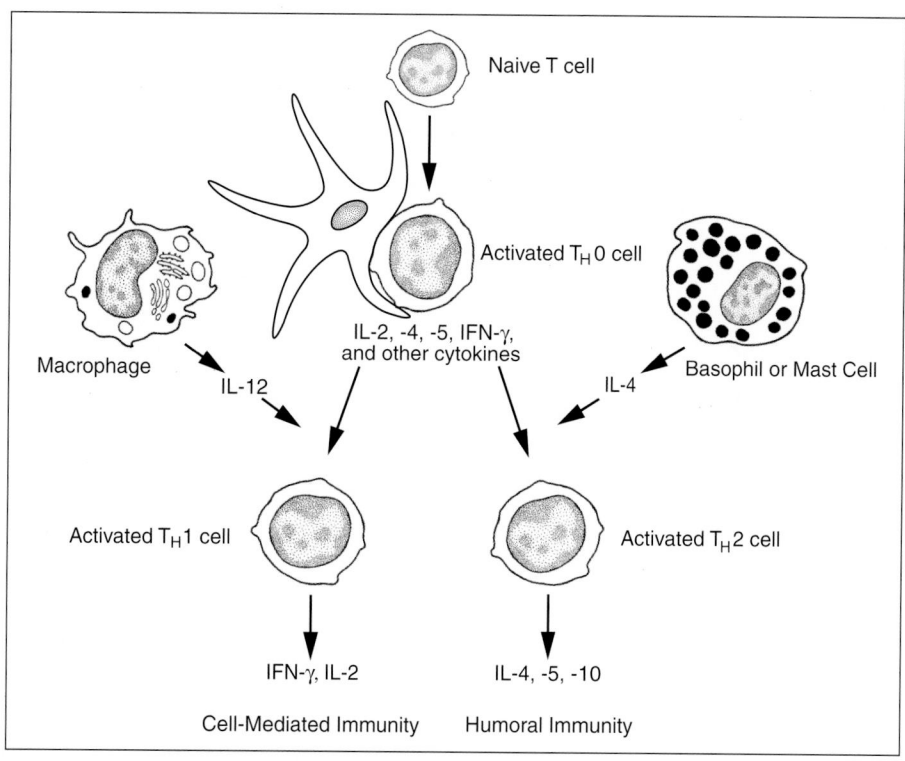

FIGURE 17.6 Pathways to cellular versus humoral immunity. A previously nonactivated ("naive") T lymphocyte is activated by an antigen-presenting cell and becomes a T_HO cell. Further differentiation depends on the cytokine environment: **IL-12** (produced by APCs and macrophages) directs the T_HO toward the T_H1 phenotype, which will direct cell-mediated immunity; **IL-4** (produced by mast cells and basophils) directs T_HO cells to the T_H2 phenotype, which will provide B cell help to humoral immunity. (Reproduced with permission from Adler SH, Gudmundsdottir H, Turka LA. Normal immune responses. In: Neilson EG, Couser WG [eds]. Immunologic renal diseases, 2nd ed. Philadelphia, PA: Lippincott Williams & Wilkins, 2001, pp. 15–46.)

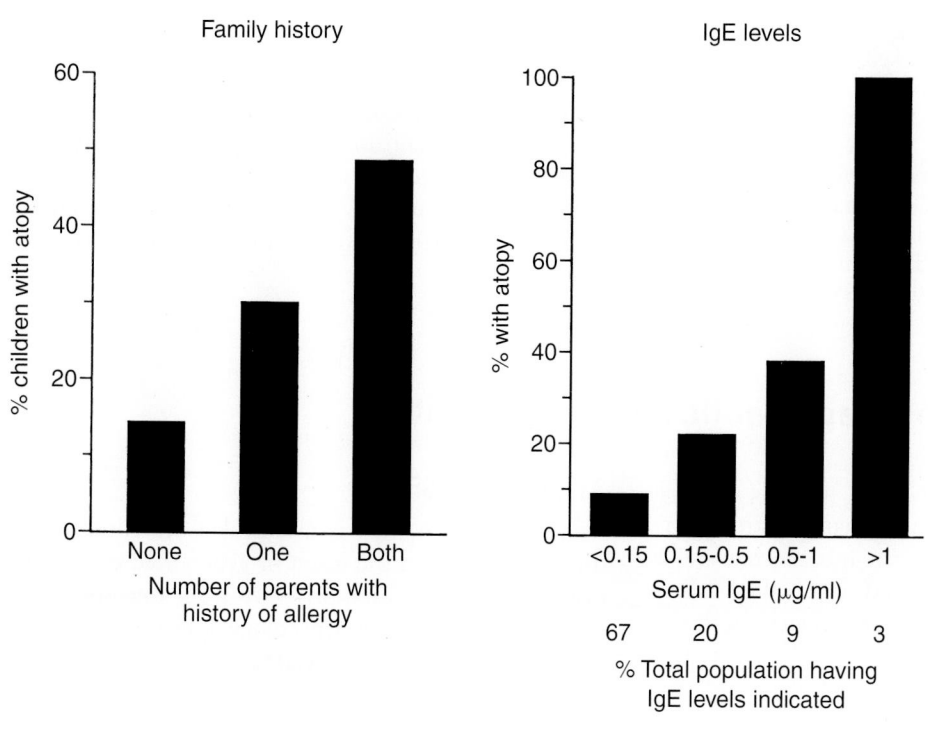

FIGURE 17.7 Risk factors in allergy. *Left:* A family history of allergy increases the risk of developing allergies. *Right:* The higher the concentration of IgE in the serum, the greater the chance of developing allergies. (Adapted with permission from [63].)

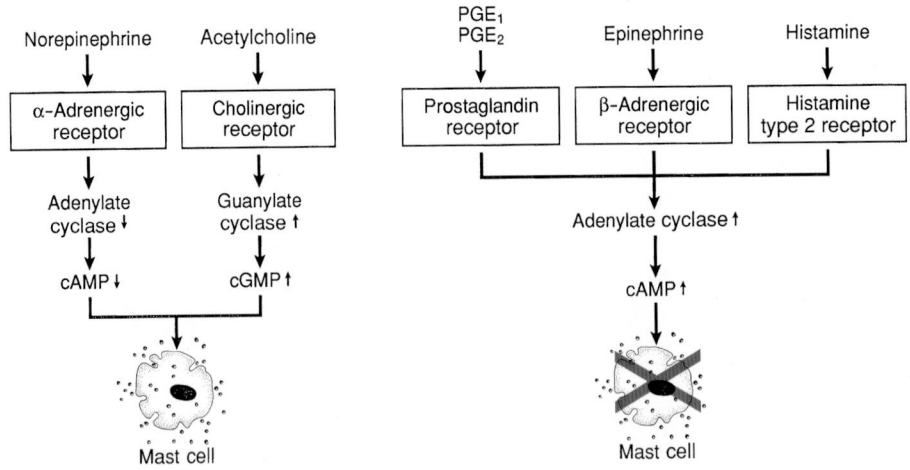

FIGURE 17.8   Modulation of mast-cell degranulation by drugs. *Left:* Release is stimulated by decreased cAMP or increased gGMP. *Right:* Release is inhibited by increased cAMP. (Adapted from 6 Immunology, VII Clinical Immunology in WebMD Scientific American ® Medicine, Dale DC, Federman DD (ed). WebMD Corporation, New York, 2003 [62].)

it. The allergen is *injected,* which is not its natural route of entry; most allergens are inhaled or swallowed and therefore penetrate the mucosal membranes. The idea is that the different route of entry will elicit a non-IgE antibody, such as IgG. Purpose: circulating IgG might be able to "grab" any antigen that penetrates the body barriers, before it can reach the IgE antibody on the mast cells (this grabbing is what is meant by "*blocking* antibodies"). There is evidence that this mechanism does work, although anaphylactic accidents (rarely) do occur during the therapy (30).

A loose end for readers with strong nerves. The authors of this book were profoundly shocked one day by reading that *anaphylaxis can be produced in mice that are congenitally deficient in mast cells* (19, 26). A reflex telephone call produced the following data. (a) These mice have *some* mast cells (less than 1 percent of normal) plus a normal amount of basophils (72): perhaps this is enough. (b) Perhaps other cells contribute to the anaphylactic response (platelets, macrophages?). (c) The central dogma of anaphylaxis "has not been demolished." So we trust.

Psychology and the mast cells. The lore on this subject includes the story of the asthmatic patient hypersensitive to the perfume of roses, who visited an art museum and developed an asthmatic attack before a painting of roses. This sequence has been confirmed experimentally. If guinea pigs hypersensitive to an antigen are submitted to a Pavlovian conditioning procedure whereby the nose is repeatedly swabbed with the antigen coupled with a smell, after some time the guinea pigs begin to release histamine into the bloodstream when presented with the smell alone (65). Similar results were obtained with rats, this time by combining the antigen with an audiovisual cue (38). These and other experiments suggest that the central nervous system may be involved in modulating mast-cell degranulation as well as in other mechanisms of mediator release: hypnotic suggestion can decrease the flare (though not the wheal) of the triple response (p. 385) (79). We will touch upon the role of the nervous system further on (p. 606).

Diseases Related to Anaphylactic Hypersensitivity

Anaphylactic shock (a whole-body response) is the most spectacular manifestation of anaphylactic hypersensitivity, but the same mast-cell IgE mechanism is shared by a number of local conditions called "allergies," such as hay fever. We will now review both the generalized and the local responses.

Anaphylactic Shock

As we have seen, this is a fearful acute clinical syndrome. It is always the result of generalized degranulation, but its manifestations vary from one species to another because the pharmacologic effects of the mediators involved are species-related.

Table 17.2 Some Ingredients of Yellow-Jacket Venom

Ingredients	Effects
Histamine, serotonin, bradykinin	Major inflammatory mediators; kinins produce pain
Histidine decarboxylase	Produces histamine
Phospholipase A and B	Initiate cascade of prostaglandin and leukotriene inflammatory mediators
Protease	Produces more inflammatory mediators by acting e.g., on complement components
Hyaluronidase	Favors spread of diffusible molecules in connective tissue
Norepinephrine, epinephrine (vasoconstrictors)[a]	Retain diffusible molecules in connective tissue

[a]The pharmacologic wisdom of yellow-jacket venom is truly diabolical, the essence of textbook inflammatory knowledge. These two ingredients are currently used in local anesthetics to hold the injected drug in place as long as possible; perhaps their purpose in yellow-jacket venom is similar. For other ingredients (e.g., cholinesterase) a rationale is not obvious.

Adapted from (60).

In humans, anaphylactic shock is well known as a result of insect stings. Note the pharmacologic wizardry displayed in yellow-jacket venom, which can do much worse than simply induce allergy (Table 17.2; Figure 17.9). Drugs can also induce anaphylactic sensitization and shock; the most frequent cause of anaphylactic shock is penicillin, with an estimated 40 deaths per year (36).

Tiny amounts of antigen may suffice for anaphylactic shock, even a vaccination. As to the clinical picture, the patient typically begins to feel faint; common symptoms are itching of the palms and soles or the genital area, and skin rashes that resemble the sting of the nettle (**urticaria**); nausea, vomiting, and diarrhea may develop within minutes. Some individuals plunge into cardio-vascular collapse: histamine causes leakage from the venules throughout the body, and the resulting loss of plasma volume causes the blood pressure to drop, while the heart rate speeds up (Figure 17.10) (71). Other victims develop air hunger from bronchial spasm or hoarseness from laryngeal edema (there are many mast cells in the larynx, and they account for some deaths). There may be a relapse after an initial improvement, surely by the mechanism of the late-phase reaction. The mortality of anaphylactic shock is about 10 percent.

In the guinea pig, the effect is essentially asphyxia. If a guinea pig is sensitized intradermally with bovine albumin and challenged intravenously 3 weeks later, it will begin to scratch its nose within seconds (itching from local degranulation); it gasps for air, collapses, and dies within minutes. Autopsy shows *overinflated* lungs—because the constricted bronchi let air in but not out—even after the lungs are removed from the body (Figure 17.11). The blood shows a *prolonged clotting time*, probably due to release of heparin into the blood, and *leukopenia,* which is attributed to leukocyte

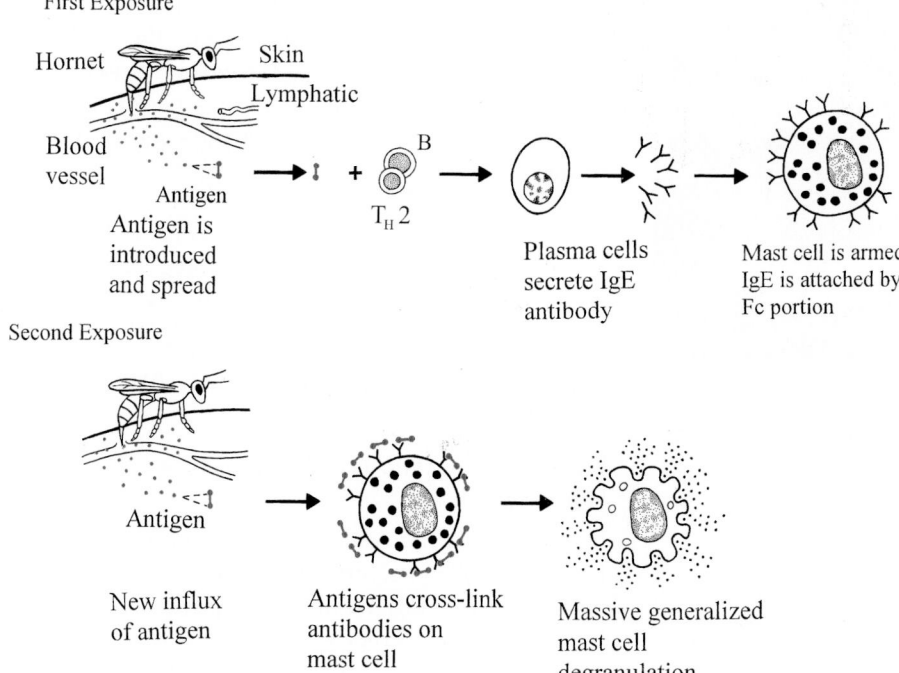

First Exposure

Plasma cells secrete IgE antibody

Mast cell is armed: IgE is attached by Fc portion

Antigen is introduced and spread

Second Exposure

New influx of antigen

Antigens cross-link antibodies on mast cell

Massive generalized mast cell degranulation

FIGURE 17.9 Mechanism of anaphylaxis after a sting (e.g., by a hornet).

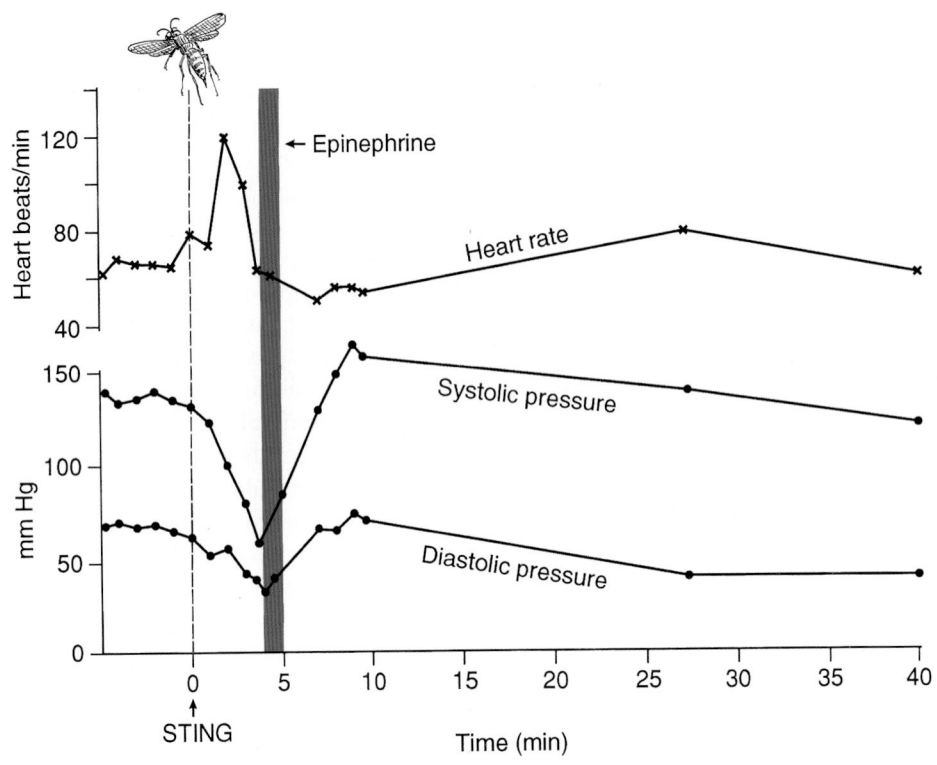

FIGURE 17.10 Effects of anaphylactic shock on human heart rate and blood pressure. This experiment was carried out in a critical care setting, with the purpose of selecting the best possible treatment. Note the very short interval between the sting by a real insect and the general effects. (Reprinted from the **Journal of Clinical Investigation,** 1980;66:1072–1080, by copyright permission of the American Society for Clinical Investigation via the Copyright Clearance Center [71].)

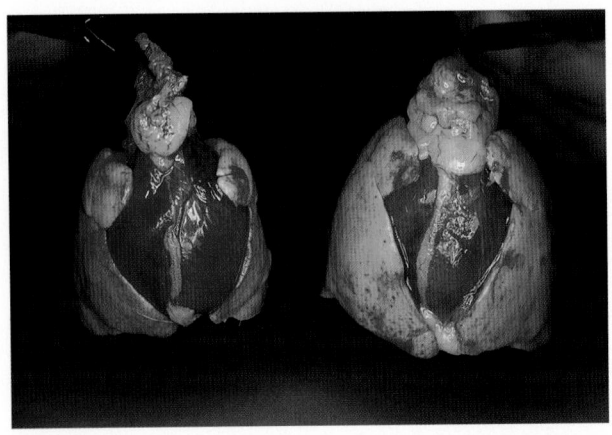

FIGURE 17.11 Heart and lungs of two guinea pigs. *Left:* This guinea pig had been sensitized with albumin and was challenged 21 days later with an intravenous dose of albumin; death from anaphylactic shock followed within 10 minutes. The lungs after dissection remained expanded due to bronchial spasm trapping air in the lungs; yet the trachea was open **patent.** *Right:* Normal guinea pig: the lungs (barely visible behind the heart) have collapsed due to their natural elasticity. Conclusion: anaphylactic shock causes spasm in the bronchi. Slightly enlarged.

clumping and retention of the clumps in the lung, an effect of platelet activating factor released by mast cells (p. 364). Thus, in the guinea pig, the effects are dominated by spasm of the bronchial musculature. Curiously, anaphylaxis in the guinea pig depends on IgG; otherwise, the mechanism is the same as in other animals.

> In the dog, the main effect is constriction of the hepatic veins, resulting in diarrhea and vomiting. In the rabbit, the critical event seems to be pulmonary hypertension and right heart failure, perhaps because too many pulmonary capillaries are blocked by leukocyte emboli (remember the platelet–leukocyte aggregates induced by PAF).

Local Manifestations of Anaphylactic Hypersensitivity

Portier and Richet could never have guessed that hay fever, food allergies, urticaria (hives), and asthma all belong to the same family as anaphylactic shock. In fact, for many years they were lumped into a mysterious category of disorders called **atopic** (a Greek term for bizarre or out of place), the reason being that—although they had the hallmarks of antigen–antibody reactions—no circulating antibody was demonstrable. Now we know why: the level of IgE antibody in the blood is very low. All these local forms of anaphylactic response follow a local application of antigen, such as pollen on the nasal mucosa.

Hay fever. Allergic rhinitis, also called hay fever, is more prevalent in developed countries, where it affects 10–15 percent of the population (74). It offers a classic example of hypersensitivity because the inhalation of harmless pollen sets up an intense and wholly unnecessary inflammatory response, creating a considerable nuisance to the patient. The mechanism of allergic rhinitis is summarized in Figure 17.12.

> Why does the sneeze come so soon after a sniff of hay? It should take time for the antigen to reach the mast cells lying under the epithelium. We have consulted some eminent immunologists, both normal and allergic, but elicited no good answer. We were told that the antigens of some allergenic particles, such as the feces of house mites, are very soluble in water and therefore quickly extracted (73); we were also reminded that some mast cells sit on the mucosa, out in the breeze (51), and may somehow accelerate the passage of the antigen. However, we found no electron microscopic proof of the statement (48) that they can increase the permeability of epithelia, as they can with venular endothelium. Someone should try to work this out.

A curious aspect of hay fever is that the nasal mucosa, constantly inflamed, eventually becomes hypertrophic and "grows out" in the form of polyps that may even appear at the nostrils (Figures 17.13, 17.14): soft, oblong masses that interfere with breathing and must be surgically removed, but may recur. We suspect that these polyps are a response to growth factors secreted by the inflammatory cells, but they carry no threat of malignant transformation. We know of only one comparable phenomenon in pathology: the outgrowth of finger-shaped "villi" from synovial membranes when they are chronically inflamed, such as in rheumatoid arthritis.

Food allergies. Allergies to food are on the rise. They are due to antigens that manage to cross the barrier of the intestinal epithelium, transcytosed by absorptive cells and by the specialized M-cells (47) that lie over Peyer's patches and solitary lymphoid follicles (Figure 17.15) (44, 49, 50). In predisposed individuals, the immune system responds by developing Type 1 hypersensitivity; mast cells armed with specific IgE appear in the intestinal mucosa and throughout the body. The antigens are commonly present in nuts, strawberries, and fish or shellfish (even cooked). Renewed ingestion of the antigen will induce a wave of mast cell degranulation; if the amount of antigen is minimal, the response can be limited to the intestinal mucosa, resulting in diarrhea; larger amounts will escape into the general circulation

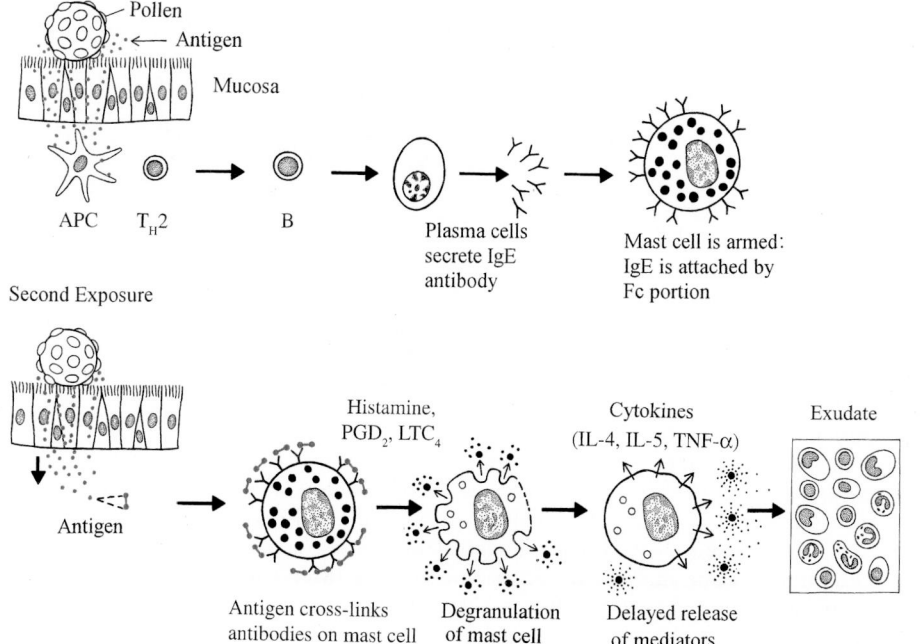

FIGURE 17.12 The mechanism of a mucosal allergy: hay fever (allergic rhinitis).

First Exposure

Pollen
Antigen
Mucosa

APC T_H2 B   Plasma cells secrete IgE antibody   Mast cell is armed: IgE is attached by Fc portion

Second Exposure

Antigen

Histamine, PGD_2, LTC_4 Cytokines (IL-4, IL-5, TNF-α)   Exudate

Antigen cross-links antibodies on mast cell   Degranulation of mast cell   Delayed release of mediators

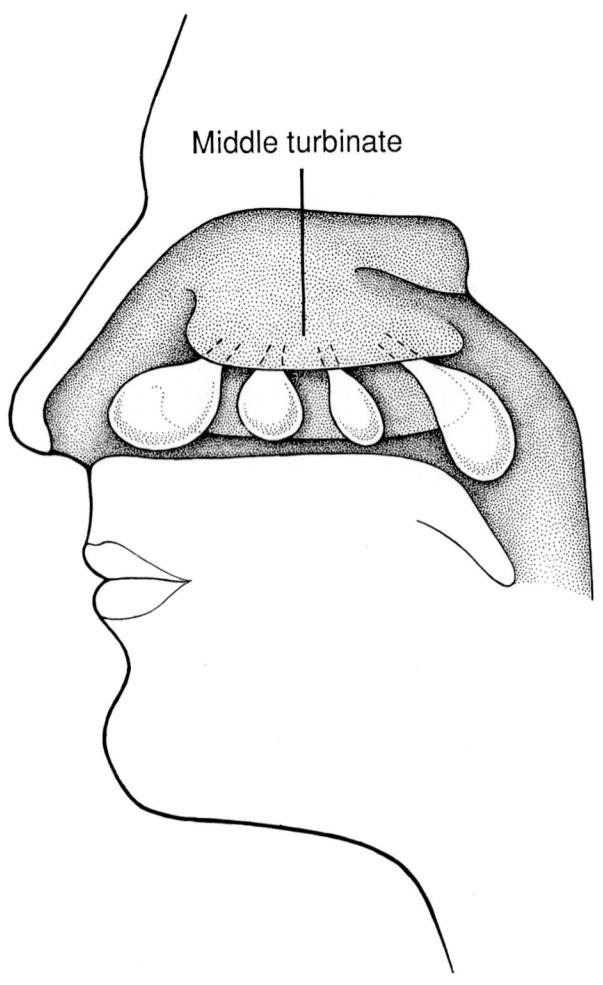

Middle turbinate

FIGURE 17.13 Nasal polyps, as seen in patients with allergic rhinitis (hay fever). Such polyps, which can completely occlude the nose, are soft structures arising from the nasal mucosa, usually beneath the middle turbinate, a shell-like bone. They are easily removed surgically but tend to recur. (Modified from [15], Copyright 1982, with permission from Elsevier.)

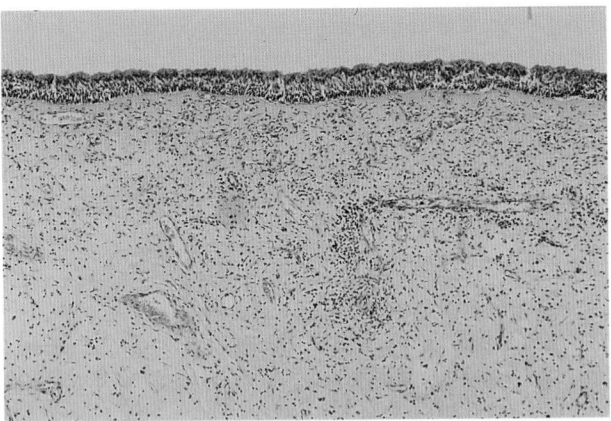

FIGURE 17.14 Histology of a nasal polyp. The surface epithelium is of the upper respiratory type; beneath it is edematous connective tissue with many vessels and a diffuse infiltrate of macrophages, lymphocytes, plasma cells, and eosinophils (not distinguishable at this enlargement). (60x)

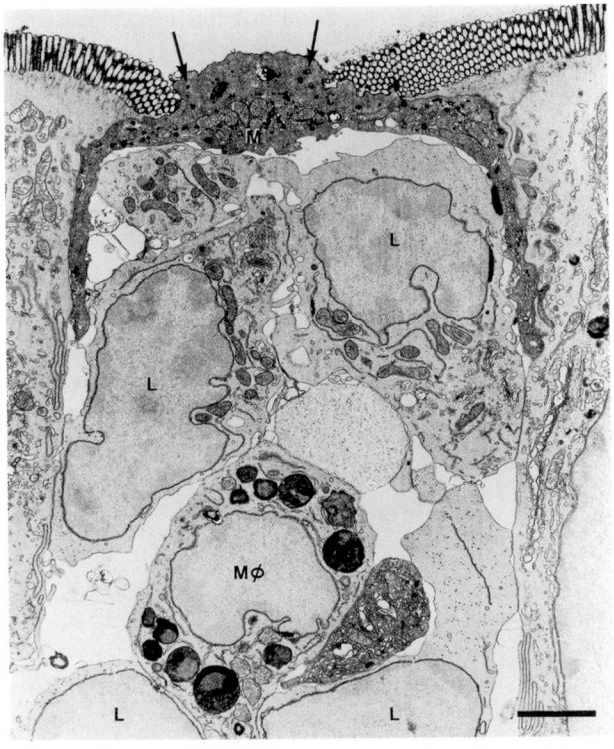

FIGURE 17.15 Macromolecular transport across the epithelium of the gut by an M cell (M) over a Peyer's patch in the mouse. Horse-radish peroxidase injected into the lumen of the gut is being transported by vesicles (arrows) into the subepithelial space. Note a macrophage (Mϕ) surrounded by lymphocytes (L). Bar = 2 μm. (Reproduced from [49] by permission from Plenum Publishing Corporation.)

and cause urticaria, asthma, and even anaphylactic shock. The most dangerous antigens are in peanuts; in the United States, they account for 1.5 million cases of allergy and 50–100 deaths per year (34a). Even a friendly kiss may cause a local reaction (20). Individuals with peanut allergy live in constant fear of unintended exposure: A deadly dose of peanuts may be lurking in any innocuous-looking sauce. These patients will surely benefit from the novel therapy with anti-IgE antibody specific for free (not cell-bound) IgE (34a, 44a).

It was a food allergy that began to clarify the basic mechanism of all atopic lesions. The breakthrough came in 1921, in Breslau. Dr. Heinz Küstner wondered why he became ill every time he ate cooked fish or shellfish. So he worked out a scientific deal with Dr. Prausnitz who, acting as guinea pig, received 0.1 ml of Küstner's serum in his skin, followed 1 day later by 0.1 ml of fish extract. Thus was born the classic Prausnitz–Küstner reaction. Interestingly, when the result was published, the gentleman who acted as the guinea pig became the senior author: the P of the PK reaction (56).

The principle of the PK reaction is to inject a minute amount of serum from the allergic subject into the skin of a normal volunteer; 24–48 hours later the suspected antigen is injected into the same site. If a wheal develops within 90 minutes, the reaction is positive. This waiting period after the serum injection allows time for the IgE antibody to become attached to the mast cells; in some cases the time can be shortened to 45 minutes. The site remains reactive for 4–6 weeks; it can also be challenged by taking the antigen by mouth. The PK reaction has dropped out of fashion because it involves the injection of human serum.

Allergic asthma. In developed countries, allergic asthma occurs in about 5 percent of adults and almost twice as many children (42); the percentage is lower in developing countries (11, 23, 37, 74).

The sequence of events leading to an allergic asthma attack is similar to that of hay fever: the bronchial mucosa contains mast cells coated with IgE antibody against a specific antigen such as horse hair; inhalation of that antigen leads to mast-cell degranulation and bronchospasm.

Recent evidence indicates that macrophages in the bronchial mucosa or free in the bronchial lumen are activated and contribute a large share of inflammatory mediators (18). The key point to remember is that the *bronchi come under multiple attack by mast-cell and macrophage mediators:* histamine, leukotrienes, prostaglandin E_2, and platelet activating factor cooperate in causing bronchospasm, vascular leakage (which means mucosal edema), hypersecretion of mucus, and an infiltrate of eosinophils and other inflammatory cells. To make matters worse, some mediators such as PAF increase the responsiveness of the bronchi to other mediators (8, 57–59). Much of the damage is caused by the eosinophils (37).

Allergic asthma tends to become chronic; when this occurs, the bronchial mucosa shows changes of chronic inflammation (p. 280), which require anti-inflammatory treatment (6).

The term *asthma* was used in Hippocratic days to mean air hunger. Today it refers to an increased responsiveness of the bronchi, which become constricted in response to stimuli that would not affect normal lungs. The stimuli are sometimes clearly antigenic, but some are nonspecific, such as cold, exercise, or stress. The lungs are abnormally distended; the combination of constricted bronchi and distended lungs recalls the findings in guinea pig anaphylaxis (p. 533). The bronchi are partially plugged by an excess of mucus secretion. They also show an eosinophilic infiltration of the mucosa, and hypertrophy of the musculature.

Urticaria. This itchy rash (also called hives) is caused by local mast-cell degranulation of any kind, not just by the IgE mechanism (Figure 17.16). We mentioned hives in relation to anaphylactic shock. The name *urticaria* comes from the latin *urtica* for nettle. The rash appears very rapidly and can disappear in less than an hour, much like the sting of the nettle. As a matter of fact, the similarity goes much deeper. The weapon of the nettle is similar to a tiny glass syringe (Figure 17.17) which pierces the skin and injects—believe it or not—histamine and serotonin plus acetylcholine, which degranulates mast cells (39). Think how many millions of years it must have taken for the nettle to work out this mix of inflammatory mediators, including the refinement of adding to the histamine an agent that degranulates mast cells (as if saying "if my histamine doesn't bother you, maybe yours will").

Atopic dermatitis (or atopic eczema). This dermatitis is a weepy sort of rash that occurs in about 3 percent of children under 5 years old, as well as in adults; it does have an allergic, IgE–mast cell component, but its pathogenesis is much more complex and includes a cell-mediated response (21).

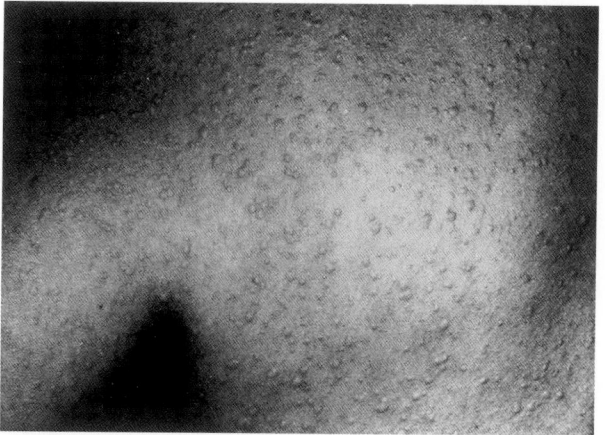

FIGURE 17.16   Close-up view of the skin in a case of severe urticaria (hives), characteristic of sudden, generalized mast-cell degranulation. In this case the degranulation was produced by an unusual mechanism: running in place for 10 minutes by a patient suffering from cholinergic urticaria. These patients are hypersensitive to cholinergic mediators; the mechanism is poorly understood. (Reproduced with permission from [28].)

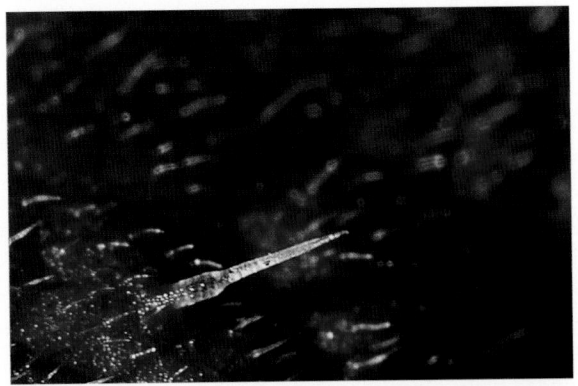

FIGURE 17.17   Stinging hair on the leaf of a nettle, a plant of the genus *Urtica*, ready to inflict *urticaria* by injecting a sophisticated mix of inflammatory mediators. (Magnification about × 25.)

Why Anaphylactic Responses Happen—Maybe

Anaphylactic responses are a nuisance at best, so why do they happen? Students never fail to ask this question, and neither do their teachers. Anaphylaxis kills and serves no purpose; asthma is crippling and sometimes fatal. Do these responses imply a wrong turn in the evolution of the immune system?

Nobody knows for sure, but here is a possible explanation: we may be dealing with an adaptation leftover from primal days when infestations with worms were prevalent. Consider the following facts: Worms tend to induce an IgE antibody response; all modern populations with a high "worm burden" also have a high plasma IgE titer and a high eosinophil count; local lesions caused by worms are rich in eosinophils, as are all anaphylactic responses (because degranulating mast cells produce chemotaxins for eosinophils); and finally, eosinophils appear to be specialized for killing worms (p. 337). Putting all this together, we can speculate that our distant, worm-ridden ancestors, having developed a high IgE titer, put it to use by evolving an IgE–mast-cell mechanism for attracting eosinophils—the best qualified cells for the job of killing such parasites. Although the worm burden has abated (at least in some places), we still respond to some environmental antigens, such as pollen instead of worms, by the same IgE–mast-cell mechanism—which has now become inappropriate.

Skeptic? Hear this. Guinea pigs attacked by ticks for the second time reject them by a basophil-related mechanism (72); whereas mice that are congenitally deficient in mast cells are unable to reject ticks, at least in one model (41).

Anaphylactoid Reactions

Red flag. This is a simple concept but a source of confusion. The key to avoiding confusion is to realize that we are momentarily stepping out of immunology: *mast cells can degranulate massively for a variety of reasons that have nothing to do with IgE or immunology.* The result is a generalized effect that *looks* anaphylactic (hypersensitivity Type 1) but is not; hence the name **anaphylactoid.** The agents capable of inducing this nonimmunologic effect are called **histamine liberators;** several hundred have been identified (31, 53).

This type of degranulation can occur in response to drugs, endogenous agents, cold, and even exercise and psychological mechanisms (2, 46). For reasons not understood, the degranulation response does not occur in all individuals. A small selection of histamine liberators is shown in Table 17.3; note that it includes complement products (anaphylatoxins). Among the drugs, note morphine; a compound called 48/80 is commonly used experimentally when it is necessary to deprive a rat of its mast cells. Remember that there are major species differences as well as local differences in the reactivity of mast cells (p. 344): *no single agent is known to degranulate them in all tissues.*

The name *anaphylactoid,* proposed by Selye in 1968 (69), means that the overall effect is virtually identical to that of anaphylaxis; in fact degranulation can be even faster (14). A classic setting is the intravenous administration of iodinated contrast media in preparation for X-ray workup (e.g., pyelography). Most patients develop acute symptoms within 1–3 minutes. Another classic setting, oddly enough, is an insect sting, which is usually cited as the typical example of the anaphylactic mechanism: bee venom contains at least three histamine liberators, melittin, phospholipase, and a "mast-cell degranulating peptide" (60). Treatment is the same as for anaphylaxis, which may explain why clinically oriented textbooks tend to ignore the anaphylactoid mechanism.

Table 17.3 Nonimmunologic Mast-Cell Degranulating Agents[a] (Histamine Liberators)

Morphine, opiates
Curare and other muscle relaxants
Radiocontrast media (intravenous)
Dextrans, iron-dextran; plasma expanders
Mannitol
Polymyxin B and other highly charged antibiotics
Many chemotherapeutic agents
Components of bee venom (MCD peptide, melittin)
Some foods (perhaps strawberries) (3)
Compound 48/80 (in experimental animals)
Egg white (intraperitoneal, in rats)

[a]These are just a few examples. Some agents (e.g., the first three items) affect only certain individuals; the reason is unknown.

From (References 3, 69, and 78).

NOTE: Two mechanisms can lead to an anaphylactoid response (7): (a) a direct effect on mast cells and (b) the intravascular activation of complement, most often due to intravenous injection of iodinated radiologic contrast media (22). Complement degranulates mast cells by means of C3a, C4a, and C5a, the so-called anaphylatoxins.

The main reason for our insistence on discussing the anaphylactoid response is that some drugs can unleash a catastrophic reaction that requires an instant response.

Dinner at a restaurant can provide a perfect example of histamine poisoning, unrelated to mast cells, and misnamed **scombroid poisoning.** It can happen with fish of the *scombridae* family (tuna, mackerel) but also with bluefish, sardines, and other fish (33, 45). Conditions required: (a) fish proteins containing much histidine; (b) sloppy fish cleaning, spilling bacteria that contain histidine decarboxylase; and (c) delayed refrigeration. A few mouthfuls (which may have a metallic or slightly peppery taste) provide the toxic dose. Symptoms: flushing, headache, racing pulse, vomiting, diarrhea, itching, swelling of the face and tongue, and sometimes wheezing. No deaths have occurred (one of us survived two episodes with tuna).

Hypersensitivity Type 2: Cytotoxic

This type of hypersensitivity is called *cytotoxic* because cells are killed, and to no good purpose. What happens is that antibody molecules become attached to specific target structures, cellular or extracellular, in the typical "claws down" or cytotoxic position. Antibodies are supposed to do just that—become attached to appropriate structures such as bacteria—and in so doing they are labeling those targets for destruction, either by complement or by leukocytes. In antibody-dependent cytotoxic hypersensitivity, *the antibodies are choosing a harmless target.*

NOTE: **How do antibodies work?** Until 2002, antibodies were thought to function mechanically, as labels conveying the message "DESTROY THIS." Then it was discovered that inside the antibody molecule is a sophisticated machinery capable of generating highly reactive oxygen species, including hydrogen peroxide and **ozone** (109a, 109b, 100a). This capacity leads us to recognize previously unsuspected mechanisms of bacterial killing—and of course also of collateral damage and autoimmune disease.

A carpet-like coating of antibody on a cell can cause at least three kinds of problems: it can cause complement to kill the labeled cell (Type 2a); it can cause leukocytes to do the same (Type 2b); and it can interfere with the function of the membrane receptors which it is covering (Type 2c).

Take another look at Table 17.1, and compare the mechanism of hypersensitivity Type 2 with Type 1. In Type 1, IgE antibodies are coating mast cells (in the cytophilic position, "claws up"). Elicitation causes mast cells to degranulate, but no cells are killed. In Type 2

the antibodies are IgG, IgM, or IgA; they are attached "claws down"; and their target is usually destroyed. Mast cells are not involved.

Hypersensitivity Reaction Type 2a: Antibody-Dependent Complement-Mediated Cytotoxicity

In this variety of cytotoxic hypersensitivity, a normal tissue component is being treated like a structure to destroy. One of the basic mechanisms for destroying bacteria or viruses is precisely to coat it with antibody. Roaming in the body fluids are two types of guardians ready to receive the message "DESTROY THIS" and to act accordingly (Figure 17.18). One is C1, the first component of complement, that beautiful flower-shaped molecule that floats around loking for microorganisms that need to be destroyed. When a molecule of C1 recognizes two properly spaced Fc segments, it becomes activated, and brings down a shower of membrane attack complexes (MACs). These MACs mercilessly perforate the labeled surface if it is a cell membrane. In the process of complement activation a split product of C3 is also produced (C3b, an opsonin) that attaches to the foreign surface and makes it more appetizing to phagocytes. So far, the carpet-of-antibody signal has brought down two curses on the labeled surface: perforation and phagocytosis. But this is not all.

Hypersensitivity Reaction Type 2b: Antibody-Dependent Cell-Mediated Cytotoxicity (ADCC)

The second type of roving guardian includes all leukocytes endowed with Fc receptors. If the invader is too large to be phagocytized in one gulp, the antibody label can take care of the matter by bringing onto the invader

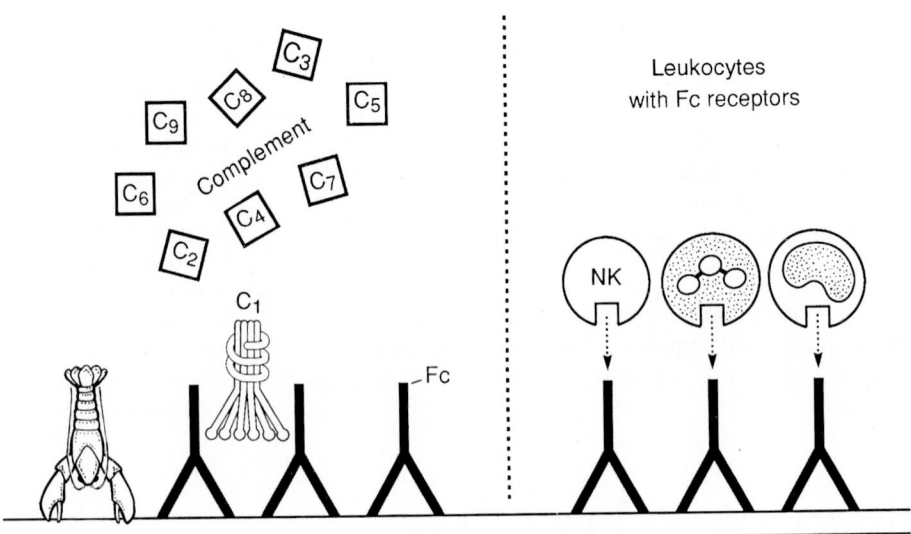

FIGURE 17.18 Surfaces coated with antibody can be attacked by two mechanisms: by complement (*left*) and by various types of leukocytes bearing receptors for the Fc portion of the globulin molecule (*right*). The result is known as antibody-dependent cytotoxicity, either complement-mediated or cell-mediated (ADCC). For these mechanisms to work, the immunoglobulin molecules must be bound "tails up."

yet other curses: NK cells, monocytes, neutrophils, and eosinophils. All these cell types bind to the carpet of Fc segments, become activated, blast it with granules and free radicals, and then crawl away to meet the next invader. ADCC, a stab-and-run mechanism, appears well suited for killing parasites too large to be phagocytized; eosinophils probably use it in their attack on worms (Figures 17.19, 17.20, and 17.21) (82, 83). This is the same phenomenon that we described earlier as *frustrated surface phagocytosis* (p. 418), which occurs when a phagocyte flattens itself against an object too large to engulf. However, it looks (to us) much more

like a purposeful kiss of death than an act of frustration. The problem with ADCC is the difficulty of proving that it actually occurs *in vivo*.

Note a cunning feature of the leukocyte Fc receptors: they bind tightly to Fc segments presented by antibodies fixed on a surface, but they bind very loosely to free antibody molecules. This is advantageous. If the surface of the leukocytes had a high affinity for Fc fragments, the leukocyte would always be coated and would lose the freedom to bind where necessary.

Hypersensitivity Reaction Type 2c: Antibody-Dependent Cellular Dysfunction

This variant of antibody-related hypersensitivity is due to the formation of antibodies (autoantibodies) against cell-membrane receptors. The receptors usually affected belong to endocrine cells or to neuromuscular junctions; *the effect of the antibody binding to the receptor can be either blocking or stimulating*. Examples will be presented in relation to autoimmune disease.

Diseases Produced by Cytotoxic (Type 2) Hypersensitivity

The binding of antibody to a surface causes disease when the surface thus marked for destruction is a normal part of the body. Examples:

ABO mismatch. In an ABO-mismatched blood transfusion, the foreign surfaces are those of the injected, mismatched red blood cells; they are recognized and coated by a natural antibody in the plasma of the ill-matched recipient, and instantly attacked by complement (Table 17.4).

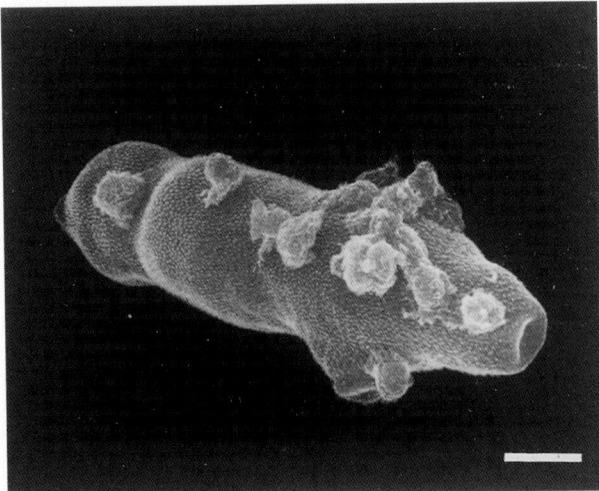

FIGURE 17.19 Scanning electron micrograph: leukocytes adhering to a schistosomulum that was preincubated in antibody and complement. **Bar** = 10 μm. (Reproduced from the **Journal of Cell Biology**, 1980;86:46–63, by copyright permission of The Rockefeller University Press [82].)

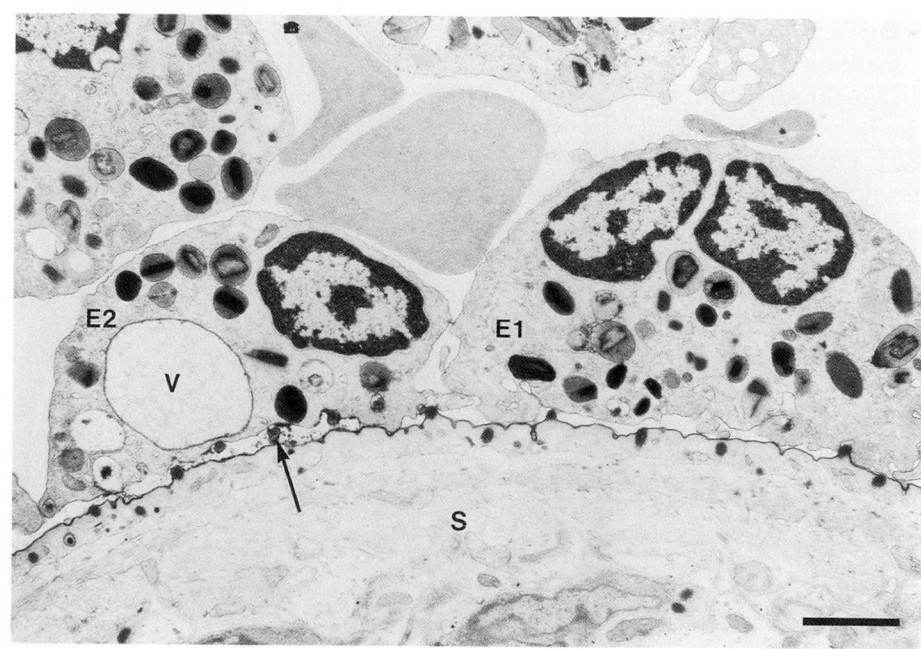

FIGURE 17.20 After 2 minutes of incubation with Schistosome larvae, two eosinophils (**E1, E2**) attacking a larva (**S**). **E1** is simply attached; **E2** has begun to degranulate against the larval surface (**arrow** points to dense material probably discharged by the eosinophil). This type of attack may lead to death of the parasite. Vacuoles such as **V** are formed by the membranes of discharged granules. **Bar** = 1 μm. (Reproduced with permission from [83], © American Society for Investigative Pathology.)

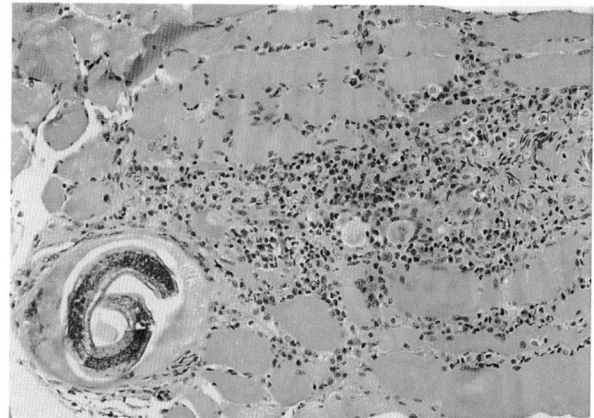

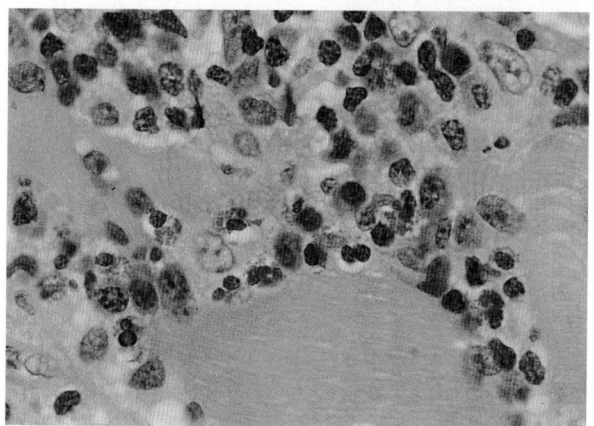

FIGURE 17.21 Striated muscle of a patient who ate raw pork as a delicacy. *Top:* Overview; the 6-shaped worm is *Trichinella spiralis.* Muscle damage and chronic inflammation. (100x) *Bottom:* Detail of the chronic inflammatory infiltrate: many plasma cells and eosinophils. (600x)

Table 17.4 Blood Groups of the ABO Series[a]

Blood Group	Contains Antigen	Contains Antibody	Will Hemolyse
A	A	Anti-B	B
B	B	Anti-A	A
AB	A & B	—	—
O	H	Anti-A & anti-B	A & B

[a]The series responsible for the most severe transfusion reactions.

The ABO system works as follows. Human red blood cells carry a number of antigens including two major ones called A and B. The red blood cells of an individual may be A, B, AB, or O (with neither antigen). Now a peculiar fact complicates the situation: individuals with type A blood also carry ready-made anti-B antibodies in their blood, type B individuals carry anti-A, type O individuals carry both anti-A and anti-B, and type AB individuals carry neither antibody. You may wonder how anyone who has never been exposed to foreign red blood cells could have antibodies against them. These antibodies are probably against antigens of the flora of the gut, which happen to be very similar to antigens on red blood cells.

With this premise, imagine an A individual receiving B blood. Because type A blood carries anti-B antibodies, the transfused B cells are greeted by instant antibody coating followed by complement activation, massive hemolysis, and generalized capillary obstruction by red blood cell aggregates. The symptoms of this major emergency resemble those of anaphylaxis because of the release of complement anaphylatoxins C5a and C3a, which cause mast-cell and basophil degranulation.

Mother-fetus mismatch (Rh hemolytic disease of the newborn). To have wiped out this disease is one of the triumphs of medicine (96). The setting, much simplified: an RhD-negative woman becomes pregnant by an RhD-positive father. If the first baby conceived is RhD positive, the normal trickle of fetal blood into the mother's blood, during the pregancy and during birth, will cause the mother to generate IgG antibodies. IgG antibodies cross the placental barrier and hemolyse the red blood cells of the fetus by a hypersensitivity Type 2 mechanism (Figure 17.22); hemolysis generates bilirubin, which is highly toxic for the fetal brain (recall the *Kernicterus,* p. 119). The firstborn may be spared, but the problem becomes worse with succeeding pregnancies. Prevention: inject the mother with anti-RhD immunoglobulin starting at the 28th week (96).

> **NOTE:** This disease is still called *erythroblastosis foetalis,* because the destruction of red blood cells causes the fetus to generate an enormous volume of immature red blood cells, *erythroblasts,* in the liver and elsewhere, and this was once thought to be the disease.

Normal surfaces become antigenic. A normal surface is sometimes made foreign by a pathologic mechanism. The most common offenders are drugs, which can combine with surface molecules of any kind of blood cells and make them antigenic; the resulting antibodies—depending on the target cell—will then deplete the patient's erythrocytes, granulocytes, or platelets (anemia, agranulocytosis, and thrombocytopenia). Why this happens in some individuals is not known.

Normal basement membranes become antigenic in Goodpasture's disease, a hemorrhagic condition of the lungs and kidneys (p. 592).

Targeting allografts. Vascular endothelium of an allograft is recognized by the recipient's immune system as foreign. Coating of the graft's blood vessels by antibody is one of the mechanisms of rejection (p. 576).

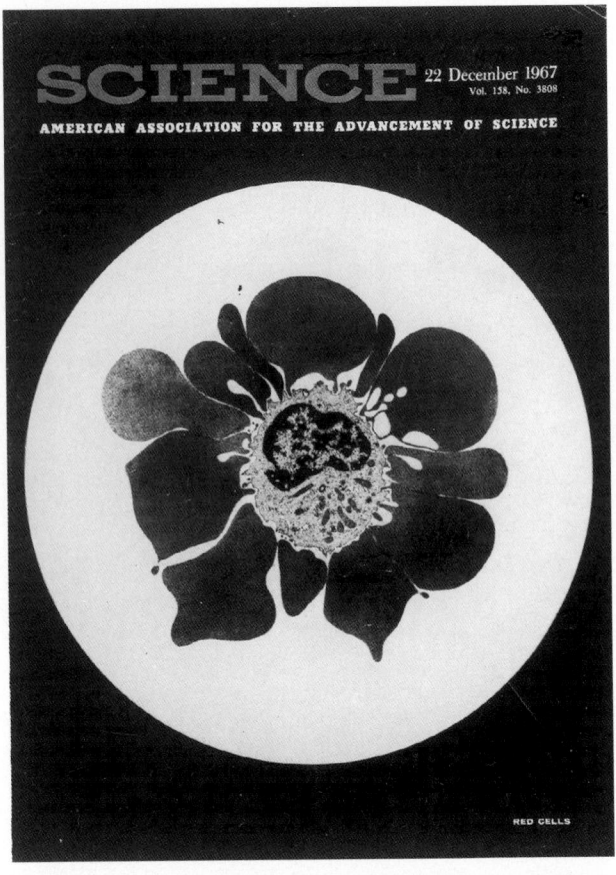

FIGURE 17.22 Classic "rosette" of red blood cells attached to a human monocyte. The mechanism: some anti-red blood cell antibodies, including autoantibodies, fix little or no complement but cause the red blood cells to become very sticky for monocytes. This sticking is followed in due time, by phagocytosis. Such is the sequence of events in *erythroblastosis foetalis,* caused by Rh incompatibility. (Reprinted by permission from [100]. Copyright 1967 by the American Association for the Advancement of Science.)

Hypersensitivity Type 3: Complex-Mediated

Type 3 hypersensitivity (Table 17.1) is based on the fact that antibodies combine with soluble antigens to form antigen–antibody *complexes* (also called immune complexes). The complexes activate complement, which attracts leukocytes, and damage occurs. Here is a paradox: complex formation is precisely what antibodies are supposed to do when they encounter bacterial products, viruses, and other antigens in solution. How does this defensive mechanism become dangerous? Very simple: when large amounts of complex are formed, large amounts of complement are activated, and large numbers of activated leukocytes appear on the scene. Activated leukocytes can be, as we have seen many times, dangerous cells. Type 3 hypersensitivity occurs when the body is flooded with antigen; in some cases the masses of complexes are large enough to plug capillaries. Too much is too much, especially when complement and leukocytes are involved.

> NOTE: *What we call "complexes" in vivo correspond to precipitates in vitro.* It follows that complex disease occurs only with those antigens that induce precipitating antibodies in the laboratory.

We may be belaboring the obvious, but let it be clear that by *complexes* we mean *antigen–antibody complexes,* not lumps of antigen.

Let us try to visualize the role of antigen–antibody complexes in a hypersensitive reaction. When large amounts of polyvalent antigens react with antibodies that are floating free in the extracellular spaces (rather than fixed to surfaces), the complexes aggregate and form fluffy masses, bristling with Fc tails (i.e., lobster tails, with the claws pointing inward, clinging to antigen). Now, as we just explained for hypersensitivity Type 2, body fluids (and especially the blood) contain two kinds of roving guardians on the lookout for carpets of antibodies: complement (C1,) and cells with Fc receptors. In Type 2 hypersensitivity, the carpets are formed on fixed substrates, mostly cell membranes, and the roving guardians focus their attacks on those cells. In Type 3, it is the outer surfaces of the antigen–antibody complexes that is attacked. Of course, attack on the complexes does no harm, but damage is caused to any cells that happen to be lying around. The main culprits are neutrophils, which in their "feeding frenzy" release their arsenal of granules and free radicals (p. 334).

To clarify these mechanisms, we will describe two classic models in which complexes are formed experimentally *in vivo.* To do so we must choose antigens capable of inducing precipitating antibodies (otherwise there will be no complexes); and the antibodies must activate complement (IgG and IgM fill the bill; IgA can activate complement by the alternative pathway).

- In the first model of complex-mediated hypersensitivity, antigen is injected *into the skin* of an animal previously immunized against that antigen; in this case the complexes form mainly *in the tissues* at the site of reinjection. This is therefore a model of *local* complex-mediated hypersensitivity.
- In the second model, antigen and antibody are caused to meet in the bloodstream; complexes therefore cause injury primarily in the *vascular system.* This is therefore a model of *general* complex-mediated hypersensitivity.

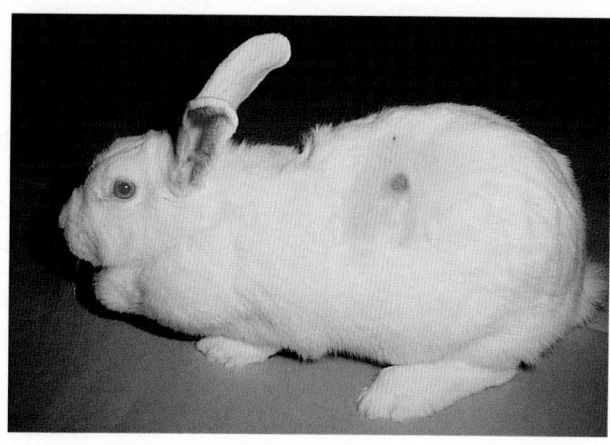

FIGURE 17.23 Arthus reaction. This rabbit was sensitized to bovine gamma globulin with six subcutaneous injections (one every 3 days, in different sites). The seventh injection produced this hemorrhagic necrosis, photographed 1 day later.

A Model of Local Complex-Mediated Hypersensitivity: The Arthus Phenomenon

The **Arthus phenomenon** consists of the development of a hemorrhagic, necrotic skin lesion where antigen has been injected into an animal previously immunized against that antigen (Figure 17.23).

We should first introduce Dr. Maurice Arthus (you may pronounce *Arthus* the English way, as long as you realize that it should be French). In the late 1800's lives were being saved by treating cases of diphtheria, tetanus, and scarlet fever with a new method discovered in 1890 by von Behring: subcutaneous injections of "antitoxins" (i.e., serum from immunized horses). When two such injections were given a few weeks apart, a local swelling sometimes appeared after the second injection. Why? In 1903 Dr. Arthus (80) tried to answer this question. Working at the Pasteur Institute in Lille, France, he injected horse serum subcutaneously and aseptically to some rabbits, 5 ml every 6 days *in different places.* A few hours after the fourth injection, a soft edema appeared at the injection site; the fifth and sixth injections produced a firmer swelling; the seventh and eighth injection caused a hemorrhagic patch (Figure 17.23) that became necrotic and eventually healed. Dr. Arthus did not study the mechanism but warned clinicians that horse serum, if injected repeatedly, could cause local necrosis. We should add that *when local changes develop, they begin to appear 4–6 hours after the injection* (we will soon see why).

Eventually the mechanism was worked out (Figure 17.24) (84, 86, 95). The injections of horse serum are absorbed, and the rabbit becomes increasingly hyperimmunized. By the seventh injection there

ARTHUS REACTION

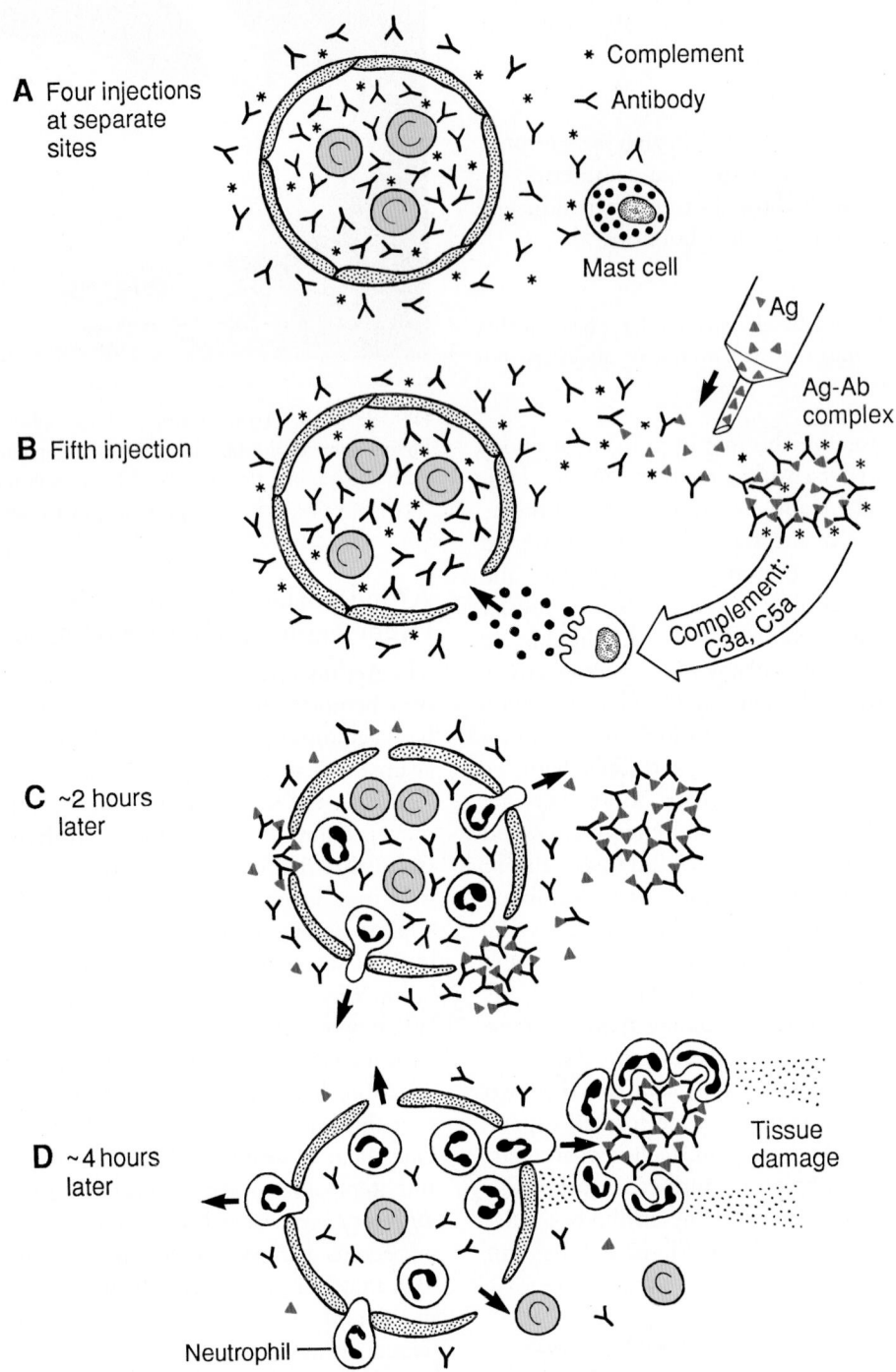

FIGURE 17.24 Mechanism of vascular injury by the Arthus reaction. **A:** Conditions that predispose to an Arthus reaction: precipitating antibodies are present in the plasma and also in the interstitium, where mast cells lie waiting. **B:** Injection of antigen at this stage creates antigen–antibody complexes, which activate complement; anaphylatoxins of complement (C3a, C4a, C5a) degranulate the mast cells, releasing histamine, which creates gaps in the venules. **C:** Antibody escapes through the venular gaps and creates massive antigen–antibody complexes. Complement activation produces chemotactic molecules, by which neutrophil emigration is initiated. **D:** Activated neutrophils phagocytize the complexes; in the process they release enzymes that cause further damage to the vascular wall and surrounding tissues. The venular basement membrane is also digested, which explains the escape of red blood cells into the tissues (hemorrhage).

is so much *antibody in the circulation and interstitial spaces* that a large subcutaneous injection of antigen can react with it and create a massive amount of antigen–antibody complex. Exactly where the initial meeting of antigen and antibody occurs has not been determined, but we believe there is enough antibody in the extracellular fluid to initiate the reaction; also, the trauma of the needle might cause some mixing of blood and injected serum. Anyway, as soon as some complex forms, the first component of complement, C1, settles on it and activates the complement cascade; anaphylatoxins are released (C3a, C4a, and C5a), the mast cells degranulate and release histamine, endothelial gaps develop in the venules, and large amounts

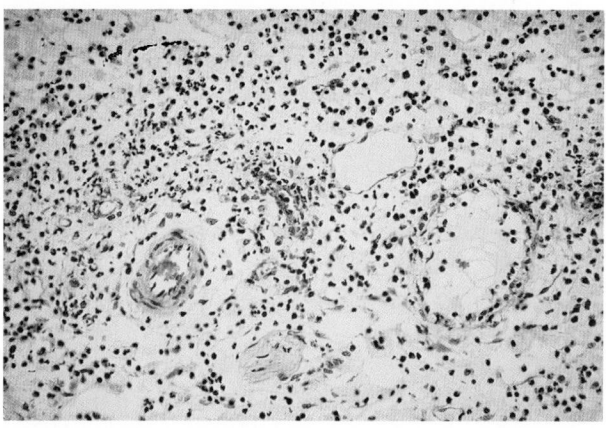

FIGURE 17.26 Typical inflammatory infiltrate of an Arthus lesion. *Right:* Dilated venule with prominent margination and diapedesis; the venular wall is on the way to destruction. *Left:* Arteriole, unaffected. From the skin of a rabbit hyperimmunized against bovine albumin, 4 hours after the seventh local injection of albumin. (Note: In the rabbit the neutrophils, which predominate here, appear as "pseudo-eosinophils.") (150x)

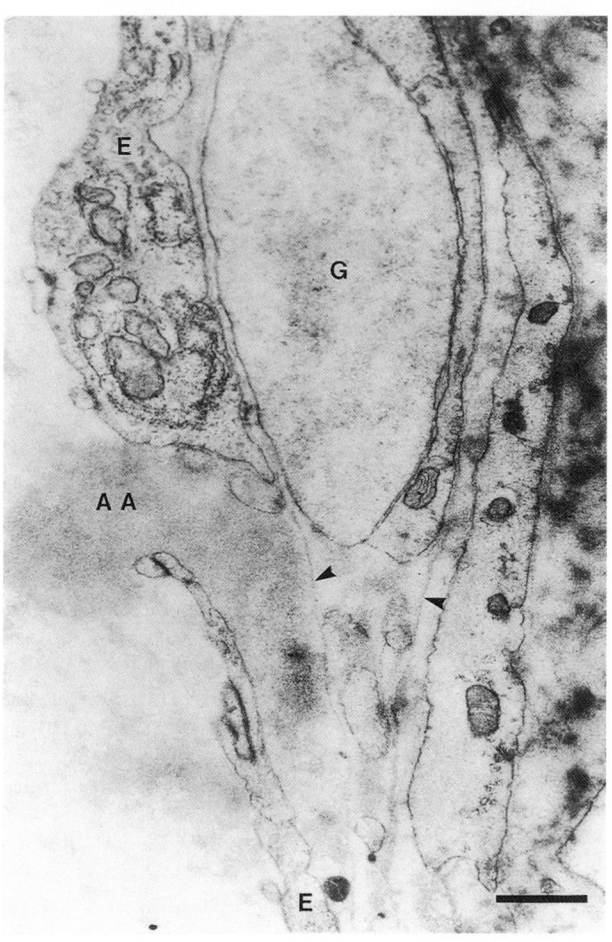

FIGURE 17.25 Electron micrograph of ongoing Arthus reaction in the wall of a rabbit venule (3 minutes after injection of antigen). Note the gap in the endothelium filled with an amorphous mass of antigen–antibody complex. **E:** Endothelium. **G:** Emigrating granulocyte. **AA:** Antigen–antibody complex. **Arrowheads:** Basement membrane. **Bar** = 1 μm. (Reproduced with permission from [102], © American Society for Investigative Pathology.)

of intravascular antibody combine with the antigen. Electron micrographs actually show fluffy masses of complex in the lumen; leukocytes are also attracted (Figure 17.25) (80, 104).

The crowd of granulocytes attracted by complement chemotaxins is remarkable; in principle the granulocytes are summoned to remove the complex, but in their fury of activation they spill enough enzymes and free radicals to destroy the venular wall as they cross it (Figure 17.26). The Arthus phenomenon was one of the first lesions to reveal the destructive power of the otherwise friendly neutrophils. *No Arthus lesion can be produced in an animal depleted of leukocytes or of complement* (86, 95, 109). As for the hemorrhage and necrosis observable with the naked eye, they are explained by the venular lesions just described; the delay of 4–6 hours is the time required for all these events to unfold.

> The Arthus phenomenon lends itself to classic immunologic games: it can be obtained as a *passive Arthus* (serum from a prepared rabbit is given intravenously to a second rabbit, which becomes immediately able to produce an Arthus reaction upon injection with antigen); or a *reversed passive Arthus* (antigen is injected intravenously, and antibody is injected locally: an Arthus lesion develops promptly if the doses are right) (95).

In a modern clinical setting, a skin reaction as Arthus described it should never be seen because proteins should not be injected locally in large amounts as they were 100 years ago. However, the basic mechanism is at work in a variety of lesions thought to be caused by complexes—for example, in the *vasculitis* produced in the "serum sickness" model of complex-induced disease, as we will now explain.

General Model of Complex-Mediated Hypersensitivity: Serum Sickness

As often happens in immunology, this mechanism of disease was first observed clinically, then worked out in the laboratory.

Clinical serum sickness. This condition used to be called "**serum fever**" or "**serum rash**" because of the clinical symptoms that appear after a *single* large subcutaneous injection of horse serum. The condition has almost vanished in its original form, because injections of horse serum are rarely indicated (99). However, serum sickness is still with us because it can be produced by a different mechanism: *a number of drugs—as a side effect—combine with plasma proteins and turn them into antigens.* The result is the same as with serum sickness: *a lot of foreign protein circulating in the blood* (94).

We hope the reader was intrigued by the "catch" planted in the previous paragraph: serum sickness was caused by a *single* injection of serum, whereas immune responses are typically induced by a second challenge. Strange but true. There is no breaking of immunologic rules. *In reading what follows, keep in mind that a single large subcutaneous injection of antigen is absorbed by the lymphatics over many days, and basically works like a series of daily injections.*

The natural history of serum sickness was worked out in 1905 by von Pirquet and Schick in the Department of Scarlet Fever and Diphtheria at the St. Anna pediatric hospital in Vienna. The work was reported in a small book called *Serumkrankheit.*

> When Dr. Schick was asked to revise the book 45 years later, he found nothing to change and so republished it as it was (108). We know of very few books that could stand that test; another is Metchnikoff's *Lectures on the Comparative Pathology of Inflammation,* which was reprinted in a paperback edition after 77 years (101).

The children in that Viennese hospital ward were treated for diphtheria or scarlet fever with antibodies from immunized horses; in practice this required huge subcutaneous doses (up to 200 ml) of horse serum. Eight to 12 days later the "Serumkrankheit" was expected; its incidence increased with the dose of serum (85 percent after 100–200 ml, 22 percent after 10–30 ml). The signs and symptoms were very much the same as those seen today in cases of drug hypersensitivity:

- A slight but painful swelling of the regional lymph nodes draining the injection site (the nodes were beginning to make antihorse-serum antibody).
- Fever and an uncomfortable itchy rash.
- Some edema, or rather fluid retention, not always visible (it was von Pirquet who first had the idea of judging the extent of edema by weighing the patient) (Figure 17.27).
- Joint pains, which were common and significant though the objective signs were minimal.
- A precipitous drop in the number of leukocytes in the peripheral blood when the symptoms appeared (presumably because the leukocytes, activated by mast-cell PAF, tend to clump, and the clumps are filtered out by the lungs).
- A mild albuminuria, but no renal disease ever developed.

Overall, *serum sickness was a nuisance but not a life-threatening event;* no patient ever died of it though two came close (107). For the Viennese team, the nuisance was acceptable because there was no alternative treatment. Antitoxic serum was the only rational therapy available. What had been tried previously was hopelessly empirical: intravenous injections of lamb blood or of milk with sugar (108). Anyway, the antisera really helped (105), and mortality by diphtheria dropped dramatically (Figure 17.28). Von Behring, the pioneer of this treatment, was rewarded with the Nobel prize.

> Test your grasp of the antibody response. Von Pirquet and Schick reported that some children had to receive *two* injections of horse serum: for example, the first to treat diphtheria, the second to treat scarlet fever. In these cases the timing of the second attack of serum sickness differed according to the interval between the first and second injection of serum. The pattern observed depended on whether the two treatments were separated by 2 to 6 weeks, 6 weeks to 6 months, or more than 6 months. Why? The answer is in Figure 17.29 (108).

Pathogenesis of Serum Sickness: Enter the Rabbit

Serum sickness remained somewhat obscure until the late 1960s. One of its puzzling features was that it broke the two-shot rule of immunology: the immune response appeared after a single injection of foreign protein. The mechanism was finally worked out by Dixon, Cochrane, and others using rabbits injected with bovine serum albumin (85, 90). The basic method of this study was to maintain, to begin with, the one-shot

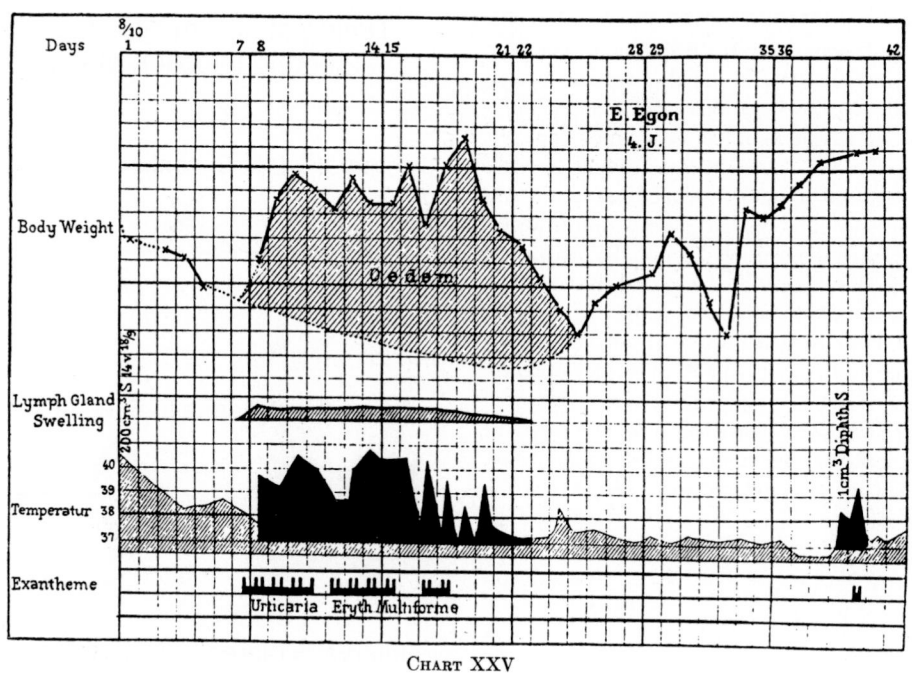

CHART XXV

FIGURE 17.27   Manifestations of serum sickness in a 4-year-old child hospitalized for diphtheria around the year 1900. Upon admission he received 200 ml of antidiphtheric serum subcutaneously. Typically, on day 8, urticaria and swelling of the lymph nodes developed. Fever appeared shortly thereafter. The skin eruption changed aspect after a few days; this also is typical. The generalized edema was assessed by changes in body weight. On the day 39, note the effect of a subcutaneous injection of 1.0 ml of "diphtheria serum for immunization." This time the response is immediate: fever and rash. See text for explanation. (Original diagram from [108].)

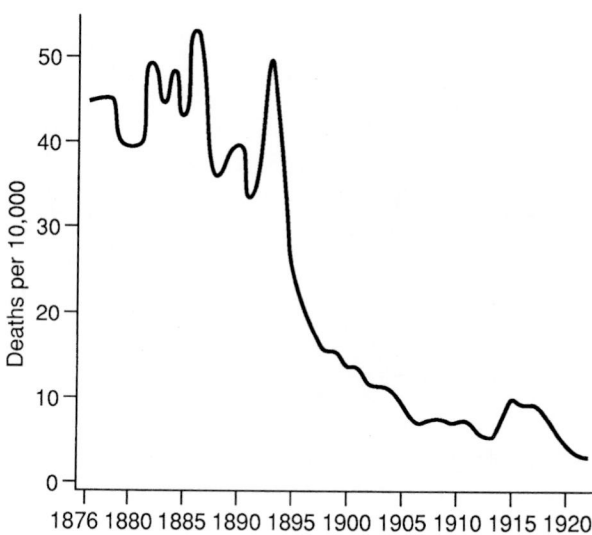

FIGURE 17.28   Drop in mortality from diphtheria coincident with the availability of anti-diphtheric serum (Prussia, about 1895; children under 15). The morbidity remained unchanged. (Redrawn from [105].)

injection but to give the dose intravenously, a more controllable route.

The main findings are summarized in Figure 17.30, which has become a classic. In essence: the amount of circulating antigen drops, slowly at first as it is phagocytized or escapes from the blood, and then faster as it is bound by increasing amounts of newly formed antibody. For 12 days no free antibody can be found because as long as antigen circulates, all the antibody is complexed. At about day 13 all the *injected antigen* has been used up (either phagocytized or complexed) and now *free antibody* appears. Morphologic injury develops (reversibly) between days 8 and 15, mainly in the "blood container" in which the complexes circulate (heart and arteries), in the blood filters (the renal glomeruli), and in the joints (reminiscent of clinical serum sickness). *The lesions are mild and reversible because the supply of antigen is limited by the one-shot approach.*

That lesions develop in the blood container seems to make sense, but then why do lesions spare the venous side? And why are the joints affected? We found no satisfactory answers.

FIGURE 17.29   This diagram answers the question, "Can one have serum sickness twice in a row?" using data reported by von Pirquet and Schick in 1905. Syringes indicate injection of horse serum; arrows indicate recurrence of serum sickness. The left part of the diagram shows that after the first injection of horse serum, serum sickness (**red square**) developed between 8 and 12 days. *Top:* If a second injection was given within 6 weeks, serum sickness reappeared immediately because the patient still had circulating antibodies. *Center:* If the second injection was given between 6 weeks and 6 months after the first, serum sickness again reappeared immediately because of some circulating antibody, and memory cells produced a third episode of serum sickness (an accelerated reaction) about a week later. *Bottom:* If the second injection was given more than 6 months after the first, no circulating antibody was left; so there was no immediate reaction, but the memory cells produced an accelerated reaction after less than a week.

Timing of serum sickness after a second injection of serum

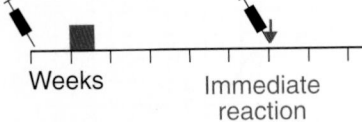

Interval = 2 to 6 weeks

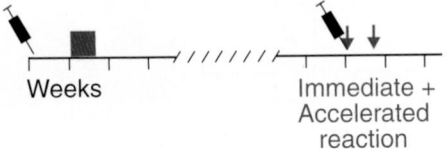

Interval = 6 weeks to 6 months

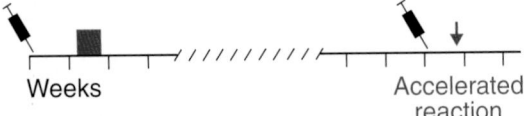

Interval = more than 6 months

FIGURE 17.30   Sequence of events in classic "one-shot" serum sickness in the rabbit. No antibody is detected in the blood before day 13 because it combines with antigen and forms complexes. After all the antigen has been complexed, antibody can be detected. Note the behavior of complement, which correlates with complex formation. The colored area indicates the time and intensity of lesions. (Redrawn with permission from [89]. Illustration by Hospital Practice.)

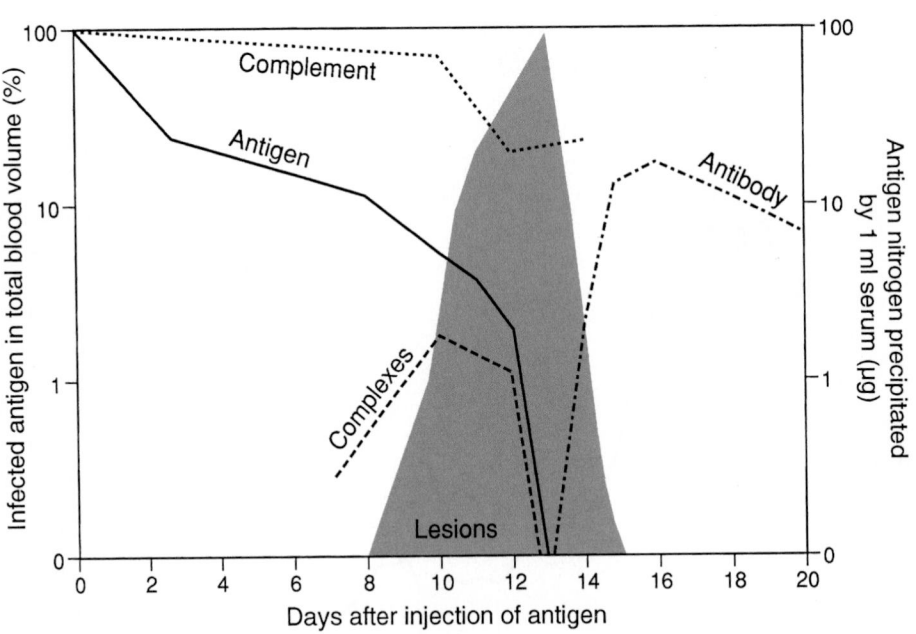

Human diseases caused by the serum-sickness mechanism are usually chronic, which means that the supply of complexes is also chronic. Therefore, a *chronic model* of experimental serum sickness was developed, by giving rabbits daily injections of antigen (91). These experiments became especially important because they showed that *the size of the complexes is critical;* and their size, as you may recall, depends on the relative concentrations of antigen and circulating antibody (Figure 17.31). This means that the size of the complexes

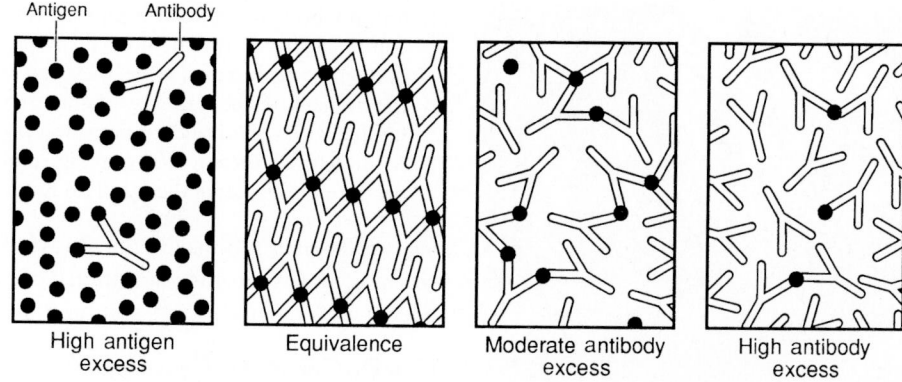

FIGURE 17.31   Antigen–antibody complexes vary in size depending on the concentration of the reactants. When complexes develop in the bloodstream, the larger complexes (formed at the equivalence point) are easily removed by the RES/MPS and cause no harm; the complexes more apt to cause damage are those of medium size, which develop in moderate antibody excess. (Adapted from 6 Immunology, VII Clinical Immunology in WebMD Scientific American ® Medicine, Dale DC, Federman DD (ed). WebMD Corporation, New York, 2003 [62].)

depends on the antibody response of the rabbit:

- *Some rabbits produce huge amounts of antibody.* Complexes formed under such conditions— antibody excess—are very large, easily removed by the littoral phagocytes of the RES (p. 316), and little or no disease ensues.

- *Other rabbits are "minimal responders,"* which leads to very small complexes as expected from the condition of antigen excess. Such complexes are too small to activate complement and to be pathogenic.

- *Medium responders are most at risk.* Their complexes are just large enough to be pathogenic but small enough to circulate for a long time; they become trapped in filtering organs, activate complement, and cause disease.

Question: why do the various rabbits respond differently? Is it not true that the immune response is programmed, and thus should proceed in a standard fashion? The unsatisfactory answer is that even though the immune response is certainly programmed, individuals have different responses, quantitatively and sometimes even qualitatively. The individual's genetic makeup is important; just consider that not everybody becomes allergic to pollen.

The lesions in experimental serum sickness are important as a model for human diseases. Because complexes are developing in the blood, lesions develop in the blood container and its main filter: the arteries, the heart, and the glomeruli. Not every detail is understood (91); surprisingly, the localization in the joints is still not explained.

Arteritis. Inflammation of the arteries is focal and hits only the small branches, especially those of the coronaries (Figure 17.32). Visualize the lesion of arteritis as a small sphere of acute inflammation encasing a short segment of an artery; typically, the wall is necrotic and infiltrated with fibrin (a combination empirically described as **fibrinoid necrosis**). Immunofluorescence shows antigen, antibody, and complement in the lesion.

There is no doubt that the medial necrosis is caused by the activated polymorphs, attracted by activated complement; but beyond this, the pathogenesis of complex-induced arteritis is not clear. Complexes are too large to cross the endothelium. To overcome this difficulty the following theoretical sequence has been proposed (81, 97): the circulating antigen induces some IgE (as well as IgG and IgM) → the IgE sensitizes mast cells and circulating basophils → some basophils settle on the arterial intima and release histamine → endothelial gaps are formed → the door opens for he complexes. As far as we know, *the basophil mechanism is purely theoretical. It has never been verified.* We prefer to believe that all the proteins involved cross the endothelium by transcytosis and then react within the arterial wall.

Cardiac lesions. Lesions are especially obvious on the valves. Small platelet masses (thrombi) attach to the luminal surfaces of the valve flaps where they come into contact when the valves snap shut: this area is thought to be prone to microtrauma, especially if the valves are distorted. It is conceivable that small patches of endothelium are removed by this mechanism; complexes could then penetrate into the underlying connective tissue, activate complement, attract leukocytes, and induce platelet deposition—but this is largely speculative. There are also diffuse mononuclear cell inflammatory infiltrates throughout the heart.

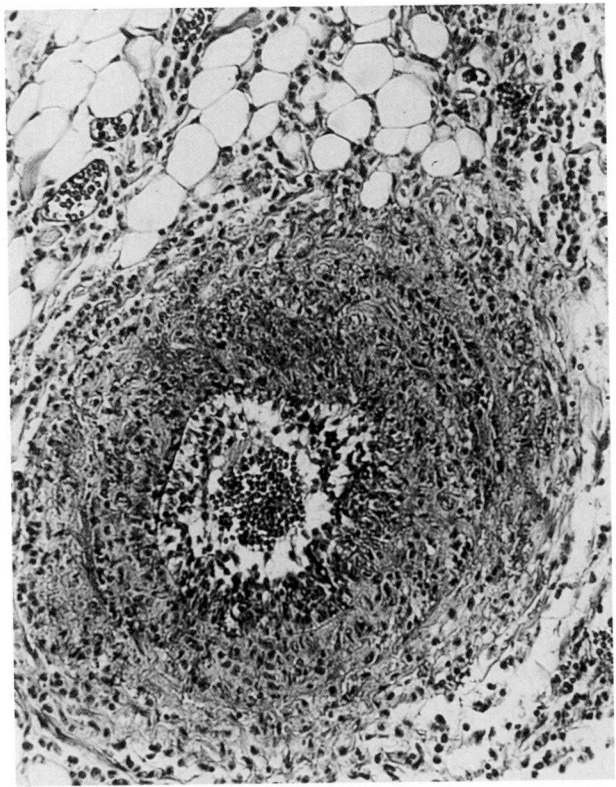

FIGURE 17.32 Arteritis in experimental serum sickness (rabbit). The intima is attacked and destroyed by leukocytes; in a more advanced stage the media is also destroyed. The main inflammatory cell is the neutrophil (not recognizable here). (Courtesy of Dr. C. G. Cochrane, Department of Immunology, Research Institute of Scripps Clinic, La Jolla, CA.)

Glomerular lesions. These lesions are partially accounted for by the filtering mechanism: lumps of protein precipitate appear along the capillary basement membrane (Figure 17.33) (p. 553). Oddly enough, electron microscopy sometimes shows them on the *outer* surface of the basement membrane, which would seem analogous to finding coffee grounds on the brew side of a coffee filter. One explanation is that antigens seep through the basement membrane filter and form complexes with antibodies where they are stopped—against the surfaces of the podocytes. However, a number of factors, such as molecular charge, affect the deposition of the complexes. Ultimately, this buildup of foreign material leads to hyperplasia of the mesangial cells (which lie outside the capillaries and phagocytize the complexes) and of the Bowman's capsule (Figure 17.34).

> Here is a challenge. Neutrophils are always attracted by complexes, yet the glomerular lesions of serum sickness are notoriously poor in neutrophils. Depletion of leukocytes abolishes arteritis but not glomerular lesions. This remains a mystery. We propose our own explanation, which has

not yet been tested: the lumps of complex do activate complement, but the chemotactic by-products are washed out with the filtrate before they can diffuse back into the lumen of the capillary. Glomerular capillaries are unique with regard to their perfusion physiology: they filter under high pressure (60 mm Hg, almost four times the pressure in skin capillaries) and do not reabsorb.

Injury of the joints. Joints are not always affected in serum sickness, but when they are, injury consists of synovial edema with fibrin deposits and mononuclear infiltrates.

How Do Complexes Cause Injury?

The most convincing experiment showing that leukocytes cause damage in complex-induced lesions is to test animals that have been depleted of leukocytes with

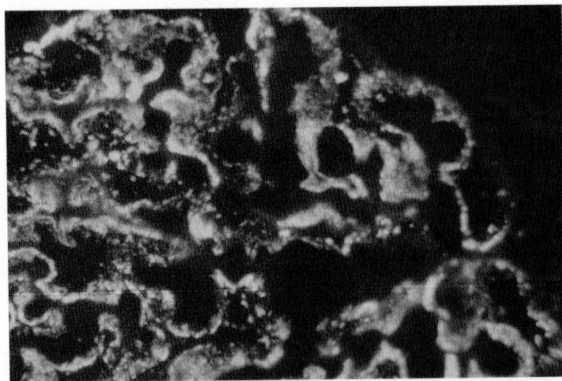

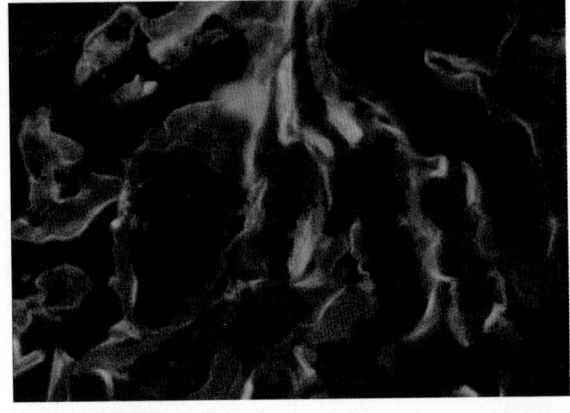

FIGURE 17.33 Glomerular tufts: Immunofluorescence staining of the glomerular basement membrane using antihuman IgG antibody. *Top:* Typical "lumpy-bumpy" pattern of fluorescence is due to clumps of antigen–antibody complexes deposited along the capillary basement membrane; from a patient with membranous glomerulonephritis (of unknown cause). *Bottom:* This linear (continuous) pattern of fluorescence occurs when the basement membrane is evenly coated with IgG antibody; from a patient with Goodpasture's disease, caused by an antibody against the glomerular basement membrane. (Courtesy of Dr. E. Galvanek, Brigham and Women's Hospital, Boston, MA.)

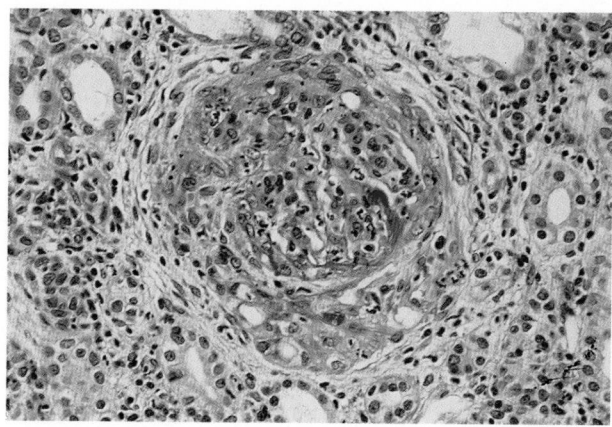

FIGURE 17.34   Glomerulus from the kidney of a rabbit in which chronic serum sickness was induced. The glomerular tuft contains many granulocytes. It has been squeezed to about half its normal size by hyperplasia of the cells lining Bowman's capsule. (250x) (Specimen kindly supplied by Dr. C. G. Cochrane, Scripps Clinic, La Jolla, CA.)

nitrogen mustard or antileukocyte serum (91). In such animals Arthus lesions, arteritis, and synovitis are suppressed even though the masses of complexes are present; the suppression occurs also if complement is depleted (84).

The mediation of glomerular injury is more complicated; it depends in part on the type of antibody involved. If rabbits are injected with IgG1 anti-glomerular–basement membrane antibodies, the resulting glomerular injury is neutrophil-dependent; with IgG2 antibodies it is not. In the latter case, the mediation of the injury is not yet known (90).

> NOTE: We should warn our readers that the mechanisms whereby complexes are deposited in the glomeruli are many and complicated (p. 552).

A basic question: how do the lesions of serum sickness relate to the Arthus lesion? Answer: they are very similar. *The neutrophil-rich lesions of serum sickness are essentially small Arthus lesions;* both types of lesion are caused by a local deposit of complex that summons a swarm of leukocytes. Remember that in both local and general models of disease, we are dealing with the same basic principle: complex-induced injury. The glomerular lesions of serum sickness are special because they depend largely on the function of filtration, but they also depend on complexes that activate complement and attract leukocytes.

Von Pirquet and Schick sometimes injected children with a second dose of serum: did this produce Arthus lesions? In fact, they did notice local redness and swelling, although not an all-out, necrotic, and hemorrhagic Arthus lesion. These local changes were noticed even a week or so after the first injection. Presumably enough antigen was left over at the injection site to react with the newly formed antibody.

Human Diseases Mediated by Antigen–Antibody Complexes

Antigen–antibody complexes are thought to participate in many human diseases. How are these diseases recognized? Microscopy is helpful: any focal arteritis or vasculitis is suspect. The next step is to analyze the lesions by immunohistochemistry: if complexes are present, they should be demonstrable with antibodies against complement and against immunoglobulin (representing antibody). The search for antigen is far more difficult because in most cases there is no clue as to what it may be. There are also methods for identifying complexes in the blood, even if the antigen is unknown (90).

The best examples of complex-mediated diseases in humans are *polyarteritis nodosa* and *glomerulonephritis;* two others, *systemic lupus erythematosus* and *rheumatoid arthritis* will be described in relation to autoimmune disease (pp. 590, 591).

Serum sickness in its classic form has almost disappeared, for obvious reasons; however, it can still develop occasionally in different clinical settings, e.g., in patients given horse antithymocyte globulin to treat aplastic anemia.

Polyarteritis nodosa. Polyarteritis nodosa (PAN) looks like an exaggerated version of serum sickness arteritis except that it tends to be deadly. It affects small and medium-sized arteries, and it is strictly segmental: *nodosa* means knotty, and the knots are spherical inflammatory foci encasing a short segment of artery, as also seen in experimental models of complex-mediated arteritis (Figures 17.35, 17.36). The inflammatory foci tend to be located at bifurcations and can progress to several complications: the inflamed arterial segments may literally blow out and bleed or simply expand into small aneurysms that can be seen on arteriograms; they can also become thrombosed and cause infarcts in the tissues downstream. Clinically, PAN prefers young adult males; it usually presents as a fever of unknown origin, accompanied by malaise and a variety of symptoms depending on the prevailing localization (often the kidney). Diagnosis depends on a biopsy taken from an organ that appears to be especially affected, such as kidney, muscle, or skin. The pathogenesis is not well understood and may be autoimmune. Antibodies against leukocytes are present, and their titer correlates with severity; 30 percent of the patients have hepatitis B antigen in the serum.

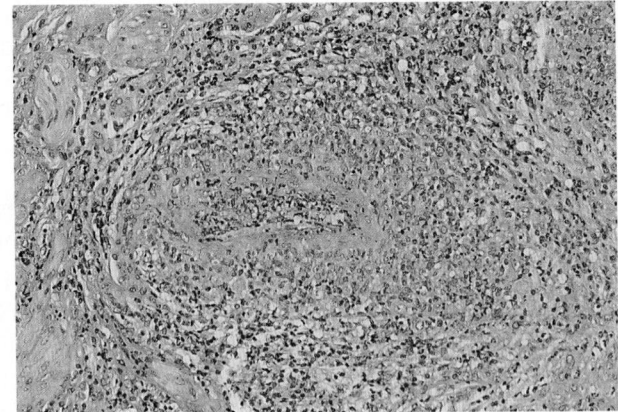 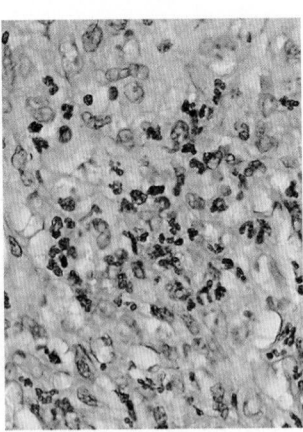

FIGURE 17.35 *Left:* Believe it or not, this was once an artery. It has been largely destroyed by periarteritis nodosa. (120x) *Right:* Cells infiltrating the artery wall are mostly neutrophils and macrophages. (350x)

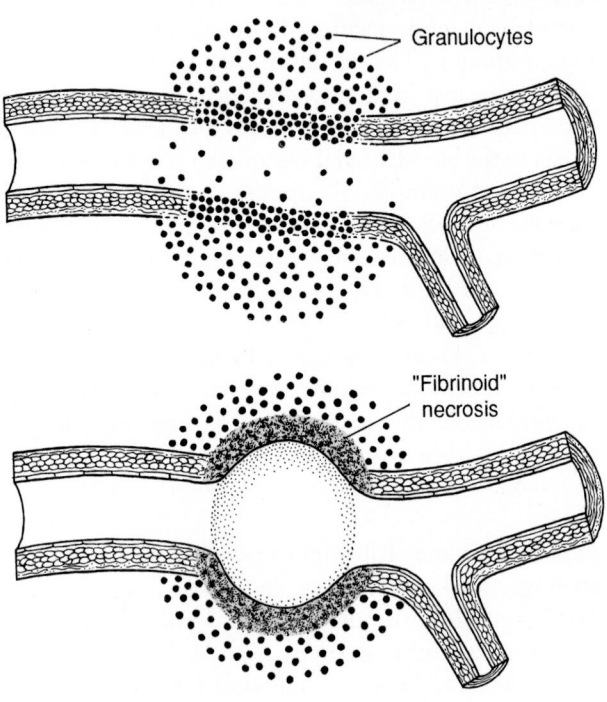

FIGURE 17.36 Structural changes in polyarteritis nodosa. *Top:* Inflammatory cells, mainly granulocytes (neutrophils and eosinophils), are attracted to a segment of the arterial media (presumably by products of complement activation caused by antigen–antibody complexes). *Bottom:* Necrosis of that segment, which becomes soaked with fibrin (fibrinoid necrosis), followed by aneurysmal dilatation.

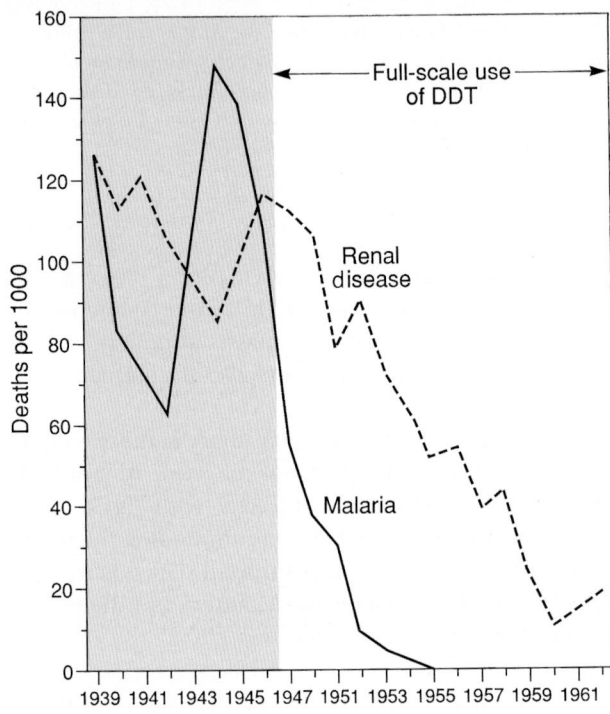

FIGURE 17.37 Evidence that malaria showers the kidney with antigen–antibody complexes, causing renal disease. In a part of British Guiana, between 1939 and 1959, the full-scale use of DDT decreased not only the number of deaths from malaria, but also the deaths from chronic renal disease due to malarial antigen–antibody complex deposition in the glomeruli. (Reproduced with permission from [93].)

Globulin and complement can be found in the lesions. Left untreated, PAN is usually fatal; corticosteroids improve the 5-year survival to 48 percent.

PAN is but one of many forms of **vasculitis,** which may affect any artery from the aorta to the microcirculation. An immune (and autoimmune) pathogenesis is often likely but not always demonstrable. The vasculitides are a vast family of lesions that are, on the whole, poorly understood (87).

NOTE: A form of mononuclear-cell vasculitis in mice depends on Type 4 (cell-mediated) hypersensitivity (103).

Glomerulonephritis. Glomerular inflammation due to showers of complexes occurs as a complication of many human diseases. All that is needed is some mechanism that injects antigens into the blood; tumors can do it, and so can many chronic infections such as syphilis (98) and malaria. In fact, it was noticed in a field study in Africa that when malaria was eradicated from a region, the associated glomerular disease tended to disappear with it (Figure 17.37) (93).

The best-known example of glomerular complex disease in man is *poststreptococcal glomerulonephritis.* The sequence begins with a throat infection with certain strains of streptococcus; streptococcal antigens are released into the blood, antibodies are formed, and the resulting complexes are retained by the glomeruli.

> The statement that "complexes are retained" may not be entirely accurate. It has been suggested that a bacterial antigen first seeps across the glomerular capillary wall and becomes deposited in the mesangium; later it is joined by the antibody. This complex then stimulates mesangial cell proliferation (Figure 17.38) (111).

> NOTE: The most common form of complex-mediated renal disease is caused, oddly enough, by complexes of IgA, the immunoglobulin that is normally secreted by mucosal surfaces (92).

The clinical effect of glomerular complexes is the so-called nephrotic syndrome; protein is lost into the urine by excessive permeability of the glomerular capillary, probably caused by the membrane-attack complex of activated complement.

Hypersensitivity pneumonitis. This is another group of diseases in which antigen–antibody complexes are thought to intervene: namely chronic lung diseases caused by organic dusts, most of them job-related. Examples are pigeon breeder's disease (inhalation of dust containing dried feces of pigeon), farmer's lung (inhalation of an *actinomyces*), humidifier lung, as well as mushroom picker's, cheese washer's, paprika slicer's, maple-bark stripper's, wood trimmer's, chicken plucker's, and even sauna-bather's disease, plus sequoiosis in the lumber industry and many others (106). The plasma of these patients contains precipitating antibodies to the various antigens as required to produce complexes and Arthus- or serum sickness-type lesions. Inhalation of the antigen causes symptoms (coughing, chills, fever, and dyspnea) with a delay of 4–12 hours, which falls between the

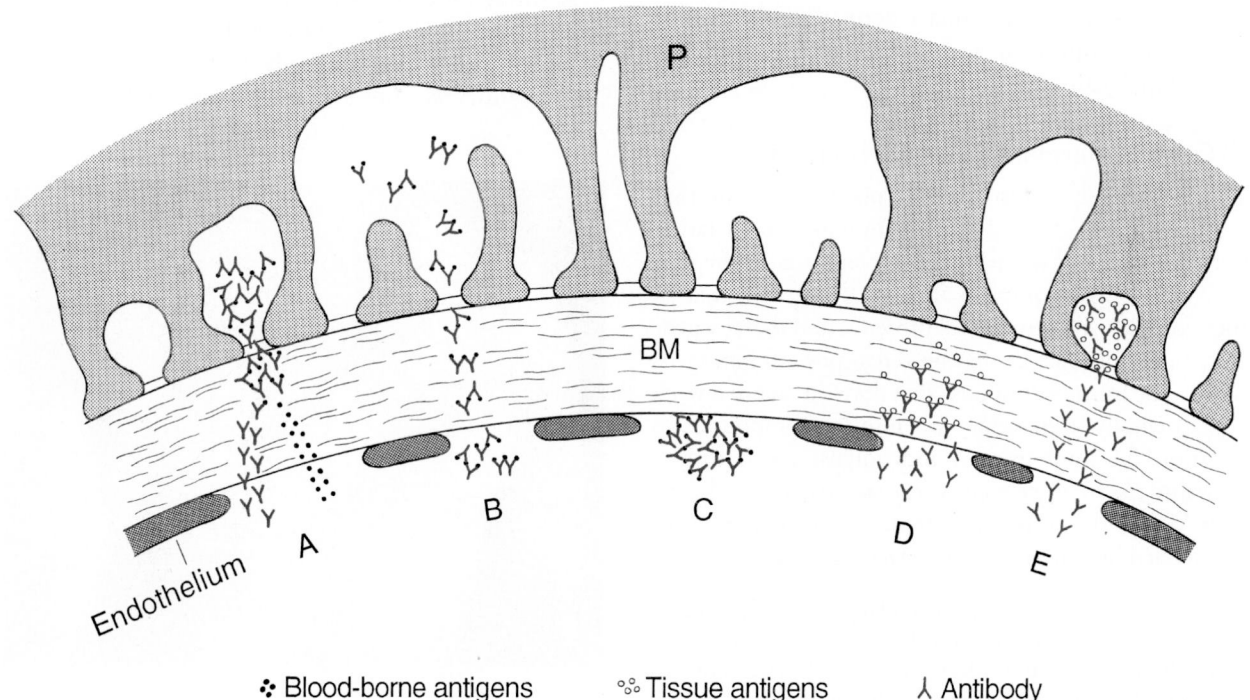

❖ Blood-borne antigens   ⸱°⸱° Tissue antigens   ⅄ Antibody

FIGURE 17.38   Various mechanisms leading to the deposition of antigen–antibody complexes against, within or beyond the glomerular basement membrane (**BM**). **A:** Antigen and antibody penetrate separately, and complexes develop within or beyond the basement membrane. **B:** Small complexes penetrate and cross the basement membrane. **C:** Large complexes are retained against the luminal (subendothelial) surface of the basement membrane. **D:** A component of the basement membrane becomes antigenic, elicits antibodies, and complexes are formed within the basement membrane. **E:** Antigens appear on the surface of the podocyte (**P**), and antibodies are trapped in that location. (Adapted with permission from [88].)

delay typical of the Arthus mechanism and that of delayed-type (cell-mediated, Type 4) hypersensitivity. The pathogenesis is not yet clear; it may include components of Type 1 hypersensitivity (allergic asthma) as well as of Type 3 (complex-mediated) and Type 4 (cell-mediated) hypersensitivity. A reminder that human classifications do not always fit with those of Nature.

Hypersensitivity Type 4: Cell-Mediated or Delayed Type Hypersensitivity (DTH)

The three types of "immediate," quick-acting hypersensitivity reactions just described are part of the price that we, vertebrates, have to pay for the privilege of using antibodies. Correspondingly, a part of the price we have to pay for using the slower, cell-mediated immunity (CMI) are the "delayed-type" hypersensitivity (DTH) reactions. Of course, DTH reactions can occur anywhere in the body, but it so happens that they are studied most easily in the skin. The host must be sensitized in a special manner (requiring 1–3 weeks), and when the skin is challenged anywhere in the body with the same antigen, a red patch appears with a delay of at least several hours. It takes this time for enough cells to gather at the spot and to produce enough cytokines to generate a visible lesion. Much of what we know about DTH was drawn from three sources: (a) contact dermatitis, (b) experiments with adjuvants, and (c) tuberculosis and the tuberculin reaction.

(1) Contact Dermatitis: A Model of DTH

The household, industrial, and plant chemicals that bring about this delayed skin reaction are not irritating in themselves, but when placed in contact with the skin they behave as incomplete antigens or *haptens*: that is, they complex with epidermal proteins, and thereby generate molecules that are recognized as powerful antigens (161). The immune response that develops about a week later is wholly unnecessary, because the compounds in question (in nonsensitized individuals) are harmless; therefore *the immune response becomes the disease*. In the New World, the everyday example of contact dermatitis is provided by poison ivy, *Toxicodendron radicans*.

This plant—native to North and South America and East Asia, but totally unknown in Europe—is truly a scourge of the outdoors and affects almost exclusively humans (142). Its only saving grace is that it is related to the Japanese lacquer tree. The harmless-looking leaves are coated with an oil that contains urushiol, the hapten; sensitization takes about 1 week. A European reader would be more likely to be familiar with the rash produced by contact with other plants (Figures 17.39, 17.40), with latex gloves, or with nickel jewelry. In any case, the clinical appearance of the skin rash is that of an extremely itchy, oozing, and slightly swollen red patch. To produce contact dermatitis experimentally, the agent often used is dimethylchlorobenzene (DMCB).

The key feature of this rash, as regards pathogenesis, is that *it does not develop in unprepared individuals*. It requires a first contact for sensitization; the second contact may occur week later or any time thereafter, whereupon the rash will develop in 12–48 hours.

Contact dermatitis may sound like a rather mundane topic, but it is important to learn about it—in the context of general pathology—because it is a perfect model of DTH, such as occurs in tuberculosis and many other infections.

A summary of its pathogenesis: in a patch of skin touched by the poison ivy leaves, Langerhans cells and other antigen-presenting cells pick up the hapten-protein antigenic complex, travel with it to the nearest

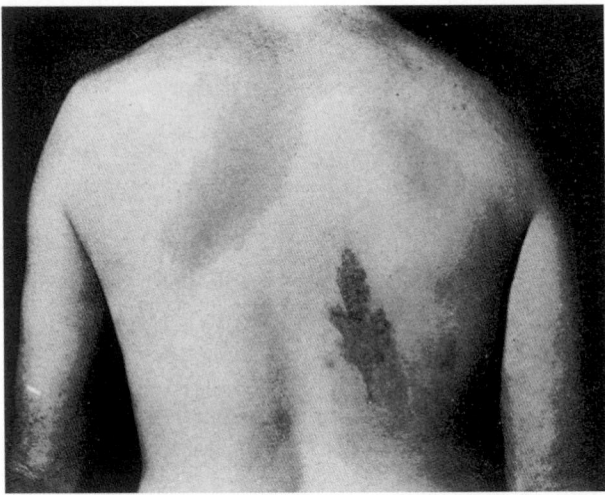

FIGURE 17.39   Contact dermatitis, a classic example of cell-mediated hypersensitivity. This gardener complained of rashes on the hands and forearms during the chrysanthemum season. A chrysanthemum leaf was strapped to his skin for 24 hours, and this is the result. There were pinhead vesicles all over the reddened area, much as with poison ivy. (Reproduced from [148].)

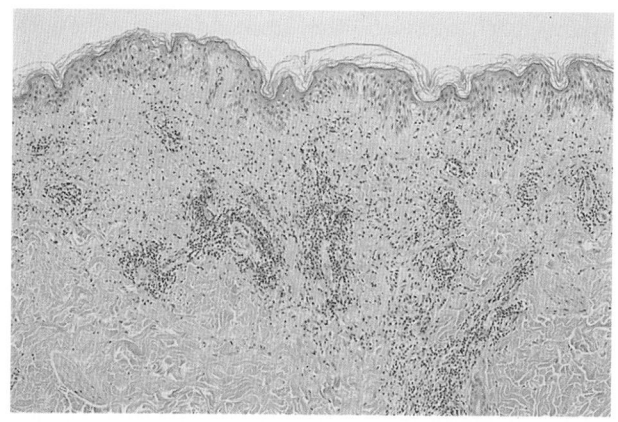

FIGURE 17.40 Contact dermatitis in human skin. The striking clinical picture (redness, itching) contrasts with these rather subdued histologic changes (mild perivenular infiltrates). (10x) (Reproduced with permission from [117], Copyright © 2001 by Dermatopathology Interactive Atlas.)

lymph nodes, and present it to the appropriate naive T-helper cells (T_H0) (Figure 17.6). A minority of these T_H0 cells become T_H2 helper cells and remain in the node; they activate B cells, which produce antibodies. But most T_H0 cells become T_H1 helper cells, which carry out cell-mediated responses (p. 530). These return to the bloodstream and *home to the target area* (where the leaves had touched). Here the T_H1 cells set up an inflammatory response, deceptively mild compared with the clinical itching: cuffs of lymphocytes around the smallest ("postcapillary") venules.

The type of cells in the perivenular cuffs depends on the species and timing. In mice there is an early neutrophil wave, but later the infiltrate consists mainly of mononuclear cells: lymphocytes and macrophages, with some basophils and eosinophils, and a scattering of neutrophils (Figure 17.41). Oddly enough the antigen-specific lymphocytes are a minority (149). The homing of lymphocytes has become an intricate field even under normal conditions, due to the interplay of chemokines, chemokine receptors, blood flow, and shear (122a).

Vascular leakage. Vascular leakage in contact dermatitis can be intense enough to produce blisters (see Figure 12.14). Electron microscopic studies have shown that leaky vessels are the superficial capillaries (182), possibly as a result of endothelial activation.

What is the purpose of this nuisance contact dermatitis reaction? None, really—but if we want to have lymphocytes capable of recognizing and attacking infectious agents and tumor cells, this is what they are likely to do in their spare time.

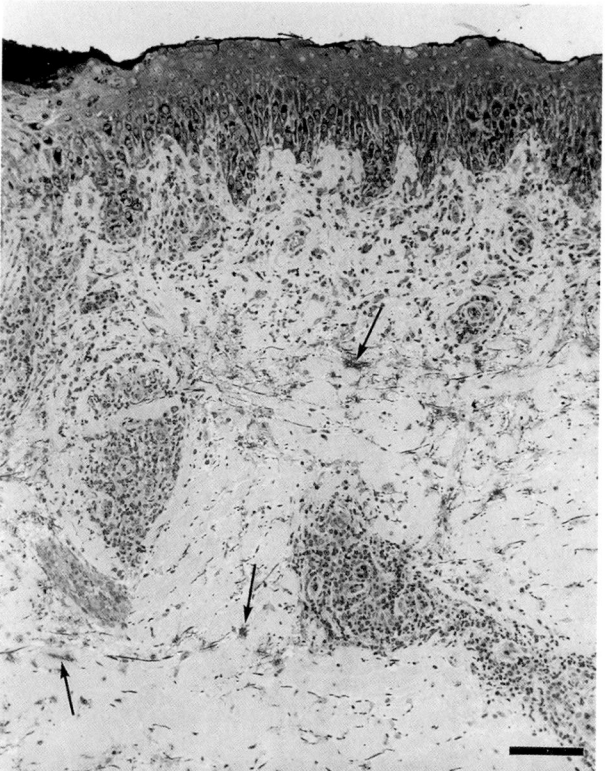

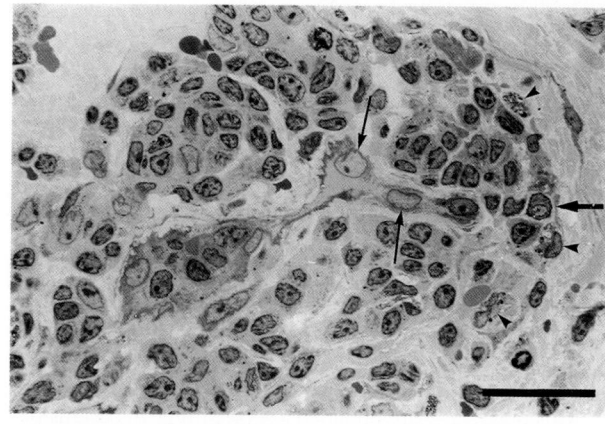

FIGURE 17.41 Foci of inflammation typical of delayed-type hypersensitivity: 72 hour contact dermatitis induced in a volunteer with dinitrochlorobenzene (essentially the same pathology as in a 72-hour **poison ivy reaction** or **tuberculin reaction**). *Top:* mononuclear cells, scattered and collected in perivenular cuffs. Note the **fibrin strands** (**arrows**), which confer the typical firmness, to this lesion. **Bar** = 100 μm. *Bottom:* Detail of a perivenular cuff. THIS IS NOT A GRANULOMA: **the causal agent is water-soluble and diffuses away; besides, granulomas have no blood vessels. Thin arrows:** thickened (activated) endothelium. **Thick arrow:** mast cell. **Bar** = 25 μm. (*Top:* Reproduced from the **Journal of Experimental Medicine,** 1973;138:686–689, by copyright permission of The Rockefeller University Press [125b]. *Bottom:* Courtesy of Dr. H. F. Dvorak, Beth Israel Hospital, Harvard Medical School, Boston, MA.)

(2) The Role of Adjuvants in Hypersensitivity

We can now ask the same kind of question that we asked in regard to IgE antibodies: why is it that some antigens induce a cell-mediated delayed type hypersensitivity (DTH)? A partial answer: if we want to *produce* DTH against a given protein, the orthodox procedure is to inject that protein mixed with an appropriate *adjuvant*. An adjuvant is "a substance that enhances, non-specifically, the immune response to an antigen" (164). So, the selected protein—say, bovine serum albumin—is mixed with a rather messy substance called *Freund's complete adjuvant,* namely a water-in-mineral oil emulsion containing heat-killed tubercle bacilli. The mixture is injected subcutaneously to a guinea pig; after 3 weeks, an intradermal injection of bovine serum albumin will produce a delayed-type response. So effective is this method that it will even pervert the immune system to react against one of the body's own tissues—if this tissue is minced, mixed with Freund's adjuvant, and injected.

This peculiar oily ritual calls for some explanation. How could anyone dream up such a nasty mixture as Freund's adjuvant?

It all began when Louis Dienes asked himself—in North Carolina in the late 1920s—why tuberculous guinea pig developed a delayed-type skin hypersensitivity to tuberculin, a mixture of proteins derived from cultures of *Mycobacterium tuberculosis* (see further) (137). Perhaps it had something to do with the peculiar tuberculous "granulation tissue"? He injected some eggwhite into the granulation tissue of his tuberculous guinea pigs; and sure enough, the guinea pigs developed a delayed tuberculin-type response also to the eggwhite. Did this depend on some action of the *live* tubercle bacilli? Dr. Dienes injected some normal guinea pigs with heat-killed *Mycobacterium tuberculosis,* which produced a strong inflammatory response. When he injected eggwhite **into this mass,** he again obtained a delayed-type hypersensitivity against eggwhite. *So the mycobacteria somehow had the property of enhancing delayed-type hypersensitivity toward an antigen injected with them.* At that time Jules Freund, a fellow Hungarian, was working with Dienes (175). In 1942 Freund and McDermott introduced the mineral oil, plus a lanolin-type solvent, which made it easier to suspend the bacilli (143). The trend to adjuvants was on.

NOTE: *Freund's adjuvant is generally used to push the immune response in the direction of DTH, and it works; but he antibody response is also increased* (150).

Actually, in recent times, adjuvants have acquired a more decorous presence. It seems clear that they work by two mechanisms: (a) they form a deposit of antigen that prolongs the contact with antigen-presenting cells; and (b) they activate antigen-presenting cells (112, 146). Some adjuvants favor cell-mediated immunity, others the antibody response (111). The list of adjuvants has become long (146); it includes liposomes (p. 225), aluminum hydroxide, and natural or modified bacterial products, such as *lipopolysaccharide* (LPS, endotoxin) and *muramyl dipeptide* (MDP), thought to be the smallest peptide sequence capable of mimicking the adjuvant effect of the tubercle bacillus (125). The hunt for bacterial adjuvants led to discover that *many of these adjuvants are ligands for the toll-like receptors* (TLRs, p. 432) (154a), whereby Freund's primitive soup of boiled bacteria in oil found its link with molecular pathology.

Then came the search for natural "adjuvanticity" in living tissues (the concept is more elegant than the name): an endogenous activator of dendritic cells was found in normal cells after repeated freezing and thawing, in cells injured by UV radiation, and in tumor cells (165a). This agent turned out to be, quite surprisingly, **uric acid.** Which means that this physiologic product of purine catabolism acquires a new function as "danger signal" to the immune system: its flag reads "CELLS ARE DYING." Heat shock proteins also behave as powerful endogenous adjuvants (113a, 117a).

The purpose of all these natural adjuvants? Perhaps to accelerate the removal of foreign material, such as infectious agents and tumor cells. We must also recall that adjuvants are an essential part of vaccines (154a).

(3) Delayed Type Hypersensitivity and Tuberculosis

The basic concepts of cell-mediated immunity (CMI), DTH, granuloma, and vaccination are so closely bound to tuberculosis, biologically and historically, that we must take a quick look at the disease (139). Tuberculosis has declined fairly steadily after 1800 (Figure 17.42), but *it is still the world's most prevalent infection;* tubercle bacilli have infected about one third of the people on the earth; 50 to 200 million cases are active; and an estimated 3 million people die of it every year (162, 174a).

One reason for the stubborn persistence of the "white plague" is that the tubercle bacillus has worked out a way to become the *nearly perfect parasite.* It does not kill quickly but rather produces slow tissue responses, mainly in the lungs, whereby the victim becomes chronically ill and can continue to cough out the agent infecting those around year after year. General symptoms are mild. The body mounts an immune

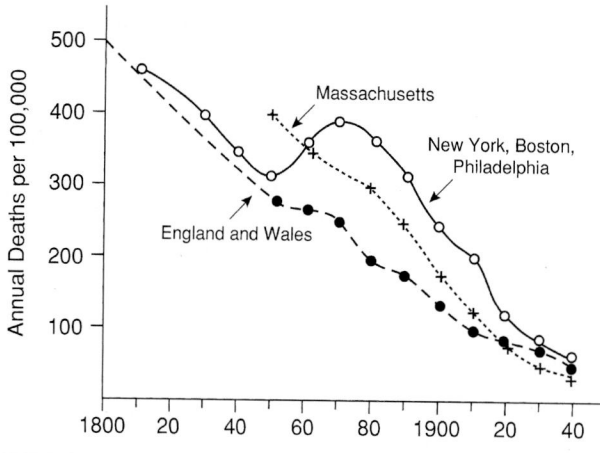

FIGURE 17.42 Mortality from pulmonary tuberculosis 1800–1940. Deaths began to decline long before specific therapy became available (streptomycin, in the 1940s). The transient increase in mortality that began around 1850 in the large cities of the United States may reflect a sudden influx of Irish immigrants. (From Dubos, René and Jean Dubos, *Tuberculosis, Man and Society.* Copyright ©1952 by René and Jean Dubos. Copyright ©1987 by Rutgers, the State University. Reprinted by permission of Rutgers University Press [139].)

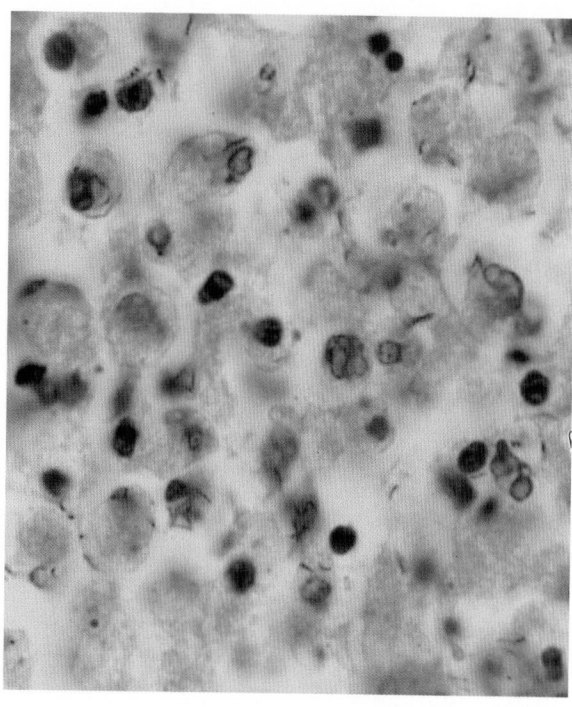

FIGURE 17.43 Histology of the lung in a case of tuberculous pneumonia. The cells are alveolar macrophages phagocytizing mycobacteria (red rods). (Acid-fast stain; 1,100x)

response that teeters on the adequate. The infected tissue occasionally melts into a necrotic semifluid mass teeming with mycobacteria (123, 126, 127, 155, 160) that helps spread the infection, but it can also heal by scarring; *progressing and healing lesions can coexist* in the same lung (136). The balance between progression and healing is poorly understood but is determined mainly by the number of bacilli present at each site.

Tuberculosis: the battle in the tissues. The tubercle bacillus, *Mycobacterium tuberculosis,* is an obligate aerobe: this is why it thrives in the lungs. It can enter the human body by several routes, but classically it is inhaled; if the infectious particles are small enough (1–3 μm), they reach the alveoli. The alveolar macrophages, probably alerted by their Toll-like receptor 2 (TLR2) (180) and other receptors (141), sense the presence of mycobacteria and phagocytize them, and the battle is on (Figure 17.43) (118, 122, 125a, 129, 132–134, 136, 155, 155a, 162, 166, 171). Cellular reinforcements are supplied by the blood, mainly monocytes; in the meantime the tubercle bacilli somehow kill off some alveolar cells (138). Within 10 days or so the immune response sets in (129, 184), and so the first **immune granuloma** develops (p. 456): a small lump of macrophages—some activated, some not—interspersed with lymphocytes.

The immune response to the mycobacterium is mainly produced by T_H1 type lymphocytes (pp. 458, 530) and

carried out by the macrophages that these helper lymphocytes activate. If the T_H2 component (always present [118, 170]) is experimentally reduced, the granulomas are smaller, and tissue damage and fibrosis are reduced (162).

If the macrophages are unable to kill all the mycobacteria, they begin to die: they are being killed (at least in part) by the tissue-damaging DTH of the immune response (133). We can visualize the cellular drama: T_H1 lymphocytes shower the macrophages with interferon gamma (IFNγ) and other cytokines, which activate them; but if some macrophages are still incapable of killing their bacterial load, cytotoxic (killer) T lymphocytes induce some of them to perform apoptosis. Ischemia from microvascular thrombosis kills other macrophages, together with the surrounding tissues. If bacillary growth is not controlled, the granuloma with its caseous core will expand into a nodule 5–15 mm in diameter visible by X-rays. To the pathologist it appears grossly as a firm, whitish lump and microscopically as a necrotic mass surrounded by a layer of viable macrophages, lymphocytes, and fibroblasts (Figure 13.23).

While the primary lesion grows, some bacilli escape along peribronchial lymphatics and seed one or more secondary infections in the hilar lymph nodes

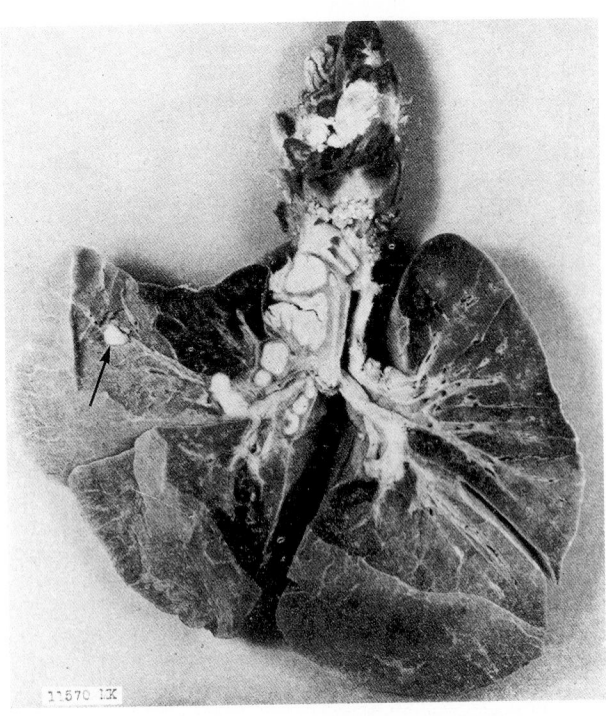

FIGURE 17.44   Rapidly progressing tuberculosis in the lungs of a 19-month-old infant. The small primary lesion in the middle lobe of the right lung (**arrow**) gave rise to greatly enlarged, caseous hilar peritracheal lymph nodes. (Reproduced by permission from [160]. Courtesy of Charles C. Thomas, Publisher, Springfield Illinois.)

(Figure 17.44, 17.45). The primary nodule in the lung with the infected nodes constitute the *primary complex* or *Ghon complex*. During all this time clinical symptoms are minimal: mild fever and weight loss, probably due to TNF-α (162).

The primary complex in most cases stops growing and "heals," sometimes with partial calcification. We used quotation marks because some bacilli probably survive in a dormant state (reminiscent of the dormant state of malignant cells); they are not replicating and therefore very difficult to kill with antibiotics (162), and they are probably responsible for maintaining a positive tuberculin test (to be explained shortly).

An individual with a "healed" primary complex may never be troubled by it again, or the disease may proceed to what is called postprimary tuberculosis, in nearby or distant sites in the body. Occasionally a large number of bacteria enter the bloodstream at the same time, probably because a mass of caseous necrosis erodes a pulmonary vein and seeds tubercle bacilli throughout the body. This is *miliary tuberculosis,* so called because the countless tiny, whitish granulomas—*all of the same size and therefore of the same age,* as seen at autopsy—suggest a comparison with millet seeds (Figure 17.45).

Caseous necrosis and hypersensitivity. Caseous necrosis deserves special attention (See Figures 13.30, 13.35) (p. 458) (136). With apologies to cheese lovers, it really

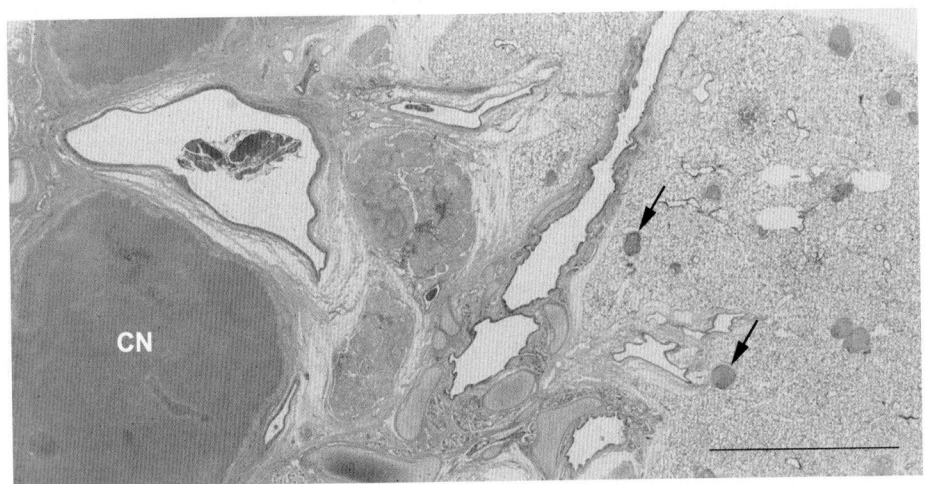

FIGURE 17.45   Lung of an undernourished infant showing progression of a tuberculous infection. *Left:* Caseous necrosis (CN) in a hilar lymph node draining a primary complex (not shown). *Right:* Lung. The small, rounded or oval masses (**arrows**) are miliary tubercles (granulomas) due to hematogenous dissemination of mycobacteria. The fact that these miliary granulomas are all roughly of the same size suggests a single episode of dissemination. **Bar = 5 mm.**

does look like semidried cream cheese. *It is biologically different from the necrosis of an infarct,* because it is saturated with mycobacterial products, which may explain why the macrophages around it do not appear eager to nibble at it. Small amounts of caseous necrosis can probably be cleared (130), but a large focus is never surrounded by a healthy scavenging layer of granulation tissue such as that around an infarct.

Caseous necrosis differs from the coagulation necrosis of an infarct also because it can expand. The cells gathered around it (mainly macrophages) die and join the necrotic mass; then a new barrier of macrophages develops just outside, and so the cycle continues. By this mechanism a tuberculous lesion can enlarge like a tumor; indeed the term *tuberculoma* is used for such expanding masses, to which the brain is especially prone.

Another peculiar feature of caseous necrosis is that in time it can undergo liquefaction, that is, become semifluid (130, 135, 136). This is a serious complication for a number of reasons: (a) the resulting creamy fluid is an excellent culture medium for mycobacteria, which may grow in it profusely; (b) accelerated growth favors the appearance of mutants, which complicates therapy; (c) when liquefaction occurs in the lung, the infectious fluid is easily aspirated and spread throughout the bronchi; and (d) the high concentration of bacteria and their tuberculin-like products tends to cause a necrotic response, much like a large dose of intradermal tuberculin may cause necrosis in the skin of a patient with active tuberculosis.

Is caseous necrosis helpful, harmful, or indifferent? After a century of speculation we seem finally to have an answer rather than a guess (131). By comparing the bacillary growth curves in rabbits, one resistant and one susceptible, M. B. Lurie (155) and A. M. Dannenberg (131) concluded that caseous necrosis is helpful because it stops the growth of bacilli: its anoxic environment chokes them. They can survive but not multiply. If liquefaction develops, of course, it is quite another matter.

As to the mechanism: caseous necrosis is generally thought to be a result of delayed-type hypersensitivity: a "mass burial" of inflammatory and parenchymal cells that are destroyed by mechanisms of immunity designed to eliminate bacteria. Several factors could contribute to the massive cell death; we will quote two, but more have been suggested (164):

- Conscientious but indiscriminate cytotoxic T-cells destroy antigen-presenting macrophages because—for the T-cells—any surface coated with specific antigen is a legitimate target.

- Cytokines are involved, especially tumor necrosis factor (TNF). It has been shown that *Mycobacterium tuberculosis* not only triggers the release of TNF, but also makes the cells of the host more sensitive to the toxicity of TNF (164).

Other mechanisms have been proposed that may contribute to caseous necrosis (130): *ischemia* due to thrombosed capillaries (128) (activated macrophages do produce procoagulant factors); *activation of complement* with damage to bystander cells (antibodies are generated in tuberculous tissue [170], but their role is uncertain); *reactive oxygen and nitrogen intermediates* relased by macrophages and neutrophils. No existing theory, however, can answer the question—*Why CASEOUS necrosis?*

A strong argument in favor of hypersensitivity as a cause of caseous necrosis is provided by other diseases characterized by granulomas with a necrotic center. A classic example is *tertiary syphilis.* At this late stage of the disease the syphilitic granulomas contain very few spirochetes, and their necrotic center is best explained as the result of a hypersensitivity reaction. Just like the caseous necrosis of tuberculosis, it tends to enlarge in tumor-like fashion.

In the past it was customary to insist on the difference between syphilitic and tuberculous necrosis. Grossly, in syphilis, the necrotic mass is firm and rubbery rather than cheesy (hence the name *gumma*); histologically, the outlines of the tissue are partially preserved. But biologically these are not very significant features. What counts is that in both diseases there is extensive focal necrosis explainable only in terms of an immune response.

Even more compelling is the comparison of tuberculous necrosis with the so-called *rheumatoid nodules,* which contain no infectious agent at all. They are found in two diseases with a strong hypersensitivity component: rheumatoid arthritis and acute rheumatic fever. Rheumatoid nodules, like tuberculous lymph nodes, can grow to tumor size (pp. 591, 593). There is no way at all to explain them—and their central necrosis—except by a hypersensitivity mechanism.

With these facts in mind, we can now return to DTH in tuberculosis.

The Tuberculin Affair

Robert Koch, who discovered the tubercle bacillus in 1882, announced 8 years later that he had discovered a cure for tuberculosis. The magic drug was **tuberculin,** actually a highly impure solution of proteins obtained by filtering mycobacterial cultures (151, 152). Perhaps he was under some pressure due to the competition from France, where Pasteur had listed another major success with the vaccination against rabies. Anyway, to understand his thinking as of 1891, we must read the description of the experiment that has gone down to history as the **Koch phenomenon** (152, 160). In Koch's own words (translated):

> If a normal guinea pig is inoculated with a pure culture of tubercle bacilli, the wound, as a rule, closes and in the first few days seemingly heals. After ten to fourteen days, however, there appears a firm nodule which soon opens, forming an ulcer that persists until the animal dies. Quite different is the result if a tuberculous guinea pig is inoculated with tubercle bacilli. For this purpose it is best to use animals that have been infected four to six weeks previously. In such an animal, also, the little inoculation wound closes at first, but in this case no nodule is formed. (Note: *Koch inadvertently omits a detail that will turn out to be crucial: this second inoculation must be superficial, i.e., in the skin, not the muscle*).
>
> On the next or second day, however, a peculiar change occurs at the inoculation site. The area becomes indurated and assumes a dark color, and these changes do not remain limited to the inoculation point, but spread to involve an area 0.5–1.0 cm in diameter. In the succeeding days it becomes evident that the altered skin is necrotic. It finally sloughs, leaving a shallow ulcer which usually heals quickly and permanently, and the regional lymph nodes do not become infected. The action of tubercle bacilli upon the skin of a normal guinea pig is thus entirely different from their action upon the skin of a tuberculous one. This striking effect is produced not only by living tubercle bacilli, but also by dead bacilli, whether killed by prolonged low temperature, by boiling, or by certain chemicals.

In essence, Koch is telling us that in a tuberculous guinea pig a second inoculation of mycobacteria leads to a sort of "accelerated rejection" of the newly infected skin; an event that might be construed as beneficial. Koch did not know that if the second injection had been deeper, in the muscle, the result would have been a rapid, massive, necrosis of the muscle, which would have made matters worse (162, 163). He proceeded to inject large doses of bacterial extract (tuberculin) into tuberculous patients. It was a disaster; some died; none was cured (168).

A warning to the reader. So what is the meaning of the Koch experiment? We spent much time trying to understand it and finally realized that there can be no more than half a dozen people in the world who can master this utterly confusing topic (121). There is a mystique about it, because it bears the name of Koch, but as published it is only a half-phenomenon; a misleading experiment that

misled even Koch. To understand where Koch went wrong, we strongly recommend two papers (147, 163).

Koch went through difficult times, but two events provided him with some consolation. He received the Nobel prize in 1905 for his overall research on tuberculosis, and in the meantime an eminent clinician, the Baron von Pirquet of serum-sickness fame (p. 546) (116), discovered that tuberculin was very useful, if not for the therapy—at least for the diagnosis of tuberculosis. Applied over a scratch in the skin of infected individuals, it produced a striking, delayed inflammatory response. This was the birth of the tuberculin test still in use, except that the somewhat messy tuberculin has been replaced by a more controlled purified protein derivative (PPD) (Figure 17.46).

And so it was that the baron von Pirquet became a pioneer of hypersensitivity reactions, both immediate in serum sickness (p. 546) and delayed in tuberculosis. In 1906 he proposed the term **allergy** to mean any altered state of reactivity, be it to tuberculin or to any other "organic, living or non-living poison" (181). The term was promptly adopted. In Europe it is generally used in the original sense of any increased state of reactivity, whatever the type of hypersensitivity, whereas in the United States its use is restricted to Type 1 hypersensitivity, that is, to allergies of the hay-fever type. The tuberculin test became crucial early in the

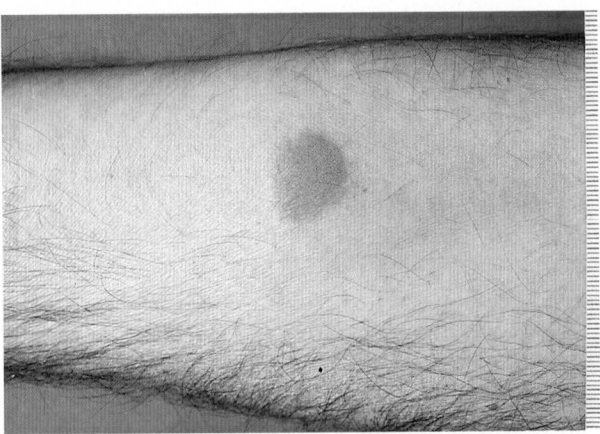

FIGURE 17.46 Strongly positive tuberculin test photographed at 48 hours, on the forearm of a 60-year-old man in good health. At age 10 he had suffered a primary tuberculous infection, which clinically healed. Despite the 50-year interval between the infection and this tuberculin injection, the local reaction at 24 hours was so intense that a red, 1 × 8 cm lymphangitic streak arose from the proximal side of the test (*right* on the figure) and advanced in the direction of lymph flow (left to right). **Scale** in millimeters.

nineteenth century for identifying and eliminating all cattle infected with bovine tuberculosis.

> There is a sad ending to the tuberculin story. The overwhelming demands of his academic career were too much for Clemens von Pirquet, who took his life in 1929, at the age of 55.

Vaccination against tuberculosis: the BCG controversy. We have lived through the disappointment of tuberculin as a cure; what about vaccination? The scene now moves to the Pasteur Institute in Lille, where the birth of the Arthus phenomenon took place in the early 1900s. By treating tubercle bacilli with ox bile, Albert Calmette and Camille Guérin managed to obtain an attenuated strain; in 1921 they proposed it as a vaccine for human use, by mouth, under the name BCG (for bacillus Calmette–Guérin) (115, 165). It was soon found that BCG causes the tuberculin test to be positive. Since then, the world is divided into two camps (159). In the United States, BCG is not used because the reported effectiveness is not obvious, and because it has the built-in drawback just mentioned: vaccinated individuals become tuberculin-positive, which makes the tuberculin test useless for diagnosing a tuberculous infection. The vaccine does not *prevent* infection; it is said to provide better protection against the disease (154), but the extent of this protection is unclear. Epidemiologic studies yielded answers ranging from 80 percent to zero (144, 178, 179). The BCG vaccine is still one of the most widely used vaccines on a global scale; the Pasteur Institute in Paris is searching for ways to improve its effectiveness. Perhaps DNA vaccines will help (120). The question is still open.

> NOTE: The BCG vaccine consists of attenuated but live bacteria; in rare cases it gives rise to a true infection, known as BCGitis (124).

The meaning of a positive PPD reaction. The PPD reaction is performed today by intradermal injection, as proposed by Charles Mantoux in 1910 ("Mantoux test"). It is considered positive if the red patch reaches at least 10 mm in diameter in 24 hours (Figure 17.46) (159) *and* is accompanied by stiffening of the skin, as tested by lifting a fold between thumb and forefinger. This feature, rarely absent (114) is especially useful when the tuberculin test is done on pigmented skin.

A positive test means that the patient has been infected with tubercle bacilli or has been vaccinated with BCG. It does not mean that there is active disease, although this is a possibility. In the United States, a positive PPD test in an individual who has not been vaccinated means that treatment for tuberculosis is recommended. Because hepatitis is a possible side-effect of that treatment and because this risk increases with age, the two risks must be weighed. *The treatment usually causes the PPD test to become negative within months or years* (184): this is the best proof available that mycobacteria do survive in the lesion.

But does a positive test tell us anything about the strength of the immune system's response to the infection? Unfortunately, it does not. A large red patch does NOT allow us to congratulate the patient for putting up an excellent fight. Patients with an active tuberculous infection may respond with a local patch of necrosis (supposedly a "Koch phenomenon"); and patients with advanced tuberculosis may develop no response at all ("**anergy**"). Rats are highly resistant to TB infection and produce a weak response to PPD; guinea pigs are easily infected and give a strong response.

To *measure* the response, we may need a different set of antigens. Remember that PPD is a selection of conveniently extractable bacterial proteins, which may have little to do with the actual tuberculous infection.

Four Types of Hypersensitivity: Some Closing Questions

We have reviewed and explained four basic mechanisms whereby the immune system reacts with vigor against harmless antigens—much like Don Quixote attacking windmills. Before proceeding any further, let us answer some pertinent questions.

(I) Why Type 1, 2, 3, or 4?

In other words: given an antigenic challenge, why should the immune system choose to respond with hypersensitivity of one type rather than another? There is no short answer to this important question. The first point is that *one type does not exclude another*. For example: poison ivy contact dermatitis is the prototype of Type 4, cell-mediated hypersensitivity; yet in some cases it induces such intense antibody formation that the patient develops "immune complex disease" (Type 3) with the related "immune complex nephropathy" (161).

Rabbits that are sensitized intravenously to produce serum sickness (Type 3, complex-mediated) when rechallenged may develop anaphylactic symptoms (Type 1). In fact, you may recall that the arteritis of serum sickness is thought by some to require the cooperation of Types 1 and 3 (p. 549). Some degree of cell-mediated hypersensitivity may also develop at the same time. *Mycobacterium tuberculosis* induces delayed-type (cell-mediated) hypersensitivity but also plenty of antibodies (especially if injected with Freund's adjuvant) but, somehow, these antibodies do not play a *known* role in the pathogenesis of the disease.

This being said, it is true that a given type tends to prevail in a given setting. Several factors are involved: the nature of the antigen, the route and manner of administration, and the animal species. For example, rubbing an antigen into the skin (across the epidermis) favors the development of a cell-mediated response, that is Type 4. Giving an antigen intravenously (so that antigen and antibody mix in high concentrations) favors the formation of complexes (Type 3); inhalation across the mucous membranes of the respiratory system, favors an anaphylactic mechanism (Type 1). Injecting an antigen mixed with Freund's adjuvant enhances the sensitization and includes a delayed response (Type 4); and different adjuvants favor different pathways.

Ultimately, of course, we are at the mercy of the dendritic cells, T-helper cells, and other minuscule creatures fluent in the cytokine language that make the important decisions for us—such as T_H1 versus T_H2. We can only hope that they are sufficiently informed of the big picture to make the right decisions.

(II) How Do Granulomas Relate to Hypersensitivity?

Of course, granulomas induced by nonantigenic foreign bodies have nothing to do with the immune response. Regarding immune granulomas, somehow the erroneous notion has crept in that they are all due to hypersensitivity, implying that the granulomatous response in general is inappropriate. Not so. *Granulomas are a life-saving product of evolution;* suffice it to see the dire effects of inhibiting the granulomatous response in tuberculosis or leprosy.

However, hypersensitivity *can* occur in immune granulomas. In tubercles, as we have just discussed, caseous necrosis is best interpreted as a manifestation of hypersensitivity. Different degrees of granulomatous response, including hypersensitivity, are well demonstrated in experimental schistosomiasis (173): live microscopic worms are injected into mouse; they settle in the roots of the portal veins and shed eggs into the liver, where they induce typical immune granulomas. A T_H1 type of cytokine environment (p. 530) prevails for about 2 weeks, followed by a mixed T_H1 and T_H2 response. If the initial T_H1 response is experimentally engineered to be excessive, it causes large granulomas to form, with destructive effects on the surrounding liver tissue. Such granulomas can be deservedly called *hypersensitivity granulomas.* A predominant T_H2 type of response has a dampening effect on the excessive inflammatory events around the granuloma.

Last, a challenge, to test the reader's understanding of granulomas and hypersensitivity. Figures 17.39–17.41 illustrate contact dermatitis, a classic example of Type 4 [cell-mediated] hypersensitivity. Figure 17.41 could very well be labeled "histology of a tuberculin reaction after 3 days." Does it show granulomas, and if not, why not? The answer is in the legend.

(III) Is There Any "Hypersensitivity" Unrelated to the Immune Response?

We know two; both are based on injecting something into a prepared animal, and both are somewhat mysterious. One is calciphylaxis (p. 259), the other is the Shwartzman phenomenon.

The Shwartzman phenomenon. This experimental phenomenon, also called the *Shwartzman reaction* is a puzzling observation dating from 1928 that is incompletely understood but still attracts attention because it relates to important themes: endotoxin damage, shock, TNF, vasculitis, and even the Koch phenomenon. It comes in two varieties, local and generalized, and works best in rabbits.

To elicit the *local Shwartzman reaction,* a small dose of endotoxin is injected intradermally into a rabbit; no visible changes appear, although microscopically the dermis shows a leukocytic infiltrate with a predominance of neutrophils (157, 171, 176). Then, 24 hours later, a second injection of endotoxin is given intravenously, and a necrotic–hemorrhagic lesion develops at the first injection site (Figure 17.47).

For the second injection, endotoxin can be replaced by zymosan, which activates complement (113). The basic question is, of course, what has changed in the tissue after the first injection? If the rabbit is depleted of leukocytes, the reaction is abolished (174), as happens with the Arthus lesion (p. 543). Other factors involved are endothelial apoptosis (153), the expression of endothelial adhesion molecules, and IL-12 as a primer that induces interferon gamma (158).

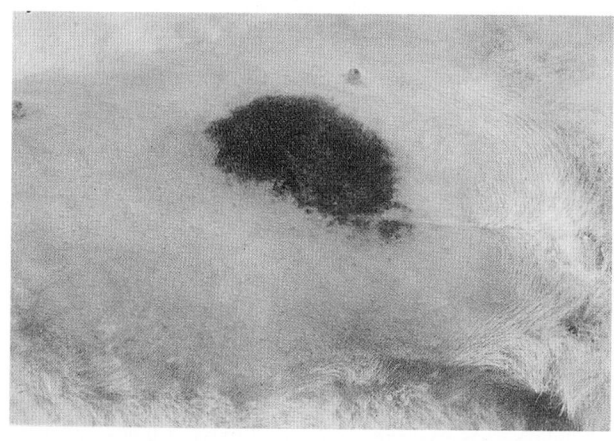

FIGURE 17.47 The local Shwartzman phenomenon. Abdominal skin of a living rabbit that received first an intradermal injection of endotoxin (meningococcus culture filtrate); then the same endotoxin was injected intravenously 24 hours later. Four hours after the second injection, this hemorrhagic lesion appeared. (Reproduced from [172]. Photograph by Mr. Harold Fowler.)

The generalized Shwartzman reaction, which should really be called the Sanarelli–Shwartzman reaction (145, 157), is produced by injecting both doses of endotoxin intravenously 24 hours apart; a disseminated intravascular coagulation follows, which may produce bilateral cortical necrosis of the kidney (Figure 17.48) and death. One theory runs as follows (167). The first injection of endotoxin produces widespread platelet destruction and release of thromboplastin, but the RES

(p. 314) manages to remove the microscopic fibrin clots. The second injection has the same effect, but this time the RES is overwhelmed ("blockaded," p. 316), and microvascular occlusion follows. *In pregnant rabbits a single intravenous injection suffices,* presumably because fibrinolysis is depressed. This may explain certain cases of bilateral cortical necrosis after septic abortions.

Another explanation (119): both local and general Shwartzman reactions are due to oversecretion of interferon gamma, and both are inhibited by antibody against interferon gamma. Once again, time will tell.

The last word to a cobra. On 21 June, 1995, the Director of the Reptile World Serpentarium in St. Cloud, Florida, was bitten by a 12-foot king cobra (177). That was not a new experience: he had been bitten by a king cobra once before, in 1987; antiserum had saved him. To any well-trained physician who might have been present at the scene of the accident it should have been obvious that there were *two* urgent problems: this latest bite was bad enough, but what about the effect of the earlier bite? Had it left the body protected, like a vaccination (by the IgG/IgM pathway), or hypersensitive and ready for anaphylaxis (by the IgE pathway)? Alas, theory could not help. As the Serpentarium director was being rushed to a hospital, I doubt that even a seasoned immunologist could have advised him on the basis of theory alone. Luckily the patient knew what to do: herpetologists may not know about IgM and IgE, but they do know by experience that immunization against snake venom requires multiple injections of venom, and that a single cobra bite offers no protection: a second bite is likely to produce anaphylactic shock. So he gave himself two shots of epinephrine. Although this was not enough to avert anaphylactic shock, he survived to tell the story—which tells us that we still have a lot to learn about the relationship between immunity and hypersensitivity.

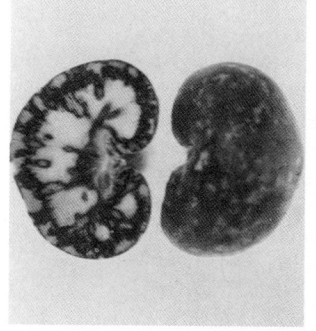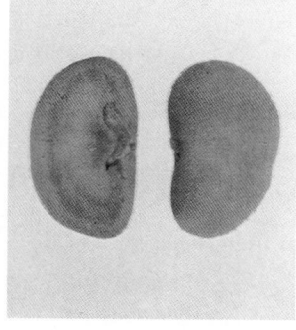

FIGURE 17.48 Generalized Shwartzman reaction. *Left:* Kidney of rabbit that received two intravenous injections of a meningococcal toxin 20 hours apart. Necrosis and hemorrhage involve large parts of the medulla and cortex. *Right:* Normal rabbit kidney. (Reproduced from the **Journal of Experimental Medicine** 1952;96: 605–624, by copyright permission of the Rockefeller University Press [176].)

References

Hypersensitivity Type 1

1. Adler SH, Gudmundsdottir H, Turka LA. Normal immune responses. In: Neilson EG, Couser WG (eds). Immunologic renal diseases, 2nd ed. Philadelphia, PA: Lippincott Williams & Wilkins, 2001, pp. 15–46.
2. Anderson SD. Exercise-induced asthma. In: Middleton E Jr, Reed CE, Ellis EF, Adkinson NF Jr, Yuninger JW, eds. Allergy principles and practice. St. Louis: CV Mosby, 1988, pp. 1156–1175.

3. Atherton DJ. Skin disorders and food allergy. J R Soc Med 1985;78(suppl 5):7–10.

4. Austen KF. The heterogeneity of mast cell populations and products. Hosp Pract 1984;19:135–146.

5. Ball TM, Castro-Rodriguez JA, Griffith KA, et al. Siblings, day-care attendance and the risk of asthma and wheezing during childhood. N Engl J Med 2000;343:538–543.

6. Barnes PJ. New aspects of asthma. J Intern Med 1992;231:453–461.

7. Bochner BS, Lichtenstein LM. Anaphylaxis. N Engl J Med 1991;324:1785–1790.

8. Braquet P, Touqui L, Shen TY, Vargaftig BB. Perspectives in platelet-activating factor research. Pharmacol Rev 1987;39:97–145.

9. Brutkiewicz RR, Welsh RM. Major Histocompatibility Complex Class I Antigens and the Control of Viral Infections by Natural Killer Cells. J Virol 1995;69:3967–3971.

10. Charlesworth EN, Hood AF, Soter NA, et al. Cutaneous late-phase response to allergen: mediator release and inflammatory cell infiltration. J Clin Invest 1989;83:1519–1526.

11. Cookson W. The alliance of genes and environment in asthma and allergy. Nature 1999;402(suppl):B5–B11.

12. Coombs RRA, Gell GH. Classification of allergic reactions responsible for clinical hypersensitivity and disease. In Gell PGH, Coombs RRA, Lachmann PJ, eds. Clinical aspects of immunology, 3rd ed. Oxford: Blackwell Scientific Publications, 1975, pp. 761–781.

13. Corry DB, Kheradmand F. Induction and regulation of the IgE response. Nature 1999;402(suppl):B18–B23.

14. de Weck AL. In: Pearce FL. Non-IgE-Mediated Mast Cell Stimulation (discussion). In: IgE, Mast Cells and the Allergic Response. Ciba Foundation Symposium 1989;147:74–92.

15. DeWeese DD, Saunders WH. Textbook of otolaryngology. St. Louis: CV Mosby, 1982.

16. Dvorak AM, Schleimer RP, Lichtenstein LM. Human mast cells synthesize new granules during recovery from degranulation. In vitro studies with mast cells purified from human lungs. Blood 1988;71:76–85.

17. Dvorak AM, Schuulman ES, Peters SP, et al. Immunoglobulin E-mediated degranulation of isolated human lung mast cells. Lab Invest 1985;53:45–56.

18. Fuller RW. Macrophages. Br Med J 1992;48:65–71.

19. Ha T-Y, Reed ND. Systemic anaphylaxis in mast-cell-deficient mice of W/W^v and Sl/Sl^d genotypes. Exp Cell Biol 1987;55:63–68.

20. Hallett R, Haapanen LAD, Teuber SS. Food allergies and kissing. N Engl J Med 2002;346:1833–1834.

21. Hanifin JM. Atopic dermatitis. J Allergy Clin Immunol 1984;73:211–222.

22. Hildreth EA. Anaphylactoid reactions to iodinated contrast media. Hosp Pract 1987;22:77–95.

23. Holgate ST. The epidemic of allergy and asthma. Nature 1999;402(suppl):B2–B4.

24. Holmes FL, Richet CR. In: Gillispie CC, ed. Dictionary of scientific biography, vol XI. New York: Charles Scribner's Sons, 1975, pp. 425–432.

25. Holt PG, Macaubas C, Stumbles PA, Sly PD. The role of allergy in the development of asthma. Nature 1999;402(suppl):B12–B17.

26. Jacoby W, Cammarata PV, Findlay S, Pincus SH. Anaphylaxis in mast cell-deficient mice. J Invest Dermatol 1984;83:302–304.

27. Kaliner MA. The late-phase reaction and its clinical implications. Hosp Pract 1987;22:73–83.

28. Kaplan AP. Urticaria and angioedema. In: Middleton E Jr, Reed CE, Ellis EF, Adkinson NF Jr, Yunginger JW, eds. Allergy. Principles and practice. St. Louis: CV Mosby, 1988, pp. 1377–1401.

29. Kay AB. Allergy and allergic diseases, part 1. N Engl J Med 2001;344:30–37.

30. Kay AB. Allergy and allergic diseases, part 2. N Engl J Med 2001;344:109–113.

31. Lagunoff D, Martin TW, Read G. Agents that release histamine from mast cells. Annu Rev Pharmacol Toxicol 1983;23:331–351.

32. Larsen GL. The pulmonary late-phase response. Hosp Pract 1987;22:155–169.

33. Lehane L, Olley J. Histamine fish poisoning revisited. Int J Food Microbiol 2000;58:1–37.

34. Leiferman KM, Fujisawa T, Gray BH, Gleich GJ. Extracellular deposition of eosinophil and neutrophil granule proteins in the IgE-mediated cutaneous late phase reaction. Lab Invest 1990;62:579–589.

34a. Leung DYM, Sampson HA, Yunginger JW, et al. Effect of anti-IgE therapy in patients with peanut allergy. N Engl J Med 2003;348:986–993.

35. Lichtenstein LM. The nasal late-phase response—an in vivo model. Hosp Pract 1988;23:105–128.

36. Lieberman P, Anderson JA (eds). Allergic diseases. Diagnosis and treatment, 2nd ed. Totowa, NJ: Humana Press, 2000.

37. Lukacs NW. Role of chemokines in the pathogenesis of asthma. Nat Rev Immunol 2001;1:108–116.

38. MacQueen G, Marshcall J, Perdue M, Siegel S, Bienenstock J. Pavlovian conditioning of rat mucosal mast cells to secrete rat mast cell protease II. Science 1989;243:83–85.

39. Maitai CK, Talalaj S, Njoroge D, Wamugunda R. Effect of extract of hairs from the herb Urtica massaica, on smooth muscle. Toxicon 1980;18:225–229.

40. Majno G. The Healing Hand: Man and Wound in the Ancient World. Cambridge, MA: Harvard University Press, 1975.

41. Matsuda H, Watanabe N, Kiso Y, et al. Necessity of IgE antibodies and mast cells for manifestation of resistance against larval Haemaphysalis longicornis ticks in mice. J Immunol 1990;144:259–262.

42. McFadden ER Jr. Pathogenesis of asthma. J Allergy Clin Immunol 1984;73:413–424.

43. McNeill WH. Plagues and peoples. Garden City, NY: Anchor Press/Doubleday, 1976.

44. Metcalfe DD, Samter M, Condemi JJ. Reactions to foods. In: Samter M, Talmage DW, Frank MM, Austen KF, Claman HN, eds. Immunological diseases, 4th ed. Boston: Little, Brown, 1988:1149–1171.

44a. Metzger H. Two approaches to peanut allergy. N Engl J Med 2002;348:1046–1048.

45. Morrow JD, Margolies GR, Rowland J, Roberts LJ II. Evidence that histamine is the causative toxin of scombroid-fish poisoning. N Engl J Med 1991;324:716–720.

46. Mrazek DA. Asthma: psychiatric considerations, evaluation, and management. In: Middleton E Jr, Reed CE, Ellis EF, Adkinson NF Jr, Yunginger JW, eds. Allergy. Principles and practice. St. Louis: CV Mosby, 1988, pp. 1176–1196.

47. Nagler-Anderson C. Man the barrier! Strategic defences in the intestinal mucosa. Nat Rev Immunol 2001;1:59–67.

48. Norman PS. Immunotherapy of IgE-mediated disease. Hosp Pract 1990;25:81–92.

49. Owen RL. Macrophage function in Peyer's patch epithelium. Adv Exp Med Biol 1982;149:507–513.

50. Owen RL, Ermak TH. Structural specializations for antigen uptake and processing in the digestive tract. Springer Semin. Immunopathol 1990;12:139–152.

51. Patterson R, McKenna JM, Suszko IM, et al. Living histamine-containing cells from the bronchial lumens of humans. Description and comparison of histamine content with cells of rhesus monkeys. J Clin Invest 1977;59:217–225.

52. Patterson R, Pruzansky JJ, Dykewicz MS, Lawrence ID. Basophil-mast cell response syndromes: a unified clinical approach. Allergy Proc 1988;9:611–620.

53. Pearce FL. Non-IgE-mediated mast cell stimulation. Ciba Found Symp 1989;147:74–92.

54. Portier P. Recherches sur les venins de coelentérés. Découverte de l'anaphylaxie. In: Notice sur les titres et travaux scientifiques de P. Portier. Paris: A. Maretheux et L. Pactat, 1936.

55. Portier P, Richet C. De l'action anaphylactique de certains venins. C R Acad Sci [D] Paris 1902;54:170–172, 548–551, 837–838.

56. Prausnitz C, Küstner H. Studien über die Ueber-empfindlichkeit. Zentralbl Bakteriol 1921;86:160–169.

57. Pretolani M, Ferrer-Lopez P, Vargaftig BB. From anti-asthma drugs to PAF-acether antagonism and back. Present status. Biochem Pharmacol 1989;38:1373–1384.

58. Pretolani M, Lefort J, Dumarey C, Vargaftig BB. Role of lipoxygenase metabolites for the hyper-responsiveness to platelet-activating factor of lungs from actively sensitized guinea pigs. J Pharmacol Exp Ther 1989;248:353–359.

59. Pretolani M, Lellouch-Tubiana A, Lefort J, Bachelet M, Vargaftig BB. PAF-acether and experimental anaphylaxis as a model for asthma. Int Arch Allergy Appl Immunol 1989;88:149–153.

60. Reisman RE. Insect allergy. In: Middleton E Jr, Reed CE, Ellis EF, Adkinson NF Jr, Yunginger JW, eds. Allergy. Principles and practice, 3rd ed. St. Louis: CV Mosby, 1988, pp. 1345–1364.

61. Richet C, Portier P. Recherches sur la toxine des Coelentérés et les phénomènes d'anaphylaxie. Résultats des Campagnes Scientifiques Accomplies sur Son Yacht par Albert Ier Prince Souverain de Monaco. Monaco, 1936.

62. Rocklin RE, Rosen FS, David J, Fearon D, Piessens WF. Clinical immunology. In: Rubenstein E, Federman DD, eds. Scientific American Medicine. New York: Scientific American, 1991, pp. 1–35.

63. Roitt IM. Essential immunology, 6th ed. Oxford: Blackwell Scientific Publications, 1988.

64. Rosen FS, Steiner LA, Unanue ER. Dictionary of immunology. New York: Stockton Press, 1989.

65. Russell M, Dark KA, Cummins RW, et al. Learned histamine release. Science 1984;225:733–734.

66. Sampson HA. Late-phase response to food in atopic dermatitis. Hosp Pract 1987;22:111–128.

67. Schadewaldt, H. La croisière du Prince Albert 1er de Monaco en 1901 et la découverte de l'anaphylaxie. In: Colloque International sur L'Histoire de la Biologie Marine. Paris: Masson & Cie, 1965, pp. 305–313.

68. Schocket AL (ed). Clinical management of urticaria and anaphaylaxis. New York, NY: Marcel Decker, Inc., 1993.

69. Selye H. Anaphylactoid edema. St. Louis: Warren H. Green, 1968.

70. Serafin WE, Austen KF. Mediators of immediate hypersensitivity reactions. N Engl J Med 1987;317:30–34.

71. Smith PL, Kagey-Sobotka A, Bleecker ER, et al. Physiologic manifestations of human anaphylaxis. J Clin Invest 1980;66:1072–1080.

72. Takafuji S, Suzuki S, Muranaka M, Miyamoto T. Influence of environmental factors on IgE production. Ciba Found Symp 1989;147:188–204.

73. Tovey ER, Chapman MD, Platts-Mills TAE. Mite faeces are a major source of house dust allergens. Nature 1981;289:592–593.

74. Turner KJ. Epidemiology of the allergic response. Ciba Found Symp 1989;147:205–209.

75. Ucker DS. Cytotoxic T lymphocytes and glucocorticoids activate an endogenous suicide process in target cells. Nature 1987;327:62–64.

76. von Mutius E, Martinez FD, Fritzsch C, et al. Prevalence of asthma and atopy in two areas of west and east Germany. Am J Respir Crit Care Med 1994;149:358–364.

77. von Mutius E, Weiland SK, Fritzsch C, Duhme H, Keil U. Increasing prevalence of hay fever and atopy among children in Leipzig, East Germany. Lancet 1998;351:862–866.

78. Wasserman SI, Marquardt DL. Anaphylaxis. In: Middleton E Jr, Reed CE, Ellis EF, Adkinson NF Jr, Yunginger JW, eds. Allergy. Principles and practice, 3rd ed. St. Louis: CV Mosby, 1988, pp. 1365–1376.

79. Ziegler-Heitbrock HWL, Möller A, Linke RP, et al. Tumor necrosis factor as effector molecule in monocyte mediated cytotoxicity. Cancer Res 1986;46:5947–5952.

Hypersensitivity Types 2 and 3

80. Arthus M. Injections répétées de sérum de cheval chez le lapin. C R Soc Biol (Paris) 1903;55:817–820.

81. Benveniste J, Henson PM, Cochrane CG. Leukocyte-dependent histamine release from rabbit platelets. The role of IgE, basophils, and a platelet-activating factor. J Exp Med 1972;136:1356–1377.

82. Caulfield JP, Korman G, Butterworth AE, Hogan M, David JR. The adherence of human neutrophils and eosinophils to schistosomula: evidence for membrane fusion between cells and parasites. J Cell Biol 1980;86:46–63.

83. Caulfield JP, Lenzi HL, Elsas P, Dessein AJ. Ultrastructure of the attack of eosinophils stimulated by blood mononuclear cell products on schistosomula of Schistosoma mansoni. Am J Pathol 1985;120:380–390.

84. Cochrane CG. The Arthus reaction. In: Zweifach BW, Grant L, McCluskey RT, eds. The inflammatory process. New York: Academic Press, 1965, pp. 613–648.

85. Cochrane CG, Koffler D. Immune complex disease in experimental animals and man. Adv Immunol 1973;16:185–264.

86. Cochrane CG, Weigle WO, Dixon FJ. The role of polymorphonuclear leukocytes in the initiation and cessation of the Arthus vasculitis. J Exp Med 1959;110:481–494.

87. Cotran RS. Pathogenesis of vasculitis: an update. In: Fenoglio-Preiser C, ed. Advances in pathology, vol 3. St. Louis: Mosby-Year Book, 1990, pp. 301–310.

88. Cotran RS, Kumar V, Robbins SL. Robbins pathologic basis of disease, 4th ed. Philadelphia: WB Saunders, 1989, pp. 1025.

89. Dixon FJ. Mechanisms of immunologic injury. In: Good RA, Fisher DW, eds. Immunobiology. Stamford, CT: Sinauer Associates, 1971, pp. 161–173.

90. Dixon FJ, Cochrane CG, Theofilopoulos AN. Immune complex injury. In: Samter M, Talmage DW, Frank MM, Austen KF, Claman HN, eds. Immunological diseases, 4th ed. Boston: Little, Brown, 1988, pp. 233–259.

91. Dixon FJ, Feldman JD, Vazquez JJ. Experimental glomerulonephritis. The pathogenesis of a laboratory model resembling the spectrum of human glomerulonephritis. J Exp Med 1961;113:899–920.

92. Emancipator SN, Lamm ME. IgA nephropathy: pathogenesis of the most common form of glomerulonephritis. Lab Invest 1989;60:168–183.

93. Giglioli G. Malaria and renal disease, with special reference to British Guiana. II. The effect of malaria eradication on the incidence of renal disease in British Guiana. Ann Trop Med Parasitol 1962;56:225–241.

94. Heckbert SR, Stryker WS, Coltin KL, Manson JE, Platt R. Serum sickness in children after antibiotic exposure: estimates of occurrence and morbidity in a Health Maintenance Organization population. Am J Epidemiol 1990;132:336–342.

95. Humphrey JH. The mechanism of Arthus reactions. II. The role of polymorphonuclear leucocytes and platelets in reversed passive reactions in the guinea-pig. Br J Exp Pathol 1955;36:283–289.

96. Jandl JH. Blaod. Textbook of hematology. Boston, MA: Little, Brown and Company, 1987.

97. Kniker WT, Cochrane CG. Pathogenic factors in vascular lesions of experimental serum sickness. J Exp Med 1965; 122:83–98.

98. Kusner DJ, Ellner JJ. Syphilis—a reversible cause of nephrotic syndrome in HIV infection. N Engl J Med 1991;324:341–342.

99. Lawley TJ, Bielory L, Gascon P, et al. A prospective clinical and immunologic analysis of patients with serum sickness. N Engl J Med 1984;311:1407–1413.

100. LoBuglio AF, Cotran RS, Jandl JH. Red cells coated with immunoglobulin G: binding and sphering by mononuclear cells in man. Science 1967;158:1582–1585.

101. Metchnikoff E. Lectures on the comparative pathology of inflammation. (Translated from the French by Starling FA, Starling, EH, 1891.) New York: Dover Publications, 1968.

102. Movat HZ, Fernando NVP. I. The earliest fine structural changes at the blood-tissue barrier during antigen-antibody interaction. Am J Pathol 1963;42:41–59.

103. Moyer CF, Strandberg JD, Reinisch CL. Systemic mononuclear-cell vasculitis in MRL/Mp-lpr/lpr mice. A histologic and immunocytochemical analysis. Am J Pathol 1987;127:229–242.

104. Rocklin RE, Rosen FS, David J, Fearon D, Piessens WF. Clinical immunology. In: Rubenstein E, Federman DD, eds. Scientific American Medicine. New York: Scientific American, 1991, pp. 1–35.

105. Schmidt H. Grundlagen der spezifischen Therapie und Prophylaxe bakterieller Infektions-krankheiten. Berlin-Grünewald: Bruno Schultz, 1940, pp. 505–506.

106. Stankus RP, Salvaggio JE. Infiltrative lung disease: hypersensitivity pneumonitis, allergic bronchopulmonary aspergillosis, and the inorganic dust pneumoconioses. In: Samter M, Talmage DW, Frank MM, Austen KF, Claman NH, eds. Immunological diseases, 4th ed. Boston: Little, Brown, 1988, pp. 1561–1585.

107. von Pirquet C, Schick B. Die Serumkrankheit. Leipzig: Franz Deuticke, 1905.

108. von Pirquet C, Schick B. Serum Sickness. Baltimore: The Williams & Wilkins Company, 1951.

109. Ward PA, Cochrane CG. Bound complement and immunologic injury of blood vessels. J Exp Med 1965;121:215–234.

109a. Wentworth P Jr, McDunn JE, Wentworth AD, et al. Evidence for antibody-catalized ozone formation in bacterial killing and inflammation. Science 2002;298:2195–2199.

109b. Wentworth P Jr, Wentworth AD, Zhu X, et al. Evidence for the production of trioxygen species during antibody-catalyzed chemical modification of antigens. PNAS 2003;100:1490–1493; published online before print as 10.1073/pnas.0437831100

Hypersensitivity Type 4

110. Abe Y, Sugisaki K, Dannanberg AM Jr. Rabbit vascular endothelial adhesion molecules: ELAM-1 is most elevated in acute inflammation, whereas VCAM-1 and ICAM-1 predominate in chronic inflammation. J Leukoc Biol 1996;60:692–703.

111. Allison AC, Byars NE. An adjuvant formulation that selectively elicits the formation of antibodies of protective isotypes and of cell-mediated immunity. J Immunol Methods 1986;95:157–168.

112. Ando M, Dannenberg AM Jr, Sugimoto M, Tepper BS. Histochemical studies relating to activation of macrophages to the intracellular destruction of tubercle bacilli. Am J Pathol 1977;86:623–633.

113. Argenbright LW, Barton RW. Interactions of leukocyte integrins with intercellular adhesion molecule 1 in the production of inflammatory vascular injury in vivo. The Shwartzman reaction revisited. J Clin Invest 1992;89:259–272.

113a. Basu S, Binder RJ, Suto R, Anderson KM, Srivastava PK. Necrotic but not apoptotic cell death releases heat shock proteins, which deliver a partial maturation signal to dendritic cells and activate the NF-κB pathway. Int Immunol 2000;12:1539–1546.

114. Beck JS. Skin changes in the tuberculin test. Tubercle 1972;72:81–87.

115. Bendiner E. Albert Calmette: a vaccine and its vindication. Hosp Pract 1992;10:113–132.

116. Bendiner E. Baron von Pirquet: the aristocrat who discovered and defined allergy. Hosp Pract 1981;16:137–158.

117. Bhawan J, Sau P, Byers D. Dermatopathology interactive atlas. Developed by Web Cottage Solutions: Delhi, India, 2001.

117a. Blachere NE, Li Z, Chandawarkar RY, et al. Heat Shock protein-peptide complexes, reconstituted in vitro, elicit peptide-specific cytotoxic T lymphocyte response and tumor immunity. J Exp Med 1997;186:1315–1322.

118. Black CA. Delayed type hypersensitivity: Current theories with an historic perspective. Dermatol Online J 1999. http://dermatology.cdlib.org/DOJvol5num1/renews/black.html

119. Billiau A. Gamma-interferon: the match that lights the fire? Immunol Today 1988;9:37–40.

120. Bloom BR, McKinney JD. The death and resurrection of tuberculosis. Nat Med 1999;5:872–874.

121. Bothamley GH, Granger JM. The Koch phenomenon and delayed hypersensitivity: 1891–1991. Tubercle 1991;72:7–11.

122. Bryk R, Lima CD, Erdjument-Bromage H, Tempst P, Nathan C. Metabolic enzymes of mycobacteria linked to antioxidant defense by a thioredoxin-like protein. Sciencexpress; published online 17 January 2002;10.1126/science.1067798

122a. Campbell JJ, Butcher EC. Chemokines in tissue-specific and microenvironment-specific lymphocyte homing. Curr Opin Immunol 2000;12:336–341.

123. Canetti G. The tubercle bacillus in the pulmonary lesion of man. New York: Springer Publishing Co., 1955

124. Casanova J-L, Blanche S, Emile J-F, et al. Idiopathic disseminated bacillus Calmette-Guérin infection: a French national retrospective study. Pediatrics 1996;98:774–778.

125. Chedid L. Muramyl peptides as possible endogenous immunopharmacological mediators. Microbiol Immunol 1983;27:723–732.

125a. Clemens DL. Characterization of the Mycobacterium tuberculosis phagosome. Trends Microbiol 1996;4:113–118.

125b. Colvin RB, Johnson RA, Mihm MC Jr, Dvorak HF. Role of the clotting system in cell-mediated hypersensitivity. I. Fibrin deposition in delayed skin reactions in man. J Exp Med 1973;138:686–698.

126. Converse PJ, Dannenberg AM Jr, Estep JE, et al. Cavitary tuberculosis produced in rabbits by aerosolized virulent tubercle bacilli. Infect Immun 1996;64:4776–4787.

127. Converse PJ, Dannenberg AM Jr, Shigenaga T, et al. Pulmonary bovine-type tuberculosis in rabbits: bacillary virulence, inhaled dose effects, tuberculin sensitivity, and Mycobacterium vaccae immunotherapy. Clin Diagn Lab Immunol 1998;5:871–881.

128. Courtade ET, Tsuda T, Thomas CR, Dannenberg AM Jr. Capillary density in developing and healing tuberculous lesions produced by BCG in rabbits. Am J Pathol 1975;78:243–260.

129. Dannenberg AM Jr. Pathogenesis of tuberculosis: native and acquired resistance in animals and humans. In: Microbiology 1984. Washington DC: Am Soc Microbiol. 1984, pp. 344–354.

130. Dannenberg AM Jr. Immune mechanisms in the pathogenesis of pulmonary tuberculosis. Rev Infect Dis 1989;11(suppl 2):S369–S378.

131. Dannenberg AM Jr. Delayed-type hypersensitivity and cell-mediated immunity in the pathogenesis of tuberculosis. Immunol Today 1991;12:228–233.

132. Dannenberg AM Jr. Immunopathogenesis of pulmonary tuberculosis. Hosp Pract 1993;1:51–58.

133. Dannenberg AM Jr. Pathogenesis and immunology: Basic aspects. In: Schlossberg D (ed). Tuberculosis, 3rd ed. New York: Springer Verlag. 1994, pp. 17–39.

134. Dannenberg AM Jr, Rook GAW. Pathogenesis of pulmonary tuberculosis: An interplay of tissue-damaging and macrophage-activating immune responses-dual mechanisms that control bacillary multiplication. In: Bloom BR (ed). Tuberculosis: Pathogenesis, protection and control. Washington, DC: American Society for Microbiology. 1994, pp. 459–483.

135. Dannenberg AM Jr, Sugimoto M. Liquefaction of caseous foci in tuberculosis. Am Rev Respir Dis 1976;113:257–259.

136. Dannenberg AM Jr, Tomashefski JF Jr. Pathogenesis of pulmonary tuberculosis. In: Fishman AP, ed. Pulmonary diseases and disorders, 2nd ed. New York: McGraw-Hill, 1988, pp. 1821–1842.

137. Dienes L. Further observations concerning the sensitization of tuberculous guinea pigs. J Immunol 1928;15:153–174.

138. Dobos KM, Spotts EA, Quinn FD, et al. Necrosis of lung epithelial cells during infection with Mycobacterium tuberculosis is preceded by cell permeation. Infect Immunity 2000;68:6300–6310.

139. Dubos R, Dubos J. The white plague: tuberculosis, man, and society. New Brunswick, NJ: Rutgers University Press, 1952.

140. Dvorak HF. Cutaneous basophil hypersensitivity. J Allergy Clin Immunol 1976;58:229–240.

141. Ernst JD. Macrophage receptors for Mycobacterium tuberculosis. Infection Immunity 1998;66:1277–1281.

142. Fisher AA, Mitchell JC. Allergic sensitization to plants. In: Rietschel RL, Fowler JF Jr (eds). Fisher's contact dermatitis, 5th ed. Philadelphia: Lippincott Williams & Wilkins. 2001, pp. 351–395.

143. Freund J, McDermott K. Sensitization to horse serum by means of adjuvants. Proc Soc Exp Biol Med 1942;49:548–553.

143a. Gallucci S, Lolkema M, Matzinger P. Natural adjuvants: endogenous activators of dendritic cells. Nat Med 1999;2:1249–1255.

144. Gheorghiu M. The present and future role of BCG vaccine in tuberculosis control. Biologicals 1990;18:135–141.

145. Good RA, Thomas L. Studies on the generalized Shwartzman reaction. II. The production of bilateral cortical necrosis of the kidneys by a single injection of bacterial toxin in rabbits previously treated with thorotrast or trypan blue. J Exp Med 1952;96:625–641.

146. Gregoriadis G. Immunological adjuvants: a role for liposomes. Immunol Today 1990;11:89–97.

147. Hernandez-Pando R, Pavön L, Arriaga K, et al. Pathogenesis of tuberculosis in mice exposed to low and high doses of an environmental mycobacterial saprophyte before infection. Infect Immunol 1997;65:3317–3327.

148. Hunter D. The diseases of occupations. London: The English Universities Press Ltd., 1969.

149. Issekutz TB, Stoltz JM, van der Meide P. Lymphocyte recruitment in delayed-type hypersensitivity. The role of IFN-γ. J Immunol 1988;140:2989–2993.

150. Kambara T, Yasaka T, Nakamura T. The role of polymorphonuclear leukocytes in delayed hypersensitivity skin reactions: suppressive effects of anti-polymorphonuclear leukocyte serum. Virchows Arch [B] 1981;37:191–198.

151. Koch R. Fortsetzung der Mittheilungen über ein Heilmittel genen Tuberculose. Dtsch Med Wochenschr 1891a;17:101–102.

152. Koch R.I. Weitere Mittheilung über das Tuberkulin. Dtsch Med Wochenschr 1891b;17:1189–1192.

153. Koide N, Abe K, Narita K, et al. Expression of intercellular adhesion molecule-1 (ICAM-1) on vascular endothelial cells and renal tubular cells in the generalized Shwartzman reaction as an experimental disseminated intravascular coagulation model. FEMS Immunol Med Microbiol 1997;18:67–74.

154. Lagranderie M, Ravisse P, Marchal G, et al. BCG-induced protection in guinea pigs vaccinated and challenged via the respiratory route. Tubercle Lung Dis 1993;74:38–46.

154a. Lien E, Golenbok DT. Adjuvants and their signaling pathways: beyond TLRs. Nat Immunol 2003;4:1162–1165.

155. Lurie MB. Resistance to tuberculosis: Experimental studies in native and acquired defensive mechanisms. Cambridge, MA: Harvard University Press, 1964.

155a. MacMicking JD, Taylor GA, McKinney JD. Immune control of tuberculosis by IFN-γ–inducible LRG-47. Science 2003;302:654-659.

156. Minton SA Jr, Minton MR. Venomous Reptiles. New York: Charles Scribner's Sons, 1969.

157. Movat HZ, Jeynes BJ, Wasi S, Movat KW, Kopaniak MM. Quantitation of the development and progression of the local Shwartzman reaction. In: Agarwal MK, ed. Bacterial endotoxins and host response. Amsterdam: Elsevier-North Holland Biomedical Press, 1980, pp. 179–201.

158. Ogasawara K, Takeda K, Hashimoto W, et al. Involvement of NK1+ T cells and their IFN-γ production in the generalized Shwartzman reaction. J Immunol 1998;160:3522–3527.

159. Reichman LB. Tuberculin skin testing. The state of the art. Chest 1979;76(suppl):764S–770S.

160. Rich AR. The pathogenesis of tuberculosis, 2nd ed. Springfield, IL: Charles C. Thomas, 1951.

161. Rietschel RL, Fowler JF Jr. Fisher's contact dermatitis 5th ed. Philadelphia: Lippincott Williams & Wilkins, 2001.

162. Rook GAW. The pathogenesis of tuberculosis. Annu Rev Microbiol 1996;50:259–284.

163. Rook GAW, Attiyah RA. Cytokines and the Koch phenomenon. Tubercle 1991;72:13–20.

164. Rosen FS, Steiner LA, Unanue ER. Dictionary of immunology. New York: Stockton Press, 1989.

165. Sakula A. BCG: who were Calmette and Guérin? Thorax 1983;38:806–812.

165a. Sauter B, Albert LA, Francisco L, et al. Consequences of cell death: exposure to necrotic tumor cells, but not primary tissue cells or apoptotic cells, induces the maturation of immunostimulatory dendritic cells. J Exp Med 2000;191:423–433.

166. Schluger NW, Rom WN. The host immune response to tuberculosis. Am J Respir Crit Care Med 1998;157:679–691.

167. Sell S. Immunology immunopathology and immunity, 4th ed. New York: Elsevier, 1987.

168. Shapiro E. Robert Koch and his tuberculin fallacy. Pharos 1983;9:19–22.

169. Shi Y, Rock KL. Cell death releases endogenous adjuvants that selectively enhance immune surveillance of particulate antigens. Eur J Immunol 2002;32:155–162.

170. Shigenaga T, Dannenberg AM Jr, Lowrie DB, et al. Immune responses in tuberculosis: antibodies and CD4-CD8 lymphocytes with vascular adhesion molecules and cytokines (chemokines) cause a rapid antigen-specific cell infiltration at sites of bacillus Calmette-Guérin reinfection. Immunology 2001;102:466–479.

171. Shima K, Dannenberg AM Jr, Ando M, et al. Macrophage accumulation, division, maturation, and digestive and microbicidal capacities in tuberculous lesions. Am J Pathol 1972;67:159–180.

172. Shwartzman G. Phenomenon of local tissue reactivity and its immunological, pathological and clinical significance. New York: Paul B. Hoeber, Inc., 1937.

173. Stadecker ML, Hernandez HC. Schistosomiasis: a model of immunologically mediated liver disease. In: Arias IM, Boyer JL, Chisari FV, et al. (eds). The Liver: Biology and pathobiology, 4th ed. Philadelphia, PA: Lippincott Williams & Wilkins, 2001, pp. 755–762.

174. Stetson CA Jr. Similarities in the mechanisms determining the Arthus and Shwartzman phenomena. J Exp Med 1951;94:347–358.

174a. Stewart GR, Robertson BD, Young DB. Tuberculosis: a problem with persistence. Nat Rev Microbiol 2003;1:97–105.

175. Taft P, Edgar B. 1991, personal communication (Dr. Piri Taft is daughter of Dr. L. Dienes).

176. Thomas L, Good RA. Studies on the generalized Shwartzman reaction. I. General observations concerning the phenomenon. J Exp Med 1952;96:605–624.

177. Thomas M. Cobra Attack! In: Reader's Digest, December 1995, pp. 128–133.

178. Tidjani O, Amedome A, ten Dam HG. The protective effect of BCG vaccination of the newborn against childhood tuberculosis in an African community. Tubercle 1986;67:269–281.

179. Tripathy SP. The case for BCG. Ann Natl Med Sci (India) 1983;19:11–21.

180. Underhill DM, Ozinsky A, Smith KD, Aderem A. Toll-like receptor-2 mediates mycobacteria-induced proinflammatory signaling in macrophages. PNAS 1999;96:14459–14463.

181. von Pirquet C. Allergie. Münch Med Wochenschr 1906;30:1–4.

182. Willms-Kretschmer K, Flax MH, Cotran RC. The fine structure of the vascular response in hapten-specific delayed hypersensitivity and contact dermatitis. Lab Invest 1967;17:334–349.

183. Youmans GP. Relation between delayed hypersensitivity and immunity in tuberculosis. Am Rev Respir Dis 1975;111:109–118.

184. Youmans GP. Tuberculosis. Philadelphia: WB Saunders, 1979.

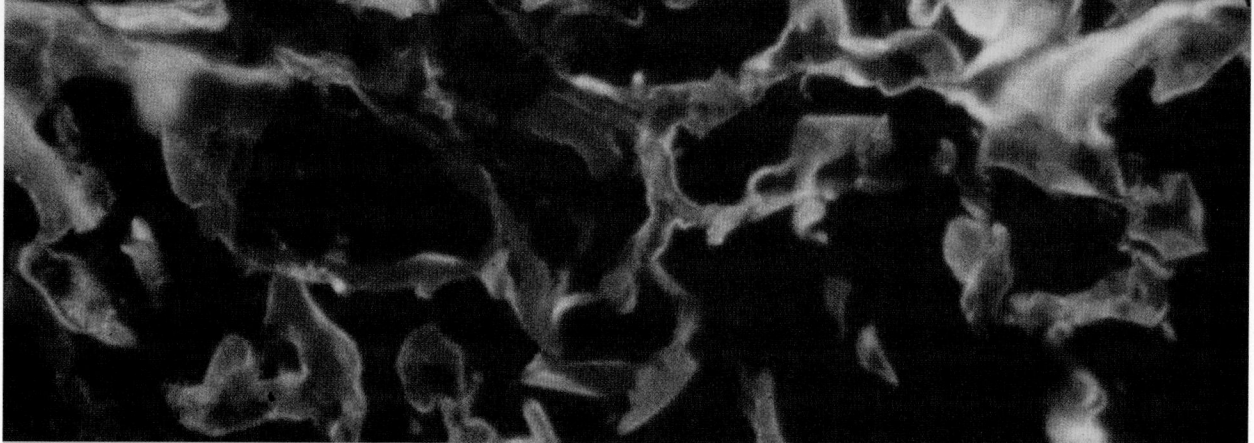

PATHOLOGY OF TRANSPLANTATION

It is a fact of life that the body is generally unwilling to accept extraneous spare parts. We owe the discovery of this law to the ever-daring surgeons (66, 83), who have tried to overcome it for some 3000 years. The first on record are the *vaidya* of ancient India, who knew that a lost nose could be rebuilt with a graft of skin from the forehead of the same patient; not from another person (51). *From the same patient:* this was the key to successful grafts. In the late 1500s the Italian surgeon Gaspare Tagliacozzi was successfully rebuilding noses using a flap of skin from the arm (88), but he made the right choice (by taking the graft from the arm of the same patient) for the wrong reason: pure convenience. In fact he was quite sure that grafts from one person to another would take. After all, he argued, it is known since Roman times that grafts can be exchanged between fig trees and olive trees, and no two people are as different as such trees. And so the surgeons kept trying. John Hunter reported in the late 1700s that he had managed to graft the spur of one cock onto the comb of another cock (we shall return to this alarming report later). The year 1906 saw the first successful grafting of a cornea from one human to another (Figure 18.1) (100); thereafter this practice became standard, although a theoretical background was not available. In 1902 Alexis Carrel, surgeon and biologist, found a method for reconnecting severed blood vessels. His motivation was sparked in 1894, when the President of the French Republic was knifed by an anarchist, and died because the surgeons were unable to suture a transected portal vein (31). Carrel used his procedure to attempt experimental grafts of limbs, kidneys, and other organs. Grafts from one part to another part of the same individual succeeded, but all others failed (16). Carrel won the Nobel prize for his surgical procedure; but after him, by and large, organ transplantation was branded hopeless. Only a "liquid" graft, blood transfusion, took hold; the ABO system was worked out in 1910, and it was soon recognized as a key to success in transfusing blood.

Why did the organ grafts fail? As early as 1910 Da Fano puzzled over the fact that the inflammatory response under rejected skin

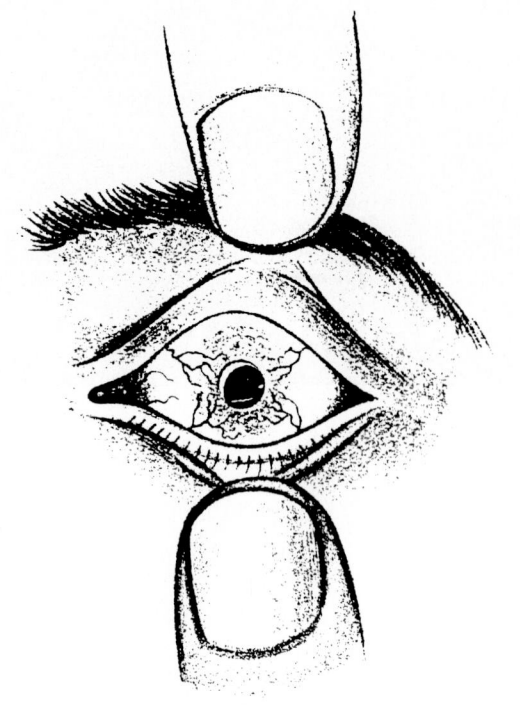

FIGURE 18.1   The first successful human allograft in 1906. The cornea was provided by an 11-year-old boy whose eye had to be enucleated because of trauma; recipient was a 45-year-old man whose eyes had been burned by quicklime 16 months earlier. (Reproduced from [100] by permission from Springer-Verlag.)

grafts consisted mainly of lymphocytes, though dead tissue is usually surrounded by polymorphonuclear leukocytes (23). He could do little with his observation because the function of lymphocytes remained a mystery until the late 1940s. During World War II, a young British zoologist, Peter Medawar, began to work out the mechanisms of graft rejection. His work was prompted, once again, by a surgical need: to find a covering for extensive burn injuries of a Royal Air Force pilot. Skin grafts from uninjured donors would have been ideal in war-time, but they would not take. Medawar discovered that the mechanism was an immune response (54–57) and won the Nobel prize in 1960.

Now is the time for some vocabulary.

- **Autograft:** graft for which donor and recipient are the same individual (also **autologous** graft).
- **Isograft:** graft between individuals of identical genetic makeup (**syngeneic**), such as identical twins or inbred animals.
- **Allograft:** graft between individuals of the same species but with different genetic makeup (**allogeneic**), such as grafts from one human being to another, or between different animals of noninbred strains. (The term *homograft* is obsolete.)
- **Xenograft:** graft between individuals of different species, such as human to mouse or baboon to human.

Graft Rejection: Role of the Immune Response

Just by observing the clinical course of graft rejection one should suspect that the underlying mechanism is an immune response; in fact this was suggested in the early 1900s by tumor researchers (83), but nobody drew the general conclusion before Peter Medawar. He and his research group, working mainly with mice bearing small patches of skin from other mice (Figure 18.2), established the following basic principles, which are valid for all grafts:

- Autografts and isografts are accepted; allografts and xenografts are rejected, xenografts sometimes in a matter of minutes (72).
- A *first* allograft begins by behaving properly: its vessels connect with those of the surrounding skin, and circulation is reestablished. However, lymphocytes and macrophages begin to appear and rapidly increase in numbers; soon the small vessels are thrombosed, necrosis sets in, and the dead graft is cast off. The initial "take" indicates that the host does not immediately recognize the graft as foreign. Such is the so-called **first-set rejection,** which requires 7–10 days.

- A *second* allograft *from the same donor* is rejected much faster and with a livelier inflammation; the drama is over in 3–4 days. Some polymorphs and plasma cells are also involved. This is **second-set rejection.**
- A *third* allograft *taken from a different donor* produces a first-set rejection, providing evidence that the rejection response is specific to the donor's tissue and therefore is consistent with an immune response. T-lymphocytes are essential to rejection. Mice that have been deprived neonatally of their thymuses, and are therefore incapable of educating their T-cells, lose the capacity to reject grafts. Conversely, if lymphocytes of a mouse that has rejected a skin graft from donor X are injected intravenously into another mouse, that mouse becomes ready to develop a second-set rejection to a first graft from donor X.

All this tells us that the rejection is based primarily on immunologic mechanisms. To understand what it is that the host recognizes as foreign, we will briefly explain the "identity cards" carried by all cells, namely the histocompatibility antigens.

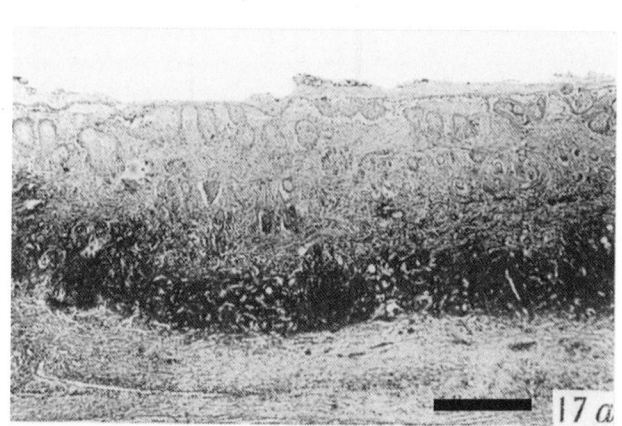
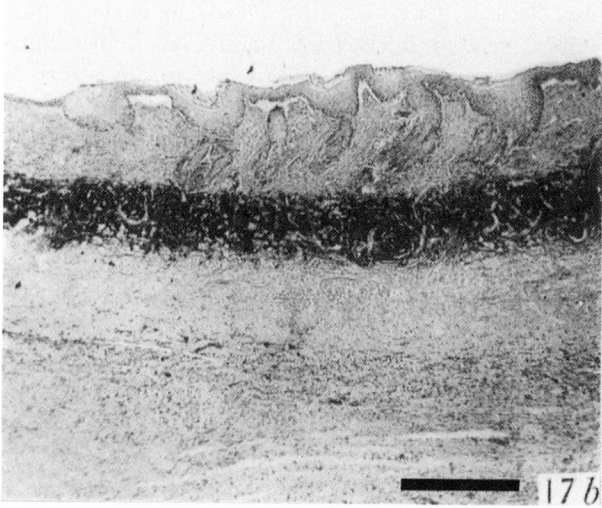

FIGURE 18.2   Allografts from the pioneer study by Peter B. Medawar in 1944. *Left:* Rabbit allograft at 8 days; the "black band" corresponds to lymphocytes. *Right:* Allograft at 16 days. **Bars** = 500 μm. (Reproduced with permission from [54].)

The Histocompatibility Antigens

Because cells have no eyes and no ears, they must recognize each other by sniffing (i.e., by chemical messengers) and by feeling each other's surfaces. If cells were covered by a pure and simple phospholipid bilayer, life would be impossible; we would be just a pile of disoriented cells. Surface identity-markers are essential. Interestingly, *while cells are choosy with regard to their outer contacts, they are poorly equipped to recognize anything foreign that has managed to get inside them.* A human cell will accept the microsurgical intrusion of a tobacco plant nucleus without a blink. A number of intracellular parasites make their living from this biological loophole; viruses, for example, have discovered that the inside of any cell and even of a bacterium is a safe place. It has been hinted that some viruses have evolved the ability to cause cell fusion so that they can pass from one cell to another without being exposed to the dangers of the outer world, where antibodies may lurk. *There are no intracellular antibodies.* Lewis Thomas wrote one of his beautiful essays on this topic: "Symbiosis as an immunological problem" (91).

Back to the surface identity-markers: All cells display one or both of two sets of surface markers (Class I and Class II); both are glycoproteins (Figure 18.3). Because immunologists (like lymphocytes) understand proteins as antigens, these surface glycoproteins are called histocompatibility *antigens.* But do remember that these surface markers have important functions when they are "at home," besides waiting to be grafted onto someone

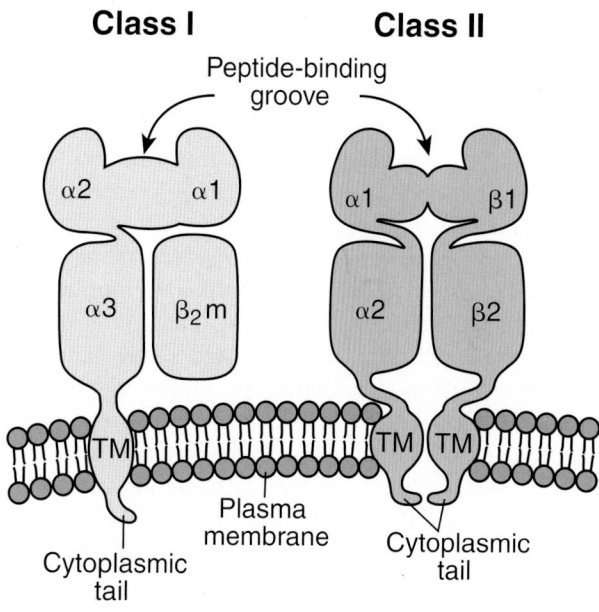

FIGURE 18.3   Two sets of surface markers for cells: HLA Class I and Class II molecules. Killer T-cells attack only cells marked by Class I molecules. The Class II molecules displayed on the surface of antigen-presenting cells enable helper T-cells to recognize them. (Reproduced with permission from: New Engl. J. Med. "Advances in Immunology: The HLA System," Klein J, Sato A. 343:702–709,2000. Copyright © 2000 Massachusetts Medical Society. All rights reserved.)

else. Because geneticists (like DNA) understand proteins as gene products, Class I and Class II histocompatibility antigens are usually explained in terms of the genes that code for them. We will follow these trends, but to remind the reader that "gene products" and "antigens" are just two other ways to say "proteins," we will temporarily confine "histocompatibility antigens" between quotation marks.

The Major Histocompatibility Complex

Now, it so happens that, in humans, the proteins that function as "histocompatibility antigens" are the products of a cluster of genes on a short segment of chromosome 6; this cluster is known as the major histocompatibility complex (MHC), or as the HLA complex (Figure 18.4) (45, 46).

> The term HLA is short for **human leukocyte antigens,** and dates from a time when it was believed that these "histocompatibility antigens" were present only on leukocytes. In mice the MHC is called H2 and it is on chromosome 17.

One factor that drastically complicates transplantation is that *the proteins coded by the HLA complex come in many variants;* in other words, for each gene in the complex there are a number of possible alleles (**alleles** are variants of a gene at a particular genetic locus).

Class I "histocompatibility antigens" are present on the surfaces of virtually all cells, including platelets, a factor that must be considered in platelet transfusions. These antigens are coded in adjacent genetic loci labeled A, B, and C (HLA-A, HLA-B, HLA-C).

Class II "histocompatibility antigens" are normally limited to cells of the immunologic family: monocytes/macrophages, dendritic cells, Langerhans cells of the epidermis, B-cells and some activated T-cells (and, for unknown reasons, spermatozoa). However, gamma-interferon (secreted by activated T-cells) causes other cells to express Class II antigens, for instance, endothelial cells and fibroblasts. Class II antigens are coded in a region of the MHC complex known as HLA-D, which includes three clusters of genes called DR, DP, and DQ.

From what we have said, it follows that *all cells that carry Class II antigens also carry Class I antigens.* This fact has its consequences: in a graft, the most antigenic cells are likely to be those that carry both classes of histocompatibility antigens, such as macrophages.

> **NOTE:** Allografts can "take" even if HLA matching is not perfect. In a series of 20,000 transplants of cadaveric kidney, one-year survival was 83.3 percent for grafts with no HLA antigens mismatched, and 77.0 for kidneys with 4 mismatches (40).

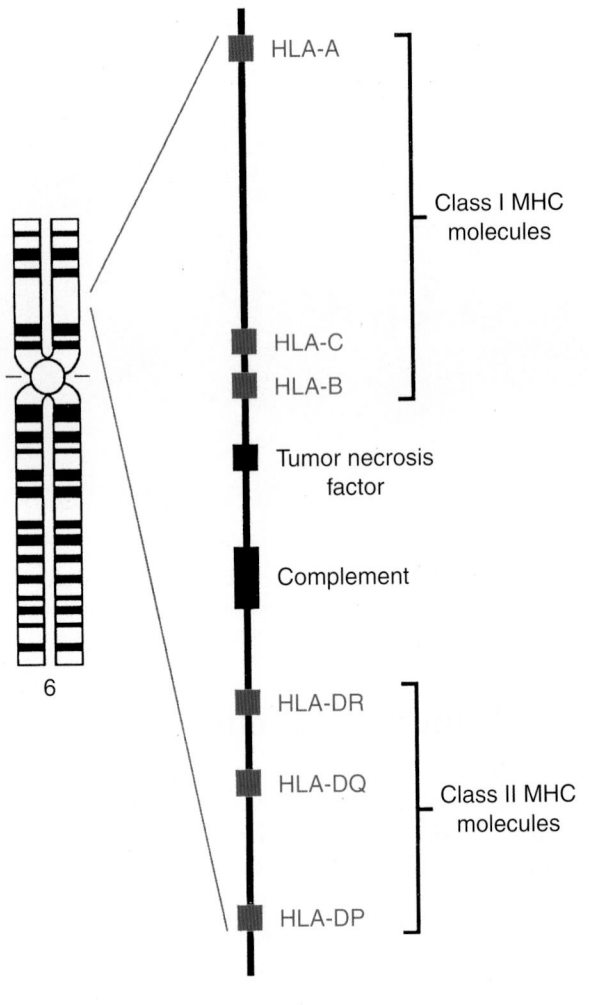

FIGURE 18.4 The best characterized loci of the human major histocompatibility complex (MHC) located in the HLA region of the short arm of chromosome 6. Inserted among the HLA genes are two genes for tumor necrosis factor and three genes for complement components. (Adapted from 6 Immunology, V Histocompatibility Antigens and Immune Response Genes in WebMD Scientific American ® Medicine, Dale DC, Federman DD (ed). WebMD Corporation, New York, 2003 [15].)

Functions of the Major Histocompatibility Complex

An elaborate system such as the HLA complex must have some profound reasons for its existence besides complicating the lives of students, teachers and surgeons. We might speculate, for example, that the tremendous variety fostered by the HLA system helps the survival of the species; if every human being carried the same HLA type, a cunning parasite able to exactly match that HLA type would escape detection and possibly wipe out the entire species. Another purpose might be to prevent mother and fetus from invading each other's tissues.

Much remains to be understood, but we can conclude that the HLA antigens are relevant (if not always useful) to three areas.

Regulation of the immune response. In several interactions between effector cells of the immune response, Class I or Class II antigens are used as "passports" (i.e., recognition molecules) sometimes accompanied by other "co-stimulatory" molecules.

Association with disease. As soon as HLA typing became possible, it turned out that many of the Class I and Class II HLA antigens are statistically associated with specific diseases (45, 46). For example, people who carry the HLA B27 antigen are 175 times more likely than normal to develop ankylosing spondylitis, a crippling disease of the spine. The known number of such associations continues to grow (30). There is even an association between the HLA antigen DR2 and narcolepsy, a disease consisting of an abnormal tendency to fall asleep (53). Most of the diseases related to HLA antigens are either inflammatory, autoimmune, or metabolic; how the correlation works is still not known, but one can speculate (99): (1) because up- or down-regulation of the immune response is a function of Class II antigens, malfunction of these antigens could lead to autoimmunity; (2) an HLA antigen might conceivably function as a receptor for a virus and therefore favor infection by that virus.

You may now wonder whether you should run to the nearest hospital and obtain your HLA type as a more reliable, albeit more expensive, substitute for palm reading. But many correlations between HLA type and disease are rather weak, and we can only estimate the relative risks because not everybody who is DR2-positive tends to fall asleep and not all sleepy individuals are DR2-positive. And anyway, do we really want to know what *might* be in store for us?

Paternity testing. The HLA system was not created for this purpose, but in practice it has become an invaluable asset for paternity testing. The principle is to compare the peripheral blood lymphocytes of mother, putative father, and child with regard to surface (HLA) antigens. The same complexity of the HLA system that decreases the chance of success of a graft increases the chance of success in identifying the father. However, in legal matters, the HLA makeup is currently not acceptable as a sole source of evidence; it must be backed by other genetic markers such as red blood cell antigens and DNA.

HLA testing is a complex matter, but in essence: human chromosome 6 carries, on each of its two strands, a string of seven HLA genes (called a *haplotype*, from *haploid genotype*). Each of us therefore expresses two haplotypes. If we are heterozygous, we can express 14 possible HLA gene products, and the polymorphism of these genes means a great variety of product combinations (Figure 18.5). To identify the HLA makeup of a given individual, blood-derived lymphocytes of that individual are exposed to one of a series of specific anti-HLA antibodies (commercially available), and then complement is added. If the antigen is present, the lymphocytes are killed by complement; then

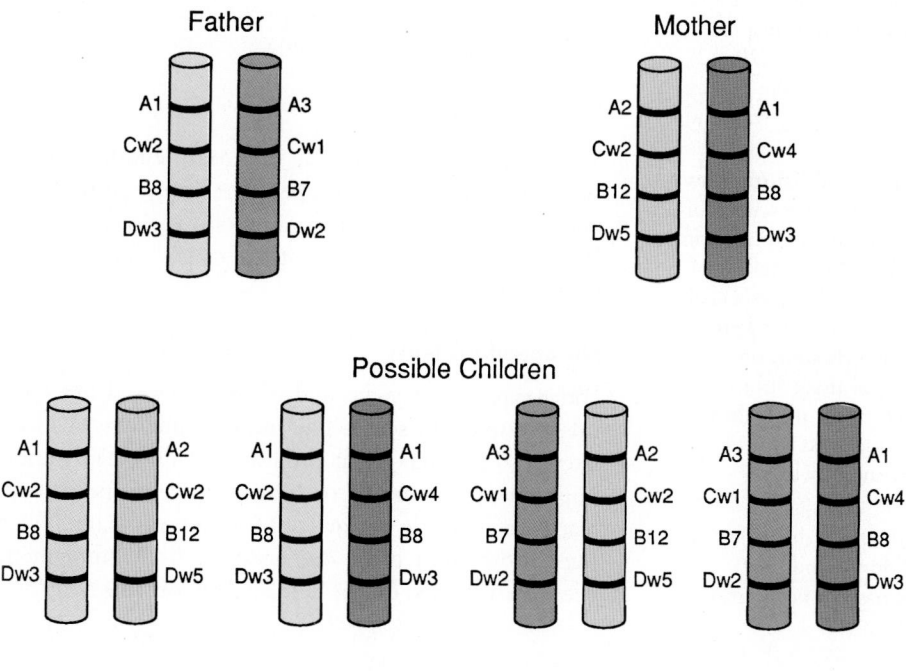

FIGURE 18.5 Haplotype combinations that may occur in the offspring of a mating. Note that the five alleles of a haplotype are always passed on together. Only five possible alleles are shown for each haplotype, but the total number recognized today is higher. (Adapted from [59] with permission from ASCP.)

the number of dead lymphocytes is counted by exposing the cell suspension to a dye (*dye exclusion test,* p. 204).

Transplantation. The very notion of HLA antigens was worked out in relation to organ transplants. In the context of organ transplants, the "HLA antigens" truly function as antigens, inducing antibody formation and cell-mediated hypersensitivity. For some organs, e.g., the kidney, the rule used to be that the closer the HLA match between donor and recipient, the greater was the chance of success (90). However, as better and better immunosuppressors became available, HLA matching became less critical, and kidney donation from living unrelated donors is now encouraged (24). Liver transplant teams can forget HLA matching altogether: it was a surprise to discover that allografts of a complex tissue such as the liver are immunologically not demanding at all. The liver survives longer than any other organ even when grafted across species barriers (92), possibly because it acts as a "killing field" for activated CD8[+] T cells (22).

Mechanisms of Graft Rejection

To be transplanted successfully, an organ must overcome four major hurdles. It must (1) be properly "harvested" (such is the term), (2) be properly preserved, (3) recover and maintain its blood flow, and (4) escape immune rejection. The loss of innervation is fortunately not critical.

Steps to Transplantation

1. **Harvesting** involves weighty ethical and technical problems; the answers are not the same everywhere. In Japan, for example, harvesting organs from cadavers is not acceptable. In the United States, some hospitals have created a Department of Transplantation and Extracorporeal Medicine.

2. **Preservation** is an art in itself (61, 66); organs are usually perfused with an elaborate fluid called Wisconsin Solution or its derivatives, and kept at 4°C (61). The procedure varies, of course, from organ to organ. In our institution a cadaver kidney is considered optimal if kept for less than 12 hours, acceptable up to 24 hours. Predictably, transplants fare better if the preservation time is short (20, 42). Preservation injury can be estimated for the kidney through urine output, and for the liver by transaminase levels in the blood (21).

3. **Reconnecting the vessels and reestablishing flow** have become routine procedures; microvascular surgeons can suture arteries with a diameter of 0.5 mm or less. However, in human allografts the reflow of blood can create serious problems, related especially to the damage due to preservation: we have here a classic situation of **ischemia–reperfusion,** one of the best-studied mechanisms of tissue injury (p. 713). As a worst-case scenario, the **no-reflow phenomenon** may occur in some areas (p. 711). Blood flow can also be lost secondarily by an immune mechanism.

4. **Immune rejection** remains the most difficult challenge. The exact interplay of donor and host immune systems, as of 2003, has not been entirely worked out. It is clear that T cells are essential (68, 79, 80, 95). Figure 18.6 summarizes two pathways of allorecognition (79, 80): a *direct pathway,* whereby host cells bump directly into donor antigen-presenting cells (APCs) and recognize them as foreign because they are coated with foreign MHC molecules; and an *indirect pathway,* whereby the graft sheds proteins that are picked up by host APCs and processed very much like microbial proteins. There has been one further step (47): the endothelium of the graft can present antigen directly to host CD8[+] T cells, bypassing the need for professional antigen-presenting cells, and possibly also the need for the primed T cells to spend some time for further "maturation" in the lymphoid organs, as is currently thought (10).

All told, if we could live the life of a kidney graft—or any other graft—from harvesting to rejection, it would probably feel like a sequence of emergencies. We will try to reconstruct it briefly.

Life Inside an Allograft

Visualize the surgical setting of a routine kidney transplant. When the surgeon opens the clamp on the renal artery and vein, and warm red blood replaces the cold Wisconsin Solution, dramatic changes occur in the oxygen-starved kidney.

Nonspecific Effects

Within minutes. Oxygen- and nitrogen-derived free radicals dominate the scene. The endothelium, as we will see later (p. 714), has spent the hours of flow deprivation building up a store of free radical precursors; as flow reappears it creates a shower of free radicals that damage the endothelium itself and nearby cells. Complement becomes activated on the damaged endothelium (4, 27),

ALLORECOGNITION
AND
GRAFT REJECTION

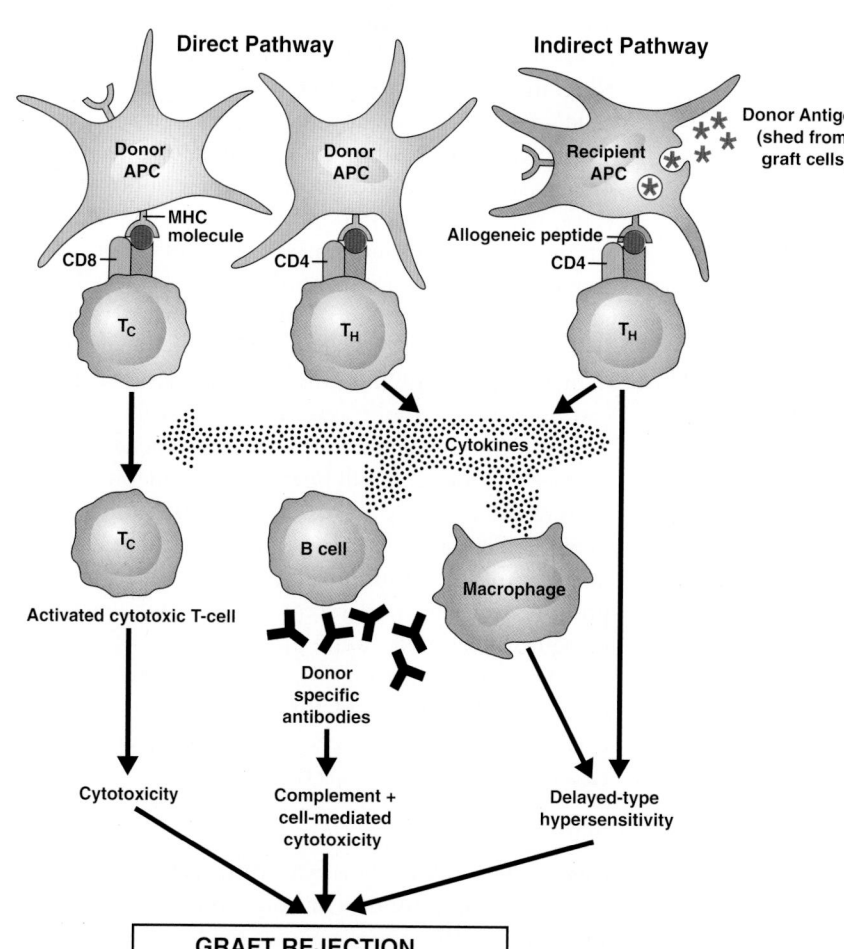

creating further injury, and attracting leukocytes; now the endothelium is activated (3, 26, 89) and more leukocytes are trapped. A vicious circle develops (49): as more and more leukocytes are trapped and emigrate, they become activated, and further activate the endothelium—which attracts more leukocytes. C-reactive protein binds to the damaged endothelial cells and contributes to activate complement (4). Damaged cells release a flood of early inflammatory mediators (histamine, arachidonic acid metabolites, platelet activating factors, etc.) and vascular leakage develops throughout the kidney.

The blood flow does not recover evenly. In some fields—which may be micro- or macroscopic—the return of the flow is delayed and may never recover (*the no-reflow phenomenon,* p. 711); the obstacles can be of many kinds, but most are leukocytes trapped in small venules or capillaries. Arteriolar spasm is also possible.

The reflow, of course, is taking place through "foreign" (allogeneic) vessels, but the leukocytes are not equipped to realize this anomaly, except the natural killer (NK) cells: they alone can recognize foreign cells without previous exposure to their antigens. The NK cells do respond to the presence of an allograft (Figure 18.7) (93); even if they kill off a few endothelial cells, the graft is not significantly affected.

Within hours. Most of the semiasphyxiated renal epithelial cells begin to recover (the fibroblasts barely noticed the emergency); some swell up and die by oncosis, releasing inflammatory materials; others die more discreetly by apoptosis. The extent of cell death depends mainly on the duration of the "cold ischemia" period (49). Within a few hours the internal *milieu* of the kidney is that of mild, diffuse, acute inflammation;

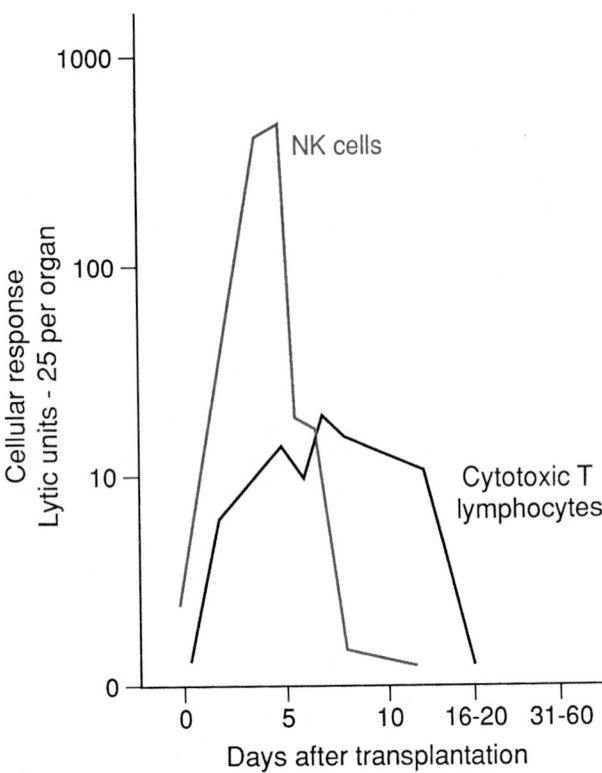

FIGURE 18.7 NK cells do participate in graft rejection. In the study here shown, their numbers exceed those of cytotoxic lymphocytes within the first few days after transplantation. (Adapted by permission from [39], © 1984 Munksgaard International Publishers Ltd., Copenhagen, Denmark.)

the corresponding fluid exudate would normally escape by the lymphatics, but all the lymphatic vessels were torn apart during harvesting. Presumably the fluid oozes out of the renal surface and is drained away by the lymphatics surrounding the surgical field. It is teeming with cells: activated neutrophils, macrophages (loaded with debris of dead kidney cells), and dendritic cells—some from the host, some from the graft where they were settled as "passenger cells."

Within days. The torn lymphatic networks have reconnected, regular lymph flow resumes. Some T cells and APCs float to the nearest lymph node, as part b of the ritual of initiating the immune response (Figure 18.6). A flood of cytokines causes them to proliferate; in mice, this means that the lymph node can double or triple its size, while blood flow increases fourfold (39). In the allograft itself, groups of cytokines and adhesion molecules appear, very similar to those induced by ischemia/reperfusion alone, without allograft (36, 49, 89). For reasons unknown, ischemia has also induced

the epithelial cells to produce more Class I and II MHC antigens, whereby the immunogenicity of the tissue should be increased (82). Endothelial damage to the arterioles heals incompletely, leaving a fibrous intimal thickening. The number of lymphocytes trapped in the allograft begins to rise after 3 days or so; thereafter, much depends on therapy.

Allorecognition amounts to a unilateral declaration of aggression against the grafted kidney: not of war, because the grafted kidney *usually* has too few weapons (immune cells) to counterattack the host (there are exceptions, to be discussed shortly). Aggression will then be carried out by the host using the same mechanisms that we discussed under hypersensitivity reactions, namely Types 2 and 3 (antibody-mediated) and Type 4 (cell-mediated). Only one mechanism is left out: Type 1, the anaphylactic pathway. Somehow it was decreed that no graft will be rejected by anaphylaxis.

Such are the early events in an allograft as we try to imagine them at the level of cells. The reader will have noticed that "nonimmune" events were given some prominence; this is a recent trend, which belatedly recognizes that graft failure proceeds in part from nonspecific events (44a, 49, 69). At the clinical level, graft failure can follow one of three major pathways, again best known for the kidney: hyperacute rejection, acute rejection, and chronic rejection.

Immune Rejection

Hyperacute rejection. This is a truly catastrophic event: rejection within minutes or hours, often on the operating table. As the surgeon allows the blood to flow, the grafted kidney becomes red and pulsatile, then turns blue, the pulsation ceases, and no urine is produced. The pace of events suggests an antibody mechanism, and such is the case: the blood of the recipient contains preformed antibodies against antigens on the endothelial surface of the graft. These antibodies bind to the endothelial antigen and thus label the endothelium for destruction; leukocytes and complement take care of this task (Type 2 hypersensitivity, p. 539). Destruction of the endothelium leads to thrombosis and blood clotting. No known treatment can help. This accident should no longer occur, because it is avoidable by proper screening of the recipient's blood.

The antibodies may belong to the ABO system, which makes the screening relatively simple. They may also the anti-HLA, produced by at least 3 mechanisms: 1) *a previous organ transplant.* 2) *Previous pregnancies.* During the trauma of birth, some fetal blood may spill into the mother's tissues; if the husband is HLA-nonidentical, the mother may generate anti-HLA antibodies. 3) *Previous*

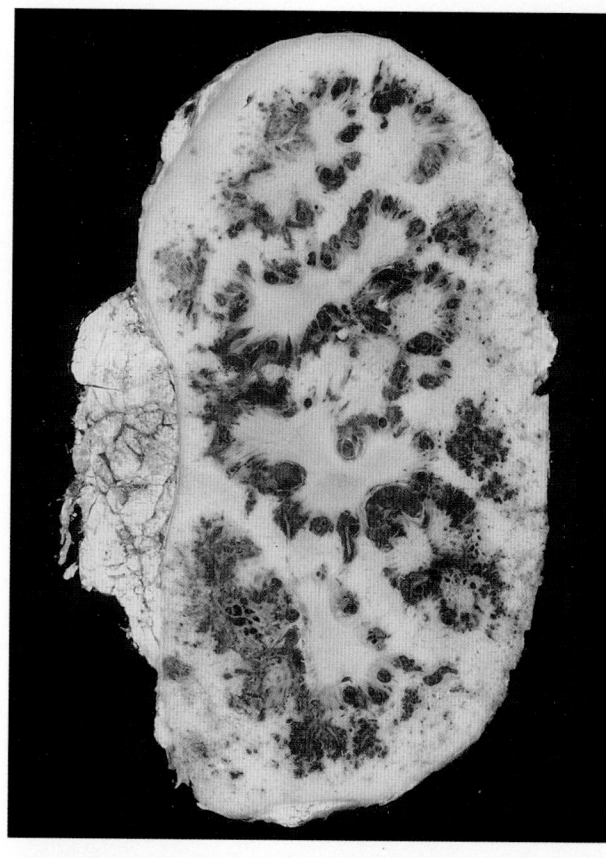

FIGURE 18.8   Acutely rejected human kidney (48 hours). The vessels are dilated and thrombosed; the parenchyma is white due to coagulation necrosis. Slightly reduced.

blood transfusions: when a patient needs a blood transfusion, there is no need to perform HLA blood typing; as a result, each transfusion from a non-identical blood donor is an opportunity to develop antibodies against allogeneic blood cells and their HLA antigens.

Acute rejection. This catastrophe occurs mostly within the first month; its frequency decreases thereafter. Grossly the kidney is mottled, with areas of congestion and necrosis (Figure 18.8). Two types of histologic damage are usually mixed, although one or the other may dominate: **vascular** and **interstitial.** *Vasculitis entails poor prognosis, because it adds one more level of threat for the kidney parenchyma: ischemia in addition to immunologic attack.* Vasculitis includes glomerular changes (acute glomerulopathy [80a]) due to antibody and complement attack. Oddly enough, some of the complement component C3 is generated by the grafted kidney (74a), whereby an innate, nonimmune mechanism contributes to renal damage. Many renal tubules are destroyed. Immunologic damage is cell-mediated and corresponds to a Type 4 hypersensitivity response; 60–80 percent of the lymphocytes are cytotoxic T cells (67). Immunofluorescence shows deposits of IgM, C1q, and C3 in the vessel walls, glomeruli, and peritubular basement membranes.

Regarding acute rejection of the heart, a sad example is shown in Figure 18.9, from a patient who chose to stop taking medicines. Others who made the same choice were more fortunate, and just lived on.

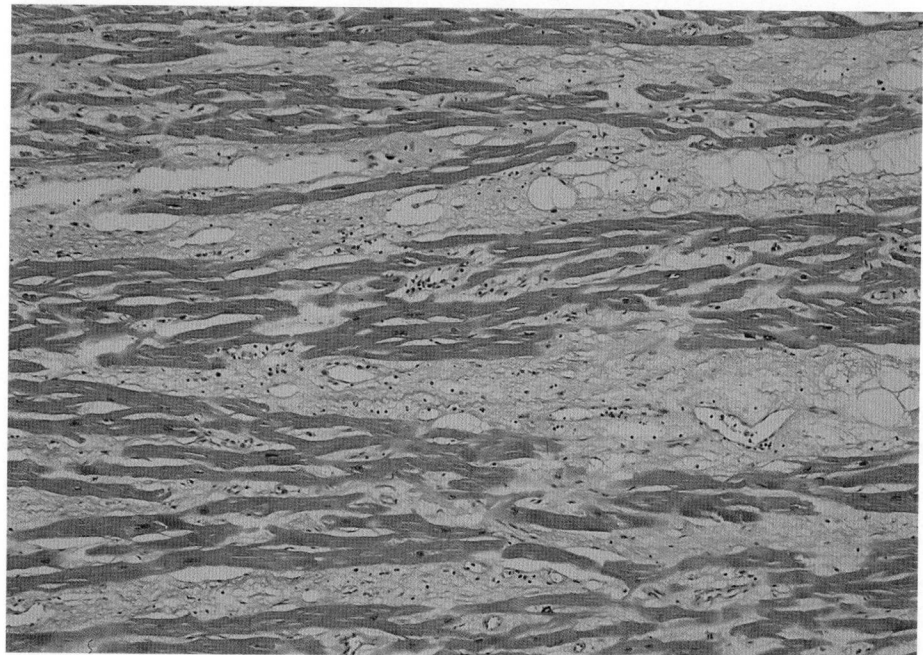

FIGURE 18.9   Rejection of a transplanted heart in a patient who chose to stop taking immunosuppressive medication. Note the diffuse edema and inflammatory infiltrate, which included only mononuclear cells (lymphocytes, macrophages, and a few plasma cells). Presumably this heart was brought to stop by cytokines. (125x)

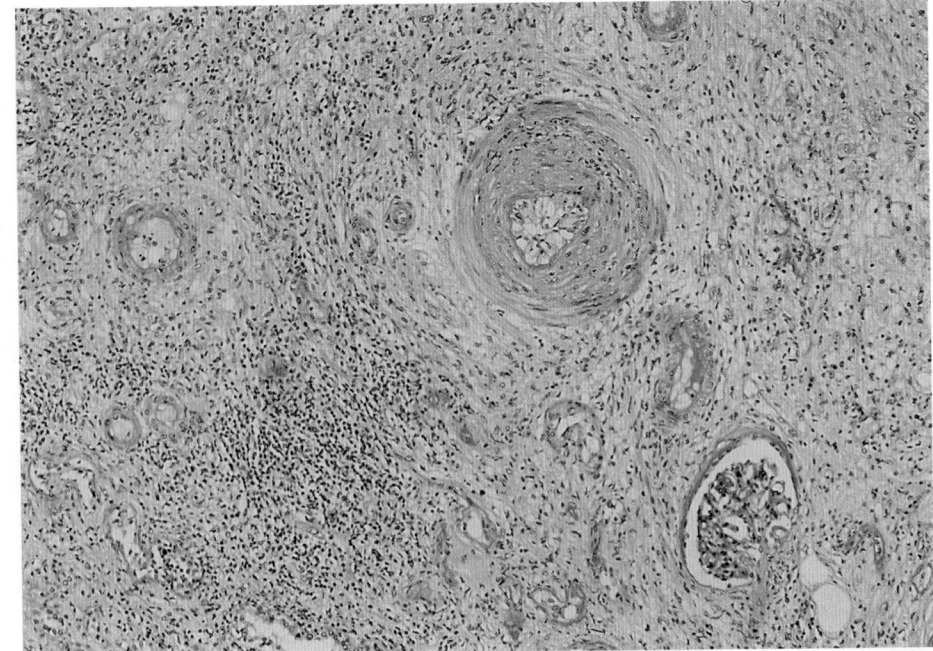

FIGURE 18.10 **Chronic allograft nephropathy.** The renal parenchyma is largely replaced by fibrosis and mononuclear cell infiltrates. Typical **transplant arteriopathy** (concentric intimal thickening with foam cells); as a cause of ischemia it is responsible for much of the parenchymal atrophy (P.A.S. stain; 125x).

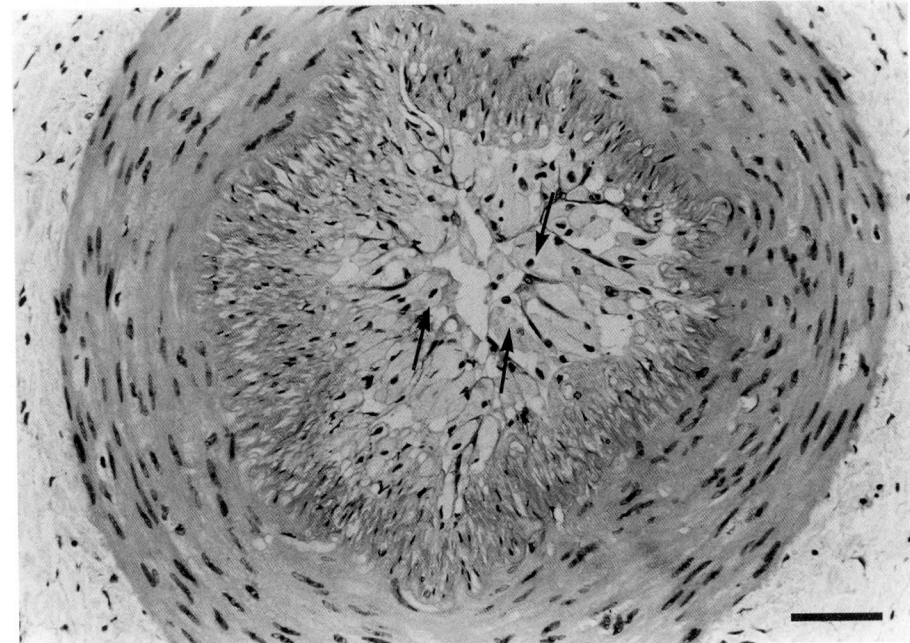

FIGURE 18.11 Typical *transplant arteriopathy* in a 90 day liver transplant. The artery is contracted, throwing the thickened intima into deep folds which contain many foam cells and obliterate the lumen. **Bar** = 250 μm. (Reproduced from [74] by permission from Elsevier Science Publishers).

Chronic rejection (of the kidney). This has been renamed **chronic allograft nephropathy,** to recognize the fact that nonimmunologic factors are also involved (60a, 69). It is a progressive, irreversible condition leading to renal failure (64). The tubules have become atrophic or have been replaced by fibrosis and mononuclear cell infiltrates (Figure 18.10). The arteries are partly obliterated by a concentric intimal thickening (**transplant arteriopathy**), which contains, oddly enough, even more foam cells than are found in atherosclerosis (Figure 18.11); they are probably due to the hypercholesterolemia induced by treatment with cyclosporin A (61). The destruction of renal parenchyma is due in large part to this arterial change, which is probably not of immune origin.

Graft-Versus-Host Disease

Ever since organ transplantation became a part of surgery, the main difficulty seemed to be that the body of the *host* would not easily accept the *graft*. But then came the grafts of bone marrow; the bone marrow is a major province of the immune system, professionally hostile to nonself. Imagine these guardian cells suddenly finding themselves grafted into a new body: **everything is nonself.** Now there are two overlapping immune systems in charge of the same body and trying to eliminate each other: this means real war. Its clinical name is graft-versus-host (GVH) disease (11, 19).

The strength of the two armies is somewhat uneven: on the side of the host, about 2 kg (44) of imunosuppressed cells; on the side of the graft, a much smaller contingent of cells that have the advantage of not being imunosuppressed, at least initially. GVH can be acute or chronic. It develops in many (or most) cases of bone marrow transplants—less in younger people, less if donor and recipient are related. Overall it is a miserable condition, and life-threatening for one-fourth to one-third of the patients (41). For reasons unknown it causes *selective epithelial damage to the target organs* (34), especially in the skin, which develops rashes (Figure 18.12), in the liver (which may produce jaundice) and in the gut (in the form of ulcerations and watery and bloody diarrhea).

Graft-versus-host disease after solid organ transplants. GVH disease after a bone marrow transplant is easily understood: since the defensive army of the host is largely disarmed by immunosuppression, the attack by a small force of embattled bone marrow can succeed. But what about transplants of solid organs? They too contain representatives of the immune system— dendritic cells, macrophages, and lymphocytes in varying numbers—and they are not immunosuppressed. Indeed, solid organs can cause a GVH disease; the small bowel and spleen, organs rich in lymphocytes, are at the top of the list (94) (the spleen is no longer grafted [25]). The kidney, we guess, cannot have much more than a couple of spoonfuls of immunocompetent cells; yet cases of kidney-related GVH disease have occurred (94). Even blood transfusions have caused GVH reactions because the transfused leukocytes were able to settle in the host (usually they just die or get killed) (81).

The **pathogenesis** of GVH disease is not fully understood; two pathways have been described: a humoral reaction (hemolysis) and a cellular response in which

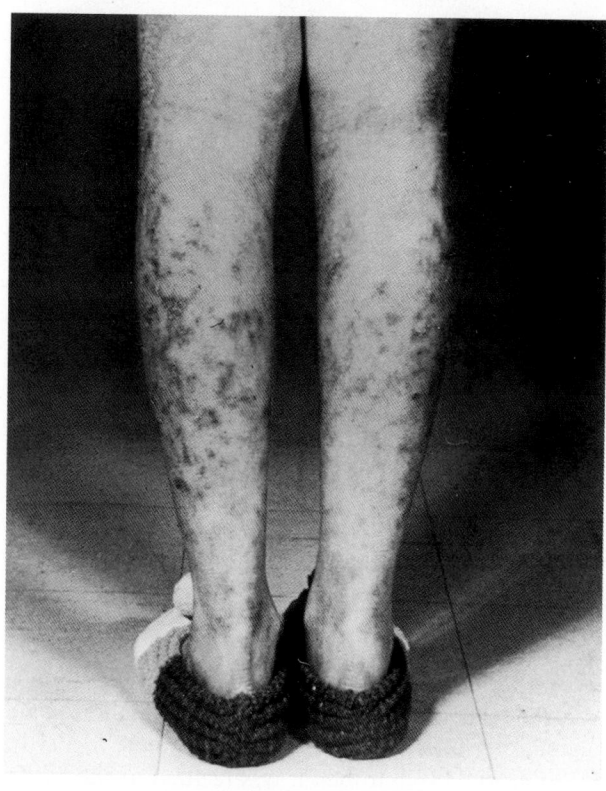

FIGURE 18.12   Graft-versus-host disease. Skin lesions in a patient who underwent a bone marrow transplant. (Courtesy of Dr. D. G. Nathan, Children's Hospital Boston, MA.)

cytotoxic T cells destroy host tisues. Some lesions show few cells, suggesting that cytokines may be responsible, possibly TNF (Figure 18.13) (70, 84).

Prevention has somewhat improved the outlook: the bone marrow graft can be depleted of T cells, or it can be replaced by a graft of hemopoietic stem cells; but GVH disease is still with us.

The graft-versus-leukemia (GVL) effect. Even an ugly happening such as GVH disease can have its positive side. If a graft of bone marrow can attack the *normal* bone marrow cells of its host, why should it not attack *leukemic* bone marrow cells of its host? In fact it does. Imagine a young woman with chronic myelogenous leukemia, treated with chemotherapy and a bone marrow graft. A relapse occurs, and *it can be treated with a simple transfusion of lymphocytes from the same donor.* This sequence has been well documented in mice and in people (5, 19).

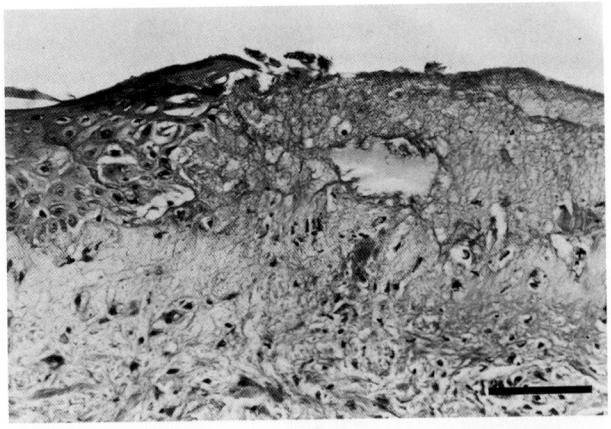

FIGURE 18.13   Biopsy of a skin lesion in graft-versus-host disease. Note the necrosis of the epidermis. The disproportion between this necrosis and the amount of inflammatory infiltrate fits with the notion that such lesions are of "toxic" nature (an effect of TNF). **Bar** = 100 μm. (Reprinted from [84], by courtesy of Marcel Dekker, Inc.)

Grafts and immunologic chimerism.   The mythical chimera had the body of a goat, the head of a lion, and the tail of a snake. Molecular chimerae include, more modestly, sheep-goats (33), but then it was realized in the 1960s that all the recipients of transplanted organs are chimerae: not only because they carry cells (and organs) of two different genotypes—sometimes more—but also because the graft and the host, at the microscopic level, exchange cells. The most spectacular chimerism follows liver transplantation: the hepatocytes and the endothelium remain where they are, but all the Kupffer cells jump ship and spread throughout the body (94). At the same time, some types of host cells migrate into the graft. This exchange occurs presumably with all grafts (9, 75); it is known as *microchimerism* (85).

Is this good, bad, or indifferent? Should microchimerism be encouraged or fought? How does it relate to tolerance? These questions have important medical implications. They inspired much research on different models, and led to different conclusions. As of 2003, the overall impression is that microchimerism matters little. It is not demonstrably related to tolerance (35, 63)—not *yet,* anyway (12).

Microchimerism does not necessarily last: 15 years after kidney transplantation only one case was positive (43). In corneal grafts, *all* cell types are usually replaced by host cells within a year or longer (98). In lung grafts, epithelia and endothelia remain, but most lymphocytes are replaced within a month (8).

Xenografts—and an afterthought on John Hunter's experiment. The shortage of human organs available for allotransplants has led to explore the possibility of harvesting organs from other mammals. Overall, this has not been a fruitful avenue of research. It is true that the immune response to some xenografts has been weaker than against allografts (72, 77): these donor-recipient combinations have been called *concordant;* but most species combinations are unfortunately *discordant.* If pig organs could be used for humans, they would be plentiful and appropriate as regards the size, but pig endothelium is coated with a carbohydrate molecule, alpha-1, 2-galactosyl (alpha-gal for short), which primates have lost—and causes a hyperacute rejection (78). The problem may be solved by genetic engineering. Some piglets that made the press (14, 48) were "knockouts" for the enzyme (alpha-1,3-galactosyltransferase) that adds the critical carbohydrate, but they are knockouts on one allele only—so they may not be the final answer.

Expectations are high, but the enthusiasm for xenografts alltogether is somewhat dimmed by the fear that they might carry some unknown virus (97). HIV, after all, was a gift of fellow primates.

In closing this section on supposedly "forbidden grafts," we should return to that historical allograft reported in the late 1700s by John Hunter: the cock's spur grafted in another cock's comb is still one of the prize exhibits of the Hunterian Museum in London. The implication of this exhibit is that we are witnessing a successful allograft. Experimental details are not available. Could this be an immunologic miracle? Or is this a 5-day result? Or maybe a horny spur is not very antigenic? In 1984 we consulted Sir Peter Medawar. His reply (58):

> I do not believe in the John Hunter story—and think it quite inconceivable that the two birds were so highly inbred as to make it possible for them to accept grafts from each other. I mean, I do not think that a natural law was suspended in Hunter's favour, though surgeons are normally quite ready to believe that such a thing can come to pass.
>
> I do think that you would be performing a public service if you persuaded a PhD student to go over the ground again.

We hope that someone will pick up that challenge. Until then, we will assume that the miraculous "graft" is just a dead spur stuck into a cock's comb, and tolerated as a thorn might be—for some time.

Grafts and the Concept of Tolerance

For the patient who needs a transplant, and for the surgical, medical, and scientific teams in charge of providing it, immunosuppression is not the ideal answer. All drugs available at this time carry the triple risk of infection, cancer, and toxicity, and besides, after 10 years, only 20 percent of the grafts are functional (76). None of this would apply if it were possible to induce at will a state of *tolerance,* defined functionally as *the survival of foreign (allogeneic or xenogeneic) tissue in normal recipients in the absence of immunosuppression* (76).

Tolerance is, of course, a natural and necessary event: almost all of our T and B cells are self-tolerant. To induce artificially the kind of therapeutic tolerance that we are invoking here will be an ambitious undertaking, but spontaneous examples are known: there are anecdotal reports of patients who for various reasons stopped taking medication and did not reject their grafts (76). More importantly, tolerance exists in Nature if you know where to look. The very notion of tolerance was born, as other concepts in immunology, of an observation in veterinary medicine (37, 65). R. D. Owen reported in 1945 that the blood of nonidentical twin calves sometimes contained red blood cells of two blood groups, one from each twin, with no pathologic effect. A twin pregnancy in cows is unusual, but when it does occur the circulation of the two placentas is mixed, so that there is free exchange of blood cells (Figure 18.14). Shortly thereafter, Burnet and Fenner (13) used this observation in an attempt to explain why the body does not build antibodies against itself; they argued that during embryonic development the body learns to recognize its own constituents and also learns how to phagocytize and digest its obsolete components without making antibodies against them. They also predicted (one wonders why they did not try the critical experiment) that if an embryo were injected with an antigen, as an adult it would not respond to that antigen. Two years later Peter Medawar proved them right: twin calves (nonidentical) would accept grafts from each other's skin. Later work showed that mice would accept skin allografts if they had been injected with the allogeneic cells in fetal life (7). Red cells of two blood groups, A and O, have been found in human twins (29).

Tolerance to Grafts: Experimental Approaches

In the search for ways to overcome graft rejection, most plans aim at modifying the response of the host; a few seek tolerance by working on the donor. As of 2003 this is still an experimental but promising field. We will select some highlights (44a, 76).

1) Grafts in "privileged sites." These are parts of the body that tolerate allografts without immunosuppression (76). They include the brain, testis, thymus, the anterior chamber of the eye, the uterus during pregnancy, and possibly the hamster cheek pouch. Several mechanisms have been suggested to explain the "privilege" of these sites, including the lack of lymphatic drainage (certainly valid for the brain) and the presence of a blood-tissue barrier, which certainly exists in the brain, the testis, and according to one source, the skin (pp. 319, 515). None of these sites is especially felicitous for a graft, but surprising observations have been made on the testis.

> In mice, allografts of testis and of [testicular] Sertoli cells survive indefinitely, even in a non-privileged site (6), and even though they are surrounded by activated, angry T cells whose purpose it is to kill allografts. It so happens that the Sertoli cells express FasL; the encounter between a Sertoli cell and a Fas-bearing T cell (which may be trying to kill it) results in apoptosis of the attacker. In essence, the killer T cells discover—too late—that their targets, the Sertoli cells, are booby-trapped. Further experiments showed that allogeneic Sertoli cells mixed with allogeneic pancreatic islets did protect the islets, but the experimental model is not yet ready for therapeutic applications (28).

As a privileged site, the *thymus* can also be exploited. The thymus is uniquely equipped for deleting self-reactive T cells. An imaginative experiment showed that antigen injected into the thymus led to deletion of all

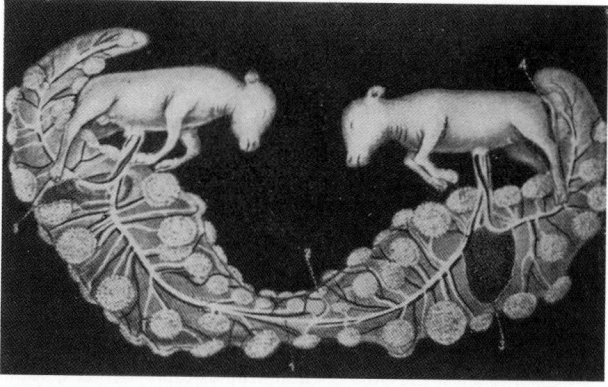

FIGURE 18.14 Nature's experiment on immune tolerance. Twin calves with a single placenta and shared circulation. See text. (**1** and **2**: vascular anastomoses.) (Reproduced from [73], after F. R. Lillie [50].)

the T cells reactive to that antigen. In human adults the thymus is involuted and therefore difficult to find, but there are infants who need cardiac transplants: an injection of bone marrow cells in their thymus prevented chronic rejection (71).

2) Producing T cell anergy. Anergy is a condition in which the T cell does not respond. This condition can be induced during antigen presentation, if the T cell is presented with a correct Signal 1 (the MHC + Peptide complex) in the absence of Signal 2 (the co-stimulatory signal, B7-1 or B7-2). When this occurs, the T cell floats away in a sort of paralyzed condition: should it meet another antigen-presenting cell, equipped with the proper signal, it will remain indifferent.

> This principle, known also as **co-stimulatory blockade,** has been tested on rats bearing kidney allografts: intravenous treatment with a protein that blocks the B7 costimulation pathway reduced functional damage (as measured by proteinuria) and prevented chronic rejection (2, 17). Unfortunately in humans it led to wholly unpredictable complications, including thrombosis (71).

3) Improving the conditions of the allograft, by eliminating the non-immune factors that affect its survival (4, 18, 49, 96). There is currently a trend to reexamine the role of non-immune factors in graft rejection. Organs obtained from cadavers suffer considerable stresses before they come to rest in their new host; the ischemic insult activates the endothelium, increases the expression of cytokines, and most surprisingly, increases the "immunogenicity" of the organ by up-regulating MHC class II antigens (18).

4) Producing tolerance by preimplantation of embryonic stem cells (1, 32). This procedure sounds like a breakthrough. In rats, embryonic stem cells injected into the portal vein induced a state of chimerism that allowed long-term acceptance of heart transplants—without irradiation or drugs. How do the stem cells escape being killed by T cells? Probably by expressing Fas ligand, whereby the T cells—as we mentioned above—eliminate themselves by a booby-trap mechanism. Now we must hope that this mechanism is not limited to rats.

5) Producing tolerance by injecting antigen in privileged site. This too sounds like a breakthrough. An antigen injected into the anterior chamber of the eye leads to *systemic* tolerization against that antigen, as well as inhibition of delayed-type hypersensitivity (DTH) against that antigen (84a). Both these changes can be interpreted as protecting the eye against excessive antibacterial inflammation. Surprising and promising.

This is but a small sample of the elegant games that can be played with antigen presentation (9a), wrestling, as it were, with the immune system. A safe, effective way of inducing tolerance will be a great gift to mankind.

What Do Plants Tell Us About Grafts?

In China the art of grafting plants was known around 1000 B.C., and also Aristotle (384–321 B.C.) knew a lot about it (38). The trees themselves, however, practiced grafting long before humans: in some species, branches pressed together tend to fuse; roots can establish grafts quite easily, sometimes even among different species. Stumps may be kept alive by this underground support, and some parasites—such as the fungus of Dutch elm disease—can spread by the same route (38). The relationship between host and graft (called *stock* and *scion*), is not the same in all cases, and anyway the rejection does not depend on phenomena that the "animal people" would call immunologic. A classic example: the quince rejects a graft of pear because the quince produces a glycoside that diffuses into the pear tissue, where it is broken down producing cyanide; so the pear cells die of cyanide poisoning (60).

Sometimes an impossible graft is made possible by an intermediate segment called *interstock,* which is compatible with both stock and scion (38); the comparison with the mammalian placenta is irresistible.

> **TO SUM UP:** Organ transplantation between humans, still a dream a few decades ago, has become a routine therapeutic procedure. Its progress has been helped by major advances in immunological theory, and the clinical experience in turn has helped formulate ever more refined immunologic concepts. Yet the most significant obstacle to transplantation, at this time, is not theoretical but social: the shortage of organs. In 1999 it was calculated that for every graft performed nine patients die while waiting for their turn (76).

References

1. Adler SH, Bensinger SJ, Turka LA. Stemming the tide of rejection. Nat Med 2002;8:107–108.
2. Azuma H, Chandraker A, Nadeau K, et al. Blockade of T-cell costimulation prevents development of experimental chronic renal allograft rejection. Proc Natl Acad Sci USA 1996;93: 12439–12444.
3. Bacchi CE, Marsh CL, Perkins JD, et al. Expression of vascular cell adhesion molecule (VCAM-1) in liver and pancreas allograft rejection. Am J Pathol 1993;142:579–581.

4. Baldwin III WM, Larsen CP, Fairchild RL. Innate immune responses to transplants: A significant variable with cadaver donors. Immunity 2001;14:369–376.

5. Barrett AJ. Mechanisms of the graft-versus-leukemia reaction. Stem Cells 1997;15:248–258.

6. Bellgrau D, Gold D, Selawry H, et al. A role for CD95 ligand in preventing graft rejection. Nature 1995;377:630–632.

7. Billingham RE, Brent L, Medawar PB. Quantitative studies on tissue transplantation immunity. III. Actively acquired tolerance. Philos Trans R Soc Lond (Biol) 1956;239:357–414.

8. Bittmann I, Dose T, Baretton GB, et al. Cellular chimerism of the lung after transplantation. An interphase cytogenetic study. Am J Clin Pathol 2001;115:525–533.

9. Bolli R. Regeneration of the human hear—no chimera? N Engl J Med 2002;346:55–56.

9a. Brent LB. Tolerance and its clinical significance. World J Surg 2000;24:787–792.

10. Briscoe DM, Sayegh MH. A rendezvous before rejection: Where do T cells meet transplant antigens? Nat Med 2002;8:220–222.

11. Burakoff SJ, Deeg HJ, Ferrara J, Atkinson K (eds). Graft-vs-Host Disease. Immunology, Pathophysiology, and Treatment. New York: Marcel Dekker, Inc., 1990.

12. Burlingham WJ. Chimerism after organ transplantation: Is there any clinical significance? Clin Transplantation 1996;10:110–117.

13. Burnet FM, Fenner F. The production of antibodies, 2nd ed. Melbourne: MacMillan and Company Limited, 1949.

14. Butler D. Xenotransplant experts express caution over knock-out piglets. Nature 2002;415:103–104.

15. Carpenter CB, David J. Histocompatibility antigens and immune response genes. In: Rubenstein E, Federman DD, eds. Scientific American medicine, 6 immunology, V. Histocompatibility antigens. New York: Scientific American, 1991, pp. 1–10.

16. Carrel A. The transplantation of organs. NY Med J 1914;99:839–840.

17. Chandraker A, Azuma H, Nadeau K, et al. Late blockade of T cell costimulation interrupts progression of experimental chronic allograft rejection. J Clin Invest 1998;101:2309–2318.

18. Chandraker A, Takada M, Nadeau KC, et al. CD28-B7 blockade in organ dysfunction secondary in cold ischemia/reperfusion injury. Kidney Int 1997;52:1678–1684.

19. Childs RW. Allogeneic stem cell transplantation. In: DeVita VT Jr, Hellman S, Rosenberg SA (eds). Cancer. Principles & Practice of Oncology, 6th ed. Philadelphia: Lippincott, Williams & Wilkins 2001, pp. 2779–2798.

20. Coffman TM. Inflammatory response to allografts. In: Norman DJ, Suki WN. Primer on Transplantation. Thorofare, NJ: American Society of Transplant Physicians, 1998, pp. 33–41.

21. Crippin J. Pathogenesis/Pathology of organ dysfunction. In: Norman DJ, Suki WN. Primer on Transplantation. Thorofare, NJ: American Society of Transplant Physicians, 1998, pp. 321–327.

22. Crispe IN, Dao T, Klugewitz K, Mehal WZ, Metz DP. The liver as a site of T-cell apoptosis: graveyard, or killing field? Immunolo Rev 2000;174:47–62.

23. Da Fano C. Zelluläre Analyse der Geschwultsim-munitätsreaktionen. Zeitschrift F. Immunitätsforsch 1910;5:1–74.

24. D'Alessandro AM, Pirsch JD, Knechtle SJ, et al. Living unrelated renal donation: The University of Wisconsin experience. Surgery 1998;124:604–611.

25. Deierhoi MH, Sollinger HW, Bozdech MJ, Belzer FO. Lethal graft-versus-host disease in a recipient of a pancreas-spleen transplant. Transplantation 1986;41:544–546.

26. Denton MD, Davis SF, Baum MA, et al. The role of the graft endothelium in transplant rejection: Evidence that endothelial activation may serve as a clinical marker for development of chronic rejection. Pediatr Transplantation 2000;4:252–260.

27. Dong J, Pratt JR, Smith RAG, Dodd I, Sacks SH. Strategies for targeting complement inhibitors in ischaemia/reperfusion injury. Mol Immunol 1999;36:957–963.

28. Duke RC, Newell E, Schleicher M, Meech S, Bellgrau D. Transplantation of cells and tissues expressing Fas ligand. Transplant Proc 1999;31:1479–1481.

29. Dunsford I, Bowley CC, Hutchison AM, et al. A human blood-group chimera. Br Med J 1953;2:81.

30. Dupont B. Immunobiology of HLA. New York: Springer-Verlag, 1989.

31. Edwards WS, Edwards PD. Alexis Carrel. Visionary Surgeon. Springfield, Illinois: Charles C. Thomas Publishers, 1974.

32. Fändrich F, Lin X. Chai GX, et al. Preimplantation-stage stem cells induce long-term allogeneic graft acceptance without supplementary host conditioning. Nat Med 2002;8:171–178.

33. Fehilly CB, Willadsen SM, Tucker EM. Interspecific chimaerism between sheep and goat. Nature 1984;307:634–636.

34. Ferrara JLM, Deeg HJ. Graft-versus-host disease. N Engl J Med 1991;324:667–674.

35. Fuchimoto Y, Yamada K, Shimizu A, et al. Relationship between chimerism and tolerance in a kidney transplantation model. J Immunol 1999;162:5704–5711.

36. Goes N, Urmson J, Ramassar V, Halloran PF. Ischemic acute tubular necrosis induces an extensive local cytokine response. Transplantation 1995;59:565–572.

37. Gowans JL. The immunology of tissue transplantation. In: Florey HW, ed. General pathology, 4th ed. Philadelphia: WB Saunders, 1970, pp. 1160–1182.

38. Hartmann HT, Kester DE, Davis FT. Theoretical aspects of grafting and budding. In: Plant propagation: principles and practices, 5th ed. New Jersey: Prentice-Hall, 1990, pp. 305–332.

39. Häyry P, von Willebrand E, Parthenais E, et al. The inflammatory mechanisms of allograft rejection. Immunol Rev 1984;77:85–142.

40. Held PJ, Kahan BD, Hunsicker LG, et al. The impact of HLA mismatches on the survival of first cadaveric kidney transplants. N Engl J Med 1994;331:765–770.

41. Holler E, Kolb HJ, Möller A, et al. Increased serum levels of tumor necrosis factor α precede major complications of bone marrow transplantation. Blood 1990;75:1011–1016.

42. Howard TK, Klintmalm GBG, Cofer JB, et al. The influence of preservation injury on rejection in the hepatic transplant recipient. Transplantation 1990;49:103–107.

43. Ishida H, Kawai T, Tanabe K, et al. Status of microchimerism in recipients 15 years after living related kidney transplantation. Transplantation 1996;62:126–128.

44. Jandl JH. Blood. Textbook of Hematology. Boston, MA: Little, Brown and Company, 1987.

44a. Kamradt T, Mitchison NA. Tolerance and autoimmunity. N Engl J Med 2001;344:655–664.

44b. Kirk AD. Location, location, location: regional immune mechanisms critically influence rejection. Nature Med 2002; 8:553–555.

45. Klein J, Sato A. Advances in immunology: The HLA system I. Review articles. N Engl J Med 2000;343:702–709.

46. Klein J, Sato A. Advances in immunology: The HLA system II. N Engl J Med 2000;343:782–786.

47. Kreisel D, Krupnick AS, Gelman AE, et al. Non-hematopoietic allograft cells directly activate CD8+ T cells and trigger acute rejection: An alternative mechanism of allorecognition. Nat Med 2002;8:233–239.

48. Lai L, Kolber-Simonds D, Park K-W, et al. Production of α-1,3-galactosyltransferase knockout pigs by nuclear transfer cloning. Science 2002;295:1089–1092.

49. Land W, Messmer K. The impact of ischemia/reperfusion injury on specific and non-specific, early and late chronic events after organ transplantation. Transplant Rev 1996;10:108–127.

50. Lillie FR. The free-martin; a study of the action of sex hormones in the foetal life of cattle. J Exp Zool 1917;23:371–452.

51. Majno G. The healing hand: man and wound in the ancient world. Cambridge, MA: Harvard University Press, 1975.

52. Malouin R. Surgeons' quest for life: the history and the future of xenotransplantation. *Perspect Biol Med 1994;37:416–428.*

53. Matsuki K, Honda Y, Juji T. HLA antigens in 206 Japanese patients with narcolepsy and 46 patients with essential hypersomnia. In: Dupont B. Immunobiology of HLA. New York: Springer-Verlag, 1989, pp. 438–440.

54. Medawar PB. The behaviour and fate of skin autografts and skin homografts in rabbits. J Anat 1944;78:176–199.

55. Medawar PB. A second study of the behaviour and fate of skin homografts in rabbits. J Anat 1945;79:157–176.

56. Medawar PB. Immunity to homologous grafted skin. II. The relationship between the antigens of blood and skin. Br J Exp Pathol 1946;27:15–24.

57. Medawar PB. The homograft reaction. Proc R Soc London B 1958;149:145–166.

58. Medawar PB. Personal letter dated 7th September 1984.

59. Miller WV, Rodey G. HLA without tears. Chicago: ASCP Press, Educational Products Division, 1981.

60. Moore R. Graft compatibility/incompatibility in higher plants. What's New in Plant Physiology 1981;12:13–16.

60a. Nankivell BJ, Borrows RJ, Fung CL-S, et al. The natural history of chronic allograft nephropathy, New Engl J Med 2003;349:2326–2333.

61. Norman DJ, Suki WN. Primer on Transplantation. Thorofare, NJ: American Society of Transplant Physicians, 1998.

62. Nowak R. Xenotransplants set to resume. Science 1994; 266:1148–1151.

63. Okasha KM, Al-Tweigeri TA, Jurado AV, Shoker AS. Analysis of the relationship between chimerism and the allogeneic humoral response. Transplantation 1998;66:1028–1034.

64. Orloff SL, Yin Q, Corless CL, et al. Tolerance induced by bone marrow chimerism prevents transplant vascular sclerosis in a rat model of small bowel transplant chronic rejection. Transplantation 2000;69:1295–1303.

65. Own RD. Immunogenetic consequences of vascular anastomoses between bovine twins. Science 1945;102:400–401.

66. Palmer R. The history of organ perfusion and preservation [on line]. International Society for Organ Preservation, 1999, retrieved October 26, 2001. URL http://www.i-s-op.org/history.htm

67. Pardo-Mindán FJ, Salinas-Madrigal L, Idoate M, et al. Pathology of renal transplatation. Sem Diagnostic Pathol 1992;9:185–199.

68. Parham P. The Immune System. New York: Garland Publishing, 2000.

69. Pascual M, Theruvath T, Kawai T, Tolkoff-Rubin N, Cosimi AB. Strategies to improve long-term outcomes after renal transplantation. N Engl J Med 2002;346:580–590.

70. Piguet P-F. The graft-versus-host disease. A search of the pathogenesis of T lymphocyte induced tissue damage. Geneva, Switzerland: University of Geneva, 1990, Thesis.

71. Platt JL, Lakkis FG. A scenic overlook on the road to clinical tolerance. Trends Immunol 2001;22:289–291.

72. Platt JL, Vercellotti GM, Dalmasso AP, et al. Transplantation of discordant xenografts: a review of progress. Immunol Today 1990;11:450–457.

73. Ponse K. La différenciation du sexe et l'intersexualité chez les Vertébrés. Facteurs héréditaires et hormones. Lausanne: F. Rouge & Cⁱᵉ, S.A., 1949.

74. Portmann BC. Histopathology of late liver graft failure: chronic rejection and other causes. In: Touraine JL, Traeger J, Bétuel H, Dubernard JM, Revillard JP, Daudon P, eds. Transplantation and clinical immunology, vol XXI. Amsterdam: Excerpta Medica, 1990, pp. 47–58.

74a. Pratt JR, Basheer SA, Sacks SH. Local synthesis of complement component C3 regulates acute renal transplant rejection. Nature Med 2002;8:582–587.

75. Quaini F, Urbanek K, Beltrami A, et al. Chimerism of the transplanted heart. N Engl J Med 2002;346:5–15.

76. Rossini AA, Greiner DL, Mordes JP. Induction of immunologic tolerance for transplantation. Physiol Rev 1999; 79:99–141.

77. Sachs DH, Bach FH. Immunology of xenograft rejection. Hum Immunol 1990;28:245–251.

78. Sandrin MS, Fodor WL, Mouhtouris E, et al. Enzymatic remodelling of the carbohydrate surface of a xenogenic cell substantially reduces human antibody binding and complement-mediated cytolysis. Nat Med 1995;1:1261–1267.

79. Sayegh MH. Why do we reject a graft? Role of indirect allorecognition in graft rejection. Kidney International 1999;56:1967–1979.

80. Sayegh MH, Turka LA. The role of T-cell costimulatory activation pathways in transplant rejection. N Engl J Med 1998;338:1813–1821.

80a. Shimizu A, Yamada K, Sachs DH, Colvin RB. Mechanisms of chronic renal allograft rejection. II. Progressive allograft glomerulopathy in miniature swine. Lab Invest 2002;82: 673–685.

81. Shivdasani RA, Haluska FG, Dock NL, et al. Brief report: graft-versus-host disease associated with transfusion of blood from unrelated HLA-homozygous donors. N Engl J Med 1993;328:766–770.

82. Shoskes DA, Parfrey NA, Halloran PF. Increased major histocompatibility complex antigen expression in unilateral ischemic acute tubular necrosis in the mouse. Transplantation 1990;49:201–207.

83. Silverstein AM. A history of immunology. San Diego: Academic Press, 1988.

84. Snover DC. The pathology of acute graft-vs.-host disease. In: Burakoff SJ, Deeg HJ, Ferrara J, Atkinson K, eds. Graft-vs.-host disease. New York: Marcel Dekker Inc., 1990:337–353.

84a. Sohn J-H, Bora PS, Suk H-J, et al. Tolerance is dependent on complement C3 fragment iC3b binding to antigen-presenting cells. Nat Med 2003;9:206–212.

85. Starzl TE, Demetris AJ, Murase N, et al. Cell migration, chimerism, and graft acceptance. Lancet 1992;339: 1579–1582.

86. Starzl TE, Demetris AJ, Murase N, et al. The changing immunology of organ transplantation. Hospital Practice October 15, 1995;31–42.

87. Storb R. Critical issues in bone marrow transplantation. Transplant Proc 1987;19:2774–2781.

88. Tagliacozzi G, 1597: Gasparis Taliacotii Bononiensis. . . De Curtorum Chirurgia per insitionem Libri Duo. Venetiis, MDXCVIII. Apud Gasparem Bindonum iuniorem. p. 59

89. Takada M, Nadeau KC, Shaw GD, Marquette KA, Tilney NL. The cytokine-adhesion molecule cascade in ischemia/reperfusion injury of the rat kidney. Inhibition by a soluble P-selectin ligand. J Clin Invest 1997;99:2682–2690.

90. Takemoto S, Terasaki PI, Cecka JM, Cho YW, Gjertson DW. Survival of nationally shared, HLA-matched kidney transplants from cadaveric donors. N Engl J Med 1992; 327:834–839.

91. Thomas L. Symbiosis as an immunologic problem. In: Neter E, Milgrom F, eds. The immune system and infectious diseases. Basel: S. Karger, 1975, pp. 2–11.

92. Thomson AW, Lu L. Are dendritic cells the key to liver transplant tolerance? Immunol Today 1999;20:27–32.

93. Touraine J-L, Moya M-J, Chargui J, Sanhadji K. Improved engraftment and chimerism by anti-NK cell treatment in allogenetic transplantation of hematopoietic stem cells. Transplant Proc 1997;29:719.

94. Triulzi DJ, Nalesnik MA. Microchimerism, GVHD, and tolerance in solid organ transplantation. Transfusion 2001;41:419–426.

95. VanBuskirk AM, Pidwell DJ, Adams PW, Orosz CG. Transplantation immunology. JAMA 1997;278:1993–1999.

96. Van Loo AA, Vanholder RC, Bernaert PR, et al. Pretransplantation hemodialysis strategy influences early renal graft function. J Am Soc Nephrol 1998;9:473–481.

97. Weiss RA. Xenografts and retroviruses. Science 1999;285: 1221–1222.

98. Wollensak G, Green WR. Analysis of sex-mismatched human corneal transplants by fluorescence in situ hybridization of the sex-chromosomes. Exp Eye Res 1999;68:341–346.

99. Zabriskie JB, Gibofsky A. Genetic control of the susceptibility to infection with pathogenic bacteria. Curr Topics Microbiol Immunol 1986;124:1–20.

100. Zirm E. Eine erfolgreiche totale Keratoplastik. Albrecht von Graefes Arch Ophthalmol 1906;64:580–593.

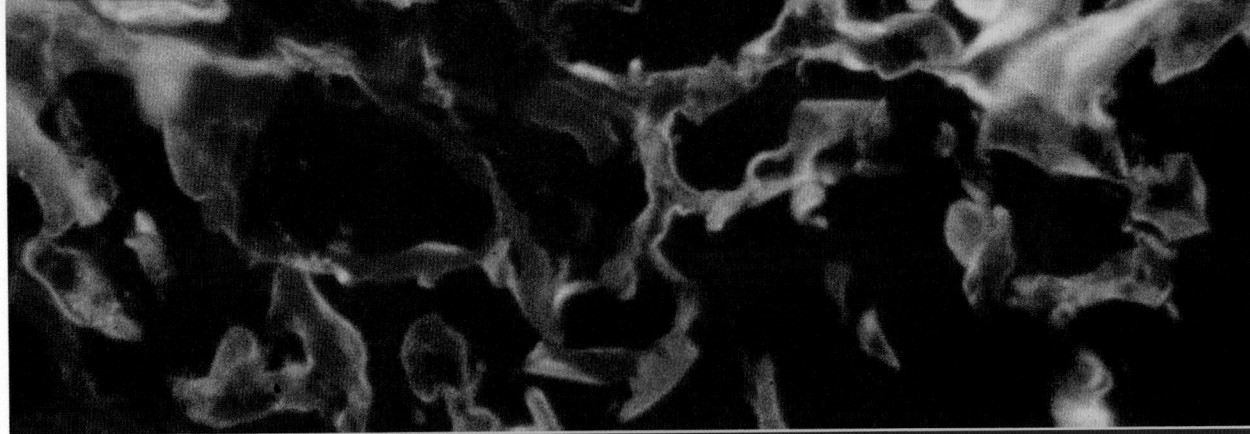

About 50 human diseases are known or suspected to be **autoimmune.** Because they are incompletely understood they are difficult to define (20, 74); but in essence, they are *chronic clinical syndromes caused by the inappropriate activation of T cells, B cells, or both against one or more bodily antigens. Microscopically their typical feature is chronic inflammation without a visible infectious cause, leading to destruction of the tissue.* Their pathogenesis draws—to varying degrees—from three sources: a malfunction of the immune system, genes, and the environment (Figure 19.1) (26).

Almost every organ of the human body has its autoimmune disease; some organs, such as the thyroid, have several. In the United States in 1996, the most common autoimmune diseases were (73): Graves' hyperthyroidism (about 3,048,000 cases), followed by rheumatoid arthritis (1,736,000), thyroiditis with hypothyroidism (1,490,000), vitiligo (1,059,000), multiple sclerosis (154,000), and insulin-dependent diabetes (147,000). The prevalence for the entire group is estimated at 3–5 percent (20, 57). Women are about 3 times more susceptible than men (47, 73). However, this does not mean that females are less immunocompetent than males; the contrary is true. In fact, females are superior survivors immunologically and otherwise (64).

The ***Natural Superiority of Women*** is the title of a book published in 1952 and updated in 1999 by the eminent anthropologist Ashley Montagu (61). Current statistics and immunology wholly support Montagu. At birth there are about 5 percent more males than females, but females outlive males by an average of 8 years. Males are more susceptible to accidents, as well as to cancer and infectious diseases. Women have slightly higher IgG and 30 percent higher IgM serum antibody levels than men, and they respond more briskly to several antigens by antibody formation. They appear to enjoy the advantage of immunoregulatory genes located on the X chromosome, of which they have two copies. This may be an evolutionary adaptation that protects females from the immunosuppression associated with childbearing (immunosuppression occurs because a fetus is essentially an allograft that has to be kept alive "against the rules"). This adaptation

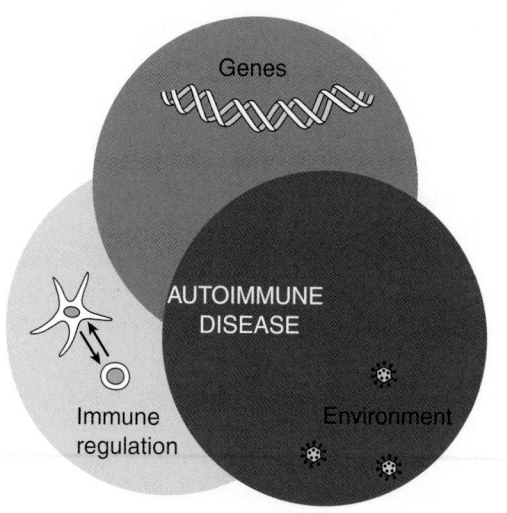

FIGURE 19.1 Requirements for the development of an autoimmune disease: a genetically predisposed individual, exposed to environmental factors, in association with defect(s) in immunoregulatory mechanisms, *may* develop an autoimmune disease. The importance of each factor may vary between individuals and diseases. (Reproduced with permission from *Nature Immunology* and Dr. C. G. Fathman [26].)

may be a two-edged sword: though females are capable of a stronger immune response to infectious agents, they are also more prone to develop autoantibodies (64). However, their tendency to develop autoimmune disorders is far outweighed by their "natural superiority." Montagu's book should be compulsory reading, for males anyway.

History and Nature of Autoimmune Disease

The concept of autoimmune diseases was slow in gaining acceptance. One reason was their imprecise name, still to be heard: **collagen diseases.** As we explained earlier (p. 266), in 1942 an eminent pathologist realized that here was a group of diseases characterized by unexplained chronic inflammation. Because inflammation occurs in connective tissue (sometimes called collagenous tissue), he called them "collagen diseases." Misled by this misnomer, other distinguished scientists were led to look for abnormal collagen and found themselves at a dead end. Autoimmunity became suspect.

> The fuzzy name of *rheumatology* did not help. It was meant to cover autoimmune diseases, the most prominent being *rheumatoid* arthritis. *Rheumatic* meant a lot to Hippocrates (55) but means nothing in modern medicine, let alone rheumat*oid*.

Another reason for skepticism was the fact that autoantibodies are found in the plasma of people that are apparently normal and tend to increase with age (79). Today this is irrelevant: a low level of autoreactivity is considered not only normal but also crucial to normal immune function (20). Last, it was objected that *autoantibodies may be a secondary phenomenon:* a well-known example are the anti-myocardium antibodies that appear after a myocardial infarction. It has even been speculated that such secondary autoantibodies might perform a useful function: by coating a bit of cell debris, they should make it stickier to macrophages and therefore easier to phagocytize (28, 34).

Today the existence of autoimmune diseases is not questioned (although occasionally one particular type may come under scrutiny as a possible misdiagnosed infection [92]). The field has been greatly strengthened by the study of natural and experimental animal models (11).

A potential source of confusion for the newcomer is the fact that *autoimmune diseases* are often classified in terms of the *diseases of hypersensitivity* (i.e., Type 2, Type 4) (see Chapter 17). In fact, the two sets of diseases can be superimposed, because they both deal with damage caused by the immune system; but (a) in diseases of hypersensitivity the immune system is inappropriately attacking *antigens introduced from the outside world* (think of pollen); whereas (b) in autoimmune diseases *the antigens come from the body itself* (e.g., basement membranes). The mechanisms of attack in (a) and (b) remain the same: antibodies and cells. Note, however, that there is no known autoimmune disease due to a Type 1 mechanism (anaphylaxis). Correspondingly, there is no Type 1 rejection of grafts.

Regarding their anatomic distribution—that is, their target organs—*autoimmune diseases form a spectrum* from the single-organ type to the systemic and multiorgan type (Table 19.1). This is simply a fact of life; it has as yet no scientific explanation. Statistics show that *developing one autoimmune disease tends to increase the risk of developing another;* therefore, a single patient may "move" along this spectrum.

We will now examine a few classic examples of autoimmune disease, emphasizing key features. The first two are based on two variants of the hypersensitivity Type 2 mechanism.

Hashimoto's thyroiditis is among the mildest autoimmune diseases. The clinical picture: typically, a woman (5–10 times more often than a man) complains of chronic fatigue; the thyroid is somewhat swollen (this is what is meant by "goiter"). *Anti-thyroglobulin* and other thyroid-specific antibodies are present in the plasma. Histology at this stage shows a focal or diffuse mononuclear cell infiltrate, mainly of lymphocytes and plasma cells, and a partial destruction of thyroid

Table 19.1 Selected Autoimmune Diseases

Disease	Target of Autoantibody
Organ-specific diseases:	
Hashimoto's thyroiditis	Thyroglobulin and microsomal antigens
Myasthenia gravis	Antiacetylcholine receptor
Graves' disease (diffuse toxic goiter)	TSH receptor
Insulin-resistant diabetes, associated with acanthosis nigricans	Insulin receptor
Insulin-resistant diabetes associated with ataxia-telangiectasia	Insulin receptor
Juvenile insulin-dependent diabetes	Islet cells; insulin
Pernicious anemia	Gastric parietal cells; vitamin B_{12}-binding site of intrinsic factor
Allergic rhinitis, asthma, functional autonomic abnormalities	β_2-adrenergic receptors
Addison's disease	Adrenal cortical cells
Idiopathic hypoparathyroidism	Antigens of parathyroid cells
Spontaneous infertility	Sperm
Premature ovarian failure	Interstitial cells; corpus luteum cells
Pemphigus	Intercellular substance of skin and mucosae
Bullous pemphigoid	Basement membrane zone of skin and mucosae
Primary biliary cirrhosis	Mitochondrial antigens
Autoimmune hemolytic anemia	Red blood cells
Idiopathic thrombocytopenic purpura	Platelets
Idiopathic neutropenia	Neutrophils
Vitiligo	Melanocytes
Chronic active hepatitis	Nuclei; hepatocyte antigens
Ulcerative colitis	Colon mucosa
Systemic diseases (non–organ-specific)	
Goodpasture's syndrome	Basement membrane (lung, kidney)
Rheumatoid arthritis	γ-globulin; EBV-related antigens
Systemic lupus erythematosus (SLE)	DNA; nucleolus; histone; lymphocytes; red blood cells; platelets; neurons; other
Sjögren's syndrome	γ-globulin; other
Scleroderma	Topoisomerase; centromere; other
Polymyositis	Nuclei; histidyl-tRNA synthetase; other
Rheumatic fever	Myocardium; heart valves; choroid plexus; neurons

Adapted with permission from (84).

follicles and cells (Figure 19.2). The damage is being done by antibodies and by killer T cells; the details are not entirely clear, but an important finding is that *antibodies can penetrate living cells* (1). Antigen–antibody complexes can be demonstrated around the follicles; some thyroid cells are probably coated with (or penetrated by) antibody and then killed by complement or by the ADCC mechanism (p. 539); others are killed by T cells. Yet the thyroid function is only mildly reduced, probably because the pituitary compensates by stimulating more thyroid hormone secretion (89). The plasma may also contain antibodies against gastric parietal cells in the absence of gastric disease; *autoimmune gastritis* may develop later, as well as pernicious anemia (because autoantibodies interfere with the absorption of vitamin B_{12}, and the lack of this vitamin leads to pernicious anemia). There is a slightly increased risk of developing lymphoma. Replacement hormone therapy enables these patients to lead normal lives.

Graves' Disease (Basedow's disease in continental Europe) is the most common form of hyperthyroidism (90). Typically, again, a woman (5–10 times more often than a man) presents with a diagnostic triad: (a) symptoms of *an excess* of thyroid hormone: sweating, palpitations, nervousness, diarrhea, and weight loss (this is what is meant by *thyrotoxicosis*); (b) protrusion of the eyes (exophthalmos) due to changes in the fat and muscle in the eye socket (29); and (c) pretibial edema (myxedema) (p. 283). The plasma contains anti-thyroglobulin antibodies as in Hashimoto's disease but also *antibodies against epitopes of the receptor for the thyroid-stimulating hormone of the pituitary;* by binding to the receptor, they are driving the cell to produce more thyroid hormone. Histologically, the typical picture of hypertrophy and hyperplasia of the thyroid follicles is no longer seen because patients are treated with anti-thyroid drugs before surgery; the diffuse chronic inflammatory infiltrate often includes typical lymphoid follicles. The peculiar changes in the orbital tissues are attributed to a cross-reactivity between the thyroid epithelium and periorbital muscles (29).

NOTE: Both these diseases are due in part to anti-thyroid antibodies, but the effect is opposite: the reason is that in Graves' disease some of the autoantibodies target a receptor and stimulate it (at last for a while) before causing its destruction. Obviously the two diseases are based on very similar mechanisms, and indeed there are cases of Hashimoto's thyroiditis that flare up into Graves' disease (*hashitoxicosis*) (89).

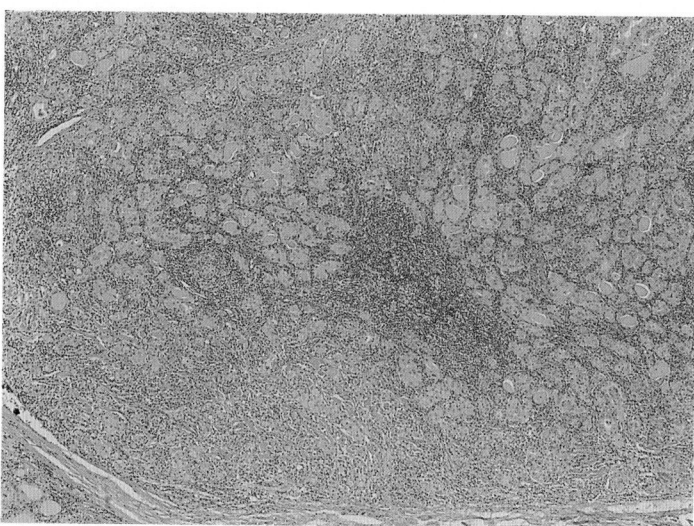
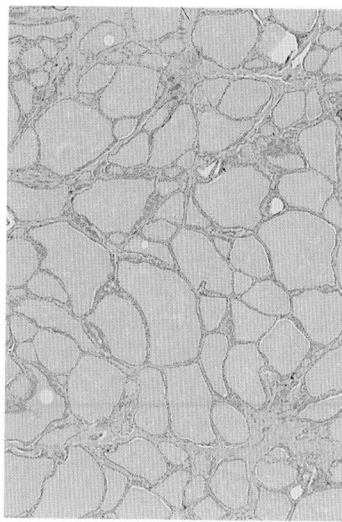

FIGURE 19.2   Comparison of diseased and normal thyroid. *Left:* Hashimoto's thyroiditis, an autoimmune disease; thyroid follicles, barely recognizable, are slowly destroyed by an intense mononuclear cell infiltrate consisting mainly of lymphocytes. *Right:* Normal thyroid. (35x)

Recently another model of pathogenesis was proposed for the autoimmune thyroid diseases: it is based on *inappropriate apoptosis of thyroid epithelial cells* by the Fas/FasL mechanism (82a). The concept is interesting but still speculative.

Sjögren's syndrome.   In this highly distressing disease, the eyes and mouth become extremely dry (*xerophthalmia, xerostomia*) because the lachrymal and salivary glands are destroyed by an infiltrate of lymphocytes, plasma cells, and fibrous tissue. Other mucosae may be involved (Figure 19.3), and other autoimmune diseases are often associated. Again, women are more often affected than men (9:1).

Diabetes.   Diabetes is not a single disease, but a group of disorders that have in common *hyperglycemia,* and affect about 5 percent of the population in Western societies (76). Over 90 percent of the patients suffer from one of two syndromes: Insulin-Dependent Diabetes Mellitus (IDDM) or diabetes Type 1, and Non–Insulin-Dependent Diabetes Mellitus (NIDDM) or diabetes Type 2, a more insidious variant (93).

> Untreated diabetics drink a lot (*polydipsia*) and therefore void much fluid, hence the name *diabetes* given or recorded by Aretaeus of Cappadocia, a Greek physician of I century AD: *diabáinein* means "to pass through," and *diabétes* means "siphon."

Long considered a low-key metabolic disease, blessed by the treatment with insulin, diabetes is moving into the third millennium as a threatening global problem in urgent need of attention. Paradoxically, this change for the worse is largely the result of human achievements in

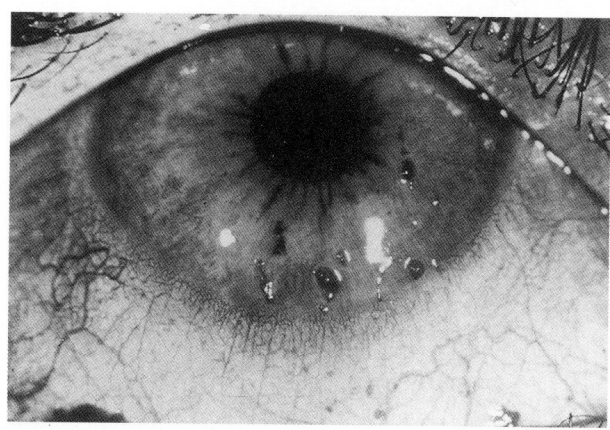

FIGURE 19.3   Cornea in severe Sjögren's syndrome has dried up and become vascularized (*keratitis filamentosa*). (Reproduced with permission from [41].)

public health and social welfare: people survive infections, live longer, move less, eat more, and become obese. And the price of obesity, very high in itself (p. 91), includes diabetes and its complications: renal failure, cataract, retinal damage, nerve damage, myocardial infarction, stroke, and amputations (13). The new term *diabesity* sums up the problem (93).

It is diabetes Type 1 that concerns us here because a large body of evidence suggests that it is an autoimmune disease (8). It is the most common chronic disease of children; insulin treatment is mandatory. It definitely has a genetic component (confirmed by its HLA associations), but its mode of inheritance is not clear. The environment also plays a role, as suggested by its geo-graphic distribution; a viral infection or a toxic agent (8) may be the triggering event. In its early stages, diabetes Type 1 is associated with chronic inflammation of the pancreatic islets (*insulitis*), which later abates, leaving the islet specifically devoid of the insulin-secreting beta cells (Figure 19.4). The consensus is that the beta cells are killed by T lymphocytes and then fail to regenerate; the plasma contains antibodies against insulin, beta cells, and other pancreatic targets, but their role in pathogenesis is not well understood. There are also abnormalities of peripheral lymphocytes. Overall, the bulk of evidence points to a T-cell–mediated disease, but lately a convincing case was made for a pathogenic role of maternal antibodies (34a, 86a).

The experimental study of diabetes is facilitated by several excellent models (8, 19, 22, 54, 63): notably the diabetes-prone BBDP/Wor rat (Figures 19.4, 19.5), the NOD (Non-Obese Diabetic) mouse from Japan (8), and the Israeli desert rat, which, if deprived of its austere desert diet in favor of hearty meals, promptly becomes obese and diabetic.

Diabetes Type 2, also called "insulin resistant," is almost 10 times more frequent. It usually appears later in life; the pancreas is free of insulitis, and insulin treatment is not always required. Both a familial and an environmental component are obvious.

Finding a cure for diabetes seems to be an attainable goal. But first we must understand the pathogenesis. Some of the world's best brains are working at it. The literature is immense; here is a sample of what was being tried in 2003.

> In the NOD mouse, a proteasome defect—specific for immune cells—interferes with the elimination of self-reactive T cells that recognize the pancreatic islets, and diabetes Type 1 develops. Injection of spleen cells from unrelated mice (plus Freund's adjuvant, p. 556) cures the diabetes permanently (48a). The islets regenerate, including the beta cells, probably by differentiation of "spleen cells" into epithelial cells. Until recently this was heresy, but no longer so. . . . We shall wait and see.

In 2001, the number of diabetics on the globe was estimated at 150 million; by 2025 the number is projected to reach 300 million, most of them Type 2 (93). The challenge is greater than that posed by tobacco, and it may be more difficult to meet: eating and sitting are more basic than smoking.

Systemic lupus erythematosus. This disease (SLE) is usually diagnosed in a young woman who complains of fever, joint pains, and skin rashes; a typical "butterfly rash" appears over the nose and cheeks (Figure 19.6) (59).

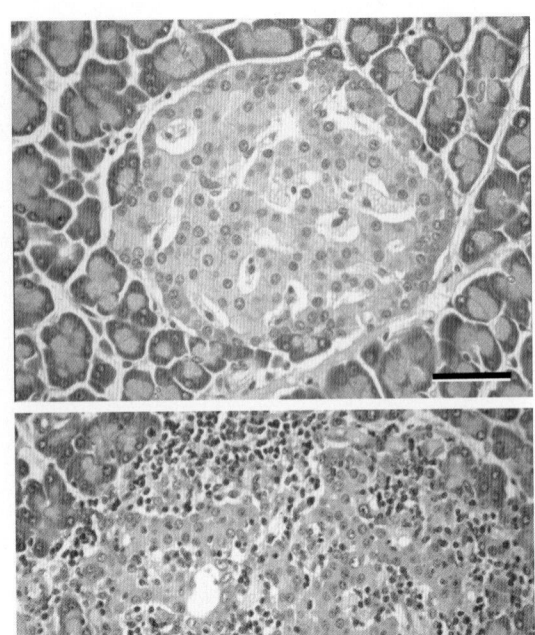

FIGURE 19.4   *Top:* Pancreatic islet of a nondiabetic, "normal" rat of the BBDP/Wor strain, which is prone to develop autoimmune diabetes. The islet is sharply defined; inflammatory cells are absent. (Reproduced with permission from [54]). *Bottom:* Inflamed islet (insulitis) in an acutely diabetic BBDP/Wor rat. The cords of islet cells are separated and distorted by the infiltrating lymphocytes. (Courtesy of Dr. A. Like, University of Massachusetts Medical School, Worcester, MA). **Bar** = 50 μm.

The name *lupus* ("wolf") is left over from the Middle Ages (82). Originally it was applied to ulcers, especially of the face, that had the appearance of having been gnawed; the classic *lupus vulgaris* was ulcerating tuberculosis of the face.

Quite unlike Graves' disease, in which a few circulating antibodies are targeted very specifically to one organ, in SLE the blood is flooded with antibodies aimed at intracellular components with no organ specificity. *Antinuclear* antibodies are typical (although not specific); they can react with the exposed nuclei of damaged or dead cells and form complexes in the renal glomeruli or along the basal surface of the epidermis (Figure 19.7), but they have also been shown to penetrate into living cells, and they may therefore contribute to the pathogenesis of SLE (36, 69). Other antibodies target red blood cells, platelets, and phospholipids which are involved with clotting (4, 5, 38);

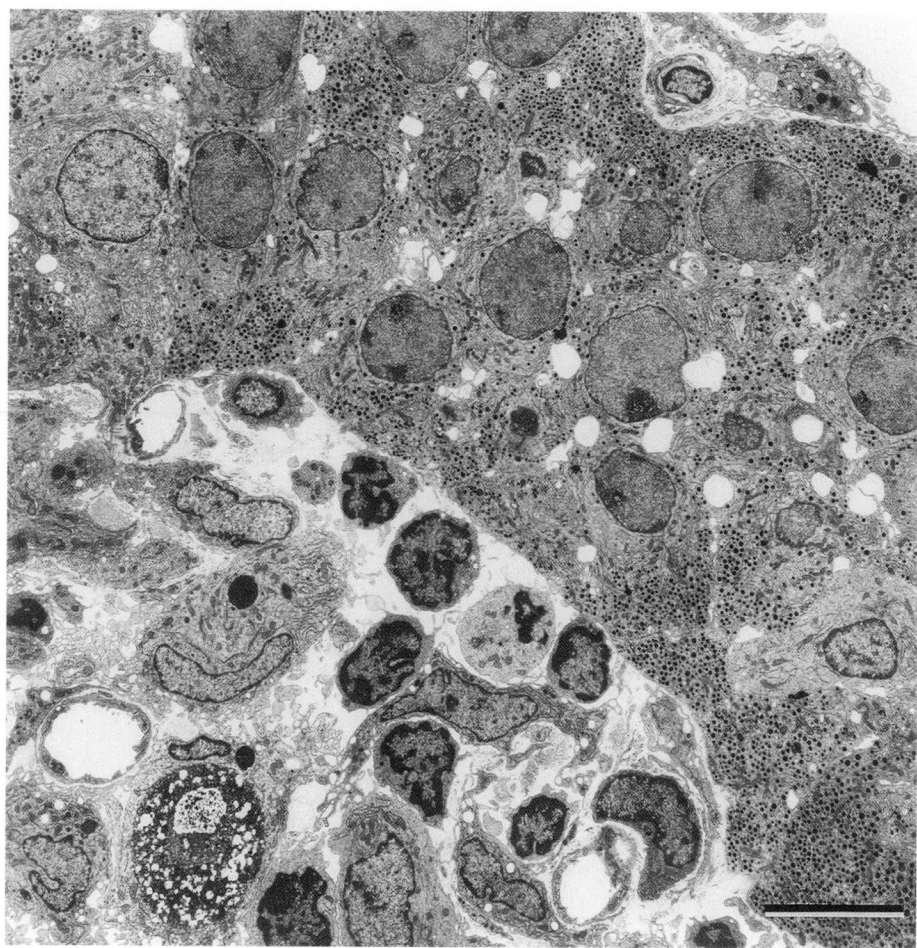

FIGURE 19.5 Low power electron micrograph of an inflamed islet from a diabetic BBDP/WO rat. The B cells, usually set in the center of the islet, are absent. The core of the islet is "hollowed out" and filled with lymphocytes and macrophages. Some of the latter contain debris of phagocytized B cells. **Bar** = 10 μm. (Reproduced with permission from [54].)

antigen–antibody complexes develop, resulting in changes recalling the "complex disease" of hypersensitivity Type 3 (p. 546). Damage can occur throughout the body, but especially in the kidneys, skin, joints, and the cardiovascular system, including "complex arteritis," which causes further damage. The clinical course is stormy; immunosuppressive therapy has improved the outcome but renal failure due to lupus glomerulonephritis remains a major threat to life. There are many experimental models, including the New Zealand mice called NZB (45, 64, 69) in which SLE develops with a sex distribution similar to the human disease—10 females to 1 male.

Rheumatoid arthritis. About 1 percent of the population worldwide is affected by *rheumatoid arthritis* (37). This is a chronic inflammatory disease of the synovium that can also affect other tissues (skin, heart, eyes, lungs); knees and hands are most often affected. The inflamed synovium contains many plasma cells; it becomes tremendously hypertrophic, up to 100 times its original

weight: a phenomenon that we have compared to the immunopathologic burgeoning of nasal polyps (p. 535). Eventually the articular cartilage is eroded and slowly replaced by a **pannus,** a sheet of connective tissue arising from the synovium. In 80 percent of these patients the blood contains an IgM autoantibody (called *rheumatoid factor*) against the patient's own IgG. The main portion of the IgG molecule that behaves as an antigen is the Fc segment (p. 289); large complexes form, consisting only of immunoglobulins that are "catching each other by the tail." The large circulating complexes may be responsible for some of the extra-articular damage typical of rheumatoid arthritis, but there are patients with no circulating rheumatoid factor, and there are normal people whose blood is positive for that factor. In the joints, however, the complexes activate complement and thereby contribute to the influx of leukocytes. Among the inflammatory cells is a high proportion of self-reactive T lymphocytes, mainly CD4$^+$ memory cells, which activate several cell types, including the endothelium; this increases the flood of

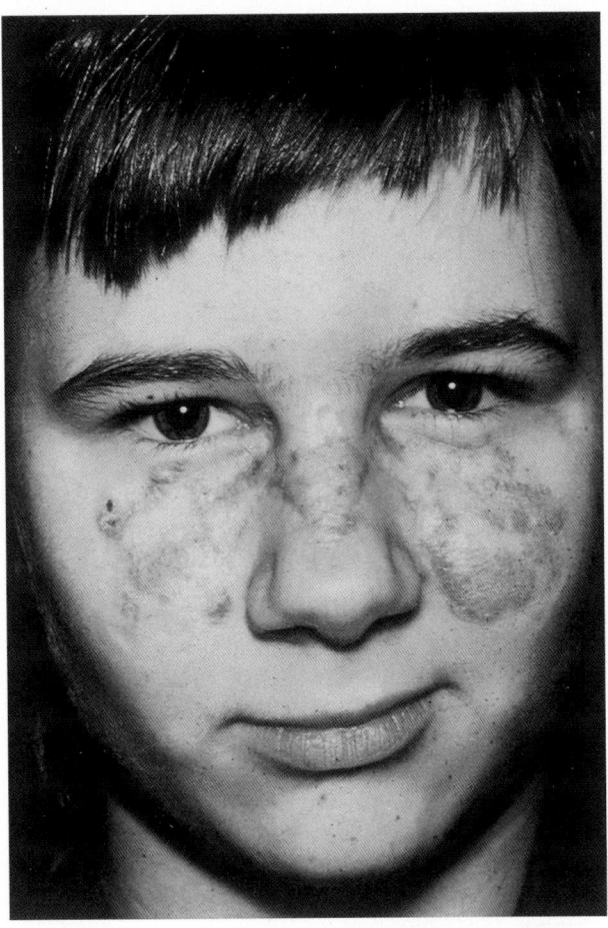

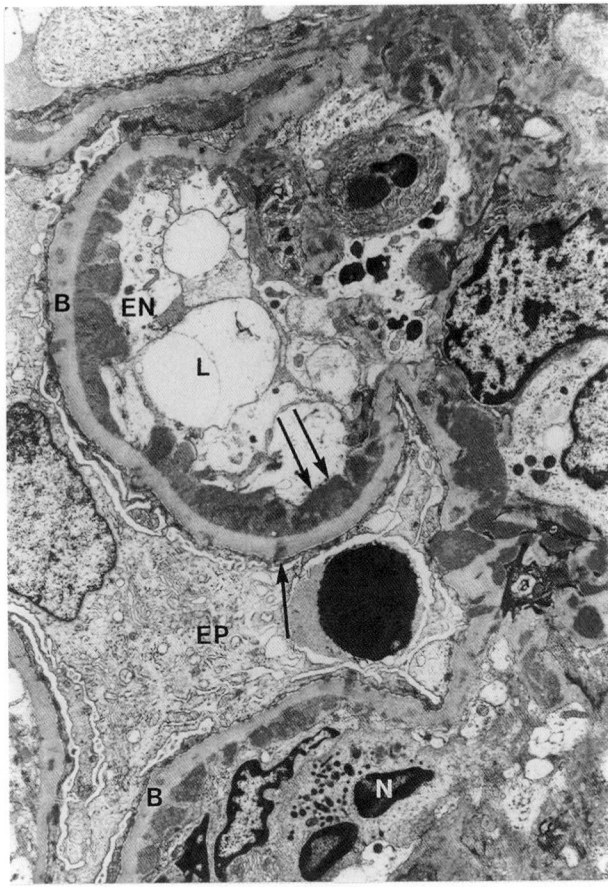

FIGURE 19.6 Typical butterfly-rash of systemic lupus in a young man aged 17. (Courtesy of Dr. J. L. Sullivan, University of Massachusetts Medical School, Worcester, MA.)

FIGURE 19.7 Deposits of antigen-antibody complexes in the capillary loops of a glomerulus, in a case of lupus nephritis (kidney biopsy). **B** = Capillary basement membrane; **EN** = endothelial cell; **EP** = visceral epithelial cell; **L** = capillary lumen; **N** = nucleus of neutrophil; **double arrow:** subendothelial deposits of antigen–antibody complexes; **single arrow:** subendothelial deposits of antigen–antibody complexes. (Courtesy of Dr. H. G. Rennke, Brigham and Women's Hospital, Harvard Medical School, Boston, MA.)

leukocytes and cytokines, which will eventually destroy the joint.

In 20–30 percent of seropositive patients, *rheumatoid nodules* appear, usually in pressure areas of the skin (Figure 19.8). A nodule is essentially an oversize granuloma with a necrotic center surrounded by "palisading" macrophages (Figure 19.9). Anticollagen antibodies do develop (against collagen Type 2), but they may be secondary to the destruction of cartilage.

It is difficult to fit all of these facts into a coherent picture. A current opinion is that rheumatoid arthritis develops in individuals who are immunogenetically predisposed and become infected with certain viruses or bacteria; candidates are Epstein-Barr virus, mycobacteria, and a few other agents (45, 73). Another lead is based on the K/BxN arthritic mouse, whose blood is loaded with pathogenic IgG antibodies against the ubiquitous enzyme glucose-6-phosphate isomerase (GPI):

the joints are selectively damaged, it seems, because they are coated with complexes of GPI plus IgG, which activate complement—and cartilage lacks complement inhibitors (57a).

Goodpasture's syndrome is essentially a two-hit, lung-kidney disease, due to autoantibodies against a collagen IV peptide in basement membranes. It can begin in either organ: if it is the lung, some injury (influenza pneumonia in the 1919 cases of Dr. E. W. Goodpasture) exposes the alveolar basement membranes; bleeding occurs, and somehow anti–basement membrane antibodies develop, which cross-react with the kidneys' glomerular and sometimes tubular basement membranes. Bleeding will then occur from the

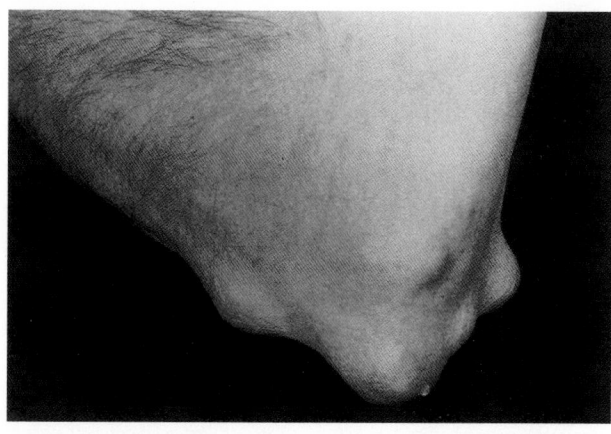

FIGURE 19.8 Elbow of a patient with rheumatoid arthritis, showing multiple subcutaneous nodules. (Reproduced with permission from [44].)

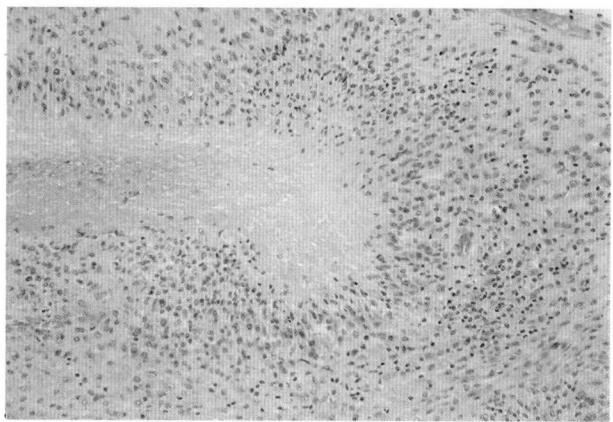

FIGURE 19.9 The mysterious rheumatoid nodule: a necrotic center surrounded by a crown of macrophages that tend to "palisade"—that is, to be radially oriented. The clinically visible nodules represent an aggregate of such structures, which tend to grow.

kidneys (hematuria due to glomerulonephritis). Why the antibodies develop is not known; a genetic background is involved (there is an 85 percent association with the HLA-DR2 allele) (65). The disease, once fatal, can now be treated successfully by plasma exchange (to eliminate the antibodies) and immunosuppression. Mysteriously, after 6–12 months, the antibodies tend to disappear (18). Two unusual features: males and females are about equaly affected; and a comparable animal model does not exist.

Systemic sclerosis is a crippling, progressive disease that manifests itself as fibrosis and stiffening of the skin (hence the older name **scleroderma**) and of internal organs, especially the lungs: pulmonary fibrosis is often the cause of death. In the early stages the fibrosis is accompanied by a scanty mononuclear infiltrate, suggesting a slow progression of inflammation to scarring, but no inflammatory agent is apparent, and the collagen deposited is chemically normal. The disease is considered to be autoimmune because the blood contains a large number of autoantibodies, mostly against nuclear components (such as the NOR [Nucleolar Organizer Region], or a topoisomerase) and other intracellular organelles (such as centromeres): yet none of these antibodies seems to correlate with manifestations of the disease, and it is not even clear that they have a pathogenetic function. A few do cross-react with viruses or bacteria and could represent molecular mimicry. Vascular changes are prominent: Raynaud's disease (p. 683) is common, and so is arteriolar pathology. It has even been suggested that the disease is produced by cycles of ischemia/reperfusion and related oxygen free radicals (75). Several T-cell anomalies can be mentioned to complicate the picture, and most intriguing is a recent report that *58 percent of skin biopsies from women with systemic sclerosis contained DNA with Y-chromosome sequences; 9 of the 11 had carried male fetuses* (3). The pathogenesis of systemic sclerosis may be one of the most frustrating topics in the medical field (31). Three good animal models are available (an avian model, and Tight Skin Mice 1 and 2) but no synthesis is in sight.

Myasthenia gravis. After the frustrating scientific mess of systemic sclerosis, the story of myasthenia gravis should provide excellent relief: it is a perfect example of laboratory work solving a clinical problem. In summary: rabbits immunized with purified acetylcholine receptors developed antibodies and became weak. This suggested that patients suffering from myasthenia gravis were weak for the same reason: antibodies were blocking their acetylcholine receptors. This mechanism was elegantly demonstrated by light and by electron microscopy of the neuromuscular junctions (Figure 19.10) (11). Oddly enough, about 12 percent of these patients develop a tumor of the thymus (thymoma) containing cells that express an antigen similar to the acetylcholine receptor (23, 47).

Vitiligo. *Vitiligo* (a name of uncertain origin) is a condition in which patches of the skin lose their melanin (Figure 19.11); it can be psychologically very distressing. The mechanism is lymphocyte attack against melanocytes, although the keratinocytes can also be damaged (Figures 19.12 and 19.13) (7).

FIGURE 19.10 Evidence that myasthenia gravis is an autoimmune disease. Samples of striated muscle obtained from patients with myasthenia gravis. Light microscopic sections (**A** and **B**) were treated by an immunohistochemical method to demonstrate the presence of C3 (**A**) and C9 (**B**). In both cases the reaction product is sharply localized at the motor endplates. **C** and **D** are electron micrographs from tissues treated in a similar manner. Localization of complement components at the motor end-plates suggests that the latter are destroyed by an autoimmune mechanism, using the membrane attack complex (MAC) as an effector. **A** and **B bars** = 25 μm; **C** and **D bars** = 10 μm. (A and C reproduced with permission from [25] *and* B and D reproduced with permission from [77].)

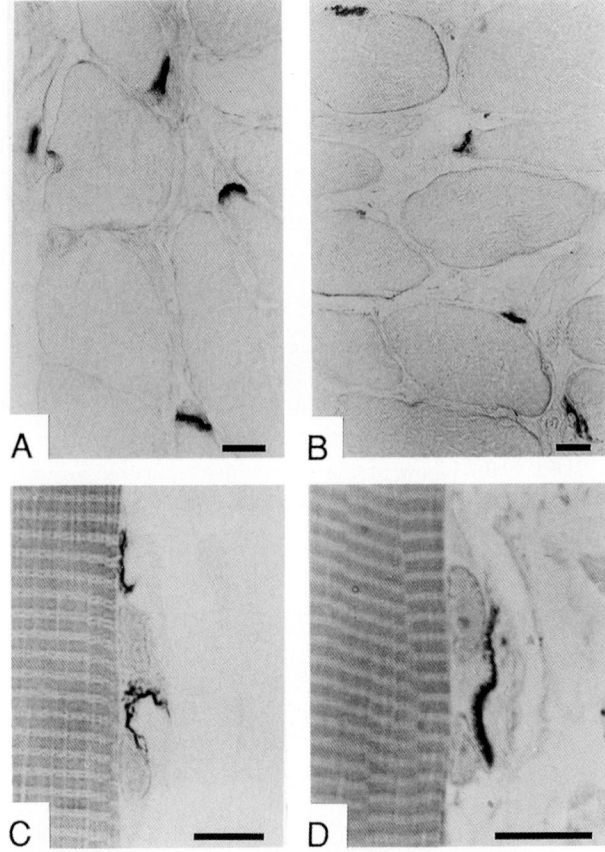

FIGURE 19.11 Vitiligo (loss of pigmentation) on the neck of a white woman. The dark dots within the area of vitiligo represent areas where repigmentation is beginning to develop; it arises from the hair follicles, under the effect of treatment (ultraviolet light plus psoralen [PUVA]). (Courtesy of Dr. J. D. Bernhard, University of Massachusetts Medical School, Worcester, MA.)

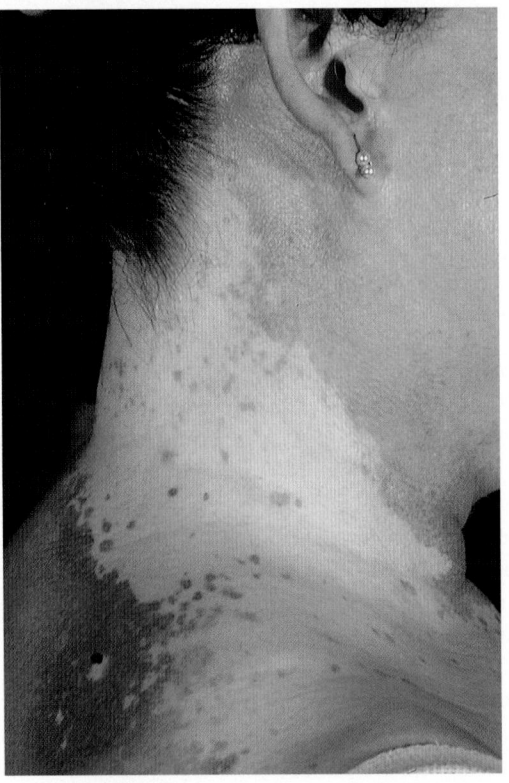

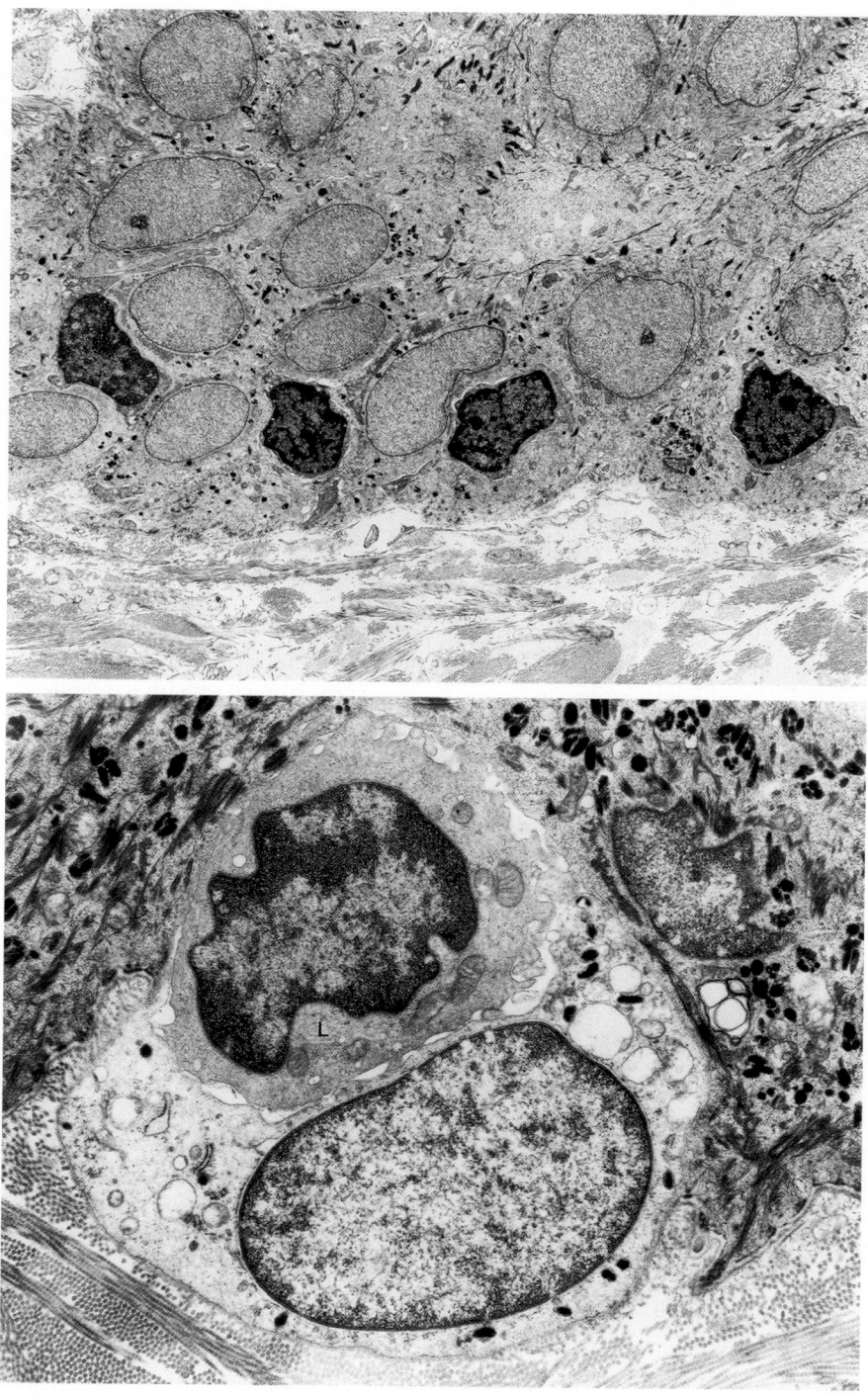

FIGURE 19.12   Skin biopsy of a dark-skinned patient affected by vitiligo. Biopsy was taken from the clinically normal skin next to the depigmented area. *Top:* Four lymphocytes invading the epidermis; they are in close contact with melanocytes. This may be interpreted as the first stage of immunologic attack. The melanocytes do not (yet) show signs of damage. *Bottom:* Lymphocyte (**L**) in close contact with a melanocyte, which shows signs of injury. (Courtesy of Dr. J. Bhawan, Boston University Medical Center, Boston, MA.)

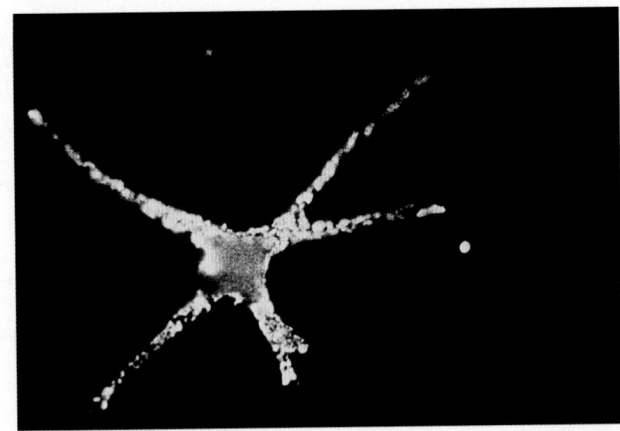

FIGURE 19.13 Human melanocyte in tissue culture, after exposure to serum from a patient with vitiligo. This immunofluorescence photomicrograph demonstrates that the melanocyte is covered with antibodies against a component of its surface. (Reprinted from [16], copyright © 1988 Alan R. Liss Inc., by permission of Wiley-Liss, a division of John Wiley & Sons, Inc.)

Pathogenesis of Autoimmune Disease

We now step into the realm of theory: no less than 14 mechanisms have been proposed to explain autoimmune diseases (73, 84). We find it convenient to group them into 3 categories: genetic, immunologic, and environmental, as shown in Figure 19.1. But whatever mechanism may be involved in any particular disease, one fact must be kept in mind: *autoimmune mechanisms are not unnatural* and may even have a function (p. 587). Autoantibodies make up a substantial part of normal plasma immunoglobulins (21). There is ample evidence that autoreactive B-cells (B-cells programmed to make autoantibody) are just sitting there waiting to be activated—but they are held in check (presumably) by suppressor mechanisms (32). Clones of autoreactive B-cells appear in mice injected with a polyclonal B-cell stimulant, such as endotoxin, PPD, some antibiotics (nystatin), some viruses, parasite components, and even some cytokines (33). As regards autoreactive T cells, their existence is also well proven in normal humans and other animals (58).

With this in mind, we now examine some of the best-known pathways to autoimmune disease.

(I) Genetic Factors

That genes play a major role in autoimmune disease is obvious. You can actually buy mice guaranteed to develop autoimmune hemolytic anemia (called New Zealand Black) or chickens that develop autoimmune thyroiditis. In humans there is a proven familial tendency to develop certain autoantibodies (70). If one identical twin develops systemic lupus, the other will be much more likely than normal to develop it (12).

For some autoimmune diseases, there is also an association with certain MHC haplotypes (80); this association has offered new hopes for therapy. If some autoimmune diseases, such as insulin-dependent diabetes, are associated with a certain Class II MHC molecule, would it be possible to devise a therapy based on antibodies against that molecule? Some positive experimental evidence is already available (85).

A pregnant woman affected by SLE can transfer some of her autoantibodies to her fetus: antibody attack against the heart may destroy the conduction system, resulting in fibrosis and congenital heart block. Other complications are possible, including placental damage (15).

(II) Immunologic Factors

(A) Release of Sequestered Antigens

Because the immune system does not "see" antigens that are sequestered inside cells, it makes sense that an immune response should develop if these antigens are suddenly released into the extracellular spaces. This is the oldest theory of autoimmune disease, and it does fit a few facts (24, 79).

- *Sympathetic ophthalmia* is the best example, even though it is not fully understood. Weeks or months after injury to one uvea (the membrane that contains the iris), a granulomatous uveitis occasionally develops in the other eye (2, 17, 68). This is thought to be an immune response to uveal tissue or pigment, and it is prevented by enucleation of the useless injured eye within 2 weeks. Antibodies to uveal tissue are not found. The response seems to be the delayed hypersensitivity type, against a common antigen of various ocular tissues.

- *Injury of the crystalline lens* follows a similar pattern. If an eye is injured and lens protein is spilled, the resulting uveitis is thought to be partly autoimmune (*uveitis phacoanaphylactica*) and may flare up in the other eye (17). Here we run, once again, into the unsettling contradictions of autoimmune disease: over 50 percent of *normal* individuals have circulating antibodies against lens protein (42).

- *Vasectomized males* often develop antisperm antibodies, but autoimmune orchitis does not follow (56, 81).

> NOTE: The antigens of sperm are unusual in that they develop at puberty and therefore miss the chance of inducing tolerance during development *in utero* (56). This might help us understand the need for a blood–testis barrier.

- *Myocardial infarction* is often followed by the appearance of antimyocardial autoantibodies (52, 53), but they seem to do no harm. They do not correlate with the puzzling post–myocardial infarct syndrome that was once thought to be an autoimmune response occurring 1–5 weeks after an infarct in 1–4 percent of the patients. These patients experienced chest pain, fever, leukocytosis, and pericardial rub due to pericardial inflammation (53).

(B) Mechanisms Related to Apoptosis

Apoptosis should prevent cell proteins from becoming antigens, but this does not always work (pp. 216, 447).

(C) An Adjuvant Effect of the Heat-Shock Proteins

The heat-shock proteins are intracellular (p. 186); when they are released and encounter the immune system they have a powerful adjuvant effect (p. 556); they activate the dendritic cells and can trigger autoimmune disease (57b).

(D) Perturbations of the Idiotype–Anti-Idiotype Network

The basic notion of idiotypes is that the variable segments of antibody molecules are themselves antigenic. In other words, the variable segments behave as epitopes, and as such they are called **idiotypes** (45). At first sight it seems absurd that an antibody should become antigenic, but remember that an antibody is after all a "unique" structure; so it stands to reason that it *could* behave like an antigen (80).

This topic is indeed as complicated as it sounds, but it was important enough to earn a Nobel prize (Niels K. Jerne, 1984), so the essentials should be understood (14, 43, 48).

The idiotype (i.e., variable segment) of an antibody molecule can be visualized as a sort of cast or negative image of the antigenic epitope. Therefore, an antibody against this idiotype (an anti-antibody) is a cast of a cast and thus should be similar to the original antigen; Jerne called it an internal image of the antigen. The series of

idiotypes continues with anti-anti-antibodies, and so on. Each new antibody molecule becomes in turn an antigen; as such it combines with specific receptors on T and B cells, resulting in either stimulation or suppression. *In this way the entire immune system can be visualized as a network of interacting components.* The basic concept is illustrated in Figure 19.14.

Mind-boggling as it is, the anti-idiotype mechanism made it possible to devise an experimental model of myasthenia gravis. The principle was to inject rabbits with an acetylcholine analog, a large molecule that behaves as an antigen when injected with Freund's adjuvant into rabbits. Read slowly: because the analog (by definition) could react with the acetylcholine receptor, an antibody against the analog (being its negative image) should not fit into the receptor. However, myasthenia-like symptoms appeared in some rabbits (88). The explanation: the antibodies had given rise to anti-antibodies, which (as negatives of negatives) reproduced the "fitting shape."

> Another intellectually satisfying product of the network concept: If anti-antibodies are made in the image of the original antigen, why not prepare vaccines consisting of anti-antibodies rather than of the original antigen? This would have several advantages, and experimentally the principle has been shown to work (14).

(III) Environmental Factors

In theory at least, the environment may contribute to an autoimmune disease in two ways: by providing it with a *cause* (such as a bacterium) or by *modulating its course* (such as sunlight enhancing the "butterfly rash" of lupus).

(A) Infection

Some anecdotal episodes are difficult to dismiss. Until the 1940s, in the far-away Faeroe Islands, multiple sclerosis had not been seen. Then an outbreak occurred, coinciding with the arrival of British troops during World War II (92). But then, if it was due to a virus, what virus could it be?

Rheumatoid arthritis is one of several autoimmune diseases that are constantly reviewed as possible infections (in this case, by mycobacterium [72]). So far no autoimmune disease has passed the test as being 100 percent infectious (6). However, it is best to keep an open mind, remembering the story of Lyme disease which was long diagnosed as a juvenile form of rheumatoid arthritis. Then the spirochete *Borrelia burgdorferi* was recognized; and it turned out that Lyme arthritis is a partially autoimmune response to an antigen on the surface of the spirochete, which shares an epitope with an important antigen from the inflamed joint: Leukocyte

FIGURE 19.14 Idiotypes and anti-idiotypes. *Top:* Structural analogy between antigen and anti-antibody. *Bottom:* Because of the structural analogy, an anti-antibody can compete with a hormone for binding with its receptor. (Adapted from information appearing in New England Journal of Medicine [14].)

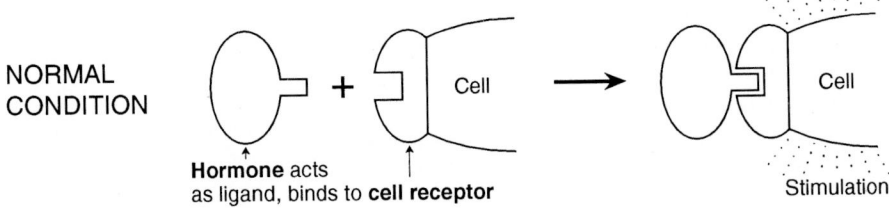

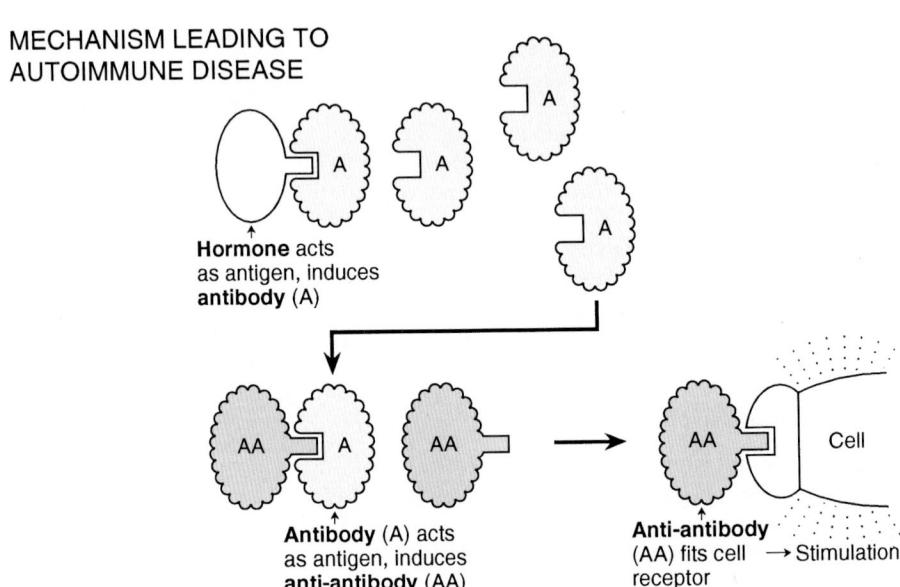

Function-associated Antigen-1 (LFA-1, also called CD11a and CD18 (26). A discovery that called for collaboration between several branches of knowledge.

(B) Molecular Mimicry

We just mentioned Lyme disease, in which the infectious agent does not produce damage by means of a toxin, but *by sharing one or more epitopes with the host;* therefore, when the host generates antibodies against the shared epitopes, it damages its own tissues as well as the infectious agent. This subtle mechanism is known as *molecular mimicry*; it is difficult to prove, but there are many examples.

The best-known human disease that is thought to arise by molecular mimicry is *acute rheumatic fever,* a heart disease that may follow a throat infection with group A streptococci. In this disease, several bacterial antigens cross-react with myocardial cells, with connective-tissue antigens of the heart valves (myocarditis and valvular damage do occur), and sometimes with antigens of the kidney and nervous tissues (Figure 19.15) (35, 91). The cross-reactions with nervous tissue are

FIGURE 19.15 Cross-reacting antigens of group A streptococci. These antigens cross-react with tissue antigens. Such reactions may explain damage to organs that are not infected. (Adapted with permission from [91].)

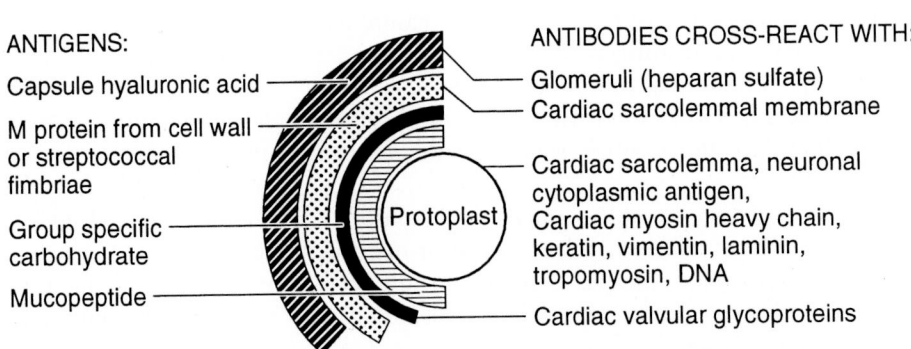

especially interesting. Symptoms of rheumatic fever include the uncontrolled movements of Sydenham's chorea, which originate from a disturbance in the subthalamic and caudate nuclei; antibodies in the serum of the patients react with the cytoplasm of neurons precisely in these nuclei.

> In acute rheumatic fever the correlations between antibodies and anatomic lesions are quite obvious, but several puzzles remain: (a) To reach their targets, the antineuron antibodies have to cross the blood–brain barrier. How could they do it? (b) In an epidemic of Group A streptococcal throat infection, only 3 percent of the victims develop rheumatic fever. Why? (c) To produce acute rheumatic fever the streptococcal infection must be in the throat (skin infections may produce glomerulonephritis). Why? (91).

Although the best example of molecular mimicry between host and parasite is offered by Group A streptococci, a more general variant of this scenario is now under study; it involves stress proteins (HSPs, p. 186). Bacteria and host may be able to synthesize stress proteins of very similar structure. In the heat of an encounter, both host and parasite would express these proteins, and an immune attack directed against bacterial stress proteins may backfire and attack the host (39, 46, 49, 83).

(C) Drugs and Toxic Agents

There are several ways for a nonantigenic body protein to become antigenic. A drug may be the culprit, and the list of possible drugs is long (9). Two examples: (a) prolonged treatment with *procainamide,* an antiarrhythmic agent, causes many patients to produce antinuclear antibodies, and even full-blown SLE; and (b) some mice develop autoimmune kidney disease if they are treated with a classic kidney poison, mercuric chloride.

The precise molecular change that makes the protein antigenic is known for rheumatoid arthritis: gamma globulins show an abnormal pattern of glycosylation, which causes them to be seen by the immune system as foreign (62). Overall, the message we need to keep in mind is that the list of chemicals (*xenobiotics*) that can cause autoimmune *responses* or autoimmune diseases in *some* animals or *some* people includes over 100 names, ranging from mercury to penicillin and cow's milk (10, 50, 51).

Some Lessons from Experimental Autoimmune Diseases

Apart from the many natural examples of autoimmune diseases, it is a fairly simple matter to produce autoimmune diseases experimentally. The basic method is to inject homogenized tissue mixed with complete Freund adjuvant (p. 556) (tissue alone is much less effective). Most organs have been tested in this manner (44, 78) and have shown that within a week or two, almost miraculously, injected thyroid produces thyroiditis, uvea produces uveitis, adrenals produce adrenalitis, peripheral nerves produce peripheral neuritis (87), central nervous tissue produces encephalomyelitis (tantalizingly similar to multiple sclerosis) (Figure 19.16) (66), and so on. Sperm produces epididymitis, perhaps because the antibodies cannot violate the blood–testis barrier (86). Incidentally, Freund's adjuvant *alone,* in rats, produces an arthritic syndrome.

Such models have been useful for working out some basic mechanisms. For example:

- Experimental autoimmune thyroiditis can be transferred from one rabbit to another with either serum or white blood cells, proving that, in this model at least, antibody-mediated and cell-mediated mechanisms are involved.

- Experimental autoimmune encephalomyelitis (EAE) can be transferred only with T cells, not with serum (40, 71).

- Rabbits can be given an autoimmune disease affecting their own central nervous system by injecting them with a single protein extracted from myelin, called myelin basic protein (MBP). MBP has been sequenced, and it turns out that it shares a sequence of six amino acids with a virus that produces encephalitis in rabbits. This suggests that a virus may initiate a brain lesion and then disappear; but nervous tissue has been damaged, and the lesion is perpetuated by endogenous MBP (30).

- Vaccination of humans against rabies is still performed in some countries with the older but cheaper method of injecting attenuated rabies virus that was grown in the brain or cords of adult animals (Semple vaccine). Roughly 1 in 400 patients develops neurologic complications, most likely due to cross-reaction between animal and human MBP (40). In fact, this clinical complication was the stimulus for trying to produce experimental allergic encephalomyelitis with rabbit brain and Freund's adjuvant.

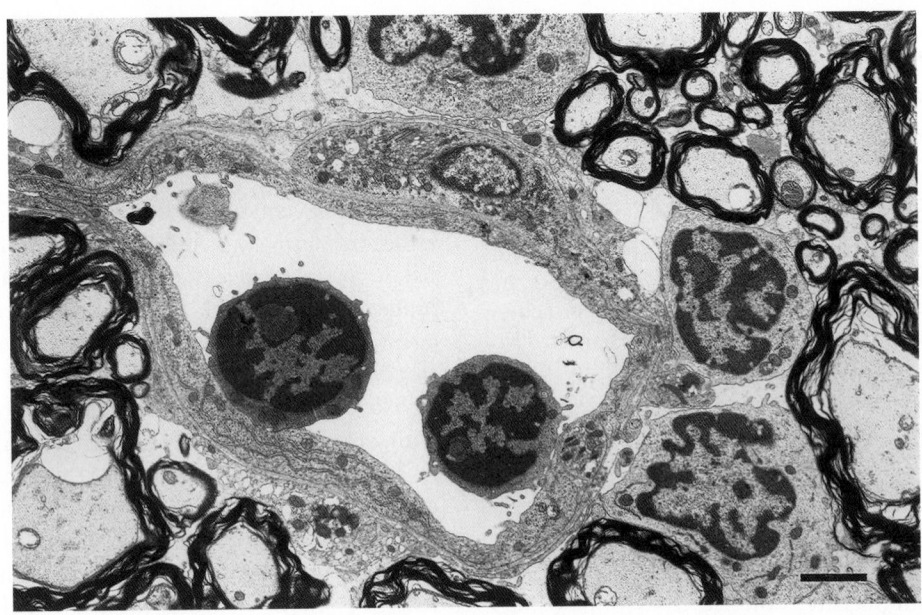

FIGURE 19.16　Early lesion of experimental allergic encephalomyelitis (EAE), the prime model for human multiple sclerosis. Two lymphocytes (probably T cells) are attached to the endothelium of the blood vessel; three others (*top and right*) have traversed the wall of the vessel and lie among myelinated nerve fibers (black rings). Interpretation: the endothelial cells presented a brain-specific antigen or a lymphocyte recognition molecule on the luminal surface; T cells with the appropriate receptors became attached, performed diapedesis, and secreted cytokines (gamma-interferon, interleukin-2) which recruited other lymphocytes. Recruited T cells produced cytokines and antibodies against the nerve tissue. Monocytes will phagocytize the debris. Mouse EAE; 15 days after sensitization with myelin. **Bar** = 2 μm. (Reproduced with permission from [67].)

Transgenic technology has been applied to this field, but mainly for working out general mechanisms of tolerance (58).

> **TO SUM UP:** Today it is common knowledge that autoimmune diseases afflict 3–5 percent of humankind. One generation ago, choosing to work in the field of autoimmunity was not a propitious choice for an academic career. Such is often the fate of scientific ideas that appear in advance of the related technology.

References

1. Alarcón-Segovia D, Ruiz-Argüelles A, Llorente L. Broken dogma: penetration of autoantibodies into living cells. Immunol Today 1996;17:163–164.
2. Albert DM, Diaz-Rohena R. A historical review of sympathetic ophthalmia and its epidemiology. Surv Ophthalmol 1989;34:1–14.
3. Artlett CM, Smith JB, Jimenez SA. Identification of fetal DNA and cells in skin lesions from women with systemic sclerosis. N Engl J Med 1998;338:1186–1191.
4. Asherson RA. Antiphospholipid antibodies and "syndromes": many questions and few answers. Isr J Med Sci 1990;26:284–286.
5. Asherson RA, Lubbe WF. Cerebral and valve lesions in SLE: association with antiphospholipid antibodies. J Rheumatol 1988;15:539–543.
6. Benoist C, Mathis D. Autoimmunity provoked by infection: how good is the case for T cell epitope mimicry? Nat Immunol 2001;2:797–801.
7. Bhawan J, Bhutani LK. Keratinocyte damage in vitiligo. J Cutan Pathol 1983;10:207–212.
8. Bieg S, Lernmark Å. Diabetes. In: Rose NR, Mackay IR (eds). The Autoimmune Diseases, 3rd ed. San Diego: Academic Press. 1998, pp. 431–457.
9. Bigazzi PE. Mechanisms of chemical-induced autoimmunity. In: Dean JH, Luster MI, Munson AE, Amos H, eds. Immunotoxicology and immunopharmacology. New York: Raven Press, 1985, pp. 277–290.
10. Bigazzi PE. Autoimmunity caused by xenobiotics. Toxicology 1997;119:1–21.
11. Bigazzi PE. Animal models of autoimmunity: spontaneous and induced. In: Rose NR, Mackay IR (eds). The Autoimmune Diseases, 3rd ed. San Diego: Academic Press. 1998, pp. 211–244.
12. Block SR, Winfield JB, Lockshin MD, D'Angelo WA, Christian CL. Studies of twins with systemic lupus erythematosus. A review of the literature and presentation of 12 additional sets. Am J Med 1975;59:533–552.

13. Brownlee M. Biochemistry and molecular cell biology of diabetic complications. Nature 2001;414:813–820.

14. Burdette S, Schwartz RS. Idiotypes and idiotypic networks. N Engl J Med 1987;317:219–224.

15. Buyon J, Szer I. Passively acquired autoimmunity and the maternal fetal dyad in systemic lupus erythematosus. Springer Semin Immunopathol 1986;9:283–304.

16. Bystryn J-C, Pfeffer S. Vitiligo and antibodies to melanocytes. Prog Clin Biol Res 1988;256:195–206.

17. Chan C-C. Relationship between sympathetic ophthalmia, phacoanaphylatic endophthalmitis, and Vogt-Koyanagi-Harada disease. Ophthalmology 1988;95:619–624.

18. Cooggins CH, Rennke HG, Rose BD. Glomerulonephritis and the nephrotic syndrome. In: Dale DC, Gederman DD (eds) Scientific American Medicine. Chpt. 10 Nephrology 1995, pp. 1–18.

19. Crisá L, Mordes JP, Rossini AA. Autoimmune diabetes mellitus in the BB rat. Diabetes Metab Rev 1992;8:9–37.

20. Davidson A, Diamond B. Autoimmune diseases. N Engl J Med 2001;345:340–350.

21. Dighiero G, Lymberi P, Guilbert B, Ternynck T, Avrameas S. Natural autoantibodies constitute a substantial part of normal circulating immunoglobulins. Ann NY Acad Sci 1986;475: 135–145.

22. Doukas J, Mordes JP. T lymphocytes capable of activating endothelial cells in vitro are present in rats with autoimmune diabetes. J Immunol 1993;150:1–11.

23. Drachman D. Myasthenia Gravis. In: Rose NR, Mackay IR (eds). The Autoimmune Diseases, 3rd ed. San Diego: Academic Press. 1998, pp. 637–662.

24. Elkon KB. Autoantibodies: their nature and significance. In: Harris EN, Exner T, Hughes GRV, Asherson RA, eds. Phospholipid-binding antibodies. Boca Raton, FL: CRC Press, 1991, pp. 60–72.

25. Engle AG, Lambert EH, Howard FM Jr. Ultrastructural localization of the terminal and lytic ninth complement gravis. J Neuropathol Exp Neurol 1980;39:160–172.

26. Ermann J, Fathman CG. Autoimmune diseases: genes, bugs and failed regulation. Nat Immunol 2001;2:759–761.

27. Federman DD. Thyroid. In: Dale DC, Federman DD (eds) Scientific American Medicine. Chpt. 3 Endocrinology, 1994, pp. 2–27.

28. Finnegan A, Needleman BW, Hodes RJ. Function of autoreactive T cells in immune responses. Immunol Rev 1990; 116:15–31.

29. Friedlaender MH, Fujishima H. Autoimmune diseases of the eye. In: Rose NR, Mackay IR (eds). The Autoimmune Diseases, 3rd ed. San Diego: Academic Press. 1998, pp. 737–758.

30. Fujinami RS, Oldstone MBA. Amino acid homology between the encephalitogenic site of myelin basic protein and virus: mechanism for autoimmunity. Science 1985;230:1043–1045.

31. Galperin C, Gershwin ME. Systemic sclerosis (scleroderma). In: Rose NR, Mackay IR (eds). The Autoimmune Diseases, 3rd ed. San Diego: Academic Press. 1998, pp. 317–342.

32. Gibson J, Basten A, Walker KZ, Loblay RH. A role for suppressor T cells in induction of self-tolerance. Proc Natl Acad Sci USA 1985;82:5150–5154.

33. Goodman MG, Weigle WO. Role of polyclonal B-cell activation in self/non-self discrimination. Immunol Today 1981;2: 54–57.

34. Grabar P. Autoantibodies and the physiological role of immunoglobulins. Immunol Today 1983;4:337–340.

34a. Greeley SA, Katsumata M, Yu L, et al. Elimination of maternally transmitted autoantibodies prevents diabetes in non-obese diabetic mice. Nature Med 2002;8:399–402.

35. Gulizia JM, Cunningham MW, McManus BM. Immunoreactivity of anti-streptococcal monoclonal antibodies to human heart valves. Am J Pathol 1991;138:285–301.

36. Hahn BH. Antibodies to DNA. N Engl J Med. 1998; 338:1359–1368.

37. Harris ED Jr. Rheumatoid arthritis. Pathophysiology and implications for therapy. N Engl J Med 1990;322:1277–1289.

38. Harris EN, Asherson RA, Hughes GRV. Antiphospholipid antibodies—autoantibodies with a difference. Annu Rev Med 1988;39:261–271.

39. Harrison LC, McColl GJ. Infection and autoimmune disease. In: Rose NR, Mackay IR (eds). The Autoimmune Diseases, 3rd ed. San Diego: Academic Press. 1998, pp. 127–140.

40. Hemachudha T, Griffin DE, Giffels JJ, et al. Myelin basic protein as an encephalitogen in encephalomyelitis and polyneuritis following rabies vaccination. N Engl J Med 1987;316: 369–374.

41. Hughes GRV. Connective tissue diseases, 3rd ed. Oxford: Blackwell Scientific Publications, 1987.

42. Jaffe NS. Cataract surgery and its complications. St. Louis: CV Mosby, 1972.

43. Jerne NK. Towards a network theory of the immune system. Ann Inst Pasteur Immunol 1974;125C:373–389.

44. Kabat EA, Mayer MM. Experimental immunochemistry, 2nd ed. Springfield, IL: Charles C. Thomas, 1964.

45. Kantor FS. Autoimmunities: diseases of "dysregulation." Hosp Pract 1988;23:75–84.

46. Kaufmann SHE. Heat shock proteins and the immune response. Immunol Today 1990;11:129–136.

47. Kirchner T, Tzartos S, Hoppe F, et al. Pathogenesis of myasthenia gravis. Acetylcholine receptor-related antigenic determinants in tumor-free thymuses and thymic epithelial tumors. Am J Pathol 1988;130:268–280.

48. Klinman DM, Steinberg AD. Idiotypy and autoimmunity. Arthritis Rheum 1986;29:697–705.

48a. Kodama S, Kühtreiber W, Fujimura S, et al. Islet regeneration during the reversal of autoimmune diabetes in NOD mice. Science 2003;302:1223–1227.

49. Koga T, Wand-Württenberger A, DeBruyn J, et al. T cells against a bacterial heat shock protein recognize stressed macrophages. Science 1989;245:1112–1115.

50. Kosuda LL, Bigazzi PE. Chemical-induced autoimmunity. In: Smialowicz RJ, Holsapple MP (eds). Experimental Immunotoxicology. Boca Raton, FL: CRC Press, 1996, pp. 419–465.

51. Kosuda LL, Hannigan MO, Bigazzi PE, Leif JH, Greiner DL. Thymus atrophy and changes in thymocyte subpopulations of BN rats with mercury-induced renal autoimmune disease. Autoimmunity 1996;23:77–89.

52. Kuch J. Autoantibodies directed against heart antigens and endocrine reactivity in patients with recent myocardial infarction. Cardiovasc Res 1973;7:649–654.

53. Liem KL, ten Veen JH, Lie KI, Feltkamp TEW, Durrer D. Incidence and significance of heart muscle antibodies in

patients with acute myocardial infarction and unstable angina. Acta Med Scand 1979;206:473–475.

54. Like AA. Spontaneous diabetes in animals. In: Volk BW, Arquilla ER, eds. The diabetic pancreas. New York: Plenum Publishing, 1985, pp. 385–413.

55. Majno G. The Healing Hand. Man and Wound in the Ancient World. Cambridge, MA: Harvard University Press, 1975.

56. Mandelbaum SL, Diamond MP, DeCherney AH. The impact of antisperm antibodies on human infertility. J Urol 1987; 138:1–8.

57. Marrack P, Kappler J, Kotzin BL. Autoimmune disease: why and where it occurs. Nat Med 2001;7:899–905.

57a. Matsumoto I, Maccioni M, Lee DM, et al. How antibodies to a ubiquitous cytoplasmic enzyme may provoke joint-specific autoimmune disease. Nature Immunol 2002;3:360–365.

57b. Millar DG, Garza KM, Odermatt B, et al. Hsp70 promotes antigen-presenting cell function and converts cell tolerance to autoimmunity *in vivo*. Nat Med 2003;9:1469–1476.

58. Miller J F A P. Transgenic models of peripheral T-cell self-tolerance and autoimmunity. In: Rose NR, Mackay IR (eds). The Autoimmune Diseases, 3rd ed. San Diego: Academic Press. 1998, pp. 29–44.

59. Mills JA. Systematic Lupus Erythematosus. N Engl J Med 1994;330:1871–1879.

60. Moller DE. New drug targets for type 2 diabetes and the metabolic syndrome. Nature 2001;414:821–827.

61. Montagu A. The Natural Superiority of Women, 5th ed. Walnut Creek: AltaMira Press, 1999.

62. Parekh RB, Dwek RA, Sutton BJ, et al. Association of rheumatoid arthritis and primary osteoarthritis with changes in the glycosylation pattern of total serum IgG. Nature 1985;316:452–457.

63. Parham P. A diversity of diabetes. Nature 1990;345:662–664.

64. Purtilo DT, Sullivan JL. Immunological bases for superior survival of females. Am J Dis Child 1979;133:1251–1253.

65. Racusen LC. Autoimmune disease in the kidney. In: Rose NR, Mackay IR (eds). The Autoimmune Diseases, 3rd ed. San Diego: Academic Press. 1998, pp. 603–621.

66. Raine CS. Analysis of autoimmune demyelination: its impact upon multiple sclerosis. Lab Invest 1984;50:608–635.

67. Raine CS. In a biological cross-fire: neuroimmunology. Sci Focus 1987;2:3–5.

68. Reed CE, Friedlaender M. Immunologic aspects of diseases of the eye. JAMA 1982;248:2692–2695.

69. Reichlin M. Systemic lupus erythematosus. In: Rose NR, Mackay IR (eds). The Autoimmune Diseases, 3rd ed. San Diego: Academic Press. 1998, pp. 283–289.

70. Roitt IM. Essential immunology, 6th ed. Oxford: Blackwell Scientific Publications, 1988.

71. Romagnani S. T cell subsets (Th1, Th2) and cytokines in autoimmunity. In: Rose NR, Mackay IR (eds). The Autoimmune Diseases, 3rd ed. San Diego: Academic Press. 1998, pp. 163–191.

72. Rook GAW, Lydyard PM, Stanford JL. A reappraisal of the evidence that rheumatoid arthritis and several other idiopathic diseases are slow bacterial infections. Ann Rheum Dis 1993;52:S30–S38.

73. Rose NR, Mackay IR (eds). The Autoimmune Diseases, 3rd ed. San Diego: Academic Press, 1998.

74. Rose NR, Mackay IR. Prelude. In: Rose NR, Mackay IR (eds). The Autoimmune Diseases, 3rd ed. San Diego: Academic Press. 1998, pp. 1–4.

75. Rosen A, Casciola-Rosen L. Environmental determinants of autoimmune disease. In: Rose NR, Mackay IR (eds). The Autoimmune Diseases, 3rd ed. San Diego: Academic Press. 1998, pp. 119–126.

76. Rossini AA, Mordes JP, Like AA. Immunology of insulin-dependent diabetes mellitus. Annu Rev Immunol 1985;3: 289–320.

77. Sahashi K, Engel AG, Lambert EH, Howard FM Jr. Immune complexes (IgG and C3) at the motor end-plate in myasthenia gravis. Mayo Clin Proc 1977;52:267–280.

78. Sell S. Immunology, immunopathology and immunity, 4th ed. New York: Elsevier, 1987.

79. Shoenfeld Y, Isenberg DA, eds. Natural autoantibodies. London: CRC Press, 1993.

80. Shoenfeld Y, Schwartz RS. Immunologic and genetic factors in autoimmune diseases. N Engl J Med 1984;311:1019–1029.

81. Shulman S. Autoimmune aspects of human reproduction. Concepts Immunopathol 1985;2:189–227.

82. Skinner HA. The origin of medical terms, 2nd ed. Baltimore: Williams & Wilkins, 1961.

82a. Stassi G, DeMaria R. Autoimmune thyroid disease: new models of cell death in autoimmunity. Nat Rev Immunol 2002; 2:195–204.

83. Strober S, Holoshitz J. Mechanisms of immune injury in rheumatoid arthritis: evidence for the involvement of T cells and heat-shock protein. Immunol Rev 1990;118: 233–255.

84. Theofilopoulos AN. Autoimmunity. In: Stites DP, Stobo JD, Wells JV, eds. Basic and clinical immunology, 6th ed. Norwalk, CT: Appleton & Lange, 1987, pp. 128–158.

85. Todd JA, Acha-Orbea H, Bell JI, et al. A molecular basis for MHC class II-associated autoimmunity. Science 1988;240: 1003–1009.

86. Tung KSK, Unanue ER, Dixon FJ. Pathogenesis of experimental allergic orchitis. II. The role of antibody. J Immunol 1971;106:1463–1472.

86a. von Herrath M, Bach J-F. Juvenile autoimmune diabetes: a pathogenic role for maternal antibodies? Nature Med 2002 8:331–333.

87. Waksman BH, Adams RD. A comparative study of experimental allergic neuritis in the rabbit, guinea pig, and mouse. J Neuropathol Exp Neurol 1956;25:293–333.

88. Wassermann NH, Penn AS, Freimuth PI, et al. Anti-idiotypic route to anti-acetylcholine receptor antibodies and experimental myasthenia gravis. Proc Natl Acad Sci USA 1982;79: 4810–4814.

89. Weetman AP. Autoimmune thyroid disease. In: Rose NR, Mackay IR (eds). The Autoimmune Diseases, 3rd ed. San Diego: Academic Press. 1998, pp. 405–430.

90. Weetman AP. Graves' Disease. N Engl J Med 2000;343: 1236–1248.

91. Williams RC Jr. Molecular mimicry and rheumatic fever. Clin Rheum Dis 1985;11:573–590.

92. Zimmer C. Do chronic diseases have an infectious root? Science 2001;293:1974–1977.

93. Zimmet P, Alberti, K G M M, Shaw J. Global and societal implications of the diabetes epidemic. Nature 2001;414:782–787.

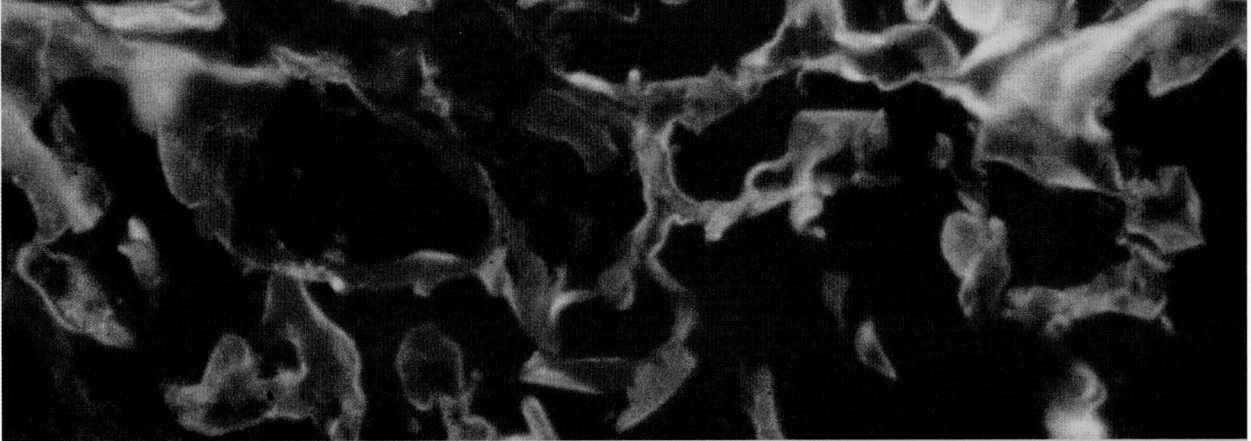

CHAPTER 20 — IMMUNOSUPPRESSION

A state of immunosuppression can be a normal condition, a goal of therapy when the immune system overreacts, an unwanted side-effect of tumor therapy, a congenital disease, or an acquired disease.

Normal Immunosuppression: Pregnancy

To survive as a species, mammals must break the rules of immunology: their pregnant females must carry an allograft until birth without rejecting it (although they do produce *paternal specific alloantibodies,* i.e., antifather antibodies). Actually, the natural mammalian fetus is only a semi-allograft (8). One might imagine that if a fetus were a full allograft it would be more antigenic, but this is not the case. A full allograft can be obtained artificially if a fetus results from fertilizing an human ovum *in vitro,* then implanting it into a surrogate mother; in this case the mother-derived genes are also allogeneic. Yet such a human fetus is immunologically so well protected that it can be carried for nine months. In other species even xenogeneic pregnancies have been achieved: a zebra can have a mare as a surrogate mother (8). Exactly how mammals accomplish this feat is still puzzling (2, 17, 23, 30). It cannot be that the uterus is exempt from the laws of immunology, because the uterine mucosa rejects experimental skin allografts (3). However, we must hurry to add that it would be a gross oversimplification to equate natural birth with the rejection of a graft. It is a more complex phenomenon, involving three individuals (mother, father, fetus), wherein the father provides half of the genes and usually also antigens as sperm (see below). The solid fact is that establishing a pregnancy is not an easy matter: in 60 percent of human pregnancies the fetus is aborted within 12 weeks. How many of these silent abortions are due to immune attack is not known. There is an established syndrome of recurrent abortion; its causes are many and the role of the immune system is not fully understood (3a).

Overall, the fetus-allograft appears to be protected by two major mechanisms: barriers between itself and the mother, and immunosuppression of the mother (Table 20.1). The principal barrier between fetus and mother is the syncytiotrophoblast, a syncytial layer that derives from the ovum and forms a continuous sheet separating the mother's blood from the placental tissues. The syncytiotrophoblast expresses neither Class I nor Class II antigens of the MHC, which makes it an immunologic no-man's-land; this is not true, however, for the rest of the trophoblast (18).

Pregnant women are partly immunosuppressed. Their lymphocytes respond less vigorously to mitogens *in vitro* (32), and their cell-mediated immunity is reduced (precisely the type of immunity most involved in graft rejection). The total number of T cells is reduced, and there is a relative loss of helper T cells (T4$^+$) (40), the same defect that occurs, much more severely, in AIDS. Certain cancers, and infections with intracellular

Table 20.1 Why Is the Baby Not Rejected? Some Proposed Mechanisms

Progesterone is immunosuppressive

Alpha-fetoprotein in amniotic fluid is immunosuppressive

Mother's plasma contains an immunosuppressive protein (PAPP-A, possibly produced by the endometrium)

Decidua and draining lymph nodes contain suppressor cells

Uterine macrophages are immunosuppressive

Endometrial epithelium loses Class I MHC antigens and replaces them with trophoblast antigens (called TLX)

Syncytiotrophoblast contains neither Class I nor Class II MHC antigens

Activated T cells are killed

TGFβ in semen is immunosuppressive

Adapted from several sources (2, 23, 35a).

parasites, carry a more severe prognosis if they occur in advanced pregnancy (32).

Current work suggests that the *proteins in semen* may help to induce the mother's tolerance. Semen is rich in TGF beta; if proteins are injected into a mouse uterus together with TGF beta, the immune response of the mouse against these proteins is depressed (35).

Therapeutic Immunosuppression

Immunosuppression as therapy is meant to protect allografts and to fight autoimmune diseases. The ideal procedure would be to render the patient tolerant to the antigen(s) of the graft or to the self-antigens in autoimmune disease, but that is still in the future. The drugs used at present (15, 21) are nonspecific immunosuppressants. They belong to three groups: (a) **corticoids,** closely related to the glucocorticoid hormones secreted by the adrenal cortex. The corticoids (e.g., *prednisone*) are essentially anti-inflammatory molecules, which perform their task by inhibiting—in a complex manner—the effect of NF-κB, the powerful nuclear transcription factor that orchestrates the transcription of many genes related to inflammation (p. 369). Main drawback: by inhibiting inflammation these drugs expose the patient to infection. (b) **Antimitotics (cytotoxic agents),** which were borrowed from cancer therapy. The rationale for antimitotics is that the immune response depends on a small number of cells that replicate to form large clones, and the antimitotics intervene at the early stage. Actually, the rationale was an afterthought; it followed the accidental observation that patients treated with antimitotics for cancer became immunosuppressed. (The prototype

of antimitotics, *cyclophosphamide,* is a byproduct of chemical warfare during World War I: it revealed its cytotoxic effect accidentally while used as "nitrogen mustard" gas.) The main drawback is that mitoses are inhibited throughout the body, including the intestine and the bone marrow, leading to life-threatening complications. (c) **Inhibitors of T cell activation,** of which **cyclosporine** is the prototype (10, 19). Cyclosporine is actually in a category of its own; it is so effective that it greatly expanded the field of transplantation. One if its many effects is to prevent T cells from secreting cytokines essential for the differentiation and proliferation of B cells and cytotoxic T cells. *Rapamycin* has similar effects (it was isolated from a bacterium of Easter Island, whereas cyclosporine comes from a Norwegian fungus). Unfortunately, no drug is free of side effects: a major drawback of cyclosporine is its toxicity for the kidney. The long-term use of immunosuppressants also increases the risk of developing cancer (6, 22 [see also p. 848]). The risk was 8.3 times as expected in patients who survived 10 or more years after bone marrow transplantation. Another risk, of course, is infection by one or more of the bacterial, viral, and fungal antigens in the environment. It is

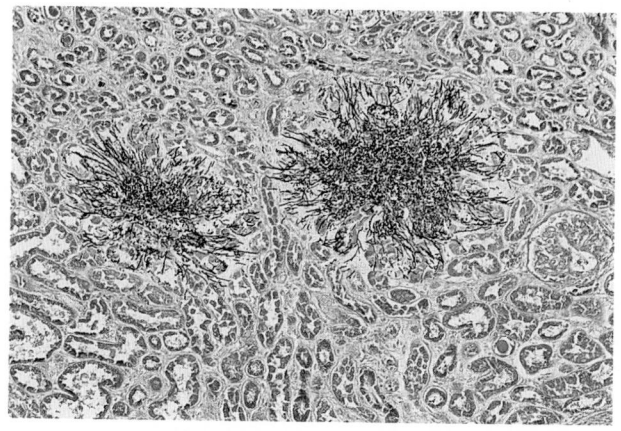

FIGURE 20.1   Two clusters of *Candida albicans,* a fungus, growing in the kidney of an immunosuppressed patient (after chemotherapy for a malignant tumor). Note the total lack of inflammatory response. (The growth of the fungi may be exaggerated during the hours between death and autopsy.) (Grocott methenamine silver stain, 80x.)

frightening to see, under the microscope, how fungi grow in the tissues of an immunosuppressed patient—as in a culture—without eliciting the slightest inflammatory response (Figure 20.1).

Congenital Immunosuppression

Congenital immunodeficiencies usually manifest themselves in infancy by an increased susceptibility to infection. Sad as they can be as diseases (antibiotics did improve the outlook), they taught us a great deal. Each one corresponds to a discrete genetic mistake in the network of defenses against infection; therefore they represent experiments of nature, which confirmed, or led us to understand, basic mechanisms of the immune system—just as lysosomal diseases helped work out the functions of the lysosomal enzymes. They can affect lymphocytes, neutrophils, macrophages, as well as the components of complement; some were reproduced by gene knockout experiments. We have described several of them as defects of inflammation (p. 520). Fortunately they are uncommon, but they are many: just those that affect lymphocytes come close to 100 (5).

Regarding lymphocytes, a deficiency can hit T cell mechanisms, B cell mechanisms, or both, in which case it is called *severe combined immunodeficiency (SCID),* pronounced "skid" (13). The clinical manifestations vary a great deal in severity. For example, *lack of IgA antibodies* (normally secreted into the intestinal lumen to control the bacterial flora) does not result in apparent intestinal disease. The *congenital lack of immunoglobulins in the serum* makes the individual susceptible to infection by viruses and by extracellular, encapsulated bacteria such as *Streptococcus pneumoniae* (which are normally opsonized by antibodies).

The congenital lack of NK cells in humans leads to severe herpesvirus infections, as might be expected from the antiviral prowess of these cells (4). Descriptions of congenital immunodeficiencies can be found in specialized textbooks (20, 29).

One of these congenital diseases was discovered in our department by the late Dr. David T. Purtilo and his collaborators. While on autopsy duty as a pathology resident, in 1969, Dr. Purtilo was called to examine a child who had died in the course of infectious mononucleosis, a viral infection not known to be lethal. No cause of death was apparent. Dr. Purtilo could have brushed off the case as a freak occurrence of death by mononucleosis, but he concluded that some important bit of information was missing and never forgot that child. Years later he autopsied another child with the same name (Duncan) who had died of lymphoma. This was the second clue on a trail that led to identifying the X-linked lymphoproliferative disease (XLP), also called *Duncan's disease* (14, 33). These children (all males) inherit a specific susceptibility to infection by the Epstein–Barr virus, the agent of infectious mononucleosis; when infected, they either succumb or develop a chronic infection (hypogammaglobulinemia) and in 25 percent of the cases a malignant lymphoma. The latter is probably a result of constant B-cell stimulation by the virus.

This episode was a sad development for the Duncan family, but it illustrates the importance of the autopsy even in our high-tech society.

Acquired Immunosuppression

Acquired immunodeficiency instantly evokes the image of AIDS, but there are other examples even closer to everyday life.

- *Aging* (which improves nothing, except perhaps wisdom in some cases) brings a decline also in the function of the immune system, especially of the T cells (42).
- *Infant prematurity* tends to correlate with inadequate immune responses, especially if the infant's problems are compounded by malnutrition. Some immunodeficient infants have developed

graft-versus-host disease after blood transfusions (7), because the transfused leukocytes became engrafted in the immunosuppressed host; in adults, the leukocytes in transfused blood can be neglected because they are almost always easily overcome by the host.

- *Severe malnutrition* is immunosuppressive, but we must recall once again the extensive literature proving that *mild* undernutrition is the one and only sure way to prolong life (p. 48).

- *Cancer,* including its treatments, tends to suppress not only inflammation (pp. 909, 912) but also the immune response.

- *Infection with the HIV-1 or -2 virus* leads almost unfailingly to the acquired immunodeficiency syndrome, AIDS, the terrifying mode of immunosuppression that appeared in 1981 (43).

The HIV virus is so powerful because it infects mainly cells of the immune system: lymphocytes, macrophages, and dendritic cells. It gains access to T-helper cells by using their C4 receptors (*in vitro,* antibodies against the C4 receptor block the infection [16]); it also uses chemokine receptors as coreceptors. Destructive cycles of virus replication and cell death continue for years. Normally there are about two T-helper cells for each cytotoxic/suppressor T cell; in AIDS, the ratio can drop to less than 1. The production of T-helper cells is also depressed (24). Eventually insufficient T-helper cells are left to produce cytotoxic T cells able to kill virus-infected cells, and the patient is overwhelmed. However, the immunosuppression of AIDS has more than one cause (37); the NK cells, although normal in number, do not function properly (37), and antigen-presenting cells may also be affected (25). On the other hand, we know that some antibody formation is maintained because it has been observed that some antigens are independent of T-cell help (T-independent antigens); in fact, AIDS patients may show *hyper*gammaglobulinemia (11).

The last forms of acquired immunodeficiency that we will consider are stress and psychological stimuli.

Psychology and the lymphocytes. It is popular knowledge that labial herpes may remain dormant for years and then erupt under stress (28) and that tuberculosis may flare up in depressed individuals. The mechanism is probably complicated, but it is proven that the immune system can be depressed by emotional factors. This is documented during bereavement. Mortality increases among widowers during the 10 years after the death of their spouses; their lymphocytes are significantly less responsive to mitogens for as long as 14 months (Figure 20.2) (36, 41). A similar depression of lymphocyte responsiveness was found in 16 psychiatry trainees taking final fellowship examinations (12).

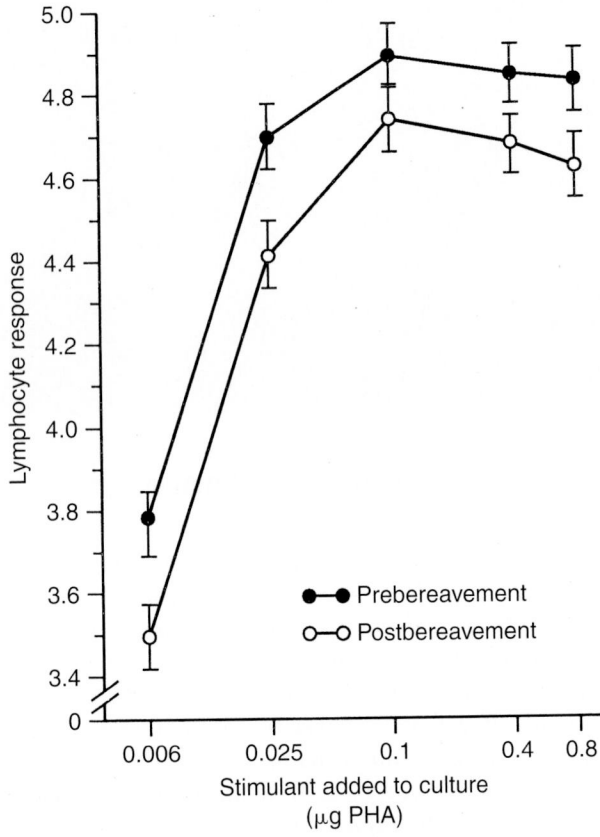

FIGURE 20.2 Depression of lymphocyte function during bereavement. The test measures the lymphocyte response after stimulation with phytohemagglutinin (PHA). (Adapted with permission from JAMA [36], Copyright 1983 American Medical Association.)

The link between stress and the immune system involves an endocrine–neuroendocrine network including ACTH, endorphins, and adrenal hormones (31).

Even more fascinating are studies showing that it is possible to "train" lymphocytes to respond to certain stimuli, recalling the pavlovian "mast cell conditioning" mentioned earlier (p. 532).

The key experiment: Cyclophosphamide, an immunosuppressant, injected intraperitoneally into rats, inhibits antibody formation and eventually kills the rats. If the rats are given saccharin-flavored water to drink in association with the injection of cyclophosphamide, after some time the saccharin drink alone—given once every three days—depresses antibody titers (9). This principle can be put to use for therapy: New Zealand mice develop systemic lupus and die within 8–14 months, unless treated with intraperitoneal injections of cyclophosphamide. If these are paired with a taste of saccharin in the drinking water, after some time just the drinks of saccharin—combined with an intraperitoneal injection of saline—prolong the life of the mice (9).

The mechanism of these conditioned responses is not well understood, but it does *not* depend on stress-induced steroids. Perhaps it is relevant that lymphatic organs receive sympathetic nerve fibers, and that neurons and leukocytes share neuroendocrine receptors (1).

What helps mice with lupus might, some day, help people with lupus.

Coda: The Immune Response at Its Best—The Pathogenesis of Influenza

In the last four chapters we have portrayed the misdeeds of the immune response. To provide our readers with a more balanced view of this lifesaving mechanism, we opted to close this section with a glimpse of the immune response at work in the course of an infectious disease. A fine example is influenza, because its pathogenesis involves an interplay of cell injury, inflammation, and regeneration, as well as T-cell and B-cell (antibody) responses. We will follow an excellent account published by P. A. Small, whose laboratory worked out many of the pertinent facts (39).

The name *influenza* is an echo of medieval Italy, when epidemics were attributed to an effect (*influenza*) of stars and planets (38). On this planet it is indeed an uncontrolled killer; in the United States alone it claims 10–20 thousand victims a year (many more in years of pandemic) and the morbidity (ratio of number of people with the disease to the total population), as everyone knows, is far greater (39).

The first step of any infection is penetration into body. Experts on infectious disease tend to see the body as a container riddled with openings (Figure 20.3); each opening has its defenses and its habitual attackers. The influenza virus invariably chooses the respiratory pathway, and once it has gained entrance it can cause three syndromes of increasing severity: (1) a simple, uncomplicated inflammation of the upper airways (*rhinotracheitis*); (2) a respiratory viral infection followed by a bacterial infection; and (3) a viral pneumonia.

1. *Rhinotracheitis.* Inflammation of the upper airways produces symptoms neatly explained by the pathologic events. Normally the epithelium of the upper respiratory tract contains mucus-secreting cells and ciliated cells (Figure 20.4); about one-third of the basement membrane is covered by basal cells, also known as *reserve cells.* Inhaled bacteria and viruses are trapped by the mucus, and the cilia sweep the whole mess, dead cells and mucus, up the trachea (we have referred to this as the "bronchial elevator") and eventually down the pharynx, unceremoniously called the tracheal toilet (39).

Inhaled virus particles hit the mucosa, penetrate into the cells via special receptors, multiply inside them, and quickly kill them. In three days the mucus-secreting cells and the ciliated cells are gone, and the basal cells spread over the basement membrane (Figure 20.4). In the meantime the underlying connective tissue (*lamina propria*) has become inflamed, and exudate oozes out through gaps between the basal cells. This explains the runny nose that is typical of this phase; the fluid is not mucus because the mucus-secreting cells are no longer there. Between 5 and 10 days after infection the basal cells differentiate into mature cells. The mucus-secreting cells reappear first; and without enough ciliated cells to move the mucus, it piles up. This

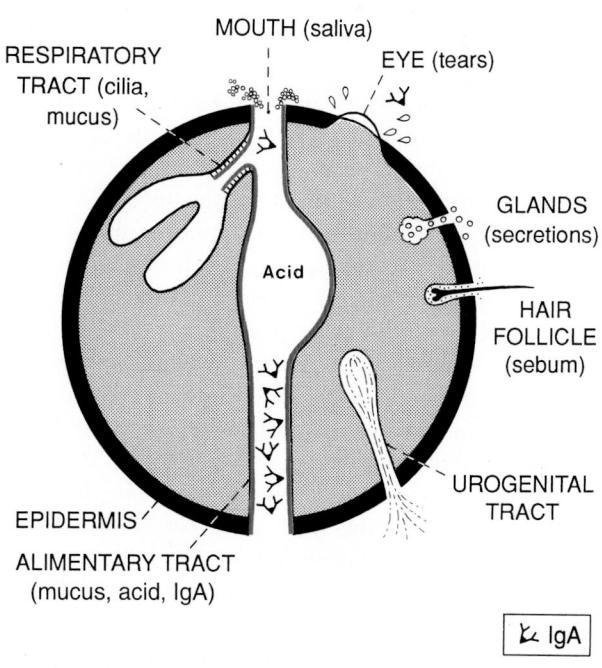

FIGURE 20.3 Schematic view of the body, indicating portals of entry for parasites, and key defenses displayed at body surfaces. (Adapted with permission from [26].)

FIGURE 20.4 Effect of influenza on the epithelium of the human trachea. *Top:* Normal, mucus-producing ciliated epithelium. *Bottom:* After 2 days of influenza infection, most of the epithelium has sloughed off; it is replaced by cuboidal, less-differentiated cells with no mucus secretion and very few cilia. One advantage of the replacement: the regenerating epithelial cells have no receptors for the influenza virus. **Bar** = 10 μm. (Reproduced by permission from [27], © Wolters-Noordhoff, Groningen, Netherlands.)

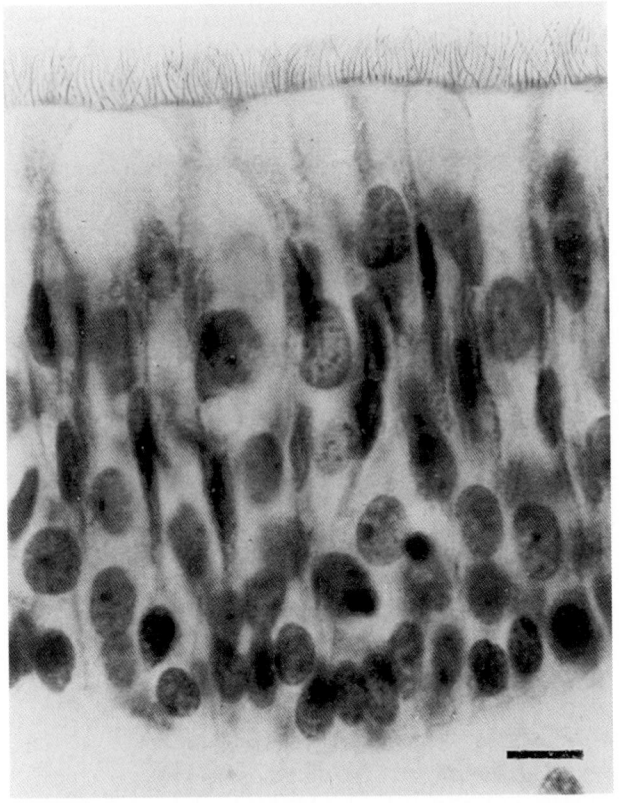

explains the snorting, nose-blowing, and coughing of this stage. The repair is complete after 2 weeks, a little earlier if the patient (as is usually the case) has suffered a previous infection. Memory cells are doing their job (to be described shortly).

Note that the regenerating basal cells have escaped the lethal attack of the influenza virus. The reason seems to be that *they have no receptors for the virus* (39). This is what saves them, and perhaps also the patient. You may recall that in discussing regeneration we mentioned that newly regenerated cells are not as "good" as mature cells (p. 33); but in the present case, immaturity is an advantage.

There is no specific cure for the rhinotracheitis of influenza, but timeless tradition prescribes rest, warmth, and lots of fluids. As it happens, this is very sensible advice: it fosters the therapeutic goal of preventing the virus from spreading beyond the upper respiratory tract. *Rest,* during which breathing is shallow, reduces the risk of inhaling the virus deeper into the lungs; *warmth* helps maintain the deeper respiratory epithelia at body temperature, which is not the optimal temperature (35°C) for influenza virus replication; and *fluid* helps mucous secretion and the elevator–toilet mechanism. Note that in this scenario fever should also help—and the traditional aspirin should not (p. 508).

2. *Viral infection followed by bacterial pneumonia.* This is the usual sequence of events: when the patient is beginning to recover, the malaise returns, the cough worsens, and the infection becomes purulent. Pus indicates the presence of leukocytes and, usually, bacterial infection. Indeed, the lack of a covering tracheo-bronchial epithelium causes bacteria to be retained (pneumococci, staphylococci, and *Haemophilus influenzae* are common offenders). Furthermore, the phagocytic function of alveolar macrophages is impaired after a bout of influenza (39).

3. *Viral pneumonia* occurs when the virus gains the upper hand and destroys the precious epithelial cells

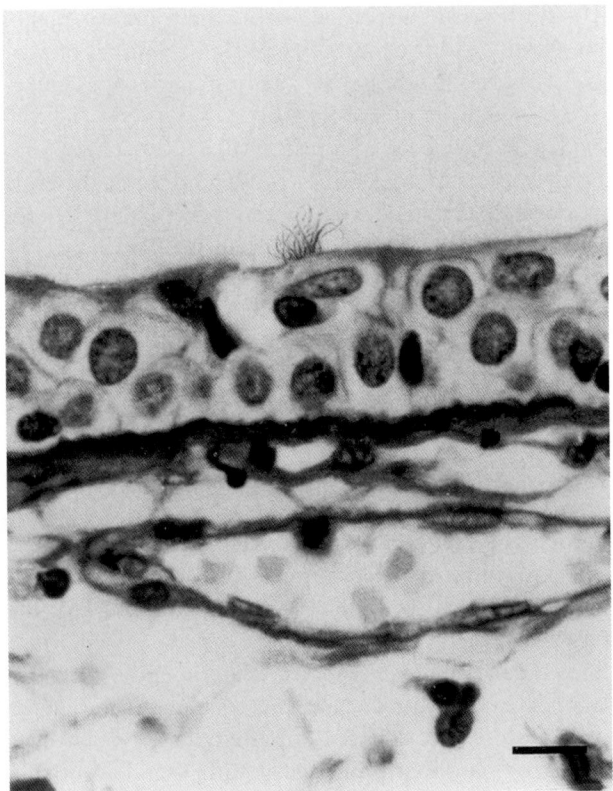

Table 20.2 Components of the Immune Response Affecting Influenza

Component	Prevention		Recovery	
	Upper Respiratory Tract	Lung	Upper Respiratory Tract	Lung
Secretory IgA	Essential	?	?	?
Systemic antibody	No role	Essential	Contributory	Contributory
Cell-mediated immunity	No role	No role	Essential	Essential

Adapted from (2, 23, 35a).

of the pulmonary alveoli, plasma leaks out of the capillaries, and pulmonary edema develops. Individuals with high capillary pressure are especially at risk—for example, in patients with mitral stenosis. A full-blown pneumonia develops.

Experiments on mice have revealed other interesting mechanisms. If the influenza virus is given as nose drops to mice anesthetized to abolish cough and gag reflexes, much of the fluid reaches the lungs immediately; and the mice die in a week. If the nose drops are given to conscious mice, the virus reaches the trachea in 3 days and the lungs in 5; thus, the lethal dose (LD50) is 2000 times greater. This experiment suggests that a slow, downward progress of the virus gives the immune system time to respond.

Blood-borne antibodies appear in infected mice, and cell-mediated immunity also develops; but neither can prevent the upper respiratory tract infection. This makes sense: the virus hides inside the epithelial cells where it is safe from antibodies. As to cell-mediated immunity, T cells and NK cells would not be expected to migrate out of the vessels to kill free virus; their proper target is represented by virus-infected cells. On the other hand, blood-borne antibodies do prevent the viral pneumonia (34); the mechanism is probably serum IgG antibody in the alveolar fluid. This type of protection is the purpose of vaccination.

We have carefully used the expression *blood borne antibodies*. Although it is true that these antibodies do not prevent the infection of the upper respiratory tract, this does not mean that all those critical epithelia go through life unprotected. They secrete their own shield as a *secretory antibody*: that is, as IgA, a special form of immunoglobulin found in almost all secretions (including those of the intestine) and is highly resistant to proteolytic attack.

What is the role of cell-mediated immunity in influenza? A good way to find out is to infect nude mice, which lack cell-mediated immunity. The result is a prolonged state of infection. Treatment with serum antibodies offers temporary help but does not cure (39).

The results from many laboratories showed that cell-mediated immunity is essential for recovery from influenza infection. This fact may help us understand the much greater mortality from influenza in persons of advanced age, whose cell-mediated immunity tends to be depressed. The higher mortality of infants is due to the lack of immunity from previous exposure.

The protective roles of the immune system in influenza are summarized in Table 20.2.

Such is, in capsule form, the pathophysiology of this viral disease. It tells us that the balance between host and parasite can be tipped by a number of factors besides the immune response—even by regeneration.

References

1. Ader R, Cohen N. Conditioned immunopharmacologic effects on cell-mediated immunity. Int J Immunopharmac 1992;14:323–327.

2. Beer AE. Immunology of reproduction. In: Samter M, Talmage DW, Frank MM, Austen KF, Claman HN, eds. Immunological diseases, 4th ed. Boston: Little, Brown, 1988:329–360.

3. Beer AE, Billingham RE. Host responses to intra-uterine tissue, cellular and fetal allografts. J Reprod Fertil 1984;(suppl)21:59–88.

3a. Benirschke K, Kaufmann P. Pathology of the human placenta. 3rd ed. New York: Springer-Verlag, 1995.

4. Biron CA, Byron KS, Sullivan JL. Severe herpesvirus infections in an adolescent without natural killer cells. N Engl J Med 1989;320:1731–1735.

5. Buckley RH. Primary immunodeficiency diseases due to defects in lymphocytes. N Engl J Med 2000;343:1313–1324.

6. Cagle PT, Lega M. Pathogenesis/Pathology of graft dysfunction. In: Norman DJ, Suki WN (eds). Primer on transplantation. Thorofare, NJ: American Society of Transplant Physicians, 1998, pp. 527–537.

7. Chandra RK. Influence of nutrition-immunity axis on perinatal infections. In: Ogra PL, ed. Neonatal infections. Nutritional and immunologic interactions. Orlando, FL: Grune & Stratton, 1984:229–245.

8. Chaouat G. The roots of the problem; the fetal allograft. In: Immunology of pregnancy. New York: CRC Press, 1993:1–17.

9. Cohen DJ, Ader R. Immunomodulation by classical conditioning. Adv Biochem Psychopharmacol 1988;44:199–202.

10. Cohen DJ, Loertscher R, Rubin MF, et al. Cyclosporine: a new immunosuppressive agent for organ transplantation. Ann Intern Med 1984;101:667–682.

11. Cohen JJ. The immune system: an overview. In: Middleton E Jr, Reed CE, Ellis EF, Adkinson NF Jr, Yunginger JW, eds. Allergy principles and practice, 3rd ed. St. Louis: CV Mosby, 1988:3–11.

12. Dorian B, Garfinkel P, Brown G, et al. Aberrations in lymphocyte subpopulations and function during psychological stress. Clin Exp Immunol 1982;50:132–138.

13. Fulop GM, Phillips RA. The *scid* mutation in mice causes a general defect in DNA repair. Nature 1990;347:479–482.

14. Grierson H, Purtilo DT. Epstein-Barr virus infections in males with the X-linked lymphoproliferative syndrome. Ann Intern Med 1987;106:538–545.

15. Halloran PF, Lui SL. Approved Immunosuppressants. In: Norman DJ, Suki WN (eds). Primer on transplantation. Thorofare, NJ: American Society of Transplant Physicians, 1998, pp. 93–102.

16. Ho DD, Pomerantz RJ, Kaplan JC. Pathogenesis of infection with human immunodeficiency virus. N Engl J Med 1987; 317:278–286.

17. Hunt JS, Orr HT. HLA and maternal-fetal recognition. FASEB J 1992;6:2344–2348.

18. Kabawat SE, Mostoufi-Zadeh M, Driscoll SG, Bhan AK. Implantation site in normal pregnancy. A study with monoclonal antibodies. Am J Pathol 1985;118:76–84.

19. Kahan BD. Cyclosporine. N Engl J Med 1989;321:1725–1738.

20. Kuby J. Immunology. 3rd ed. New York: W.H. Freeman and Company, 1997.

21. Leichtman AB, Rossi SJ. Pharmacotherapy in solid organ transplant recipients. In: Norman DJ, Suki WN (eds). Primer on transplantation. Thorofare, NJ: American Society of Transplant Physicians, 1998, pp. 123–138.

22. Locker J, Nalesnik M. Molecular genetic analysis of lymphoid tumors arising after organ transplantation. Am J Pathol 1989; 135:977–987.

23. Makrigiannakis A, Zoumakis E, Kalantaridou S, et al. Corticotropin-releasing hormone promotes blastocyst implantation and early maternal tolerance. Nat Immunol 2001;2: 1018–1022.

24. McCune JM. The dynamics of CD4+ T-cell depletion in HIV disease. Nature 2001;410:974–979.

25. Miedema F, Tersmette M, van Lier RAW. AIDS pathogenesis: a dynamic interaction between HIV and the immune system. Immunol Today 1990;11:293–297.

26. Mims CA. The pathogenesis of infectious disease. London: Academic Press. 1976.

27. Mulder J, Hers JFP. Influenza. Groningen, The Netherlands: Wolters-Noordhoff Publishing, 1972.

28. Parham P. The immune system. New York: Garland Publishing, 2000.

29. Paul WE. Fundamental immunology. 4th ed. Philadelphia, PA: Lippincott-Raven Publishers, 1999.

30. Pearson H. Immunity's pregnant pause. Nature 2002;420: 265–266.

31. Plotnikoff NP, Murgo AJ. Enkephalins-endorphins: stress and the immune system. Introduction. Fed Proc 1985;44:91.

32. Purtilo DT, Hallgren HM, Yunis EJ. Depressed maternal lymphocyte response to phytohaemagglutinin in human pregnancy. Lancet 1972;1:769–771.

33. Purtilo DT, Yang JPS, Cassel CK, et al. X-linked recessive progressive combined variable immunodeficiency (Duncan's disease). Lancet 1975;1:935–941.

34. Ramphal R, Cogliano RC, Shands JW Jr, Small PA Jr. Serum antibody prevents lethal murine influenza pneumonitis but not tracheitis. Infect Immun 1979;25:992–997.

35. Robertson SA, Ingman WV, O'Leary S, Sharkey DJ, Tremellen KP. Transforming growth factor beta—a mediator of immune deviation in seminal plasma. J Reprod Immunol 2002;57:109–128.

35a. Samter M, Talmage DW, Frank MM, Austen KF, Claman HN, eds. Immunological diseases, 4th ed. Boston: Little, Brown, 1988.

36. Schleifer SJ, Keller SE, Camerino M, Thornton JC, Stein M. Suppression of lymphocyte stimulation following bereavement. JAMA 1983;250:374–377.

37. Sirianni MC, Tagliaferri F, Aiuti, F. Natural killer cell deficiency in AIDS. Immunol Today 1990;11:81–82.

38. Skinner HA. The origin of medical terms, 2nd ed. Baltimore: Williams & Wilkins, 1961.

39. Small PA Jr. Influenza: pathogenesis and host defense. Hosp Pract 1990;25:51–62.

40. Sridama V, Pacini F, Yang S-L, et al. Decreased levels of helper T cells. A possible cause of immunodeficiency in pregnancy. N Engl J Med 1982;307:352–356.

41. Stein M. Bereavement, depression, stress, and immunity. In: Guillemin R, Cohn M, Melnechuk T, eds. Neural modulation of immunity. New York: Raven Press, 1985:29–44.

42. Weigle WO. Effects of aging on the immune system. Hosp Pract 1989;24:112–119.

43. Weiss RA. Gulliver's travels in HIV land. Nature 2001; 410:963–967.

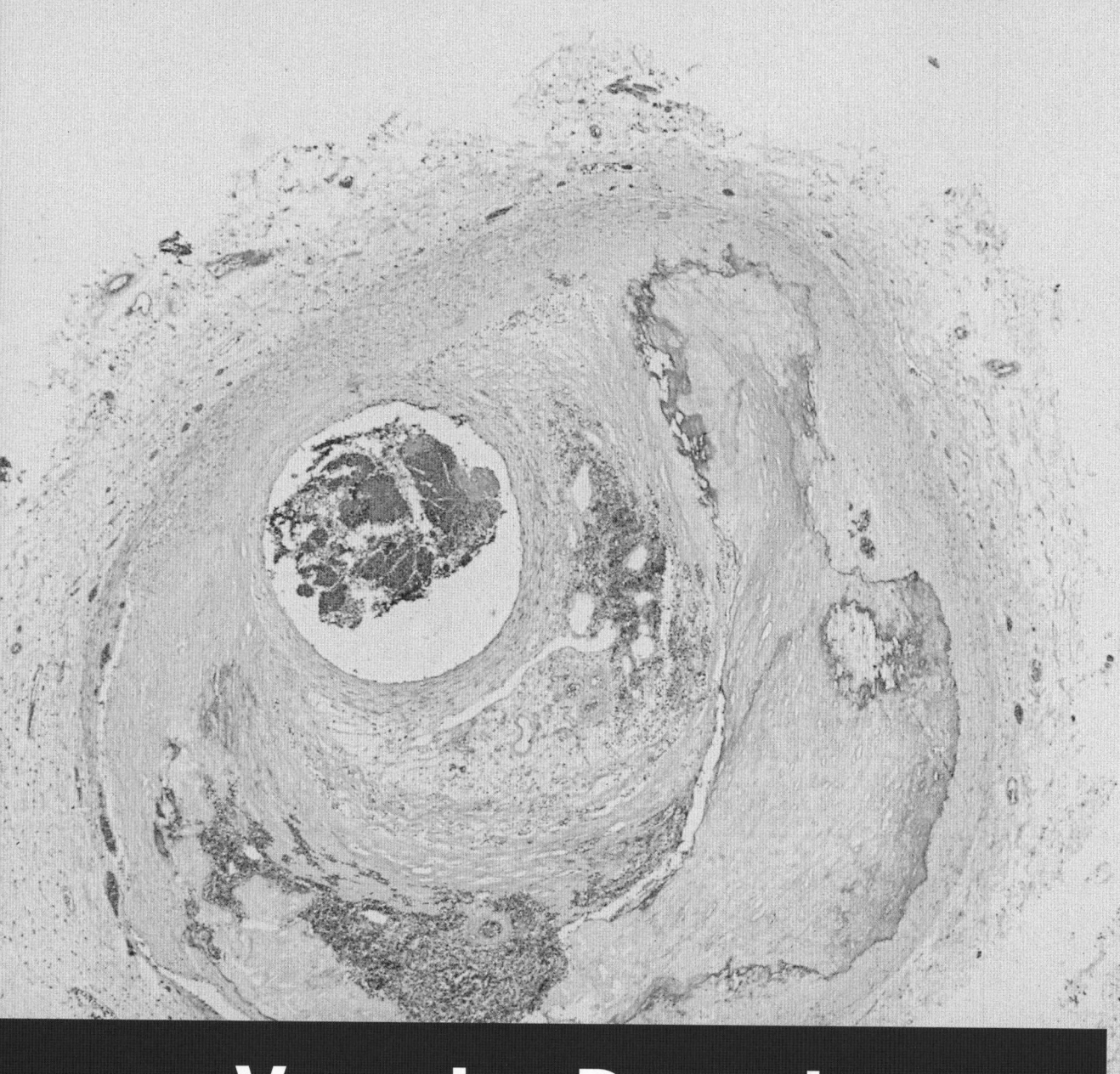

PART IV **Vascular Disturbances**

DISTURBANCES OF FLUID EXCHANGE

CHAPTER 21

- Endothelium: The Primal Frontier
- Normal Fluid Exchanges Across Capillary Endothelium
- Hyperemia
- Edema

Cells that lead solitary lives, such as amoebae in a swamp, must survive at the mercy of their environment. At the opposite extreme are the cells of vertebrates: they live in a fluid environment that they collectively maintain and control. This implies that vertebrates must generate, and supply to every corner of the body, a master fluid with very complex properties (namely blood) contained in a closed system of vessels equipped with a pump, and assisted by another complete system of vessels, the lymphatics. That this is not an easy task is proven by human mortality statistics. In industrialized countries the principal cause of death is failure of the system's tubing, such as atherosclerosis, or of the pump, such as myocardial infarcts (Figure 21.1). Furthermore, blood vessels are involved, directly or indirectly, in almost every disease. Inflammation is largely a vascular phenomenon, and tumors survive on their blood supply. This is why vessels deserve a section of their own in General Pathology.

Seen from the perspective of function, the vascular system consists, broadly speaking, of two parts, both made essentially of tubing lined with endothelium. One part, visible to the naked eye, consists of large tubing (arteries and veins) and a pump. This part is a *plumbing system for delivering blood to the other part,* the microcirculation, where the exchanges between blood and tissues take place; this has been called the "business end" of the vascular system. Correspondingly, some types of malfunction—such as obstruction—can happen to either part of the vascular system, whereas other malfunctions are characteristic of one part or the other. For example: problems of wall maintenance (atherosclerosis) prevail in large arteries, which are unique in having thick walls devoid of "maintenance equipment" such as capillaries and macrophages; valvular failures are prominent in the heart, which is unique in being a pump with chambers connected by valves; and disorders of fluid exchange are a major feature of microcirculatory pathology.

Endothelium: The Primal Frontier

Before plunging into vascular pathology we should acknowledge the key function of the endothelium, which lines the entire container of the blood (Figure 21.2). It is so thin that its existence was denied up to 1865 (24), yet it has become one of the most studied cell types (35, 36, 46, 47). It can secrete an amazing variety of products, and since its total weight has been estimated at one kilogram (43), it is by far the largest endocrine gland. The molecules it secretes (52) include collagen and elastin, factors opposing or favoring the clotting of blood, prostaglandins, cytokines, vasodilators and vasoconstrictors including the powerful endothelins (34) and nitric oxide (23), free radicals, and adhesion molecules. Much of this was learned from endothelial cells grown *in vitro*. Studies of the endothelium *in vivo* have taught us that *its structure and function differ slightly from one organ to another, and even along the same vessel from arteriole to capillary to venule* (48, 49).

A controversy of nearly epic proportions raged for decades concerning the endothelium as a permeability barrier; it was a classic example of hard morphologic facts not fitting with neat mathematical calculations (24), as we recalled in Chapter 10. The dust has not entirely settled (27, 33), but those who believe in demonstrable facts agree that endothelial cells do perform active transport by means of the vesicles or *caveolae* discovered by George Palade at the dawn of cell biology, in 1951. Palade postulated that the system of caveolae ferried fluid and particles across the endothelium. This mechanism was called *transcytosis* by Nicolae Simionescu (Figure 21.3)(45).

Note this key point: the system of *caveolae* functions slowly and selectively, almost molecule by molecule (e.g., by binding and ferrying albumin). *The events of inflammatory exudation and hydrostatic transudation that occur in pathology take place on a much larger scale.* The **inflammatory exudate** of "vascular leakage" flows out of endothelial gaps that are huge compared with the *caveolae*. **Transudates** are ultrafiltrates of plasma; they consist of fluid and of molecules (up to about 20 Å) that flow out of the intercellular junctions (30). Whether the two systems—transcytosis versus flow—relate to eachother is not known. There is no known disease affecting transcytosis (although Cav-1 knockout mice that lack the marker protein *caveolin-1,* are fascinating [32a]).

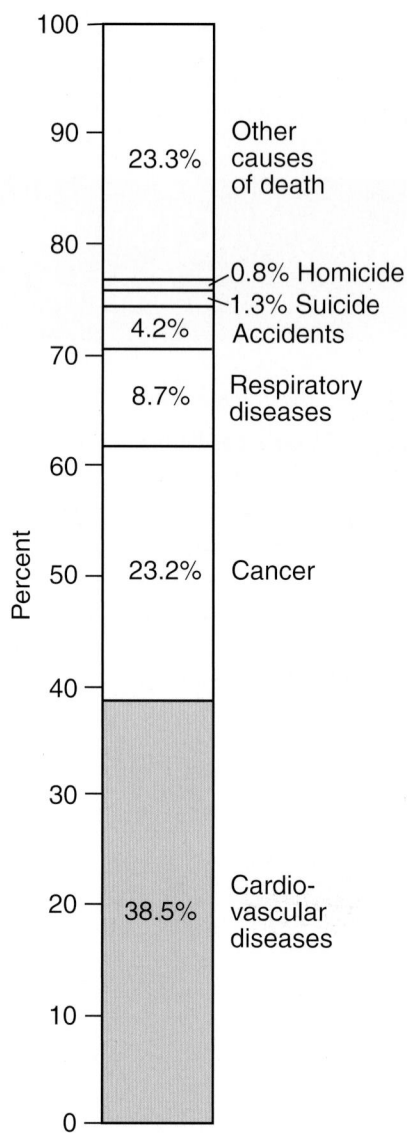

FIGURE 21.1 Cardiovascular disease is the single most important cause of death in the United States. (Adapted with permission from [12].)

TO SUM UP: The Starling equilibrium, as we reviewed it (p. 387), can probably afford to ignore transcytosis, because exudates and transudates deal with barrels of water, and transcytosis with teaspoons of brine.

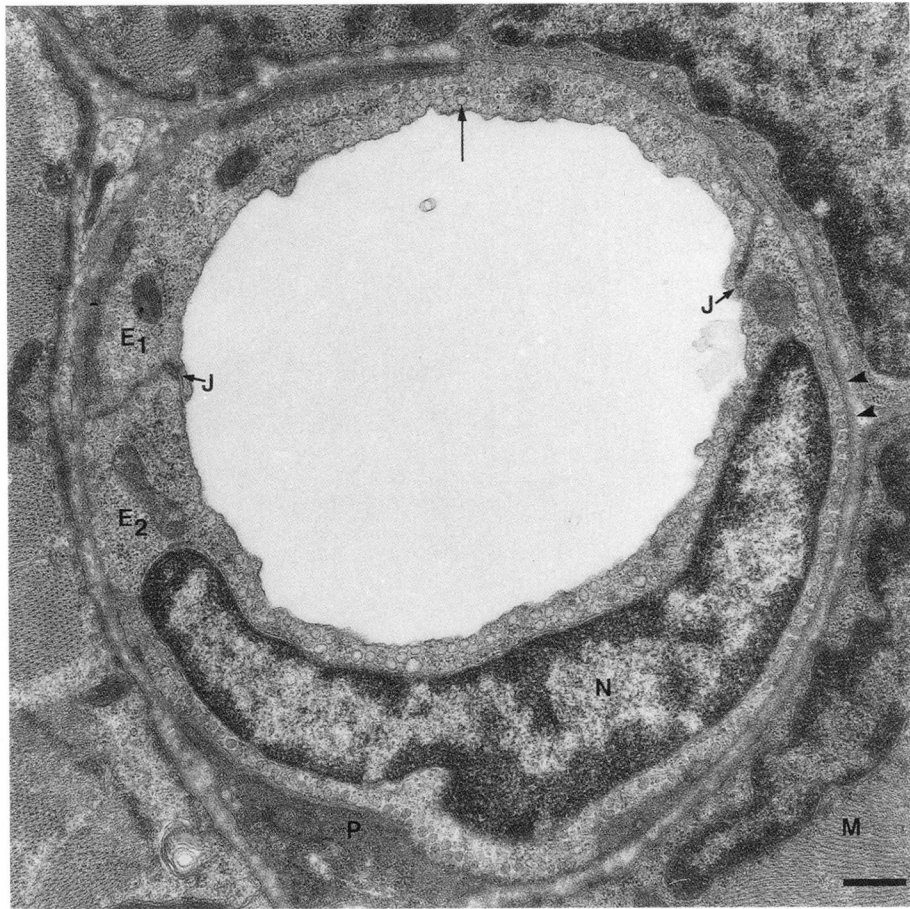

FIGURE 21.2 Capillary in rat striated muscle, fixed by perfusion under physiologic pressure. The capillary is lined by two endothelial cells (E_1, E_2); J = junctions between E_1 and E_2; N = nucleus of endothelial cell; P = part of a pericyte; M = striated muscle cell; **arrow** = micropinocytic vesicle; **arrowheads** = pericapillary basement membrane. **Bar** = 0.5 μm.

Normal Fluid Exchanges Across Capillary Endothelium

All extracellular fluids exist in a state of equilibrium with the plasma; exchanges between the two compartments occur across the "capillary" wall. (The quotation marks are there to remind us that in this particular instance the term *capillary* is meant to include the venules; although venules differ from capillaries with regard to structural details and pharmacologic responses, their walls are about as thin as those of capillaries and are in fact more permeable [48, 49].) The physiologic exchanges of fluid between blood and tissues are governed by Starling's equilibrium, as summarized in Chapter 10 and Table 10.1.

Our purpose now is to point out some less known facts about the Starling equilibrium.

The phenomenon of negative tissue pressure. It is certainly not intuitive that there should be a vacuum in the tissues (i.e., a pressure lower than atmospheric pressure);

in fact, practically all textbooks to this day define the tissue pressure as negligible or positive with a value of a few millimeters Hg. Yet the evidence for negative pressure is crystal clear. To prove the point, one has to find a suitable experimental model: namely, a tissue space large enough so that a fine needle connected to a manometer can obtain a reliable measurement. A simple solution was found in 1960 by A. C. Guyton and his co-workers (Dr. Guyton is a surgeon turned physiologist) (13, 15, 16). They took standard ping-pong balls or other hollow plastic spheres, perforated them with some 200 holes (Figure 21.4), and implanted them aseptically into the subcutaneous tissue or other tissues of dogs. Several weeks later, when inflammation had subsided, granulation tissue had developed around the spheres; it had also lined the inner surface of the spheres, leaving the central space permanently free and filled with fluid (Figure 21.5). At this point the

FIGURE 21.3 Endothelial transcytosis, demonstrated in pulmonary capillaries of a rat. The lungs were perfused with a solution of albumin molecules bound to particles of colloidal gold; the latter are visible here as black dots. *Top:* At 3 minutes, the albumin–gold particles are adsorbed to uncoated pits and to plasmalemmal vesicles open to the surface. *Center:* After 5 minutes, some particles are being ferried across by transcytosis, others are being unloaded toward the albuminal surface. *Bottom:* At 35 minutes, many gold particles have been discharged across the endothelium into the albuminal space. **Bars** = 0.1 μm. (*Top:* Reproduced with permission from [44]. *Center* and *Bottom:* Reproduced from the **Journal of Cell Biology,** 1986; 102:1304–1311, by copyright permission of The Rockefeller University Press [9].)

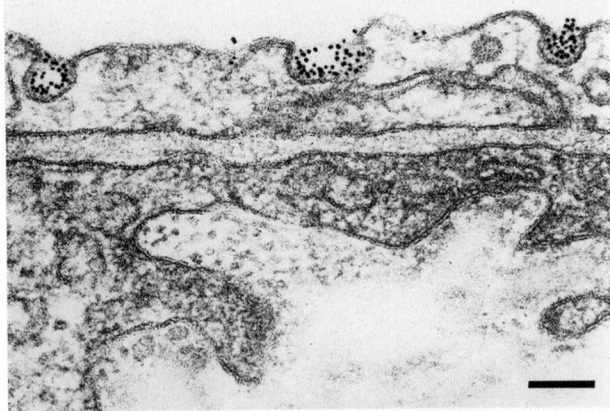

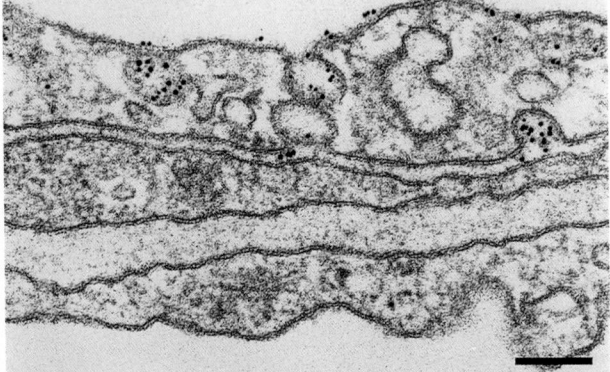

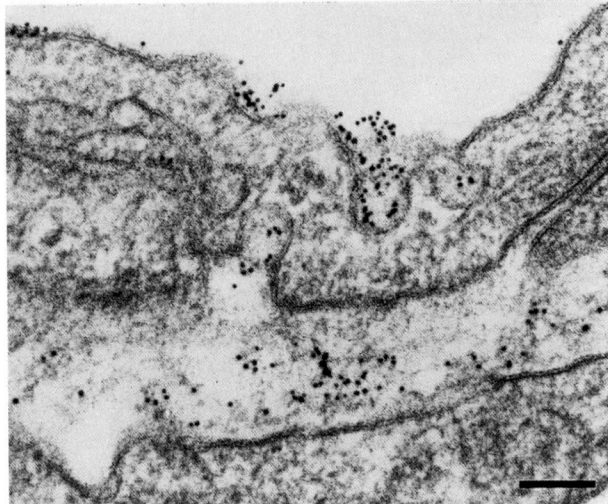

central cavity could be considered as an expansion of the normal tissue spaces and in equilibrium with them. *A needle inserted into that cavity consistently found a negative pressure* with readings of −4 to −6 mm Hg. Strange as this may seem, this fits a number of other observations; for example, note the pressures measured in other expanded tissue spaces (14):

Pleural space	−8 mm Hg;
Joints	−4 to −8 mm Hg;
Epidural space	−4 to −7 mm Hg.

Exceptions to the rule of negative interstitial pressure include the very special environments of the eye and of the cerebrospinal fluid (16).

This partial vacuum is maintained by two forces: the osmotic suction of the plasma and the pumping action of the lymphatics, which remove fluid as well as osmotically active proteins. As we will see, this vacuum is an important safety factor against edema.

Guyton's concept is gaining acceptance only very slowly, even though it is nothing new in the big picture of biology. The negative pressures in animal tissues are minuscule compared with those in the sap of desert plants, which are of the order of −40 to −60 atmospheres (42). If a drop of liquid is placed on a cut in the xylem of a transpiring tree, the drop will be sucked in. The negative pressures recorded in the sap are 1000 times greater overall than those recorded in animal tissues (42).

Role of the lymphatics. Starling's law implies that the fluid escaping along the arterial end of the capillary is reabsorbed along the venous end. This is true for about 90 percent of the filtered fluid; the remaining 10 percent is drained away by the lymphatics. But how can the lymphatics act as a drain in an environment with a negative pressure?

In fact, the tissue spaces are under negative pressure *because* they are drained by the lymphatics. The lymphatic capillaries are equipped with valves. Every time the tissue is squeezed by body movement, a tiny amount of fluid is squirted downstream across the valves, which snap shut as soon as the pressure abates.

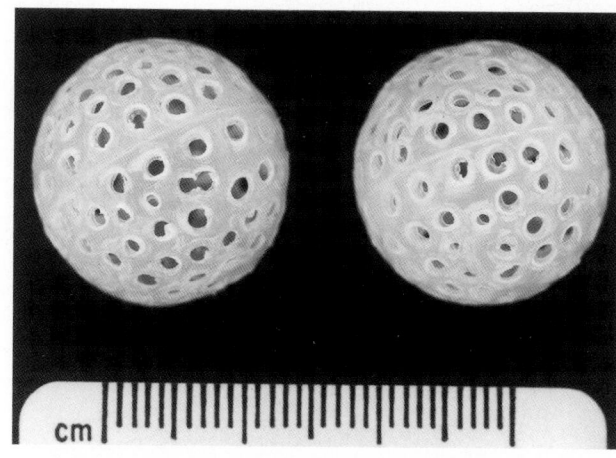

FIGURE 21.4   One of many types of perforated plastic spheres used by Guyton and collaborators for their measurements of hydrostatic pressure in the interstitial fluid. **Scale** in centimeters. (Courtesy of Dr. A. C. Guyton, University of Mississippi School of Medicine, Jackson, MS.)

Active contraction of the lymphatic itself is thought to be another pumping device (14).

The concept of edema safety factor. Starling's law, narrowly interpreted, suggests that fluid exchanges in the tissues are in precarious equilibrium. The capillaries ooze a little more fluid than they can reabsorb, but the providential lymphatics carry away the excess. This situation suggests that the slightest increase in venous pressure would upset the balance; more fluid would escape, less would be re-absorbed, and edema would develop. In reality, negative pressure comes to the rescue: no fluid can accumulate in the tissues as long as the interstitial pressure is negative. The excess fluid is sucked away by the lymphatics and by the oncotic pressure of the plasma proteins, and edema cannot begin to develop until the interstitial pressure rises from −6 or −5 mm Hg to zero (14).

This is why the reader, who is presumably in a sitting position while perusing these lines, is not developing edema of the buttocks.

All these mechanisms will help understand the pathophysiology of hyperemia and edema.

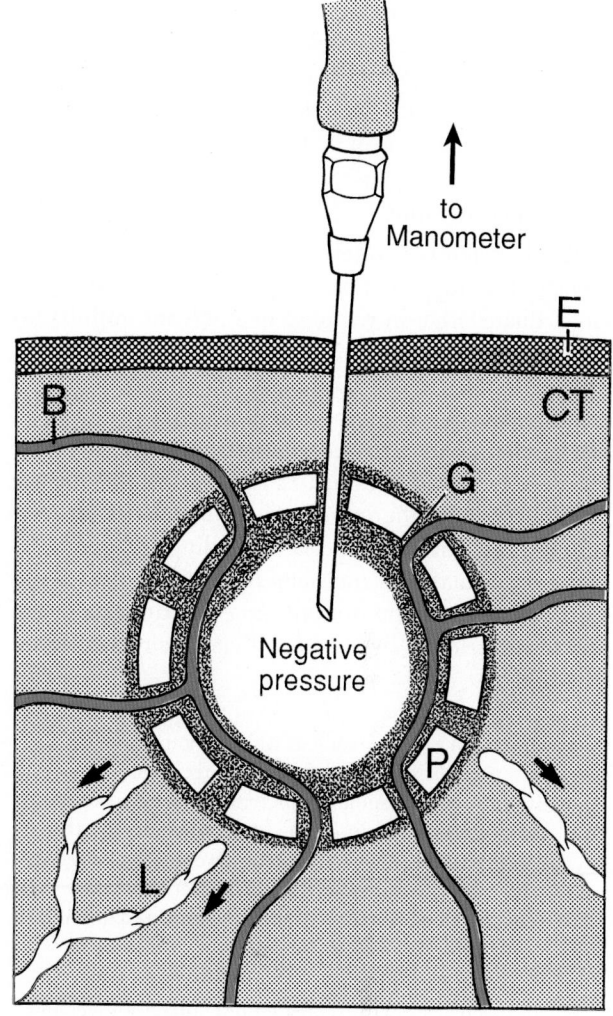

FIGURE 21.5   Demonstrating the negative interstitial pressure, using one of the perforated capsule as shown (**P**) in the preceding figure. Over 3 weeks the capsule becomes covered and partly lined with granulation tissue (**G**), which includes a network of blood capillaries (**B**). Lymphatics have not been demonstrated in this granulation tissue, but of course they exist (**L**) in the surrounding tissues. The negative pressure is maintained by a combination of forces: removal of fluid and proteins by the lymphatics (**arrows**), and the suction provided by the oncotic pressure of the plasma proteins. **T** = Connective tissue, **E** = epidermis. (Adapted from [14].)

Hyperemia

Although blood is life-giving, vessels overfilled with blood spell trouble. This fact was recognized, however dimly, by the Hippocratic physicians, who blamed "congestion" for many ills and bled their patients accordingly. **Hyperemia** is the term used to mean that *the vessels of the microcirculation contain more blood than normal.*

Hyperemia can be of two kinds. A red face is hyperemic and so are the dusky blue fingernails of a patient in congestive heart failure. In both cases the vessels are overfilled, but the redness and the blueness point to different situations: *blood flow is either increased (active hyperemia) or decreased (passive hyperemia-congestion).* Correspondingly, the temperature of hyperemic skin is either abnormally warm or abnormally cool.

Active Hyperemia

Active hyperemia is often harmless or even beneficial. In fact, it is taught as a part of physiology that the arterioles dilate either in response to a nervous impulse (as in blushing) or as a result of functional demand (as in exercising muscle). In both cases, the microcirculation is flushed with more blood under higher pressure; all the capillaries are perfused whereas normally they take turns. The raised pressure causes an increase in the amount of fluid filtering out of the capillaries (*transudation*), but without necessarily leading to edema because the situation is transient and the lymphatics can take care of it. We do not puff up every time we blush.

However, even hyperemia offers plenty of pathophysiology.

- Strenuous exercise, such as running a marathon, brings about an intense and prolonged muscular hyperemia. Transudation increases and may exceed the draining capacity of the lymphatics. Under these conditions, tissue pressure can rise enough to impair blood flow, with results that are sometimes irreversible. This scenario is called the **compartment syndrome** (p. 684).

- Persistent active hyperemia appears to be a stimulus for vascular growth. Increased flow places a mechanical stress on the microcirculation, and the small vessels respond by enlarging and adapting to the increased function (40, 41). The arterioles become arteries, some capillaries become arterioles, and the venules become small veins. This may be one of the mechanisms whereby collateral circulation develops (Figure 21.6). We have seen this mechanism at work also in the active hyperemia of acute inflammation (p. 396).

- In poorly controlled diabetes, hyperemia is one of the earliest and possibly the earliest vascular change (54). Blood flow is increased in the skin, retina and kidney, and capillary pressure is pathologically raised (51). This hyperemia is brought about by hyperglycemia, as can be proven experimentally by infusing glucose to normal humans or animals for 4–5 hours (54). The mechanism sounds paradoxical (54); tissues perceive hyperglycemia as hypoxia ("pseudo-hypoxia"), and react accordingly by vasodilatation and increased blood flow.

In hypoxic tissues the ratio NADH/NAD is increased: NADH increases because there is not enough oxygen to oxidize it to NAD. In diabetes the ratio of NADH/

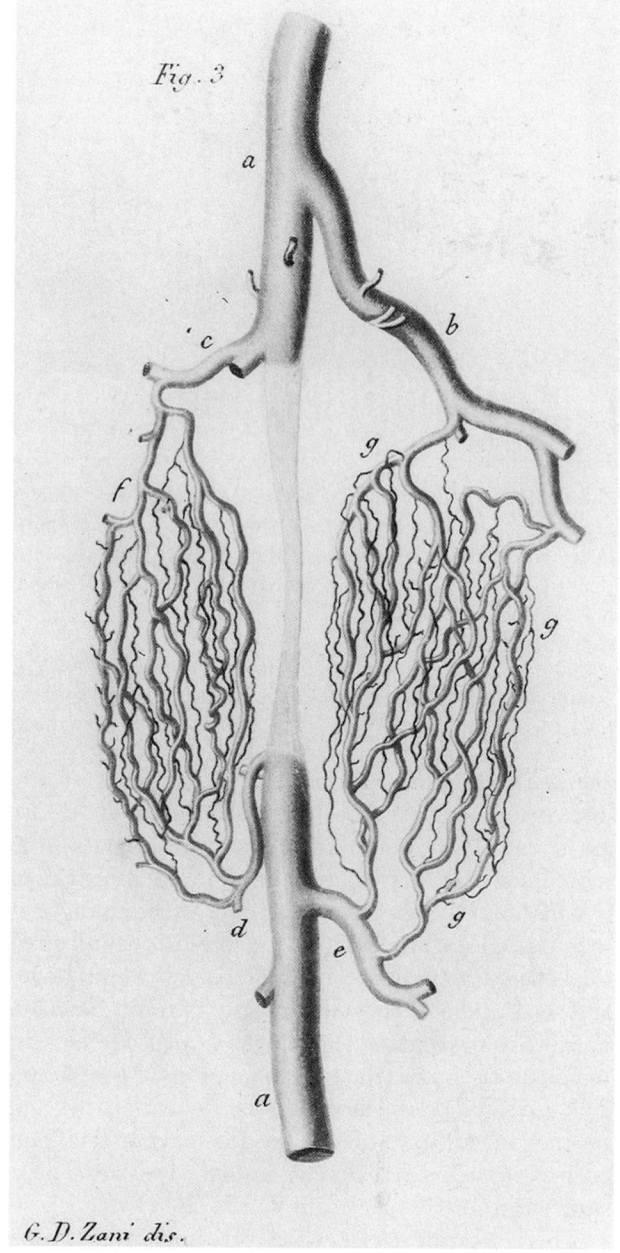

FIGURE 21.6 Development of collateral circulation, demonstrated by L, Porta in Italy in 1845. A segment of the femoral artery (**a**) of a dog was tied off; 3 months later, dissection shows how the collateral circulation has developed. Branches (**b, c**) upstream from the tie have enlarged or acquired connections (**f, g**) with branches distal to the ligature (**d, e**). (Reproduced from [32].)

NAD is also increased, because more NADH is produced—due to the increased oxidation of sorbitol coupled to the reduction of NAD to NADH.

This persistent vasodilatation in diabetics is important, because the microvascular pathology typical of diabetes, including a thickened capillary basement membrane, may be a consequence of this early malfunction (51).

- Bone fractures in children, especially those between the ages of 2 and 10, may cause an increase in the length of the fractured bone (25). This is attributed to increased blood flow to the fractured bone; indeed, a similar overgrowth can occur as a result of a congenital or accidental arteriovenous fistula (an abnormal communication between an artery and vein) or of large hemangiomas (tumors composed of blood vessels) (7).

Passive Hyperemia (Congestion)

Passive hyperemia, also known as **congestion,** is much more damaging. Less blood flow means less oxygen, less substrates, and less removal of waste products. Congested tissues may develop edema (20). Causes can be local, such as an obstructed vein, or general, such as congestive heart failure.

Congested organs enlarge due to overfilling with blood. Eventually, over weeks and months, they become firmer because of diffuse fibrosis.

The fibrosis of chronic congestion is especially obvious in the liver and lung. Why it should develop is not clear, except that fibroblasts function optimally in a slightly anoxic environment (p. 467). It is also a fact that persistent edema of the skin leads to fibrosis.

The color of congested organs in bluish or purple rather than red; *cyanotic* is the technical term (Greek *kyanós,* blue). The blueness is due in part to a change in the color of the blood; sluggish flow leads to greater oxygen extraction, and thus to a decrease in the ratio of bright red oxyhemoglobin to dusky red carboxyhemoglobin. Cyanosis of the skin, however, calls for a more complex physical explanation.

Congested white skin appears blue for the same basic reason that the sky is blue; so the experts tell us (2, 8). The color of the skin normally depends on the light absorbed by various pigments (mainly melanins, plus oxidized and reduced hemoglobin) and on the light returned to the viewer by reflection and diffraction ("remittance"). A vein under the skin appears blue because most of the light is absorbed by the red blood cells, and the component that remains visible is mainly the blue light diffracted by the epidermis and dermis by a Tyndall effect. A similar phenomenon explains the blueness of deep-seated melanotic nevi ("blue nevi"). The normal color of the skin would actually be much redder were it not for the superimposed bluish diffraction just mentioned. Reduced hemoglobin has an absorption spectrum slightly displaced toward the red, which allows the remittance of more blue. It is the absolute concentration of reduced hemoglobin that appears as cyanosis; it must be at least 5 gm per 100 ml (normal total hemoglobin is 14 gm per 100 ml). This means that a severely anemic person will surely be pale but may never have enough reduced hemoglobin, in absolute amounts, to become cyanotic.

The effects of chronic congestion on the structure and function of organs depend on the tissues. To illustrate this, we will discuss congestion in three organs of very different structures: liver, lungs, and spleen.

Congested liver. Liver congestion is a classic result of heart failure (Figure 21.7). Normally, the liver lies

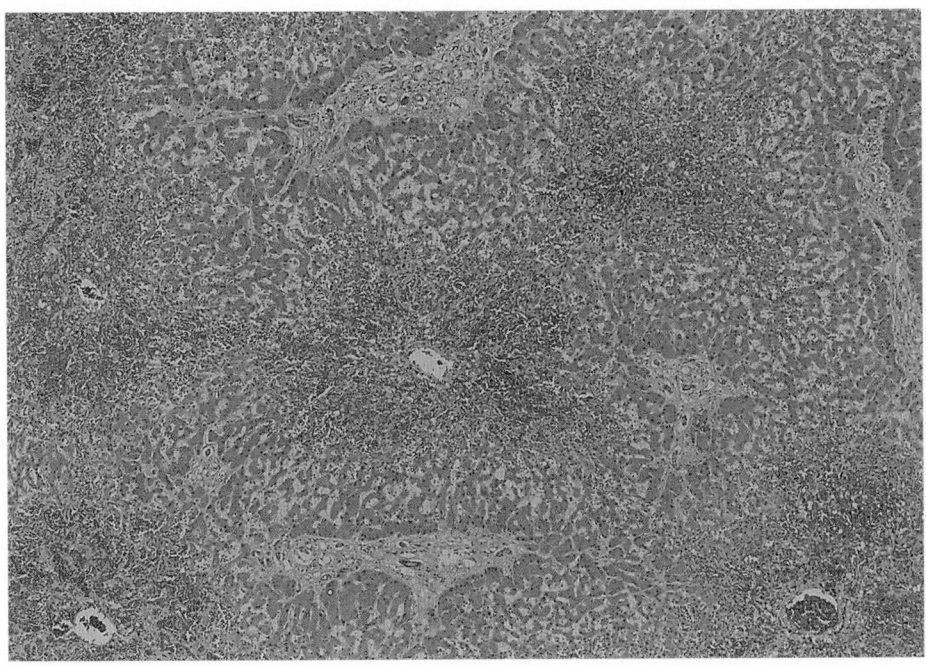

FIGURE 21.7 Severe congestion of the liver due to heart failure. To understand this slide, orientation is critical: **centrolobular veins** are in the center of "hemorrhagic" areas; **portal spaces** have much more connective tissue; **blood flows** from the periphery to the center of the lobules (see text). (45x)

against the diaphragm, just centimeters below the heart; if the right ventricle fails, blood is backed up in the liver, which can swell to 3000 gram, double its weight. The pathologic effect on liver tissue is best understood by remembering that the liver lobule, in the traditional interpretation of liver structure, functions like a funnel in the sense that the blood flows toward the central vein. In this system, sluggish flow means that only the cells at the periphery of the lobule receive an adequate amount of oxygen and nutrients; these cells may show no change. The cells in the middle third of the lobule will be anoxic, and the reader will hopefully remember that the classic effect of anoxia on liver cells is steatosis (p. 86). The centrolobular cells become atrophic or just die and disappear, leaving space for a pool of blood under pressure.

> In extreme cases only the cells surrounding the portal spaces survive, because life-supporting arterial blood comes from there; all the rest of the liver is necrotic. At this point the liver still appears as if it were made of lobules, but these are *pseudolobules,* centered by portal spaces (not by portal veins) supporting a few liver cells, surrounded by a red sea of congestion: hence the descriptive French name of "inverted liver" (38).

To the naked eye, the cut surface of the congested liver shows a mottled pattern of red dots on a yellowish background, hence the name *nutmeg liver,* a very appropriate term to anyone who has seen the cut surface of a nutmeg (Figure 21.8). In the long run, a mild degree of fibrosis creeps in (*cardiac cirrhosis*).

Overall, congestion in the liver causes mainly parenchymal changes, with a fairly minor connective tissue response.

Congested lungs. Lungs become congested when a malfunction of the left heart causes the blood to back up in the pulmonary circulation. A typical acute setting (hours) is the sudden failure of the left ventricle due to an extensive myocardial infarct. As blood backs up in the pulmonary circulation, the congested capillaries bulge into the alveoli, allowing transudate to escape, at first into the connective tissue spaces. Luckily for the patient, the lymphatics of the lung are extremely efficient and can drain away a great deal of fluid, preventing further trouble. However, if congestion persists, the transudate eventually spills into the air spaces. The bulging alveolar capillaries can also burst, thereby mixing the transudate with plasma and red blood cells (Figure 21.9). The result is a frothy pink edema fluid that can suffocate the patient.

With these facts in mind, one can anticipate the effects of chronic congestion: a classic setting is stenosis (constriction) of the mitral valve, which causes a persistent backing up of blood in the lungs. The alveolar walls respond to chronic interstitial edema by developing a *diffuse fibrosis.* Spilled red blood cells are picked up by the resident alveolar macrophages, which become loaded with typical rusty-colored granules of hemosiderin (Figure 21.10). These helpful macrophages—there may be several in each alveolus—are known for obvious reasons as *heart failure cells;* eventually, they can be coughed out by the patient, who will notice a rusty-colored sputum.

Congested lungs become clinically less compliant (stiffer) and at autopsy appear firm and brown (brown induration).

Congested spleen. This is a wholly different matter, because—when it is chronic—congestion of the spleen

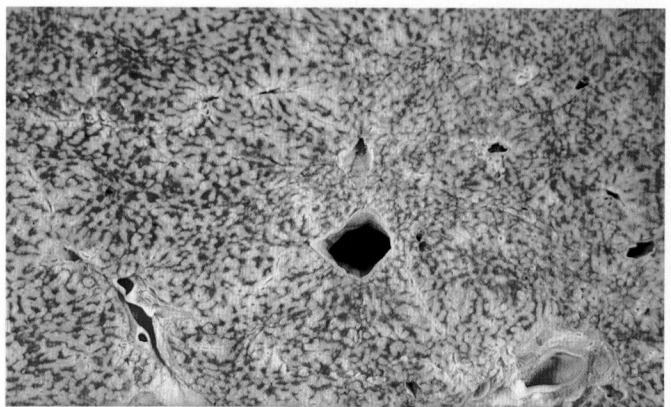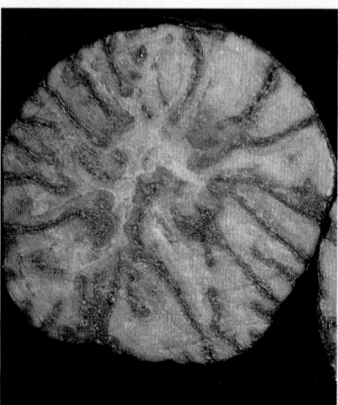

FIGURE 21.8   *Left:* The "nutmeg liver" typical of chronic congestion. The liver is filled with blood (hence the red background) and studded with yellow dots and streaks corresponding to the centers of the lobules. The steatosis responsible for the yellow discoloration is caused by anoxia. *Right:* The polished surface of a nutmeg justifies the comparison (~2x actual size).

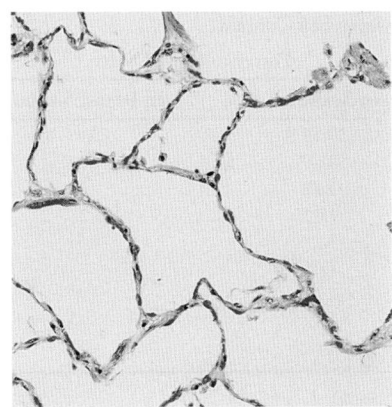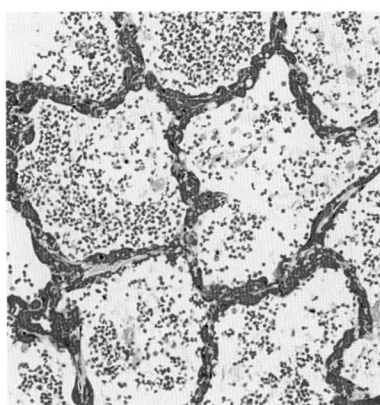

FIGURE 21.9 *Left:* Normal lung (control). *Right:* Lung with severe acute congestion of the alveolar capillaries. Note hemorrhage into the alveolar spaces. (140x)

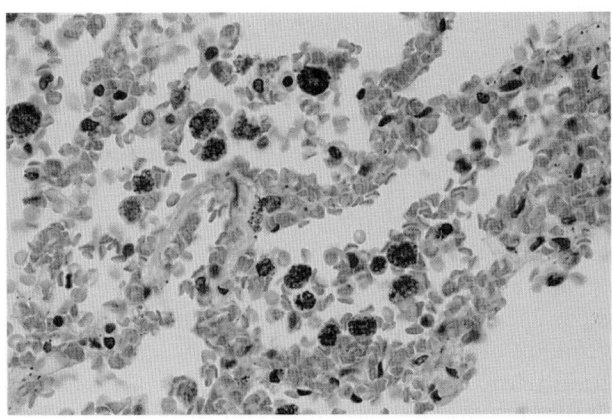

FIGURE 21.10 Human lung with acute congestion: note red blood cells spilled into the alveolar spaces, and macrophages loaded with hemosiderin ("heart failure cells"). The congestion has not lasted long enough to induce a change typical of chronic congestion: fibrosis of the alveolar walls.

leads to hypertrophy and thereby to *increased* function. Recall that the splenic vein empties into the portal vein; so whenever the portal flow through the liver is impaired (e.g., by cirrhosis), the increased venous pressure in the portal vein is transmitted to the splenic vein. Over months and years, the "overblown" spleen responds by increasing its mass: it undergoes true hypertrophy. This enlargement of the spleen leads to the syndrome called *hypersplenism,* defined by reduced numbers of circulating red cells, white cells, and platelets. The mechanism appears to involve an excessive trapping of circulating blood cells in the splenic sinusoids and an excessive number of splenic macrophages ready to devour these cells.

The main point here is the interesting paradox of congestion leading to increased function, but to no advantage.

Congested lower limbs. Chronic congestion of the lower limbs due to heart failure causes a vicious circle: the large veins, submitted to increased hydrostatic pressure, dilate to such a point that their valves become incompetent, thus producing varicose veins and worsening the congestion. The chronically congested skin becomes edematous, ulcers develop about the ankles (and heal poorly), and the surrounding skin tends to become brownish from microscopic hemorrhages (21). Fibrin cuffs develop around some capillaries, presumably from chronic seepage of plasma (53); but overall, the pathogenesis of stasis ulcers is not yet well understood (31).

> Migraine headaches may be somehow related to hyperemia; the mechanism is still not clear (37).

Edema

Edema is an excess of extracellular fluid—except in the brain, where the excess may be either intra- or extracellular.

> For some reason, intracellular edema is not known in the "lower organs," as neuropathologists are apt to call anything below the brain. Intracellular edema of these organs may exist, but its consequences would not be as drastic as

for the brain, which is locked in a box of bone and cannot afford to expand.

The body of a normal adult contains about 40 liters of water (14); most of it (25 liters) is sequestered in cells, including 2 liters in red blood cells; about 12 liters are in the extracellular spaces and 3 more in the plasma. The volume of water retained in each of these three

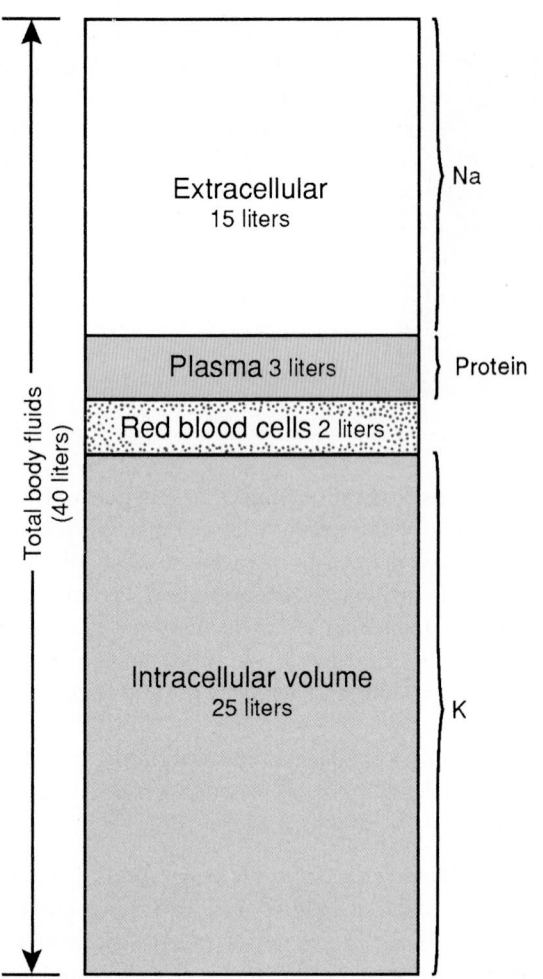

FIGURE 21.11 Body fluids. Diagram shows volumes of intracellular and extracellular fluid, blood, and total body fluids. (Adapted from [14], Copyright 1986, with permission from Elsevier.)

Table 21.1   Blood and Seawater: Salt Content

Electrolyte	Percent of Total Salts	
	In Seawater	In Blood Serum
Na	30.59	39
Mg	3.79	0.4
Ca	1.20	1
K	1.11	2.7
Cl	55.27	45
SO_4	7.66	—
CO_3	0.21	12
Br	0.19	—
P_2O_5	—	0.4

Adapted from (17).

and cause it to swell; the ancient Greek *óidema* actually means swelling. It can also fill preformed spaces and create pockets of free fluid; these pockets have special names according to the organ in which they occur. Accumulations of fluid in the pleura, pericardium, or joints are called *hydrothorax, hydropericardium,* or *hydrarthrosis;* in the peritoneum they are called *ascites.* A severe generalized edema is called *anasarca* or *dropsy,* the latter from the ancient Greek *hydrops.*

The nature of the fluid itself must also be considered. Recall: a protein-poor fluid resulting from ultrafiltration of plasma across the capillary wall is called a **transudate.** A protein-rich fluid due to increased endothelial permeability is called an **exudate** (p. 434). When the nature of a collection of fluid is not clear, we use the convenient and noncommittal term **effusion.**

Local Edema

From the basic rules of capillary filtration and reabsorption and of endothelial permeability it is not difficult to understand the various clinical settings of edema. The mechanisms, however, are often multiple.

Local edema can be due to venous obstruction, lymphatic obstruction, or acute inflammation.

Local venous obstruction. Venous obstruction can be produced, for example, by a tight cast or by a venous thrombus, particularly in the lower limbs. In terms of the Starling equilibrium, this type of edema is due to increased venous pressure leading to excessive filtration (*transudative edema*). The edema is recognized clinically by pressing a finger firmly on the skin: a little depression or "pit" is produced (p. 626).

Lymphatic obstruction. Lymphedema is a reminder of the low-key but essential task of the lymphatic vessels. The obstruction can be purely functional: paraplegics sometimes suffer from edema of the paralyzed limbs, presumably because the lymphatics cannot perform their

spaces depends closely on one particular solute: *potassium* in the intracellular space, *sodium* in the extracellular space, and *proteins* (mainly albumin) in the plasma (Figure 21.11). The main electrolytes in plasma maintain roughly the same relative concentrations as in seawater, our ancestral plasma (Table 21.1).

Extracellular water is held in the tissue almost entirely as a gel by large, feathery, proteoglycan molecules (p. 282). As mentioned earlier, without these molecules all the extracellular fluid would run into the legs and feet in a matter of hours; in fact, when the amount of extracellular fluid exceeds the reserve capacity of the proteoglycans (they can imbibe an additional 30–50 percent above normal), it floods any available space. It can accumulate in the *loose connective tissue*

draining function without the pumping effect of muscular contraction. More commonly, the obstacle along the lymphatic pathways is iatrogenic. Treatment for breast tumor often includes removal or irradiation of the axillary lymph nodes; the lymphatic pathways are therefore interrupted (in the case of radiation therapy, by fibrosis) and lymphedema of the arm is a distressing consequence (Figure 21.12).

An extreme example of chronic lymphatic obstruction is the tropical disease filariasis, which is caused by the nematode *Wuchereria bancrofti* and presently affects over 250 million people. It is appropriately called *elephantiasis* (Figure 21.13) (6, 26). The threadlike worms live coiled together in human lymphatics, where they somehow choose to dwell (Figure 21.14); there they cause a chronic inflammatory reaction, especially when they die, leading to obstruction and lymphedema. The swollen tissues respond by permanent expansion, therefore this edema is nonpitting. The mechanism, however,

is complicated (19a). In temperate climates a venereal disease, *lymphogranuloma venereum,* that destroys the local and regional lymph nodes can lead to genital elephantiasis in both men and women. It is due to a *Chlamydia,* an intracellular organism larger than a virus.

Congenital malformations of the lymphatics lead to lymphedema in rare conditions.

Acute inflammatory edema. This edema can be recognized by the cardinal signs of acute inflammation: redness, heat, pain, and swelling. The pitting phenomenon is absent, presumably because the fibrin network of inflammation acts as a gel and traps the fluid. This type of local edema is caused, as we already know, by increased microvascular permeability (p. 387).

General Edema

Body-wide mechanisms of edema can operate in two principal ways: by raising the pressure in the entire

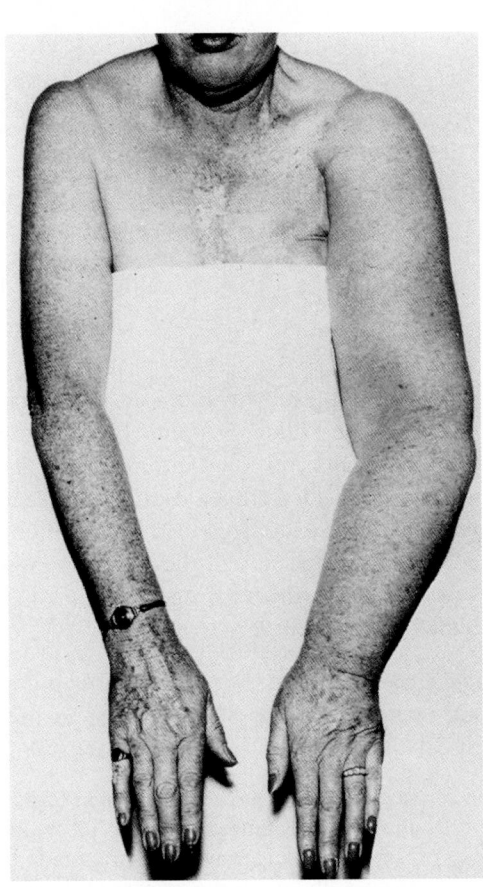
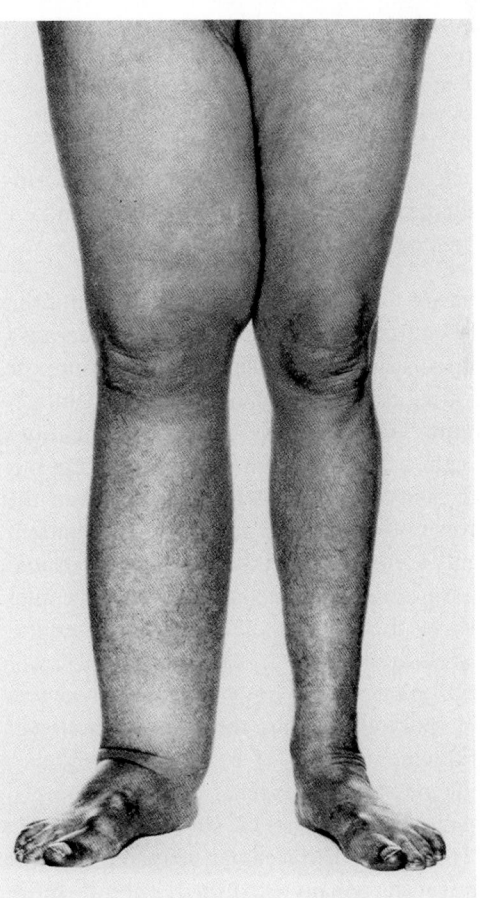

FIGURE 21.12   Two examples of iatrogenic lymphedema. *Left:* Lymphedema of the left arm after mastectomy; edema had been mild for 9 years, then increased suddenly. *Right:* Lymphedema after inguinal dissection and irradiation for a malignant melanoma that involved regional nodes; edema increased gradually over 30 years and was then treated surgically. (Reproduced from [19].)

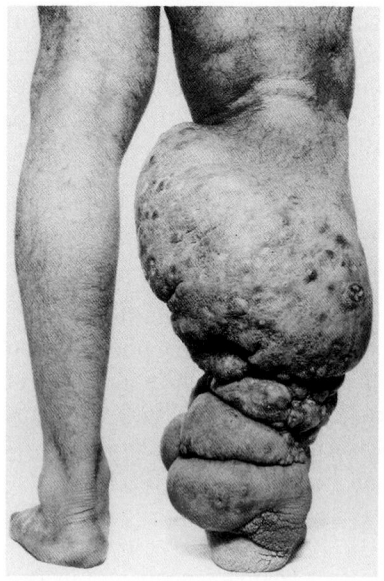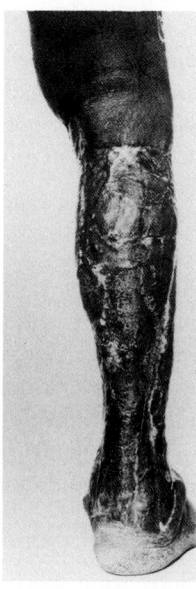

FIGURE 21.13   Advanced tropical elephantiasis in a native of Iraq. *Left:* Normal left leg. *Center:* Affected right leg before surgery. *Right:* Right leg 6 weeks after an operation using free grafts of healthy skin taken from the patient's back and from the opposite thigh. (Reproduced from [19].)

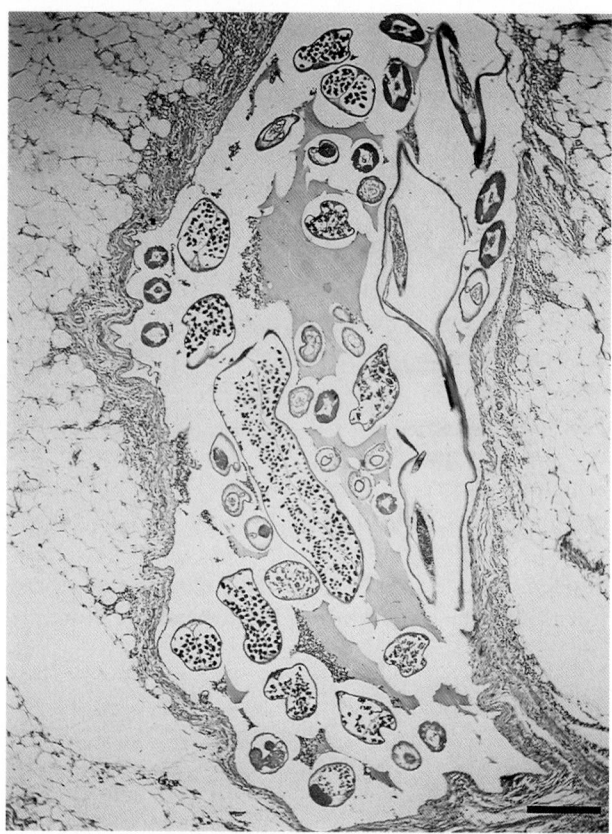

FIGURE 21.14   Male and female worms in a dilated lymphatic. This is *Wuchereria bancrofti,* a common cause of lymphedema in tropical countries. **Bar** = 250 μm. (Reproduced with permission from The Pathology of Tropical and Extraordinary Diseases, MIS # 70-6688 [26].)

venous tree, either pulmonary or systemic, which happens when the heart fails; or by decreasing the oncotic pressure of the plasma proteins.

Cardiogenic edema. This is by far the most common. The basic mechanics are easily grasped by considering a map of the circulatory system (Figure 21.15). Suppose that there is a failure of the left side due to an infarct of the left ventricle; edema develops only in the lungs because the right heart pumps blood into the lungs but the left heart cannot forward it adequately. When the failure involves both ventricles, it leads to generalized congestion and edema. In this case the edema is related to overfilling the large veins; the pressure in the venules is highest where the column of blood is the tallest. Therefore, excess fluid begins to seep out into the lower or "dependent" parts of the body (*dependent edema*): the ankles in walking patients, the skin of the lower back in bedridden patients.

The pathogenesis of cardiogenic edema is complicated by many factors. First of all, remember (see Figure 21.11) that the extracellular space is "sodium space," and it can remain expanded only if more sodium is provided. More sodium is indeed provided, and by several mechanisms. To begin, the kidney is involved. Reduced renal blood flow leads to more complete reabsorption of the glomerular filtrate by the

proximal tubules; furthermore, being inadequately perfused, the kidney responds by secreting renin; the renin–angiotensin system in turn causes the adrenals to secrete more aldosterone, leading to further sodium retention and thus to expanded blood volume and more edema. Although not all the details are worked out, it should be clear that cardiogenic edema is more than a hydrostatic disturbance.

Nephrogenic edema. Edema can be induced by the kidney in several ways, depending on the underlying disease:

- *By a glomerular mechanism.* Protein (principally albumin) is lost through leaky capillary loops, thereby reducing the oncotic pressure of the plasma. Because albumin is the smallest of the plasma proteins, it contributes most to the oncotic pressure of the plasma (see Table 10.2). Leaky glomeruli occur in any inflammatory disease of the glomerulus (glomerulonephritis).

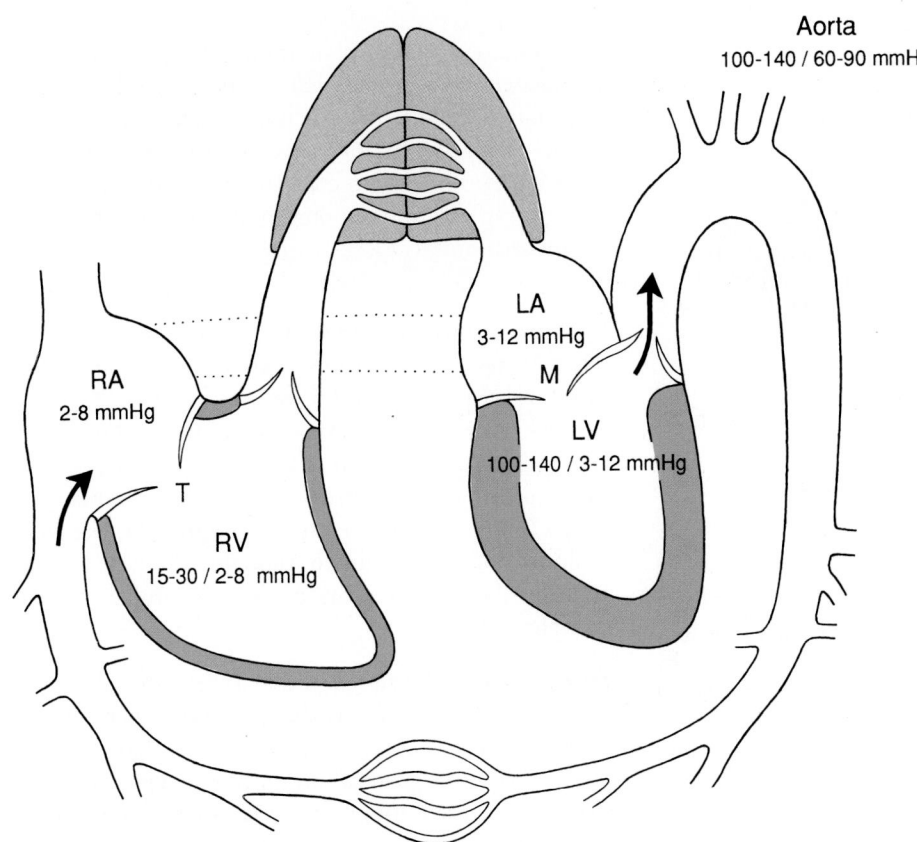

Aorta
100-140 / 60-90 mmHg

LA
3-12 mmHg

M

LV
100-140 / 3-12 mmHg

RA
2-8 mmHg

T

RV
15-30 / 2-8 mmHg

FIGURE 21.15 Map of the greater and lesser circulations. For clarity, the two sides of the heart are shown as separated. **LA:** Left atrium. **LV:** Left ventricle. **RA:** Right atrium. **RV:** Right ventricle. **M:** Mitral valve. **T:** Tricuspid valve. Dotted lines connecting the atria indicate that the wall between the atria in that area is a thin fibrous membrane, called the *foramen ovale*. In 10–20 percent of all individuals the fibrous membrane acts as a flap-valve. This is the route taken by paradoxical emboli. (Courtesy of Dr. H. F. Cuénoud, University of Massachusetts Medical School, Worcester, MA.)

- *By constriction of the afferent arterioles.* Constriction reduces the glomerular filtrate and leads to greater reabsorption of sodium and water by the proximal convoluted tubules.
- *By secreting renin.* This causes the adrenals to secrete more aldosterone, which increases the reabsorption of sodium; the retained sodium produces edema by expanding the blood volume.
- *By failing to excrete salt and water.* As fluid intake continues, the blood volume expands. This occurs in acute renal failure, which has a variety of causes including ischemia, massive infection, and obstruction of the urinary pathways.

Nephrogenic edema is rarely severe; it tends to affect the eyelids first and then the genitalia and ankles. This is usually explained by the fact that the subcutaneous tissue in these sites is loose.

Edema associated with liver cirrhosis. This edema is a combination of local and general causes (3). The cirrhotic liver is criss-crossed by a meshwork of fibrous strands that slowly contract and strangle the parenchyma; fluid weeps from the liver surface and accumulates in the peritoneal cavity; the belly can protrude to grotesque proportions. The condition is called **ascites.**

Interestingly, the name ascites comes from *askós* for "wine bag." The Greeks carried wine and water in pouches made of animal skins; the method is still used in Africa, and we are told that it works very well. The protruding belly of cirrhotic (and perhaps alcoholic) patients reminded the Greeks of their wine-bags. They also knew that the belly was full of fluid; in fact, a Hippocratic book explains how to drain it.

Although ascites has been with us for so long, its pathogenesis is still debated (4). The traditional explanation is based on the "backward" mechanism, that is, on the backup of portal blood due to an obstacle in the liver; its main components are the following:

- The roots of the portal veins are strangled, which increases portal pressure.
- The lymphatics of the liver are also strangled.
- Portal pressure is further increased by arteriovenous anastomoses; nodules of regenerating liver do develop, but they do not have the proper vascular architecture, with the result that arterial blood feeds directly into the roots of the portal vein.
- Insufficient albumin is synthesized by the liver.
- Aldosterone is inadequately inactivated by the malfunctioning liver cells, which normally conjugate it; this results in salt and water retention.

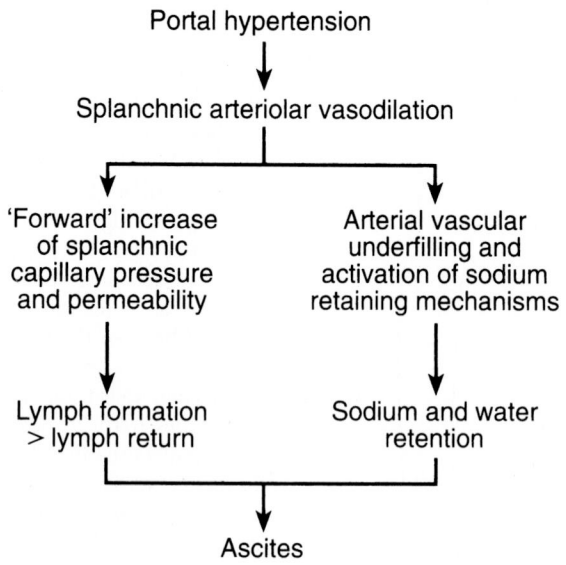

Portal hypertension

↓

Splanchnic arteriolar vasodilation

'Forward' increase of splanchnic capillary pressure and permeability | Arterial vascular underfilling and activation of sodium retaining mechanisms

Lymph formation > lymph return | Sodium and water retention

↓

Ascites

FIGURE 21.16   Pathogenesis of ascites in the course of liver cirrhosis, according to the "forward theory." (Reproduced by permission of Arroyo V. in "Oxford Textbook of Clinical Hepatology," J. Bircher, J-P. Benhamou, N. McIntyre, M. Rizzetto, J. Rodés (eds), 1999 [4], and by permission of Oxford University Press.)

• The kidney responds by activating the renin–angiotensin system, as if blood volume were reduced.

As if all this were not enough, high abdominal pressure from the ascitic fluid can create an obstacle to venous return from the lower limbs, where edema may also develop.

According to the "forward" mechanism, the arterioles in the splanchnic (intestinal) area are dilated in response to the portal hypertension and contribute to it, while flow to the kidney, muscles, skin, and brain is reduced; the steps are shown in Figure 21.16.

Whatever the mechanism of ascites, there is more trouble in store: the increased abdominal pressure creates an obstacle to venous reflow from the lower limbs, where edema may also develop.

NOTE: Ascites can also develop without liver cirrhosis if the peritoneal cavity is seeded with tumors (carcinomatosis of the peritoneum). This type of ascites is best explained by the fact that tumors produce permeability-increasing factors (p. 764), which presumably affect the entire peritoneal surface. Some experimental tumors are

maintained by transplantation in the peritoneum, precisely because they have a special tendency to produce ascites, in which they grow (p. 762); their capacity to increase vascular permeability in the peritoneum is comparable to an intraperitoneal injection of a potent inflammatory mediator, serotonin (28).

Hypoalbuminemia. Insufficient albumin can lead to edema if the concentration of albumin drops from the normal 4.5 percent to 2.5 percent or less. There is a normal loss of albumin to the gastrointestinal tract, and this fraction can be increased in many diseases. These protein-losing enteropathies can be inflammatory, neoplastic, infectious, or of cardiac origin. The edema of malnutrition was originally thought to reflect hypoalbuminemia, but the mechanism is probably more complex (10).

Edema from sundry causes. Edema brought about by *glucocorticoid treatment* is due to several mechanisms, including salt retention and possibly a change in the connective tissue ground substance; the typical localization to the face ("moon face") is not explained. *High altitude* causes cerebral as well as pulmonary edema (mountain sickness); the pathogenesis is still debated (5, 18). An even greater mystery is *idiopathic cyclic edema* whereby a patient suffers from periodic episodes of local or generalized edema that can be severe enough to cause shock if untreated.

Effects of Edema on Tissues

Skin. Edema of the skin can cause a great deal of discomfort, but it is painless unless it is caused by inflammation. In subcutaneous tissue, the excess fluid is initially free to move about, hence the clinical phenomenon of pitting; a finger pressed firmly on edematous skin for a few seconds leaves a depression that disappears in about one minute (Figure 21.17). This free-moving fluid facilitates infection. Bacteria, even if suspended in fluid, can easily perform their aggressive functions such as multiplying and producing toxins, whereas leukocytes are helpless because they crawl but do not swim. For these reasons, injuries of edematous skin, even minor ones, can lead to severe and rapidly spreading infections. If edema persists for weeks or longer, connective tissue produces new cells and new fibers to fill the extra spaces, and the swelling becomes permanent.

Edema is critically dangerous in two organs: the lung and the brain.

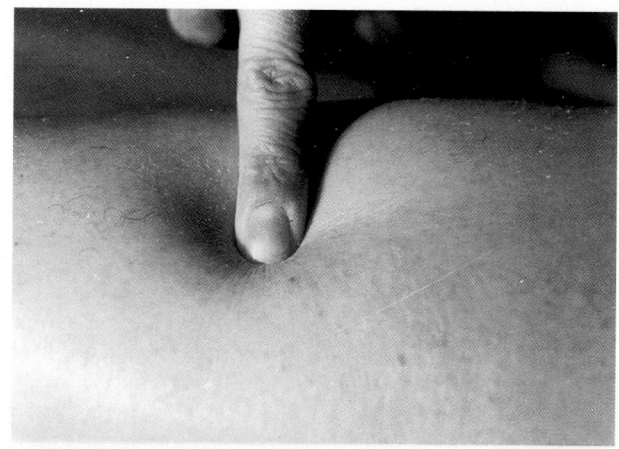

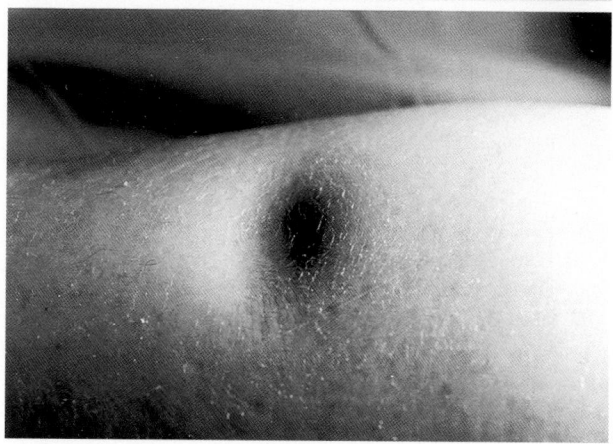

FIGURE 21.17 Pitting edema in the leg of a patient suffering from right ventricular heart failure. Firm pressure with a finger, sustained for a few seconds, leaves a depression that disappears in about a minute. If the edema is the result of chronic lymphatic obstruction (lymphedema), the pitting phenomenon cannot be elicited. (Courtesy of Dr. H. F. Cuénoud, University of Massachusetts Medical School, Worcester, MA.)

Lung. Edema of the lung has a pathophysiology of its own. It can be transudative as well as exudative; its causes, besides heart failure, include infection, toxic agents, pure oxygen, and paradoxically, anoxia, as in high-altitude disease. Most of these agents damage the alveolar capillary, which becomes leaky and produces a protein-rich edema.

Physiologists have calculated that the edema safety factor in the lung is higher than in other tissues: 21 mm Hg, a reassuring fact, considering that pulmonary edema, unlike edema in most other organs, can be quickly fatal (14). Due to the large capacity of the lung's lymphatics and to the pumping action of respiratory movements, the efficiency of lymphatic drainage is very high and can increase tenfold in chronic edema. At first the edema fluid accumulates in the narrow space

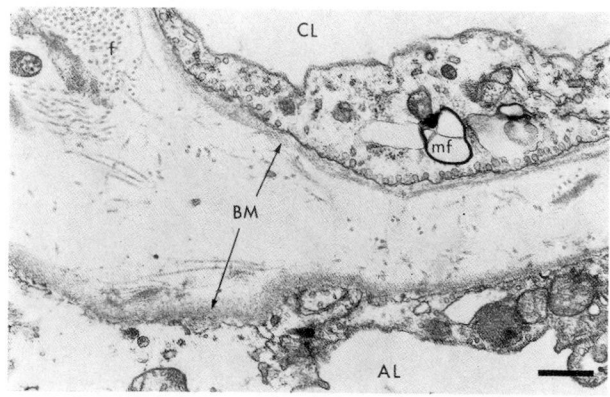

FIGURE 21.18 Electron micrograph: Edema of the alveolar wall, in the lung of a patient who had breathed oxygen at high concentration for 3 days (oxygen pneumonitis or respirator-lung syndrome). The basement membranes (**BM**), which are normally very close or in direct contact, are separated by edema. Note damage in the endothelium and epithelium. **CL:** Capillary lumen, **AL:** Alveolar lumen, **mf:** myelin figure. **Bar** = 1 μm. (Reproduced by permission from [11], © by The US & Canadian Academy of Pathology, Inc.)

between the capillary and the alveolar epithelium (interstitial edema) (Figure 21.18) (11); then it pours out into the alveolar space (alveolar edema). If the patient survives, the alveolar fluid may become secondarily infected from inhaled bacteria.

Pulmonary edema is visible by X-rays, because it replaces air with water, which is much more radio-opaque (Figure 21.19).

Cerebral edema. The brain has no lymphatic drainage and little room to expand within the skull. Thus, if it does swell, the increased volume of the brain produces dramatic shifts of tissue, with compression of blood vessels and distortion of vital centers. Parts of the brain may protrude (herniate) through several anatomical openings, such as the *foramen magnum* leading to the spinal cord. After head injury, acute cerebral edema develops almost immediately and can be lethal. Early symptoms include headache, nausea, and vomiting. Neuropathologists recognize many forms of cerebral edema (1), but for our purposes it suffices to mention two major mechanisms:

- *Intracellular edema* (also called cytotoxic edema), which is typically seen as a result of ischemia; this corresponds to the hypoxic cellular swelling already discussed (p. 203).
- *Vasogenic edema,* which is due to diffuse damage to the blood–brain barrier (e.g., after trauma or around focal lesions such as tumors or abscesses).

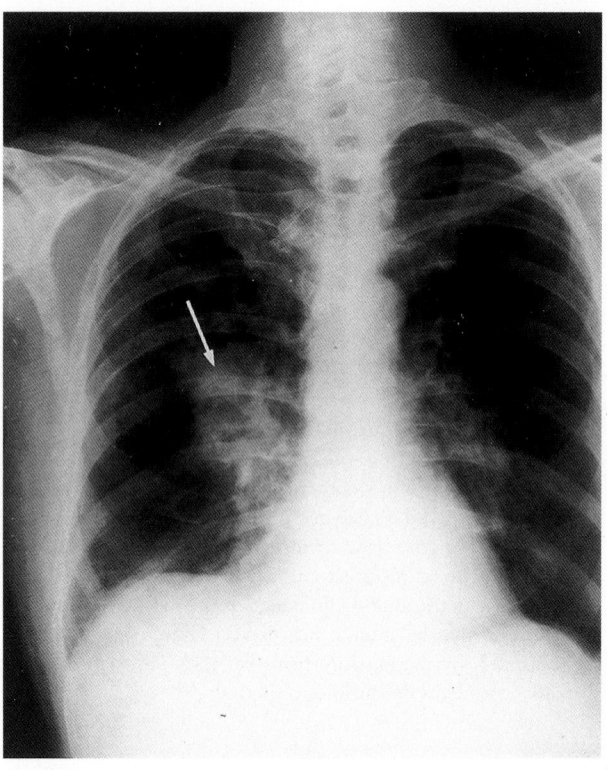

FIGURE 21.19 Arrow: a patch of pulmonary edema caused by high altitude, in the typical pattern of "cotton balls." A side effect of a lecture delivered at 14,000 feet in Cuzco, Peru.

The fluid accumulates mainly in the extracellular spaces of the white matter and can lead to myelin breakdown. Cerebral edema can be recognized by computerized tomography and by magnetic resonance imaging (MRI) even when mild, such as in early mountain sickness (22).

TO SUM UP: The principal actor in this chapter is the endothelium. In the early 1900s, it was not even certain that the endothelium existed, and if it did exist it could only be an inert semipermeable membrane. By the late 1900s, this dull, flat tissue had become a factory of mediators, cytokines, and growth factors, not to mention dozens of adhesion molecules that direct the traffic of lymphocytes in their normal travels and the recruiting of all leukocytes in inflammatory diseases, including—as we will see—atherosclerosis; tumors cannot grow if the endothelium does not supply capillaries, grafts will not take if the endothelium is not compatible, and blood will clot if the endothelium misbehaves. In other words, the endothelium has become a central issue in biology and medicine.

References

1. Adams JH, Corsellis JAN, Duchen LW, eds. Greenfield's neuropathology, 4th ed. New York: John Wiley & Sons, 1984.
2. Anderson RR, Parrish JA. The optics of human skin. J Invest Dermatol 1981;77:13–19.
3. Arroyo V, Bernardi M, Epstein M, et al. Pathophysiology of ascites and functional renal failure in cirrhosis. J Hepatol 1988;6:239–257.
4. Arroyo V, Ginés P, Planas R, Rodés J. Pathogenesis, diagnosis, and treatment of ascites in cirrhosis. In: Oxford textbook of clinical hepatology, Vol I, 2nd ed. Oxford: Oxford University Press, 1999, pp. 697–731.
5. Bäertsch P, Maggiorini M, Ritter M, et al. Prevention of high-altitude pulmonary edema by nifedipine. N Engl J Med 1991;325:1284–1289.
6. Binford CH, Connor DH, eds. Pathology of tropical and extraordinary diseases, vol 2. Washington, DC: Armed Forces Institute of Pathology, 1976.
7. Coleman SS. Lower limb length discrepancy. In: Lovell WW, Winter RB, eds. Pediatric orthopaedics, vol 2, 2nd ed. Philadelphia: JB Lippincott, 1986, pp. 781–863.
8. Edwards EA, Duntley SQ. The pigments and color of living human skin. Am J Anat 1939;65:1–33.
9. Ghitescu L, Fixman A, Simionescu M, Simionescu N. Specific binding sites for albumin restricted to plasmalemmal vesicles of continuous capillary endothelium: receptor-mediated transcytosis. J Cell Biol 1986;102:1304–1311.
10. Golden MHN, Golden BE, Jackson AA. Albumin and nutritional oedema. Lancet 1980;1:114–116.
11. Gould VE, Tosco R, Wheelis RF, Gould NS, Kapanci Y. Oxygen pneumonitis in man. Ultrastructural observations on the development of alveolar lesions. Lab Invest 1972;26:499–508.
12. Greenlee RT, Hill-Harmon MB, Murray T, Thun M. Cancer statistics, 2001. CA Cancer J Clin 2001;51:15–36.
13. Guyton AC. A concept of negative interstitial pressure based on pressure in implanted perforated capsules. Circ Res 1963; 12:399–414.
14. Guyton AC. Textbook of medical physiology, 7th ed. Philadelphia. WB Saunders, 1986.
15. Guyton AC, Armstrong GG, Crowell JW. Negative pressure in the interstitial spaces. Physiologist 1960;3:70.
16. Guyton AC, Granger HJ, Taylor AE. Interstitial fluid pressure. Physiol Rev 1971;51:527–563.
17. Henderson LJ. The fitness of the environment; an inquiry into the biological significance of the properties of matter. Boston: Beacon Press, 1958.
18. Johnson TS, Rock PB. Acute mountain sickness. N Engl J Med 1988;319:841–845.
19. Kinmonth JB. The lymphatics. London: Edward Arnold, 1982.
19a. Lammie PJ, Cuenco KT, Punkosdy GA. The pathogenesis of filarial lymphedema: is it the worm or is it the host? Ann NY Acad Sci 2002;979:131–142.
20. Landis EM, Jonas L, Angevine M, Erb W. The passage of fluid and protein through the human capillary wall during venous congestion. J Clin Invest 1932;11:717–734.

21. Leu HJ. Morphology of chronic venous insufficiency—light and electron microscopic examinations. VASA Band 1991;20:330–342.

22. Levine BD, Yoshimura K, Kobayashi T, et al. Dexamethasone in the treatment of acute mountain sickness. N Engl J Med 1989;321:1707–1713.

23. Lloyd-Jones D, Bloch KD. The vascular biology of nitric oxide and its role in atherogenesis. Annu Rev Med 1996;47:365–375.

24. Majno G. The capillary then and now: an overview of capillary pathology. Mod Pathol 1992;5:9–22.

25. McCullough FL. Skeletal trauma in children. Orthop Nurs 1989;8:41–46.

26. Meyers WM, Neafie RC, Connor DH. Bancroftian and Malayan filariasis. In: Binford CH, Connor DH, eds. Pathology of tropical and extraordinary diseases, vol 2. Washington, DC: Armed Forces Institute of Pathology, 1976, pp. 340–355.

27. Michel CC, Curry FE. Microvascular permeability. Physiol Rev 1999;79:703–716.

28. Nagy JA, Herzberg KT, Masse EM, Zientara GP, Dvorak HF. Exchange of macromolecules between plasma and peritoneal cavity in ascites tumor-bearing, normal, and serotonin-injected mice. Cancer Res 1989;49:5448–5458.

29. National Cancer Institute. Cancer statistics review 1973–1986. Washington, DC: US Department of Health and Human Services, National Institutes of Health, 1989.

30. Palade GE. The microvascular endothelium revisited. In: Simionescu N, Simionescu M, eds. Endothelial cell biology in health and disease. New York: Plenum Press, 1988, pp. 3–22.

31. Partsch H. Investigations on the pathogenesis of venous leg ulcers. Acta Chir Scand Suppl 1988;544:25–29.

32. Porta L. Delle Alterazioni Patologiche delle Arterie per la Legatura e la Torsione. Esperienze ed Osservazioni. Milano: Tipografia di Giuseppe Bernardoni di Gio, 1845.

32a. Razani B, Combs TP, Wang XB, et al. Caveolin-1-deficient mice are lean, resistant to diet-induced obesity, and show hypertriglyceridemia with adipocyte abnormalities. J Biol Chem 2002;277:8635–8647.

33. Renkin EM. Transport pathways and processes. In: Simionescu N, Simionescu M, eds. Endothelial cell biology in health and disease. New York: Plenum Press, 1988, pp. 51–68.

34. Rubanyi GM, Botelho LHP. Endothelins. FASEB J 1991;5:2713–2720.

35. Rubanyi GM, Dzau VJ. The endothelium in clinical practice: Source and target of novel therapies. New York: Marcel Dekker, 1997.

36. Ryan US. Endothelial cells, vol 1. Boca Raton, FL: CRC Press, 1988.

37. Sacks O. Migraine. Understanding a common disorder. Berkeley, CA: University of California Press, 1985.

38. Sandritter W, Thomas C. Histopathologie. Stuttgart: F.K. Schattauer Verlag, 1977.

39. Schaper W. Tangential wall stress as a molding force in the development of collateral vessels in the canine heart. Experientia 1967;23:595–596.

40. Schaper W, Sharma HS, Quinkler W, et al. Molecular biologic concepts of coronary anastomoses. J Am Coll Cardiol 1990;15:513–518.

41. Scheel KW, Fitzgerald EM, Martin RO, Larsen RA. The possible role of mechanical stresses on coronary collateral development during gradual coronary occlusion. A simulation study. In: Schaper W, ed. The pathophysiology of myocardial perfusion. Amsterdam: Elsevier/North-Holland Biomedical Press, 1979, pp. 489–518.

42. Scholander PF, Hargens AR, Miller SL. Negative pressure in the interstitial fluid of animals. Science 1968;161:321–328.

43. Simionescu M. Receptor-mediated transcytosis of plasma molecules by vascular endothelium. In: Simionescu N, Simionescu M, eds. Endothelial cell biology in health and disease. New York: Plenum Press, 1988, pp. 69–104.

44. Simionescu M, Ghitescu L, Fixman A, Simionescu N. How plasma macromolecules cross the endothelium. News Physiol Sci 1987;2:97–100.

45. Simionescu N. The microvascular endothelium: segmental differentiations, transcytosis, selective distribution of anionic sites. In: Weissmann S, Samuelson B, Paoletti R, eds. Advances in inflammation research, vol 1. New York: Raven Press, 1979, pp. 61–70.

46. Simionescu N, Simionescu M, eds. Endothelial cell biology in health and disease. New York: Plenum Press, 1988.

47. Simionescu N, Simionescu M, eds. Endothelial cell dysfunctions. New York: Plenum Press, 1992.

48. Simionescu N, Simionescu M, Palade GE. Structural basis of permeability in sequential segments of the microvasculature of the diaphragm. I. Bipolar microvascular fields. Microvasc Res 1978a;15:1–16.

49. Simionescu N, Simionescu M, Palade GE. Structural basis of permeability in sequential segments of the microvasculature of the diaphragm. II. Pathways followed by microperoxidase across the endothelium. Microvasc Res 1978b;15:17–36.

50. Tooke JE, Östergren J, Adamson U, Fagrell B. The effects of intravenous insulin infusion on skin microcirculatory flow in type 1 diabetes. Int J Microcirc Clin Exp 1985;4:69–83.

51. Tooke JE, Shore AC. The regulation of microvascular function in diabetes mellitus. In: Pickup JC, Williams G, eds. Textbook of diabetes, vol 2. Oxford: Blackwell Scientific Publications, 1991, pp. 546–553.

52. Vane JR, Änggård EE, Botting RM. Regulatory functions of the vascular endothelium. N Engl J Med 1990;323:27–36.

53. Vanscheidt W, Laaff H, Wokalek H, Niedner R, Schöpf E. Pericapillary fibrin cuff: a histological sign of venous leg ulceration. J Cutan Pathol 1990;17:226–268.

54. Williamson JR, Chang K, Frangos M, et al. Hyperglycemic pseudohypoxia and diabetic complications. Diabetes 1993;42:801–813.

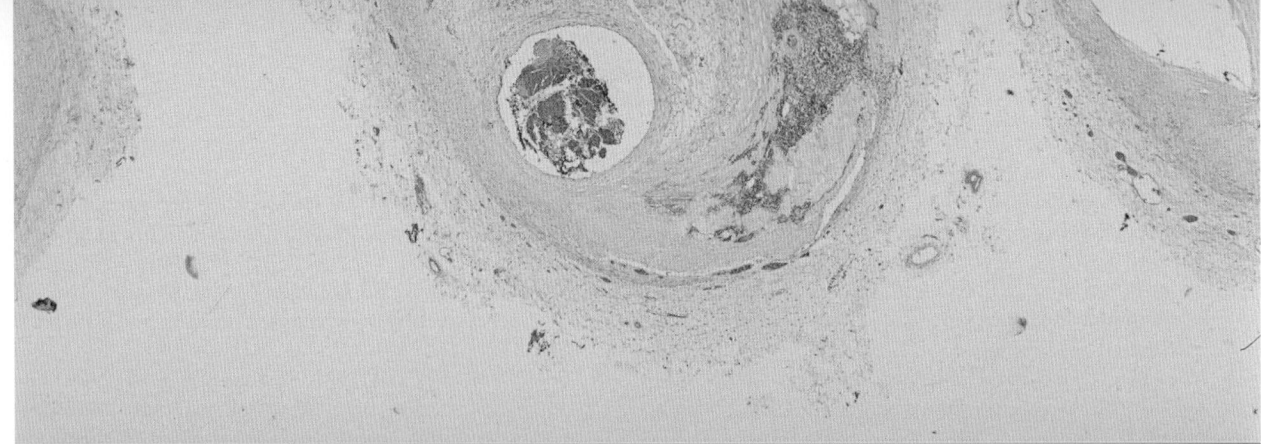

CHAPTER 22 HEMOSTASIS AND THROMBOSIS

Injury, as we mentioned earlier, creates three kinds of problems of different urgency: bleeding, infection, and destruction of tissues (see Figure 8.1). Nature counters with three processes: hemostasis, inflammation and regeneration. *Hemostasis* (*"stopping of blood"*) is the fastest: it has to act within seconds because blood is the essence of life. One of the hemostatic devices provided by evolution is clotting, a process by which blood becomes a solid mass as soon as it makes contact with connective tissue, *while remaining fluid in the container itself.* Now imagine the engineering problem of creating a fluid with these properties. To be effective, the clotting mechanism must be hair-triggered; but at the same time it must be kept from firing inappropriately because then the whole mass of circulating blood might clot. This feat is achieved by means of an intricate system of checks and balances in which clotting agents are controlled by inhibitors that are controlled by inhibitors of inhibitors—while a parallel system (fibrinolysis) destroys the clots as fast as they are forming. The intricacy of this system for Nature, and for those who attempt to understand it, is measured by the fact that the plasma concentration of control molecules, both anticlotting and antifibrinolysis, is much greater than that of the clotting factors (109). Again, because the system is so complicated it can misfire and create unwanted and dangerous intravascular solid or semi-solid masses called *thrombi.* Before we proceed any further, it is essential to learn the basic terminology of this field.

Basic Terminology

- **A clot** is the end-product of the activated clotting mechanism, which can operate *in vitro* as well as *in vivo.*

Blood clotting is based upon the appearance of a three-dimensional network of threads which imprisons the red blood cells. The threads are made of the protein *fibrin.* For blood to coagulate, the clotting system must be activated to produce the enzyme **thrombin,** which acts on **fibrinogen,** a plasma protein, thereby generating **fibrin.**

- A **thrombus** *is any solid object developing from the blood* IN VIVO *and within the vascular system.* This includes the same type of red clot that can be obtained *in vitro;* we will call such masses *red thrombi,* to emphasize that they were formed *in vivo* (p. 644).

- **Thrombosis** *includes more than clotting:* the "solid objects derived from the blood *in vivo*" include clumps of pure platelets, masses of fibrin, or mixtures of platelets and fibrin, which develop during hemostasis but not when whole blood coagulates

in a test tube. It may be helpful to remember that thrombosis has been defined as "*hemostasis in the wrong place*" (75).

- A **hematoma** is a mass of spilled blood that creates a swelling.
- An **ecchymosis** is a sheet of blood spilled in the tissues, without creating significant swelling.
- A **petechia** (pronounced pe-TEE-kia) is a tiny hemorrhage, 1–2 mm in diameter.
- **Blood spilled into a body cavity** (the pleura, the pericardium, the peritoneum, or a joint) gives rise to conditions known as **hemothorax, hemopericardium, hemoperitoneum,** and **hemarthrosis.**

Hemostasis: The Control of Bleeding

Let us assume that we sever a small artery (50–500 μm in diameter) in the omentum of a rat and follow what happens by light and electron microscopy (26, 48, 49, 63, 91). We will witness a three-step process (Figure 22.1):

1. *The severed artery contracts immediately*—not enough to stop the bleeding, but enough to lower the pressure downstream. (In severed veins this contraction is virtually absent, but it is also unnecessary, because venous blood pressure is much lower.) This response is important: in rabbits treated with an anticoagulant, hemostasis in a wound depends solely on vasoconstriction; bleeding abates but then resumes as soon as the vasoconstriction has worn off (26).

   Arterial constriction is probably due at first to trauma. Later it is reinforced or maintained by products of the platelets deposited on the mouth of the severed vessel, especially serotonin and thromboxane A_2.

2. *A plug of platelets develops at the mouth of the vessel and beyond* (49). As the hemorrhage continues, red blood cells stream by, but platelets stick to the traumatized part of the artery and to the connective tissue outside it. This creates a fragile but quickly growing *platelet plug,* which may become thick enough to occlude the vessel and contain the bleeding (Figure 22.2). At this stage the plug consists almost entirely of platelets. Although a few fibrin filaments begin to develop on the surface of the platelet plug, they are still too thin to stabilize the mass (117). This is the *primary hemostatic plug;* it forms within seconds and minutes after the trauma (16, 58, 105).

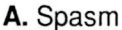

A. Spasm

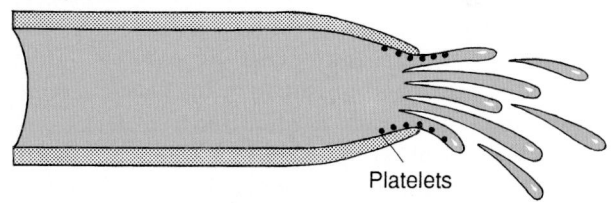

Platelets

B. Primary plug

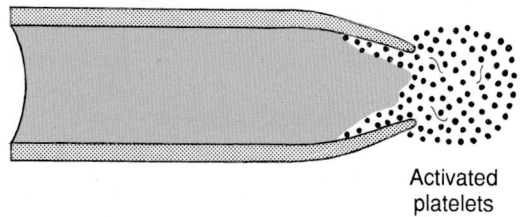

Activated platelets

C. Secondary plug

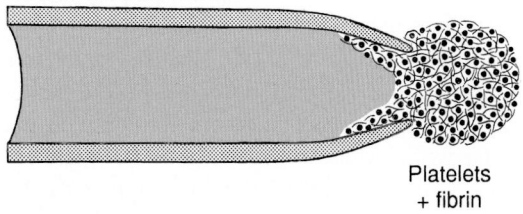

Platelets + fibrin

FIGURE 22.1 The three steps of hemostasis in a small artery that has just been severed. The entire sequence occurs in a few minutes.

FIGURE 22.2 Hemostatic plug from a severed enteric artery of a dog; electron micrographs. The sites from which the sections were taken are shown in the diagrams of the plug in the upper left-hand corners. **A:** Severed artery. **H:** Hemostatic plug. *Top:* This part of the plug consists of packed platelets. *Bottom:* At the periphery of the plug the platelets in contact with collagen are swollen and degranulated. The small dark patches represent fibrin. **Bars** = 0.5 μm. (Reproduced with permission from [91].)

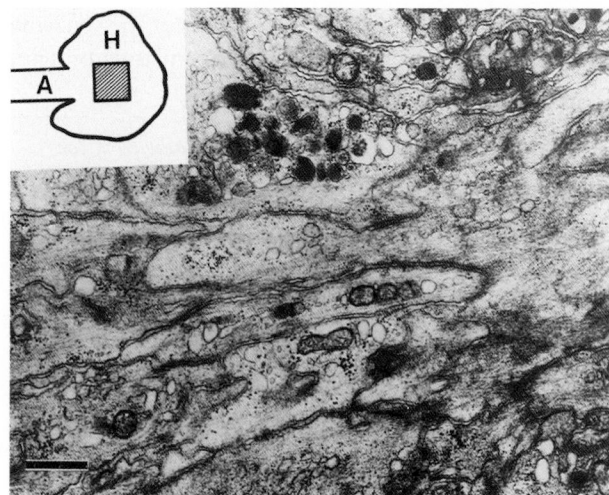

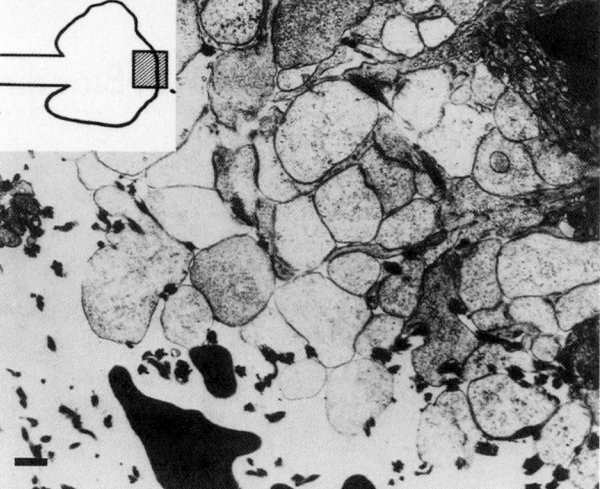

3. *Fibrin filaments stabilize the platelet plug and the mass of red blood cells in the tissues beyond it.* The crumbly platelet plug is now reinforced by a network of fibrin and becomes a *secondary hemostatic plug.* In human volunteers this stage was reached at 30 minutes (117). The emergency is over.

From this point on the stage is set for a process similar to wound healing: this secondary hemostatic plug is destined to be organized, that is, slowly reabsorbed and replaced by granulation tissue, and eventually by a tiny scar. The fibrin, blood cells and debris are cleared away by macrophages.

All three steps of hemostasis are essential (109), especially steps 2 and 3. Patients with platelet counts below 10,000 or with nonfunctional platelets lack step 2, the pure platelet plug. Hemophiliacs lack step 3; they have normal platelets but impaired blood clotting and therefore cannot produce fibrin.

This overview of hemostasis taught us that three actors are involved in hemostasis: the platelet, the process of blood clotting, and the vascular wall. We will now consider each in some detail.

The Platelet in Hemostasis

Considering that platelets are just flat little discs a micron or two in diameter and without a nucleus, they are extraordinarily complex (Figure 22.3). Normal platelets are stiff and do not stick, but their secret is that they can be activated within seconds to an almost explosive performance, which includes becoming sticky and helping the blood to clot (Figure 22.4). Platelet activators include, first of all, *collagen surfaces*—which makes sense because injury brings platelets in contact with the extravascular world where collagen abounds. There are also soluble activators: *thrombin,* which signals to the platelets that the clotting sequence is activated; adenosine diphosphate (*ADP*), which is released by activated platelets and injured red cells and helps amplify the platelet response; *epinephrine;* and some *prostaglandins.*

Fully activated platelets swell into sticky, branching spheres and die (63). This process depends on the coordinated action of membrane, granules, and cytoskeleton; it can be subdivided somewhat artificially into four phases, which tend to overlap:

1. Adhesion (to other surfaces)
2. Aggregation (with other platelets)
3. Swelling
4. Secretion

The first part of the activation program, adhesion and early aggregation, is reversible; the subsequent steps are not. Platelet response varies somewhat depending on the stimulus, but ADP causes platelets to swell maximally in 5–10 seconds (63).

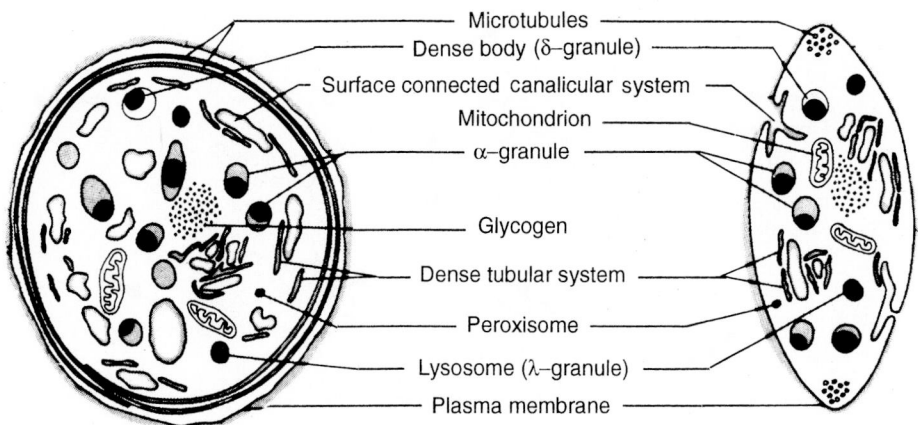

FIGURE 22.3 Diagram of a human platelet (face and profile) showing components visible by electron microscopy and cytochemistry. (Reproduced with permission from [14].)

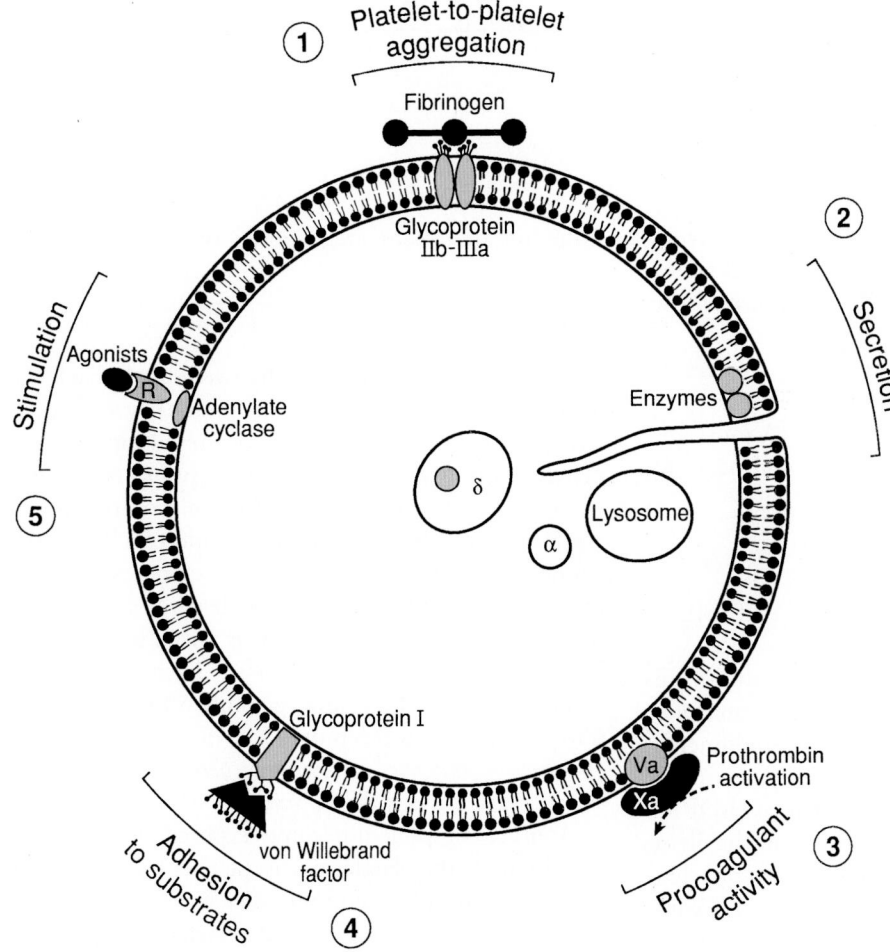

FIGURE 22.4 Platelets, small as they are, are equipped to perform at least five functions: (1) Binding to fibrinogen, which acts as a glue with other platelets (*aggregation*). (2) *Secretion* originates from the membrane (enzymatic production of thromboxane) as well as by extrusion of granule contents through the canalicular system. (3) *Prothrombin activation,* a key step in the clotting mechanism. (4) *Adhesion to nonplatelet surfaces,* by means of specific receptors for von Willebrand factor. (5) *Stimulation by agonists,* such as thrombin, epinephrine, or ADP which lead to aggregation and secretion. (Adapted with permission from [111].)

Adhesion

Adhesion refers to the sticking of platelets to certain tissue surfaces, not to each other (95). Platelets do not stick except fleetingly to normal endothelium, and it is uncertain whether they will stick to it if it is injured.

However, they are equipped with ligands that make them stick instantly to subendothelium: that is, to the basement membrane or the collagenous tissue that is exposed if the endothelium is removed. Some of these ligands are specific for molecules of von Willebrand

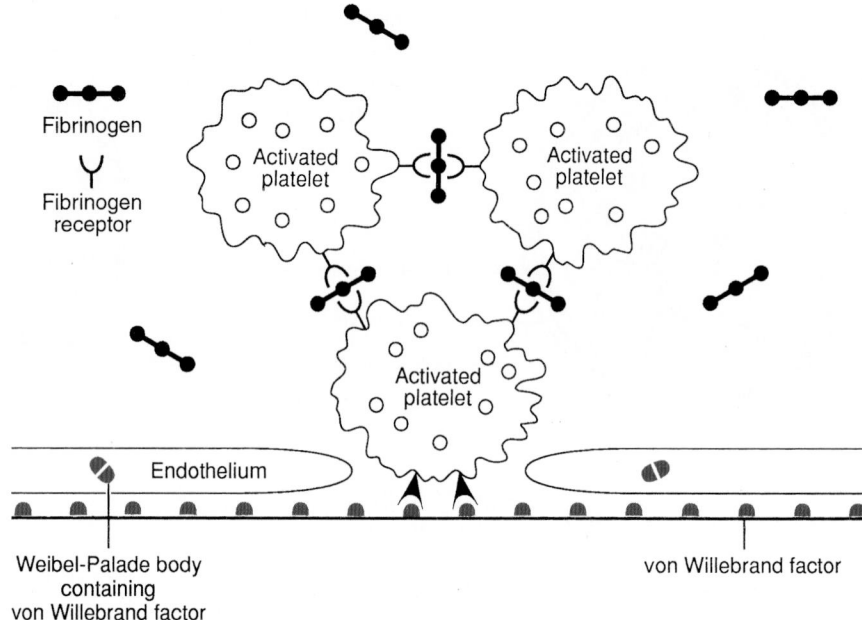

factor (vWF) adsorbed to the subendothelial structures (Figure 22.5). Recall that von Willebrand factor is concentrated in the Weibel–Palade bodies of the endothelium; endothelial cells secrete some of it toward their basement membrane (100), where it becomes bound to collagen, ready to attract a layer of platelets in case of endothelial damage. Almost instantly after adhesion the platelets spread and begin to degranulate.

Aggregation

Aggregation is the sticking of platelets to each other; this is how a hemostatic plug grows.

It has been very instructive to study aggregation with the aggregometer, proposed by the British pharmacologist G. V. R. Born (18). This is actually a turbidometer. A ray of light is passed through a suspension of platelets, and an aggregating agent such as ADP is added to the suspension. The intensity of the light transmitted by the suspension increases as platelets aggregate. On the same principle, fog seen out of a window is opaque, rain is not (63). With a low dose of ADP the aggregation is reversible, and with a higher dose the aggregation curve is biphasic. That is, the first wave of aggregation is caused by the added ADP, the second by the ADP released by the aggregating platelets themselves (Figure 22.6).

Depending on the activator, aggregating platelets change shape and turn into spiny or hairy little spheres.

Adhesion molecules are exposed on their threadlike extensions.

Swelling

Seen by electron microscopy the swelling of platelets is obvious (Figure 22.2). As the membrane is stretched, its charges spread out, decreasing the repulsion between platelets, and *fibrinogen* adhesion receptors are exposed. These receptors consist of a pair of glycoproteins and are known by the inconvenient name of GP-IIb-IIIa complex (Figure 22.4) (99). This complex (on one platelet) seizes a fibrinogen molecule while another part of the same fibrinogen molecule is seized by a GP-IIb-IIIa complex of another platelet. Each platelet has about 50,000 of these sites, possibly a record concentration of adhesion receptors (30). In essence, *the main glue among platelets is fibrinogen; between platelets and endothelium it is von Willebrand factor* (Figure 22.5).

Another component becomes exposed on the platelet membrane as the platelet swells: platelet factor 3 (PF3), which is a phospholipid that takes part in the clotting mechanism. Now the activated platelet is helping the clotting sequence, which produces thrombin, which in turn activates more platelets.

Secretion

Finally, the cytoskeleton of the platelet gathers itself into a "noose"—or rather, a basket that tightens around a cluster of granules in the center of the platelet. As a

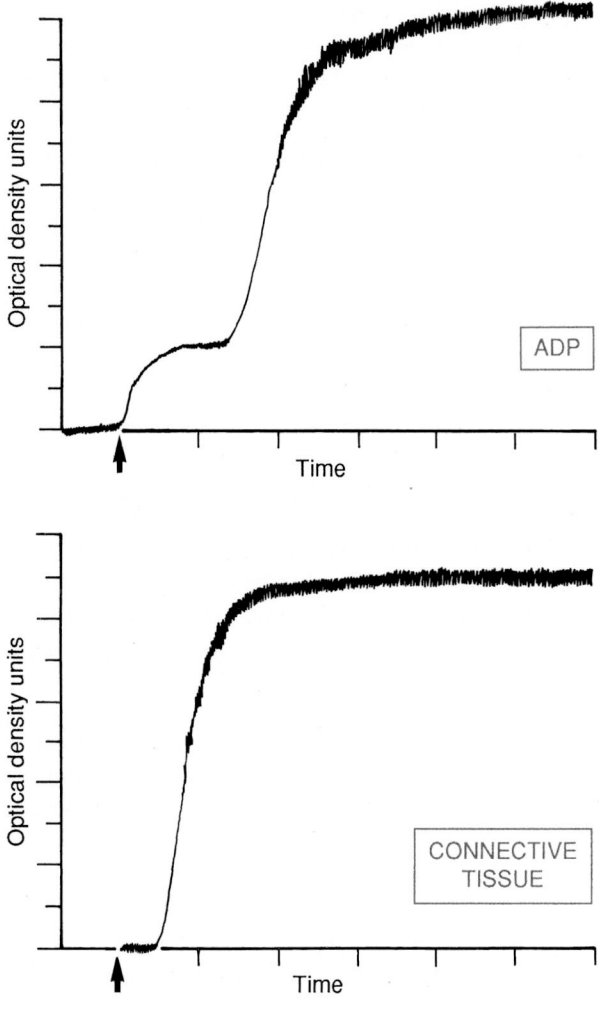

result, the content of the granules is squeezed out through the tubular system. The alpha granules contribute, among much else, two factors that help clotting: some ready-made fibrinogen (which will add to the fibrin ultimately produced by the clotting cascade) and an anti-anticoagulant, namely platelet factor 4. *Delta granules* (delta for *dense,* see Figure 22.3) release ADP, which activates more platelets.

In addition, the dying platelet manages, in its last gasp, to actively synthesize and secrete an arachidonic acid metabolite: *thromboxane* A_2, a powerful aggregator of platelets.

In the context of a hemostatic plug, these latest events help the plug to grow. Both ADP and thromboxane A_2 induce aggregation and thereby recruit more platelets; the secretion of fibrinogen and the assistance given to clotting by platelet factor 3 make sure that fibrin filaments appear right inside the plug, where they are needed for mechanical strengthening, rather than in the extracellular spaces at random.

Such is the story of the *platelet plug* in the hemostatic process. Now we can examine another major contributor to the hemostatic process: the blood clotting mechanism.

The Clotting Mechanism

Like the complement system, clotting is a system of fine-tuned checks and balances. We will sketch the essentials; specialized textbooks (31, 63) will satisfy any further appetite.

In clotting, the blood is stiffened into a solid mass by a three-dimensional network of fibrin (see Figure 9.31), which derives from a circulating precursor, fibrinogen. The basic purpose of the clotting cascade is to produce fibrin. Each unit of the fibrin polymer is a fibrinogen molecule from which four short peptides have been cleaved (Figure 9.32) (p. 360); the enzyme responsible for the cleaving is thrombin. Therefore, the basic reaction of the clotting system is

$$\text{Fibrinogen} \xrightarrow{\text{thrombin}} \text{fibrin}$$

Obviously, thrombin cannot circulate in its active state or blood would be a solid. The critical point, then, is how to activate thrombin. This is achieved by an array of circulating molecules that are numbered from I to XIII (in the order of discovery, not in the order of function: experts have no pity for the outsiders). Most of these molecules were identified in patients who congenitally lacked one or another. Most but not all are proenzymes, which must be activated; each proenzyme activates the next and amplifies the effect, much as happens with the complement system. This is why the coagulation mechanism is also referred to as a cascade. (We will just comment that the term *cascade,* "waterfall," is not very proper; no waterfall becomes thousands of times larger as it plunges.)

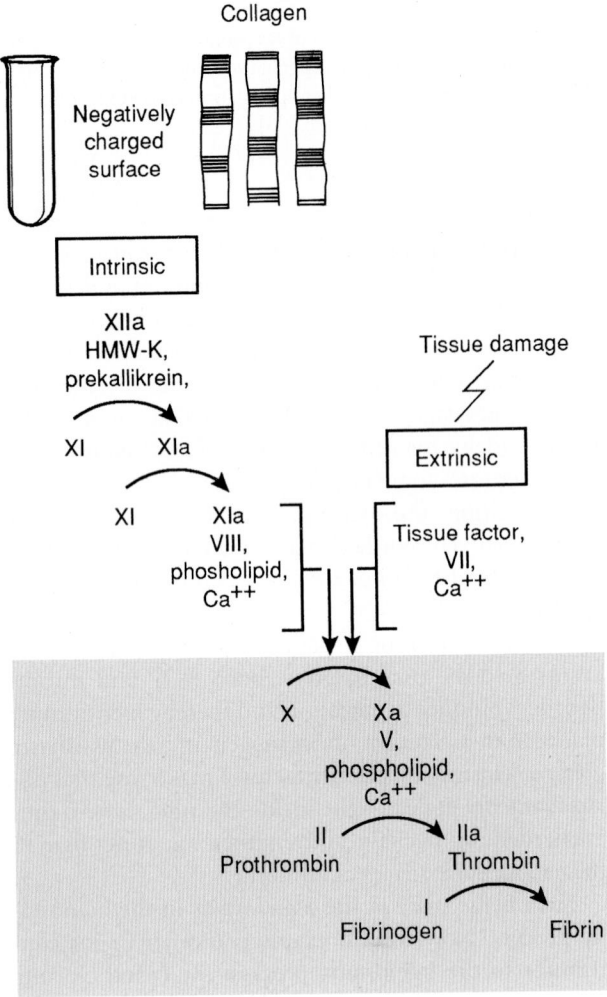

Collagen

Negatively charged surface

Intrinsic

XIIa
HMW-K,
prekallikrein,

XI   XIa

XI   XIa
          VIII,
          phospholipid,
          Ca++

Tissue damage

Extrinsic

Tissue factor,
VII,
Ca++

X   Xa
         V,
         phospholipid,
         Ca++

II   IIa
Prothrombin   Thrombin

I
Fibrinogen   Fibrin

FIGURE 22.7   The coagulation cascade. The intrinsic and extrinsic pathways meet at the level of factor X.

A simplified version of the clotting cascade, Figure 22.7, shows the following characteristics:

- *Clotting occurs by either of two converging pathways;* note the analogy with activation of the complement system.
- *Besides the clotting factors there are some cofactors, notably phospholipids and calcium.* The phospholipids act as surfaces. The advantage of assembling the reagents on a surface, as usual, is to favor the reaction by concentrating and positioning the reagents. An example: to produce thrombin (factor IIa) factors Va and Xa attach to a special domain on the surface of an activated platelet (Figure 22.8). In this favorable position and with the help of calcium, factor X can activate in 2 minutes the amount of prothrombin that it could activate in 1 year if it were floating free (63).

Just for comparison: the complement cascade has no lipid factors, but it uses the "surface trick" from the very start: C1 becomes attached to the surface of the cell destined to be perforated (p. 354).

At several steps there are feedback loops that either inhibit or accelerate the reaction. This maddening complication is part of the essential fine tuning of the clotting/anticlotting balance.

Blood can clot also in the absence of platelets, but not as well. The surface of activated platelets exposes a lipid domain, platelet factor 3, that greatly accelerates the clotting process (it intervenes at two steps of the cascade). If platelet-rich-plasma is allowed to clot and examined by scanning electron microscopy, filaments of fibrin seem to emerge from platelet clumps (Figure 22.9). Macrophages can also act as centers of fibrin formation, by means of fibrin receptors on their plasma membrane (Figure 22.10). Modern photographs of this event are virtually identical to the drawing published in 1882 by Bizzozero, in the paper that first proposed the name *platelet* (Figure 22.11).

Why are there two pathways for clotting? It is important to realize that the two pathways were discovered and defined *in vitro*. Early studies showed that blood clotting could be triggered experimentally in two ways: (a) By pouring the blood into a glass container. It turned out that the property of the glass responsible for this effect was its negative surface charge; other surfaces with that property would have the same effect, including collagen. (b) By mixing blood with tissue extracts. These extracts contained a clotting "tissue factor," later identified as thromboplastin. When the entire clotting sequence was worked out, it became apparent that the two clotting mechanisms set in motion different clotting factors, leading to chain reactions that converge at the level of factor X (Figure 22.7).

It is traditional to point out that the longer pathway, activated by negative surfaces, functions with factors that are contained in the blood: hence its name, *intrinsic pathway*. The shorter pathway needs an extra "tissue factor" supplied from outside; hence it is called the *extrinsic pathway*. But this distinction is not sharp at all. For instance, the typical activator of the extrinsic mechanism—the complex [thromboplastin + factor VII]—also activates factor IX of the intrinsic pathway.

How are the two pathways triggered in vivo? The intrinsic pathway requires a negatively charged surface, a condition that can be fulfilled without breaking open any vessel if the endothelium is lost by trauma or some other mechanism. The subendothelium is strongly

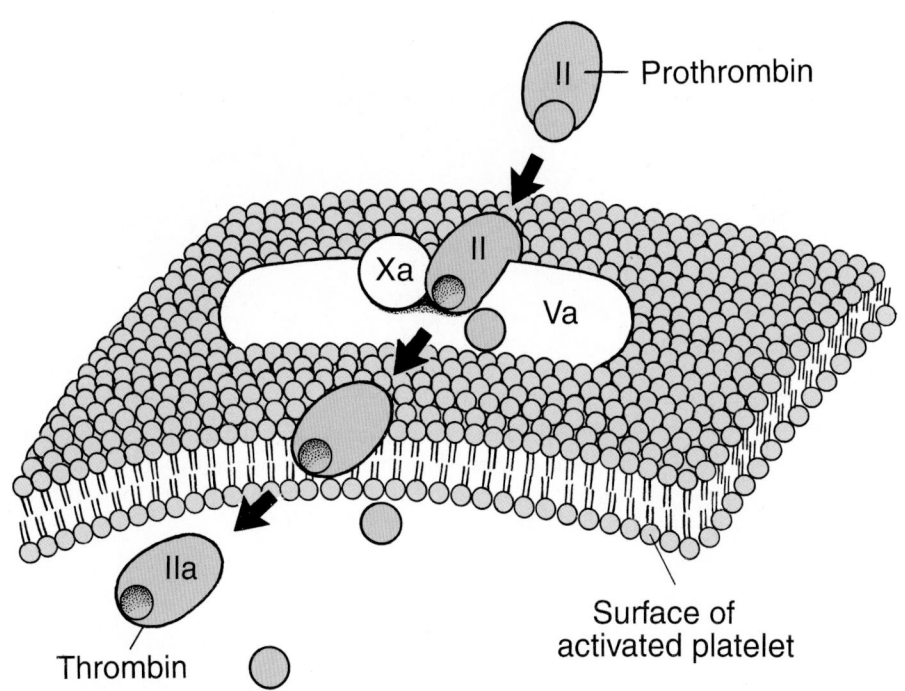

FIGURE 22.8 A critical step near the end of the clotting cascade: activation of prothrombin to thrombin. This reaction is greatly accelerated by the surface of activated platelets, which holds in place the activating complex formed by Xa and Va. (Adapted with permission from [93].)

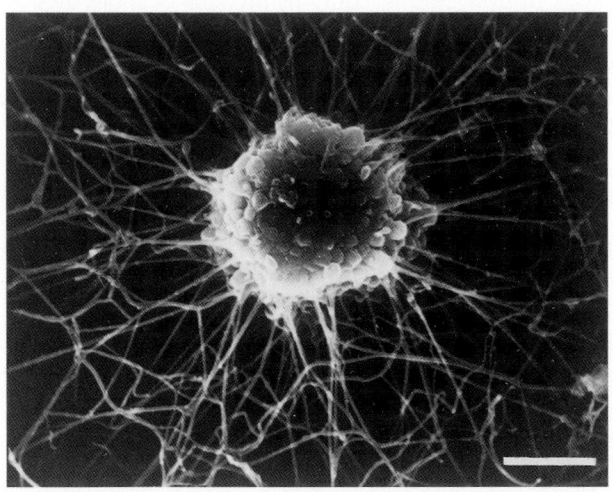

FIGURE 22.9 Clot developing *in vitro* from platelet-rich plasma (scanning electron micrograph). A cluster of platelets appears to be tugging at the surrounding network of fibrin. **Bar** = 5 μm. (Reproduced from [13] by permission from Elsevier Science Publishers.)

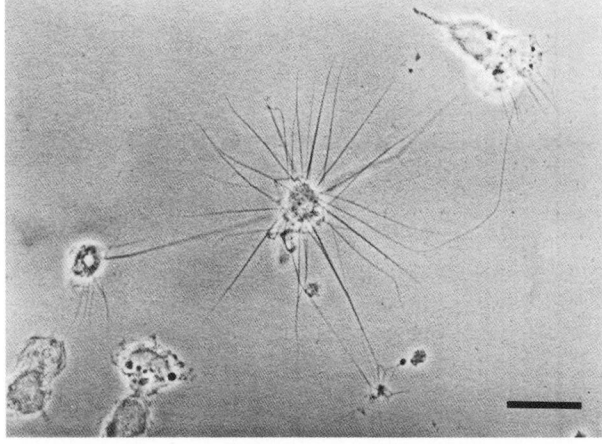

FIGURE 22.10 Needles of fibrin arising from the surface of cultured human monocytes after 10 minutes of incubation with plasma. Receptors for fibrin and fibrinogen are present on the surface of monocytes. Phase microscopy. **Bar** = 10 μm. (Reproduced from the **Journal of Experimental Medicine** 1983;157:473–485, by copyright permission of The Rockefeller University Press [60].)

thrombogenic, thanks especially to its collagen fibers and to the basement membrane, although not everybody agrees about the latter (68). It follows that the Hageman factor (factor XII) becomes fixed and activated on de-endothelialized surfaces.

If blood is spilled out of the vessels, which is by far the most common situation, the extrinsic pathway is triggered by injured cells, which release thromboplastin; while the Hageman factor operates alongside, being activated by collagen.

Thromboplastin (tissue factor) is a membrane-spanning protein; some tissues produce it constitutively (fibroblasts, smooth muscle cells, cardiac valve stromal cells, placental

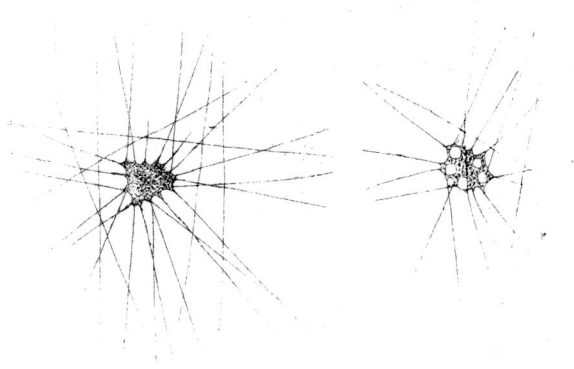

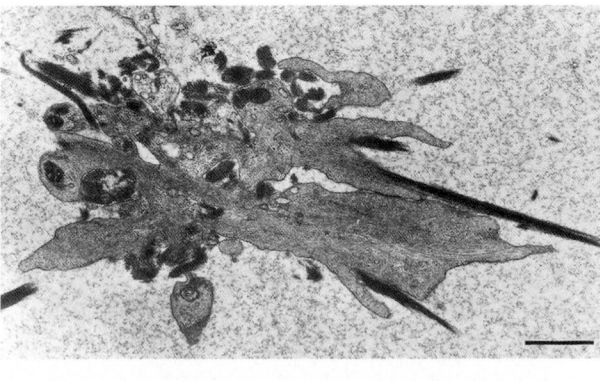

FIGURE 22.11   Role of platelets in coagulation as illustrated by G. Bizzozero in 1882. Dog blood examined for 2–3 minutes: platelets have aggregated into clumps from which radiate fine filaments of fibrin. (Reproduced from [16].)

FIGURE 22.12   Platelet during clot formation (electron micrograph). The dark filaments of fibrin appear to be firmly attached to the platelet. **Bar** = 1 μm. (Reproduced from [13] by permission from Elsevier Science Publishers.)

trophoblast, probably brain), some produce it if properly stimulated (endothelium, monocytes, and macrophages, stimulated for example by endotoxin), and some produce little or none (lymphocytes, neutrophils) (6, 39, 92). Thromboplastin is present in high concentration in the brain, perhaps because in this organ even the slightest hemorrhage can be hazardous (38). Histochemistry shows thromboplastin in many extravascular cells, especially in the outer vascular coat (adventitia)—as if constituting a hemostatic envelope ready to activate clotting (38).

How do the two pathways share the job in vivo? There is much evidence that they always operate together. Indeed, bleeding disorders develop in patients deficient with regard to one or the other pathway (63).

Given that the two pathways, *in vivo,* work in unison, we do not know if either one contributes differently from the other in any particular situation. The extrinsic pathway is shorter and may be slightly faster; perhaps it is called upon when the blood mixes with a great deal of crushed tissue that supplies tissue factor. Note the *difference between the two pathways of clotting and the two pathways of complement;* those of complement really have two separate functions. The alternative pathway offers the advantage of killing bacteria in the absence of antibody (p. 356).

Retraction of the Clot-Oozing Serum

After a clot forms, it contracts (contraction and retraction in this context mean the same thing). This amazing phenomenon, also called **syneresis,** is easily observed *in vitro.* If you pour fresh blood into a test tube, it will clot; and within about 2 hours the red mass will shrink while oozing out a yellowish fluid called **serum** (see Figure 15.5).

NOTE: Do not confuse serum with plasma. *Plasma is a physiologic fluid; serum is not:* it has lost its fibrinogen and contains myriads of molecules released during clotting.

The clotted red mass shrinks to about half its original volume; it cannot shrink further because red blood cells take up almost half of the total blood volume. In contrast, if plasma that contains platelets is poured into a test tube, it will form a diffuse whitish clot, which will shrink to about one-tenth of the fluid volume. *In the absence of platelets, the plasma will clot but not contract.*

These experiments tell us that retraction must have something to do with platelets. It does: electron microscopy has shown that while platelets are dying they cling to the filaments of fibrin by their membrane receptors, and their inner actin–myosin system keeps pulling (Figure 22.12) (29).

The mechanism of clot contraction is basically the same as in muscle contraction; in fact, a blood clot shaped like a strip can be made to respond *in vitro* very much like smooth muscle (76). There is a puzzle, however. Although the contractile mechanism is based on actin–myosin as in muscle, no known muscle can contract to one-tenth of its original length. Perhaps the platelets twist the filaments around themselves (Figure 22.13) (89), but we are more inclined to believe in a hand-over-hand type of pull such as we have described for fibroblasts (p. 488) (13). As a matter of fact, platelets can be replaced by fibroblasts for inducing the retraction of the fibrin clot (94).

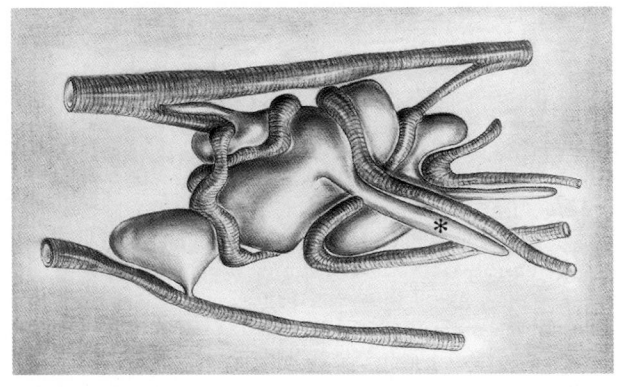

FIGURE 22.13 Reconstruction, from serial sections, of platelet–fibrin contacts during clot retraction. This electron microscopic image suggests that clot retraction may occur by shortening platelet pseudopodia (**asterisk**) and by adhesion of twisted fibrin filaments to the body of the contracting platelet. (Reprinted with permission from [89], Copyright 1984, with permission from Elsevier.)

An Odd Alliance: The Clotting–Kinin Connection

What is the purpose of clot retraction? Common sense suggests that retraction may toughen the hemostatic plug by squeezing out fluid; it might conceivably help in pulling together the sides of small wounds, but firm evidence is lacking (102).

> There is an experiment of Nature in this regard: rare individuals are born with platelets that lack receptors for fibrinogen (Glanzmann's thrombasthenia, which means "platelet weakness"). Clot retraction is impaired, and the patients do suffer from bleeding disorders and prolonged bleeding after surgery (63).

An Odd Alliance: The Clotting–Kinin Connection

In describing the mediators of inflammation, we mentioned a blood-borne kinin precursor that binds to negative surfaces just like the Hageman factor does: high molecular weight kininogen (HMWK, p. 351). Therefore, when a negatively charged surface is exposed to plasma, two types of molecules will attach to it: Hageman factor and HMWK (Figure 9.23). The point of this peculiar association becomes obvious when we learn that HMWK floats around in plasma loosely bound to two other molecules. One is factor XI of the clotting system, precisely the molecule that the Hageman factor is supposed to activate: so HMWK very helpfully delivers substrate to the Hageman factor. The other molecule that is bound to HMWK is prekallikrein; this is the precursor of kallikrein, the enzyme that HMWK needs for cleaving kinins. The result is that we have Hageman factor and prekallikrein side by side, and they are programmed to activate each other with a double effect: the clotting cascade is activated and kinins are released.

We still need to explain why Nature has chosen to combine these two functions, clotting and kinin generation. Kinins do not clot blood; they are inflammatory mediators. As such they are potent stimulators of smooth muscle, including the medial smooth muscle of severed arteries. We therefore venture to guess that the two molecules delivered by HMWK carry a double message to the Hageman factor: "clot the blood, but also turn off the spouts."

> *A Hageman puzzle.* For readers with strong nerves, here is a puzzling but interesting fact. It is dogma that the Hageman factor (factor XII) triggers the intrinsic pathway, together with the kinin and fibrinolytic cascades. This factor was named after a gentleman who lacked it: Mr. John Hageman, a railroad brakeman whose bleeding time was unusually long but who was otherwise asymptomatic (102). Besides the puzzling fact that he did not suffer from spontaneous bleeding problems, Mr. Hageman confused posterity by dying of thromboemboli (103), thereby proving that his intrinsic clotting cascade was functional. Clearly, besides the Hageman factor, there must be some other way to trigger the intrinsic mechanism *in vivo*. One possibility: the surfaces of activated platelets activate factor XI independently of the Hageman factor (63).

Factors that Oppose Clotting

Clotting is potentially dangerous. Here are some of the mechanisms that tend to limit it (Table 22.1).

- *Dilution of clotting factors by blood flow* is the most important. Consider a successful hemostatic plug;

Table 22.1 Natural Plasma Inhibitors of Coagulation (*) and Fibrinolysis

Inhibitors	Normal Plasma Concentration (mg/dL)	Major Enzymes Inhibited	Hereditary Deficiency States
*Antithrombin III (heparin cofactor)	18–30	Factor IX_a, factor X_a, thrombin	Thrombosis
*Protein C	0.4	Factor Va_1, factor VIII_a	Thrombosis
α-Macroglobulin	150–350	Kallikrein, thrombin, plasmin	?
α_1-Antitrypsin	200–400	Factor X, elastase	Pulmonary emphysema
α_2-Plasmin inhibitor (α_2-antiplasmin)	5–7	Plasmin	Bleeding tendency
C1 inactivator (C1 esterase inhibitor)	15–35	Factor XII_a, factor XII, kallikrein	Hereditary angioneurotic edema

Adapted from (32) and (109).

the clotting mechanism has worked, but some mechanism must stop the plug from growing to fill the entire vascular system. Local blood flow does this by washing away and diluting the clotting factors, which are eventually removed by the liver and other provinces of the RES (p. 315).

- *Natural anticoagulants,* namely factors that oppose the formation of fibrin, in contrast with others that destroy it after it has formed (fibrinolysis; see later). Understandably, these anticlotting agents are designed to be especially effective on the surface of the endothelium, which must be protected from being embroiled in clotting. The major anticoagulants are antithrombin III and proteins C and S. Their story is complex but important: individuals who lack one or the other suffer from episodes of thrombosis. We will briefly describe these two anticoagulants as an example of Nature's complex ways.

Antithrombin III (AT III), also called heparin cofactor, is made by the endothelium, the liver, and megakaryocytes. In contact with heparin, or with heparinlike molecules such as those that coat the endothelium, AT III becomes 1000 times more effective, blocking thrombin as well as four other activated clotting factors (Figure 22.14). Antithrombin III has its own opponents: platelet factor 4 (not surprising because platelets on the whole favor coagulation) and three adhesive proteins that bind heparin (von Willebrand factor, thrombospondin, and laminin).

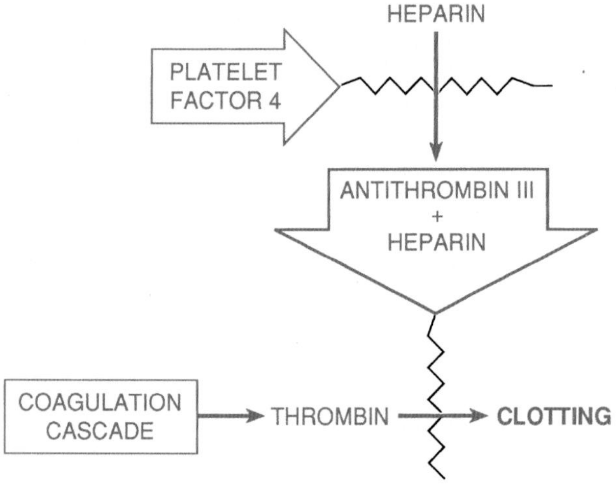

> NOTE: **Heparin,** a proteoglycan, is extensively used for therapeutic purposes; but whether it is present in normal plasma is not certain (20). It is the major constituent of mast cell granules, and it is released during degranulation (p. 343). Its molecular size and properties vary a great deal in different preparations. For our purposes it is important to remember that, in the clotting process, the "heparinlike" molecules on the surface of the endothelium (heparan sulfate) behave like heparin.

Protein C is a proenzyme that circulates, waiting for its chance; this comes when thrombin hits the endothelial surface and is bound by thrombomodulin. The complex (thrombomodulin + thrombin) activates protein C, which selectively inactivates factors V and VIII (Figure 22.15) (7, 28, 45) whereby the generation of thrombin is reduced. **Protein S** (for Seattle) is made by the endothelium and modulates the process.

Fibrinolysis

Fibrin is a precious stop-gap material, but it is never there to stay. It has a built-in, short-term obsolescence. Macrophages recognize it as something to eliminate and break it down. It is also destroyed by free-floating enzymes: this is fibrinolysis. Interestingly, the split products of fibrin inhibit blood clotting.

The simplest way to demonstrate fibrinolysis is to let some blood stand in a test tube at room temperature: within minutes it clots; within a couple of hours the

FIGURE 22.14 Inhibition of thrombin generated by the coagulation cascade. "Heparin" combines with antithrombin III to oppose the clotting effect of thrombin ("heparin" includes heparin-like molecules bound to the surface of the endothelium). Note that thrombin has an ally in platelet factor 4 (released by stimulated platelets), which prevents heparin from combining with antithrombin III. (Adapted with permission from [98].)

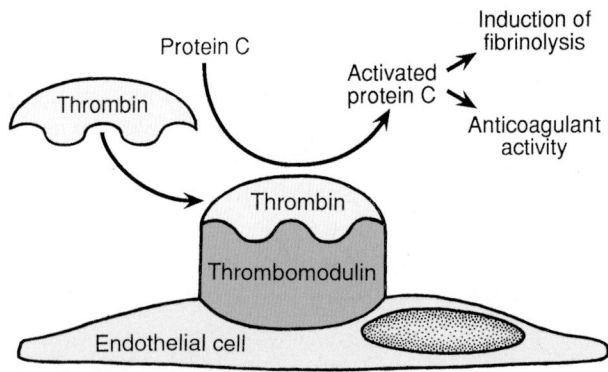

FIGURE 22.15 Contributions of the endothelium to anticlotting mechanisms. Thrombin is inactivated by binding to thrombomodulin; the complex then activates protein C, which initiates both anticoagulation and fibrinolysis. (Adapted from the **Journal of Clinical Investigation,** 1 70:127–134, by copyright permission of the American Society for Clinical Investigation via Copyright Clearance Center [33].)

clot retracts, and by the end of the day it dissolves and becomes unclottable. The same sequence occurs in the blood vessels after death.

"Animals who are run very hard, and killed in such a state, have not . . . their blood coagulated; and the effect . . . is in proportion to the cause" (69). So wrote John Hunter in 1794, in his famous treatise *On the Blood, Inflammation, and Gun-shot Wounds*. It is now well-established that the fibrinolytic activity of plasma is increased by exercise (122); perhaps this is related to the beneficial effect of exercise in decreasing the risk of coronary thrombosis. Fibrinolysis is also increased in venous blood when flow is sluggish, another logical arrangement. For these effects we must be grateful, as we will see, to the endothelium.

NOTE: The stress of surgery also increases fibrinolysis, but after surgery fibrinolytic activity drops and remains low for 7–10 days (fibrinolytic shutdown [63]); this coincides with the increased postoperative risk of thrombosis and of peritoneal adhesions (p. 451).

The enzyme responsible for fibrinolysis is **plasmin**, a very active serine protease that is also capable of hydrolyzing many other substrates. Plasmin circulates as an inactive precursor, plasminogen (a liver product), together with its activator (tissue plasminogen activator, tPA), which is also inactive. tPA is synthesized by a number of cells, including the endothelium.

Plasminogen must be activated. In the blood-stream this happens automatically, and most conveniently, when tPA attaches to fibrin filaments, where it also finds its substrate: both plasminogen and its activator have a high affinity for fibrin (Figure 22.16). Another mechanism for activating plasminogen is the Hageman factor, which switches on the two opposing processes: clotting and fibrinolysis.

Plasminogen activator (tPA) is secreted by the endothelium, especially and very appropriately under conditions of sluggish flow; it is released from a complex with tPA-inhibitor (63). Other cell types also produce tPA:

- *Mesothelial cells and activated macrophages* (25, 73); this is important for dissolving fibrinous adhesions in the inflamed peritoneum and pleura (108).
- *The lining of the uterus.*
- *Many malignant tumors,* which may also do the opposite, that is, secrete clotting factors.

ACTORS | SEQUENCE OF EVENTS

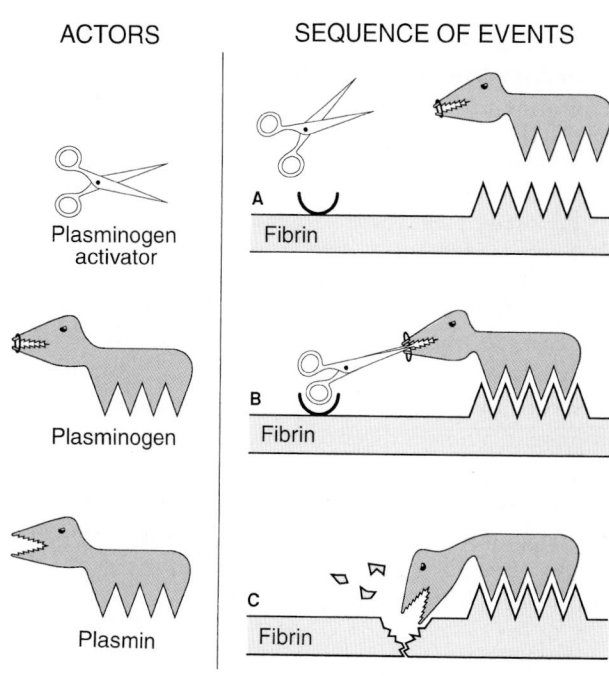

FIGURE 22.16   A cartoon version of some molecular interactions in fibrinolysis. **A:** Both plasminogen and its activator settle on a filament of fibrin. The animal-like features of plasminogen are fanciful, but the "paws" symbolize the lysin-binding sites critical in binding to fibrin. **B:** Plasminogen activator transforms plasminogen into an active enzyme, plasmin. **C:** Plasmin breaks down the fibrin. (Simplified and reproduced with permission from [73].)

Urokinase is a plasminogen activator found in urine, where it may have the function of keeping the renal tubules open (66). Urokinase is synthesized by a variety of cells including cultured endothelium (17). Both tPA and urokinase are also different from streptokinase, another plasminogen activator obtained from streptococci.

The current great interest in plasminogen activators is due to their therapeutic use: they all lead to the dissolution of fibrin and therefore of thrombi and thromboemboli. The first activators to be tried were streptokinase and urokinase; both work, but they also attack fibrinogen in its fluid phase and therefore cause a general depletion of fibrinogen, which is a hazard. Another drawback of streptokinase is that it is antigenic. In contrast, tPA has a much higher affinity for fibrin and therefore acts much more specifically where it is needed (15); it can be given intravenously, and it is not antigenic. This is why the production of recombinant tPA for antithrombotic therapy was hailed as a major step forward. It was obtained from a human melanoma, a rare therapeutic use of a malignant tumor (113).

> Nothing is perfect, however; tPA cannot distinguish between fibrin in a thrombus and fibrin in a purposeful hemostatic plug. Therefore, a major complication is hemorrhage (74, 83).

To demonstrate fibrinolysis microscopically, a simple method is to cut a section of fresh tissue, overlay it with a thin layer of fibrin (which always has plasminogen adsorbed to it), and incubate it at 37°C. Wherever tPA is present, a hole is digested in the fibrin overlay, which is easily shown by staining (Figure 22.17). According to this test the endothelium induces fibrinolysis—but strangely, not everywhere. Even in the cross section of a single vessel, one side may produce fibrinolysis, the other not. The reason is not known (59).

> Inhibitors of fibrinolysis are mainly alpha-2-antiplasmin, alpha-1-antitrypsin, alpha-2-macroglobulin, and plasminogen activator inhibitor (PAi). The endothelium, which secretes tPA, also secretes a tPA inhibitor.

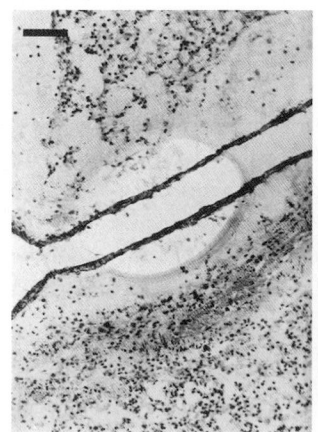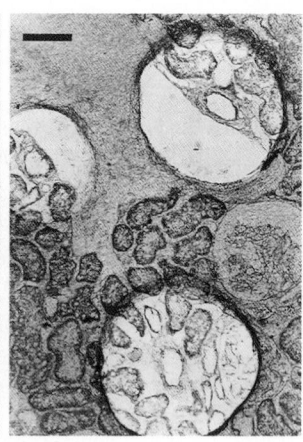

FIGURE 22.17   Demonstration of fibrinolysis by the endothelium in frozen sections of unfixed rat tissues. Each section is overlaid with a thin layer of fibrin, incubated at 37°C for 20 minutes, and stained with hematoxylin and eosin. Clear circular zone indicates fibrinolysis. *Left:* Longitudinal section of a small vein. Why the fibrinolysis is limited to one segment of the vein (a common finding) is not known. **Bar** = 100 μm. *Right:* Renal cortex. The three circles of fibrinolysis are centered on veins. **Bar** = 100 μm. (Reproduced with permission from [50].)

Role of the Vascular Wall in Hemostasis

If we think of the vascular system in terms of container and content, the content performs the main tasks in hemostasis: platelets form a plug, the blood clots. However, the vascular wall is not passive. As we have seen, the arterial media contracts (little is known about contraction of veins and capillaries), and the subendothelium acts as a trap for platelets. We still need to discuss the key role of the endothelium in clotting (51, 52).

Normally, the endothelium is one of the very few cell types that can live with the blood without clotting it; only the leukocytes, platelets, and red blood cells can do the same. This property frustrates the makers of artificial blood vessels, who have found it very difficult to copy it.

The endothelial surface is extremely complex. It turns out that the endothelium performs a *balancing act* between opposing and favoring the clotting mechanism. At first sight it seems mind-boggling that the endothelium should ever be programmed to favor clotting and thrombosis (Figure 22.18); this conflicting behavior has been labeled schizophrenic (34). However, such are the facts, and there are times when intravascular clotting might be life-saving—for example, to limit the spread of infection.

In adopting M. Gimbrone's diagram of the endothelial balancing act concept (Figure 22.18) (52), we have taken the liberty of tilting the balance toward the anticlotting action because we find it difficult to accept that the endothelium is always on the verge of betrayal. We will now briefly comment on these opposing endothelial tendencies, using Figure 22.18 as a guideline.

Endothelial Mechanisms that Inhibit Intravascular Clotting and Thrombosis

At least six protective mechanisms are known (see Figure 22.18). They inhibit key steps of the thrombotic process, beginning with platelet aggregation.

The endothelium opposes platelet aggregation

- Secretion of prostacyclin (PGI_2) begins as soon as the endothelial cell is exposed to thrombin, a platelet aggregator. Prostacyclin is a powerful inhibitor of platelet aggregation and the most powerful vasodilator known. Vasodilatation increases blood flow, which tends to wipe away the platelets. PGI_2 is secreted by the endothelium when it is injured or stimulated by a number of agents (pp. 347, 359).
- Adenosine diphosphate (ADP), a strong aggregator secreted by platelets, is converted by the endothelium to adenine nucleotides, which inhibit platelet aggregation (19).
- Secretion of endothelium-derived relaxing factor (nitric oxide) (80).

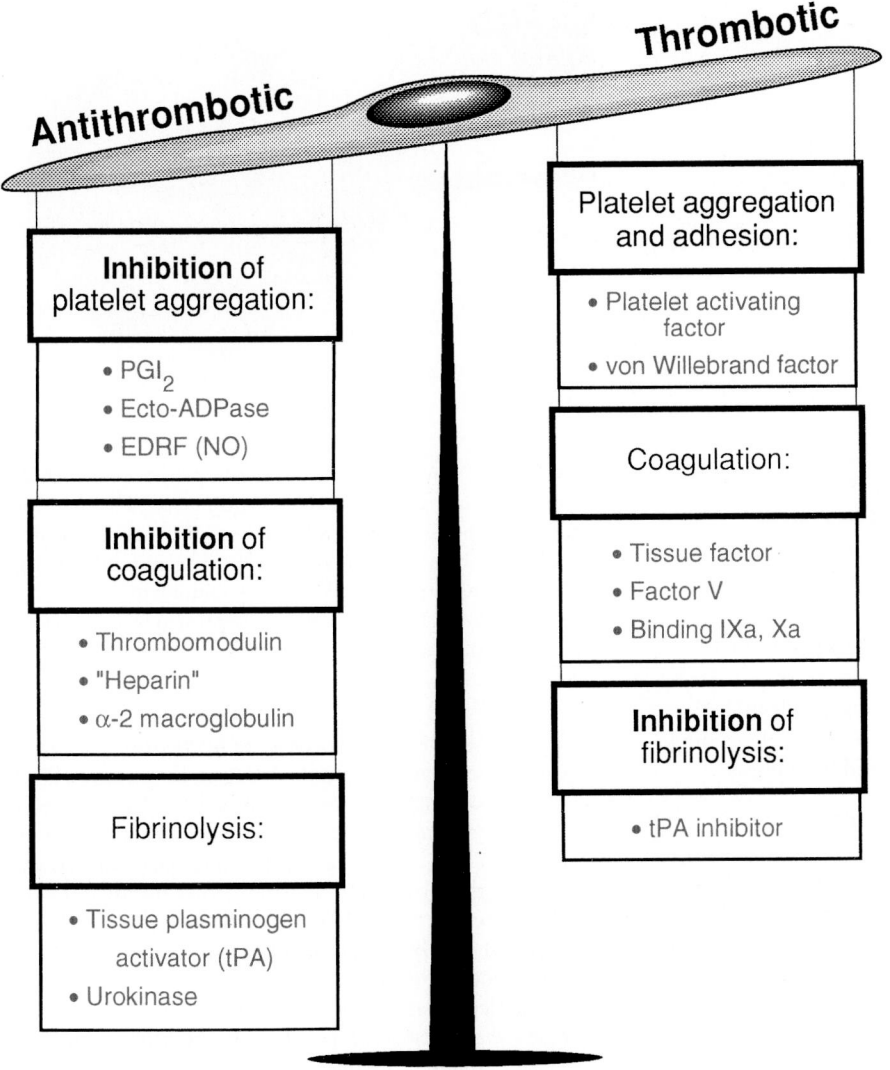

Antithrombotic

Thrombotic

Inhibition of
platelet aggregation:

- PGI$_2$
- Ecto-ADPase
- EDRF (NO)

Inhibition of
coagulation:

- Thrombomodulin
- "Heparin"
- α-2 macroglobulin

Fibrinolysis:

- Tissue plasminogen activator (tPA)
- Urokinase

Platelet aggregation
and adhesion:

- Platelet activating factor
- von Willebrand factor

Coagulation:

- Tissue factor
- Factor V
- Binding IXa, Xa

Inhibition of
fibrinolysis:

- tPA inhibitor

FIGURE 22.18 The endothelial balance. The surface of the endothelial cells can either favor or inhibit thrombosis, depending on its functional condition. (Modified from [52], Copyright 2003, with permission from Elsevier.)

The endothelium opposes thrombin
- Thrombin is captured by thrombomodulin, a protein on the endothelium, and the resulting complex activates plasma protein C, a powerful anticoagulant.
- Thrombin generation is reduced: heparin-like molecules on the endothelial surface conspire with plasma antithrombin II to inactivate all clotting factors from IXa to IIa.

The endothelium favors fibrinolysis. It secretes two plasminogen activators, tPA and urokinase.

Endothelial Mechanisms that Favor Intravascular Clotting

The *clotting activities* of the endothelium are aimed at the same targets as above, but with opposite intent.

The endothelium favors platelet aggregation
- von Willebrand factor (vWF), stored in the Weibel–Palade bodies, is the "glue" that enables platelets to stick to the subendothelium.
- The endothelium can be induced to secrete that omnipotent inflammatory mediator platelet activating factor (PAF), at least *in vitro.*

The endothelium favors the coagulation cascade
- Factors V, IX, and X bind to the endothelial surface.
- Tissue factor (thromboplastin), the very source of the extrinsic coagulation mechanism, is expressed by endothelial surfaces. This response is induced by agents such as interleukin-1 and tumor necrosis factor; it requires some time (hours) to take effect because it requires protein synthesis.

The endothelium opposes fibrinolysis

- The accumulation of fibrin is encouraged by an endothelium-derived inhibitor of tPA, called plasminogen activator inhibitor (PAI).

The Hemostatic Mechanism: A Capsule Overview

In summary, here is the sequence of events that stop bleeding:

- Blood comes in contact with connective tissue.
- Hageman factor is activated by collagen.
- Hageman factor activates the clotting, fibrinolytic and kinin cascades.
- Fibrin is formed.
- Platelets adhere to collagen and become activated.
- Activated platelets help the clotting process.
- Platelets pile up to form a mechanical plug.
- Severed arteries contract (due to platelet products, probably also kinins).
- Fibrin binds plasminogen and tissue plasminogen activator (tPA).
- tPA is activated by binding and digests fibrin.
- Fibrin may or may not continue to form, depending on the relative rates of clotting and fibrinolysis.

Such is, greatly simplified, the intricate story of hemostasis. There are still many holes to fill. For example, anyone who sees—for the first time—a surgical scalpel parting human skin is impressed by the scanty hemorrhage, other than a couple of "bleeders" that may require a hemostat. Millions of capillaries are severed; yet after the cut has been dabbed with a swab or two, it remains dry. Exactly how the capillaries are plugged is not clear; an old light-microscopic study suggests that many are sealed much as a plastic tube is sealed by heat (64).

We will close with an episode of clotting history we find especially interesting, also because it links the beach and the laboratory, in the tradition of Metchnikoff.

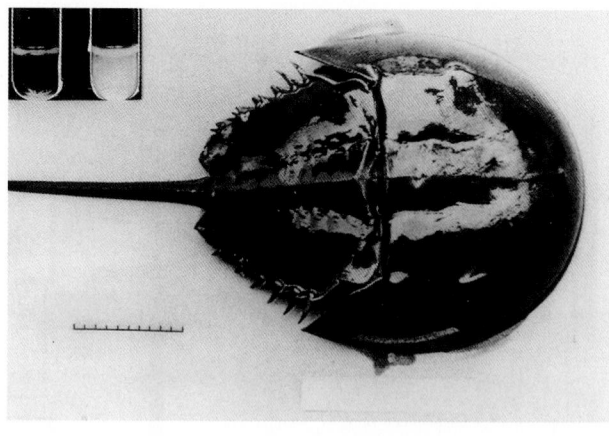

FIGURE 22.19   A dorsal view of *Limulus polyphemus,* the horseshoe crab, much reduced (**scale** in centimeters). The inset illustrates the Limulus test: the test tube at left contains a lysate of Limulus amebocytes; it does not clot. The test tube at right shows clotting after the addition of endotoxin. (From [71], Copyright © 1985 Alan R. Liss. Inc. Reprinted by permission of John Wiley & Sons, Inc.)

The horseshoe crab (***Limulus polyphemus***) lives on the eastern seaboard of North America (Figure 22.19). Its blood contains only one type of cell, called amebocyte. Amebocytes congregate at a site of injury and degranulate, recalling the behavior of platelets; they release a protein that (by itself) does not cause limulus blood to coagulate (Figure 11.12) (72). One day, about 1956, the biologist F.B. Bang had the opportunity to autopsy some horseshoe crabs that had died of an unknown cause. He noticed that the blood had massively coagulated; the crabs were also infected by an endotoxin-producing vibrio. Pursuing the matter, Levin and Bang showed that the protein secreted by the amebocytes had been clotted by endotoxin. The current practice of testing plasma and cerebrospinal fluid for endotoxin by assaying them with Limulus blood (the *Limulus test*) was born in this manner.

Thrombosis: A Definition

Sometimes the normal hemostatic mechanisms are turned on inappropriately, and solid clumps (**thrombi**) develop in the blood vessels or in the heart. The basic components of thrombi and those of hemostatic plugs are the same—platelets, fibrin, and red and white blood cells—but they are put together differently because they form under different conditions.

To qualify as a thrombus, a solid intravascular clump must fulfill three conditions: it must be formed (a) within the heart or vessels, (b) from constituents of the blood, and (c) during life.

The purpose of these qualifications is to exclude extravascular clots that develop from spilled blood, and clots that form in vessels after death.

What kinds of solid masses could arise from the blood? Because a thrombus represents a malfunction of the clotting mechanism, we can expect—alone or in combination—(a) platelet aggregates, (b) clotted blood, and (c) fibrin. They will be called, respectively, **platelet thrombi, red thrombi,** and **fibrin thrombi** (also called white or grey thrombi).

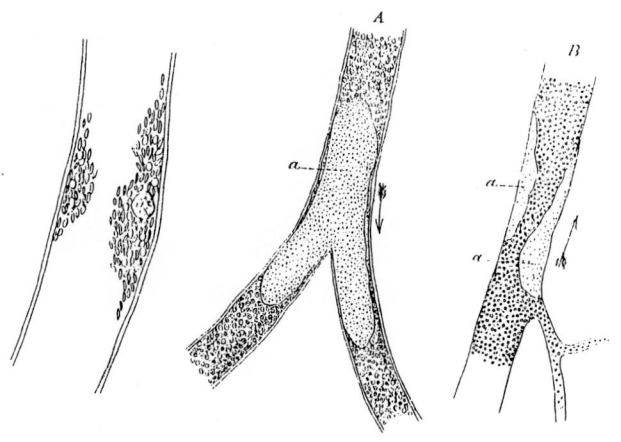

FIGURE 22.20 First illustration of thrombosis as observed in living guinea pig mesentery by Bizzozero (1882). *Left:* Parietal thrombus consisting of platelets and occasional leukocytes, in an arteriole after it was gently pressed with a needle. *Center:* Arteriole embolized at the level of a bifurcation; this embolus (**a**) later disintegrated and vanished (compare with the retinal embolus shown in Figure 23.11). *Right:* Two parietal thrombi consisting of platelets, in a small vein. (Reproduced from [16].)

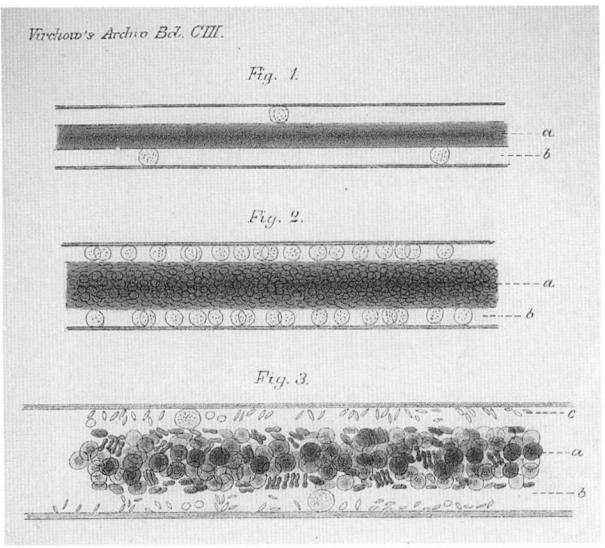

FIGURE 22.21 Early vascular changes in inflammation observed in the omentum of a living dog "about one foot high," as studied in 1886. *Top:* "A vessel" (probably a venule) with accelerated blood flow. The axial stream is obvious; it flows so fast that the individual red blood cells cannot be identified. In the clear plasma zone, occasional leukocytes can be seen rolling along. *Center:* Small vein in which flow is beginning to slow; the red blood cells are now identifiable. Many white blood cells adhere to the wall. *Bottom:* More advanced stasis in another venule. Not only leukocytes but also platelets adhere to the wall (early thrombosis). These observations were made 19 years after Cohnheim and just after the discovery of platelets. Cohnheim (1867) had missed the platelets; perhaps his microscope was not as powerful. (Reproduced from [41].)

A perennial source of confusion to students is that an honest red clot, formed in the living vascular system by the regular clotting mechanism, is not called a clot; it is called a red thrombus. This terminology was introduced by pathologists working in autopsy rooms, where it is essential to find out whether "clots" happened before or after death. The word thrombus is meant to convey instantly the notion "formed *in vivo*." An acceptable alternative to red thrombus might be a *red clot formed while the patient was still alive,* but red thrombus is shorter.

Many physicians who need to explain an occluded coronary artery in lay terms will tell their patients "you had a clot." This is acceptable for purposes of communication.

Today our interpretation of thrombosis seems self-evident, but in Virchow's time it seemed logical that a thrombus was an inflammatory secretion of the vascular wall. The first illustration showing that thrombi and emboli could be formed by platelets came from the hand of Bizzozero in 1882 (Figure 22.20) (16). His observations were made not on slides but on living transparent membranes, obviously an advantage for the study of dynamic events. This technical detail, together with improved optics, made it possible to discover that margination—known to occur with leukocytes—also applied to platelets (Figure 22.21).

Mechanisms of Thrombosis: "Virchow's" Triad

It was Virchow, once again, who adopted the ancient term *thrómbos* (lump or clot) to represent a new concept. Tradition also credits Virchow with pronouncing, in 1845, the law that thrombosis depends on three kinds of changes:

- Changes in the vascular wall (intimal damage)
- Changes in flow (slow or turbulent)
- Changes in the blood (hypercoagulability)

This is the famous **"triad of Virchow,"** still perfectly valid, and now firmly rooted in National Board exams. However, we feel compelled to introduce it between quotation marks, because there is no mention of a "triad" in any of Virchow's papers.

This arcane trinity was a gift of posterity. In truth, Virchow did discuss each of the three factors in various writings, beginning with the second lecture he ever gave, at age 23.

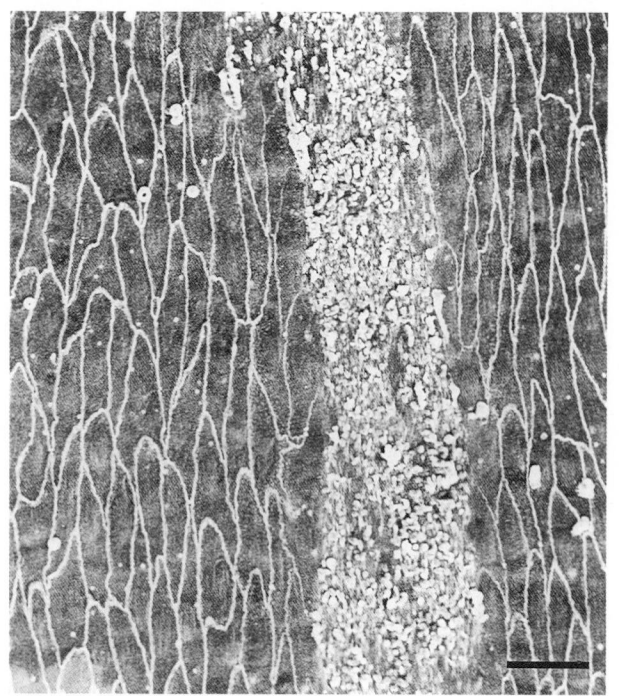

FIGURE 22.22   Carpet of platelets has been deposited on the denuded surface 15 minutes after it was scratched with a nylon filament. Scanning electron microscopy after staining with silver. **Bar** = 25 μ.m. (Reproduced by permission from [104], by © The US Canadian Academy.)

The manuscript of this 1845 lecture, which was perceived as revolutionary, was rediscovered in Germany in 1966 by two American scholars, Kenneth Brinkhous and Elizabeth Sommer. As far as we know, it has not been translated (22, 23). Anyway, this episode confirms that whatever Virchow said tended to become a law, even if he did not say it.

The Triad

What is still not so clear is how the triad theory should be interpreted. Does it mean that all three factors are necessary? Let us examine the evidence.

Intimal damage. It is easy to study the role of intimal damage by removing the endothelium. A microscopic scratch in the aorta of a rat is almost immediately carpeted with a thin layer of platelets (Figure 22.22), which swell and degranulate (Figure 22.23). The same result is obtained if a whole vessel, artery or vein, is deprived of endothelium by the technique called *ballooning:* a surgical catheter tipped with a small inflatable balloon (as used for embolectomy) is introduced in the vessel; then the balloon is inflated and the catheter is pulled out. In so doing the endothelium is wiped off (Figure 22.24).

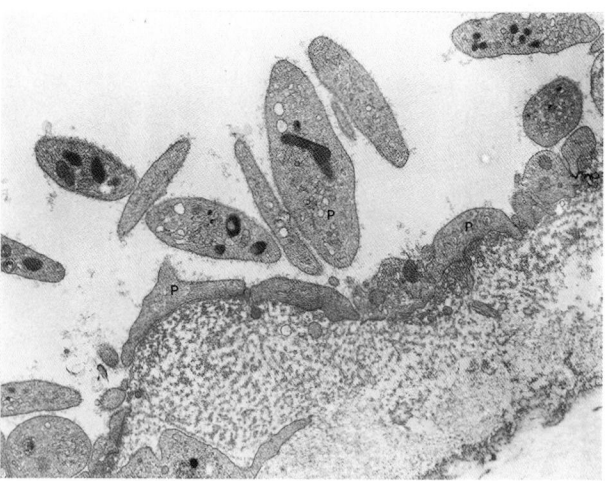

FIGURE 22.23   Electron microscopy of a rat aorta, 15 minutes after it was gently scratched with a nylon thread, removing the endothelium. A carpet of platelets (**P**) has covered the denuded intima; a second, incomplete layer of platelets has formed just above the first. (Courtesy of Dr. Michael A. Reidy, University of Washington, Seattle, WA.)

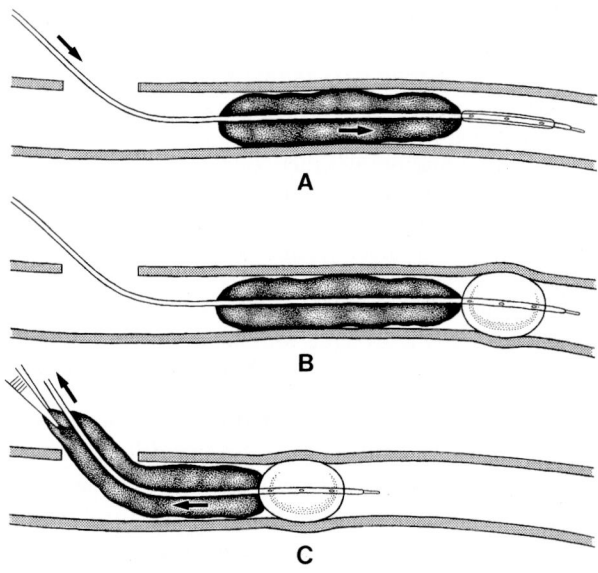

FIGURE 22.24   Extraction of an arterial embolus with the Fogarty catheter. **A:** Catheter is pushed through the embolus. **B:** Balloon is inflated. **C:** Catheter is retrieved, pulling the embolus with it. (Adapted from [47] by permission from SURGERY GYNECOLOGY & OBSTETRICS.)

Platelets adhere to the subendothelium for the same reason that they form hemostatic plugs: their surface receptors interlock with factor VIII (vWF) bound to the matrix. In arteries these carpet-like platelet thrombi do

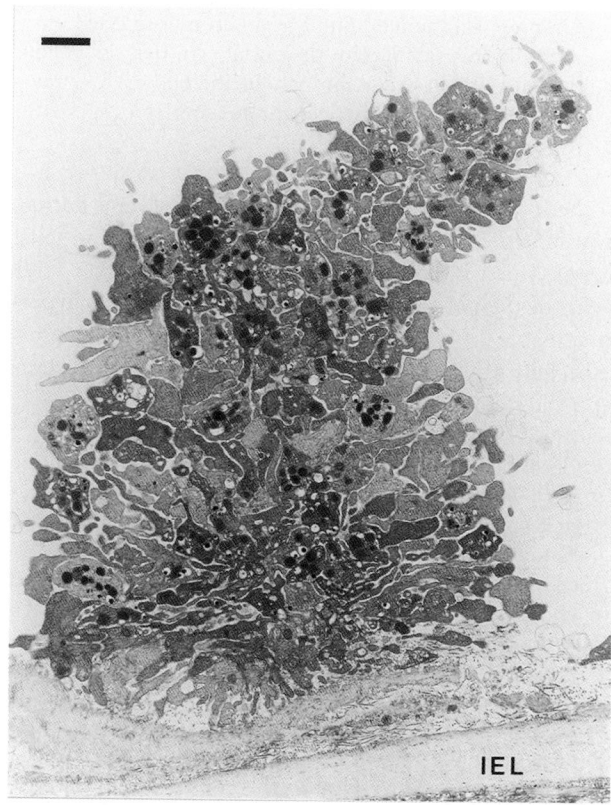

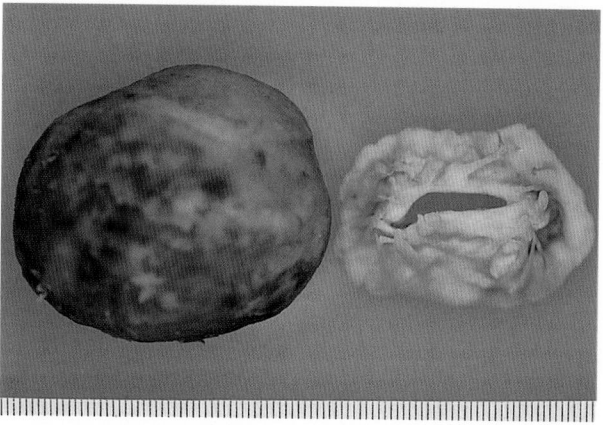

FIGURE 22.25 Typical platelet thrombus, produced *in vitro* by circulating blood for 10 minutes over a rabbit aorta deprived of its endothelium. Note that the platelets at the surface of the thrombus still contain some granules, whereas the platelets that were first in contact with the internal elastic lamina (**IEL**) have degranulated. **Bar** = 1 μm. (Reproduced with permission from [8].)

FIGURE 22.26 *Left.* Ball thrombus about the size of a plum. This free thrombus was removed surgically from the left atrium of a patient who suffered from stenosis and insufficiency of the mitral valve, which was also excised (*right*). **Scale** in millimeters. (Courtesy of Dr. H. F. Cuénoud, University of Massachusetts Medical School, Worcester, MA.)

not grow because the swift current washes away the platelets and the chemical mediators that activate them; small clusters of platelets that are torn off may be small enough to avoid becoming emboli downstream. By contrast, if an artery is deprived of its endothelium and perfused *in vitro* at a low rate of flow, substantial thrombi will develop (Figure 22.25) (86). Overall, we have learned that intimal damage alone can generate thrombi, modulated by flow.

Clinically, intimal damage occurs in many settings: after trauma or surgery, in infected tissues, in immune responses (such as in grafts), and on the surfaces of atherosclerotic plaques when they break open.

Sluggish flow. Sluggish flow gives platelets a better chance to stick and clotting factors a better chance to act. This explains why thrombosis is much more frequent in veins than in arteries (there is even a special word for venous thrombosis, *phlebothrombosis*); furthermore, the valves

in the veins favor thrombosis because they produce eddies and pockets of stagnant blood.

The power of sluggish flow in creating thrombi is illustrated by a spectacular condition all too familiar to cardiologists, the so-called *ball thrombus* (Figure 22.26).

If the mitral valve becomes stenotic, blood is retained in the left atrium, where it forms an eddy. In the long run a free, spherical thrombus can form in this eddy: under these conditions a change in the endothelial surface is probably not involved (the thrombus can be visualized by echocardiography and surgically removed).

Hypercoagulability. The third item of Virchow's triad is obvious but hard to define. There is no doubt that hypercoagulability exists: there are at least 48 conditions—ranging in seriousness from cancer through pregnancy to prolonged air travel—known to be associated with an increased risk of thrombosis (7, 67, 110). Considering the large number of natural clotting and anticlotting agents that could malfunction, this long list of risky situations should not come as a surprise. However, no single blood change can account for all the hypercoagulable states; there is no single laboratory test for hypercoagulability.

Experimental Thrombosis

Experimentally, the best way to show the importance of this rather evanescent factor of thrombogenesis-hypercoagulability is to follow a series of classical experiments performed in the 1950s under the name of *serum-induced thrombosis* (35, 118, 121).

Serum-induced thrombosis. What happens in a vein when blood stops flowing? To find out, anesthetize a rabbit, and carefully expose about 5 cm of a jugular vein. Gently apply two clamps on the vein about 4 cm apart. An hour or so later, slit the vein between the clamps: surprise! The blood in the isolated segment is still fluid. This shows that *stasis alone cannot initiate the clotting process.* Any clotting factors that were released into the vein by the surgical procedure have been successfully opposed by the anticlotting mechanisms of the vein's endothelium. Remember that stasis induces the endothelium to favor fibrinolysis by secreting more plasminogen activator (tPA).

It may have been a surprise to learn that the blood between two ligatures is still fluid after 1 hour, but F. Zahn knew in 1875 that it is still fluid after 5 days (124).

Now let us add one more of Virchow's three factors: hypercoagulability. In another rabbit (as a control) expose a jugular vein without clamping it, and inject into the bloodstream (using a different vein) 1.3 ml of fresh serum per kg of body weight. Human serum will do. This serum (remember the definition of serum, p. 638) is loaded with activated clotting factors; yet no adverse reaction occurs in the rabbit even though its blood, if tested, is more prone than normal to clot (35). Then, within 1 minute, apply the two clamps to the jugular vein; 10 minutes later the blood in the jugular is clotted. Why? Because the clotting factors contained in the injected serum have no effect where the blood is circulating; but where the blood is held in complete stasis, they make it clot. This method can be used also for producing experimental pulmonary emboli, using two clamps on a peripheral vein (120).

An interesting addendum: if fresh serum is injected intravenously in a rabbit with the portal vein tied off, venous thrombosis will occur throughout the body. This proves that the liver is very active in removing clotting factors from the blood (35, 67).

Serum-induced thrombosis relates to several human conditions. In pregnancy, phlebothrombosis of the lower limbs is not uncommon: pressure on the large veins of the pelvis creates stasis, and the blood is hypercoagulable (67). The same is true for bedridden patients, especially after surgery; their leg veins suffer from stasis and their blood is notoriously hypercoagulable.

Clinically, a few mechanisms of hypercoagulability are clear, especially among the inherited disorders, such as lack of antithrombin III (88) or proteins C or S (28). Among the acquired disorders, increased platelet stickiness (platelet hyperreactivity) is best known. Increased aggregability of platelets in the morning is associated with an increased frequency of myocardial infarction in the morning (114). Smoking activates the Hageman factor (factor XII) (10); pregnancy and recent surgery are accompanied by increased levels of fibrinogen (an acute-phase reactant, p. 505). The pathogenesis of atherosclerosis appears to include a unique pathway to thrombosis: a high level of the plasma protein lipoprotein(a), which interferes with fibrinolysis (56, 85).

> **TO SUM UP:** Virchow's triad is here to stay, even if Virchow never heard about it. Clinical and experimental data show that two of the three factors are enough to trigger thrombosis.

Life History of a Thrombus

Knowing the three basic conditions that favor thrombosis, we will now follow, step by step, the development of an actual thrombus (as well as we understand it) in a deep vein in the calf of a bedridden, postsurgical patient (Figure 22.27).

Genesis of a Thrombus

Platelet Adhesion and Aggregation

As platelets flow along the vein, they are more concentrated along the endothelium, because they are the smallest formed elements in the blood (Figure 22.21). Recall the river analogy: rocks roll in the center of the stream, sand is deposited along the banks. Because we are dealing with a postoperative patient, the platelets aggregate more easily than normal. As they flow past a valve in a vein, they are caught in the eddy behind it, aggregate, and settle on the wall. This step is not well understood.

Here we pause for an admission of ignorance. Nobody has ever proven that the endothelium is damaged in the veins of the calf in a bedridden patient. To the contrary, histology and even electron microscopy (5) of early venous thrombi show that the endothelium is structurally intact (61). The same is true for microscopic thrombi that may develop secondarily in a focus of aseptic inflammation (Figure 22.28). Yet the platelets are telling us, by sticking to it, that the surface of the endothelium is not normal. We must conclude that *the change in the vascular wall that favors thrombosis may be functional.* Perhaps in a bedridden patient the endothelium of some large veins is functionally abnormal or somehow activated by the mild trauma

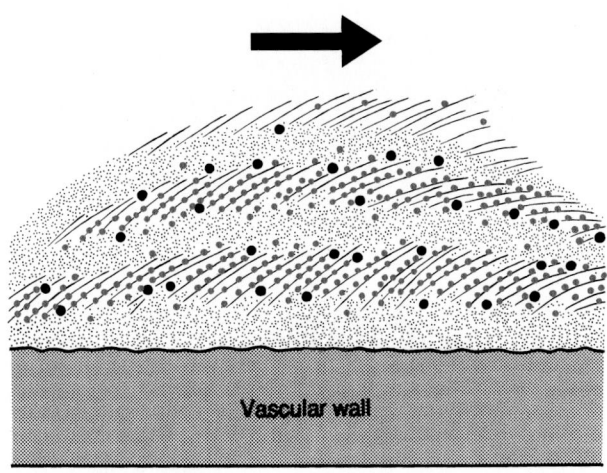

FIGURE 22.27 Layered growth of a mixed thrombus. The first layer, whitish to the naked eye, consists of platelets; its surface favors coagulation and gives rise to filaments of fibrin that entrap red blood cells and a few white blood cells. This new (red) layer is thrombogenic and causes the deposition of a new layer of platelets; and so the cycle repeats. Black dots (•) = leukocytes trapped in the fibrin.

of continued pressure (activated endothelium expresses tissue factor and starts the clotting cascade, p. 720).

Once attached to the wall, the platelets are activated, swell, spread out, and become sticky; more platelets pile over them, favored by the eddy.

Fibrin Formation

Then comes a new event: threads of fibrin grow out of the platelet layer just as in a hemostatic plug; visualize

them swaying in the lazy current, trapping red blood cells (Figure 22.27). In this way a fluffy, red carpet is laid over the platelets (red because of the entrapped red blood cells). The surface of this fibrin layer is thrombogenic because platelets stick to nascent fibrin, so the fibrin layer is soon buried under another layer of platelets; then these platelets generate their own carpet of fibrin filaments and red cells; and so the process continues. Note the behavior of the leukocytes, which tend to stick to the surfaces of the platelet layers, perhaps in response to chemotactic factors released by the platelets (21).

> Platelets stick to fibrin while it is being generated, but not when it is fully cross-linked. Neutrophils inhibit platelet activation, while red blood cells enhance it—mechanisms unclear (80).

Lines of Zahn

In the way just described, *the thrombus develops as a laminated structure,* which makes it very different from clots formed after death or *in vitro*. The layering is rarely as regular as shown in our diagram because flow conditions are irregular, but red and white parts are always recognizable, hence the name **mixed thrombus** (Figure 22.29). The two components are visible to the naked eye on a cut surface of a thrombus; the layers of platelets are whitish, and sandwiched between them are red layers of fibrin and entrapped red blood cells. These layers are known as the **lines of Zahn** (Figure 22.30). Sometimes the lines run perpendicular to the surface; in this case the white layers of platelets stand out as white ripples alternating with sunken red lines (the latter have undergone clot retraction or syneresis, p. 638).

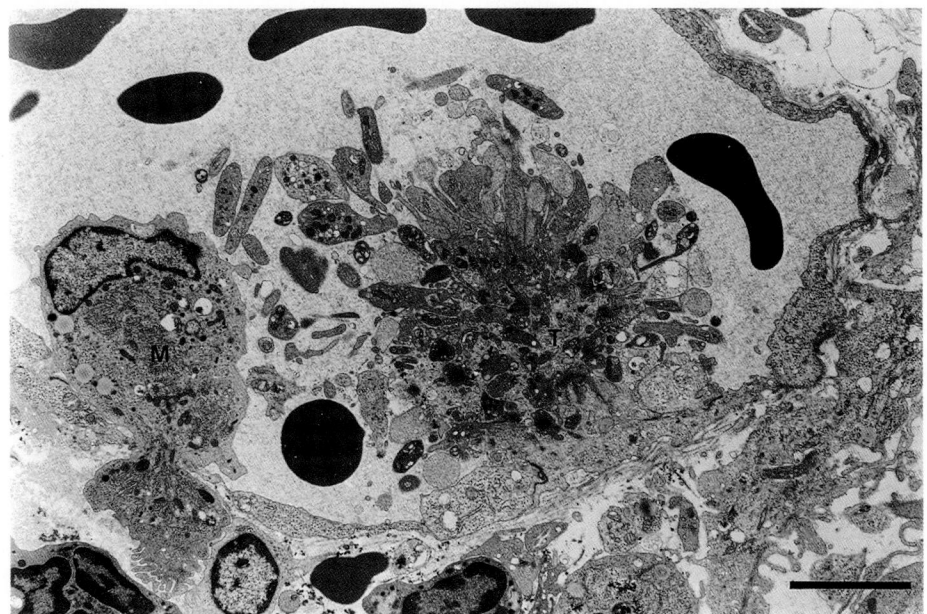

FIGURE 22.28 Microscopic parietal thrombus (**T**) in a rat venule, in a focus of aseptic inflammation 48 hours old. Thrombi are common in inflamed tissues. Note the macrophage (**M**) performing diapedesis. **Bar** = 5 μm.

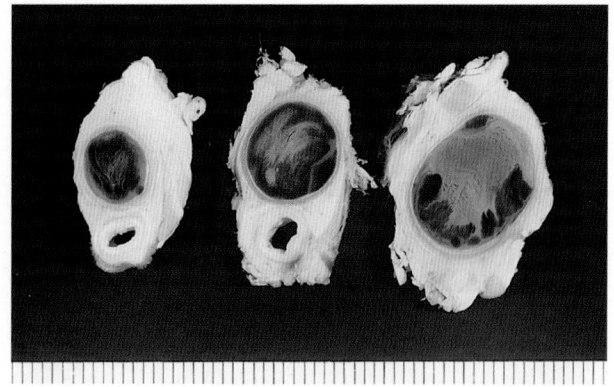

FIGURE 22.29 Occluding thrombi in the popliteal and femoral veins (*above*). The thrombi are mixed, i.e., red and "white"—actually light brown. Note that the accompanying artery is not thrombosed. From a patient who died of adenocarcinoma of the stomach. **Scale** in millimeters.

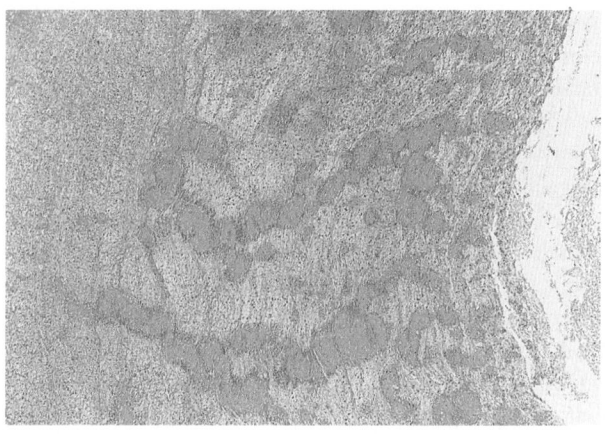

FIGURE 22.30 Mixed thrombus in a large vein. Lumen at *right*. The heavy pink lines are classic *lines of Zahn,* consisting mainly of platelets; hanging between them are threads of fibrin, much like festoons, with entrapped red blood cells. *Left:* The deep side of the thrombus, where it is attached to the intima, is just out of sight. The dense population of cells in this area included fibroblasts, indicating that the thrombus had been there for about a week. (25x)

It has been aptly said that the white ripples of compacted platelets on the surface of a thrombus are "not unlike geological strata which reach the surface of a thrombus as an outcrop" (Figure 22.31) (61). Some thrombi have few if any orderly lines, but it is still clear that they are composed of white and red parts.

> Friedrich Zahn described his ripples, if not his lines, over a century ago at the Institute of Pathology in Geneva, Switzerland. Zahn was probably the first to define thrombi as red, white, or mixed (124). On cross sections of mixed

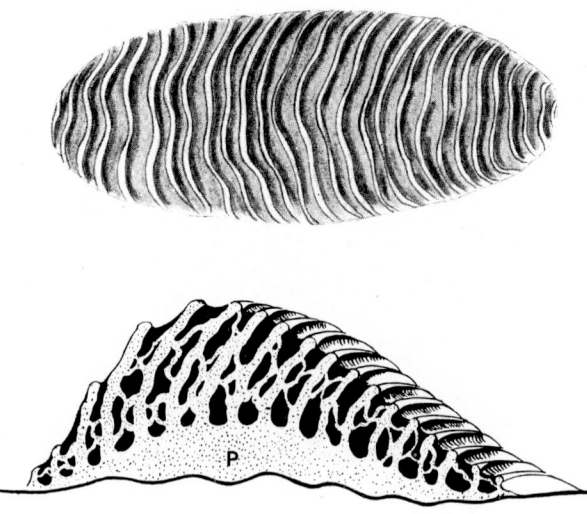

FIGURE 22.31 Layered thrombus. *Top:* Surface of a thrombus as it appears through a magnifying glass. The ridges, perpendicular to the direction of flow, are the original "ripple lines" of Zahn and consist of aggregated platelets. *Bottom:* Cross section shows that the layers of platelets (**P**) are interconnected between them are strands of fibrin containing red blood cells (**black areas**). Thrombi of this appearance are rare, but they help understand the correlation between surface ridges and lines of Zahn. (Reproduced by permission from [55].)

thrombi he noticed that white and red material formed irregular layers rather than a neat onion-skin pattern, "perhaps due to disturbed axial direction of blood flow" (Figure 22.32). Later he observed that the surfaces of some mixed thrombi were rippled. He compared these ripples with the ripples in the mud on the bank of the river Arve, along which he walked on the way to work. He actually suggested that the ripples on the thrombi and the river bank might develop by the same hydrodynamic mechanism. The great German pathologist Ludwig Aschoff tried to prove the hydrodynamic explanation, but his experiments were inconclusive (4). The mechanism of layering, as we now see it, is a result of platelet physiology interacting with blood flow. From what we have said, it should be clear that the surface rippling (Figure 22.31, *top*) is a continuation of the layering of the thrombotic mass.

The Many Fates of a Thrombus

The thrombus continues to grow until the vessel is occluded or until antithrombus forces gain the upper hand. If the thrombus merely restricts the lumen, it is called **parietal** (Figure 22.33); if it fills the lumen completely, it is called **occlusive** (Figure 22.29). Occlusion is a critical step, because flow is the major defense against the clotting factors oozing from the thrombus: the blood in the segment of vein containing the thrombus will clot. Fortunately, the clotting will not extend to the

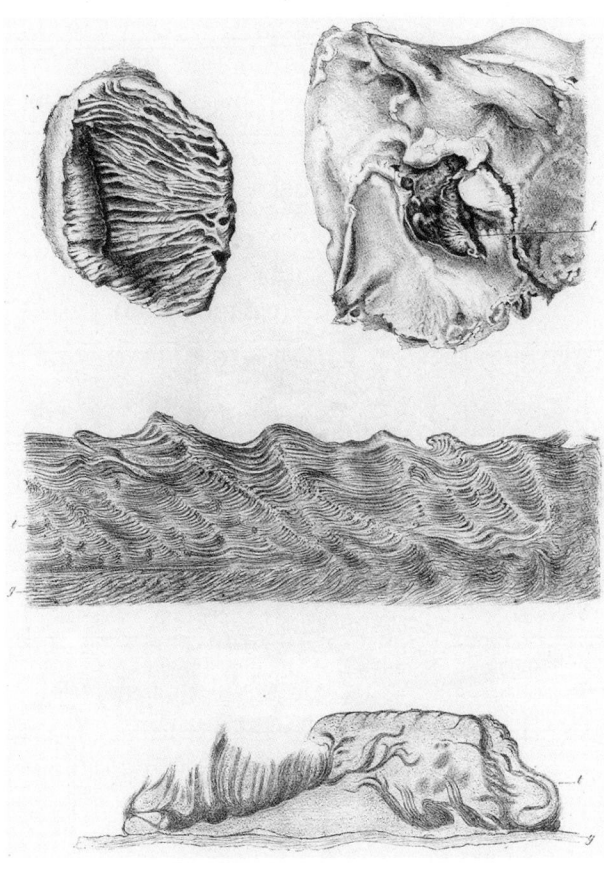

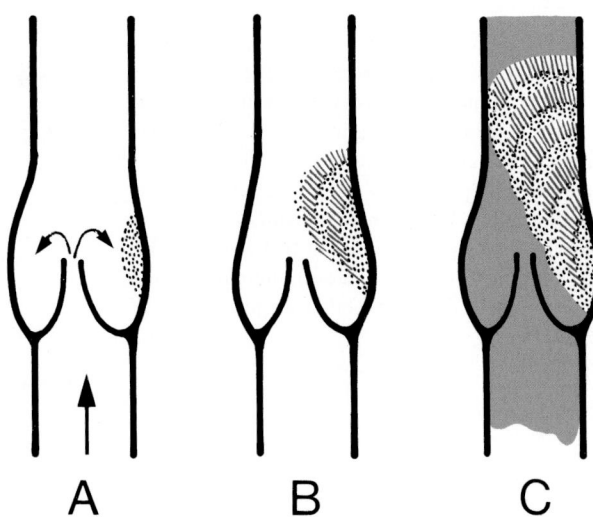

FIGURE 22.33   Stages in the progression of a venous thrombus. **A:** Typically, the thrombus begins in the recess behind a valve. **B:** The thrombus grows downstream by a succession of white layers (platelets) and red layers (fibrin with entrapped red cells). If the lumen is occluded by the growing mixed thrombus (**C**), the blood will clot proximally and distally to the obstruction. At this stage the entire thrombus consists of a mixed (i.e., white and red) **head,** attached to the wall, and one or two red **tails** filling the lumen. The formation of tails depends on the local conditions of flow as determined by the vein's branching pattern. See the following figure. (Adapted with permission from [12]. Copyright © 1969 by the American Society of Clinical Pathologists.)

FIGURE 22.32   Structure of thrombi as illustrated by Zahn in 1891. *Top and center:* Thrombi with a typical rippled surface. *Bottom:* Cross section shows banded structures (lines of Zahn). (Reproduced from [125].)

- *A thrombus may be dissolved* in a matter of hours, probably with the help of enzymes from trapped leukocytes; fibrinolysis is accomplished by plasmin adsorbed to the fibrin filaments. The mass breaks up into microscopic fragments that cause no significant damage as they embolize the lungs.

- *A thrombus may break off* and become an embolus (see Chapter 23).

- *A thrombus may become covered by cells and organized.* This process has not been adequately studied. Oddly enough, few studies have focussed on this basic process. Two facts are clear: (a) *The surface of the thrombus is slowly covered by large, flat mononuclear cells,* which have the effect of stopping the deposition of platelets. Most of these cells appear to derive from the bloodstream; as such they would be well qualified for the task of stopping the deposition of platelets, because their own surface must be non-thrombogenic. They have been called monocytes-macrophages, possibly able to turn into endothelial cells or myofibroblasts. This covering process can be seen with hours (65) but in large venous thrombi it may require weeks for completion (112). (b) *The mass of platelets is reabsorbed by mononuclear cells of uncertain origin* (the vascular

whole circulatory system, because veins have many connections, and flow will find a new path around the obstacle. At this point the laminated head of the thrombus will be prolonged by one or two tails of clotted blood (red thrombi) (55). The red tail (or tails) point downstream, upstream, or both ways, depending on the location of the branches and the course of blood flow (Figure 22.34).

> NOTE: The head of a thrombus is the only part that is attached to the wall, often to the valve; the tails are free, especially after clot retraction has occurred, which makes them especially prone to break loose. A thrombus filling a superficial vein can be palpated or rather felt (*very gently!*) through the skin.

The further life history of a thrombus is illustrated in Figure 22.35. The following description applies to both venous and arterial thrombi.

FIGURE 22.34   Role of the vein's branching pattern in stopping the growth of a thrombus. *Top:* Platelet thrombi begin to develop in the recesses of a valve. *Center:* An occluding grey thrombus has formed, and the blood flowing through the vein will clot both proximally and distally, creating two red thrombi. The branches maintain the flow thereby diluting the clotting factors. *Bottom:* The red thrombi contract (syneresis) and dangle dangerously in the flowing blood, ready to break off as emboli.

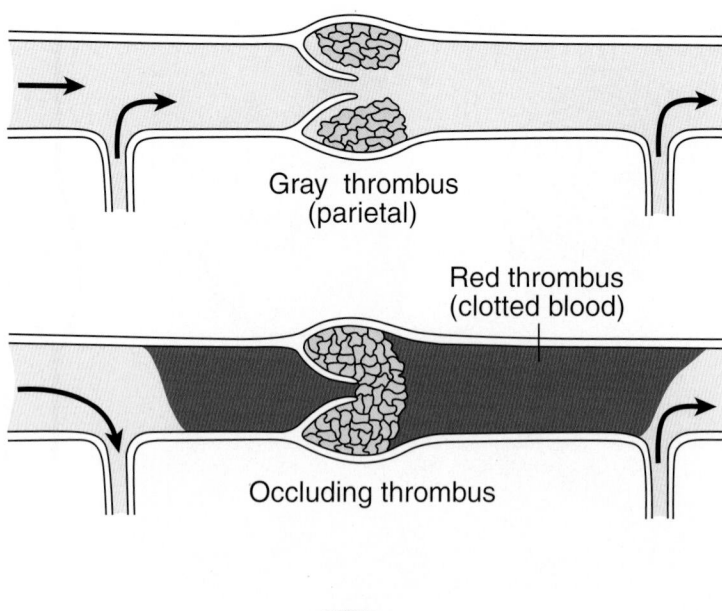

Gray thrombus
(parietal)

Red thrombus
(clotted blood)

Occluding thrombus

low flow

Syneresis

FIGURE 22.35 Fates of a thrombus. In **F,** no vessel is shown running all the way across the thrombus ("recanalizing" the occlusion) because this event is not proven.

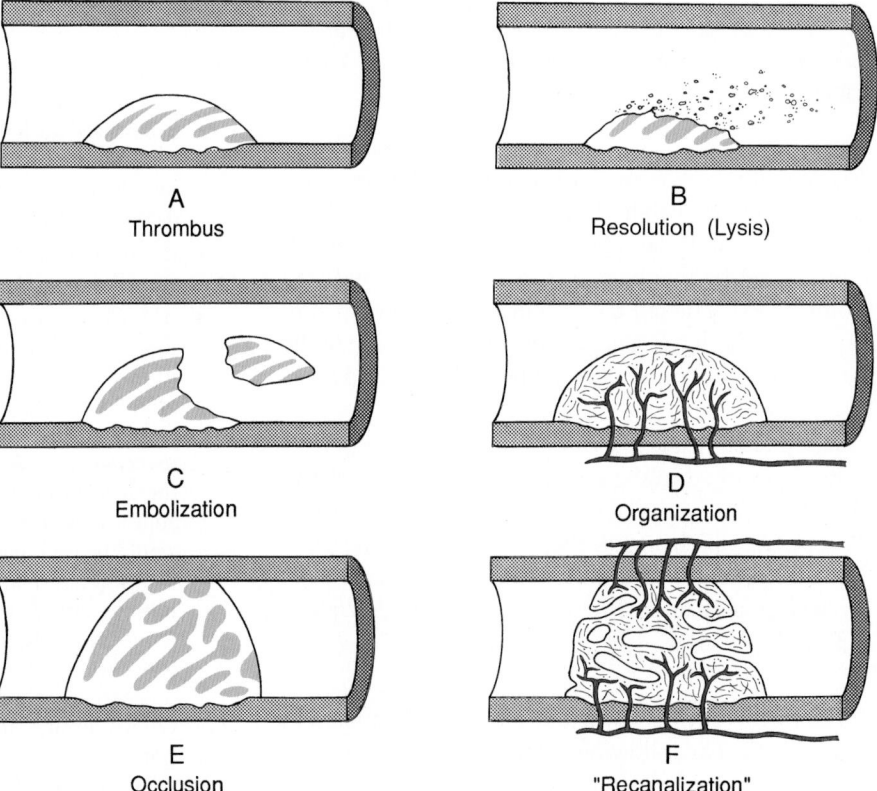

blood flow ➡

A
Thrombus

B
Resolution (Lysis)

C
Embolization

D
Organization

E
Occlusion

F
"Recanalization"

wall, the blood, or both). In large veins these thrombi are reabsorbed with help from cells and vessels supplied by the perivascular microcirculation; which means that some chemical message from the thrombus has alerted the microcirculation surrounding the vein. All these studies should now be repeated using markers to identify the "mononuclear cells" involved in the various phases of thrombus growth and reabsorption. They may very well include stem cells. How the medial smooth muscle cells participate is not known. Once organized, a parietal thrombus leaves on the wall of the vessel a fibrous scar, pigmented for some time with hemosiderin. An organized occluding thrombus appears in cross section like a fibrous mass perforated by vessels (see Figure 22.35F) (36, 61).

Amyloid is sometimes found in old thrombi, perhaps because plasma precursors of amyloid are deposited in the thrombus and macrophages turn them into amyloid (p. 289) (53, 54).

It is said that an occluding thrombus may be organized and "recanalized." Experimentally, venous thrombi are said to recanalize much more extensively than arterial thrombi (46). **Recanalization** is supposed to mean that new channels, lined with endothelium, are running across the occlusion and restoring blood flow. This favorable outcome may well occur, but it could be demonstrated only by studying serial sections of a thrombus; as far as we know, this has not been done. The presence of many small vessels in a thrombus suggests that we are looking at adventitial vessels that have simply organized the thrombus. It is unlikely that adventitial vessels would communicate with the lumen of the occluded vessel (36), especially if it is an artery: the ingrowing adventitial capillaries would have a pressure of roughly 20 mm Hg against a pressure about four times greater in the artery.

- *A thrombus may partially* calcify like any mass of necrotic material.

For obscure reasons, little white beads of calcium salts 3 or 4 mm in diameter are commonly seen in the pelvis by radiologists; they are called *phleboliths* because they are assumed to represent calcified thrombi. Pathologists find them quite often loose in the pelvis, and assume that they were generated in veins. Everybody, surgeons included, has learned to disregard them as insignificant oddities, but it is annoying that something so common be unexplained. According to an inquisitive Genevan surgeon they are not phleboliths at all, but necrotic, calcified epiploic appendages.

Differences between Arterial and Venous Thrombi

Arterial thrombi develop under conditions of high shear; they are more compact and white and tend to

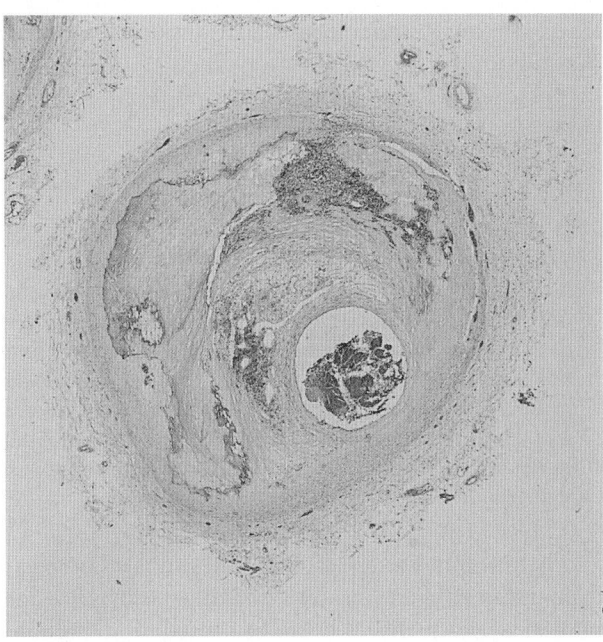

FIGURE 22.36   Cross section of a coronary artery with severe atherosclerosis. The diameter of the lumen (*lower right*) is reduced to about one third. The wall contains calcified masses with a basophilic rim. *Left of lumen:* Intramural hemorrhage. Red thrombus in lumen was cause of death. (10x)

remain parietal. Lamination may therefore be missing. Thrombi in small arteries are more dangerous than venous thrombi because arteries are much less anastomosed than veins. In arteries, occlusive thrombi usually form over an atherosclerotic plaque that has cracked open; they are not much larger than the head of a match, but in a coronary artery they can kill (Figure 22.36).

Endarterectomy. In view of what we have said about thrombi, the surgical procedure of scraping away—from inside—the intima and much of the media of carotid arteries, which lead directly into the brain, would seem absurd: the surgery exposes to blood flow *collagenous tissue,* a classic activator of platelets! The answer is twofold: (a) flow in the carotids is so fast that thrombi can barely develop; and (b) anticoagulation does the rest: the incidence of embolic complications is "only" 1 percent. . . .

Aneurysms. Arterial thrombi lead us to a brief discussion of aneurysms. An **aneurysm** is a local dilatation of an artery due to a weakening of its wall. The weakening mechanism in large arteries is almost always atherosclerosis. Similar local dilatations occur in veins; they are known as **varices.** Aneurysms can be shaped like a sac (*saccular*) or like a spindle (*fusiform*). Saccular aneurysms of the aorta may appear as bulging, hemispherical pockets 10–15 cm in diameter; they are usually lined, and sometimes filled, with thrombus.

> ***Dissecting aneurysms*** are mentioned here for completeness but they are of special nature. They occur virtually only in the aorta and its major branches. The inner layer of the arterial wall suddenly tears open; blood rushes into the tear and proceeds to dissect (separate) the media into two layers, sometimes along the entire length of the aorta. The blood may then find its way back into the lumen through a second tear. All this may take place in a matter of minutes. Survival is rare but possible.

The thrombus in a saccular aneurysm is a compact, firm, rubbery mass that has patently been there for months or years. Bits of it can be carried off as emboli, but the mass itself may help survival because it prevents the thin aneurysmal pocket from bursting under the aortic pressure. These massive thrombi have one unusual characteristic: they never become organized, they simply "sit" on the thinned arterial wall, which tolerates them with the utmost indifference. Why? Platelets are loaded with inflammatory mediators, and organization could be helpful by reinforcing the paper-thin wall and anchoring the thrombus. The answer, we believe, is that no chemical message ever reaches the adventitia in concentrations large enough to be perceived. As the aneurysm begins to form, over months and years, all mediators arising in the thrombus are washed away by the torrential arterial flow; furthermore, platelets do not stick on old, fully cross-linked fibrin (p. 649), and the muscular media of large arteries is a major obstacle to outward diffusion. Later the wall thins, but by then the thrombus has grown so thick (up to several centimeters) that outward diffusion from freshly deposited platelets becomes negligible.

Gross Aspects of Thrombi

In the setting of a medicolegal autopsy, it can be critical to distinguish between a red thrombus and a postmortem clot.

Differences between thrombi and postmortem clots. Typical *mixed thrombi* are laminated (lines of Zahn) and adhere to the intimal surface; even if the lamination is not present, a mixture of red and white parts is the signature of a mixed thrombus. Pure *platelet thrombi* are whitish and tend to crumble. *Red thrombi* are the real challenge to

pathologists, but usually they are attached at some point to a mixed thrombus. *Postmortem clots* are rubbery, shiny, and usually red. They are never laminated because lamination requires blood flow, and nowhere are they attached to the intima.

A peculiar feature of postmortem clots is that they can be made of two superimposed layers, one red and one white. This is a result of erythrocyte sedimentation after death (Figure 15.5). When the heart stops, the blood within it clots very slowly, and the red blood cells have the time to settle, perhaps more so if the patient's sedimentation rate was high. When clotting finally occurs, the upper part of the blood mass, which is free of red blood cells, clots into a yellowish, gelatinous mass that has the time-honored but somewhat repulsive name of ***chicken fat clot.*** The point of this distinction is to prevent confusion of this peculiar postmortem artifact with a white thrombus.

Vegetations. Traditionally, a thrombus on a cardiac valve is called a vegetation. The name is well chosen because these thrombi often develop as branching structures attached to a base on the valve, rather like a bush (Figure 22.37). They may grow to a length of 2–3 cm, with branches that easily break off and embolize. Vegetations develop most frequently on the valves of the left heart, especially if misshapen due to congenital or acquired disease. The reason: normally, the mitral and aortic valves slam shut under pressures that are at least four times greater than those of the corresponding valves on the right side; if in addition they are deformed and *insufficient* (unable to close completely) their surface is exposed to greatly increased flow velocities (5–6 m/sec instead of 1–2 m/sec) and thus to increased shear stress. The result is microtrauma to the endothelium, and exposure of the subendothelial tissue, which is thrombogenic and becomes covered with platelets.

Infected thrombi. Infected thrombi can occur anywhere, but the prototypes are infected vegetations, especially on the mitral valve. Emboli arising from these thrombi carry, of course, a double threat: infarction and infection. The interaction of platelets and bacteria is variable and not fully understood. They tend to stick together; in some experimental models this tends to protect the host, in others it helps disseminate the bacteria (57, 97, 123). Activated platelets do release a potent platelet microbicidal protein (PMP) (123), but once they have fired that shot in the context of a thrombus the surviving bacteria can form true colonies (Figure 22.38), surrounded by fibrin filaments (Figure 22.39) (3, 40) that probably act as a shield against leukocyte attack.

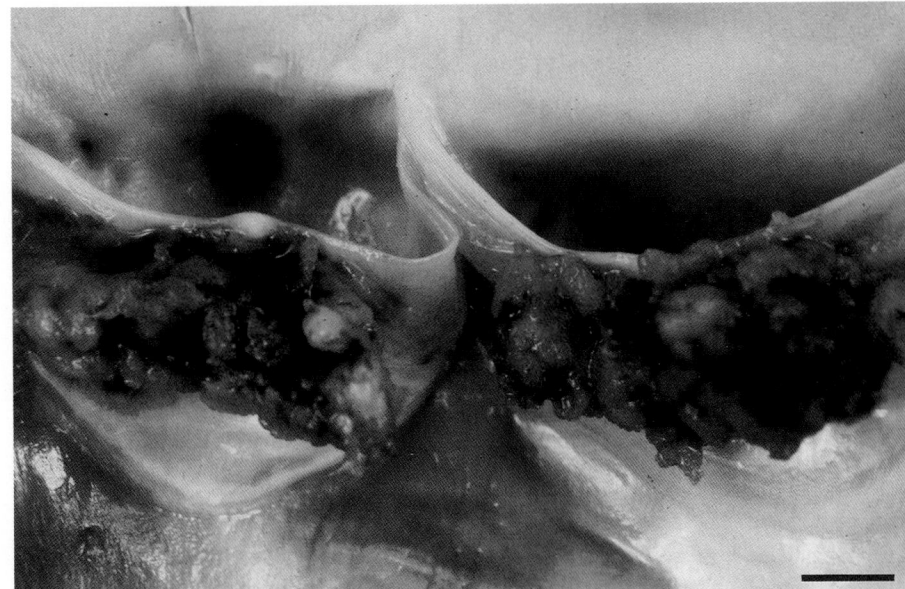

FIGURE 22.37 "Vegetations": Thrombi on the aortic valves in a debilitated leukemic patient who had undergone a bone marrow transplant. This is non-infectious endocarditis. **Bar** = 5 mm. (Courtesy of Dr. W. D. Edwards, Department of Laboratory Medicine and Pathology, The Mayo Clinic, Rochester, MN.)

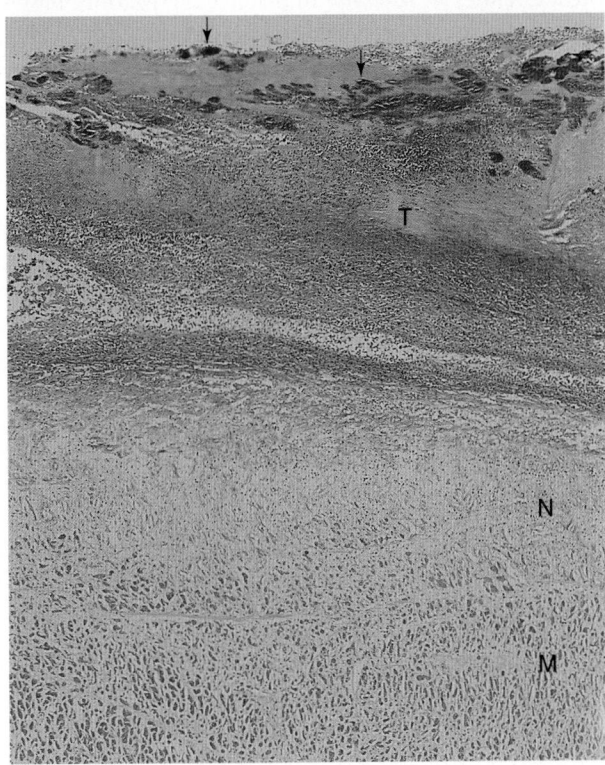

FIGURE 22.38 An infected thrombus on the inner surface of the heart (left ventricle). *Lower half:* Myocardium (**M**). A thin horizontal slit separates it from the thrombus. The upper half of the myocardium is necrotic (loss of structure) (**N**); it may have been killed (a) by the overlying thrombus (anoxia and lack of nutrients) or (b) by infarction followed by thrombosis. *Upper half:* Thrombus (**T**), seeded with bacterial cultures (purple spots) (**arrowheads**). The infection must have come from the lumen. Swarms of blue dots = leukocytes attracted by the bacteria. Such thrombi shed septic emboli. (30x)

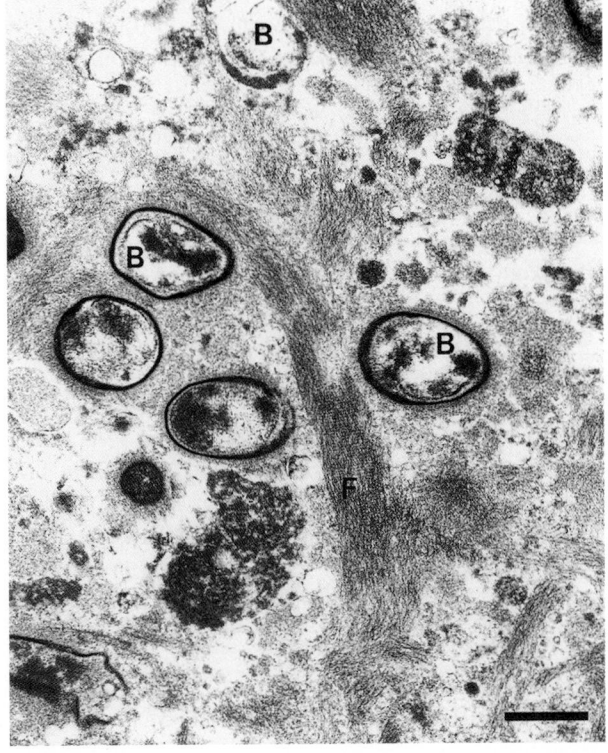

FIGURE 22.39 Electron micrograph of an infected thrombus on a mitral valve, from a case of bacterial endocarditis. **F** = fibrin strands; **B** = bacteria. The platelets that originally built up this thrombus have long since broken up. **Bar** = 0.5 μm.

Clinical Aspects of Thrombosis

The yearly incidence of thrombosis in the United States, including symptomless cases, could be of the order of half a million to a million, possibly more (90); firm figures are not available. One way to reach an estimate is to start with pulmonary thromboembolism, which is a reflection of thrombosis. The number of new cases of pulmonary thromboembolism per year in the United States is estimated at 170,000, plus 99,000 cases of recurrent disease (2). Yearly deaths from pulmonary emboli are estimated at 50,000 to 200,000 (11). Considering that there are many times more pulmonary emboli than fatal ones and that some thrombi never embolize, the high estimate seems reasonable.

Most dangerous as sources of emboli are the thrombi in the *large veins of the lower limbs: femoral, iliac, and popliteal.* The deep veins of the calf thrombose easily but seem to pose less threat; the superficial veins, including the large saphenous vein, can thrombose but rarely produce emboli. *Many thrombi are symptomless.*

> A study of symptomless thrombosis was carried out, using radioactive fibrinogen, on patients who had had two common, low-risk operations: hernia and prostatectomy. In the legs of patients over 50, thrombi developed in 25 and 50 percent, respectively (107).

Pain. Pain could be a useful warning sign of thrombosis, but it is not always present. Occasionally, thrombosis of a superficial vein is accompanied by dramatic symptoms: edema, sometimes redness, pain, and fever. This is thrombophlebitis, an enigmatic condition described by Trousseau in Paris as *phlegmasia alba dolens* (white painful inflammation) (115). There are in fact two enigmas: why does thrombosis occur in the first place? and why does the vein become inflamed?

> There is usually a predisposing factor such as lying in bed after surgery, a malignant tumor, or pregnancy. As to the inflammation, bacteria are rarely involved. We will propose an explanation: platelets are loaded with inflammatory mediators (21). If the thrombus becomes occlusive and the platelets continue to de-granulate, their mediators would no longer be washed away but should be able to diffuse through the thin venous wall and cause inflammation, including pain. This would account for the aseptic nature of the process. This hypothesis should not be too difficult to test.

Aspirin and thrombi. Among the many virtues of aspirin is that of being antithrombogenic. It irreversibly acetylates in platelets an enzyme of prostaglandin metabolism (prostaglandin G/H synthase), with the result that platelets can no longer produce thromboxane A_2, a platelet activator. Inevitably, the same enzyme is inhibited also in the endothelium, which uses it to produce prostacycline, an *inhibitor* of platelet aggregation. However, platelets cannot synthesize new enzyme for as long as they live (8–10 days), so the inhibition is permanent, whereas the endothelium can quickly recover (96). As a result, the anti-platelet effect of aspirin prevails, the formation of the hemostatic plug is inhibited, and bleeding time is prolonged. Still, much effort is concentrated on finding drugs that inhibit thromboxane synthesis without affecting the helpful endothelial production of prostacyclin (27, 28).

> Anticoagulants, which block the clotting cascade, are the most effective antithrombotic agents, especially for venous thrombi, because fibrin is the glue that stabilizes thrombi. There is, of course, a trade-off between the dangers of hemorrhage and those of thrombosis and its complications. The anticoagulants most used are heparin (116), warfarin (which has no connection with warfare; it stands for Wisconsin Alumni Research Foundation, Inc.), and inhibitors of the glycoprotein IIb/IIIa receptor complex, which is the ultimate common pathway for platelet-to-platelet aggregation (85a).

Disseminated Intravascular Coagulation

Imagine the blood clotting throughout the circulatory system. This catastrophe occurs almost daily in hospitals, as a life-threatening event known as disseminated intravascular coagulation (DIC) (70). *It never occurs as a disease in itself but as a complication* to some primary event that triggers generalized blood clotting. This primary event can be **sepsis,** especially gram-negative sepsis (Gram-negative bacteria produce endotoxin, which activates the intrinsic clotting cascade); *severe trauma* (especially to the brain, which is especially rich in thromboplastin); a complication of *childbirth* (amniotic fluid embolism, a retained dead fetus); **shock;** a *tumor;* the bite of a rattlesnake; and much else. The mechanism leading to generalized coagulation is not always the same and not always clear.

Of course, if a large amount of thromboplastin is introduced into the circulation, the blood clots everywhere and death is almost immediate. This is what a

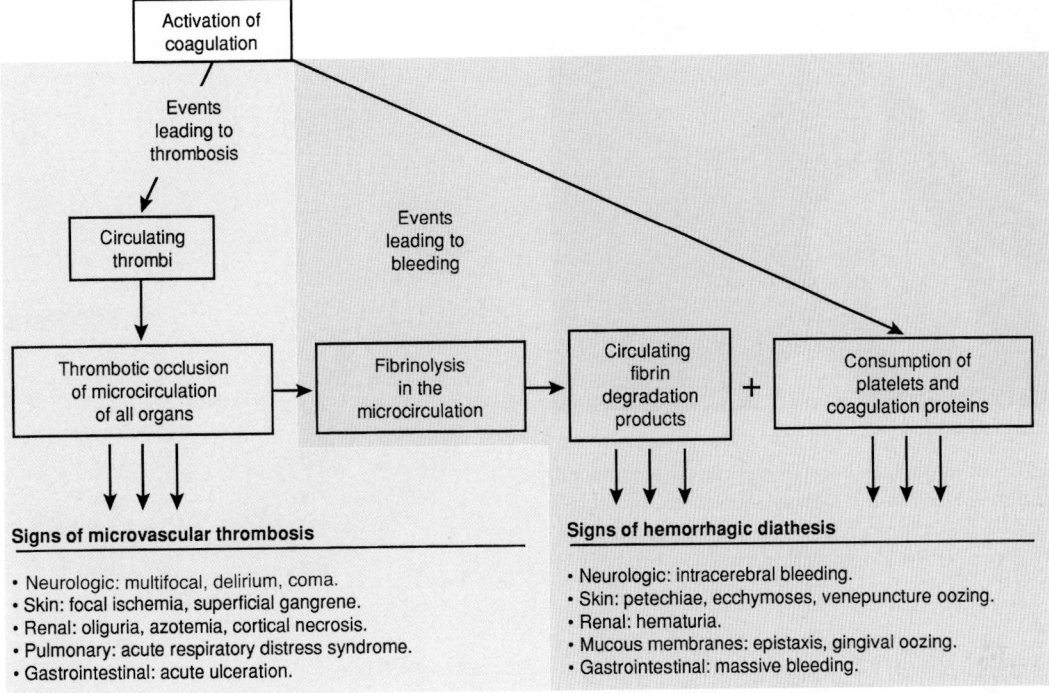

FIGURE 22.40   During disseminated intravascular coagulation (DIC), two conflicting sets of events develop: one set leads to coagulation and thrombosis (*left*); the other to fibrinolysis and bleeding (*right*). (Adapted with permission from [81].)

Frenchman reported to the Paris Academy of Medicine in 1834 (102). He had injected a generous amount of mashed brain intravenously into experimental animals, thereby triggering the extrinsic pathway of coagulation. Later, with smaller doses of intravenous tissue, it was found that the animal could survive; but then the blood had become incoagulable. It had been, as we now say, defibrinated. This is a key feature of DIC: a combination of clotting and nonclotting, leading to thromboembolic problems as well as to hemorrhage. Hence DIC is also known by the oxymoronic name (as Jandl puts it) of *hemorrhagic microthrombosis* (63). Bleeding is inevitable because the clotting factors are being used up, which accounts for another name, **consumption coagulopathy** (Figure 22.40) (81).

DIC is a complicated and varied syndrome, but in the acute form *the cascade of events is initiated when an activator of the clotting system finds its way into the blood.* It may be an endogenous factor, such as thromboplastin, or an exogenous factor, such as endotoxin. In either case, thrombin is produced on a large scale, with three main effects:

1. Loose microscopic aggregates of fibrin develop in the bloodstream and embolize the arterioles and capillaries throughout the body (large thrombi do

not form [102]). Some microthrombi may originate in the capillaries, but this is not clear.

2. Platelets are activated and form aggregates that become microemboli. Some of these are removed by the littoral phagocytes of the liver, but others occlude arterioles and capillaries throughout the body. In parallel, *thrombocytopenia* develops.

3. Endothelial cells exposed to thrombin and to fibrin filaments respond by secreting a plasminogen activator. So the plasmin (fibrinolytic) system is also activated, and fibrin/fibrinogen degradation products (FDP) are released; in fact they are the classic markers of DIC. FDP have further pernicious effects: some act as anticoagulants or damage the endothelium and increase vascular permeability.

The red cells are not spared. Imagine them ramming at high speed into capillaries partially clogged by meshes of fibrin filaments. Some red cells break up, and others are sliced into smaller pieces, which continue to circulate as "schistocytes," "helmet cells," or the like (Figure 22.41).

This complication is known as *microangiopathic hemolytic anemia.* The same predicament can befall red blood cells in other situations, such as when they are forced through an angioma or a malignant tumor.

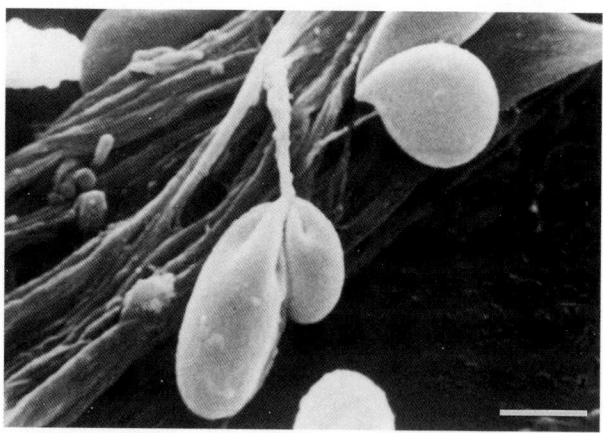

FIGURE 22.41   Fibrin threads in capillaries can slice red blood cells. This scanning electron micrograph shows a red blood cell being "hanged" across a fibrin strand. From a clot prepared *in vitro*. **Bar** = 2 μm. (Reproduced with permission from [24].)

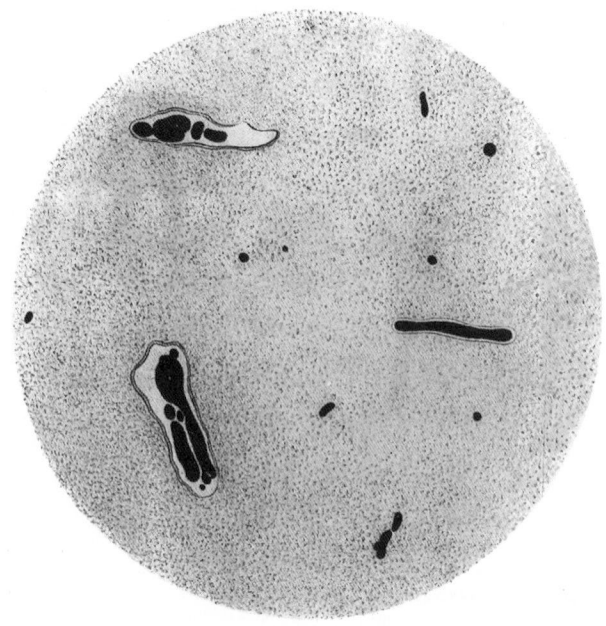

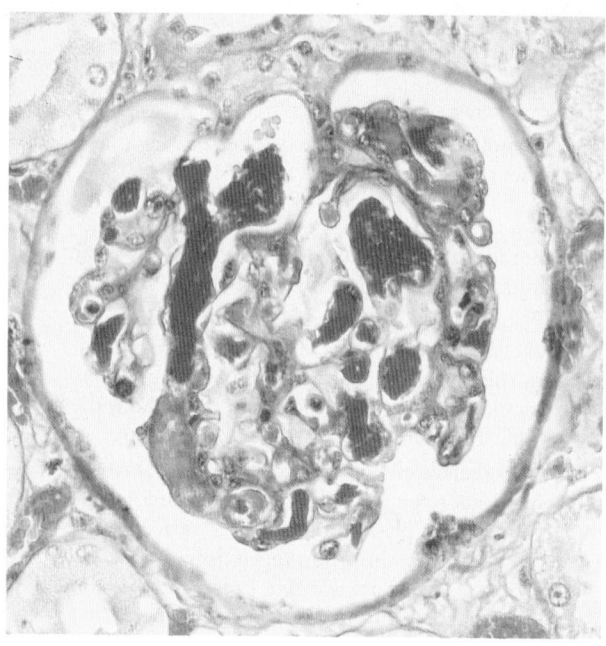

FIGURE 22.42   A result of disseminated intravascular coagulation: platelet-fibrin thrombi in the glomerular capillaries, in the kidney of a 34-year-old man with AIDS who died 3 days after a bout of pneumonia with gram-negative bacteria. (Fraser-Lendrum stain; 270x). (Reproduced with permission from: New Engl. J. Med. "Images in Clinical Medicine: Disseminated Intravascular Coagulopathy", Bastacky S, Lee R.E. 345:1394,2001. Copyright © 2001 Massachusetts Medical Society. All rights reserved.)

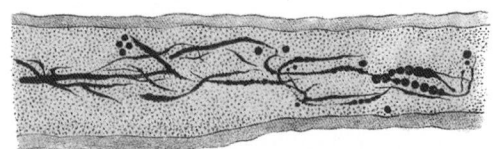

FIGURE 22.43   Fibrin thrombi in brain capillaries of a patient who died of meningitis and bronchopneumonia, presumably accompanied by terminal sepsis and disseminated intravascular coagulation. This illustration appeared in *Virchows Archiv* in 1892. *Top:* Brain tissue with vessels occluded by fibrin thrombi (either formed locally or embolized). *Bottom:* Detail showing vessel containing filaments of fibrin. (Reproduced from [77].)

A great deal of damage is caused by microthrombi and microemboli. Most affected is the kidney because of its function as a filter (Figure 22.42). In the brain, microthrombi or emboli of fibrin (which were seen as early as 1892) often cause death (Figure 22.43). In the skin, large patches of hemorrhagic infarction may turn to gangrene. In the gastrointestinal tract, ulceration and hemorrhage are common (82). The infarcted tissues release thromboplastin and thereby create a vicious circle. The platelets, which might check the bleeding, are severely depleted by aggregation and by adhesion to the fibrin thrombi. Other clotting factors are also depleted. This anomalous mixture of clotting and hemorrhage is a therapeutic nightmare. The optimistic version: trying to think up a way to stop the vicious circle is an interesting intellectual challenge.

The solution is another paradox. To stop the bleeding, the best weapon is an anticoagulant; a controlled infusion of heparin, together with other measures such as the replenishment of exhausted clotting factors, may sometimes be effective. We will return to DIC in relation to shock.

TO SUM UP: The unique feature of cardiovascular pathology is the precarious balance between two contrasting needs: the blood must remain fluid to feed the tissues, and it must clot to prevent blood loss. The endothelium in this setting peforms superbly, but we still need to find an artificial membrane capable of behaving—at the very least—as a non-clottable container. We need to learn more about the healing of thrombi: how real is recanalization? Do the circulating stem cells contribute? Exactly how do platelets retract the clot? At the cellular level we find most intriguing the comparison between the retraction of the fibrin clot by the platelets and the retraction of collagen fibrils by fibroblasts in wound healing.

References

1. Alexander CJ. Chair-sitting and varicose veins. Lancet 1972; 1:822–824.

2. Anderson FA Jr, Wheeler HB. Venous thromboembolism. Risk factors and prophylaxis. Clin Chest Med 1995;16:235–251.

3. Archer GL. Experimental endocarditis. In: Duma RJ (ed), Infections of Prosthetic Heart Valves and Vascular Grafts. Baltimore: University Park Press, 1977, pp. 43–59.

4. Aschoff L. Lectures on Pathology. New York: Paul B. Hoeber, Inc., 1924.

5. Ashford TP, Freiman DG. The role of the endothelium in the initial phases of thrombosis. Am J Pathol 1967;50:257–273.

6. Bach RR. Initiation of coagulation by tissue factor. CRC Crit Rev Biochem 1988;23:339–368.

6a. Bastacky S, Lee RE. Images in clinical medicine: Disseminated intravascular coagulopathy. N Engl J Med 2001; 345:1394.

7. Bauer KA. Hypercoagulability—A New Cofactor in the Protein C Anticoagulant Pathway. N Engl J Med 1994;330:566–567.

8. Baumgartner HR. The role of blood flow in platelet adhesion, fibrin deposition, and formation of mural thrombi. Microvasc Res 1973;5:167–179.

9. Baumgartner HR, Muggli R. Adhesion and aggregation: morphological demonstration and quantitation in vivo and in vitro. In: Gordon JL (ed), Platelets in Biology and Pathology. Amsterdam: North-Holland Publishing Company, 1976, pp. 23–60.

10. Becker CG, Dubin T. Activation of factor XII by tobacco glycoprotein. J Exp Med 1977;146:457–467.

11. Becker DM. Venous thromboembolism: epidemiology, diagnosis, prevention. J Gen Intern Med 1986;1:402–411.

12. Beckering RE Jr, Titus JL. Femoral-popliteal venous thrombosis and pulmonary embolism. Am J Clin Pathol 1969;52:530–537.

13. Behnke, O. The blood platelet. A potential smooth muscle cell. In: Perry SV, Margreth A, Adelstein RS (eds), Contractile Systems in Non-Muscle Tissues. Amsterdam: North-Holland Publishing Company, 1976, pp. 105–115.

14. Bentfeld-Barker ME, Bainton DF. Identification of primary lysosomes in human megakaryocytes and platelets. Blood 1982;59:472–481.

15. Bergmann SR, Fox KAA, Ter-Pogossian MM, Sobel BE, Collen D. Clot-selective coronary thrombolysis with tissue-type plasminogen activator. Science 1983;220:1181–1183.

16. Bizzozero J. Ueber einen neuen Formbestandtheil des Blutes und dessen Rolle bei der Thrombose und der Blutgerinnung. Virchows Arch Pathol Anat 1882;90:261–332.

17. Booyse FM, Osikowicz G, Feder S, Scheinbuks J. Isolation and characterization of a urokinase-type plasminogen activator ($M_r = 54,000$) from cultured human endothelial cells indistinguishable from urinary urokinase. J Biol Chem 1984;259: 7198–7205.

18. Born GVR, Cross MJ. The aggregation of blood platelets. J Physiol 1963;168:178–195.

19. Born GVR, Honour AJ, Mitchell JRA. Inhibition by adenosine and by 2-chloroadenosine of the formation and embolization of platelet thrombi. Nature 1964;202:761–765.

20. Brandt KD. Glycosaminoglycans. In: Kelley WN, Harris ED, Ruddy S, Sledge CB (eds), Textbook of Rheumatology, vol. 1, 2nd ed. Philadelphia, W.B. Saunders Company, 1985.

21. Braunstein PW, Cuénoud HF, Joris I, Majno G. Platelets, fibroblasts and inflammation. Tissue reactions to platelets injected subcutaneously. Am J Pathol 1980;99:53–62.

22. Brinkhous KM. The problem in perspective. In: Sherry S, Brinkhous KM, Genton E, Stengle JM (eds), Thrombosis. Washington, DC: National Academy of Sciences, 1969, pp. 335–338.

23. Brinkhous KM, Sommer E. Why Virchow became a physician. Arch Pathol 1968;85:331–334.

24. Bull BS, Kuhn IN. The production of schistocytes by fibrin strands (a scanning electron microscope study). Blood 1970; 35:104–111.

25. Chapman HA Jr, Vavrin Z, Hibbs JB Jr. Macrophage fibrinolytic activity: identification of two pathways of plasmin formation by intact cells and of a plasminogen activator inhibitor. Cell 1982;28:653–662.

26. Chen TI, Tsai C. The mechanism of haemostasis in peripheral vessels. J Physiol 1948;107:208–288.

27. Clarke RJ, Mayo G, Price P, FitzGerald GA. Suppression of thromboxane A_2 but not of systemic prostacyclin by controlled-release aspirin. N Engl J Med 1991;325:1137–1141.

28. Clouse LH, Comp PC. The regulation of hemostasis: the protein C system. N Engl J Med 1986;314:1298–1304.

29. Cohen I, Gerrard JM, White JG. Ultrastructure of clots during isometric contraction. J Cell Biol 1982;93:775–787.

30. Coller BS. Platelets and thrombolytic therapy. N Engl J Med 1990;322:33–42.

31. Colman RW, Hirsh J, Marder VJ, Salzman EW (eds). Hemostasis and Thrombosis: Basic Principles and Clinical Practice, 2nd ed. Philadelphia: JB. Lippincott Company, 1987.

32. Colman RW, Marder VJ, Slazman EW, Hirsh J. Overview of hemostasis. In: Colman RW, Hirsh J, Marder VJ, Salzman EW

(eds), Hemostasis and Thrombosis: Basic Principles and Clinical Practice, 2nd ed., Philadelphia: JB. Lippincott Company, 1987, pp. 3–17.

33. Comp PC, Jacocks RM, Ferrell GL, Esmon CT. Activation of protein C in vivo. J Clin Invest 1982;70:127–134.

34. Cotran RS, Kumar V, Robbins SL. Robbins Pathologic Basis of Disease, 5th ed. Philadelphia: WB. Saunders Company, 1994.

35. Deykin D. The role of the liver in serum-induced hypercoagulability. J Clin Invest 1966;45:256–263.

36. Dible JH. The Pathology of Limb Ischaemia. St. Louis: Warren H. Green, Inc., 1966.

37. Donati MB, Curatolo L, Borgia R, Balconi G, Morasca L. Fibrin clot retraction by cultured human fibroblasts. In: de Gaetano G, Garattini S (eds), Platelets: A Multidisciplinary Approach. New York: Raven Press, 1978, pp. 149–158.

38. Drake TA, Morrissey JH, Edgington TS. Selective cellular expression of tissue factor in human tissues. Implications for disorders of hemostasis and thrombosis. Am J Pathol 1989; 134:1087–1097.

39. Drake TA, Pang M. Effects of interleukin-1, lipopolysaccharide, and streptococci on procoagulant activity of cultured human cardiac valve endothelial and stromal cells. Infect Immun 1989;57:507–512.

40. Durack DT, Beeson PB. Experimental bacterial endocarditis. I. Colonization of a sterile vegetation. Br J Exp Pathol 1972;53:44–49.

41. Eberth CJ, Schimmelbusch C. Experimentelle Untersuchungen über Thrombose. Virchows Arch Pathol Anat Physiol Klin Med 1886;103:39–87 and 105:331–350.

42. Eberth CJ, Schimmelbusch C. Die Thrombose nach Versuchen und Leichenbefunden. Stuttgart: Ferdinand Enke, 1888.

43. Esmon CT. Regulation of protein C activation by components of the endothelial cell surface. In Gimbrone MA Jr (ed), Vascular Endothelium in Hemostasis and Thrombosis. Edinburgh: Churchill Livingstone, 1986, pp. 99–119.

44. Esmon CT. The regulation of natural anticoagulant pathways. Science 1987;235:1348–1352.

45. Feigl W, Susani M, Ulrich W, et al. Organisation of experimental thrombosis by blood cells: Evidence of the transformation of mononuclear cells into myofibroblast and endothelial cell. Virchow Arch (Pathol Anat) 1985;406:133–148.

46. Flanc C. An experimental study of the recanalization of arterial and venous thrombi. Br J Surg 1968;55:519–524.

47. Fogarty TJ, Cranley JJ, Krause RJ, Strasser ES, Hafner CD. A method for extraction of arterial emboli and thrombi. Surg Gynecol Obstet 1963;116:241–244.

48. French JE. The structure of natural and experimental thrombi. Ann R Coll Surg Engl 1965;36:191–200.

49. French JE, MacFarlane RG, Sanders AG. The structure of haemostatic plugs and experimental thrombi in small arteries. Br J Exp Pathol 1964;45:467–474.

50. Fuchs U, Graff J. Gefässwand und Fibrinolyse—Pathologische Aspekte. Folia Haematol 1986;113:176–183.

51. Gimbrone MA Jr (ed), Vascular Endothelium in Hemostasis and Thrombosis. Contemporary Issues in Haemostasis and Thrombosis, vol. 2. Edinburgh: Churchill Livingstone, 1986a.

52. Gimbrone MA Jr. Vascular endothelium: nature's blood container. In: Gimbrone MA Jr (ed), Vascular Endothelium in Hemostasis and Thrombosis. Contemporary Issues in Haemostasis and Thrombosis, vol. 2. Edinburgh: Churchill Livingstone, 1986b, pp. 1–13.

53. Glenner GG, Osserman EF, Benditt EP, et al. (eds), Amyloidosis. New York: Plenum Press, 1986.

54. Goffin YA, Gruys E, Sorenson GD, Wellens F. Amyloid deposits in bioprosthetic cardiac valves after long-term implantation in man. A new localization of amyloidosis. Am J Pathol 1984;114:431–442.

55. Hadfield G. Thrombosis. Ann R Coll Surg Engl, 1950; 6:219–234.

56. Hajjar KA, Gavish D, Breslow JL, Nachman RL. Lipoprotein (a) modulation of endothelial cell surface fibrinolysis and its potential role in atherosclerosis. Nature 1989;339: 303–305.

57. Hawiger J. Adhesive interactions of blood cells and the vessel wall. In: Colman RW, Hirsh J, Marder VJ, Salzman EW (eds), Hemostasis and Thrombosis, 2nd ed. Philadelphia: JB Lippincott Company, 1987, pp. 182–209.

58. Hayem G. Sur le mécanisme de l'arrêt des hémorrhagies. CR Acad Sci (Paris) 1882;95:18–21.

59. Hedner U, Nilsson IM. The role of fibrinolysis. Clin Haematol 1981;10:327–342.

60. Hogg N. Human monocytes are associated with the formation of fibrin. J Exp Med 1983;157:473–485.

61. Hume M, Sevitt S, Thomas DP. Venous Thrombosis and Pulmonary Embolism. Cambridge: Harvard University Press, 1970.

62. Hunter J. A Treatise on the Blood, Inflammation, and Gun-Shot Wounds. London: John Richardson, 1794.

63. Jandl JH. Blood: Textbook of Hematology. Boston: Little, Brown and Company, 1987.

64. Jorgensen L, Borchgrevink CF. The platelet plug in normal persons. 1. The histological appearance of the plug 15 to 20 minutes and 24 hours after the bleeding and its rôle in the capillary haemostasis. Acta Pathol Microbiol Scand 1963; 57:40–56.

65. Joris I, Braunstein PW Jr. Platelets and endothelium: Effect of collagen-induced platelet aggregates on pulmonary vessels. Exp & Molec Pathol 1982;37:393–405.

66. Kane KK. Fibrinolysis—a review. Ann Clin Lab Sci 1984;14:443–449.

67. Kitchens CS. Concept of hypercoagulability: a review of its development, clinical application, and recent progress. Semin Thromb Hemost 1985;11:293–315.

68. Kozin F, Cochrane CG. The contact activation system of plasma: biochemistry and pathophysiology. In: Gallin JI, Goldstein IM, Snyderman R (eds), Inflammation: Basic Principles and Clinical Correlates. New York: Raven Press, 1988, pp. 101–120.

69. Leu HJ, Feigl W, Susani M. Angiogenesis from mononuclear cells in thrombi. Virchows Arch A 1987;411:5–14.

70. Levi M, Cate HT. Disseminated intravascular coagulation. N Engl J Med 1999;341:586–592.

71. Levin J. The history of the development of the limulus amebocyte lysate test. Prog Clin Biol Res 1985;189:3–28.

72. Levin J, Bang FB. Clottable protein in limulus: its localization and kinetics of its coagulation by endotoxin. Thromb Diath Haemorrh 1968;19:186–197.

73. Lijnen HR, Collen D. Interaction of plasminogen activators and inhibitors with plasminogen and fibrin. Semin Thromb Hemost 1982;8:2–10.

74. Loscalzo J, Braunwald E. Tissue plasminogen activator. N Engl J Med 1988;319:925–931.

75. Macfarlane RG. Haemostasis: introduction. Br Med Bull 1977;33:183–185.

76. Majno G, Bouvier CA, Gabbiani G, Ryan GB, Statkov P. Kymographic recording of clot retraction: effects of papaverine, theophylline and cytochalasin B. Thromb Diath Haemor 1972;28:49–53.

77. Manasse P. Ueber hyaline Ballen und Thromben in den Gehirnegefässen bei acuten Infectionskrankheiten. Virchows Arch Pathol Anat Physiol Klin Med 1892;130:217–233.

78. Mann KG, Fass DN. The molecular biology of blood coagulation. In: Fairbanks VF (ed), Current Hematology, vol. 2. New York: John Wiley & Sons, Inc., 1983.

79. Marcus AJ. Platelets and their disorders. In: Ratnoff OD, Forbes CD (eds), Disorders of Hemostasis. Philadelphia: W.B. Saunders Company, 1991.

80. Marcus AJ, Safier LB. Thromboregulation: multicellular modulation of platelet reactivity in hemostasis and thrombosis. FASEB J 1993;7:516–522.

81. Marder VJ. Microvascular thrombosis. In: Lichtman MA (ed), Hematology and Oncology. New York: Grune & Stratton, 1980, pp. 230–234.

82. Marder VJ, Martin SE, Colman RW. Clinical aspects of consumptive thrombohemorrhagic disorders. In: Colman RW, Hirsh J, Marder VJ, Salzman EW (eds), Hemostasis and Thrombosis: Basic Principles and Clinical Practice. Philadelphia: J.B. Lippincott Company, 1982, pp. 664–693.

83. Marder VJ, Sherry S. Thrombolytic therapy: current status. (Second of two parts). N Engl J Med 1988;318:1585–1595.

84. McGehee WG, Rapaport SI, Hjort PF. Intravascular coagulation in fulminant meingococcemia. Ann Intern Med 1967;67:250–260.

85. Miles LA, Fless GM, Levin EG, Scanu AM, Plow EF. A potential basis for the thrombotic risks associated with lipoprotein(*a*). Nature 1989;339:301–303.

85a. Miller WL, Reeder GS. Adjunctive therapies in the treatment of acute coronary syndromes. Mayo Clin Proc 2001;76:391–405.

86. Millet J, Theveniaux J, Pascal M. A new experimental model of venous thrombosis in rats involving partial stasis and slight endothelium alterations. Thromb Res 1987;45:123–133.

87. Mills JA. Aspirin, the ageless remedy? N Engl J Med 1991;325:1303–1304.

88. Moake JL. Hypercoagulable states: new knowledge about old problems. Hosp Pract 1991;26:31–42.

89. Morgenstern E, Korell U, Richter J. Platelets and fibrin strands during clot retraction. Thromb Res 1984;33:617–623.

90. Moser KM. Pulmonary embolism: where the problem is not. JAMA 1976;236:1500.

91. Mustard JF, Packham MA. Normal and abnormal haemostasis. Br Med Bull 1977;33:187–192.

92. Nemerson Y, Bach R. Tissue factor revisited. Prog Hemost Thromb 1982;6:237–261.

93. Nesheim ME, Hibbard LS, Tracy PB, et al. Participation of factor Va in prothrombinase. In: Mann KG, Taylor FB Jr (eds), The Regulation of Coagulation. New York: Elsevier North-Holland, 1980.

94. Niewiarowski S, Regoeczi E, Mustard JF. Adhesion of fibroblasts to polymerizing fibrin and retraction of fibrin induced by fibroblasts. Proc Soc Exp Biol Med 1972;140:199–204.

95. Packham MA, Mustard JF. Platelet adhesion. Prog Hemost Thromb 1984;7:211–288.

96. Patrono C. Aspirin as an antiplatelet drug. N Engl J Med 1994;330:1287–1294.

97. Polack B, Delolme F, Peyron F. Protective role of platelets in chronic (Balb/C) and acute (CBA/J) *plasmodium berghei* murine malaria. Haemostasis 1997;27:278–285.

98. Puszkin EG, Aledort LM. Platelets: biochemistry and physiology. In: Root WS, Berlin NI (eds), Physiological Pharmacology, vol. 5. New York: Academic Press, 1974, pp. 177–198.

99. Pytela R, Pierschbacher MD, Ginsberg MH, Plow EF, Ruoslahti E. Platelet membrane glycoprotein IIb/IIIa: member of a family of Arg-Gly-Asp-specific adhesion receptors. Science 1986;231:1559–1562.

100. Rand JH, Gordon RE, Sussman II, Chu SV, Solomon V. Electron microscopic localization of factor-VIII-related antigen in adult human blood vessels. Blood 1982;60:627–634.

101. Ratnoff OD. The evolution of knowledge about hemostasis. In: Ratnoff OD, Forbes CD (eds), Disorders of Hemostasis. Orlando: Grune & Stratton, Inc., 1984, pp. 1–21.

102. Ratnoff OD. Disseminated intravascular coagulation. In: Ratnoff OD, Forbes CD (eds), Disorders of Hemostasis. Orlando: Grune & Stratton, Inc., 1984, pp. 289–319.

103. Ratnoff OD, Busse RJ Jr, Sheon RP. The demise of John Hageman. N Engl J Med 1968;279:760–761.

104. Reidy MA, Schwartz SM. Endothelial regeneration. III. Time course of intimal changes after small defined injury to rat aortic endothelium. Lab Invest 1981;44:301–308.

105. Robb-Smith AHT. Why the platelets were discovered. Br J Haematol 1967;13:618–637.

106. Roberts HR, Lozier JN. New perspectives on the coagulation cascade. Hosp Pract 1992;1:97–112.

107. Rubenstein E. Thromboembolism. In: Rubenstein E, Federman DD (eds), Scientific American Medicine, pt. 1 Cardiovascular Medicine, Sect. XVIII. New York: Scientific American, Inc., 1991, pp. 1–10.

108. Ryan GB, Grobéty J, Majno G. Mesothelial injury and recovery. Am J Pathol 1973;71:93–112.

109. Saito H. Normal hemostatic mechanisms. In: Ratnoff OD, Forbes CD (eds), Disorders of Hemostasis. Orlando: Grune & Stratton, Inc., 1984, pp. 23–42.

110. Seghatchian MJ, Samama MM, Hecker SP (eds). Hypercoagulable states: fundamental aspects, acquired disorders, and congenital thrombophilia. Boca Raton: CRC Press, 1996.

111. Shattil SJ, Bennett JS. Platelets and their membranes in hemostasis: physiology and pathophysiology. Ann Intern Med 1980;94:108–118.

112. Tanaka K, Hirst AE, Smith LL. Rate of endothelialization in venous thrombi. Arch Surg 1982;117:1045–1048.

113. The TIMI Study Group. Comparison of invasive and conservative strategies after treatment with intravenous tissue plasminogen activator in acute myocardial infarction. Results of the thrombolysis in myocardial infarction (TIMI) phase II trial. N Engl J Med 1989;320:618–627.

114. Trip MD, Cats VM, van Capelle FJL, Vreeken J. Platelet hyperreactivity and prognosis in survivors of myocardial infarction. N Engl J Med 1990;322:1549–1554.

115. Trousseau A. Phlegmatia alba dolens. In: Clinique Médicale de Hôtel-Dieu de Paris, vol. 3, 2nd ed. Paris: Balliere, 1865, pp. 654–712.

116. Turpie AGG, Robinson JG, Doyle DJ, et al. Comparison of high-dose with low-dose subcutaneous heparin to prevent left ventricular mural thrombosis in patients with acute transmural anterior myocardial infarction. N Engl J Med 1989; 320:352–357.

117. Wester J, Sixma JJ, Geuze JJ, Heijnen HFG. Morphology of the hemostatic plug in human skin wounds. Transformation of the plug. Lab Invest 1979;41:182–192.

118. Wessler S. Studies in intravascular coagulation. III. The pathogenesis of serum-induced venous thrombosis. J Clin Invest 1955;34:647–651.

119. Wessler S, Cohen S, Fleischner FG. The temporary thrombotic state. N Engl J Med 1956;254:413–419.

120. Wessler S, Freiman DG, Ballon JD, et al. Experimental pulmonary embolism with serum-induced thrombi. Am J Pathol 1961;38:89–101.

121. Wessler S, Reiner L, Freiman DG, et al. Serum-induced thrombosis. Studies of its induction and evolution under controlled conditions in vivo. Circulation 1959;20:864–874.

122. Williams RS, Logue EE, Lewis JL, et al. Physical conditioning augments the fibrinolytic response to venous occlusion in healthy adults. N Engl J Med 1980;302:987–991.

123. Yeaman MR, Sullam PM, Dazin PF, Bayer AS. Platelet microbicidal protein alone and in combination with antibiotics reduces *Staphylococcus aureus* adherence to platelets in vitro. Infect Immun 1994;62:3416–3423.

124. Zahn FW. Untersuchungen über Thrombose. Bildung der Thromben. Virchows Arch Pathol Anat Physiol Klin Med 1875;62:81–124.

125. Zahn FW. Ueber die Rippenbildung an der freien Oberfläche der Thromben. Int Beitr Wissenschaftlichen Med 1891;2: 201–215. Festschrift Rudolf Virchow, Berlin, 1891.

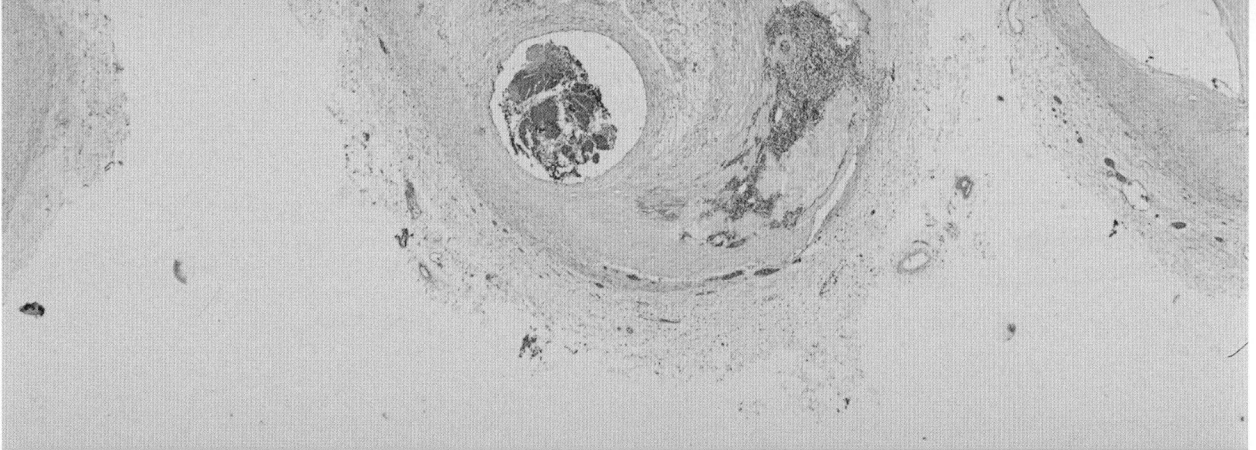

- Obstacles Arising in the Lumen: Emboli
- Obstruction by Changes in the Vascular Wall
- Obstruction by Compression
- Obstructions at the Capillary Level

Inadequate blood flow—**ischemia**—is one of the major threats to life; ischemic tissues become atrophic or die. It is therefore important to understand the many causes of impaired flow. No other topic illustrates better Virchow's definition of pathology as "physiology with obstacles" (p. 14).

Blood flow through a vessel can be impaired by three local mechanisms (Figure 23.1): an obstacle arising in the lumen; a thickening of the vessel's wall; and compression of the vessel from outside. A fourth, body-wide calamity—failure of the pump, leading to circulatory shock—will be discussed later. We will now review the three local mechanisms (Table 23.1).

Obstacles Arising in the Lumen: Emboli

Obstacles to flow that arise in the lumen can be thrombi (already discussed) or emboli. **Emboli are solid, liquid, or gaseous objects carried by the blood that cannot mix with the blood, and that are large enough to become impacted in the downstream lumen.** It follows that an embolus can exist as such only for 5 or 6 seconds: the time it takes to travel and to become impacted. **Embolism** is the impaction of an embolus.

Emboli: Sources and Impaction

The concept of embolism is attributed to Virchow, but it actually surfaced soon after Harvey published his discovery of the circulation in 1628 (17). Observations made at autopsies led the Swiss physician Jakob Wepfer (1620–1695) to conclude that solid bodies formed in the blood could break loose and obstruct arteries; and the Florentine physician–scientist Francesco Redi (1626–1698) showed experimentally that animals can be killed by introducing air into their circulation, thereby "interrupting the pulse." There were many other pioneers. However, it was certainly Virchow who

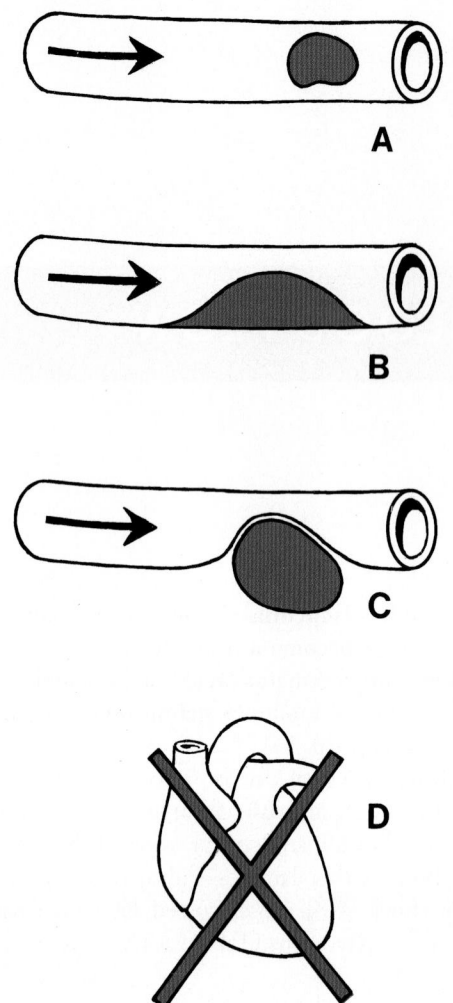

FIGURE 23.1 Four mechanisms that impair blood flow. **A:** Obstruction carried by the bloodstream (embolus). **B:** Intrinsic obstacle due to a change in the vascular wall. **C:** Extrinsic obstacle compressing the vessel. **D:** Malfunction of the cardiac pump.

codified the notion that thrombi can become emboli. (A **thrombus**—recall—is any solid mass that arises in the bloodstream *in vivo* from components of the blood.) Virchow also chose the ancient word *embolus* (from the Greek *en-bállein,* in-throw).

> Virchow did not know about the observations of his ancient predecessors, but he certainly became the champion of embolism, as we are about to prove. The fateful year 1848 saw him as a young revolutionary in Berlin (he was 26), siding with those who were fighting on the barricades in the name of democracy. One day of that same year, working as a prosector, he happened to meet Schoenlein, court physician and a political adversary, to discuss an autopsy. The cause of death was supposed to have been cerebral hemorrhage, but Virchow pointed out an

Table 23.1 Obstacles to Blood Flow
Obstructions arising in the lumen
Thrombi
Arterial thrombi
Venous thrombi
Emboli
Thromboemboli
Paradoxical emboli
Emboli of atheroma
Emboli of fat or bone marrow
Gas emboli
Amniotic fluid emboli
Therapeutic emboli
Sundry emboli
Obstructions by changes in the vascular wall
Arteriosclerosis
Atherosclerosis
Arteriolosclerosis
Mönckeberg's disease
Arterial spasm
Obstructions by external compression
Increased tissue pressure
Compartment syndrome
Torsion
Increased pressure on body parts
Pressure sores

embolus that had obstructed a cerebral artery. Whereupon Schoenlein, only half in jest, retorted: "Really, you see barricades everywhere!" (127).

Most emboli arise from thrombi (hence the term **thromboembolism**); however, a single red or white blood cell can also embolize a capillary under some circumstances (p. 687). Emboli can also be droplets of body fat, fragments of bone marrow (usually mobilized by trauma), the content of atheromatous plaques, fragments of tumors, parasites, bubbles of air or other gases, debris injected intravenously, trophoblast cells, bits of brain or liver after accidents, runaway cardiac catheters (164), and even bullets.

Rules of Embolism

Where is an embolus likely to become impacted? The rules are best understood with an example:

- *Emboli arising from the peripheral veins* end in the lungs, with the rare exception of paradoxical emboli (see further). Example: drug addicts who inject into their veins all manner of unclean preparations fill their lungs with foreign body granulomas.

- *Emboli arising in arterial blood* (pulmonary veins, left heart, aorta, and branches) end up in arteries anywhere in the body, including the lungs: theoretically at least, the lungs—which have a double circulation—could receive emboli in the bronchial and in the pulmonary arteries, but we have never heard of emboli in the *bronchial* arteries (pulmonary emboli typically settle in the *pulmonary* arteries).

- *Emboli arising in the mesenteric veins* (colon, rectum, small intestine, etc.) end up in the liver, because the mesenteric and hepatic venous systems are arranged in series (this explains the love affair of the worm *Schistosoma mansoni:* male and female settle in the mesenteric veins and copulate in there for months, shedding thousands of eggs that embolize the liver). These are the only VENOUS EMBOLI known to us.

Thromboemboli in Pulmonary Arteries

Pulmonary thromboemboli in human pathology are common. Clinically, the yearly incidence in the United States is of the order of 600,000 cases (5); about 10 percent of these patients die within 1 hour (142). Pulmonary emboli are commonly found postmortem: in our experience, about once every 8–10 autopsies. Large emboli that become lodged astride the bifurcation of the pulmonary artery (**saddle emboli**) are usually lethal (Figure 23.2)

About 80 percent of all thromboemboli arise from thrombi in the deep veins of the thigh and from the popliteal vein (10, 69); the main risk factors for developing the initial thrombosis include a history of (previous) pulmonary embolism, age over 40, major surgery, cancer, obesity, and multiple trauma (5). Visualize these thrombi as soft, oblong masses of clotted blood mixed with irregular whitish layers of platelets; such thrombi often fill a vein and form a cast of its lumen, even extending into its branches. Pieces of such thrombi can

become detached; these emboli can be longer and thicker than pencils. Because of their size, it is possible to stop them in their tracks by placing an umbrella-shaped metal filter in the inferior vena cava (Figure 23.3). When emboli become impacted in the pulmonary arteries, they are often doubled up or coiled. After the impact, some blood flow can usually trickle past (109); in so doing it may deposit fresh platelets on the embolus, until it becomes fully occlusive.

The various fates of an embolus are shown in Figure 23.4. As has been proven with serial arteriograms, *most pulmonary emboli undergo complete lysis and disappear* within 2–3 weeks (47, 164). The next most common fate is reabsorption, i.e., organization. An embolus is organized very much like a thrombus: the embolus is covered first by a carpet of flattened monocytes and later by endothelium (79); the underlying mass is then slowly reabsorbed, probably with the assistance of monocytes activated to macrophages. Smooth muscle cells are thought to creep out of the arterial media, colonize the embolus, and secrete collagen, elastin, and ground substance; the final result is a special kind of scar that is probably without fibroblasts because there are none in the arterial intima and media. The overall shape of the scar may be that of a patch flattened against the arterial

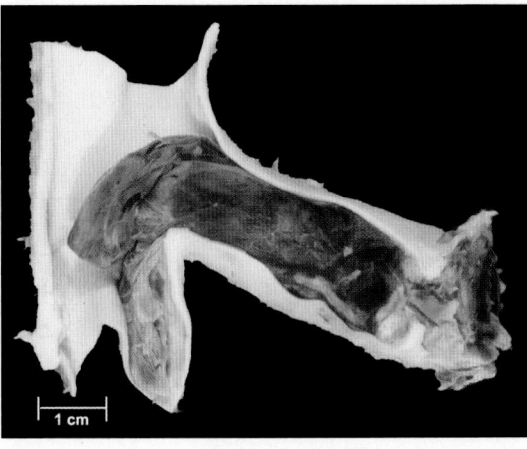

FIGURE 23.2 Saddle embolus occluding both branches of the pulmonary artery. The size and shape of this embolus indicate that it came from a large vein of the lower limb. Direction of flow: *from top left* (common pulmonary artery) to *bottom left* (left pulmonary artery) and *right* (right pulmonary artery).

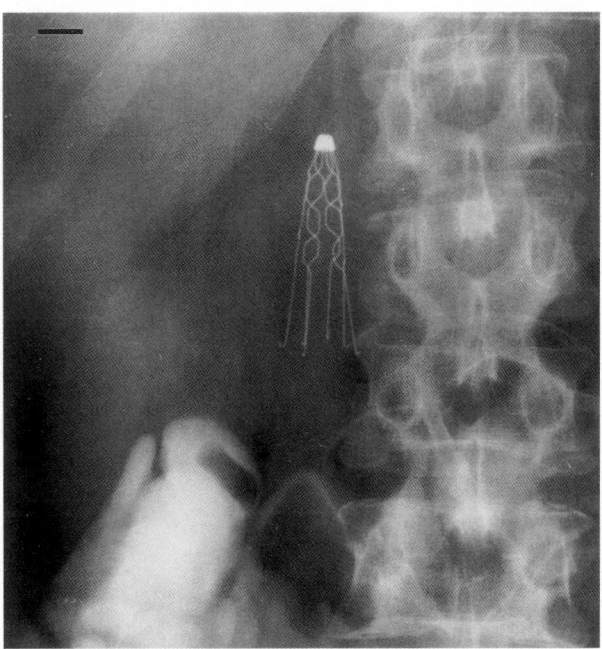

FIGURE 23.3 X-ray of the abdomen in a patient who had been implanted with a metallic "umbrella" (Greenfield filter) in the inferior vena cava as a protection against thromboemboli. **Bar** = 1 cm. (Courtesy of Dr. A. Davidoff, University of Massachusetts Medical School, Worcester, MA.)

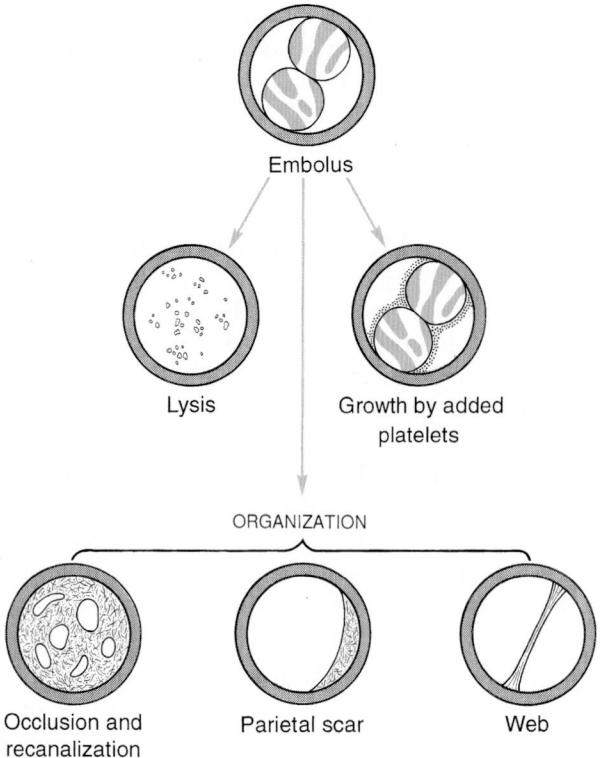

FIGURE 23.4 Fates of an embolus consisting of thrombotic material (thromboembolus).

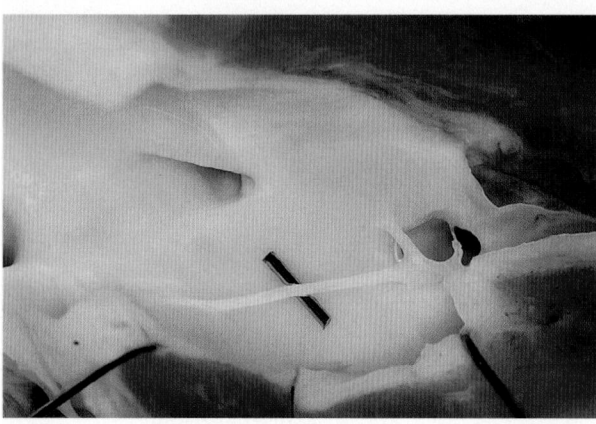

FIGURE 23.5 Webs in a pulmonary artery. These stringlike structures represent the end-stage of organized, healed emboli. A metal rod (**black**) was slipped beneath the longest web. Slightly enlarged.

wall, a solid plug perforated by canals, or a free strand (called a **web**) crossing the lumen (Figure 23.5). Webs are often found at autopsy in the larger branches of the pulmonary arteries (88); they are harmless but interesting as evidence of previous emboli.

Thromboemboli in Systemic Arteries

To become impacted in the systemic circulation, an embolus must arise from the left heart or from lesions of the aorta (e.g., thrombi in aneurysms). The left heart is a rich source of thromboemboli for four reasons:

- Infarcts affect especially the left ventricle, and a common complication of these infarcts is thrombosis in the ventricular cavity (p. 705). Thrombi inside a beating heart are of course easily turned into emboli.

- Thrombosis affects the mitral valve much more frequently than the tricuspid; these thrombi, called vegetations, are extremely prone to break off and embolize.

- Atrial fibrillation leads to decreased atrial contraction, dilatation of the left atrium, and stagnation of the blood with formation of thrombi. Fibrillation is a condition of disorderly contraction of the myocardial fibers, leading to ineffective pulsation.

- Loose thrombi can develop in a dilated left atrium. The classic example is the so-called **ball thrombus** (20). Imagine a stenotic, stiffened mitral valve that can neither open nor close properly (Figure 22.26); under these conditions, at each systole of the left ventricle blood is pumped back into the left atrium through the insufficient mitral valve. The left atrium expands, and the systolic reflux creates a permanent eddy in which a free-standing thrombus can develop and grow to a diameter of several centimeters. As mentioned earlier, this is the best proof that thrombosis can occur in the absence of endothelial injury because the ball thrombus is loose in the lumen.

All these sources of thrombi can produce emboli that are pumped into the aorta; their journey can end anywhere, but especially in the lower limbs (39).

It is sometimes feasible to remove an embolus impacted in an artery, using the Fogarty catheter (Figure 22.24) (44). Note the paradox: the Fogarty catheter is also used experimentally to produce endothelial damage (denudation). The rationale for its use in embolectomy is that the embolus is much more dangerous than endothelial denudation by the catheter.

Paradoxical Emboli

These rule-breaking emboli arise in the systemic veins; but instead of ending in the lungs, they embolize the systemic arteries. They bypass the lung in one of two ways:

- Small emboli pass through the arteriovenous anastomoses in the pulmonary circulation. Experiments using intravenous injections of microspheres have shown that normal lungs contain arteriovenous shunts that are 20–40 times the diameter of a capillary (61). This pathway is certainly used by embolic fat droplets and probably also by small air bubbles (84).

- Larger emboli must find a right-to-left passage in the heart (78, 95, 165). A congenital defect (a gap) in the interventricular septum can provide such a pathway; this is rare, but about 10–20 percent of all normal hearts have a *foramen ovale* patent enough to allow the passage of a probe (95).

The *foramen ovale* is a leftover from the intricacies of cardiac embryology. Imagine an oval gap between the atria about the size of a small coin. Now close that gap with a fibrous membrane a little wider than the gap, applied in the left atrium and soldered all around. The membrane remains pressed against the rim of the gap by the slightly higher pressure in the left atrium. However, in one of every 5 or 10 humans, the rim and the membrane are not wholly soldered; thus, at autopsy, a probe can be slipped across the gap; this is called a **patent foramen ovale.**

If the pressure in the right heart is momentarily raised, such as by coughing or straining, some blood can be ejected across a patent *foramen ovale,* together with any embolus that may be floating by.

Bad luck does exist, but it is statistically almost impossible to conceive that a huge embolus may come along precisely at the time that the patient is coughing or straining. A cardiologist-pathologist, Dr. H. Cuénoud,

advised us that paradoxical embolism is likely to be a two-stage event: first, a long embolus becomes entangled in the retaining tendons (*chordae tendineae*) of the tricuspid valve; and when the patient happens to develop a bout of high pressure that squirts blood across the *foramen ovale,* an end of the thrombus is sucked into the gap (Figure 23.6).

Some emboli trapped in the passage can actually be caught in the act, either at autopsy or *in vivo* by echocardiography (Figure 23.6) (20, 165, 176). This calamity is rare, but its incidence is probably underestimated because *patients with stroke are four times more likely to have a patent foramen ovale,* compared with the general population (94).

Astute clinicians have made the diagnosis during life (123); a suspicious setting is an ischemic stroke in a young adult (78, 94).

Paradoxical emboli are rare, but they do occur; it is well to remember that *even a small bubble of air injected intravenously has a chance of skipping the lungs and ending in the brain or in a coronary.*

Emboli of Atheroma

Atheroma is the gruel-like necrotic material contained in atherosclerotic plaques; it is released into the blood when a plaque breaks open. This accident happens spontaneously and during catheterization or surgery on atherosclerotic arteries, whereby plaques are inevitably traumatized (Figure 23.7). Cholesterol crystals and necrotic debris usually embolize small arteries of the

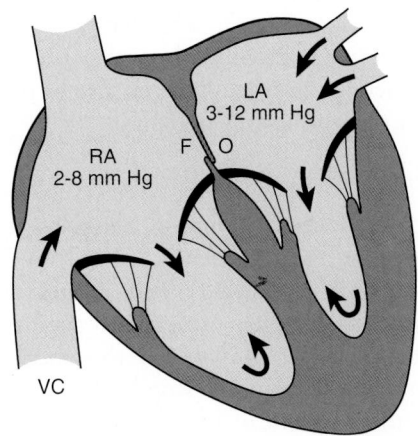 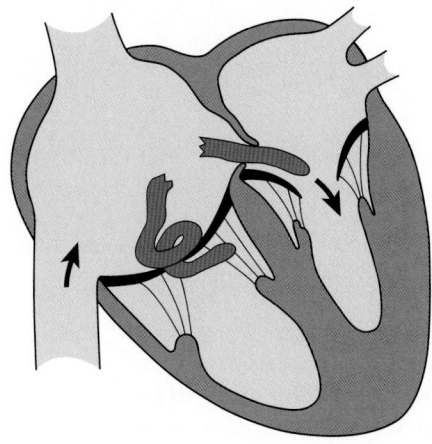

FIGURE 23.6   Mechanism of paradoxical thromboembolism. *Left:* Normal heart. **RA, LA** = right, left atrium; **VC** = inferior vena cava. The atria are separated in part by a fibrous membrane (*foramen ovale*), which, in 6 percent of the population, behaves as a flap valve. Normal pressure within the atria in the **LV.** *Right:* A long, branching venous thrombus, arrived from the vena cava minutes/hours ago and has become entangled in the tricuspid valve, occluding it for a few seconds and thereby raising the pressure in the **RA.** This is enough to distend the **RA,** open the flap valve of the *foramen,* and allow part of the thrombus to slip into the **LA.**

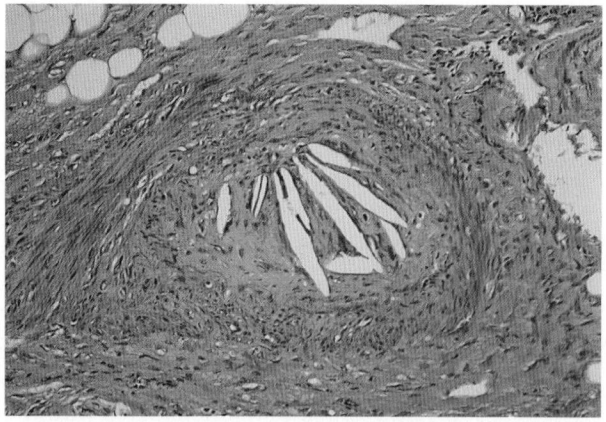

FIGURE 23.7   A small mesenteric artery obliterated by an embolus of atheroma, probably from the aorta. Of the embolus only the cholesterol crystals remain (white slits); the rest of the lumen is filled with reactive cells supplied by the arterial wall (endothelium, smooth muscle) and by the blood (macrophages). These features suggest that the embolism occurred at least weeks earlier. (60x)

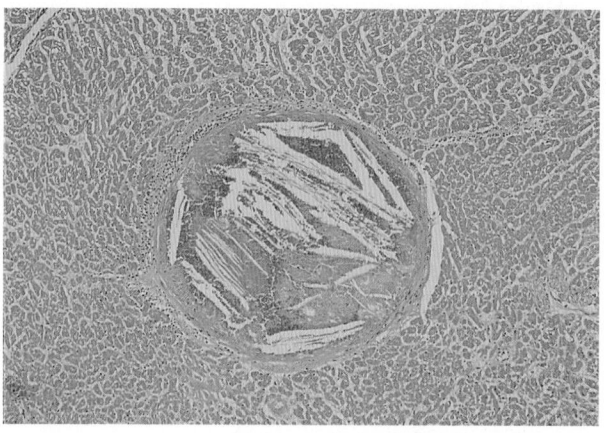

FIGURE 23.8   Branch of a coronary artery obstructed by an embolus of atheromatous material and surrounded by necrotic myocardium. The slits in the lumen are the negative image of cholesterol crystals. The patient died of a myocardial infarction 2 days after coronary artery bypass graft surgery. (60x)

order of 1–2 mm or less (188); an infarct may follow (Figure 23.8). Favorite target organs are the kidney, spleen, brain, intestine (Figures 23.9, 23.10), and skin. Many cholesterol emboli are symptomless; but when symptoms do arise, they are often misinterpreted because they can mimic a number of unrelated conditions (32) from belly pain to a skin disease.

NOTE: Besides the microemboli of crystals, ulcerated atheromatous plaques covered with platelets can shed microemboli consisting mainly of platelets (90, 91).

Transient ischemic attacks. It was the notion of microscopic atheroembolism to the brain that led to the concept of the transient ischemic attack (TIA). TIAs are episodes of neurologic dysfunction that appear suddenly, last minutes or hours, and—by definition—disappear. If they do not disappear, the diagnosis shifts to a stroke. Herein lies the dilemma posed by TIAs: *their causes and clinical manifestations overlap with those of strokes.* Recent reviews point out that the former tendency to consider TIAs as benign, as opposed to strokes, is misleading (1a, 43a): 10–20 percent of patients who suffered a TIA have a stroke in the next 3 months (1a). Therefore, waiting for 24 hours for the reversal is much too long; one hour is the recommended limit. *TIAs are best considered as medical emergencies, which offer a rare chance to stave off a stroke (1a).*

As for the mechanism: originally the TIAs were attributed to transient spasm of cerebral arteries, until an ophtalmologist in the early 1960s happened to examine the retina of a patient during an episode of transient monocular blindness (**amaurosis fugax**). He saw a whitish material plugging a retinal arteriole; as it was cleared away, the blackout also disappeared (Figure 23.11) (196). This observation suggested that TIAs are also due to microscopic atheromatous emboli or platelet emboli arising upstream, e.g., in the internal carotid arteries or in a fibrillating heart. From the point of view of pathophysiology, they teach us that reversible ischemic injury can happen also in the highly vulnerable central nervous system.

Emboli of Fat and Bone Marrow

Fat embolism is common, being largely a complication of bone fractures: that is, fat cells in the bone marrow break up; oily droplets float around and coalesce; and some droplets are sucked into gaping venules torn by the fracture, from which they begin a complicated journey—with a first stop in the lung. All this happens within the time of a few heartbeats, as was documented in victims of a helicopter crash (130).

Liposuction has caused several deaths from massive fat embolism (54). Milder fat embolism is known to occur after bone surgery, after trauma or surgery involving adipose tissue, in fat necrosis from acute pancreatitis (130, 144), and

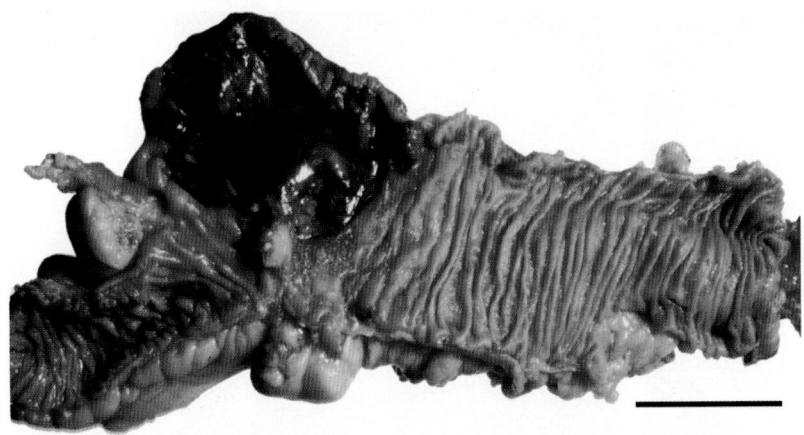

FIGURE 23.9   Hemorrhagic infarct of the cecum (*top left*) due to multiple emboli of atheroma from the aorta. *Center right:* Ascending colon; *bottom left:* small intestine. The clinical diagnosis, understandably, was acute appendicitis. **Bar** = 5 cm.

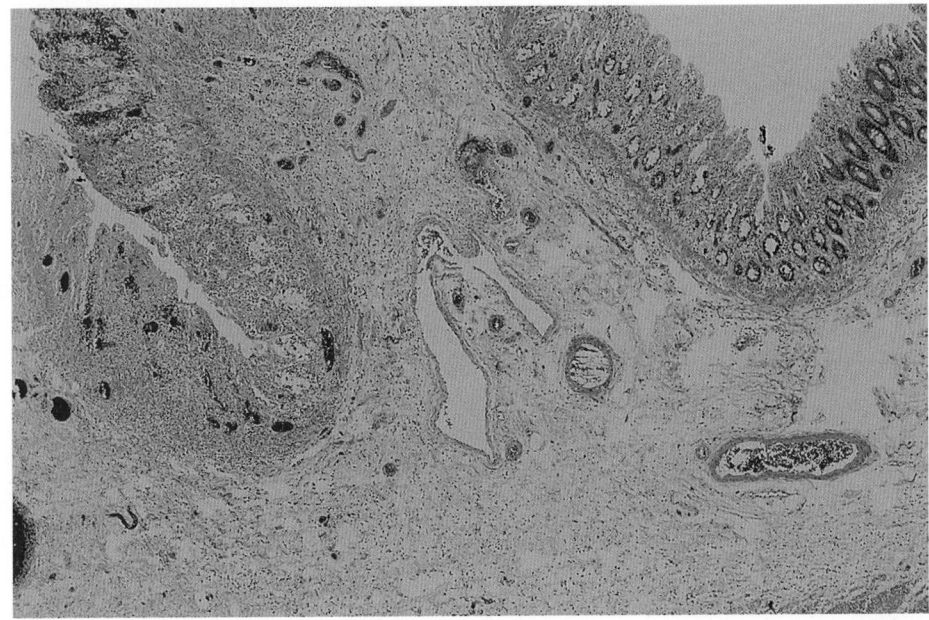

FIGURE 23.10   Histology of the junction between live and dead mucosa of the colon (see previous figure). *Mucosa, top right:* Relatively normal glands: live tissue. *Mucosa, left:* Dead glands, partially autolyzed. Scattered dilated venules with no plasma. Note the arteriole containing an embolus of atheroma (cholesterol crystals). (35x)

even from fatty livers of chronic alcoholics (Figure 23.12) (37, 102). The development of microemboli from intravenous fat emulsions used for parenteral nutrition has been contested (148).

Almost every fracture is accompanied by some degree of fat embolism; but clinically, only about 1 percent of patients with a single fracture develop pulmonary and systemic symptoms (the proportion rises to 5–10 percent of patients with pelvic or multiple long-bone fractures) (155). After blunt trauma, the fat emboli arise from subcutaneous fat tissue (120). The symptoms—typically delayed by 1–3 days—are mainly respiratory distress and lethargy or other signs pointing to brain damage. The mortality from systemic fat embolism is of the order of 10–15 percent. It is clearly important to

work out the pathogenesis in order to plan a rational therapy.

One part of the story of fat embolism is simple: namely, the mechanical part. The oily droplets embolize the lung, where they cause subclinical hypoxemia (133, 140) and sometimes overt respiratory distress; then some droplets emerge from the lung and embolize the systemic circulation. Some of these systemic droplets may have squeezed through the alveolar capillaries, but the larger ones surely have passed through the arteriovenous anastomoses mentioned earlier. Thanks to this second pathway, it is quite possible that many droplets repeat their circular journey over and over until they are broken up (153). In the meantime, the lung, showered with microemboli, can

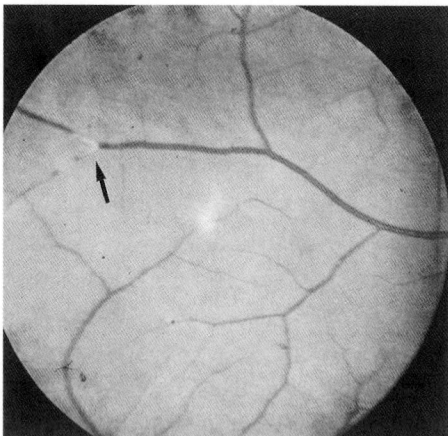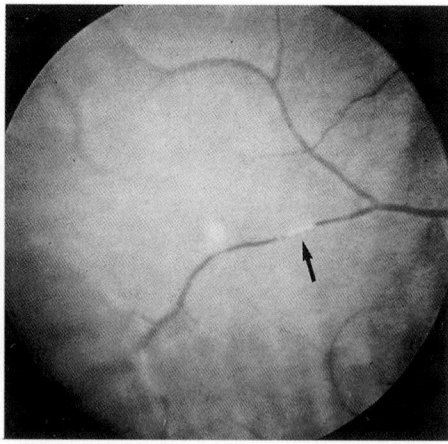

FIGURE 23.11 *Left:* Small thromboembolus photographed as it slowly passed through the retinal circulation (**arrow**). The patient was having an attack of *amaurosis fugax* (transient blindness). The embolus moved along for a few minutes, paused at a bifurcation, and became smaller as it reached the retinal periphery. Such emboli usually arise from thrombi in the carotid artery or from a thrombosed mitral valve. *Right:* Similar embolus pausing at a bifurcation. (*Left:* Courtesy of Dr. R.W.R Russell, St. Thomas' Hospital, London, UK. *Right:* Reproduced with permission from [145].)

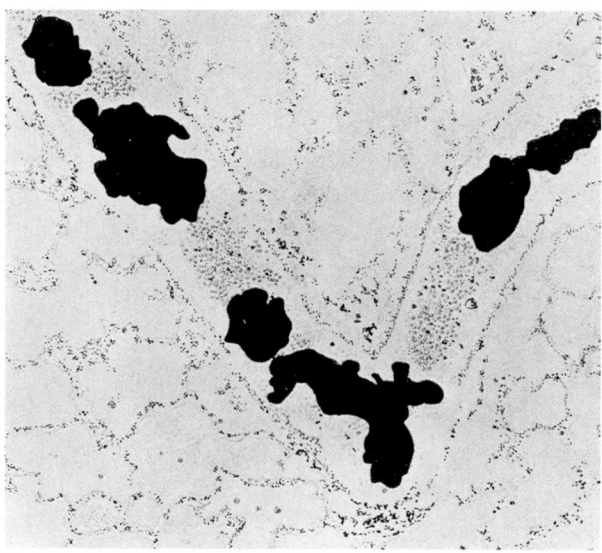

FIGURE 23.12 Multiple fat emboli (black masses) in a small pulmonary artery (section of lung stained with osmium tetroxide). This patient, an alcoholic, had a 2600-g fatty liver and died from a superimposed carbon tetrachloride intoxication. The fat globules were presumably released by necrotic liver cells. (Reproduced with permission from [102], © American Society for Investigative Pathology.)

develop a capillary leak syndrome—or *acute respiratory distress syndrome* (ARDS) (p. 722)—which explains the clinical respiratory failure and hypoxemia (140). The lung damage may be due to activated neutrophils (122).

In the systemic circulation, the main target organs of fat emboli are: the *brain,* where each embolus can produce a tiny infarct surrounded by a "ring hemorrhage" (153), enough to prove that fat embolism can produce serious damage; the *kidney* (droplets of fat are commonly found in the urine, showing that some glomeruli have been damaged by the emboli); and the *skin,* where the presence of emboli may be betrayed by small petechiae (minute round spots of hemorrhage) recalling those of the brain: the conjunctiva is a good place to look for them. Droplets of fat can also be found in the sputum.

Some loose ends related to fat embolism (60, 74). (a) *Fatty acids* have been drawn into the picture. In the lung, digestion of the fat emboli by macrophages could release fatty acids, which are toxic and could contribute to the local damage (132). Normally the plasma fatty acids are carried by albumin, but after trauma the load of free fatty acids could exceed the carrying capacity of circulating albumin (117). (b) It has been suggested that fatty acids could arise systemically (*even in the absence of trauma*) because stress releases adrenaline, which increases lipolysis and thereby the amount of circulating free fatty acids. All this is possible but unproven. (c) Occasional fat emboli have been reported in nontraumatic settings such as diabetes and inhalation anesthesia (155). It seems that lipoproteins can become unstable and aggregate. Rabbits treated with cortisone develop fat emboli (103). Perhaps occasional fat emboli arise by this physico-chemical mechanism.

Bone marrow emboli arise like fat emboli: whole chunks of hemopoietic bone marrow are mobilized

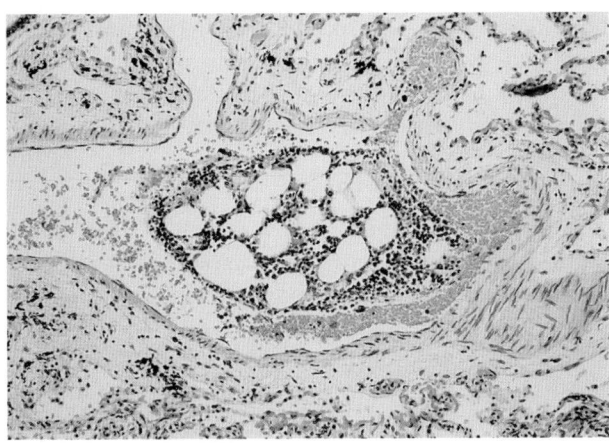

FIGURE 23.13 *Center:* Embolus of bone marrow in the lumen of a small artery: a result of rib fracture during cardiopulmonary resuscitation (CPR). The embolus is an oval mass of fat cells and hematopoietic cells (the latter not recognizable at this power).

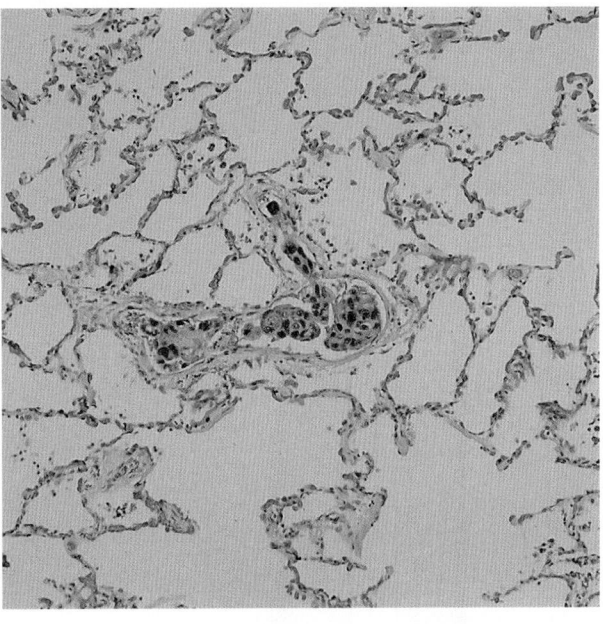

FIGURE 23.14 Emboli of a hepatoma in a pulmonary arteriole. These emboli were pumped into the lung by vigorous efforts at cardiopulmonary resuscitation (CPR) in a patient whose liver was found later to contain a large hepatoma. (60x)

from the site of a fracture, sometimes with spicules of bone. Today, marrow emboli are a routine histologic finding in the small pulmonary arteries of patients who died after vigorous efforts of cardiopulmonary resuscitation (CPR) (Figure 23.13). These emboli are clinically insignificant. However, we saw one case in which an unrecognized hepatoma (liver tumor) had showered the lungs with microscopic metastases, apparently as a result of CPR (Figure 23.14).

Gas Emboli

There are hints in Morgagni's work that in past centuries air was blown into the jugular veins to dispatch large animals (164). Smaller volumes of air and other gases introduced into the bloodstream block the microcirculation because bubbles with a diameter of 30–60 μm have enough surface tension to behave like solid beads; they probably also damage the endothelium and activate the clotting system (111, 135). Gas emboli are best known as a complication of diving, but they also occur as a side effect of medical care: a recent review lists at least *17 medical-surgical specialties—and many more procedures—that can cause gas emboli* (120a).

Iatrogenic gas emboli. Air can find its way into the circulatory system, for example, through an intravenous catheter or an extracorporeal-bypass pump. If the volume of air is large (50–100 cc) a frothy mixture may fill the heart, embolize to the lungs and cause death; smaller amounts of air can be tolerated, but one should not forget the possibility of small bubbles passing

through an open foramen ovale and embolizing to the brain. Air can also enter a carotid artery accidentally in the course of an endarterectomy. More difficult to prevent is air embolism during procedures such as arthroscopy or laparoscopy, in which air is blown into a cavity to create space for inspection or for surgery; a significant improvement has been to replace air with CO_2 which is more soluble. On a happier note, tiny air emboli can be useful because they are strikingly visible by echocardiography: such "microbubbles" are now used in cardiology for diagnostic purposes (46).

Medical students should keep in mind at least one critical setting. *There is a negative pressure in the veins of the head, neck, and chest during inspiration in the upright position;* therefore these veins can draw in air. Trauma of the neck and chest can be fatal for this reason.

The caisson syndrome. Better known as *decompression sickness,* this syndrome concerns—beyond workers in *caissons*—sport divers and occasional pilots and astronauts who transfer too fast from high to low pressure (111, 135). The French word *caisson* refers to a boxlike chamber large enough to hold one or more workers; it is lowered into the water open side down, so that it remains filled with compressed air. Whoever is inside it can walk, for example, on the bottom of the sea while

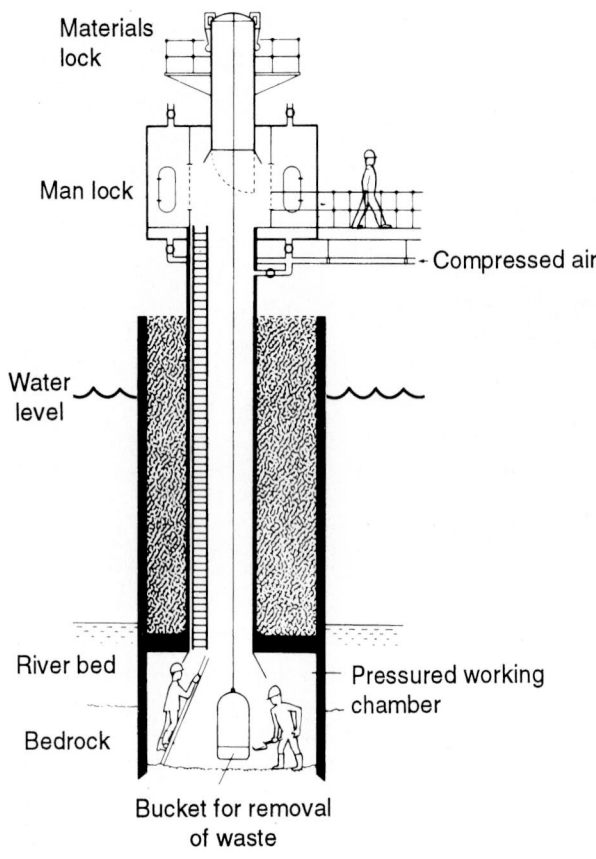

Materials lock

Man lock

Compressed air

Water level

River bed

Bedrock

Pressured working chamber

Bucket for removal of waste

FIGURE 23.15   Modern version of the caisson, a pressurized chamber for working under water. (Reproduced with permission from [174].)

most of the body is in air (Figure 23.15). The physiologic principle exploited by the caisson is sound and is now applied to scuba diving: *in order to breathe under water, air must be delivered to the lungs at the same pressure as that of the surrounding water.* Thus, all body tissues and blood become saturated with gas at high pressure (about one additional atmosphere for every ten meters of depth). If a diver resurfaces too quickly, the dissolved gases come out of solution and are released massively within the body as bubbles (much the same happens when you open a bottle of champagne). The bubbles distort the tissues and act as emboli in the blood, causing endothelial damage and platelet aggregation (189), as happens with fat emboli. Nitrogen is the main culprit because it is fat-soluble but poorly soluble in tissue fluids; thus, it creates persistent bubbles in lipid-rich tissues, most importantly the central nervous system. Treatment is prompt recompression in a special chamber while breathing pure oxygen. (111). Chronic effects are mainly epiphyseal necrosis in some long

bones, resulting in secondary osteoarthrosis. The pathogenesis is still not completely understood, and the disease is still with us, since modern versions of the ancient caissons are used for deep-sea drilling (64, 175).

Amniotic Fluid Embolism

Amniotic fluid embolism is a rare but catastrophic event that occurs as a complication of labor and cesarean section. Its clinical presentation is the mother's sudden respiratory distress, cyanosis, and collapse (114, 136). The syndrome is unleashed by penetration of amniotic fluid into the circulation, presumably through a tear in the amniotic membranes. Microscopic emboli of fetal origin are found in the lung (epithelial squames, lanugo hair, fat and mucus droplets, meconium) but not in quantities to cause cardiorespiratory failure. It is more likely that the syndrome depends on other mechanisms such as anaphylaxis (26, 27) or disseminated intravascular coagulation and/or pulmonary arterial spasm due to a prostaglandin of the spasmogenic F series (PGF_2 alpha), which is found in the amniotic fluid (114).

Sundry and Therapeutic Emboli

Embolism by microscopic foreign bodies in the lung is a common complication of drug addiction. Drugs on the illicit market are diluted with inert fillers such as talcum, which is innocuous if taken by mouth but becomes a foreign body when injected intravenously. Less dangerous are microscopic fragments of filters and other materials related to cardiopulmonary bypass surgery, hemodialysis, and other interventions (125, 164, 183). Pulmonary emboli of placental cells are a normal and harmless occurrence (Figure 23.16).

The ultimate fate of these small foreign objects has a peculiar twist. They become covered by monocytes and eventually create a granuloma, and the arterial elastica interna beneath the granuloma breaks up. Then, it is thought, the granuloma is slowly extruded into the lung tissue, perhaps aided by arterial pressure, while the arterial wall rebuilds itself behind it (164).

Therapeutic emboli are presently in the news, since a Canadian group from the University of Alberta devised a protocol whereby diabetics Type 1 can be freed of insulin injections: a suspension of human (cadaver) islets is injected into the portal vein (145a, 153a). Figure 23.17 shows an early experiment proving that human islets embolized into the liver through the portal vein of a diabetic mouse could survive and restore normomglycemia.

Therapeutic emboli have also been used for destroying tumors *in vivo*. Favorite targets have been

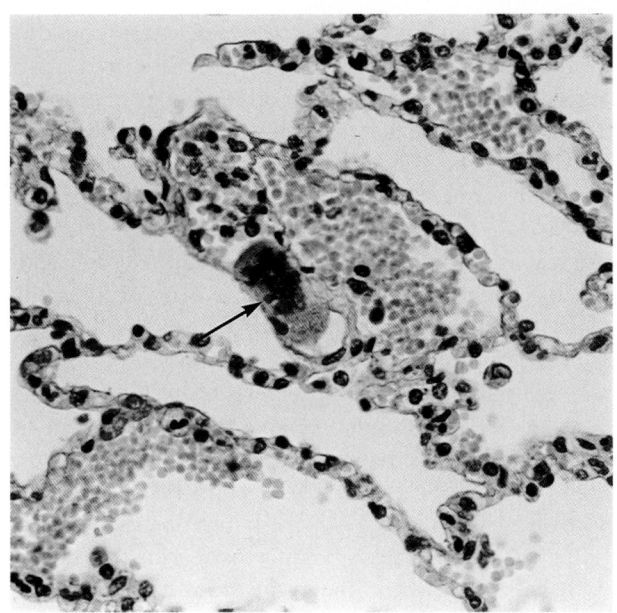

FIGURE 23.16   A normal event: placental giant cell (syncytiotrophoblast) (**arrow**) that embolized to the lung. Autopsy finding in a young woman who died of infected abortion at 16 weeks. (Courtesy of Dr. K. Benirschke, University of California, San Diego, CA.)

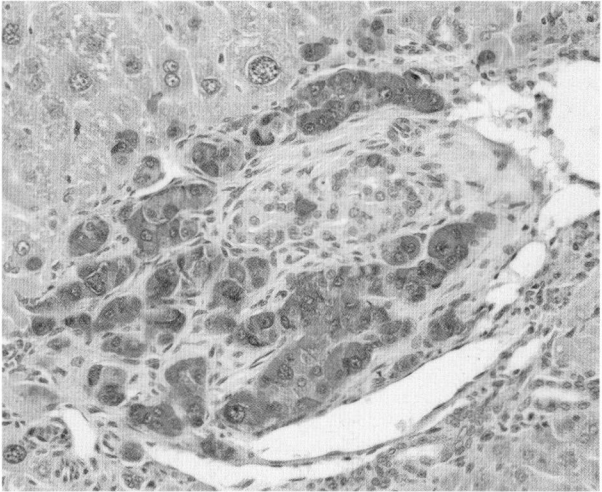

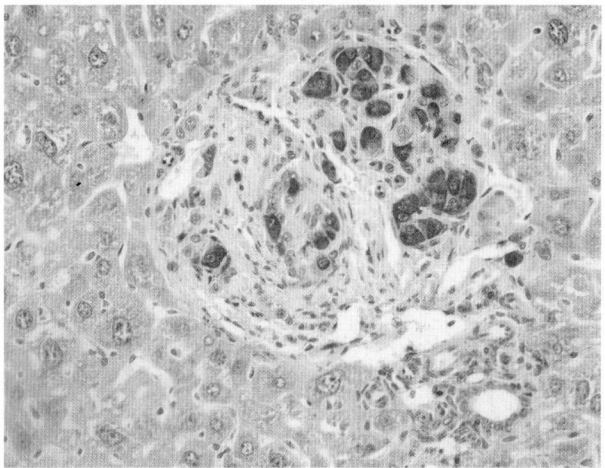

FIGURE 23.17   Liver with islet emboli. Functional therapeutic emboli, such as these isolated human islets injected into the portal vein of mice with chemically induced diabetes, restored these mice to normoglycemia. (Insulin immunoperoxidase and methyl green stain; 470x) (Courtesy of Drs. A. Rossini and M. Appel, University of Massachusetts Medical School, Worcester, MA.)

carcinomas of the kidney. Emboli introduced by catheter into the renal artery have varied from minced autologous muscle to plastic microspheres, and even lead shot. Pain is a major problem, and the complications are many (110). However, there is one hopeful lead: it seems that embolization of a renal carcinoma may favor the regression of metastases (169). We are drawn to speculate that the necrosis of a tumor within the body is a very different biological process from the sudden disappearance of a tumor by surgical removal.

Obstruction by Changes in the Vascular Wall

Impaired blood flow can result from changes in the vascular wall. The two main culprits are atherosclerosis and arterial spasm. Both lead to stenosis of the arterial lumen.

Biophysicists have given us a general and somewhat reassuring law about stenosis: *flow through a stenosed tube or artery is not significantly affected until the lumen is reduced by 70–80 percent* (Figure 23.18) (100, 112). This does not mean that a 65 percent stenosis of a coronary artery has no effect; the functional reserve is decreased. Should the heart require more blood as a result of exercise, that extra demand may not be met—also because at higher flow rates a stenosis produces a relatively greater flow reduction (100).

Atherosclerosis

Although special diseases are not considered in this book, we will touch briefly on two forms of arteriosclerosis, because—as a cause of ischemia—they are common enough to represent a basic problem.

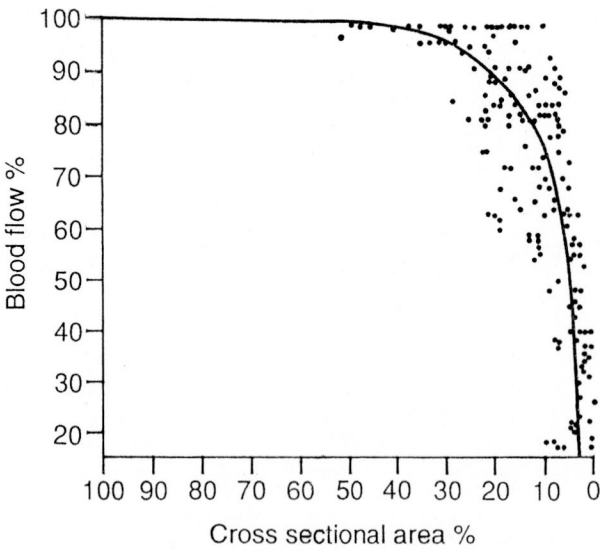

FIGURE 23.18   Surprisingly, the flow through a stenotic artery is not seriously affected until the stenosis has reduced the cross-sectional area of the lumen by 70–80 percent. (Adapted with permission from [112].)

Arteriosclerosis is a broad term that means "hardening of the arteries." It includes three diseases that decrease arterial elasticity in different ways (Table 23.1):

- *Atherosclerosis,* a disease of the large and medium-sized arteries; it begins in the intima, where it produces "plaques" filled with a necrotic, gruel-like material (*athére* is Greek for gruel or porridge); *this is the disease that laymen mean when they say "arteriosclerosis";*
- *Arteriolosclerosis,* affecting the small arteries, to be discussed later; and
- *Mönckeberg's disease,* rather uncommon, a calcification of the media of large arteries.

The following discussion refers to **atherosclerosis.** In the Western world, no disease kills more people; its impact on the adult population in terms of myocardial infarcts and stroke has no match. *Among the risk factors that predispose to atherosclerosis, nutrition and high blood cholesterol rank highest;* almost all experimental models of atherosclerosis are animals (even birds) maintained on a high cholesterol diet. Although a high level of blood cholesterol should affect all blood vessels, pathologic changes develop only in large and medium-sized arteries, and then only parts of those arteries: the basic lesion is the *plaque,* typically a centimeter or so in diameter. Therefore, to understand atherosclerosis, we must understand the structure and the genesis of the plaque.

A typical early plaque, e.g., on the inner surface of a human aorta, is a smooth, slightly raised lesion; a cut across it shows that it contains a small mass of necrotic-looking material (*atheroma*) containing tiny brilliant flakes that represent cholesterol crystals; the atheroma is covered by a thin lid known as *fibrous cap.* The genesis of the plaque, as it was worked out experimentally in the 1980s (Figure 23.19), was based largely on feeding animals a high cholesterol diet: by that time it was agreed that the lipid in the plaques comes from plasma lipoproteins (mainly low-density lipoproteins [LDL]), and that high plasma cholesterol is a major factor.

In the birth of a plaque, the first change visible with the electron microscope is the appearance of submicroscopic lipid droplets (liposomes) and LDL particles beneath the endothelium (Figure 23.20). This can be seen in rabbits and hamsters after only 1–2 weeks on a high-cholesterol diet (113, 159, 160). Because the endothelium is intact, the likeliest interpretation is that LDL particles are being transcytosed into the subendothelial space, where they come to lie, either intact or degraded to liposomes.

At about the same time monocytes and some lymphocytes adhere to the endothelium overlying the lipid deposit (Figure 23.21), perform diapedesis, and take residence beneath the endothelium (Figure 23.22). This emigration is initiated by adhesion molecules expressed by the endothelium, including VCAM-1 and ICAM-1 (30, 30a, 43, 98, 135b) and by chemotactic molecules released by the growing plaque. Once they have settled, the *monocytes* become *macrophages,* pick up much of the lipid that has rained into the subendothelial space, and change name once again: they become *foam cells* (p. 92) (Figure 23.23) (82, 143). The cellular population is further increased by smooth muscle cells that migrate from the media into the intima.

At this point, seen by scanning electron microscopy, the intimal lesion appears as a hill stretched in the direction of flow; it is covered with endothelium and may have a few mononuclear cells sticking to it (Figure 23.24). This is called a **fatty streak.**

The fatty streak continues to grow, by continued immigration of monocytes and lymphocytes and by proliferation of intimal and medical smooth muscle cells. Some of these join the foam cells and even phagocytize lipid. Others grow as a layer beneath the endothelium, constituting a sort of roof, reinforced by collagen, elastin, and other matrix proteins; this becomes the so-called fibrous cap. At this stage the lesion is called a **fibrofatty plaque.** Eventually, the core of the plaque, filled with foam cells and smooth muscle cells, becomes necrotic and turns into atheroma (Figure 23.25).

As to the time frame: with the extremely high levels of hypercholesterolemia that can be reached in experimental animals, the process just described can occur over several months. In humans it takes years.

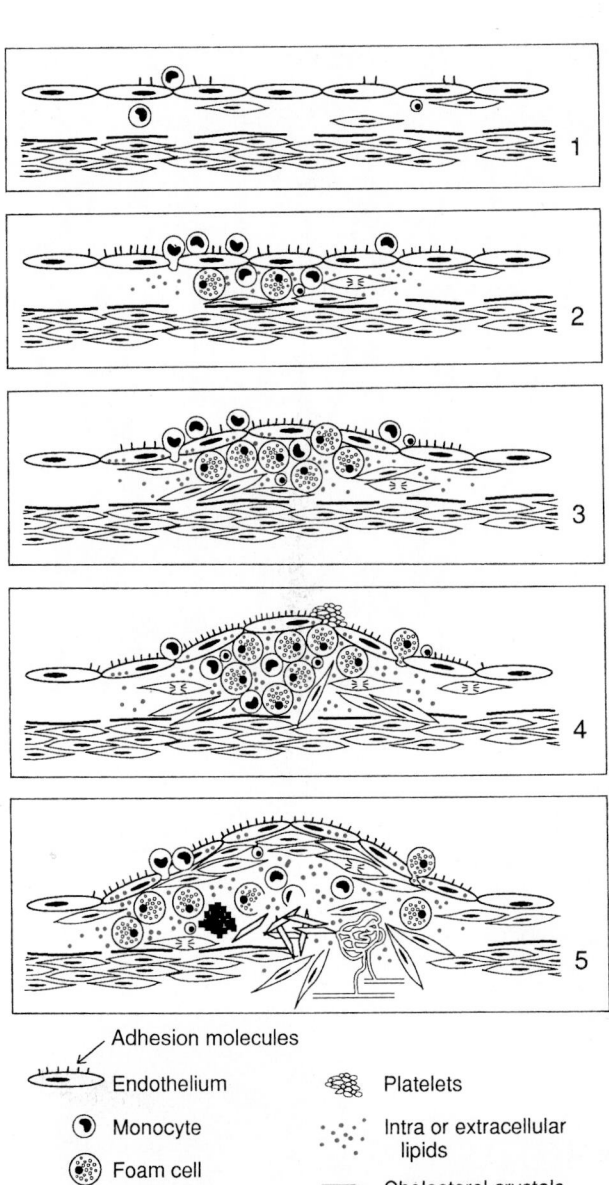

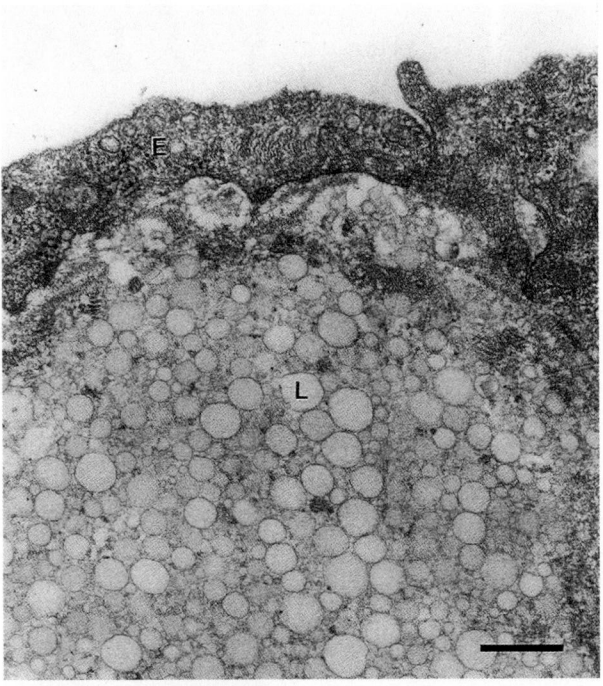

FIGURE 23.19 Birth, growth, and development of an atherosclerotic plaque as seen in experimental hypercholesterolemic animals. *1*: Normal arterial wall with endothelial cells, subendothelial space, interrupted elastic lamina, and smooth muscle cells of the media. Occasional macrophages and lymphocytes migrate into the subendothelial space. *2*: The two earliest events detectable: the transendothelial passage of lipid droplets (which accumulate as liposomes) and the transendothelial migration of monocytes (which turn into foam cells). *3*: Crowded foam cells cause the endothelium to bulge. Some foam cells may return to the bloodstream. Smooth muscle cells arise from the media. *4*: Growth of the plaque by increase in the number of foam cells and smooth muscle cells. Platelets adhere where endothelial cells allow gaps to develop. *5*: Necrosis occurs in the plaque, followed by development of cholesterol crystals, calcification, and vascularization from the adventitia. (Adapted from [105].)

FIGURE 23.20 Evidence of transendothelial transport in early atherosclerosis. Electron micrograph of a guinea pig aortic valve after 1 week on a hypercholesterolemic diet. **L:** Mass of rounded bodies (liposomes) composed of lipid that must have crossed the intact epithelium. **E:** Endothelium. **Bar** = 0.5 μm. (Courtesy of Drs. M. and N. Simionescu, Institute of Cellular Biology and Pathology, Bucharest, Romania.)

Foam cell puzzles. Foam cells are at center stage in atherosclerosis, but their role is not entirely clear. Are they part of the problem or part of the solution? Electron microscopy has suggested that some of them migrate back into the bloodstream (53), in which case they would be performing a laudable function. But what would they do in the bloodstream? Their size is such that they would become microemboli and break up. Nor is it clear why foam cells die in the plaque. Perhaps the core of the plaque suffers from anoxia, or perhaps some lipid has a toxic effect. Another puzzle has been that monocytes incubated with particles of native LDL did not phagocytize them. They do so only if the particles are oxidized or otherwise modified (p. 94)—hence the theory that the endothelium modifies (oxidizes) the LDL particles as it transmits them to the subendothelium (131).

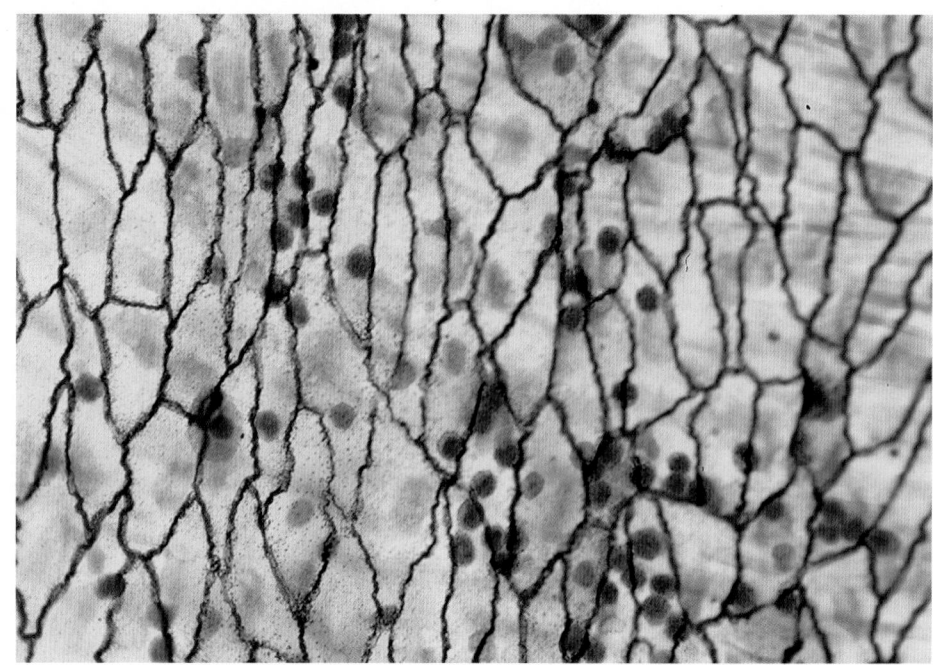

FIGURE 23.21 Inner surface of the aorta of a rat after 8 weeks on a hypercholesterolemic diet. The network of black lines represents junctions between endothelial cells. Many mononuclear cells are sticking to the endothelial surface; those that are faintly stained have migrated beneath the endothelium. (Silver nitrate and hematoxylin stain; 570x)

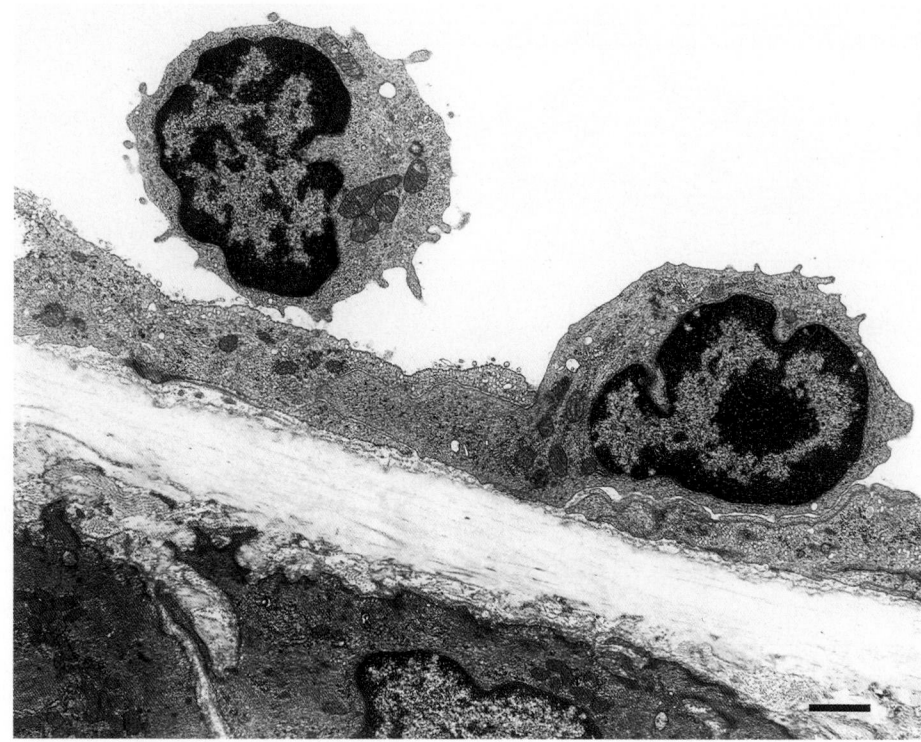

FIGURE 23.22 Margination and diapedesis of monocytes along the aortic intima of a rat after 11 weeks on a high-cholesterol diet. **Bar** = 1 μm. (Reproduced with permission from [82], © American Society for Investigative Pathology.)

This oxidation mechanism is important scientifically (oxidized lipoproteins are related to monocyte sticking [23]) and clinically, as a possible target for therapy of atherosclerosis by means of antioxidants (13). A new family of atherogenic oxidized phospholipids was found in plaques and promotes foam cell formation (135a).

Final puzzles: some foam cells are *dendritic cells* stuffed with lipid granules. What are they doing there? (12a). And why is the plaque secreting *ozone?* (168a).

Life history of the plaque. An early plaque as we described it in the rat (Figure 23.25), with a thickness of 1–2 mm,

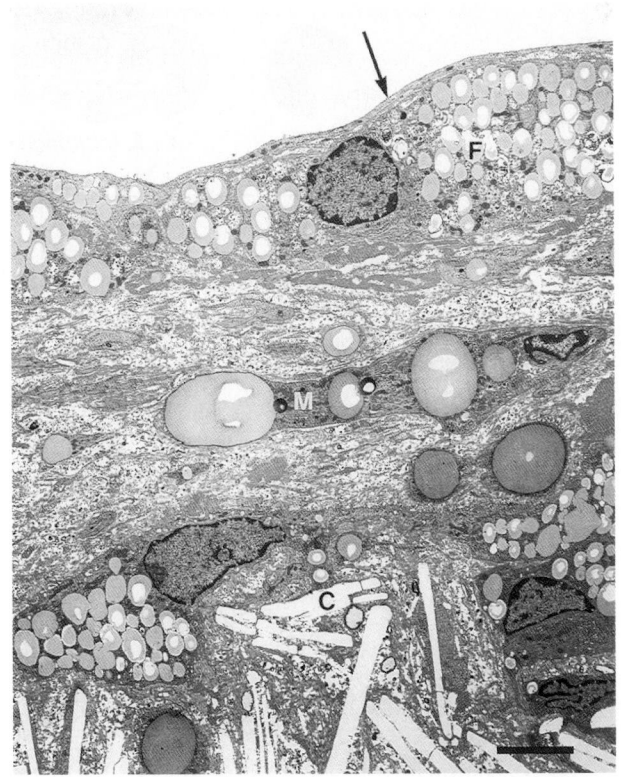

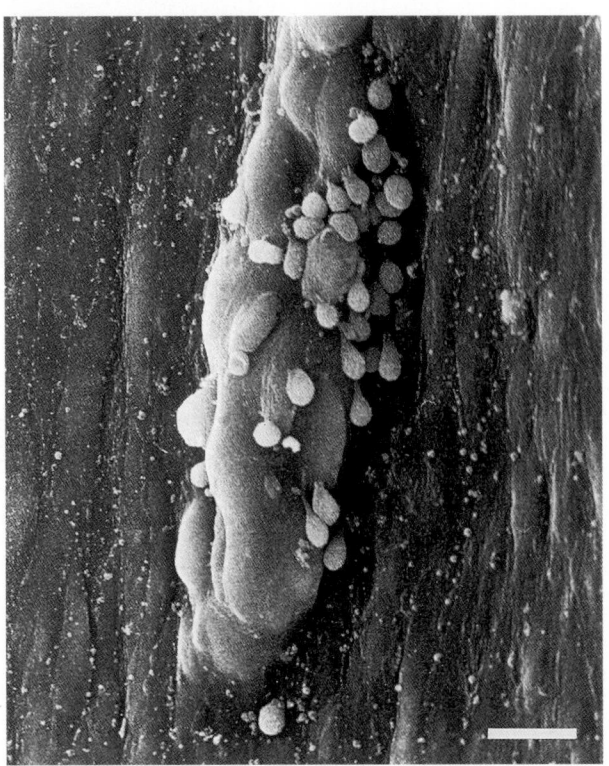

FIGURE 23.23   Various aspects of lipid deposition in the aortic intima of a rat after 1 year of hypercholesterolemia. **Arrow:** Very thin endothelial layer. **F:** Macrophage-derived foam cell. **M:** Smooth muscle cell, containing fewer and larger droplets. **C:** Crystals of cholesterol among necrotic debris. **Bar** = 5 μm. (Reproduced with permission from [82], © American Society for Investigative Pathology.)

FIGURE 23.24   Early fatty streak in the aorta of a rat after 8 weeks on a hypercholesterolemic diet (scanning electron micrograph). The elongated bulge is due to foam cells packed beneath the endothelium. Its surface appears to be selectively sticky for other leukocytes, mostly monocytes. **Bar** = 25 μm. (Reproduced with permission from [106].)

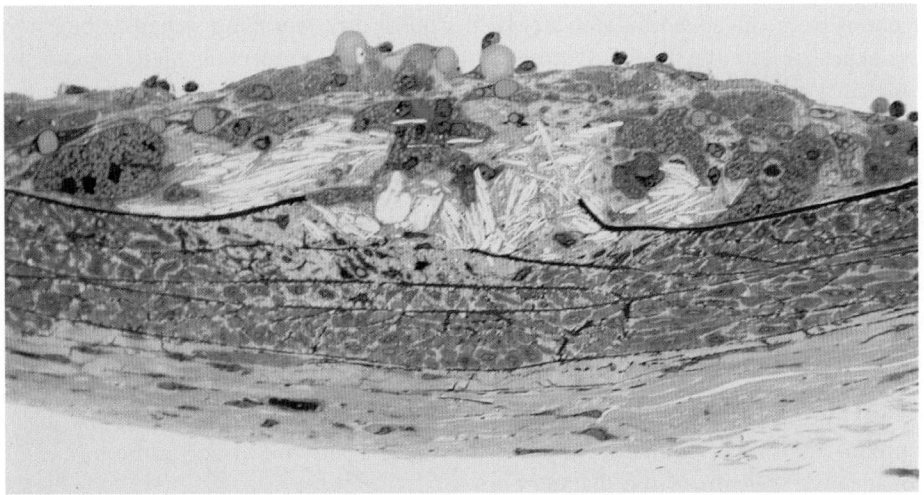

FIGURE 23.25   Miniature atherosclerotic plaque in the aorta of a rat maintained for 11 months on a high cholesterol diet. *Center:* Note break in the internal elastic membrane (**dark blue line**), which normally separates intima from media. *Center:* The intima has thickened, forming a plaque with necrotic core (cholesterol crystals). Mononuclear cells are attached to the endothelium. Among the subendothelial foam cells, cells with few, large droplets are derived from smooth muscle cells. (350x)

FIGURE 23.26 A proposed mechanism of thrombosis in atherosclerosis. The initiating factor is an excess of the lipoprotein called Lp(a). Lp(a) competes with plasminogen for a shared binding site on the surface of endothelial cells; this interferes with the normal activation of the fibrinolytic pathway. Impaired fibrinolysis leads to fibrin formation and thrombosis. (Reprinted by permission from [150]; Copyright © 1989 Macmillan Magazines Limited.)

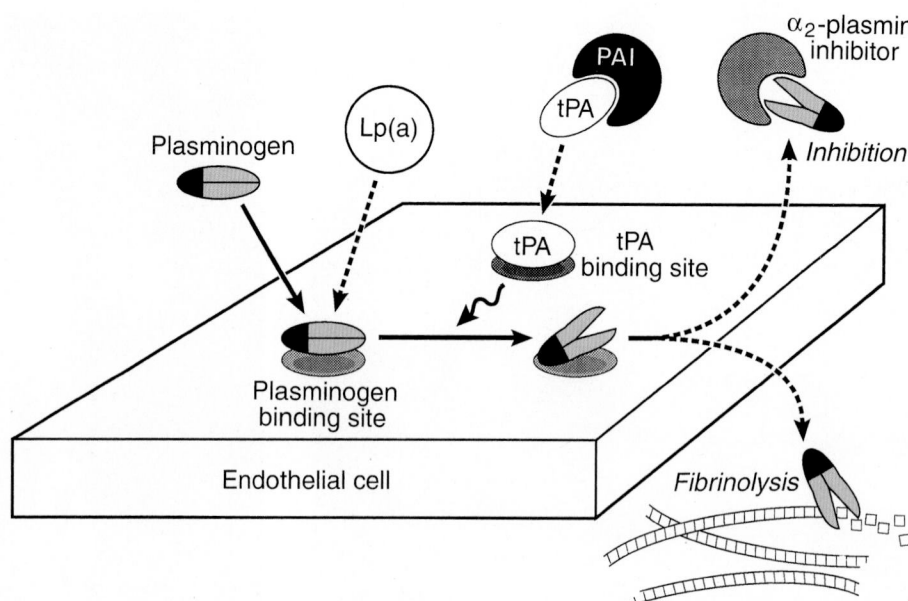

tends to grow and to develop a series of *complications:* stenosis of the lumen, calcification, hemorrhage, ulceration, thrombosis, release of atheromatous emboli, with consequences that are more threatening in relatively small arteries, such as the coronaries. These complications depend primarily on the behavior of the fibrous cap, which consists of collagen, smooth muscle cells and endothelium. It may retain its components indefinitely; it may also calcify, or become thin and break down quite suddenly. This catastrophe is best known in the coronary arteries. Normally the media contains no vessels. However, the necrotic core of a plaque can stimulate angiogenesis from the adventitia and newly-formed capillaries penetrate into the plaque. Occasionally one such vessel may bleed into the plaque: a thin cap may burst open, exposing the necrotic core to flowing blood, and within minutes a thrombus develops. The lumen is occluded, and the patient—who may have been quite unaware of having a problem of this nature—suffers a "heart attack."

This episode points to the fibrous cap as a critical structure. Now that the early stages of atherosclerosis are fairly well understood, much research is focussed on this late phase (98a, 99). The stability of the plaque depends a great deal on the cells involved and on the cytokine environment that they maintain, especially regarding the collagenous skeleton of the plaque. For example: interferon-gamma secreted by T cells can inhibit collagen synthesis, whereas T cells, smooth muscle cells, and macrophages secrete collagenase and other matrix-destroying enzymes. Knowing these enzymatic

effects may offer a new handle for preventing a plaque-driven crisis.

The breakdown of the fibrous cap and its dramatic clinical consequences point to a typical feature of atherosclerosis: *for most of its course it is a totally silent disease.* When symptoms do appear as a result of plaque complications—a myocardial infarct, a stroke—it is often too late to do much about it. Prevention is the answer.

Other features of atherosclerosis. (1) *Thrombosis may develop even on structurally intact endothelium.* This possibility was long debated, but it now seems well supported: abnormally high levels of a lipoprotein called LP(a) can lead to thrombosis by the mechanism shown in Figure 23.26 (7a, 72). (2) Thrombi may release vasoconstrictors that induce *spasm* at the site of the plaque.

Reversibility. Everybody agrees that fatty streaks in humans and experimental animals are the predecessors of plaques; that they cause no immediate harm; and that they can regress completely with lipid-lowering diets and drugs (165a). Plaques may shrink very slightly but they do not disappear (165a) even though treatment can improve clinical conditions and mortality rate. Once again, prevention is the way.

We had to dedicate all this space and time to explain how atherosclerosis can become an obstacle to flow. We shall end with a challenging question: on the basis of the last two or three pages, *what type of disease is*

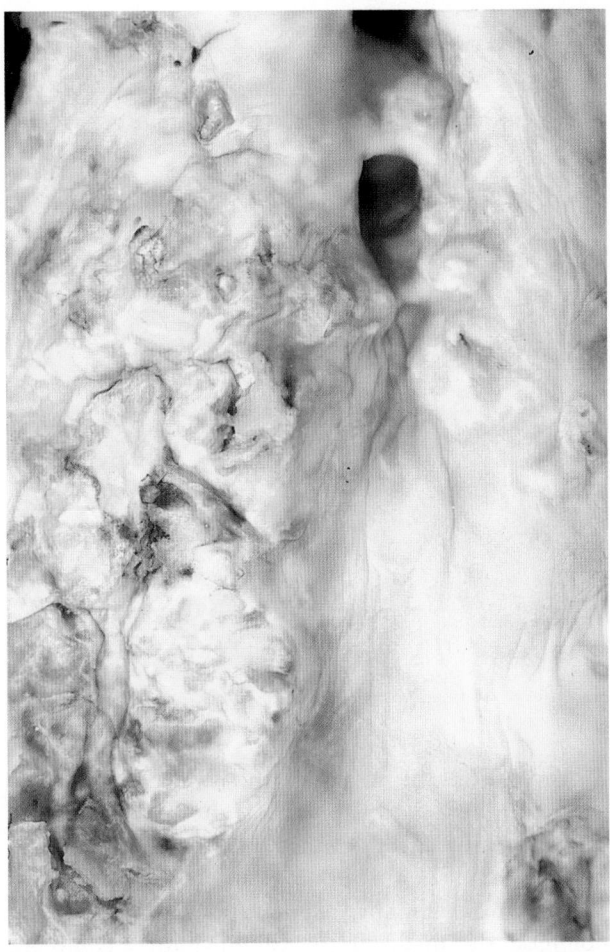

FIGURE 23.27 Inner surface of the aorta of a 65-year-old man. *Left:* Confluent ulcerated plaques. The yellowish material is atheroma; it is not covered by thrombi because the swift aortic flow prevents the deposition of platelets. A common finding at our institution. Slightly enlarged.

atherosclerosis? It used to be called a "degenerative" disease, because the affected arteries look ulcerated, calcified, and generally unfit to function (Figure 23.27). But "degenerative" has no scientific meaning (p. 165). In 1983 we worked on the early changes of atherosclerosis induced in the rat by a high cholesterol diet, and concluded that atherosclerosis could be interpreted as inflammation applied to large arteries (82). A similar conclusion was reached by others (143).

At first this concept was accepted with skepticism, because the arterial wall lacks a microcirculation, which is considered the anatomical basis for the RUBOR TUMOR CALOR of inflammation. In the advanced lesions of atherosclerosis (Figure 23.27) the inflammatory nature of the lesion is drowned out by secondary and tertiary changes, but the components of the *early* lesions include *adhesion.*

The components of atherosclerosis includes *adhesion proteins, margination, diapedesis, phagocytosis, collagen synthesis and breakdown,*—all features of inflammation; hence there is no surprise in the 2002 suggestion that *"atherosclerosis can be considered to represent an inflammatory response of macrophages and lymphocytes to 'invading' pathogenic lipoproteins in the arterial wall"* (97a). This is true, but hypercholesterolemia comes first; atherosclerosis as an inflammatory disease *"is initiated by and progresses in the context of hypercholesterolemia"* (165b).

To understand the mechanism of atherosclerosis is essential, because pathology can be a guide for planning therapy. Blood cholesterol is not the only villain in atherosclerosis (147a). Current research is aimed at defining different types of *vulnerable plaques* and correlating them with different types of *vulnerable patients* (121a). New therapeutic goals include stabilizing plaques and controlling angiogenesis (98b). The concept of atherosclerosis as an inflammatory disease has led to discover that it produces an increase in C-reactive protein (139a) (p. 505). The latest newcomers to the pathogenesis of atherosclerosis include NF-κB (28a), heat shock proteins (106a) and autoimmunity (141a).

Arteriolosclerosis

This "hardening of the arterioles" is common but poorly understood. It has little or no connection with atherosclerosis. Two varieties are known.

Hyaline arteriolosclerosis means that the arteriolar wall is stuffed with blood-borne macromolecules (Figure 7.1), especially lipoproteins: this "hyalin" stains for fat. This condition is common in the kidney, spleen, and other organs, it increases with age, and it is aggravated by hypertension; it has little clinical significance, although it can produce small foci of atrophy in the kidney. Why the arteriolar endothelium becomes leaky is not known.

Hyperplastic arteriolosclerosis means that the arteriolar muscular cells have undergone hyperplasia at the expense of the lumen and stiffening the wall (Figure 23.28). This condition is usually the result of severe hypertension; it affects arterioles throughout the body but especially those of the kidney.

Arterioles are the principal resistance vessels, hence diffuse arteriolosclerosis can cause hypertension; conversely, hypertension is known to cause or aggravate arteriolosclerosis. Despite these important connections, this aspect of vascular pathology has received little attention.

Arterial Spasm

There is no standard definition of spasm, but we may consider it as an *intense persistent vasoconstriction.* The time frame may be hours or days. Arterial spasm can be

FIGURE 23.28 Two types of arteriolar changes in rat "remnant kidneys" (after removal of one kidney and ⅚ of the other). *Left:* Necrosis of the wall. *Right:* Hyperplastic thickening of the vascular wall with great reduction of the lumen. **Bars** = 25 μm. (Reproduced with permission from [149], © American Society for Investigative Pathology.)

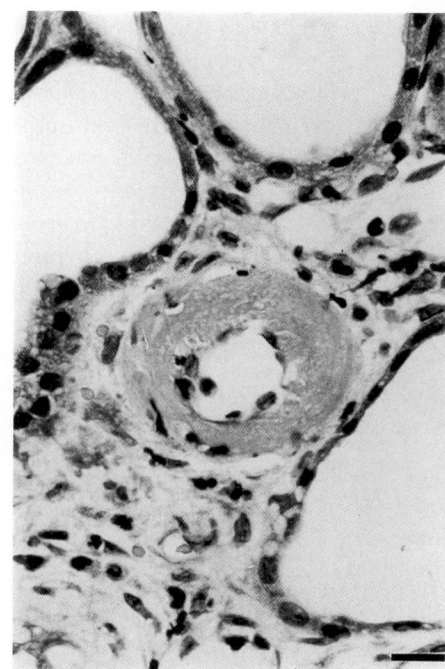
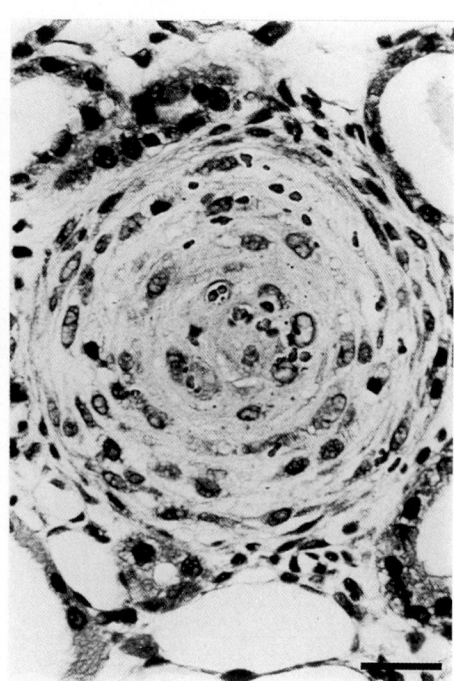

useful as a first line of defense against hemorrhage, but then, why should an artery become spastic for hours or days to the point of creating an infarct?

This aberrant behavior of arteries occurred in epidemic proportions during the Middle Ages. After rye bread came into the general diet, tens of thousands of people saw their nose, hands, and feet shrivel up and blacken with dry gangrene and burning pain, "as if charred by St. Anthony's fire" (now called **ergotism**). The reason was that the rye was contaminated with the fungus **ergot** (*Claviceps purpurea*) (Figure 23.29), and it so happens that ergot alkaloids are potent vasoconstrictors (16). The modern equivalent of St. Anthony's fire may be cocaine abuse; it also can induce (among other damage) necrosis of the skin, presumably by vasospasm (Figure 23.30) (198).

We should mention that arteriolar spasm is at the root of at least one **physiologic infarct:** the monthly shedding of the endometrium (24, 154).

Pathophysiology of spasm. In small arteries—known in physiology as the stopcocks of the circulation—the lumen can be constricted to the point of obliteration (Figure 23.31) (157). The mechanism is shown in Figure 23.31.

A possible cause of arterial spasm was suggested by a single autopsy: a patient known to suffer from coronary spasm had 5–6 times more mast cells in the adventitia of the spastic artery, compared with controls (45). Mast cells produce at least three kinds of coronary constrictors: histamine, prostaglandin D_2, and leukotrienes.

A major link in the pathogenesis of spasm was discovered in 1980 and is known as the **Furchgott phenomenon:** the media cannot relax in the absence of endothelium. The first inkling came from experiments *in vitro.* Acetylcholine, a powerful vasodilator, could not relax the media if the endothelium was absent. Then the mechanism was found. When the endothelium is stimulated by acetylcholine (or by many other agents), it produces a relaxing factor, nitric oxide (NO)(Figure 23.32). Now it is possible to understand the spasm of an artery denuded of its endothelium and lined with platelets (179).

Other surprising facts turned up later. In experimental hypercholesterolemia and in atherosclerosis, the endothelial response is perverted. That is, *when the media is stimulated with vasodilators, it contracts instead of relaxing* (179), in pigs as well as in humans (101). This may explain why coronary spasm tends to occur in segments already stenosed by atherosclerotic plaques (50, 156).

Electron microscopy has shown that spasm has a built-in potential for a vicious circle. We have found experimentally that a *tightly contracted artery traumatizes its own endothelium* (80). Indeed, there seems to be a flaw in the design of the arterial wall. When the media contracts concentrically, the intima cannot reduce its caliber except by forming many longitudinal folds, rather like an accordion (Figure 23.33). As a result, the endothelium inside the folds is unavoidably

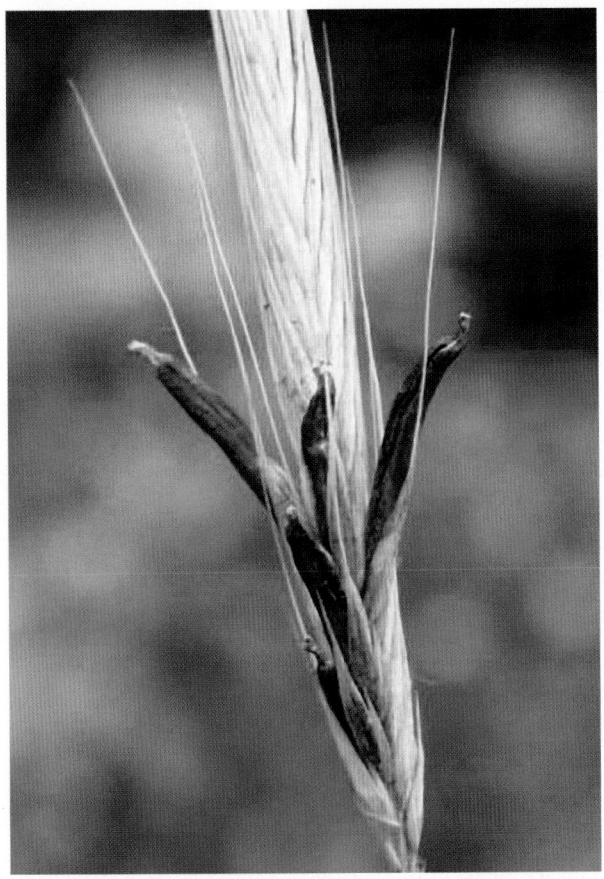

FIGURE 23.29   Winter rye parasitized by the fungus *Claviceps purpurea*. Several kernels are replaced by a purple-brown structure (sclerotium) shaped like a spur. Its alkaloids, derivatives of lysergic acid, are potent vasoconstrictors; they induce persistent arterial spasms and gangrene (*ergotism,* from the French *ergot,* spur). (Courtesy of Dr. H. F. Cuénoud, University of Massachusetts Medical School, Worcester, MA.)

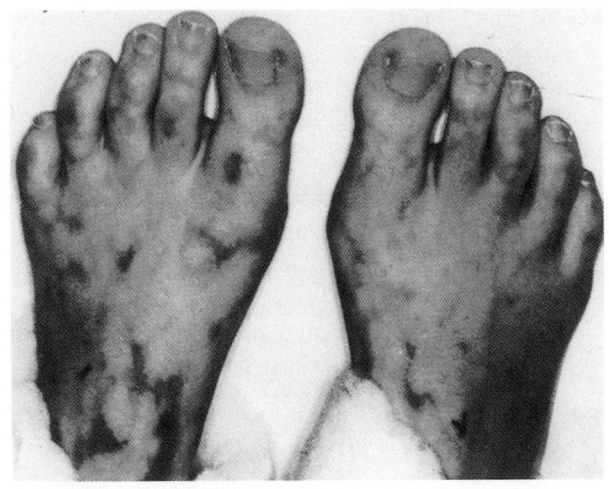

FIGURE 23.30   Effect of spasm in the small arteries: necrotizing lesions in the skin of a patient after inhalation of cocaine (crack). (Reproduced with permission from [198].)

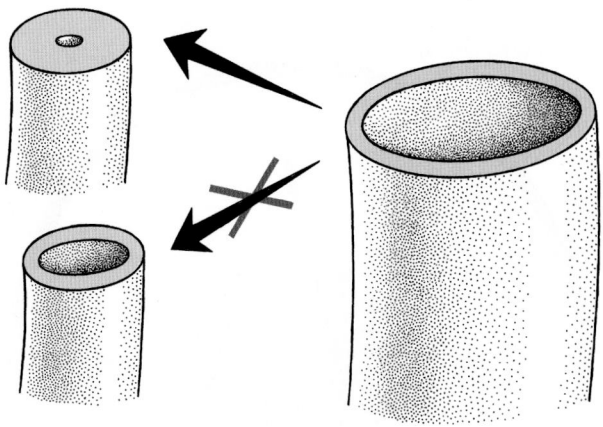

FIGURE 23.31   When an artery contracts the lumen shrinks proportionately more than the outer diameter. The reason: as the media contracts, it also becomes thicker. (Adapted with permission from [157].)

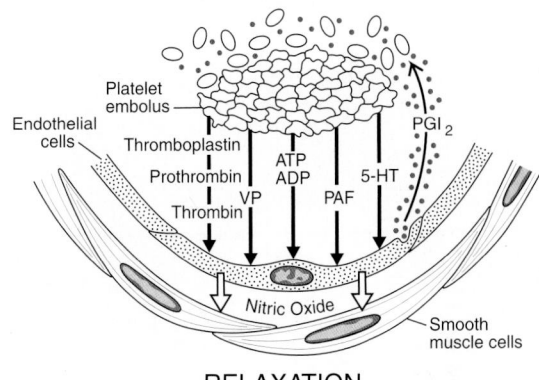

RELAXATION

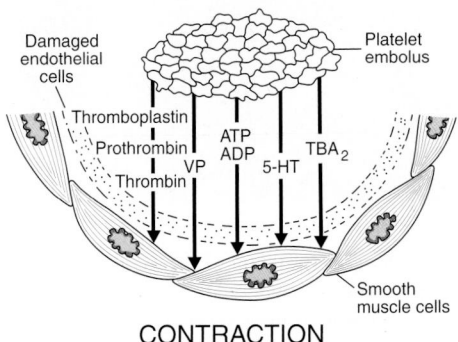

CONTRACTION

FIGURE 23.32   The **Furchgott phenomenon.** *Top:* Factors released by a platelet thrombus cause a normal artery to relax. The endothelium responds by secreting PGI_2, which opposes thrombus formation, and nitric oxide (NO), a powerful vasodilator. *Bottom:* If the same platelet factors are released in an artery deprived of endothelium, no nitric oxide is generated, and the artery contracts. (Adapted with permission from [179]. Original illustration by I. Arbel.)

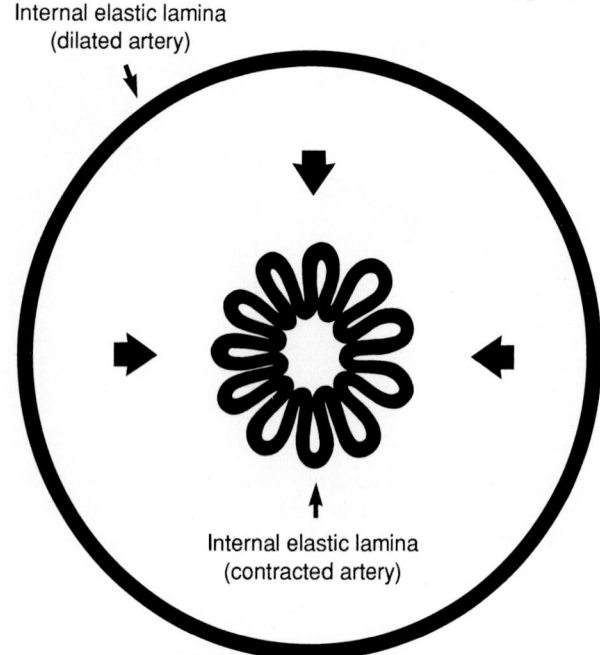

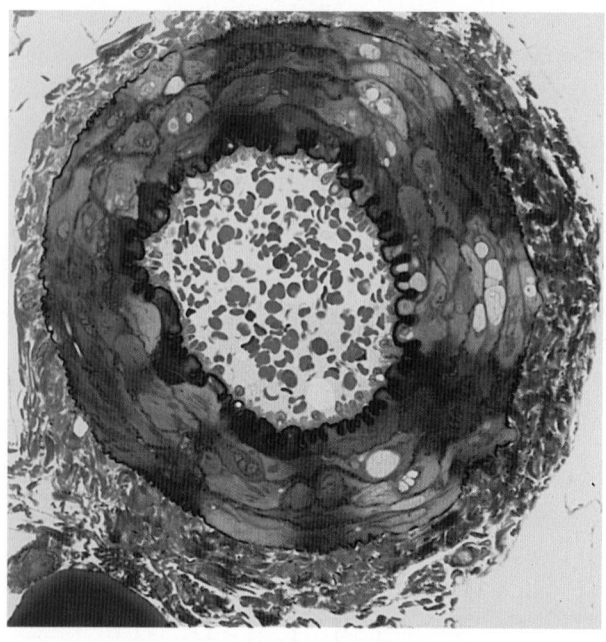

FIGURE 23.33 *Top:* Diagram of the internal elastic lamina of a small artery, and its change after full contraction. Because the elastic membrane cannot shorten, it is thrown into tight longitudinal folds. *Bottom:* Arterial spasm, shown in cross section of a spermatic artery of a rat, contracted by a local application of norepinephrine. The dark wavy line along the inner surface is the internal elastic lamina, thrown into folds by the medial contraction. The cartwheel pattern of the media is due to zones of hypercontraction alternating with noncontracted vacuolated zones. The vacuoles represent herniations of one cell into another. (370x)

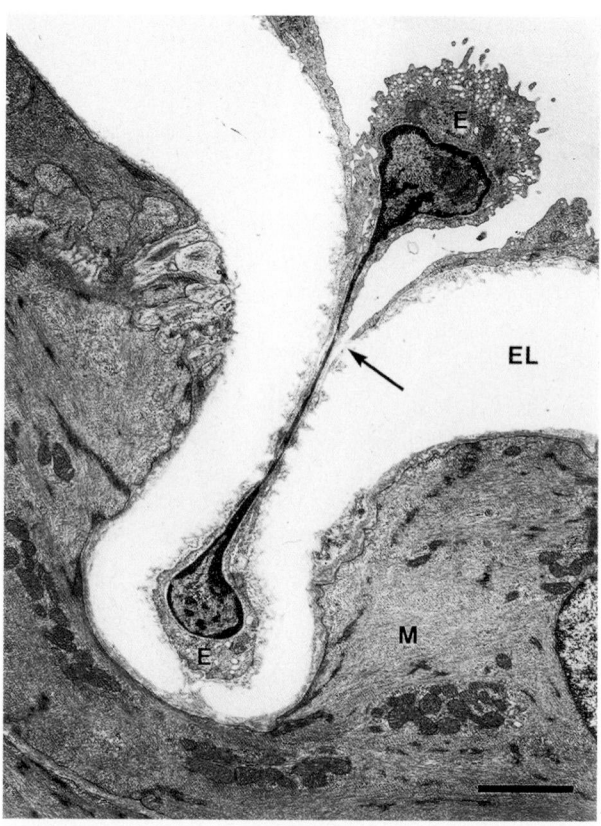

FIGURE 23.34 Intima of a spastic artery; electron microscopic detail. Endothelial cell (**E**) squeezed almost to vanishing thinness in a tight fold of the internal elastic lamina (**EL**). Endothelial breaks can develop under such conditions; a small break is shown by the **arrow. M:** Part of a smooth muscle cell. **Bar =** 2 μm. (Reproduced with permission from [80], © American Society for Investigative Pathology.)

squeezed (Figure 23.34), and some endothelial damage occurs (11, 80).

Another self-inflicted injury occurs in the spastic media: smooth muscle cells develop cell-to-cell herniae that appear as vacuoles (p. 78) (81). This is not a serious injury as a single event, but chronic effects have not been studied.

Spasm in human disease. Spasm is a known cause of disease, especially in the heart and brain.

• *Coronary spasm.* Some individuals suffer from severe chest pain (angina pectoris) even at rest without any stress. This so-called variant angina or Prinzmetal angina has been convincingly shown to be the result of coronary spasm (Figure 23.35) (15). Myocardial infarcts due to spasm are rare but well documented (11, 15, 25, 182). *A reflex coronary spasm due to cold hands is a recognized hazard of snow shoveling:* dipping a hand in ice-cold water is the **cold pressor test** used in cardiology for producing a reflex, not

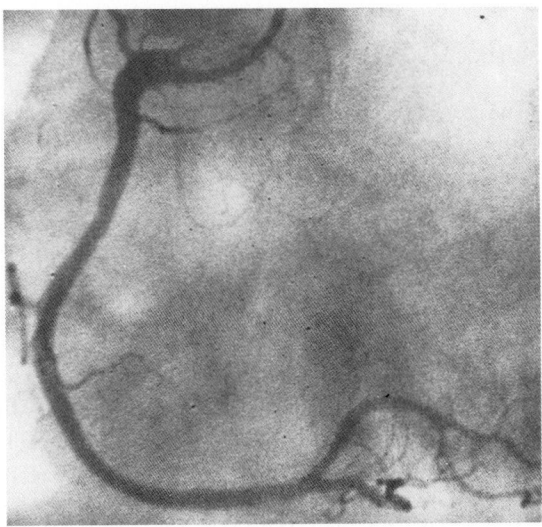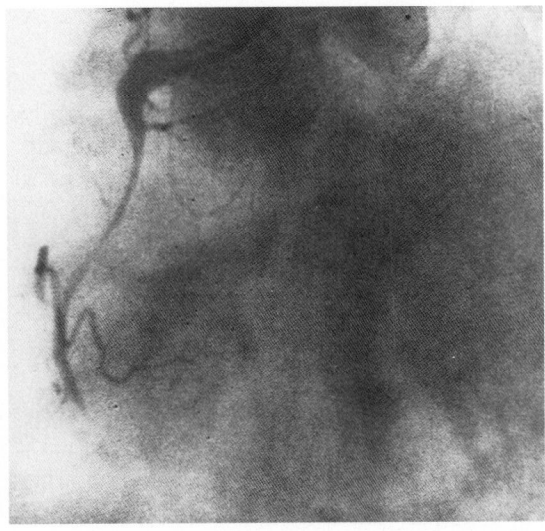

FIGURE 23.35   Arterial spasm can be intense enough to stop the flow of blood. *Left:* Arteriogram of the right coronary artery in a patient who suffered from episodes of chest pain due to coronary spasm (the so-called Prinzmetal angina). The image shows only mild narrowings, insufficient to cause ischemia. *Right:* Four minutes after an intravenous injection of a vasoconstrictor (ergonovine), the same artery shows a long segment of severe narrowing followed by total obstruction. At this point the patient experienced chest pain; after administration of a vasodilator (nitroglycerine) the artery dilated and the pain disappeared: (Courtesy of Dr. F. A. Heupler, Director, Cardiac Catheterization Laboratory, The Cleveland Clinic Foundation.)

without danger, constriction of the coronary arteries. Interestingly, the vasoconstrictor ergonovine, currently used by cardiologists for coronary testing, is a direct descendant of ergot, the cause of St. Anthony's fire.

- *Cerebral arterial spasm.* This is a feared complication of subarachnoid hemorrhage; it occurs with a delay of 4–14 days and can cause severe neurologic deficits (3). One of its peculiar features is its long duration, which is probably due to the fact that free hemoglobin, released at the site of hemorrhage, inhibits the endothelium-dependent relaxation of the arteries. In addition, hemoglobin itself is a vasoconstrictor (85).

- *Raynaud's phenomenon* is a three-stage event seen most often in young women (63). A feeling of cold or an emotional upset trigger a bilateral spasm in the fingers, which become white; then cyanotic. The event comes to an end with a phase of reactive hyperemia (redness) (Figure 23.36). This may be the only trouble, but occasionally there is an underlying disease, such as rheumatoid arthritis or a hematologic abnormality (2, 19).

- Transient blindness of one eye can be due to arterial spasm (18).

- Sudden death by cocaine abuse may be related to coronary spasm (86, 115).

- A genetically induced cardiomyopathy of the hamster produces scattered foci of necrosis, attributed to spasm in small arteries (40).

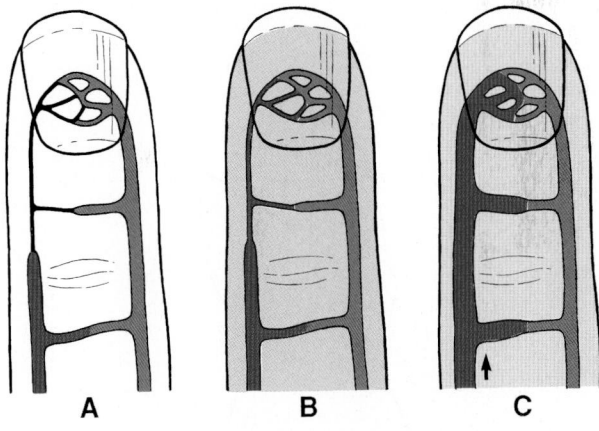

FIGURE 23.36   Three phases of Raynaud's phenomenon: **A:** White phase, due to spasm of the small arteries. **B:** Blue phase, when limited arterial flow permits pooling of poorly oxygenated blood. **C:** Red phase, when the spasm ends and oxygenated blood flows back into the finger (**arrow**). (Adapted from [166]. Illustration by H. Greenfield.)

- The pathogenesis of *acute* stress ulcers of the stomach probably includes a component of vasoconstriction, but the mechanism is more complex (96).

- Venous spasm may occur (93), but it is not a known cause of disease.

Obstruction by Compression

Obstacles to flow due to compression affect primarily the veins because they have the lowest pressure and the thinnest walls. This means that the pathogenesis of pressure damage begins in the veins. Veins may be squeezed from within (by increased tissue pressure) or from without (by external pressure).

Compression by Increased Tissue Pressure: The Compartment Syndrome

The compartment syndrome is a painful ischemic accident that happens, as the name implies, to organs contained within a tight "container" with little leeway for expansion—typically the muscles of the limbs, which are snugly packed in fibrotendinous wrappings (*fasciae*) (Figure 23.37) (107, 119, 134). The fasciae create anatomic and functional compartments. (Another typical setting is the abdominal cavity; see below). Whenever the content of a compartment swells rapidly because of edema, inflammation, or hemorrhage, tissue pressure can rise above venous pressure, and a vicious circle is set in motion, leading to infarction.

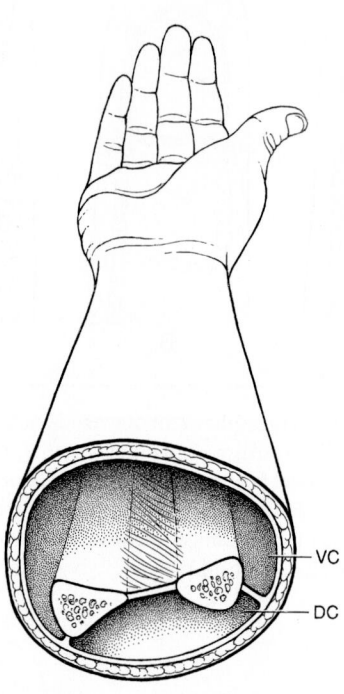

FIGURE 23.37   The two compartments of the forearm, which explain the development of compartment syndromes in this area. **DC:** Dorsal compartment. **VC:** Volar (anterior) compartment. (Adapted with permission from [107].)

The case of the Marathon runner.   The nature of the compression problem is best illustrated by the case of an inexperienced runner determined to win a marathon. Right from the start the muscles of the calf call for more blood. This is perfectly normal; the arterioles dilate, and the microcirculation is perfused more fully and under higher pressure (hyperemia). Now the volume of the muscle has increased a little, but there is still room for it in the distended fascia. Because capillary pressure has increased, more transudate is formed; for a time the lymphatics are able to drain it. The runner presses on. The hyperemia increases, the transudate increases. Tissue pressure begins to rise, but the fascia surrounding the muscle cannot be distended any further. The small veins and the lymphatics begin to be squeezed. The muscle begins to ache. Now a vicious circle sets in:

> Increased tissue pressure → compression of the veins and lymphatics (while high-pressure arterial inflow continues) → congestion of the tissues → increased transudation from the capillaries → anoxic swelling of the muscle fibers → increased tissue pressure → more compression of the veins → . . .

Pain is the warning. If the runner takes heed, the situation is reversible; if not, the vicious circle can be interrupted only by releasing the tissue pressure. This means surgery: the fascia has to be slit open (fasciotomy) (118).

> We have heard about a well-known athlete whose performance was greatly improved after bilateral fasciotomy of the calf. Apparently, the operation created more space also for muscle hypertrophy.
>   The term *shin splints,* incidentally, covers a number of injuries, including compartment syndromes (8, 77).

Clinical signs are a throbbing, unrelenting pain, out of proportion with the clinical setting; weakness of the muscles affected, and, eventually, numbness of the part due to compression of the nerves. The muscles feel tense and swollen; in some orthopedic services the degree of tissue pressure is evaluated with manometric devices; criteria vary, but a value above 35–45 mm Hg usually calls for decompression.

The case of the tight cast.   Another classic setting for the compartment syndrome is a tight cast on a fractured limb. *Severe pain should sound the alert.* If the pressure is not released, the muscle is infarcted and replaced by a slowly contracting fibrous mass. The notorious deformation of the forearm called Volkmann's contracture,

Obstructions at the Capillary Level

Obstacles to flow can develop, obviously, also in the capillaries; however, little is known about capillary pathology altogether (104). Here are some highlights.

The Hyperviscosity Syndromes

Flow in the microcirculation, and especially in the capillaries, can be hampered by increased viscosity of the blood, a problem that does not affect larger vessels. Hyperviscous blood interferes with the function of virtually every organ. The symptoms are therefore quite varied: fatigue, blurred vision, headache, dizziness, and bleeding from the gums and nose. The ophthalmoscope can show quite strikingly the congested microcirculation (Figure 23.41)(147).

How does the blood become too viscous? It may contain too many red blood cells (polycythemia), too many white blood cells (leukemia), stiff or distorted cells, or high concentrations of proteins that tend to aggregate (76):

- *Polycythemia* can be secondary (to anoxia, as in chronic mountain sickness, or in cases of renal carcinomas secreting an excess of erythropoietin); or it can be primary, a red-cell equivalent of leukemia, although it is not as malignant.

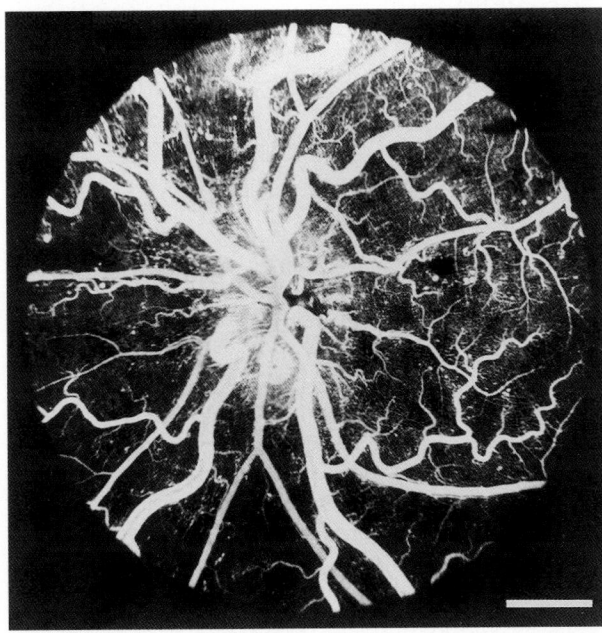

FIGURE 23.41 Dilated retinal arteries and veins in a case of hyperviscosity syndrome. **Bar** = 1 mm. (Reproduced from [147], copyright 1992 by Appleton & Lange, with permission from The McGraw-Hill Companies.)

- The role of *leukemia* as a cause of hyperviscosity will be discussed below.

- *Plasma proteins that increase viscosity* are found in multiple myeloma, especially when the product of the monoclonal neoplastic plasma cells is IgG3, which tends to form complexes (especially at cool temperatures), or IgA, which tends to form elongated polymers. Waldenström's macroglobulinemia is another B-cell malignancy in which the hypersecreted protein is IgM; in many cases the IgM precipitates develop in the cold (hence the name *cryoglobulin, krýos* = "icy cold"). This explains the clinical appearance of Raynaud's phenomenon in cold weather (p. 683). Cryoglobulins are typically associated with *Mycoplasma* pneumonia.

Capillary Pathology

Complete obstruction can occur in capillaries as in any other vessel, but little is known about it. In fact, little is known about capillary pathology altogether (104). The capillaries have long been considered to be privileged vessels, spared by most diseases except diabetes. It used to be said that "blood never clots in capillaries," which is surely wrong; but it is a fact that clots in capillaries are rarely found *postmortem,* probably because the fibrinolytic activity of the endothelium destroys them. It is also true that no known vasoactive agent affects capillary function, whether it relates to contractility, caliber, or permeability. Perhaps evolution has deprived them of the necessary receptors because they should remain aloof: their unimpeded function is critical.

We have summarized in Figure 23.42, and in the following list, the principal mishaps known to occur in capillaries; most of them are obstacles to flow (104):

1. *Impaction of leukocytes.* It seems strange that nature should have made leukocytes larger than most capillaries (p. 713); this can lead to capillary plugging and cause leukostasis. This is common in leukemia, especially myelocytic leukemia; in such cases it may cause complications in the brain and lungs, and even death from microcirculatory failure (121, 147). *Leukostasis* is now receiving much attention because it is implicated in the pathogenesis of reflow after ischemia (p. 712), shock (p. 720) (22), and other conditions (56, 73, 137). The normal tendency of leukocytes to become temporarily impacted in the capillaries (36) can be exaggerated by several mechanisms: trapping by adhesion proteins, increased stiffness due to activation (197), and increased size (in leukemia).

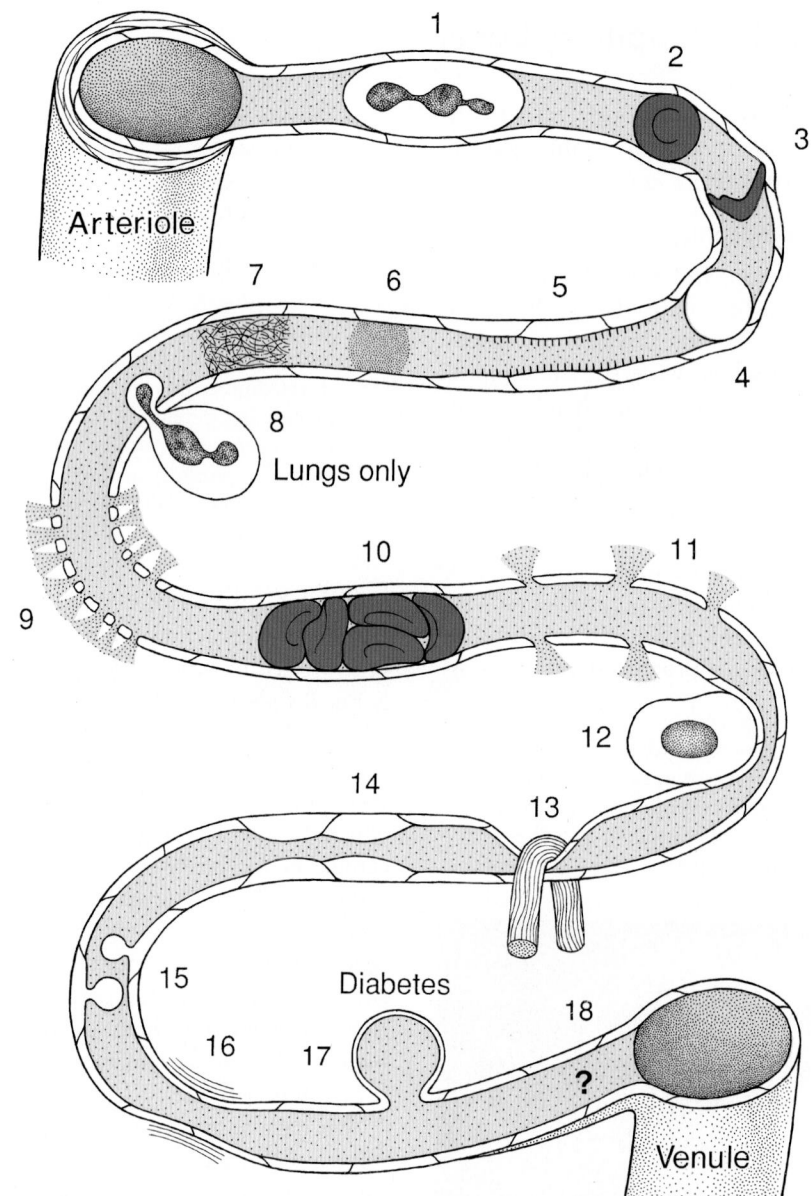

FIGURE 23.42   Pathologic mechanisms that may affect *capillary* structure and function. **1:** Plugging by leukocytes. **2:** Plugging by stiffened erythrocytes, as in acidosis. **3:** Plugging by abnormally shaped erythrocytes, as in sickle cell disease. **4:** Plugging by fat droplets. **5:** Activation of the endothelium, with expression of adhesion molecules. **6:** Plugging by immunoglobulin precipitates (as in *Mycoplasma* pneumonia) or by antigen/antibody complexes. **7:** Plugging by fibrin, either embolized or locally generated. **8:** Sticking of leukocytes followed by diapedesis (in lung capillaries only). **9:** Direct injury of the capillary wall. **10:** Stasis of red blood cells, as occurs when plasma is lost. **11:** Late capillary leakage, as it occurs in inflammation. **12:** Compression by swollen extravascular cells, such as occurs with anoxic glial cells. **13:** Kinking over a collagen fiber. **14:** Swelling of endothelial cells, as in eclampsia. **15:** Blebbing of endothelial cells. **16:** Stenosis by a multilayered, thickened basement membrane. **17:** Microaneurysms, as in diabetes. **18:** Open for future discoveries.

2. *Impaction of red blood cells.* Red blood cells can become impacted when their rigidity and volume are increased by acidosis (29, 35, 152). Ischemic tissues are acid. The red blood cells of diabetics are stiffer than normal and may cause flow disturbances (161).

3. *Impacted sickle cells in sickle cell anemia.* Two mechanisms have been proposed. (a) Sickled red blood cells are deformed by the internal crystallization of the abnormal hemoglobin S. Under normal circumstances, red blood cells flowing through the microcirculation of the spleen have to squeeze through very tight

passages; sickled cells are held up and can impede flow to the point of causing complete infarction of the spleen (*autosplenectomy*) (Figure 23.43) (168). A similar sequence can lead to multiple organ failure (124). (b) In sickle cell anemia, even nonsickled cells tend to stick to the endothelium (71).

4. *Embolism by fat droplets.*
5. *Activation of the endothelium.* This may lead to leukocyte sticking, clotting, and other changes.
6. *Plugging by immunoglobulin precipitates* (as in *Mycoplasma* pneumonia) or by antigen–antibody precipitates.
7. *Plugging by fibrin clots,* embolized or formed locally.
8. *Temporary occlusion during diapedesis in alveolar capillaries.*
9. *Direct injury to the capillary* (as produced by oxygen overdose in the lungs) leads to diffuse, prolonged capillary leakage.

10. *Stasis of red blood cells (massive impaction)* due to fluid loss.
11. *Capillary leakage* by vascular remodeling as seen after 24–48 hours of inflammation (p. 396).
12. *Extrinsic compression by swollen cells,* such as in ischemic brain (p. 711).
13. *Kinking over a collagen fiber,* in tissues swollen by edema.
14. *Endothelial swelling,* as in the renal glomeruli in eclampsia (70).
15. *Endothelial blebbing,* as seen in ischemia.
16. *Repeated duplication of basement membranes,* which may lead to capillary stenosis in diabetes and other conditions (p. 281).
17. *Microaneurysms,* as occur in diabetes; it seems that the endothelial wall is "blown out" because the pericytes have died (Figure 23.44) (48, 177, 193).
18. Open for new discoveries.

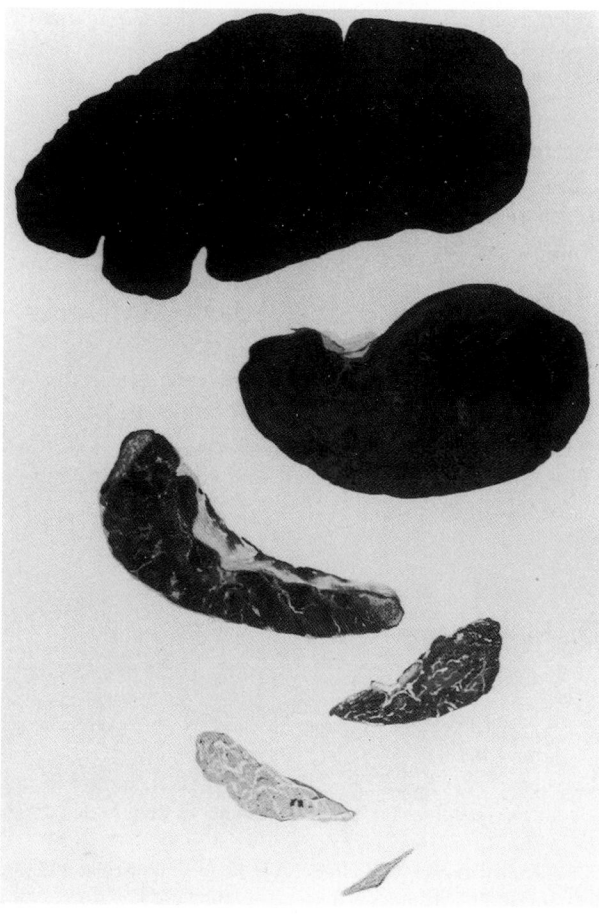

FIGURE 23.43 Human spleens illustrating the progressive atrophy that occurs in sickle cell anemia. The sickle cells become jammed in the microcirculation and impair blood flow; this may lead to autosplenectomy. Slightly enlarged. (Reproduced from [151] by permission of Oxford University Press.)

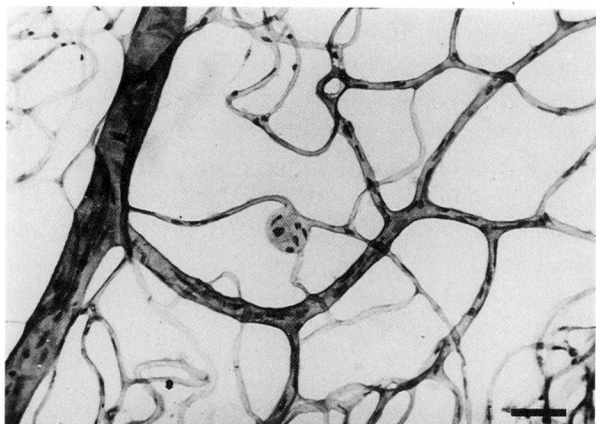

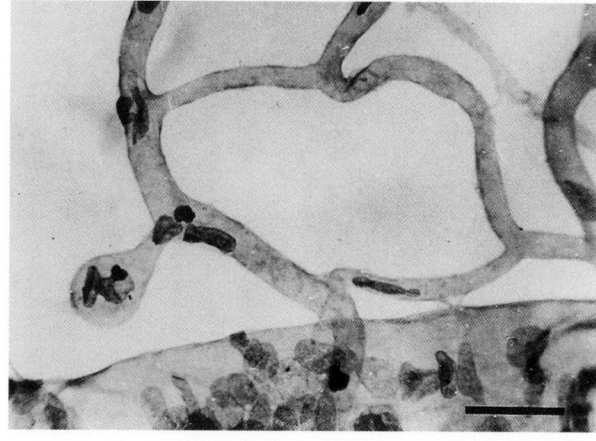

FIGURE 23.44 Microaneurysms in the retina of a diabetic patient. The entire vascular network of the retina was freed from other tissues by trypsinization, then laid out flat and photographed. *Top:* **Bar** = 500 μm. *Bottom:* **Bar** = 50 μm. The aneurysmal dilatations are thought to represent areas of weakness due to loss of pericytes. (Reproduced from [48] by permission from Springer-Verlag.)

Let it be clear that flow through a *single* capillary may be impaired by *several* defects of structure and function. The microcirculation in diabetes offers a maddening example: its causes of malfunction include changes in the endothelium (increased permeability, increased production of von Willebrand factor, decreased production of plasminogen activator), a thickened and biochemically abnormal basement membrane, microaneurysms due to pericyte loss, increased stickiness of the platelets, stiffening of the red blood cells, and the list is not complete (89, 186).

Vascular plugging in plants. Obstacles can develop also in the vessels of apple trees and tomato plants (59, 187), and infarcts develop, although plant pathologists do not call them by that name ("wilting" is one of the alternatives). Infection and other types of injury cause vessels to become occluded by a mechanism that seems to be purposeful, like thrombosis in animals; this type of vascular occlusion is achieved by large cellular protrusions called tyloses (from the Greek *týlos*, lump or knob) (Figure 23.45). These **tyloses** resemble what animal pathologists call blebbing: the capillary-occluding mechanism listed as #13 in the figure just described. Nature plays themes and variations.

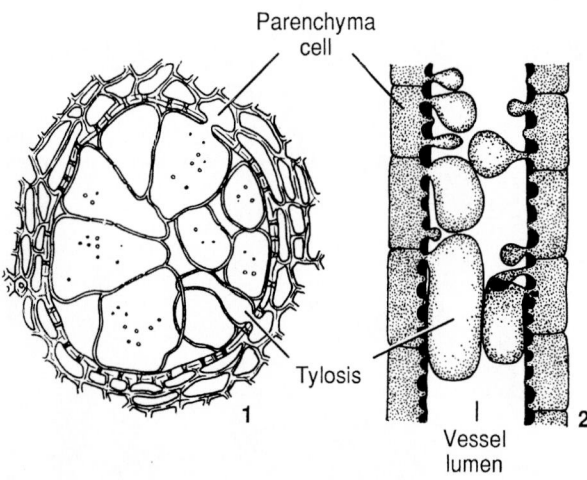

FIGURE 23.45   Example of plant pathology reminiscent of human pathology: namely, the blebbing and herniation of perivascular cells into the lumen, resulting in vascular occlusion. These plant protrusions are called tyloses. *Left:* Cross section of a vessel of *Robinia pseudacacia. Right:* Longitudinal section of a vessel of the vine tree *Vitis vinifera.* (Reprinted with permission from [41], Copyright 1967, Pergamon Press Ltd.)

TO SUM UP: The variety of obstacles that may develop in the circulatory system reflects the problems that may develop in any plumbing system, but there are some oddities due to the subdivision of the vascular system into three sections—arteries, veins, and capillaries. In arteries, flow runs from large to smaller vessels, so that a variety of objects carried by the blood in large arteries will become impacted into smaller arteries. In veins, the blood runs from smaller to larger vessels, hence embolization cannot occur; objects carried by the blood will go through the heart and embolize the pulmonary arteries. Venous flow is slow, which favors thrombosis. Capillary circulation is threatened by many types of malfunction, including obstruction by white or red blood cells, all of which are normally larger than the capillary lumen. In the microcirculation, several obstructive mechanisms can be at work at the same time, notably in diabetes.

Arteries suffer from a major disease related to age and to plasma cholesterol: atherosclerosis. We cannot explain why it has no counterpart in veins, but we can speculate. The arterial wall (notably the media) is designed for maximal toughness; the main components of the media are elastin and collagen, plus smooth muscle cells to synthesize both. When the media is infiltrated by plasma cholesterol it has no means to get rid of it: the media contains no macrophages and no capillaries to carry it away. Cholesterol cannot be broken down. The result is atherosclerosis.

It seems that the arterial wall was not designed for our current diet.

References

1. Agrios GN. Plant pathology, 3rd ed. New York: Academic Press, 1988.

1a. Albers GW, Caplan LR, Easton JD, et al. Transient ischemic attack—proposal for a new definition. N Engl J Med 2002; 347:1713–1716.

2. Allen EV, Barker NW, Hines EA Jr. Peripheral vascular diseases, 3rd ed. Philadelphia: WB Saunders, 1962.

3. Allen GS, Ahn HS, Preziosi TJ, et al. Cerebral arterial spasm—a controlled trial of nimodipine in patients with subarachnoid hemorrhage. N Engl J Med 1983;308:619–624.

4. Allman RM. Pressure ulcers among the elderly. N Engl J Med 1989;320:850–853.

5. Anderson FA, Wheeler HB. Venous thromboembolism: risk factors and prophylaxis. Clin Chest Med 1995;16:235–251.

6. Anderson JB, Williamson RCN. Testicular torsion in Bristol: a 25-year review. Br J Surg 1988;75:988–992.

7. Anderson RH, Wilcox BR, Becker AE. Anatomy of the normal heart. In: Hurst JW, Anderson RH, Becker AE, Wilcox BR. Atlas of the heart. New York: Gower Medical Publishing, 1988, pp. 1.1–1.20.

7a. Ariyo AA, Thach C, Tracy R. Lp(a) lipoprotein, vascular disease, and mortality in the elderly. N Engl J Med 2003; 349:2108–2115.

8. Armstrong RB. Muscle damage and endurance events. Sports Med 1986;3:370–381.

9. Bartsch RC, McConnell EE, Imes GD, Schmidt JM. A review of exertional rhabdomyolysis in wild and domestic animals and man. Vet Pathol 1977;14:314–324.

10. Beckering RE Jr, Titus JL. Femoral-popliteal venous thrombosis and pulmonary embolism. Am J Clin Pathol 1969;52: 530–537.

11. Benacerraf A, Scholl JM, Achard F, Tonnelier M, Lavergne G. Coronary spasm and thrombosis associated with myocardial infarction in a patient with nearly normal coronary arteries. Circulation 1983;67:1147–1150.

11a. Berde CB, Sethna NF. Analgesics for the treatment of pain in children. N Engl J Med 2002;347:1094–1103.

12. Biegelsen ES, Loscalzo J. Endothelial function and atherosclerosis. Coronary Artery Dis 1999;10:241–258.

12a. Bobryshev YV, Watanabe T. Subset of vascular dendritic cells transforming into foam cells in human atherosclerotic lesions. Cardiovasc Pathol 1997;6:321–331.

13. Bocan TMA, Mueller SB, Brown EQ, Uhlendorf PD, Mazur MJ, Newton RS. Antiatherosclerotic effects of antioxidants are lesion-specific when evaluated in hypercholesterolemic New Zealand white rabbits. Exp Mol Pathol 1992;57:70–83.

14. Bove FJ. The story of ergot. Basel: S. Karger, 1970.

15. Braunwald E, ed. Heart disease. A textbook of cardiovascular medicine, 3rd ed. Philadelphia: WB Saunders, 1988.

16. Brazeau P. Oxytocins. Oxytocin and ergot alkaloids. In: Goodman LS, Gilman A, eds. The pharmacological basis of therapeutics, 4th ed. New York: Macmillan, 1970, pp. 893–907.

17. Buess H. Zur Geschichte des Embolie-Begriffs bis auf Virchow. In: Leuch O, Merkelbach O, eds. Schweizerisches Medizinisches Jahrbuch 1946. Basel: Benno Schwabe & Co., 1946, pp. 57–69.

18. Burger SK, Saul RF, Selhorst JB, Thurston SE. Transient monocular blindness caused by vasospasm. N Engl J Med 1991;325:870–873.

19. Cardelli MB, Kleinsmith DM. Raynaud's phenomenon and disease. Med Clin North Am 1989;73:1127–1141.

20. Chartier L, Béra J, Delomez M, et al. Free-floating thrombi in the right heart. Circulation 1999;99:2779–2783.

21. Cheitlin MD, McAllister HA, de Castro CM. Myocardial infarction without atherosclerosis. JAMA 1975;231:951–959.

22. Chien S, Sung K-LP, Schmid-Schönbein GW, et al. Rheology of leukocytes. Ann NY Acad Sci 1987;516:333–347.

23. Chisolm GM. Oxidized lipoproteins and leukocyte-endothelial interactions: growing evidence for multiple mechanisms. Lab Invest 1993;68:369–371.

24. Christiaens GCML, Sixma JJ, Haspels AA. Hemostasis in menstrual endometrium: a review. Obstet Gynecol Surv 1982;37:281–303.

25. Cipriano PR, Koch FH, Rosenthal SJ, et al. Myocardial infarction in patients with coronary artery spasm demonstrated by angiography. Am Heart J 1983;105:542–547.

26. Clark SL. New concepts of amniotic fluid embolism: a review. Obstet & Gynecol Survey 1990;45:360–368.

27. Clark SL, Hanakins GDV, Dudley DA, Dildy GA, Porter TF. Amniotic fluid embolism: analysis of the national registry. Am J Obstet Gynecol 1995;172:1158–1169.

28. Clinton SK, Libby P. Cytokines and growth factors in atherogenesis. Arch Pathol Lab Med 1992;116:1292–1300.

28a. Collins T, Cybulski MI. NF-κB: pivotal mediator or innocent bystander in atherogenesis? J Clin Invest 2001; 107:255–264.

29. Crandall ED, Critz AM, Osher AS, Keljo DJ, Forster RE. Influence of pH on elastic deformability of the human erythrocyte membrane. Am J Physiol 1978;235:C269–C278.

30. Cybulsky MI, Gimbrone MA Jr. Endothelial expression of a mononuclear leukocyte adhesion molecule during atherogenesis. Science 1991;251:788–791.

30a. Cybulsky MI, Iiama K, Li H, et al. A major role for VCAM-1, but not ICAM-1, in early atherosclerosis. J Clin Invest 2001;107:1255–1262.

31. Daniel RK, Priest DL, Wheatley DC. Etiologic factors in pressure sores: an experimental model. Arch Phys Med Rehabil 1981;62:492–498.

32. Darsee JR. Cholesterol embolism: the great masquerader. South Med J 1979;72:174–180.

33. Davies PF, Robotewskyj A, Griem ML, Dull RO, Polacek DC. Hemodynamic forces and vascular cell communication in arteries. Arch Pathol Lab Med 1992;116:1301–1306.

34. DePaola N, Gimbrone MA Jr, Davies PF, Dewey CF Jr. Vascular endothelium responses to fluid shear stress gradients. Arterioscler Thromb 1992;12:1254–1257.

35. Dintenfass L. Microrheology of blood in health and disease. In: Onogi S, ed. Proceedings of the Fifth International Congress on Rheology, vol 2. Tokyo: University of Tokyo Press, 1970, pp. 27–59.

36. Doerschuk CM, Beyers N, Coxson HO, Wiggs B, Hogg JC. Comparison of neutrophil and capillary diameters and their relation to neutrophil sequestration in the lung. J Appl Physiol 1993;74:3040–3045.

37. Durlacher SH, Meier JR, Fisher RS, Lovitt WV Jr. Sudden death due to pulmonary fat embolism in chronic alcoholics with fatty livers. J Forensic Sci 1959;4:215–228.

38. Edmonds CR, Barbut D, Hager D, Sharrock NE. Inoperative cerebral arterial embolization during total hip arthroplasty. Anesthesiology 2000;93:315–318.

39. Elliott JP Jr, Hageman JH, Szilagyi DE, et al. Arterial embolization: problems of source, multiplicity, recurrence, and delayed treatment. Surgery 1980;88:833–845.

40. Factor SM, Minase T, Cho S, Dominitz R, Sonnenblick EH. Microvascular spasm in the cardiomyopathic Syrian hamster: a preventable cause of focal myocardial necrosis. Circulation 1982;66:342–354.

41. Fahn A. Plant anatomy. Oxford: Pergamon Press, 1967.

42. Falk E, Shah PK, Fuster V. Coronary plaque disruption. Circulation 1995;92:657–671.

43. Faruqi RM, DiCorleto PE. Mechanisms of monocyte recruitment and accumulation. Br Heart J 1993:S19–S29.

43a. Fischer CM. Transient ischemic attacks. N Engl J Med 2002;347:1642–1643.

44. Fogarty TJ, Cranley JJ, Krause RJ, Strasser ES, Hafner CD. A method for extraction of arterial emboli and thrombi. Surg Gynecol Obstet 1963;116:241–244.

45. Forman MB, Oates JA, Robertson D, et al. Increased adventitial mast cells in a patient with coronary spasm. N Engl J Med 1985;313:1138–1141.

46. Forsberg F, Merton DA, Liu JB, Needleman L, Goldberg BB. Clinical applications of ultrasound contrast agents. Ultrasonics 1998;36:695–701.

47. Fred HL, Axelrad MA, Lewis JM, Alexander JK. Rapid resolution of pulmonary thromboemboli in man. JAMA 1966;196:121–123.

48. Fuchs U, Tinius W, vom Scheidt J, Reichenbach A. Morphometric analysis of retinal blood vessels in retinopathia diabetica. Graefe's Arch Clin Exp Ophthalmol 1985;223:83–87.

49. Galpin JE, Chow AW, Bayer AS, Guze LB. Sepsis associated with decubitus ulcers. Am J Med 1976;61:346–350.

50. Ganz P, Alexander RW. New insights into the cellular mechanisms of vasospasm. Am J Cardiol 1985;56:11E–15E.

51. Garfin SR. Historical review. In: Mubarak SJ, Hargens AR, eds. Compartment syndromes and Volkmann's contracture. (Saunders monographs in clinical orthopaedics, vol III). Philadelphia: WB Saunders, 1981, pp. 6–16.

52. Gelberman R. Volkmann's contracture of the upper extremity: pathology and reconstruction. In: Mubarak SJ, Hargens AR, eds. Compartment syndromes and Volkmann's contracture. (Saunders monographs in clinical orthopaedics, vol III). Philadelphia: WB Saunders, 1981, pp. 183–193.

53. Gerrity RG, Naito HK. Lipid clearance from fatty streak lesions by foam cell migration. Artery 1980;8:215–219.

54. Ginsberg MM, Gresham L. Deaths related to liposuction. N Engl J Med 1999;341:1000.

55. Gershuni DH. Volkmann's contracture of the lower extremity: pathology and reconstruction. In: Mubarak SJ, Hargens AR, eds. Compartment syndromes and Volkmann's contracture. (Saunders monographs in clinical orthopaedics, vol III). Philadelphia: WB Saunders, 1981, pp. 194–208.

56. Goldblum SE, Cohen DA, Gillespie MN, McClain CJ. Interleukin-1-induced granulocytopenia and pulmonary leukostasis in rabbits. J Appl Physiol 1987;62:122–128.

57. Goldhaber SZ. Pulmonary embolism. N Engl J Med 1998;339:93–104.

58. Goldhaber SZ. A contemporary approach to thrombolytic therapy for pulmonary embolism. Vasc Med 2000;5:115–123.

59. Goodman RN, Király Z, Wood KR. The biochemistry and physiology of plant disease. Columbia, MO: University of Missouri Press, 1986.

60. Gossling HR, Donohue TA. The fat embolism syndrome. JAMA 1979;241:2740–2742.

61. Gossling HR, Pellegrini VD Jr. Fat embolism syndrome. A review of the pathophysiology and physiological basis of treatment. Clin Orthop 1982;165:68–82.

62. Gott AM. Lipid lowering, regression, and coronary events. Circulation 1995;92:646–656.

63. Greenfield H. Raynaud's phenomenon: the cold facts. Harvard Health Letter 1992;17(3):1–2.

64. Gregg PJ, Walder DN. Caisson disease of bone. Clin Orthop 1986;210:43–54.

65. Gutstein WH, Anversa P, Guideri G. Spasm of small coronary arteries and ischemic myocardial injury induced by hypothalamic stimulation in the rat. Am J Pathol 1987;129:287–294.

66. Haigh JC, Stewart RR, Wobeser G, MacWilliams PS. Capture myopathy in a moose. J Am Vet Med Assoc 1977;171:924–926.

67. Hajjar KA, Gavish D, Breslow JL, Nachman RL. Lipoprotein(a) modulation of endothelial cell surface fibrinolysis and its potential role in atherosclerosis. Nature 1989;309:303–305.

68. Hamilton TA, Major JA, Chisolm GM. The effects of oxidized low density lipoproteins on inducible mouse macrophage gene expression are gene and stimulus dependent. J Clin Invest 1995;95:2020–2027.

69. Having O. Deep vein thrombosis and pulmonary embolism. An autopsy study with multiple regression analysis of possible risk factors. Acta Chir Scand Suppl 1977;477:1–120.

70. Heaton JM, Turner DR. Persistent renal damage following pre-eclampsia: a renal biopsy study of 13 patients. J Pathol 1985;147:121–126.

71. Hebbel RP. Blockade of adhesion of sickle cells to endothelium by monoclonal antibodies. N Engl J Med 2000;342:1910–1912.

72. Howard GC, Pizzo SV. Biology of disease: lipoprotein (a) and its role in atherothrombotic disease. Lab Invest 1993;69:373–386.

73. Howard RJ, Crain C, Franzini DA, Hood I, Hugli TE. Effects of cardiopulmonary bypass on pulmonary leukostasis and complement activation. Arch Surg 1988;123:1496–1501.

74. Hulman G. Pathogenesis of non-traumatic fat embolism. Lancet 1988;1:1366–1367.

75. Inano H, English D, Doerschuk CM. Effect of zymosan-activated plasma on the deformability of rabbit polymorphonuclear leukocytes. J Appl Physiol 1992;73:1370–1376.

76. Jandl JH. Blood. Boston: Little, Brown, 1987.

77. Jones DC, James SL. Overuse injuries of the lower extremity: shin splints, iliotibial band friction syndrome, and exertional compartment syndromes. Clin Sports Med 1987;6:273–290.

78. Jones HR Jr, Caplan LR, Come PC, Swinton NW Jr, Breslin DJ. Cerebral emboli of paradoxical origin. Ann Neurol 1983;13:314–319.

79. Joris I, Braunstein PW Jr. Platelets and endothelium: effect of collagen-induced platelet aggregates on pulmonary vessels. Exp Mol Pathol 1982;37:393–405.

80. Joris I, Majno G. Endothelial changes induced by arterial spasm. Am J Pathol 1981;102:346–358.

81. Joris I, Majno G. Medial changes in arterial spasm induced by L-norepinephrine. Am J Pathol 1981;105:212–222.

82. Joris I, Zand T, Nunnari JJ, Krolikowski FJ, Majno G. Studies on the pathogenesis of atherosclerosis. I. Adhesion and emigration of mononuclear cells in the aorta of hypercholesterolemic rats. Am J Pathol 1983;113:341–358.

83. Judson R. Pressure sores. Med J Aust 1983;1:417–422.

84. Jungbluth A, Erbel R, Darius H, Rumpelt H-J, Meyer J. Paradoxical coronary embolism: case report and review of the literature. Am Heart J 1988;116:879–885.

85. Kanamaru K, Waga S, Kojima T, Fujimoto K, Niwa S. Endothelium-dependent relaxation of canine basilar arteries. Part 2: inhibition by hemoglobin and cerebrospinal fluid from patients with aneurysmal subarachnoid hemorrhage. Stroke 1987;18:938–943.

86. Karch SB, Billingham ME. The pathology and etiology of cocaine-induced heart disease. Arch Pathol Lab Med 1988; 112:225–230.

87. Kerstell J, Hallgren B, Rudenstam C-M, Svanborg A. I. The chemical composition of the fat emboli in the post-absorptive dog. Acta Med Scand Suppl 1969;499:3–18.

87a. Kolodgie FD, Gold HK, Burke AP, et al. Intraplaque hemorrhage and progression of coronary atheroma. N Engl J Med 2003;349:2316–2324.

88. Korn D, Gore I, Blenke A, Collins DP. Pulmonary arterial bands and webs: an unrecognized manifestation of organized pulmonary emboli. Am J Pathol 1962;40:129–151.

89. Korthius RJ, Fuselier SP, Jerome SN. Diabetic microangiopathy. In: Mortillaro NA, and Taylor AE. The pathophysiology of the microcirculation. Boca Raton: CRC Press, Inc., 1994, pp. 141–160.

90. Kyrle PA, Minar E, Hirschl M, et al. High plasma levels of factor VIII and the risk of recurrent venous thromboembolism. N Engl J Med 2000;343:457–462.

91. Lam JYT, Chesebro JH, Steele PM, Badimon L, Fuster V. Is vasospasm related to platelet deposition? Relationship in a porcine preparation of arterial injury in vivo. Circulation 1987;75:243–248.

92. Lapuk S, Woodbury DF. Volkmann's ischemic contracture. A case report. Orthop Rev 1988;17:618–624.

93. Lawrie GM. Spasm of saphenous veins used as conduits for aortocoronary bypass grafting. Am J Cardiol 1988;61:675.

94. Lechat P, Mas JL, Lascault G, et al. Prevalence of patent foramen ovale in patients with stroke. N Engl J Med 1988;318: 1148–1152.

95. Leonard RCF, Neville E, Hall RJC. Paradoxical embolism. A review of cases diagnosed during life. Eur Heart J 1982; 3:362–370.

96. Levinson MJ. Gastric stress ulcers. Hosp Pract 1989;24:59–68.

97. Lewis RJ, Chalmers GA, Barrett MW, Bhatnagar R. Capture myopathy in elk in Alberta, Canada: a report of three cases. J Am Vet Med Assoc 1977;171:927–932.

97a. Li AC, Glass CK. The macrophage foam cell as a target for therapeutic intervention. Nat Med 2002;8:1235–1242.

98. Li H, Cybulsky MI, Gimbrone MA Jr, Libby P. An atherogenic diet rapidly induces VCAM-1, a cytokine-regulatable mononuclear leukocyte adhesion molecule, in rabbit aortic endothelium. Arterioscler Thromb 1993;13:197–204.

98a. Libby P. Molecular bases of the acute coronary syndromes. Circulation 1995;91:2844–2850.

98b. Libby P, Aikawa M. Stabilization of atherosclerotic plaques: new mechanisms and clinical targets. Nature Med 2002; 8:1257–1262.

99. Libby P, Geng YJ, Aikawa M, et al. Macrophages and atherosclerotic plaque stability. Curr Opin Lipidol 1996;7:330–335.

100. Logan SE. On the fluid mechanics of human coronary artery stenosis. IEEE Trans Biomed Eng BME 1975;22:327–334.

101. Ludmer PL, Selwyn AP, Shook TL, et al. Paradoxical vasoconstriction induced by acetylcholine in atherosclerotic coronary arteries. N. Engl J Med 1986;315:1046–1051.

102. MacMahon HE, Weiss S. Carbon tetrachloride poisoning with macroscopic fat in the pulmonary artery. Am J Pathol 1929;5:623–630.

103. Mahley RW, Gray ME, LeQuire VS. Role of plasma lipoproteins in cortisone-induced fat embolism. Am J Pathol 1972; 66:43–64.

104. Majno G. The capillary then and now: an overview of capillary pathology. Mod Pathol 1992;5:9–22.

105. Majno G, Cuénoud HF, Joris I. Arteriosclerosis 1988: the cellular events. New Trends in Arrhythmias 1989;5:33–40.

106. Majno G, Zand T, Nunnari JJ, Kowala MC, Joris, I. Intimal responses to shear stress, hypercholesterolemia, and hypertension. Studies in the rat aorta. In: Simionescu N, Simionescu M, eds. Endothelial cell biology in health and disease. New York: Plenum Press, 1988, pp. 349–367.

106a. Maron R, Sukhova G, Faria AM, et al. Mucosal administration of heat shock protein-65 decreases atherosclerosis and inflammation in aortic arch of low-density lipoprotein receptor-deficient mice. Circulation 2002;106:1599–1601.

107. Matsen FA III, Winquist RA, Krugmire RB Jr. Diagnosis and management of compartmental syndromes. J Bone Joint Surg 1980;62A:286–291.

108. McEwen SA, Hulland TJ. Histochemical and morphometric evaluation of skeletal muscle from horses with exertional rhabdomyolysis (typing-up). Vet Pathol 1986;23:400–410.

109. McIntyre KM, Sasahara AA. The hemodynamic response to pulmonary embolism in patients without prior cardiopulmonary disease. Am J Cardiol 1971;28:288–294.

110. Miller FJ, Mineau DE. Transcatheter arterial embolization—major complication and their prevention. Cardiovasc Intervent Radiol 1983;6:141–149.

111. Moon RE, Vann RD, Bennett PB. The physiology of decompression illness. Sci Am 1995;70–77.

112. Moore WS, Malone JM. Effect of flow rate and vessel calibre on critical arterial stenosis. J Surg Res 1979;26:1–9.

113. Mora R, Lupu F, Simionescu N. Prelesional events in atherogenesis: colocalization of apolipoprotein B, unesterified cholesterol and extracellular phospholipid liposomes in the aorta of hyperlipidemic rabbit. Atherosclerosis 1987;67:143–154.

114. Morgan M. Amniotic fluid embolism. Anaesthesia 1979;34: 20–32.

115. Morris DC. Cocaine heart disease. Hosp Pract 1991;26: 83–92.

116. Morrow DA, Ridker PM. C-reactive protein, inflammation, and coronary risk. Med Clin North Am 2000;84: 149–161.

117. Moylan JA, Birnbaum M, Katz A, Everson MA. Fat emboli syndrome. J Trauma 1976;16:341–347.

118. Mubarak SJ. Etiologies of compartment syndromes. In: Mubarak SJ, Hargens AR, eds. Compartment syndromes and Volkmann's contracture. (Saunders monographs in clinical orthopaedics, vol III). Philadelphia: WB Saunders, 1981, pp. 71–97.

119. Mubarak SJ, Hargens AR, eds. Compartment syndromes and Volkmann's contracture. (Saunders monographs in clinical orthopaedics, vol III). Philadelphia: WB Saunders, 1981.

120. Mudd KL, Hunt A, Matherly RC, et al. Analysis of pulmonry fat embolism in blunt force fatalities. J Trauma Inj Inf Crit Care 2000;48:711–715.

120a. Muth CM, Shank ES. Gas embolism. N Engl J Med 2000;342:476–482.

121. Myers TJ, Cole SR, Klatsky AU, Hild DH. Respiratory failure due to pulmonary leukostasis following chemotherapy of acute nonlymphocytic leukemia. Cancer 1983;51:1808–1813.

121a. Naghavi M, Libby P, Falk E, et al. From vulnerable plaque to vulnerable patient: a call for new definitions and risk assessment strategies: Part I Circulation. 2003;108:1664–1772.

122. Nakata Y, Dahms TE. Triolein increases microvascular permeability in isolated perfused rabbit lungs: role of neutrophils. J Trauma Inj Inf Crit Care 2000;49:320–326.

123. Nellessen U, Daniel WG, Matheis G, et al. Impending paradoxical embolism from atrial thrombus: correct diagnosis by transesophageal echocardiography and prevention by surgery. J Am Coll Cardiol 1985;5:1002–1004.

124. Noguchi CT, Schechter AN. The intracellular polymerization of sickle hemoglobin and its relevance to sickle cell disease. Blood 1981;58:1057–1068.

125. Orenstein JM, Sato N, Aaron B, Buchholz B, Bloom S. Microemboli observed in deaths following cardiopulmonary bypass surgery: silicone antifoam agents and polyvinyl chloride tubing as sources of emboli. Hum Pathol 1982;13:1082–1090.

126. Osegbe DN. Testicular torsion in a hot country. N Engl J Med 1988;318:1129–1130.

127. Osler W. Rudolf Virchow, the man and the student. Boston Med Surg J 1891;125:425–427.

128. Owen CA. Clinical diagnosis of acute compartment syndromes. In: Mubarak SJ, Hargens AR, eds. Compartment syndromes and Volkmann's contracture. (Saunders monographs in clinical orthopaedics, vol III). Philadelphia: WB Saunders, 1981a, pp. 98–105.

129. Owen CA. The crush syndrome. In: Mubarak SJ, Hargens AR, eds. Compartment syndromes and Volkmann's contracture. (Saunders monographs in clinical orthopaedics, vol III.) Philadelphia: WB Saunders, 1981b, pp. 166–182.

130. Palmovic V, McCarroll JR. Fat embolism in trauma. Arch Pathol 1965;80:630–635.

131. Parthasarathy S. Modified lipoproteins in the pathogenesis of atherosclerosis. Austin, RG In Landis Company, 1994.

132. Peltier LF. Fat embolism. III. The toxic properties of neutral fat and free fatty acids. Surgery 1956;40:665–670.

133. Peltier LF. Fat embolism. A perspective. Clin Orthop 1988;232:263–270.

134. Perry MO. Compartment syndromes and reperfusion injury. Surg Clin North Am 1988;68:853–864.

135. Phillips JL. The bends: Compressed air in the history of science, diving, and engineering. New Haven: Yale University Press, 1998.

135a. Podrez EA, Poliakov E, Shen Z, et al. A novel family of atherogenic oxidized phospholipids promotes macrophage foam cell formation via scavenger receptor CD36 and is enriched in atherosclerotic lesions. J Biol Chem 2002;277:38517–38523.

135b. Poston RN, Haskard DO, Coucher JR, Gall NP, Johnson-Tidey RR. Expression of intercellular adhesion molecule-1 in atherosclerotic plaques. Am J Pathol 1992;140:665–673.

136. Price TM, Baker VV, Cefalo RC. Amniotic fluid embolism. Three case reports with a review of the literature. Obstet Gynecol Surv 1985;40:462–475.

137. Redl H, Dinges HP, Schlag G. Quantitative estimation of leukostasis in the posttraumatic lung—canine and human autopsy data. Prog Clin Biol Res 1987;236A:43–53.

138. Resnick N, Collins T, Atkinson W, Bonthron DT, Dewey CF Jr. Platelet-derived growth factor B chain promoter contains a cis-acting fluid shear-stress-responsive element. Proc Natl Acad Sci 1993;90:4591–4595.

139. Reuler JB, Cooney TG. The pressure sore: patho-physiology and principles of management. Ann Intern Med 1981;94:661–666.

139a. Ridker PM, Rifai N, Rose L, Buring JE, Cook NR. Comparison of C-reactive protein and low-density lipoprotein cholesterol levels in the prediction of first cardiovascular events. N Engl J Med 2002;347:1557.

140. Riseborough EJ, Herndon JH. Alterations in pulmonary function, coagulation and fat metabolism in patients with fractures of the lower limbs. Clin Orthop 1976;115:248–267.

141. Rogers MC. Do the right thing. Pain relief in infants and children. N Engl J Med 1992;326:55–56.

142. Rosenow EC III, Osmundson PJ, Brown ML. Pulmonary embolism. Mayo Clin Proc 1981;56:161–178.

143. Ross R. Atherosclerosis: a problem of the biology of arterial wall cells and their interactions with blood components. Arteriosclerosis 1981;1:293–311.

144. Ross RM, Johnson GW. Fat embolism after liposuction. Chest 1988;93:1294–1295.

145. Russell RWR. Carotid artery disease and *Amarousis Fugax*. In: Miller S, ed. Clinical ophthalmology. Bristol: Wright, 1987, pp. 524–532.

145a. Ryan EA, Lakey JR, Paty BW, et al. Successful islet transplantation: continued insulin reserve provides long-term glycemic control. Diabetes 2002;51:2148–2157.

145b. Saggi BH, Sugerman HJ, Ivatury RR, Bloomfield GL. Abdominal compartment syndrome. J Trauma 1998;45:597–609.

146. Saiura A, Sata M, Hirata Y, Nagai R, Makuuchi M. Circulating smooth muscle progenitor cells contribute to atherosclerosis. Nat Med 2001;7:382–383.

147. Sanders MD, Graham EM. Ocular disorders associated with systemic diseases. In: Vaughn D, et al. eds. General ophtalmology, 13th ed. Norwalk, CT: Appelton & Lange, 1992, p. 311.

147a. Savia U. At the heart of atherosclerosis. Special focus on atherosclerosis. Nat Med 2002;8:1207–1262.

148. Schröder H, Paust H, Schmidt R. Pulmonary fat embolism after intralipid therapy—a post-mortem artifact? Light and

electron microscopic investigations in low-birth-weight infants. Acta Paediatr Scand 1984;73:461–464.

149. Schwartz MM, Bidani AK, Lewis EJ. Glomerular epithelial cell function and pathology following extreme ablation of renal mass. Am J Pathol 1987;126:315–324.

150. Scott J. Thrombogenesis linked to atherogenesis at last? Nature 1989;341:22–23.

151. Serjeant GR. Sickle cell disease. Oxford: Oxford University Press, 1985.

152. Sevick EM, Jain RK. Effect of red blood cell rigidity on tumor blood flow: increase in viscous resistance during hyperglycemia. Cancer Res 1991;51:2727–2730.

153. Sevitt S. The significance and pathology of fat embolism. Ann Clin Res 1977;9:173–180.

153a. Shapiro AM, Lakey JR, Ryan EA, et al. Islet transplantation in seven patients with type 1 diabetes mellitus using a gluco-corticoid-free immunosuppressive regimen. N Engl J Med 2000;343:230–238.

154. Shaw ST Jr, Roche PC. Menstruation. In: Finn CA, ed. Oxford reviews of reproduction biology. Oxford: Clarendon Press, 1980, pp. 41–96.

155. Shier MR, Wilson RF. Fat embolism syndrome: traumatic coagulopathy with respiratory distress. Surg Annu 1980; 12:139–168.

156. Shimokawa H, Tomoike H, Nabeyama S, et al. Coronary artery spasm induced in atherosclerotic miniature swine. Science 1983;221:560–562.

157. Shipley RE, Gregg DE. The effect of external constriction of a blood vessel on blood flow. Am J Physiol 1944;141:289–296.

158. Silverstein MC, Heit JA, Mohr DN, et al. Trends in the incidence of deep vein thrombosis and pulmonary embolism. Arch Intern Med 1998;158:585–593.

159. Simionescu N. Prelesional changes of arterial endothelium in hyperlipoproteinemic atherogenesis. In: Simionescu N, Simionescu M, eds. Endothelial cell biology in health and disease. New York: Plenum Press, 1988, pp. 385–429.

160. Simionescu N, Mora R, Vasile E, et al. Prelesional modifications of the vessel wall in hyperlipidemic atherogenesis. Extracellular accumulation of modified and reassembled lipoproteins. Ann NY Acad Sci 1990;598:1–16.

161. Simpson LO. Intrinsic stiffening of red blood cells as the fundamental cause of diabetic nephropathy and microangiopathy: a new hypothesis. Nephron 1985;39:344–351.

162. Skoglund RW, McRoberts JW, Ragde H. Torsion of the spermatic cord: a review of the literature and an analysis of 70 new cases. J Urol 1970;104:604–607.

163. Snyder AB, Barone JG, DiGiacomo JC, Barone JE. Postoperative pulmonary leukostasis. Crit Care Med 1990; 18:116–117.

164. Spencer H. Pathology of the lung, 4th ed. Oxford: Pergamon Press, 1985.

165. Srivastava TN, Payment MF. Paradoxical embolism—thrombus in transit through a patent foramen ovale. N Engl J Med 1997;337:681.

165a. Stein Y, Stein O. Does therapeutic intervention achieve slowing of progression or bona fide regression of atherosclerotic lesions? Arterioscler Thromb Vasc Biol 2001;21:183–188.

165b. Steinberg D. Atherogenesis in perspective: hypercholesterolemia and inflammation as partners in crime. Nat Med 2002;8:1211–1217.

166. Stephenson J. Raynaud's phenomenon: the cold facts. Harvard Health Letter 1992;17(3):1–4.

167. Strock PE, Majno G. Vascular responses to experimental tourniquet ischemia. Surg Gynecol Obstet 1969;129: 309–318.

168. Stuart J, Johnson CS. Rheology of the sickle cell disorders. Baillieres Clin Haematol 1987;1:747–775.

169. Swanson DA, Wallace S. Surgery of metastatic renal cell carcinoma and use of renal infarction. Semin Surg Oncol 1988; 4:124–128.

170. Taylor C, Lillis C, LeMone P. Fundamentals of nursing: the art and science of nursing care. Philadelphia: JB Lippincott, 1989.

171. Taylor DC, Salvian AJ, Shackleton CR. Crush syndrome complicating pneumatic antishock garment (PASG) use. Injury 1988;19:43–44.

172. Templeman D, Lange R, Harms B. Lower-extremity compartment syndromes associated with use of pneumatic antishock garments. J Trauma 1987;27:79–81.

173. Thomas DP, Gurewich V, Ashford TP. Platelet adherence to thromboemboli in relation to the pathogenesis and treatment of pulmonary embolism. N Engl J Med 1966;274:953–956.

174. Thomas IH. Studies relating to the aetiology of caisson disease of bone. Newcastle-upon-Tyne, UK: University of Newcastle-upon-Tyne, 1983a, thesis.

175. Thomas IH. Caisson disease of bone. The seed and the soil. J R Coll Surg Edinb 1983b;28:347–360.

176. Thompson T, Evans W. Paradoxical embolism. Q J Med 1930;23:134–150.

177. Tilton RG, Faller AM, Hoffmann PL, Kilo C, Williamson JR. Acellular capillaries and increased pericyte degeneration in the diabetic extremity. Front Diabetes 1987;8:186–189.

178. van Buchem MA, te Velde J, Willemze R, Spaander PJ. Leucostasis, an underestimated cause of death in leukaemia. Blut 1988;56:39–44.

179. Vanhoutte PM. The endothelium and control of coronary arterial tone. Hosp Pract 1988;23:67–84.

180. Vanhoutte PM, Shimokawa H. Endothelium-derived relaxing factor and coronary vasospasm. Circulation 1989;80:1–9.

181. Vichinsky EP, Neumayr LD, Earles AN, et al. Causes and outcomes of the acute chest syndrome in sickle cell disease. N Engl J Med 2000;342:1855–1865.

182. Vincent GM, Anderson JL, Marshall HW. Coronary spasm producing coronary thrombosis and myocardial infarction. N Engl J Med 1983;309:220–223.

183. Vogler C, Sotelo-Avila C, Lagunoff D, et al. Aluminum-containing emboli in infants treated with extracorporeal membrane oxygenation. N Engl J Med 1988;319:75–79.

184. Wakamatsu M, Wolf P, Benirschke K. Bilateral torsion of the normal ovary and oviduct in a young girl. J Fam Pract 1989;28:101–102.

185. Walco GA, Cassidy RC, Schechter NL. Pain, hurt, and harm: the ethics of pain control in infants and children. New Engl J Med 1994;331:541–544.

186. Walker JD, Viberti GC. Pathophysiology of microvascular disease: an overview. In: Pickup JC, Williams G (eds). Textbook of diabetes. Oxford: Blackwell Scientific Publications 1992;2, pp. 526–533.

187. Wallis FM, Truter SJ. Histopathology of tomato plants infected with *Pseudomonas solanacearum,* with emphasis on ultrastructure. Physiol Plant Pathol 1978;13:307–317.

188. Warren BA. Atheroembolism. Boca Raton, FL: CRC Press, 1986.

189. Warren BA, Philp RB, Inwood MJ. The ultrastructural morphology of air embolism: platelet adhesion to the interface and endothelial damage. Br J Exp Pathol 1973;54:163–172.

190. Weisse AB. The Nibelungen Sitzfleisch syndrome: a new clinical entity? Hosp Pract April 15, 1998, p. 51.

190a. Wentworth Jr P, Nieva J, Takeuchi C, et al. Evidence for ozone formation in human atherosclerotic arteries. Science 2003;302:1053–1056.

191. Willerson JT. Clinical diagnosis of acute myocardial infarction. Hosp Pract 1989;24:65–77.

192. Williamson JR, Chang K, Rowold E, Kilo C, Lacy PE. Islet transplants in diabetic Lewis rats prevent and reverse diabetes-induced increases in vascular permeability and prevent but do not reverse collagen solubility changes. Diabetologia 1986;29:392–396.

193. Williamson JR, Chang K, Tilton R, Kilo C. Etiopathogenesis of diabetic microangiopathy. An integrated view. Front Diabetes 1987;8:58–66.

194. Willms-Kretschmer K, Majno G. Ischemia of the skin. Electron microscopic study of vascular injury. Am J Pathol 1969; 54:327–353.

195. Witkowski JA, Parish LC. Histopathology of the decubitus ulcer. J Am Acad Dermatol 1982;6:1014–1021.

196. Wolf PA. Transient ischemic attacks locating the source. Hosp Pract 1985;20:35–43.

197. Worthen GS, Schwab III B, Elson EE, Downey GP. Mechanics of simulated neutrophils: cell stiffening induces retention in capillaries. Science 1989;245:183–186.

198. Zamora-Quezada JC, Dinerman H, Stakecker MJ, Kelly JJ. Muscle and skin infarction after free-basing cocaine (crack). Ann Intern Med 1988;108:564–566.

199. Zand T, Majno G, Nunnari JJ, et al. Lipid deposition and intimal stress and strain: a study in rats with aortic stenosis. Am J Pathol 1991;139:101–113.

ISCHEMIA AND SHOCK

Having run through a long list of obstacles to blood flow, we are ready to examine the downstream effect of those obstacles, namely inadequate blood flow or *ischemia*. Inadequate flow may be limited to a small part of an organ; it may also affect the body as a whole, in which case the result is called *shock*. We will begin with local ischemia.

Ischemia vs. Anoxia

Not surprisingly, it was Virchow—the barricade expert—who coined the word *ischemia* by combining the Greek *iskho,* I hold back, with *háima,* blood. He wisely chose the verb "to hold back" rather than "to stop" because the concept of ischemia includes insufficient blood flow as well as total lack of flow. The term **anoxia,** strictly speaking, should be used only to mean *absence of oxygen;* however, it tends to be used rather loosely to mean **hypoxia,** insufficient oxygen.

This being said, which is worse for the cells: ischemia or hypoxia?

Consider that a tissue deprived of oxygen suffers *one* loss; whereas a tissue deprived of blood flow suffers *three:*

- *The supply of oxygen,* which is not stored in significant amounts
- *The supply of substrates* for metabolic and synthetic processes
- *The removal of waste products*

Therefore, we can expect ischemia to be more damaging than hypoxia. Ischemia will always have a component of hypoxia, but there are situations of *pure hypoxia without ischemia.* Three examples: (1) **high-altitude sickness,** the *soroche* of The Andes, is brought about by pure hypoxia (59) (2). In victims of **drowning,** as long as the heart beats, the brain and all other organs are perfused—which explains why such individuals (especially children) can be rescued after they have been submerged for longer than three minutes, the period said to be critical for successful cardio-pulmonary resuscitation (3). The brain damage of **pearl and sponge divers,** who hold their breath for several minutes, is anoxic—but not ischemic.

> In the Polynesian islands the pearl divers' disease has many names including *Nou-nou parau* (pearl shell insanity); it ranges from transient functional impairments to permanent paralysis and dementia (28).

The difference between anoxia and ischemia can be illustrated with cell cultures. We have grown bovine endothelial cells *in vitro* under conditions of complete anoxia for as long as 4 days with no visible adverse effects; the tissues were presumably surviving on anaerobic glycolysis. But if we also removed glucose to obtain a kind of "ischemia *in vitro,*" cells began to die within an hour (37).

Cells that are metabolically more demanding, such as heart cells, do show injury after an hour or two of incubation in nitrogen: mitochondrial and cellular swelling, as well as blebs, still reversible (Figures 24.1, 24.2).

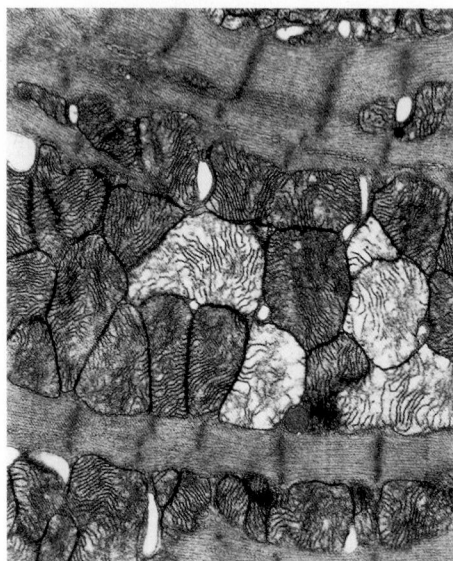
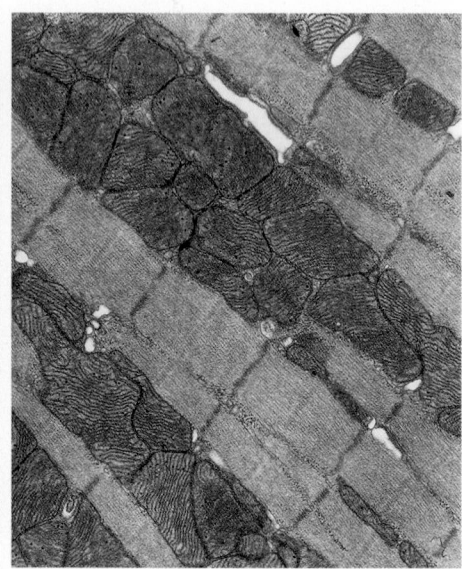

FIGURE 24.1   *Left:* Anoxic rat heart cell after 1 hour incubation in culture medium. Note some mitochondrial swelling, loss of matrix granules, and shortening of the sarcomeres. *Right:* Recovery from 60 minutes of anoxia after 30 minutes of reoxygenation. The mitochondria appear normal and have reacquired their matrix granules. The sarcomeres are more relaxed. (Reproduced with permission from [126], © American Society for Investigative Pathology.)

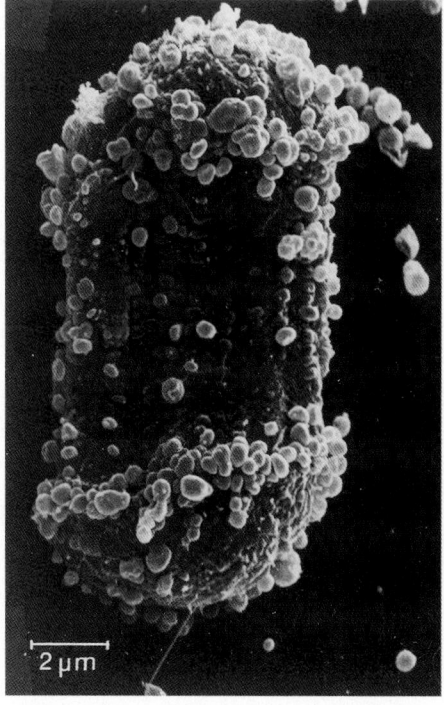
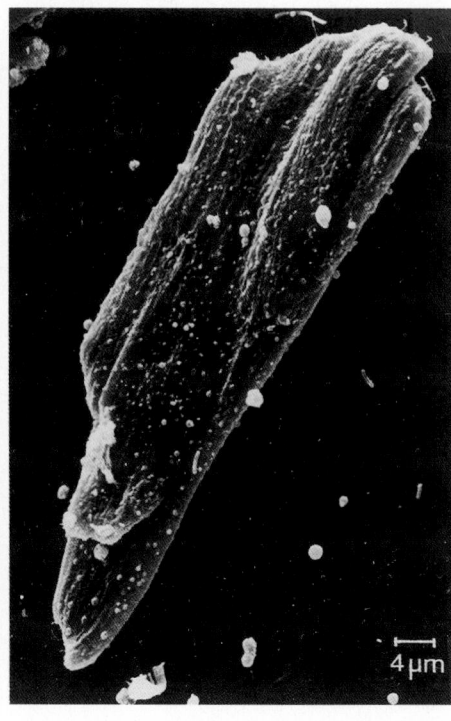

FIGURE 24.2   *Left:* Anoxic rat heart cell after 2 hours of incubation with nitrogen. Note many microscopic blebs and contraction of the cell. *Right:* Recovery from 2 hours of anoxia by 30 minutes of reoxygenation. The blebs have almost disappeared, and the cell has become more elongated. (Reproduced with permission from [126], © American Society for Investigative Pathology.)

Types of Anoxia

Anoxia is a common mechanism of disease (69). If we catalog the obstacles that can interfere with the cell's use of oxygen, we come up with five groups (physiology textbooks have more complex schemes): **anoxic anoxia** means that oxygen is absent in the atmosphere (such is the case of a housefly in pure nitrogen: it can survive 12–24 hours [69]); **hypoxic anoxia** occurs when the supply of oxygen to the pulmonary alveoli is curtailed (as in asthma); **anemic anoxia** means that the oxygen-carrying capacity of the blood is reduced (e.g., in severe anemia); **circulatory anoxia** is due to inadequate supply of [normal] blood to the tissues; and in **toxic anoxia** a toxic agent prevents the cell's metabolism from utilizing oxygen. Whenever the cells are submitted to one or more of these challenges, they can react in two opposite ways: (a) by turning on those genes that can help them survive (99) and (b) by giving up and triggering apoptosis (78).

Cellular Adaptations to Anoxia

Hypoxia sensors are a well know feature of yeasts, but in recent years we have learned that several cell types of mammalian cells share this privilege. The peripheral arm of the system are oxygen sensor molecules distributed in the cytoplasm (33, 148); they record the level of oxygen, and convey it to a family of **hypoxia inducible factors** (**HIF 1, 2, 3,** discovered in 1992 [128, 129]). The HIF then dive into the nucleus and activate the pertinent genes (Figure 24.3).

The HIF proteins are heterodimers; under normal oxygen conditions the alpha moiety is retained in the cytoplasm, ubiquinated and degraded by proteasomes; if hypoxia occurs, ubiquitination stops, and the alpha moiety is allowed to join the beta moiety in the nucleus, where the complete HIF binds to the appropriate DNA sequences (Figure 24.3) (33). The genes that are activated under low-oxygen emergency conditions include, understandably, those for *erythropoietin* (which will increase the synthesis of red blood cells), for *vascular endothelial growth factor (VEGF),* and for *glucose transport* (128, 156).

> NOTE: Under conditions of *hyper*oxia, the nuclear factor NF-κB is activated, resulting in increased transcription of inflammatory genes (TNF, IL-8) (33).

The genetic "reflex" of responding to anoxia by producing VEGF, and thereby stimulating angiogenesis, is probably common to all ischemic tissues (90, 91, 98). But would this increase the blood supply? The research group of J. and W. Schaper points out that angiogenesis is a microvascular phenomenon (VEGF, after all, stands for vascular *endothelial* growth factor). Its effect is to enrich the capillary network and to better distribute the available blood, but the total blood supply is not significantly increased. The task of increasing blood flow is accomplished by previously existing small arteries, which enlarge under the stimulus of increased pressure and shear stress—a phenomenon that the Schapers have called **arteriogenesis** (19, 66, 143). The final result is the development of a *collateral circulation* (see Figure 21.6).

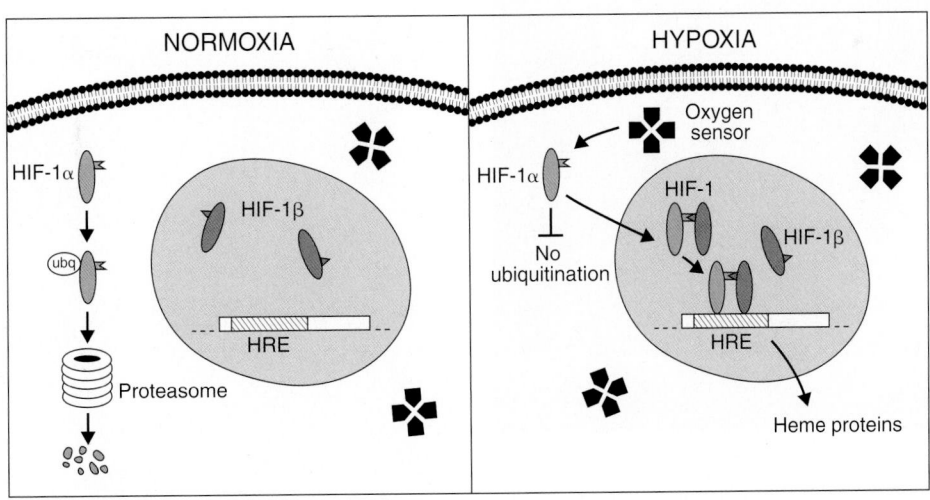

FIGURE 24.3 The activation of genes by hypoxia depends on a hypoxia-inducible factor (HIF), a heterodimer. Under normal conditions of oxygenation its alpha moiety in the cytosol is constantly ubiquinated and destroyed by proteasomes. When the oxygen sensor molecules (not yet well defined) signal hypoxia, ubiquination stops and the alpha moiety is allowed to meet its beta moiety in the nucleus. The dimeric HIF then binds to the Hypoxia Response Elements (HRE) of the appropriate genes. (Reprinted from Molec Genetics Metabol 71, D'Angio CT, Finkelstein JN. Oxygen regulation of gene expression: a study in opposites, pp. 371–380, Copyright 2000, with permission from Elsevier Science.)

Local Ischemia and Infarction

When an artery or a vein is obstructed, some pathologic effect may be expected on the tissues downsteam (for an artery) or upstream (for a vein)—depending on a long list of conditions. In practice, each organ has its own set of vascular peculiarities, but there are also some general rules of ischemia and infarction. (Recall that *a mass of tissue that died of inadequate blood flow is called an infarct.*)

Arterial obstruction. Arteries can be tied off or otherwise occluded if their function can be taken over without delay by branches (anastomoses) connecting them to neighboring vascular fields. Arteries lacking such connections are called **terminal;** if any one is occluded, an infarct will develop downstream without delay. Such are the renal, coronary, cerebral, and retinal arteries (Figure 24.4). We are not aware of any advantage for the organs supplied by terminal arteries.

Venous obstruction. Veins are much more interconnected than arteries and can be tied off with few exceptions. There are, however, veins with a tree-like arrangement such as that of terminal arteries (e.g., the renal vein); if they are tied off, the result will be an infarct—upstream of the occlusion.

Chronic ischemia. If a terminal artery is obstructed gradually (e.g., by a slowly growing atherosclerotic plaque), the neighboring arterial fields may be able to stave off ischemic damage by developing a **collateral circulation,** as described above. This is typical of the heart; in other organs, notably in the kidney, the effect is **atrophy.** The parenchymal cells become atrophic and gradually disappear; the final result, after weeks or months, is a fibrous scar (Figure 24.5).

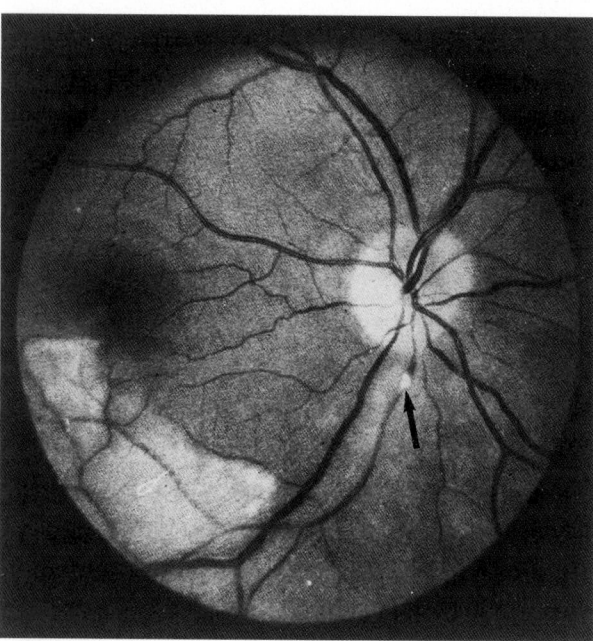

FIGURE 24.4   Retinal vessels are a natural window to the microcirculation. The **arrow** points to a small calcified embolus, originating from a thrombus on the mitral or aortic valve (subacute bacterial endocarditis). The white patch at the bottom left represents the corresponding zone of retinal infarction. (Reproduced from [122], copyright 1992 by Appleton & Lange, with permission from The McGraw-Hill Companies.)

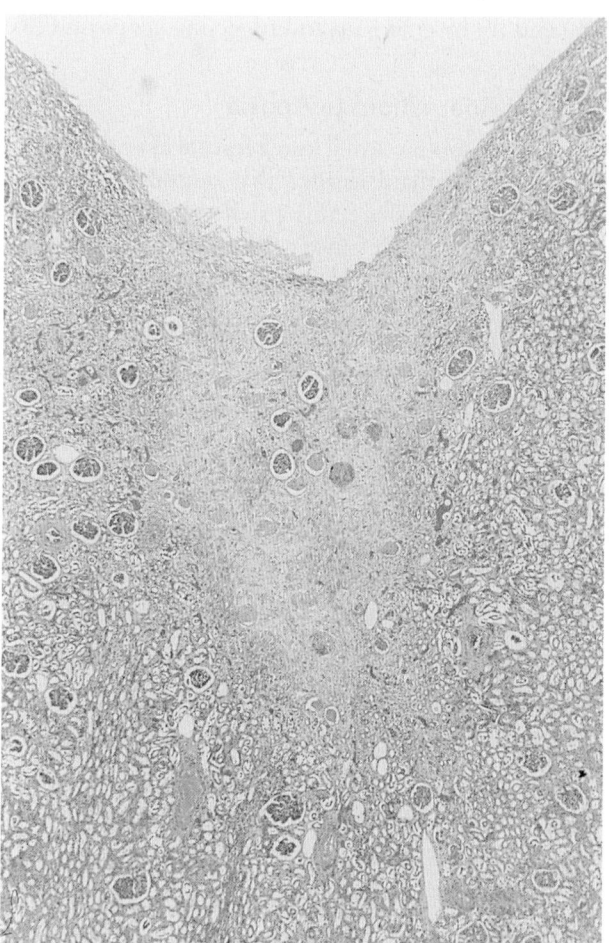

FIGURE 24.5   Small scar in the renal cortex from chronic ischemia due to arteriolosclerosis. *Top:* The surface of the kidney is depressed because renal parenchyma has disappeared and was replaced by connective tissue; some glomeruli have survived. The scar of a small infarct due to embolism would be very similar. (15x)

Chronic ischemia of the kidney has been studied a great deal because it has a unique functional effect: **hypertension.** The experimental method is to constrict the renal artery with an adjustable clamp, a device that made Dr. H. Goldblatt famous (55). After this example, Goldblatt

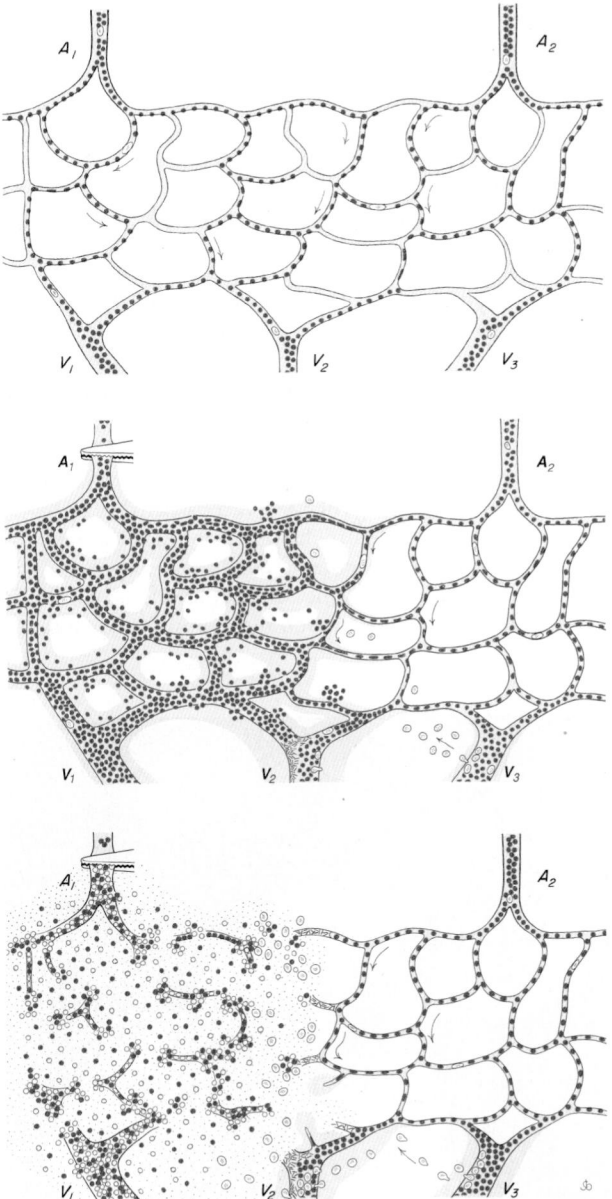

FIGURE 24.6 Microcirculatory changes in and around an infarct. *Top:* Capillary network fed by two terminal arterioles, A_1, A_2. *Center:* A_1 has been clamped; its downstream capillaries become anoxic, leaky, and paralyzed (distended); A_2 can supply some blood to fill them up, but not to maintain flow. Edema and microscopic bleeding occur (minutes/hours). *Bottom:* The two capillary fields break apart; the field of A_2 seals off, its venules supply leukocytes to scavenge the debris of A_1 (days).

clamps were applied to many other arteries, but nobody else became famous—until Dr. J. F. R. Kerr applied a simple ligature to a branch of the portal vein, produced ischemic atrophy of the liver, and discovered apoptosis.

Acute ischemia: pathogenesis of an infarct. Consider the classic case of a renal infarct. An embolus from the left heart settles in a branch of a renal artery; within seconds, the *blood pressure downstream from the embolus drops to near zero* and remains there, because there are no anastmoses to the surrounding arterial branches. The capillary networks, however, are interconnected (see diagram of Figure 24.6), so there will be a trickle of blood into the infarct from the surrounding capillary network—but not enough to keep the tissue alive. Within minutes the infarct fills with blood. To the naked eye, it will be turgid and bright red; this is called **a red infarct,** best seen in the lung (Figures 24.7, 24.8). In the meantime the infarcted tissues die and become a mass of denatured proteins (p. 205); all the cells die, including those of the capillary walls. Within a couple of days the red blood cells trapped in the infarct hemolyze, the hemoglobin diffuses away, and the whiteness of the denatured protein is revealed (Figure 24.8; see also Figure 5.21). The mass of dead tissue releases a vast number of inflammatory mediators; eventually the whole infarct will be surrounded by a barrier of inflammation and in time it will be reabsorbed ("organized", p. 446). The end result will be a scar (Figure 24.9).

Red and white infarcts. From the description above, it follows that *in the beginning infarcts are red*—or at least cyanotic—and then become white as the hemoglobin

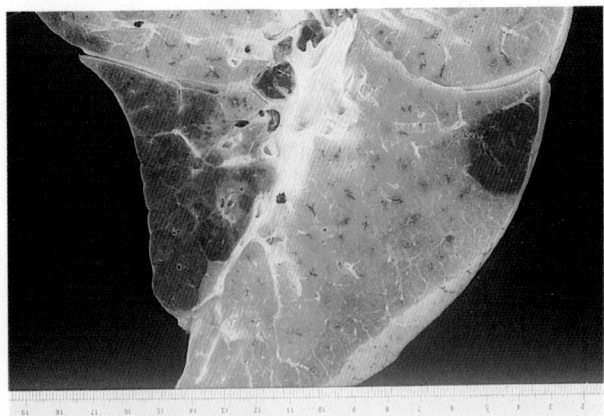

FIGURE 24.7 Slice of a human lung showing two recent infarcts still at the red stage. On a chest X-ray they would have appeared roughly as triangles with the base on the pleura. **Scale** in centimeters.

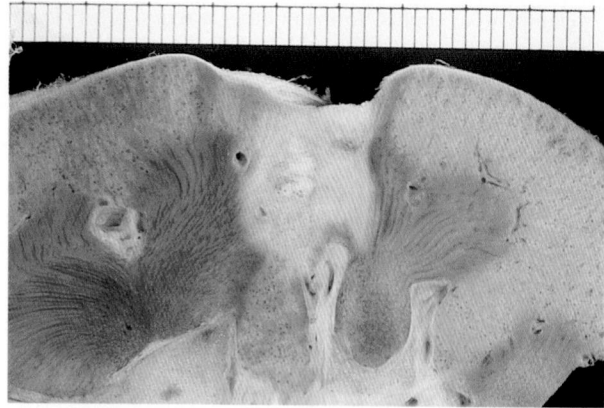

FIGURE 24.8 Cut surface of a kidney; the white area indicates infarction. The depressed surface indicates that removal of necrotic tissue has been taking place for several weeks. Some necrotic tissue is still present. From a patient with a defective prosthetic aortic valve that had been shedding thromboemboli. **Scale** in millimeters.

diffuses away. In the heart, the red (purple) phase is visible experimentally, but the greenish color of the myoglobin tends to mask it. In brain infarcts the red phase is sometimes missing: reason unknown. Some textbooks explain the red and white infarcts as different kinds of infarcts, not as different stages; it is true that the lung with its double circulation produces spectacular red infarcts, but the timing is the main factor.

The name **infarct** is very appropriate: the latin *infarcire* means "to stuff in," here referring to the tissues stuffed with blood.

At autopsy, the gross diagnosis of a recent myocardial infarct is a recurrent problem because visible changes do not appear until many hours or even a day after infarction. The diagnosis can be helped by dipping slices of tissue in triphenyltetrazolium chloride, a dye that stains normal myocardium brick red (TTC test) (79). Infarcts older than 3 hours remain unstained, and so do 50 percent of 30-minute infarcts (146). The principle: a myocardial dehydrogenase becomes nonfunctional in the infarcted area (Figure 24.10). (The TTC test is a gift from botany: it was devised in 1942 to distinguish live and dead parts of seeds [62, 89].)

Infarcts without obstacles to flow. Here are two classic examples.

- *A myocardial infarct can occur with patent coronaries.* Suppose that the aortic valve is constricted (*aortic stenosis*): the left ventricle will be obliged to pump against increased resistance and becomes hypertrophic. Meanwhile, the coronary arteries that arise from the aorta just beyond the stenosis receive less

FIGURE 24.9 Cross section of a heart showing the scar (**S**) of a myocardial infarct in the wall of the left ventricle (**LV**). Normally the thickness of the ventricular wall should be the same all around. The scar consists of fibrous tissue that tends to give way over the years and may bulge like an aneurysm. **RV:** right ventricle. (Courtesy of Dr. W. D. Edwards, Mayo Clinic, Rochester, MN.)

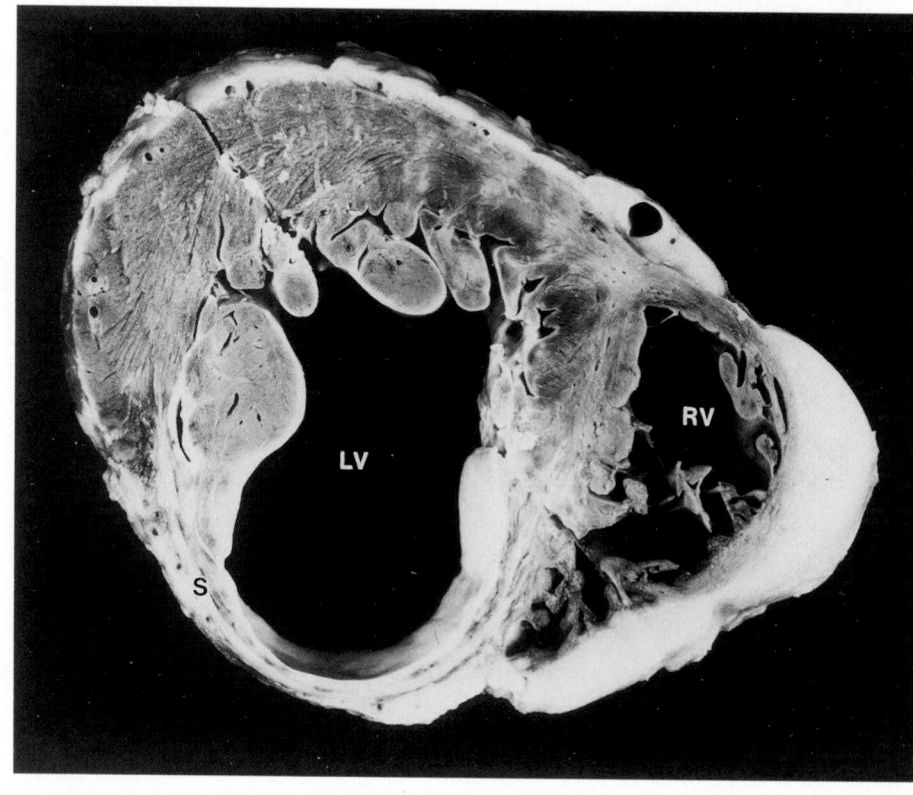

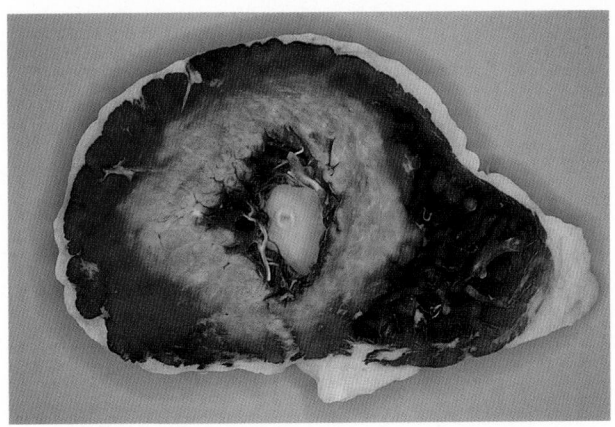

FIGURE 24.10 Slice of a human heart, unfixed and stained by the TTC method (see text; red = normal; lack of stain = recent infarct). *Left ventricle* at left; the tip of the right ventricle is barely visible at right. Lack of stain around the left ventricle shows an extensive, circumferential infarct beneath the endocardium of the left ventricle. *There was no coronary occlusion.* This type of infarct (without coronary occlusion) develops when the heart is insufficiently perfused, as may happen in shock. (Courtesy of Dr. H. F. Cuénoud, University of Massachusetts Medical School, Worcester, MA.)

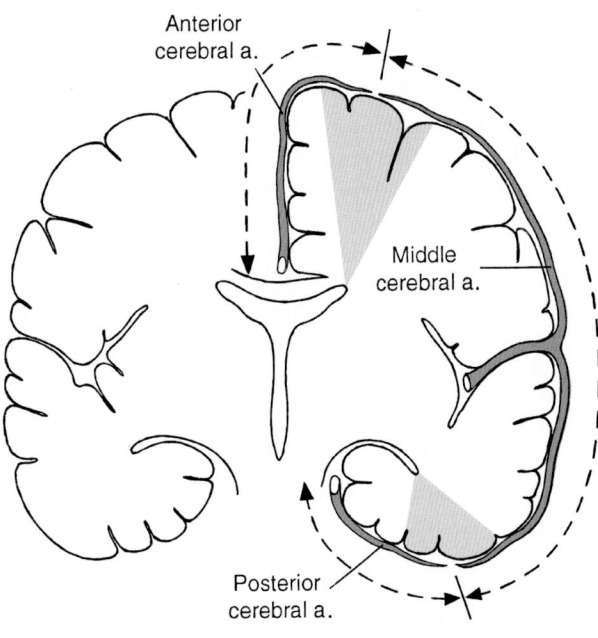

FIGURE 24.11 Parts of the brain most susceptible to ischemia and infarction: the so-called watershed zones (pink) between the territories supplied by the anterior, middle, and posterior cerebral arteries. (Adapted from [2], Copyright 1988, with permission from Elsevier.)

blood. Now, if the left ventricle is placed under a sudden strain and needs more blood than it can receive, it may develop an infarct (22).

- *Watershed lesions* are fairly common in the brain and the colon; as the name suggests, they are areas of ischemia at the junction of territories supplied by two arteries (139). In the brain, watershed lesions are seen in survivors of cardiac arrest (Figure 24.11). The mechanism of this type of infarction is probably as follows: when the heart resumes pumping, two adjacent cerebral arteries do not immediately supply the periphery of their territories. (In the colon, ischemic damage tends to develop at the junction of the transverse and the descending colon, the watershed between the territories of the superior and inferior mesenteric arteries [121].)

Factors that Modulate Ischemic Damage

Many studies in this area aim at improving organ preservation for transplant surgery. The major variables are:

The nature of the cells and tissues. Epithelia, for example, are more delicate than connective tissues; a chronically ischemic kidney will lose most of its nephrons, but the fibroblasts that replace them show no sign of ischemic damage.

Temperature of the tissue. Higher temperatures increase tissue damage. This is why many surgeons choose to

cool the heart during surgery for bypass (101) and why drowning in cold water can be followed by recovery if the submersion lasted 40 minutes, or even longer (34, 46). Children are the best survivors of drowning, probably because they cool faster; but it is a fact that immature brains are more resistant to anoxia (142).

Abnormally viscous blood. Whatever the cause, blood that is too thick can lead to brain damage; a hematocrit above 46 percent increases the risk (16). Conversely, a low leukocyte count (in dogs) reduces the size of myocardial infarcts (116).

Blood glucose. Hypoglycemia causes brain lesions similar to those of anoxia. The effects of hyperglycemia are somewhat controversial. Intuitively, one might think that—for ischemic cells—glycolysis, although inefficient, would be better than nothing in terms of energy production. On the other hand, glycolysis produces lactic acid, and local acidosis is detrimental (75, 109, 134). The damage may be self-limiting because acidosis poisons the glycolytic mechanism (84, 115). Local acidosis also increases the rigidity of red blood cells, making the blood more viscous (111). There are occasional dissenting voices: under certain conditions, acidosis is said to protect against ischemic damage (93, 131).

Myocardium that is depleted of glycogen before ischemia makes a better recovery (109). Clinical studies concluded that the outcome of cerebrovascular accidents was worse in hyperglycemic patients, but experimental results have been contradictory (40).

The hour of the day bears some relationship to myocardial infarction, which is much more frequent at 8–9 AM than at 5 PM. It seems that the blood level of catecholamines is higher and that the platelets are stickier in the early morning (107). Insomniacs may want to read an article on the dangers of going to bed (9).

Ischemia in Organs with Double Blood Supply

The two main examples are the lungs and liver. **The lungs** receive most of their blood under low pressure from the pulmonary arteries and some blood under high pressure from the bronchial arteries. The two networks are connected. For this reason, occlusions in the bronchial arteries do not produce ischemia (the bronchial arteries are not reconnected in the course of lung transplants). Occlusions of the pulmonary arteries by emboli are commonplace. Depending on the size of the occluded artery and on the function of the heart, *occlusion may produce a transient hemorrhage, an infarct, or no effect at all.* Here are the somewhat bewildering facts:

- *Massive bilateral embolism.* If 60 percent or more of the pulmonary flow is cut off, the result is instant death. Many clinicians have experienced the shock of seeing a patient rise from bed only to keel over without uttering a sound. The cause is usually a single massive embolus astride the pulmonary artery bifurcation (*saddle embolus*) (see Figure 23.2). Death being so sudden, there is of course no infarction. (The mechanism of death: occlusion of the pulmonary arteries interrupts the circulation, whereby the heart stops beating.)

- *Sudden obstruction of a single, main pulmonary artery.* The sudden and total occlusion or constriction of the right or left pulmonary artery produces only minimal cardiocirculatory effects (120). There is no infarction. Virchow was the first to face this rather surprising effect (36), and he correctly argued that the lung has two circulations: when the pulmonary flow is cut off, the bronchial arteries take over. This has been abundantly confirmed.

- *Emboli in peripheral branches of the pulmonary arteries.* Emboli in arteries that are less than 3 mm in diameter (140) can produce two kinds of lesions: intraalveolar hemorrhage without necrosis (Figure 24.12) or hemorrhagic infarct.

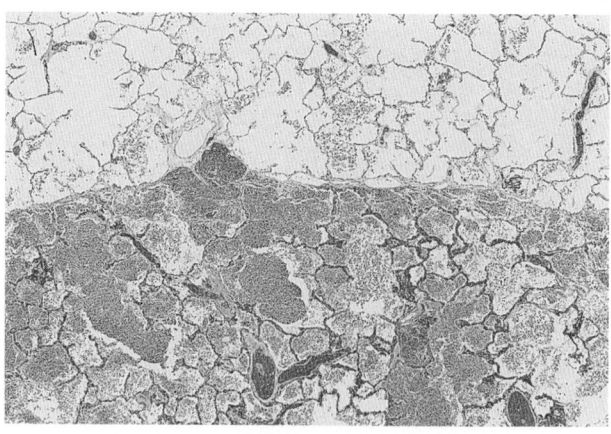

FIGURE 24.12   *Below:* Lung tissue just after embolism. Diffuse congestion and hemorrhage into the alveolar spaces may or may not proceed to necrosis. The sharp limit between hemorrhagic and normal lung (*above*) corresponds to an interlobular septum. (25x)

So we are faced with a paradox: emboli in the smaller pulmonary arteries are more dangerous to lung tissue than occlusion of the large arteries. We are embarrassed to say that, despite much thinking by the experts (31), there is no proven explanation.

Here is a possibility: if the arteries of the pulmonary and bronchial circulation anastomose about half-way between the hilus and the pleura, emboli in the proximal (larger) pulmonary arteries can be made harmless by the bronchial circulation; emboli in the smaller arteries cannot.

We also need to understand the nature of the pulmonary hemorrhage and how it relates to a hemorrhagic infarct. Schematically, we see the problem as follows (61):

- *Pathogenesis of the hemorrhage.* A branch of the pulmonary artery is occluded; the tissue downstream begins to suffer, but the bronchial circulation succeeds, just barely, in keeping it alive. Some ischemic capillaries break down, hence the hemorrhage, but eventually the bronchial circulation improves (arterial dilatation?) and the tissue survives. Macrophages clean up the spilled blood.

- *Pathogenesis of a hemorrhagic infarct.* A branch of the pulmonary artery is occluded, and the tissue downstream dies because the bronchial circulation is unable to rescue it; bronchial artery blood just trickles into the dead tissue, so the infarct is hemorrhagic.

In other words, the hemorrhage represents an early and reversible stage of infarction; it is an *incomplete infarct* (61). These purely hemorrhagic and reversible lesions really exist (see Figure 24.12); the best proof is supplied by serial chest X-rays after a pulmonary embolism, which show an infiltrate in the lung that fades away within a week or less. This cannot represent an infarct (31) because only 50 percent of infarcts clear within 3 months (102).

A pulmonary infarct and a hemorrhage are clinically indistinguishable except by following their progression on chest films: a shadow that disappears in 2–4 days must be a hemorrhage (61). Many lung infarcts are silent; the classic symptoms are chest pain, dyspnea, hemoptysis, and systemic hypotension (117). The pain is probably due to an acute inflammatory response in the parietal pleura. Remember that *deep lesions (within the lung itself) are painless:* people walk around without feeling their pneumonia.

Why do some emboli in normal lungs produce hemorrhage and others an infarct, even though they lodge in arteries of similar caliber?

We can offer two answers; the first is based on traditional experience:

- *In the lungs of patients with heart disease, infarcts are much more frequent than hemorrhages.* This can be explained. In a patient with left ventricular failure, an embolus in a branch of a pulmonary artery creates downstream a territory of congested vessels, perhaps even some hemorrhage; if the heart were functioning normally, the bronchial circulation would intervene to relieve this congestion, but since the left heart is failing, the bronchial circulation is also failing and cannot rescue the embolized territory, which becomes an infarct (31).
- The different effect of emboli that lodge in arteries of the same size may depend on the completeness of occlusion. In an angiographic study, the degree of occlusion varied between 13 and 68 percent (mean 37 percent) (111). Infarcts are reportedly more common than hemorrhage in cases of shock, pulmonary edema, pneumonia, and malignancy (140).

A teaser: what happens when an embolus lands in a grafted lung? In lung transplants the bronchial circulation

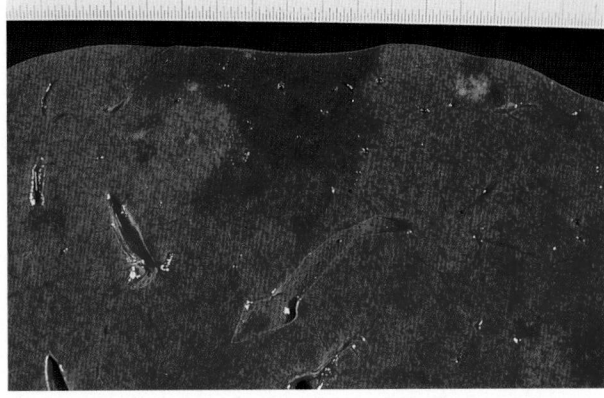

FIGURE 24.13   Typical Zahn infarct of the liver in a patient with generalized carcinoma. Such infarcts (limited to the liver) are caused by thrombosis in a branch of the portal vein; in this case the thrombosis was probably related to the carcinoma. *Top right:* A small whitish metastasis. **Scale** in centimeters.

is not reconnected; therefore all emboli should produce infarcts. So far nobody has reported a higher incidence of infarcts in grafted lungs, and there may be a good reason: in dogs with grafted lungs, the neglected bronchial artery seems to reconnect itself on its own (104).

The liver receives arterial blood from the hepatic artery and venous blood from the portal vein; blood from the two sources is mixed at the microcirculatory level. Because some oxygen and all necessary nutrients can be supplied by the portal vein, infarcts by arterial occlusion are rare; but they do occur. If a small branch of the portal vein is occluded, necrosis does not develop; liver tissue simply becomes atrophic. Smaller cells and wider sinusoids produce a red, depressed area called a *Zahn infarct* (11, 155). The venous obstruction is usually a thrombus of the kind that may develop in the presence of generalized cancer or other debilitating condition (Figure 24.13). Clinically it is not significant.

Examples of Infarction

The natural history of an infarct varies depending on the organ involved. It makes a great difference whether the organ beats, thinks, or conveys feces.

Myocardial Infarcts

Myocardial infarcts are special for many reasons, besides the fact that they kill many humans, and correspondingly more is known about them. Here is a partial list.

Infarction occurs in a contractile tissue. Therefore, one of the earliest effects of acute myocardial ischemia is local paralysis. This phenomenon can be witnessed as it occurs in the exposed heart of a dog or pig: the ischemic area becomes purplish within 5–15 seconds, then ceases to beat and bulges passively at every systole (115). Within 40 minutes most of the myocardial cells are irreversibly injured (115). (Release of enzymes by myocardial infarcts was discussed on p. 225.)

Because the heart beats, the paralyzed myocardial fibers become stretched and wavy. Stretched and wavy fibers ("**wavy fibers**" for short) therefore become a sign of infarction before necrosis sets in (13). The traditional way to diagnose a myocardial infarct histologically was to look for signs of necrosis, which means that the infarct could not be detected before it was at least 8 hours old. The wavy fibers develop much earlier, possibly within 30 minutes of the onset of ischemia (Figure 24.14) (14).

We observed the wavy fibers in Geneva as a result of a challenge by the World Health Organization. The WHO was planning to establish worldwide statistics of death by myocardial infarction and needed a histological marker more sensitive than outright necrosis. We simply looked at many sections of clinically recent myocardial infarcts, and noticed that many of these hearts contained foci of thin and wavy fibers. The mechanism: as ischemia sets in, the ischemic fibers stop contracting; but they are connected to the living fibers outside of the infarct, which continue to beat. Therefore, the paralyzed fibers are rhythmically tugged; in the process they become long, thin, and wavy, while still retaining their nuclei. Preliminary work on dogs showed that wavy fibers are present at 3 hours (29). The wavy fibers seem to have escaped recognition because they look "more beautiful" than normal straight ones. Yet a moment's reflection is enough to realize that a wavy fiber could not possibly beat to produce contraction. By shortening, it would just straighten.

Contraction bands are another hallmark of ischemic damage in contractile cells; they are transverse bands of hypercontracted sarcomeres (Figure 24.15). By electron microscopy, groups of sarcomeres appear to be packed together almost as if telescoped (Figure 24.16). The pathogenesis is not clear (3, 50), but it requires ATP (141) and it is related to calcium overload. A similar change occurs in ischemic striated muscle.

The infarct may contact flowing blood. This happens when infarction reaches the inner surface of the heart. Dying cells release thromboplastin, with the result that a thrombus may cover the infarcted area. Imagine the fate of a thrombus on the wall of a beating left ventricle: fragments may become detached and produce emboli in the systemic arteries.

The infarct may burst under pressure, leading to **cardiac tamponade** (French term meaning that blood spilling into the pericardium acts as a "tampon" or "stopper" on the heart). This happens because the infarcted tissue becomes soft; in fact an old name for a myocardial infarct was *myomalacia,* muscle softening (157). This tenderizing of dead myocardial cells is helped by the enzymes of leukocytes, which rush to the scene. There is no apparent usefulness to the acute phase of this inflammatory

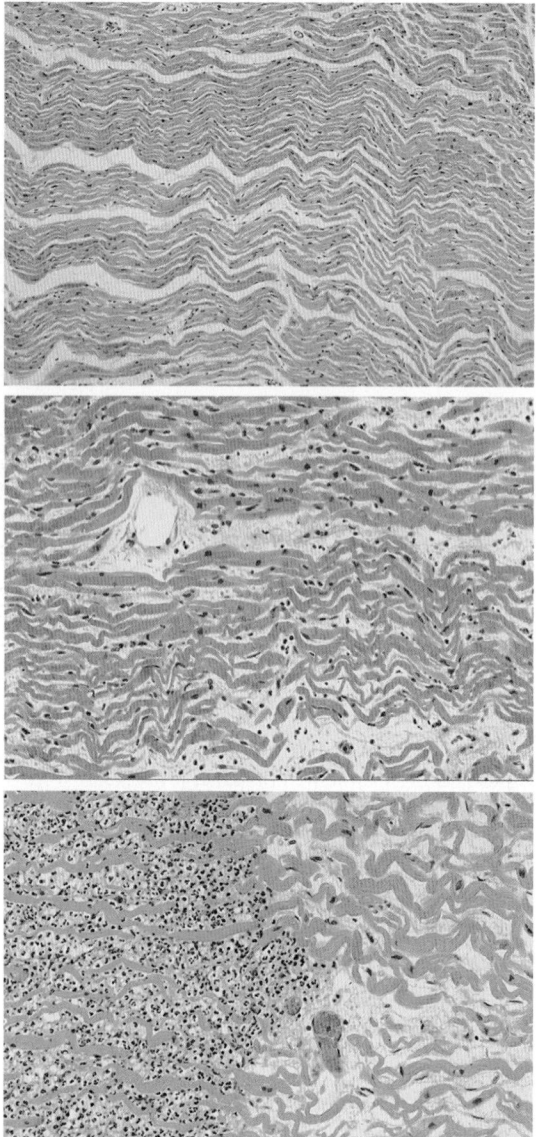

FIGURE 24.14   Myocardial wavy fibers. *Top:* Edge of an infarct. Imagine the myocardial tissue at far left pulsating and tugging at the paralyzed fibers to the right, which are becoming thin and wavy. Nuclei still well-defined. *Center:* Recent infarct. The fibers are not only wavy but also stretched very thin. Nuclei still present. *Bottom:* Patch of dead wavy fibers, most without nuclei, invaded by leukocytes (coming from the left). (*Bottom:* Courtesy of Dr. H. F. Cuénoud, University of Massachusetts Medical School, Worcester, MA.)

response (p. 433); it finds no bacteria to destroy. One could argue that it does more harm than good.

In dogs, some antiinflammatory agents (inhibitors of prostaglandin metabolism) do reduce the size of myocardial infarcts; they also inhibit the local release of the leukotriene LTB_4, a powerful leukotactic agent (123).

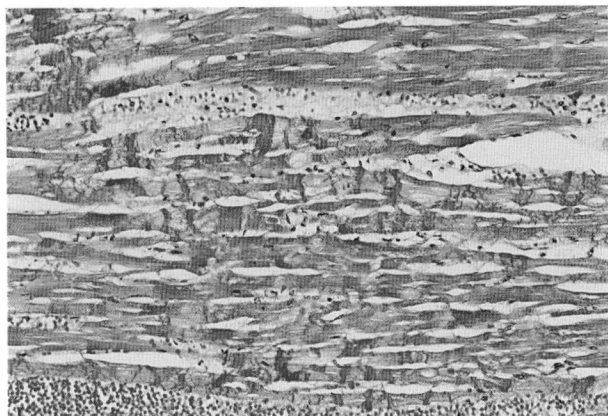

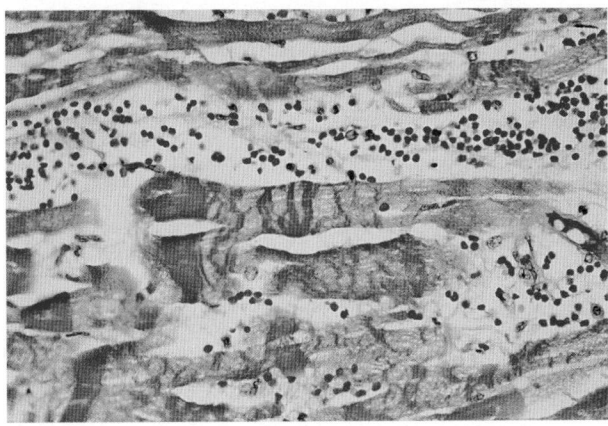

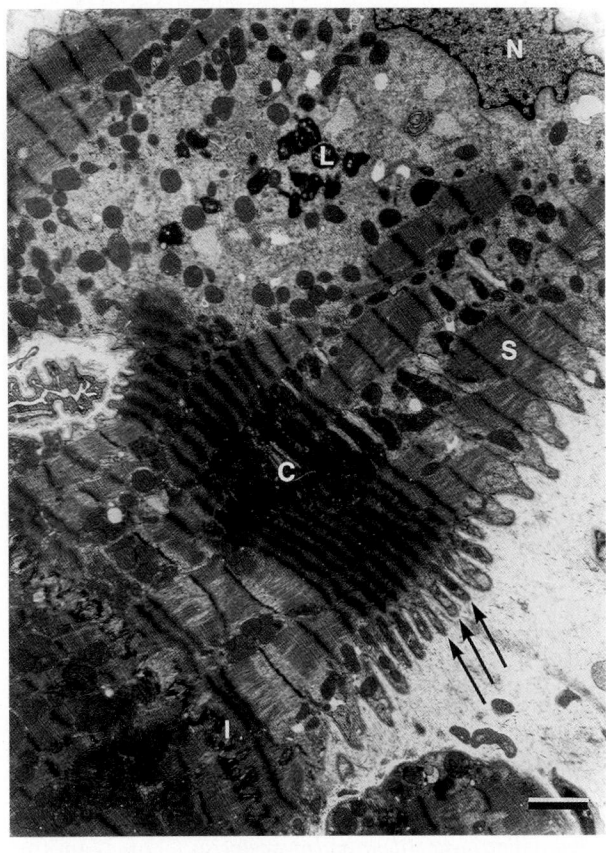

FIGURE 24.15   *Top:* Myocardial contraction bands (dark red bands across myocardial fibers): a hallmark of ischemia, produced only in living tissue. Specimen taken near an infarct, which explains the inflammatory cells and the spilled red blood cells (120x). *Bottom:* Contraction bands seen at a higher power. (230x)

FIGURE 24.16   Contraction bands are typical of ischemia; this one (**C**) was found in a biopsy of human heart (electron micrograph). The sarcomeres (**S**) on either side are relatively normal; in the contraction band they appear to be telescoped. Note the corresponding tight folds in the sarcolemma (**arrows**). **L:** lipofuscin, **I:** intercalated disk, **N:** nucleus. **Bar** = 2 μm.

Infarcts become hemorrhagic if reperfused. Usually the red phase of a myocardial infarct is mild and brief; but if the infarct is reperfused 45 minutes or more after coronary occlusion, the infarct becomes hemorrhagic (51). The mechanism: reperfusion came too late, and the reflow of blood simply spills into dead tissue (Figure 24.17). Whether this makes things worse—as regards local healing—is not certain (94).

Reperfusion of a recent myocardial infarct can be attempted by two means: coronary bypass surgery and thrombolysis (68, 144). Thrombolysis is achieved by injecting tissue plasminogen activator (tPA) or streptokinase intravenously within 3–6 hours (71, 149). To the nonexpert it may seem futile to attempt reperfusion after several hours when it is known that myocardial cells are dead after 40 minutes. The experts have two answers: there may be a salvageable border zone around the infarct (this is controversial) (10); and experiments on dogs show that infarction starts beneath the endocardium and proceeds like a wavefront toward the endocardium (73), a process that takes 3–6 hours (Figure 24.18). Therefore, the window of opportunity for thrombolysis lasts longer than 40 minutes. Ultimately, the rationale for thrombolysis stands on the bare fact that—statistically—it can help (15, 58, 77).

Normally, capillary perfusion is most difficult beneath the endocardium. In the left ventricle of the dog during systole, the interstitial pressure averages 121 ± 10 mm Hg compared with 93 ± 7 beneath the epicardium (6). It follows that an acute reduction in coronary flow will affect first the subendocardial capillaries. This explains why the subendocardial zone in humans is so susceptible to infarction (see Figure 24.10).

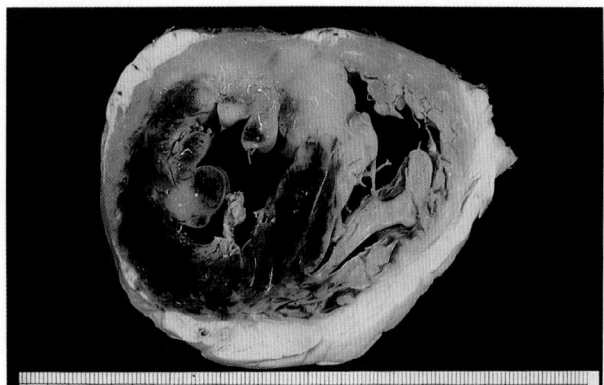

FIGURE 24.17   Cross section of a heart, showing an extensive hemorrhagic infarction of the left ventricular wall (*left*). The hemorrhagic filling (dark brown) of the necrotic tissue is due to the special circumstances of this infarction, as explained by the clinical history. Ten hours after surgery for triple bypass, the blood pressure of the patient dropped. When resuscitation efforts failed, the chest was reopened. One of the grafts was found to be occluded, and a new anastomosis was performed. The patient died 20 hours after the second operation. The hemorrhagic aspect of the infarct is clearly due to reperfusion of nonviable myocardium. (Heart fixed in formalin.) **Scale** in centimeters.

Hibernating myocardium and myocytolysis. This is another aspect of myocardial ischemia, namely *prolonged ischemia followed by slow recovery* (23). Cardiologists are familiar with the fact that a portion of the left ventricle may not be contracting properly, even for months or years (47, 83). Then this zone may happen to receive more blood as a result of bypass surgery; it emerges from hibernation and gradually resumes normal beating (150). On their part, pathologists are familiar with bunches of myocardial fibers that look empty, as if their fibrils had melted away (hence the name *myocytolysis*) (Figure 24.19). These fibers are neither dead nor shrunken. They are assumed to be suffering from chronic ischemia, and could not possibly be capable of beating without a period of "better feeding." The *myocytolytic* fibers are interpreted as the histologic equivalent of hibernating, chronically ischemic myocardium (133, 150) and therefore a special kind of atrophy.

> Normally, capillary perfusion is most difficult beneath the endocardium. In the left ventricle of the dog during systole, the interstitial pressure averages 121 ± 10 mm Hg compared with 93 ± 7 beneath the epicardium (8). It follows that an acute reduction in coronary flow will affect first the subendocardial capillaries. This explains why the subendocardial zone in humans is so susceptible to infarction (see Figure 24.10).

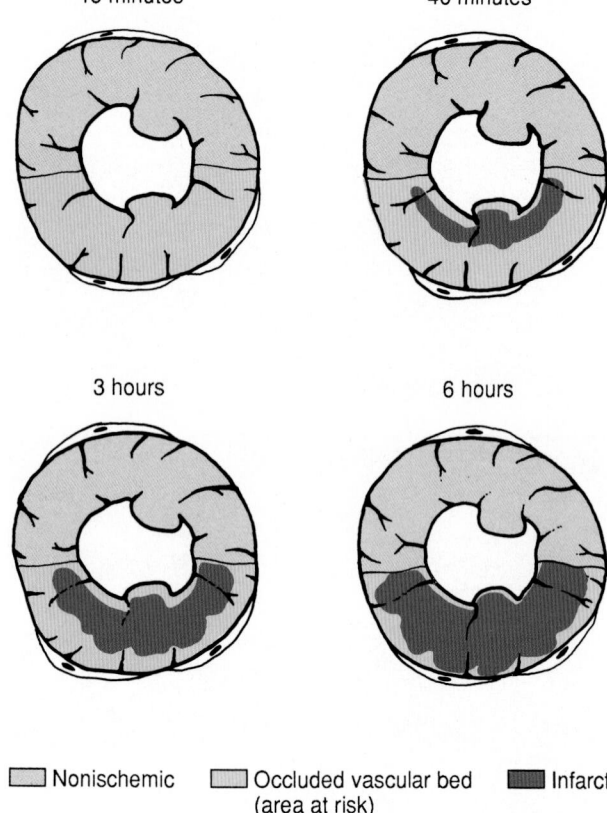

15 minutes	40 minutes
3 hours	6 hours

☐ Nonischemic   ☐ Occluded vascular bed   ■ Infarct
(area at risk)

FIGURE 24.18   **Wave front phenomenon** in myocardial infarction. After occlusion of the left circumflex coronary artery, cell death always occurs first in the subendocardium, later extends to involve the middle and outer portions of the myocardium. The full extent of myocardial infarction is achieved by 6 hours. Because of this phenomenon, it makes sense to attempt to reperfuse a myocardial infarct even after 40 minutes, the time it takes for a myocardial cell to die of ischemia. (Adapted with permission from [73]. Illustration by R. Margulies.)

Stunned myocardium. In everyday life, "stunning" lasts less than hibernation, and indeed stunning represents yet another but short-term effect of myocardial ischemia. Experimentally, if a coronary artery of a dog is occluded for less than 20 minutes, *and then reperfused,* no necrosis follows, but the corresponding myocardium remains depressed or "stunned" for hours or days, and finally recovers on its own. A similar disturbance can follow thrombolytic therapy (80). The mechanism is probably related to calcium overload and free radical generation (12, 83).

> *The calcium paradox and the "stone heart."* Experimentally, if a heart is first perfused with a calcium-free medium and then reperfused with calcium, the return of the calcium initiates massive, explosive tissue disruption,

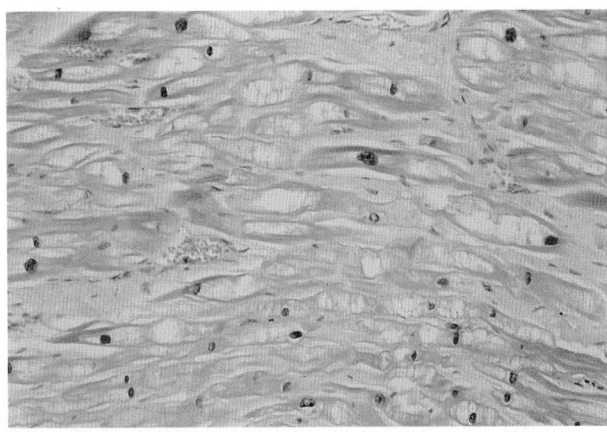

FIGURE 24.19 Myocytolysis, the effect of chronic ischemia on myocardial cells. The cells swell, their organelles are dissolved; eventually only an empty basement membrane remains. Longitudinal section. (120x)

enzyme release, and a firm contracture of the whole heart (81, 114, 158). The mechanism is uncertain, but it seems likely that the first perfusion with calcium-free medium causes mild membrane damage; then when calcium returns, it penetrates the fibers and sets off the response: contraction bands develop (141). This **calcium paradox** recalls the oxygen paradox set off by returning oxygen to ischemic tissue (63). There is, alas, a clinical equivalent to the calcium paradox: sometimes a patient undergoing a cardiopulmonary bypass dies on the operating table with the heart irreversibly contracted in systole. This has been called the "stone heart" (27).

Therapy for myocardial infarction has taxed the imagination of many researchers (21). Attempts to counteract different steps in the pathogenesis have included antiinflammatory drugs (48), calcium channel blockers (not useful), aspirin and anticoagulants (useful) (7), hyaluronidase (rationale unclear), and even retrograde perfusion through the veins (60). Other remedies for ischemic cell death have been discussed earlier (p. 209).

Infarction of Other Tissues

Infarcts can occur in any organ, including the very small hypophysis. The following selection illustrates the many possible consequences of infarction.

Nervous tissue. Infarcts of the brain differ from infarcts of other tissues in their tendency to liquefy (pp. 208, 229). They can be seen by nuclear magnetic resonance imaging even before that stage (Figure 24.20). The extent of brain destruction can be impressive (Figure 24.21), yet brain infarcts, dreadful as they may be, are painless.

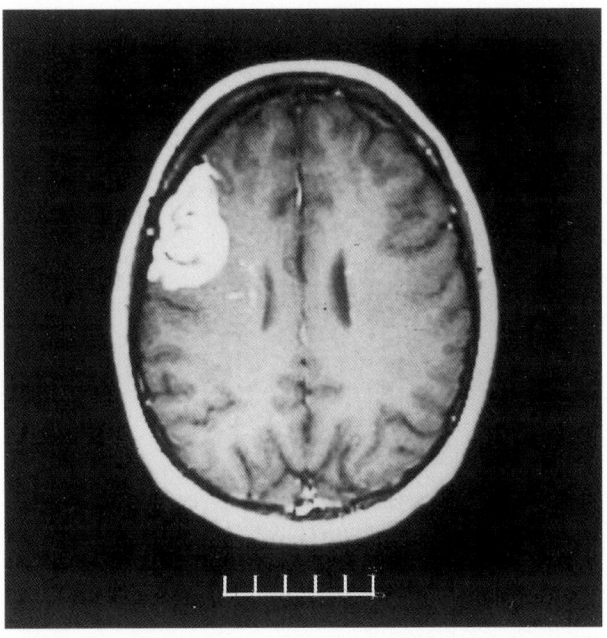

FIGURE 24.20 Cerebral infarct 2 days old (white area *at left*). Viewed by nuclear magnetic resonance (NMR) in a young woman suffering from systemic lupus. **Scale** in centimeters. (Courtesy of Dr. G. Gerard, Winthrop University Hospital, Mineola, New York.)

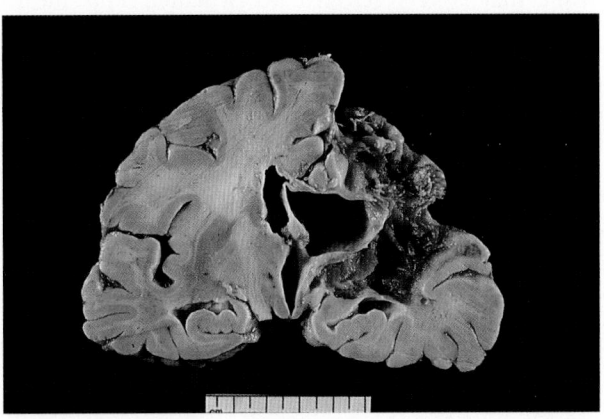

FIGURE 24.21 Extensive infarction of the right hemisphere due to occlusion of the middle cerebral artery. The destruction and reabsorption of cerebral tissue occurred over months and years. **Scale** in centimeters. (Courtesy of Dr. T. W. Smith, University of Massachusetts Medical School, Worcester, MA.)

Some cerebral infarcts are hemorrhagic (Figure 24.22). Experimental work suggests that this happens when a phase of ischemia (~6 hr) is followed by reperfusion (127). In human infarcts reperfusion could be due to a sudden rise of blood pressure or to lysis or contraction of a thromboembolus. In other words, the

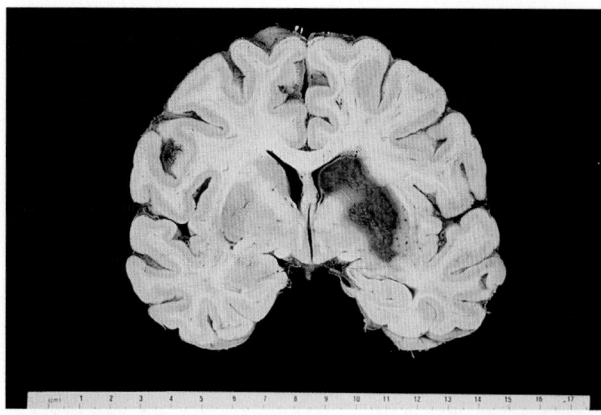

FIGURE 24.22 Hemorrhagic infarct in the right hemisphere, due to obstruction of small branches arising from the middle cerebral artery. **Scale** in centimeters. (Courtesy of Dr. T. W. Smith, University of Massachusetts Medical School, Worcester, MA.)

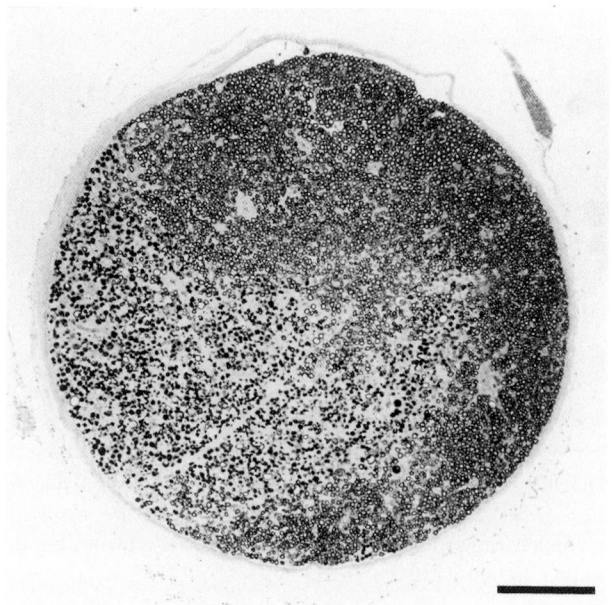

FIGURE 24.23 Cross section of a rat sciatic nerve, showing the effect of infarction 7 days after experimental embolization. Microspheres were injected into the arteries supplying the nerve. Note loss of myelinated fibers. Stain was phenylenediamine. **Bar** = 200 μm. (Reproduced with permission from [110], © American Society for Investigative Pathology.)

mechanism of damage in hemorrhagic infarction in the brain is the same as in myocardial red infarcts after iatrogenic reperfusion.

Ischemia of the nervous tissue is special for two reasons: (a) *ischemia is currently recognized as an important complication of trauma, especially to the spinal cord,* a tissue that is very sensitive to ischemia. This means that the treatment of such injuries must also address an ischemic component. (b) *The pathogenesis of ischemic damage to nervous tissue involves excitotoxins,* neurotransmitters with excitatory properties (p. 228) (108).

For brain cells the order of decreasing vulnerability to ischemia is as follows (86):

1. Neurons (with local variations)
2. Oligodendroglia
3. Astroglia
4. Microglia (i.e., macrophages)
5. Connective tissue structures

We mentioned earlier that the incidence of cerebral infarction was reported to be greater if the hematocrit is higher than 46 percent (normal values are 45–52 percent in males, 37–48 percent in females) (138a). Of the 500,000 strokes per year in the United States, 75 percent are infarcts; the others are due to hemorrhage, that is, rupture of atherosclerotic arteries (1).

Nerve ischemia is thought to be the mechanism of diabetic neuropathy, a result of microcirculatory derangements including increased blood viscosity (Figure 24.23) (20, 42).

Intestine. Infarcts of the intestine can be the result of arterial occlusion (emboli, atherosclerosis) or venous occlusion (by thrombosis, volvulus, or strangulated hernia). They are especially dangerous because the whole thickness of the wall is affected: peristalsis stops; bacterial growth in the lumen goes unchecked, producing gas, which dilates the intestine and dangerously stretches its inert wall; eventually bacteria cross the wall, even before it breaks down, causing peritonitis.

Kidneys and spleen. Embolization of these organs causes red infarcts that soon become white (see Figures 5.21 and 24.8). These infarcts may cause pain, but many are clinically silent and have little significance. Computed tomography can visualize 75 percent of splenic infarcts (44, 72).

Lung. The lung is a special case because it has a double circulation (see p. 704).

Bones. Bones suffer infarcts in *caisson* disease (p. 671). In sickle cell anemia, targets of infarction (by impacted red blood cells) are the vertebrae and the head of the femur, which may slowly cave in under pressure and become deformed.

Whole limbs. Almost invariably, the *lower* limbs are involved. The most common cause is atherosclerosis (often complicated by diabetes), and the precipitating factor is a thrombus over an atherosclerotic plaque.

When a limb is affected in this manner, the dead tissue is exposed to the outer world; the possible consequences (p. 221) are two: (a) The tissue may dry out and turn into *dry gangrene,* a relatively benign development because bacteria do not grow in dried tissue; this allowed the Hippocratic physicians—who did not amputate—to watch a blackened limb fall off bit by bit over 2–3 months (95). (b) If the limb becomes infected, it turns greenish and foul-smelling; this is the sinister *wet gangrene.*

Ischemia and Reperfusion

Until the 1980s, the topic of reperfusion after ischemia was largely a matter of academic interest. Today it is common knowledge that reperfusion can cause much damage, and the field is growing fast, driven largely by the hope of improving several aspects of therapy: (a) *organ transplantation,* an ever-expanding enterprise, has created a variety of "ischemia-reperfusion" situations that need to be better understood; the harvested organs are maintained under conditions comparable to ischemia, and the problems that arise after tranplantation are not exclusively immunologic. (b) *Septic shock:* medical and surgical progress allow more and more patients to survive conditions that used to be lethal; many of these patients now face the prospect of septic shock, which involves, as we will see, all the basic elements of ischemia and reperfusion. (c) *The hope of reperfusing infarcts:* stroke and myocardial infarcts are still among the top killers, and the damage they inflict could probably be reduced if there were some way to reperfuse the affected tissues.

The study of ischemia-reperfusion has led to two interrelated sets of observations: (a) the no-reflow phenomenon, namely the fact that reflow is not necessarily complete; and (b) the fact that most of the tissue damage does not occur during ischemia, but during reflow.

The No-Reflow Phenomenon

Reflow after a short period of ischemia (seconds or minutes, depending on the organ) is a simple matter: nothing bad happens beyond functional changes, and accordingly the topic is taught by physiologists. Consider a tourniquet: if the circulation is cut off for a few minutes and then released, there is a phase of active hyperemia, which is attributed to metabolic products acting on the arterioles, especially adenosine (76). This is a fine arrangement: the ATP of ischemic tissues cannot be regenerated; instead, it is degraded to adenosine diphosphate, then to monophosphate, and finally to simple adenosine, which is a vasodilator that tends to correct the ischemia. Note that *prolonged* ischemia, to the contrary, leads to the formation of *vasoconstrictor* eicosanoids (106).

Reflow after prolonged ischemia involves a great deal of pathophysiology. The first rule is that reflow through *dead* tissue is not possible.

The pioneer experiments on reflow were done by Cohnheim in 1872 (25, 26). His procedure was to tie off the tongue of a frog; if the ligature is released after more than 3 days—he writes—"the blood . . . barely forces its way into the commencement of the arteries and a little distance in advance of the point of ligature, and . . . no more blood reaches the small arteries to say nothing of the capillaries and veins" (26). After shorter periods of ischemia (12–60 hours) reflow did occur; but the tongue became swollen, congested, and inflamed. With ischemic rabbit ears the results were the same, but the sequence was much faster.

To demonstrate the lack of reflow through dead tissue, let us repeat the experiments of Sheehan and Davis of Liverpool, performed almost a century after Cohnheim (132). First, clamp the artery and vein of a rabbit kidney for 3 hours; at this point the kidney is dead (the limit for irreversible renal ischemia in the rat is 1 hour for two-thirds of the animals [97]). Now release the clamp; the kidney quickly becomes congested and stuffed with blood. There is a trickle of blood out of the renal vein, but after half an hour or so it stops, and the kidney looks like a typical red infarct. What stops the flow of blood? Sheehan and Davis listed seven possibilities and were pleased with none. In retrospect, the basic mechanism may be fairly straightforward. We would expect our readers to work it out before reading the answer.

The answer: the ischemic endothelium breaks down; when blood flow returns, plasma escapes from the vessels, which remain filled with a sludge of red blood cells that cannot be pushed along. Tissue pressure rises (the kidney is wrapped in a tight capsule); the veins are thereby compressed, while the overfilled capillaries expand and bleed. In the meantime, thromboplastin is released by all the dead cells, and whatever plasma is left in the vessels clots, permanently blocking the path to reflow.

So much for the reperfusion of dead tissue. *The reperfusion of tissues that are ischemic but still alive* can be tested with the same experimental models. We explored this topic in the 1960s by testing reflow in the globally ischemic rabbit brain. To visualize reflow we infused a suspension of carbon black. We could see with our naked eyes that reperfusion was not complete

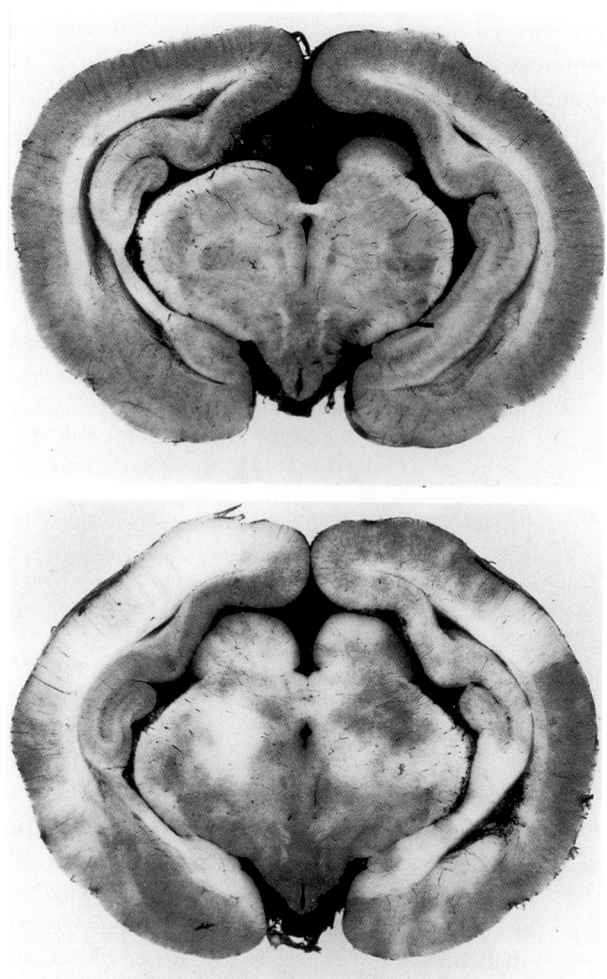

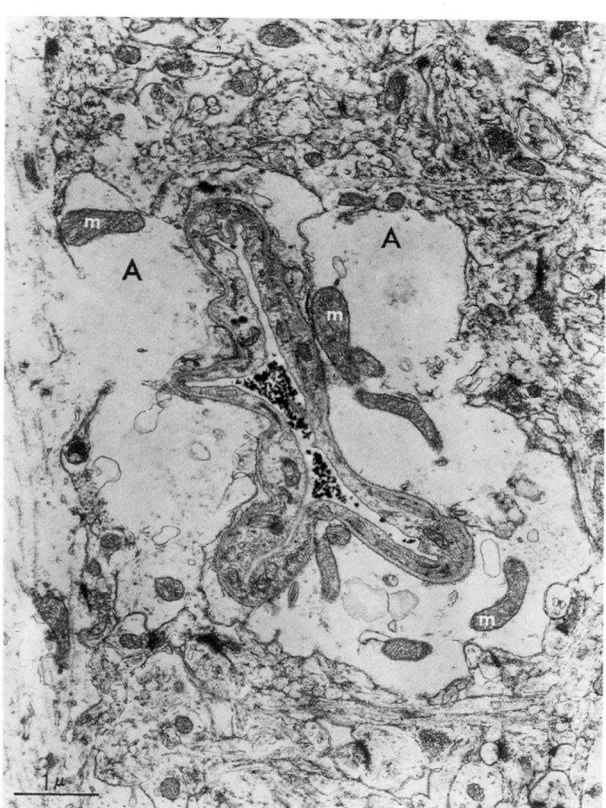

FIGURE 24.25 A mechanism of no-reflow in the brain of a rabbit infused with carbon and killed after 15 minutes of ischemia. The "feet" of astrocytes (**A**) surrounding a capillary are greatly swollen; the lumen, which contains some carbon black particles, is reduced to a slit. **m:** Astrocytic mitochondria. **Bar** = 1 μm. (Reproduced with permission from [24], © American Society for Investigative Pathology.)

FIGURE 24.24 The no-reflow phenomenon illustrated in the rabbit brain. *Top:* Section through a normal rabbit brain after perfusion with carbon black. The white matter stands out clearly because it contains fewer capillaries. *Bottom:* Rabbit brain submitted to 7.5 minutes of ischemia followed by carbon perfusion 30 minutes later. Notice the spotty distribution of non-perfused white areas representing the no-reflow phenomenon. **Scale** in millimeters. (Reproduced with permission from [5], © American Society for Investigative Pathology.)

even after a period of ischemia as short as 5 minutes (Figure 24.24). The hind limb of the rat, made ischemic by a tourniquet, showed patchy reflow after 30 minutes. We called this incomplete reperfusion *the no-reflow phenomenon* (5, 85, 96, 136, 137, 151). Similar results were obtained by others with the kidney (138), the heart (53, 54, 81), the skin (99a), and other organs. We concluded that *some obstacle or obstacles had developed in or around the vessels of the ischemic tissues.* Seventeen known possibilities are shown in Figure 23.42. In our material (rabbit brain) the swelling of the perivascular

glial cells was spectacular. These cells are exquisitely sensitive to anoxia or ischemia (24, 52); they swell selectively and thereby compress the capillaries (Figure 24.25).

A great deal of further work from many laboratories has shown that *the microcirculatory obstacles caused by ischemia vary from tissue to tissue,* and that they develop by three mechanisms: compression from outside, endothelial damage, and capillary plugging by leukocytes. The brain offers the most obvious example of compression (Figure 24.25); no other tissue has a comparable structural arrangement of pericapillary cells prone to swell by anoxia. Endothelial changes are not striking during total ischemia, as mentioned above, but a functional change—not apparent even by electron microscopy—is important: *endothelial activation,* manifested by the appearance of adhesion molecules. This mechanism accounts for much of the **capillary plugging** by leukocytes (57). Even under normal

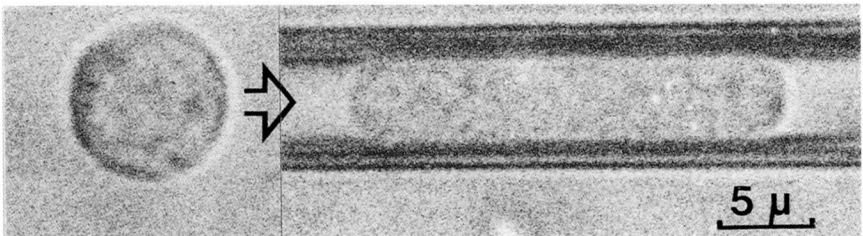

FIGURE 24.26   Deformation of a granulocyte that was sucked into a pipette. Actual photograph. In this case, the estimated increase of the surface area of the leukocyte is 35 percent. The leukocyte at the left, about to be sucked into the pipette, serves as a control for the shape and size of a normal granulocyte. (Reproduced from [161] by permission from S. Karger AG, Basel.)

conditions, a leukocyte passing through a capillary is squeezed into a cylindrical shape (Figures 24.26, 24.27) (57, 125, 135). In an ischemic tissue, both the leukocyte and the endothelium (49) become more sticky. A fascinating corollary: in cats, it has been possible to inhibit the damage of reflow by pretreating the animal with an *antibody* against the leukocyte adhesion complex CD18, the same molecular complex that we encountered in discussing margination and diapedesis (65). Now we can understand why myocardial infarcts in dogs depleted of neutrophils are 43 percent smaller than those in controls (116).

> *Two thoughts about leukocyte plugging.* (1) If leukocytes stick in capillaries even under normal conditions, it makes sense that diapedesis in inflammation should be planned to occur in the venules: the larger diameter of the venules allows blood to flow even if a few leukocytes are stuck to the endothelium. (2) *But why should capillaries hold up the leukocytes?* Red blood cells whip through the microcirculation in 1–2 seconds. Perhaps a delay gives the leukocytes more time to sniff out messages (e.g., cytokines) from the extracellular world, and to react accordingly.

Last, we should mention that a new feature has been added to the pathogenesis of the no-reflow phenomenon: after the ischemic period, when reflow begins, at first the perfusion may be complete, but obstacles may develop progressively thereafter (82).

Damage Caused by Ischemia-Reperfusion

Now we will consider the problem of ischemia from a different point of view. The no-reflow phenomenon emphasizes the *lack* of reperfusion after ischemia; it tells a surgeon that when opening the vascular clamp on a transplanted kidney, not all the kidney parenchyma may receive the blood. Here we are examining those post-ischemic areas that *do* receive blood, and we are faced with the paradox that these are the tissues where damage does develop.

We must briefly philosophize on this point, because it may seem intellectually repulsive that total lack of

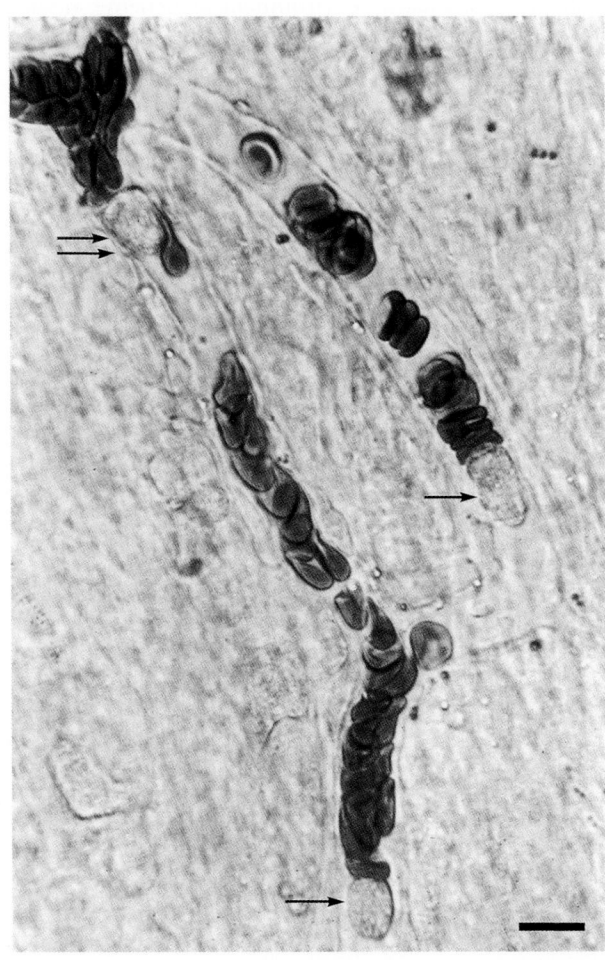

FIGURE 24.27   Three leukocytes (**arrows**) holding up the red cell traffic in skin capillaries of a human volunteer. **Double arrows:** Red cell squeezing past the impacted leukocyte. **Bar =** 10 μm. (Reproduced from [174] by permission from S. Karger AG, Basel.)

flow produces no visible damage. In reality, the damage is there, but latent. In the middle of an infarct the cell membranes are slowly falling apart, but without flow there is little to see—except for some blebbing. Mast cells may be releasing histamine, but without flow there can be no vascular leakage. The tissue is soaked with cytokines and chemotactic mediators, but the leukocytes are too far away to receive the call. The leakage of autolytic enzymes from the lysosomes (in most organs) is slow. Overall, as we mentioned in relation to cell death, this is a fortunate circumstance for the pathologist. When the whole body dies, most of the cells die in a matter of hours, but under the microscope they still look "normal." If their true damage were revealed, the microscopic findings at an autopsy 12 or more hours after death would be drowned in chaos.

In the asphyxiating environment of ischemic tissue, the arrival of flow is like a match in a box of fireworks. Oxygen means life but also free radicals; and free radicals are a major factor in the pathology of reperfusion. Now we must take you to Alabama, where the breakthrough occurred.

Free radicals and reperfusion damage. Dr. D. N. Granger and co-workers were studying ischemic damage to the intestine of the cat (74), using a model of *low flow* (i.e., local reduction of blood pressure to 30–40 mm Hg.) Note the interesting choice of a *low-flow* model rather than a model of total ischemia. In the previous paragraph we have emphasized that visible tissue damage does not occur during total ischemia, but during reflow. *In a model of low flow, ischemia and reflow are occurring at the same time.*

And so, after an hour of low flow, the vessels became leaky. The experimenters tried to protect them by *pretreatment* with antihistamines: no effect. They tried an inhibitor of prostaglandin synthesis: no effect. They tried a free-radical scavenger, superoxide dismutase (SOD): it worked.

The Alabama group then proposed an hypothesis to explain the generation of free radicals in their system; this mechanism is now widely accepted as the principal key to reperfusion damage (Figure 24.28) (18, 45, 100).

The theory is fairly simple. Ischemic cells accumulate an *excess of a substrate and of an enzyme,* which—if they reacted together—would destroy the cells. However, the reaction cannot take place because it requires oxygen which, by definition, is absent in ischemic tissue. When oxygen is supplied by reflow, the time bomb goes off.

> The substrate accumulated by ischemic cells is hypoxanthine. During ischemia, ATP breaks down to ADP, then to AMP, then to adenosine, to inosine, and finally to hypoxanthine (76). The enzyme is xanthine oxidase, generated as follows: the ischemic cell imbibes an excess of calcium, which activates proteolytic enzymes set free by ischemia. These proteases act on the innocuous enzyme xanthine dehydrogenase and convert it to xanthine oxidase.

> When reflow comes, molecular oxygen comes with it. The xanthine oxidase then acts on hypoxanthine and produces uric acid, with superoxide (O_2^-) as a byproduct. Superoxide is not very dangerous, but as we learned earlier, superoxide dismutase acts on superoxide to produce H_2O_2, whereupon superoxide and H_2O_2 react to produce the highly toxic hydroxyl radical (p. 196).

> A vast number of facts fit this theory (56). Reactive oxygen species are produced by the endothelium and by the leukocytes. A key role is played by the endothelium, which is both damaged and activated. Damage leads to reduced NO synthase activity, which in turn can induce most of the changes produced by reflow: in the arterioles, impaired endothelium-dependent dilatation; in the capillaries, leukocyte plugging, fluid loss; in the venules, leukocyte rolling, diapedesis, fluid loss. Hence the possibility of several vicious circles. Further confirmation is provided by experiments with genetically engineered mice (e.g., deficient in adhesion molecules, or overexpressing superoxide dismutase). The severity of endothelial damage correlates with the number of adherent and emigrated leukocytes; the neutrophil protease most damaging to the endothelial barrier function was found to be elastase. One word of caution, however: *the local "mediator soup" and its effects vary from tissue to tissue.* It is still dangerous to generalize; NO, for example, has been reported to be protective in some tissues and deleterious in others (87, 105).

> A few examples of therapeutic attempts against ischemia-reperfusion injury in experimental animals: in the liver, reperfusion damage was reduced by IL-13, which suppresses cytokine synthesis by macrophages (154); in the kidney, protection was obtained by blocking an adhesion molecule, P-selectin (135); in the rabbit ear, protection was given by intravenous antibodies against the adhesion protein CD18 (145); in the myocardium (153), **growth factors** helped; the latter have helped in several organs. Another successful approach is **ischemic preconditioning:** the organ to be made ischemic is prepared by being submitted to several short bouts of ischemia (113).

Ischemia-reperfusion (I/R) after local injury is attracting a great deal of attention; in fact, I/R is being used as a basic form of injury for testing therapeutic agents. This line of research will help understand also the systemic variety of ischemia-reperfusion, namely circulatory shock, which we will now consider.

ISCHEMIA

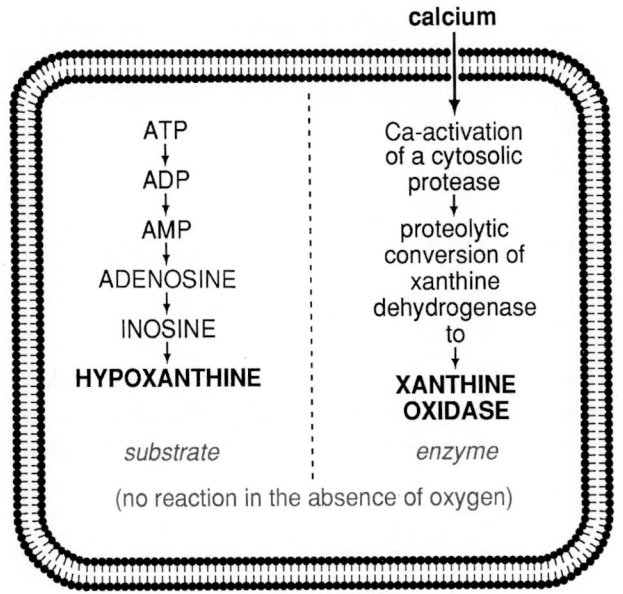

FIGURE 24.28 A mechanism to explain the tissue damage produced by reperfusion after ischemia. *Top:* Ischemia. During the ischemic interval the cells (endothelial and other cells) produce an enzyme and a substrate that cannot react with each other in the absence of oxygen. *Bottom:* Reperfusion. When flow returns, and oxygen is supplied, the enzyme (an oxidase) attacks the substrate and produces injurious free radicals.

REPERFUSION

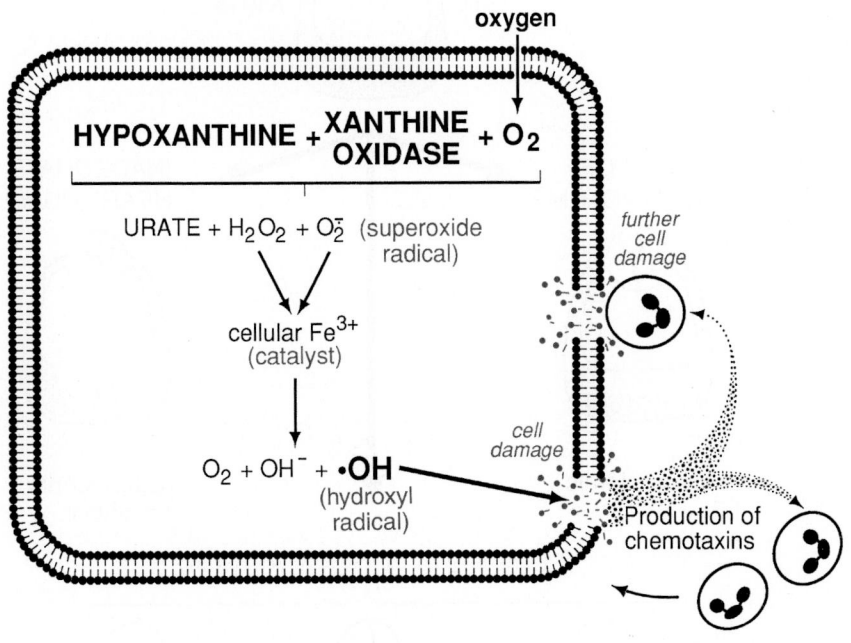

General Ischemia: Shock

Shock is best defined as *a condition of whole body hypoperfusion.* It is not a disease of its own but a complication of some other serious disease. **Anyone suffering from shock is also suffering from some other major problem,** which is responsible for creating the situation of hypoperfusion. This makes shock difficult to diagnose and to treat; *its clinical picture must always be seen through the signs and symptoms of the precipitating disease,* be it trauma, a myocardial infarct, surgery, sepsis, or the like.

Shock is obviously a cardiovascular problem, at least initially; it should not be confused with **coma,** which concerns the nervous system. ***Coma is a sleeplike condition with unresponsiveness to stimuli, however intense.*** No patient could ever say "I am in a coma," whereas many patients in shock are alert. It is true, however, that prolonged shock can lead to coma.

The concept of shock as inadequate perfusion was slow in developing. At first, the word shock was the translation of the French *secousse,* used in 1731 to describe the impact of a bullet as a "jarring of the nervous system." As late as World War I, *hemorrhagic* shock was attributed to a toxin. Finally, in 1940, Minot and Blalock opened the era of shock as "a peripheral circulatory failure resulting from a discrepancy in the size of the vascular bed and the volume of intravascular fluid" (202).

Classification of Shock

Consider the cardiovascular system as consisting of a pump, a fluid, and two tubes connected to a microvascular network (Figure 24.28): insufficient flow through this system can result from three major mechanisms, which may overlap:

THE FLUID LEVEL IS LOW due to loss of blood volume.

THE PUMP IS WEAK due to heart malfunction.

THE CONTAINER IS TOO LARGE by vasodilatation.

This broad picture, represented in Figure 24.29, allows us to understand the three major clinical settings of shock: (a) *Hypovolemic shock* is due to low blood volume

---

FIGURE 24.29 Explaining the decreased perfusion in different types of shock. *Top:* Normal circulatory system, represented as a pump connected by two channels (arteries and veins) to a container (the peripheral circulation). *Three heavy arrows:* Mechanisms that lead to low flow. *Left: The blood volume is too small* (typically by hemorrhage). *Right: The pump is inadequate* (typically because of a myocardial infarct; there is also loss of fluid to the tissues.) *Bottom row: The container has become too large* by peripheral vasodilatation, often complicated by loss of fluid to the tissues.

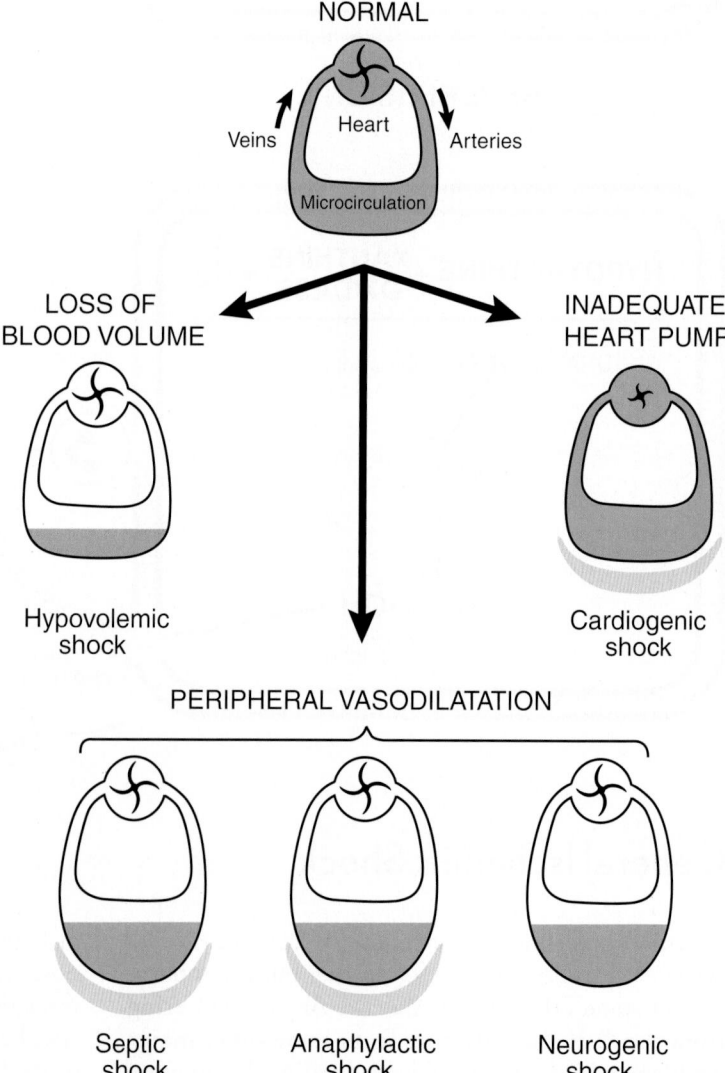

in the system. The underfilling may be the effect of losing whole blood (hemorrhagic shock), plasma alone (e.g., by severe burns), or fluid alone by persistent vomiting or diarrhea. (b) *Cardiogenic shock* (pump failure) occurs when the function of the heart is impaired. The heart itself may have suffered an infarct, or the pulmonary circulation may be severely impaired by an embolus in the pulmonary artery, which acts like a clamp on the entire circulatory system. (as shown in Figure 24.29, cardiogenic shock may include a component of fluid loss). (c) *Shock by generalized vasodilatation,* also called "distributive shock" (221). This situation of "container too large" occurs in three main settings of vasodilatation: *neurogenic shock,* a complication of general anesthesia, involving pure vasodilatation with no loss of fluid; *anaphylactic shock* (e.g., by the sting of a bee), which implies some degree of vascular leakage; and *septic shock,* in which a significant amount of fluid is lost to the extravascular spaces; this means that two major mechanisms are contributing to the state of shock: the container is too large and the content is insufficient.

ANY FORM OF SHOCK CAN PROGRESS TO SEPTIC SHOCK, because all forms of shock include, by definition, hypoperfusion of the intestine: this leads to ischemia and necrosis of the intestinal mucosa, allowing toxins and bacteria to seep into the bloodstream.

In all forms of shock, the organs and tissues suffer— some more, some less—by at least five mechanisms, just as happens in *local* hypoperfusion, described earlier in this chapter: lack of oxygen, lack of substrates, lack of waste removal, damage from low flow, and damage from inflammation. To these we may add damage from bacterial toxins, limited to septic shock.

Damage from low flow is a critical concept. Low flow is the main characteristic of shock. As mentioned earlier, low flow has two components, which makes it— paradoxically—more damaging than no flow at all: **because the flow is *inadequate* there is ischemic damage; and because *some flow persists,* the perfused ischemic tissue also develops reperfusion damage** (free-radical damage, inflammation, leukocyte plugging).

From Bleeding to Sepsis

Each type of shock has its peculiarities. We will offer a brief analysis of hemorrhagic shock, because it is the best understood, and it illustrates very clearly the progression to septic shock.

About 10 percent of the blood volume can be lost without a decrease in blood pressure or cardiac output, but with greater losses both functions drop; they reach zero with a blood loss of 35–45 percent. As hypotension develops, correcting reflexes intervene immediately (Figure 24.30). A sympathetic response is initiated by the baro-receptors (pressure sensors): (a) the arterioles constrict (hence the cold skin), thereby increasing the peripheral resistance; (b) the veins constrict, helping to restore blood volume; and (c) the heart rate increases. The vasomotor reflexes do not affect the heart and the brain, which are therefore the main beneficiaries of the protective reflexes (199).

At this stage the clinical picture includes rapid, shallow breathing; cold, clammy, and cyanotic skin; constricted veins; fast, shallow pulse; low blood pressure; and low or nil urine output; the patient may be fully conscious (248). This is the stage of *compensated hypotension* (187).

The immediate reflexes are followed, in a matter of hours, by slower corrective responses. The kidney, for example, responds to anoxia by activating the renin– angiotensin–aldosterone system, leading to salt and water conservation; the secretion of vasopressin, a vasoconstrictor, helps correct the hypotension.

Up to a point—and *which* point is the crucial issue—it is still possible to reverse the downhill trend by restoring the blood volume, even with a plasma substitute. If this is not done, and the compensatory mechanisms fail, the circulatory functions begin to deteriorate: the vasomotor center is depressed, the peripheral vessels dilate, and the blood pressure drops. All tissues suffer. In the liver and gut the circulation is further impaired by a selective **arterial spasm** (159, 239). Now a series of vicious circles are set in motion, so that shock breeds more shock (200).

> NOTE: The seminal work on hemorrhagic shock, both **reversible and irreversible,** was done in the 1940s and 1950s by a scholarly Boston surgeon, Dr. Jacob Fine (188). His approach was to remove from a dog a known amount of blood, and to reinfuse it later. In this model the reversibility of shock can be determined quite precisely, but the results are of course not applicable to humans. After Dr. Fine, the emphasis on the point of irreversibility faded away, also because it tends to remove hope.

Vicious Circles in Shock

Vicious circles are typical of shock of all kinds (Figure 24.31). Here are some examples:

- *Poor perfusion of the heart* impairs myocardial function, with further impairment of cardiac output,

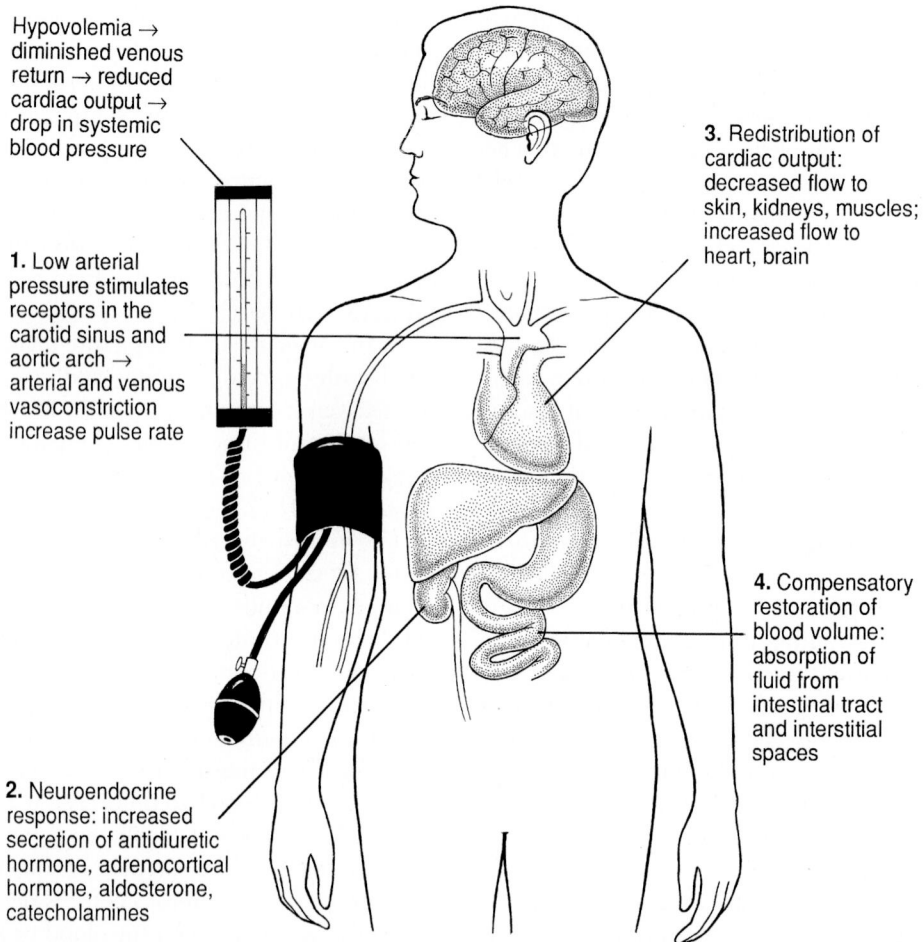

Hypovolemia → diminished venous return → reduced cardiac output → drop in systemic blood pressure

1. Low arterial pressure stimulates receptors in the carotid sinus and aortic arch → arterial and venous vasoconstriction increase pulse rate

3. Redistribution of cardiac output: decreased flow to skin, kidneys, muscles; increased flow to heart, brain

4. Compensatory restoration of blood volume: absorption of fluid from intestinal tract and interstitial spaces

2. Neuroendocrine response: increased secretion of antidiuretic hormone, adrenocortical hormone, aldosterone, catecholamines

FIGURE 24.30   Major compensating mechanisms in hypovolemic shock. (Adapted from [177].)

and therefore reduced perfusion of all organs including the heart itself.

- *Poor perfusion of the pancreas* induces the pancreas to produce peptides that further de press cardiac function (205); a circulating myocardial depressant factor (MDF) has actually been demonstrated in shock patients (Figure 24.32) (219).

- *Poor perfusion of the liver* places it in double jeopardy because the liver receives its blood from two sources: 40 percent from the hepatic artery and 60 percent from the portal vein (230). The liver is the site where most of the lactic acid is broken down; now it is presented with an excess of it, but being anoxic it cannot handle it, so the liver becomes a producer of lactate (206); this worsens the acidosis, which impairs cardiovascular function (202, 231). Under these conditions the liver becomes unable to inactivate all the chemical mediators that flood the circulation, thus creating another vicious circle.

- *Poor perfusion of the kidneys* impairs renal function and thereby the excretion of acid metabolites, which worsens the acidosis; reduced blood perfusion may lead to tubular necrosis, with further retention of toxic metabolites.

- *Poor perfusion of the lungs* contributes to the genesis of the "shock lung" (see later), which further impairs the oxygenation of the blood.

- *Poor perfusion of the gut* causes a breakdown of the mucosal barrier (the gut is very sensitive to ischemia); bacteria reach the blood (188, 229), setting the stage for septic shock; sloughing of the mucosa causes bleeding and further fluid loss, aggravating the poor perfusion throughout the body.

While these vicious circles are developing, blood tests convey some worrisome news: *the plasma is being loaded with inflammatory mediators,* molecules that are not supposed to be there except as traces and then only

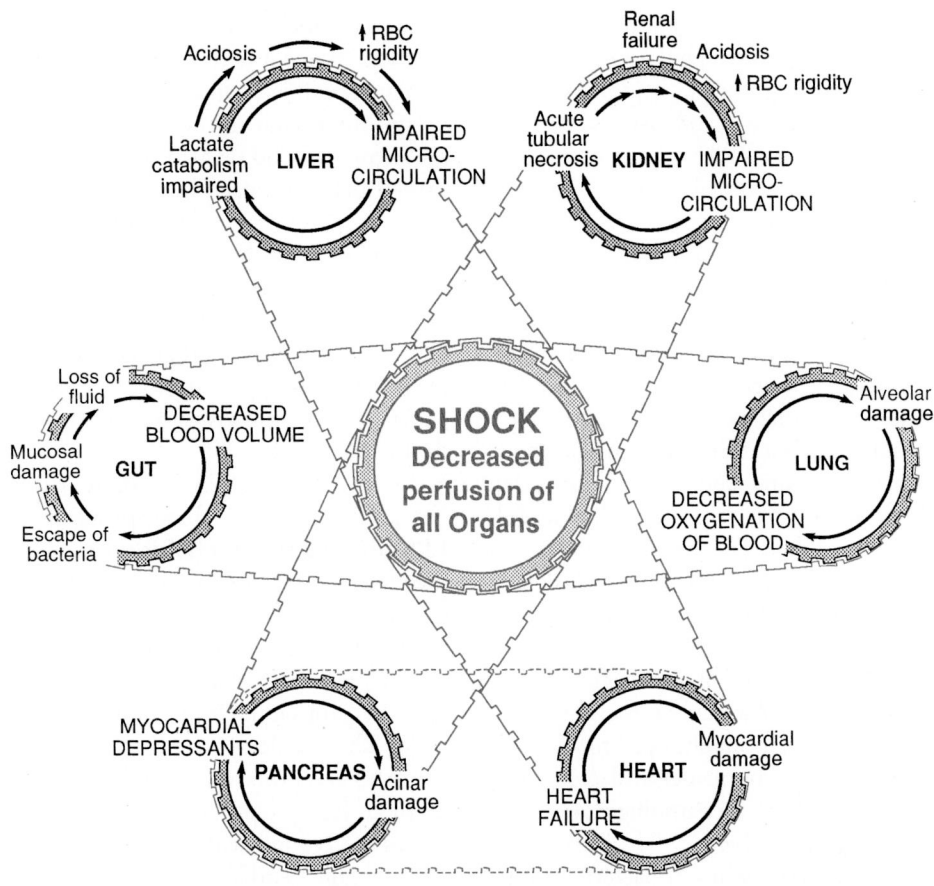

FIGURE 24.31   Some of the vicious circles that occur in shock. The condition of shock (decreased perfusion) is represented in the center. When this wheel begins to turn, it activates many other wheels, creating conditions that in turn aggravate shock. Some of the secondary wheels activate each other (*bottom*). Other vicious circles can be proposed, such as microvascular occlusion by leukocytes as a result and as a cause of decreased perfusion.

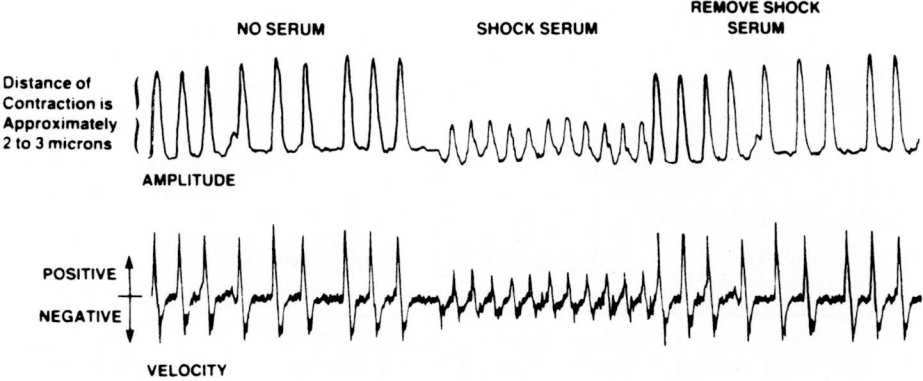

FIGURE 24.32   Demonstrating a myocardial depressant substance in serum from a patient during the acute phase of septic shock. The serum was applied to a culture of rat myocardial cells contracting spontaneously in a petri dish: it depressed both the extent (*top*) and the velocity (*bottom*) of cell shortening. (Adapted from the **Journal of Clinical Investigation,** 1985;76:1539–1553, by copyright permission of the American Society for Clinical Investigation via Copyright Clearance Center [220].)

to be quickly inactivated. In patients and in experimental animals, virtually all the known mediators have been found in the plasma during shock, beginning with histamine, serotonin, and kinins (168, 169, 170, 181, 185). Platelet activating factor (PAF), anaphylatoxins, and a variety of cytokines, especially tumor necrosis factor (TNF) and interleukins 1 and 8 (IL-1, IL-8), which can be considered as proinflammatory, and IL-6, mainly anti-inflammatory (226). All of these molecules are pharmacologically very active (this is, after all, their original purpose) and their superimposed effects create a *syndrome of generalized inappropriate inflammation*. Normally, of course, inflammation is a local phenomenon, elicited by mediators; but if the mediators are generated in inordinate amounts and poured into the blood stream, responses that are normally useful become life-threatening. There are two components to an inflammatory exudate: fluid from vascular leakage, and cells from diapedesis. In advanced shock, vascular leakage occurs throughout the body; blood volume is lost, aggravating the situation of hemorrhagic (hypovolemic) shock. *Leukocytes are activated,* marginate in venules hampering the circulation, clump, embolize all organs, obstruct capillaries. The reader will recognize here—vastly multiplied—the same pathologic events of *local hypoperfusion* described earlier.

The situation becomes even worse if bacterial products are included. This is to be expected if hemorrhagic shock lapses into septic shock; clinical indications of this step—not always obvious—may include fever, a flush and warmer skin, hence the term "warm shock" for this stage.

Septic shock is usually due to bacteria and toxins that are "translocated" (the customary term) across the ischemic, damaged intestinal mucosa to the mesenteric lymph nodes and to the blood; gram-negative bacteria are involved in 60 percent of the cases, gram-positive in 20–40 percent; anaerobes and fungi in the rest. If the agent is a gram-negative bacterium, **endotoxin** (also known as Lipopolysaccharide or LPS) can be expected to appear in the blood.

LPS (Figure 24.33) is an amazing molecule, a foreign, bacterial product that can pose as the *prima donna* of inflammatory mediator: a tiny amount injected into experimental animals can reproduce the entire syndrome of shock.

In the plasma, LPS is bound to a carrier protein (actually an acute phase protein [p. 504]) called **LPS-binding protein (LBP);** for some time, the theory held that the LPS-LBP complex binds to monocytes and macrophages via their CD14 receptor, and activates both cells to secrete TNF and IL-1, with drastic effects on the endothelium and leukocytes (162). But CD14 lacks an intracellular "tail": how could it activate any cell at all? The problem was solved when another family of powerful receptors was found, the now-famous TLRs, Toll-like Receptors, including one for LPS (p. 432); it acts as co-receptor with CD14 (180a).

Now the endothelium and the leukocytes are activated throughout the system; the endothelium becomes leaky (probably also by direct damage) and expresses adhesion molecules, as it would in a focus of local inflammation (186, 195, 225, 246). The endothelium is also misled into expressing tissue factor,

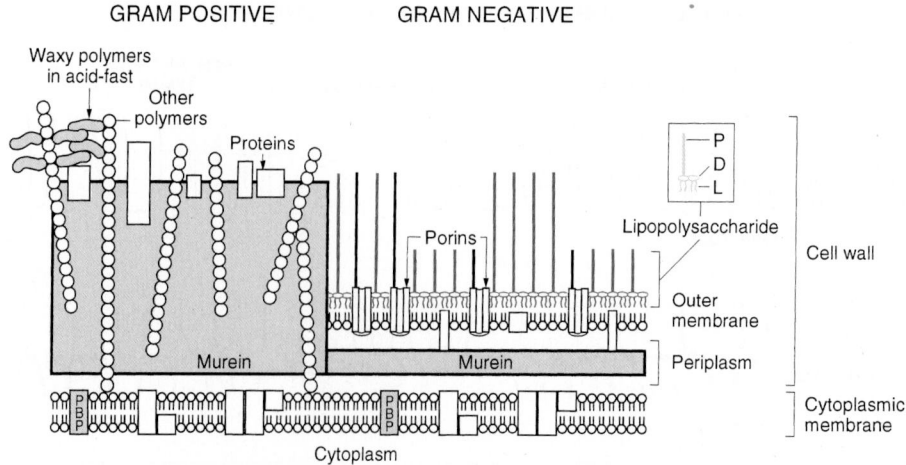

FIGURE 24.33   Endotoxin (lipopolysaccharide, LPS). Inset: a molecule of LPS, consisting of a polysaccharide moiety of variable length (**P**), two disaccharide units (**D**) and a lipid moiety (**L**: four fatty acids). The main figure shows the position of LPS in the wall of gram-negative bacteria: the wall of gram-positive bacteria is shown for comparison. (Adapted from [237], Copyright 1991, with permission from Elsevier.)

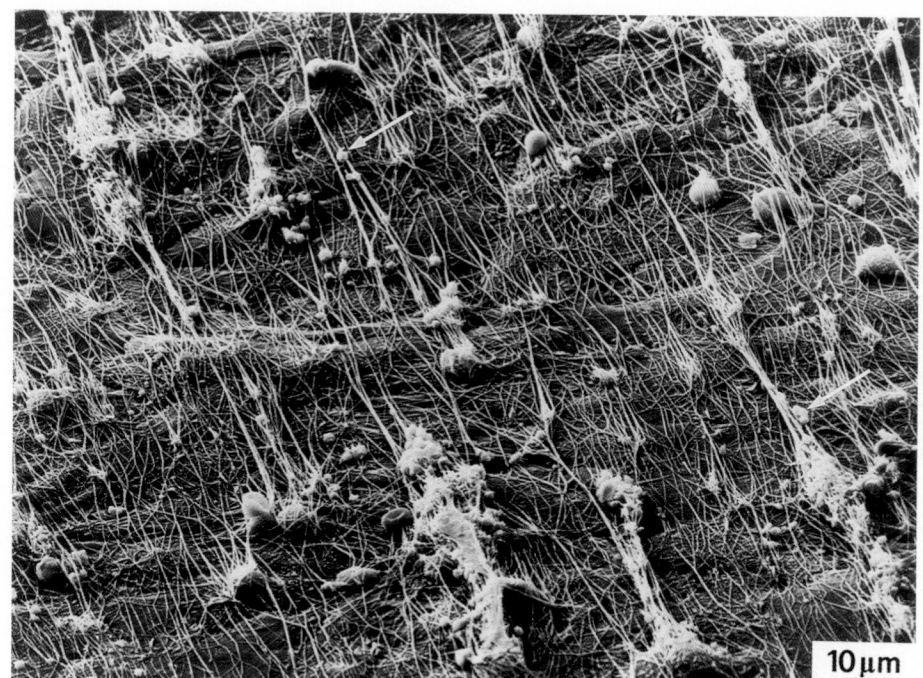

FIGURE 24.34 Cultured human endothelium perverted by endotoxin into producing clots. Scanning electron micrograph. The filaments are fibrin. Endothelial cultures were incubated 4–18 hours with endotoxin and then superfused with freshly drawn human blood for 5 minutes. Fibrin strands are deposited only at low shear rates, such as could occur in veins. Platelets (**arrows**) adhere to the fibrin. (Reproduced with permission from [180].)

10 μm

whereby filaments of fibrin develop on its surface (Figure 24.34): intravascular clotting is very bad news. The platelets, also activated by LPS, clump and embolize the lung capillaries, where they release their arsenal of inflammatory mediators. Another effect of endotoxin is almost diabolical: low-density lipoprotein (LDL) tends to protect the endothelium against endotoxin, which is fat-soluble and dissolves into the LDL particles. But then, the endothelial cells transport the endotoxin-loaded LDL particles to the tissue spaces, where they can trigger an inflammatory response (216). There is more: *endotoxin activates the complement cascade* (243), *the coagulation cascade, the fibrinolytic cascade, and the kinin cascade.* This is truly incendiary behavior.

> It is instructive to remember that back in the 1950s, when Dr. Fine—whom we mentioned above—announced that his dogs in advanced hemorrhagic shock were dying of endotoxin poisoning, he was ridiculed: how could a toxin explain a hydraulic phenomenom such as hemorrhagic shock?

The drastic role of endotoxin as a local and general irritant eventually inspired the literature: it became the topic of two masterly essays by the late Lewis Thomas (233, 234), a pathologist who achieved fame also as a writer. Thomas describes the effect of endotoxin in apocalyptic terms: all our cells seem to dread this ancient molecule, which turns on all our defenses in a manner that appears "unnecessary, panic-driven." And indeed, the situation does call for biochemical panic: in

addition to the effects of endotoxin, failure of the microcirculation leads to impaired utilization of substrates, first of glucose and then of fat and protein (249). Because oxygen is lacking, mitochondrial respiration is down, and anaerobic glycolysis is up, leading to acidosis. In striated muscle, proteolysis is greatly increased: sepsis is associated with Z-band disintegration followed by breakdown through the ubiquitin-proteasome pathway (247).

Among the mishaps in the microcirculation, the escape of fluid into the tissues (Figure 24.35) becomes more and more difficult to compensate, while the plugging of capillaries by leukocytes creates another vicious circle by aggravating the ischemia (160, 163, 164, 241, 242).

As the patient approaches the bitter end, one or more organs begin to fail; this stage was originally defined as *multiple organ failure syndrome* (MOF), later changed to *multiple organ dysfunction syndrome* (MODS) to allow for varying degrees of failure. The gut, always loaded with gram-negative bacteria, can be seen as the "motor of multiple organ failure" (189, 190), but any organ can be hit, also the brain—leading to coma (166). The sequence is more often lungs → liver → intestine → kidney (184). Few patients survive the failure of three organs. Each failing system calls for support, creating a therapeutic nightmare. The *coup de grâce* may come in the guise of disseminated intravascular coagulation (DIC), the paradoxical syndrome of combined clotting and bleeding that we described in Chapter 22.

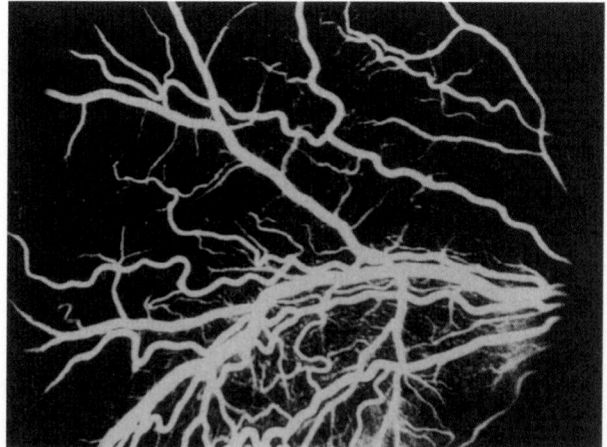

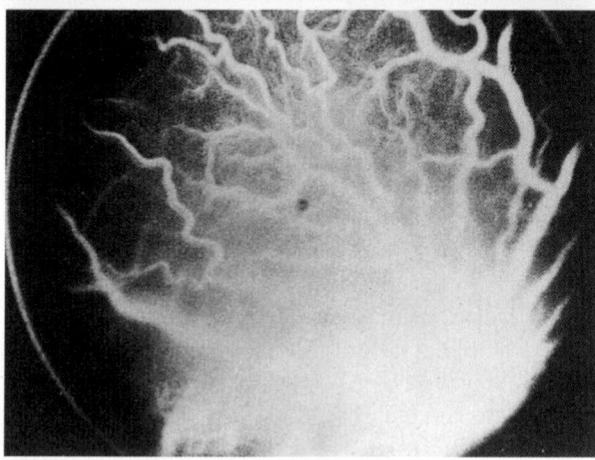

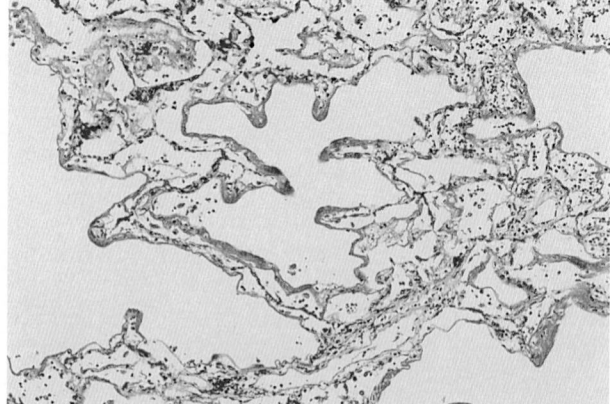

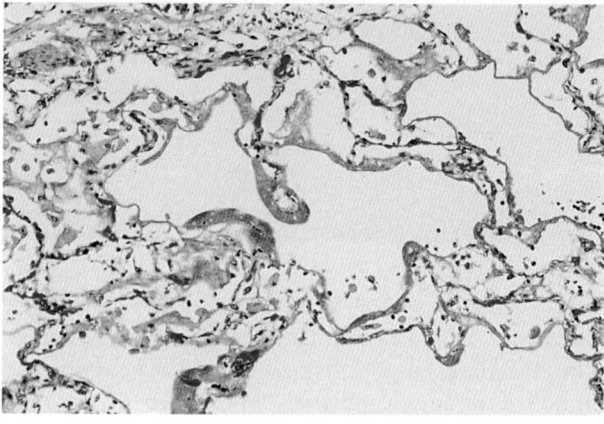

FIGURE 24.35   *Top:* Retinal angiogram of a normal dog. The vessels, demonstrated by an intravenous injection of fluorescein, are sharply outlined because the dye does not leak out. *Bottom:* Fluorescein was injected 6 hours after infusion of *Escherichia coli:* note extensive vascular leakage. (Reproduced with permission from [238]. *Copyright © 1983, American Medical Association.* All rights reserved.)

Organ Changes in Shock

All organ changes in shock are potentially reversible, except those of the brain (202).

- *The lungs* develop changes typical enough to deserve the name of **shock lungs,** corresponding to the clinical condition now called *diffuse alveolar damage* (DAD). It was long known as the acute respiratory distress syndrome (ARDS) (245). This is a major complication.

   In DAD the gas exchanges in the lung are severely curtailed; the alveolar capillaries are leaky, the alveolar lining is partly necrotic and replaced by a fibrin ("hyalin") membrane; many alveoli are filled with exudate. Clinically, the patient develops an acute respiratory insufficiency, the heart rate accelerates, and cyanosis appears. Oxygen therapy is of

FIGURE 24.36   *Top:* Lung in an early stage of adult respiratory distress syndrome (ARDS) caused in this case by oxygen therapy for 4 days. Some alveoli are lined by thick, hyalin, eosinophilic membranes consisting of necrotic cells and fibrin. Many alveoli contain inflammatory cells. (80x) *Bottom:* Detail, showing alveoli wholly or partially lined by hyalin membranes. (120x)

little help. X-rays show a diffuse infiltration, and at autopsy the lung appears heavy and congested.

   Microscopically, part of the alveolar lining is replaced by hyaline membranes (Figure 24.36), which consist of fibrin and debris of dead alveolar epithelium. The capillaries in the alveolar wall are damaged and leaky, hence the fibrin in the membranes.

   The mechanism of alveolar damage (both epithelial and capillary) is probably multiple (217, 245). Because it can develop in the course of oxygen therapy ("*respirator lung*") the mechanism was thought to be toxic, due to the oxygen-derived free radicals; this is probably true, but another source of damage is the forced mechanical expansion of the alveoli (245). In septic shock the injury appears to originate within the alveolar capillaries: activated neutrophils are trapped and release free radicals and enzymes, and the endothelial and epithelial cells are damaged or killed. Neutrophils are activated by endotoxin itself, as well as by activated complement and other chemotaxins (leukotriene B_4, platelet

activating factor). Remember that activated leukocytes tend to aggregate, and therefore to become microemboli; the tendency of leukocytes to stick is
also increased (235, 236, 244).

What happens next? The alveoli become filled
with semifluid exudate; fibroblasts migrate into it
and organize it (Figure 24.37). Surprisingly, some
patients recover even from this stage: the alveolar
filling is reabsorbed and air flows back into the
alveoli.

- *The liver* shows necrosis, which is centrolobular at
first but can also be massive; more than one-fourth
of the liver may die (183) justifying the term *liver
infarction* (Figure 24.38). On the other hand, the
leukocyte infiltration can be severe enough to call
for the diagnosis of *hypoxic hepatitis* (64). Jaundice
may develop (232).

- *The kidneys* can cease to function altogether.
The Achilles heel of the nephron is the convoluted ascending limb in the medulla, which is
hypoxic already under normal conditions, due to
its heavy energy requirements for the work of
urinary concentration: the oxygen pressure
there is 10–20 mm Hg, as opposed to ~50 in
the cortex (176).

- *The heart* shows subendocardial hemorrhages
(mechanism unclear); in addition, pathologists at
Duke University have described a myocardial
change in hemorrhagic shock that is almost specific:
the "**zonal lesion**" (Figure 24.39) (207–209, 224).
The change affects a small "zone" of the myocardial
cell; the fibrils normally attached to the intercalated
disc seem to have torn away from it, and the adjacent sarcomeres are supercontracted. In dogs this

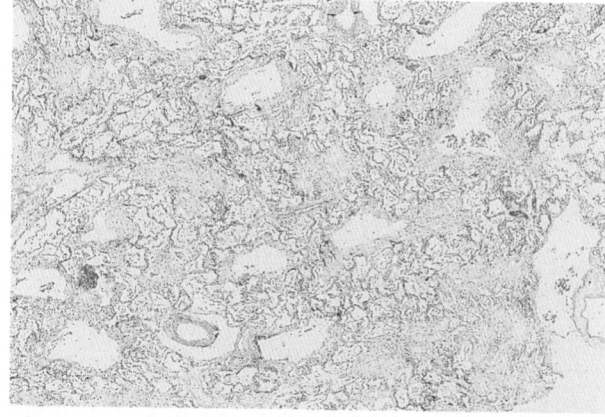

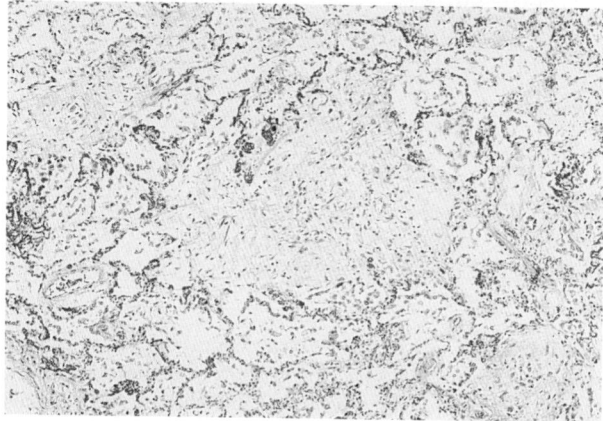

FIGURE 24.37 Advanced ARDS. *Top:* Few alveoli contain air;
most are filled with inflammatory cells, not identifiable at this
enlargement. (30x) *Bottom:* Detail showing that the alveoli contain fibroblasts (elongated cells) in addition to macrophages.
The exudate has been organized, resulting in obliteration of the
air space. (60x)

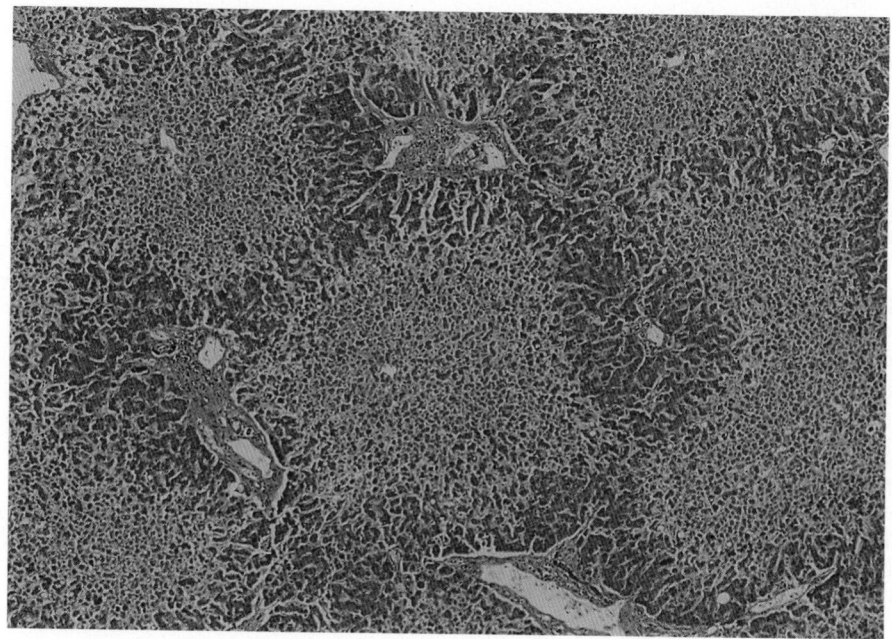

FIGURE 24.38 Liver in a case of
septic shock: extensive centrolobular necrosis, interpreted as a result
of hypoxia and arterial spasm
superimposed on portal endotoxemia. (50x)

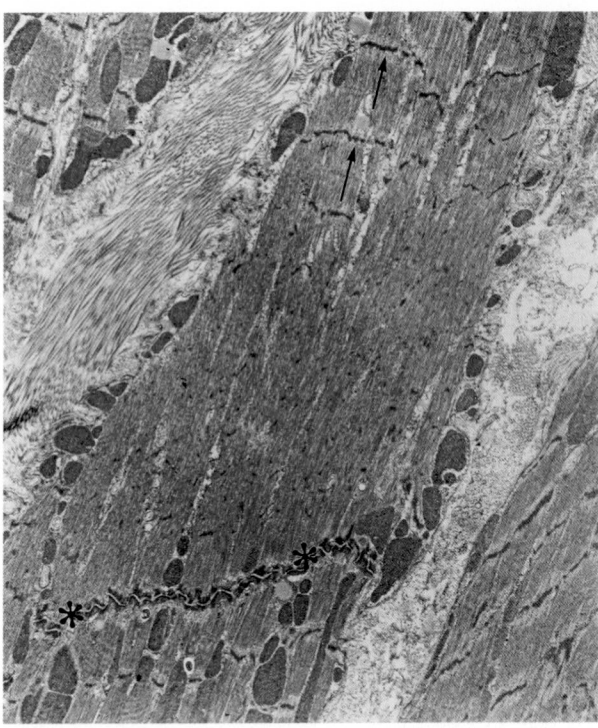

FIGURE 24.39 Myocardial zonal lesion, typical of shock. **Arrows:** Z bands. The sarcomeres above the intercalated disk (**asterisks**) are no longer distinguishable because the Z bands have been pulled out of shape. From a papillary muscle of a cat in hemorrhagic shock. (Courtesy of Dr. N. B. Ratliff Jr., The Cleveland Clinic Foundation, Cleveland, OH.)

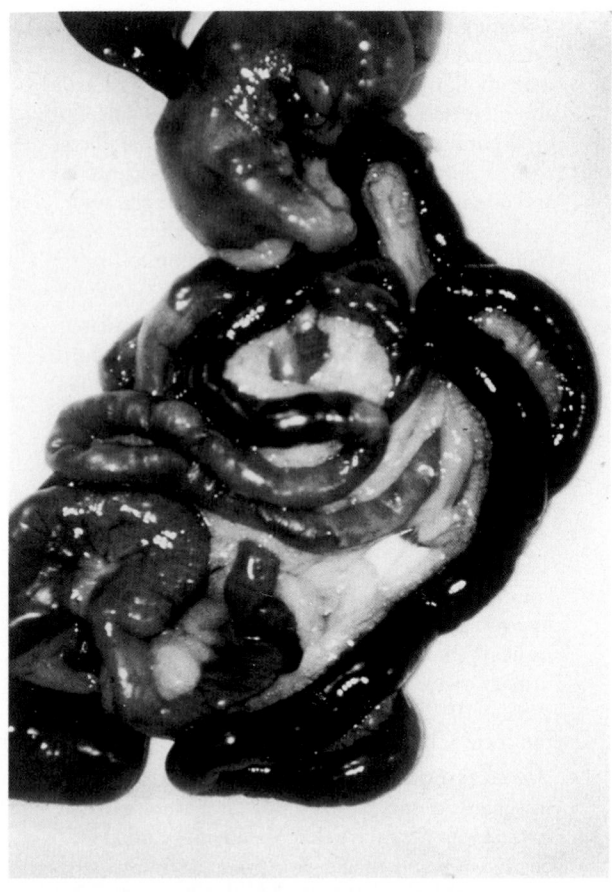

FIGURE 24.40 Effect of tumor necrosis factor (TNF) on the gastrointestinal tract of a rat. These hemorrhagic changes, typical of shock, were present 4 hours after infusion of TNF into the tail vein. (Reproduced by permission from [240]. Copyright 1986 by the American Association for the Advancement of Science.)

occurred within 15–45 minutes of hemorrhagic shock. In humans it has been seen only "in situations where the heart is beating strongly and rapidly" (178).

Today this lesion is best interpreted in the light of a similar change found in "septic" rats (16 hours after cecal ligation and puncture): a disruption of the Z-bands, associated with a calcium-dependent release of myofibrils in the cytoplasm (247). This cellular pathology helps understand the severe atrophy and catabolism of muscles during and after septic shock.

- *The pancreas* can develop small patches of self-digestion with the typical fat necrosis (p. 230). Occasionally the full-blown picture of acute pancreatic necrosis is a surprise finding at autopsy: this is usually an extremely dramatic and painful episode, but it can escape notice if the patient is terminally ill.
- *The gut* becomes edematous, congested, and hemorrhagic (Figure 24.40); the mucosa tends to slough off and bleed. As a virtually endless source of bacteria and toxins seeping into the blood, the gut certainly deserves its reputation of "motor of the

multiple organ failure syndrome." Two drastic experiments illustrate this point: in rats, ischemia of the gut by occlusion of the splanchnic artery produces a severe form of shock (201), and conversely, enterectomy (the removal of the entire small and large intestines) improves survival (179).

- Damage to the *brain* can be generalized and result in coma, but localized lesions can develop in the watershed areas mentioned earlier (196). The main problem is that hypoxia and ischemia of the brain lead to cellular swelling (i.e., to intracellular edema). This raises the intracranial pressure, which creates a further obstacle to blood flow, which causes more ischemic swelling, and so on: another vicious circle. The ultimate anatomic catastrophe is the "respirator brain," a swollen, semiliquid mass that represents essentially autolysis of the brain *in vivo;* fragments of cerebellum float away in the cerebrospinal fluid and can be found attached to the spinal cord.

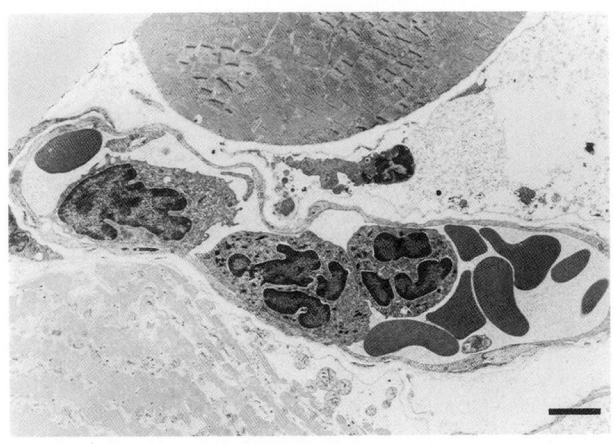

FIGURE 24.41   Three leukocytes plugging a small postcapillary venule after 3 hours of hemorrhagic shock (rat maintained at a mean arterial pressure of 40 mm Hg). **Bar** = 2 μm. (Courtesy of Drs. J. Barroso-Aranda and G. W. Schmid-Schönbein, University of California, San Diego, La Jolla, CA.)

• *The microcirculation* must be mentioned here, because it is present in all tissues, and although it has—almost by definition—a low visibility, it is one of the principal players in all ischemic conditions (212, 213).

Inappropriate activation of the endothelium can be disastrous; the same is true for leukocytes. Plugging of capillaries by leukocytes may *look* benign (Figure 24.41) but

functionally it can lead to total ischemia. Generalized arteriolar dilatation could kill by itself. Missing at this time is a quantitative evaluation of these critical factors.

Septic Shock without Bacteria: New Perspectives

By 1980, the battle against septic shock had been fought for two decades with antibacterial, anti-endotoxin approaches. Mortality had not changed much. Furthermore, some cases that appeared clinically as "septic shock" showed no evidence of bacteremia or endotoxinemia; rather, they were characterized by extensive tissue destruction; acute pancreatitis was the best example. Could it be (223) that—sometimes—*the whole syndrome is due not to the bacteria, but to the inflammatory response to the bacteria—or even to aseptic, dead tissue?*

Shocking as it was, we must admit that also in terms of General Pathology the new theory made very good sense; dying and necrotic tissue, as we have abundantly discussed, does elicit a lively aseptic inflammation (p. 446). In 1992 a Consensus Conference Committee of the American College of Chest Physicians and the Society for Critical Care Medicine published a report (172, 173) recognizing that a syndrome similar or identical to "sepsis" can arise in the absence of infection; this new syndrome was named *systemic inflammatory response syndrome,* or SIRS (171). Figure 24.42 shows a set of three overlapping conditions (from left to right): infection

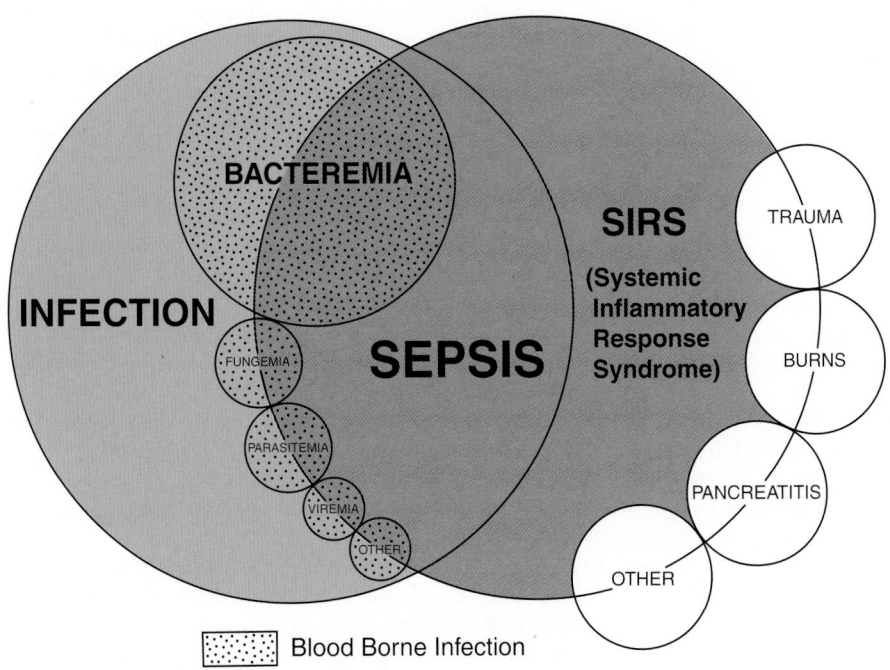

FIGURE 24.42   The overlapping concepts of infection, sepsis, and the systemic inflammatory response syndrome. Note that SIRS (including shock) can occur in the absence of infection. (Adapted with permission from [173].)

without shock, infection with shock (sepsis), and a "septic syndrome" of shock without infection.

And so there followed a decade of anti-inflammatory treatment of shock. Alas, a thorough review of the literature in 1999 (192, 193) showed that mortality, once again, had not changed significantly. Therapy for septic shock according to the SIRS concept seemed to work in animal models, but not in humans. Explanations were sought: (a) Perhaps there are too many mediators to fight all at once. (b) Agents like endotoxin, IL-1, or TNF cause cascades of changes; it may be hopeless to fight downstream events. (c) The protocols of animal experiments may not duplicate closely enough the human condition.

All of the above may be true, but a better answer is that pure anti-inflammatory therapy must be combined with anticoagulant therapy: this can be done by treating with activated protein C, a natural anticoagulant which has also anti-inflammatory properties (211) (see Figure 22.15). In a large international study, mortality dropped from 30.8 to 24.7 percent. Not a huge gain, unless you happen to be in the fortunate 6.1 percent.

As of early 2003, there is further hope from other therapeutic approaches: high doses of insulin; and low doses of corticoids (neither has a clear-cut rationale) (180a).

> TO SUM UP: With the syndrome of shock we have reached a level of disease that encompasses virtually all organs and tissues. And yet, in each facet of its all-encompassing pathogenesis, shock teaches us that the underlying problem is still a problem of the cell, the elementary patient.

References

Ischemia

1. Adams JH, Corsellis JAN, Duchen LW, eds. Greenfield's neuropathology, 4th ed. New York: John Wiley & Sons, 1984.

2. Adams JH, Graham DI. An introduction to neuropathology. Edinburgh: Churchill Livingstone, 1988, p. 72.

3. Adomian GE, Laks MM, Billingham ME. The incidence and significance of contraction bands in endomyocardial biopsies from normal human heart. Am Heart J 1978;95:348–351.

4. Al-Mehdi A, Shuman H, Fisher AB. Fluorescence microtopography of oxidative stress in lung ischemia-reperfusion. Lab Invest 1994;70:579–587.

5. Ames A III, Wright RL, Kowada M, Thurston JM, Majno G. Cerebral ischemia. II. The no-reflow phenomenon. Am J Pathol 1968;52:437–453.

6. Ames III A, Maynard KI, Kaplan S. Protection against CNS ischemia by temporary interruption of function-related processes of neurons. J Cereb Blood Flow Metab 1995;15:433–439.

7. Antman EM, Braunwald E. Acute MI management in the 1990s. Hosp Pract 1990;25:65–82.

8. Armour JA, Randall WC. Canine left ventricular intra-myocardial pressures. Am J Physiol 1971;220:1833–1839.

9. Asher RAJ. The dangers of going to bed. Br Med J 1947;2: 967–968.

10. Axford-Gately RA, Wilson GJ. The "border zone" in myocardial infarction. An ultrastructural study in the dog using an electron-dense blood flow marker. Am J Pathol 1988;131: 452–464.

11. Bellesi G, Santini F. Sull'atrofia congestizia circoscritta del fegato (cosidetto infarto di Rattone-Zahn). Profilo anatomo-patologico e problematica della patogenesi. Arch De Vecchi Anat Patol 1966;47:913:930.

12. Bolli R, Marban E. Molecular and cellular mechanisms of myocardial stunning. Physiol Rev 1999;79:609–634.

13. Bouchardy B, Majno G. Histopathology of early myocardial infarcts. Am J Pathol 1974;74:301–318.

14. Bouchardy B, Majno G. A new approach to the histologic diagnosis of early myocardial infarcts. Cardiology 1971/72;56: 327–332.

15. Bowers TR, O'Neill WW, Grines C, et al. Effect of reperfusion on biventricular function and survival after right ventricular infarction. N Engl J Med 1998;338:933–942.

16. Brierley JB, Graham DI. Hypoxia and vascular disorders of the central nervous system. In: Adams JH, Corsellis JAN, Duchen LW, eds. Greenfield's neuropathology, 4th ed. New York: John Wiley & Sons, 1984, pp. 125–207.

17. Bruick RK, McKnight SL. Oxygen sensing gets a second wind. Science 2002;295:807–808.

18. Bulkley GB. Free radical-mediated reperfusion injury: a selective review. Br J Cancer 1987;55(suppl VIII):66–73.

19. Buschmann I, Schaper W. The pathophysiology of the colleral circulation (arteriogenesis). J Pathol 2000;190:338–342.

20. Cahill BE, Kerstein MD. Ischemic neuropathy. Surg Gynecol Obstet 1987;165:469–474.

21. Campbell CA, Przyklenk K, Kloner RA. Infarct size reduction: a review of the clinical trials. J Clin Pharmacol 1986;26:317–329.

22. Cheitlin MD, McAllister HA, de Castro CM. Myocardial infarction without atherosclerosis. JAMA 1975;231:951–959.

23. Chen C, Ma L, Dyckman W, et al. Left ventricular remodeling in myocardial hibernation. Circulation 1997;96(suppl II): II-46–II-50.

24. Chiang J, Kowada M, Ames A III, Wright RL, Majno G. Cerebral ischemia. III. Vascular changes Am J Pathol 1968;52: 455–465.

25. Cohnheim J. Untersuchungen üeber die Embolischen Processe. Berlin: Verlag von August Hirschwald, 1872.

26. Cohnheim J. Lectures on general pathology, sect I. The pathology of the circulation. London: The New Sydenham Society, 1889.

27. Cooley DA, Reul GJ, Wukasch DC. Ischemic contracture of the heart: "stone heart." Am J Cardiol 1972;29:575–577.

28. Cross ER. Taravana. Diving syndrome in the Tuamotu diver. In: Rahn H, ed. Physiology of breath-hold diving and the AMA

of Japan. Washington, DC: National Academy of Sciences, 1965, pp. 207–219.

29. Cuénoud HF. Unpublished data.

30. Cursio R, Gugenheim J, Ricci JE, et al. A caspase inhibitor fully protects rats against lethal normothermic liver ischemia by inhibition of liver apoptosis. FASEB J 1999; 13:253–261.

31. Dalen JE, Haffajee CI, Alpert JS, et al. Pulmonary embolism, pulmonary hemorrhage and pulmonary infarction. N Engl J Med 1977;296:1431–1435.

32. D'Amico M, Di Filippo C, Solito E, et al. Lipocortin 1 reduces myocardial ischemia-reperfusion injury by affecting local leukocyte recruitment. FASEB J 2000;14:1867–1869.

33. D'Angio CT, Finkelstein JN. Oxygen regulation of gene expression: a study in opposites. Mol Genet Metabol 2000;71: 371–380.

34. Daviss B. Cold water to the rescue. Science 1985;85(June):72.

35. Dell'Italia L. Reperfusion for right ventricular infarction. N Engl J Med 1998;338:978–980.

36. Dexter L. A brief history of venous thrombosis and pulmonary embolism. In Dalen JE, ed. Pulmonary embolism. New York: Medcom Press, 1972, pp. 1–5.

37. Doukas J, Cutler AH, Boswell CA, Joris I, Majno G. Reversible endothelial cell relaxation induced by oxygen and glucose deprivation. Am J Pathol 1994;145:211–219.

38. Downing S. Transmyocardial laser revascularization. N Engl J Med 2000;342:436–438.

39. DuBose TD Jr. Metabolic Acidosis. In: Braunwald E, Fauci AS, Kasper DL, et al. (eds). Harrison's principles of internal medicine. 15th ed. New York: McGraw Hill, 2001, pp. 283–291.

40. Duverger D, MacKenzie ET. The quantification of cerebral infarction following focal ischemia in the rat: influence of strain, arterial pressure, blood glucose concentration, and age. J Cereb Blood Flow Metab 1988;8:449–461.

41. Dvorak HF, Brown LF, Detmar M, Dvorak AM. Vascular permeability factor/vascular endothelial growth factor, microvascular hyperpermeability, and angiogenesis. Am J Pathol 1995;146:1029–1039.

42. Dyck PJ. Hypoxic neuropathy: does hypoxia play a role in diabetic neuropathy? The 1988 Robert Wartenberg Lecture. Neurology 1989;39:111–118.

43. Eppinger M, Deeb GM, Bolling, SF, Ward PA. Mediators of ischemia-reperfusion injury of rat lung. Am J Pathol 1997;150: 1773–1784.

44. Federle M, Moss AA. Computed tomography of the spleen. CRC Crit Rev Diagn Imaging 1983;19:1–16.

45. Fehér J, Csomós G, Vereckei A. Free radical reactions in medicine. Berlin: Springer-Verlag, 1987.

46. Felix WR, MacDonnell KF, Jacobs L. Resuscitation from drowning in cold water. N Engl J Med 1981;304:843–844.

47. Ferrari R. Ischaemic heart disease: clinical improvement with metabolic approach. Rev Port Cardiol 2000;19 Suppl 5:V7–V20.

48. Flynn PJ, Becker WK, Vercellotti GM, et al. Ibuprofen inhibits granulocyte responses to inflammatory mediators. A proposed mechanism for reduction of experimental myocardial infarct size. Inflammation 1984;8:33–44.

49. Formigli L, Manneschi LI, Adembri C, et al. Expression of E-selectin in ischemic and reperfused human skeletal muscle. Ultrastruct Pathol 1995;19:193–200.

50. Ganote CE. Contraction band necrosis and irreversible myocardial injury. J Mol Cell Cardiol 1983;15:67–73.

51. Garcia-Dorado D, Théroux P, Solares J, et al. Determinants of hemorrhagic infarcts. Histologic observations from experiments involving coronary occlusion, coronary reperfusion, and reocclusion. Am J Pathol 1990;137:301–311.

52. Garcia JH, Liu K-F, Yoshida Y, Chen S, Lian J. Brain microvessels: factors altering their patency after the occlusion of a middle cerebral artery (Wistar rat). Am J Pathol 1994;145: 728–740.

53. Gavin JB, Humphrey SM, Herdson PB. The no-reflow phenomenon in ischemic myocardium. Int Rev Exp Pathol 1983a; 25:361–383.

54. Gavin JB, Thomson RW, Humphrey SM, Herdson PB. Changes in vascular morphology associated with the no-reflow phenomenon in ischaemic myocardium. Virchows Arch (Pathol Anat) 1983b;399:325–332.

55. Goldblatt H. Studies on experimental hypertension: V. The pathogenesis of experimental hypertension due to renal ischemia. Ann Intern Med 1937;11:69–103.

56. Granger DN. Ischemia-reperfusion: mechanisms of microvascular dysfunction and the influence of risk factors for cardiovascular disease. Microcirculation 1999;6:167–178.

57. Granger DN, Schmid-Schönbein GW. Physiology and pathophysiology of leukocyte adhesion. New York: Oxford University Press, 1995.

58. Gusto Angiographic Investigators. The effects of tissue plasminogen activator, streptokinase, or both on coronary-artery patency, ventricular function, and survival after acute myocardial infarction. N Engl J Med 1993;329:1615–1622.

59. Hackett PH, Roach RC. High-altitude illness. N Engl J Med 2002;345:107–114.

60. Haendchen RV, Corday E, Meerbaum S. Hypothermic synchronized retroperfusion of the coronary veins for the treatment of acutely ischemic myocardium. Compr Ther 1982;8:7–15.

61. Hampton AO, Castleman B. Correlation of postmortem chest teleoroentgenograms with autopsy findings with special reference to pulmonary embolism and infarction. Am J Roentgenol Rad Ther 1940;43:305–326.

62. Hartmann HT, Kester DE, Davies FT Jr. Plant propagation: principles and practices, 5th ed. Englewood Cliffs, NJ: Prentice Hall, 1990.

63. Hearse DJ, Humphrey SM, Bullock GR. The oxygen paradox and the calcium paradox: two facets of the same problem? J Mol Cell Cardiol 1978;10:641–668.

64. Henrion J. Ischemia/reperfusion injury of the liver: pathophysiologic hypotheses and potential relevance to human hypoxic hepatitis. Acta Gastroenterol Belg 2000;63:336–347.

65. Hernandez LA, Grisham MB, Twohig B, et al. Role of neutrophils in ischemia-reperfusion-induced microvascular injury. Am J Physiol 1987;253:H699–H703.

66. Hershey JC, Baskin EP, Glass JD, et al. Revascularization in the rabbit hindlimb: dissociation between capillary sprouting and arteriogenesis. Cardiovasc Res 2001;49:619–625.

67. Herskowitz A, Choi S, Ansari AA, Wesselingh S. Cytokine mRNA expression in postischemic/reperfused myocardium. Am J Pathol 1995;146:419–428.

68. Higginson LAJ, White F, Heggtveit HA, et al. Determinants of myocardial hemorrhage after coronary reperfusion in the anesthetized dog. Circulation 1982;65:62–69.

69. Hochachka PW, Lutz PL, Sick T, Rosenthal M, van den Thillart G (eds). Surviving hypoxia. Mechanisms of control and adaptation. Boca Raton FL: CRC Press, 1993.

70. Inglott FS, Mathie RT. Nitric oxide and hepatic ischemia-reperfusion injury. Hepato-Gastroenterol 2000;47:1722–1725.

71. ISAM Study Group. A prospective trial of intravenous streptokinase in acute myocardial infarction (ISAM). Mortality, morbidity, and infarct size at 21 days. N Engl J Med 1986; 314:1465–1471.

72. Jaroch MT, Broughan TA, Hermann RE. The natural history of splenic infarction. Surgery 1986;100:743–749.

73. Jennings RB, Reimer KA. Pathobiology of acute myocardial ischemia. Hosp Pract 1989;24:89–107.

74. Kalimo H, Garcia JH, Kamijyo Y, Tanaka J, Trump BF. The ultrastructure of "brain death." II. Electron microscopy of feline cortex after complete ischemia. Virchows Arch B Cell Pathol 1977;25:207–220.

75. Kalimo H, Rehncrona S, Söderfeldt B, Olsson Y, Siesjö BK. Brain lactic acidosis and ischemic cell damage: 2. Histopathology. J Cereb Blood Flow Metab 1981;1:313–327.

76. Katori M, Berne RM. Release of adenosine from anoxic hearts. Relationship to coronary flow. Circ Res 1966;19:420–425.

77. Kennedy JW. Streptokinase for the treatment of acute myocardial infarction: a brief review of randomized trials. J Am Coll Cardiol 1987;5:28B–32B.

78. Khan S, Cleveland RP, Koch CJ, Schelling JR. Hypoxia induces renal tubular epithelial cell apoptosis in chronic renal disease. Lab Invest 1999;79:1089–1099.

79. Klein HH, Puschmann S, Schaper J, Schaper W. The mechanism of the tetrazolium reaction in identifying experimental myocardial infarction. Virchows Arch A Pathol Anat 1981; 393:287–297.

80. Kloner RA. Do neutrophils mediate the phenomenon of stunned myocardium? J Am Coll Cardiol 1989;13: 1164–1166.

81. Kloner RA, Przylkenk K, Campbell CA. Coronary reperfusion following experimental myocardial infarction. J Cardiol Surg 1987;2:291–297.

82. Kloner RA, Rude RE, Carlson N, et al. Ultrastructural evidence of microvascular damage and myocardial cell injury after coronary artery occlusion: which comes first? Circulation 1980;62:945–952.

83. Kloner RA, Bolli R, Marban E, Reinlib, Braunwald E and participants. Medical and cellular implications of stunning, hibernation, and preconditioning. An NHLBI workshop. Circulation 1998;97:1848–1867.

84. Kost GJ. Surface pH of the medial gastrocnemius and soleus muscles during hemorrhagic shock and ischemia. Surgery 1984;95:183–190.

85. Kowada M, Ames A III, Majno G, Wright RL. Cerebral ischemia. An improved experimental method for study; cardiovascular effects and demonstration of an early vascular lesion in the rabbit. J Neurosurg 1968;28:150–157.

86. Krainer L. Pathological effects of cerebral anoxia. Am J Med 1958;25:258–266.

87. Kurose I, Wolf R, Grisham MB, Granger DN. Modulation of ischemia/reperfusion-induced microvascular dysfunction by nitric oxide. Circ Res 1994;74:376–382.

88. Lahiri S, Prabhakar NR, Forster II RE (eds). Oxygen sensing. Molecule to man. Adv Exp Med and Biol, Vol 475. New York: Kluwer Academic/Plenum Publishers, 2000.

89. Lakon G. The topographical tetrazolium method for determining the germinating capacity of seeds. Plant Phys 1949;24:389–394.

90. Lee J-M, Zipfel GJ, Choi DW. The changing landscape of ischaemic brain injury mechanisms. Nature 1999;399:A7–A14.

91. Lee SH, Wolf PL, Escudero R, et al. Early expression of angiogenesis factors in acute myocardial ischemia and infarction. N Engl J Med 2000;342:626–633.

92. Lemasters JJ, Bond JM, Currin RT, et al. Reperfusion injury to heart and liver cells: protection by acidosis during ischemia and a "pH paradox" after reperfusion. In: Hochachka PW, Lutz PL, Sick T, Rosenthal M, van den Thillart G (eds). Surviving hypoxia. Mechanisms of control and adaptation. Boca Raton FL: CRC Press, 1993, pp. 495–507.

93. Levene CI, Kapoor R, Heale G. The effect of hypoxia on the synthesis of collagen and glycosaminoglycans by cultured pig aortic endothelium. Atherosclerosis 1982;44:327–337.

94. Little WC, Rogers EW. Angiographic evidence of hemorrhagic myocardial infarction after intracoronary thrombolysis with streptokinase. Am J Cardiol 1983;51:906–908.

95. Majno G. The Healing Hand. Man and Wound in the Ancient World. Cambridge, MA: Harvard University Press, 1975.

96. Majno G, Ames A III, Chiang J, Wright RL. No reflow after cerebral ischaemia. Lancet 1967;2:569–570.

97. Marshall V, Jablonski P, Howden B, et al. Recovery of renal function in the rat after warm ischaemia: functional and morphological changes. In: Pegg DE, Jacobsen IA, Halasz NA, eds. Organ preservation: basic and applied aspects. Lancaster: MTP Press Limited, 1982, pp. 69–76.

98. Marti HJH, Bernaudin M, Bellail A, et al. Hypoxia-induced vascular endothelial factor expression precedes neovascularization after cerebral ischemia. Am J Pathol 2000;156:965–976.

99. Maxwell PH, Dachs GU, Gleadle JM, et al. Hypoxia-inducible factor-1 modulates gene expression in solid tumors and influences both angiogenesis and tumor growth. Proc Natl Acad Sci USA 1997;904:8104–8109.

99a. May JW Jr, Chait LA, O'Brien BM, Hurley JV. The no-reflow phenomenon in experimental free flaps. Plast Reconst Surg 1978;61:256–267.

100. McCord JM. Oxygen-derived free radicals in post-ischemic tissue injury. N Engl J Med 1985;312:159–163.

101. McDonagh PF, Laks H. Use of cold blood cardioplegia to protect against coronary microcirculatory injury due to ischemia and reperfusion. J Thorac Cardiovasc Surg 1982;84:609–618.

102. McGoldrick PJ, Rudd TG, Figley MM, Wilhelm JP. What becomes of pulmonary infarcts? Am J Roentgenol 1979; 133:1039–1045.

103. McIntyre DM, Sasahara AA. The hemodynamic response to pulmonary embolism in patients without prior cardiopulmonary disease. Am J Cardiol 1971;28:288–294.

104. Mégevand R, Cruchaud A, Kapanci Y. Etude de l'action de différents médicaments immuno-suppresseurs appliqués aux allogreffes pulmonaires chez le chien. Helv Chir Acta 1968;35:327–330.

105. Messina A, Knight KR, Dowsing BJ, et al. Localization of inducible nitric oxide synthase to mast cells during ischemia/reperfusion injury of skeletal muscle. Lab Invest 2000;80:423–431.

106. Mullane KM. Eicosanoids in myocardial ischemia/reperfusion injury. Adv Inflam Res 1988;12:191–214.

107. Muller JE, Tofler GH. Circadian variation and cardiovascular disease. N Engl J Med 1991;325:1038–1039.

108. Nedergaard M. Mechanisms of brain damage in focal cerebral ischemia. Acta Neurol Scand 1988;77:81–101.

109. Neely JR. Metabolic disturbances after coronary occlusion. Hosp Pract 1989;24:81–96.

110. Nukada H, Dyck PJ. Microsphere embolization of nerve capillaries and fiber degeneration. Am J Pathol 1984;115:275–287.

111. Paljärvi L, Rehncrona S, Söderfeldt B, Olsson Y, Kalimo H. Brain lactic acidosis and ischemic cell damage: quantitative ultrastructural changes in capillaries of rat cerebral cortex. Acta Neuropathol 1983;60:232–240.

112. Pe'er J, Shweiki D, Itin A, et al. Hypoxia-induced expression of vascular endothelial growth factor by retinal cells is a common factor in neovascularizing ocular diseases. Lab Invest 1995;72:638–645.

113. Peralta C, Perales JC, Bartrons R, et al. The combination of ischemic preconditioning and liver Bcl-2 overexpression is a suitable strategy to prevent liver and lung damage after hepatic ischemia-reperfusion. Am J Pathol 2002;160:2111–2122.

114. Przyklenk K, Kloner RA. Superoxide dismutase plus catalase improve contractile function in the canine model of the "stunned myocardium." Circ Res 1986;58:148–156.

115. Reimer KA, Jennings RB. Myocardial ischemia, hypoxia, and infarction. In: Fozzard HA, Jennings RB, Haber E, Katz Am, Morgan HE, eds. The heart and cardiovascular system, vol 2. New York: Raven Press, 1986, pp. 1133–1201.

116. Romson JL, Hook BG, Kunkel SL, et al. Reduction of the extent of ischemic myocardial injury by neutrophil depletion in the dog. Circulation 1983;67:1016–1023.

117. Rosenow EC III, Osmundson PJ, Brown ML. Pulmonary embolism. Mayo Clin Proc 1981;56:161–178.

118. Royds JA, Dower SK, Qwarnstrom EE, Lewis CE. Response of tumour cells to hypoxia: role of p53 and NFkB. Mol Pathol 1998;51:55–61.

119. Rollwagen FM, Li Y-Y, Pacheco ND, Dick EJ, Kang Y-H. Microvascular effects of oral interleukin-6 on ischemia/ reperfusion in the murine small intestine. Am J Pathol 2000;156:1177–1182.

120. Sabiston DC Jr. Pathophysiology, diagnosis, and management of pulmonary embolism. Am J Surg 1979;138:384–391.

121. Saegesser F, Roenspies U, Robinson JWL. Ischemic diseases of the large intestine. Pathobiol Annu 1979;9:303–337.

122. Sanders MD, Graham EM. Ocular disorders associated with systemic diseases. In: Vaughn D, et al. eds. General ophtalmology, 13th ed. Norwalk, CT: Appelton & Lange, 1992, p. 310.

123. Sasaki K, Ueno A, Katori M, Kikawada R. Detection of leukotriene B_4 in cardiac tissue and its role in infarct extension through leucocyte migration. Cardiovasc Res 1988;22:142–148.

124. Schaper W, Schaper J. (eds). Collateral circulation. Boston: Kluwer Academic Publishers, 1993.

125. Schmid-Schönbein GW. Capillary plugging by granulocytes and the no-reflow phenomenon in the microcirculation. Fed Proc 1987;46:2397–2401.

126. Schwartz P, Piper HM, Spahr R, Spieckermann PG. Ultrastructure of cultured adult myocardial cells during anoxia and reoxygenation. Am J Pathol 1984;115:349–361.

127. Seki H, Yoshimoto T, Ogawa A, Suzuki J. Hemodynamics in hemorrhagic infarction—an experimental study. Stroke 1985;16:647–651.

128. Semenza GL. Hypoxia-inducible factor I: control of oxygen homeostasis in health and disease. Pediatr Res 2001;49:614–617.

129. Semenza, GL, Agani F, Feldser D, et al. Hypoxia, HIF-1, and the pathophysiology of common human diseases. In: Lahiri S, Prabhakar NR, Forster II RE (eds). Oxygen sensing. Molecule to man. Adv Exp Med and Biol, Vol 475. New York: Kluwer Academic/Plenum Publishers, 2000, pp. 123–130.

130. Serafín A, Roselló-Catafau J, Prats N, et al. Ischemic preconditioning increases the tolerance of fatty liver to hepatic ischemia-reperfusion injury in the rat. Am J Pathol 2002;161:587–601.

131. Shanley PF, Johnson GC. Calcium and acidosis in renal hypoxia. Lab Invest 1991;65:298–305.

132. Sheehan HL, Davis JC. Renal ischaemia with failed reflow. J Pathol Bacteriol 1959b;78:105–120.

133. Shen Y-T, Kudej RK, Bishop SP, Vatner SF. Inotropic reserve and histological appearance of hibernating myocardium in conscious pigs with ameroid-induced coronary stenosis. Basic Res Cardiol 1996;91:479–485.

134. Siesjö BK. Acidosis and ischemic brain damage. Neurochem Pathol 1988;9:31–88.

135. Singbartl K, Green SA, Ley K. Blocking P-selectin protects from ischemia/reperfusion-induced acute renal failure. FASEB J 2000;14:48–54.

136. Strock PE, Majno G. Vascular responses to experimental tourniquet ischemia. Surg Gynecol Obstet 1969a;129:309–318.

137. Strock PE, Majno G. Microvascular changes in acutely ischemic rat muscle. Surg Gynecol Obstet 1969b;129:1213–1224.

138. Summers WK, Jamison RL. The no reflow phenomenon in renal ischemia. Lab Invest 1971;25:635–643.

138a. Tohgi H, Yamanouchi H, Murakami M, Kameyama M. Importance of the hematocrit as a risk factor in cerebral infarction. Stroke 1978;9:369–374.

139. Torvik A. The pathogenesis of watershed infarcts in the brain. Stroke 1984;15:221–223.

140. Tsao M-S, Schraufnagel D, Wang N-S. Pathogenesis of pulmonary infarction. Am J Med 1982;72:599–606.

141. Vander Heide RS, Angelo JP, Altschuld RA, Ganote CE. Energy dependence of contraction band formation in perfused hearts and isolated adult myocytes. Am J Pathol 1986;125:55–68.

142. van Hof MW, Wildervanck de Blécourt EMW. Early brain damage due to hypoxia. In: Almli CR, Finger S, eds. Early brain damage, vol 1. Research orientations and clinical observations. New York: Academic Press, 1984, pp. 81–91.

143. van Royen N, Piek JJ, Buschmann I, et al. Stimulation of arteriogenesis: a new concept for the treatment of arterial occlusive disease. Cardiovasc Res 2001;49:543–553.

144. Vander Salm TJ, Pape LA, Price J, Burke M. Hemorrhage from myocardial revascularization. J Thorac Cardiovasc Surg 1981;82:768–772.

145. Vedder NB, Winn RK, Rice CL, et al. Inhibition of leukocyte adherence by anti-CD18 monoclonal antibody attenuates reperfusion injury in the rabbit ear. Proc Natl Acad Sci USA 1990;87:2643–2646.

146. Vivaldi MT, Kloner RA, Schoen FJ. Triphenyltetrazolium staining of irreversible ischemic injury following coronary artery occlusion in rats. Am J Pathol 1985;121:522–530.

147. Walz W. (ed). Cerebral Ischemia: Molecular and Cellular Pathophysiology. Totowa, NJ: Humana Press, 1999.

148. Wenger RH. Mammalian oxygen sensing, signaling and gene regulation. Exp Biol 2000;203:1253–1263.

149. White HD, Norris RM, Brown MA, et al. Effect of intravenous streptokinase on left ventricular function and early survival after acute myocardial infarction. N Engl J Med 1987;317:850–855.

150. Wijns W, Vatner SF, Camici PG. Hibernating myocardium. N Engl J Med 1998;339:173–181.

151. Willms-Kretschmer K, Majno G. Ischemia of the skin. Electron microscopic study of vascular injury. Am J Pathol 1969;54:327–353.

152. Yamazaki T, Seko Y, Tamatani T, et al. Expression of intercellular adhesion molecule-1 in rat-heart with ischemia/reperfusion and limitation of infract size by treatment with antibodies against cell adhesion molecules. Am J Pathol 1993;143: 410–418.

153. Yellon DM, Baxter GF. Reperfusion injury revisited: is there a role for growth factor signaling in limiting lethal reperfusion injury? Trends Cardiovasc Med 1999;9:245–249.

154. Yoshidome H, Kato A, Miyazaki M, Edwards MJ, Lentsch AB. IL-13 activates STAT6 and inhibits liver injury induced by ischemia/reperfusion. Am J Pathol 1999;155:1059–1064.

155. Zahn FW. Ueber die Folgen des Verschlusses der Lungenarterien und Pfortaderäste durch Embolie. Verh Ges Dtsch Naturforsch Ärzte 1898;69:9–11.

156. Zhang J-Z, Behrooz A, Ismail-Beigi F. Regulation of glucose transport by hypoxia. Am J Kidney Dis 1999;34:189–202.

157. Ziegler E. Ueber Myomalacia cordis. Virchows Arch Pathol Anat Physiol Klin Med 1882;90:211–212.

158. Zimmerman ANE, Daems W, Hülsmann WC, et al. Morphological changes of heart muscle caused by successive perfusion with calcium-free and calcium-containing solutions (calcium paradox). Cardiovasc Res 1967;1:201–209.

Shock

159. Bailey RW, Brengman ML, Fuh KC, et al. Hemodynamic pathogenesis of ischemic hepatic injury following cardiogenic shock/resuscitation. Shock 2000;14:451–459.

160. Bagge U, Amundson B, Lauritzen C. White blood cell deformability and plugging of skeletal muscle capillaries in hemorrhagic shock. Acta Physiol Scand 1980;180:159–163.

161. Bagge U, Skalak R, Attefors R. Granulocyte rheology. Experimental studies in an *in vitro* micro-flow system. Adv Microcirc 1977;7:29–48.

162. Bannerman DD, Goldblum SE. Direct effects of endotoxin on the endothelium: barrier function and injury. Lab Invest 1999;79:1181–1199.

163. Barroso-Aranda J, Schmid-Schönbein GW. Transformation of neutrophils as indicator of irreversibility in hemorrhagic shock. Am J Physiol 1989;257:H846–H852.

164. Barroso-Aranda J, Schmid-Schönbein GW, Zweifach BW, Engler RL. Granulocytes and no-reflow phenomenon in irreversible hemorrhagic shock. Circ Res 1988;63:437–447.

165. Barroso-Aranda J, Zweifach BW, Mathison JC, Schmid-Schönbein. Neutrophil activation, tumor necrosis factor, and survival after endotoxic and hemorrhagic shock. J Cardiovasc Pharmacol 1995;25(Suppl):S23–S29.

166. Baue AE, Chaudry IH. Prevention of multiple systems failure. Surg Clin North Am 1980;60:1167–1178.

167. Bernard GR, Vincent J-L, Laterre P-F, et al. Efficacy and safety of recombinant human activated protein C for severe sepsis. N Engl J Med 2001;344:699–709.

168. Bond RF. Mediator mechanisms in shock. Fed Proc 1985; 44:273–274.

169. Bone RC. Multiple system organ failure and the sepsis syndrome. Hosp Pract 1991a;26:101–126.

170. Bone RC. The pathogenesis of sepsis. Ann Intern Med 1991b;115:457–469.

171. Bone RC. Toward a theory regarding the pathogenesis of the systemic inflammatory response syndrome: what we do and do not know about cytokine regulation. Crit Care Med 1996;24:163–172.

172. Bone RC, Balk RA, Cerra FB, Dellinger RP. Definitions for sepsis and organ failure and guidelines for the use of innovative therapies in sepsis. Chest 1992;101:1644–1655.

173. Bone RC, Sibbald WJ, Sprung CL. The ACCP-SCCM consensus conference on sepsis and organ failure. Chest 1992; 101:1481–1483.

174. Brånemark PI. Intravascular anatomy of blood cells in man. Basel: S. Karger, 1971.

175. Braunwald E, Faci AS, Kasper DL, et al. (eds). Harrison's Principles of Internal Medicine. 15th ed. New York: McGraw Hill, 2001.

176. Brezis M, Rosen S. Hypoxia of the renal medulla— its implications for disease. N Engl J Med 1995;332:647–655.

177. Carey LC. Shock: differential diagnosis and immediate treatment. Hosp Med 1975;11:68–93.

178. Chang J, Hackel DB. Comparative study of myocardial lesions in hemorrhagic shock. Lab Invest 1973;28:641–647.

179. Chang T-W. Improvement of survival from hemorrhagic shock by enterectomy in rats: finding to implicate the role of the gut for irreversibility of hemorrhagic shock. J Trauma 1997;42:223–230.

180. Clozel M, Kuhn H, Baumgartner HR. Procoagulant activity of endotoxin-treated human endothelial cells exposed to native human flowing blood. Blood 1989;73:729–733.

180a. Cohen J. The immunopathogenesis of sepsis. Nature 2002;420:885–891.

181. Colman RW. The role of plasma proteases in septic shock. N Engl J Med 1989;320:1207–1209.

182. Czermak BJ, Breckwoldt M, Ravage ZB, et al. Mechanisms of enhanced lung injury during sepsis. Am J Pathol 1999;154:1057–1065.

183. Dal Nogare AR. Southwestern Internal Medicine Conference: septic shock. Am J Med Sci 1991;302:50–65.

184. Deitch EA. Multiple organ failure: pathophysiology and potential future therapy. Ann Surg 1992;216:117–134.

185. Dinarello CA. The proinflammatory cytokines interleukin-1 and tumor necrosis factor and treatment of the septic shock syndrome. J Infect Dis 1991;163:1177–1184.

186. Doherty DE, Zagarella L, Henson PM, Worthen GS. Lipopolysaccharide stimulates monocyte adherence by effects on both the monocyte and the endothelial cell. J Immunol 1989;143:3673–3679.

187. Ferguson DW, Abboud FM. The pathophysiology, recognition, and management of shock. In: Hurst JW, ed. The heart, 7th ed. New York: McGraw-Hill Information Services Company, 1990, pp. 442–461.

188. Fine J. The bacterial factor in traumatic shock. Springfield, IL: Charles C. Thomas, 1954.

189. Fink MP, Cohn SM, Lee PC, et al. Effect of lipopolysaccharide on intestinal intramucosal hydrogen ion concentration in pigs: evidence of gut ischemia in a normodynamic model of septic shock. Crit Care Med 1989a;17:641–646.

190. Fink MP, Rothschild HR, Deniz YF, Cohn SM. Complement depletion with *Naje haje* cobra venom factor limits prostaglandin release and improves visceral perfusion in porcine endotoxic shock. J Trauma 1989b;29:1076–1085.

191. Fischer JE. Metabolism in surgical patients: protein, carbohydrate, and fat utilization by oral and parenteral routes. In: Townsend CM, Beauchamp RD, Evers BM, Mattox KL (eds). Sabiston Textbook of Surgery, 16th ed. Philadelphia: W.B. Saunders Company, 2001, pp. 90.

192. Fischer CJ, Agosti JM, Opal SM, et al. Treatment of septic shock with tumor necrosis factor receptor:Fc fusion protein. N Engl J Med. 1996;334:1697–1702.

193. Freeman BD, Eichacker PQ, Natanson C. The role of inflammation in sepsis and septic shock: a meta-analysis of both clinical and preclinical trials of anti-inflammatory therapies. In: Gallin JI, Snyderman R. (eds). Inflammation: Basic Principles and Clinical Correlates. 3rd ed. Philadelphia: Lippincott Williams & Wilkins, 1999.

194. Freeman BD, Natanson C. Anti-inflammatory therapies in sepsis and septic shock. Expert Opinion Investigational 2000;9:1651–1663.

195. Fries JW, Williams AJ, Atkins RC, et al. Expression of VCAM-1 and E-selectin in an *in vivo* model of endothelial activation. Am J Pathol 1993;143:725–737.

196. Garcia JH. Morphology of global cerebral ischemia. Crit Care Med 1988;16:979–987.

197. Gitlin N, Serio KM. Ischemic hepatitis: widening horizons. Am J Gastroenterol 1992;87:831–836.

198. Goris RJA, Boekholtz WKF, van Bebber IPT, Nuytinck JKS, Schillings PHM. Multiple-organ failure and sepsis without bacteria. Arch Surg 1986;121:897–901.

199. Guyton AC. Textbook of medical physiology, 7th ed. Philadelphia: WB Saunders, 1986.

200. Hackel DB, Ratliff NB, Mikat E. The heart in shock. Circ Res 1974;35:805–811.

201. Hayward R, Lefer AM. Time course of endothelial-neutrophil interaction in splanchnic artery ischemia-reperfusion. Am J Physiol 1998:275:H2080–H2086.

202. Hardaway RM. Shock: the reversible stage of dying. Littleton, MA: PSG Publishing Commpany, 1988.

203. Harlan JM, Harker LA, Reidy MA, et al. Lipopolysaccharide-mediated bovine endothelial cell injury *in vitro*. Lab Invest 1983;48:269–274.

204. Kistler EB, Hugli TE, Schmid-Schönbein GW. The pancreas as a source of cardiovascular cell activating factors. Microcirculation 2000;7:183–192.

205. Lefer AM. Interaction between myocardial depressant factor and vasoactive mediators with ischemia and shock. Am J Physiol 1987;252:R193–R205.

206. Lindberg B. Liver circulation and metabolism in haemorrhagic shock. Acta Chir Scand Suppl 1977;476:1–18.

207. Martin AM Jr, Green WB, Simmons RL, Soloway HB. Human myocardial zonal lesions. Arch Pathol 1969;87:339–342.

208. Martin AM Jr, Hackel DB. The myocardium of the dog in hemorrhagic shock. A histochemical study. Lab Invest 1963;12:77–91.

209. Martin AM Jr, Hackel DB, Kurtz SM. The ultrastructure of zonal lesions of the myocardium in hemorrhagic shock. Am J Pathol 1964;44:127–140.

210. Matthay MA. The acute respiratory distress syndrome. N Engl J Med 1996;334:1469–1470.

211. Matthay MA. Severe sepsis—a new treatment with both anticoagulant and antiinflammatory properties. N Eng J Med 2001;344:759–762.

212. Mazzoni MC, Schmid-Schönbein GW. Mechanisms and consequences of cell activation in the microcirculation. Cardiovasc Res 1996;32:709–719.

213. McCuskey RS, Urbaschek R, Urbaschek B. The microcirculation during endotoxemia. Cardiovasc Res 1996;32:752–763.

214. Mitsouka H, Kistler EB, Schmid-Schönbein. Generation of *in vivo* activating factors in the ischemic intestine by pancreatic enzymes. PNAS 2000;97:1772–1777.

215. Munford RS. Sepsis and Septic Shock. In: Braunwald E, Fauci AS, Kasper DL, Hauser SL, Longo DL, Jameson JL. (eds). Harrison's Principles of Internal Medicine. 15th ed. New York: McGraw Hill, 2001, pp. 799–804.

216. Navab M, Hough GP, Van Lenten BJ, Berliner JA, Fogelman AM. Low density lipoproteins transfer bacterial lipopolysaccharides across endothelial monolayers in a biologically active form. J Clin Invest 1988;81:601–605.

217. Ognibene FP, Martin SE, Parker MM, et al. Adult respiratory distress syndrome in patients with severe neutropenia. N Engl J Med 1986;315:547–551.

218. Opal SM, Huber CE. Sepsis. Chapter 30, Section 7. WebMD, Scientific American Medicine, 2001.

219. Parrillo JE. The cardiovascular pathophysiology of sepsis. Annu Rev Med 1989;40:469–485.

220. Parrillo JE, Burch C, Shelhamer JH, et al. A circulating myocardial depressant substance in humans with septic shock. J Clin Invest 1985;76:1539–1553.

221. Parrillo JE, Parker MM, Natanson C, et al. Septic shock in humans: advances in the understanding of pathogenesis, cardiovascular dysfunction, and therapy. Ann Intern Med 1990;113:227–242.

222. Parrillo J. Pathogenetic mechanisms of septic shock. N Engl J Med 1993;328:1471–1477.

223. Pinsky MR, Matuschak GM. A unifying hypothesis of multiple system organ failure: failure of host defense homeostasis. J Crit Care 1990;5:108–114.

224. Ratliff NB, Kopelman RI, Goldner RD, Cruz PT, Hackel DB. Formation of myocardial zonal lesions. Am J Pathol 1975;79:321–334.

225. Redl H, Dinges HP, Buurman WA, et al. Expression of endothelial leukocyte adhesion molecule-1 in septic but not traumatic/hypovolemic shock in the baboon. Am J Pathol 1991;139:461–466.

226. Redl H, Schlag G, Bahrami S, et al. The cytokine network in trauma and sepsis: TNF and IL-8. In: Schlag G, Redl H (eds). Pathophysiology of shock, sepsis, and organ failure. Berlin: Springer-Verlag, 1993, pp. 468–490.

227. Schlag G, Redl H. (eds). Pathophysiology of Shock, Sepsis, and Organ Failure. Berlin: Springer-Verlag, 1993.

228. Schlag G, Redl H, Khakpour Z, Davies J, Pretorius J. Hypovolemic-traumatic shock models in baboons. In: Pathophysiology of Shock, Sepsis, and Organ Failure. Berlin: Springer-Verlag, 1993, pp. 384–402.

229. Schweinburg FB, Frank HA, Fine J. Bacterial factor in experimental hemorrhagic shock. Evidence for development of a bacterial factor which accounts for irreversibility to transfusion and for the loss of the normal capacity to destroy bacteria. Am J Physiol 1954;179:532–540.

230. Seeley HF. Pathophysiology of haemorrhagic shock. Br J Hosp Med 1987;37:14–20.

231. Shapiro JI. Functional and metabolic responses of isolated hearts to acidosis: effects of sodium bicarbonate and carbicarb. Am J Physiol 1990;258:H1835–H1839.

232. Sherlock S. Diseases of the liver and biliary system, 8th ed. Oxford: Blackwell Scientific Publications, 1989.

233. Thomas L. The lives of a cell. New York: The Viking Press, 1974.

234. Thomas L. The youngest science. New York: The Viking Press, 1983.

235. Till GO, Hatherill JR, Tourtellotte WW, Lutz MJ, Ward PA. Lipid peroxidation and acute lung injury after thermal trauma to skin. Evidence of a role for hydroxyl radical. Am J Pathol 1985;119:376–384.

236. Till GO, Morganroth ML, Kunkel R, Ward PA. Activation of C5 by cobra venom factor is required in neutrophil-mediated lung injury in the rat. Am J Pathol 1987;129:44–53.

237. Tipper DJ. Antibiotic inhibitors of bacterial cell wall biosynthesis. In: Encyclopedia of Human Biology, Volume 1. New York: Academic Press Inc., 1991, pp. 271–285.

238. Tom WW, Villalba M, Szlabick RE, et al. Fluorophotometric evaluation of capillary permeability in gram-negative shock. Arch Surg 1983;118:636–641.

239. Toung T, Reilly PM, Fuh KC, Ferris R, Bulkley GB. Mesenteric vasoconstriction in response to hemorrhagic shock. Shock 2000;13:267–273.

240. Tracey KJ, Beutler B, Lowry SF, et al. Shock and tissue injury induced by recombinant human cachectin. Science 1986;234:470–474.

241. Vedder NB, Fouty BW, Winn RK, Harlan JM, Rice CL. Role of neutrophils in generalized reperfusion injury associated with resuscitation from shock. Surgery 1989;106:509–516.

242. Vedder NB, Winn RK, Rice CL, Harlan JM. Neutrophilmediated vascular injury in shock and multiple organ failure. Prog Clin Biol Res 1989;299:181–191.

243. Vukajlovich SW, Hoffman J, Morrison DC. Activation of human serum complement by bacterial lipopolysaccharides: structural requirements for antibody independing activation of the classical and alternative pathways. Mol Immunol 1987;24:319–331.

244. Ward PA, Till GO, Hatherill JR, Annesley TM, Kunkel RG. Systemic complement activation, lung injury, and products of lipid peroxidation. J Clin Invest 1985;76:517–527.

245. Ware LB, Matthay MA. The acute respiratory distress syndrome. N Engl J Med 2000;342:1334–1349.

246. Whisler RL, Cornwell DG, Proctor KVW, Downs E. Bacterial lipopolysaccharide acts on human endothelial cells to enhance the adherence of peripheral blood monocytes. J Lab Clin Med 1989;114:708–716.

247. Williams AB, Decourten-Myers GM, Fischer JE, et al. Sepsis stimulates release of myofilaments in skeletal muscle by a calcium-dependent mechanism. FASEB J 1999;13:1435–1443.

248. Wyngaarden JB, Smith LH, eds. Cecil textbook of medicine, vol 1, 16th ed. Philadelphia: WB Saunders, 1982.

249. Zimmerman JJ, Dietrich KA. Current perspectives on septic shock. Pediatr Clin North Am 1987;34:131–163.

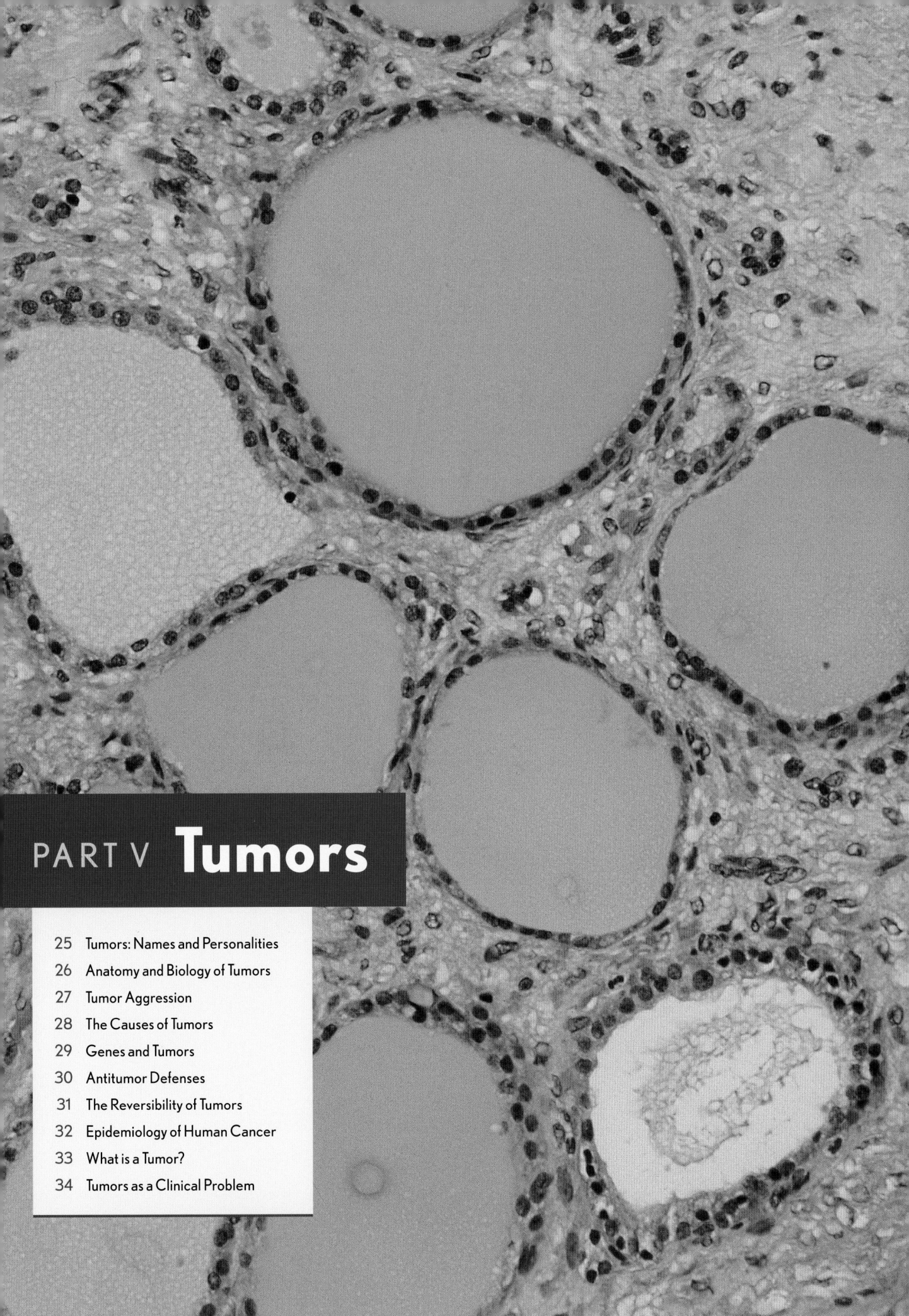

PART V **Tumors**

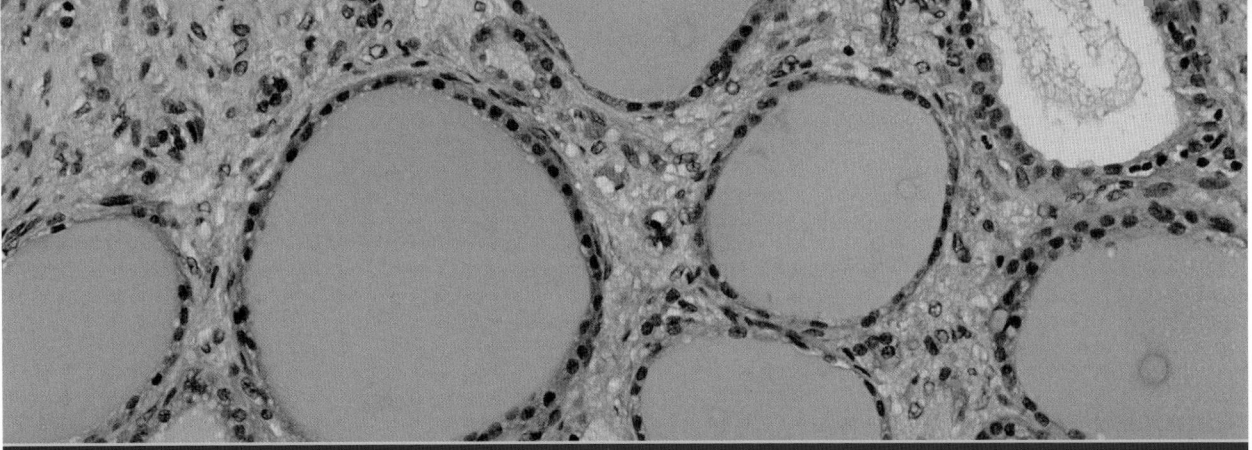

TUMORS: NAMES AND PERSONALITIES

In multicellular animals and plants, all organs live and function thanks to the planned, harmonious, highly disciplined cooperation of different types of cells. One of the accidents that can disrupt this harmony is the focal, purposeless overgrowth of one of the cellular components: this is, in essence, a **tumor.**

It is fortunate that we are writing this chapter well after 1976. Before that year, the world of tumors—as seen by the nonexpert—was quite depressing. Tumor cells were outlaws, cells gone mad. They seemed to follow no rules. The subject of tumors contrasted sharply with other topics of general pathology, which have a neat internal logic of their own: vascular disturbances are almost as logical as plumbing problems, inflammation reads like an epic of self-defense, diapedesis is beautiful and we know what it means. Nothing was intellectually beautiful about tumors, and little was predictable; in fact, the eminent Mexican pathologist Ruy Pérez Tamayo once said very aptly that no generalization could be made about tumors, except this one—namely, that no generalization could be made.

Then it was realized, almost overnight, that many tumors are driven by *normal* growth-related genes that are expressed inappropriately (**oncogenes**); and other tumors are triggered by the loss of genes that *normally* repress growth (**suppressor genes**). So, tumor cells are neither outlaws nor mad; they are ordinary cells that are simply obeying the wrong orders. In some cases they are even ready to mend their ways if the internal driving message can be corrected. Because there are so many types of cells—about 200 in humans—and so many genes as sources of orders (about 30,000 genes [3]) the variety of tumors is so great that the underlying unity is hard to discern; in humans the types of tumors that the pathologist's microscope can distinguish is on the order of 600 and growing. Thus the novice will probably continue to be struck more by the variety than by the unity. However, the important point is that at long last we have the tools to work out some basic rules of the game, at the level of the genes.

And so the story of tumors has developed into a huge web of hard facts, overlapping all other chapters of general pathology and reaching, more than any other type of disease, into all facets of human life: from the embryo and genetics to worldly professions, nutrition, sex, toxicology, and the environment of our planet.

Tumors: A Working Definition

As a start, we must be content with a working definition of a tumor, because a flawless one does not exist. We will be better prepared to answer the question "What is a tumor?" at the end of this section (p. 945).

Henry Pitot, author of an excellent book on tumors (19), proposed this sober statement: *A tumor is a heritably altered, relatively autonomous growth of tissue.* Everyone would accept that tumors represent a *growth,* as long as we add that some tumors stop growing for years. *Heritable* means passed on from tumor cell to daughter cell, not from parents to children, although that happens too. The reference to *tissue* is meant to imply that tumors are a curse of multicellular creatures, be they animals or plants (21). Nature imposes a "tumor burden" (a standard expression of oncologists) even on corals (1), oysters, fruit flies (Figure 25.1) (9, 10), and salmon (Figure 25.2).

> Is it really true that unicellular organisms are spared? Paramecia exposed to carcinogens develop peculiar shapes (6, 17). Also, we could visualize a science-fiction horror story of amoebae in a pond proliferating out of control like a monstrous leukemia and perhaps metastasizing to other ponds. Somehow this does not happen, but we consulted some yeast experts, and learned the following. Normal yeast cells are very sensitive to food deprivation; when food supplies become scarce, they withdraw from the cell cycle and dramatically reduce their metabolic activity. If they are transfected with the *ras*2 oncogene (homologous to the various human *ras* oncogenes) they proliferate out of control, and when nutrients run out they just die. It seems to us that this condition is not far removed from a yeast leukemia (6, 17).

Tumors in general, including benign and malignant varieties, differ from other types of growth in at least four ways:

- *They are purposeless,* meaning that, in the human perspective, they are of no conceivable use to the host. In the perspective of certain viruses, of course, a tumor serves a vital purpose.
- *They tend to be atypical,* which means that their microscopic patterns and their individual cells are structurally and functionally abnormal to varying degrees.

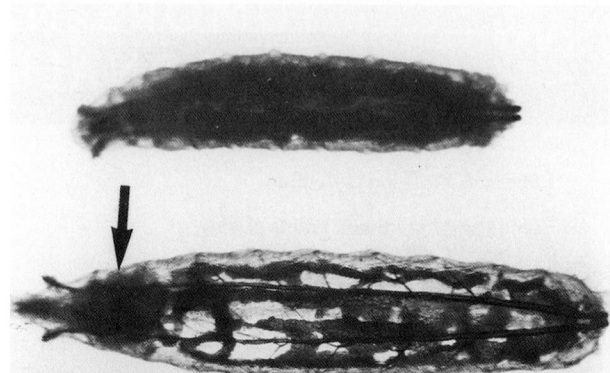

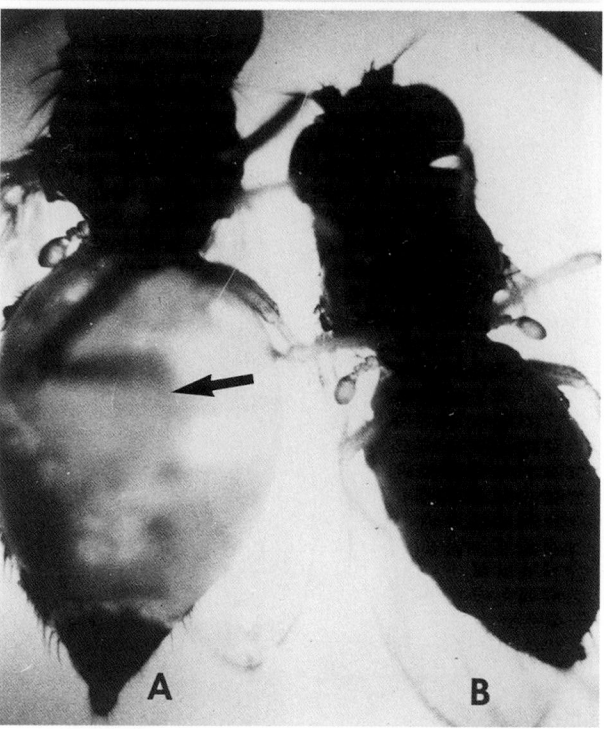

FIGURE 25.1   Tumor in the fruit fly, *Drosophila melanogaster.* *Top:* Normal larva and a larger mutant larva containing a tumorous mass in the frontal part (neuroblastoma, **arrow**). *Bottom* **A:** Bloated adult, which has been injected with tumorous brain tissue (*Drosophila* neuroblastoma) that is now growing in the abdomen (**arrow**), as was confirmed by histology. **B:** Control. (Reproduced with permission from [9].)

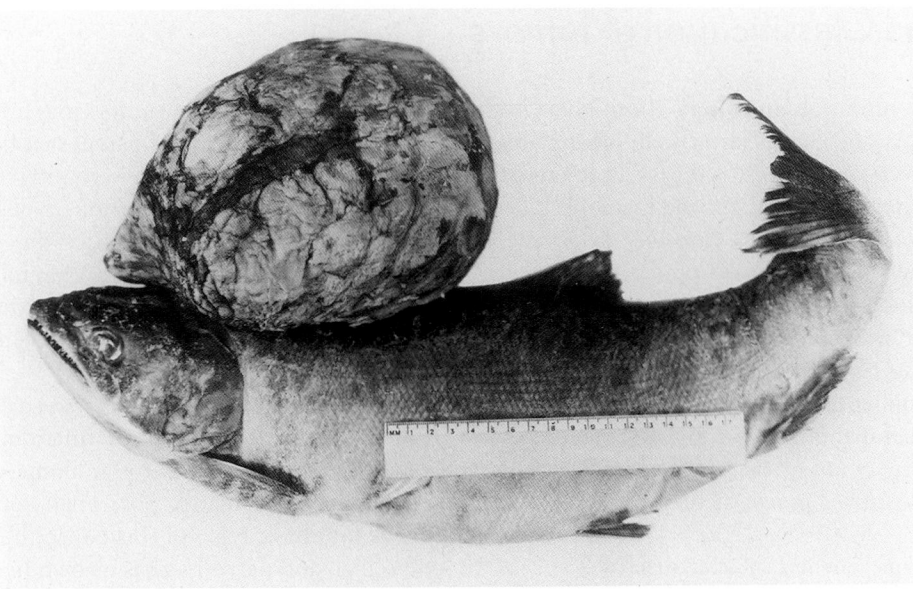

FIGURE 25.2   Coho salmon with a fibrolipoma. (Courtesy of Dr. J. C. Harshbarger, Smithsonian Institute, Washington, DC.)

- *They tend to be autonomous;* that is, they escape the controls that regulate growth (they only *tend* to escape; fortunately for many patients, some tumors do respond to controlling hormones).
- *They tend to be aggressive;* that is, they invade the host.

TO SUM UP: Tumors are purposeless growths of tissue that tend to be atypical, autonomous, and aggressive.

Benign and Malignant: Points of View

The reader should be ready for a surprise. Whereas "everybody knows" that some tumors are benign and others are malignant, experts in tumor biology do not. They mostly ignore benign tumors and almost never talk about them. The experimental production of a tumor is called **carcinogenesis,** which means production of **cancer,** a malignant tumor. To our knowledge, there is not even a book about benign tumors. We consulted some experts, and the upshot was that when they speak of tumors in general they are referring to malignant tumors, because *they assume that all tumors are malignant or on their way to becoming malignant.* So-called benign tumors are just beginning to have a place in the current theories of carcinogenesis, as a facultative step on the way to malignancy (see Figure 29.8); an occasional oddity that is not easily explained. We shall return more than once to this important point (pp. 952, 770, 782).

However, we must advise worried readers that in real life (of people, as opposed to experimental animals), benign-behaving tumors do exist, as a clinical reality if not as a scientific entity. It is everyday clinical experience that some human tumors behave *predictably* as benign; fibroadenomas of the breast and most lipomas fall into this category. After they have been removed, the patients can forget about them; exceptions are extremely rare.

Regarding the text that follows, we want our position to be clear. *When discussing human tumors,* we will use the traditional distinction between "benign" tumors (slowly growing, noninfiltrating, not fatal) and "malignant" tumors (more rapidly growing, infiltrating, metastasizing, and—if untreated—fatal). *When discussing experimental carcinogenesis,* we will follow the party line of the experts: tumors are malignant or on the way to malignancy. In the end, we will attempt to reconcile these views.

Names and Classification of Tumors

The science of tumors is **oncology** (from the Greek *ónkos,* a mass). As oncologists know well, talking about tumor causes great anxiety because the world at large still believes that tumors are mysterious and incurable killers. Therefore, the technical terms *neoplasm* or *neoplasia* (new growth) are sometimes used professionally in the hope that bystanders will not understand. In antiquity the term *tumor* was much less frightening because it meant a swelling of any kind, including the pregnant abdomen; remember that *tumor* is one of the four cardinal signs of inflammation. This is a good time to point out that a *swelling or lump may correspond to a variety of disturbances other than a tumor,* such as:

- A bacterial infection (e.g., abscess, tuberculosis)
- An inflammatory response to other pathogens (e.g., parasites, fungi, viruses)
- A rheumatic nodule
- An enlarged lymph node
- A hematoma (spilled blood)
- An aneurysm
- A hernia
- A bone callus (healed fracture)
- A malformation

Cancer is synonymous with malignant tumor; the Latin *cancer* is actually a literal translation of the Greek *karkínos* for crab, a common creature on Mediterranean shores. In the Hippocratic books, *karkínos* and *karkínoma* are used for conditions that we would almost certainly call *carcinoma* (epithelial cancer) or, more generally, *cancer.* There seem to have been many reasons for borrowing the image of the crab, and the choice was extraordinarily successful: the name of the innocent crustacean has become a sinister metaphor, even for the destructive ills ("cancers") of society (24).

> In the second century A.D., Galen explained that "cancer of the breast is so called because of the fancied resemblance to a crab given by the lateral prolongations of the tumor and the adjacent distended veins" (20). Radiating dilated veins often do appear over and around a bulging tumor. In the sixteenth century, Gabriele Falloppio (of Fallopian tube fame) reviewed the ancient origins of the name, gave the explanations that we have mentioned, and added one more: cancers are "extremely hard, rough tumors, resembling a crab in this respect as well" (20). Today the claws of the Greek crab describe just as effectively what we see of breast cancer through the microscope or on mammograms: ominous offshoots with which a cancerous mass seems to "grab" the surrounding tissues.

The nomenclature of tumors is as untidy as might be expected of a collection of names that began 2500 years ago. After it was realized—around 1885 (20)—that each type of tumor represents one type of cell, an effort was made to name all tumors accordingly; but tradition could not be wholly displaced. What follows is the ABC of tumor terminology; we can not discuss dozens of tumors of different types without being familiar with their names (Table 25.1).

Note first that the ending *-oma* usually denotes a tumor, just as *-itis* denotes inflammation. The inevitable exceptions include granuloma, atheroma, glaucoma, and neuroma (p. 30). Then consider that each of the four basic types of tissue—epithelial, connective, muscular, and nervous—has its own benign and malignant tumors.

> A molecular classification of tumors based on gene expression and microarray technology is not yet available, but the first steps have been taken (11, 16). Some pathologists worry that their microscopes may be replaced by computers and maps of genes (16). We doubt that this will happen; in the history of pathology new technologies have added depth to the old ones without displacing them. However, it will be fascinating to see how the new classification of tumors will fit with the time-honored histologic classification.

Tumors of Epithelia

Tumors of epithelial origin represent about 80 percent of all tumors.

Benign. Benign tumors of epithelium can arise from glands or surface linings. Those that arise *from glands,* whether exocrine or endocrine, are called **adenomas** (from *adén,* gland). Examples are pancreatic adenoma, salivary gland adenoma, and sweat gland adenoma (the last two also have more fanciful Greek names: *sialoadenoma* and *hydroadenoma*). Adenomas riddled with cavities (cysts) are called *cystadenomas.*

Benign epithelial tumors arising *from surfaces* are more readily seen and have earned colorful descriptive names referring to their shapes (Figure 25.3). A club-shaped tumor arising (or dangling) from a surface by means of a stalk is called a **polyp** (Figures 25.4, 25.5); if the polyp lacks a stalk it is called a *sessile polyp,* which means "sitting" (as in the word *session*). In either case the neoplastic part is only the covering epithelium; the core is just connective tissue stroma. If a polyp also contains some glandular growth, we speak of an *adenomatous polyp.*

Table 25.1 Nomenclature of Tumors

Cell/Tissue of Origin	Benign Tumor	Malignant Tumor
Tumors of Epithelia		
Covering epithelia	**Polyp, papilloma**	**Carcinoma, papillary carcinoma**
Squamous stratified	Squamous cell papilloma	Squamous cell carcinoma
Basal cells	Seborrheic keratosis*	Basal cell carcinoma
Mesothelial cells	Fibrous mesothelioma (rare)	Mesothelioma
Urinary (transitional epithelium)	Transitional cell papilloma	Transitional cell carcinoma
Glandular epithelia	**Adenoma**	**Adenocarcinoma**
	Cystadenoma	**Cystadenocarcinoma**
	Papillary adenoma	**Papillary adenocarcinoma**
Liver cells	Liver cell adenoma	Hepatoma
Renal tubules	Renal cell adenoma	Renal cell carcinoma (formerly hypernephroma)
Testicular tubules	▇	Seminoma
		Embryonal carcinoma
Placental epithelium	Hydatidiform mole	Choriocarcinoma
Tumors of Connective Tissues		
Fibroblasts	Fibroma	Fibrosarcoma
Immature (fetal) fibroblasts	Myxoma	Myxosarcoma
Fat cells (lipoblasts)	Lipoma	Liposarcoma
Chondrocytes	Chondroma	Chondrosarcoma
Osteoblasts	Osteoma	Osteosarcoma
Meningeal cells	Meningioma	Malignant meningioma
Synovial cells	▇	Synoviosarcoma
Endothelium: blood vessels	Hemangioma	Hemangiosarcoma
Endothelium: lymphatics	Lymphangioma	Lymphangiosarcoma
Erythroblasts	▇	Erythroleukemia
Myeloblasts		Myeloblastic leukemia
Monoblasts		Monocytic leukemia
Lymphocytes		Lymphomas, myeloma, lymphocytic leukemia
Tumors of Muscular Tissues		
Striated muscle	Rhabdomyoma (rare)	Rhabdomyosarcoma
Smooth muscle	Leiomyoma	Leiomyosarcoma
Tumors of Neural Origin		
Astrocytes	Astrocytoma	Glioblastoma
Oligodendrocytes	Oligodendroglioma	Malignant oligodendroglioma
Ependymal cells	Ependymoma	Malignant ependymoma
Schwann cells	Schwannoma	Malignant schwannoma
Neuroblasts	Ganglioneuroma†	Neuroblastoma
Melanocytes	Nevus	Melanoma
Mixed Tumors (two or more cell types but from one germ layer)		
Salivary glands	Pleomorphic adenoma	Malignant mixed tumor of salivary gland
Renal blastoma	▇	Wilms' tumor (nephroblastoma)
Teratomas (several cell types representing all three embryonal germ layers)		
Totipotential cells	Mature teratoma, dermoid cyst	Teratocarcinoma

A display of the somewhat erratic tumor terminology. The red blocks emphasize the peculiar fact that some malignant tumors have no benign counterpart; other benign counterparts are indicated as rare.

*Strange names are common in dermatology. This one applies to a very common warty growth that has nothing to do with seborrhea.

†Ganglioneuroma as a benign tumor is unusual: instead of being a precursor of the corresponding malignant tumor (as many benign tumors are), it arises by differentiation of the malignant form.

Polyps appear as soft, fleshy masses growing out of the skin or a mucosa. Their appearance explains the name, which takes us back to the sunny shores of Greece: it means octopus (*poly*-pus, many feet, is an imprecise version of *octo*-pus, eight feet). Figure 25.6 shows an ancient Greek representation of an octopus; its body even recalls the peduncle of a typical polyp (*peduncle* = stalk).

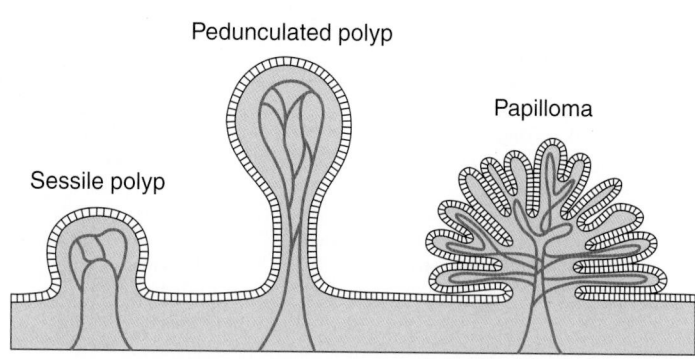

FIGURE 25.3 Nomenclature of epithelial tumors protruding from the skin or from a mucosal surface. NOTE: both polyps and papillomas can be either sessile or pedunculated. A pedunculated papilloma (not shown in the diagram) is illustrated in Figure 25.5. In common parlance these benign growths are often lumped together as "polyps."

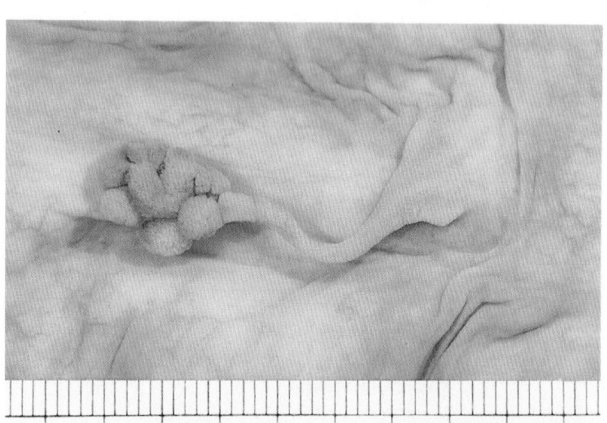

FIGURE 25.4 Typical "polyp" of the colon found incidentally at autopsy. Note the long peduncle, which favors twisting and thereby bleeding. **Scale** in millimeters.

A **papilloma** is also an outgrowth from an epithelial surface, but it has long, thin branches (*papillae*) (Figures 25.7, 25.8, 25.9). There is a good reason for distinguishing polyps from papillomas. Simple geometry tells us that a papilloma has more epithelial surface and therefore more tumor mass than a polyp of comparable size. This means that papillomas tend to grow more actively than polyps; malignant tumors arise from papillomas more often than from polyps.

> NOTE: If the papillae are packed tightly together, a papilloma may look like a polyp (Figure 25.10). A fitting comparison is that of a cauliflower; only a lengthwise cut reveals its branching structure.

You may wonder why the epithelium of a papilloma should grow outward and create branches, rather than grow downward and create blind canals. The latter does happen, and the result is called an *inverted papilloma,* a

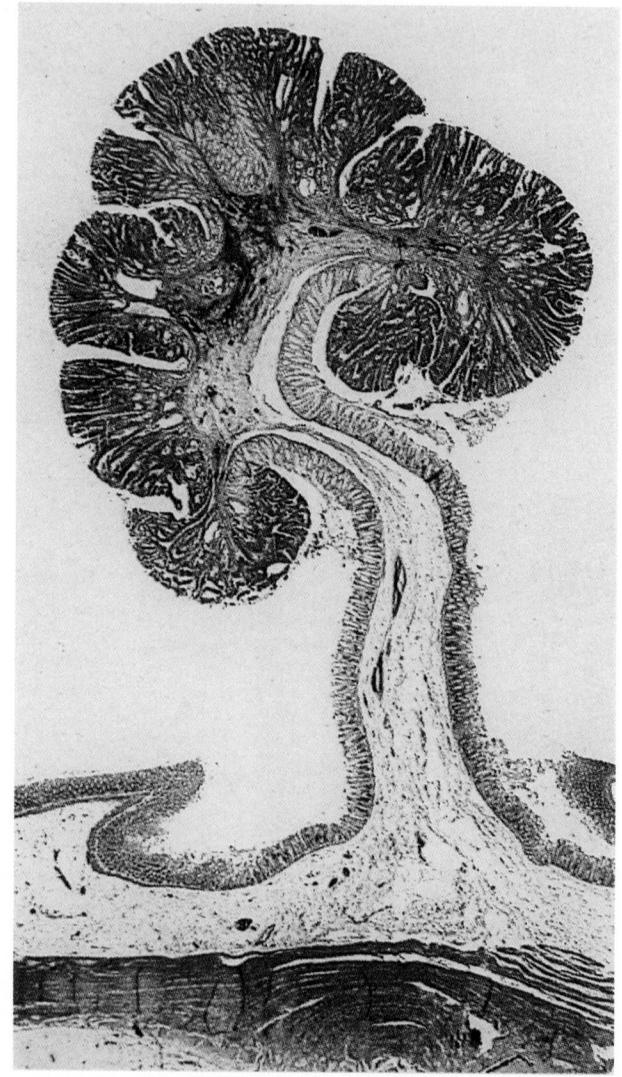

FIGURE 25.5 Cross section of a typical colorectal "polyp" (actually pedunculated papilloma). The tumor is found lying on the mucosa as shown in Figure 25.4; its head tends to be dragged along by the stools, and as it is stretched and twisted, it may easily bleed. (Reproduced with permission from [7].)

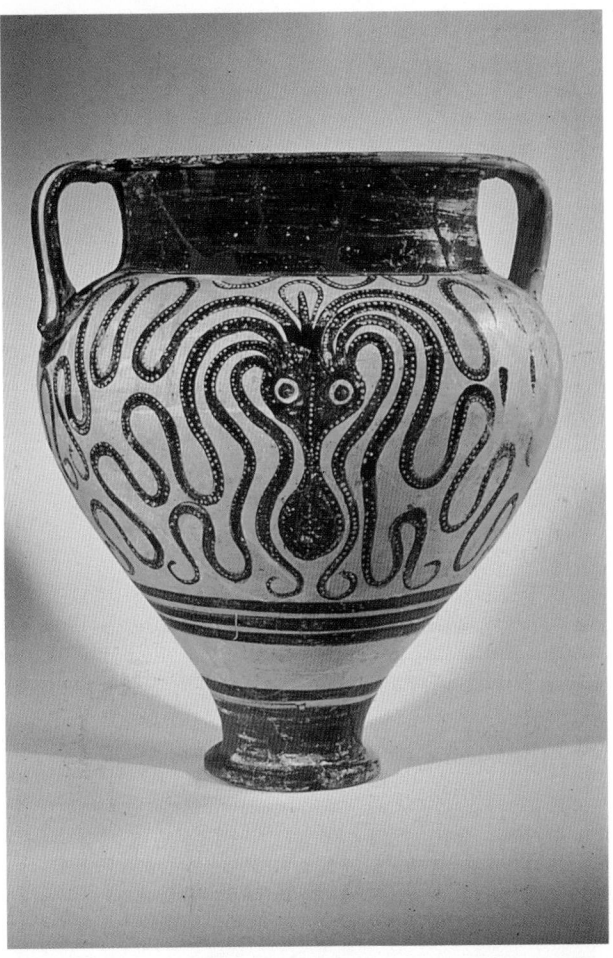

FIGURE 25.6 *Polyp* comes from the Greek word for "octopus." This is how the Greeks saw an octopus; the oblong, pear-shaped body is actually very similar to what we now call a pedunculated polyp. From a Mycaenean vase, about 1350 BC. (Courtesy of the Trustees, British Museum, London, England.)

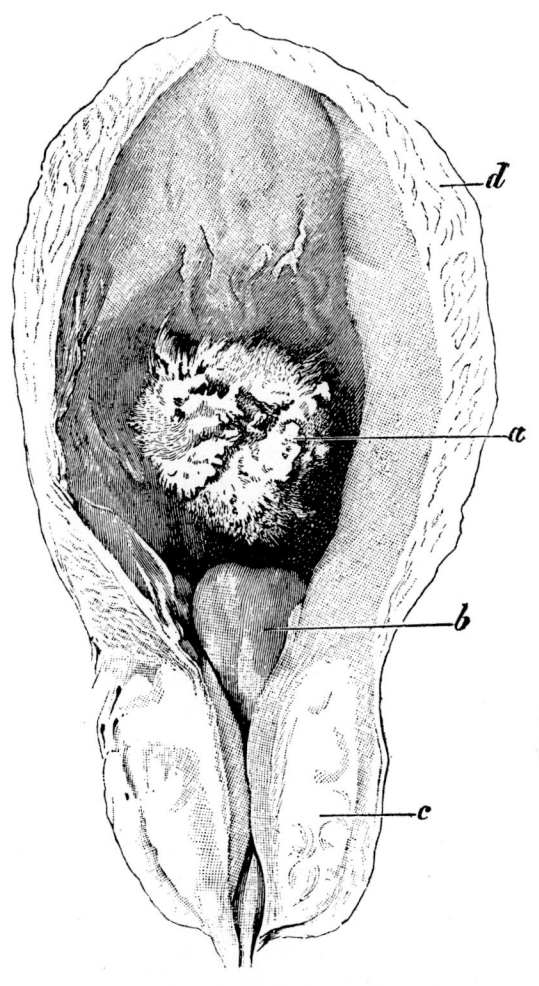

FIGURE 25.7 Papilloma of the urinary bladder as illustrated in 1908. **a:** Papilloma. **b, c:** Enlarged prostate. **d:** Thickened wall of the urinary bladder (the smooth muscle layer developed hypertrophy in response to the resistance caused by the enlarged prostate). (Reproduced from [25].)

rare occurrence. Such papillomas arise in the nose and in the bladder.

Malignant. Malignant epithelial tumors are called **carcinomas;** those that arise from glands are **adenocarcinomas.** The basic names carcinoma and adenocarcinoma are often qualified by descriptive terms that indicate the cell of origin (basal cell carcinoma, squamous cell carcinoma), the structure (papillary carcinoma, cystadenocarcinoma, cystic papillary adenocarcinoma), or the function (mucus-secreting adenocarcinoma).

Tumors of Connective Tissues

Tumors of connective tissues have acquired a more orderly set of names. For benign tumors, the basic rule is to add *-oma* to the proliferating cell type:

fibroblasts	fibroma
fat cells	lipoma
blood vessels	hemangioma
lymphatic vessels	lymphangioma
bone	osteoma
cartilage	chondroma
embryonal fibroblasts	myxoma
bone marrow	myeloma

Myelomas are malignant; this is the inevitable exception to the rule. In Figure 25.11, a myeloma of the tibia appears on cross section as a soft lump—soft but capable of eroding its bony casing.

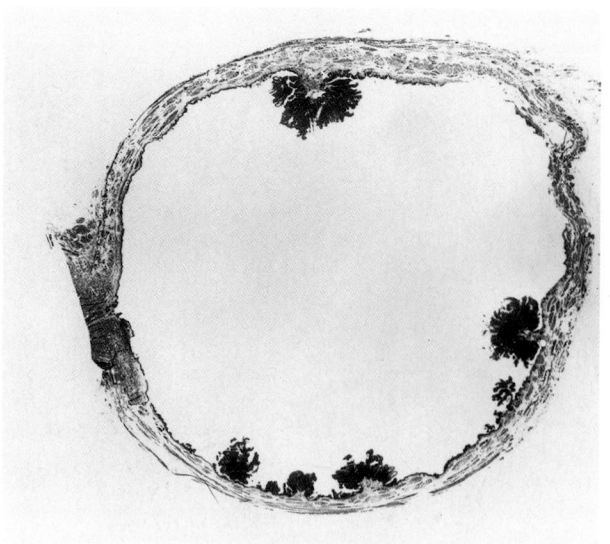

FIGURE 25.8   Section through an entire human bladder showing multiple papillary carcinomas of the "recurrent" type (recurrence does not necessarily occur at the same site as the primary tumor). (Courtesy of Dr. R. O. K. Schade, Dr. L. G. Koss and of the Armed Forces Institute of Pathology. (Reproduced with permission from [15].)

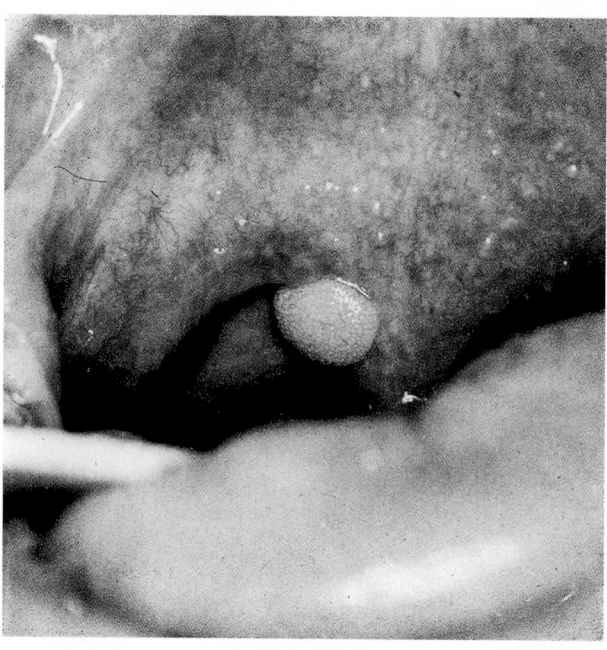

FIGURE 25.10   Papilloma of the soft palate in a 59-year-old man. The papillae appear as tiny white dots; they are too tightly packed to be seen as separate branches. (Courtesy of Dr. G. Fiore-Donno, School of Dentistry, Geneva, Switzerland.)

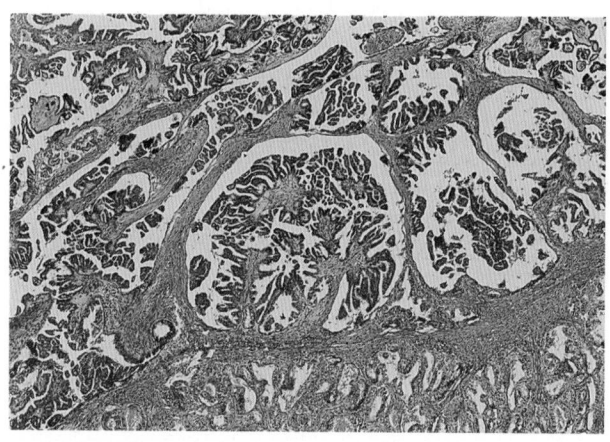

FIGURE 25.9   Architecture of a papillary cystadenocarcinoma. Cysts are rounded spaces lined by epithelium and filled with fluid; if the epithelium produces malignant papillae, the tumor is called papillary cystadenocarcinoma (see Figure 26.29). *Center:* Typical cyst containing at least two branching papillae arising from the wall (*bottom*). The papillae are cut either lengthwise or transversally. (30x)

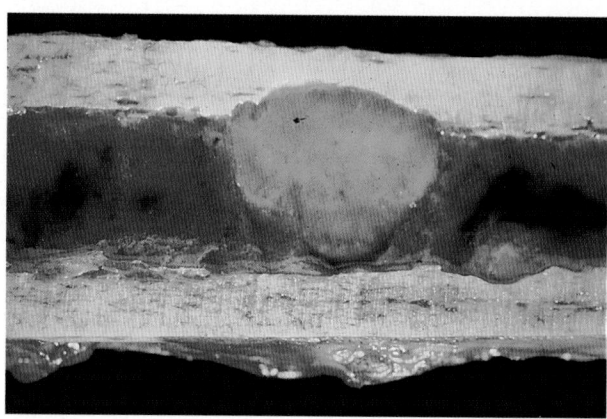

FIGURE 25.11   Tibia cut lengthwise; the patient died of multiple myeloma. *Center:* A lump of malignant plasma cells arising in the bone marrow. Although soft, it has managed to erode the thick bone (*top*).

A *hemangioma* of the liver (Figure 25.12) appears as a dark-red mass embedded in the liver; the single thin-walled vessels are obvious on the cut surface. *Myxomas* are so called because they produce a "myxoid," i.e., "mucuslike" ground substance.

Malignant tumors of connective tissues are called **sarcomas:** hence fibrosarcoma, liposarcoma, chondrosarcoma, and so on. The tumors of lymphoid organs have special names such as *leukemias* (which deserve a special name as the only "liquid" tumors); *lymphomas,* so named even though they are malignant (they used to be called lymphosarcomas); *Hodgkin's disease;* and so on (see Table 25.1).

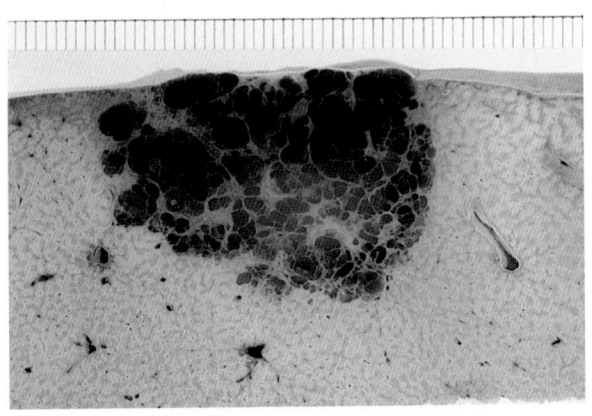

FIGURE 25.12 Hemangioma of the liver, discovered accidentally at autopsy. This is a typically benign tumor, despite the obvious lack of encapsulation. **Scale** in millimeters.

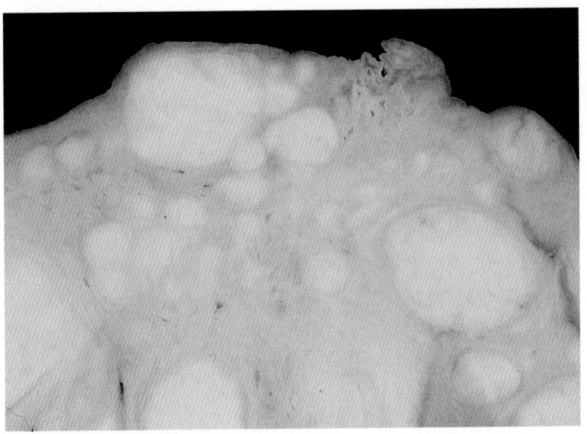

FIGURE 25.13 Cross section of the muscular wall of a uterus containing multiple leiomyomas (this condition is known as *leiomyomatosis* of the uterus). Magnification approximately × 2.

Tumors of Muscle Tissues

Muscle tumors are camouflaged by Greek names. A *leiomyoma* is a benign tumor of smooth muscle (*léios*, smooth; *mys*, muscle); the very common *leiomyomas* of the uterus appear in cross section as pale, firm, spherical masses embedded in the uterine wall (Figure 25.13). A benign tumor of striated muscle is called a *rhabdomyoma* on the grounds that the striations are equated microscopically to little bars or rods; *rhábdos* means rod or wand (as in rhabdomancy). The malignant counterparts are *leiomyosarcoma* and *rhabdomyosarcoma*.

Tumors of Nervous Tissues

Tumors of nervous tissue are easily understood from Table 25.1. You will be interested to discover that there

exists a *ganglioneuroma*, a tumor of neurons; it has a distinctive natural history (p. 922). Note that a malignant glial tumor is not called a gliosarcoma but a *glioblastoma;* the ending *-blastoma* usually refers to a poorly differentiated cell of embryonic type (which is correspondingly more malignant).

Tumors of Mixed Cell Types

Tumors of more than one cell type (mixed tumors) are not uncommon; we must assume that they derive from immature cells that can still differentiate in several directions. Some classic examples:

- The benign, mosaic-like tumors of connective tissues: e.g., fibrolipomas, angiofibrolipomas.
- The so-called *pleomorphic adenomas* of the salivary glands, which are bizarre but common (*pleomorphic is just another way of saying polymorphic*). These tumors contain a mixture of epithelial tubules and bundles of mesenchymal-appearing cells; both have now been shown to derive from epithelium (5a).
- The common *fibroadenoma of the breast;* here the proliferating glands are surrounded by a mantle of special connective tissue that many believe to be a layer of benign mesenchymal tumor surrounding the sheets of benign epithelial tumor (Figure 25.14). There is no doubt that something similar occurs in another and more worrisome breast tumor called *cystosarcoma phyllodes,* which means leaflike; sheets of epithelium intersect a sarcomatous mass, so that the tumor (when cut open) displays a leaflike structure, as if it were made of compressed papillae. This is but one of the many bizarre patterns that tumors can display.

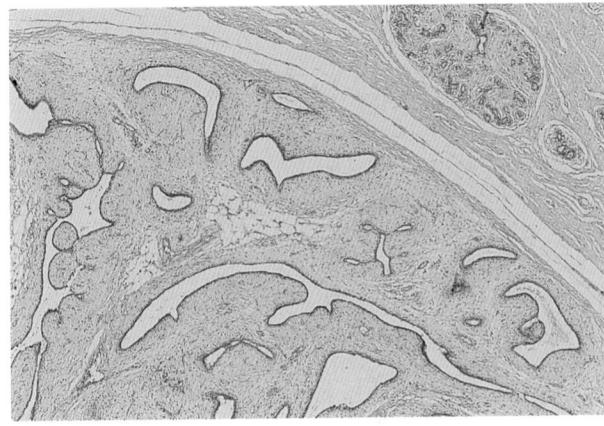

FIGURE 25.14 Fibroadenoma of the breast. Its pattern of long slits in fibrous tissue bears only a vague resemblance to the glandular pattern of the normal breast (*top right corner*). (30x)

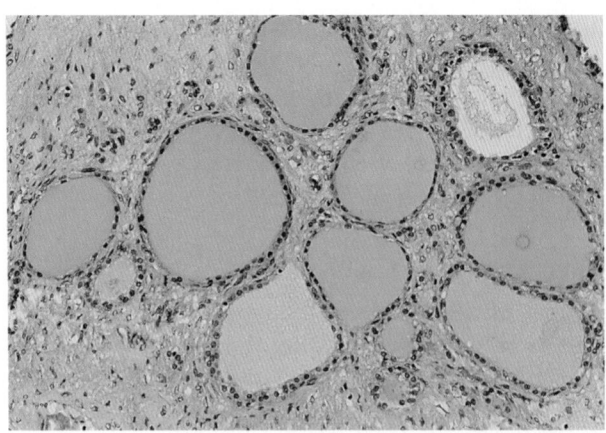

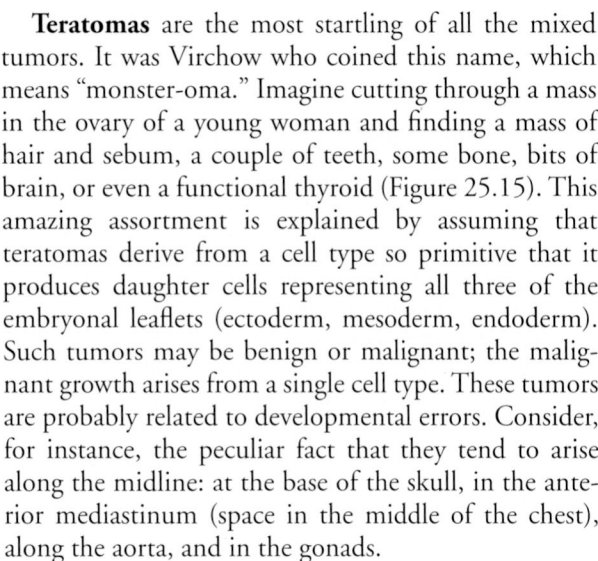

FIGURE 25.15   Typical thyroid follicles in a teratoma of the ovary (*struma ovarii*). Such inclusions of thyroid tissue can be functional and can even produce hyperthyroidism. (120x)

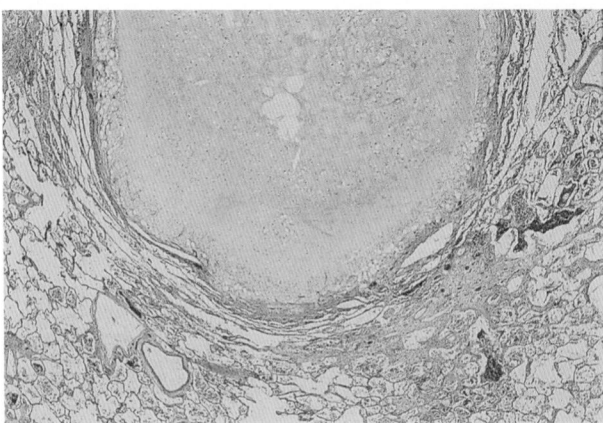

FIGURE 25.16   Typical hamartoma of the lung: a sharply defined mass of hyalin cartilage. The surrounding lung is somewhat compressed, but there is no invasion. (10x)

Teratomas are the most startling of all the mixed tumors. It was Virchow who coined this name, which means "monster-oma." Imagine cutting through a mass in the ovary of a young woman and finding a mass of hair and sebum, a couple of teeth, some bone, bits of brain, or even a functional thyroid (Figure 25.15). This amazing assortment is explained by assuming that teratomas derive from a cell type so primitive that it produces daughter cells representing all three of the embryonal leaflets (ectoderm, mesoderm, endoderm). Such tumors may be benign or malignant; the malignant growth arises from a single cell type. These tumors are probably related to developmental errors. Consider, for instance, the peculiar fact that they tend to arise along the midline: at the base of the skull, in the anterior mediastinum (space in the middle of the chest), along the aorta, and in the gonads.

Tumor-Like Lumps

A **hamartoma** is not really a tumor, although it may appear so to the naked eye; it is a lump of tissues that belong to the organ in which the lump is found but have been "wrongly assembled" in the course of development. We still recall the sudden anxiety of a 22-year-old student, a heavy smoker, when a routine chest X-ray showed a round 3-cm mass in the left lung. Surgery produced a firm, sharply limited mass of cartilage,

smooth muscle, and epithelium, which you will recognize as typical components of bronchi (Figure 25.16). Hamartomas are present at birth and grow with the individual. Their name derives from *hamartía,* scribal error or mistake, as if the body, while assembling the lung, ended up with a lump of leftovers and just buried them. Another type of hamartoma worries surgeons who, while operating on the abdomen, discover a sprinkling of small, round, whitish, slightly raised spots on the liver, which suggest metastases from an unknown cancer. A biopsy will show the reassuring image of hamartoma made of peaceful-looking bile ducts.

Choristomas are little lumps of normal tissue that do not belong in the organ where the lump is found. For example, a small mass of pancreatic tissue may be found in the duodenal mucosa (often called a *pancreatic inclusion*); or tiny accessory spleens may be found in the abdominal cavity. The term *choristoma* seems to be going out of fashion; it is being replaced by the more understandable expression *ectopic tissue.*

At this point it will help to review Table 25.1 and related comments. Note two oddities: there is a *nearly total lack of benign tumors of lymphoid tissue.* As to *fibromas,* they are listed, but fibroblasts, which are so ready to multiply in healing tissues, rarely produce benign tumors.

Tumors Have Personalities

Being able to name a tumor according to its cell of origin and/or its structure is important, but it is not enough for predicting the tumor's biology and behavior

(in other words, "adenoma" or "carcinoma" are not as fully descriptive as "daisy" or "sparrow"). Tumors of one morphologic type—such as papillomas or adenocarcinomas—behave differently in different organs, which surely reflects differences in the tissue of origin. For example:

- An angioma of the liver is a quiet neoplasm that almost never disturbs its bearer. It is usually discovered at autopsy. By contrast, an angioma of the skin in the newborn may develop into an awful-looking mass (p. 922) and then regress and disappear. Other angiomas persist and are very difficult to treat.
- A "papilloma" should be benign (indeed, a papilloma of the skin is utterly benign). But a papilloma of the larynx is a worrisome tumor that tends to recur; it may kill by suffocation even if benign, but it may also heal by itself. A papillomatous tumor of the urinary bladder is often malignant.
- An adenocarcinoma is a malignant tumor of a gland. However, if it arises from the prostate, the patient may live for years; if it concerns the pancreas, most patients die within 3 months of the diagnosis.

Even the part of the organ in which a tumor arises can make a difference in a tumor's behavior, especially for tumors of the skin. A pigmented mole almost anywhere on the body is of no concern, except for cosmetic reasons, whereas a pigmented mole on the palms of the hands or on the soles of the feet is prone to undergo malignant transformation and must be removed, preferably in childhood if it is observed.

Why the part of an organ should make a difference is probably explained by the fact that normal cells of the same type can differ according to their location. This is well proven for endothelial cells, mast cells (p. 342), fibroblasts (5, 8, 18), adipocytes (2, 4a, 13, 23), and liver cells in the lobule (12).

To the medical student, this means that it will be necessary to learn the personality of the most common human tumors, as determined statistically, while keeping in mind that the aggressiveness of a tumor in any particular case may vary unpredictably. A mesothelioma of the pleura may kill one patient within a year and allow another patient to survive 5 years. These differences are not yet explainable, but they are compatible with current knowledge of tumors: *the original molecular defect need not be identical,* and the body's responses are also variable. Even the attitude of the patient is a factor (22). All of this amounts to saying that at the molecular as well as the clinical level, *each tumor must be thought of as a potentially different disease.*

For this reason, predicting the life span of a patient is unwise to say the least, and robbing a patient of hope is inexcusable.

References

1. Bigger CH, Hildemann WH. Cellular defense systems of the coelenterata. In Cohen N, and Sigel MM eds. The Reticuloendothelial System. A Comprehensive Treatise, vol. 3, Phylogeny and Ontogeny. New York: Plenum Press, 1982, pp. 59–87.
2. Björntorp P. Development of adipose tissue *in vivo* and *in vitro*. In Angel A, Hollenberg CH, and Roncari DAK eds. The Adipocyte and Obesity: Cellular and Molecular Mechanisms. New York: Raven Press, 1983, pp. 33–39.
3. Bork P, Copley R. Filling in the gaps. Nature 2001;409: 818–820.
4. Burck KB, Liu ET, Larrick JW. Oncogenes. An Introduction to the Concept of Cancer Genes. New York: Springer-Verlag, 1988.
4a. Cahill GF Jr, Renold AE. Adipose tissue: a brief history. In Angel A, Hollenberg CH, Roncari DAK eds., The adipocyte and obesity: cellular and molecular mechanisms. New York: Raven Press, 1983, pp. 1–7.
5. Conrad GW, Hart GW, Chen Y. Differences *in vitro* between fibroblast-like cells from cornea, heart, and skin of embryonic chicks. J Cell Sci 1977;26:119–137.
5a. Debiec-Rychter M, Van Valckenborgh I, Van den Broeck C, et al. Histologic localization of PLAG1 (pleomorphic adenoma gene 1) in pleomorphic adenoma of the salivary gland: cytogenetic evidence of common origin of phenotypically diverse cells. Lab Invest 2001;81:1289–1297.
6. El-Mofty MM, Abdelmeguid N, Michael AE, El-Marhouni KM. A quick test for screening the carcinogenity of certain chemicals, using various protozoan parasites. Folia Morphol 1988;36:350–356.
7. Fenoglio-Preiser CM, Hutter RVP. Colorectal polyps: pathologic diagnosis and clinical significance. CA Ca J Clin 1985;35:322–344.
8. Gabbiani G, Hirschel BJ, Ryan GB, Statkov PR, Majno G. Granulation tissue as a contractile organ. A study of structure and function. J Exp Med 1972;135:719–734.
9. Gateff E. Malignant neoplasms of genetic origin in *Drosophila melanogaster*. Science 1978a;200:1448–1459.
10. Gateff E. The genetics and epigenetics of neoplasms in *Drosophila*. Biol Rev 1978b;58:123–168.
11. Golub TR, Slonim DK, Tamayo P, et al. Molecular classification of cancer: class discovery and class prediction by gene expression monitoring. Science 1999;286:531–536.
12. Gumucio JJ. Functional organization of the liver. In: Bircher J, Benhamou JP, McIntyre N, Rizzetto M, Rodes J (eds). Oxford Textbook of Clinical Hepatology. 2nd ed. New York: Oxford University Press, 1999, pp. 437–445.
13. Hollenberg CH, Roncari DAK, Djian P. Obesity and the fat cell: future prospects. In Angel A, Hollenberg CH, and Roncari DAK eds. The adipocyte and obesity: cellular and molecular mechanisms. New York: Raven Press, 1983, pp. 291–300.
14. Kaiser HE. Animal neoplasms—a systematic review. In Kaiser HE ed. Neoplasms—comparative pathology of growth in animals, plants, and man. Baltimore: Williams & Wilkins, 1981, pp. 747–812.

15. Koss LG. Atlas of tumor pathology, 2nd ser, fasc 11. Tumors of the urinary bladder. Washington, DC: Armed Forces Institute of Pathology, 1975.

16. Ladanyi M, Chan WC, Triche TJ, Gerald WL. Expression profiling of human tumors: The end of surgical pathology? J Mol Diagn 2001;3:92–97.

17. Mottram JC. The problem of tumours. London: HK Lewis & Co Ltd, 1942.

18. Phipps RP. Pulmonary fibroblast heterogeneity. Boca Raton: CRC Press Inc, 1992.

19. Pitot HC. Fundamentals of oncology, 3rd ed. New York: Marcel Dekker Inc, 1986.

20. Rather LJ. The genesis of cancer. Baltimore: The Johns Hopkins University Press, 1978.

21. Scharrer B, Lockhead MS. Tumors in the invertebrates: a review. Cancer Res 1950;10:403–419.

22. Siegel BS. Love, medicine and miracles. New York: Harper & Row, 1986.

23. Smith U. Regional differences and effect of cell size on lipolysis in human adipocytes. In Angel A, Hollenberg CH, Roncari DAK eds. The adipocyte and obesity: cellular and molecular mechanisms. New York: Raven Press, 1983, pp. 245–250.

24. Sontag S. Illness as metaphor and AIDS and its metaphors. New York: Doubleday, 1990.

25. Ziegler E. General pathology. New York: William Wood and Company, 1908.

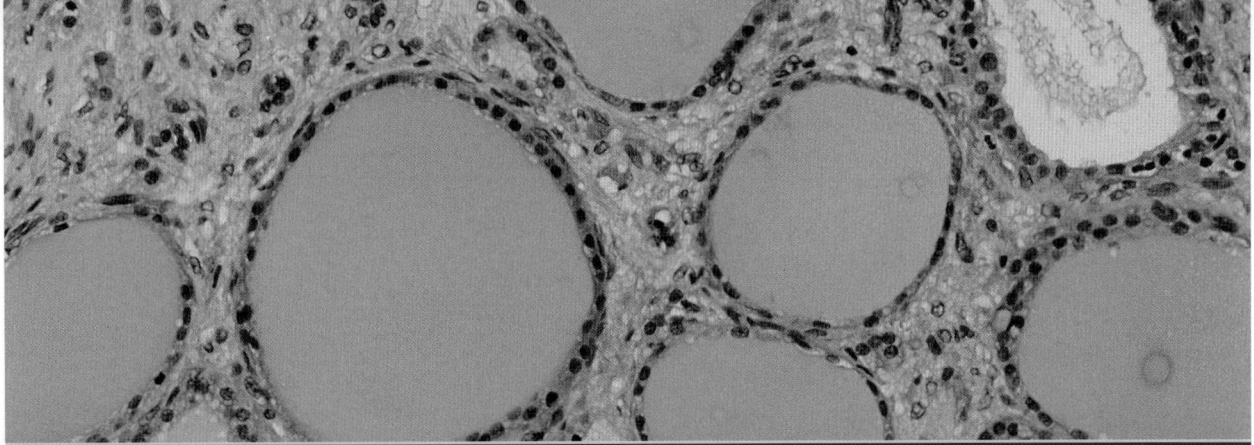

ANATOMY AND BIOLOGY OF TUMORS

Tumors were once thought to consist of nondescript "deposits." The news that they were made of cells was rushed into print by Johannes Müller (Virchow's teacher) in 1838, the very same year that saw the birth of the cell theory (Figure 26.1). That was no coincidence: the young Theodor Schwann, pioneer of the cell theory, was working in Müller's laboratory (196, 197). The next most urgent question, then, became: What is the difference between a normal cell and a tumor cell? The better part of two centuries has gone by, but nobody has rushed into print with an answer valid for all tumors; the few who have tried were proved wrong. We have learned, however, that tumor cells are characterized by *defects in their DNA,* well below the limit of visibility even for electron microscopes; these molecular defects usually translate as changes in the structure and/or function of the tumor cells. It is true that *we cannot mention a single change that is common to all tumor cells;* so, whenever the DNA defect is defined, we must face the task of correlating this defect with any change that the cell may show.

To explain the nature of tumors, we will follow this sequence: (a) the cells of the tumor, (b) the tumor as a whole, (c) the birth and growth of the tumor, (d) the tumor as an aggressor, and (e) the causes of tumors, which will lead us into the world of DNA, oncogenes, and suppressor genes.

The Tumor Cell

The most informative way to follow the change from normal cell to malignant cell would be to examine cell cultures in which this change is expected to occur. However, it took a long time to realize that malignancy ("*transformation*") can occur *in vitro.*

In the 1940s, W. R. Earle and collaborators treated fibroblast cultures with methylcholanthrene and found that some cells took on a

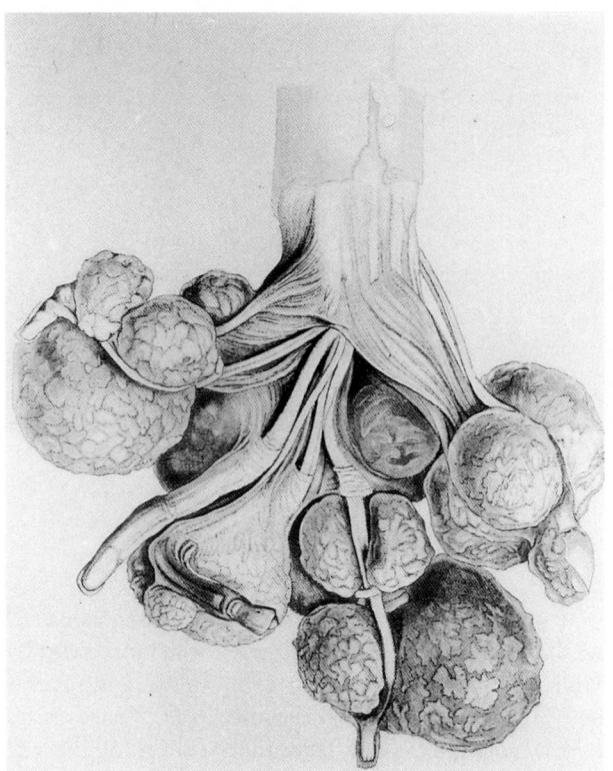

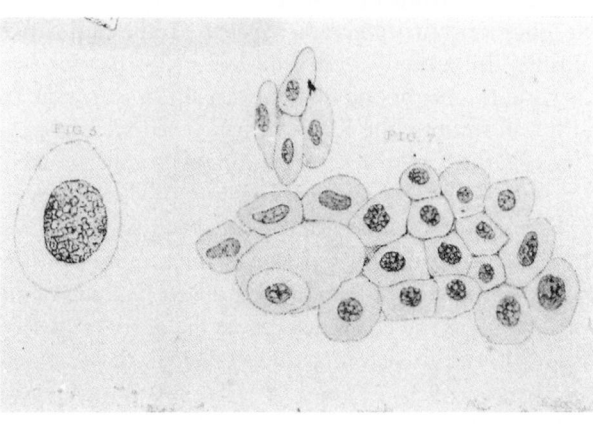

FIGURE 26.1 The first illustration of tumor cells. In 1840, Johannes Müller took samples from a museum specimen (*top*) showing multiple cartilaginous tumors of the hand (enchondromas). *Bottom:* The microscope showed that the tumors consisted of cells with irregular nuclei. (Adapted from [177].)

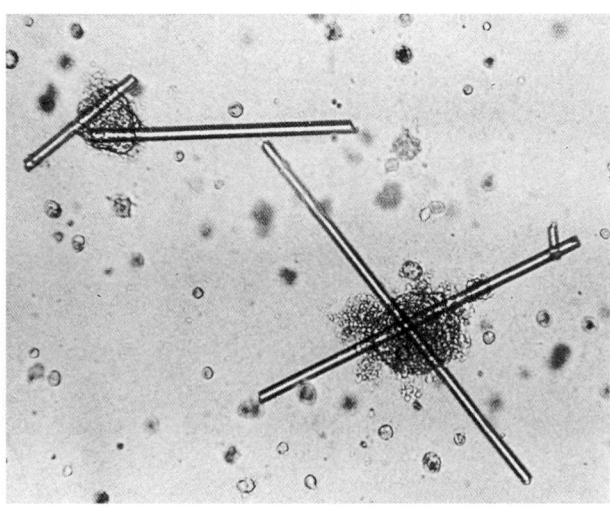

FIGURE 26.2 The phenomenon of anchorage-dependent growth of normal cells. Cells of a hamster cell line, freely suspended in agar, fail to grow (note lack of free clusters); but those cells that take a foothold on microscopic glass fibrils succeed in forming colonies. (From [222], Copyright © 1968 Alan R. Liss. Reprinted by permission of Wiley-Liss, Division of John Wiley & Sons, Inc.)

malignant phenotype; when implanted into mice these cells formed sarcomas that killed the host (64, 65). This pioneer work was forgotten for 20 years (202), partly because it seemed to have a flaw: fibroblasts from untreated cultures also produced sarcomas in 8 percent of the animals. Today this would not surprise anybody: it is an accepted fact that a malignant phenotype can occasionally spring up spontaneously in cultures of cell lines.

We just used the word *transformation.* To the average person this is a very vague term; hence it is surprising to see it used in tumor language to mean a change as definitive as *switch to malignancy of cultured cells.* However, a vague term may be appropriate, because the change itself—in a population of growing cells—is difficult to pinpoint (6, 88). The two absolute requirements for defining a cell as transformed are (a) *immortality* (but not all immortal cell lines are transformed) and (b) *the ability to form malignant tumors when transplanted into a suitable host.*

The concept of transformation is imprecise enough, but beware of another source of confusion: *the so-called transforming growth factors (TGFs) do not transform:* at least not in the sense of causing malignancy. These polypeptides, originally discovered as products of tumors, are able to induce some types of normal cells to grow dispersed in agar, as *anchorage-independent* cells, whereas most normal cells prefer to grow safely anchored to a surface (Figure 26.2) (151). We now know that TGFs are produced also by normal tissues, that other growth factors such as PDGF can induce anchorage-independent growth, and that the change is always reversible. Thus platelets, for example, contain large amounts of TGF-beta—which does not mean, of course, that platelets are carcinogenic.

The first classic study concerning the steps of transformation came in 1970: Barbara Barker and Katherine

Sanford (11) watched a variety of cell lines as they grew in culture and identified a sequence of five cytologic features that announce transformation: when injected *in vivo,* the cultures that had tested positive under the microscope (on the scale from 1 to 5) gave rise to sarcomas, in increasing numbers. The progressive changes were:

1. Increased cytoplasmic basophilia
2. Increased number and size of nucleoli
3. Increased nuclear-cytoplasmic ratio
4. Retraction of the cytoplasm
5. Formation of clusters and cords of cells

Today, if we were to draw up a composite picture of the malignant cell, it would be as in the following pages.

The details vary from one cancer to another and in the same cancer they may change with time: as a pessimist might guess, the change is usually from bad to worse, although a rare malignant tumor may turn benign. Malignant features can be found in all aspects of cell biology: structure, behavior, function, and biochemistry.

Structural Differences

To visualize a cancer cell, begin with the corresponding normal cell and make it

- Less differentiated,
- With some features of a rapidly growing cell, and
- With some additional anomalous features (*atypia*)

Lack of differentiation. Lack of differentiation means that the special features of the normal cell are imperfectly expressed: a ciliated cell will have fewer cilia, a secretory cell less secretion, and so on. This fact has given rise to the common and synonymous terms *anaplasia* and *dedifferentiation,* both implying that the cancer cell has somehow regressed to a lesser state of differentiation. However, it seems unlikely that tumors consist of mature cells that regress. The current concept of carcinogenesis is that tumors contain undifferentiated stem cells whose progeny fail to mature. In other words, the tumor cell is born in a state of low differentiation and does not become immature by dedifferentiating itself.

This concept needs to be qualified. (a) Some kind of "backward differentiation" does indeed occur in malignant tumors as they change from bad to worse, a phenomenon known (backwardly) as *tumor **progression*** (p. 781). (b) In some malignant tumors, such as squamous cell carcinoma of the epidermis, full differentiation does occur here and there; in fact, this observation gave rise to the theory that cancer may be a disease of differentiation (p. 947).

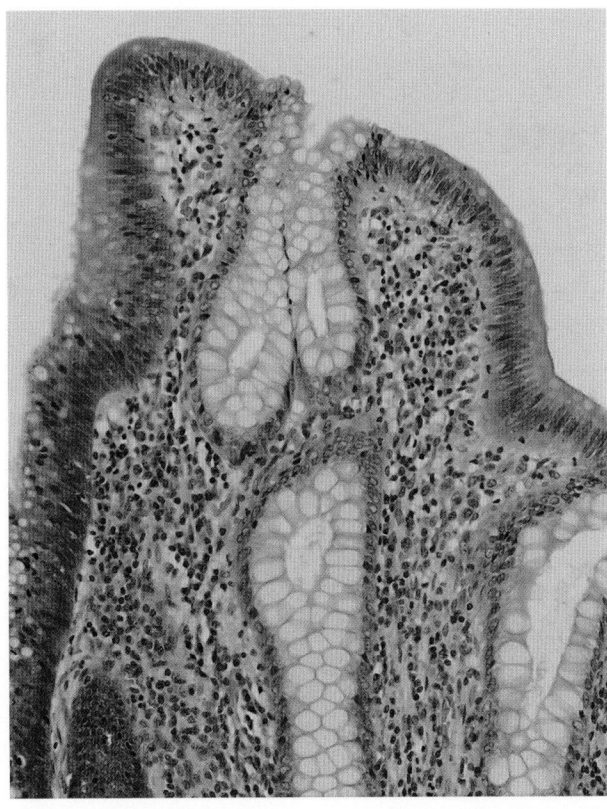

FIGURE 26.3 Part of a benign polyp, in a case of *polyposis coli,* illustrating the differences between normal and neoplastic epithelium. *Top center:* Two normal mucus-secreting glands. Follow their epithelium upward, where it meets neoplastic epithelium, and note the cellular differences: size, shape and basophilia of the cells and nuclei, mucus secretion. (120x)

Fast growth. Features of fast-growing cells are easy to grasp:

- *Cytoplasmic basophilia is increased,* which means more RNA and thus more active protein synthesis (Figure 26.3). (Needless to say, this rule does not apply to slow-growing malignant tumors.) The electron microscope shows many free ribosomes, which correspond to the fact that the cell is busy making "more of itself" rather than producing proteins for export.
- *Nucleoli increase in size and number* (remember that RNA is synthesized within them), and the nucleolar organizer region may be abnormal.

When stained with silver, interphase nuclei show tiny black dots which look like artefacts but they are not (Figure 26.4): they correspond to a small collection of proteins related to ribosomal genes, hence the name AgNOR (for nucleolar organizer region). They can be quntitated to estimate the rate of tumor proliferation (51, 52); with some exceptions, abundant AgNOR tends to correlate with poor survival (188).

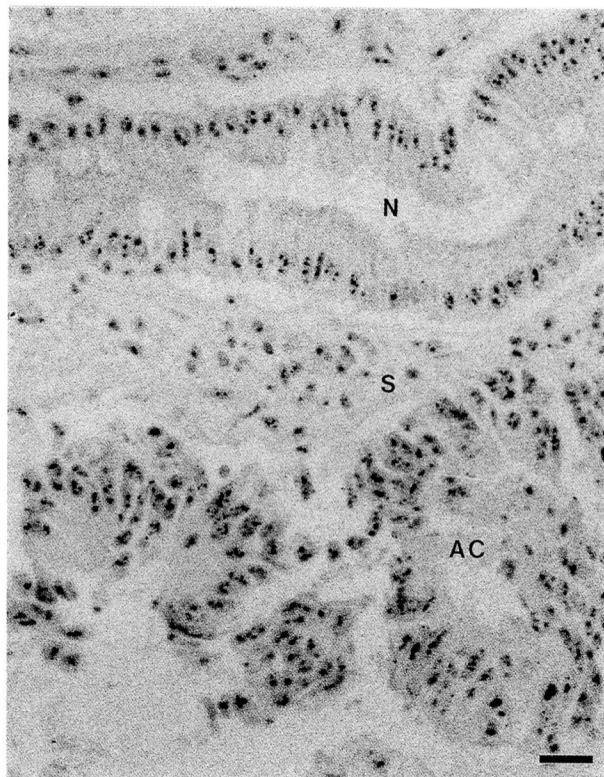

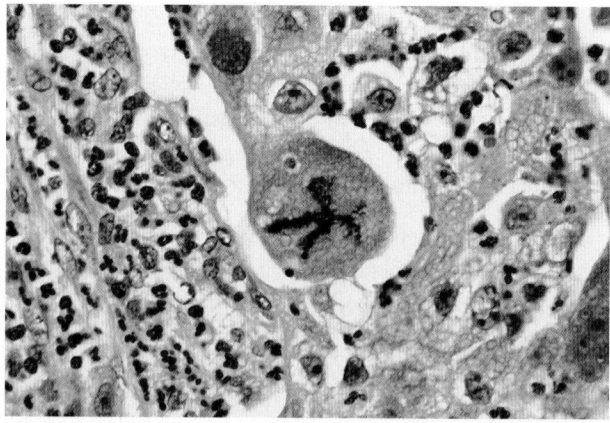

FIGURE 26.5   Tetrapolar mitosis in a squamous cell carcinoma of the cervix. (370x)

FIGURE 26.4   Histologic section of an adenocarcinoma of the colon (**AC**), stained with silver to demonstrate the nucleolar organizer region (NOR). **N:** Normal gland. Neoplastic cells contain more NORs than normal epithelial cells or cells within the stroma (**S**). The quantitative difference between normal and cancerous cells, however, is not always as clear-cut as in this example. **Bar** = 25 μm. (Courtesy of Dr. M. Derenzini, Department of Experimental Pathology, University of Bologna, Italy.)

- *Nucleoporin 88 (Nup88) is increased.* This is a recent finding (101).

  The nuclear pores are crossed by an intense two-way traffic, controlled by a ring of 50–100 proteins called nucleoporins (Nup). An antibody against Nup88 was found to stain almost all malignant tumors and premalignant dysplasias and some fetal tissues but not benign tumors. It may be that the protein is rubbed off by the heavy molecular traffic and spilled into the cytoplasm. This may become one of the best histochemical markers of malignancy.

- *Glycogen content is high,* as it is in embryonic cells. This abundance of glycogen correlates with the anaerobic glycolysis typical of embryonic as well as of tumor cells.

Atypical features. The features of atypia are especially important because *atypia tends to parallel the degree of*

aggressiveness. It can hit virtually every aspect of cellular structure. For example:

- *Size and shape of the cell are abnormal.* Typically, a malignant cell is more rounded and tends to be irregular. Today these changes begin to make sense: malignancy is linked to cytoskeletal disturbances, which lead to internal disarray as well as to mechanical effects on cell shape (p. 865).

- *The shape of the nucleus is irregular.* This is one of the most reliable criteria of malignancy, especially when the size and shape of the nucleus vary from cell to cell: but why so? Ingenious experiments on cultures of cancer cells have provided the answer (97): most of the abnormal nuclei contained abnormal chromosomes, ring-shaped, dicentric, or with other defects. Thus, abnormalities in nuclear shape can be considered primarily as signs of genetic instability.

- **Mitoses** are too numerous and some may be abnormal (Figure 26.5). Organizing the mitotic spindle is the responsibility of the **centrosomes,** which are now under scrutiny. Indeed, in tumor cells the centrosomes can show a number of anomalies (152, 180). Multiple centrosomes are often associated with the lack of a powerful tumor suppressor gene, *p53;* the lack of this controlling gene could allow centrosomes to replicate when they should not (163). Multiple centrosomes could well result in multipolar mitoses. Furthermore, by increasing the frequency of mitotic errors, the centrosomes could also confer a mutator phenotype to tumors (152, 163).

- *Cell-specific organelles are distorted or lost,* as best seen by electron microscopy. A good example are the sarcomeres of striated muscle: in rhabdomyosarcomas they are rudimentary (Figure 26.6) or disappear altogether.

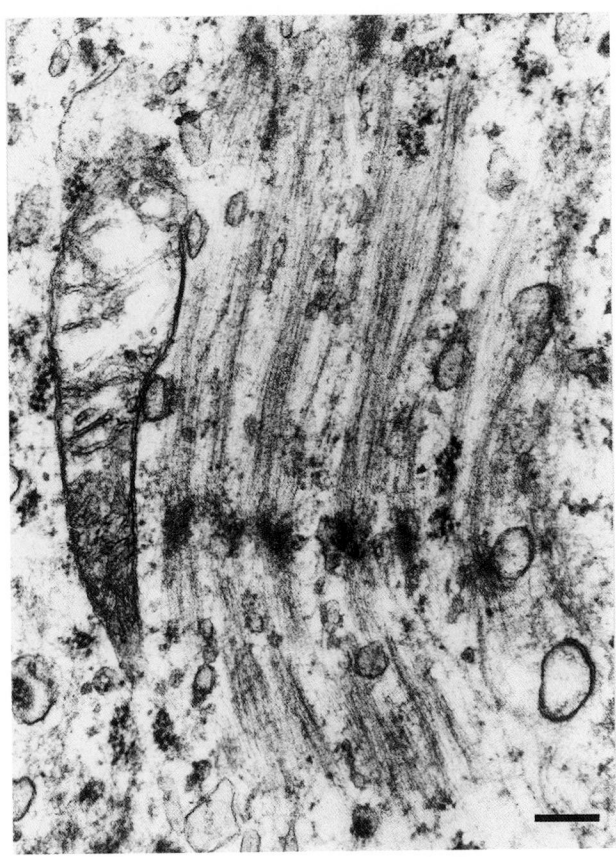

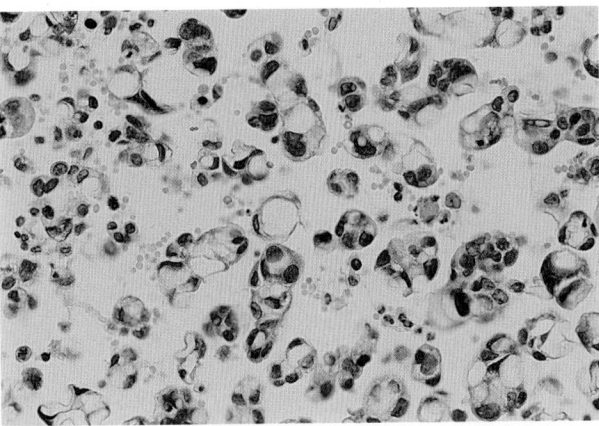

FIGURE 26.7   Typical signet-ring cells in the ascitic fluid of an 80-year-old woman with bilateral ovarian metastases from a mucus-secreting adenocarcinoma of the stomach. The ascitic fluid was spun down and the pellet was embedded and cut as if it were a piece of tissue. The signet-ring appearance is due to a large intracellular droplet of mucus; the "stone" of the ring is the compressed nucleus. (270x)

FIGURE 26.6   Bundles of fibrils representing sketchy sarcomeres in a cell from a rhabdomyosarcoma (in the nasal cavity of a 26-year-old woman). The family history of this patient was intriguing: a sister had died of an osteosarcoma at age 12; both parents had worked in a uranium reprocessing plant for 9 years. **Bar** = 0.2 μm. (Reprinted from [115], Copyright 1986, with permission from Elsevier.)

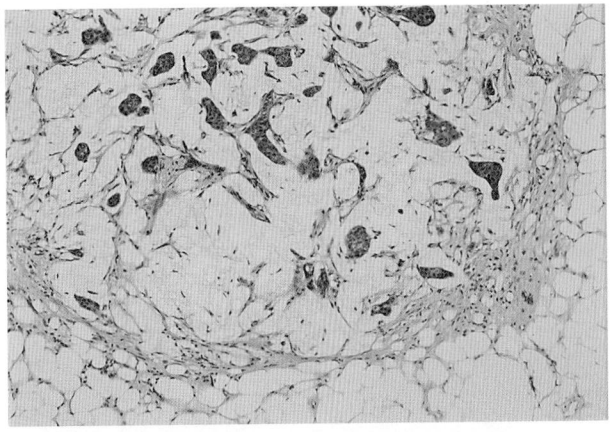

FIGURE 26.8   Mucus-secreting carcinoma of the breast: Clumps of deeply basophilic carcinomatous cells are surrounded by pools of mucus that they have secreted. In other parts of this tumor mucus secretion was absent. (60x)

*The case for "**mitochondriomas.**"* We refer the reader to p. 138, where we discussed the bizarre intracellular "tumors" consisting of mitochondria that proliferate until they fill the cell. No other organelle shows this behavior, presumably because no other organelle shares the bacterial ancestry of mitochondria. And correspondingly, no other organelle besides the nucleus contains DNA.

- *Secretion becomes irregular,* as best seen in mucus-secreting cells. Mucus may not be produced at all, or it may be retained as a large droplet that distends the cell (Figure 26.7); it may also be secreted indiscriminately into the tissue spaces, so the cells find themselves floating in their own product (Figure 26.8).
- *The cell surface often bristles with a large number of microvilli* (Figure 26.9) (55), perhaps another manifestation of cytoskeletal disturbances.
- *Sundry abnormalities may appear,* too many to list. For example, epithelial cells that normally surround

a glandular lumen can develop an internal lumen (Figure 26.10) (213). However, intracytoplasmic lumina are occasionally seen in non-neoplastic cells (108). Occasionally, a new type of organelle appears, which is unexplained but may be useful as a marker for a particular type of tumor; such is the *ribosome–lamella complex* of the so-called hairy-cell leukemia (Figure 26.11) (135). Another classic example is the Auer rod of acute myelogenous leukemia; it represents an abnormal neutrophil granule (Figure 26.12).

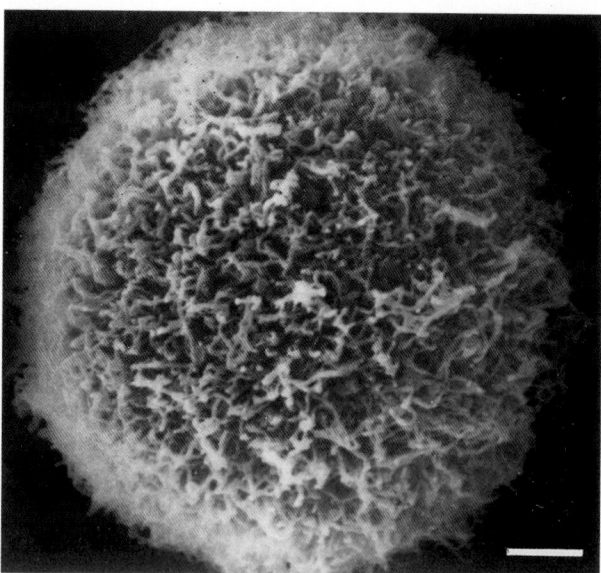

FIGURE 26.9   Cell from a carcinoma of the breast, suspended in a pleural effusion, covered with microvilli. **Bar** = 500 μm. (Reproduced with permission from [55].)

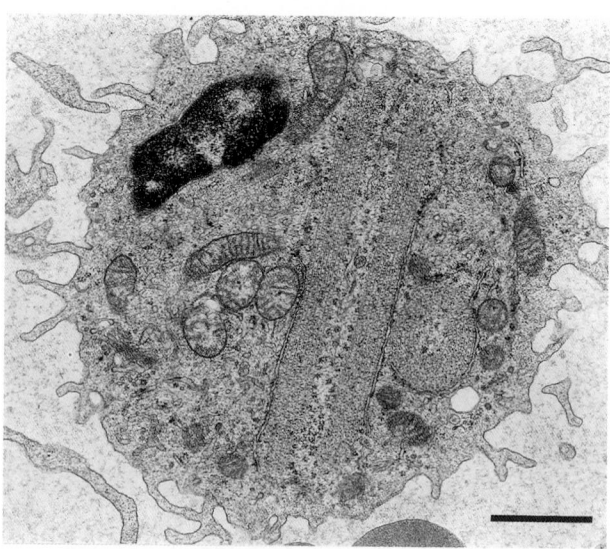

FIGURE 26.11   The "ribosome–lamella complex," one of the peculiar inclusions found in some malignant cells. This rod-shaped structure (shown in longitudinal and in transverse section) is typical, although not entirely characteristic, of hairy-cell leukemia. It can be seen also by light microscopy. **Bar** = 1 μm. (Reproduced from [135].)

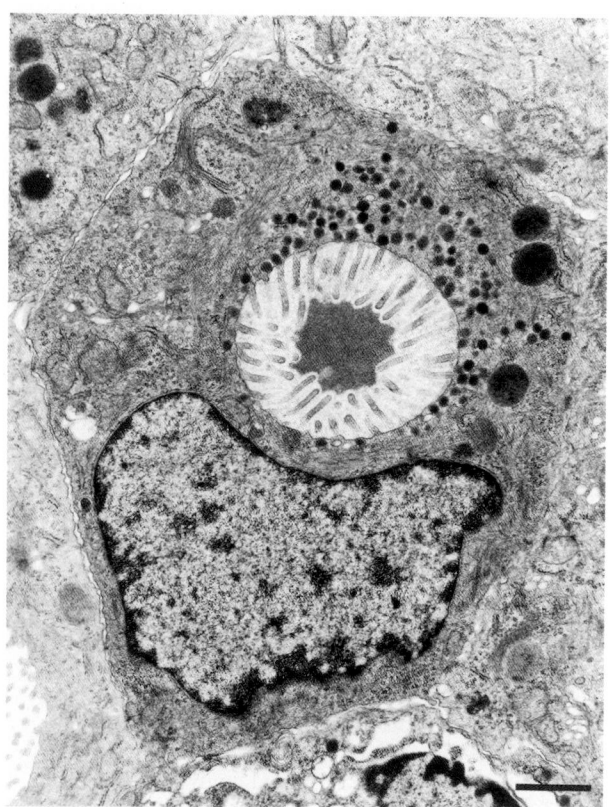

FIGURE 26.10   A bizarre form of cellular atypia: An intracellular lumen, complete with microvilli, in an epithelial cell of an invasive lobular carcinoma of the breast. **Bar** = 1 μm. (Copyright 1986. From [213]. Reproduced by permission of Taylor & Francis, Inc, http://www.routledge-ny.com)

Behavior in Culture

A number of behavioral changes characterize transformed cells.

Immortality. Transformed cells can grow forever. A sadly famous lady named Henrietta Lacks died in 1951 of a cervical carcinoma; cells from her tumor, the ubiquitous HeLa cells (p. 824), are still growing relentlessly in laboratories throughout the world. Note that this immortality does not compare with the immortality of bacteria: in real life, every strain of "immortal" malignant cells dies when it kills its host unless it is cultured like the HeLa cells. *Every case of cancer is therefore a "new" disease.*

Why are cancer cells immortal? The answer appears to hinge on the telomere-telomerase mechanism, which we discussed in Chapter 2: linear chromosomes must be capped by telomeres, which are progressively eroded (a lethal pathway for the cell) unless they are rebuilt by the enzyme telomerase. Virtually all tumors express telomerase (247), but telomerase expression by itself does not imply transformation (130), witness the telomerase-positive stem cells. Expression of the human telomere gene is regulated by the immortalizing oncoprotein Myc, which is up-regulated in most human cancers (48): could this mean that telomerase

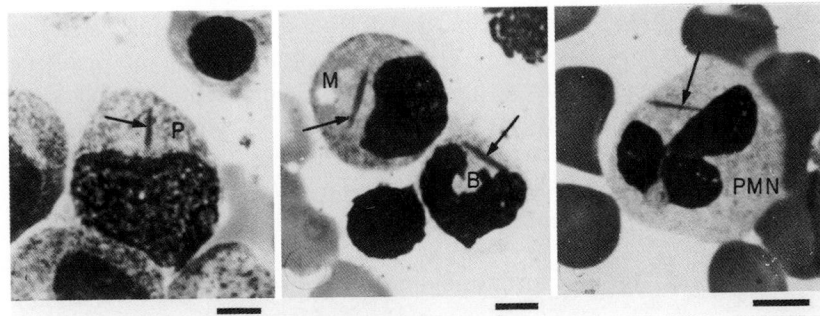

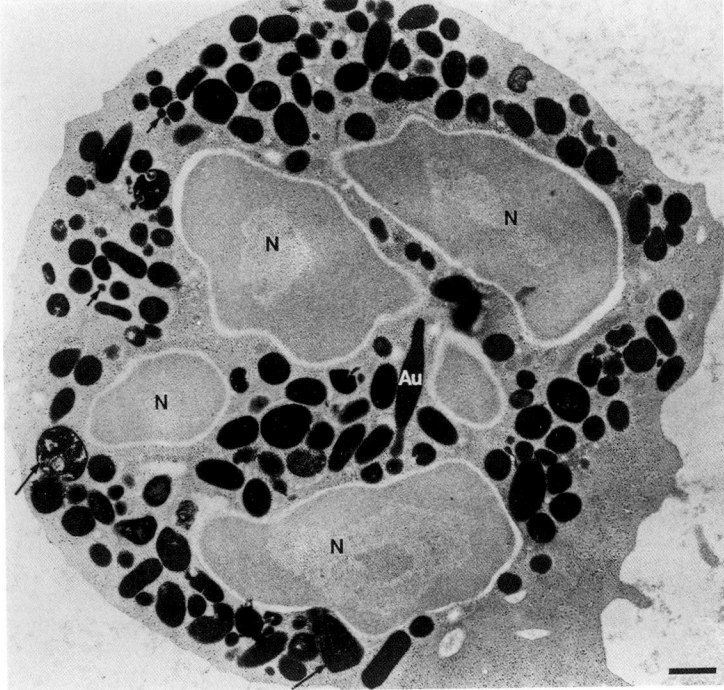

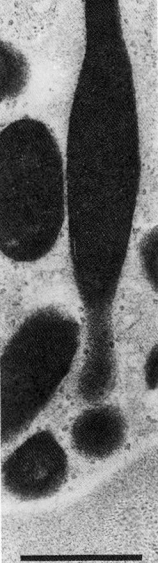

FIGURE 26.12 Abnormalities in the granules of neutrophils in acute myelogenous leukemia. *Top:* **Arrows** point to elongated azurophilic granules (Auer rods) in a promyelocyte (**P**), a myelocyte (**B**), a metamyelocyte (**M**), and a mature polymorphonuclear neutrophil (**PMN**). Wright stain; **bars** = 5 μm. *Bottom left:* Mature neutrophil reacted for peroxidase. The nucleus (**N**) is subdivided into five lobes. All granules are peroxidase-positive and thus azurophilic; some are abnormally small or defective (**arrows**); one is elongated (**Au:** Auer rod). Peroxidase-negative specific granules are missing. **Bar** = 0.5 μm. *Bottom right:* Detail of the Auer rod shown at left. **Bar** = 0.5 μm. (Reproduced with permission from [8].)

expression is an accidental byproduct of Myc up-regulation? Or could it be that tumors express telomerase because they derive from stem cells that are telomerase positive (102)? What would be the effect of telomerase inhibitors on cancer patients? Answers are surely on the way—bringing more questions.

Loss of anchorage dependence. As mentioned earlier, *normal* cells prefer to grow on a surface; they become attached to it, spread out, and begin to replicate (see Figure 26.2) (222). In contrast, transformed cells can also do well in a fluid medium such as soft agar, in which they maintain a more rounded shape. Cytoskeletal changes are probably involved (202).

Loss of contact inhibition. Transformed cells grow to cover all available space, then continue to grow and pile up over each other haphazardly (p. 852). Normal cells usually stop when they contact each other, at which point they constitute a confluent sheet with little or no cell overlap.

The term *contact inhibition* has been used in various ways; for some it has meant inhibition of movement and for others inhibition of growth, hence the current tendency to replace the phrase *loss of contact inhibition* with the cumbersome *decreased density-dependent inhibition of growth* (202).

Loss of orientation on an oriented substrate. This less known feature is illustrated in Figure 26.13. In essence, malignant cells growing on a surface with a distinctive pattern have partially lost the ability to align themselves accordingly. This is, we presume, another consequence of a faulty cytoskeleton.

Decreased requirement for growth factors. Normal cells tend to be fussy about the medium in which they are

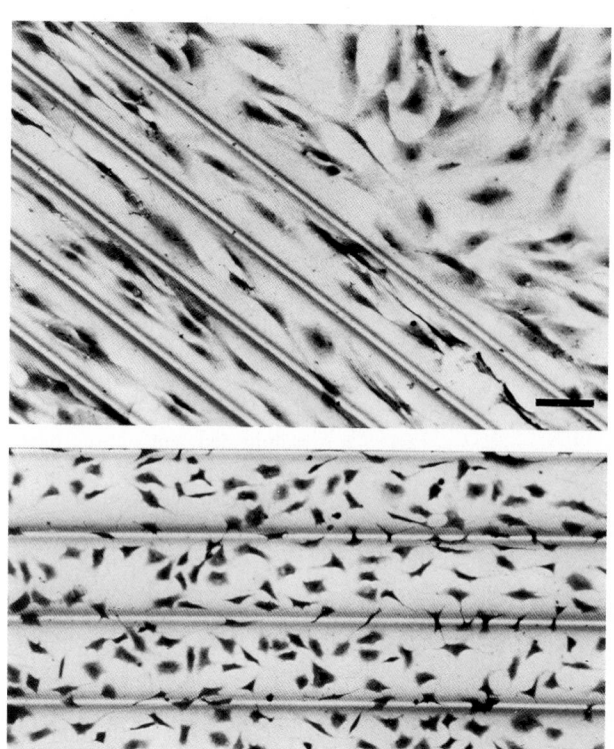

FIGURE 26.13   *Top:* Normal mouse fibroblasts that had been seeded 24 hours earlier on a surface, partly flat (*top right*) and partly etched (*lower left*). Where grooves were present, the fibroblasts oriented themselves accordingly. *Bottom:* Transformed fibroblasts show very little tendency to become oriented along the grooves. **Bars** = 50 μm. (Reproduced with permission from [239].)

nurtured; special mixtures of growth factors must be worked out for each type. Transformed cells are much easier to grow and require less serum (i.e., fewer growth factors). The reason is now apparent: malignant cells supply their own growth factors by a curious property known as autocrine secretion (p. 35).

Behavior upon Transplantation

For transplants to succeed they must be performed on animals that do not reject them. The choice lies between syngeneic, immunosuppressed, or congenitally immunodeficient animals. The latter include the SCID mice (p. 605) and the sorry-looking nude mice, which (besides having no hair) have no thymus and therefore lack the ability to reject a graft. The basic procedure is to inject a suspension of the tumor cells subcutaneously; one million is usually enough. If the cells are

malignant, they form a palpable nodule usually within weeks. *Normal* adult cells injected in this manner either die or survive without significant growth; this is the general rule for all grafts of normal tissues, with one startling exception: one way to produce a very malignant teratoma in the mouse is to graft normal but embryonic tissue into the testis (p. 925).

Functional and Biochemical Changes

Motility and chemotaxis. Many types of cancer cells can move around rather like amoebae, although their normal counterparts may be stationary. This characteristic helps us understand the mechanism of invasiveness; it was actually shown *in vitro* that the fastest moving cells are the most invasive (103). Moreover, some cancer cells secrete a factor that accelerates their motion and even directs it by chemotaxis (p. 816) (which sounds like a cellular version of "pulling oneself up by one's bootstraps").

Surface-related changes. Such changes are many; they are summarized in Figure 26.14 and the following list. Of course, they vary from tumor to tumor.

- *Decreased adhesion between cells.* In a classic experiment D. R. Coman of Philadelphia showed in 1944 that cells of a carcinoma are more easily pulled apart than their normal counterparts (Figure 26.15). The experiment was criticized as too simple, but since then it has been abundantly proven that malignant cells in general have fewer intercellular contacts and fewer attachments to the stroma (166, 249) because actin-to-membrane attachments are one of the prime targets of transformation-related disturbances (173). This reduced cohesion helps to understand the invasiveness of malignant cells (p. 814).

- *Altered intercellular communication* (112). Overall, it seems that *decreased* communication between cells favors cell proliferation (139, 184, 251): for example, mice lacking connexin32 (a gap junction protein of liver cells) spontaneously developed 8 times more liver tumors than control mice (232). Some carcinogens decrease intercellular communication across gap junctions (147). Some transformed cells stop growing when they establish contact with normal cells (167); needless to say, if all tumor cells did this, there would be no tumors. Junctions between normal and neoplastic cells have long been observed by electron microscopy (236).

Of course, gap junctions (communicating junctions) also exist between the neoplastic cells of a given tumor. These channels allow the passage of molecules as large as 2 kilodaltons; growth-controlling signals might follow this route (167). This story is becoming more interesting since it turned out that the famed *src*

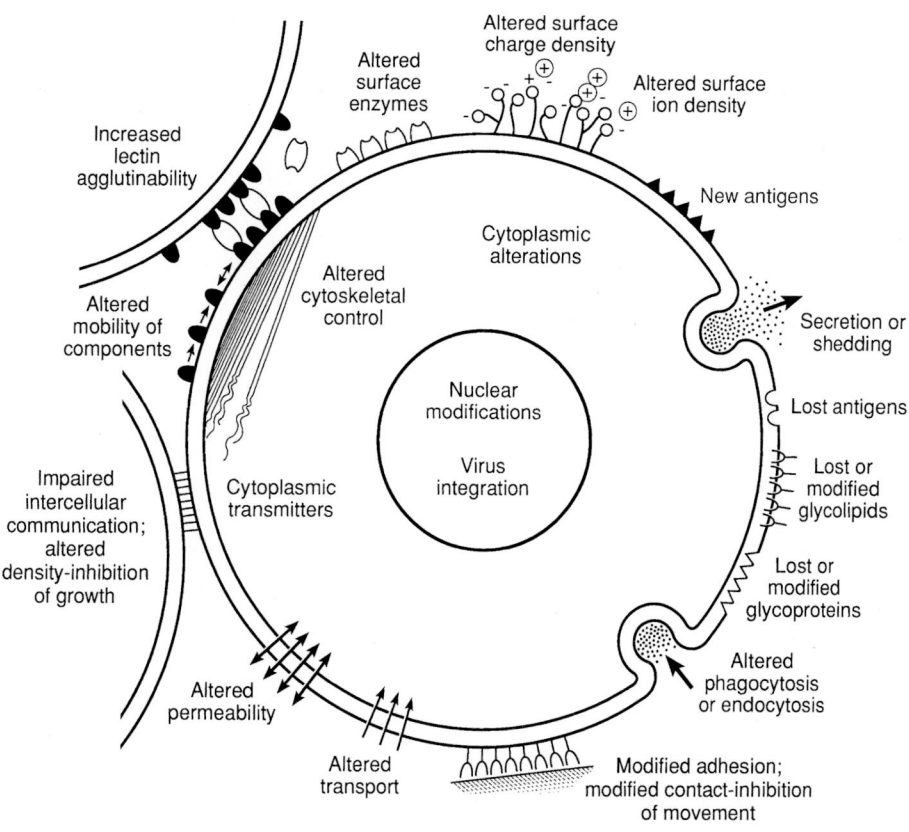

FIGURE 26.14 Some of the cell surface alterations found in tumor cells. (Adapted from [179] with permission from Elsevier Science Publishing.)

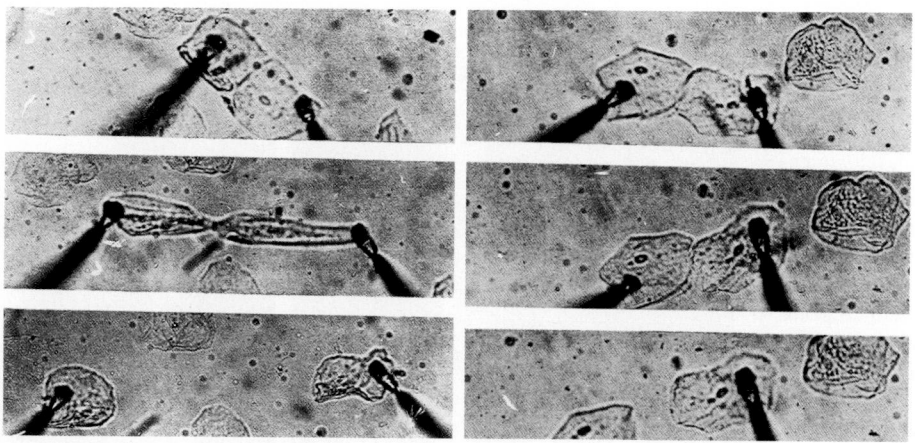

FIGURE 26.15 Coman's classic experiment demonstrating the loose connection between cancerous epithelial cells. *Left:* A pair of normal, living squamous epithelial cells from the lip; as they are drawn apart by microneedles they stretch because they cling to each other tenaciously. *Right:* A pair of living squamous epithelial cells from a carcinoma of the lip. As the needles just begin to move apart, the cells detach with little deformation. This simple experiment drew attention to the decreased adhesion between malignant cells. (Reproduced with permission from [39].)

oncogene regulates intercellular communication and growth (156).

- *Increased susceptibility to agglutination by lectins* (carbohydrate-binding proteins, p. 135) such as concanavalin A. In other words, lectins that recognize and agglutinate normal cells only after mild proteolytic digestion, agglutinate untreated malignant cells (15). This is merely a laboratory tool for detecting an abnormality of cancer cells; it tells us that specific carbohydrate sites on transformed cells are somehow more "exposed" than normal on the cell surface (15). Because surface carbohydrates are key factors in cell recognition, we can assume that a change in their arrangement affects the "social relations" of malignant cells.

- *Tendency to shed surface molecules,* including proteins, glycoproteins, and enzymes. This has many implications (24). Shedding enzymes such as collagenase can help the malignant cell work its way through the extracellular matrix (p. 815). Shedding tissue factor, fibronectin, or other macromolecules may lead to exaggerated clotting (60). Conversely, shedding plasminogen activator generates plasmin, a trypsin-like enzyme that digests fibrin and may perhaps extricate cells from fibrin clots; it is an old observation that malignant cells *in vitro* dissolve plasma clots whereas normal cells do not (Figure 26.16) (226). (Plasminogen circulates with the blood and is always available in low concentration in the extracellular fluid.)

  Some of the shed molecules can be found in the blood and are therefore available as tumor markers, a useful device for diagnosing the presence of a particular type of tumor or for monitoring its response to therapy (p. 955). The shedding of tumor

antigens may help the tumor cell escape immune attack: the immune system is kept busy destroying these loose molecules while the tumor cells are left intact.

This type of shedding is a military strategy. During World War II, Allied airplanes shed clouds of metal leaflets, which looked like targets on radar and kept the flak busy, while the planes went on with their mission.

Biochemical changes follow the general rule that there are no general rules—but a limited number of tumors do show biochemical differences than can be exploited as a target for therapy. The classic example: some tumor cells require more exogenous **asparagine** than normal cells do. Treatment with L-asparaginase (obtained from bacteria) depletes the asparagine supply and starves the tumor cells. This works best for acute lymphocytic and myelocytic leukemias; anaphylactic reaction to the enzyme limits its usefulness. The degree of **DNA methylation** is currently pursued as a basic aspect of tumor biology with therapeutic possibilities (p. 891) but it is too early to tell. Another biochemical change that we find potentially important, and which seems to apply to many tumors, is that rhodamine 123, a fluorescent dye, localizes in the mitochondria of living cells; normal cells release it within a few hours whereas epithelial tumors retain it for 2–5 days (Figure 26.17) (19). Efforts are under way to exploit this phenomenon (34).

Other differences will be discussed in relation to oncogenes; a longer list can be found in specialized textbooks. Currently the bottom line is that *many of the biochemical and physiological differences described for*

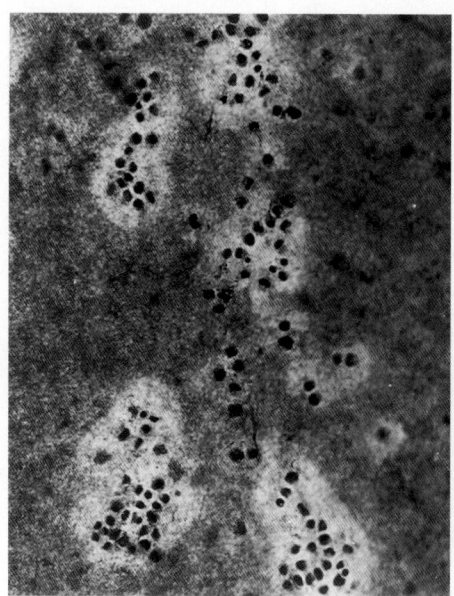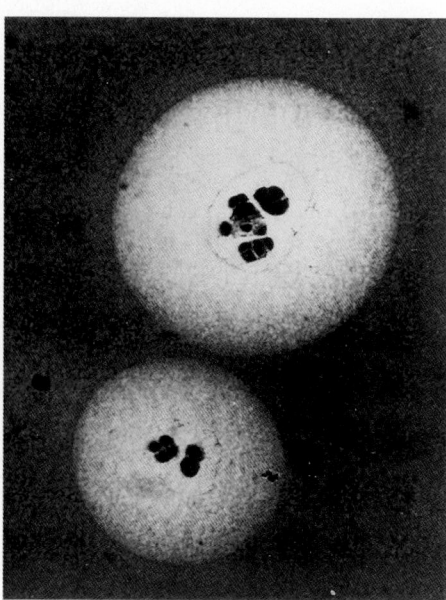

FIGURE 26.16 Demonstrating the secretion of tissue plasminogen activator (tPA) by tumor cells. Low and high power. The dark dots are rat ascites tumor cells seeded onto a fibrin film that contains plasminogen naturally adsorbed to the fibrin. The clear areas represent digested fibrin; they would not develop in the absence of plasminogen. (Courtesy of Dr. K. Tanaka, Kyushu University, Fukuoka, Japan.)

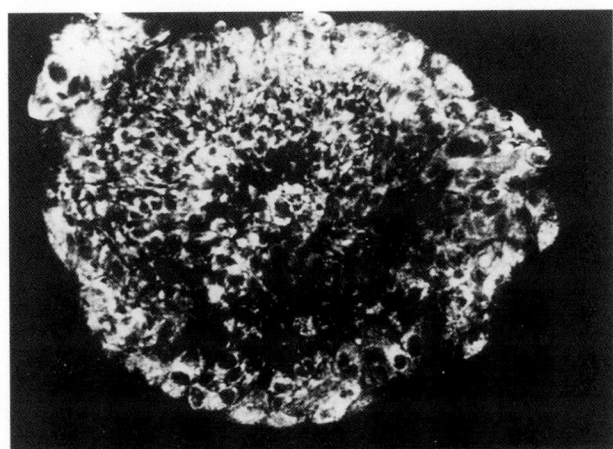

FIGURE 26.17   An abnormality of mitochondria in some tumors. *Top:* Fluorescence photomicrograph; culture of a human colon carcinoma stained with the fluorescent dye rhodamine 123 for 10 minutes and left in dye-free medium for 24 hours. Much dye is retained. *Bottom:* Lack of rhodamine 123 retention by a culture of normal human colonic epithelium, treated as above. (From [34], Copyright © 1990 John Wiley & Sons. Reprinted by permission of John Wiley & Sons, Ltd.)

malignant cells reflect accelerated growth or immaturity, not the neoplastic condition. Tumor cells grow fast and tend to be immature: two properties that they share with embryonic, fetal, or fast-growing cells.

The classic proof of this point is the theory of Otto Warburg (244), a pioneer in the study of respiratory enzymes, which led him to the Nobel prize in 1931. In a monograph published in 1930 (243) Warburg pointed out that slices of normal tissues incubated in the presence glucose produced lactic acid only if they were deprived of oxygen (*anaerobic glycolysis*), whereas slices of tumors produced lactic acid also if they were supplied with oxygen (*aerobic glycolysis*). He concluded that tumors suffered from an irreversible disturbance of their respiratory metabolism. The observations were perfectly correct, but the theory did not stand the test of time (118). It remains true that aerobic glycolysis is common in tumors, but it is merely one of many features that tumor cells share with immature cells (185, 248). An extensive review of tumor mitochondria produced a long list of biochemical anomalies, but none was specific to tumors (185).

TO SUM UP: From this chapter onward, the reader should begin to put together a portrait of the cancer cell. The portrait that *we* are trying to convey is that of an abnormal, but not radically abnormal, cell. Despite the pathologic connotation of behaviors such as *invasion* and *metastasis,* the malignant phenotype is not entirely "new" in biology. Some of its features are those of immature, embryonic-type cells. Even "invasion" is typical of the normal trophoblast and of leukocytes in the course of their defensive expeditions. All this fits with the present notion that malignant cells, in some cases, can be reprogrammed to resemble their normal counterparts (p. 924).

The Structure of Tumors

To understand the gross and microscopic aspect of tumors, it is essential to realize that all tumors consist of two components: (a) a population of neoplastic cells that is supported and nourished by (b) connective tissue and vessels supplied by the host. In other words, every solid tumor contains a neoplastic **parenchyma** (the distinctive tissue of an organ) lying in a non-neoplastic **stroma** (the supporting framework of an organ). *Stroma* is a Greek word well suited to this use; it is related to *straw* and means *bed:* a bed for the parenchymal cells. This dual composition is best appreciated in microscopic sections; in epithelial tumors (such as adenomas and carcinomas) the parenchymal epithelial structures stand out quite clearly against the connective tissue stroma. It is not as easy to recognize the two components in sections of connective tissue tumors such as sarcomas; the contrast between tumor and stroma is minimal because both are mesenchymal (Figure 26.18).

With the naked eye the diagnosis of sarcoma versus carcinoma is not easy. Because sarcomas lack the contrast

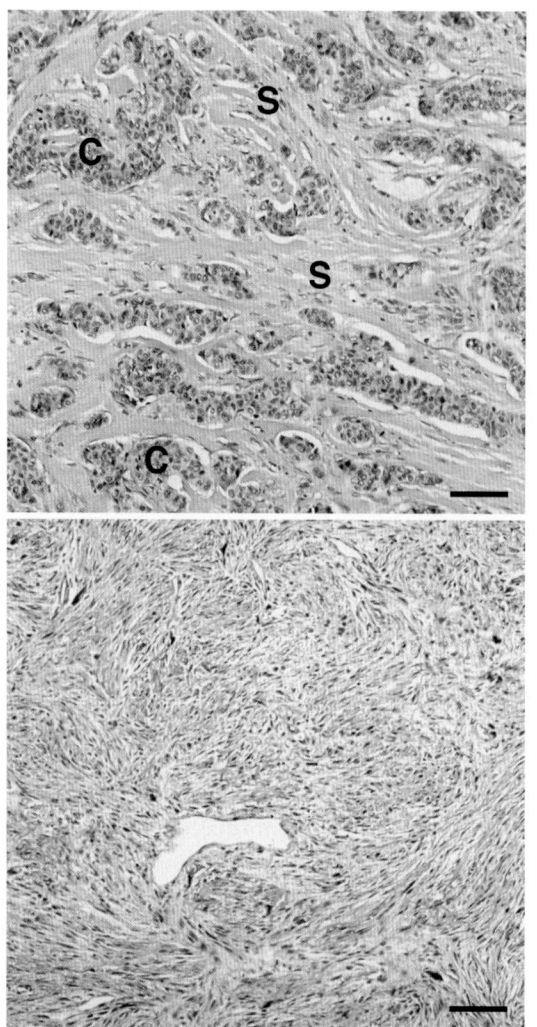

Gross Features of Tumors

Most tumors look like lumps, but there are some major exceptions. Some appear as hollow craters (ulcers); there are even some liquid tumors.

The Tumor–Host Interface

Regarding those tumors that do appear as lumps, it is a general rule that benign tumors tend to have sharply defined edges whereas malignant tumors tend to have branches reaching into their surroundings. However, there are many exceptions. Above all, beware of the legend that "benign tumors are encapsulated, malignant ones not." This is a gross oversimplification. Many benign tumors have no capsule at all, such as leiomyomas of the uterus, hemangiomas of the skin (Figure 26.19) or liver, and fibrohistiocytomas of the skin (which actually look infiltrating). It is also true that benign tumors are sometimes surrounded by a thin fibrous capsule, perhaps laid down by the surrounding tissues as a response to pressure (Figure 26.20). On the other hand, some very malignant tumors may have a capsule; it is usually incomplete and the tumor breaks through it (Figure 26.21). Fast-growing malignant tumors have a special way of surrounding themselves with a fibrous coat: as they rapidly expand within parenchymal organs such as the kidney or liver, the parenchymal cells are squeezed out of existence, and their stroma alone remains to surround the tumor. This has been called a *pseudocapsule* (162). Its genesis is obvious in renal cell carcinomas because atrophic glomeruli remain to tell the story (Figure 26.22).

FIGURE 26.18 *Top:* A "classic" carcinoma (adenocarcinoma of the breast). The difference between the cords of carcinoma (**C**) and the stroma (**S**) is easily seen. *Bottom:* Malignant tumor of mesenchymal cells (fibrous histiocytoma of the skin). The (normal) vessel in the center is obvious, but elsewhere it is difficult or impossible to distinguish between tumor cells and their supporting stroma. **Bars** = 100 μm.

between epithelium and stroma, they appear smoother on cross sections; hence the traditional—but not too convincing—comparison of sarcomas with fish flesh (*sarx* is Greek for flesh).

The concept that all tumors have a *vascularized* stroma supplied by the host means that, to a large extent, the body cooperates with the aggressor. This is a fact; tumors could not exist if they were unable to induce *angiogenesis* (pp. 481, 490, 774).

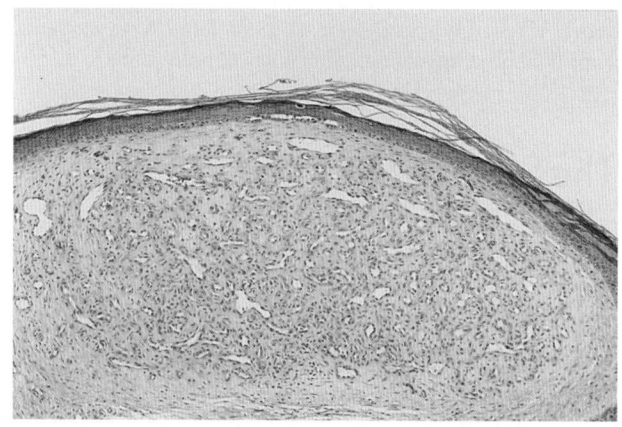

FIGURE 26.19 Capillary hemangioma of the skin, a benign tumor excised for cosmetic reasons—essentially a tangle of capillaries. There is no capsule. *Top:* Epidermis. (60×)

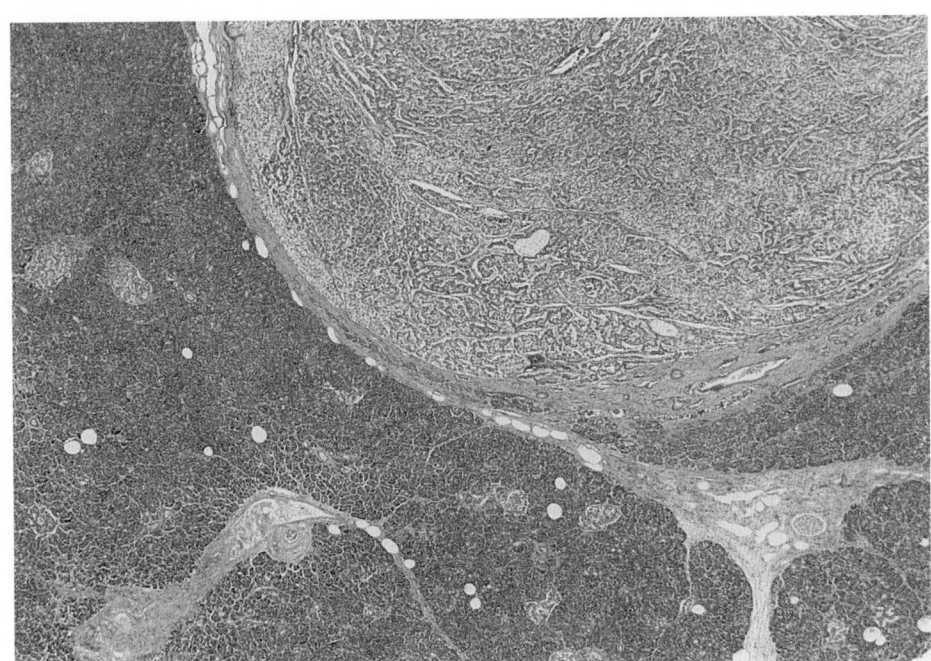

FIGURE 26.20   *Top right:* A benign tumor of the endocrine pancreas (adenoma), surrounded by a thin fibrous capsule. *Bottom left:* Pancreatic tissue including several islets of Langerhans. (20x)

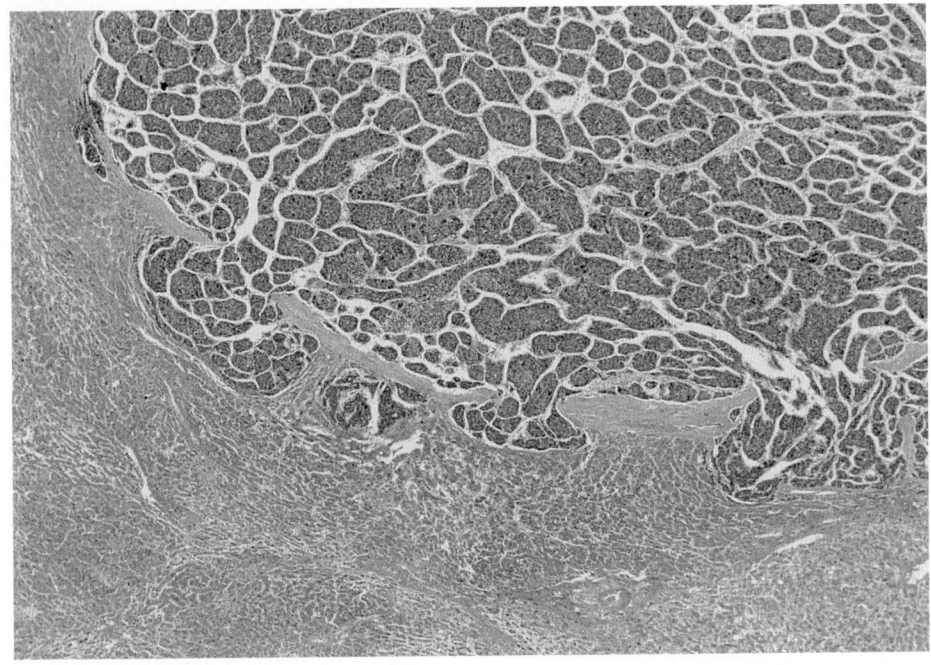

FIGURE 26.21   A carcinoma of the liver (Hepatoma, *top*) expanding into liver tissue (*bottom*). Tumor and liver are separated by a thin fibrous capsule, but at two points this capsule is perforated by mushroom-shaped masses of tumor. Note pressure atrophy of the liver. (20x)

The capsule issue has practical relevance for surgery. Certain benign tumors such as the fibroadenoma of the breast can be removed with little or no surrounding tissue because they are surrounded by a capsule or by a clear-cut cleavage plane; occasionally they can even be "shelled out." In contrast, infiltrating malignant tumors must be removed along with a generous layer of the surrounding tissue.

Regarding the pseudocapsules of renal cell carcinomas and other large malignant tumors, their outer surface often carries large tortuous veins. Why these superficial

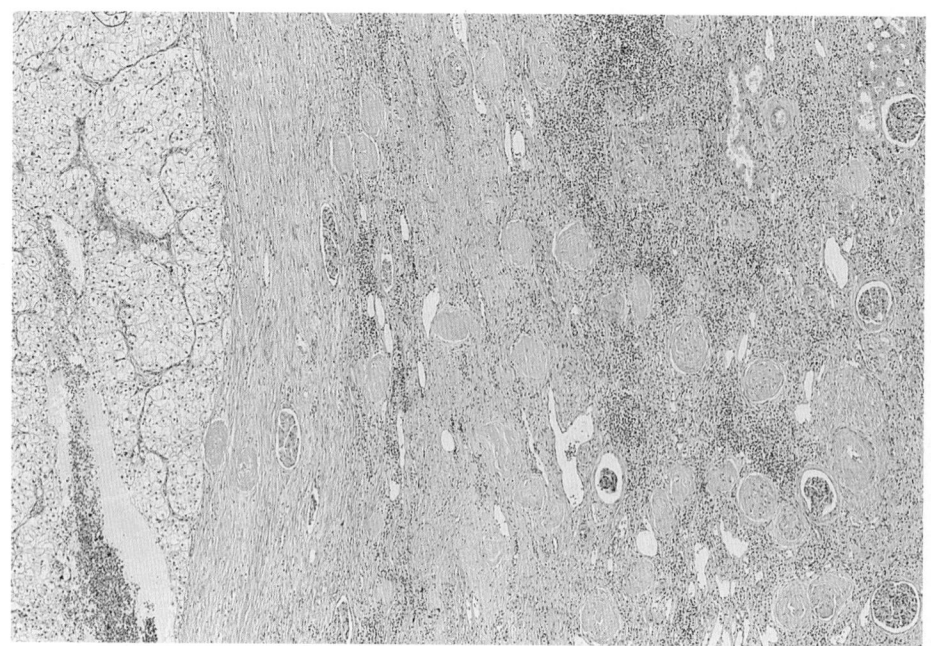

FIGURE 26.22 The concept of "pseudocapsule" around a tumor. *Left:* Renal cell carcinoma. *Right:* Kidney tissue. Between the two is atrophic kidney parenchyma, which constitutes the pseudocapsule: i.e., what is left of the kidney tissue after it has been squeezed out of existence by the advancing tumor. This mechanism is proved by the many atrophic, flattened glomeruli contained in the pseudocapsule. (50x)

veins grow so large is not clear. Perhaps they expand under the stimulus of growth factors in the blood that they drain out of the tumor. Needless to say, they do not even remotely recall a crab sitting on the tumor with claws extended, as someone fancied long ago (p. 738).

Ulcerated Tumors

Tumors that arise from a bacterially contaminated surface (such as the skin or gut) tend to become ulcerated (Figure 26.23). In the gut this is due to bacterial infection, with some help from digestive enzymes. At first the surface of the tumor is eroded by mechanical friction; then bacteria colonize it, and persist (tumors have abnormal vessels, and correspondingly generate a poor inflammatory response). The result is an ulcer that does not heal. Malignant tumors are especially prone to ulcerate, and when they do, they can be difficult to recognize: are we dealing with an ulcer or with an ulcerated tumor? A raised edge (also called a rolled edge), as shown in Figure 26.24, strongly suggests an ulcerated tumor. When radiologists examine X-rays of questionable gastric ulcers, taken after a barium swallow, they can actually see the raised edge as a negative image. However, the diagnosis of tumor versus ulcer can be made only by the microscope. Witness Figure 26.24, which defies all classic teaching about raised edges.

Another site where tumors may typically be present as ulcers is the face, or any part of the skin exposed to the sun (Figure 26.25). Any skin ulcer that persists for longer than 3–6 weeks is suspect. An everyday example is the basal cell carcinoma of the face, a malignancy with a very

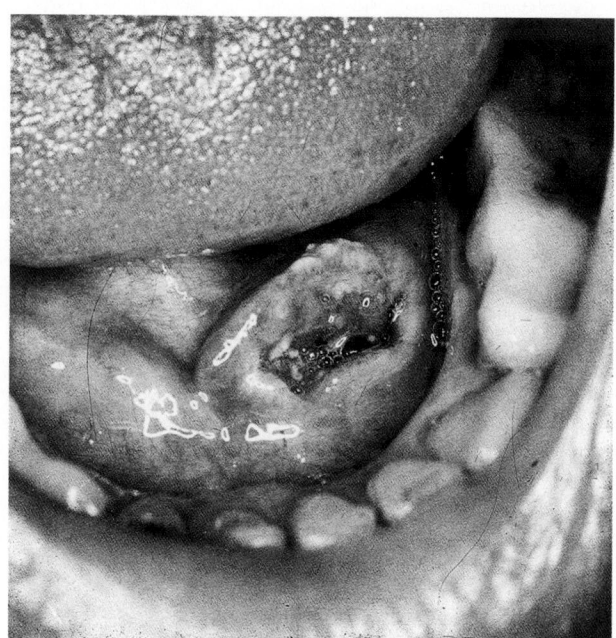

FIGURE 26.23 Craterlike ulcerated carcinoma from the floor of the mouth in a 40-year-old-woman. The raised edges are characteristic of an ulcerated tumor as opposed to a simple ulcer. (Courtesy of Dr. G. Fiore-Donno, School of Dentistry, Geneva, Switzerland.)

distinctive personality: it grows slowly but tends to ulcerate so relentlessly that its ancient Latin name was *ulcus rodens*, the gnawing ulcer (Figure 26.26). Such persistent "ulcers" are best removed as a whole rather than biopsied;

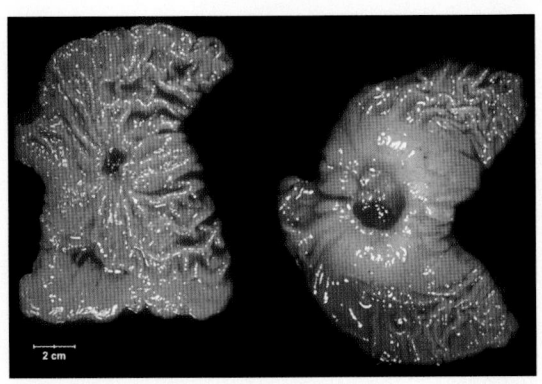

FIGURE 26.24 Gastric ulcer or ulcerated cancer? The naked eye can mislead. *Left:* Ulcer without "rolled edges" and with radiating mucosal folds, suggestive of a chronic process. *Right:* Ulcer with greatly swollen margins, suggesting cancer. Microscopic examination showed an ulcerated carcinoma (*left*) and a gastric ulcer (*right*). (Courtesy of Dr. R. Lattes, Columbia University, New York, NY.)

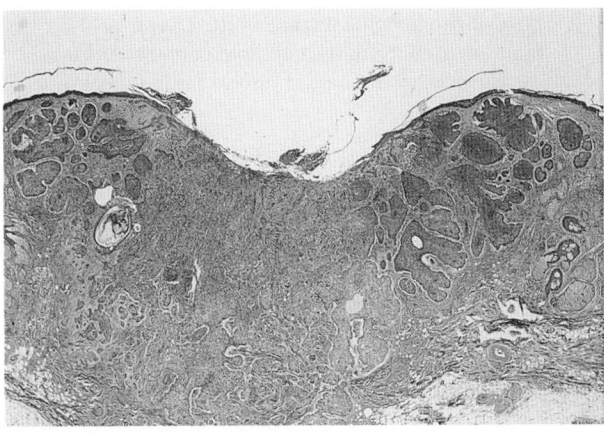

FIGURE 26.26 Ulcerated basal cell carcinoma of the face, similar to that shown in Figure 26.25. The cords of basal cells are obvious at *top right* and *left;* their connection with the epidermis is best seen at higher powers. (10x)

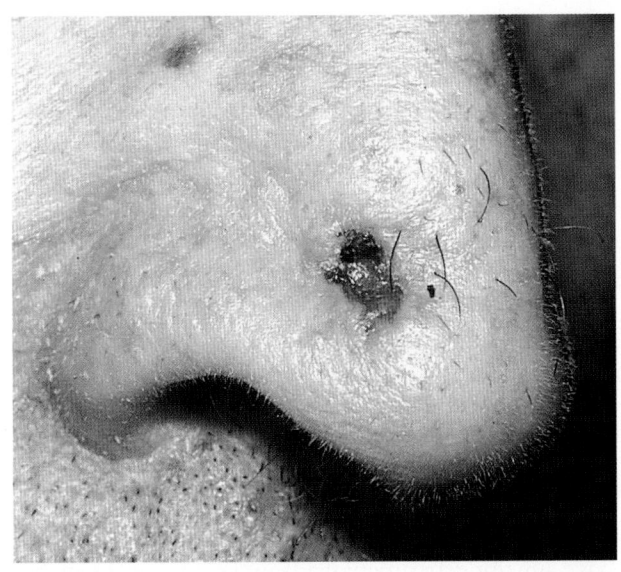

FIGURE 26.25 Basal cell carcinoma. The small ulcer on the nose of this 76-year-old man has been present for about 3 months. This presentation is typical of a basal cell carcinoma. (Courtesy of Dr. R. A. Johnson, New England Deaconess Hospital, Boston, MA.)

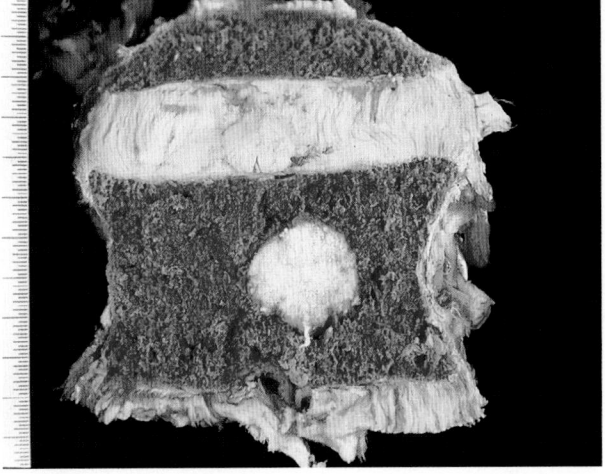

FIGURE 26.27 Metastasis of a carcinoma of the breast in a human vertebra. **Scale** in centimeters.

called scirrhous carcinomas (from the Greek *skirrhós,* hard). Epithelial tumors with little stroma are soft or medullary (which means marrowlike). Carcinomas of both kinds occur, for example, in the breast.

The Cut Surface of a Tumor

A cut surface provides a lot of information:

- *Tumor tissue tends to be white* (Figure 26.27), whether benign or malignant, and even in areas that are clearly not necrotic. This is bizarre because no

they almost invariably turn out to be basal cell carcinomas; and once removed, they pose no further threat.

The Consistency of Tumors

Most tumors feel firm, even hard, especially those with a large amount of connective tissue stroma. The latter are normal parenchyma is truly white, except for the brain on account of its high lipid content. As far as we know, the whiteness of tumors has not been explained.

We have submitted this problem to several experts, who offered three excellent solutions. (a) The late biochemist Albert Szent-Györgyi, twice Nobel laureate, suggested that oxidative processes in tumors are low, and on the whole "oxidation tends to entail colored products." Aerobic glycolysis (p. 757) is typical of tumors. (b) Quite independently, a similar suggestion was made by Dr. H. Pitot. In tumors, he wrote, there is a "relative lack of cytochromes which are tan, orange, beige or even brown and a dramatic increase in nucleic acids . . . which are white or very light yellow in visible light." (c) Dr. P. Gullino (who made important contributions to studies of the vascularization of tumors) noted that tumors are less vascularized than the normal corresponding tissue; this may be the principal mechanism (the interstitial pressure in tumors is high (p. 788); this would tend to compress the blood vessels).

> NOTE: The whiteness of tumor tissue is unrelated to the whiteness of necrosis. A liver adenoma, white to the naked eye, is free of necrosis and can be histologically very similar to normal liver tissue.

Of course, some tumors contain pigments. Melanomas can be extraordinarily black, even in fish (Figure 3.53); angiomas are red with blood; and hepatomas can be green with bile.

- *The margin of the tumor* may blend with the normal tissue around it; this suggests infiltration, an aggressive feature typical of malignancy. A sharp margin is compatible with benign behavior, albeit with the reservations mentioned earlier.
- *Foci of necrosis* usually mean bad news because *necrosis is much more common in malignant tumors and correlates statistically with poor prognosis* (Figure 26.28) (171). Necrosis is usually of the coagulative type and may be accompanied by hemorrhage. The mechanisms of necrosis in tumors will be discussed later (p. 767).
- *Large spaces filled with fluid (cysts) suggest that the tumor is epithelial.* The mechanism: if the tumor contains secreting glands, the secretion has no way out and therefore expands the lumen of the glands (Figure 26.29).

The Special Case of Liquid Tumors

It is sometimes said that leukemias are liquid tumors; this is not completely accurate because the circulating leukemic cells come from the bone marrow, which is

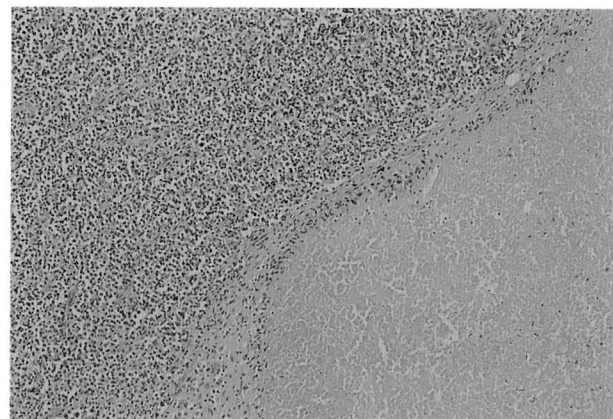

FIGURE 26.28 Poor inflammatory response in tumors. *Bottom right:* Coagulative necrosis, presumably ischemic, in a lymphoma. A thin layer of reactive cells, mainly fibroblasts, has developed along the demarcation line with the tumor, but there is no granulation tissue. The lymphoma (*left*) appears typically as a "sea of lymphocytes." (60x)

very soft but not truly fluid, even though it can be aspirated with a needle. The term is quite appropriate, however, for the experimental tumors called **ascites tumors,** extensively studied by George and Eva Klein at the Karolinska Institute (140). Many transplantable tumors of rats and mice can be induced (some more easily than others) to grow freely in the peritoneal cavity where they induce an exudate (**ascites**) and thrive within it like bacteria in a broth, without invading the peritoneal surfaces, at least initially. The ascitic fluid is presumably caused by factors increasing vascular permeability that are secreted by the tumor cells (p. 787). The biological change of cells to ascites tumor behavior is irreversible; it may be a manifestation of tumor progression. Ascites tumors are an artefact, but they do have a major experimental advantage in that the malignant cells are easily harvested.

The Microscopic Structure of Tumors

The basic principle of tumor structure, which is sufficiently established to resemble dogma, is that *tumors tend to reproduce the cellular type and the architectural pattern of the parent tissue.* There is a corollary: Benign tumors are relatively faithful imitations of the original tissue, malignant tumors are rather caricatures.

Considering that the human body contains roughly 200 types of cells and that tumors tend to create fanciful variants, it is easy to grasp that the microscopic patterns of tumors number in the hundreds. Because pathologists must memorize them, they are sometimes

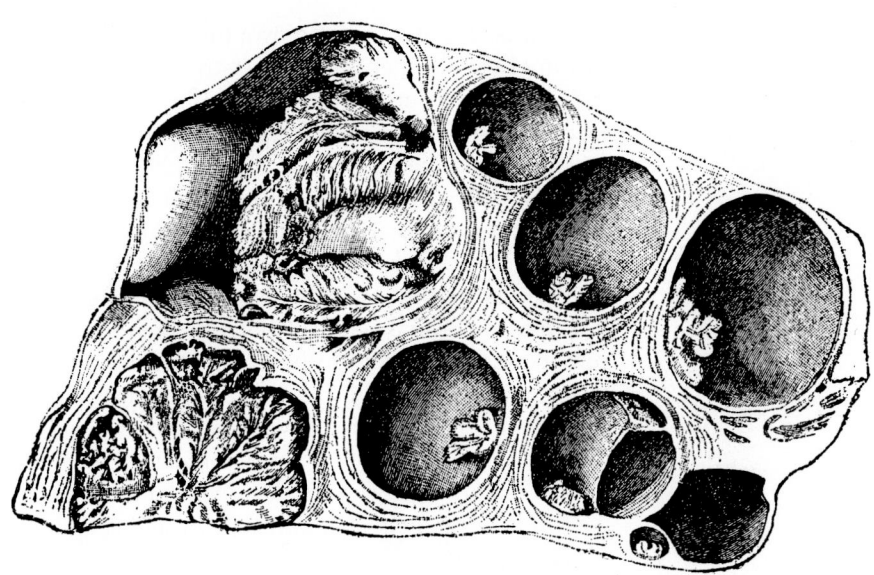

FIGURE 26.29 A papillary cystadenocarcinoma of the ovary seen in cross section. Drawn from a specimen ca. 1900. (Reproduced from [257].)

teased as "stamp collectors." We will offer two examples, comparing a normal tissue with its benign and malignant counterpart (Figures 26.30, 26.31).

The first step in working out the structure of tumors is to distinguish the non-neoplastic stroma from the tumor cells.

The Stroma of Tumors

All tumors have a stroma consisting of connective tissue, vessels, a moderate inflammatory infiltrate (61), and sometimes, myofibroblasts (211). The amount of each component varies greatly; the scirrhous tumors just mentioned are packed with collagen fibers but, oddly enough, also with elastic fibers (235).

> Even more odd is the fact that some of the elastin in human breast cancers is produced by the neoplastic epithelial cells as well as by fibroblasts and microvascular endothelium. This was found by means of *in situ* hybridization of mRNA for human elastin (146)

The intimate contact between tumor and stroma exposes the stromal cells to a variety of enzymes, growth factors, and other secretions of the tumor cells. As a result, the fibroblasts in the stroma of a tumor can be functionally quite abnormal (100, 209). The overproduction of collagen by fibroblasts of scirrhous tumors is probably a response to tumor cell products (133). The stroma can also affect the tumor, for example, by sequestering positive or negative growth factors; matrix-degrading enzymes secreted by stromal fibroblasts can dock on the tips of tumor cell pseudopodia, become activated, and help the tumor's invasive activity (153, 220).

In colorectal carcinomas the c-*myc* gene is expressed by the tumor cells as well as by the stromal cells; the latter are probably responding in this manner to epidermal growth factor (EGF) produced by the tumor cells (164).

Many more examples could follow (10, 90, 183), but the key point is that there is a great deal of cross-talk between tumor cells and stroma, enough to be considered as a possible target for anti-tumor therapy (66, 153).

Not only stromal cells but any tissue near a tumor is exposed to an overdose of growth factors; for example, the thickening of the gastric mucosa surrounding a gastric carcinoma is attributed to EGF secreted by the tumor (150).

The blood vessels of tumors, in theory at least, can derive from two sources: some may be produced anew by angiogenesis, others may represent preexisting microcirculation incorporated by the growing tumor (187). As expected, their density varies greatly from tumor to tumor and between different areas of the same tumor; values published for various rat and mouse tumors, relating to relative volume occupied by the vessels, range from 1 to 50 percent (4, 75, 107, 253). But whatever their density, the key point to remember is that *the blood supply of a tumor is less than to the corresponding normal tissue* (186, 187).

Transmission and scanning electron microscopy of tumor vessels show many abnormal features (63, 113). Tumor vessels tend to have an irregular diameter and branching pattern; they do not fit well into the standard classification of arterioles, capillaries, and venules; and even large vessels have thin walls and incomplete cellular coats (113). The endothelial cells can be

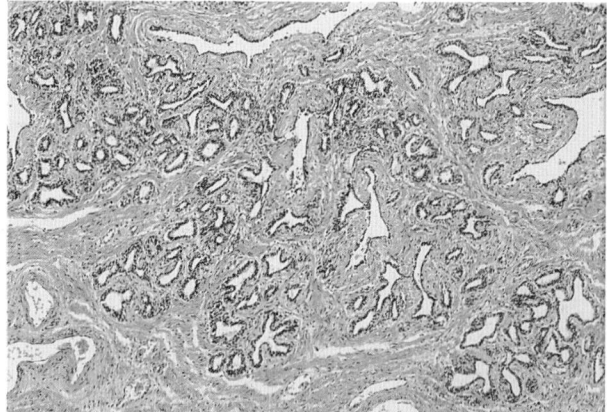

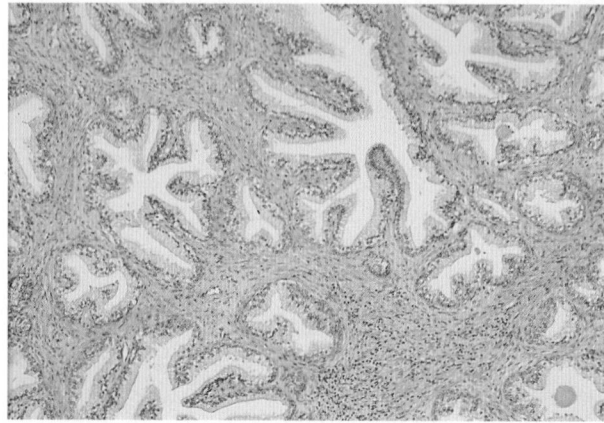

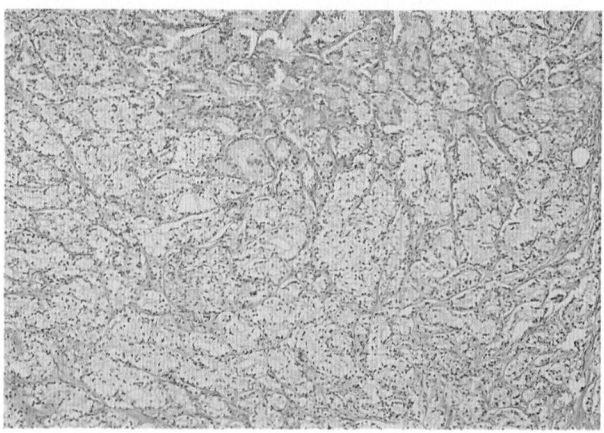

FIGURE 26.30 Comparing normal prostatic glands (*top*) with glands of prostatic hypertrophy (*center*) and with an adenocarcinoma of the prostate (*bottom*). In the latter, the glandular structure is preserved but barely apparent. (60x)

disorganized, loosely connected, with aberrant projections that can even cross the lumen; most importantly, they have intercellular and sometimes transcellular gaps, through which tumor cells could easily crawl.

All these features fit the known functional properties of tumor vessels: they react poorly to vasoactive agents (186), and many are leaky (9a, 63). If dyes are injected intravenously in tumor-bearing mice, parts of the tumors can be stained, especially the rim (99). The vessels leak not only because their lining is incomplete but also because tumor cells secrete factors that increase permeability (Figure 26.32) (31, 58, 63, 143). It is noteworthy that the *vascular permeability* factor (VPF) described by Dvorak and collaborators in experimental tumors was later found to be also a potent *angiogenic* factor produced by many fetal and adult tissues, including human tissues, especially under anoxia: hence its double name VPF/VEGF (for vascular endothelial growth factor) (58). Vascular leakage in tumors has its good side: it can help chemotherapy by allowing drugs to seep out (62).

Another feature of tumor vessels that should help tumor chemotherapy is that their endothelium has a high mitotic rate: its labeling index (p. 784) is 20–2000 times higher than normal (Figure 26.33) (49, 50). This should allow chemotherapy to hit "cycling" blood vessels as well as "cycling" tumor cells (49).

The vessels of brain tumors tend to maintain a blood-brain barrier, which means that they retain a significant level of normality. It also means that they complicate therapy because to reach brain tumors with chemotherapeutic agents it is necessary to break down the blood-brain barrier temporarily; this can be done, for example, by injecting hypertonic mannitol into the carotid artery.

A controversy is currently raging over the fine structure of vessels in certain tumors (72, 202a). One group of researchers has reported that retinal melanomas contain channels bordered by tumor cells only, without endothelium, and thus without "angiogenesis" in the current sense. They called it *vasculogenic mimicry*. Another highly reputable group could not confirm the findings. Time will tell.

The process whereby tumor vessels are generated—tumor angiogenesis—is a story in itself; we will tell it in relation to tumor growth (p. 774). Inflammation in tumors will be discussed on p. 787.

The Neoplastic Component of Tumors

After tumor cells are identified, two questions must be answered: where do they come from? and how aggressive are they?

The ancestry of tumor cells is often quite clear because tumors tend to reproduce the original cell and tissue. See, for example, an adenoma of the endocrine

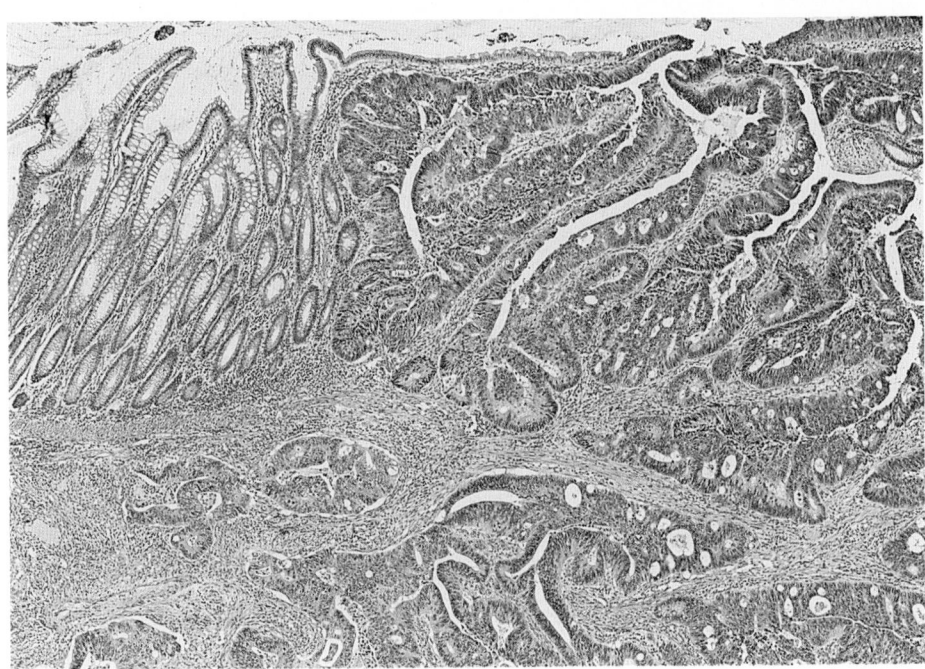

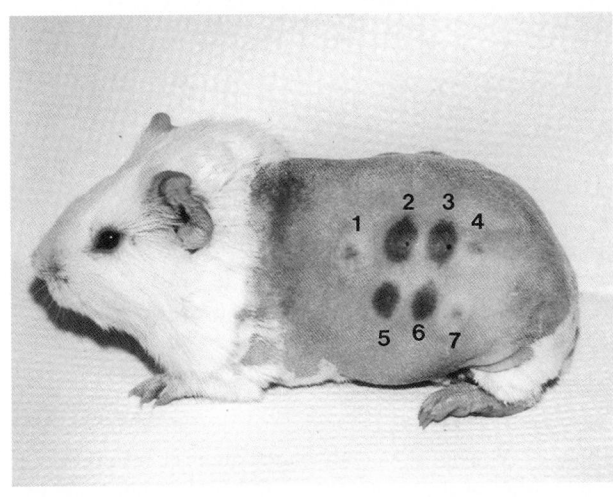

FIGURE 26.32 Evans blue test demonstrating vascular permeability factors (VPF) produced by an ascites tumor. Actually, this experiment marks the discovery of the very important VEGF (vascular endothelial growth factor). The seven skin sites of this otherwise normal guinea pig were injected with **1:** Antibody against VPF (control, negative); **2:** VPF from *Line 10* ascites tumor (strongly positive); **3:** VPF plus an unrelated antibody (strongly positive); **4:** VPF plus specific neutralizing antibody (negative, neutralized); **5:** VPF from a different ascites tumor (*Line 1*) (strongly positive); **6:** VPF plus unrelated antibody (strongly positive); **7:** VPF plus specific antibody, again showing neutralization of the VPF factor. (Courtesy of Drs. D. R. Sanger and H. F. Dvorak, Department of Pathology, Beth Israel Hospital, Boston, MA.)

pancreas (Figure 26.20) or a leiomyoma of the uterus (Figure 25.13). Even if the tumor is so undifferentiated that it has lost all identifiable structural features, it usually retains some cell-specific antigen that can be recognized by a specific antibody. Antibodies can also be helpful for distinguishing look-alikes (Figure 26.34).

The question of aggressiveness can be answered by studying abnormalities of the cells and abnormalities of tissue architecture. These are the cornerstones of tumor diagnosis.

Cellular abnormalities. The malignant phenotype has already been portrayed; in summary, when diagnosing a tumor, the following criteria must be kept in mind.

- *Lack of differentiation.* Whereas normal cells have set characteristics that define their state of maturity (differentiation), tumor cells tend to be, and to look, less differentiated. For example, a mucus-secreting cell in a tumor may contain minimal amounts of mucus and a fat cell may contain many small droplets of fat (like embryonic fat) rather than a single larger drop (Figure 26.35). *Highly undifferentiated cells suggest a very aggressive tumor.* We will learn later that one way to treat malignant tumors is to encourage them to differentiate.
- *Cytologic atypia,* that is, abnormal size, shape, or content of cells.
- *Pleomorphism (polymorphism).* Cellular atypia goes hand in hand with cellular pleomorphism because the

FIGURE 26.33 Comparing the turnover of endothelial cells in various mouse tissues by injecting tritiated thymidine every 8 hours for 7 days. The rate is highest for the placenta, high for five types of mouse tumor, very low for nine normal adult tissues. (Adapted and reproduced with permission from [49], © 1984 Munksgaard International Publishers Ltd, Copenhagen, Denmark.)

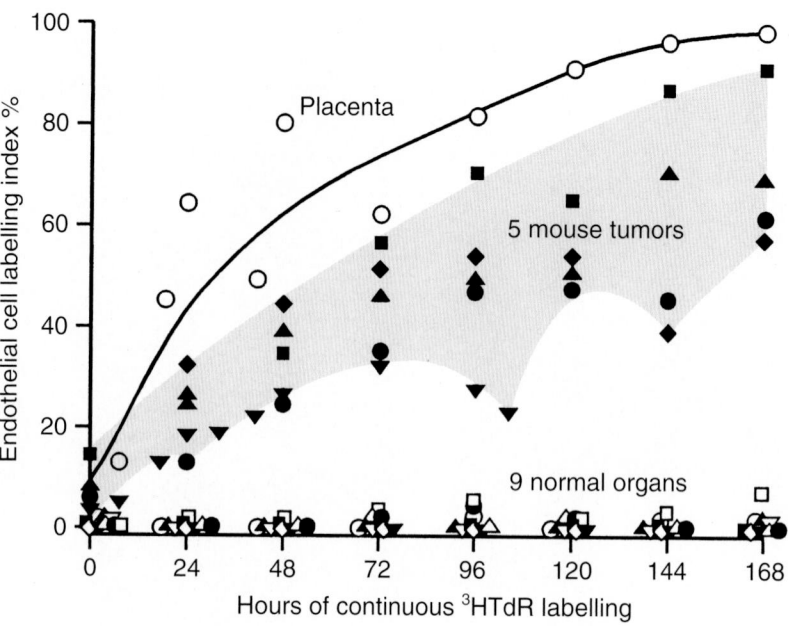

FIGURE 26.34 Illustrating the limits of histology in diagnosing tumors. **A:** Normal smooth muscle (human myometrium). **B:** Leiomyoma of the uterus. **C:** Tumor of Schwann cells (Schwannoma). Most of such "lookalikes" are solved by immunohistochemistry. **Bar** = 100 μm.

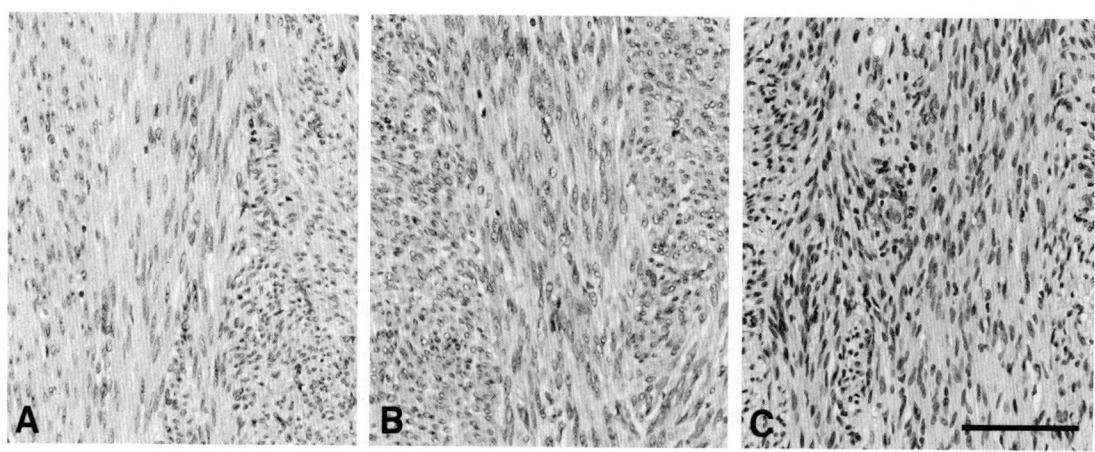

degree of atypia tends to vary from one cell to another and from one microscopic field to another. The sight of a tissue with nuclei of different sizes and shapes is immediately suspect (Figure 26.36). Assessing pleomorphism is often a subjective, almost artistic judgment. It can be made quantitative by deferring the judgment, for example, to the fluorescence-activated cell sorter (FACS) (p. 15); however, the verdicts of the FACS are time-consuming, expensive, and virtually limited to "liquid tumors."

Abnormalities of architecture. Architectural atypia. By this we mean abnormal cellular pattern. This feature is best

seen in glandular tumors, in which beautiful normal patterns give way to disorderly structures of varying degrees of ugliness and, correspondingly, of threat (Figure 26.37).

Infiltration (local invasion) means that tumor tissue invades its neighboring tissues. *Infiltration is a nearly absolute sign of malignancy* (Figures 26.38, 26.39).

Secondary Changes in Tumors

Because tumors are poorly planned structures, they tend to develop mishaps. One of these is ulceration (p. 760); others are listed below.

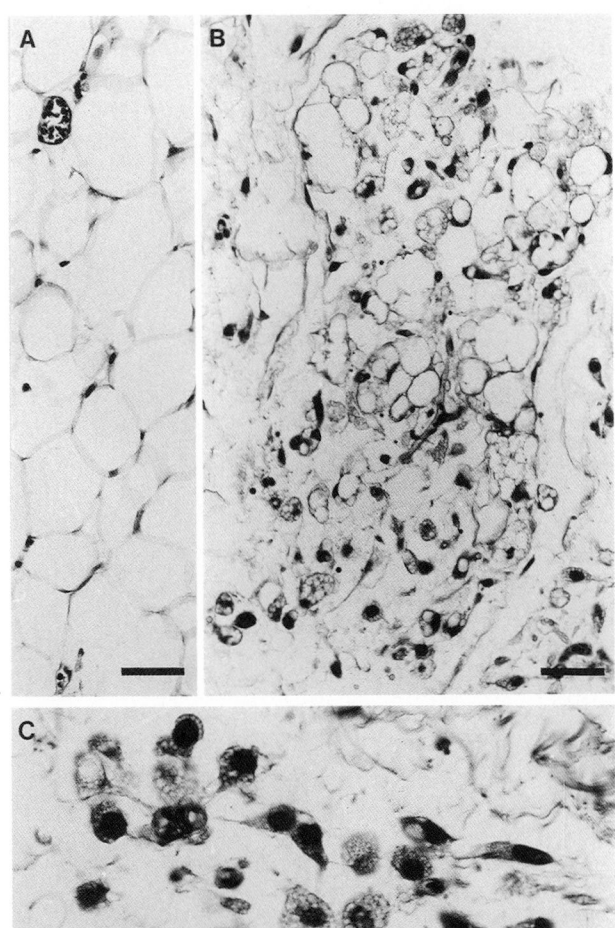

FIGURE 26.35   **A:** Normal adipose tissue. **B:** Malignant tumor of adipose tissue (liposarcoma). The cells are irregular; many contain small, multiple pockets of fat, as better shown at higher power in **C. Bars** = 50 μm.

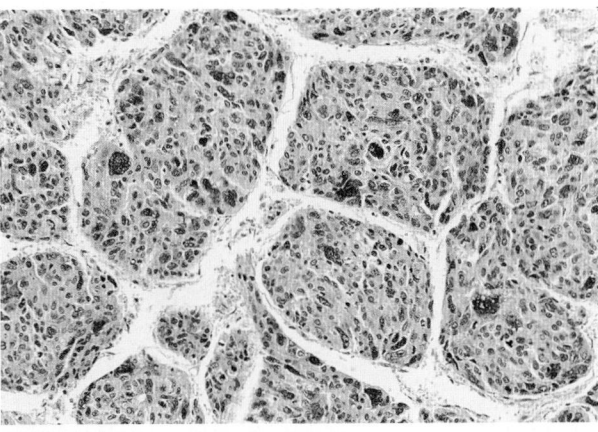

FIGURE 26.36   Malignant tumor of liver tissue (hepatoma). This tumor can be interpreted as a caricature of normal liver tissue: it consists of cords of epithelial cells. Note the variations in nuclear size and shape. (120x)

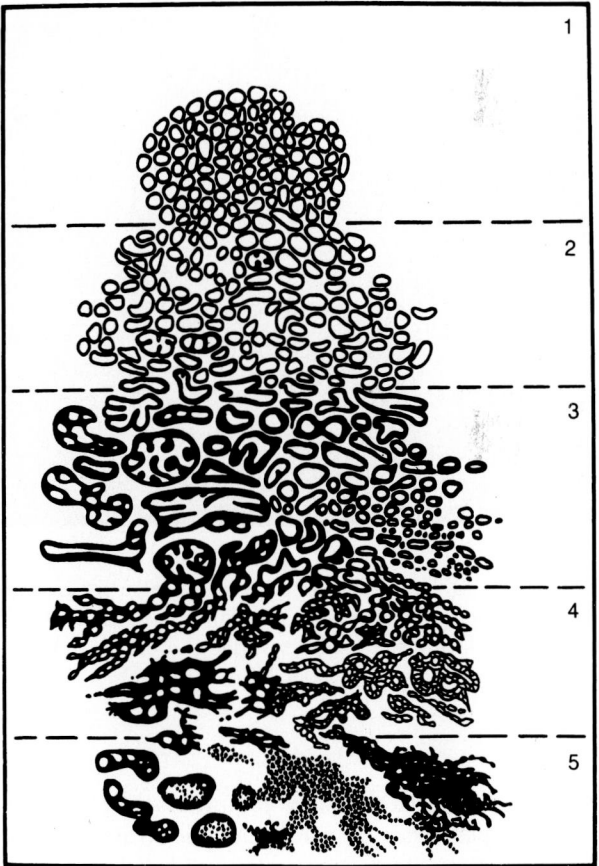

FIGURE 26.37   A simplified drawing of the so-called Gleason grading system for prostatic adenocarcinoma. As the glandular structure departs more and more from the original pattern (**1**) and as glandular atypia increases, the prognosis becomes worse. (Reproduced with permission from [98a], © Lea & Febiger, 1977.)

Necrosis

Necrotic masses, so common in malignant tumors, develop in two ways. (a) *Ischemia* is the reason for the massive central necrosis almost invariably seen in large malignant tumors (Figure 26.40), and sometimes in large benign tumors. It is best explained by the impairment of blood flow caused by high tissue pressure (p. 788). (b) *Programmed cell death* leading to the massive pileup of necrotic cells is seen in many epithelial tumors (28, 171). Consider the epithelium of the skin: normally the basal cells multiply, move upward, die, and slough off. The same program operates in cancers of the skin, but most of the cells that slough off have no outlet: the tumor is not a flat surface but a tangle of

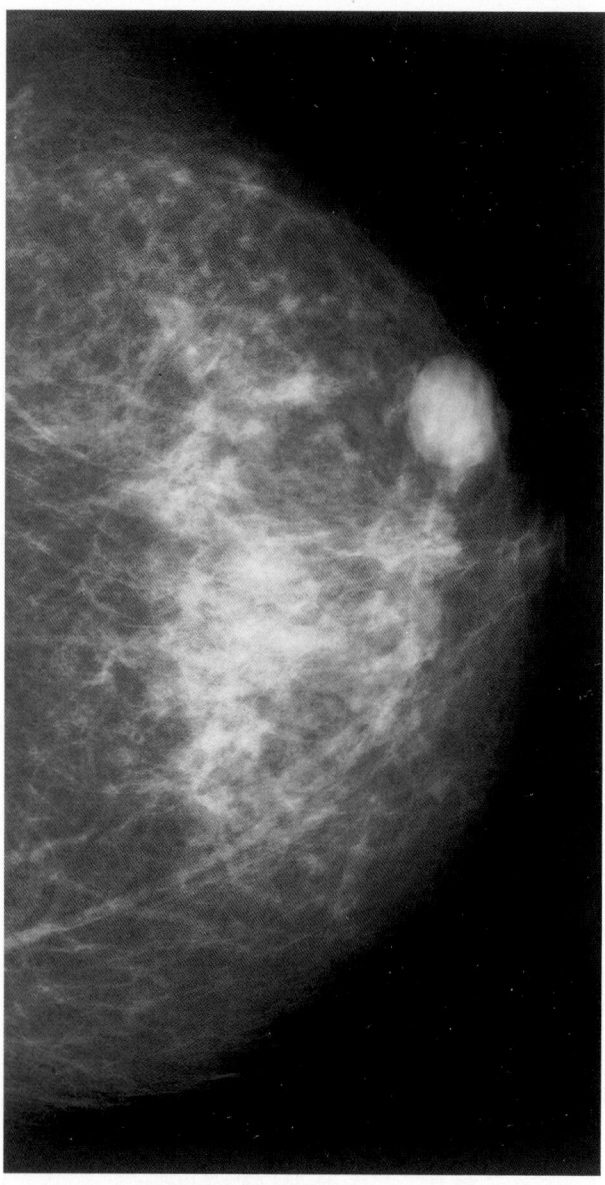

FIGURE 26.38 Mammogram showing a benign tumor with sharp outlines (fibroadenoma). The diffuse mass at the left is normal glandular tissue. (Courtesy of Dr. C. D'Orsi, University of Massachusetts Medical School, Worcester, MA.)

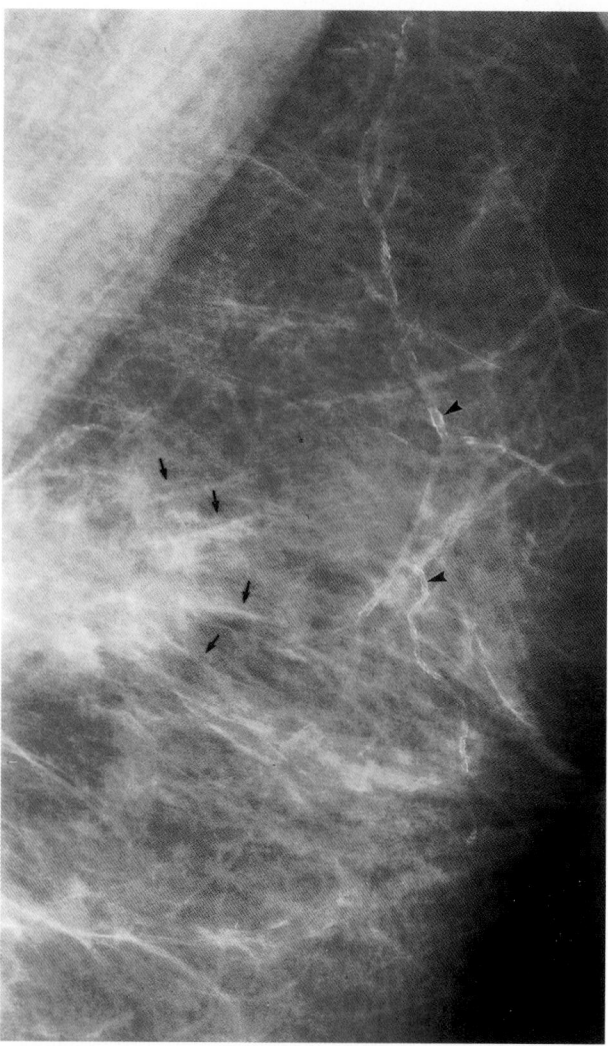

FIGURE 26.39 Mammogram showing a typical malignant tumor (carcinoma) in a 66-year-old woman. **Arrows:** Streaks suggestive of infiltration. *Top left:* Pectoral muscle to which the mass was clinically adherent. Note the calcified arteries (**arrowheads**). (Courtesy of Dr. C. D'Orsi, University of Massachusetts Medical School, Worcester, MA.)

roots. So, the cells that have completed their cycle remain trapped inside the tumor and pile up as a necrotic mass. This is the genesis of the "epithelial pearls" of squamous cell carcinoma (Figure 26.41).

NOTE: Cell death by apoptosis occurs throughout all tumors, malignant or not (pp. 216, 786, 891); here we are dealing only with secondary necrosis.

Calcification

Calcification usually develops in dead cells or necrotic masses. For reasons unknown, the cells of some carcinomas have a special propensity to calcify, especially in the breast and ovary; the resulting tiny, gritty calcifications have suggested a comparison with sand, hence the name *psammomas* for these tumors (Greek *psámmos,* sand) (Figures 26.42, 26.43). In the breast, tiny calcifications are so common that mammography exploits them as an early warning of possible malignancy.

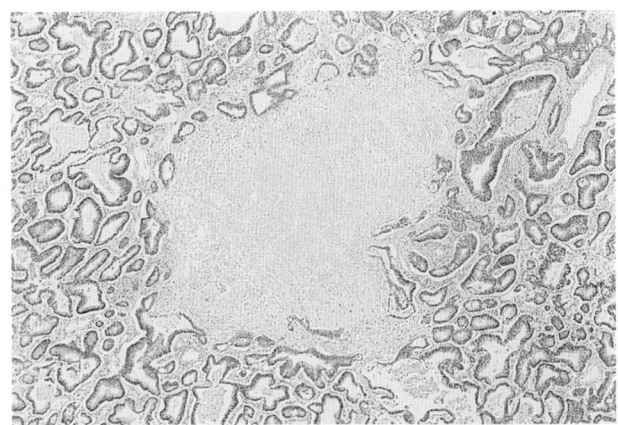

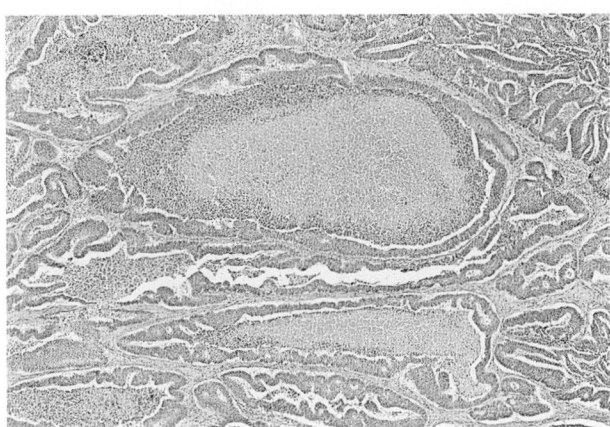

FIGURE 26.40   Necrosis in carcinomas: two mechanisms. *Top:* A focus of ischemic necrosis. The tissue died in bulk; faint outlines of the original structures are visible (adenocarcinoma of the lung). *Bottom:* In adenocarcinoma of the colon, atypical glands shed their epithelium into the lumen (programmed cell death, usually via apoptosis). (25x)

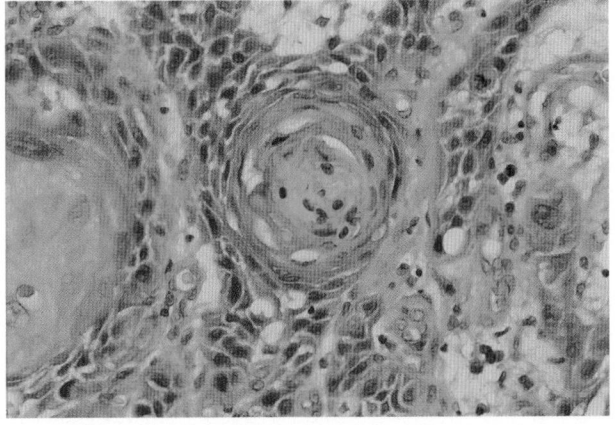

FIGURE 26.41   Typical epidermal "pearl" characteristic of squamous cell carcinoma of the skin. Pearls consist of squamous cells that have reached maturation (keratinization) but cannot slough off because they lie deep in the tumor. (230x)

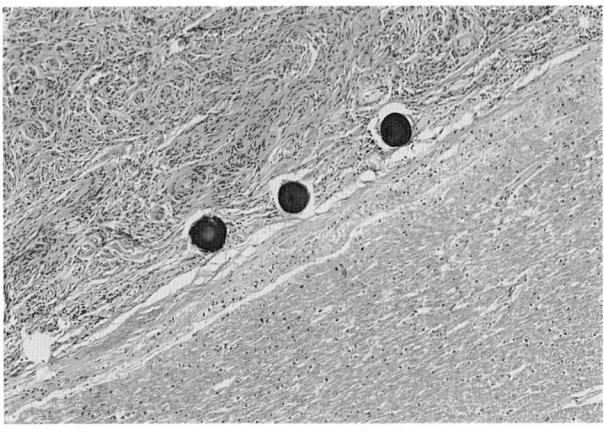

FIGURE 26.42   Microscopic calcifications in a tumor. Three "psammoma bodies" at the periphery of a meningioma (*top left*). *Lower right:* White matter. (Specimen courtesy of Dr. Thomas W. Smith, University of Massachusetts Medical School, Worcester, MA.)

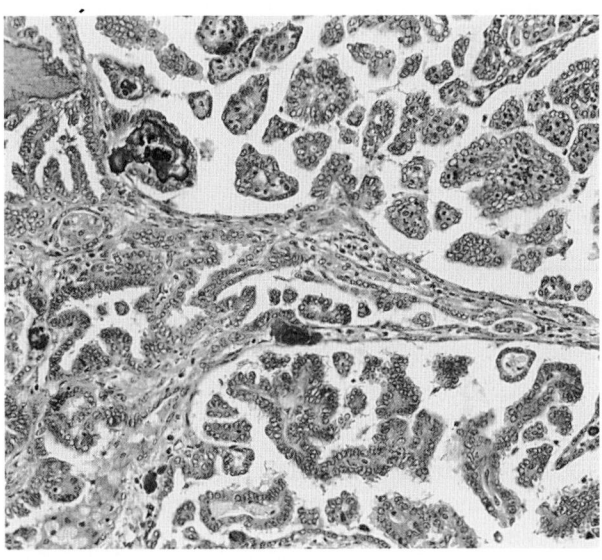

FIGURE 26.43   Microscopic calcifications (*psammoma bodies*) tend to develop in some tumors, e.g., in this papillary cystadenocarcinoma of the ovary. The "isolated" structures are actually cross sections of branching papillae; some are calcified (basophilic material). (120x)

Unfortunately, benign lesions also calcify, and there is no way yet to distinguish them.

The genesis of microscopic psammoma bodies needs more study; it may differ from tumor to tumor (21). A strange mechanism has been observed in carcinomas of the breast: the calcification of secretions within an intracellular lumen (Figure 26.44) (2).

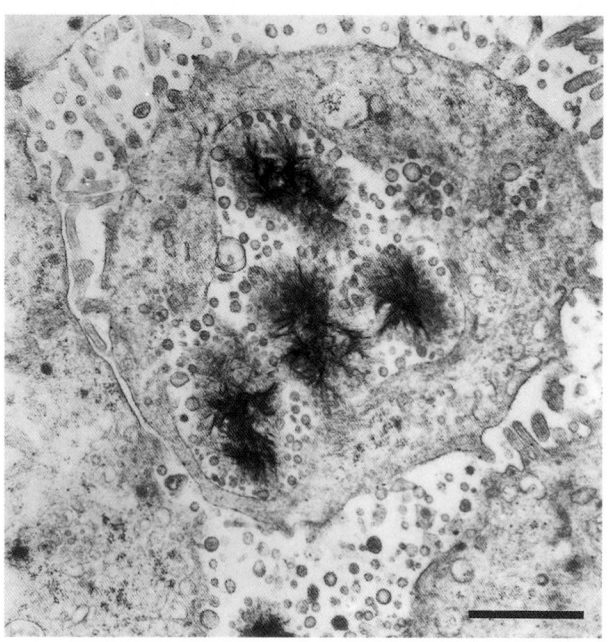

FIGURE 26.44   Example of calcification in carcinoma of the breast. Four clusters of apatite crystals have formed in what appears to be an intracellular lumen. **Bar** = 1 μm. (From [2], Copyright © 1975. Reprinted by permission of John Wiley & Sons, Ltd.)

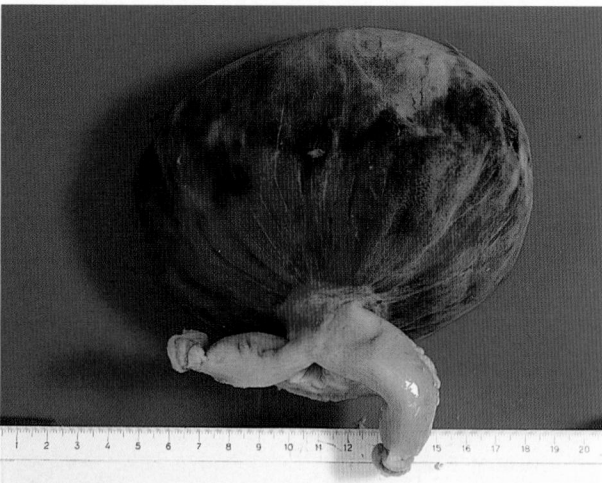

FIGURE 26.45   Infarction of a benign tumor by torsion. This leiomyoma, bulging from the outer wall of the small intestine, twisted itself around its peduncle; as it became necrotic it caused enough inflammation and pain to mimic appendicitis. (The original color was deep purple from venous congestion.) **Scale** in centimeters. (Courtesy of the Department of Pathology, Geneva, Switzerland.)

Leiomyomas sometimes calcify, and this seems to have been true also 5000 years ago: a rounded calcified mass about 5 cm in diameter, found in a neolithic burial site in Switzerland, was diagnosed as "presumed calcified leiomyoma of the uterus" (145).

Torsion

Torsion is an accident that besets pedunculated tumors, be they benign or malignant. Ovarian tumors are especially susceptible. As might be expected, the veins in the twisted stalk are compressed first, while the arteries still manage to pump blood beyond the stricture. The result is a red infarct: the tumor has killed itself (Figure 26.45).

Differences Between Benign and Malignant Tumors: A Summary

We have mentioned the key principles for recognizing a "malignant tumor": the degree of malignancy tends to correlate with atypia; local invasiveness suggests malignancy; **metastasis proves malignancy.** In addition to these guidelines, there are many finer criteria, summarized in Table 26.1. All are helpful, but they are only suggestive and therefore must be interpreted with a grain of salt. Mitoses, for example, are plentiful not only in malignant tumors but also in regenerating tissues.

Afterthoughts on tumor diagnosis. Identifying tumors "benign" or "malignant" under the microscope is more complex than matching a pattern with a name. Earlier we resorted to the term *ugliness* in relation to malignant

Table 26.1 Comparison of Various Features in Benign and Malignant Tumors

Feature	In Benign Tumors	In Malignant Tumors
Rate of growth	Slow	Fast
Mode of growth	Expansile	Infiltrative
General effects	Uncommon (except endocrine)	Common
Metastases*	—	Common
Recurrence after removal	Rare	Common
Gross:		
Capsule	Common	Pseudocapsule
Necrosis	Rare	Common
Ulceration	Rare	Common
Microscopic:		
Atypia	Mild	Severe
Pleomorphism	Mild	Severe
Mitoses	Few	Many
Nuclear/cytoplasmic ratio	Normal	Increased
Nucleolus	Normal	Prominent
Ploidy	Often normal	Usually abnormal

*Most reliable criterion.

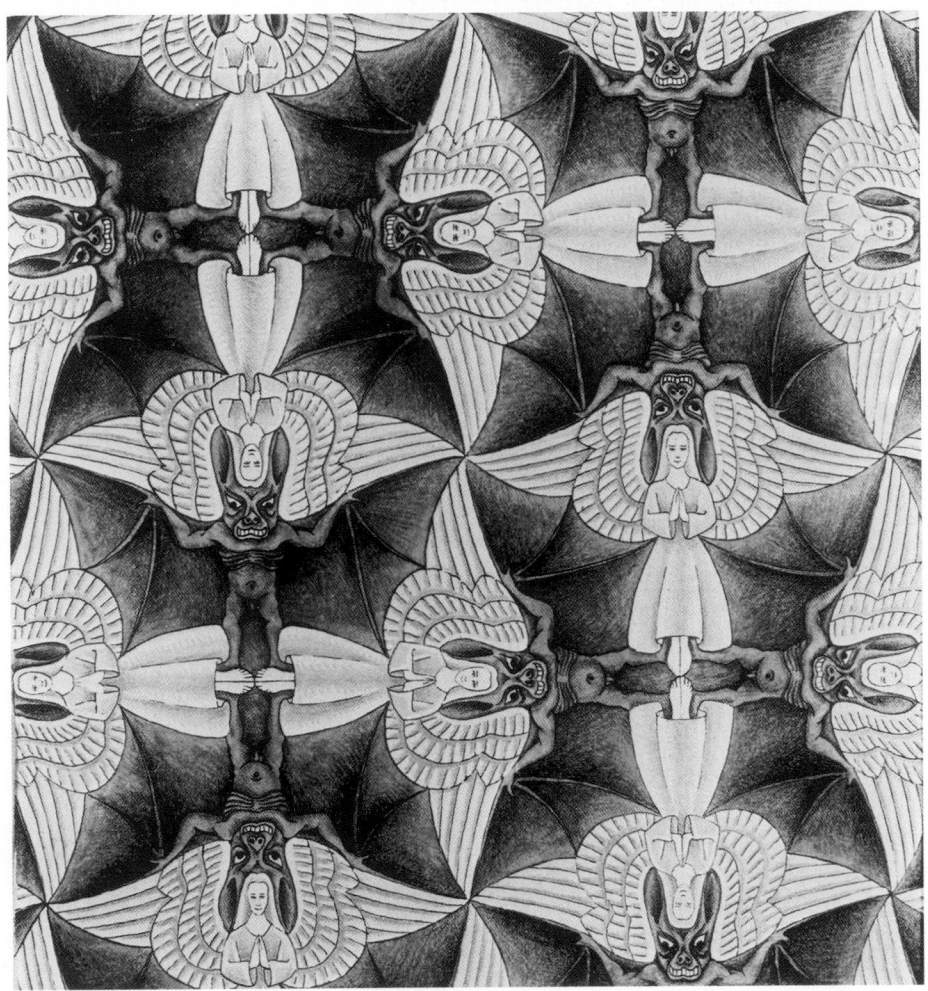

FIGURE 26.46   Interwoven angels and devils, the nightmare of a pathologist who feels that malignancy may be lurking behind a generally benign appearance (according to the rules, the final diagnosis hinges on the *worst* finding). The composition is by Dutch artist M. C. Escher (1941). (Reproduced by permission from [69], M. C. Escher's "Study of Regular Division of the Plane with Angels and Devils" © 2003 Cordon Art B.V. —Baarn—Holland. All rights reserved.)

cells. We did so because the concepts of atypia and polymorphism require a certain degree of aesthetic judgment, and to this degree the diagnosis is tinged by the personality of the observer. This is why pathology, like all of medicine, is science as well as art. Medical students traditionally anguish over tumor diagnosis: how much atypia is required for the verdict of malignancy? Only experience can tell. Pathologists anguish too over certain tumors. There are some known traps, such as leiomyomas that look perfectly benign and yet metastasize, thus earning the paradoxical name of *metastasizing leiomyomas* (43). There are bland-looking thyroid "adenomas" that have already metastasized to the bone when they are first seen. And

then there are tumors that could be labeled either benign or malignant for equally valid reasons. The worried pathologist who studies such slides feels as if contemplating the intertwined angels and devils of Escher (Figure 26.46).

To maximize the reliability of microscopic diagnosis there are specific guidelines for each type of tumor, based on statistics and experience. The internationally recognized authority is represented by the fascicles published by the U.S. Armed Forces Institute of Pathology (A.F.I.P.) which also functions as a diagnostic consulting service worldwide. The A.F.I.P. has long been one of the most important, effective, peaceful, and welcome ambassadors of the United States.

Birth and Growth of a Tumor

The key ingredient, in order to produce a tumor, is a cell type capable of dividing; today this means virtually any cell type, since the dogma of permanent cells has fallen (see Chapter 2). Even the cells of the crystalline lens, which appeared utterly incompatible with replication, have yielded to the oncogene wizards: true carcinomas of the lens have been produced in transgenic mice, using the gene for the lens protein alpha-A-crystallin combined with a coding sequence from the oncogenic virus SV40 (Figures 26.47, 26.48) (158, 178).

Which Cells Generate Tumors?

It is now believed that tumors arise from undifferentiated stem cells, which retain the capacity of differentiating into more mature forms. This concept originated about a century ago; it was suggested by the structure of teratomas, which contain a great variety of tissues, all of which can be proven to derive from a single cell (142, 144). Microscopically the existence of stem cells is not difficult to prove in epithelia, where they can actually be seen as reserve cells squatting on the basement membrane. Besides teratomas, the concept fits with the pathogenesis of certain leukemias (73, 202); but for most tissues the concept remains hypothetical. The main reason is that it is extremely difficult to identify a cell that qualifies as a stem cell in connective tissues.

How Many Cells Are Needed to Start a Tumor?

Most tumors are born, like people, from one cell, which means that a 75-kg human being, made of somewhere near 75,000,000,000,000 cells, can be felled by the misbehavior of "one renegade cell" (247).

NOTE: The following discussion concerns only the monoclonal versus polyclonal *birth* of tumors. It has nothing to do with the fact that all malignant tumors tend to *become* polyclonal in their advanced stages, by the phenomenon of progression (p. 781).

The evidence for tumor monoclonality comes from several sources. In mice, leukemia can be transmitted by injecting one leukemic cell (215). Furthermore, if all the cells in a tumor (human or other) carry a specific, recognizable chromosomal defect that is not present in the normal cells of the same individual, they must have inherited it from a single ancestor. This is the case of the

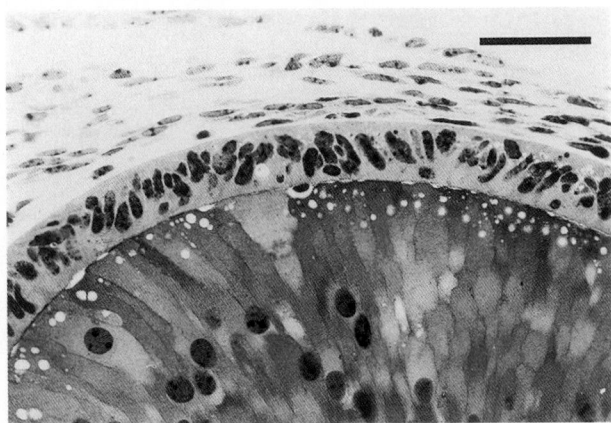

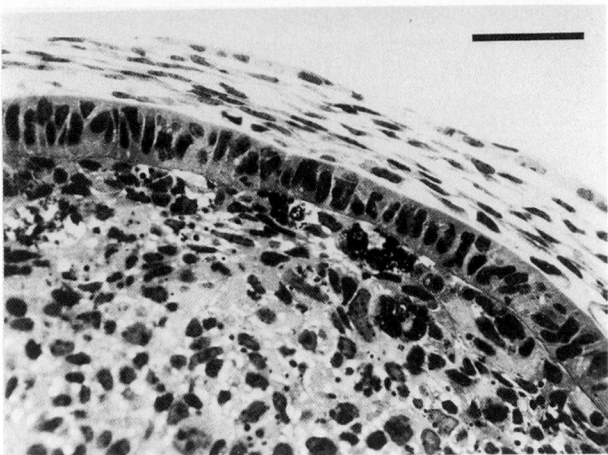

FIGURE 26.48   *Top:* Section through the normal crystalline lens of a mouse. *Bottom:* Lens of a transgenic mouse developing a malignant tumor. The overall structure is preserved, but there is extensive cellular atypia. **Bars** = 50 μm. (Reproduced with permission from [178].)

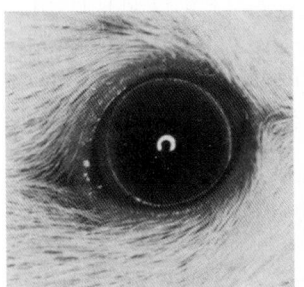 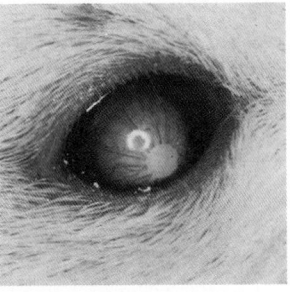

FIGURE 26.47   *Left:* Eye of a normal mouse. *Right:* Eye of a transgenic mouse developing a tumor of the lens. (Reprinted with permission from [158]. Copyright 1987 by the American Association for the Advancement of Science.)

historic Philadelphia chromosome present in chronic myelogenous leukemia (p. 895).

Another approach to studying the clonality of tumors is offered by individuals who are chimeras; if their tumors are not chimeric, this suggests that the tumors derived from a single cell. Accordingly, there has been much interest in tumors of women who are heterozygous for glucose-6-phosphate dehydrogenase (G6PD), an experiment of nature that has been much used for studies of monoclonality. Simply stated, G6PD comes in many variants (isoenzymes) and is encoded by a gene on the X chromosome. Women have two X chromosomes, one of maternal and the other of paternal origin. Now it so happens that in all female embryos, at the blastocyst stage, all cells are submitted to a random inactivation of one X chromosome; in some cells the maternal chromosome is inactivated, in others the paternal. This means that all the adult woman's organs will be a mosaic of cells bearing either the maternal or the paternal X chromosome; and if, by chance, the isoenzymes encoded by the two chromosomes are different, as happens most often in women of African origin, all organs contain both enzymes. What about tumors? Most tumors, benign or malignant, produce only one enzyme, suggesting a monoclonal origin (73, 252). However, this type of evidence is not flawless. It could also indicate that the tumor began as a polyclonal growth, but later a more successful clone crowded out the others.

A rather spectacular example of chimeras are the so-called allophenic mice, obtained by combining two blastocysts. If the embryos are selected from a white and a black mouse, the striped adults are chimeras even to the naked eye (Figure 26.49) (170). Most but not all tumors in these chimeric mice are monoclonal (40, 121).

If methylcholanthrene is used to produce fibrosarcomas in mice, low and high doses tend to produce monoclonal and polyclonal tumors, respectively (252).

There is nothing intrinsically bizarre about tumors being polyclonal. Multiple tumors do exist side by side; one uterus may contain dozens of myomas. Therefore, a polyclonal tumor can be considered, conceptually, as the fusion of two adjacent tumors (114). A good example is the common basal-cell carcinoma of the skin, which when studied histologically is often multicentric; that is, it appears to start at several points along the epidermis (Figure 26.50). One venereal wart (*condyloma acuminatum*) was found to arise from 4000–5000 cells (73).

The best evidence for tumor monoclonality comes from hematologic or mesenchymal tumors; the best examples

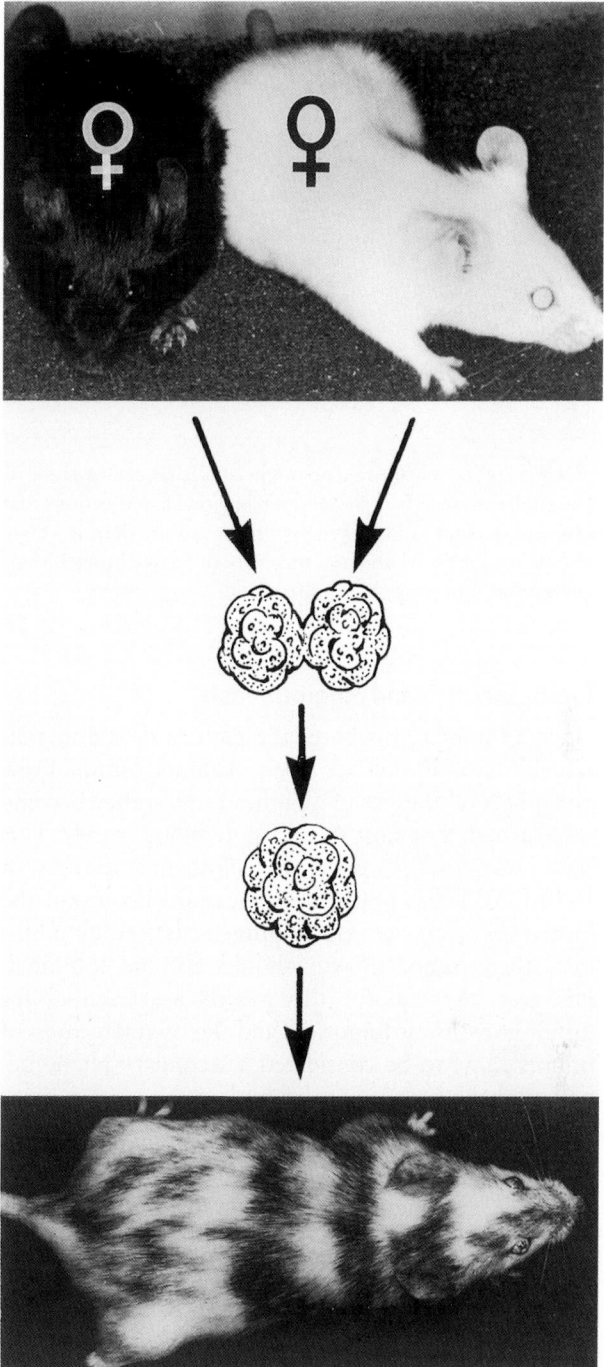

FIGURE 26.49 *Bottom:* Allophenic mouse derived from the fusion of two embryos, one from a black mouse, another from a white one. (Adapted with permission from [169].)

of polyclonality come from epithelia. This makes sense. Epithelia are located in the body as shields against chemical and physical carcinogens, which offers greater opportunities for clusters of mutagenic events (114). Remember that 80 percent of tumors are epithelial.

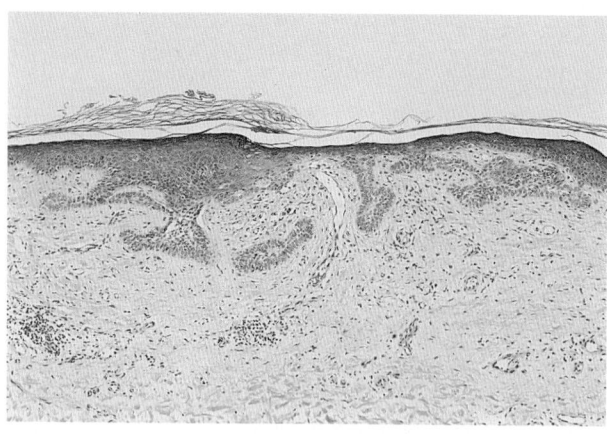

FIGURE 26.50   Multicentric origin of a basal cell carcinoma. The epidermis seen here shows several epithelial projections that represent distinct points of ingrowth toward the dermis. (Slide courtesy of Dr. R. Malhotra, University of Massachusetts Medical School, Worcester, MA.) (60x)

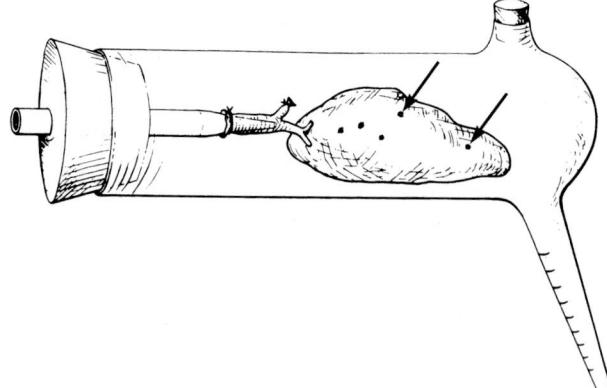

FIGURE 26.51   A thyroid gland maintained by perfusion *in vitro*, and metastasized with a suspension of melanoma cells. The metastases (**arrows**) do not grow beyond 1–2 mm in diameter, because under the conditions of this experiment new vessels cannot develop. (Reproduced with permission from [77].)

Tumor Growth and Angiogenesis

Once a tumor cell is born, the path to developing an actual tumor is not yet open. Tumors cannot grow much beyond the size of a pinhead unless they become vascularized. The host must supply blood vessels. This "law" was first expressed in Cohnheim's lectures in 1889 (35). It has practical implications because if the formation of new vessels (**angiogenesis**) can be inhibited, then tumor growth should also be inhibited. However, the concept that vessels are essential for tumor growth was forgotten, and the vascularization of tumors came to be considered a secondary phenomenon, perhaps a reaction to necrosis.

The Rediscovery of Angiogenesis

Tumor angiogenesis was rediscovered in the 1940s (245) and then became a science on its own, thanks to the systematic studies of Dr. Judah Folkman, an extremely imaginative surgeon–biologist. This tale is worth recounting.

Dr. Folkman's first encounter with experimental tumors was not planned as such. His purpose at the time was to find some effective blood substitutes. To test the effectiveness of some candidates, he perfused isolated dog thyroids to find out how long they could be kept alive. Under the best conditions the thyroids seemed to survive longer than 1 week; but would the same blood substitutes also support growth? To check this point Dr. Folkman mixed some mouse melanoma cells into the perfusing fluid, thinking that the black melanoma cells would be good indicators of new growth. Indeed, tiny black melanomas did appear on the perfused thyroids. At first they grew very fast, but then—surprisingly—they all stopped growing at the same stage, when they reached a diameter of 1–2 mm (Figure 26.51) (77, 78).

An important byproduct of this study was the discovery by Dr. Michael Gimbrone that the endothelium of perfused capillaries breaks down *unless platelets are added to the perfusing medium* (93). This fits well with an old clinical observation: when the number of circulating platelets drops below 10,000/mm³, tiny hemorrhages (petechiae) appear. The mechanism of this classic bit of pathophysiology may be explained at long last: the factor supplied by the platelets to the endothelium appears to be lysophosphatidic acid (91).

Dr. Folkman then tested the following hypothesis: perhaps *tumors cannot grow beyond 1–2 mm unless they are supported by ingrowth of new capillaries,* which could not occur in the perfusion system. To test this idea he had to find a living system in which tumor cells could be made to grow with or without blood vessels; his choice was the anterior chamber of the rabbit eye. Rabbit tumor cells injected into that space grew, within 2 weeks, into free-floating **spheroids** with a volume of about 0.5 mm³; thereafter, the spheroids persisted without further growth. However, if they were manually seated against the iris, which is highly vascularized, they grew in 3 days to 16,000 times the original volume; their growth curve shot up almost at a right angle (96) (Figure 26.52). The behavior of the floating spheroids may be a clue to the phenomenon of tumor dormancy observed clinically (78, 96); for example, a mastectomy scar, may remain normal for years until suddenly a spheroids serve as models of nodular tumors, minus the influence of the host; they can also be used to test the effects of chemotherapy.

Another model used by the Folkman group was the rabbit cornea (94), which has no blood vessels. Tiny bits of rabbit tumor inserted into a flat pocket created in the thickness of the cornea could not grow as spheres (due to the tight quarters) but formed a sheet; as the sheet advanced toward the edge of the cornea, capillaries began to grow toward it, advancing as much as 1 mm per day. When they reached the tumor, it began to grow so fast that in 4 weeks it was as large as the eye (81). This type of experiment suggested that the capillaries might be growing in response to a powerful call, perhaps a diffusible factor. A tumor angiogenesis factor was soon obtained from a variety of tumors; it was tested by "loading" it into plastic pellets implanted into the cornea (Figure 26.54).

> The modern industry of plastic pellets for slow delivery of drugs was greatly boosted as a by-product of this work (84). The idea to use pellets of plastic as slow-release devices came through a chance observation. As a resident, Dr. Folkman had noticed that the silicone rubber tubing of a laboratory pump became stained with a dye added to the fluid. Almost anyone else would have considered this a nuisance; to Dr. Folkman it meant that if the silicone rubber picked up the dye it might also pick up a drug, and also release it. It did both.

Now admire the latest, much simpler, and cheaper model for studies of angiogenesis on a large scale: fertilized eggs are incubated for 3–4 days and then poured out on a Petri dish, where the embryo continues to grow (admittedly rather flat) for up to 3 weeks (Figure 26.55). Small objects laid on the vascular chorioallantoic membrane can be tested for angiogenic and anti-angiogenic substances. In this way it was confirmed that cartilage produces an inhibitory factor to angiogenesis (Figure 26.56) (30, 67, 68, 81). Cartilage was tested because it is usually spared by advancing tumors. Tradition held that the obstacle was mechanical, but the mechanism turned out to be more subtle: cartilage contains a protein that inhibits angiogenesis *in vivo* and *in vitro;* it also inhibits collagenases (174).

The natural history of tumor angiogenesis *in vivo* is much the same as that of wound healing (p. 481). Sprouts come from capillaries and venules whose endothelial cells secrete proteolytic enzymes, which help them escape their cage of basement membrane. The new cells emigrate, and eventually multiply and form tubes (Figure 26.57). If the stimulus ceases, the vessels break up and disappear (7, 76). *In vitro,*

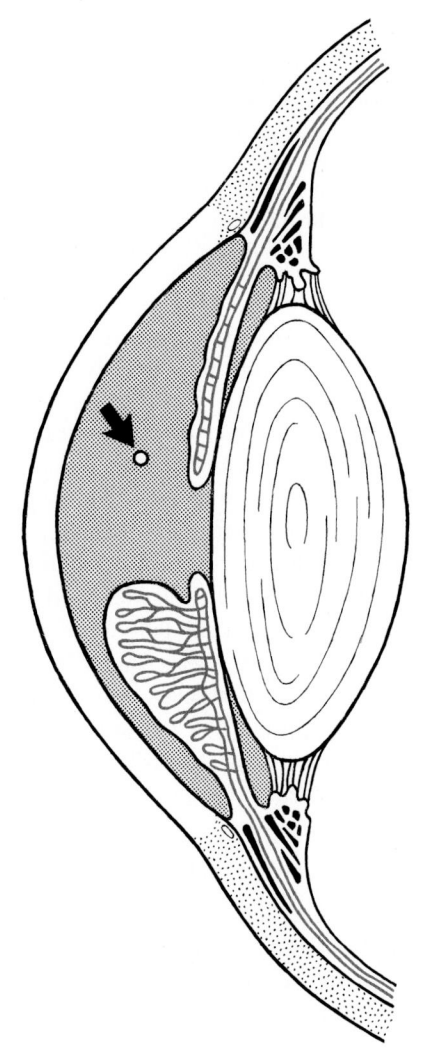

FIGURE 26.52 Malignant tumor cells, introduced into the anterior chamber of the rabbit's eye and left floating there, survive but stop growing before they reach the diameter of 1 mm (**arrow**). If this avascular "spheroid" is placed in contact with the iris (*bottom*), it is invaded by new vessels and grows. Diagram of an experiment by J. Folkman (1974). (Reproduced with permission from [75].)

cancerous nodule grows in it, presumably from cells that had remained quiescent since surgery.

Spheroids are an established tool for tumor research (Figure 26.53) (1, 57, 82, 110, 176, 224). Tumor cells maintained in stirred culture media tend to grow as rounded aggregates. Under ideal conditions with continuously renewed medium, these spheroids grow to a maximal diameter of 3–4 mm, at which point they contain a necrotic center surrounded by about 1 million cells. In contrast, the two-dimensional growth of a standard tumor culture *in vitro* is limitless; diffusion is not restricted. The

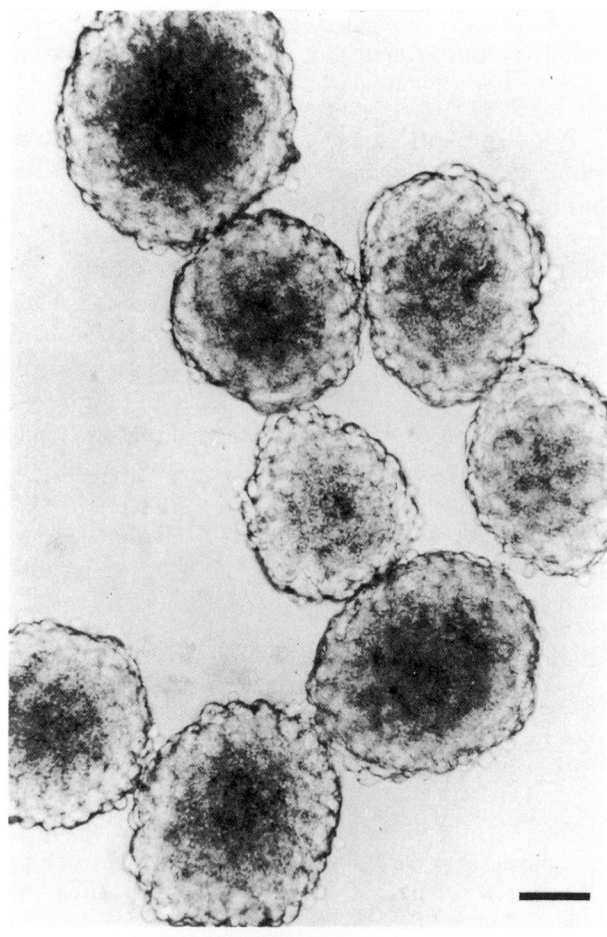

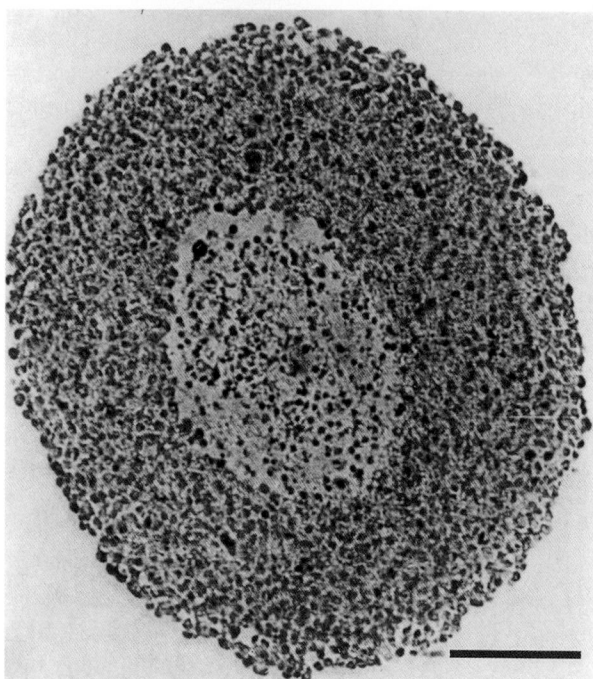

FIGURE 26.53 Spheroids that developed *in vitro* in a spinning suspension of hamster lung carcinoma cells. These spheroids can be used as models for the study of tumor growth. *Top:* Whole mount showing a "squash preparation" of spheroids. *Bottom:* Histological cross section through the center of a spheroid. The thickness of the viable rim is about 120 micrometers. **Bars** = 100 μm. (Reproduced with permission from [224].)

endothelial cells respond to angiogenic stimuli, in most cases, by moving around more actively (Figure 11.27) (255) and by dividing.

Different tumors produce different combinations of factors. For example, induction of angiogenesis may precede neoplastic transformation, so the appearance of blood vessels may be the first sign of malignancy; this fact was first established by implanting fragments of normal hyperplastic, preneoplastic, and malignant mouse mammary tissue in the rabbit eye, (78, 85, 86, 95, 223). The stimulus to tumor angiogenesis may not come only from the tumor cells; anoxic macrophages, as we now know (pp. 481, 490), can also contribute. Hence the paradox that *the inflammatory response within a tumor may help it grow.*

Angiogenesis Factors and Inhibitors

When Folkman's studies began, polypeptide growth factors were almost unknown except for their forerunner, nerve growth factor. Today so many angiogenesis factors have been purified or otherwise described in

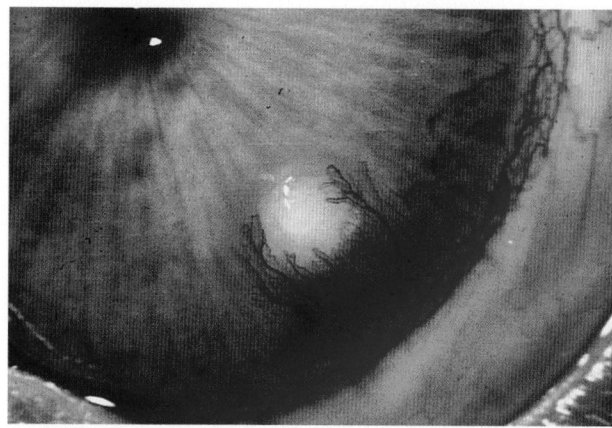

FIGURE 26.54 Tumor angiogenesis factor was impregnated into a 1 mm³ slow-release plastic pellet. Implanted in the cornea, the pellet, 11 days later, has induced vascular growth. (Courtesy of Dr. J. Folkman, Harvard Medical School, Boston, MA.)

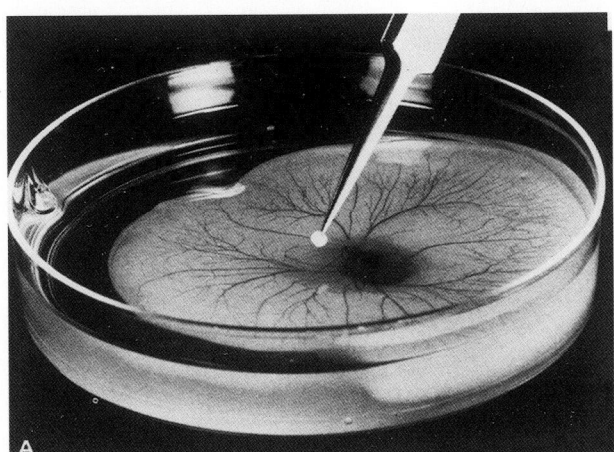

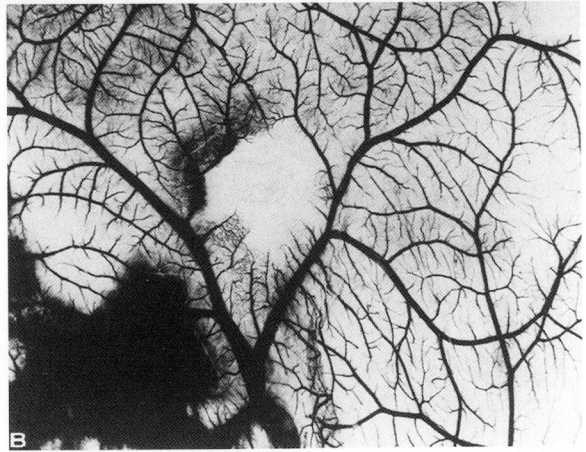

FIGURE 26.55 Chorioallantoic membrane method for studying the microcirculation. A yolk bearing a chick embryo is poured into a petri dish, where it becomes flat and convenient for microscopic study between days 6 and 10. The chick does not hatch. *Top:* Disc of methylcellulose loaded with an antiangiogenic substance is about to be implanted on the membrane. *Bottom:* Avascular zone that has developed 48 hours later. The vessels have been injected with India ink. The disc contained heparin and 11 α-epicortisol. (Reproduced with permission from [78].)

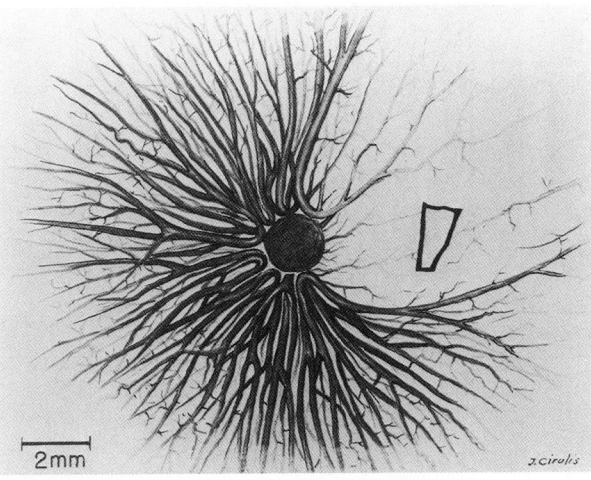

FIGURE 26.56 Inhibition of angiogenesis by cartilage: Diagram of an experiment in which a dose of tumor angiogenesis factor (**disk in center**) and a fragment of cartilage (*right*) were implanted on a chorioallantoic membrane. Growth of new vessels induced by TAF was inhibited around the cartilage. (Reproduced from the **Journal of Experimental Medicine**, 1975;141:427–439, by copyright permission of The Rockefeller University Press [30].)

so many laboratories that we are puzzled by their abundance (83, 256). They have been obtained from tumors, activated macrophages, some classes of lymphocytes (78), platelets, endothelium, from ischemic tissues (91a) and from many normal tissues (44)—but not from neutrophils (172).

Some were hiding among well-known molecules: VEGF (vascular endothelial growth factor) and TGF-beta (transforming growth factor beta), which, most confusingly, stimulates angiogenesis *in vivo* but inhibits endothelial cells *in vitro* (194). Also paradoxical is the effect of TNF-alpha (tumor necrosis factor alpha): injected intravenously, it causes tumors to become necrotic, as expected, but injected locally into normal tissues, it stimulates angiogenesis. **Angiogenin,** the first angiogenic factor to be sequenced, presents yet another puzzle: it has no effect on endothelial cells grown *in vitro*. Some prostaglandins are angiogenic, especially E_1 and E_2 (45, 131, 256).

Eventually a pattern emerged: many angiogenic factors are chemically bound to heparin, a property that is exploited for extracting them. There is much heparin in the connective tissue matrix and in basement membranes; this means that the angiogenic factors, held in these sites in ready-to-act form, can be supplied almost instantly after a local injury.

Considering this plethora of angiogenic factors, it seemed for a short time that the original question— what makes angiogenesis start—was reversed: why is it that blood vessels do not grow all the time?

In the absence of tissue injury and repair, angiogenesis in the normal adult is minimal. It is part of normal function only in the female; menstruation, ovulation, and placentation are akin to physiologic wounds, which require new capillaries (74). We should add, however, that new capillaries are made whenever we build more tissue, such as adipose tissue by overeating or striated muscle by exercise.

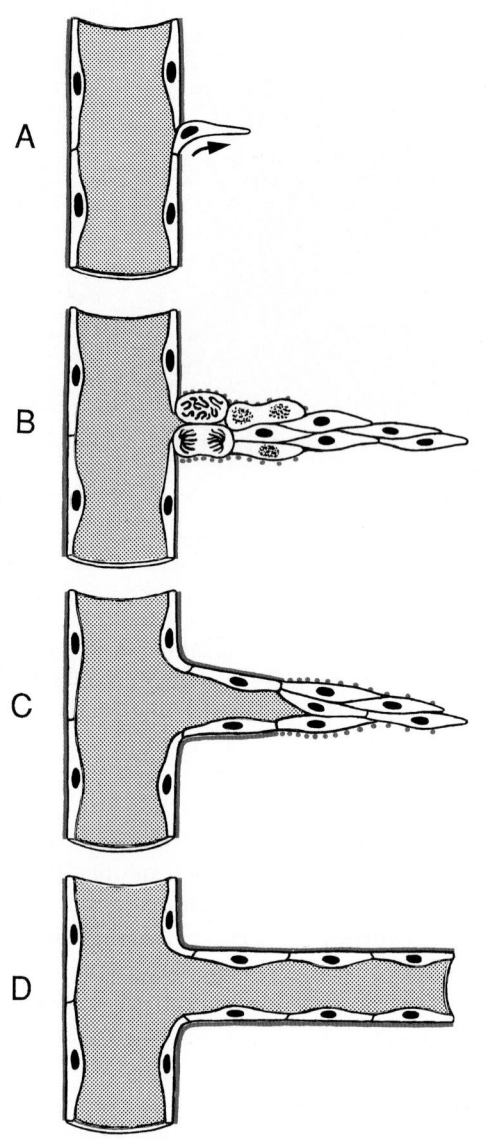

FIGURE 26.57 The basic steps of angiogenesis, originating from venules or capillaries. **A:** Pseudopod from an endothelial cell perforates the basement membrane (red line) and becomes the bridgehead for further growth. **B:** Endothelial cells multiply and a capillary sprout begins to form, surrounded by incomplete basement membrane. **C:** Lumen begins to appear in the sprout. **D:** Mature new blood vessel is formed. (Adapted with permission from [12].)

The intricate story of angiogenesis became clearer when Dr. Folkman's group found that the growth of new vessels depends on a **balance between stimulating and inhibiting factors** (137). The existence of inhibiting factors had long been surmised, but they did not yield their secret easily. It turned out that they had been created along a different plan: instead of being performed, they were built into larger, apparently quite unrelated molecules: *angiostatin* came from plasminogen, *endostatin* from Type 18 collagen, *vasostatin* from calreticulin, and so on. Proteolytic enzymes are needed to release them (136). This new set of findings suggested that early tumors, still free of vessels, are able to activate an **angiogenesis switch** at the appropriate time: certainly when they reach a maximum diameter of 1–2 mm.

The "balance" concept helps us understand the behavior of metastases after the surgical removal of a primary tumor: sometimes they regress, other times they burst into growth. Perhaps they were maintained with the help of angiogenin, or held in check by angiostatin (79, 80, 151a).

After three decades of basic science, clinical trials are under way to test over 24 drugs (136). Expectations are high; we can only speculate. In theory, anti-angiogenic drugs should be capable only of *stopping* the progression of a tumor, holding it in a sort of dormancy; combined treatment with chemotherapy and/or radiotherapy may be needed. A single case of a 5-year-girl with a rapidly growing tumor of the mandible, treated with an anti-angiogenic drug (interferon alpha-2a), was completely healed for as long as 3 years (132). Anti-angiogenic therapy should be nontoxic, but protein drugs have other problems, including the production of antibodies (136).

While the world is waiting, a book on "Dr. Folkman's war" appeared (41). The outcome of this 30-year war will surely appear in the daily news.

Lymphangiogenesis

We introduce this topic after angiogenesis because the titles suggest a certain symmetry, but the two fields have developed quite asymmetrically. Progress in the physiology and pathology of lymphatics has been slow ever since the lymphatics were discovered in 1621, and it was not accelerated in our days by the fact that tumors contain no lymphatics (217). Still, the general phenomenon of lymphangiogenesis was illustrated in chronic inflammation decades before the word was coined (see Figure 12.15).

Interest in the field increased abruptly after 2000 with the discovery of *histochemical markers* specific or nearly specific for lymphatic endothelium and of *growth factors* able to induce lymphangiogenesis. Three of these belong, interestingly, to the VEGF molecular family: VEGF-C, VEGF-D, and VEGF-F (134, 195, 217). Their ligands are receptors VEGFR-1, VEGFR-2, and VEGFR-3 (33a). Studies using these molecular tools have confirmed that tumors, by and large, are surrounded by lymphatic vessels but contain few or none. There are, of course, lymphatic vessels *around* tumors; in melanomas, tumor cells may permeate preexisting lymphatics (54). Yet, lymphangiogenic factors are produced by tumor cells and by tumor-associated macrophages (208). In either case, the production of these factors correlates with an *increase in lymphatic metastases* (217). This suggests that antibodies against the lymphangiogenesis factors or their ligands may be tried as a new approach to cancer therapy.

Progress in this field was hampered by the lack of a reliable experimental model of lymphangiogenesis not associated with angiogenesis. The Folkman group may have solved the problem (33b) by modifying the corneal pocket method (p. 775): in mice, implants of bFGF in very low dose produce lymphangiogenesis alone; lymphatics are dramatically stained red, blood vessels yellow.

Because tumors have no lymphatic system, what functional effects may be expected? The answer will be found shortly (p. 788).

The Theory of Tumor Initiation, Promotion, and Progression

As soon as it became possible to produce tumors experimentally by means of chemical carcinogens, in particular by painting tar on the back of mice, two facts became apparent: first, carcinogenesis in these models is an extremely slow process; it is one of the slowest biological processes known. The reason is still unclear. Second, carcinogenesis occurs in these models by separate, sudden steps, from a reversible hyperplasia to a benign tumor to a malignant tumor of increasing aggressiveness.

The concept that tumors develop by steps was born in the 1930s, in the laboratory of Peyton Rous at the Rockefeller Institute. Working on rabbit tumors produced by a virus (200) or tar (201), Rous and his coworkers noticed that the *path to malignancy was not a continuous slope.* At first they obtained hyperplastic lesions that behaved as benign warts or papillomas; but then these papillomas did not become globally more and more atypical until they could be called cancers. Instead, most cancers arose quite suddenly and *only in a part of a papilloma, as a wholly new and different event.*

Intensive work on the multistep theory soon produced a dogma: tumor production occurs in two main phases, **initiation** and **promotion**, followed by a relentless, stepwise increase in malignancy called *progression.* (The British oncologist Leslie Foulds who coined

the term **progression** in the 1940s meant it to include the whole life history of the tumor; today it is restricted to the terminal phase.) We will now take a closer look at these concepts.

Initiation and Promotion

A puzzling fact had been reported off and on since the 1920s: if the skin of an experimental animal is painted with tar and then biopsied for microscopic study, tumors often arise at the site of the biopsy (157). This phenomenon was studied extensively in the 1940s, again in the laboratory of Peyton Rous. The basic plan was to tar rabbit ears "throughout a period somewhat less than is ordinarily required to elicit growths," and then to wound the ear. The results were clear; wounding was enough to encourage latent neoplastic cells. "The medicolegal bearing of these facts," wrote the authors, "is obvious." The tar had somehow initiated the neoplastic process, and the wound promoted it.

> We must note in passing that the medicolegal implications (tumors elicited by trauma on a prepared tissue) did not really materialize. Human tumors following trauma are rare (p. 854).

Then came variations on the theme (18, 26, 27). The principle of initiation by a subcarcinogenic dose was retained, but wounding as a promoter was replaced with a local irritant; the choice was croton oil (16, 175), a dreadfully irritating drug from India that had been used medically for centuries, if not millennia (p. 61). This technique of promotion became more "scientific" when two laboratories, one in Germany, the other in New York, independently isolated the irritating principle of croton oil and named it, respectively, *phorbol myristate acetate* (PMA) and *tetradecanoyl phorbol acetate* (TPA)—the latter name seems to have won. Many other initiators and promoters were proposed, but the most popular of the promoters remains TPA (Figure 26.58).

Eventually the basic rules of the initiation–promotion routine were worked out. To begin, *promotion before initiation produces no tumors.* The permutations are best explained graphically (Figure 26.59) (26).

What are the cellular and subcellular equivalents of initiation and promotion?

The current interpretation is that the birth of a tumor cell requires at least two successive events. First, an initiator strikes the DNA of a cell and introduces a "suitable" defect. (At this point the cell is potentially a cancer cell but is somehow held in check.) Second, a promoter causes the cell to multiply and to generate a tumor, thus revealing the latent curse of the initiated

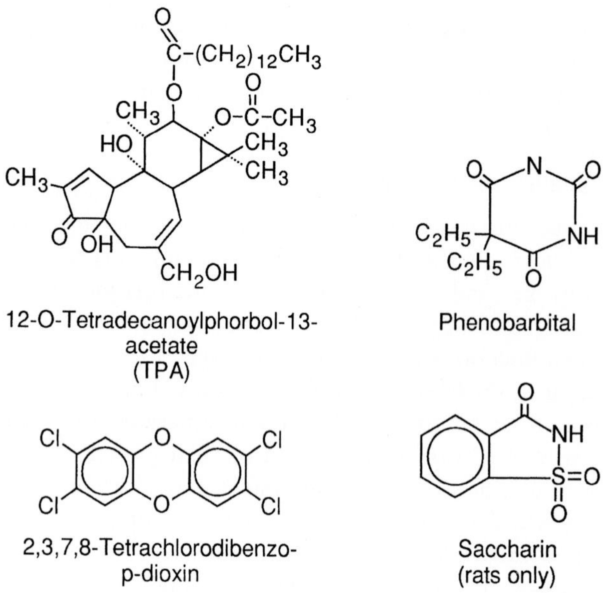

FIGURE 26.58 Chemical structure of some typical tumor promoters. (Adapted from [5].)

■			Tumors
■	PPPPPPP		Tumors
▪	PPPPPPP		Tumors
▪		PPPPPPP	Tumors
▪			No tumors
None	PPPPPPPPPPPPPPPPPPPPP		No tumors
PPPPPPP ▪			No tumors

■ Initiator, single large dose
▪ Initiator, subcarcinogenic dose
P = Promoter

FIGURE 26.59 Distinction between initiation and promotion. The effect of initiation depends in part on the dose of the initiator. **Large square:** Full carcinogenic dose. **Small square:** Subcarcinogenic dose, e.g., of methylcholanthrene. Each **P** represents one dose of promoter (such as phorbol ester, 2–5 applications per week). The scheme is largely derived from painting carcinogens on the skin of mice; the time is in the range of 1–2 years. (Adapted with permission from [204]. Copyright 1971 Massachusetts Medical Society. All rights reserved.)

cell. Note, however, the possible hitch: why didn't the DNA-repair enzymes correct the defect? The answer is that they will correct the defect—unless mitosis occurs promptly to make the defect "permanent" (38, 71).

It is obvious that initiation and promotion are seen as very different processes:

- *Initiation* is conceived as a quick, almost instantaneous process; if it is repeated, the effect on the tissue is additive. It may take place even in minutes (17), and once it has happened the effect is **nearly permanent.** In the mouse the effect of initiation may last as long as a year (87). In the long run, however, the effect does wane (210). This should be good news for smokers, who continually initiate their bronchial mucosa. Those who quit can look forward to recovering a safe bronchial mucosa within a few years. Overall, these findings about initiation fit with the notion of an agent that damages DNA. Initiators can be chemical, physical, or biological. They do not cause cell proliferation; in fact, carcinogens in general are (somewhat paradoxically) inhibitors of cell proliferation (71). Initiated cells are morphologically indistinguishable from normal cells, at least to the present.
- *Promotion* is viewed as a slow process; its effect is **reversible** and nonadditive. Many promoters cause cells to multiply; in fact, there is some consensus that hyperplasia is a typical effect of promoters (Figure 26.60) (141). However, it is not the only effect; it has been claimed that "most all" promoters (27) eliminate metabolic cooperation between adjacent cells by destroying the gap junctions (238). Phorbol esters (the classic tumor promoters) have a vast array of effects. Quite a stir greeted the discovery that TPA activates protein kinase C; this gives TPA the key to a number of intracellular processes (p. 61). Some promoters have a certain degree of organ specificity: for example, saccharin (*in rats*) for the bladder (190, 216). For saccharin, the carcinogenic mechanism in rat bladder is now understood (p. 951).

As regards our daily lives, the initiation–promotion theory means that we may be surrounded by "innocent" promoters that can play a nasty role if we have been unknowingly prepared by some toxin, radiation, or other initiating agent. Experimentally, promoters include mitogens as physiologic as hormones (154) and as innocuous as physiologic saline instilled into initiated bronchi (3, 155).

Where do we stand today with regard to the theory of initiation and promotion? In the sixth edition of De Vita's huge treatise on cancer (2001), it is mentioned only in passing. Perhaps this means that it is taken for granted. Anyway, we must acknowledge that the theory fits very well with the current concepts of carcinogenesis by oncogenes and suppressor genes. It is generally agreed that carcinogenesis is a multistep sequence, with the single exception of "acute transforming viruses" such as the Rous sarcoma virus, which

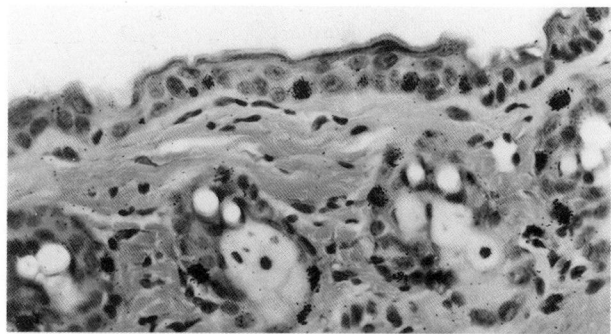

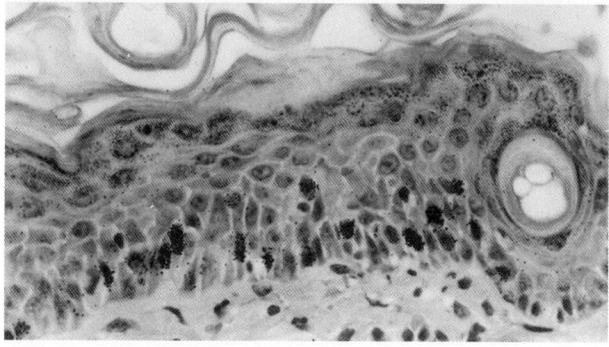

FIGURE 26.60 Demonstrating the hyperplastic effect of a classic tumor promoter, TPA. Histologic sections and autoradiographs of mouse skin. *Top:* Control; mitoses are indicated by clusters of black (silver) grains. *Bottom:* 48 hours after a local application of 2 micrograms of TPA. Note hyperplasia, increased cornification, and increased number of mitoses. (Courtesy of Dr. A. J. P. Klein-Szanto, Fox Chase Cancer Center, Philadelphia, PA.)

seems to work in one step. The theory also fits with many human cancers (191). Besides, nobody would think of disagreeing with the concept of progression, an everyday reality of cancer wards.

However, the theory of initiation and promotion has its flaws, as all theories do (233, 237). It was derived largely from experiments based on painting mouse skin, a somewhat limited sample of carcinogenesis. The diagram of Figure 26.59 looks neat, but it should not be taken too literally: it does not convey the exceptions. *Most carcinogens are initiators as well as promoters,* a fact that is brushed off by deciding that these are "complete carcinogens" (27, 190). Furthermore, *some promoters can also produce tumors.* Last, the initiation–promotion scheme *requires a mutagen,* whereas it is now well known that many cancers arise without mutagens. In essence, then, the facts appear to tell us that the initiation–promotion theory offers a satisfactory paradigm for interpreting some, and perhaps most cancers of the skin and other sites (189, 192, 193, 210), but not all cancers. We shall return to this topic on p. 950, where an additional mechanism is proposed.

Tumor Progression

Once malignant tumors have started to grow, they tend to "go from bad to worse": this is how Rous and Kidd described in 1941 what is now called *tumor progression,* the third phase in the initiation–promotion–progression paradigm (190, 191, 201). The term implies a drive toward increasing malignancy of the tumor itself and of its metastases. Occasionally a step in this evolution can be appreciated even with the naked eye by a change in color: a heavily pigmented melanoma may produce colorless metastases; a hepatoma may produce metastases that are greenish, because they can still produce bile, as well as pale ones that have lost that ability. The basic mechanism is thought to be a **genetic instability** of neoplastic cells, a concept proposed around 1902 by the German geneticist T. Boveri (9) and then again in 1976 by P. C. Nowell of Philadelphia (56, 181, 182).

> Dr. Nowell had discovered in 1960 the Philadelphia chromosome typical of chronic myelogenous leukemia (p. 895). He conceived "genetic instability" at first as a result of *chromosomal* flaws that caused the cell to slip from a euploid to an aneuploid karyotype (p. 890); progression is now understood more broadly as the effect of disturbances that may occur anywhere from chromosome to gene to DNA structure.

The role of clones in progression is illustrated in Figure 26.61. After a single cell is transformed, new clones continue to appear; under constant evolutionary pressures, some cells are eliminated because of a biological disadvantage, others succeed because they are progressively less demanding of growth factors, less sensitive to drugs and X-rays, more invasive, more metastatic, . . . The final result is a polyclonal tumor.

The heterogeneity of tumor cell populations has major clinical implications. It means, for example, that tumors should be treated as early as possible, when their population is most homogeneous; drugs should be varied to discourage the development of specific drug resistance; and drugs given jointly should be chosen among those that induce different mechanisms of drug resistance—such as enhanced repair of DNA damage versus decreased transport across the cell membrane (207).

> After having read, a few pages back, that most tumors are *born* monoclonal, the notion that established malignant tumors are found to be typically polyclonal may seem to be something of a paradox. As a matter of fact, this concept was not easily accepted; in 1977 it was considered so outlandish that a manuscript proposing it was refused by a journal. The authors eventually won the battle; one of their arguments was that, after all, they themselves (just as the referees) were polyclonal creatures that had progressed from monoclonal beginnings (116).

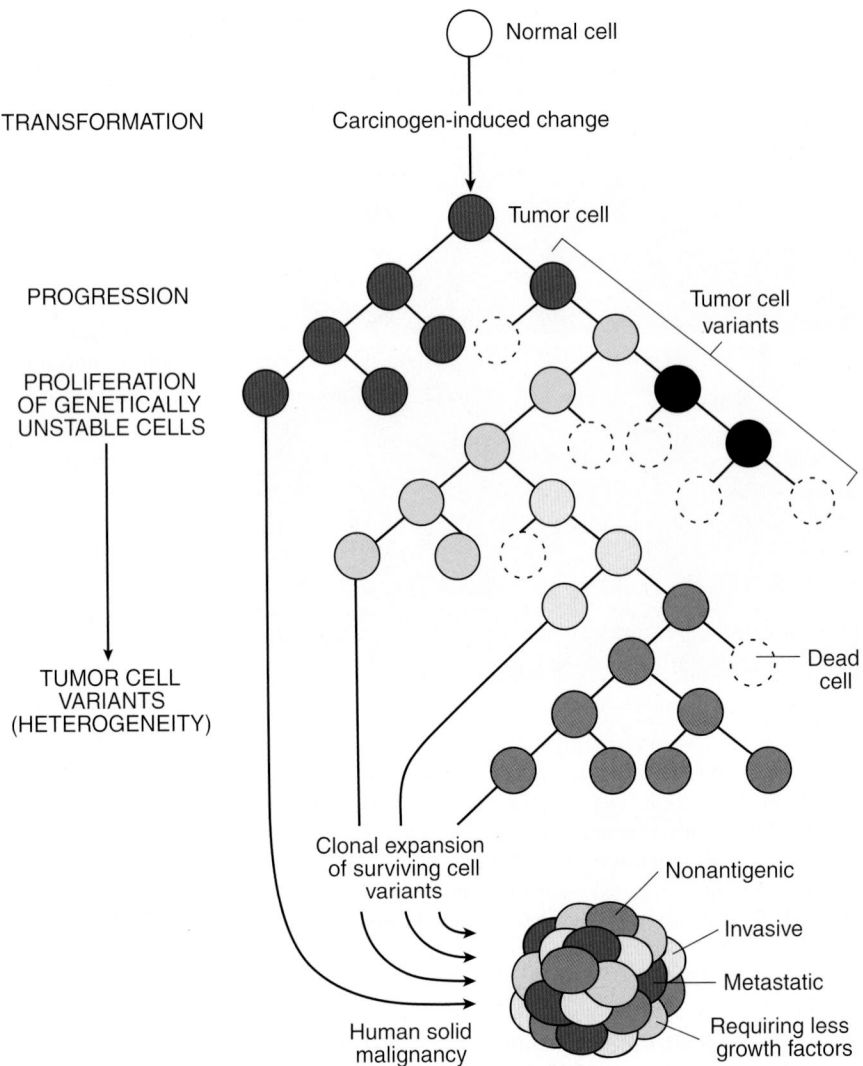

FIGURE 26.61 Clonal development of a tumor, starting from a single cell. Each division produces cells that differ with regard to survival and aggressive behavior; many die, the fittest carry on. The final result is a *polyclonal* mass. (Reproduced by permission from Nancy Lou Gahan Riccio [artwork] and I. Tannock [230].)

Within figure:

Normal cell

TRANSFORMATION

Carcinogen-induced change

Tumor cell

PROGRESSION

Tumor cell variants

PROLIFERATION OF GENETICALLY UNSTABLE CELLS

Dead cell

TUMOR CELL VARIANTS (HETEROGENEITY)

Clonal expansion of surviving cell variants

Nonantigenic

Invasive

Metastatic

Requiring less growth factors

Human solid malignancy

One unsolved problem regarding progression is the *existence of a benign-tumor stage before the appearance of a malignancy* (pp. 737, 901). In most experimental tumors (especially skin tumors) a benign stage is evident; however, in some cases a carcinoma seems to develop directly from "normal" epidermis without an intermediate stage of papilloma (87); is this simply an accelerated variant of the usual scheme? In humans, a stepwise evolution of melanomas is sometimes seen (117); in other species the malignancy seems to strike out of the blue, without benign precursor (199). Many researchers still believe that most human cancers develop without a benign precursor. However, this may be due to our own inadequate observation; by the time an inner cancer is recognized, it may have erased its benign precursor, as happens with colonic polyps. When more facts are available, it may turn out that most human

malignant tumors do indeed have benign precursors. We will return to the topic of progression in relation to genes (p. 890) and to precancerous lesions on p. 897.

How Fast Do Tumors Grow?

The rate of tumor growth is a question of great practical importance because most anticancer treatments now available suppress cell proliferation. Therefore, while we wait for more specific and really anti*cancer* drugs (as opposed to antiproliferative drugs), therapy remains centered around the kinetics of tumor cell division.

Volume Doubling Time

The volume doubling time of a whole tumor is easily measured in mice; for transplanted tumors it is of the order of 1–5 days (231). For human tumors, it is

Table 26.2 Doubling Times of Human Tumors (reported from six sources)

Site	No. of Measurements	Median Volume-Doubling Time (days)	Range (days)
Lung metastases	86	40	4–745
Lung metastases	24	40	11–164
Lung metastases from colon or rectum	25	96	34–210
Primary bronchial carcinomas	22	105	27–480
Primary bronchial carcinomas	12	62	17–200
Primary skeletal sarcomas	6	75	21–366

Adapted from (218).

convenient to remember a number that is 30 times greater: 1–5 months (Table 26.2). The record for short doubling time probably belongs to a mouse carcinoma called Ehrlich ascites tumor; when this tumor is seeded into the peritoneum, its cell population doubles in 21 hours (20). Nobody knows why tumors grow so fast in mice (p. 952).

The actual doubling times reported for humans are of the order of 50–100 days, with extremes of 1 week and 1 year (123, 218). Note that we are referring to volumes, not diameters. Tumors that are highly sensitive to chemo- or radiotherapy are also those that grow fastest—which makes sense because both properties depend on a high mitotic rate. Data for human tumors have been difficult to obtain because the results can be affected by treatment. Most of the figures available were obtained by studying serial X-rays of primary and metastatic tumors of the lung, but keep in mind that metastases tend to grow faster than the primary tumor (Figure 26.62).

The Gompertzian Curve

The doubling times reported are in a sense misleading because the rate of growth of a tumor changes throughout its life. Until 1964, tumor growth rates offered a confusing picture. It was found that some tumors seemed to grow exponentially, like young bacterial cultures; but applying this exponential curve to certain slowly growing tumors led to the absurd conclusion that the tumors had started before conception (165). Clearly something was wrong with the measurements, or with the assumptions. A breakthrough came when Anna Laird of the Argonne National Laboratory found that *tumor growth is an exponential process that is limited by an exponential retardation;* this function was

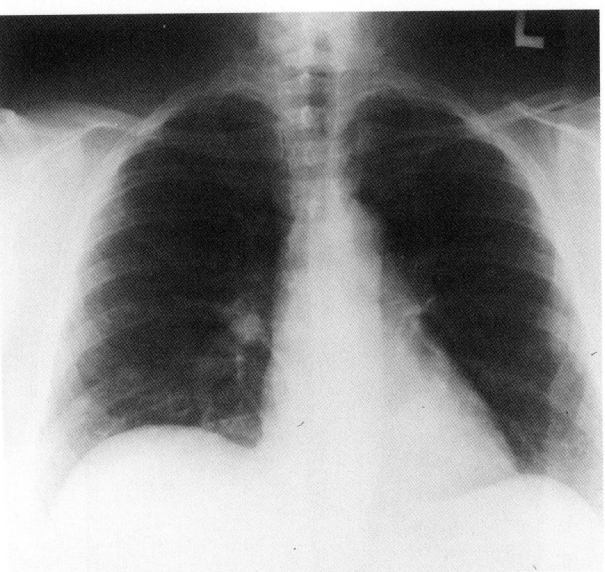

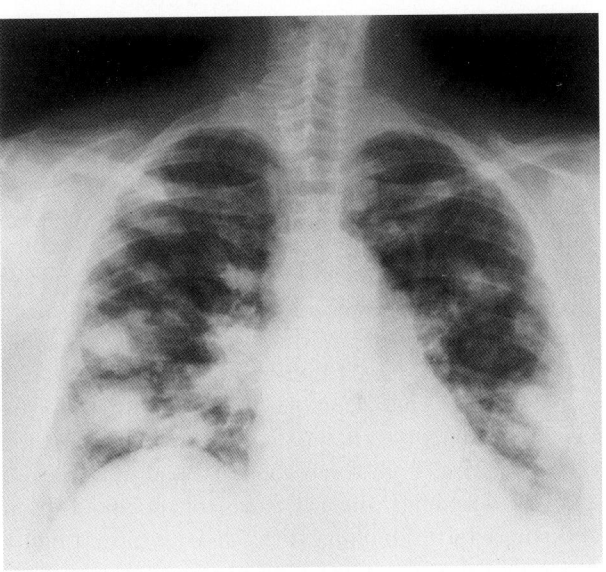

FIGURE 26.62 The growth of metastases in the lung can be exceedingly rapid: These two X-rays were taken only 43 days apart. Undifferentiated carcinoma of the ovary. (Courtesy of Dr. A. Davidoff, University of Massachusetts Medical School, Worcester, MA.)

defined by the mathematician Benjamin Gompertz (1779–1865) (92) and is now widely known as the Gompertzian curve (148, 149). Interestingly, this curve also describes the rate of growth of the human fetus (Figure 26.63) (165, 214). In simple terms: tumor growth is fast at the outset, then it declines.

Why so?

In the fetus, the retarding force is probably differentiation (214). In tumors, it must be the decrease in

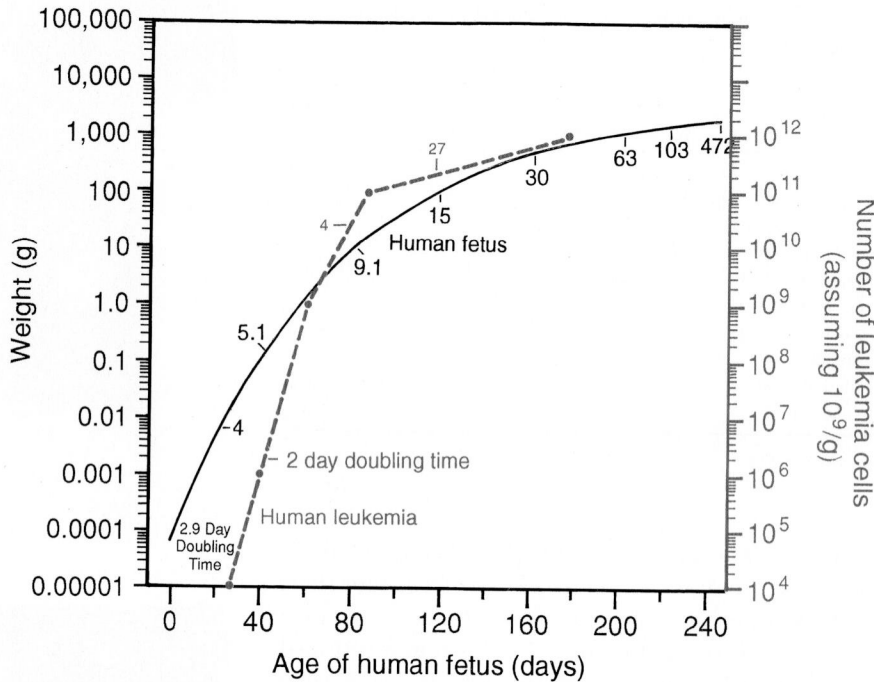

FIGURE 26.63 Demonstrating that the growth curve of tumor tissue (in this study, human leukemia) approaches the growth curve of the human fetus. In either case, the curve fits the so-called Gompertzian equation. (Adapted with permission from [214].)

blood supply relative to size; the tumor grows faster than the vessels. The respective growth rates of capillary endothelium and tumor cells have actually been compared in a mouse tumor. They show that as capillary growth falls behind, the mean intercapillary distance increases, whereby many tumor cells should become anoxic as well as starved and should die (228).

Now see the tangible implications of the Gompertzian curve. It has long been known that a tumor, starting from a cell about 10 μm in diameter, takes 30 doublings to reach a mass of roughly 1 gram and another 10 doublings to reach 1 kg (36), a figure often quoted as the upper limit of the "tumor burden" that is compatible with life. This means that when we discover a tumor about 1 cm in diameter—an early tumor by clinical standards—it is indeed a small tumor; but *most of its growth in terms of cell doublings has already occurred.* It is high on the Gompertzian curve, and its cells are no longer multiplying very fast; for this reason the most propitious time for anticancer therapy has already gone by (Figure 26.64). Interestingly, if a few cells are taken from a tumor at an advanced stage of growth and implanted elsewhere, they start a new tumor that resumes growth according to a new Gompertzian curve (221).

The Gompertzian curve has also blown apart a dangerous myth: an overoptimistic idea (which we used to teach) that tumors, when discovered clinically, had been there for 10–20 years and that therefore there was no great urgency to remove them. Now it seems likely that most tumors detected clinically have developed in 2 years or less (221).

Number of Replicating Cells

The study of tumor growth at the cellular level (as opposed to the tissue level) probes deeper into the biology of the tumor. The key is to measure the number of replicating cells, which can be done in several ways. The basic result is that *tumor cells grow—in general—more slowly than their normal counterparts.* (13).

There are four standard methods for measuring cell growth in tumors.

- *Counting mitoses in histologic sections.* This procedure, when applied to experimental tumors, is easier if the animal is injected with a microtubular poison such as colchicine, which stops all mitoses in metaphase (p. 159). The percentage of cells in mitosis then provides the *mitotic index.*

- *Histochemical demonstration of dividing cells,* e.g.: using antibodies against cell-cycle related proteins (109).

- *Radioactive labeling of dividing cells* in vivo. A tumor-bearing animal is injected with tritiated thymidine, which is incorporated into the DNA of cells preparing to divide. Microscopic sections of the tumor are then overlaid with an X-ray emulsion, whereby autoradiographs are produced: silver grains develop over each dividing cell (Figure 26.65). The

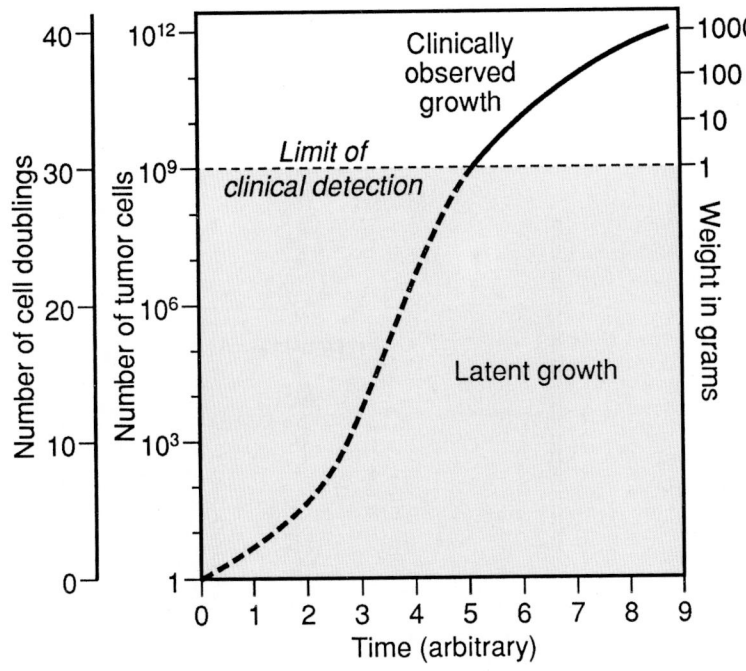

FIGURE 26.64   A depressing curve. To reach a palpable size (1 gram), a tumor requires 30 cell doublings; only 10 more doublings are needed to reach one kilogram. Skin tumors are an exception: They can be detected well before they weigh 1 gram. (Adapted from [231].)

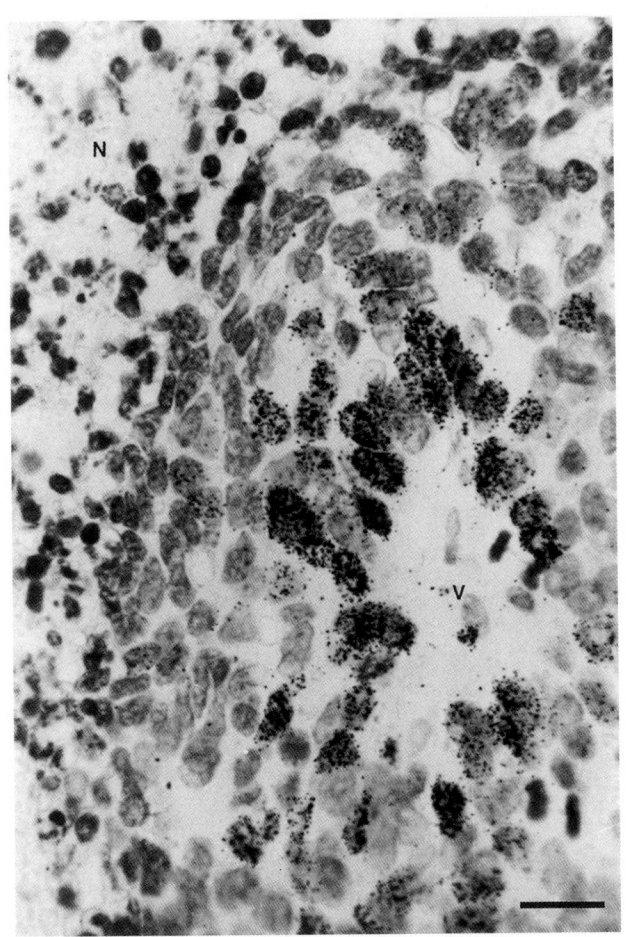

FIGURE 26.65   Autoradiograph from a malignant tumor labeled with thymidine; note the intense labeling adjacent to a blood vessel (**V**). This particular tumor, a mouse adenocarcinoma, contained regions of necrosis (**N**) through which ran cords of viable tissue such as the one shown here in cross section. **Bar** = 25 μm. (Reproduced with permission from [227].)

percentage of labeled cells found in this manner is the *labeling index.*

- *By the cell-sorter* (p. 15), which can be loaded with a suspension of tumor cells treated with a DNA stain and then instructed to count those that are in the S-phase of the cell cycle.

On histologic sections, the labeling method is more sensitive and more accurate than the mitotic count because labeled cells are easier to identify than mitoses. Labeled cells are also more numerous because the DNA synthesis (S-phase) of the cell cycle lasts much longer than mitosis. Furthermore, counting mitoses can be misleading. Suppose that the mitoses in a given tumor were normal in number but lasted twice as long as in the control tissue; the net result would be a doubling of the visible mitoses, which could falsely suggest an increased mitotic rate (13).

For tumors in rodents the percentage of replicating cells, as shown by the labeling index, is in the range of 2–8 percent. In human tumors the same index is generally lower than 10 percent, and lower than in normal

Table 26.3 Cell-Cycle Times of Various Normal Tissues
and Tumors in Humans

Tissue	Cell-Cycle Time (hr)
Bone-marrow precursor cells	18
Colon, epithelium of crypt cells	39
Rectum, epithelium of crypt cells	48
Bronchus, epithelial cells	220
Carcinoma of stomach	72
Acute myeloblastic leukemia	80–84
Chronic myeloid leukemia	120
Carcinoma of bronchus	196–260

epithelia such as the lining of the intestinal mucosa
(index about 16 percent) (231). As to the cell cycle
(160) studies available on human tumors also show
times longer than normal: 20 hours for leukemias,
60 hours for superficial solid tumors (Table 26.3)
(231). All this goes to say that cell replication inside a
tumor (with a few exceptions) is far from a frenzy. It is
actually depressed, but unfortunately not depressed
enough.

Cell Loss: Apoptosis and Other Mechanisms

(*For apoptosis in tumors, see p. 216 and p. 891.*)

Overall, data show that the apparent slow growth of
tumors has little to do with the duration of the cell cycle:
cell loss is a major factor. *A tumor grows because there is
an excess of cell production over cell loss* (Figure 26.66).
Tumor cells can be lost by several pathways:

1. *Apoptosis,* usually the main factor (p. 216),
2. *Differentiation* (p. 947),
3. *Ischemic cell death* (p. 203)
4. *Antitumor defenses,* (p. 909), and
5. *Escape into the bloodstream* (usually a small minority,
   p. 812).

The overall cell loss varies greatly, but can be estimated: knowing (by experiment) the cycling time of
the cells in a given tumor and the labeling index, it is
possible to calculate the *theoretical* doubling time of the
tumor. The *actual* doubling time is shorter. From the
difference one can estimate the amount of cell loss,
which can be of the order of 50 percent or more (218).

Anyway, in terms of replication, tumors contain four
populations of neoplastic cells (Figure 26.67) (214):
population A, cycling cells; population B, cells that can
be recruited into cycling but are temporarily quiescent
(at the G_o stage); population C, cells that are permanently unable to divide (e.g., because they have differentiated); and population D, dead and dying cells.

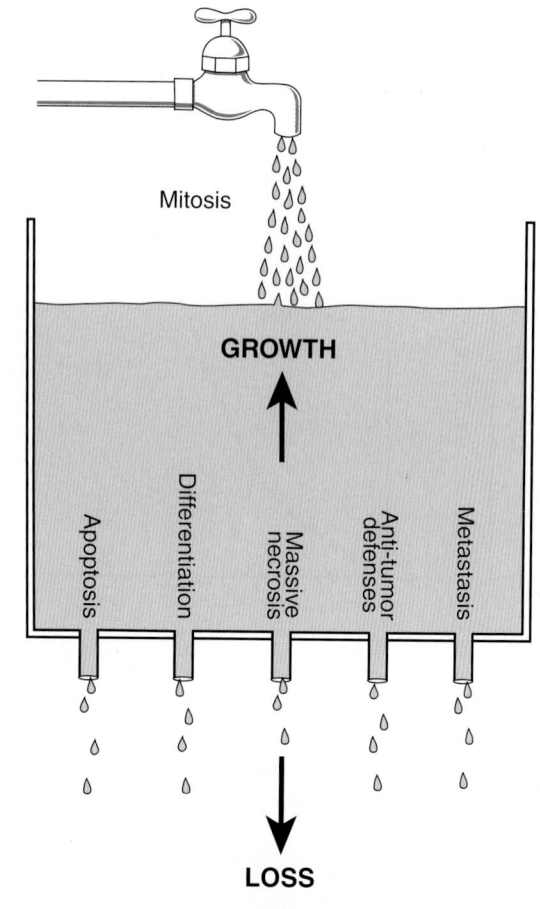

FIGURE 26.66 Diagram showing that tumors grow by an imbalance between cell production and cell loss. (Modified from
[219].)

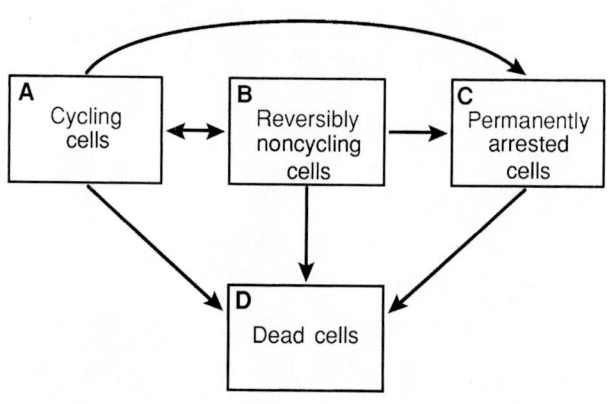

FIGURE 26.67 The neoplastic cells of a tumor belong to four
growth populations (**A, B, C, D**). The purpose of current cancer
therapy is to move tumor cells from **B** to **A**, because chemotherapeutic agents are most effective against cycling cells. (Adapted
from [221].)

The existence of different cell populations in a tumor is critical for planning therapeutic strategies. Population A is the main target of anticancer agents because such agents are most effective against cycling cells; therefore, the ideal procedure is to kill off the cells in population A and then move as many cells as possible from B to A. An empirical but effective way to do this is to reduce the mass of the tumor, a procedure known in surgery as "debulking." Somehow debulking prods the noncycling cells into a spurt of growth, and while they are cycling, they become targets for another therapeutic attack (221).

Growth of tumor cells can be inhibited by contact with normal cells, at least *in vitro* (22, 167). We have already mentioned this curious phenomenon in relation to cell-to-cell communications (p. 754); for the time being it is an intriguing curiosity worthy of more study.

Last: *how does the tumor maintain its critical slight margin of growth against cell deletion by apoptosis and other mechanisms?* Presumably, clones of cells that cannot maintain this pace never become tumors.

> **TO SUM UP:** The popular image of a tumor tends to be that of a monstrous creature that grows unrestrained. This is a myth. Tumors grow fast enough to kill, but their growth is fraught with obstacles.

Life Inside a Tumor

Tumor cells have to live and grow in their own self-made environment: an untidy assembly of connective tissue and vessels that they have extorted from the host but not properly planned. It turns out to be a hostile environment: like that of some fast-growing cities, it is haphazard, polluted, and lacking in services. Oncologists, whose aim is to wipe out its inhabitants, exploit these environmental faults as best they can.

What life must be like for the cells of a malignant tumor we can but dimly perceive (23). Most of their neighbors are other malignant cells; this means competition for scarce nutrients, but also a free supply of paracrine growth factors. Because a tumor's vessels are leaky, the surrounding *milieu* is rather similar to an inflammatory exudate, and some of the surrounding cells are in fact inflammatory cells.

Inflammation in Tumors

Summoned by chemotactic messages, a variety of host cells migrate into the tumor. They include natural killer cells as well as T-lymphocytes; both are potential enemies of tumor cells (B-lymphocytes are largely ineffective, as we will see in Chapter 30). Many of the immigrant cells are macrophages, drawn in by chemokines secreted by the tumor itself (161). How many macrophages? Counts in rodent tumors yielded numbers averaging 10–30 percent of the cell population within the tumor (70, 225). Their function is ambiguous (42a); they could make themselves useful by scavenging dead tumor cells, although this task is overwhelming when massive necrosis occurs. Overall the inflammatory response to injury *within* the tumor is poor; true granulation tissue rarely if ever develops around a necrotic core (Figure 26.28). Experiments on tumors of rats and mice have shown that a cotton thread placed in tumor tissue elicits a minimal response compared with that of normal tissues (159). True, some types of human tumors do elicit a hefty inflammatory (immune) response, but they are the exception; some tumors actually depress the inflammatory response (p. 912). Tumor cells also produce a variety of molecules that cause **vascular leakage** (Figure 26.32) (31, 59, 151a). For example, if a suspension of tumor cells is injected subcutaneously into an experimental animal, within hours the cells become embedded in a gel of fibrin. This means that fibrinogen leaked out of the vessels and then clotted, presumably as a result of a tumor procoagulant activity. What this may mean to the tumor cell, however, is not certain because tumor cells can also induce the opposite effect fibrinolysis.

Inflammatory carcinoma of the breast. This is an uncommon (1–3 percent) and still unexplained presentation of breast cancer. The skin is red and hot, typically with *peau d' orange* features; the breast may be swollen, often without a palpable mass, and therefore may suggest the diagnosis of mastitis. Histology shows a poorly differentiated ductal carcinoma diffusely infiltrating the lymphatics. The prognosis was very poor but has improved (120). Perhaps these [adeno-]carcinomas secrete an irritant?

The Internal Milieu of Tumors

The basic data on the aqueous internal environment of tumors, their **internal milieu,** were obtained by P. M.

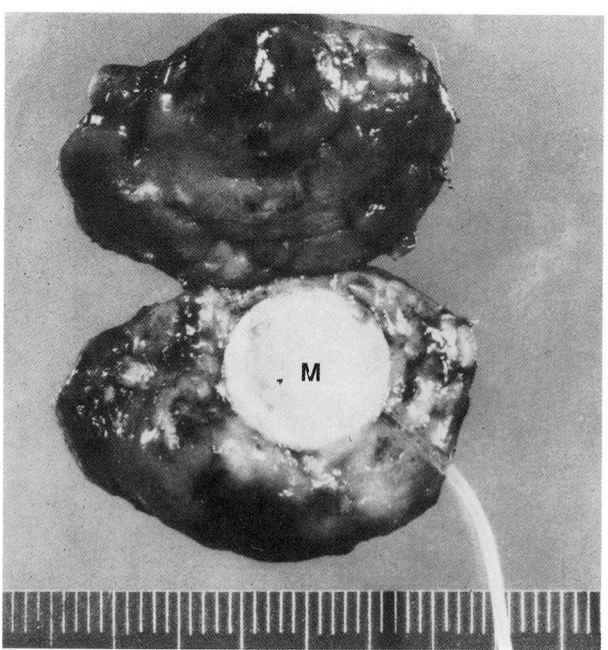

FIGURE 26.68 A method for studying the internal milieu of a tumor: A carcinoma of the rat is grown around a micropore chamber (**M**) equipped with a draining catheter. **Scale** in millimeters. (Reproduced with permission from [106].)

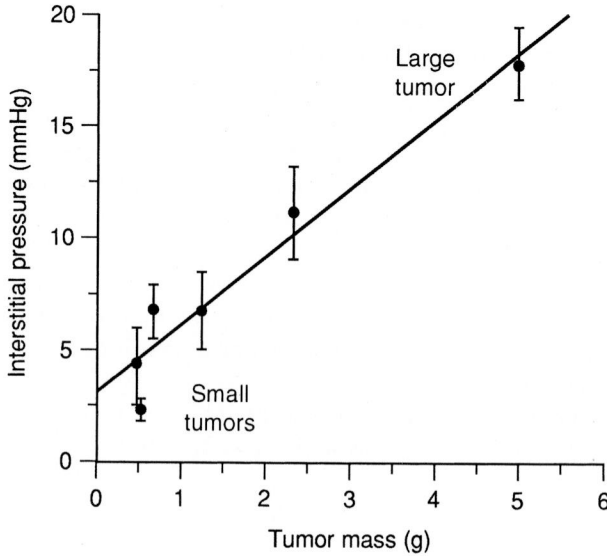

FIGURE 26.69 Values of tissue pressure measured in the center of mouse transplantable tumors (Walker 256 carcinoma). (Adapted with permission from [25].)

Gullino and co-workers by means of a small plastic chamber permanently implanted into an experimental tumor (Figure 26.68); interestingly, no granulation tissue developed around the sampling device (104), confirming the inadequate inflammatory response within tumor tissue. These and later studies showed that the medium in which the tumor cells live is quite pathologic (89, 104). Although derived basically from plasma, the medium is almost free of glucose (105) and is polluted with enzymes released from dead cells; it may therefore act as a tenderizer, dissociating the live tumor cells and thereby perhaps helping invasion (p. 815). It is also acid, in the range of pH 6.7–7.0 (104, 241), and in many parts hypoxic due to the poor distribution of blood vessels (126).

Another peculiarity of this acid fluid is that it flows as a slow current toward the tumor's surface. The genesis of this current is twofold: lack of lymphatics, and leaky blood vessels.

Lymphatics are Missing

Whether malignant tumors have few lymphatics or none at all matters little, because *functionally* we are dealing with a system devoid of lymphatic drainage. In other words, we can consider malignant tumors as an experiment of nature to show what happens when lymphatics are missing. The experiment is in itself a puzzle, because malignant tumors can produce both angio- and lymphangiogenetic factors, yet respond much more intensely to the first. What does happen in malignant tumors, as might be guessed, is that the fluid seeping out of the capillaries and venules into a confined environment distends the tissue spaces and raises the tissue pressure. In most normal tissues, the pressure is negative (p. 615). In tumors, especially the larger ones, tissue pressure is positive (33, 104, 119, 124, 129); the highest pressure is in the center (14, 128, 129), where it can be as much as 30 mm Hg (Figure 26.69), even 45 mm in human melanomas (126). Due to the high tissue pressure, blood flow in the centers of the tumor is impaired (127). This phenomenon is surely related to the typical central necrosis of malignant tumors, which is usually and rather glibly explained by stating that "tumors outgrow their vessels."

Blood Vessels Are Leaky

The source of the fluid that oozes from the tumor is, of course, the microcirculation: many vessels—as we have seen—are leaky. The amount of this fluid is considerable. A porous chamber inserted into an experimental tumor drains 4–5 times as much fluid as one inserted into normal skin (33). Obviously, this fluid has to go somewhere. In fact, the interstitial fluid inside a tumor continues to move toward the surface at a velocity

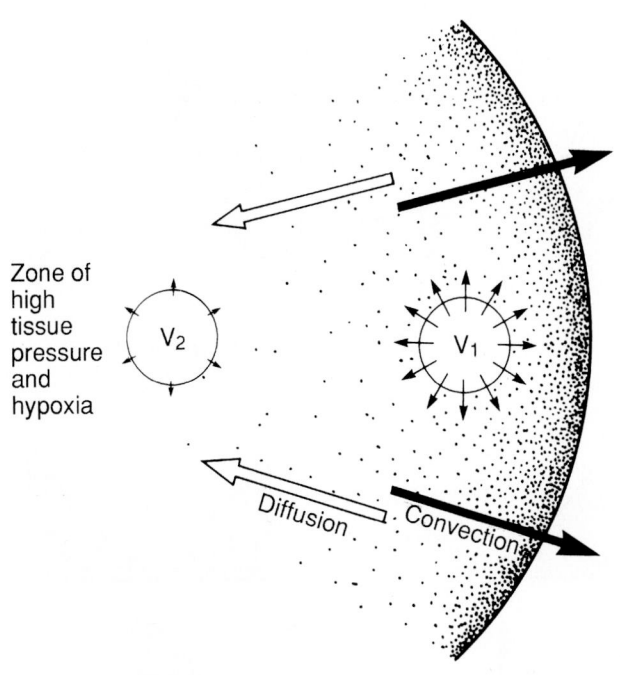

Zone of
high
tissue
pressure
and
hypoxia

V_2

V_1

Diffusion Convection

FIGURE 26.70 Schematic cross section of a tumor illustrating some aspects of tumor fluid dynamics. Interstitial pressure is assumed to decrease from the center to the periphery. The two circles ($\mathbf{V}_1$ and $\mathbf{V}_2$) represent microscopic vessels; **arrows** emerging from the vessels indicate filtration pressure. The pressure gradient leads to a radial, outward convection (**black arrows**), which opposes the radial, inward diffusion (**open arrows**). In the center of the tumor, the interstitial pressure being higher, the microvascular transudation of fluid and of macromolecules (**small dots**) is lower. (Adapted with permission from [129].)

calculated at 6–12 μm per minute, and then drains out into the surroundings at the respectable rate of about 0.2 ml per hour per gram of tissue, as measured in a rat carcinoma (33, 125).

These simple facts of hydraulics mean a lot to the oncologist (127, 128). Because flow in the center of the tumor is poor (as well as uneven), chemotherapeutic agents have to diffuse into that zone from the well-perfused outer shell; but this diffusion is opposed by the outward convection (Figure 26.70) (14, 126). This convection also flushes out any autocrine chemoattractants that the tumor may secrete (p. 816), with the result that mobile or mobilized tumor cells are attracted outward (this, however, is pure speculation).

Brain tumors should offer a special opportunity to study the oozing phenomenon because the lack of lymphatics in the brain itself should trap the edema fluid around the tumor. The topic is complicated by the blood–brain barrier, which is usually (but capriciously) incomplete in primary brain tumors. Edema of the white matter around a glioma is common; around meningiomas it is "classic" (203). This topic needs further study.

The loss of plasma from the vessels into the tumor raises the intravascular hematocrit, which impairs flow by raising the viscosity of the blood (212). Other factors also conspire to increase the viscosity: sluggish flow favors the aggregation of red blood cells into rouleaux (p. 506), and the acidic tumor environment increases the rigidity of red blood cells (p. 688) (124).

Hypoxia

Hypoxia threatens any tumor cell that moves too far away from the blood vessel(s). We will call this "hypoxia" to go along with current terminology, but actually cells too far from the blood supply suffer from lack of oxygen, lack of substrates, and loss of waste removal—that is, from ischemia. The critical distance is of the order of 100 μm; in one pioneer study no tumor cell was found alive at 180 μm distance from a vessel (234).

Tumor cords. The effects of ischemia are best studied, quantitatively, in some fast-growing tumors (mostly epithelial) that develop in the shape of cords. Each cord is made of a capillary surrounded by a sleeve of tumor cells. The reverse pattern is also possible: a cord of tumor cells surrounded by capillaries. In either case, mitoses occur close to the blood vessel(s) and decrease centrifugally, which means that there is a constant displacement of cells from the vascular core toward the necrotic never-never land (Figure 26.71) (219, 227).

The radius of the cord depends on the partial pressure of oxygen, the diameter of the vessel, the coefficient of diffusion of oxygen, and the rate of oxygen consumption by the tumor cells. It was found to be 98.7 ± 11.9 μm in retinoblastomas and 104 μm in squamous cell carcinomas. The cord pattern, prevalent in retinoblastomas, occurs also in other tumors, such as squamous cell carcinomas of the lung (34 percent) and of the cervix (14 percent) (32).

This pathophysiology of tumor cords has practical consequences: most tumor therapies are cell-cycle dependent; therefore, they hit the cycling perivascular cells but tend to spare those beyond, which are alive but anoxic and not cycling. As the perivascular cells are killed by the treatment and disappear, their places in the cord are taken by the noncycling cells that have survived the "cure." Now these newcomers, having moved closer to the capillary, have a second chance to grow—and therefore to be hit by the next dose of therapy (229).

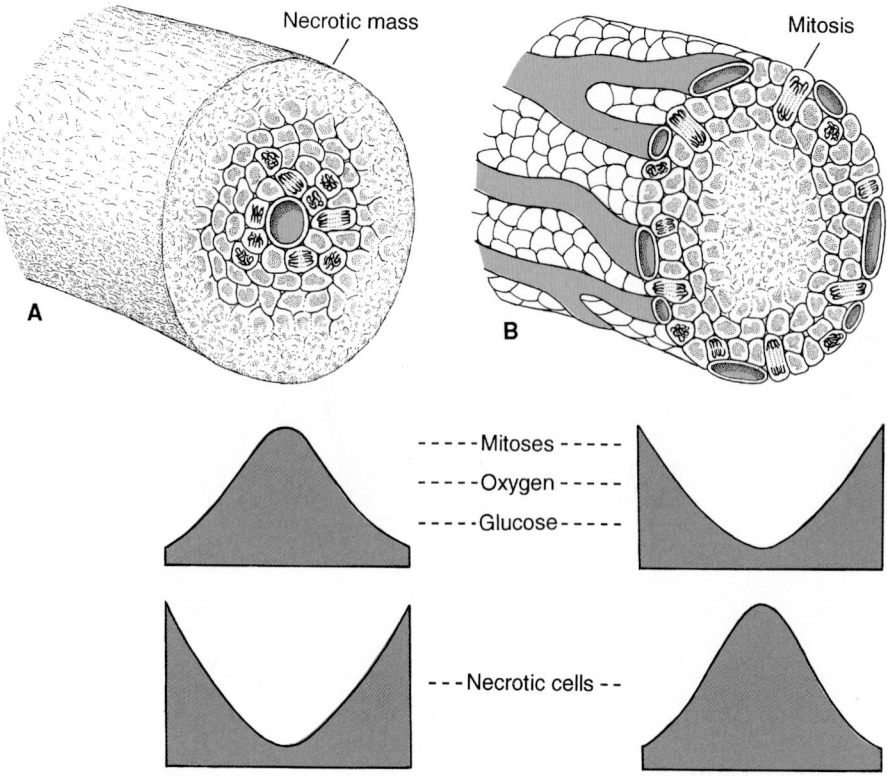

FIGURE 26.71 Two patterns of tumor growth. **A:** Sleeve of tumor cells around a central longitudinal vessel. Mitoses are more numerous near the center, necrotic cells prevail at the periphery. **B:** Mass of tumor cells surrounded by blood vessels. Mitoses prevail at the periphery, necrosis in the center. (Adapted from [171] by permission of Oxford University Press.)

How do the necrotic tumor cells disappear? Do they all disappear? Do they completely disappear? This is not clear. All malignant tumors contain macrophages (250), but it is obvious that there are not enough macrophages around to phagocytize the whole necrotic mass. Our impression is that dead tumor cells undergo a combination of autolysis and denaturation, whereby a part of the mass shrivels away. This would explain the depressed surface of subcapsular tumor metastases in the liver (see Figure 27.14).

The growth of tumors has a lot to do with hypoxia. Because hypoxia is a typical "accident" in the life of a cell, we would expect hypoxic tumor cells to die by the mechanism typical of accidental cell death as seen in infarcts, namely with swelling (oncosis). Oddly enough, many hypoxic tumor cells die by suicide (apoptosis); as a result, hypoxia selects for survival those tumor cells that are *less* apt to commit suicide—thereby favoring the progression of the tumor toward ever greater malignancy. We shall return to this topic in discussing oncogenes.

Hypoxia poses another challenge for the oncologists: it makes the cells more resistant to radiation. It takes 2–3 times the normal dose of radiation to kill them compared with well-oxygenated cells (37); remember that the mechanism of cell killing by X-rays depends in part on the formation of *oxygen-derived* free radicals. Solving such problems requires a close collaboration between cell biologist, pathologist, and oncologist.

What if the necrotic masses were digested away by bacteria? This was tried on tumor-bearing mice: intravenous injection of *Clostridium novyi* spores combined with chemotherapy caused most of the tumors to become entirely necrotic, and half of the mice were cured (46).

TO SUM UP: Tumors are mistaken organs in more than one way, caricatures of real organs, built of genetically flawed cells sustained by an abnormal microcirculation. The resulting *milieu intérieur* of the tumor is actually hostile to the tumor cell (240); but unfortunately not hostile enough to kill it.

References

1. Acker H, Carlsson J, Durand R, Sutherland RM, eds. Spheroids in cancer research. Recent results in cancer research, vol 95. Berlin: Springer-Verlag, 1984.
2. Ahmed A. Calcification in human breast carcinomas: ultrastructural observations. J Pathol 1975;117:247–251.
3. Akaza H, Murphy WM, Soloway MS. Bladder cancer induced by noncarcinogenic substances. J Urol 1984;131:152–155.
4. Algire GH, Chalkley HW. Vascular reactions of normal and malignant tissues in vivo. I. Vascular reactions of mice to wounds and to normal and neoplastic transplants. J Natl Cancer Inst 1945;6:73–85.

5. Archer MC. Chemical carcinogenesis. In: Tannock IF, Hill RP, eds. The basic science of oncology. New York: Pergamon Press, 1987, pp. 89–105.

6. Armed Forces Institute of Pathology. Atlas of tumor pathology, 2nd series, fasc 1. Washington, DC: Universities Associated for Research and Education in Pathology, Inc, 1967.

7. Ausprunk DH, Falterman K, Foldman J. The sequence of events in the regression of corneal capillaries. Lab Invest 1978;38:284–294.

8. Bainton DF, Friedlander LM, Shohet SB. Abnormalities in granule formation in acute myelogenous leukemia. Blood 1977;49:693–704.

9. Balmain A. Cancer genetics: from Boveri and Mendel to microarrays. Nat Rev Cancer 2001;1:77–82.

9a. Baluk P, Morikawa S, Haskell A, Mancuso M, McDonald DM. Abnormalities of basement membrane on blood vessels and endothelial sprouts in tumors. Am J Pathol 2003;163:1801–1815.

10. Barcellos-Hoff MH, Ravani SA. Irradiated mammary gland stroma promotes the expression of tumorigenic potential by unirradiated epithelial cells. Cancer Res 2000;60:1254–1260.

11. Barker BE, Sanford KK. Cytologic manifestations of neoplastic transformation *in vitro*. J Natl Cancer Inst 1970;44:39–63.

12. Barnhill RL, Wolf JE Jr. Angiogenesis and the skin. J Am Acad Dermatol 1987;16:1226–1242.

13. Baserga R. The cell cycle. N Engl J Med 1981;304:453–459.

14. Baxter LT, Jain RK. Transport of fluid and macromolecules in tumors. I. Role of interstitial pressure and convection. Microvasc Res 1989;37:77–104.

15. Ben-Bassat H, Inbar M, Sachs L. Changes in the structural organization of the surface membrane in malignant cell transformation. J Membrane Biol 1971;6:183–194.

16. Berenblum I. The cocarcinogenic action of croton resin. Cancer Res 1941;1:44–48.

17. Berenblum I. Sequential aspects of chemical carcinogenesis: skin. In: Becker FF, ed. Cancer. A comprehensive treatise, vol 1. New York: Plenum Press, 1975, pp. 323–344.

18. Berenblum I, Shubik P. A new, quantitative approach to the study of the stages of chemical carcinogenesis in the mouse's skin. Br J Cancer 1947;1:383–391.

19. Bernal SD, Lampidis TJ, McIsaac RM, Chen LB. Anticarcinoma activity in vivo of rhodamine 123, a mitochondrial-specific dye. Science 1983;222:169–172.

20. Bertalanffy FD, Schachter R, Ali J, Ingimundson JC. Mitotic rate and doubling time of intraperitoneal and subcutaneous Ehrlich ascites tumor. Cancer Res 1965;25:685–691.

21. Berthezene F, Greer MA. Studies on the composition of the thyroid psammoma bodies of chronically iodine-deficient rats. Endocrinology 1974;95:651–659.

22. Bertram JS, Faletto MB. Requirements for and kinetics of growth arrest of neoplastic cells by confluent 10T½ fibroblasts induced by a specific inhibitor of cyclic adenosine $3':5'$-phosphodiesterase. Cancer Res 1985;45:1946–1952.

23. Bissell MJ, Radisky D. Putting tumours in context. Nat Rev Cancer 2001;1:46–54.

24. Black PH. Shedding from the cell surface of normal and cancer cells. Adv Cancer Res 1980;32:75–199.

25. Boucher Y, Baxter LT, Jain RK. Interstitial pressure gradients in tissue-isolated and subcutaneous tumors: implications for therapy. Cancer Res 1990;50:4478–4484.

26. Boutwell RK. Some biological aspects of skin carcinogenesis. Prog Exp Tumor Res 1964;4:207–250.

27. Boutwell RK. Tumor promoters in human carcinogenesis. In: DeVita VT, Hellman S, Rosenberg SA, eds. Important advances in oncology 1985. Philadelphia: JB Lippincott, 1985, pp. 16–27.

28. Bowen ID. Laboratory techniques for demonstrating cell death. In: Davies I, Sigee DC, eds. Cell ageing and cell death. Cambridge: Cambridge University Press, 1984, pp. 5–40.

29. Bowen ID, Bowen SM. Programmed cell death in tumours and tissues. London: Chapman and Hall, 1990.

30. Brem H, Folkman J. Inhibition of tumor angiogenesis mediated by cartilage. J Exp Med 1975;141:427–439.

31. Brown LF, Berse B, Jackman RW, et al. Increased expression of vascular permeability factor (vascular endothelial growth factor) and its receptors in kidney and bladder carcinomas. Am J Pathol 1993;143:1255–1262.

32. Burnier MN, McLean IW, Zimmerman LE, Rosenberg SH. Retinoblastoma. The relationship of proliferating cells to blood vessels. Invest Ophthalmol Vis Sci 1990;31:2037–2040.

33. Butler TP, Gullino PM. Quantitation of cell shedding into efferent blood of mammary adenocarcinoma. Cancer Res 1975;35:512–516.

33a. Cassella M, Skobe M. Lymphatic vessel activation in cancer. Ann NY Acad Sci 2002;979:120–130.

33b. Chang I, Kaipainen A, Folkman J. Lymphangiogenesis. New mechanisms. Ann NY Acad Sci 2002;979:111–119.

34. Chen LB, Rivers EN. Mitochondria in cancer cells. In: Carney D, Sikora K, eds. Genes and cancer. Chichester: John Wiley & Sons, 1990, pp. 127–135.

35 Cohnheim J. Lectures on general pathology. Section II: the pathology of nutrition. London: The New Sydenham Society, 1889.

36. Collins VP, Loeffler RK, Tivey H. Observations on growth rates of human tumors. Am J Roentgenol 1956;76:988–1000.

37. Coleman CN. Hypoxia in tumors: a paradigm for the approach to biochemical and physiologic heterogeneity. J Natl Cancer Inst 1988;80:310–317.

38. Columbano A, Rajalakshmi S, Sarma DSR. Requirement of cell proliferation for the initiation of liver carcinogenesis as assayed by three different procedures. Cancer Res 1981;41:2079–2083.

39. Coman DR. Decreased mutual adhesiveness, a property of cells from squamous cell carcinomas. Cancer Res 1944;4:625–629.

40. Condamine H, Custer RP, Mintz B. Pure-strain and genetically mosaic liver tumors histochemically identified with the β-glucuronidase marker in allophenic mice. Proc Natl Acad Sci USA 1971;68:2032–2036.

41. Cooke R. Dr. Folkman's war. New York: Random House, 2000.

42. Cotran RS, Kumar V, Collins T: Robbins pathologic basis of disease. Philadelphia: W.B. Saunders Company, 1999.

42a. Coussens LM, Werb Z. Inflammation and cancer. Nature 2002;420:860–867.

43. Cramer SF, Meyer JS, Kraner JF, et al. Metastasizing leiomyoma of the uterus. S-phase fraction, estrogen receptor, and ultrastructure. Cancer 1980;45:932–937.

44. D'Amore PA. Growth factors, angiogenesis and metastasis. Prog Clin Biol Res 1986;212:269–283.

45. D'Amore PA, Thompson RW. Mechanisms of angiogenesis. Annu Rev Physiol 1987;49:453–464.

46. Dang LH, Bettegowda C, Huso DL, Kinzler KW, Vogelstein B. Combination bacteriolytic therapy for the treatment of experimental tumors. Proc Natl Acad Sci USA 2001;98:15155–15160.

47. De Baetselier P. Neoplastic progression by somatic cell fusion. In: Liotta LA, ed. Influence of tumor development on the host. Dordrecht: Kluwer Academic Publishers, 1989, pp. 112–120.

48. De Lang T, DePinho RA. Unlimited mileage from telomerase? Science 1999;283:947–949.

49. Denekamp J. Vascular endothelium as the vulnerable element in tumours. Acta Radiol Oncol 1984;23:217–225.

50. Denekamp J, Hobson B. Endothelial-cell proliferation in experimental tumours. Br J Cancer 1982;46:711–720.

51. Derenzini M, Pession A, Trerè D. Quantity of nucleolar silver-stained proteins is related to proliferating activity in cancer cells. Lab Invest 1990;63:137–140.

52. Derenzini M, Ploton D. Interphase nucleolar organizer regions in cancer cells. Int Rev Exp Pathol 1991;32:149–192.

53. D'Errico A, Garbisa S, Liotta LA, et al. Augmentation of type IV collagenase, laminin receptor, and Ki67 proliferation antigen associated with human colon, gastric, and breast carcinoma progression. Mod Pathol 1991;4:239–246.

54. de Waal RMW, van Altena MC, Erhard H, et al. Lack of lymphangiogenesis in human primary cutaneous melanoma. Am J Pathol 1997;150:1951–1957.

55. Domagala W, Koss LG. Configuration of surfaces of human cancer cells in effusions. A scanning electron microscopic study of microvilli. Virchows Arch B [Cell Pathol] 1977;26:27–42.

56. Donehower LA. Genetic instability in animal tumorigenesis models. In: Cancer surveys, Vol. 29. Checkpoint controls and cancer. Plainview, NY, Cold Spring Harbor Laboratory, 1997, pp. 329–352.

57. Durand RE. Multicell spheroids as a model for cell kinetic studies. Cell Tissue Kinet 1990;23:141–159.

58. Dvorak HF. Brown LF, Detmar M, Dvorak AM. Vascular permeability factor/vascular endothelial growth factor, microvascular hyperpermeability, and angiogenesis. Am J Pathol 1995;146:1029–1039.

59. Dvorak HF, Orenstein NS, Carvalho AC, et al. Induction of a fibrin-gel investment: an early event in line 10 hepatocarcinoma growth mediated by tumor-secreted products. J Immunol 1979;122:166–174.

60. Dvorak HF, Quay SC, Orenstein NS, et al. Tumor shedding and coagulation. Science 1981;212:923–924.

61. Dvorak HF. Tumors: wounds that do not heal. Similarities between tumor stroma generation and wound healing. N Engl J Med 1986;315:1650–1659.

62. Dvorak HF, Nagy JA, Dvorak AM. Structure of solid tumors and their vasculature: implications for therapy with monoclonal antibodies. Cancer Cells 1991;3:77–85.

63. Dvorak HF, Nagy JA, Dvorak JT, Dvorak AM. Identification and characterization of the blood vessels of solid tumors that are leaky to circulating macromolecules. Am J Pathol 1988;133:95–109.

64. Earle WR. Production of malignancy in vitro. IV. The mouse fibroblast cultures and changes seen in the living cells. J Natl Cancer Inst 1943;4:165–212.

65. Earle WR, Nettleship A. Production of malignancy in vitro. V. Results of injections of cultures into mice. J Natl Cancer Inst 1943;4:213–227.

66. Egeblad M, Werb Z. New functions for the matrix metalloproteinases in cancer progression. Nat Rev Cancer 2002;2:161–174.

67. Eisenstein R, Kuettner KE, Neapolitan C, Soble LW, Sorgente N. The resistance of certain tissues to invasion. III. Cartilage extracts inhibit the growth of fibroblasts and endothelial cells in culture. Am J Pathol 1975;81:337–348.

68. Eisenstein R, Sorgente N, Soble LW, Miller A, Kuettner KE. The resistance of certain tissues to invasion. Penetrability of explanted tissues by vascularized mesenchyme. Am J Pathol 1973;73:765–774.

69. Escher MC, Locher JL. The world of M.C. Escher. New York: Harry N. Abrams, 1974.

70. Evans R, Lawler EM. Macrophage content and immunogenicity of C57BL/6J and BALB/cByJ methylcholanthrene-induced sarcomas. Int J Cancer 1980;26:831–835.

71. Farber E. Chemical carcinogenesis. A biologic perspective. Am J Pathol 1982;106:269–296.

72. Fausto N. Vasculogenic mimicry in tumors. Fact or artifact? Am J Pathol 2000;156:359.

73. Fialkow PJ. Clonal origin and stem cell evolution of human tumors. Prog Cancer Res Ther 1977;3:439–453.

74. Findlay JK. Angiogenesis in reproductive tissues. J Endocrinol 1986;111:357–366.

75. Folkman J. Tumor angiogenesis factor. Cancer Res 1974;34:2109–2113.

76. Folkman J. What is the role of endothelial cells in angiogenesis? Lab Invest 1984;51:601–604.

77. Folkman J. Toward an understanding of angiogenesis: search and discovery. Perspect Biol Med 1985a;29:10–36.

78. Folkman J. Tumor angiogenesis. Adv Cancer Res 1985b;43:175–203.

79. Folkman J. Angiogenesis in cancer, vascular, rheumatoid and other disease. Nature Med 1995;1:27–31.

80. Folkman J. Angiogenesis inhibitors generated by tumors. Molec Med 1995;1:120–122.

81. Folkman J, Cotran R. Relation of vascular proliferation to tumor growth. Int Rev Exp Pathol 1976;16:207–248.

82. Folkman J, Hochberg M. Self-regulation of growth in three dimensions. J Exp Med 1973;138:745–753.

83. Folkman J, Klagsbrun M. Angiogenic factors. Science 1987;235:442–447.

84. Folkman J, Long DM. The use of silicone rubber as a carrier for prolonged drug therapy. J Surg Res 1964;4:139–142.

85. Folkman J, Watson K, Ingber D, Hanahan D. Induction of angiogenesis during the transition from hyperplasia to neoplasia. Nature 1989a;339:58–61.

86. Folkman J, Weisz PB, Joullié MM, Li WW, Ewing WR. Control of angiogenesis with synthetic heparin substitutes. Science 1989b;243:1490–1493.

87. Foulds L. Neoplastic development, vol 2. London: Academic Press, 1975.

88. Freeman AE, Huebner RJ. Problems in interpretation of experimental evidence of cell transformation. J Natl Cancer Inst 1973;50:303–306.

89. Freitas I, Baronzo GF, Bono B, et al. Tumor interstitial fluid: misconsidered component of the internal milieu of a solid tumor. Anticancer Res 1997;17:165–172.

90. Frisch SM, Ruoslahti E. Integrins and anoikis. Curr Opin Cell Biol 1997;9:701–706.

91. Gainor JP, Morton CA, Bell DR, Vincent PA, Minnear FL. Platelet phospholipids decrease vascular endothelial permeability via a novel signaling pathway independent of cAMP/protein kinase A. In: Goetzl EJ, Lynch KR (eds). Lysophospholipids and eicosanoids in biology and pathophysiology. New York: New York Academy of Sciences, 2000, pp. 315–318.

91a. Galloway AC, Pelletier R, D'Amore PA. Do ischemic hearts stimulate endothelial cell growth? Surgery 1984;96:435–439.

92. Gillispie CC, ed. Dictionary of scientific biography, Gomperta, B., 1972. New York: Scribner, 1970–1980.

93. Gimbrone MA, Aster RH, Cotran RS, et al. Preservation of vascular integrity in organs perfused *in vitro* with a platelet-rich medium. Nature 1969;222:33–36.

94. Gimbrone MA Jr, Cotran RS, Leapman SB, Folkman J. Tumor growth and neovascularization: an experimental model using the rabbit cornea. J Natl Cancer Inst 1974;52:413–427.

95. Gimbrone MA Jr, Gullino PM. Neovascularization induced by intraocular xenografts of normal, preneo-plastic, and neoplastic mouse mammary tissues. J Natl Cancer Inst 1976a;56:305–318.

96. Gimbrone MA Jr, Leapman SB, Cotran RS, Folkman J. Tumor dormancy in vivo by prevention of neovascularization. J Exp Med 1972;136:261–276.

97. Gisselsson D, Björk J, Höglund M, et al. Abnormal nuclear shape in solid tumors reflects mitotic instability. Am J Pathol 2001;158:199–206.

98. Gittes RF. Carcinoma of the prostate. N Engl J Med 1991;324:236–245.

98a. Gleason DF. Histologic grading and clinical staging of prostatic carcinoma. In: Tannenbaum M. Urologic Pathology: The Prostate. Philadelphia: Lea & Febiger, 1977, pp. 171–198.

99. Goldacre RJ, Sylvén B. On the access of blood-borne dyes to various tumour regions. Br J Cancer 1962;16:306–322.

100. Goldberg ID, Rosen EM (eds). Epithelial-mesenchymal interactions in cancer. Basel: Birkhauser Verlag, 1995.

101. Gould VE, Orucevic A, Zentgraf H, et al. Nup88 (karyoporin) in human malignant neoplasms and dysplasias: correlations of immunostaining of tissue sections, cytologic smears, and immunoblot analysis. Hum Pathol 2002;33:536–544.

102. Greaves M. Is telomerase activity in cancer due to selection of stem cells and differentiation arrest? TIG 1996;12:127–128.

103. Grimstad IA. Direct evidence that cancer cell locomotion contributes importantly to invasion. Exp Cell Res 1987;173:515–523.

104. Gullino PM. The internal milieu of tumors. Prog Exp Tumor Res 1966;8:1–25.

105. Gullino PM. Extracellular compartments of solid tumors. In: Becker FF, ed. Cancer, vol 3. New York: Plenum Publishing, 1975, pp. 327–354.

106. Gullino PM. Influence of blood supply on thermal properties and metabolism of mammary carcinomas. Ann NY Acad Sci 1980;335:1–21.

107. Gullino PM, Grantham FH. The vascular space of growing tumors. Cancer Res 1964;24:1727–1732.

108. Hagiwara H, Ohwada N, Fujimoto T. Intracytoplasmic lumina in human oviduct epithelium. Ultrastruct Pathol 1997;21:163–172.

109. Hall PA, Levinson DA, Woods AL, et al. Proliferating cell nuclear antigen (PCNA) immunolocalization in paraffin sections: an index of cell proliferation with evidence of some deregulated expression in some neoplasms. J Pathol 1990;162:285–294.

110. Hamilton G. Multicellular spheroids as an in vitro tumor model. Cancer Lett 1998;131:29–34.

111. Hanahan D, Weinberg RA. The hallmarks of cancer. Cell 2000;100:57–70.

112. Hanna EA, Umhauer S, Roshong SL, et al. Gap junctional intercellular communication and connexin43 expression in human ovarian surface epithelial cells and ovarian carcinomas *in vivo* and *in vitro*. Carcinogenesis 1999;20:1369–1373.

113. Hashizume H, Baluk P, Morikawa S, et al. Openings between defective endothelial cells explain tumor vessel leakiness. Am J Pathol 2000;156:1363–1380.

114. Heim S, Mandahl N, Mitelman F. Genetic convergence and divergence in tumor progression. Cancer Res 1988;48:5911–5916.

115. Henderson DW, Papadimitriou JM, Coleman M. Ultrastructural appearances of tumours, 2nd ed. Edinburgh: Churchill Livingstone, 1986.

116. Heppner GH. Tumor heterogeneity. Cancer Res 1984;44:2259–2265.

117. Herlyn M, Clark WH, Rodeck U, Mancianti ML, Jambrosic J, Koprowski H. Biology of tumor progression in human melanocytes. Lab Invest 1987;56:461–474.

118. Hill RP. Metastasis. In: Tannock IF, Hill RP, eds. The basic science of oncology. New York: Pergamon Press, 1987, pp. 160–175.

119. Hori K, Suzuki M, Abe I, Saito S. Increased tumor tissue pressure in association with the growth of rat tumors. Jpn J Cancer Res (Gann) 1986;77:65–73.

120. Hortobagyi GN, Singletary SE, Strom EA. Treatment of locally advanced and inflammatory breast cancer. In: Harris JR, Lippman ME, Morrow M, Osborne CK (eds). Diseases of the breast. 2nd ed. Philadelphia: Lippincott Williams & Wilkins, 2000, pp. 645–660.

121. Iannaccone PM, Gardner RL, Harris H. The cellular origin of chemically induced tumours. J Cell Sci 1978;29:249–269.

122. Iozzo RV. Tumor stroma as a regulator of neoplastic behavior. Lab Invest 1995;73:157–160.

123. Iversen OH. Kinetics of cellular proliferation and cell loss in human carcinomas. A discussion of methods available for *in vivo* studies. Eur J Cancer 1967;3:389–394.

124. Jain RK. Determinants of tumor blood flow: a review. Cancer Res 1988;48:2641–2658.

125. Jain RK. Delivery of novel therapeutic agents in tumors: physiological barriers and strategies. J Natl Cancer Inst 1989;81: 570–576.

126. Jain RK. Vascular and interstitial barriers to delivery of therapeutic agents in tumors. Cancer Metastasis Rev 1990;9: 253–266.

127. Jain RK. Barriers to drug delivery in solid tumors. Scient Am 1994;271:58–65.

128. Jain RK. Delivery of molecules, particles and cells to solid tumors (Whitaker Lecture). Annal of Biomed Eng 1996;24: 457–473.

129. Jain RK, Baxter LT. Mechanisms of heterogeneous distribution of monoclonal antibodies and other macromolecules in tumors: significance of elevated interstitial pressure. Cancer Res 1988;48:7022–7032.

130. Jiang X-R, Jimenez G, Chang E, et al. Telomerase expression in human somatic cells does not induce changes associated with transformed phenotype. Nat Genet 1999;21:111–114.

131. Joseph-Silverstein J, Rifkin DB. Endothelial cell growth factors and the vessel wall. Semin Thromb Hemost 1987;13: 504–513.

132. Kaban LB, Mulliken JB, Ezekowitz RA, et al. Antiangiogenic therapy of a recurrent giant cell tumor of the mandible with interferon alpha-2a. Pediatrics 1999;103:1145–1149.

133. Kao RT, Hall J, Engel L, Stern R. The matrix of human breast tumor cells is mitogenic for fibroblasts. Am J Pathol 1984; 115:109–116.

134. Karkkainen M, Mäkinen T, Alitalo K. Lymphatic endothelium: a new frontier of metastasis research. Nat Cell Biol 2002;4:E2–E5.

135. Katayama I, Nagy GK, Balogh K Jr. Light microscopic identification of the ribosome-lamella complex in "hairy cells" of leukemic reticuloendotheliosis. Cancer 1973;32:843–846.

136. Kerbel RS. Tumor angiogenesis: past, present and the near future. Carcinogenesis 2000;21:505–515.

137. Kerbel R, Folkman J. Clinical translation of angiogenesis inhibitors. Nat Rev Cancer 2002;2:727–739.

138. Keski-Oja J, Postlethwaite AE, Moses HL. Transforming growth factors in the regulation of malignant cell growth and invasion. Cancer Invest 1988;6:705–724.

139. Klaunig JE, Ruch RJ. Role of inhibition of intercellular communication in carcinogenesis. Lab Invest 1990;62:135–146.

140. Klein G, Klein E. Conversion of solid neoplasms into ascites tumors. Ann NY Acad Sci 1955;63:640–661.

141. Klein-Szanto AJP. Morphological evaluation of tumor promoter effects on mammalian skin. In: Slaga TJ, ed. Mechanisms of tumor promotion, vol II. Boca Raton, FL: CRC Press, 1984, pp. 41–72.

142. Kleinsmith LJ, Pierce GB Jr. Multipotentiality of single embryonal carcinoma cells. Cancer Res 1964;24:1544–1551.

143. Kohn S, Nagy JA, Dvorak HF, Dvorak AM. Pathways of macromolecular tracer transport across venules and small veins. Lab Invest 1992;67:596–607.

144. Kondo S. Carcinogenesis in relation to the stem-cell-mutation hypothesis. Differentiation 1983;24:1–8.

145. Kramar C, Baud C-A, Lagier R. Presumed calcified leiomyoma of the uterus. Morphologic and chemical studies of a calcified mass dating from the neolithic period. Arch Pathol Lab Med 1983;107:91–93.

146. Krishnan R, Cleary EG. Elastin gene expression in elastotic human breast cancers and epithelial cell lines. Cancer Res 1990;50:2164–2171.

147. Krutovskikh VA, Mesnil M, Mazzoleni G, Yamasaki H. Inhibition of rat liver gap junction intercellular communication by tumor-promoting agents in vivo. Lab Invest 1995;72:571–577.

148. Laird AK. Dynamics of tumor growth. Br J Cancer 1964; 18:490–502.

149. Laird AK. Dynamics of tumour growth: comparison of growth rates and extrapolation of growth curve to one cell. Br J Cancer 1965;19:278–291.

150. Lee EY, Wang TC, Clouse RE, DeSchryver-Kecskemeti K. Mucosal thickening adjacent to gastric malignancy: association with epidermal growth factor. Mod Pathol 1989;2:397–402.

151. Leof EB, Proper JA, Getz MJ, Moses HL. Transforming growth factor type β regulation of actin mRNA. J Cell Physiol 1986;127:83–88.

151a. Liekens S, De Clercq E, Neyts J. Angiogenesis: regulators and clinical applications. Biochem Pharmacol 2001;61:253–270.

152. Lingle WL, Salisbury JL. Altered centrosome structure is associated with abnormal mitoses in human breast tumors. Am J Pathol 1999;155:1941–1951.

153. Liotta LA, Kohn EC. The microenvironment of the tumor-host interface. Nature 2001;411:375–379.

154. Lipsett MB. Interaction of drugs, hormones, and nutrition in the causes of cancer. Cancer 1979;43:1967–1981.

155. Little JB, McGandy RB, Kennedy AR. Interactions between polonium-210 α-radiation, benzo(a)pyrene, and 0.9% NaCl solution instillations in the induction of experimental lung cancer. Cancer Res 1978;38:1929–1935.

156. Loewenstein WR, Azarnia R. Regulation of intercellular communication and growth by the cellular src gene. Ann NY Acad Sci 1988;551:337–346.

157. MacKenzie I, Rous P. The experimental disclosure of latent neoplastic changes in tarred skin. J Exp Med 1941;73:391–416.

158. Mahon KA, Chepelinsky AB, Khillan JS, et al. Oncogenesis of the lens in transgenic mice. Science 1987;235:1622–1628.

159. Mahoney MJ, Leighton J. The inflammatory response to a foreign body within transplantable tumors. Cancer Res 1962; 22:334–338.

160. Malumbres M, Barbacid M. To cycle or not to cycle: a critical decision in cancer. Nat Rev Cancer 2002;1:222–231.

161. Mantovani A. Tumor-associated macrophages in neoplastic progression: a paradigm for the in vivo function of chemokines. Lab Invest 1994;71:5–16.

162. Martinez-Hernandez A. The extracellular matrix and neoplasia. Lab Invest 1988;58:609–612.

163. Marx J. Do centrosome abnormalities lead to cancer? Science 2001;292:426–429.

164. Matsumura T, Dohi K, Takanashi A, Ito H, Tahara E. Alteration and enhanced expression of the c-myc oncogene in human colorectal carcinomas. Pathol Res Pract 1990;186: 205–211.

165. McCredie JA, Inch WR, Kruuv J, Watson TA. The rate of tumor growth in animals. Growth 1965;29:331–347.

166. McNutt NS. Ultrastructural comparison of the interface between epithelium and stroma in basal cell carcinoma and control human skin. Lab Invest 1976;35:132–142.

167. Mehta PP, Bertram JS, Loewenstein WR. Growth inhibition of transformed cells correlates with their junctional communication with normal cells. Cell 1986;44:187–196.

168. Meyerson M, Counter CM, Eaton EN, et al. hEST2, the putative human telomerase subunit gene, is upregulated in tumor cells and during immortalization. Cell 1997;90:785–795.

169. Mintz B. Allophenic mice of multi-embryo origin. In Daniel JC Jr, ed. Methods in mammalian embryology. San Francisco: WH Freeman, 1971, pp. 186–214.

170. Mintz B, Illmensee K. Normal genetically mosaic mice produced from malignant teratocarcinoma cells. Proc Natl Acad Sci USA 1975;72:3585–3589.

171. Moore JV. Death of cells and necrosis of tumours. In: Potten CS, ed. Perspectives on mammalian cell death. Oxford: Oxford University Press, 1987, pp. 295–325.

172. Moore JW III, Sholley MM. Comparison of the neovascular effects of stimulated macrophages and neutrophils in autologous rabbit corneas. Am J Pathol 1985;120:87–98.

173. Morré DJ. Membrane alterations in neoplasia. In: Sirica AE, ed. The pathobiology of neoplasia. New York: Plenum Press, 1989, pp. 323–344.

174. Moses MA, Sudhalter J, Langer R. Identification of an inhibitor of neovascularization from cartilage. Science 1990;248:1408–1410.

175. Mottram JC. A developing factor in experimental blastogenesis. J Pathol Bacteriol 1944;56:181–187.

176. Mueller-Klieser W. Three-dimensional cell cultures: from molecular mechanisms to clinical applications. Am J Physiol 1997;273 (Cell Physiol 42):C1109–C1123.

177. Müller J. On the nature and structural characteristics of cancer, and of those morbid growths which may be confounded with it. London: Sherwood, Gilbert and Piper, 1840.

178. Nakamura T, Mahon KA, Miskin R, et al. Differentiation and oncogenesis: phenotypically distinct lens tumors in transgenic mice. New Biol 1989;1:193–204.

179. Nicolson GL. Trans-membrane control of the receptors on normal and tumor cells. II. Surface changes associated with transformation and malignancy. Biochim Biophys Acta 1976;458:1–72.

180. Nigg EA. Centrosome aberrations: cause or consequence of cancer progression? Nat Rev Cancer 2002;2:1–11.

181. Nowell PC. The clonal evolution of tumor cell populations. Science 1976;194:23–28.

182. Nowell PC. Cytogenetics of tumor progression. Cancer 1990;65:2172–2177.

183. Olumi AF, Grossfeld GD, Hayward SW, et al. Carcinoma-associated fibroblasts direct tumor progression of initiated human prostatic epithelium. Cancer Res 1999;59:5002–5011.

184. Pauli BU, Weinstein RS. Cell junctional alterations in cancer. In: Liotta LA, ed. Influence of tumor development on the host. Dordrecht: Kluwer Academic Publishers, 1989, pp. 121–132.

185. Pedersen PL. Tumor mitochondria and the bioenergetics of cancer cells. Prog Exp Tumor Res 1978;22:190–274.

186. Peterson H-I. Vascular and extravascular spaces in tumors: tumor vascular permeability. In: Peterson H-I, ed. Tumor blood circulation: angiogenesis, vascular morphology and blood flow of experimental and human tumors. Boca Raton, FL: CRC Press, 1979, pp. 77–85.

187. Peterson H-I. The microcirculation of tumors. In: Orr FW, Buchanan MR, Weiss L, eds. Microcirculation in cancer metastasis. Boca Raton, FL: CRC Press, 1991, pp. 277–298.

188. Pich A, Chiusa L, Margaria E. Prognostic relevance of AgNORs in tumor pathology. Micron 2000;31:133–141.

189. Pitot HC. The natural history of neoplastic development: the relation of experimental models to human cancer. Cancer 1982;49:1206–1211.

190. Pitot HC. Fundamentals of oncology, 4th ed. New York: Marcel Dekker, Inc., 2002.

191. Pitot HC. Stages in neoplastic development. In: Schottenfeld D, Fraumeni JF Jr (eds). Cancer epidemiology and prevention, 2nd ed. New York: Oxford University Press, 1996, pp. 65–79.

192. Pitot HC, Goldsworthy T, Moran S, Sirica AE, Weeks J. Properties of incomplete carcinogens and promoters in hepatocarcinogenesis. Carcinogenesis 1982;7:85–98.

193. Pitot HC, Sirica AE. The stages of initiation and promotion in hepatocarcinogenesis. Biochim Biophys Acta 1980;605:191–215.

194. Piulats J, Mitjans F. Angiogenesis switch pathways. In: Bronchud MH, Foote MA, Peters WP, Robinson MO (eds). Principles of molecular oncology. Totowa, NJ: Humana Press, 2000.

195. Plate K. From angiogenesis to lymphangiogenesis. Nat Med 2001;7:151–152.

196. Rather LJ. The genesis of cancer: a study in the history of ideas. Baltimore: The Johns Hopkins University Press, 1978.

197. Rather LJ, Rather P, Frerichs JB. Johannes Müller and the nineteenth-century origins of tumor cell theory. Science History Publications, 1986.

198. Reed JC. Dysregulation of apoptosis in cancer. J Clin Oncol 1999;17:2941–2959.

199. Ross PM. Apparent absence of a benign precursor lesion: implications for the pathogenesis of malignant melanoma. J Am Acad Dermatol 1989;21:529–538.

200. Rous P, Beard JW. The progression to carcinoma of virus-induced rabbit papillomas (Shope). J Exp Med 1935;62:523–548.

201. Rous P, Kidd JG. Conditional neoplasms and subthreshold neoplastic states. A study of the tar tumors of rabbits. J Exp Med 1941;73:365–390.

202. Ruddon RW. Cancer biology, 2nd ed. New York: Oxford University Press, 1987.

202a. Ruoslahti E. Specialization of tumour vasculature. Nat Rev Cancer 2002;2:83–90.

203. Russell DS, Rubinstein LJ. Pathology of tumours of the nervous system, 5th ed. Baltimore: Williams & Wilkins, 1989.

204. Ryser HJ-P. Chemical carcinogenesis. N Engl J Med 1971;285:721–734.

205. Sachs L. Constitutive uncoupling of pathways of gene expression that control growth and differentiation in myeloid leukemia: a model for the origin and progression of malignancy. Proc Natl Acad Sci USA 1980;77:6152–6156.

206. Sager R, Gadi IK, Stephens L, Grabowy CT. Gene amplification: an example of accelerated evolution in tumorigenic cells. Proc Natl Acad Sci USA 1985;82:7015–7019.

207. Schnipper LE. Clinical implications of tumor-cell heterogeneity. N Engl J Med 1986;314:1423–1431.

208. Schoppmann SF, Birner P, Stöcki J, et al. Tumor-associated macrophages express lymphatic endothelial growth factors and are related to peritumoral lymphangiogenesis. Am J Pathol 2002;161:947–956.

209. Schor SL. Fibroblast subpopulations as accelerators of tumor progression: The role of migration stimulating factor. In: Goldberg ID, Rosen EM (eds). Epithelial-mesenchymal interactions in cancer. Basel: Birkhäuser Verlag, 1995, pp. 273–296.

210. Scribner JD, Süss R. Tumor initiation and promotion. Int Rev Exp Pathol 1978;18:137–198.

211. Seemayer TA, Lagacé R, Schürch W, Tremblay G. Myofibroblasts in the stroma of invasive and metastatic carcinoma. A possible host response to neoplasia. Am J Surg Pathol 1979;3:525–533.

212. Sevick EM, Jain RK. Effect of red blood cell rigidity on tumor blood flow: increase in viscous resistance during hyperglycemia. Cancer Res 1991;51:2727–2730.

213. Shousha S, Bull TB, Burn I. Alveolar variant of invasive lobular carcinoma of the breast: an electron microscopic study. Ultrastruct Pathol 1986;10:311–319.

214. Skipper HE, Perry S. Kinetics of normal and leukemic leukocyte populations and relevance to chemotherapy. Cancer Res 1970;30:1883–1897.

215. Skipper HE, Schabel FM Jr, Wilcox WS. Experimental evaluation of potential anticancer agents. XIV. Further study of certain basic concepts underlying chemotherapy of leukemia. Cancer Chemother Rep 1965;45:5–28.

216. Slaga TJ, Fischer SM, Weeks CE, et al. Specificity and mechanism(s) of promoter inhibitors in multistage promotion. Carcinog Compr Surv 1982;7:19–34.

217. Stacker SA, Achen MG, Jussila L, Baldwin ME, Alitalo K. Lymphangiogenesis and cancer metastasis. Nat Rev Cancer 2002;2:573–583.

218. Steel GG. Cell loss as a factor in the growth rate of human tumours. Eur J Cancer 1967;3:381–387.

219. Steel GG. Growth kinetics of tumours. Oxford: Clarendon Press, 1977.

220. Sternlicht MD, Werb Z. How matrix metalloproteinases regulate cell behavior. Annu Rev Cell Dev Biol 2001;17:463–516.

221. Stockdale FE. Cancer growth and chemotherapy. In: Rubenstein E, Federman DD, eds. Scientific American Medicine. Oncology. New York: Scientific American, 1987, pp. 1–13.

222. Stoker M, O'Neill C, Berryman S, Waxman V. Anchorage and growth regulation in normal and virus-transformed cells. Int J Cancer 1968;3:683–693.

223. Strum JM. Angiogenic responses elicited from chorioallantoic membrane vessels by neoplastic, preneoplastic, and normal mammary tissues from GR mice. Am J Pathol 1983;111:282–287.

224. Sutherland RM, McCredie JA, Inch WR. Growth of multicell spheroids in tissue culture as a model of nodular carcinomas. J Natl Cancer Inst 1971;46:113–120.

225. Talmadge JE, Key M, Fidler IJ. Macrophage content of metastatic and nonmetastatic rodent neoplasms. J Immunol 1981;126:2245–2248.

226. Tanaka K, Kohga S, Kinjo M, Kodama Y. Tumor metastasis and thrombosis, with special reference to thromboplastic and fibrinolytic activities of tumor cells. GANN Monogr Cancer Res 1977;20:97–119.

227. Tannock IF. The relation between cell proliferation and the vascular system in a transplanted mouse mammary tumour. Br J Cancer 1968;22:258–273.

228. Tannock IF. Population kinetics of carcinoma cells, capillary endothelial cells, and fibroblasts in a transplanted mouse mammary tumor. Cancer Res 1970;30:2470–2476.

229. Tannock IF. Oxygen distribution in tumours: influence on cell proliferation and implications for tumour therapy. Adv Exp Med Biol 1976;75:597–603.

230. Tannock IF. Biology of tumor growth. Hosp Pract 1983;18:81–93.

231. Tannock IF. Tumor growth and cell kinetics. In: Tannock IF, Hill RP, eds. The basic science of oncology. New York: Pergamon Press, 1987, pp. 140–159.

232. Temme A, Buchmann A, Gabriel H-D, et al. High incidence of spontaneous and chemically induced liver tumors in mice deficient for connexin32. Curr Biol 1977;7:713–716.

233. Tennant R. What is a tumor promoter? Environ Health Perspect 1999;107:A390–A391.

234. Thomlinson RH, Gray LH. The histological structure of some human lung cancers and the possible implications for radiotherapy. Br J Cancer 1955;9:539–549.

235. Tremblay G. Elastosis in tubular carcinoma of the breast. Arch Pathol 1974;98:302–307.

236. Tremblay G, Babai F. Intercellular junctions between Novikoff hepatoma cells and hepatic cells. Exp Cell Res 1972;74:355–358.

237. Trosko JE. Commentary: is the concept of "tumor promotion" a useful paradigm? Mol Carcinogen 2001;30:131–137.

238. Trosko JE, Yotti LP, Warren ST, Tsushimoto G, Chang C-C. Inhibition of cell-cell communication by tumor promoters. Carcinogenesis 1982;7:565–585.

239. Vasiliev JM, Gelfand IM. Morphogenetic reactions and locomotor behaviour of transformed cells in culture. In: Weiss L, ed. Fundamental aspects of metastasis. Amsterdam-Oxford: North Holland Publishing Company, 1976, pp. 71–98.

240. Vaupel P, Kallinowski F, Kluge M. Pathophysiology of tumors in hyperthermia. Recent Results Cancer Res 1988;107:65–75.

241. Vaupel P, Müller-Klieser W. Interstitieller Raum und Mikromilieu in malignen Tumoren. Mikrozirk Forsch Klin 1983;2:78–90.

242. Volpe JPG. Genetic instability of cancer: why a metastatic tumor is unstable and a benign tumor is stable. Cancer Genet Cytogenet 1988;34:125–134.

243. Warburg O. The metabolism of tumours. London: Constable & Co. Ltd., 1930.

244. Warburg O. On the origin of cancer cells. Science 1956;123:309–314.

245. Warren BA, Shubik P. The growth of the blood supply to melanoma transplants in the hamster cheek pouch. Lab Invest 1966;15:464–478.

246. Weinberg RA. Racing to the beginning of the road. New York: W.H. Freeman & Co., 1996.

247. Weinberg RA. One renegade cell. New York: Basic Books, 1998.

248. Weinhouse S. Changing perceptions of carbohydrate metabolism in tumors. In: Arnott MS, van Eys J, Wang Y-M, eds. Molecular interrelations of nutrition and cancer. New York: Raven Press, 1982, pp. 167–181.

249. Weinstein RS, Merk FB, Alroy J. The structure and function of intercellular junctions in cancer. Adv Cancer Res 1976; 23:23–89.

250. Weiss L. Principles of metastasis. New York: Academic Press, 1985.

251. Welsch F. Teratogens and cell-to-cell communication. In: De Mello WC, ed. Cell intercommunication. Boca Raton, FL: CRC Press, 1990, pp. 133–160.

252. Woodruff MFA. Tumor clonality and its biological significance. Adv Cancer Res 1988;50:197–229.

253. Yamaura H, Sato H. Quantitative studies on the developing vascular system of rat hepatoma. J Natl Cancer Inst 1974; 53:1229–1240.

254. Yuspa SH, Shields PG. Etiology of cancer: chemical factors. In DeVita VT Jr., Hellman S, Rosenberg SA (eds). Cancer: Principles & practice of oncology. Philadelphia: Lippincott Williams & Wilkins, 2001, pp. 179–193.

255. Zetter BR. Migration of capillary endothelial cells is stimulated by tumour-derived factors. Nature 1980;285:41–43.

256. Zetter BR. Angiogenesis. State of the art. Chest 1988;93 (suppl):159S–166S.

257. Ziegler E. General pathology. New York: William Wood and Company, 1908.

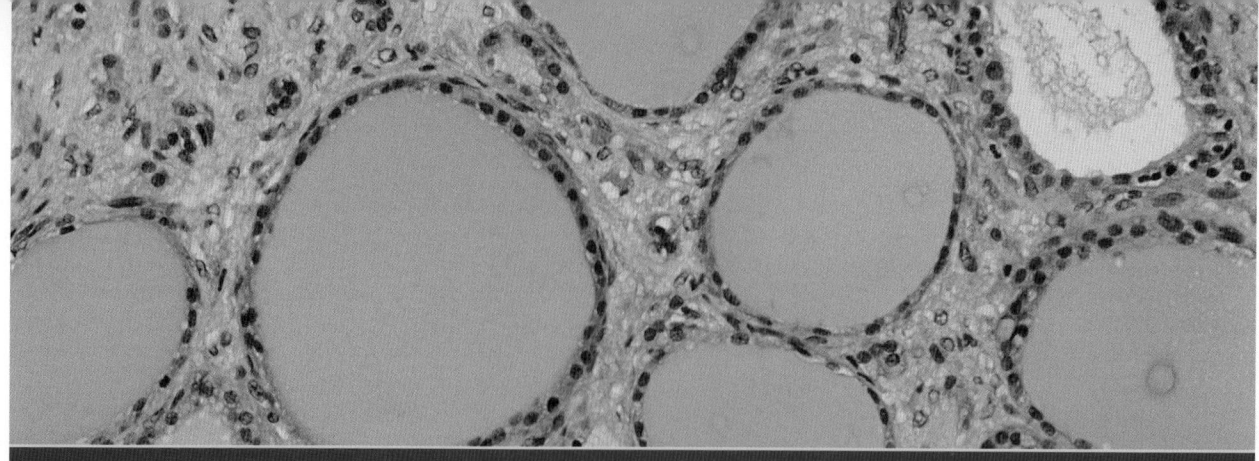

S ooner or later, malignant tumors trespass into the vital space of other tissues. They do so by several mechanisms: they infiltrate their surroundings; they seed into any open space; they find their way into the blood or lymph and set up distant colonies. All this recalls the behavior of a parasite, except that tumors arise within their host, and die with it.

The Biology of Tumor Aggression

We will begin with local infiltration: If it is true that the name *cancer* refers to claws reaching out to grasp surrounding tissues, the ability of cancer to invade was observed some 2500 years ago.

Local Invasion

In fairness to the tumor cell, the strategies of invading and even of metastasizing are part of normal life. We were all born thanks to the ability of the trophoblast to invade the uterine wall, a process still incompletely understood. As regards metastases, trophoblastic cells normally embolize the lung (see Figure 23.16). Even the life-saving inflammatory process resorts to "infiltration"; the leukocytes are true invaders, and tumor cells, as we will see, use some of their techniques.

Invasion by malignant tumors can be seen with the naked eye. For example, scirrhous carcinomas of the breast seen in cross section are star-shaped, or perhaps we should say crab-shaped, with claws reaching out to the skin and to the muscle, so that the tumor is anchored (Figure 27.1). The resulting lack of mobility of the mass over the deeper planes is an ominous clinical sign. Histologically the infiltration corresponds to cords of tumor cells embedded in strands of fibrous connective tissue containing fibroblasts and myofibroblasts (Figure 27.2); these fibrous structures tend to retract, hence the retraction of the nipple, another sign of poor prognosis (Figure 27.3).

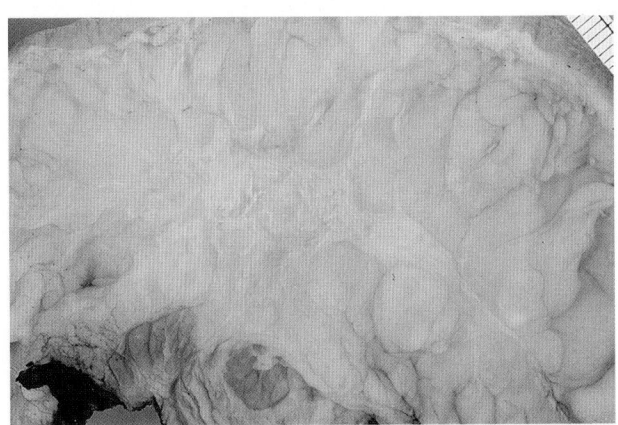

FIGURE 27.1   Cut surface of a carcinoma of the breast, before fixation in formalin. The pale pink tumor mass and its extensions do not offer much contrast against the yellow background of fat tissue, but they are much firmer to the touch. Some of the branches extend toward the muscle (*lower left*) and toward the skin, not visible here. **Scale** in millimeters (Courtesy of T. M. Turner, University of Massachusetts Medical School, Worcester, MA.)

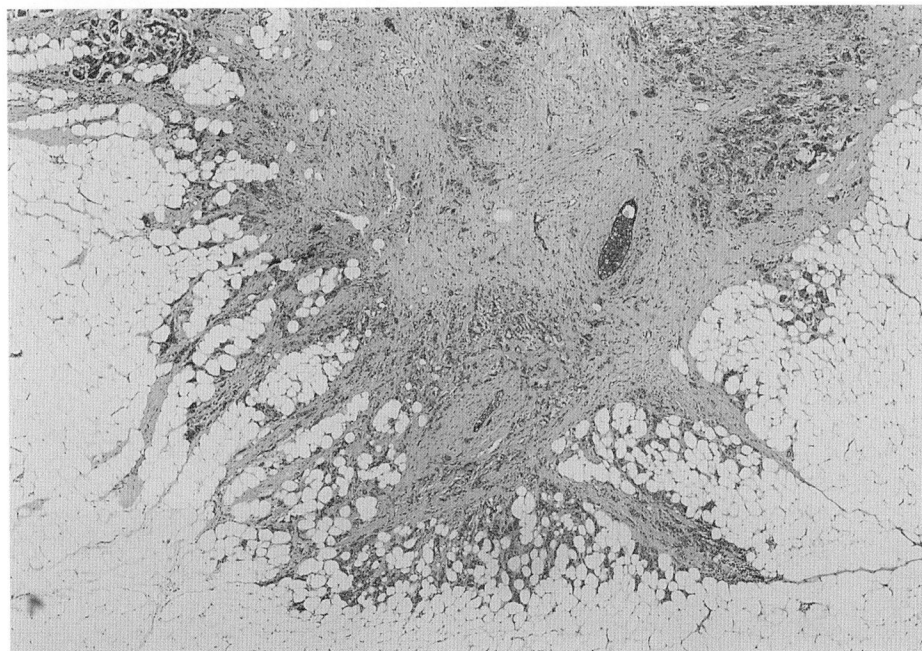

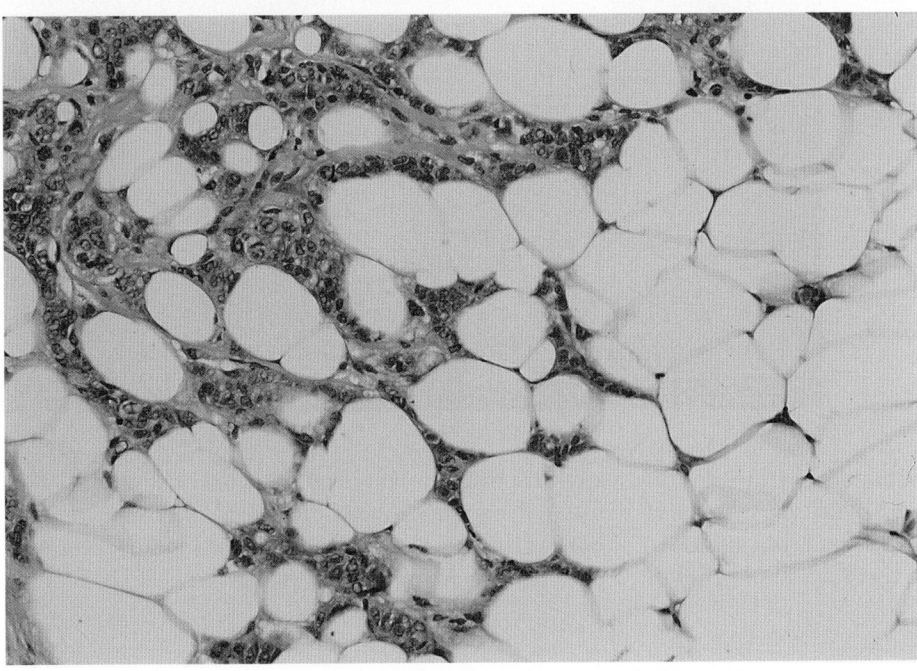

FIGURE 27.2   Typical pattern of invasion by a carcinoma of the breast. *Top:* The tumor advances by infiltrating the extracellular spaces in the adipose tissue. At a later stage, it induces an intense connective tissue response. (20x) *Bottom:* Detail showing carcinoma cells advancing between the fat cells. (180x)

FIGURE 27.3   Retraction of the nipple, caused by an underlying carcinoma of the breast. The retraction is probably due to myofibroblasts in the stroma of the tumor. The fine puckering of the skin (*peau d'orange*) visible below the nipple is indicative of lymphatic invasion. (Reproduced from [24] by permission of Oxford University Press.)

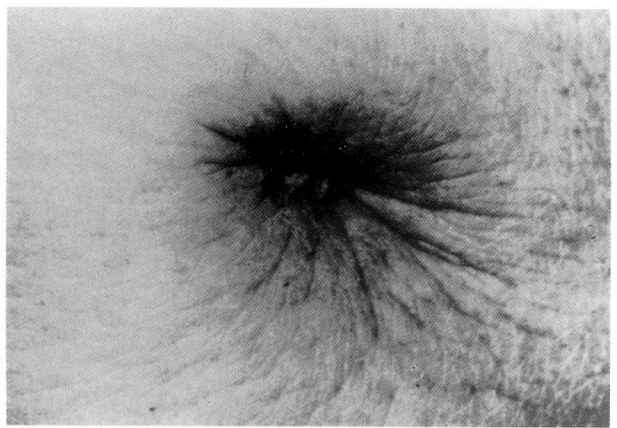

FIGURE 27.4   Invasion by a squamous cell carcinoma of the lip. *Top left:* Epithelium of the lip. Proceeding to the right, the epithelium plunges into the subjacent connective tissue spaces, which respond with a mild lymphocytic infiltrate. This tumor seems to lack any tendency to grow outward. (60x)

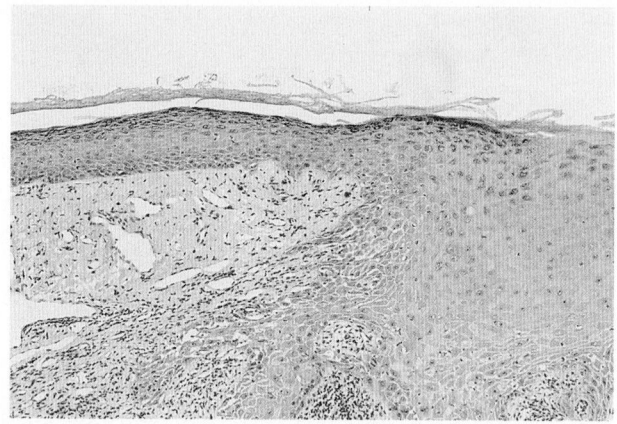

FIGURE 27.5   Cross section of a human heart. The left ventricle is almost filled with a white mass: a large subendocardial metastasis from a carcinoma of the kidney. Metastases to the heart are uncommon; amazingly, this one produced no symptoms and was diagnosed only at autopsy. (Courtesy of Dr. H. F. Cuénoud, University of Massachusetts Medical School, Worcester, MA.)

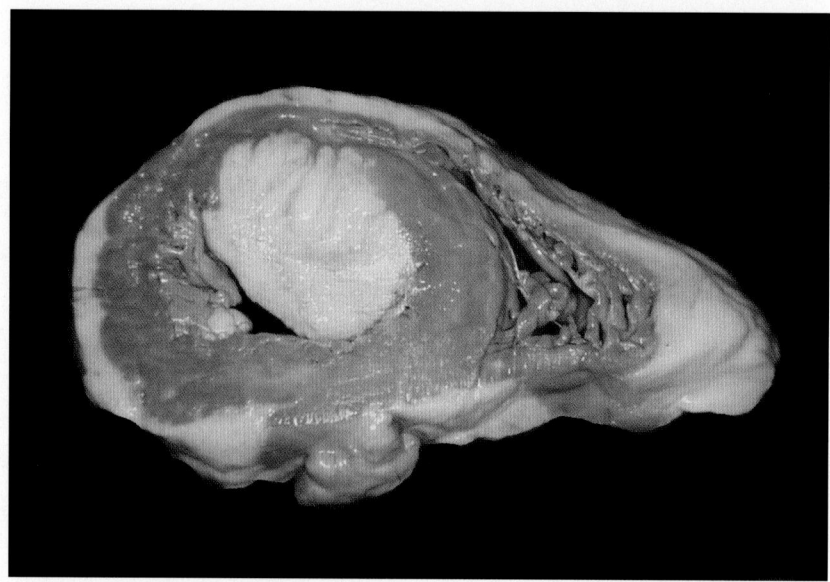

At the level of histology, the concept of invasion is best appreciated by examining the transition between a squamous epithelium and a squamous cell carcinoma (Figure 27.4). As the malignant tissue advances, almost any structure that happens to be in the way can be infiltrated and destroyed (Figure 27.5). Even compact bone can be eroded (see Figure 25.11), but for this purpose the advancing mass of malignant cells recruits the

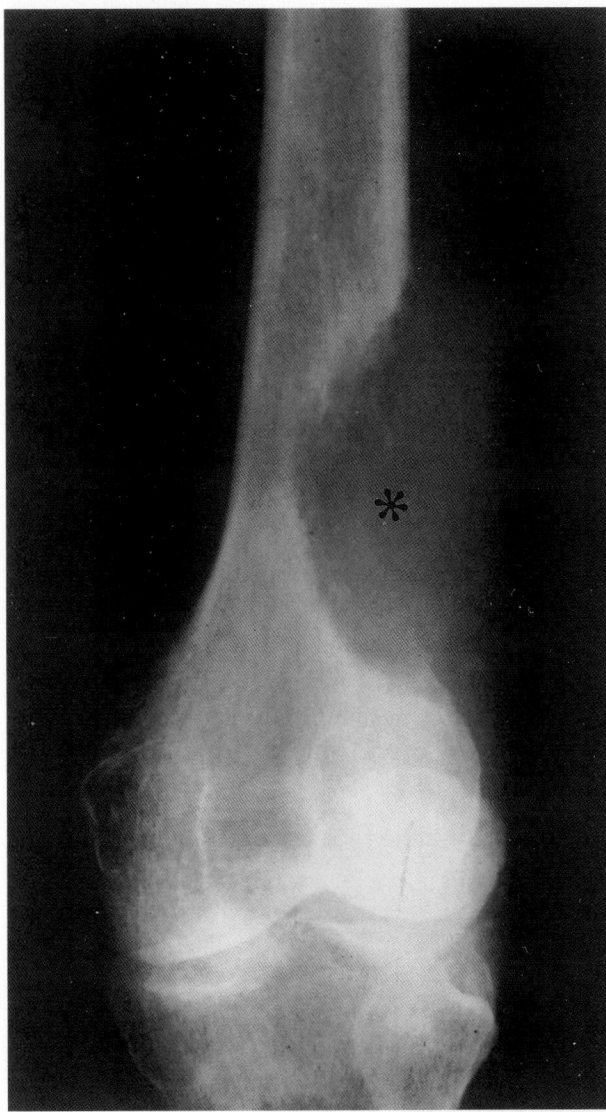

FIGURE 27.6 Metastasis of a carcinoma of the breast to the femur; this is an osteolytic metastasis (**asterisk**), a very aggressive one because the bone has had no time to react with condensation. (Courtesy of Dr. A. Davidoff, University of Massachusetts Medical School, Worcester, MA.)

help of cells that are programmed to excavate bone tissue: osteoclasts and macrophages (161). However, invaded cancellous bone may also respond to invasion with a burst of *osteogenesis,* thereby becoming more dense. Radiologists see these two opposite effects very clearly and refer to them as *osteolytic* and *osteoblastic* responses (Figures 27.6, 27.7).

> Tumor cells can also destroy bone directly, as was shown by incubating human breast cancer cells with fragments of bone that had been devitalized and therefore contained no osteoclasts (53). The dissolution of bone tissue releases growth factors that can stimulate tumor growth (114). Conversely, some tumors secrete osteoclast-stimulating factors (122). Two of these tumor-derived activators of osteoclasts are transforming growth factor-alpha (80) and prostaglandin E_2 (65). This prostaglandin connection has an amazing corollary: in rats, aspirin inhibits bone destruction by a tumor (159).

Tumor cells advancing in tissue spaces sometimes follow the paths of least resistance, such as the perineurial spaces (Figure 27.8); if they reach a serosal surface they may "fall into" the serosal space and produce the phenomenon of **seeding.** *Hyaline cartilage and arterial walls are rarely invaded;* an intact abdominal aorta may be surrounded by a ring of pancreatic

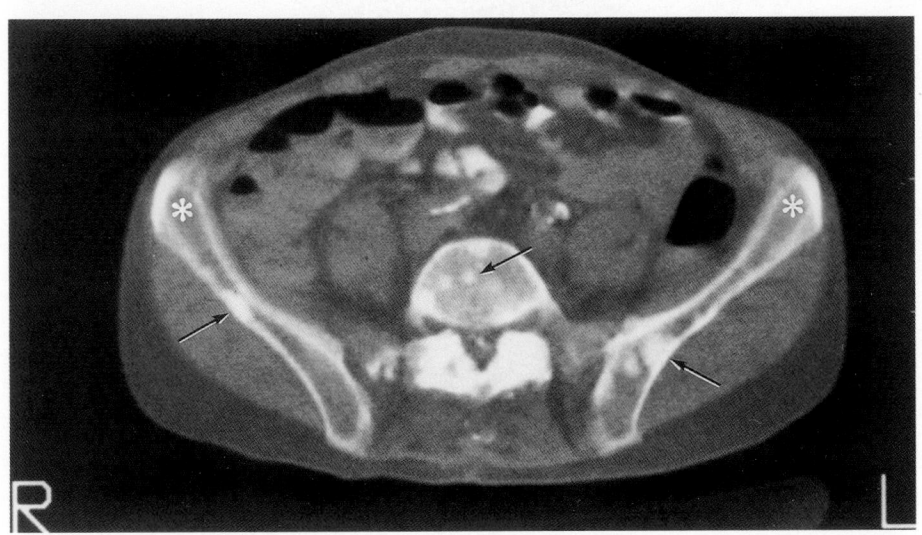

FIGURE 27.7 Osteoblastic metastases from a carcinoma of the prostate, seen in a CT scan of the pelvic region. The dense areas (**arrows**) represent new bone formation induced by the presence of the tumor. **Asterisks** Iliac bones. (Courtesy of Dr. A. Davidoff, University of Massachusetts Medical School, Worcester, MA.)

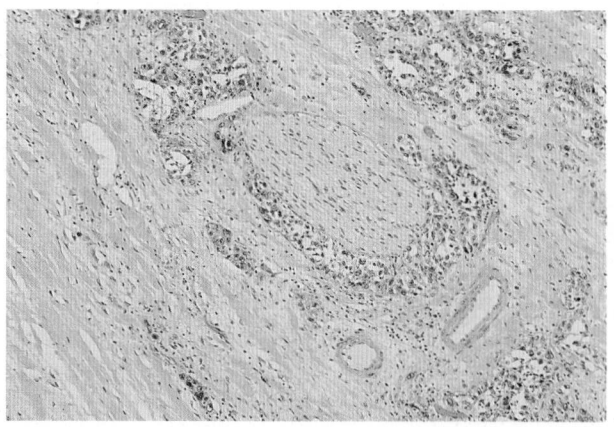

FIGURE 27.8   Carcinoma of the prostate invading a nerve (*center*). The mass of tumor cells around the nerve is actually filling the perineurial space, a path of least resistance. (60x)

carcinoma. It used to be said that both these tissues escape invasion because they are mechanically tough, but the mechanisms may be more subtle: It has been possible to extract from hyalin cartilage a low-molecular weight "anti-invasion factor" that inhibits angiogenesis (this may explain why normal cartilage contains no vessels), while also inhibiting proteolytic enzymes and tumor cell growth (152, 154). As for arteries, they contain a lot of elastin, and malignant tumors which clear the way with collagenase do not contain much elastase (116). In cancer of the colon, *bacterial products* may be a factor in tumor invasion: peptides produced by bacteria stimulated cancer cell mobility and invasiveness, tested on a collagen gel (141a).

Metastases

A *metastasis* is a secondary tumor that grows separately from the primary and has arisen from detached, transported cells (209). In essence, it is a colony of the primary tumor. The "seed" that starts a metastatic growth can be transported by the blood or lymph, or by fluid in tissue spaces. Metastases represent the most lethal expression of malignancy and the most important concern of the treating physician. By the time the diagnosis of cancer is made, over half of the patients already have microscopic metastases (58) and will die of them, because there is, overall, little hope for cure at that stage.

Metastases via the Bloodstream

Tumor cells have several options for gaining access to the bloodstream (Figure 27.9), but the most common portals of entry are probably the capillaries and venules, which have very thin walls (Figure 27.10) (97).

FIGURE 27.9   Four possible pathways for tumor cells to reach the bloodstream: (**1**) direct infiltration by the tumor, (**2**) invasion by individual tumor cells, (**3**) shedding into spaces lacking endothelial lining (doubtful), and (**4**) penetration into the lymphatics.

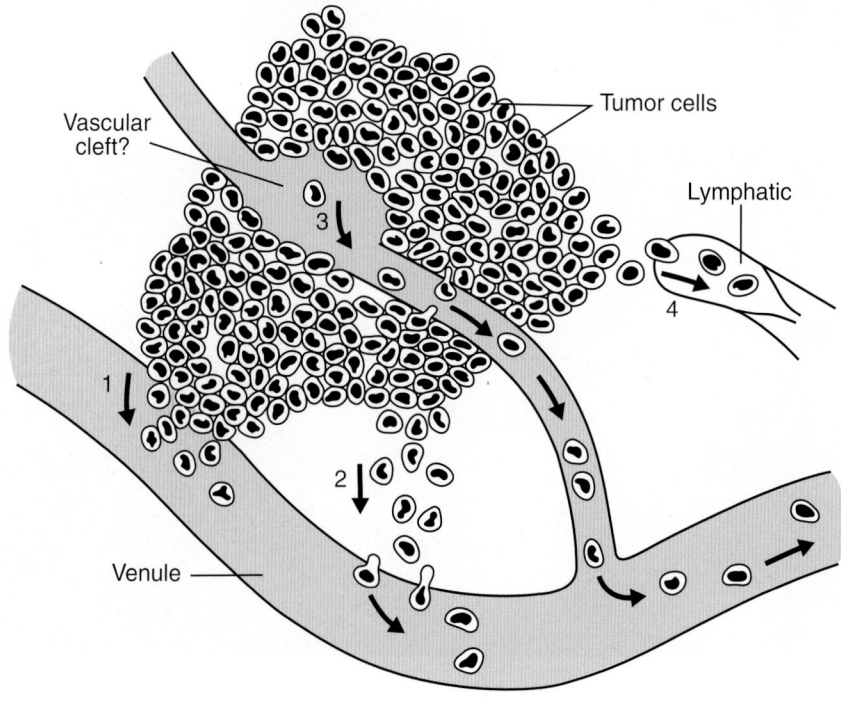

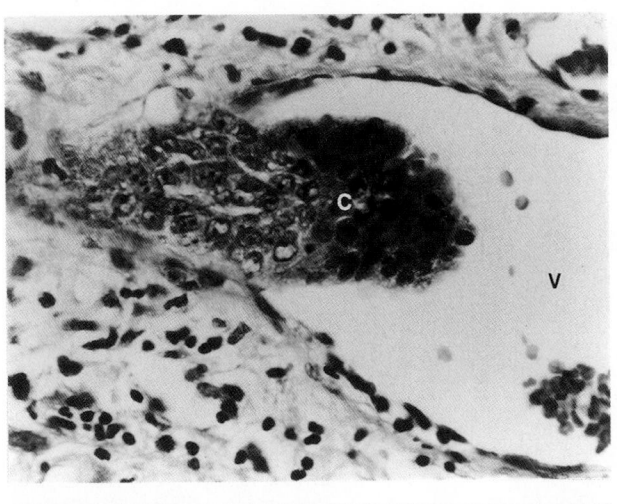

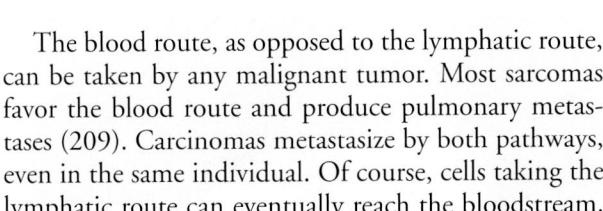

FIGURE 27.10   A mass of malignant cells from a transitional cell carcinoma of the bladder (**C**) invading the wall of a venule (**V**). (Reproduced by permission from [97], © by The US & Canadian Academy of Pathology, Inc.)

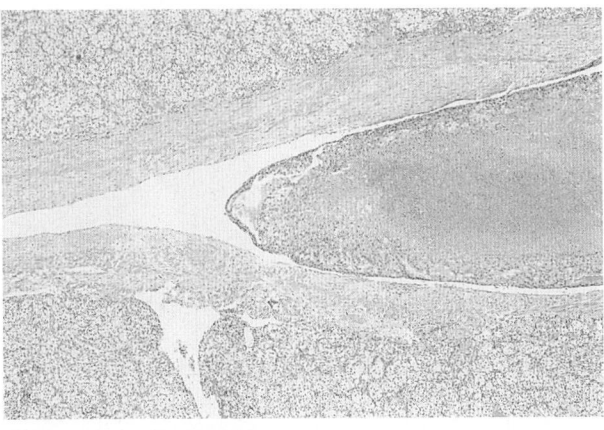

FIGURE 27.11   A threatening sight, typical of renal cell carcinomas. A renal vein, cut along its axis, contains a bullet-shaped mass of carcinomatous tissue advancing from right to left (the clear space is venous lumen). Such growths can reach as far as the heart. (25x)

The blood route, as opposed to the lymphatic route, can be taken by any malignant tumor. Most sarcomas favor the blood route and produce pulmonary metastases (209). Carcinomas metastasize by both pathways, even in the same individual. Of course, cells taking the lymphatic route can eventually reach the bloodstream.

Occasionally, a malignant tumor breaches into a large vein and grows within it as a continuous rootlike extension of the tumor; this behavior is typical of renal cell carcinomas, which tend to invade the renal vein and form a plug that can grow along the inferior vena cava and into the right heart (Figure 27.11).

There are no exceptions to the rule that metastases are malignant, even though some may look deceptively benign under the microscope (hence such improper names as "metastasizing adenoma" and "metastasizing leiomyoma"). However, it is true that some malignant tumors metastasize rarely (p. 812).

Normal cells introduced into the bloodstream may embolize and survive but they do not turn into tumors. Pancreatic islets, injected into the portal vein embolize the liver and—with some help—survive in experimental animals as well as humans (p. 672).

To the naked eye a single metastasis may look like a primary tumor, but when metastases are multiple, as often occurs in the liver or lung, the diagnosis is clear. In the liver they can be seen radiologically by computerized tomography (Figure 27.12). They may be so many as to defy counting. Even experienced pathologists shudder at the common sight of a liver so full of metastases that little normal tissue is left.

Perhaps because they tend to grow faster than primary tumors, metastases tend to be spherical (Figure 27.13): this is why on chest X-rays they are sometimes described as a "coin lesion" if single, or as "cannon balls" if multiple. Liver metastases of carcinomas usually become necrotic in their centers; therefore, as seen on the liver surface, they have a depressed central zone (Figure 27.14).

Metastases can generate more metastases (35, 79, 196, 197): this can be proven experimentally (Figure 27.15). It follows that *there can be a cascade of metastases of several orders;* for example, a metastasis to the kidney from a carcinoma of the rectum is probably a third-order metastasis (Figure 27.16) (43, 44).

Organ distribution of blood-borne metastases. This has been a long-standing puzzle. If blood-borne metastases were distributed geographically according to the plain laws of embolism, it should be possible to predict the target organs simply by considering the anatomy of the vascular system. However, this criterion works, in a general way, only for tumors of organs drained by the portal system: they do metastasize primarily to the liver (201, 202). Tumors arising in other parts of the body show organ preferences that cannot be explained on anatomical grounds alone. For example:

- Carcinomas of the breast usually metastasize to the skeleton.
- The kidneys act as filters and receive 20–25 percent of the cardiac output, yet they develop far fewer metastases than the much smaller adrenals.

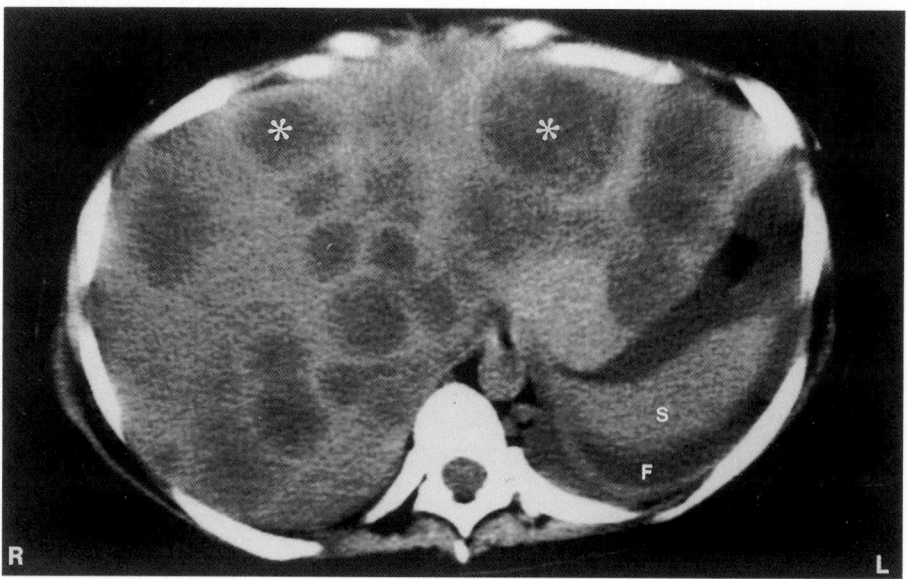

FIGURE 27.12 Liver metastases from a carcinoma of the pancreas seen in a CT scan. The metastases (**asterisks**) appear more translucent than the liver. Note the absence of metastases in the spleen (**S**) and the presence of fluid (**F**) in the peritoneum, indicating ascites. The latter could be due to portal obstruction as well as to peritoneal metastases. (Courtesy of Dr. A. Davidoff, University of Massachusetts Medical School, Worcester, MA.)

FIGURE 27.13 Cannonball type of metastases in the lung. These spherical, sharply circumscribed metastases are typical of sarcomas. The French term for this X-ray appearance is more poetic: *lâcher de ballons,* release of balloons. From a case of malignant schwannoma developing in a patient with neurofibromatosis. **Scale** in millimeters.

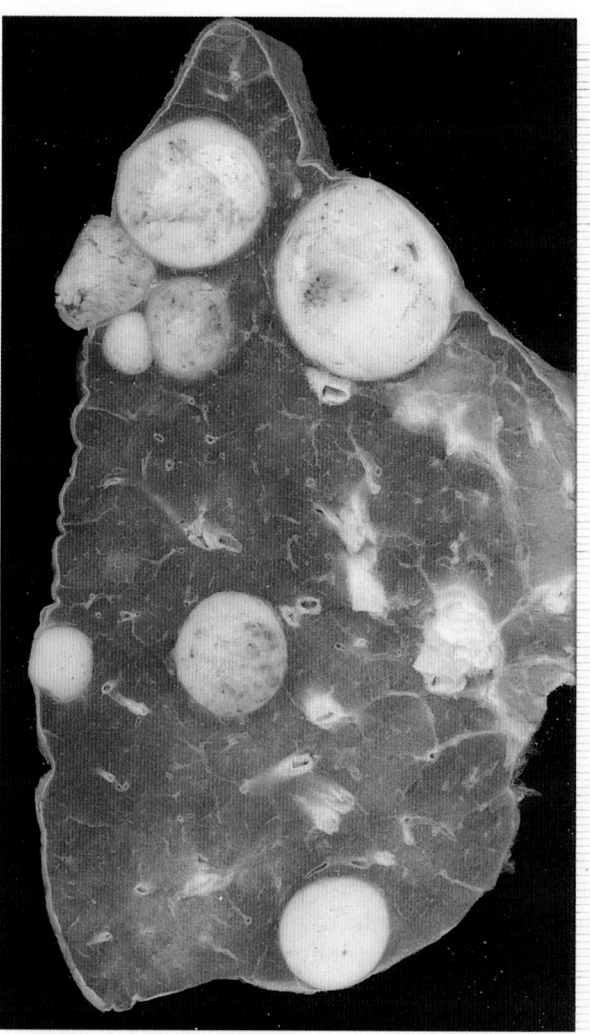

- The adrenals are favorite targets of bronchial carcinomas.
- The myocardium is rarely metastasized, and the same is true for striated muscles, although they represent some 40 percent of the body mass.
- Some carcinomas of the gastrointestinal tract favor the ovaries; bilateral metastatic tumors of the ovaries are a classic condition known as "Krukenberg tumor."
- The intestine receives 10 percent of the cardiac output, yet it receives few metastases, although melanomas of the skin sometimes produce a single metastasis to the small intestine.
- Hepatomas never metastasize to the skin, whereas sarcomas do.

The spleen is often cited as an organ that is relatively spared by metastases, but this is controversial (181). The spleen is certainly a favorite target of lymphomas and leukemias; and it is said that, at the microscopic level, metastases are much more frequent than observation with the naked eye would suggest (181). Our own impression is that grossly visible splenic metastases from carcinomas are rare; perhaps their growth is inhibited. The spleen is rich in NK cells, which can kill tumor cells.

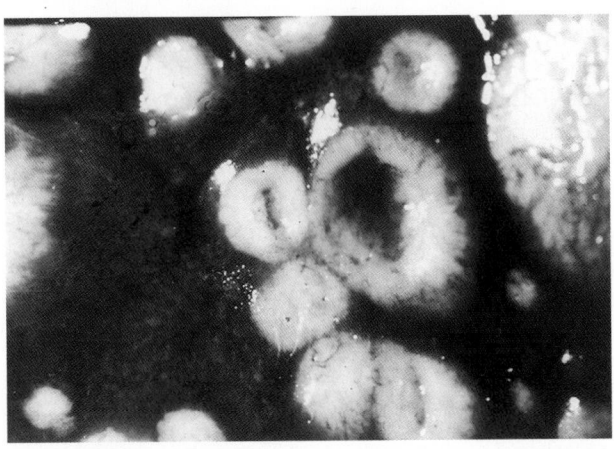

FIGURE 27.14 Surface of a liver riddled with metastases from a carcinoma. The center of several metastases is umbilicated (i.e., depressed) due to necrosis of the central portion. Natural size. (Courtesy of Dr. L. S. Gottlieb, The Mallory Institute of Pathology, Boston, MA.)

To explain the long list of metastases in unexpected organs, it was proposed a century ago that the selection in any given case was due to special properties of either the "seed" or the "soil" (145, 216). It is clear that in some cases the purely mechanical embolic mechanism is at work; in others the "seed" or the "soil" determine the result: adhesion molecules play a major role (p. 821). Not surprisingly, different rules apply to different tumors.

A subset of unexpected blood-borne metastases, especially in the vertebrae, can be explained by the existence of a system of veins in and around the spine known as the Batson venous system.

The Batson venous system. This system, also called the vertebral venous plexus (14, 15, 32, 43, 64), is a special

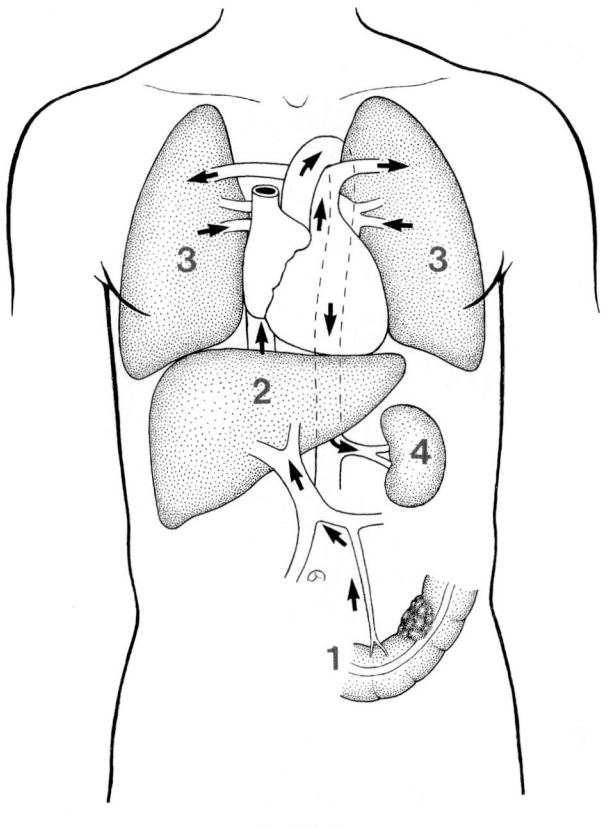

FIGURE 27.16 Sequence of metastases postulated for a carcinoma of the large intestine. The primary tumor (**1**) metastasizes to the liver (**2**) which then metastasizes to the lungs (**3**). Nodules in the lung then metastasize by the general circulation, for example to the kidney (**4**).

two-way thoroughfare of anastomosed veins—*without valves*—disposed around the vertebrae and running from the neck to the pelvis (Figure 27.17). After death the collapsed veins are hard to see, but in life they form a large reservoir. The relationship between this venous

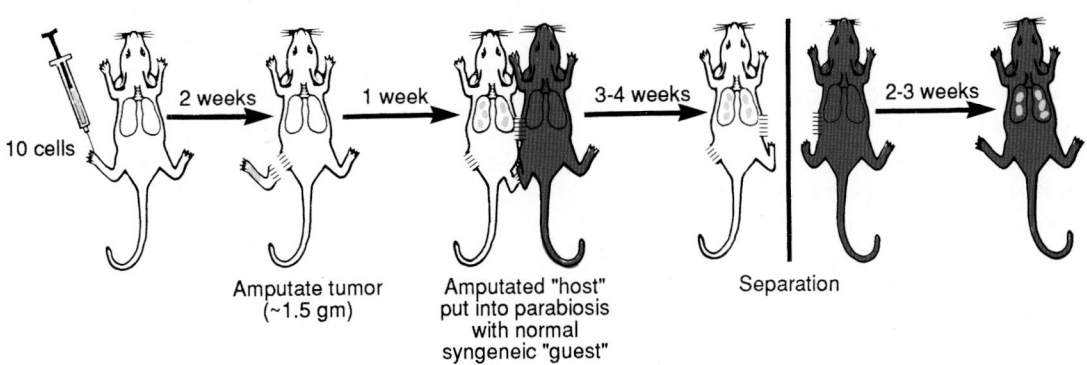

FIGURE 27.15 Experimental proof that metastases can give rise to further metastases. (Adapted from [79].)

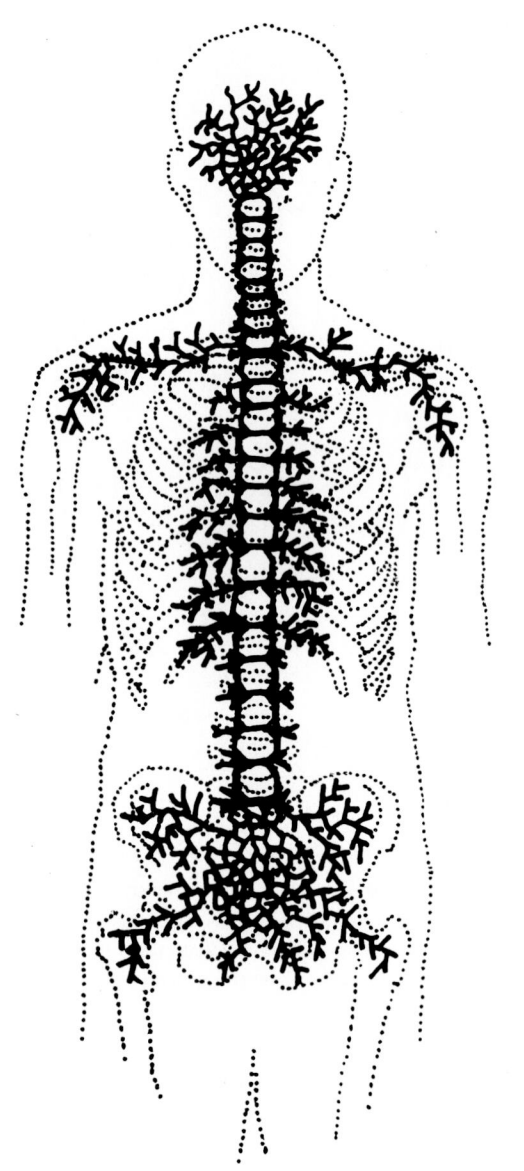

malignant cells injected into a femoral vein in rats and rabbits produced tumors almost exclusively in the lungs; but if the abdominal pressure was raised during the injection, tumors appeared mostly in the vertebrae (32).

What was happening? The *valveless veins* that run along the abdominal surface of the vertebrae are exposed to intraabdominal and intrathoracic pressure; they are connected to the caval system as well as to veins within the vertebrae, which drain toward the spinal cord. When the abdominal pressure is raised (such as by coughing, straining, or lifting a weight) blood is squeezed out of the caval system, through the anastomoses, into the deeper part of the Batson system. Malignant cells floating in this blood are pushed into the deep plexus and then float or drain up as far as the skull without passing through the heart or the lungs, where they might be mechanically destroyed.

The Batson system can explain many "aberrant" metastases such as a cranial metastasis from an adrenal tumor, and especially the high incidence of vertebral involvement in tumors of the thyroid, prostate, and breast.

> For example: tumor cells from a breast cancer can drain into the intercostal veins; if intrathoracic pressure is raised by coughing, the blood in these veins is squeezed back into the vertebral system. As to the physiologic *raison d'être* of the Batson system, it may act as a reservoir to prevent deep veins from bursting when thoracic and abdominal pressures are abruptly raised by physical effort.

Spread via the Lymphatics

The lymphatic pathway is a favorite of carcinomas. The long-standing dogma that *sarcomas rarely metastasize to the lymph nodes* is true overall, except for rhabdomyosarcomas (209). Malignant cells wandering out of the primary tumor penetrate the surrounding loosely structured lymphatic capillaries without destroying the endothelium (25); thereafter they probably float up to the next lymph node, where they settle in the peripheral sinus and grow (Figure 27.19). Eventually they may invade the entire node (Figure 27.20) and grow downstream or upstream into the lymphatic network. The result is literally a solid cast of the lymphatics; the individual vessels are often so distended that they can be seen with the naked eye.

This pattern of lymphatic invasion is also known as **lymphatic permeation.** Carcinomas of the breast can permeate the lymphatics of the overlying skin (Figure 27.21); presumably as a result of lymphatic obstruction, the skin becomes slightly edematous and puckered, hence the name *peau d'orange* (Figure 27.3).

FIGURE 27.17   Anatomical layout of the Batson system (vertebral venous system). (Reproduced with permission from [43].)

system and the caval and portal systems is shown schematically in Figure 27.18.

To understand the relevance of the Batson system to metastasis it is helpful to know how it was discovered. Oscar V. Batson was professor of anatomy in Philadelphia. By injecting radioopaque media into the dorsal vein of the penis in cadavers and in monkeys, he found that, if the abdominal pressure was raised, the material penetrated the lumbar spine rather than the caval system, mimicking the distribution of metastases from prostatic carcinoma. This mechanism works also *in vivo:*

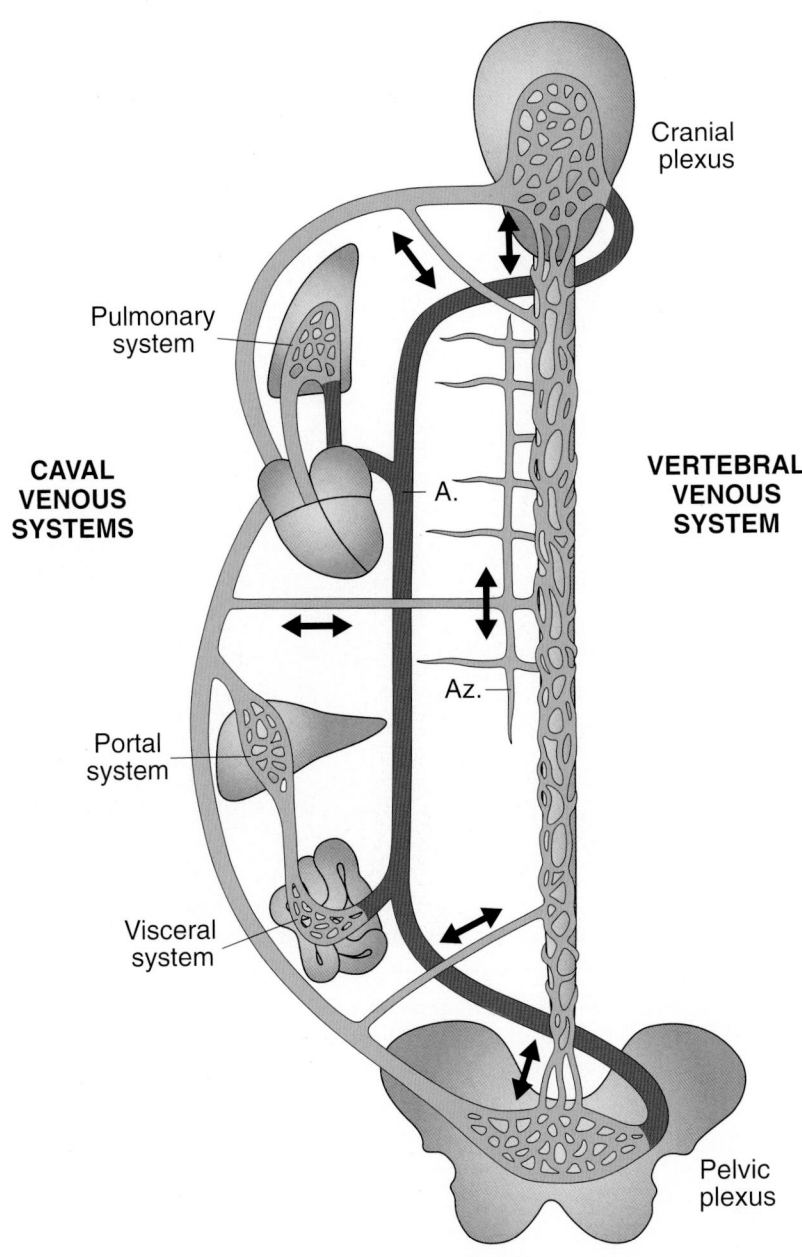

Cranial
plexus

Pulmonary
system

**CAVAL
VENOUS
SYSTEMS**

A.

**VERTEBRAL
VENOUS
SYSTEM**

Az.

Portal
system

Visceral
system

Pelvic
plexus

FIGURE 27.18   Batson's vertebral venous system: overall view. Notice how malignant cells released from a carcinoma in the pelvic region could reach the skull without ever passing through the caval system or the lungs. **A:** Aorta. **Az:** Azygos vein.

Both primary and metastatic carcinomas of the lung can produce an extensive filling of the lymphatics: thin whitish threads visible to the naked eye appear on the pleura and on the diaphragm (Figures 27.22, 27.23); within the lung itself, lymphatic permeation tends to follow the periarterial lymphatics and is usually accompanied by fibrosis (Figure 27.24). Perhaps the pumping action of respiration has something to do with the tendency of carcinomas to permeate the lymphatics of the lung. However, it seems more likely that we are dealing with a biologic peculiarity of certain malignant cells: there are reported cases of gastric carcinomas producing lymphatic invasion almost throughout the body (209).

NOTE: lymph nodes downstream from a tumor can swell even before they have received metastatic cells. Antigens and other irritating materials leach out of the tumor, especially if it contains much necrosis and even more so if it is ulcerated and infected. When the lymph node receives these antigenic and chemical messengers it responds by swelling, due in part to extensive

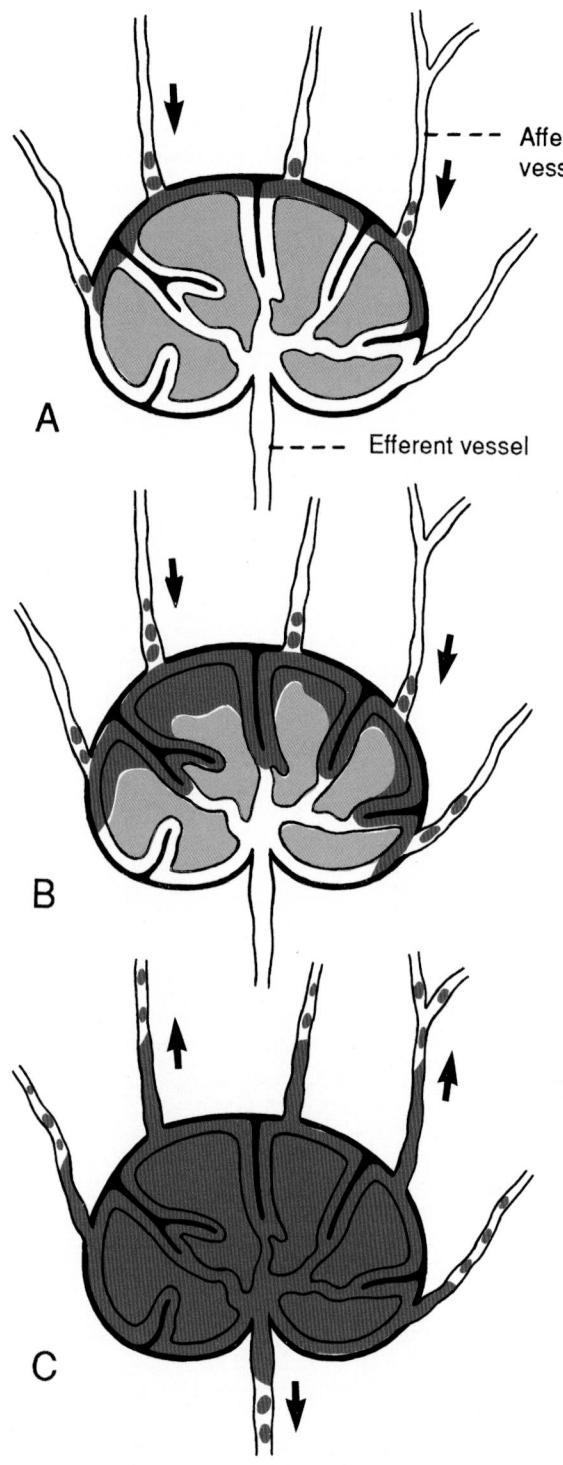

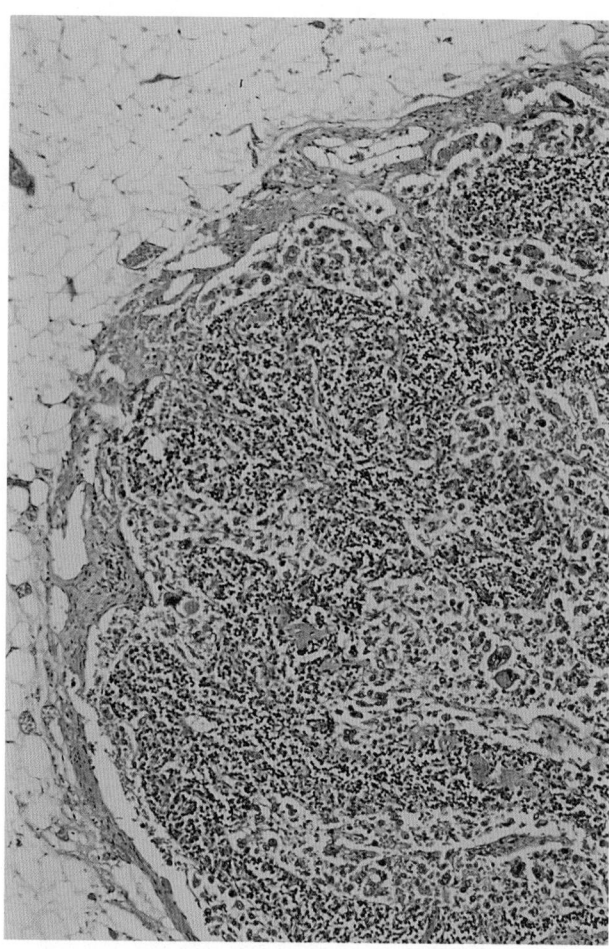

FIGURE 27.20   Invasion of a lymph node by a carcinoma. Between masses of lymphatic tissue (with its small darkly stained lymphocytes) are dilated sinuses filled with cells, some of which can be recognized as atypical (especially at *lower right*). (60x)

FIGURE 27.19   Steps in the metastasization of a lymph node by a carcinoma. **A:** Malignant cells reach the node from the afferent lymphatics and fill the peripheral sinus. **B:** The entire lymph node is invaded by the carcinoma. **C:** The lymph node has ceased to function as such and becomes a center for tumor growth. Solid cords of tumor cells grow into the afferent and efferent lymphatics. (Adapted with permission from [96].)

hyperplasia of the cells in the sinuses; the resulting microscopic pattern is known as *sinus histiocytosis* (26, 197). Clinically, swollen lymph nodes downstream from a tumor are very worrisome; only the microscope can distinguish between a metastasis and an innocent reaction.

We would like to report that the lymph nodes are very effective filters of metastatic tumor cells as they are of inert particles (p. 438), but the experimental evidence is not very reassuring. In one of the few studies on this topic, tumor cells were injected into the footpad of the rat; from there they drained into the popliteal lymph node and were briefly held up, but by 5 days

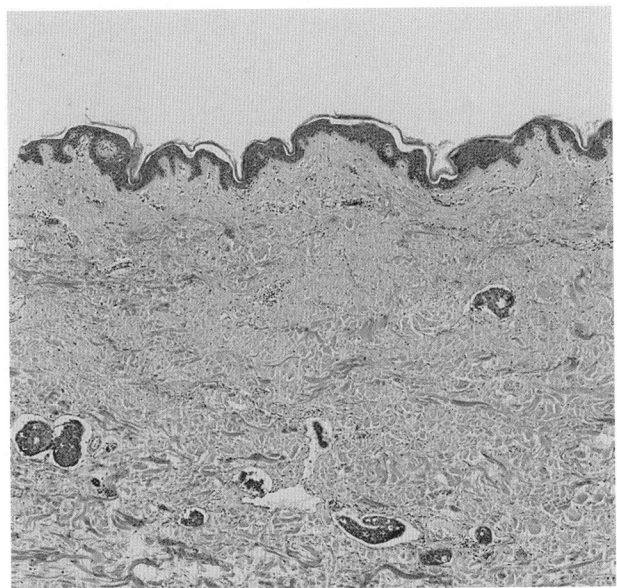

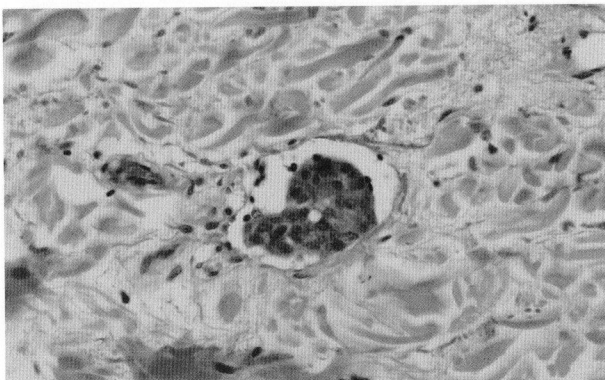

FIGURE 27.21 Lymphatic infiltration by tumor cells in the skin overlying a carcinoma of the breast. *Top:* The small masses of malignant cells should be visualized in three dimensions as casts of the lymphatic network. *Bottom:* Detail of infiltrated and dilated lymphatic.

they had already reached the next lymphatic station, namely the paraaortic node (26). If a dose of BCG was injected into the footpad (thereby inflaming the lymph node) 1 week before the injection of tumor cells, the metastatic destruction of the node was delayed, but there was little effect on the progression of the malignant cells to the next node.

The behavior of the lymph nodes toward metastatic cells is of course very important to the surgeon who has to decide whether to remove the lymph nodes draining a primary tumor. Microscopically there are no obvious signs of an aggressive antitumor-cell campaign in the lymph node (25). However, there is statistical evidence that some metastases do die in the nodes (181).

This statistical evidence was obtained by comparing the frequency of microscopic axillary metastases from carcinoma of the breast (40 percent in one series) with the development of clinically positive nodes in a parallel series of patients whose axillary nodes were not removed (15 percent): these figures suggest that about two-thirds of the microscopic metastases did not grow.

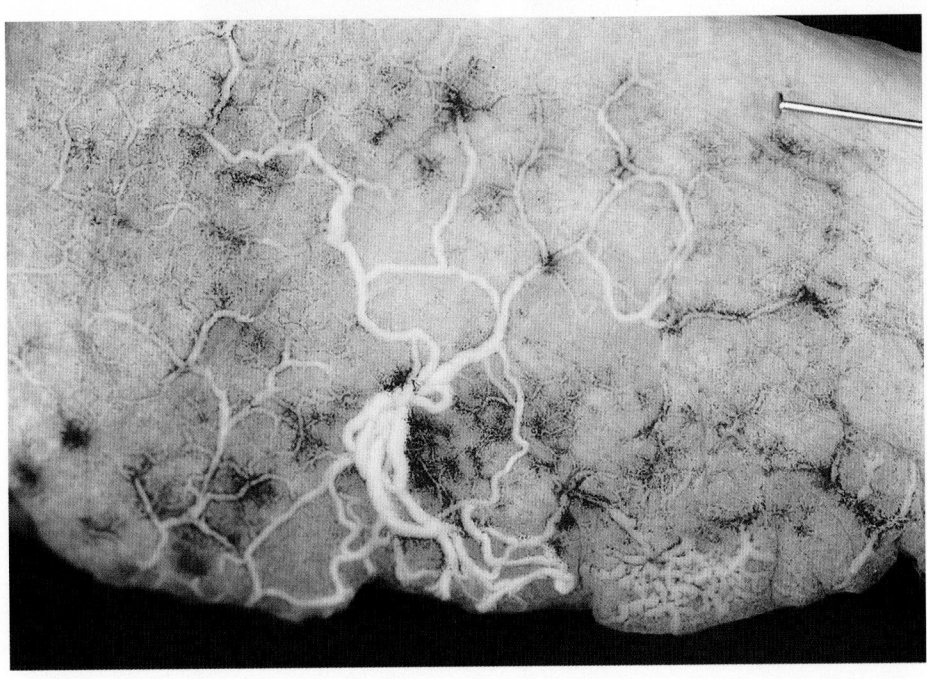

FIGURE 27.22 Neoplastic invasion of the pleural lymphatics by a carcinoma of the colon with metastases to the lung. The whitish irregular lines represent dilated lymphatics filled with carcinoma. The pin provides the scale.

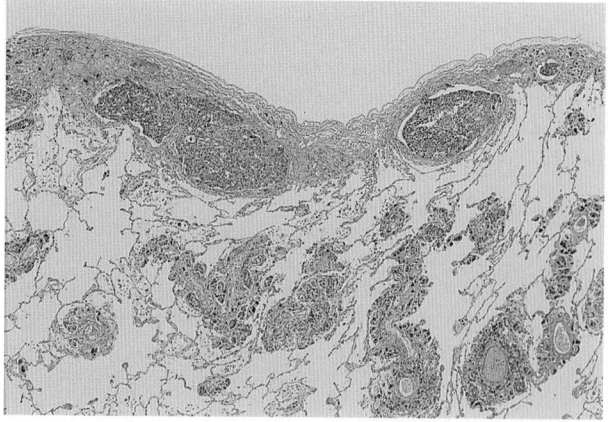

FIGURE 27.23   Lung (pleural surface at top) showing lymphatic permeation by a carcinoma. In this case, besides the pleural lymphatics, also the intrapulmonary lymphatics are involved; they surround the small arteries. Note central necrosis in some of the tumor masses. (30x)

As is usual with tumors, there can be no general rule; with regard to melanomas, for example, it may or may not be useful to excise the regional lymph nodes, depending on the size and thickness of the primary tumor (Figure 27.25).

(For lymphatics in tumors, see p. 788; for lymphangiogenesis, see pp. 439, 778.)

Seeding in Body Cavities

This event is common in the peritoneum as a complication of malignancies in abdominal organs. Hundreds of metastatic nodules can develop (Figure 27.26). The seeding is usually more severe in the pelvic recesses, presumably because the cells tend to settle there by gravity; the result is a stiffening of the peritoneal lining that can be felt by rectal or vaginal examination. Sometimes the omentum is seeded extensively, and the fibrous reaction induced by the invading cells causes it to retract and shrivel into a firm mass that can be palpated in the upper abdomen. Peritoneal seeding is usually accompanied by ascites (free fluid in the abdomen); adhesions may also develop. Some cells remain free and grow in the ascitic fluid, forming microscopic clusters or **spheroids** (p. 775).

The pathogenesis of malignant ascites and other malignant effusions needs more study. Probable mechanisms: tumors produce several factors that induce vascular leakage (p. 787), and these could diffusely affect the peritoneal membrane; furthermore, fluid oozes from the surfaces of malignant tumors (p. 788).

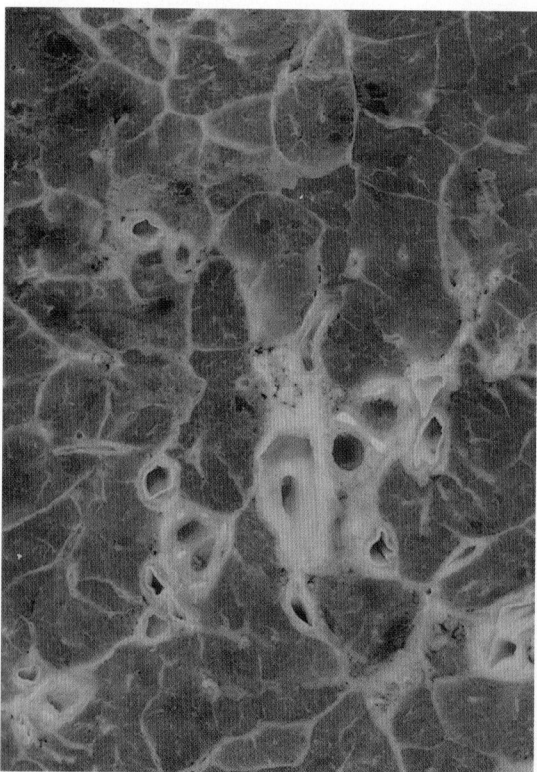 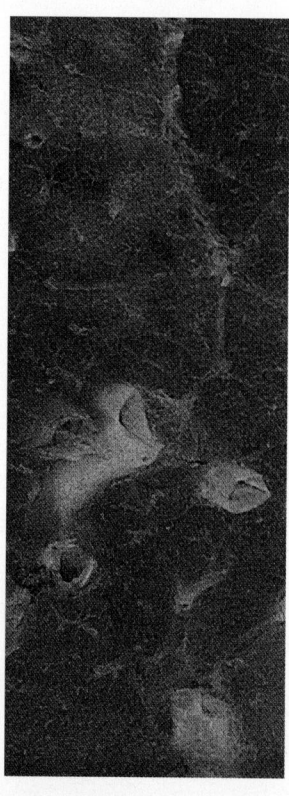

FIGURE 27.24   *Left:* The mosaic pattern of this lung is due to carcinomatous invasion of the lymphatics in the septa between pulmonary lobules. A strong fibrous reaction accompanies the invading cells. *Right:* Cut surface of normal lung.

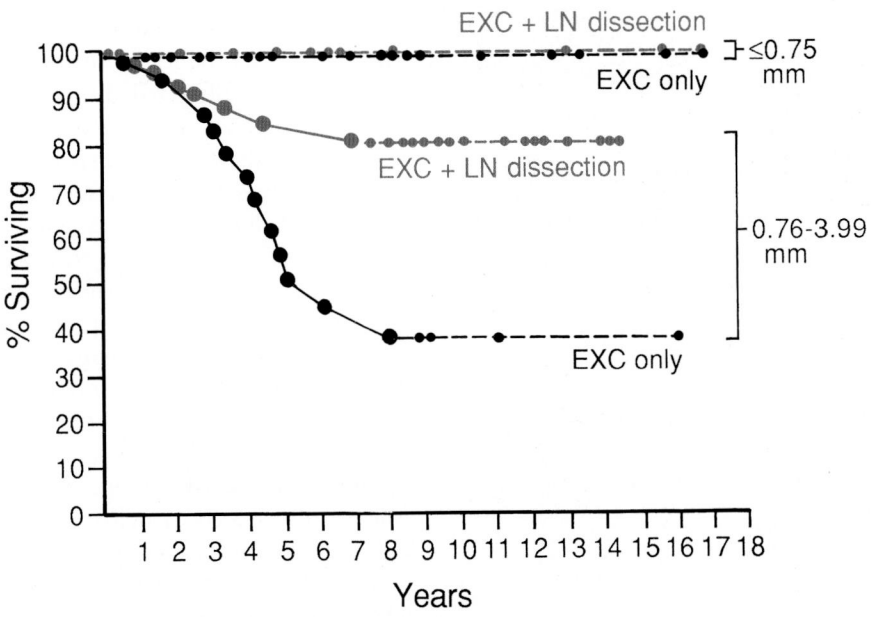

FIGURE 27.25   Survival curves of patients with melanoma: one group with thin (<75 mm) melanomas and one with melanomas of intermediate thickness (0.76–3.99 mm). In each group, patients were operated with or without lymph node (**LN**) dissection. Excision (**EXC**) of the lymph nodes was helpful for thin melanomas; for melanomas thicker than 4 mm the advantage disappeared (data not shown). Such studies indicate that the dissection of lymph nodes must be tailored to the primary tumor. (Reproduced with permission from [11].)

Seeding via the cerebrospinal fluid can occur with tumors of the central nervous system (mainly malignant gliomas): tumor cells shed into the cerebrospinal fluid settle and give rise to nodules in the ventricles or in the leptomeningeal spaces (168).

Implantation on epithelial surfaces is rare: a carcinoma of the gut protruding above the surface does not produce "seedlings" where it rubs against normal mucosa. Epithelial surfaces are inhospitable, being covered by mucus, cornified cells, and even bacteria. However, there have been reports of carcinomas implanted from one vocal cord to the other, from the cervix to the vagina, from tongue to cheek, from one side of the esophagus to the opposite side, from the renal pelvis to the bladder, and so on (209). In such cases it is obviously difficult to rule out metastasis by the lymphatic or hematogenous pathway. Yet we should recall once again the precedent of the trophoblast, which is able to implant itself on an epithelial surface, and a foreign one at that. If the trophoblast can do it, tumors should be able to do it too; but if they ever do become implanted on an epithelial surface, it must be a rare event.

Which Tumors Metastasize—and When?

In theory, malignant tumors might be capable of metastasizing from day one, but there seems to be a delay. Perhaps they do start on day one, but success of the

metastatic colonies is hampered by two factors: it takes many metastatic cells (thousands, possibly millions) to produce one successful colony, and a very small tumor might not have enough cells to shed; also, the ability of tumor cells to produce successful metastases increases as a result of tumor progression.

We expect important news from microarray analysis. A sample: it appears that gene expression profiles of a breast cancer can predict the disease outcome (192a).

The size of the primary tumor (which implies a time factor) tends to correlate with the presence of metastases, hence the constant effort to detect smaller and smaller primary tumors, especially of the female breast. Melanomas of the skin are measured with regard to thickness on histologic sections; it was found that fractions of a millimeter count: if the thickness is less than 0.76 mm, the cure rate is 100 percent; between 0.76 and 4.00 mm there is an increasing risk (up to 80 percent) of metastases; above 4.00 mm there is an 80 percent risk of metastases at the time of observation (10). This is a reminder that very small tumors can also metastasize.

There are many exceptions to the correlation between size or thickness of a primary tumor and presence of metastases. Some melanomas of the skin metastasize before the

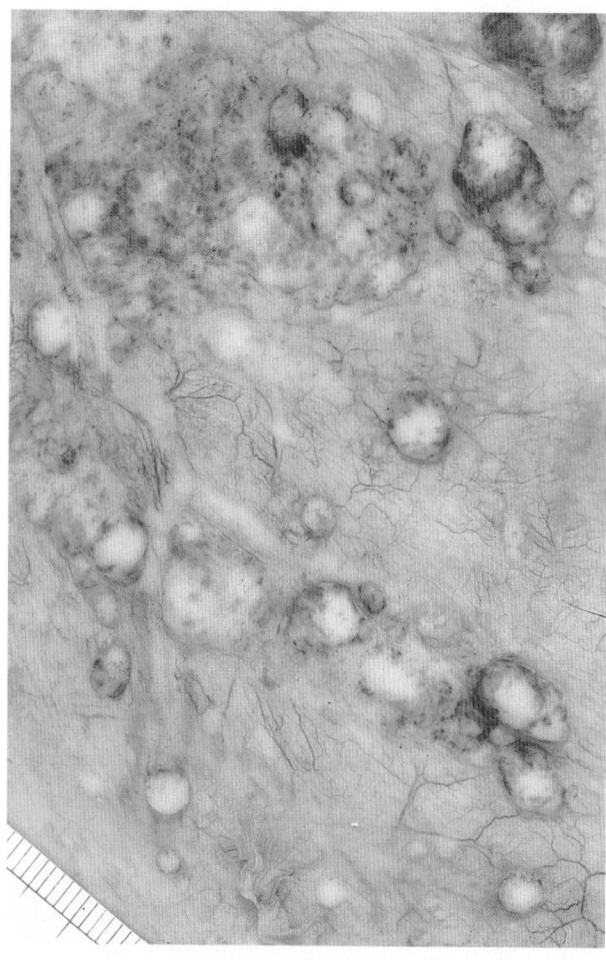

FIGURE 27.26   Peritoneal seeding of a carcinoma of the pancreas; these nodules developed on the peritoneal surface of the diaphragm. **Scale** in millimeters.

patient has noticed them; occasionally they even regress and disappear, leaving only the metastases as proof of their brief existence.

There is also a malignant tumor that almost never metastasizes: the very common basal cell carcinoma of the skin. This tumor appears typically on areas of the skin exposed to sunlight, especially the face, as a small crusty lesion that does not heal (see Figure 26.25). It is

locally invasive and if allowed to grow it can destroy half the face, yet the rest of the body is spared. Medical students are usually puzzled by the fact that this tumor is called malignant although the cure rate by surgery is 100 percent: the reason is that *if* it is allowed to grow it kills by invasion. Metastases are so rare that if one occurs it is still publishable as news.

Tumors of the central nervous system rarely produce metastases to the rest of the body, probably because they develop in a closed space and therefore kill the host before visceral metastases are large enough to be detected. Although metastases to the lungs, bones, and other organs have been described, the average pathologist may see one or two examples in a lifetime (168).

Dormant metastases are the nightmare of many "successfully treated" patients. In some cases, metastatic cells lie dormant for 5–10 years or even 35 years (209), then suddenly start to grow. The latent phase may be related to lack of angiogenesis (62); it might also represent a balance between cell birth and death (59). Trauma can wake up dormant cells: it has been shown in the rat that intraportal injection of malignant cells did not produce tumors; but nodules developed after the liver was traumatized (59).

Mother-to-fetus metastases do occur, but very rarely (28, 125). Malignant tumors in pregnant women are not uncommon, but published cases of metastases to the placenta are only 40, half of which concern melanomas. Two cases of maternal melanoma and four cases of maternal leukemia have been associated with the same tumor in the infants, all of which died of it. It has been speculated that these cases may not represent metastases but viral transmission. There is one known case of placental metastasis from a fetal neuroblastoma.

Iatrogenic metastases occur by several mechanisms. Chemotherapy may cause wide dissemination; the reason is not clear (126, 181); it may be related to endothelial injury (142). Surgical trauma may wake up dormant metastases; on the other hand, the intraoperative release of tumor cells into the bloodstream, however worrisome, has no measurable effect (p. 818). Implantation along a needle track, after biopsy, is exceedingly rare (211).

Mechanisms of Invasion and Metastasis

The Metastatic Cascade
From the point of view of the malignant cell, invasion and metastasis require the ability to overcome a series of obstacles, which have been aptly compared to a decathlon, named the *metastatic cascade* (Figure 27.27)

(118, 136, 143, 207). To produce a hematogenous metastasis a cell must separate itself from the tumor mass and move in the right direction; it must digest its way through the intercellular matrix, and then through a vascular basement membrane to penetrate the lumen of a

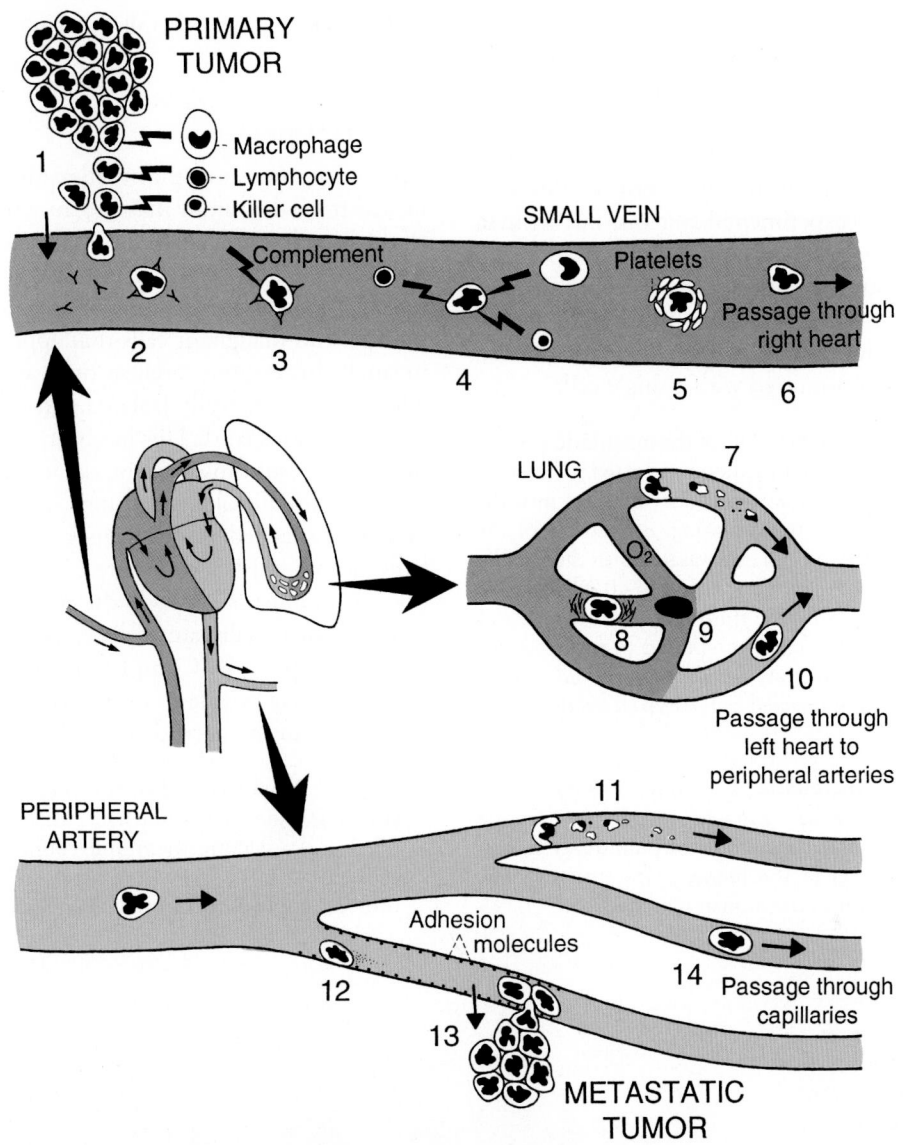

FIGURE 27.27 Cancer cells that travel in the bloodstream experience a series of adventures that are—from the point of view of the cancer cell—bad, good, or indifferent. (**1**) Encounters with killer cells of various types on the way toward a blood vessel. (**2**) Coating with antibody and (**3**) killing by complement. (**4**) Intravascular killing by various types of killer cells. (**5**) Coating with platelets, which may supply the cancer cell with growth factors. (**6**) Passage through the heart. (**7**) Impaction and breakup in a lung capillary. (**8**) Arrest in the alveolar capillaries. (**9**) Exposure to toxic levels of oxygen. (**10**) Return toward the systemic circulation. (**11**) Impaction and breakup in the peripheral capillaries. (**12**) Margination in vessels of the microcirculation. (**13**) Trapping in the microcirculation followed by metastatic growth. (**14**) Return toward the heart. The circuit (without stops) takes about 1 minute.

vessel; once there, it must escape the various defensive systems of the blood, including antibodies, complement, macrophages, killer cells of various sorts, oxygen, and even blood clotting; when it reaches a vessel small enough to be embolized, it must survive the impact and the mechanical squeeze; then it must proceed in reverse, penetrate the endothelium and the basement membrane,

escape a new set of dangerous cells (macrophages, lymphocytes), multiply, induce angiogenesis, and finally establish a tumor. In view of all these difficulties, it is not surprising that many tumor cells fail. At each step of the metastatic cascade the metastatic cells are selected by a basic principle: survival of the fittest (59), which contributes to the phenomenon of tumor progression.

Despite the undeniable threat of tumor progression, we can sum up with a mildly optimistic statement: *the metastatic process is highly inefficient* (200). Many cells try but few succeed. Clumps of about four cells are more likely to "take" than single cells (105). It is usually stated that metastatic takes are on the order of 0.1–0.01 percent; this applies to experimental systems, but in man the efficiency can be even less than 10^{-7} (p. 818).

All this may sound reassuring, but of course even if one cell survives it is one too many. We should also remember that in some models of experimental leukemia the disease can be transmitted with a single cell.

Actual data on the "inefficiency" of the metastatic cascade vary, of course, according to the model used. The latest figures produced using melanoma cells injected into the mouse *portal vein* gave the following: 80 percent of the melanoma cells survived and extravasated into the liver by the third day; of these survivors, only 1 in 40 cells grew to form micrometastases by the third day, and of these micrometastases only 1 percent progressed to form macroscopic tumors. Most micrometastases disappeared, and by day 13, 36 percent of injected cells survived as "dormant" (113).

Genetic control of metastasis. According to Ohtaki et al. (141), a human gene, *KiSS-1,* encodes a peptide (*metastin*) that reduces the number of pulmonary metastases of a melanoma in the mouse. Most interestingly, metastin is abundant in the human placenta.

Data are available for all the steps of the metastatic cascade.

(1) Detachment

There is no question that malignant cells become detached from the tumor mass because they can be found in the bloodstream, single or in clusters (see later); one such cluster ready to be carried away was shown in Figure 27.10. In tissue sections of carcinomas, it is common to find malignant cells that appear to be single or in small clusters, but serial sections are needed to show whether they are really isolated and not a cross section of a continuous cord. This has been done for several tumors. The result: most of the isolated clumps of tumor cells seen in histologic sections are cross sections of branches attached to the tumor mass, but a few are truly detached islands (Figure 27.28). The next question, then, must be: how do the cells become detached?

Recall that malignant cells tend to be more loosely connected (p. 754). Complete detachment from their neighbors may be due to proteolytic enzymes diffusing outward from the necrotic core of the tumor.

Leonard Weiss has studied this mechanism by punching cores out of normal mouse livers, then incubating them at 37 degrees, shaking them and counting the number of cells released (197, 198). Extracts of necrotic parts of tumors, applied to normal liver, increased the release.

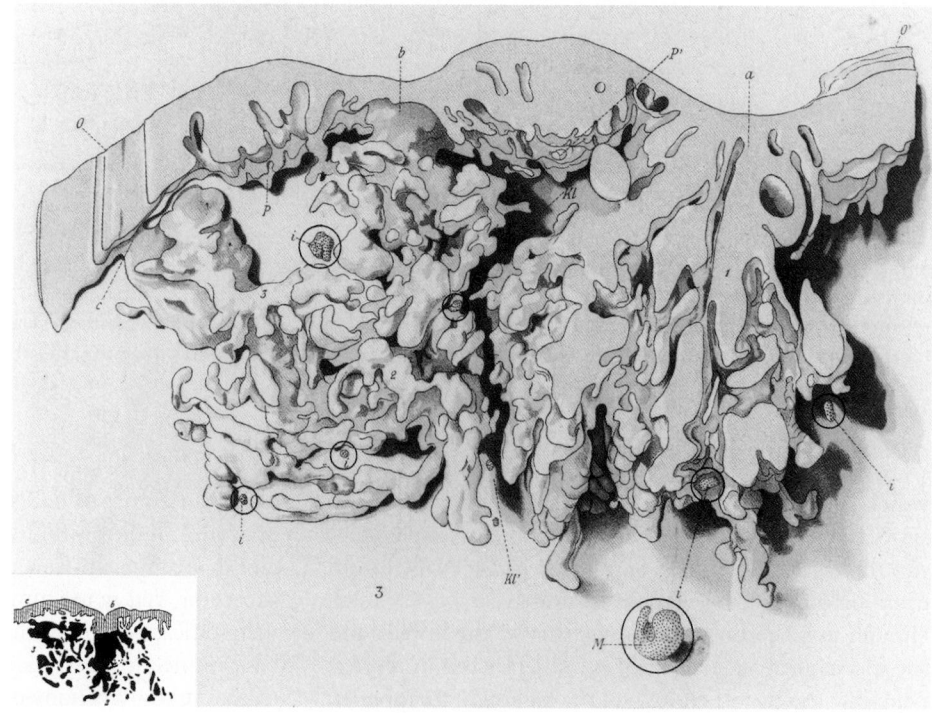

FIGURE 27.28 Model of a small squamous cell carcinoma of the scrotum, reconstructed from serial sections. A schematic view of a histologic section is shown in the *inset.* According to the reconstructed model, the tumor masses that appear histologically (*inset*) as isolated are actually connected to the tumor mass. Only a few small clumps of tumor tissue are free standing (*circles*). The mass **M** was 6 mm from the main tumor mass and was considered to be a metastasis. (Reproduced from [155].)

Interestingly, regenerating livers released more cells than normal controls. The tumor extracts also brought about the detachment of cells from cell masses grown *in vitro* (198, 203).

Tumor cells can also become detached because their adhesion molecules are not properly expressed. Epithelial cells, for example, are connected by *adhaerens* junctions, in which E-(*epithelial*) cadherins and catenins collaborate almost literally as in a zipper; in tumors, many types of mutations can affect the cadherin and catenin genes, contributing to tumor progression and invasiveness. In a mouse transgenic model of pancreatic carcinoma, the loss of E-cadherin coincided with the transition from well-differentiated adenoma to invasive carcinoma (12). Conversely, on cultured cells, E-cadherin has invasion-suppressing properties (78). Another fascinating experiment: *in vitro,* in a breast cancer line, tamoxifen suppressed the invasive phenotype and restored cadherin expression (12).

Active motility of tumor cells could also favor the detachment process, and there is ample proof that many types of malignant cells do show ameboid motion (see further).

Massage of tumors has long been known to favor the seeding process (59, 106, 192) as we illustrated earlier (see Figure 23.14). However, let it be clear that malignant tumors need no massage for releasing cells into the bloodstream: a mammary tumor of the rat, that required 10 million cells for a 100 percent successful inoculum, shed that number of cells every day into the bloodstream (23, 74) (see further).

(2) Invasion

The interface between tumor and host is currently visualized as a zone of intense enzymatic activity: a band of matrix soaked in enzymes and their products, as well as growth factors and other cytokines. This is where the advance of the tumor is decided: hence this busy area may become the target for "stromal therapy" (102). The enzymes are contributed by the tumor cells (135, 137) and by activated stromal cells (151, 191) in varying proportions. The malignant cells must digest their way through this gelatinous layer, using heparanase (60, 193) and collagenase specific for collagen fibrils and for basement membranes; they do so in part by appropriating stromal enzymes and using them mounted on their own surface (17). The enzymes critical for tumor invasion are proteases (**matrixins or matrix metalloproteinases [MMPs]**), of which about 25 are known (17, 80, 210). Mixed with these enzymes are their products, which can affect many different

processes and thereby greatly complicate the issue. Elastin fragments include angiostatin, and collagen XVIII yields endostatin, a suppressor of tumor growth, which means that inhibiting these enzymes may suppress as well as enhance tumor growth (17, 52, 183).

A definitive proof of active invasion is the sight of cancer cells penetrating the fibers of skeletal muscle (Figure 27.29) (98). Invasiveness can be tested and measured *in vitro,* by placing tumor cells on a membrane of human amnion relined with endothelium (Figure 27.30) (87, 169). Another *in vitro* test has gladiatorial connotations: the principle is to place normal and malignant cells face to face. This is called *confrontation* (45). However, confrontation experiments based on tissue culture (a two-dimensional system) can be misleading because all the cells participating in the

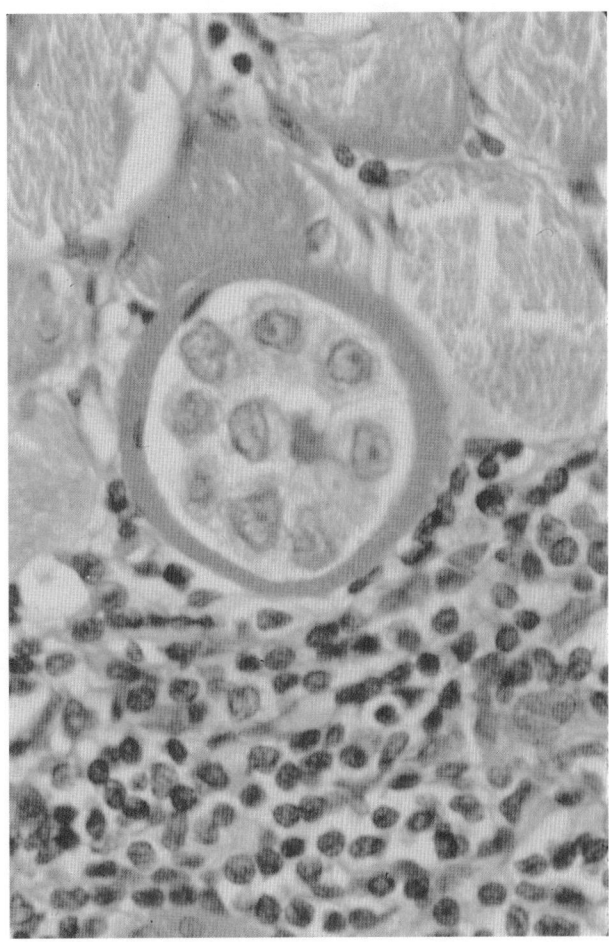

FIGURE 27.29   An extreme case of tumor infiltration. The circular structure is a muscle fiber greatly expanded by invading malignant tumor cells from an adenocarcinoma of the breast. Above it are parts of noninvaded fibers. (Reproduced with permission from [98].)

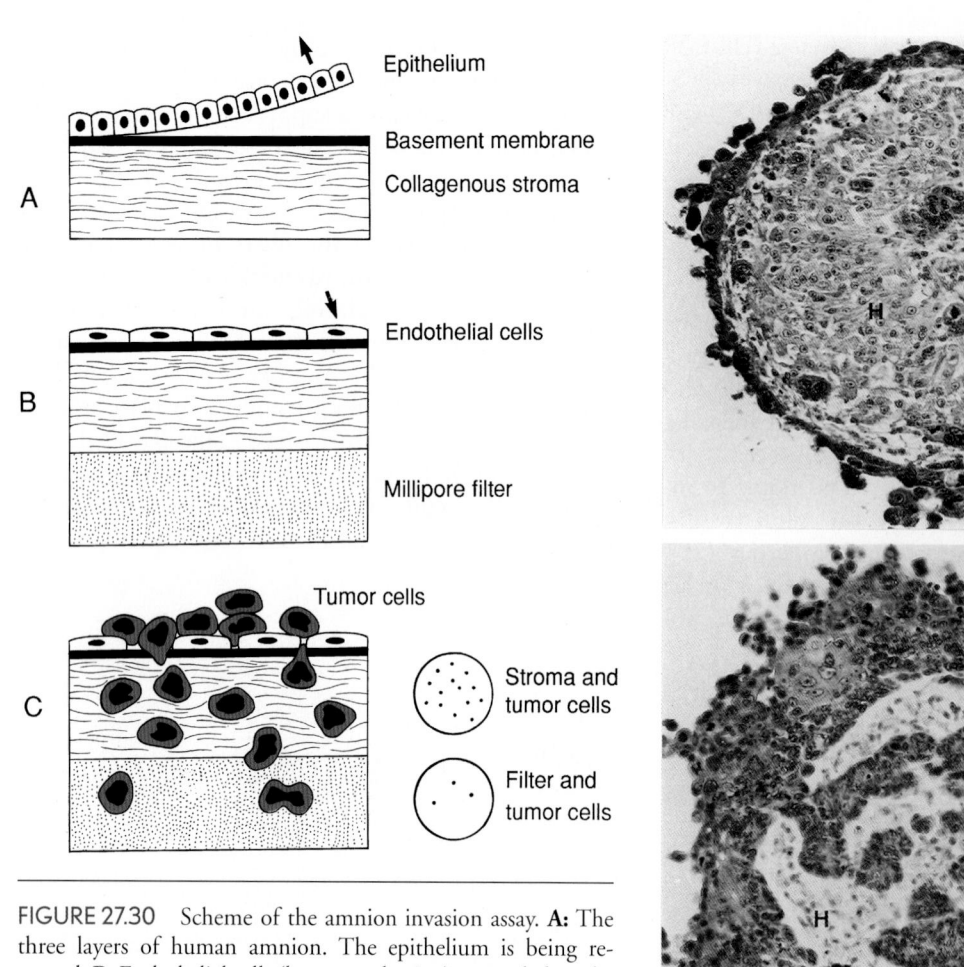

FIGURE 27.30 Scheme of the amnion invasion assay. **A:** The three layers of human amnion. The epithelium is being removed. **B:** Endothelial cells (human or bovine) are seeded on the amnion and grown to confluence; a millipore filter is placed between the amnion. **C:** Tumor cells seeded over the surface cross the endothelium and invade the stroma and filter. Stroma and filter are then peeled apart, stained, and examined under a microscope. Counting the tumor cells measures their invasiveness. (Reproduced from [169].)

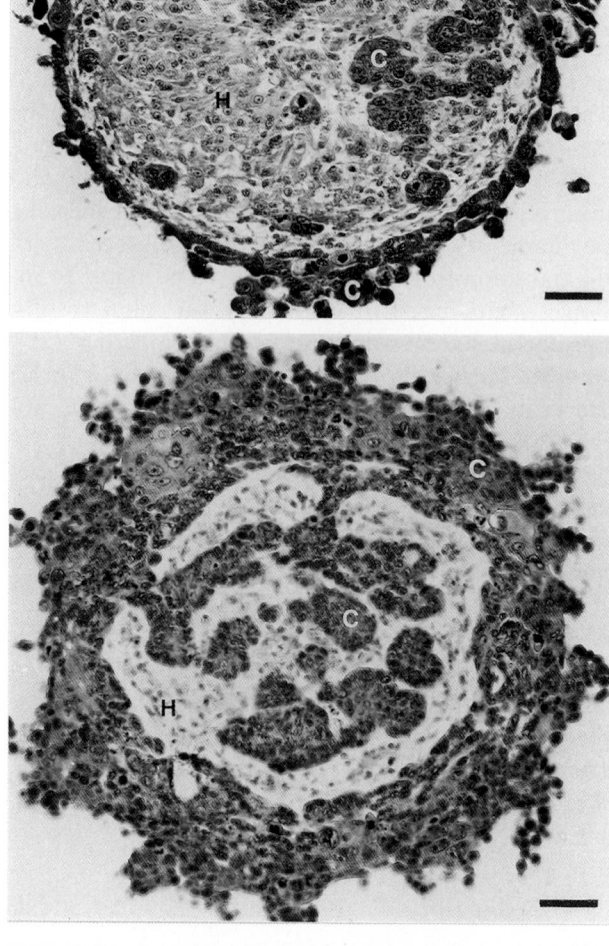

FIGURE 27.31 Histologic sections of spheroids, obtained by confronting—in three-dimensional culture—embryonic chick heart (**H**) and a line of malignant epithelial cells derived from a rat bladder carcinoma (**C**). The spheroids were fixed after 7 days (*top*) and 14 days (*bottom*). Note how the mass of heart cells is progressively invaded by the tumor cells. **Bars** = 50 μm. (Reproduced from [173] by permission of S. Karger AG, Basel.)

test are attached to a fixed substrate, unlike the situation *in vivo* (115). More telling results are obtained by confronting small three-dimensional tumor spheroids with normal tissues, as shown in Figure 27.31 (117): malignant spheroids become attached to benign tissues and invade them (117, 119, 120).

How do cancer cells force their way into surrounding tissues? *Growth pressure* might be exploited by cancer cells forcing their way into the surroundings, but it cannot be the only mechanism because invasion can be demonstrated *in vitro* by the confrontation method, which rules out this factor (117).

Active motility of cancer cells is well proven. It was calculated as far back as 1916 that the speed of cells observed *in vitro* would enable malignant cells to crawl from the breast to the axillary lymph nodes in 4 weeks (196). Several movies have been made also *in vivo*

(33a, 116, 213). Furthermore, Liotta and co-workers extracted a factor from human melanoma cells that increases the rate of motion of the same cells (*chemokinesis*) and also attracts them; it does not attract neutrophils (Figure 27.32) (107). This *autocrine motility factor* means that tumor cells have joined the family of chemotactic cells. But there is more: there are reports that tumor cells respond to chemotactic stimuli with increased adhesiveness and release of hydrolytic enzymes: these are typical leukocyte responses (188).

FLOW OF INTERSTITIAL FLUID

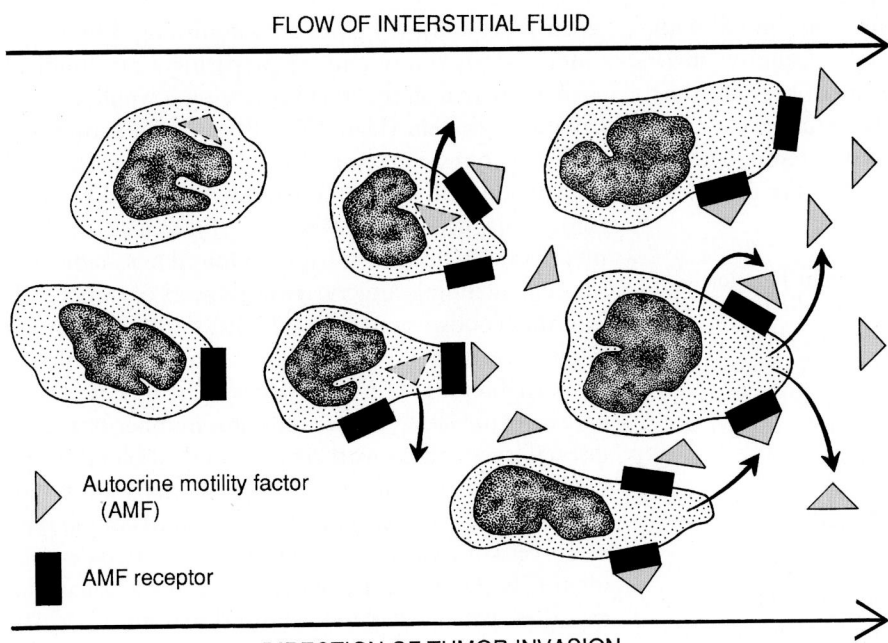

▷ Autocrine motility factor
   (AMF)

■ AMF receptor

DIRECTION OF TUMOR INVASION

FIGURE 27.32 Proposed role of tumor autocrine motility factor. Tumor cells secrete the factor, which binds to their own surface receptors and stimulates random as well as directed motility. The flow of interstitial fluid in the tumor tends to sweep the factor to the periphery and presumably contributes to the invasive process. (From [104], copyright © 1986 Alan R. Liss. Adapted and reprinted by permission of Wiley-Liss, Inc., a subsidiary of John Wiley & Sons, Inc.)

Some inflammatory mediators are chemotactic for some tumor cells. As to tumor products, chemotactic as well as antichemotactic factors have been described (107, 108). Some of the breakdown products of the enzymatic digestion of the matrix are chemotactic for some tumor cells (137).

The resistance of cartilage to invasion was discussed earlier (p. 775).

What happens when a malignant cell contacts a normal cell? This should be the crucial confrontation in the drama of aggression by tumors, but not much is known about it except that the cells of invaded tissue tend to disappear. Pressure atrophy is surely one explanation (27, 63, 90), but there must be other, more subtle mechanisms. Electron microscopy shows pseudopods of tumor cells pushing their way into host liver cells (Figure 27.33); phagocytosis of cell debris by macrophages and tumor cells was sometimes observed (63). Actual destruction of invaded tissue was seen *in vitro* when

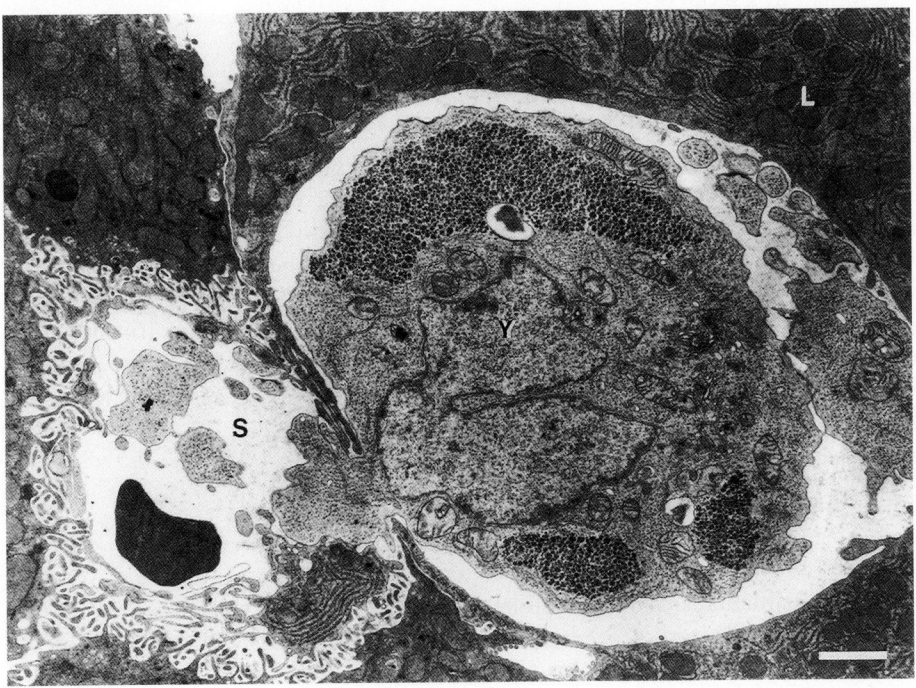

FIGURE 27.33 Active infiltration by a malignant cell. A cell of the so-called Yoshida sarcoma (**Y**) injected into the portal vein and actively escaping through the wall of the sinusoid (**S**); in so doing, it creates a deep indentation in the neighboring liver cell (**L**). **Bar** = 2 μm. (Reproduced with permission from [90].)

fragments of nervous tissue were confronted with malignant cells (116). A tantalizing possibility: there are increasing rumors of possible "marriage" (fusion) between normal and malignant cells in tumors (p. 929). This mechanism sounds extremely interesting; it has not created headlines—yet, but we had the good fortune to find a very likely example (p. 930).

> Electron microscopy has shown that tight junctions develop between normal and malignant cells (9, 27, 48, 132). This too could be important because chemical messages related to growth control could be exchanged. We have already mentioned the strange fact that some transformed cells stop growing when they make contact with normal cells (p. 754).

(3) Penetration into the Blood Vessels

It should be easier for the tumor cells to invade the vessels of the tumor itself rather than the preformed vessels around it: the perivascular basement membrane of the tumor vessels is incomplete, and the endothelium may be riddled with holes—as we have seen. But anyway, the invading tumor cells must be prepared to perform what amounts to *reverse diapedesis*. They surely have many ways to solve the problem, but a basic three-step mechanism has been proposed by Liotta and collaborators (110): attachment, lysis, and invasion. When tumor cells reach the perivascular basement membrane, they attach to it by means of laminin receptors (laminin is an adhesive molecule that reinforces basement membranes (13)); then the tumor cells secrete collagenase Type 4, specific for the collagen of the basement membrane (Figure 27.34), and eventually move through. In a series of elegant experiments, Liotta and others have proven all these points for a variety of tumors. For example, metastatic efficiency has been correlated with collagenase secretion (66, 103). Others have shown experimentally that protease inhibitors oppose metastasis (137).

Tumor cells may not always need this arsenal of molecular tools to reach the bloodstream: vessels in tumors are often defective and may lack basement membrane (204). Scanning electron microscopy has shown that the invading cell may punch its way through an endothelial cell, creating a temporary migration pore. This has been shown for leukemia cells, which are simply doing what normal leukocytes do when they leave bone marrow (39), but it is also true for melanoma cells, which somehow "learned" how to do it (Figures 27.35, 27.36) (40).

(4) Transport in the Bloodstream

Tumor cells are found in the blood of experimental animals as well as in humans (Figure 27.37). In either case it is possible to count the number released during a given time, and the figures are astonishing. Butler and Gullino devised a system for preparing a rat tumor in such a way that all the blood perfusing it would emerge from a single vein (Figure 27.38); by cannulating that vein they found that every day each gram of tissue shed 3.2 million cells, i.e., about the volume of a pinhead (23). This occurred *before* the appearance of lung metastases. In humans it has been found repeatedly that trauma, including surgery, sends showers of tumor cells into the bloodstream (Figure 27.39) (70). The number rarely exceeds 1000 per milliliter. This figure still appears frightening, but there seems to be no correlation between circulating cancer cells and number of metastases. Glaves and co-workers (64) studied blood in the renal veins in 10 patients with renal cell carcinoma; 8 of the 10 subjects' blood contained tumor cell emboli (i.e., single cells or clusters) numbering 140–73,090 per milliliter (71). From the size of the tumors it was calculated that these patients had been exposed to some 3.7×10^7 tumor cell emboli per day for at least 180 days; yet only 3 of the 10 patients had extraperitoneal metastases at the time of surgery, and only one developed metastases within 35 months. This amounts to an efficiency of less than 10^7 (71, 206).

> An amazing report was published in 1984 (186). A patient suffering from an inoperable ovarian carcinoma developed severe ascites. After 257 liters of fluid had been removed, it was decided to install a venous shunt whereby the ascitic fluid was reinfused directly into the bloodstream. Relief was immediate. When the patient died 27 months later, the peritoneum was covered with tumor implants, as anticipated, but elsewhere there was not a single metastasis despite the daily infusion of malignant cells for over 2 years.

Hazards encountered by tumor cells in the blood are many (see Figure 27.27): coating with antibodies followed by lysis with complement, encounters with killer cells of various kinds and, according to recent studies, exposure to a toxic concentration of oxygen (3). The only possible advantage for the tumor cell might be the coating with platelets, which in some experimental systems seems to help the metastatic process (68, 89, 185). And then, within seconds of gaining entry into the bloodstream, tumor cells face the trauma of embolization, which can be their demise.

(5) Embolization Followed by Cell Death

Most tumor cells injected intravenously are killed by biomechanical trauma in minutes (205, 206). Very few are viable after 24 hours. The mechanical impact of embolism is fatal to many tumor cells because they are larger and less deformable than leukocytes (57, 199);

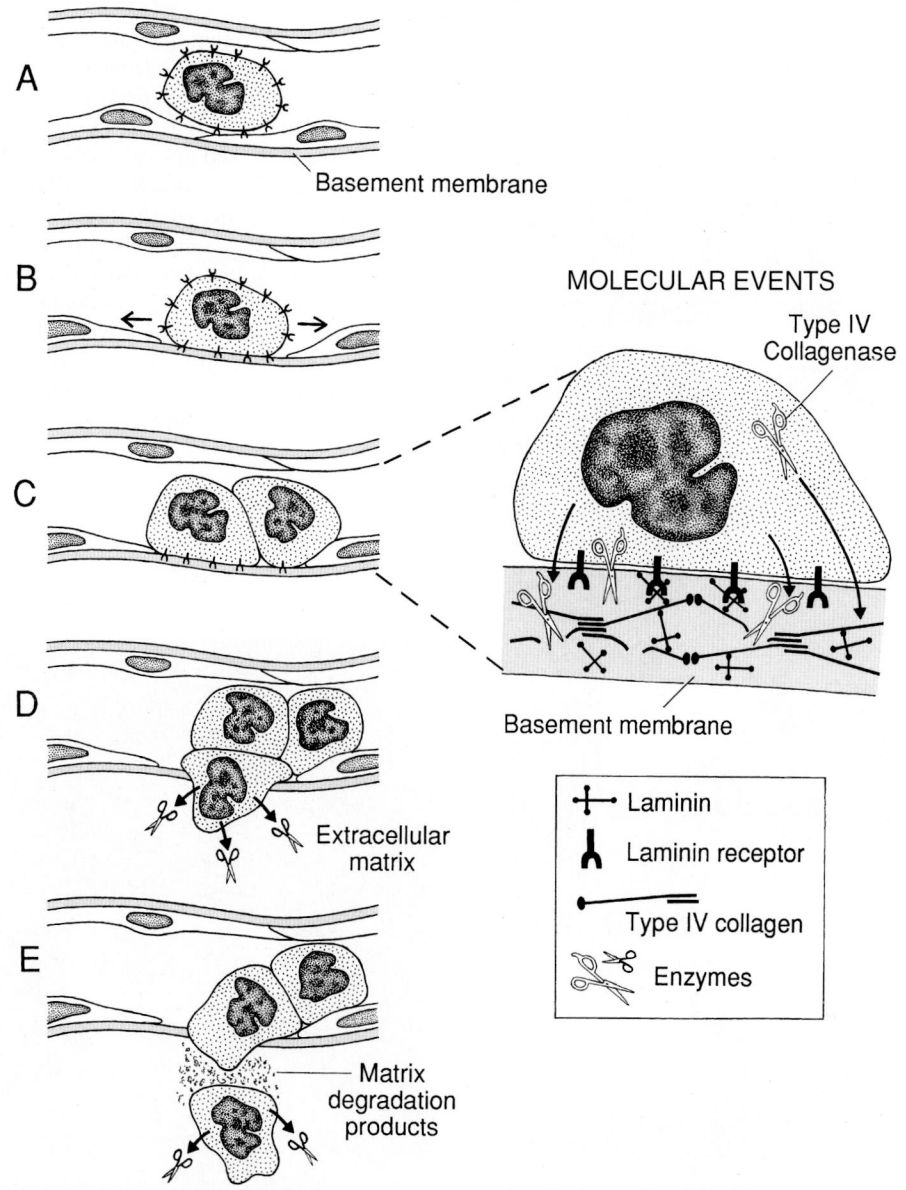

FIGURE 27.34   Development of a metastasis from a malignant cell in a capillary. **A:** Tumor cell trapped in a capillary either by embolization or by adhesion molecules (not shown). **B:** The surrounding endothelial cells retract (actively?), enabling the tumor cell to attach to the basement membrane by its laminin receptors. **C:** The tumor cell divides. **D:** A tumor cell digests its way through the basement membrane by means of collagenase and other hydrolytic enzymes. **E:** Some matrix degradation products are chemotactic, so other tumor cells follow the same path. (Adapted, with permission from the Annual Review of Biochemistry, vol. 55, © 1986 by annual Reviews Inc. [108].)

experiments with filters of various pore sizes have proven that cells less capable of changing shape are especially liable to be killed by filtration (172). Biomechanical trauma must be especially severe in the heart where capillaries receive a hefty squeeze at every beat, i.e., more than once per second (204). Similar effects apply to skeletal muscle. Now we begin to understand why the heart and the large mass of muscular tissue are rarely metastasized.

In an experiment on normal and denervated muscles in the rat, 87 percent of control muscles developed metastases compared with 31 percent in electrically stimulated muscles and 100 percent in denervated and stimulated muscles (206).

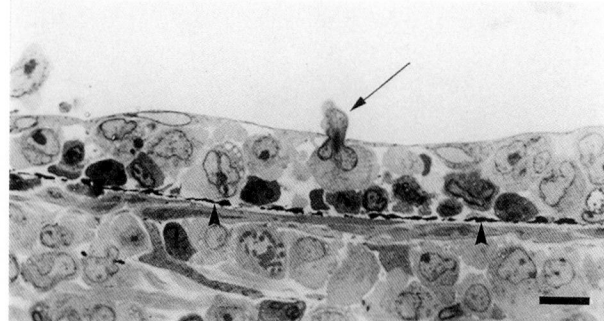

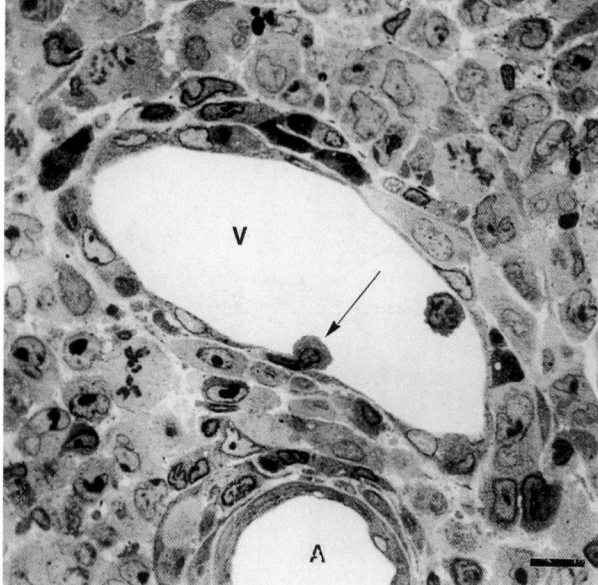

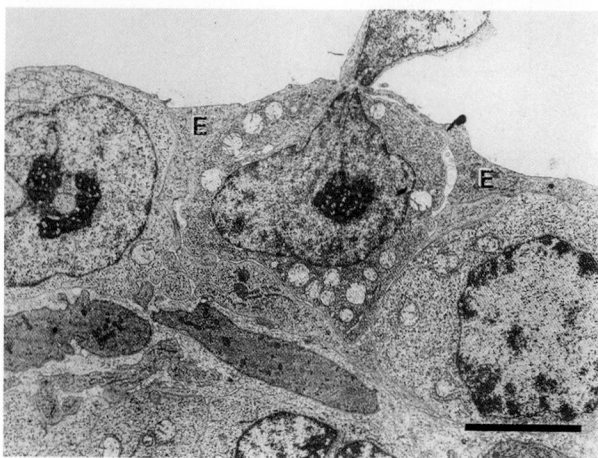

FIGURE 27.35　Penetration of malignant cells into the lumen of blood vessels (reverse diapedesis) illustrated with a malignant rat tumor (myeloma). *Top:* From a graft of tumor over a large branch of the femoral vein (**V**). One tumor cell is poking (**arrow**) through the endothelial surface (*). **Arrowheads** point to the internal elastic lamina. **Bar** = 10 μm. *Center:* A tumor cell (**arrow**) passing through the endothelium of a venule (**V**). Because the vessel is completely surrounded by tumor cells (note the mitoses), it is most likely that the direction of cell movement is from the tumor into the lumen. Another malignant cell is already in the lumen attached to the endothelium. **A:** Arteriole. **Bar** = 10 μm. *Bottom:* Electron microscopic view suggestive of reverse diapedesis. **E:** Endothelium. **Bar** = 2 μm. (Reprinted from [40], Copyright 1982, with permission from Elsevier.)

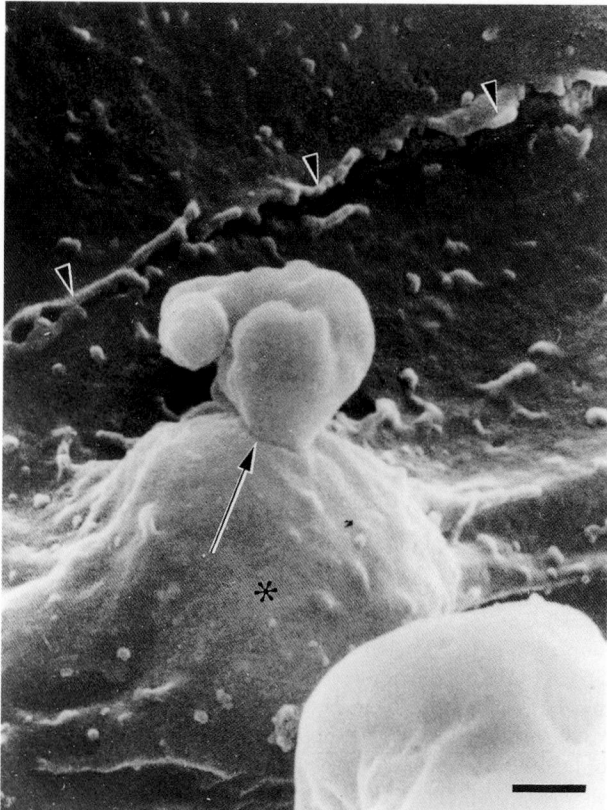

FIGURE 27.36　Intima of a venule inside a malignant rat tumor (same as in the previous figure). The bulge (**asterisk**) represents a subendothelial malignant cell that appears to squirt out of a migration pore at the top of the bulge (**arrow**). Note that this reverse diapedesis does not occur along the junction between two endothelial cells (**arrowheads**). **Bar** = 1 μm. (Reprinted from [40], Copyright 1982, with permission from Elsevier.)

In theory, a squeezing effect occurs also in the lung where inspiration, by distending the alveoli and their capillaries, should traumatize any metastatic cell in transit (204). Unfortunately the lung remains a favorite site for metastases, but it may be that without the biomechanical trauma of breathing and squeezing, the number of lung metastases would be even greater.

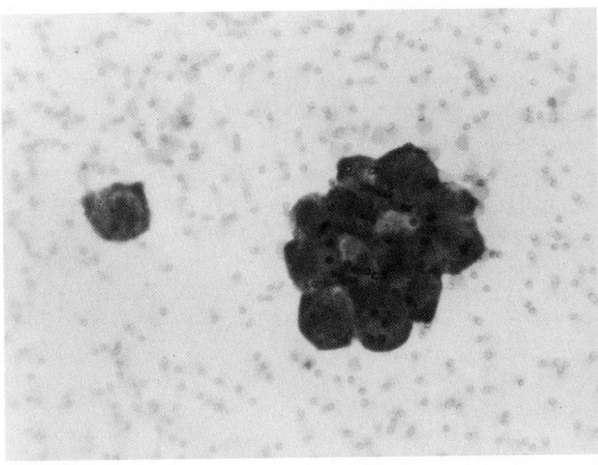
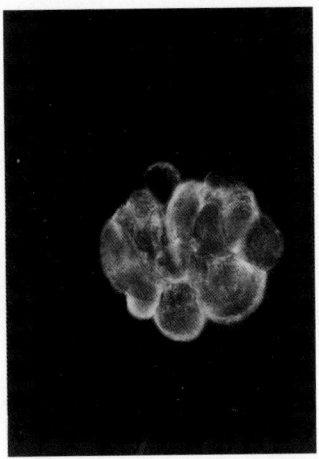

FIGURE 27.37   Blood-borne cancer cells. *Left:* Cells of mouse lung carcinoma obtained from right ventricular blood by centrifugation. *Right:* Cells of a human renal cell carcinoma spun out from the blood of the renal vein prior to a nephrectomy; stained by immunofluorescence with antibody to cytokeratin. The kidney tumor measured 10 cm in diameter; in removing it, great care was taken (as always) to minimize the surgical trauma and associated release of cells. No metastases were found 5 years after surgery. (Courtesy of D. Glaves, Roswell Park Memorial Institute, New York; reproduced with permission from [71].)

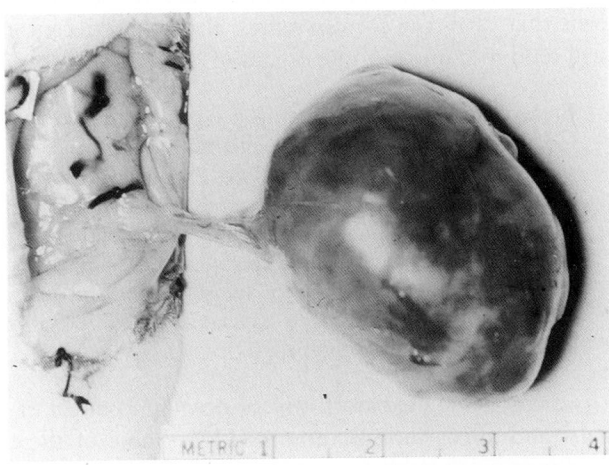

FIGURE 27.38   Method for growing a rat tumor in such a way that the blood supply comes from a single source through a peduncle. This carcinoma (Walker 256) was first implanted in the ovary, which was then pulled out of the abdominal cavity, sutured into a subcutaneous space, and surrounded by a paraffin bag. To take this photograph the paraffin bag was removed, and the tumor was pulled away from the host to show the peduncle containing the ovarian artery and vein, now supplying the tumor. (Reproduced with permission from [75], copyrighted 1980 New York Academy of Science, USA.)

Biomechanical trauma in capillaries of the lung and of the general circulation seems to account for the inefficiency of the metastatic process. In patients with advanced breast cancer, Méhes et al. (123) found that most circulating cancer cells were apoptotic.

(6) Embolization Followed by Growth

The embolic episode has been recorded cinematographically *in vivo*, quite a technical feat (213, 215). It was shown that some tumor cells survive embolic trauma and continue to circulate (57, 215).

The development of a successful tumor embolus is best shown by electron microscopy (Figure 27.40) (29, 35, 86, 93, 177, 184). Details vary with experimental model (158). The malignant cell or cluster settles in a capillary or precapillary vessel where it is always tightly apposed to the endothelial surface; it is often associated with platelets (which may act as a supply of growth factors) and with some strands of fibrin (194). Within a few hours the malignant cell (be it isolated or part of a cluster) sends a pseudopod between the endothelial cells or through them and makes contact with the basement membrane, while flow may resume. Thereafter the cell may exit from the vessel and pursue its career outside or divide and grow into a metastatic lump that occludes the lumen (204). Seen by electron microscopy the diapedesis of a tumor cell appears surprisingly similar to that of a leukocyte. New vessels may begin to sprout toward the metastasis after 24 hours (213), and a tumor vascular network is visible at 4 days (105).

Organ Selection

Mechanisms of organ selection by metastases are being studied intensively (149, 167, 216). As mentioned earlier, some organs appear to be selected by a purely mechanical mechanism, simply because they drain the

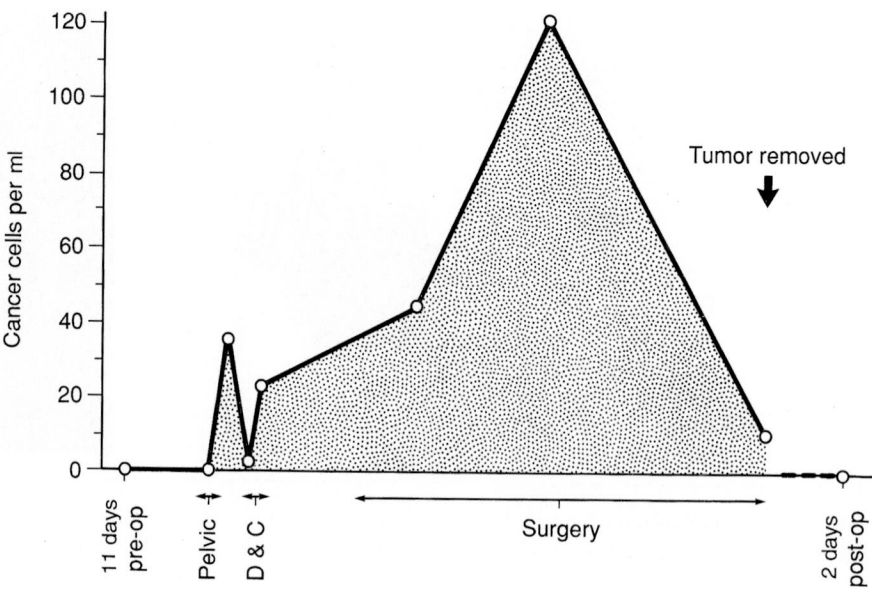

FIGURE 27.39   Number of cancer cells released into the blood by pelvic examination, cervical dilatation and curettage (D&C), and tumor resection. The patient suffered from an ovarian carcinoma. (Reproduced with permission from [166].)

blood of the primary tumor (such is the case of the liver as a target for metastases from the colon); more often, the selection is based on subtle properties of the seed and/or of the soil. However, it should not be forgotten that some bizarre localizations might still occur as random embolism by cells that have escaped capillary filters. By injecting microspheres intravenously it was shown that the lungs contain arteriovenous bypasses larger than 500 μm (136), and the same is true for other organs.

Several mechanisms of organ selection have been suggested.

Local injury. Selection of injured tissue is fairly easy to understand (142, 181). If mouse lungs are damaged by exposure to oxygen (1) or by activating complement, which leads to neutrophil-mediated injury (pp. 357, 447, 469) (144), tumor cells injected intravenously show greater retention in the lungs. Injury might also be produced by repeated tumor embolization (195). Whatever the cause of injury, it seems likely that exposed basement membranes would offer an easier foothold to the neoplastic cells (137). There are many examples of mechanical trauma as a localizing agent; in fact it has been proposed that the recurrence of a tumor in a postoperative scar is not necessarily the result of a surgical accident, as surgeons tend to think, but rather the effect of a biological, embolic event beyond surgical control (46, 61).

Chemotactic factors. Here is a perfect example. An international team tested the hypothesis that some organs secrete a specific chemokine into the blood, and cancer cells that carry the corresponding chemokine receptor will tend to home in those organs (129). It worked.

Breast cancer cells of varied sources expressed the receptor CXCR4 (normal breast tissue did not), and the corresponding chemokine CXCL12 was expressed in several organs commonly selected by breast cancer metastases: lymph nodes, bone marrow, and lung. In a mouse model of breast cancer, antibodies against CXCR4 significantly reduced metastases to regional lymph nodes and lung, suggesting that some day this mechanism might possibly be used for chemoprevention (102).

Chemotactic mediators exist or develop in target organs and affect various tumors (137). Some of these materials are breakdown products of matrix proteins (fibronectin, laminin, collagen, elastin, and bone) (216) and are generated by tumor-derived enzymes. The matrix can affect tumor cell adhesion in yet another way: endothelial cells, grown *in vitro* on a substrate that contains an extract of the stroma of a given organ, become particularly sticky for tumor cells that tend to home on that organ (149, 153).

Growth factors and growth inhibitors. Such factors contained in target organs may condition the take of a metastasis. For example, cells of prostatic carcinomas that reached the vertebrae via the Batson system grow faster there than in the primary tumor: they may be stimulated by a growth factor produced in bone marrow (216).

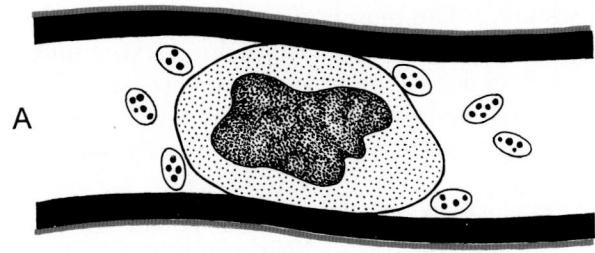

Tumor cell is arrested.

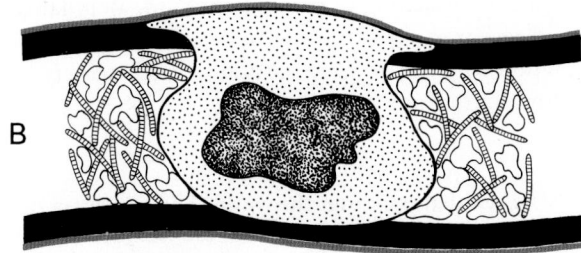

4-16 hours: thrombosis.
Endothelium is perforated.

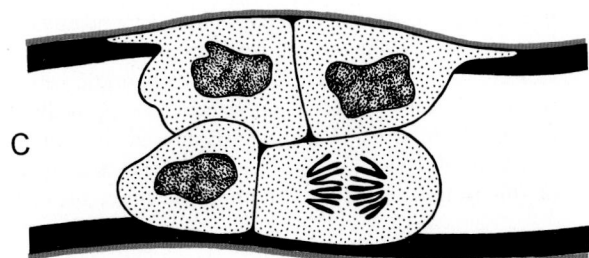

24-48 hours: tumor cells proliferate.

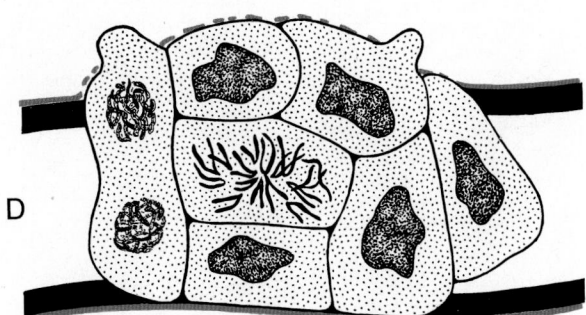

3-5 days: tumor nodule is formed.
Basement membrane is dissolving.

FIGURE 27.40   Steps in the arrest and extravasation of metastatic cancer cells; a scheme based on experimental findings. **A:** Initial arrest, with close (selective?) contact between tumor cell and endothelium; some platelets aggregate. **B:** Further platelet aggregation and formation of fibrin; separation of endothelial cells and contact between tumor cell and basement membrane. **C:** Lysis of platelet thrombus; intravascular proliferation of the tumor cells. **D:** Further expansion of the tumor mass; dissolution of the subendothelial basement membrane. Red line = Basement membrane. (Adapted with permission from [34].)

Surface recognition mechanisms. Tumor cells can come to a halt in selected organs by means of adhesion molecules, very much like leukocytes in inflammation (12, 16). The most obvious example is that of lymphoma cells, which metastasize to lymph nodes by means of the normal lymphocyte homing receptor, key to the normal lymphocyte recirculation (8, 146, 163). There is a mouse melanoma that ordinarily metastasizes to the lung; it also metastasizes into pieces of mouse fetal lung (but not of other tissues) implanted and revascularized in the thigh. This indicates that the metastatic cells "choose" the lung not only by a passive embolic process, but also by a selective mechanism (35) (Figure 27.41). Many studies have addressed this topic, both *in vitro* and *in vivo* (42, 149, 150). For example, it has been shown *in vitro* that activated human endothelium (obtained by exposure to IL-1, TNF, or endotoxin) is more adhesive for human melanoma cells (41, 164): an interesting link between inflammation and tumors. The preferential adhesion of metastatic cells to the endothelium of particular organs has been studied in several ways. An elegant approach has been to prepare endothelial monolayers from the microcirculation of mouse brain, lung, and ovary, and then expose them to dispersed cells from glioma, hepatoma, lymphoma, and other mouse tumors: some (alas not all) of the adhesion preferences coincided with known *in vivo* metastatic behavior of the tumors (7).

The intercellular adhesion molecule ICAM-1, which is involved in leukocyte adhesion, is absent on normal melanocytes and the cells of small melanomas that are thinner than the critical figure of 0.76 mm (p. 811) but present in most larger melanomas and their metastases (85). Now here is an attempt to exploit tumor adhesion molecules for therapy: knowing that laminin and fibronectin are involved in tumor cell adhesion and knowing that the specific sequences for their adhesive properties are repetitive structures such as Arg-Gly-Asp (RGD), synthetic polypeptides of the poly(RGD) type were

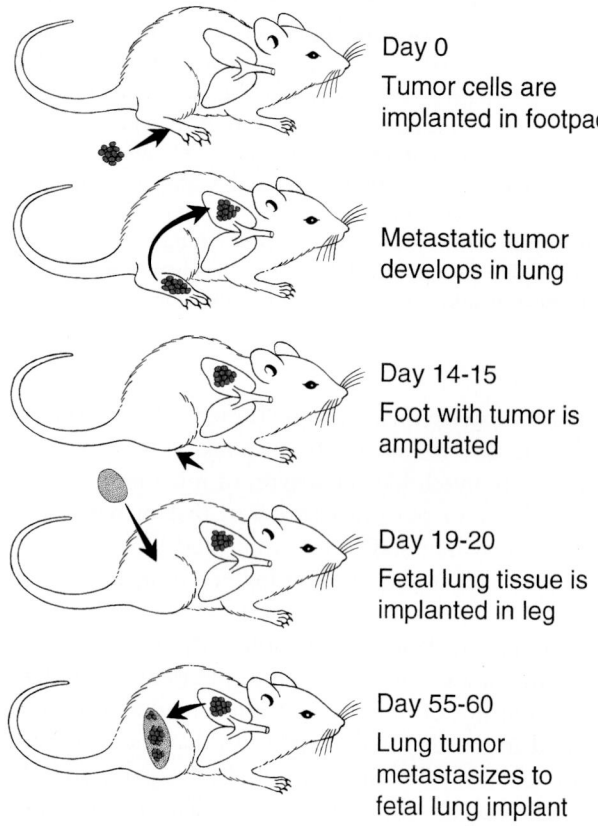

Day 0
Tumor cells are implanted in footpad

Metastatic tumor develops in lung

Day 14-15
Foot with tumor is amputated

Day 19-20
Fetal lung tissue is implanted in leg

Day 55-60
Lung tumor metastasizes to fetal lung implant

FIGURE 27.41   Experiment in the mouse to demonstrate that a tumor that usually metastasizes to the lung also metastasizes to fetal lung tissue (from a syngeneic animal) implanted intramuscularly in a thigh. This suggests that the metastatic preference for lung tissue is not based simply on the filtering mechanism of the lung but also on the nature of lung tissue. (From [36], Copyright © 1986 Alan R. Liss. Reprinted by permission of Wiley-Liss, Inc., a subsidiary of John Wiley & Sons, Inc.)

prepared: injected intravenously in mice they reduced the number of lung metastases, and *in vitro* they inhibited the adhesion of tumor cells to fibronectin substrates. The poly(RGD) molecules had blocked the tumor receptors (171).

The mechanisms involved in the expression of metastatic or antimetastatic genes are just beginning to be studied (92, 101, 109, 138, 216); a gene (*nm23*) that reduces metastatic potential has been identified in carcinomas of mice and humans (19); transfected into cells of a highly metastatic murine melanoma it reduced their ability to metastasize (99).

This whole discussion of metastases is based on the assumption that they derive from migrant cells. Conceivably, in the case of virus-induced tumors some secondary tumors could arise from the spread of the virus

itself (197). This must be kept in mind as a theoretical possibility (197). For example, in chickens infected with Rous sarcoma virus, wounds lead to tumor formation with a frequency near 100 percent (176), but these growths should be considered new primary tumors.

TO SUM UP: The successful metastatic cell that has completed its decathlon must be the result of a Darwinian selection process that has given it major advantages for growth and invasion over its nonmetastatic counterparts: appropriate receptors for attaching to the endothelium, abundance of receptors for extravascular matrix components, and the ability to produce and secrete a variety of matrix-degrading enzymes.

The cell that took over the world. The capacity of tumor cells to invade is even greater than can be appreciated with the microscope. It was October 4, 1951, when Henrietta Lacks died of a highly aggressive carcinoma of the cervix; from this tumor was obtained the first dependable line of human malignant cells. For all laboratories involved in cancer research, throughout the world, HeLa cells became an indispensable tool. The cells responded by overtaking—unnoticed—many other cell types that were being grown in culture. In 1968 the cell bank at the American Type Culture Collection, where samples of important cell cultures are preserved, had in its custody 34 supposedly different cell lines. Careful checking showed that 24 were HeLa cells (Figure 27.42) (72). The impact and the cost of this tumor-related catastrophe were never measured.

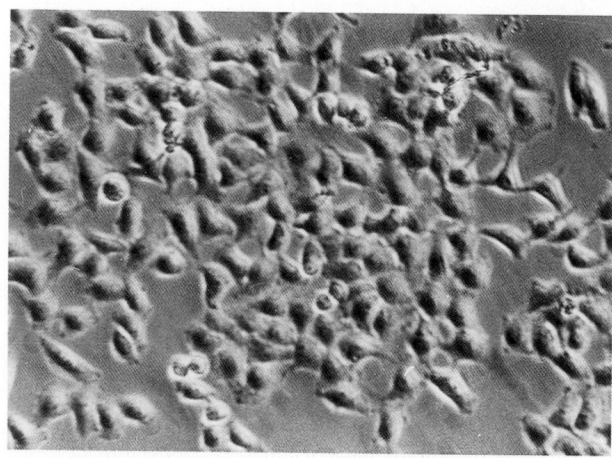

FIGURE 27.42   Culture of HeLa cells. (Courtesy of A. H. Cutler, University of Massachusetts Medical School, Worcester, MA.)

Effects of Tumors on the Host

All tumors are harmful to some degree, just by their bulk or by more subtle biological mechanisms. The harm can be local or distant.

Local Effects

Local effects are common even with benign tumors. Bulky lesions are especially hazardous in the skull, where space is limited and the anatomical structures are delicate. For example, cerebrospinal fluid produced in the cerebral ventricles flows through narrow passages; a small benign tumor, even a cyst, strategically located in one of these passages can obstruct the flow and cause one or all of the ventricles to dilate; the surrounding brain tissue shrinks accordingly (Figure 27.43). A small benign tumor of the hypophysis can bulge above the bony recess in which the hypophysis lies and damage the optic chiasm from which the optic nerves arise. Occlusion of a lumen can occur anywhere in the body when a tumor arises in a tubular or other hollow structure. Ulceration is another common effect of tumors bulging from a body surface (p. 760). The result is infection, bleeding, or both (the bleeding, however, can be clinically useful as a sign of a hidden tumor, e.g., of the bladder).

Some local effects are more subtle. The mucosa that surrounds cancers of the colon and rectum often shows

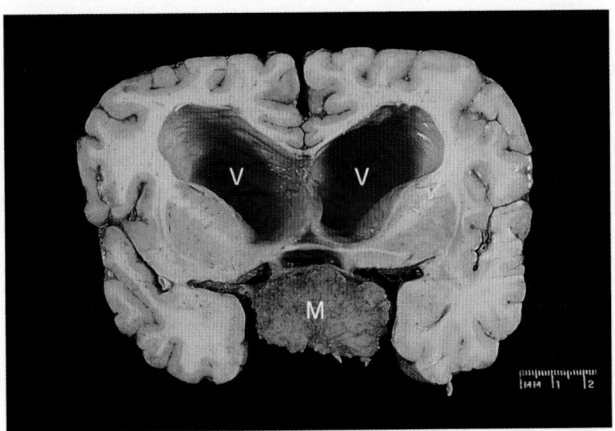

FIGURE 27.43 Example of damage caused by a benign tumor in the human brain. Most of the cerebrospinal fluid is produced in the lateral ventricles (**V**) and drains out through an aqueduct not visible here. Pressure by a meningioma (**M**) on the aqueduct has caused a dilatation of the lateral ventricles with corresponding atrophy of the cerebral tissue. **Scale** in centimeters. (Courtesy of Dr. T. W. Smith, University of Massachusetts Medical School, Worcester, MA.)

hyperplasia and angiogenesis, most likely due to factors secreted by the tumor (95); this reminds us of the many functional and structural effects of the tumor on its own stroma. When a malignant tumor invades the pleura it usually produces an effusion: this is attributed to vascular permeability factor/vascular endothelial growth factor (VPF/VEGF) generated by the tumor cells (214).

There is virtually no limit to the local trouble malignant tumors can cause. Because they can infiltrate, they can destroy tissues that are in their way; in the abdomen they can mat all the organs into a solid inextricable mass, constrict or erode any part of the gut, or cause fistulae (abnormal communications) between gut and skin, bladder and rectum, or any two hollow viscera. We have seen a colon cancer erode its way into the heart.

Distant Effects: The Paraneoplastic Syndromes

Tumors—benign or malignant—can produce remote effects by purely humoral mechanisms unrelated to invasion and metastasis. These provide a long list of symptom complexes observed in man and virtually all animal species (130). The variety is astounding: a tumor may come to the patient's attention disguised as rheumatoid arthritis (157), as a disease of an endocrine gland, of the skin, muscle, blood, or nervous system; even as ischemia of the fingers (187).

Tumor-derived hormones are only one of the mechanisms. It was realized in the 1960s that there is, beside hormones, a vast array of "humors from tumors" (81) capable of affecting every tissue in the body: cytokines, prostaglandins, enzymes, growth factors, and other polypeptides, not to mention antigens and molecules still unspecified (22). Today, the name *paraneoplastic syndrome* is given to all those symptom complexes that accompany tumors and concern distant targets (skin, nerves, muscle, blood, etc.) whether the mechanisms be hormonal, toxic, immunologic, or unknown. These syndromes usually disappear if the tumor is removed or destroyed, but some lesions are irreversible (e.g., in the nervous system). The two best known mechanisms are hormonal and immunologic.

How common are the paraneoplastic syndromes? This is difficult to establish from current data, but we have seen figures ranging from 7 to 50 percent of all cancer patients. Whatever their incidence, these syndromes must be kept in mind for practical reasons: they may be the first sign of a hidden cancer; they may mimic metastases; they may cause unnecessary discomfort; and they may help follow the regression or recurrence of the tumor.

Table 27.1 Selected Hormones Formed Ectopically and Their More Common Clinical Effects[a]

Tumor	Hormone	Symptoms	Biochemical
Small cell carcinoma of lung, pancreatic tumors	Antidiuretic hormone	Confusion, convulsions, coma	$\downarrow$ Na$^+$
Small cell carcinoma of lung, carcinoid, islet-cell carcinoma of pancreas, medullary thyroid carcinoma	Adrenocorticotrophic hormone or corticotrophin-releasing hormone	Proximal muscle weakness, polyuria, edema, pigmentation changes	$\downarrow$ K$^+$ $\uparrow$ Blood sugar
Multiple myeloma	Osteoclast activity factor		
Squamous cell carcinoma of lung, renal carcinoma, hepatoma	Parathyroid hormone	Constipation, polyuria, polydipsia, vomiting, psychosis, coma	$\uparrow$ Ca^{++}
Breast carcinoma	Prostaglandins		
Renal carcinoma, hepatoma, bronchogenic carcinoma, adrenal carcinoma	Human chorionic gonadotropin	Precocious puberty in boys, irregular menses	

[a]Very rare examples of the ectopic secretion by tumors of almost all nonsteroid hormones have been documented. Reproduced from (182).

Descriptions of a few common paraneoplastic syndromes follow (Table 27.1). The best known fall into six groups: endocrine, hematologic, gastrointestinal, renal, cutaneous, and neurologic. A few examples follow; details may be found in clinical texts (6).

Endocrine Disturbances

These are the best understood of all paraneoplastic syndromes. Nobody should be surprised to learn that a tumor of a parathyroid gland, benign or malignant, can produce hypercalcemia: this is in line with the function of the normal parathyroid. But then it was realized that many malignant tumors secrete hormones quite unrelated to the tissue of origin. On second thought, this too is not surprising: the genes for producing hormones are present in all cells; they just have to be turned on. Malignant tumors can be expected to do so.

This phenomenon is named *ectopic hormone secretion*. It is possible that all malignant tumors secrete ectopic hormones in small amounts (139, 140). The most common offenders are carcinomas of the lung: the standard explanation being that the lung derives from the endoderm, and therefore its carcinomas express genes that are activated in other endodermal derivatives such as the hypophysis or the parathyroids (134). *Paraneoplastic hypercalcemia* is found in 10–20 percent of cancer patients (81). But beware: tumors can produce hypercalcemia in many ways.

Hypercalcemia of neoplastic origin can be caused by: (a) parathyroid tumor; (b) extensive metastatic bone destruction such as occurs with multiple myeloma (the powerful osteolytic effect of this tumor is attributed to a cytokine named *osteoclast activating factor,* OAF) (67, 111); (c) a parathyroid-hormone-like peptide (21a); (d) prostaglandin E_2 (160, 179) (other prostaglandins are osteoblastic) (210); (e) tumor necrosis factor beta

(*lymphotoxin*); (f) interleukin-1 (124); (g) transforming growth factor alpha, which is also thought to play a role in the self-stimulation of tumor growth (22).

Hypocalcemia is actually more common than hypercalcemia as a paraneoplastic effect in patients with lytic (destructive) lesions of the skeleton (6).

The ectopic secretion of ACTH or of its precursor ("big ACTH" or pro-opiocortin) may lead to Cushing's syndrome: hypertension, weight loss, hypokalemia, hyperglycemia, muscle atrophy, and sometimes the typical "moon face" (81). Other classic associations are the bizarre production of insulin by mesotheliomas and sarcomas (22, 38) and of erythropoietin by renal cell carcinomas: the latter can produce a high hematocrit (above 55 for men and 50 for women) with resulting symptoms related to high blood viscosity (p. 687).

These hormone-related paraneoplastic syndromes are so common that they inspired an aphorism (100):

> If there is overproduction of a hormone, look for a tumor;
>
> If there is a tumor, look for evidence of hormone overproduction

Hematologic Disturbances

Hypercoagulable state. As many as 90–95 percent of cancer patients have been reported to have abnormalities of the clotting system (50, 56, 162, 170, 175): shortened clotting time, elevated fibrin/fibrinogen split products, elevated fibrinogen thrombocytosis. This is perhaps an overcompensation for a constant, low-grade intravascular coagulation (22).

The tendency to develop thrombosis in cases of cancer is attributed to four main mechanisms (19a, 112, 133, 148): (a) platelets are activated by tumor products such as ADP or by tumor-induced thrombin generation; (b) tumors secrete procoagulants such as tissue factor or factor X activators; they can also shed fibronectin (20) and other procoagulant materials from the cell surface (51); **the mucin secreted by adenocarcinomas is thrombogenic** (156, 165); (c) activated monocytes and macrophages in the tumor or in the RES secrete tissue factor and other procoagulants; (d) the liver secretes less anticoagulants such as antithrombin III and protein C (reasons unclear).

These abnormalities help understand the clinical thrombotic or hemorrhagic complications that occur in 9–15 percent of cancer patients (133). At autopsy, the number of thrombotic events found is even greater, especially in the form of thromboemboli. The four most important cardiovascular and hematologic complications of tumors are outlined below.

Migratory thrombophlebitis. The name refers to bouts of thrombophlebitis in multiple locations without an apparent predisposing factor such as bed rest or varicose veins. Back in the 1860s a great French clinician, Armand Trousseau, realized that this clinical sequence often reveals an underlying cancer, hence the current term *Trousseau's syndrome* (190). An occult cancer, especially of the pancreas, lung, or stomach, should be suspected in any case of thrombosis in an upper limb unrelated to trauma, or in cases of pulmonary embolism and deep venous thrombosis below the age of 50 (73, 165).

Trousseau's memorable passage reads as follows: "If you feel uncertain about the nature of a disease of the stomach, and hesitate between a chronic gastritis, a simple ulcer and a carcinoma, a *phlegmasia alba dolens* appearing in the leg or arm will dispel your indecision, and you will be permitted to take a positive stand regarding the existence of the cancer" (190). The Latin term *phlegmasia alba dolens* (literally *white painful inflammation*), still used by some physicians, refers to thrombophlebitis with pain and edema.

Nonbacterial thrombotic endocarditis. Marantic endocarditis (from *marasmus*, "wasting of the body") consists of small, warty-looking masses of platelets and fibrin, sometimes too small to be seen by echocardiography but large enough to throw emboli to the brain, kidney, and other viscera (Figure 27.44).

Microangiopathic hemolytic anemia. Microangiopathic hemolytic anemia is a peculiar but not uncommon situation in which red blood cells, forced to squeeze through tight places or fibrin meshes, break up or are sliced into smaller pieces called *schistocytes* or *helmet cells,* easily identified on smears; they seal up and continue to circulate for a few days (84).

Actually, not all the hazards facing the red blood cells in patients with malignant tumors are well understood (4). Several mechanisms of damage have been proposed: (a) narrow capillaries or intravascular fibrin strands within the tumor itself; (b) narrowing of pulmonary arterioles by embolized neoplastic cells and fibrin, which would explain the association with metastatic carcinoma (77); (c) the fibrin thrombi of DIC, the ultimate manifestation of hypercoagulability in cancer (p. 656). Massive "slicing" of red blood cells can occur in hemangiomas.

Anemia. Anemia is another classic complication of advanced cancer. Unlike microangiopathic anemia just mentioned, it is normocytic (the red blood cells are

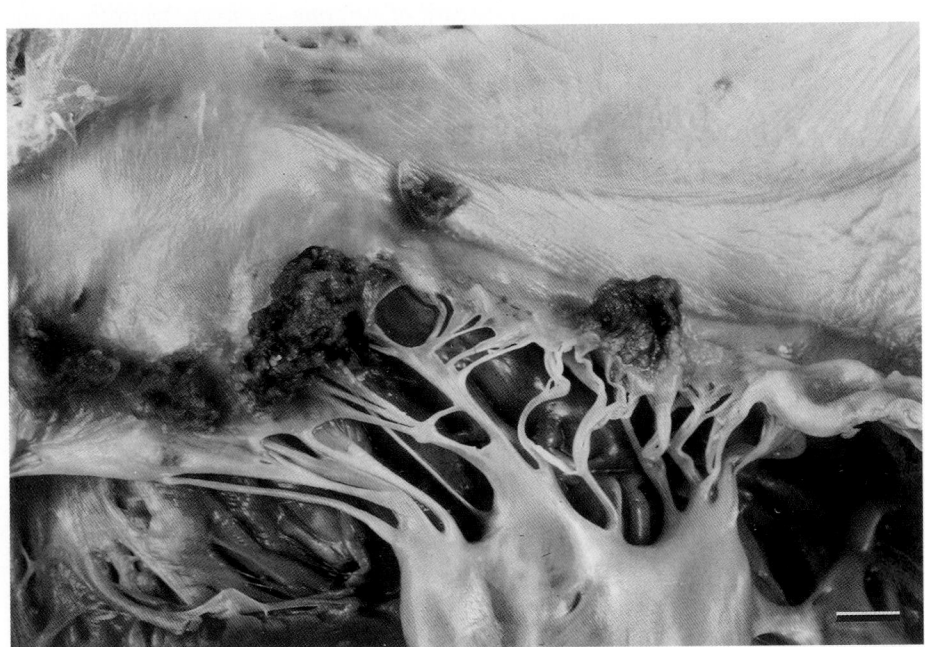

FIGURE 27.44 Thrombi on the mitral valve: an example of noninfective, "marantic" vegetations. The patient was a 46-year-old man who died of a mucin-producing gastric carcinoma, a known cause of hypercoagulability. **Bar** = 5 mm. (Courtesy of Dr. W. D. Edwards, Department of Laboratory Medicine and Pathology, The Mayo Clinic, Rochester, MN.)

normal in shape) as well as normochromic (the amount of hemoglobin per cell is normal). Long unexplained (10 mechanisms had been proposed) (22), anemia turns out to be another misdeed of cachectin/TNF (128), a cytokine that has a great deal to do with cancer patients (see further). The red blood cells are produced at a lower rate and have shorter life spans. Erythropoietin levels are also low (127).

Not to be forgotten are microcirculatory disturbances due to increased blood viscosity: renal cell tumors, for example, secrete erythropoietin, which stimulates bone marrow to produce excess red blood cells, whereby the viscosity of the blood is increased; leukemia can lead to leukocyte plugging of capillaries with similar consequences (p. 687).

> Other hematologic effects of cancers include granulocytosis related to the secretion of a colony-stimulating factor (CSF), granulocytopenia (due to an inhibitor?), thrombocytosis, and, paradoxically, thrombocytopenia, often related to therapy.

Gastrointestinal Syndromes

Protein-losing enteropathy. These patients typically suffer from cancer in some part of the gastrointestinal tract or from Hodgkin's disease; they lose excessive amounts of plasma protein from the gastrointestinal mucosa (the normal loss is about 10 percent) and develop hypoproteinemia, usually without drastic general symptoms (edema). The excessive loss is attributed to discrete cellular changes of the gastrointestinal mucosa or to lymphatic obstruction.

Renal Complications

The kidneys can be affected by distant tumors in many ways (Table 27.2) (147). Classic mechanisms of renal damage in tumor-bearing patients are: (a) glomerular damage caused by tumor antigens complexed with antibodies and deposited along the basement membrane (pp. 550, 553); (b) glomerular damage caused by amyloid deposits, in cases of multiple myeloma; (c) if severe hypercalcemia is present, it may lead to calcification of the renal parenchyma (nephrocalcinosis) (p. 256); (d) again in multiple myeloma, the tubules may become clogged with casts containing immunoglobulins and other proteins (31).

Skin Changes

Another long list, headed by *acanthosis nigricans,* a symmetric, brown, warty hyperpigmentation with hyperkeratosis of the axilla and other flexural areas (Figure 27.45). More than half of the cases represent the

Table 27.2　Renal Damage with Extrarenal Cancer: Study of 344 Malignant Tumors

Cancer	Number	Percentage
Lymphomas and leukemias	47	15.0
Multiple myeloma	10	3.1
Renal metastases (nonleukemia)	25	8.0
Hydronephrosis	18	5.7
Pyelonephritis	20	6.4
Acute tubular necrosis	44	14.0
Infarction	7	2.2
Disseminated intravascular coagulation	4	1.3
Nephrocalcinosis	9	2.9
Amyloid	6	1.9
Bence-Jones nephropathy	7	2.2
"Bile nephrosis"	10	3.2
Herpes with lymphoma	1	0.3
Glomerulonephritis	5	1.6
Radiation nephritis	1	0.3

Adapted from (147).

warning sign of an internal malignancy, especially a carcinoma of the gastrointestinal tract. Many of the cutaneous paraneoplastic syndromes are proliferative lesions, and growth factors have been implicated but not nailed down as causal agents (54).

Neurologic Disorders

Although rare, these paraneoplastic disorders have revealed a new facet of autoimmune disease (1). They can hit the nervous system almost anywhere, from the retina (83) to the cerebellum (49) or the spinal cord, but this is not how they really start. As a rule, *the patient is unaware of carrying a tumor, typically of the breast, ovary, or lung.* This tumor happens to express a gene that is normally expressed in some well-defined part of the nervous system, behind the blood-brain barrier. The immune system has never "seen" this protein; it reacts against it as if it were foreign, and floods the bloodstream with antibodies and cytotoxic T cells, which somehow reach behind the blood-brain barrier and destroy the tissue that expressed the fatal protein. Of course the reaction is also directed against the tumor, and so intensely that in a few recorded cases it is destroyed (37).

Miscellaneous Effects

Strange but not rare is the bizarre clubbing of the fingers called hypertrophic pulmonary osteopathy when the bone is also thickened. Finger clubbing is known in French as *hippocratisme digital* because it is mentioned in the Hippocratic books as a condition associated with chronic pulmonary disease (Figure 27.46): the

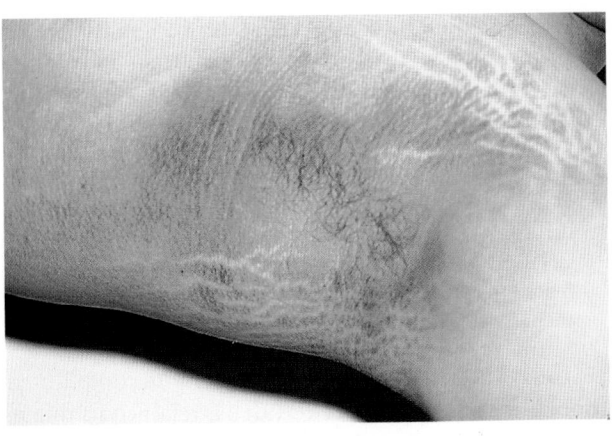

FIGURE 27.45 Velvety, brown-black, excessively cornified (hyperkeratotic) plaques of *acanthosis nigricans* in the armpit of an obese 21-year-old man. This lesion, which tends to develop in skin folds, may accompany malignancy as well as obesity, diabetes, and other conditions. (Courtesy of Drs. E. Gonzalez and J. D. Bernhard, University of Massachusetts Medical School, Worcester, MA.)

association is perfectly correct and today we include cancer, but the pathogenesis remains a frustrating mystery (22). Low serum albumin affects over 90 percent of cancer patients: it is probably a part of the acute phase response (p. 505) caused by the release of TNF by tumor macrophages.

Cachexia

Wasting of the whole body is the ultimate paraneoplastic syndrome. Its ancient name, from a Greek word for "being in a bad way," echoes the dread of malignant tumors, which can reduce the body to skin and bones. It affects most cancer patients, especially those with cancer of the stomach and pancreas. Anorexia plays a key role, together with a loss of the sense of taste (47); we recall a starved-looking patient with a cancer of the pancreas, contemplating a tasty meal and sadly stating that "he saw no reason to eat it." The two main theories to explain cachexia before 1986 were the following: (a) *Tumors produce some sort of toxin.* Perhaps they do, but research on "toxohormones" has attracted little interest (121, 131, 183). (b) *The tumor acts as a "nitrogen trap,"* i.e., it traps the nutrients and starves the host. This is too simplistic, and anyway, overfeeding does not cure cachexia (55).

Then, as so often happens, a new insight burst on the scene, from a wholly "unrelated" line of research.

Dr. Anthony Cerami of Rockefeller University was interested in therapy for sleeping sickness, which affects both humans and cattle in parts of Africa. Field observations in Africa led him to observe the profound cachexia of the affected cattle, a condition that contrasted with the small number of circulating trypanosomes (Figure 27.47). Back in New York, in 1980, Rouzer and Cerami chose to study the mechanism of cachexia in rabbits infected with

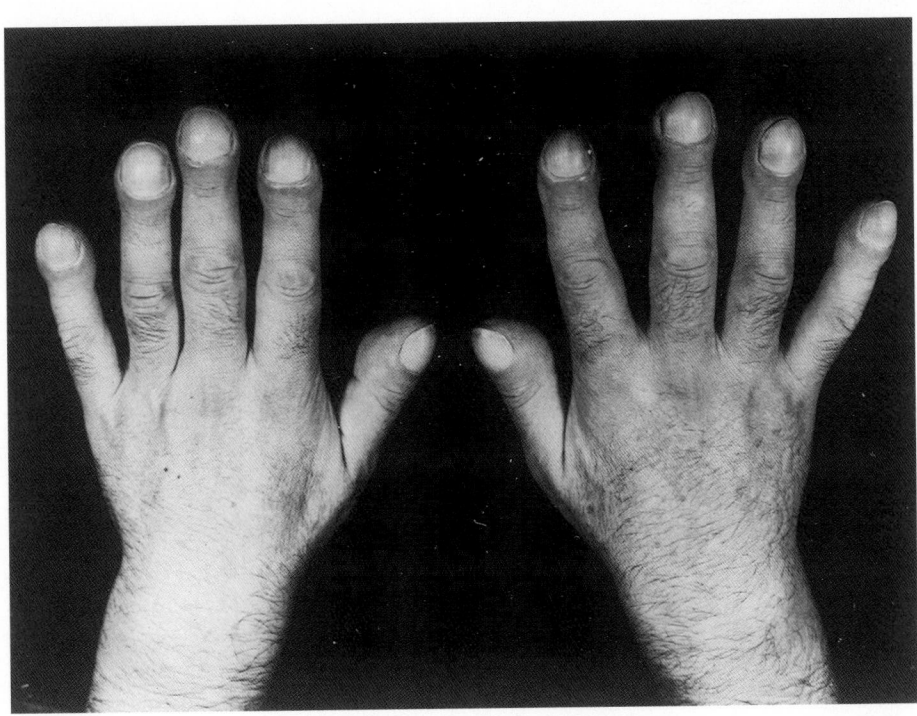

FIGURE 27.46 Clubbing of the fingers: a peculiar consequence of chronic lung disease, including cancer. The mechanism is not well understood. (Reproduced with permission from [69].)

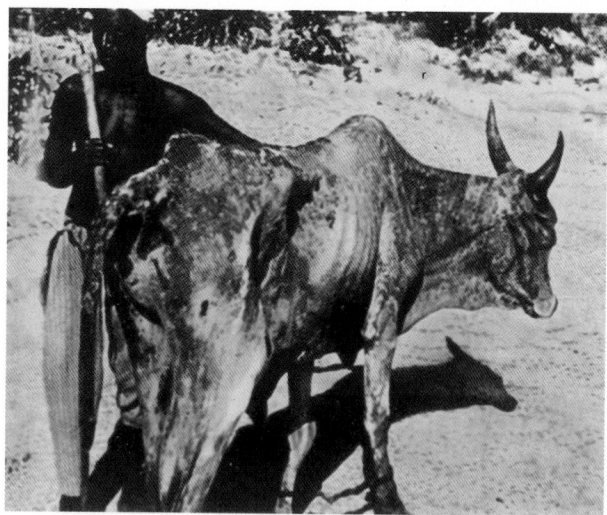

FIGURE 27.47   In parts of Africa sleeping sickness affects cattle and humans. This extreme cachexia contrasts sharply with the small number of trypanosomes in the blood of these animals. In tracking the mechanism of this cachexia, Dr. Anthony Cerami and collaborators discovered "cachexin," which turned out to be tumor necrosis factor. (Courtesy of the Wellcome Foundation, Inc., London, England, and of Dr. A. Cerami, Rockefeller University, New York, NY.)

trypanosoma: the rabbits lost 50 percent of their weight, yet they too had very few parasites in the blood and mild internal lesions. Curiously, the blood became intensely lipemic, suggesting a defect in the degradation of triglycerides. It was concluded that the cachexia reflected an exaggerated host response, rather than a virulent aggression by the parasite. A further study on mice made cachectic with injections of endotoxin showed that cachexia was associated with inhibition of lipoprotein lipase (91). Using this inhibition as a guide, the researchers isolated, from the blood of the mice, a protein which they called cachectin. When they sequenced it—surprise!—it turned out to be identical to the recently isolated TNF, tumor necrosis factor, a product of macrophages (18). Antibodies against TNF reduced the cachexia in tumor-bearing mice (178).

Today the story has become much more complicated (does it ever do otherwise?). TNF has retained its role in cachexia and even its alternative name, *cachectin*. As we have seen in an earlier chapter, it has also become a key player in septic shock. But as regards cachexia it has come to share the guilt with other cytokines, mainly IL-1 and IL-6 (5, 189), while other cytokines have turned out to be anti-cachectic—mainly IL-4, IL-10, and IL-13. In the meantime, we have learned a few other essential facts: there are major differences between starvation and cachexia. Starvation mobilizes mainly fat and spares skeletal muscle. Cachexia draws on both (21). Cachexia shrinks muscle by at least two mechanisms: the ubiquitin-proteasome pathway is activated (33), and current research in mice suggests that the hormone **myostatin** is also involved (217). Cattle breeders had long been familiar with this hormone, indirectly, because its absence generates *double-muscled cattle;* myostatin knockout mice develop a huge muscle mass (217).

How Does Cancer Kill?

Statistics are few, but by comparing four sources ranging from 1971 to 2001 (3, 82, 94, 174), a few salient points emerge.

- *Infection* is at the top of the list; in the three earlier studies, it accounts for 32, 36, and 47 percent of the deaths. This fits with the anti-inflammatory nature of both cancer and anticancer therapy. *The microorganisms change:* in the 1960s–1970s, gram-negative microorganisms predominated; in the 1970s–1980s, gram-positive microorganisms took over; today filamentous fungi are a major threat, especially in patients with prolonged neutropenia (174). *The portal of entry is often gastrointestinal:* the mucosa of the gastrointestinal tract is damaged by chemotherapy and radiation, so that bacteria can escape into the intestinal wall and beyond. Mucosal injury is followed by loss of the antibacterial agents secreted by various cells, including the epithelium (lactoferrin, lysozyme, phospholipase A$_2$, defensins) (174).

- *Hemorrhage and thromboembolic phenomena* accounted for 10–20 percent of all cancer deaths in the three earlier studies. Hemorrhage alone was a significant cause of death only in acute leukemia.

- *Cachexia* was not given a major role (1 percent of deaths in the first series). The remaining deaths were attributed to respiratory failure, renal failure and sundry causes.

Tumors can also kill when the die—if they die by the **tumor lysis syndrome.** We mentioned this phenomenon in relation to cell death (p. 227). In essence, if a tumor is very sensitive to chemo- or radiotherapy, it may die suddenly and massively under treatment, and release life-threatening amounts of potassium (which can cause a fatal arrhythmia) and of phosphate (which can lead to renal failure). The larger the tumor, the greater is the danger. Burkitt's lymphoma is often involved (p. 872). Dialysis may be required, but fortunately the condition is limited to 5–7 days because the wave of cell death comes to an end (30, 31).

TO SUM UP: We have reviewed the aggressive behavior of tumor cells; how does it compare with that of conventional parasites? There are definite similarities; both multiply, both can infiltrate locally, both can spread by invading blood and lymphatic vessels, and both tend to kill the host. There is one major difference. Professional parasites inherit their aggressive tools shaped by millions of years of evolutionary experience. Tumor cells cannot learn or improve their performance by experience, because every tumor dies with its host. For this we should be grateful.

References

1. Albert ML, Darnell JC, Bender A, et al. Tumor-specific killer cells in paraneoplastic cerebellar degeneration. Nat Med 1998; 4:1321–1324.

2. Alexander P. The biology of metastases. In: Carney D, Sikora K, eds. Genes and cancer. Chichester: John Wiley & Sons, 1990, pp. 313–328.

3. Ambrus JL, Ambrus CM, Mink IB, Pickren JW. Causes of death in cancer patients. J Med 1975;6:61–64.

4. Antman KH, Skarin AT, Mayer RJ, Hargreaves HK, Canellos GP. Microangiopathic hemolytic anemia and cancer: a review. Medicine 1979;58:377–384.

5. Argilés JM, López-Soriano FJ. The role of cytokines in cancer cachexia. Med Res Rev 1999;19:223–248.

6. Arnold SM, Lowy AM, Patchell R, Foon KA. Paraneoplastic syndromes. In: DeVita VT Jr, Hellman S, Rosenberg SA (eds). Cancer: principles & practice of oncology, 6th ed. Philadelphia: Lippincott Williams & Wilkins. 2001, pp. 2511–2536.

7. Auerbach R, Lu WC, Pardon E, et al. Specificity of adhesion between murine tumor cells and capillary endothelium: an *in vitro* correlate of preferential metatasis *in vivo*. Cancer Res 1987;47:1492–1496.

8. Azzarelli B, Easterling K, Norton JA. Leukemic cell-endothelial cell interactions in leukemic cell dissemination. Lab Invest 1989;60:45–64.

9. Babai F, Tremblay G. Ultrastructural study of liver invasion by Novikoff hepatoma. Cancer Res 1972;32:2765–2770.

10. Balch CM, Murad TM, Soong SJ, et al. A multifactorial analysis of melanoma: prognostic histopathological features comparing Clark's and Breslow's staging methods. Ann Surg 1978;188:732–742.

11. Balch CM, Soong SJ, Murad TM, Ingalls AL, Maddox WA. A multifactorial analysis of melanoma. II. Prognostic factors in patients with stage I (localized) melanoma. Surgery 1979;86: 343–351.

12. Bani MR, Giavazzi R. Invasion and metastasis. In: Bronchud MH, Foote M, Peters WP, Robinson MO (eds). Principles of molecular oncology. Totowa, NJ: Humana Press 2001, pp. 297–321.

13. Barsky SH, Rao CN, Hyams D, Liotta LA. Characterization of a laminin receptor from human breast cacinoma tissue. Breast Cancer Res Treat 1984;4:181–188.

14. Batson OV. The function of the vertebral veins and their rôle in the spread of metastases. Ann Surg 1940;112:138–149.

15. Batson OV. The vertebral vein system. Am J Roentgenol Radium Ther Nucl Med 1957;78:195–212.

16. Belloni PN, Tressler RJ. Microvascular endothelial cell heterogeneity: interactions with leukocytes and tumor cells. Cancer Metastasis Rev 1989/90;8:353–389.

17. Bergers G, Coussens LM. Extrinsic regulators of epithelial tumor progression metalloproteinases. Curr Opin Genet & Dev 2000;10:120–127.

18. Beutler B, Cerami A. Cachectin and tumour necrosis factor as two sides of the same biological coin. Nature 1986;320: 584–588.

19. Bevilacqua G, Sobel ME, Liotta LA, Steeg PS. Association of low nm23 RNA levels in human primary infiltrating ductal breast carcinomas with lymph node involvement and other histopathological indicators of high metastatic potential. Cancer Res 1989;49:5185–5190.

19a. Bick RL. Cancer-associated thrombosis. N Engl J Med 2003; 349:109–111.

20. Black PH. Shedding from normal and cancer-cell surfaces. N Engl J Med 1980;303:1415–1416.

21. Body J-J. Metabolic sequelae of cancers (excluding bone marrow transplantation). Curr Opin Clin Nutr Metab Care 1999; 2:339–344.

21a. Broadus AE, Mangin M, Ikeda K, et al. Humoral hypercalcemia of cancer. Identification of a novel parathyroid hormone-like peptide. N Engl J Med 1988;319:556–563.

22. Bunn PA Jr, Ridgway EC. Paraneoplastic syndromes. In: DeVita VT Jr, Hellman S, Rosenberg SA, eds. Cancer: principles & practice of oncology, 3rd ed. Philadelphia: JB Lippincott, 1989, pp. 1896–1940.

23. Butler TP, Gullino PM. Quantitation of cell shedding into efferent blood of mammary adenocarcinoma. Cancer Res 1975; 35:512–516.

24. Calman KC. Clinical aspects of invasion. In: Mareel MM, Calman KC, eds. Invasion: experimental and clinical implications. Oxford: Oxford University Press, 1984, pp. 1–23.

25. Carr I, Carr J, Dreher B. Lymphatic metastasis of mammary adenocarcinoma. An experimental study in the rat with a brief review of the literature. Invasion Metastasis 1981;1: 34–53.

26. Carr I, McGinty F. Lymphatic metastasis and its inhibition: an experimental model. J Pathol 1973;113:85–95.

27. Carr I, McGinty F, Norris P. The fine structure of neoplastic invasion: invasion of liver, skeletal muscle and lymphatic vessels by the Rd/3 tumour. J Pathol 1976;118:91–99.

28. Catlin EA, Roberts DJ, Erana R, et al. Transplacental transmission of natural-killer-cell lymphoma. N Engl J Med 1999; 341:85–91.

29. Chew EC, Josephson RL, Wallace AC. Morphologic aspects of the arrest of circulating cancer cells. In: Weiss L, ed. Fundamental aspects of metastasis. Amsterdam: North Holland Publishing Company, 1976, 121–150.

30. Cohen LF, Balow JE, Magrath IT, Poplack DG, Ziegler JL. Acute tumor lysis syndrome. A review of 37 patients with Burkitt's lymphoma. Am J Med 1980;68:486–491.

31. Cohen AH, Border MD. Myeloma kidney. An immunomorphogenetic study of renal biopsies. Lab Invest 1980;42:248.

32. Coman DR, deLong RP. The role of the vertebral venous system in the metastasis of cancer to the spinal column. Experiments with tumor-cell suspensions in rats and rabbits. Cancer 1951;4:610–618.

33. Combaret L, Rallière C, Taillandier D, Tanaka K, Attaix D. Manipulation of the ubiquitin-proteasome pathway in cachexia: pentoxifylline suppresses the activation of 20S and 26S proteasomes in muscles from tumor-bearing rats. Mol Biol Rep 1999;26:95–101.

33a. Condeelis J, Segall JE. Intravital imaging of cell movement in tumours. Nat Rev Cancer 2003;3:921–930.

34. Crissman JD, Hatfield JS, Menter DG, Sloane B, Honn KV. Morphological study of the interaction of intravascular tumor cells with endothelial cells and subendothelial matrix. Cancer Res 1988;48:4065–4072.

35. Crissman JD, Hatfield JS, Schaldenbrand M, Sloane BF, Honn KV. Arrest and extravasation of B16 amelanotic melanoma in murine lungs. A light and electron microscopic study. Lab Invest 1985a;53:470–478.

36. Crissman JD, Hatfield JS, Honn KV. Clinical and experimental morphologic parameters predictive of tumor metastasis. Prog Clin Biol Res 1986;212:251–265.

37. Darnell RB. Onconeural antigens and the paraneoplastic neurologic disorders: at the intersection of cancer, immunity, and the brain. Proc Natl Acad Sci USA 1996;93:4529–4536.

38. Daughaday WH, Emanuele MA, Brooks MH, et al. Synthesis and secretion of insulin-like growth factor II by a leiomyosarcoma with associated hypoglycemia. N Engl J Med 1988;319: 1434–1440.

39. De Bruyn PPH, Cho Y. Entry of metastatic malignant cells into the circulation from a subcutaneously growing myelogenous tumor. J Natl Cancer Inst 1979;62:1221–1227.

40. De Bruyn PPH, Cho Y. Vascular endothelial invasion via transcellular passage by malignant cells in the primary stage of metastases formation. J Ultrastruct Res 1982;81: 189–201.

41. Dejana E, Bertocchi F, Bortolami MC, et al. Interleukin 1 promotes tumor cell adhesion to cultured human endothelial cells. J Clin Invest 1988;82:1466–1470.

42. Dejana E, Martin-Padura I, Lauri D, et al. Endothelial leukocyte adhesion molecule-1-dependent adhesion of colon carcinoma cells to vascular endothelium is inhibited by an antibody to Lewis fucosylated type I carbohydrate chain. Lab Invest 1992;66:324–330.

43. del Regato JA. Pathways of metastatic spread of malignant tumors. Semin Oncol 1977;4:33–38.

44. del Regato J. Physiopathology of metastasis. In: Weiss L, Gilbert HA, eds. Pulmonary metastasis. Boston: GK Hall & Co, 1978, pp. 104–113.

45. de Ridder L, Mareel M, Vakaet L. Invasion of malignant cells into cultured embryonic substrates. Arch Geschwulstforsch 1977;47:7–27.

46. DerHagopian RP, Sugarbaker EV, Ketcham A. Inflammatory oncotaxis. JAMA 1978;240:374–375.

47. DeWys WD. Anorexia as a general effect of cancer. Cancer 1979;43:2013–2019.

48. Dingemans KP, Roos E, van den Bergh Weerman MA, van de Pavert IV. Invasion of liver tissue by tumor cells and leukocytes: comparative ultrastructure. J Natl Cancer Inst 1978;60: 583–598.

49. Dropcho EJ, Whitaker JN. Cerebellar ataxia as a paraneoplastic syndrome. Hosp Pract 1989;24:69–84.

50. Dvorak HF. Thrombosis and cancer. Hum Pathol 1987;18: 275–284.

51. Dvorak HF, Quay SC, Orenstein NS, et al. Tumor shedding and coagulation. Science 1981;212:923–924.

52. Egeblad M, Werb Z. New functions for the matrix metalloproteinases in cancer progression. Nat Rev Cancer 2002;2: 161–174.

53. Eilon G, Mundy GR. Direct resorption of bone by human breast cancer cells in vitro. Nature 1978;276:726–728.

54. Ellis DL, Kafka SP, Chow JC, et al. Melanoma, growth factors, acanthosis nigricans, the sign of Leser-Trélat, and multiple acrochordons. A possible role for alpha-transforming growth factor in cutaneous paraneoplastic syndromes. N Engl J Med 1987;317:1582–1587.

55. Evans WK, Makuch R, Clamon GH, et al. Limited impact of total parenteral nutrition on nutritional status during treatment for small cell lung cancer. Cancer Res 1985;45: 3347–3353.

56. Falanga A, Donati MB. Pathogenesis of thrombosis in patients with malignancy. Int J Hematol 2001;73:137–144.

57. Fidler IJ. Metastasis: quantitative analysis of distribution and fate of tumor emboli labeled with ^{125}I-5-Iodo-2′-deoxyuridine. J Natl Cancer Inst 1970;45:773–782.

58. Fidler IJ. Introduction. Ciba Found Symp 1988;141:1–4.

59. Fidler IJ, Gersten DM, Hart IR. The biology of cancer invasion and metastasis. Adv Cancer Res 1978;28:149–250.

60. Finkel E. Potential target found for antimetastasis drugs. Science 1999;285:33–34.

61. Fisher B, Fisher ER, Feduska N. Trauma and the localization of tumor cells. Cancer 1967;20:23–30.

62. Folkman J. Angiogenesis in cancer, vascular, rheumatoid and other disease. Nature Med 1995;1:27–31.

63. Gabbert H, Gerharz CD, Ramp U, Bohl J. The nature of host tissue destruction in tumor invasion. An experimental investigation on carcinoma and sarcoma xenotransplants. Virchows Arch Cell Pathol 1987;52:513–527.

64. Galasko CSB. The anatomy and pathways of skeletal metastases. In: Weiss L, Gilbert HA, eds. Bone metastasis. Boston: GK Hall Medical Publishers, 1981.

65. Galasko CSB, Bennett A. Relationship of bone destruction in skeletal metastases to osteoclast activation and prostaglandins. Nature 1976;263:508–510.

66. Garbisa S, Pozzatti R, Muschel RJ, et al. Secretion of type IV collagenolytic protease and metastatic phenotype: induction by

transfection with c-Ha-*ras* but not c-Ha-*ras* plus Ad2-E1a. Cancer Res 1987;47:1523–1528.

67. Garrett IR, Durie BGM, Nedwin GE, et al. Production of lymphotoxin, a bone-resorbing cytokine, by cultured human myeloma cells. N Engl J Med 1987;317:526–532.

68. Gasic GJ. Role of plasma, platelets, and endothelial cells in tumor metastasis. Cancer Metastasis Rev 1984;3:99–116.

69. Ginsburg J. Clubbing of the fingers. In: Hamilton WF, Dow P, eds. Handbook of physiology, sect 2, vol III. Washington, DC: American Physiological Society, 1965, pp. 2377–2389.

70. Glaves D. Detection of circulating metastatic cells. Prog Clin Biol Res 1986;212:151–165.

71. Glaves D, Huben RP, Weiss L. Haematogenous dissemination of cells from human renal adenocarcinomas. Br J Cancer 1988;57:32–35.

72. Gold M. A conspiracy of cells. Albany, NY: State University of New York Press, 1986.

73. Goldberg RJ, Seneff M, Gore JM, et al. Occult malignant neoplasm in patients with deep venous thrombosis. Arch Intern Med 1987;147:251–253.

74. Gullino PM. *In vivo* release of neoplastic cells by mammary tumors. GANN Monogr Cancer Res 1977;20:49–55.

75. Gullino PM. Influence of blood supply on thermal properties and metabolism of mammary carcinomas. Ann NY Acad Sci 1980;335:1–21.

76. Heppner KJ, Matrisian LM, Jensen RA, Rodgers WH. Expression of most matrix metalloproteinase family members in breast cancer represents a tumor-induced host response. Am J Pathol 1996;149:273–282.

77. Hilgard P, Gordon-Smith EC. Microangiopathic haemolytic anaemia and experimental tumour-cell emboli. Br J Haematol 1974;26:651–659.

78. Hirohashi S. Inactivation of the E-cadherin-mediated cell adhesion system in human cancers. Am J Pathol 1998;153:333–339.

79. Hoover HC, Ketcham AS. Metastasis of metastases. Am J Surg 1975;130:405–411.

80. Ibbotson KJ, Twardzik DR, D'Souza SM, et al. Stimulation of bone resorption in vitro by synthetic transforming growth factor-alpha. Science 1985;228:1007–1009.

81. Ihde DC. Paraneoplastic syndromes. Hosp Pract 1987;22:105–124.

82. Inagaki J, Rodriguez V, Bodey GP. Causes of death in cancer patients. Cancer 1974;33:568–573.

83. Jacobson DM, Thirkill CE, Tipping SJ. A clinical triad to diagnose paraneoplastic retinopathy. Ann Neurol 1990;28:162–167.

84. Jandl JH. Blood. Boston: Little, Brown, 1987.

85. Johnson JP, Stade BG, Holzmann B, Schwäble W, Riethmüller H. *De novo* expression of intercellular-adhesion molecule 1 in melanoma correlates with increased risk of metastasis. Proc Natl Acad Sci USA 1989;86:641–644.

86. Jones DS, Wallace AC, Fraser EE. Sequence of events in experimental metastases of Walker 256 tumor: light, immuno-fluorescent, and electron microscopic observations. J Natl Cancer Inst 1971;46:493–504.

87. Kalebic T, Williams JE, Talmadge JE, et al. A novel method for selection of invasive tumor cells: derivation and character-

ization of highly metastatic K1735 melanoma cell lines based on *in vitro* and *in vivo* invasive capacity. Clin Exp Metastasis 1988;6:301–318.

88. Karkkainen M, Mäkinen T, Alitalo K. Lymphatic endothelium: a new frontier of metastasis research. Nat Cell Biol 2002;4:E2–E5.

89. Karpatkin S, Pearlstein E. Role of platelets in tumor cell metastases. Ann Intern Med 1981;95:636–641.

90. Kawaguchi T, Nakamura K. Analysis of the lodgement and extravasation of tumor cells in experimental models of hematogenous metastasis. Cancer Metastasis Rev 1986;5:77–94.

91. Kawakami M, Cerami A. Studies of endotoxin-induced decrease in lipoprotein lipase activity. J Exp Med 1981;154:631–639.

92. Kerbel RS. Growth dominance of the metastatic cancer cell: cellular and molecular aspects. Adv Cancer Res 1990;55:87–132.

93. Kinjo M. Lodgement and extravasation of tumour cells in blood-borne metastasis: an electron microscope study. Br J Cancer 1978;38:293–301.

94. Klastersky J. Daneau D, Verhest A. Causes of death in patients with cancer. Eur J Cancer 1972;8:149–154.

95. Kuniyasu H, Yasui W, Shinohara H, et al. Induction of angiogenesis by hyperplastic colonic mucosa adjacent to colon cancer. Am J Pathol 2000;157:1523–1535.

96. Kurokawa Y. Experiments on lymph node metastasis by intralymphatic inoculation of rat ascites tumor cells, with special reference to lodgment, passage, and growth of tumor cells in lymph nodes. GANN 1970;61:461–471.

97. Larsen MP, Steinberg GD, Brendler CB, Epstein JI. Use of *Ulex europaeus* agglutinin I (UEAI) to distinguish vascular and "pseudovascular" invasion in transitional cell carcinoma of bladder with lamina propria invasion. Mod Pathol 1990;3:83–88.

98. Lasser A, Zacks SI. Intraskeletal myofiber metastasis of breast carcinoma. Hum Pathol 1982;13:1045–1046.

99. Leone A, Flatow U, King CR, et al. Reduced tumor incidence, metastatic potential, and cytokine responsiveness of nm23-transfected melanoma cells. Cell 1991;65:25–35.

100. Liddle GW, Ball JH. Manifestations of cancer mediated by ectopic hormones. In: Holland JF, Frei E III, eds. Cancer medicine. Philadelphia: Lea & Febiger, 1973, pp. 1046–1057.

101. Liotta LA. Cancer cell invasion and metastasis. Sci Am 1992;266:54–63.

102. Liotta LA. An attractive force in metastasis. Nature 2001;410:24–25.

103. Liotta LA, Garbisa S, Tryggvason K. Biochemical mechanisms involved in tumor cell penetration of the basement membrane. In: Liotta LA, Hart IR, eds. Tumor invasion and metastasis. The Hague: Martinus Nijhoff Publishers, 1982, pp. 319–333.

104. Liotta LA, Guirguis RA, Schiffman E. Tumor autocrine motility factor. Prog Clin Biol Res 1986;212:17–22.

105. Liotta LA, Kleinerman J, Saidel GM. Quantitative relationships of intravascular tumor cells, tumor vessels, and pulmonary metastases following tumor implantation. Cancer Res 1974;34:997–1004.

106. Liotta LA, Kleinerman J, Saidel GM. The significance of hematogenous tumor cell clumps in the metastatic process. Cancer Res 1976;36:889–894.

107. Liotta LA, Mandler R, Murano G, et al. Tumor cell autocrine motility factor. Proc Natl Acad Sci USA 1986;83:3302–3306.

108. Liotta LA, Rao CN, Wewer UM. Biochemical interactions of tumor cells with the basement membrane. Annu Rev Biochem 1986;55:1037–1057.

109. Liotta LA, Steeg PS. Clues to the function of Nm23 and Awd proteins in development, signal transduction, and tumor metastasis provided by studies of *Dictyostelium discoideum.* J Natl Cancer Inst 1990;82:1170–1172.

110. Liotta LA, Wewer U, Rao NC, et al. Biochemical mechanisms of tumor invasion and metastasis. Anti-Cancer Drug Design 1987;2:195–202.

111. Luben RA. An assay for osteoclast-activating factor (OAF) in biological fluids: detection of OAF in the serum of myeloma patients. Cell Immunol 1980;49:74–80.

112. Luzzatto G, Schafer AI. The prethrombotic state in cancer. Semin Oncol 1990;17:147–159.

113. Luzzi KJ, MacDonald IC, Schmidt EE, et al. Multistep nature of metastatic inefficiency. Am J Pathol 1988;153:865–873.

114. Manishen WJ, Sivananthan K, Orr FW. Resorbing bone stimulates tumor cell growth. A role for the host microenvironment in bone metastasis. Am J Pathol 1986;123:39–45.

115. Mareel MM. Is invasiveness in vitro characteristic of malignant cells? Cell Biol Int Rep 1979;3:627–640.

116. Mareel MM. Recent aspects of tumor invasiveness. Int Rev Exp Pathol 1980;22:65–129.

117. Mareel MM, Bruyneel E, Storme G. Attachment of mouse fibrosarcoma cells to precultured fragments of embryonic chick heart. An early step of invasion in vitro. Virchows Arch B Cell Pathol 1980;34:85–97.

118. Mareel MM, De Baetselier P, Van Roy FM. Mechanisms of invasion and metastasis. Boca Raton, FL: CRC Press, 1991.

119. Mareel MM, De Bruyne GK, Vandesande F, Dragonetti C. Immunohistochemical study of embryonic chick heart invaded by malignant cells in three-dimensional culture. Invasion Metastasis 1981;1:195–204.

120. Mareel MM, Van Roy FM, De Baetselier P. The invasive phenotypes. Cancer Metastasis Rev 1990;9:45–62.

121. Masuno H, Yoshimura H, Ogawa N, Okuda H. Isolation of a lipolytic factor (toxohormone-L) from ascites fluid of patients with hepatoma and its effect on feeding behavior. Eur J Cancer Clin Oncol 1984;20:1177–1185.

122. McDonald DF, Schofield BH, Prezioso EM, et al. Direct bone resorbing activity of murine myeloma cells. Cancer Lett 1983;19:119–124.

123. Méhes G, Witt A, Kubista E, Ambros PF. Circulating breast cancer cells are frequently apoptotic. Am J Pathol 2001;159:17–20.

124. Meikle MC. Hypercalcaemia of malignancy. Nature 1988;336:311.

125. Mesonero CE. Appearance of neoplasms during pregnancy. In: Levine AS, ed. Etiology of cancer in man. Dordrecht: Kluwer Academic Publishers, 1989, pp. 102–114.

126. Milas L, Tofilon PJ, Brock WA. Assessment of antitumor (antimetastatic) efficacy of cytotoxic agents. Prog Clin Biol Res 1986;212:305–320.

127. Miller CB, Jones RJ, Piantadosi S, Abeloff MD, Spivak JL. Decreased erythropoietin response in patients with the anemia of cancer. N Engl J Med 1990;322:1689–1692.

128. Moldawer LL, Marano MA, Wei H, et al. Cachectin/tumor necrosis factor-α alters red blood cell kinetics and induces anemia in vivo. FASEB J 1989;3:1637–1643.

129. Müller A, Homey B, Soto H, et al. Involvement of chemokine receptors in breast cancer metastasis. Nature 2001;410:50–56.

130. Nagourney RA, Woolley PV. Paraneoplastic syndromes. In: Liotta LA, ed. Influence of tumor development on the host. Dordrecht: Kluwer Academic Publishers, 1989, pp. 214–227.

131. Nakahara W, Fukuoka F. Toxohormone: a characteristic toxic substance produced by cancer tissue. GANN 1949;40:45–69.

132. Nakamura K, Kawaguchi T, Asahina S, et al. Electronmicroscopic studies on extravasation of tumor cells and early foci of hematogenous metastases. GANN Monogr Cancer Res 1977;20:57–71.

133. Nand S, Messmore H. Hemostasis in malignancy. Am J Hematol 1990;35:45–55.

134. Nathanson L, Hall TC. Lung tumors: how they produce their syndromes. Ann NY Acad Sci 1974;230:367–377.

135. Nicolson GL. Cancer metastasis. Organ colonization and the cell-surface properties of malignant cells. Biochim Biophys Acta 1982;695:113–176.

136. Nicolson GL. Cancer metastasis: tumor cell and host organ properties important in metastasis to specific secondary sites. Biochim Biophys Acta 1988;948:175–224.

137. Nicolson GL. Metastatic tumor cell interactions with endothelium, basement membrane and tissue. Curr Opin Cell Biol 1989;1:1009–1019.

138. Nicolson GL. Molecular mechanisms of cancer metastasis: tumor and host properties and the role of oncogenes and suppressor genes. Curr Opin Oncol 1991;3:75–92.

139. Odell WD, Wolfsen AR. Hormones from tumors: are they ubiquitous? Am J Med 1980;68:317–318.

140. Odell W, Wolfsen A, Yoshimoto Y, et al. Ectopic peptide synthesis: a universal concomitant of neoplasia. Trans Assoc Am Physicians 1977;40:204–227.

141. Ohtaki T, Shintani Y, Honda S, et al. Metastasis suppressor gene KiSS-1 encodes peptide ligand of a G-protein-coupled receptor. Nature 2001;411:613–617.

141a. Oliveira MJ, Van Damme J, Lauwaet T, et al. Beta-casein-derived peptides, produced by bacteria, stimulate cancer cell invasion and motility. EMBO J. 2003;22:6161–6173.

142. Orr FW. The influence of endothelial injury and inflammatory processes on metastasis. In: Orr FW, Buchanan MR, Weiss L, eds. Microcirculation in cancer metastasis. Boca Raton, FL: CRC Press, 1991, pp. 239–255.

143. Orr FW, Buchanan MR, Weiss L, eds. Microcirculation in cancer metastasis. Boca Raton, FL: CRC Press, 1991.

144. Orr FW, Warner DJA. Effects of systemic complement activation and neutrophil-mediated pulmonary injury on the retention and metastasis of circulating cancer cells in mouse lungs. Lab Invest 1990;62:331–338.

145. Paget S. The distribution of secondary growths in cancer of the breast. Lancet 1889;1:571–573.

146. Pals ST, Horst E, Ossekoppele GJ, et al. Expression of lymphocyte homing receptor as a mechanism of dissemination in non-Hodgkin's lymphoma. Blood 1989;73:885–888.

147. Pascal RR. Renal manifestations of extrarenal neo-plasms. Hum Pathol 1980;11:7–17.

148. Patterson WP, Ringenberg OS. The pathophysiology of thrombosis in cancer. Semin Oncol 1990;17:140–146.

149. Pauli BU, Augustin-Voss HG, El-Sabban ME, Johnson RC, Hammer DA. Organ-preference of metastasis. The role of endothelial cell adhesion molecules. Cancer Metastasis Rev 1990;9:175–189.

150. Pauli BU, Johnson RC, El-Sabban ME. Organotypic endothelial cell surface molecules mediate organ preference of metastasis. In: Simionescu N, Simionescu M, eds. Endothelial cell dysfunctions. New York: Plenum Press, 1991.

151. Pauli BU, Knudson W. Tumor invasion: a consequence of destructive and compositional matrix alterations. Hum Pathol 1988;19:628–639.

152. Pauli BU, Kuettner KE. The regulation of invasion by a cartilage-derived anti–invasion factor. In: Liotta LA, Hart IR, eds. Tumor invasion and metastasis. The Hague: Martinus Nijhoff Publishers, 1982, pp. 291–308.

153. Pauli BU, Lee C-L. Organ preference of metastasis. The role of organ-specifically modulated endothelial cells. Lab Invest 1988;58:379–387.

154. Pepper MS, Montesano R, Vassalli J-D, Orci L. Chrondrocytes inhibit endothelial sprout formation in vitro: evidence for involvement of a transforming growth factor-beta. J Cell Physiol 1991;146:170–179.

155. Peterson W. Beiträge zur Lehre vom Carcinom. I. Ueber Aufbau, Wachstum und Histogenese der Hautcarcinome. Beitr Klin Chir 1902;32:543–660.

156. Pineo GF, Brain MC, Gallus AS, Hirsh J, Hatton MWC, Regoeczi E. Tumors, mucus production, and hyper-coagulability. Ann NY Acad Sci 1974;230:262–270.

157. Pines A, Kaplinsky N, Olchovsky D, Frankl O. Rheumatoid arthritis-like syndrome: a presenting symptom of malignancy. Report of 3 cases and review of the literature. Eur J Rheum Inflam 1984;7:51–55.

158. Poste G, Fidler IJ. The pathogenesis of cancer metastasis. Nature 1980;283:139–146.

159. Powles TJ, Clark SA, Easty DM, Easty GC, Neville AM. The inhibition by aspirin and indomethacin of osteolytic tumour deposits and hypercalcaemia in rats with Walker tumour, and its possible application to human breast cancer. Br J Cancer 1973;28:316–321.

160. Powles TJ, Dowsett M, Easty DM, Easty GC, Neville AM. Breast-cancer osteolysis, bone metastases, and anti-osteolytic effect of aspirin. Lancet 1976;1:608–610.

161. Quinn JM, McGee JO, Athanasou NA. Human tumour-associated macrophages differentiate into osteoclastic bone-resorbing cells. J Pathol 1998;184:31–36.

162. Rasche H, Dietrich M. Hemostatic abnormalities associated with malignant diseases. Eur J Cancer 1977;13;1053–1064.

163. Renkonen R, Paavonen T, Nortamo P, Gahmberg CG. Expression of endothelial adhesion molecules in vivo: increased endothelial ICAM-2 expression in lymphoid malignancies. Am J Pathol 1992;140:763–767.

164. Rice GE, Gimbrone MA Jr, Bevilacqua MP. Tumor cell-endothelial interactions. Increased adhesion of human melanoma cells to activated vascular endothelium. Am J Pathol 1988;133:204–210.

165. Rickles FR, Edwards RL. Activation of blood coagulation in cancer: Trousseau's syndrome revisited. Blood 1983;62: 14–31.

166. Roberts SS, Watne AL, McGrew EA, et al. Cancer cells in the circulating blood. Surg Forum 1958;8:146–151.

167. Ruoslahti E, Giancotti FG. Integrins and tumor cell dissemination. Cancer Cells 1989;1:119–126.

168. Russell DS, Rubinstein LJ. Pathology of tumours of the nervous system, 5th ed. Baltimore: Williams & Wilkins, 1989.

169. Russo RG, Foltz CM, Liotta LA. New invasion assay using endothelial cells grown on native human basement membrane. Clin Exp Metastasis 1983;1:115–127.

170. Sack GH, Levin J, Bell WR. Trousseau's syndrome and other manifestations of chronic disseminated coagulopathy in patients with neoplasms: clinical, patho-physiologic, and therapeutic features. Medicine 1977;56:1–37.

171. Saiki I, Murata J, Iida J, et al. Antimetastatic effects of synthetic polypeptides containing repeated structures of the cell adhesive Arg-Gly-Asp (RGD) and Tyr-Ile-Gly-Ser-Arg (YIGSR) sequences. Br J Cancer 1989;60:722–728.

172. Sato H, Suzuki M. Deformability and viability of tumor cells by transcapillary passage, with reference to organ affinity of metastasis in cancer. In: Weiss L, ed. Fundamental aspects of metastasis. Amsterdam-Oxford: North Holland Publishing Company, 1976, pp. 311–317.

173. Schroyens W, Bruyneel R, Tchao R, et al. Comparison of invasiveness and non-invasiveness of two epithelial cell lines in vitro. Invasion Metastasis 1984;4:160–170.

174. Segal BH, Walsh TJ, Holland SM. Infections in the cancer patient. In: Cancer. Principles and practice of oncology, 6th ed. Philadelphia: Lippincott Williams & Wilkins, 2001, pp. 2815–2686.

175. Seghatchian MJ, Samama MM, Hecker SP (eds). Hypercoagulable States: fundamental aspects, acquired disorders, and congenital thrombophilia. Boca Raton, FL, CRC Press, 1996.

176. Sieweke MH, Thompson NL, Sporn MB, Bissell MJ. Mediation of wound-related Rous sarcoma virus tumorigenesis by TGF-β. Science 1990;248:1656–1660.

177. Sindelar WF, Tralka TS, Ketcham AS. Electron microscopic observations on formation of pulmonary metastases. J Surg Res 1975;18:137–161.

178. Sherry BA, Gelin J, Fong Y, et al. Anticachectin/tumor necrosis factor-α antibodies attenuate development of cachexia in tumor models. FASEB J 1989;3:1956–1962.

179. Sherwood LM. The multiple causes of hypercalcemia in malignant disease. N Engl J Med 1980;303:1412–1413.

180. Stetler-Stevenson WG, Kleiner DE Jr. Molecular biology of cancer: invasion and metastases. In: DeVita VT Jr, Hellman S, Rosenberg SA (eds). Cancer: principles and practice of oncology, 6th ed. Philadelphia: Lippincott Williams & Wilkins, 2001, pp. 123–136.

181. Sugarbaker EV. Patterns of metastasis in human malignancies. Cancer Biol Rev 1981;2:235–278.

182. Sutherland DJ. Hormones and cancer. In: Tannock IF, Hill RP, eds. The basic science of oncology. New York: Pergamon Press, 1987, pp. 204–222.

183. Sylvén B, Holmberg B. On the structure and biological effects of a newly-discovered cytotoxic polypeptide in tumor fluid. Eur J Cancer 1965;1:199–202.

184. Tanaka K, Kohga S, Kinjo M, Kodama Y. Tumor metastasis and thrombosis, with special reference to thromboplastic and fibrinolytic activities of tumor cells. GANN Monogr Cancer Res 1977;20:97–119.

185. Tanaka NG, Tohgo A, Ogawa H. Platelet-aggregating activities of metastasizing tumor cells. V. In situ roles of platelets in hematogenous metastases. Invasion Metastasis 1986;6: 209–224.

186. Tarin D, Vass ACR, Kettlewell MGW, Price JE. Absence of metastatic sequelae during long-term treatment of malignant ascites by peritoneo-venous shunting. A clinico-pathological report. Invasion Metastasis 1984;4:1–12.

187. Taylor LM Jr, Hauty MG, Edwards JM, Porter JM. Digital ischemia as a manifestation of malignancy. Ann Surg 1987;206: 62–68.

188. Terranova VP, Hic S, Diflorio RM, Lyall RM. Tumor cell metastasis. CRC Crit Rev Oncol Hematol 1986;5:87–114.

189. Tisdale MJ. Biology of cachexia. J Natl Can Inst 1997;89: 1763–1773.

190. Trousseau A. Phlegmatia alba dolens. Clinique Médicale de L'Hotel-Dieu de Paris, vol 3, 2nd ed. Paris: J-B Ballière et Fils, 1865, pp. 654–712.

191. Tryggvason K, Höyhtyä M, Salo T. Proteolytic degradation of extracellular matrix in tumor invasion. Biochim Biophys Acta 1987;907:191–217.

192. Tyzzer EE. Factors in the production and growth of tumor metastases. J Med Res 1913;28:309–332.

192a. Van't Veer LJ, Weigelt B. Road map to metastasis. Nat Med 2003;9:999–1000.

193. Vlodavsky I, Goldshmidt O, Zcharia E, et al. Mammalian heparanase: involvement in cancer metastasis, angiogenesis and normal development. Semin Cancer Biol 2002;12:121–129.

194. Wallace AC, Chew E-C, Jones DS. Arrest and extravasation of cancer cells in the lung. In: Weiss L, Gilbert HA, eds. Pulmonary metastasis. Boston: GK Hall & Co., 1978, pp. 26–42.

195. Warren BA. Cancer cell-endothelial reactions: the microinjury hypothesis and localized thrombosis in the formation of micrometastases. In: Donati MB, Davidson JF, Garattini S, eds. Malignancy and the hemostatic system. New York: Raven Press, 1981, pp. 5–25.

196. Weiss L. Fundamental aspects of metastasis. Amsterdam-Oxford: North Holland Publishing Company, 1976.

197. Weiss L. Cell detachment and metastasis. GANN Monogr Cancer Res 1977;20:25–35.

198. Weiss L. Some mechanisms involved in cancer cell detachment by necrotic material. Int J Cancer 1978;22:196–203.

199. Weiss L. The hemodynamic destruction of circulating cancer cells. Biorheology 1987;24:105–115.

200. Weiss L. Metastatic inefficiency. Adv Cancer Res 1990;54: 159–211.

201. Weiss L, Grundmann E, Torhorst J, et al. Haematogenous metastatic (sic) patterns in colonic carcinoma: an analysis of 1541 necropsies. J Pathol 1986;150:195–203.

202. Weiss L, Haydock K, Pickren JW, Lane WW. Organ vascularity and metastatic frequency. Am J Pathol 1980;101: 101–114.

203. Weiss L, Holmes JC. Some effects of tumor necrosis on components of active cell movement. In: Sträuli P, Barrett AJ, Baici A, eds. Proteinases and tumor invasion. New York: Raven Press, 1980, pp. 181–200.

204. Weiss L, Orr FW, Honn KV. Interactions of cancer cells with the microvasculature during metastasis. FASEB J 1988;2: 12–21.

205. Weiss L, Orr FW, Honn KV. Interactions between cancer cells and the microvasculature: a rate-regulator for metastasis. Clin Exp Metastasis 1989;7:127–167.

206. Weiss L, Schmid-Schönbein GW. Biomechanical interactions of cancer cells with the microvasculature during metastasis. Cell Biophys 1989;14:187–215.

207. Welch DR, Bhuyan BK, Liotta LA, eds. Cancer metastasis: experimental and clinical strategies. Prog Clin Biol Res, vol 212. New York: Alan R. Liss, 1986.

208. Westermarck J, Kähäri VM. Regulation of matrix metalloproteinase expression in tumor invasion. FASEB J 1999;13: 781–792.

209. Willis RA. The spread of tumours in the human body, 3rd ed. London: Butterworth, 1973.

210. Wold LE, Pritchard DJ, Bergert J, Wilson DM. Prostaglandin synthesis by osteoid osteoma and osteoblastoma. Mod Pathol 1988;1:129–131.

211. Wolinsky H, Lischner MW. Needle track implantation of tumor after percutaneous lung biopsy. Ann Intern Med 1969; 71:359–362.

213. Wood S. Pathogenesis of metastasis formation observed in vivo in the rabbit ear chamber. Arch Pathol 1958;66:550–568.

214. Yano S. Shinohara H, Herbst RS, et al. Production of experimental malignant pleural effusions is dependent on invasion of the pleura and expression of vascular endothelial growth factor/vascular permeability factor by human lung cancer cells. Am J Pathol 2000;157:1893–1903.

215. Zeidman I. The fate of circulating tumor cells. I. Passage of cells through capillaries. Cancer Res 1961;21:38–39.

216. Zetter BR. The cellular basis of site-specific tumor metastasis. N Engl J Med 1990;322:605–612.

217. Zimmers TA, Davies MV, Koniaris LG, et al. Induction of cachexia in mice by systemically administered myostatin. Science 2002;296:1486–1488.

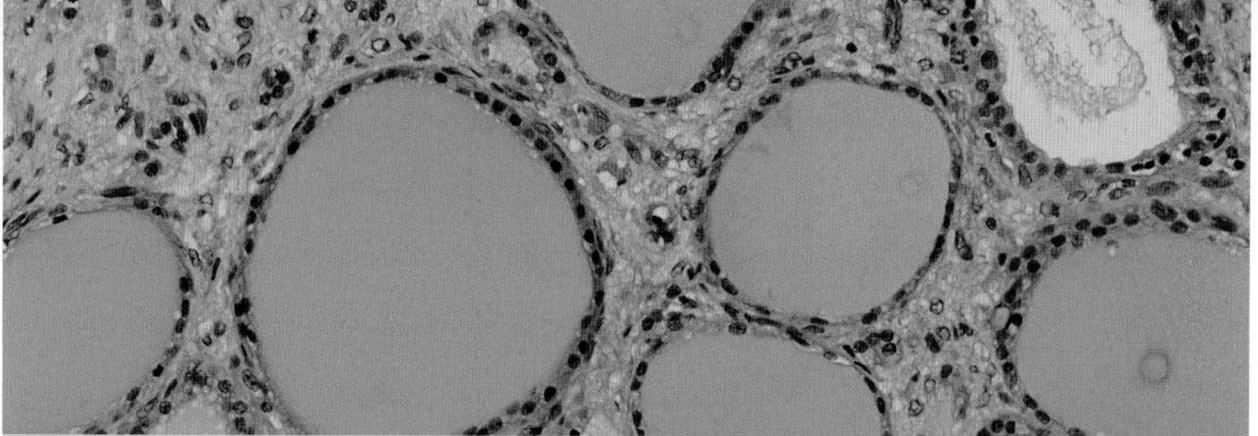

Contrary to the popular belief that we do not know "the cause of cancer," we know, if anything, too many causes: predisposing, initiating, promoting, perpetuating; physical, chemical, viral, bacterial, parasitic; dietary, environmental, occupational, and related to lifestyle (Figure 28.1). We have also learned that we will never find "the cause" of cancer, because, like other diseases, tumors never have a single cause. This is part of the ABC of medicine in general. Even a simple fracture may have a long list of causes. This concept was beautifully stated by Alan Gregg, an eminent physician and educator (97):

> We ought to use the word "why" in the plural, and ask, "Whys is this patient [ill]?". . . . A particular case of a fractured jaw in a sailor may be the result of convergent causes—no letters from home, too much alcohol, the loan of a car by a friend, a dark night, an oncoming car on a road covered with ice at a curve, the fact that the left-hand rule is used in the British Isles, new brake linings, a skid, and a telephone pole. These constitute the whys, not the why, of a fractured jaw. It is a cataract of consequences. Take out any one of these whys and the accident would not have occurred.

Gregg did not exaggerate in attributing 11 causes to a fractured jaw. There is a human carcinoma that is supposedly caused by aflatoxin, a fungal poison; a careful search into the genesis of this tumor brings up 10 contributing causes: ethnic, social, dietary, ecological, botanical, physiological, biochemical, genetic, infectious, and immunologic; eliminate any one and no tumor develops. The causation of cancer—and of disease in general—should be seen as a chain of many links, as illustrated on p. 946.

With this in mind we must begin to analyze the possible causes of cancer. The basic fact in this field—to many it will come as a surprise—is that on a worldwide basis *most cancers are related to the environment or to human behavior* (60, 133) (see Figure 28.1). We will therefore begin our study with environmental causes. History tells us that they belong to three groups: chemical (the

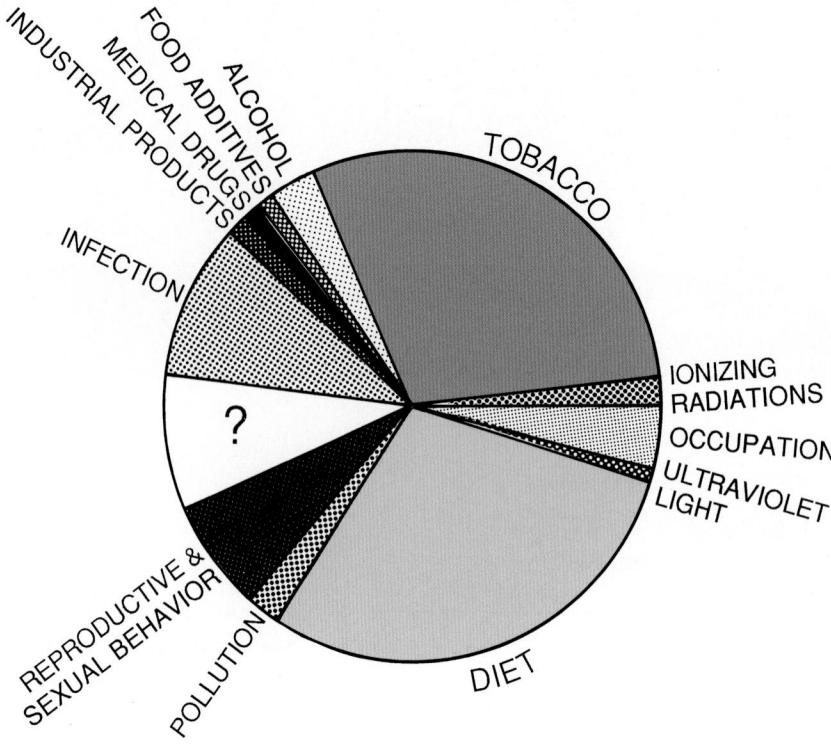

FIGURE 28.1 Principal causes of human cancer. (Reprinted with permission from Nature [132], copyright 1983 Macmillan Magazines Limited.)

largest), physical, and biological. Do they have anything in common? Yes: most of the agents in these three groups have the ability to damage the DNA chain permanently and are therefore called *genotoxic*; some, however, are definitely non-genotoxic. This apparent dilemma will be addressed in due time (p. 951).

Chemical Causes of Tumors

Chemical causes of tumors were the first to be recognized because some chemicals produce obvious occupational diseases; today chemicals are responsible for most human tumors, estimated as 80–90 percent of the total. The list of hazardous agents is so varied that this chapter may seem like a patchwork of unrelated topics: what does tar have to do with diet, or mustard gas with lubricating oil? The answer is that the DNA chain can be nonspecifically damaged by an enormous variety of chemicals, related, as we will see, by the broad physicochemical property of being electrophilic.

In addition to this physicochemical *Leitmotif*, this section on chemical carcinogenesis will be punctuated by another recurring theme: many leads to the discovery of cancer-producing chemicals came from practicing physicians. The experiments were run by society or by nature, and an alert clinician blew the whistle; laboratory experiments came later (268, 269).

Milestones on the Trail of Chemical Cancer: From Snuff to Benzpyrene

Tobacco. Very appropriately, tobacco begins our story, back in 1761.

For well-to-do Englishmen in the mid-1700s tobacco smoking was no longer subject to the death penalty, but it was considered vulgar; the approved habit was to inhale it as snuff. And so the first warning against tobacco came from a prominent figure in eighteenth century London, a scholarly physician–botanist named John Hill (who also coined the term *paramecium*). In 1761 Dr. Hill published a little book describing the ill effects of snuff powder, including "polypusses," which could turn into terrible, ulcerated cancers (206). The latter diagnosis was not easy: in Hill's day the biological nature of cancer was still unknown. Incidentally, the cancer-causing agents in snuff are not tar components but nitrosamines (201).

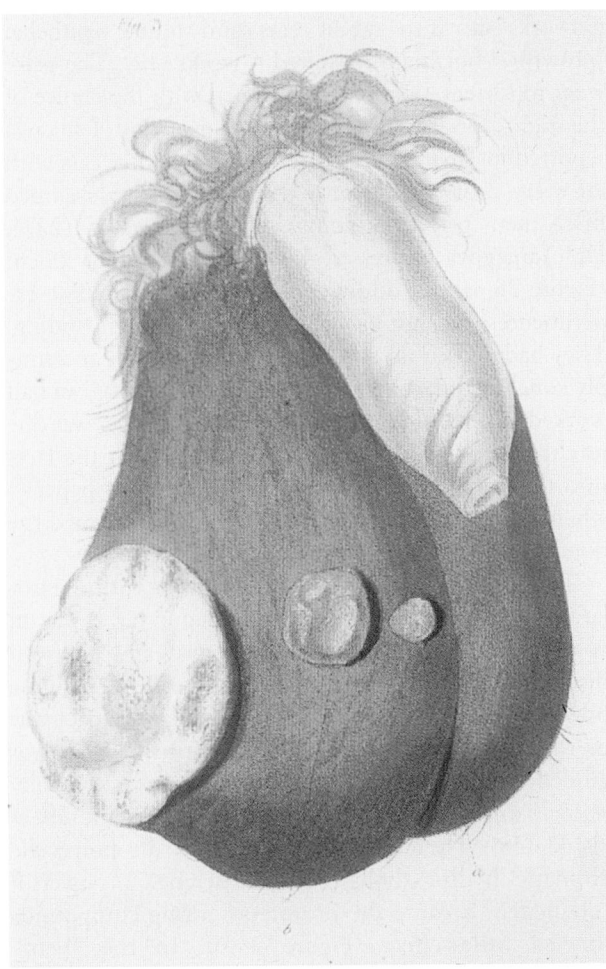

FIGURE 28.2 Chimney-sweeper's cancer as illustrated in 1841 by a British surgeon, Sir Astley Cooper. Three stages are shown. *Right:* Early stage, much like a wart. *Left:* Advanced stage; the tumor has grown into an ulcerated mass. *Center:* Intermediate stage. (Adapted from [51].)

Soot. Only a few years later, in 1775, another London physician, Sir Percivall Pott, Fellow of the Royal Society, published his *Chirurgical Works* (196, 279). In Volume 3, besides more "Remarks on the Polypus of the Nose," he tells of chimney sweeps who had come to his attention because of scrotal cancer (Figure 28.2). Chimneys, at that time, were built in such a way as to allow the passage not only of a sweeping tool but of a whole—small—human being armed with a brush and surely also with a desperate need to survive. In the words of Sir Percivall:

It is a disease which always makes its first attack on, and its first appearance in the inferior part of the scrotum; where it produces a superficial, painful, ragged, ill-looking sore,

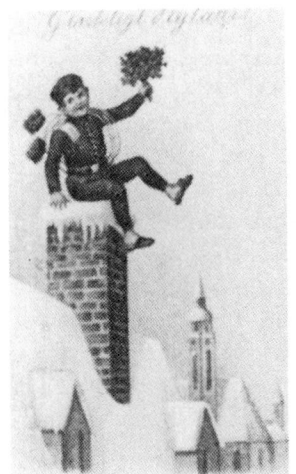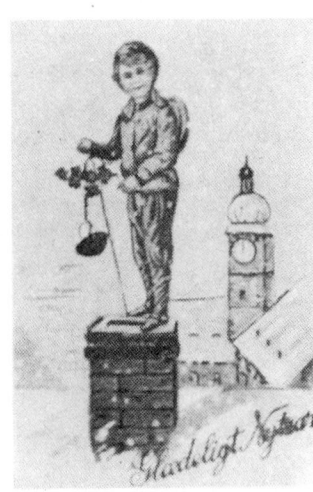

FIGURE 28.3 Children employed as chimney sweeps in nineteenth century Denmark. From a New Year greeting card of the time. (Reproduced with permission from [104].)

with hard and rising edges. The trade call it the soot-wart. I never saw it under the age of puberty (203).

The last remark tells a great deal: chimney sweeps began climbing into chimneys as small children, even at the tender age of four years (38) (Figure 28.3). "The disease, in these people," wrote Sir Percivall, "seems to derive its origin from a lodgement of soot in the rugae of the scrotum." After many years of exposure, superficial "soot warts" began to appear, and eventually one of these turned into invasive cancer. The delay after the first exposure was on the order of 20–30 years or more (38). Although the soot wart was considered almost like a trademark, a puzzling feature was its rarity in continental Europe; a study in 1892 suggested that the difference was due to protective clothing and the habit of frequent bathing, which removed the soot from the deep rugae of the scrotum (38). Sir Percivall, oddly enough, makes no reference to the preventive possibilities of soap and water (198). So, half a century later, Sir Astley Cooper could still illustrate the soot wart in his surgical treatise (Figure 28.2). The Danes, however, saw the connection: tradition has it that three years after Sir Percivall's paper the Danish Chimney-Sweeper's Guild urged its members to take daily baths (160).

Tar and its derivatives. Sir Percivall was writing at the eve of the American Revolutionary war; the British, unable to keep their ships watertight with wood tar from their former Colonies, turned to the old German method of preparing tar by heating coal in the absence of air. A few years later came the idea of producing street-lighting gas by the same method. Now a great deal of tar was generated as by-product. The next problem was what to do with that abundance of black, sticky material: there had to be some industrial use for it besides tarring ships and occasional sailors. By the mid-1800s, distillation products of tar began to find uses, for instance, as solvents (which allowed Charles Mackintosh to make his first rainproof mackintoshes). Then came phenol, the first antiseptic; dyes derived from aniline; myriads of new organic compounds such as benzene (the famous 6-carbon ring was described by Kekulé in 1866). Soon a powerful German distillation industry was born.

Those were the 1860s. It takes 20–25 years of exposure for most cancers to develop. In 1895, a German surgeon, L. Rehn, noticed three cases of bladder cancer among 45 workers who had been preparing fuchsin dyes from aniline for 15 to 29 years (207): bladder cancer is rare enough to make such a cluster highly suspect. Similar "aniline bladder cancers" were soon discovered in other countries. Actually, aniline itself is not directly the culprit; several of its derivatives, aromatic amines, turned out to be highly carcinogenic with a delay of 5–30 years. The worst offender is betanaphthylamine (Figure 28.4) (90); before its use was discontinued, as many as 100 percent of exposed workers developed bladder cancer (49). More recently, exposure to benzene itself has been linked with leukemia (47, 210).

Tar as a tool of oncology. While tar products continued to claim more victims, several attempts were made to produce experimental tumors with it, but failed because the experimental design was wrong (228). An Englishman, for example, narrowly missed the mark: he injected

gasworks tar into rabbit ears and found epithelial "growths," but he only waited 4 weeks (12). The prize went to Oriental patience combined with the choice of the right species. In 1915, Yamagiwa and Ichikawa reported in Japanese that after painting rabbit ears with tar every 2 or 3 days for a year, papillomas developed first, then true carcinomas with metastases (227). Dr. Yamagiwa expressed his joy in a haiku poem (Figure 28.5), but oddly enough, the two Japanese experimenters did not give much weight to their finding. They had chosen tar as a "nonspecific" irritant and simply concluded that Virchow (with whom Yamagiwa had worked for several years [269]) was right: cancer was due to chronic irritation. Their concern was to fit the facts into the known pattern. However, their short paper—when it was published in English (1918):—opened the flood-gates: the era of tar-painting had begun.

The next major step came in the 1930s with the isolation of specific carcinogens contained in tar. It was an epic of chemistry: Sir Ernest Kennaway and his team distilled 2 tons of tar down to 7 grams of crystalline powder. Just as the Curies were guided by radioactivity in their extraction of radium, the British group was guided by a fluorescence spectrum that was empirically known to be associated with the carcinogenic effect (133, 228). The culprits turned out to be polycyclic aromatic hydrocarbons; 3,4-benzpyrene, a powerful carcinogen, became the prototype; 3-ring compounds showed little effect (Figure 28.6). In the "benz-pyromania" that followed (228), attention was turned to natural polycyclic compounds, and a potent carcinogen, 3-methycholanthrene, was soon prepared from bile acids (50) and became a standard tool for producing tumors (77). However, it is no longer thought to be generated *in vivo* (15).

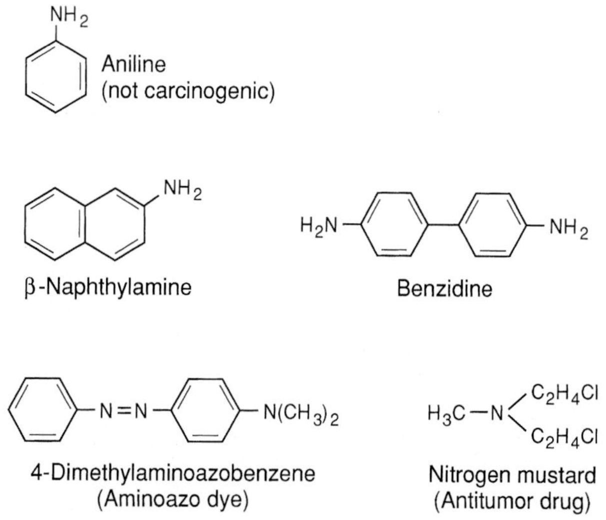

NH$_2$

Aniline
(not carcinogenic)

NH$_2$

β-Naphthylamine

H$_2$N — NH$_2$

Benzidine

N=N — N(CH$_3$)$_2$

4-Dimethylaminoazobenzene
(Aminoazo dye)

H$_3$C — N < C$_2$H$_4$Cl / C$_2$H$_4$Cl

Nitrogen mustard
(Antitumor drug)

FIGURE 28.4   Some carcinogens and related molecules.

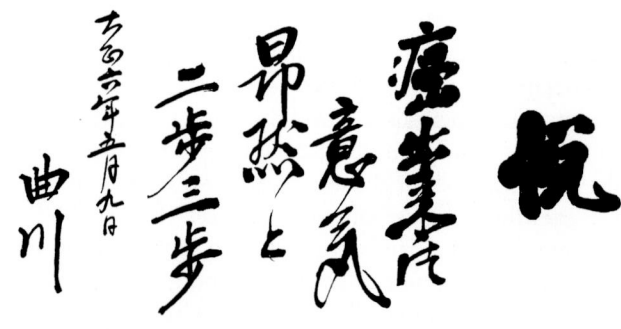

FIGURE 28.5   Haiku composed by Dr. Yamagiwa on a silk scroll in 1917 to celebrate the first skin cancer produced by painting tar on a rabbit ear. In essence it means: "Cancer was produced! Proudly I walk a few steps," but in Japanese it is much more poetic. (Reproduced with permission from [227].)

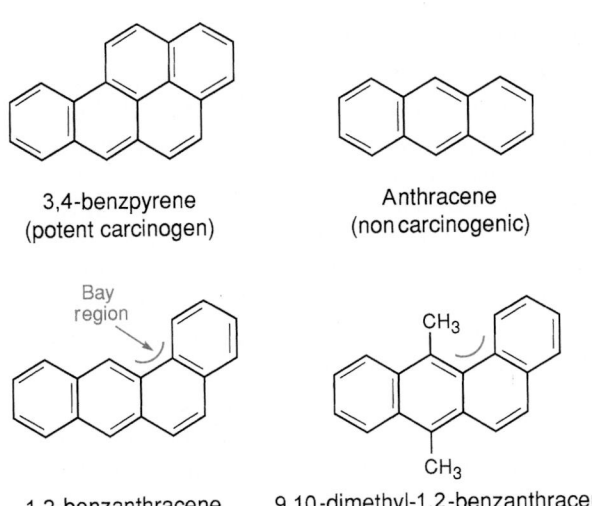

3,4-benzpyrene
(potent carcinogen)

Anthracene
(non carcinogenic)

Bay
region

1,2-benzanthracene
(borderline carcinogen)

CH₃

CH₃

9,10-dimethyl-1,2-benzanthracene
(very potent carcinogen)

FIGURE 28.6   Formulae of polycyclic hydrocarbons, including three carcinogens.

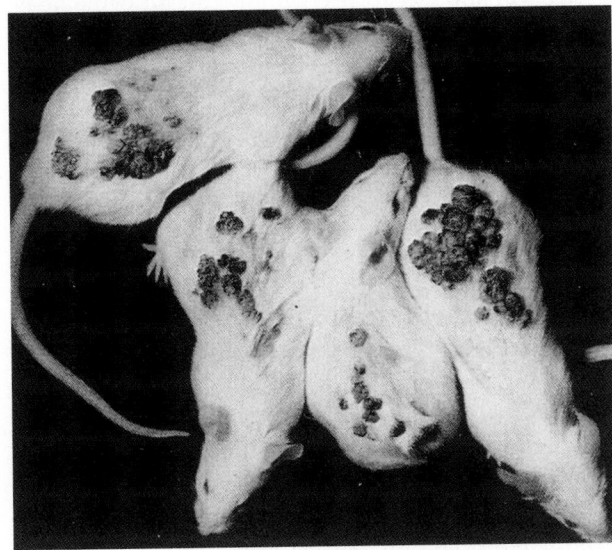

FIGURE 28.7   Papillomas on the back of mice after a 12-week induction–promotion program: a single application of dimethyl benzanthracene (DMBA) followed by croton oil twice a week. (Reproduced with permission from [27].)

Skin tumors produced by tar or by purified carcinogens were studied primarily in mice (Figure 28.7) and rabbits (279). In the early experiments, a nonspecific dermatitis appeared first, followed by loss of hair and excessive keratinization (*hyperkeratosis*). Then wartlike papillomas developed; some regressed, others continued to grow. If painting was discontinued, these benign epidermal growths usually regressed, but if painting was resumed they reappeared faster and in greater numbers. Eventually a carcinoma developed in one area, rarely in two or three (82, 216, 217). Endless variations were tried on the theme of painting-plus-some-other-treatment. Today the paintbrush is replaced by more precise methods of application (257), but the basic results are the same. An important by-product of all this work was the construction of a theory on cancer development, through the stages of initiation, promotion, and progression.

The Nature of Chemical Carcinogens

Before we leave tar for other carcinogens, we should briefly examine the property that makes a molecule carcinogenic.

Electrophilic agents. Over 12 families of carcinogens are known at this time. They include molecules as simple as elemental chromium or as complex as aflatoxin. A unifying thread through this chemical melange was proposed in 1969 by Elizabeth and James Miller (160–163). Their theory is that a carcinogenic molecule must be an *electrophilic reactant;* i.e., it must have a relatively electron-deficient site; *this makes it seek nucleophilic sites*—that is, atoms that have easily shared electrons such as exist in amino groups, with which they form a covalent bond (Figure 28.8) (203). Such nucleophilic groupings are very common—even water qualifies—but the critical point is that they are relatively abundant on DNA, RNA, and protein (159).

This rule proposed by the Millers applies to chemical agents classified as genotoxic; non-genotoxic

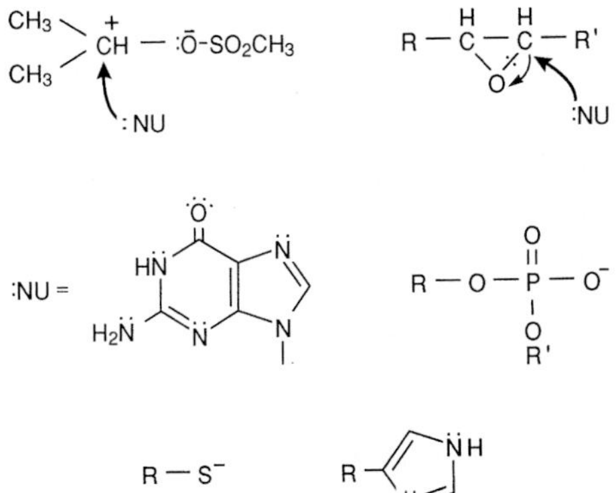

FIGURE 28.8   Examples of strong electrophilic reactants (positive ions or uncharged molecules with electron-deficient atoms) and their reactions with nucleophiles (:NU) through sharing of electron pairs of electron-rich atoms. (Reproduced with permission from [160].)

carcinogens, as we will see, interfere with cells in a different way. Although there are exceptions (159) the electrophilic requirement is so consistent that it is now possible to predict with reasonable accuracy the carcinogenic potential of a molecule (159). The electrophilic hypothesis has an important corollary: in their native states, few carcinogens are electrophilic. They are inactive, and are activated in the body.

Metabolic activation of carcinogens. As soon as a variety of carcinogens was available for experimentation, it became obvious that some, such as tar derivatives, act *at the site* where they are applied, whereas most of the others elicit tumors *in distant organs* and each one always affects the same organ(s), no matter how it is administered. This suggested that some carcinogens must be modified within the body before they become effective (270), and it is now an established fact that most carcinogens are inactive in their native state. The Millers proposed that the inactive carcinogens (procarcinogens) are metabolized stepwise to one or more "proximate" carcinogens and eventually to the ultimate carcinogen, the electrophilic species. The metabolic activation can be performed by enzymes of the endoplasmic reticulum such as the P-450 cytochromes (p. 142), but other enzyme systems may also be involved (70, 107), including enzymes of pathogenic bacteria and of the normal flora. Enzyme actions are easily modulated; we are therefore closer to understanding a number of puzzles:

- The organ selectivity of carcinogens may depend on the presence, absence, or balance of appropriate enzymes. As an example, di-methylnitrosamine given orally to rats induces liver cancer. If the rats are kept on a low-protein diet, liver enzymes drop below the critical level, making more carcinogen available to the kidney; then only kidney tumors develop (154).
- Individual differences in susceptibility to cancer could depend on differences in enzyme activity or amounts due to age, diet, or exposure to xenobiotics other than the carcinogen. An example: the carcinogenicity of several aromatic amines can be completely prevented by phenobarbital, a powerful inducer of liver enzymes (70).
- Species differences may also reflect different enzymes and/or enzyme levels.

So much about the nature of carcinogens. The reader should be aware that there are substances that work as cocarcinogens, which enhance the effect of carcinogens though by themselves they have no carcinogenic effect. Fortunately, other molecules work as **anticarcinogens;** such are tannic acid (57) and vitamins A, E, and C (p. 846).

The Chemical Carcinogens

This title promises some chemistry, but the key fact that we want to convey is a matter of psychology: *although most human cancers are caused by chemicals, these chemicals are mainly self-inflicted.*

Cancer from *industrial pollution* certainly exists, but it is not the main aspect of environmental decay: it has been estimated that industrial pollution contributes only 4 percent of all cancer deaths (60). We hurry to add that "only" 4 percent really means 16,000 human beings lost every year in the United States alone, a large figure, which in theory should be reducible to zero. However, new chemicals appear faster than they can be tested for carcinogenic activity. Considering that it takes about 20 years for a new carcinogen to manifest itself on cancer incidence curves, we can anticipate that the list of industrial and environmental carcinogens will continue to grow. Yet it is sobering to realize that the air in the house of a smoker can be more polluted than the city air outside (32).

We will now cite six overlapping categories of chemical carcinogens that are especially relevant to man: (a) related to smoking and other pursuits of pleasure, (b) dietary, (c) hormonal, (d) occupational, (e) therapeutic, and (f) sundry (234a). The only comforting message of this list is that many of these deadly substances are avoidable, at least in theory.

Carcinogens on the road to pleasure. It is mind-boggling that **tobacco** was barely questioned as a cause of cancer before 1950 (285). Yet, in the words of the Surgeon General of the United States, if we consider all the tobacco-related diseases, "Cigarette smoking is the chief [ ] avoidable cause of death in our society" (262). Figures are too large to grasp: half a million deaths per year, one in every four to five American deaths (Figure 28.9) (262)—let alone the millions killed abroad by exported tobacco (56). Nor is cancer the only ill effect of smoking. And yet tobacco is produced in 21 states and Puerto Rico; it brings 2.1 billions of dollars to its growers (280); and it is heavily subsidized by the same federal government that employs the Surgeon General. We tried to obtain hard numbers on the amount of this federal subsidy, but they are buried in such deep strata of paper that even the experts have no grasp of the facts (263).

Anyway, it has been calculated that life is shortened by 14 minutes for every cigarette smoked (31). So much for tobacco.

Alcohol is not itself a carcinogen, but it leads to cancer in two ways. Alcohol abuse, as everyone should know by now, leads to *cirrhosis of the liver.* In this condition the liver tissue is strangled in a three-dimensional network of contracting connective tissue;

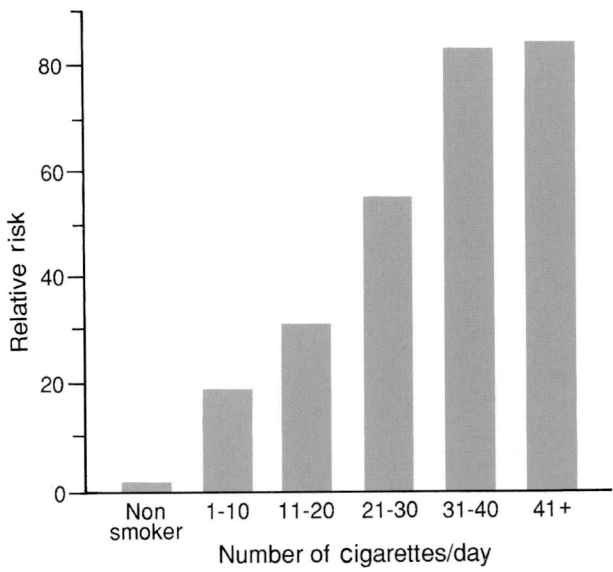

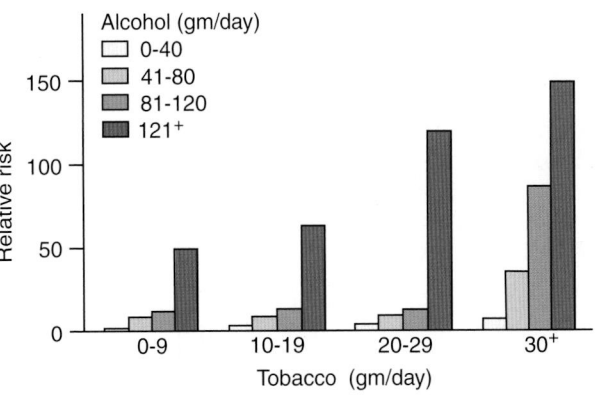

FIGURE 28.10 Alcohol and tobacco interact to influence the risk of esophageal cancer. (Adapted from [252] with permission from Editions Scientifiques Elsevier.)

FIGURE 28.9 Correlation between number of cigarettes smoked and the risk of developing lung cancer in males. (Adapted with permission from [286].)

in the meshes the liver tissue attempts to regenerate, so that on cross sections a cirrhotic liver appears as a mesh of fibrous tissue riddled with small nodules of regenerating cells (see Figures 13.44, 13.45). In the long run, one of the regenerating nodules may become neoplastic. Furthermore, alcohol in large doses increases the risk for cancer of the mouth, pharynx, larynx, esophagus, lung (in nonsmokers) and rectum (192, 211). More worrisome but also unexplained is the fact that a very moderate consumption (half a drink or more daily) increases the risk of breast cancer in women by about 30 percent (211). The 57 percent of American women who consume alcohol will have to weigh this risk against the tempting advantage that moderate alcohol intake reduces the risk of myocardial infarction (171).

And *alcohol plus tobacco* is a bad combination: they somehow interact to increase the risk of esophageal cancer (Figure 28.10). Perhaps alcohol favors the uptake of carcinogens across epithelial linings.

Diet and cancer. Diet relates to cancer in many ways, some of which are understood, others not (6, 93, 192, 211). That diet in general is somehow related to cancer is best shown by the Seventh Day Adventists, who do not drink alcohol or smoke, and about 50 percent of whom also refrain from using coffee, tea, or spices (188). Their mortality for cancers *unrelated* to smoking or drinking is 30–50 percent lower than that of the general population, with two exceptions: the risk among Seventh Day Adventists was higher for the prostate and for the endometrium (164).

Another example of diet-related cancer statistics is that of Japanese immigrating to the United States: their offspring shift from the typical Japanese pattern of cancer prevalence (high for the stomach, low for the colon) to the American pattern (low for the stomach, high for the colon) (102, 211). Besides diet, different enteric bacteria have been shown to secrete a factor able to increase the motility of colon cancer cells *in vitro* (179a).

Total caloric intake is definitely a factor: rodents on a restricted diet live 20–50 percent longer than controls on a non-restricted diet, *and* have less cancer, *and*—if treated with carcinogens—develop fewer tumors (2). In *p53*-knockout mice on a calorie-restricted diet, the appearance of tumors is delayed (124).

The consumption of fat has been somewhat difficult to evaluate as a risk factor for cancer, because it is not easy to extricate it from the effect of total caloric intake. However, a direct relationship was found between total fat intake and cancer of the colon and rectum (Figure 28.11) (230). A similar correlation with cancer of the breast has not held up (259).

The role of fiber was brought to light in the 1970s by an extraordinarily thoughtful and dedicated British surgeon-missionary-epidemiologist, Denis Burkitt (Figure 28.12), who spent most of his professional life in Africa, where he also discovered "Burkitt's tumor." He had no research grants, and opened the field of "fiber" as a factor in cancer epidemiology with observations as simple as the following:

It is noticeable that the stools of those eating high residue diets are almost invariably bulky, soft and non-odorous [...]. The relative absence of fetid smell in the stools of people in developing communities and in the stools of wild animals [...] is also significant and is believed to indicate a lower rate of bacterial decomposition compared to that occurring in Western countries (36).

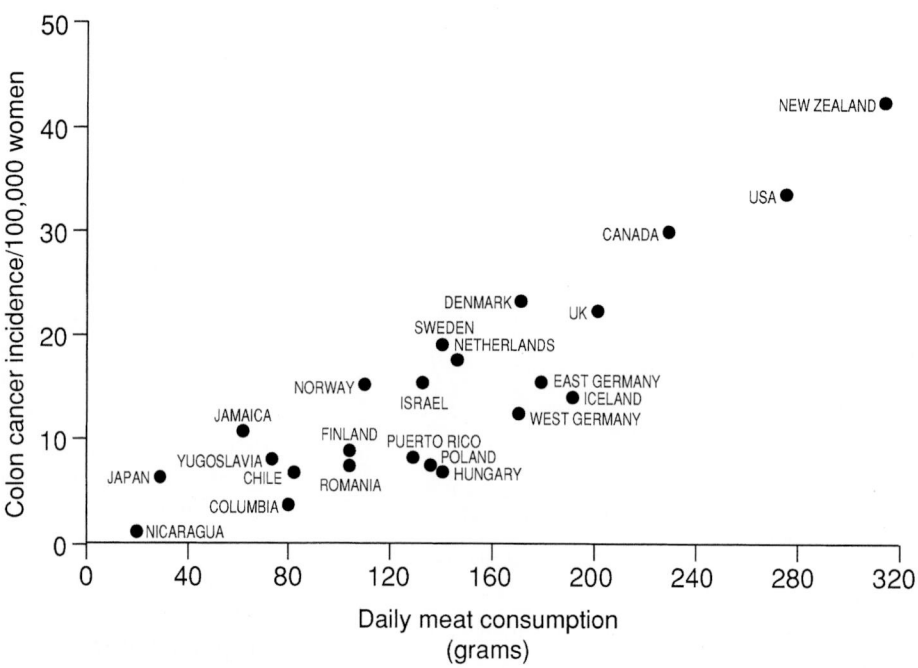

FIGURE 28.11 Correlation between colon cancer in women and daily meat consumption in 23 countries. (From [7], Copyright © 1975. Adapted by permission of Wiley-Liss, a division of Wiley & Sons, Inc.)

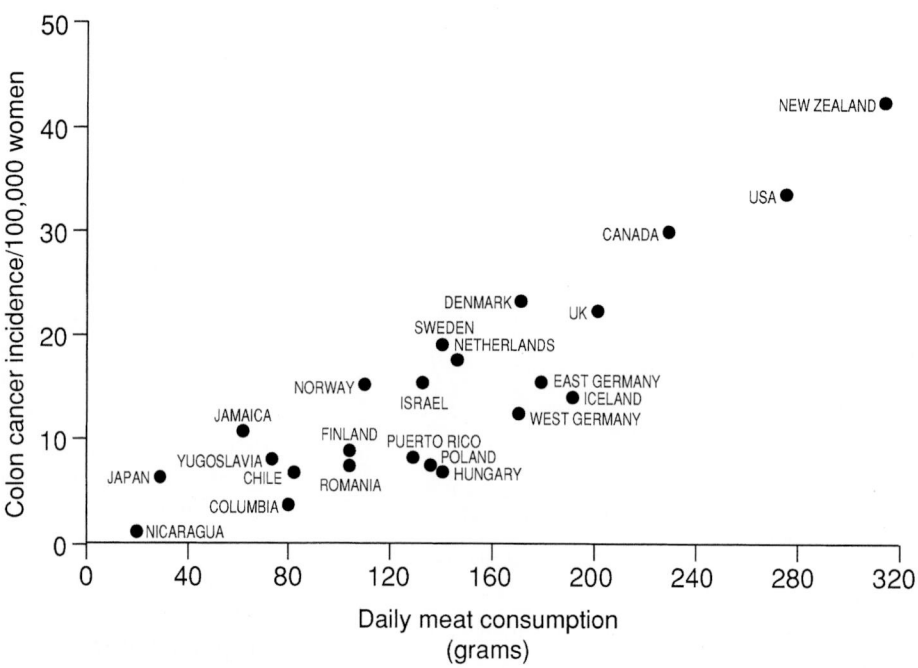

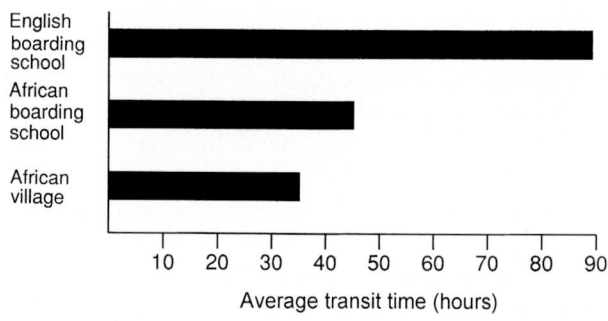

FIGURE 28.13 Differences in the transit time of stools in three populations. Denis Burkitt, who pointed out this phenomenon, correlated it with the geographic differences in the incidence of colon cancer. (Reproduced from [36].)

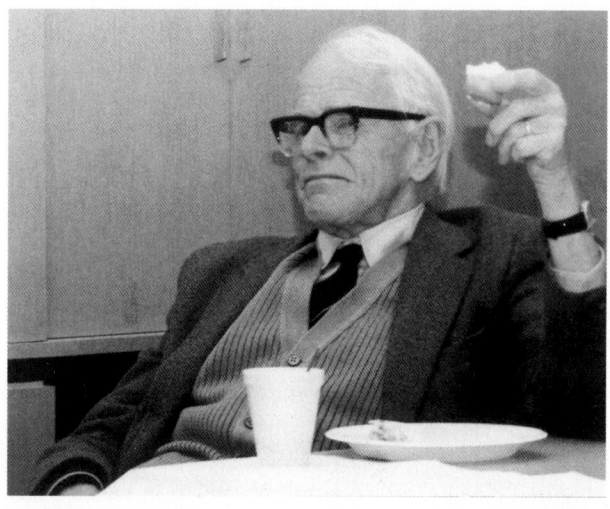

FIGURE 28.12 The late Dr. Denis Burkitt submitted to a fiber-poor diet while visiting the University of Massachusetts Medical School in 1990. (With kind permission from Dr. D. P. Burkitt, Bisley, United Kingdom.)

Burkitt also noticed that colon cancer is rare in all animals and in people who consume less processed food. He pointed out the striking difference between the intestinal transit time in people on refined and unrefined diets (Figure 28.13). The incidence of cancer along the colon and rectum certainly increases in the direction of fecal progress, suggesting a role for contact time between mucosa and feces (and we now know that fecal mutagens are generated in the colon). Today the field of "fiber" has become very complicated (no surprise), because, to begin, it is very difficult to define what is meant by this term (211, 230). Many epidemiologic studies have confirmed the effect of fiber (234a), others have not (197) (Figure 28.14). It may be that high intake of fiber is correlated with other protective dietary factors or habits (276). But anyway, the example—and the message—of Dr. Burkitt goes far beyond the consumption of fiber.

Besides Burkitt's tumor and the fiber story, Dr. Burkitt made another set of observations that is less known. As he practiced surgery for most of his life in rural Africa, he noticed that many diseases that the Western world takes

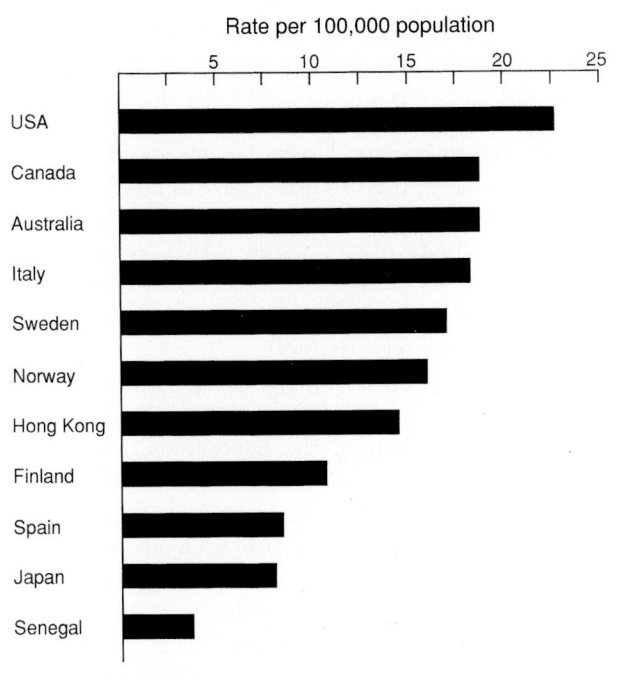

Rate per 100,000 population

| | 5 | 10 | 15 | 20 | 25 |

USA

Canada

Australia

Italy

Sweden

Norway

Hong Kong

Finland

Spain

Japan

Senegal

FIGURE 28.14 International variations in the incidence of colon cancer. (Adapted with permission from [264a].)

NITROSAMINES

$$R_2N-N=O \qquad CH_3-N-CH_3$$

Basic structure   Dimethylnitrosamine

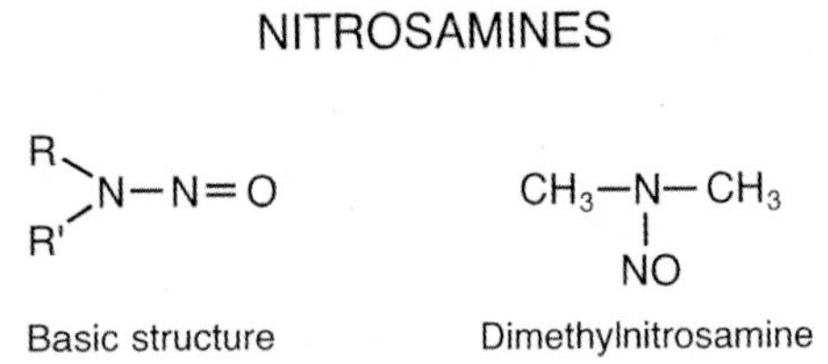

FIGURE 28.15 Nitrosamines: the basic structure, and an aliphatic nitrosamine. (Reproduced from [277], copyright 1986 by Macmillan, with permission from The McGraw-Hill Companies.)

for granted were rare or missing altogether: varicose veins, diverticulosis, hemorrhoids, hiatus hernia, appendicitis, just to mention a few. According to Dr. Burkitt's concept, all these "Western diseases can be traced to the Western diet, which reduces stool volume, prolongs transit time (leading to constipation), and requires more straining for defecation." These factors conspire to increase pressure in the abdomen, and consequently also in the veins of the lower limbs (248, 249). Food for thought.

Dietary carcinogens. There is of course no limit to the carcinogens that can be eaten with food or can develop while digesting or metabolizing it; oral and bacterial flora, vitamins, cholesterol, and bile acids introduce other variables. It is unsettling to find out that, *after tobacco,* the major source of environmental carcinogens is the diet (96). Over 99 percent of these carcinogens are natural or produced during the preparation of food. Additives and the like account for less than 1 percent. After preparing this chapter, the only advice we can give is to stop eating.

Of special concern are the **nitrosamines,** the most omnipotent carcinogens in the sense that they affect the broadest range of species, including humans (Figure 28.15) (143, 201). The principal theory to explain gastric cancer is based on nitrosamine formation in the stomach (166). Nitrosamines are formed by a reaction between nitrous acid (HNO_2) and secondary amines (165) (*nitrosation*):

$$2\ HNO_2 \rightarrow N_2O_3 + H_2O$$
$$R_2NH + N_2O_3 \rightarrow R_2N \cdot NO + HNO_2$$

Sodium nitrite is used as a food additive in cured meat and fish to improve taste and appearance. Nitrites are also used in pathology museums to preserve the color of fixed specimens: nitrosohemoglobin is attractively pink (165). Nitrites are also invaluable for protecting against the lethal *Clostridium botulinum* (128). The necessity of adding nitrites to food has been questioned because plenty of nitrites are contained in unprocessed foods. Plant foods contain nitrates that oral bacteria reduce to nitrites (240). *The reaction between nitrites and secondary amines is inhibited by adding ascorbic acid to food* (165, 166); fruit and vegetables in the diet have the same effect. Nitrosamines, as mentioned earlier, are present also in tobacco smoke.

Natural dietary carcinogens are produced by bacteria and plants (117), which means that fans of natural foods are not necessarily safe from dietary cancer. In 1960 and 1961, two epidemics (*epizootics* would be the proper term) killed thousands of turkeys in England and devastated the rainbow trout production in Idaho (282). The epidemics were traced to peanut meal, imported from South Africa, that was contaminated with the common fungus *Aspergillus flavus;* fed to rats it produced hepatomas. The chemical culprit was *aflatoxin B_1,* one of the most potent carcinogens known; it is thought to be major factor in the high incidence of liver cancer in many countries where grain is stored in warm and humid conditions (Africa and Asia) (33). The aflatoxin may not act alone but in conjunction with hepatitis B virus, which is also associated with liver cancer (9). We have chosen the "aflatoxin hepatoma" as an example of a typical multifactorial cancer (p. 946).

The cycad nut (117) cannot be a staple of our readers' diet unless they live in southwest Japan, but the effects of its consumption do convey an important message: it produces cancer of the liver and kidneys in ordinary laboratory rats but not in bacteria-free rats. The ultimate carcinogen, in this case cycasin, a relative of the nitrosamines, is released by intestinal bacteria (141). The ways of cancer are infinite.

Dietary anticarcinogens. It is time for some good news, supplied overwhelmingly by vegetables and fruit (6, 96, 211, 276). Besides fiber, diets contain a variety of agents that have shown anticarcinogen effects in epidemiologic studies and/or *in vitro*. The cheerful yellow-orange and yellow-red color of vegetables are due mainly to carotenoids, which have cancer-preventing virtues; one of these carotenoids, lycopene—abundant in tomatoes—decreases the risk of prostate, lung, and stomach cancer. Garlic contains organosulfides, which may be smelly but have several anticarcinogenic effects. Much can be said in praise of broccoli, cauliflower, cabbage, and Brussels sprouts.

Vitamin A and other retinoids have been reported as anticarcinogenic for several organs (skin, breast, and bladder). Vitamin C, taken orally, does protect against nitrosamines, but two thorough studies have failed to show any general anticancer effect (278). Vegetarians enjoy lower rates of cancer of the breast, colon, and prostate; epidemiologic studies suggest a protective effect of certain seeds (maize, corn, beans). **Protease inhibitors** are abundant component of all seeds; in fact, a soybean protease inhibitor was found to be anticarcinogenic *in vivo* and *in vitro* (134, 288).

This is known as the Bowman-Birk Inhibitor; it may help understand the different incidence of cancers in Asian and Westen populations (17, 39, 96, 247).

Hormones as carcinogens. Hormones are not likely to be genotoxic, that is, they do not behave as DNA poisons. Yet they have many links with tumors. The hormonal status of the body plays a major role in experimental carcinogenesis (89). As we will see later, even virus-induced mammary tumors of the mouse can be prevented by ovariectomy (p. 859).

Endocrine tumors in rodents are easily produced by *overstimulation of a gland*. For example, if the thyroid is atrophied by irradiation, the hypophysis oversecretes thyrotropic hormone, enlarges, and eventually becomes neoplastic (85–88). The carcinogenic effect of endocrine overstimulation has also been proven by an imaginative experiment that takes advantage of the fact that estrogens are inactivated in the liver (22, 23, 87). In the normal female rat and mouse, the pituitary stimulates the gonads, which respond by secreting estrogens, and the blood level of estrogen serves as a "brake" (a feedback loop that controls pituitary stimulation). Now, abolish this feedback by removing one ovary and implanting the other into the spleen, so that it releases its estrogen into the splenic vein and thence into the liver, where it is inactivated. The pituitary, now deprived of this estrogen feedback, responds by overproducing gonadotropin, which causes a hyperplasia of the granulosa cells in the ovary (Figure 28.16). This hyperplastic response can produce first a benign tumor

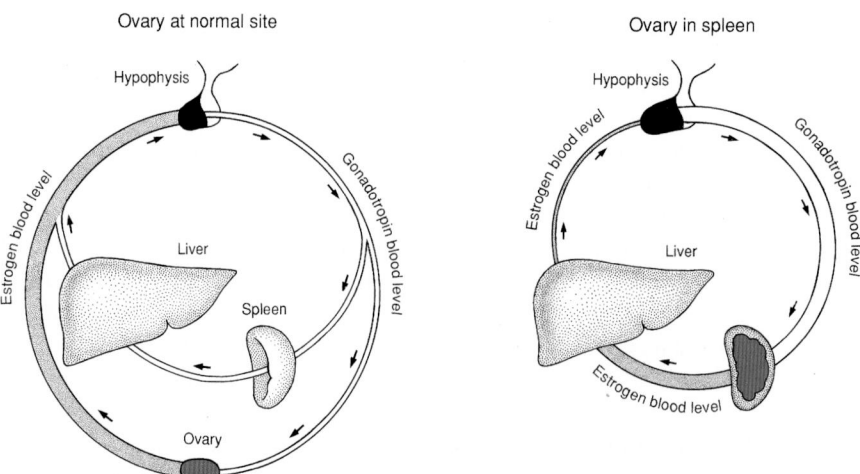

FIGURE 28.16   Example of hormonal carcinogenesis in the rat. *Left:* In the normal rat, estrogens secreted by the ovary reach the hypophysis and regulate the blood level of gonadotrophin. *Right:* If the ovary is implanted into the spleen, blood from the spleen drains into the liver where the estrogens are inactivated; therefore the hypophysis perceives an ovarian insufficiency and increases the secretion of endotrophin. As a result there is a hypertrophy of the hypophysis and an enlargement of the ovarian implant in the spleen that can become neoplastic. (Adapted with permission from [86].)

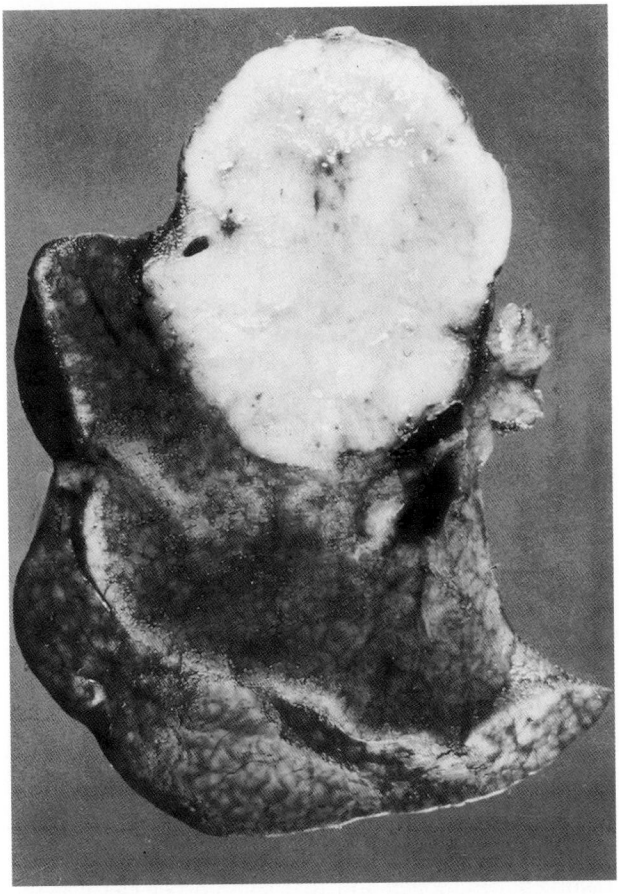

FIGURE 28.17 Carcinogenesis in rat liver by initiation with diethylnitrosamine, followed by promotion with stilbestrol for 20 weeks; the stilbestrol dose was about 200 times the usual contraceptive dose in humans. The white mass is a tumor that appeared 29 weeks after the end of the treatment. Diameter about 3 cm. (Reproduced by permission from [260], © by The US & Canadian Academy of Pathology, Inc.)

that cannot be transplanted successfully and finally a transplantable malignant tumor (95). Note the classic progression: hyperplasia → benign tumor → malignant tumor.

Also, in rats, if the liver is submitted to an initiation of carcinogenesis, estrogens are effective tumor promoters (Figure 28.17).

In humans, certain tumors (breast, ovary, endometrium, and prostate) correlate with hormonal levels (108, 159). Endogenous estrogens are the link between obesity (276) and cancer of the endometrium: adipose tissue converts androgens to estrogens (p. 40). Therapeutic levels of estrogens in postmenopausal women increase the risk of endometrial cancer, whereas contraceptive doses in premenopausal women induce, oddly enough, liver adenomas (62, 260).

The high incidence of cancer of the breast in nuns could also be mentioned under occupational diseases. Two major risk factors for breast cancer are being nulliparous and being overweight (108, 276). This correlation, first observed in nuns, appeared in 1700 in the pioneering treatise *De morbis artificum* (On the Diseases of Workers) by Bernardino Ramazzini:

> Every city in Italy has several religious communities of nuns, and you can seldom find a convent that does not harbor this accursed pest, cancer, within its walls. Now why is it that the breasts suffer for the derangements of the womb, whereas other parts of the body do not suffer in this way or so frequently? It is certainly because there is between them a mysterious sympathy that so far has escaped the researches of prosecutors, though perhaps the course of time will reveal it, since the whole domain of Truth has not yet been conquered. (204, 283)

The reverse of the coin, giving birth to a child at early age, protects against breast cancer. These facts can be reconciled as follows: we know from the study of carcinogenesis that the more a cell is differentiated, the less it is susceptible to malignant transformation (224); ostensibly the epithelium of the mammary gland becomes fully differentiated only in the course of lactation (224).

> We can now add, or rather delete, another piece of the puzzle: after several years of political, rather than scientific, debate, we can safely conclude that induced abortion does NOT increase the risk of breast cancer (176).

However, the natural history of breast cancer includes more than hormones, as we will see later.

Occupational carcinogens. After the soot wart, another scrotal cancer appeared in Scotland early in the twentieth century; it was due to mineral oil (232). Workers in the cotton industry attended the "mule," a machine that carried rotating spools and had to be lubricated constantly. As mule spinners leaned over the edge of the machine, oil soaked into their clothes at the level of the groin, eventually causing scrotal cancer in many workers.

In more recent times (1974), the physician of a chemical plant where *polyvinyl chloride resins* were manufactured was alerted by the fact that three workers in two years had died of angiosarcoma of the liver, a rare tumor (54). The cause of this bizarre cluster was quickly traced to vinyl chloride, the plastic monomer (145, 195). The worker's exposure had lasted from 2 to 18 years; in laboratory rodents the latent period is less than a year (194).

Asbestos was discovered to be a carcinogen in 1960, thanks to maps of cancer mortality. An exceptionally high incidence of lung cancer in white males of coastal Georgia was correlated with work in shipyards during World War II (26). The inhaled fibers produce fibrosis and eventually malignant tumors of the mesothelium of the pleura, pericardium, and peritoneum (see Figures 13.47, 13.48). The fibers, although insoluble, are both cytotoxic and genotoxic by generating free radicals; they have been shown to damage DNA and disturb mitosis (255). Asbestos acts synergistically with cigarette smoke (172).

Nickel and *chromium* correlate with the incidence of cancer of the lung, and nickel also with the incidence of cancer of the nasal sinuses (59, 237). The same tissues are affected in leather workers and in manufacturers of hardwood furniture, but the carcinogen is unknown. Again, it was a general practitioner who noticed this connection. Dr. John Jones of Clydach, South Wales, diagnosed two cases of carcinoma of the ethmoid sinus in a single year (237).

> The molecular mechanisms of carcinogenesis by nickel shows how complicated oncology can be. Possible effects of nickel ions include chromosome damage, mutagenesis, formation of left-handed DNA (Z-DNA), inhibition of DNA excision–repair, tumor promotion, and enhancement of tumor progression by inhibition of NK cells (236).

Therapeutic carcinogens. An irony of tumor therapy is that our most powerful antitumor agents produce tumors. This may be inescapable at present; *carcinogens and our current anticarcinogens aim at the same target: the DNA molecule* (187). And so, as of 2002, **second cancers** are six to ten percent of all new cancers diagnosed in the USA every year (or 95,000 of about 1.2 million); they are **the 4th or 5th most common type of cancer** (15a). Survivors of childhood cancers are at an increased risk of developing a second primary cancer when compared to the general population. Both chemotherapy as well as radiotherapy are risk factors (15a). Overall, however, these results are interpreted as not outweighing the benefits of therapy (40, 183, 250).

The therapeutic use of *diethylstilbestrol* became, unfortunately, a *cause célèbre* in 1971 (Figure 28.18) (110–112, 156). This episode shows the importance of the alert practitioner as a watch against unexpected carcinogens.

> Adenocarcinoma of the vagina is a rare tumor, usually seen in women over 50. Suddenly, between 1966 and 1969, seven young women 15–22 years old came to the same gynecologist, A. L. Herbst, with an adenocarcinoma of the vagina. Suspecting an unknown carcinogen, Dr. H. Ulfelder, the epidemiologist of the clinical team, took

$$HO \text{—} \langle \text{ring} \rangle \text{—} \underset{\underset{C_2H_5}{|}}{\overset{\overset{C_2H_5}{|}}{C}} = C \text{—} \langle \text{ring} \rangle \text{—} OH$$

Diethylstilbestrol

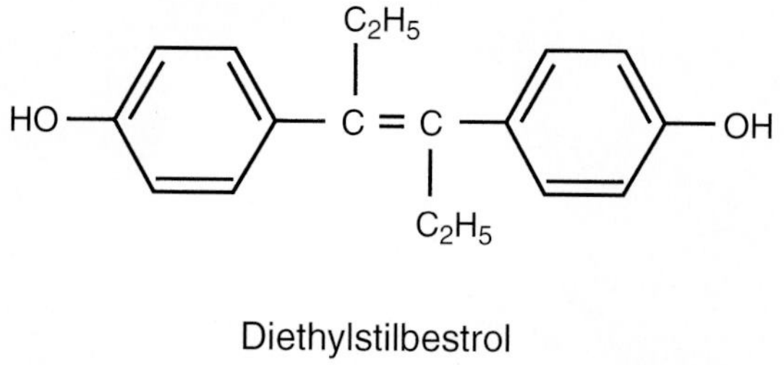

FIGURE 28.18   The formula of diethylstilbestrol.

careful, detailed histories from each patient. Nothing unusual surfaced. Finally one patient, because she was so young, came with her mother, who volunteered her own strong belief: she was sure that the culprit was a drug she had been given during pregnancy. This hint was not followed up, but when a second mother offered the same suggestion, Dr. Ulfelder investigated. The drug turned out to be diethylstilbestrol, customarily given to stop bleeding during pregnancy.

After the first few cases, hundreds more came to light, and thousands of young women whose mothers were treated during pregnancy are still living with this threat. Fortunately, their risk up to age 34 is fairly low, 1 in 1000, which suggests that diethylstilbestrol is not a complete carcinogen and that some other factor is involved (156). Alas, a review in the year 2000 adds a further risk for high-grade squamous cell carcinoma of the cervix and vagina (105, 106). Much less is known about males exposed to DES *in utero;* disorders of the reproductive tract have been reported (239) but cancer risk is probably not increased (235).

Immunosuppression for therapeutic purposes is another pathway to cancer (p. 604).

Sundry carcinogens. Free radicals can certainly injure DNA strands. They are involved in the well-known carcinogenesis by ionizing radiations (81). But what about endogenous sources of free radicals, such as activated leukocytes? Is it thinkable that leukocytes could be carcinogenic (13)? The concept has been proposed, and the evidence, although indirect, is impressive. In one study, mouse fibroblasts were exposed to activated human leukocytes and then were injected into nude mice; they produced tumors (274).

> The ability of a substance to cause mutations can be tested with a large number of assays on bacteria. Human leukocytes exposed to bacteria do cause bacterial mutations; and the free-radical scavenger, superoxide dismutase, inhibits the mutations. Heat-killed cells, lymphocytes, and

leukocytes from a patient with chronic granulomatous disease, which cannot mount a respiratory burst (pp. 420, 520), did not cause mutations (273). Activated human leukocytes exposed to mammalian cells caused visible chromosomal changes (272).

All this occurs *in vitro;* what happens *in vivo* remains to be seen. Perhaps this free radical mechanism is involved in carcinogenesis by plastic sheets (p. 855) and possibly by asbestos.

Among carcinogens discovered by accident (228) are the potent fluorenamides (N-2-fluorenylacetamide, 2-FAA),

patented in 1940 as insecticides. Their use ended abruptly when their carcinogenic effects on rats were discovered. Interestingly, guinea pigs are immune to this carcinogen because they do not metabolize the molecule to its ultimate form (man does, as was found using trace doses in volunteers with advanced cancer). The effect of *urethane* was discovered at the National Cancer Institute in experiments on the effects of radiation. The mice had to be maintained under sedation for prolonged periods, wherefore the standard veterinary solution of urethane was used. Lung tumors appeared in 26 of 29 mice, and the urethane, not the radiation, was found to be the cause.

Physical Causes of Tumors

Besides ultraviolet and ionizing radiation, the physical causes of cancer include burns, physical trauma (a minor but interesting category), and a bizarre but fascinating phenomenon: carcinogenesis by plastic sheets, which led to the concept of solid-state carcinogenesis.

Radiation

Considering the vast range of the electromagnetic spectrum to which we are exposed, including radio waves (256), it is fortunate that only the ultraviolet and ionizing radiations are carcinogenic (Figure 3.52) (221a, 255).

Magnetic fields need not be feared as a cause of leukemia in children through residential exposure (144) and cellular telephone users are temporarily safe from brain tumors, but long-range studies on heavy users are needed (127, 246).

Ultraviolet light is the major source of skin cancer, but the risk is highly dependent on skin pigmentation (p. 937). It is difficult to find precise figures for the incidence, because most of UV-caused skin cancers are the benevolent (if not benign) basal cell carcinomas, which are treated almost casually, often not reported and thus not even included in cancer statistics. In 1996 non-melanoma skin cancers in the USA were about 800,000, of which 80 percent were basal cell and 20 percent were squamous cell carcinomas, definitely more aggressive.

The incidence of melanoma is inversely related to latitude (66), which clearly implicates sunlight; in fact even the number of sunspots have been said to affect the statistics of human melanoma (119). The increase in melanoma since 1935 implicates, we hope, only a behavioral trend: the otherwise innocent practice of

sun-worship (Figure 28.19). So we are probably dealing, once again, with a large number of theoretically avoidable cancers. We introduce a note of uncertainty in this statement because a further increase in the incidence of melanoma might implicate a more threatening cause—the thinning of the ozone layer (152).

As to the pathogenesis of UV cancer: UV light has been subdivided into three bands, named A, B and C (see Figure 3.52), of which Type B is the most carcinogenic.

Type A penetrates into the skin more deeply than B, but it is weakly absorbed by DNA and is carcinogenic indirectly, by releasing free radicals with secondary damage to DNA. *Type B* is responsible for most of UV cancers; *Type C* produced by mercury lamps used for sterilizing (255) is absorbed by the atmosphere.

Non-melanoma skin cancer develops on areas of the skin most exposed to sunlight; melanoma, by contrast, appears to develop as a result of acute sunburns: a history of 5 or more acute sunburns in adolescence doubles the risk of melanoma (92, 255) and a single neonatal sunburn will produce melanoma in mice (178). As a malignant tumor, melanoma is distinctive also because it offers one of the best-documented examples of progression from a benign lesion to a fully aggressive, metastasizing tumor. The six steps now recognized are: mature melanocyte → common nevus → melanocytic dysplasia → radial growth phase (RGP) melanoma → vertical growth phase (VGP) melanoma → metastatic melanoma (113).

Experimentally, UV rays behave as complete carcinogens, but repeated exposures are needed. Treatment with a promoter such as phorbol ester accelerates the response *in vivo* in *in vitro* (169, 205). At the molecular

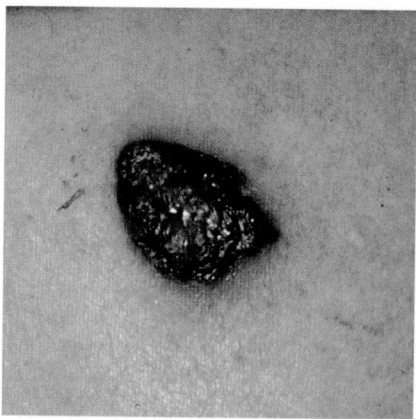

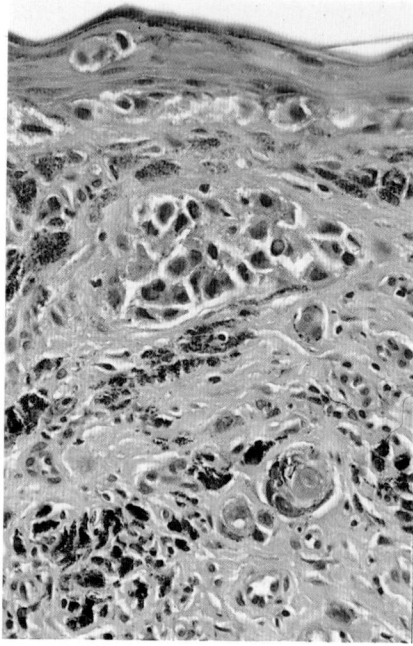

FIGURE 28.19   *Top:* Melanoma of the back in a 58-year-old white man without a history of sunburns. The lesion, not ulcerated, has been present for several months. *Bottom:* Histologic aspect: groups of atypical cells loaded with melanin. At top left corner, note the small cluster of malignant cells invading the epidermis (100x). (Reproduced with permission from [16], Copyright © 2001 by Dermatopathology Interactive Atlas.)

level, UV rays do not have enough energy to ionize their targets, but they raise them to a short-lived excited state and thereby damage DNA strands by forming dimers and crosslinks (205). It may be relevant that *UV radiation tends to depress the immune system;* a mild sunburn depresses the viability and function of circulating lymphocytes for as long as 24 hours (152).

The effect of UV radiation on leukocytes is an intriguing topic. Some UV rays reach as deep as the capillaries, and

about 5 percent of cardiac output flows through the skin. The white color of leukocytes, it has been said (220), protects these cells against DNA injury because it reflects the entire spectrum; but later work showed that UV radiation does damage the leukocytes' DNA (168).

Ionizing radiations. Ionizing radiations are part of our natural environment, but as carcinogens they are to a large extent a man-made problem. Figure 28.20 shows the sources of ionizing radiations to inhabitants of the United States; the largest share is the radiation background (cosmic rays and terrestrial radiation), whereas 18 percent is due to medical or industrial sources. Some ionizing radiations are electromagnetic (X-rays and gamma rays) and others are particulate (electrons, protons, alpha and beta particles) (Figure 3.52).

Radiation cancer claimed its first known victims as an occupational disease long before the discovery of ionizing radiation (121, 264). It was known for centuries that Czech and German miners working on either side of the Erz mountains were being killed by a mysterious "mountain disease" (*Bergsucht*). The mines first yielded silver, later nickel and other metals, and finally uranium; the ore was the same as that in which Mme. Curie dicovered radium. The mysterious "pneumonia" of the miners was not recognized as cancer until 1929 when the first autopsies were performed (189); the culprit was radon gas, a decay product of radium (149).

In 1895 Roentgen discovered X-rays and dedicated them to the benefit of mankind (he did not patent his X-ray machine); seven years later the first report of a case of skin cancer in a radiologist was published. Many more followed, and industrial exposure became an added hazard (Figure 28.21). Between 1929 and 1943 ten times more radiologists died of leukemia than other physicians: a difference that has since disappeared (137, 149).

For the discovery of radium, Pierre and Marie Curie received the Nobel prize in 1904, but the award came at a high price: both Mme. Curie and her daughter Irene died of leukemia (184). Radium claimed many other victims; it was used to make fluorescent paint for the dials of watches. The women who painted the dials ingested radium by licking their brushes to make fine points. Many of these women developed osteosarcomas of the mastoid and carcinomas of the nasal sinuses (Figure 28.22) (122), while their employers denied any responsibility. The story of the "radium girls" is worth reading (45).

The true hazards of radiation (137) were not perceived until recently; both authors of this book remember shoe shops in which customers stepped onto an X-ray box to admire the snug fit of their new shoes.

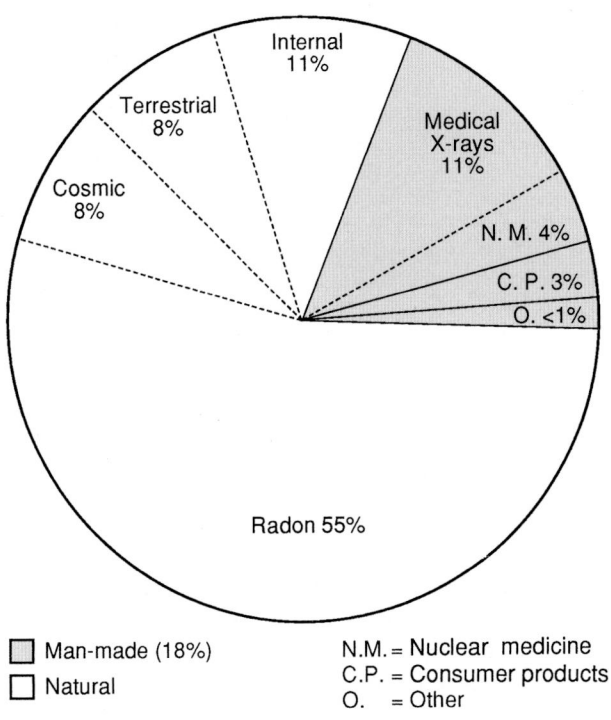

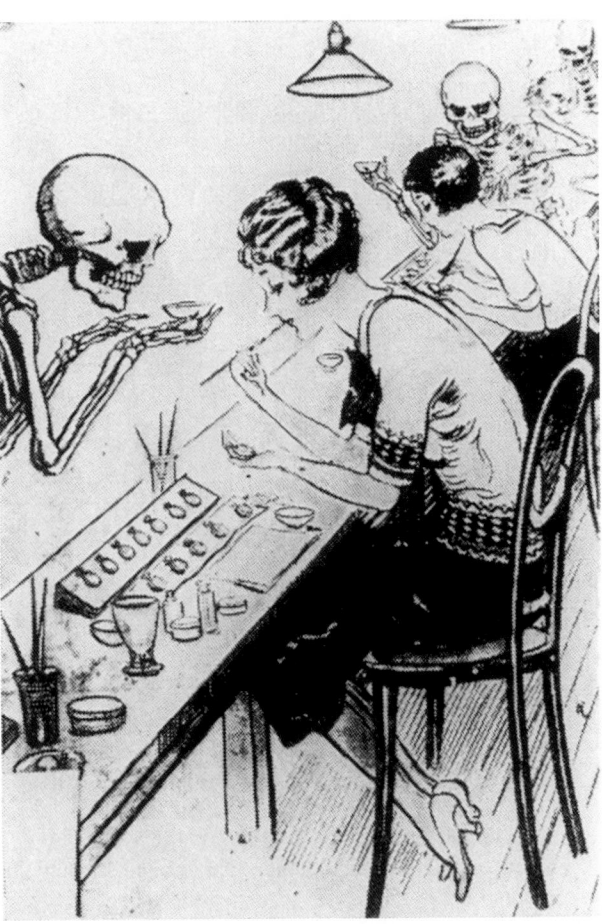

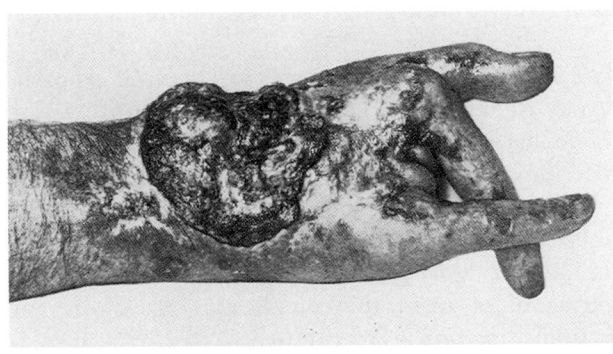

FIGURE 28.20 Percentage contribution of various sources of radiation to the total average effective dose (U.S. population). (Reproduced with permission from the NCRP [174].)

FIGURE 28.22 A famous cartoon in a New York newspaper: Death holding a dish of mesothorium paint to a technician, who applies it to the watch dial. Note how the technician is drawing the brush to a point with her lips. (Reproduced from [122].)

FIGURE 28.21 Carcinoma of the back of the hand in a 57-year-old man who worked for 27 years in the manufacture of X-ray apparatus, in the early days of radiology. By 1922 about 100 radiologists had died from malignant disease due to their occupation. (Reproduced from [122].)

This casual use of radiation produced some medical disasters.

For example, in the 1940s and 1950s, children were irradiated routinely to reduce the size of the tonsils or of the thymus, which were perceived as too large (today the latter is a nondisease). In one series, cancer of the thyroid developed in 8 percent with a delay of 20–30 years (72, 149). Other children, perhaps 200,000 worldwide, had their scalps submitted to the very "handy" X-ray epilation for a common fungal infection; the cost was an increase in the incidence of tumors of the scalp, brain, parotid, neck and thyroid, plus some mental illness (3, 116, 167). The parotid is similarly affected by X-ray treatment for acne, still current (37, 199). Radioactive thorium dioxide ("Thorotrast") was used after 1928 as a contrast medium in radiology to visualize arterial trees. After its quick performance in the arteries it continued to circulate until it was all picked up and removed by the RES, including the Kupffer cells (p. 314) (see Figure 8.12). Predictably, the liver suffered most from the prolonged exposure to thorium radiation: the first angiosarcoma of the liver was diagnosed at autopsy 12 years later (150, 261). By 1999, 454 primary liver cancers were recorded (258).

FIGURE 28.23 Radiation effects on mitosis in cultured cells (mouse lymphoma). (**a**) Anaphase with two bridges. (**b**) Anaphase with loss of a chromosome. The lost chromosome will give rise to a micronucleus. (Reproduced with permission from [223].)

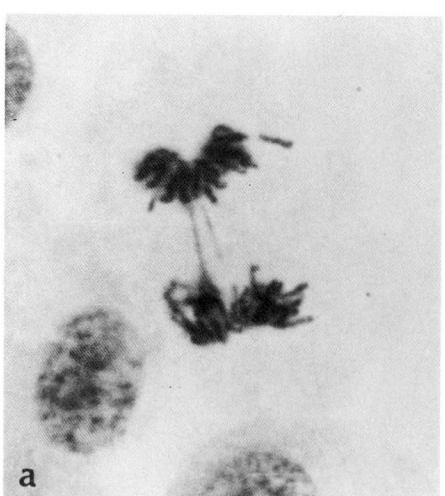

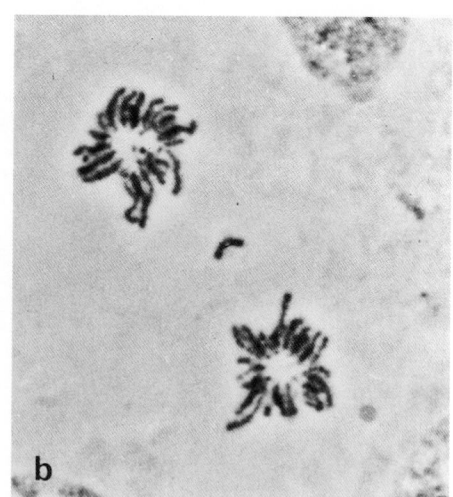

Ionizing radiations have been called *universal carcinogens* because, unlike chemical carcinogens, they induce cancers in virtually all tissues of all species at all ages, possibly including the fetus.

The amount of energy absorbed by irradiated matter is expressed in a unit called a *rad* (100 ergs deposited per gram); however, rads tell nothing about ionization density, which is expressed as LET (linear energy transfer: energy lost per unit of distance traveled in kiloelectron volts per micrometer) (150).

For a given dose, highly ionizing radiations (high-LET) are more carcinogenic, suggesting that ionization is an important factor. Unlike UV rays, a single exposure to ionizing radiation is enough to cause cancer, as demonstrated by the survivors of the Nagasaki and Hiroshima atomic bombs; leukemia appeared after about 6 years, whereas other solid tumors increased after 20 years (48, 116). This difference in latency between leukemias and solid tumors is a general rule (137). The tumors, benign and malignant, caused by radiation are similar to spontaneous tumors and tend to develop at the customary age (137), with one peculiarity: chronic lymphatic leukemia does not seem to develop from radiations of any kind.

Some individuals are especially prone to radiation cancer. The classic example is the familial form of retinoblastoma (251). We shall explain this condition further on p. 887.

The molecular damage due to radiation can occur anywhere in a cell; but because the protoplasm is 80 percent water, the main direct target is water, which breaks into free radicals that cause indirect damage. Another source of free radicals is molecular oxygen, hence the difficulty of killing the hypoxic parts of tumors (p. 789). DNA can undergo single or double-stranded breaks, loss of bases, or formation of abnormal bonds between adjacent bases (which become dimers). The half-time for repair of this damage, measured in the epithelium of rat skin, was estimated at 3 ± 1 hours (37). Sometimes one or more chromosomes go astray during mitosis (Figure 28.23) and then set up their own separate home in a "micronucleus" (Figure 28.24).

The biological effect of radiation damage can manifest itself at a metabolic, genetic, or cellular level. Irradiated cells may survive but suffer so-called *reproductive death:* they can no longer divide. Sometimes they become gigantic (Figure 28.25). The most studied aspect of radiation injury is shortened cell survival, which is exploited for tumor radiotherapy. Most sensitive are bone-marrow cells and intestinal epithelium, cells that have high mitotic rates.

It is certainly a paradox that radiation, which typically shortens cell survival, should also be capable of immortalizing cells by conferring malignant transformation on them; this complication of radiotherapy is studied *in vitro* in cell cultures.

Transformation *in vitro* is invaluable for testing potential cancer-preventing agents (205). The standard method is to grow cells of an appropriate type in Petri dishes until they are confluent; often used in the line of mouse embryo fibroblasts called 3T3. These cells are not normal because they are aneuploid and immortal. However, they remain contact inhibited, and they are not considered neoplastic because they do not form tumors when injected into suitable recipient animals. They are perhaps on the way to becoming neoplastic because they occasionally give rise to foci of transformed cells that are tightly packed (Type 1 foci) or have lost contact inhibition and pile up over each other (Type 2 and 3 foci) (Figure 28.26) (208). To return to the assay: Petri dishes with confluent cells are irradiated

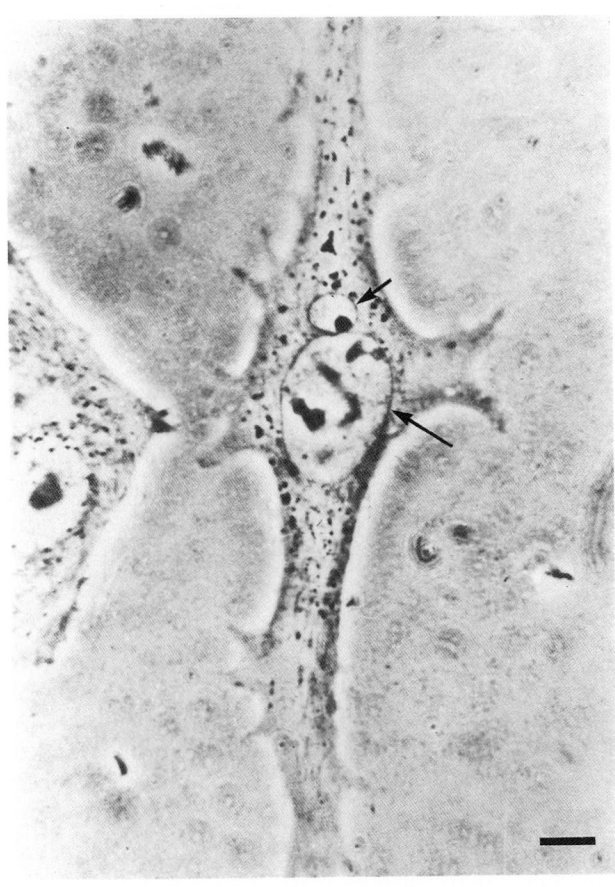

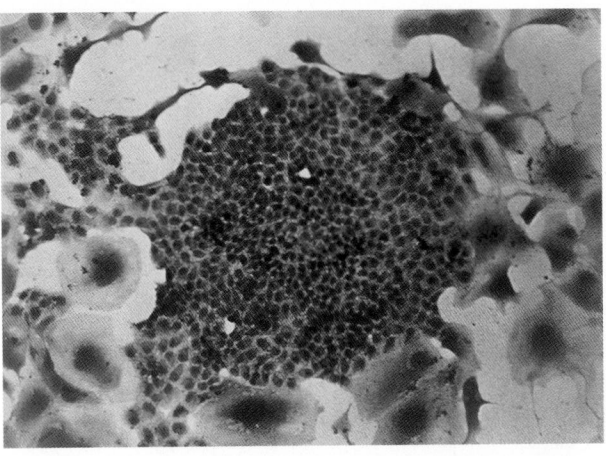

FIGURE 28.25 Cell mutations induced by irradiation in cultured HeLa cancer cells. The large "monster" cells have lost their reproductive capacity but carry on metabolic functions. (Reproduced with permission from [202].)

FIGURE 28.24 Cultured irradiated cell with a main nucleus (**long arrow**) and a micronucleus (**short arrow**), the latter deriving from a lost chromosome fragment. **Bar** = 10 μm. (Reproduced with permission from [100].)

and then kept for 4–6 weeks, after which they are fixed, stained, and the transformed foci are counted (Figure 28.27). With this number as a baseline, it is fairly simple to test agents that increase the number of foci (such as the cancer promoting phorbol esters) or inhibit them (such as protease inhibitors, selenium, and vitamin A, C, or E) (146).

Physical Trauma

Mechanical trauma is usually ruled out as a cause of tumors, but this point of view should be reexamined. A

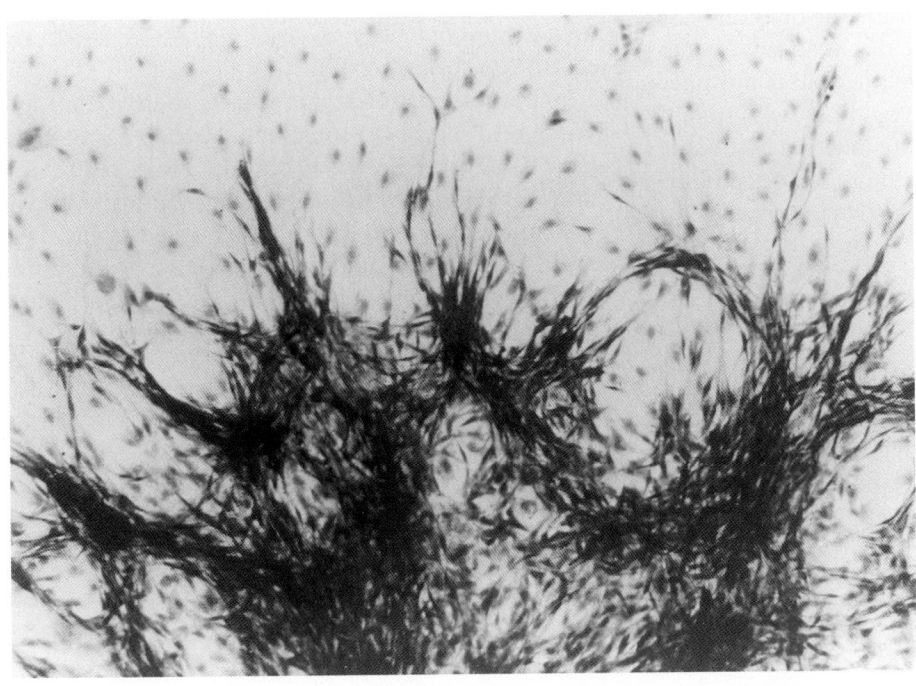

FIGURE 28.26 Edge of a focus of transformed fibroblasts 6 weeks after irradiation. Compared with normal cells (*top*), transformed cells are highly basophilic and tend to overlap. (Courtesy of Dr. A. R. Kennedy, University of Pennsylvania, Pittsburgh, PA.)

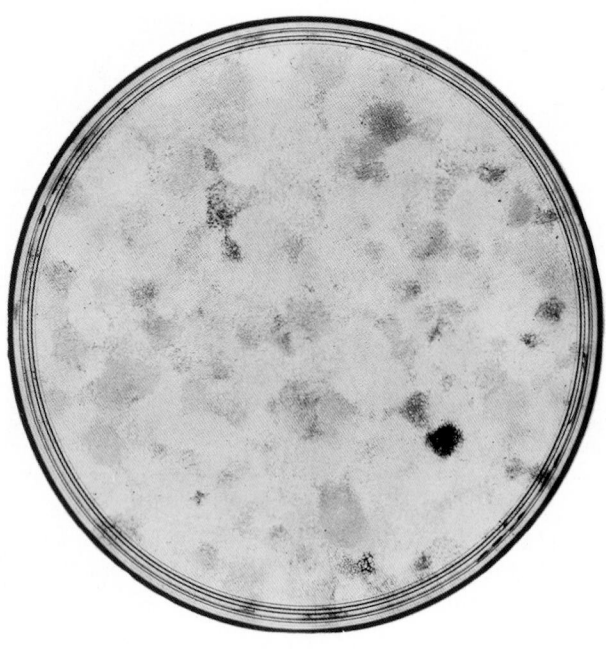

FIGURE 28.27 Mouse fibroblasts growing in a Petri dish, stained with methylene blue 6 weeks after irradiation. A large focus of piled-up transformed cells stands out on a background monolayer of nontransformed cells. (Courtesy of Dr. A. R. Kennedy, University of Pennsylvania, Philadelphia, PA.)

single trauma on *normal* tissues is indeed unlikely to produce a tumor, because the short burst of mitoses that comes with repair is *statistically* unlikely to produce a malignant mutation. However, two other settings are possible: (a) a single traumatic lesion does not heal and becomes chronic, usually as a result of infection, thereby prolonging the period of mitotic divisions; and (b) a single trauma hits a tissue that is already predisposed to develop a tumor. This mechanism is illustrated by the classic experiments by Peyton Rous, who studied rabbit skin prepared with a noncarcinogenic dose of tar, and showed that malignant tumors developed predictably wherever the prepared skin was traumatized by biopsy (p. 859).

> We had the opportunity to study a patient who appeared to illustrate the first modality. A 26-year-old construction worker was hit in a cheek by a swinging hook; the wound never healed and 9 years later gave rise to a squamous cell carcinoma. In this case the lack of healing (although unexplained) provided a powerful link between trauma and cancer. The insurance company chose to settle out of court.

A computer search for titles combining *scar* and *tumor* brought up a wealth of recent reports of carcinomas (not sarcomas) arising in scars. The incidence seems to be greater outside North America (142).

Many of the scars that developed tumors derived from mechanical injuries, including surgical scars (126) and burns (1, 8), but the list included venipuncture (after 6 months; the original puncture site never healed) (275), frostbite (68), snake bite (142), and even a surgical wound of the thigh from which skin grafts had been taken 6 weeks previously to cover a burn (103). A study of 1774 basal cell carcinomas found a history of trauma in 7.3 percent (177).

It is clear that carcinomas sometimes arise in scars and even in recent wounds; fibrosarcomas are almost never seen except after irradiation (131). The real issue is their frequency. As just mentioned, there may be differences among populations. In the wake of World War I, the Germans rated the incidence of malignancies (in 3,710,371 hospital-treated wounds) as 5.3 per million; the French estimate was 10 times higher (121). In burn wounds the incidence of malignancy is probably higher than in mechanical wounds.

Chronic irritation such as that in ulcers is a special form of trauma. Malignant tumors arising on persistent ulcers, especially after burns, are sometimes mentioned in surgical circles as Marjolin's ulcer (80). Quite apart from the fact that Professor Marjolin never described such an event (233), the occurrence is so rare that even one case is publishable (219). In a recent review of 46 cases of squamous cell carcinoma after a burn the latent period averaged 43 years. It was concluded by the reviewers that the incidence of this complication is dropping, perhaps because the care of burns has greatly improved (63). Occasionally a tumor develops around a foreign body. A man, who may have been the last victim of World War I, died of a sarcoma developing around fragments of a German grenade, 65 years later. Sarcomas around Dacron aortic grafts have also been reported (see below) (107).

Esophageal strictures after caustic injury (from ingesting acids or alkali) sometimes develop carcinomas after 30–45 years; the stenosis causes gastric reflux and chronic irritation, which may be the culprit (55, 221).

Meningiomas represent a peculiar exception: they are the only tumors statistically associated with a history of trauma (head trauma) and even foreign bodies such as bullets (218). We have no explanation.

> The so-called scar carcinomas of the lung are probably not carcinomas in scars, but rather desmoplastic carcinomas, that is, carcinomas that induce a dense, fibrous stroma (65).

Besides causing tumors, trauma relates to tumors in other ways. It has been shown many times in experimental animals that mechanical, chemical, or surgical trauma can localize metastases (79, 173); this mechanism may also apply to surgical wounds (p. 822).

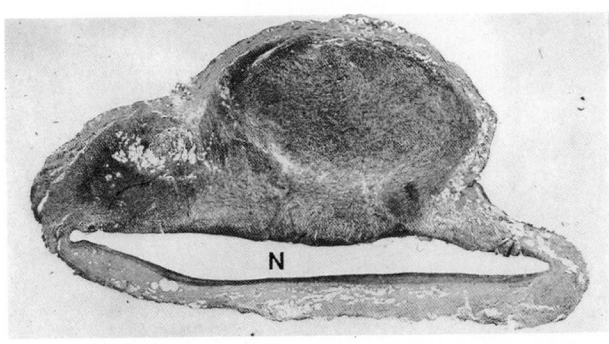

FIGURE 28.28 Example of the mysterious plastic sheet sarcoma. A square of nylon film (**N**) was implanted subcutaneously in a rat; 22 months later a fibrosarcoma developed over the film **Bar** = 1 mm. (Reproduced from [181].)

Dormant cancer cells can be awakened: in rats injected with as few as 50 malignant cells in the liver, repeated laparotomy and exploration of the liver greatly accelerates the appearance of tumors (78). Trauma can also localize a circulating virus: rabbit papilloma virus injected intravenously creates papillomas where the skin has been shaved; the mechanism has not been studied.

The Puzzle of Plastic Sheet Sarcomas (Solid State Carcinogenesis)

This is a strange story (18, 29) although time has wiped away most of the mystery.

In 1941 it was reported that disks of bakelite (a plastic) implanted subcutaneously in rats produced sarcomas. Nobody picked up the trail. In 1948, Oppenheimer and co-workers (180) were producing hypertension in rats by wrapping one kidney in cellophane. This procedure causes a fibrous reaction that strangles the kidney, which becomes ischemic and responds by producing renin, and thereby hypertension. It was found quite accidentally that sarcomas had developed around some of the cellophane wrappings. Further work showed that virtually any plastic sheet implanted under the skin—including nylon, dacron, saran, and many others—induces sarcomas in rats and mice. The percentage of implants that produced tumors varied between 7 and 50 percent. The latent period ranged from 7 months to 2½ years (181). If the plastic sheet was removed after 6 months, the carcinogenic effect persisted (Figure 28.28).

Then came variations on the theme. It was found that the plastic sheets (or disks) have to be of a certain size, of the order of 2 × 3 cm; if they are cut into small pieces or pulverized, the effect disappears. Smooth surfaces work much better than rough ones (11). One of the experimenters, with whom we spoke, was particularly bewildered by finding that sarcomas failed to appear if the sheets had become accidentally folded during implantation or if they were perforated. Millipore filters with small pores induce tumors; those with large pores do not (94). The mystery spread beyond plastic: sheets of gold and silver and steel also produce sarcomas, and so do many other inert substances (18), including plates of glass and quartz; but powdered glass or quartz will not do.

The name *solid-state carcinogenesis* seems well justified. But how does it work? The mere presence of *any* foreign body will not do: sarcomas around surgical prostheses in humans, happily, are in the "nearly never" category. One theory blamed the macrophages: free radicals, produced by macrophages activated on the surface of a foreign body, might be able to damage the DNA of surrounding fibroblasts and create malignant mutations. We prefer to take the hint offered by the study of **carcinogenesis by asbestos fibers.** It is now apparent that these "inert" fibers are not inert at all: their surface can generate free radicals (287), especially where the fibers are broken, exposing unsaturated valences (84).

A positive, if somewhat worrisome, result of this research is that biomaterials in routine clinical use have been proposed for the study of sarcomas, much as tar painting of the skin has been used for carcinomas (125 of 490 rats produced grossly visible tumors after 26–110 weeks) (135).

We close this section on physical carcinogenesis with a word of praise for granulation tissue. This exuberant variety of connective tissue, teeming with mitoses, is an almost everyday companion because it develops at virtually all sites of injury. It flourishes in millions of ulcers worldwide. Yet its growth is so well controlled that, in humans, it almost never lapses into a sarcoma. The worst it does is produce a keloid, which may or may not be a tumor. Only genetic engineering was able to break down this wonderful "self-control" of granulation tissues: there are transgenic mice in which healing wounds lapse into fibrosarcomas (222).

Biological Causes of Tumors and the Revolution of 1976

On a worldwide basis about 16 percent of all cancers are due to infection (9 percent in the USA, 21 percent in developing countries (147, 185, 190).

Note that infectious agents can induce tumors by three mechanisms: *genetic,* by perverting the cellular DNA (as in papillomas produced by viruses), *inflammatory,* by

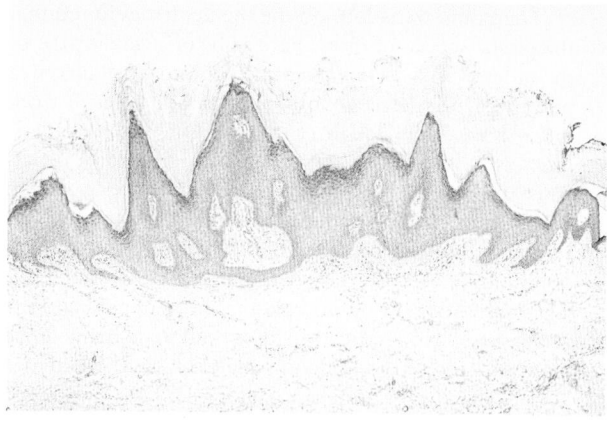

FIGURE 28.29 Common wart, the result of epidermal infection by a papilloma virus. Note the hyperplasia of the epidermis (its normal thickness is represented at the extreme right) as well as the exaggerated production of keratinized cells (hyperkeratosis).

inducing a chronic response that lapses into neoplastic growth (as in gastric cancers due to *Helicobacter pylori*), and immunosuppressive (as in Kaposi's sarcoma in AIDS patients) (190). Historically, the idea that bacteria might be the cause of cancer surfaced with the birth of bacteriology in the late 1800s; it was soon abandoned, in part because cancer did not appear to be contagious.

The first tumors that were attributed to infectious agents included human warts and plant galls.

Galls, Warts and Other Puzzles

Viruses were surmised as "filterable agents" before they could be seen. They were discovered in association with another killer, tobacco. The first disease to be proven of viral origin, in 1892, was the so-called **mosaic disease** of the tobacco plant. Shortly thereafter it was shown that the common wart, a benign tumor (Figure 28.29), is transmissible from one human volunteer to another, confirming a fact that most school children know. In 1908 two Danish veterinarians, Ellermann and Bang, showed that fowl leukemia can also be transmitted by a cell-free filtrate (64). This was a milestone in cancer research, but it did not come through as such: the authors themselves shared the current belief that leukemia had little to do with "real tumors," and their suggestion that leukemia in general is an infectious disease did not have much data to support it. Indifference and skepticism were also the lot of Peyton Rous when he announced in 1911 that he had succeeded in transmitting from hen to hen a solid malignant tumor with a cell-free filtrate (213, 214): it was a sarcoma, unquestionably malignant (Figure 28.30), but it was easy to object that hens are not mammals, and, after all, everybody

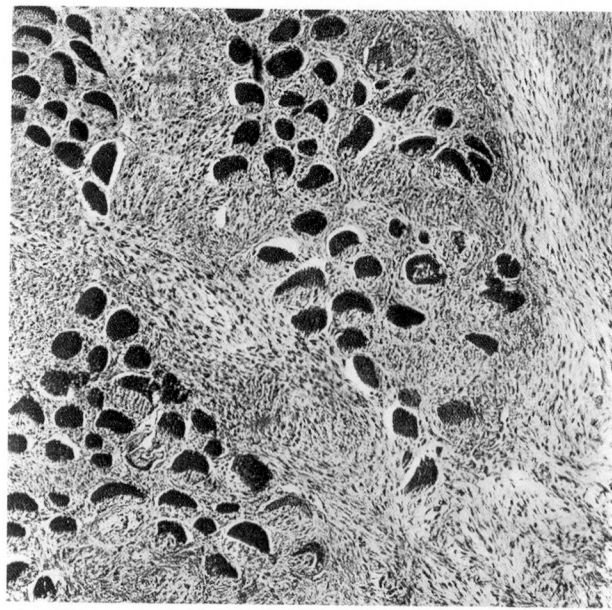

FIGURE 28.30 A historical event: This sarcoma was obtained by injecting into the breast muscle of a chicken a cell-free extract of a chicken tumor (now known as Rous sarcoma). The muscle fibers (dark masses) are dissociated by swarms of tumor cells. (Reproduced from the **Journal of Experimental Medicine,** 1911;13:397–411, by copyright permission of The Rockefeller University Press [214].)

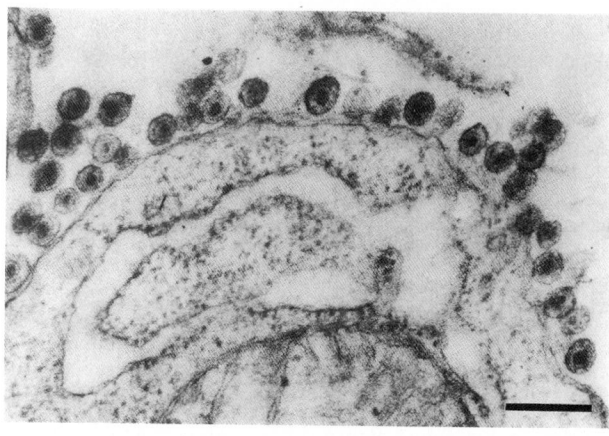

FIGURE 28.31 Particles of Rous sarcoma virus grown on a chorioallantoic membrane of a chick embryo. A characteristic row of virus particles on the surface of the plasma membrane. **Bar** = 0.3 μm. (Reproduced by permission from [99]. Electron micrograph prepared by Haguenau F, Febvre H, Arnoult J from J. Microscopie 1:445,1962.)

knew that cancer was not contagious. Rous was actually told by Simon Flexner that good science includes knowing when to quit (109). The electron microscope, which could have easily demonstrated the virus in the tumor (Figure 28.31), did not yet exist. So Rous

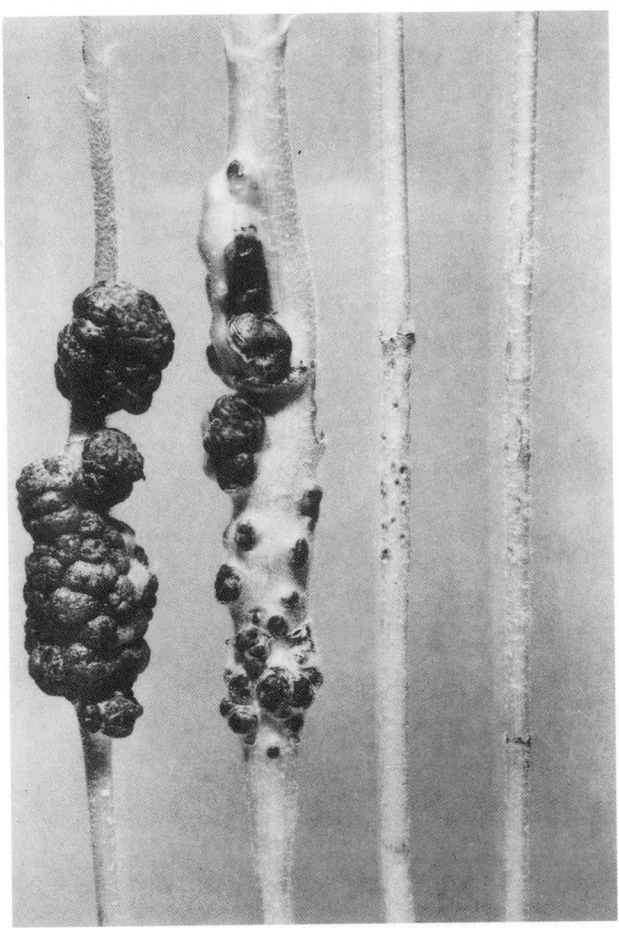

FIGURE 28.32   Plant tumor caused by a bacterium. Sunflower stems inoculated with virulent strains of *Agrobacterium tumefaciens* (*left*) and with two control strains. (Reproduced with permission from [130].)

decided to quit. Thanks to his longevity, he received his Nobel prize anyway—55 years later.

The crown gall, a bacterial tumor.   Another major discovery had just flashed by, unnoticed by the medical world because it concerned tumors in plants. In 1908, two plant pathologists of the U.S. Department of Agriculture, Smith and Townsend, showed that certain natural growths (crown galls) on the Paris daisy were caused by a soil bacterium, now called *Agrobacterium tumefaciens* (Figure 28.32) (231). This bacterium carries a bit of DNA in the shape of a ring (a plasmid); a specific part of this plasmid is somehow inserted into the DNA of a plant cell, whereupon growth is initiated; from that point on the bacterium is no longer necessary (30). This is a perfect example of natural genetic engineering; but of course it could not be appreciated in 1908 (284). Since then we have learned that a bacterium,

Helicobacter pylori, produces gastric cancer in humans by a wholly different mechanism: chronic irritation (83, 182, 254) (see p. 905).

Worms: the Fibiger epic.   In the meantime a novel kind of oncologic adventure was beginning to unfold in Copenhagen. Johannes Fibiger, a distinguished pathologist, happened to autopsy three rats who had died at the same time in the same cage. All three had papillomatous growths in their fore-stomachs. Histology showed that they contained some sort of worm. The pursuit of this worm, which Fibiger thought to be the cause of the tumor, turned into a consuming endeavor (41, 76, 179, 271).

Because nobody could diagnose the worm, Fibiger reconstructed it from 900 serial sections. It was an unknown nematode. To find a live one he had 1100 rats trapped in Copenhagen, but they all had the wrong worms and no gastric tumors. The supplier of the original three rats had gone out of business. Anyone else would have given up, but not Fibiger. Perhaps there was another stage of that worm in some other host. In an old 1824 paper he found that certain cockroaches were a possibility. But where would rats and cockroaches live together? Bakeries, decided Fibiger. For years he dissected bakery cockroaches, in vain. He was close to despair when someone told him of a sugar refinery with a different, American cockroach; he raided that refinery and finally came up with 61 rats of which 40 had worms and 9 had gastric tumors. Triumphantly he named the worm *Spiroptera neoplastica* (later *Gongylonema neoplasticum*), reconstructed its life cycle and studied the tumors in greater detail. Just in time, the sugar refinery went up in flames with all its rats, worms, and roaches (179).

For his 19-year pursuit of the cancer-causing worm Fibiger received in 1926 the Nobel Prize, the first one to be awarded for cancer research. Then came the critics (118). Fibiger had fed his bakery rats just white bread and water, clearly a vitamin-deficient diet. It was claimed that his "tumors" were just a hyperplastic response to lack of vitamin A and that his metastases were not real metastases. His results could not be duplicated, yet his slides are still there to see; papillomas, at least, are undeniable (118). In the midst of this storm, Fibiger died of cancer.

Today, all the fuss about Fibiger's data makes little sense. There is nothing unusual about a worm causing cancer or about the difficulty of duplicating results with a different strain or a different diet. However, Nobel prizes for cancer research were shelved for 40 years.

Trematodes (flatworms) are clearly associated with cancer in man and other mammals; liver flukes (*Clonorchis sinensis*), for example, live in the bile ducts, which respond with hyperplasia, adenomatous hyperplasia and sometimes, eventually, with cancer (cholangiocarcinoma). Another flatworm, *Schistosoma haematobium,* is associated with squamous cell carcinoma of the bladder (44); the adult worm happens to seek refuge in the pelvic veins, including those of the bladder, where it sets up a chronic inflammation. In parts of Africa the disease is so common that bloody urine was once thought to be a manifestation of puberty.

> Exactly how the bladder carcinomas are produced by *Schistosoma* is not clear; carcinogens may be involved (91), but the constant regeneration of the bladder epithelium is surely a factor (46, 200). The worm *Spirocerca lupi* is associated with esophageal sarcomas in the dog (245).

Viruses: On the Trail of Oncogenes

Cancer research rolled on, while the experts continued to argue whether the study of viruses was relevant to human tumors. We pick up the trail at the Rockefeller Institute in New York, where Dr. Rous was trying to forget his "filterable sarcoma."

Shope's horned rabbits. A hunter from Cherokee, Iowa, visiting the laboratory of Richard Shope around 1933, advised his host that "horned rabbits" were common in his part of the country (229). Shope obtained some live specimens. The horns turned out to be papillomas: filiform or branching structures consisting of a thin vascular core coated by epidermis. Because cornified cells continued to form but did not slough off, the tumors appeared as tough horns (Figure 28.33). This is the mystery of the horned rabbits still displayed as jackalopes in curio shops and museums in the Mississippi valley. But how could such tumors be endemic? Shope prepared some glycerinated extracts and applied them to the scarified skin of other rabbits; they produced papillomas. If he injected the extract intravenously, papillomas developed only in scarified areas. This was the first virus-induced tumor to be described in a mammal.

Shope's laboratory at the Rockefeller Institute was next door to the laboratory of Rous. Shope had already acquired fame for the discovery of two mammalian tumors transmitted by viruses (he had also described a "filterable" rabbit myxoma), and felt rather sorry for the sad end of Rous's chicken sarcoma 22 years earlier. So he suggested to Rous that he take over the study of the rabbit papilloma (103). Rous was delighted. Using cell-free extracts, he tried to transfer the tumor from cottontail to domestic rabbits, and discovered that the rather harmless Shope papillomas could progress in less than a year to carcinomas. This was the first unequivocal proof of tumor progression. It produced another landmark paper by Rous in 1935 (Figure 28.34) (82, 215).

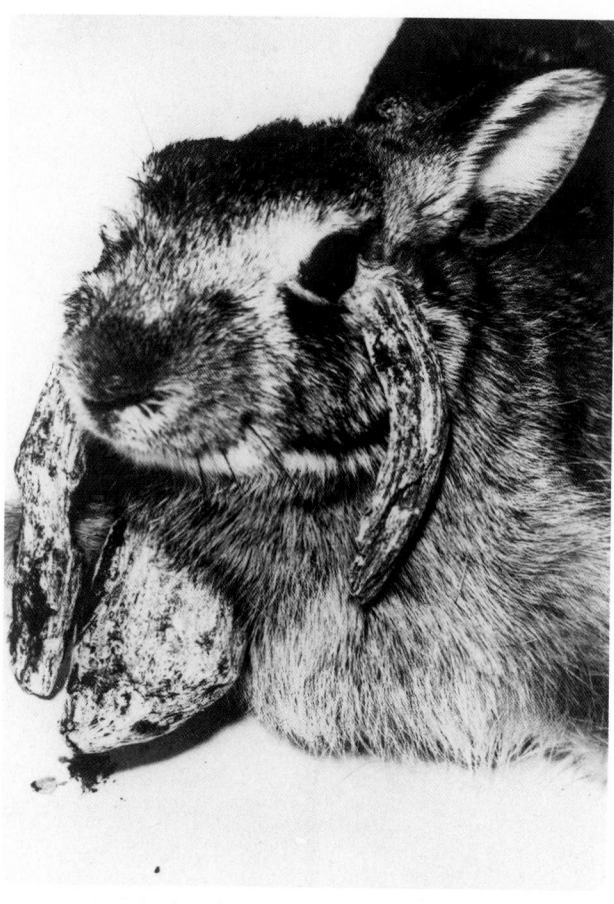

FIGURE 28.33 "Horned rabbit": A naturally infected Kansas cottontail rabbit bearing multiple Shope papillomas. (Reproduced with permission from [138], copyright 1980 Cold Spring Harbor Laboratory.)

Bittner's milk factor. The year 1936 saw yet another landmark. John Bittner at the Jackson Memorial Laboratory in Maine was studying a strain of mice with an inherited predisposition to develop mammary cancer (Figure 28.35). How was this trait transmitted? Bittner hit upon the idea of trying "foster nursing": newborn female pups from a control strain were fostered by mothers from the cancerous line, and 90 percent of them developed mammary cancer. Female pups from the cancerous strain were promptly assigned to normal foster mothers; only 10 percent developed cancer. Clearly some agent was being transmitted by the milk; the lactating female did not have to be cancerous, as long as she belonged to the cancerous strain. Later the "milk factor" was identified as an RNA virus and called mouse mammary tumor virus (MMTV) (Figure 28.36).

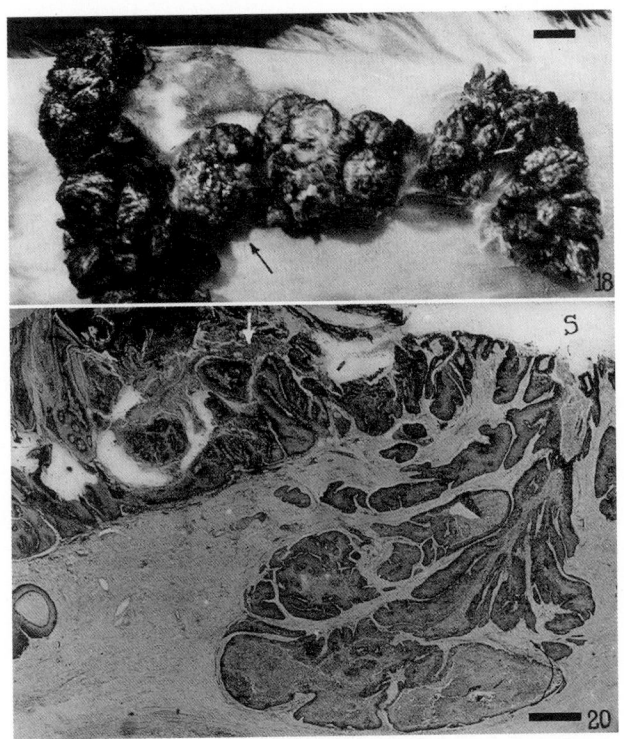

FIGURE 28.34   Progression of the virus-induced Shope papilloma to carcinoma. *Top:* Gross aspect of the papilloma on the back of a rabbit. **Arrow:** Site of the biopsy. **Bar** = 10 mm. *Bottom:* Benign papilloma (**white arrow**); at right, the downgrowth denotes malignancy. From a classic 1935 paper by Rous and Beard. **Bar** = 1 mm. (Reproduced from the **Journal of Experimental Medicine,** 1935;62:523–548, by copyright permission of The Rockefeller University Press [215].)

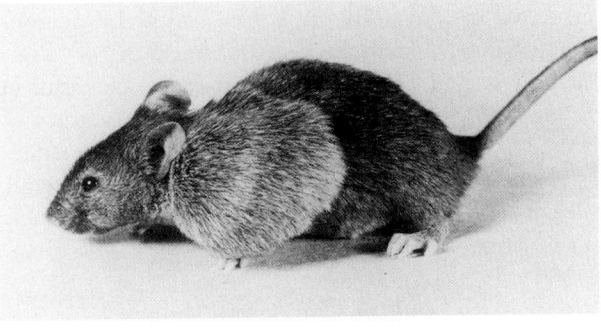

FIGURE 28.35   Spontaneous mammary carcinoma in a 7½-month-old C3H female mouse. (Reproduced with permission from [99].)

Remember Bittner's mammary tumor as a perfect example of the multifactorial nature of cancer: MMTV alone is harmless. To produce a mammary carcinoma three conditions must be present:

(1) The presence of the virus, (p. 874)
(2) An inherited predisposition, and
(3) A certain hormonal environment. In ovariectomized females no tumors develop, whereas males develop tumors if treated with estrogen (24, 25).

Mouse leukemia virus. Ludvik Gross demonstrated this virus in 1951 in New York, thanks to a new experimental twist. Gross had at hand two strains of mice in which all adults developed leukemia. The condition

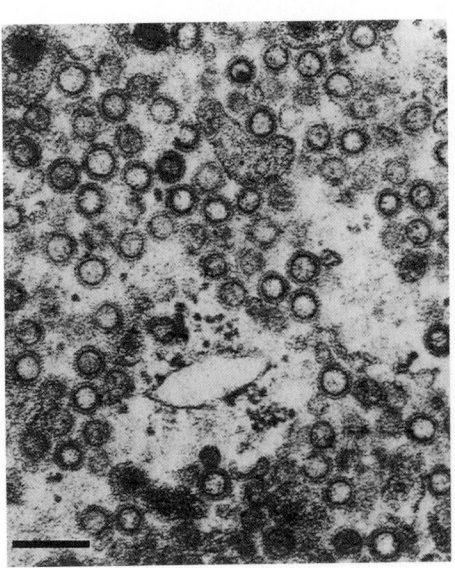

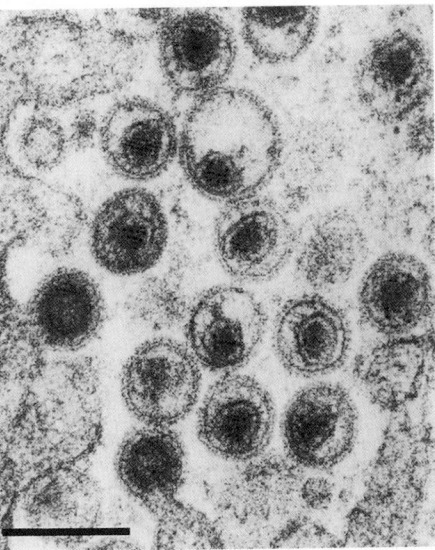

FIGURE 28.36   Virus particles from the spontaneous mammary carcinoma of a C3H mouse. *Left:* So-called type A particles in the cytoplasmic matrix. They are 650–750 Å in diameter, have 2 concentric membranes and no internal nucleoid. *Right:* Type B particles in the intercellular spaces. They have an average diameter of 1000–1050 Å. Most of them contain an electron-dense nucleoid surrounded by a membrane. **Bars** = 0.2 μm. (Reproduced with permission from [99].)

suggested a viral agent, but none could be demonstrated. Knowing that the transmission of Rous sarcoma and of Shope tumors was more successful in young animals, Gross injected a cell-free extract of leukemic cells into newborns of a leukemia-free strain; as adults, about half of these mice became leukemic (98). This very simple method is now applied routinely for isolating tumor viruses (225).

Retroviruses and the Oncogene Theory

By the 1950s it was clear that the pursuit of tumor viruses was interesting, but the facts at hand also suggested that human tumors as a whole did not fit into the picture of a viral disease. Nobody could have predicted that the next major breakthrough in the understanding of tumors, human or other, would come through study of Rous's chicken sarcoma, which dedicated scientists had kept transmitting throughout World War II. It so happens that the Rous sarcoma is caused by an RNA virus or **retrovirus,** and these viruses have some very special properties. We need to consider them briefly.

RNA viruses and reverse transcriptase. A unique feature of all viruses, oncogenic or not, is that they contain either RNA or DNA but not both (with minor exceptions). All other organisms contain both: they carry their genetic information encoded in DNA and transcribe it into RNA as needed. The Rous sarcoma virus, for example, contains only RNA.

When a virus of any kind infects a cell, it must take over some of the cell's machinery for protein synthesis because its own is incomplete. To do this it must supply instructions to the cell. For DNA viruses this is not a problem: they just insert their DNA into the DNA of the cell. But what about RNA viruses? Some have opted to skip the DNA phase and just translate their RNA into protein by using the cell's enzymes. However, there is another possibility, which was envisioned in 1962 by Howard Temin of the University of Wisconsin. Temin's inspired guess was that *some RNA viruses have evolved the ability to transcribe their RNA backwards into DNA.* In ordinary cells this is not possible; transcription always runs from DNA to RNA. Temin's prophetic concept was borne out: the necessary enzyme, *reverse transcriptase,* was discovered in 1970 in Temin's laboratory, encoded in virions of the Rous sarcoma (241). The same discovery was made independently at the Massachusetts Institute of Technology, in the laboratory of David Baltimore, using mouse leukemia virus. This led to a shared Nobel prize in 1975.

Retroviruses, the new name for this group of RNA viruses, changed the face of biology. Their reverse transcriptase became a tool for the new science of genetic engineering: it made it possible to synthesize DNA from any RNA. Retroviruses also turned out to be the oldest thieves on record. They have been stealing cellular genes since time immemorial (Figure 28.37); and the stolen genes were changed into cancer genes. We will now see how this was discovered, thanks to a chain

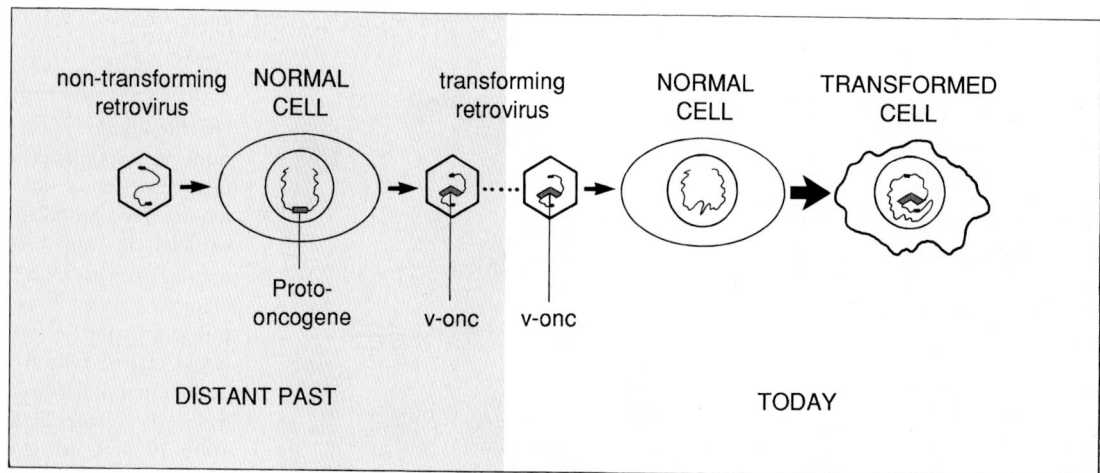

FIGURE 28.37 Scheme of the theft (transduction) of a gene (proto-oncogene) by a retrovirus. In the first step of this process, an ancestral virus integrates its genome in the chromosomes of an infected cell. This viral genome then transduces a cellular proto-oncogene, which therefore comes under the control of the virus. A normal cell infected by this recombinant virus can no longer control the transduced, activated genetic fragment (oncogene) and is condemned to multiply out of control. (Adapted with permission from [234].)

of events that R. A. Weinberg—one of the pioneers—later called the Revolution of 1976 (268).

Birth of the term oncogene. The term *oncogene*, literally "gene that produces cancer," was already around at the time of the discovery of the retroviruses in the early 1970s. It has been chosen for a theory proposed in 1969 by Huebner and Todaro of the National Cancer Institute (120). The theory as it was proposed is obsolete, but recounting it helps to understand why the term *oncogene* is something of a misnomer. Most, and perhaps all, cells, so went the theory, contain a viral genome capable of turning the cell into a cancer cell. This genome is normally latent, but stimuli such as X-rays or carcinogens can cause it to be expressed. Howard Temin elaborated on this theory and proposed that the oncogenic viral genome was produced within the cell by a phenomenon he called "misevolution" (242). In essence, he saw the cell as a mother of carcinogenic viruses ready to be inherited and activated. It was a near miss.

The discovery of oncogenes in retroviruses. Now we move to the laboratory of Michael Bishop and Harold Varmus at the University of California in San Francisco in 1976 (19–21). The plan was to prove or, more likely, disprove the oncogene theory just mentioned by looking for the supposed tumor-causing gene in the nucleus. A critical experiment was possible thanks to a new tool: a mutant strain of Rous sarcoma virus that had lost the ability to cause sarcomas. The lost piece of viral genome was precisely the sarcoma-producing gene (called v-*src*: v for viral, *src* for sarcoma-producing; pronounced v-sarc). Using this fact, a junior member of the team, Dominique Stehelin, synthesized a radioactive copy of the critical gene as a single-stranded bit of DNA. The next task was to check whether v-*src* was present in any cell, neoplastic or not. This was accomplished by exploiting the tendency of single strands of DNA to seek and combine with complementary strands of DNA, a process known in molecular biology as *hybridization* (Figure 28.38) (20). To the amazement of everyone, the radioactive v-*src* hybridized with fragments of *normal* chicken DNA, as well as of DNA from other normal birds, fishes, and mammals, including man—not to mention sponges and slime molds. This meant that *the sarcoma-producing gene, or a gene very similar to it, is a part of the normal cellular genome*, as c-*src* (c stands for cellular) (268, 269).

A closer analysis of the *src* gene of the virus showed that it contains introns, noncoding segments, which identify it as a cellular gene rather than a viral gene. Conclusion: the Rous sarcoma virus has pirated a

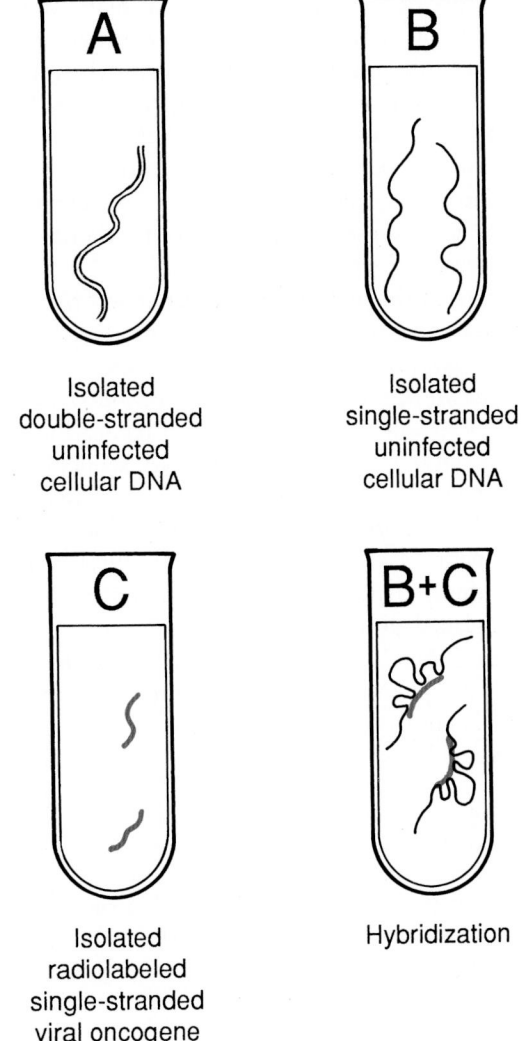

FIGURE 28.38   This is how the viral oncogene v-*src* was identified in cellular DNA. **A:** Double-stranded chicken DNA. **B:** Double strands are denatured and have become single strands. **C:** Separately, single-stranded DNA containing the *src* oncogene are isolated from Rous sarcoma virus and radioactively labeled **B + C:** When B is mixed with C, some of the viral DNA strands hybridize with normal chicken DNA strands, establishing the presence of a chicken oncogene (c-*src*) homologous to the viral oncogene (v-*src*). (Adapted from [20]. Original illustration by B. Tagawa.)

cellular gene sometime during its evolution. The original oncogene theory was therefore turned upside down; we are not dealing with cells that produce oncogenic viruses, but with viruses that steal (the technical term is *transduce*) normal cellular genes. These normal precursors of oncogenes are called *proto-oncogenes* (see Figure 28.37).

The story of v-*src* has been repeated many times in discoveries of tumor-producing retroviruses from a variety of birds and mammals. Each retrovirus usually has one pirated oncogene (34) and occasionally the same oncogene is found in more than one virus. Perhaps we are beginning to see the end of the list of proto-oncogenes that can be stolen by retroviruses (140). When did these gene thefts occur? We have consulted several experts; nobody knows.

The search for more viral oncogenes and their normal proto-oncogene counterparts has produced a basic fact: *the viral copies of the cellular genes are not perfect; their flaws are due to the fact that reverse transcription is a highly error-prone mechanism.* At each replication cycle as many as 0.5 percent of the RNA sequences are copied incorrectly into DNA (34). These errors play a role in the generation of tumors, as we will see.

The name *proto-oncogene* for the cellular counterparts of the viral oncogenes is not a good name because these so-called proto-oncogenes are not wicked genes just sitting there waiting for the chance to produce a tumor. They are normal genes with important growth-related functions in a cell's normal activity. The name *mitogenes* has been suggested (67).

> The name *proto-oncogene* is also a source of confusion for yet another reason. Keep in mind that even a perfectly normal gene can be "oncogenic" if it is expressed in excess or inappropriately. Should we call such a gene a proto-*oncogene*, although it does not need to be modified? Probably not—but this may explain why the term oncogene is often used rather loosely to include proto-oncogene.

At this point the reader will want to know how oncogenes produce cancer, but first we must pay tribute to another line of research: oncogenes can be discovered without the help of retroviruses.

Oncogenes discovered by transfection. Although it was fashionable in the late 1970s to chase oncogenes in retroviruses, some teams of researchers (52, 140, 226, 266) took a different tack: is it possible to find oncogenes in tumors that are not produced by retroviruses? The approach was to extract *DNA from tumors* (human or experimental, obtained with chemical carcinogens) and insert it by transfection (see below) into the genomes of cultured cells. The appearance of transformed cells would indicate that the inserted DNA contained an oncogene (the reader will recall that foci of transformed cells can be detected with the naked eye, p. 854). Cells of a focus can be cloned, grown, and injected into a suitable animal to test whether they produce a tumor. This method, too, struck gold; more oncogenes were discovered in this way than in retroviruses (53, 268, 269).

Transfection (gene transfer) is literally a trick whereby DNA is sneaked across a living cell's membrane into its nucleus, bypassing the natural tendency of the cell to phagocytize and digest any material presented to it. The DNA to be transfected into the nucleus is coprecipitated with crystals of calcium phosphate; the mixture is then allowed to settle on a monolayer of cultured cells. This is a cardinal method in molecular biology, yet nobody really knows how it works. Although in theory it is very inefficient (the yield depends on the type of cell and is of the order of one or a few cells per million) (52), the important point is that *some* cells are transfected.

Not all tumors yield transfectable oncogenes (perhaps because the method for finding them is not perfect), but it was certainly amazing to discover that transfecting DNA from a human bladder carcinoma into mouse fibroblasts produces a fibrosarcoma (140). Every tumor oncogene found by this method had its counterpart DNA sequence in the normal cellular genome, just as had been found for oncogenes discovered with retroviruses. Some of the oncogenes discovered by transfection turned out to be the same oncogenes previously identified in retroviruses. This showed that a proto-oncogene could lead to cancer by at least two mechanisms, viral and nonviral. But there was another surprise in store.

The DNA of normal cells can also produce tumors. Yes. DNA from normal human embryos, from chick embryos, and other sources also produced tumors (52). This suggests that normal cells contain genes (proto-oncogenes) that can be activated as a consequence of DNA rearrangements, as may be produced by transfection.

What kinds of genes are liable to become oncogenes? Because each gene is best defined by its product, much effort is concentrated in finding out what proteins are coded by the proto-oncogenes. Despite many loose ends, a picture is emerging: *the gene products of proto-oncogenes are either growth factors, growth-factor receptors, or links in an intracellular network through which external stimuli induce cell proliferation* (Figure 28.39). This picture helps us understand how tumor cells grow *in vitro* without added growth factors: they are able to stimulate themselves by produce their own growth factors and receptors, an autocrine phenomenon (281).

The four main categories of proto-oncogene products are the following:

- *Growth factors.* The best example of a virus that produces this category of oncogene product is a simian sarcoma virus endowed with an oncogene called v-*sis*. This oncogene codes for a protein that is very similar to the B chain of platelet-derived growth factor (PDGF); v-*sis* was probably derived from a

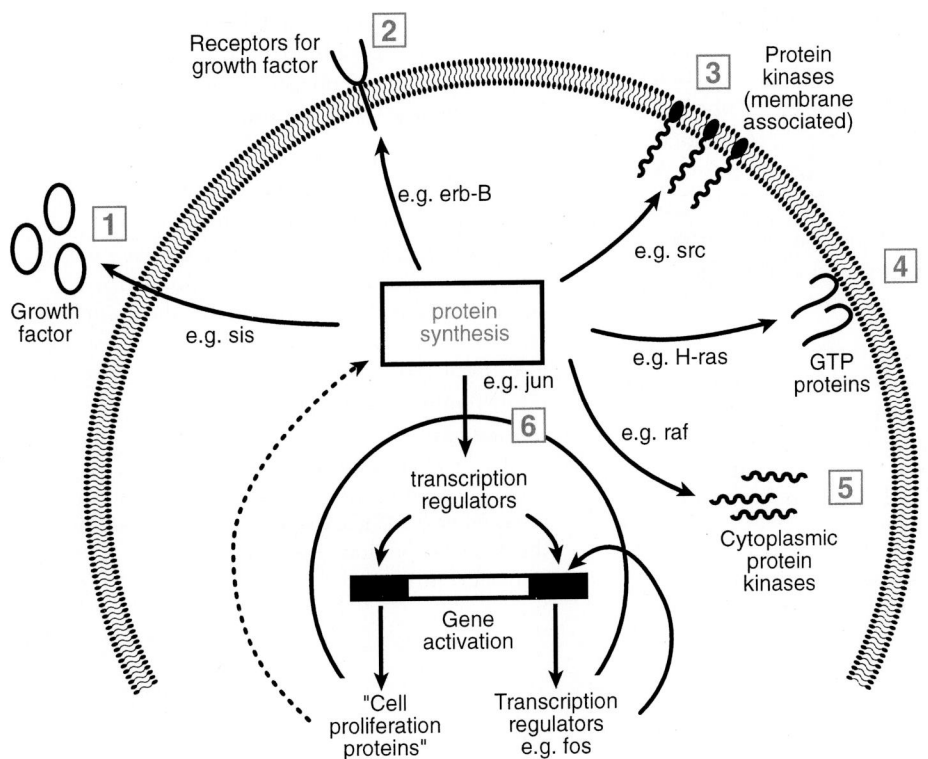

FIGURE 28.39 Diagram of a cell, indicating the six major classes of oncogene products: (1) secreted; (2), (3), (4) associated with the cell membrane; (5) active in the cytoplasm; (6) active on the nucleus. (Adapted with permission from [4].)

normal cell's c-*sis,* which codes for PDGF (34). This is the only known example of a *secreted* oncogene product (34). PDGF alone does not cause "transformation," but cells that constantly secrete PDGF are probably self-stimulating; a number of human tumors do produce PDGF-like molecules. Imaginative readers might conclude that antibodies against pseudo-PDGF should stop the growth of cells transformed by v-*sis; in vitro* the experiment works, but only sometimes.

- *Growth factor receptors and other transmembrane proteins.* All these gene products are inserted into the cell membrane; most of them represent defective, truncated receptors for growth factors: epithelial growth factor (EGF), macrophage colony-stimulating factor (CSF-1), and the insulin receptor. Normally the intracellular domain of these normal molecules functions as a tyrosine kinase, and this function persists in the oncogene version. Protein kinases transfer phosphate groups from themselves to other proteins, thus regulating their activity. It seems clear that tyrosine phosphorylation plays an important role in cell growth and differentiation (34), but exactly how the defective gene products lead to transformation is not clear. Conceivably a defective growth-factor receptor remains in a permanent state of activation and misinforms the cell accordingly.

- *Membrane-related, guanine triphosphate (GTP)–binding proteins (ras-proteins).* These gene products are related to the family of G-proteins, which transduce signals from growth-factor receptors to the phospatidyl inositol second-messenger cascade (34). They are coded by three varieties of *ras* genes, the first to be related to human tumors, but originally isolated from a murine sarcoma. (The product of the *ras* gene of beer yeast, *Saccharomyces cerevisiae,* is 90 percent homologous to human p21 [see later].) Proto-oncogenes must perform very basic functions to have deserved this tremendous degree of evolutionary conservation.

Ras genes code for 21-kilodalton proteins called p21, which are located in cell membranes, bind guanine nucleotides (GTP and GDP), and function as GTP-ases. About 15 percent of human solid tumors contain one or more *ras* genes with single-base alterations. Activated *ras* genes have also been found in premalignant and malignant lesions induced experimentally with carcinogens.

- *Nuclear proteins.* The special feature of these gene products is the tendency to localize in the nucleus where they probably take part in regulating gene expression. Some have a very short half-life, even minutes, which would agree with such a function. Several oncogenes of this group are known to be activated during normal cell replication: for example, c-*fos,* c-*myc,* and *p53* are activated sequentially during liver regeneration (244).

Finally, we can proceed to the basic question.

How are proto-oncogenes activated? To pervert a normal proto-oncogene into an oncogene, two basic options are available, and may be applied jointly: (1) to make it encode a *defective, "hyperactive" protein,* and (2) to make it encode *too much* protein (Figure 28.40). In other words, the structure *and/or* the function of a proto-oncogene may be disturbed. Descriptions of four mechanisms follow (Figure 28.40):

1. *A defective protein can result from a point mutation,* the simplest possible coding defect in an oncogene. This is a change in a single nucleotide that affects the coding for a single amino acid in the protein product (267). Note, however, that not all point mutations lead to tumor growth: to do so they must hit a specific gene in a specific way.

Example: the *ras* proto-oncogenes code for GTP-binding proteins. A point mutation creates a defective

protein that is no longer able to hydrolyze and deactivate GTP but traps it in such a way that it continues to transmit growth stimuli (267). (The comparison with a jammed doorbell is irresistible.)

2. *Overproduction of a normal protein can result from gene amplification:* multiple copies of the same gene are produced, sometimes as many as 50–100.
3. *Overproduction of a normal protein can result from abnormal activity of the oncogene.* Assume that a chromosomal rearrangement occurs; the normal regulatory sequence of the proto-oncogene has been lost (misplaced) and is replaced by another that calls for inappropriate stimulation.
4. *A defective protein may be a "fusion protein,"* the result of two abnormally combined genes. This is a result of chromosomal rearrangement: an oncogene is placed next to an actively transcribed gene, and the two gene products merge into a single "monster" protein.

PROTO-ONCOGENE:

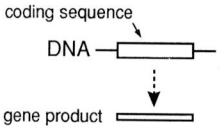

1. DELETION OR POINT MUTATION IN CODING SEQUENCE	2. GENE AMPLIFICATION
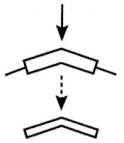 Hyperactive protein made in normal amounts	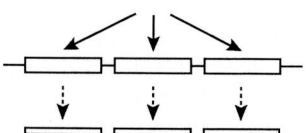 Normal protein greatly overproduced
3. CHROMOSOME REARRANGEMENT	4. CHROMOSOME REARRANGEMENT
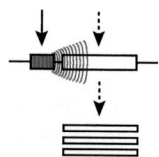 Nearby strong enhancer causes normal protein to be overproduced	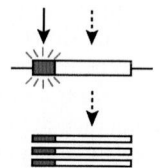 Fusion to actively transcribed gene greatly overproduces "fusion protein" or the fusion protein is hyperactive

FIGURE 28.40   Four mechanisms of oncogene activation. (Modified with permission from [4].)

How does an oncogene produce cells with a malignant pheno-type? Because proto-oncogenes are involved in growth control, it is not surprising that they can be pushed to induce excessive cell growth. But why should the cells also *look* malignant and *behave* as malignant? The answers are just beginning to come in. Here are a few telling experiments, introduced by the questions they ask:

- *How can the oncogene products affect the shape of the cell?* A few oncogene products have been visualized by means of labeled antibodies. It appears that the product of the *src* oncogene carried by the Rous sarcoma virus tends to be localized along the cell membrane (Figure 28.41) (19) and especially in attachment plaques (Figure 28.42) (19, 212). This suggests that this particular oncogene product affects the cytoskeleton and therefore alters the shape of the cell. The rounded or abnormal shape of some malignant cells and their propensity to lose their attachments may have this simple explanation (123).

A few more details on this observation. The oncogene of the Rous sarcoma, v-*src*, codes for a protein called pp60/v-*src*, which belongs to the group of transmembrane proteins. It was surprising at first to find it residing so far from the nucleus: how could it affect cell growth from that remote location? Then it was discovered that its intracytoplasmic tail functions as tyrosine kinase and that this enzyme probably phosphorylates the common cytoskeletal protein *vinculin*, among other substrates. Vinculin is part of the adhesion plaques, which are domains of the cell membrane

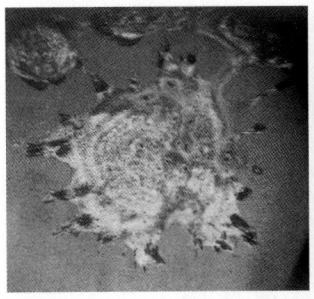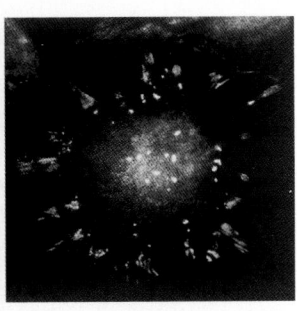

FIGURE 28.42 Example of the correlation between cytoskeleton and oncogene products: *Left:* Cell transformed by the oncogene *src* and attached to the supporting surface by means of adhesion plaques. These surface specializations appear dark in this micrograph, taken by interference-reflection photography. *Right:* The same cell treated with an antibody to the oncogene pp60v-*src* labeled with a fluorescent dye. Under ultraviolet light it is obvious that most of the oncogene product is localized in the adhesion plaques. (Reproduced with permission from [19]. Photographs courtesy of Dr. L. R. Rohrschneider, Fred Hutchinson Research Center, Seattle, WA.)

reinforced by cytoskeletal components. Adhesion plaques enable cells to grasp their substrate and spread over it; and because pp60/v-*src* is also localized there, one could conceive a scenario in which the defective pp60/v-*src* disturbs the complicated assembly of the adhesion plaque, thereby accounting for the rounded shape of neoplastic cells (Figure 28.43) (123).

- *What happens if the protein product of an oncogene is injected into a normal cell?* This has been done many times. For example, the normal, human *ras* proto-oncogene protein injected into normal cells has little effect, but injecting the corresponding oncogene product induces a burst of mitoses and dramatic morphologic changes in the injected cells. Within 24 hours the cells return to normal, presumably because the injected protein has been metabolized (74).

- *What if an antibody to an oncogene product is microinjected into a tumor cell?* The answer, so far, is that the malignant cell resumes a normal appearance (34).

- *Can neoplastic cell behavior be linked to a single enzymatic activity?* Here is a beautiful example (170). Transgenic mice expressing a polyoma virus oncogene (mT) develop endothelial tumors, namely hemangiomas. Endothelial cells of these tumors, grown *in vitro* three-dimensionally in fibrin gels, form cystic structures recalling hemangiomas. They also express high fibrinolytic activity. When this proteolytic activity is neutralized by appropriate inhibitors, the endothelial cells correct their behavior and develop into normal-looking, capillary tubules (Figure 28.44).

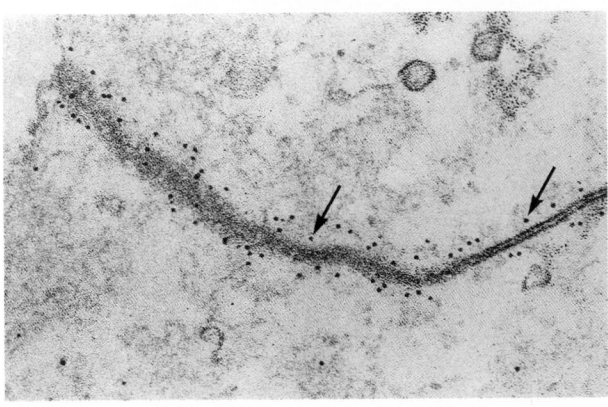

FIGURE 28.41 The preferential location of oncogene products along the cell membrane. Electron micrograph showing the junction between two cells infected with the Rous sarcoma. The section was treated with a rabbit antibody to the oncogene product pp60v-*src*; the antibody was linked with ferritin so as to make it visible by electron microscopy. It is obvious that the grains of ferritin (**arrows**) are located along the cell membranes. (Reproduced with permission from [19]. Photographs courtesy of Dr. M. C. Willingham, National Cancer Institute, Bethesda, MD.)

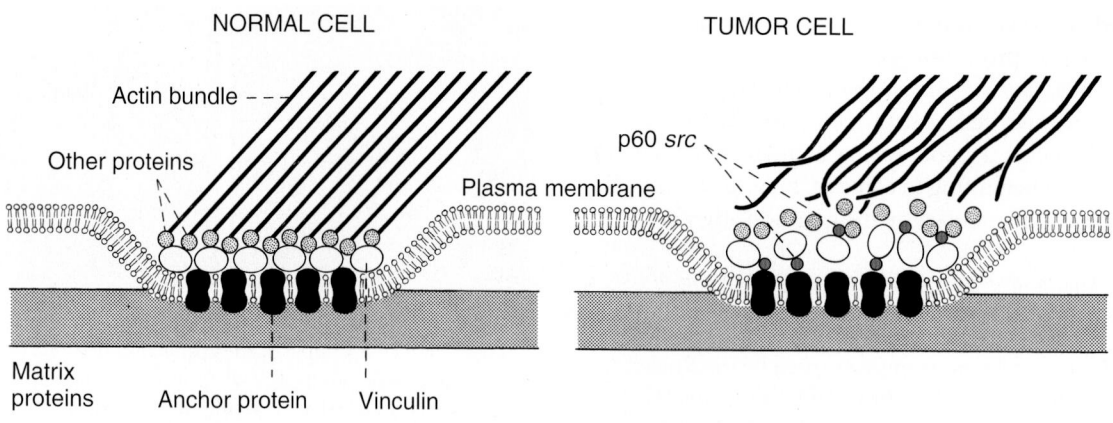

NORMAL CELL   TUMOR CELL

FIGURE 28.43 *Left:* Adherent plaque in a normal cell (schematic). *Right:* Cell transformed by the Rous sarcoma virus; p60v-*src* appears in the adhesion plaque, and vinculin is found to be phosphorylated on tyrosine. Phosphorylation by p60v-*src* may disrupt the vinculin link and thereby contribute to the typical disorganization of actin bundles in transformed cells. (Adapted with permission from [123].)

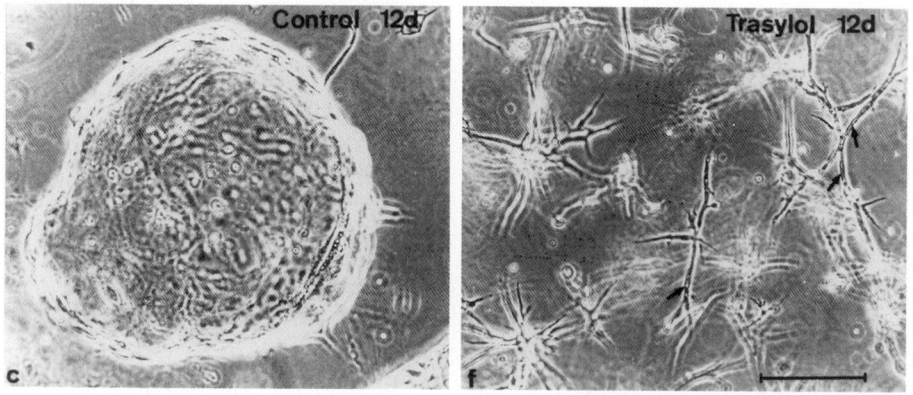

FIGURE 28.44 How do oncogenes produce tumors? Here is a fascinating example, the hemangioma of transgenic and chimeric mice expressing the polyoma virus mT oncogene. *Left:* Hemangioma-like sac produced by incubating for 12 days hemangioma cells suspended in a fibrin gel. *Right:* Hemangioma cells incubated for 12 days in a fibrin gel *and* in the presence of Trasylol, a protease inhibitor. The cells have formed thin, branching cords, partly hollow, resembling normal capillary sprouts (**arrows**). Conclusion: proteolytic activity may be responsible for the aberrant morphogenetic behavior of the hemangioma cells. **Bar** = 200 μm. (Reproduced by permission from [170], Copyright by Cell Press.)

The natural history of tumors includes much more than oncogenes. In the next two chapters we will recount the discovery of the **suppressor genes,** which normally *oppose* cell growth, and in this regard behave as a mirror image of oncogenes. But before we do so we will explore the essentials of oncogenesis by viruses.

Oncogenic Viruses: An Overview

The genetic information carried by viruses, as mentioned earlier, may be encoded in DNA or RNA; correspondingly there are two classes of oncogenic viruses, with distinct characteristics. Many oncogenic viruses exist in nature as hitchhikers in selected hosts in which they do not usually cause tumors, whereas they may cause tumors in other hosts.

A frightening lesson was learned from New World monkeys. At the New England Regional Primate Center it was discovered in 1971 that squirrel monkeys and spider monkeys (*Saimiri sciureus* and *Ateles geoffroyi*) each live in apparent harmony with their own particular strain of herpes virus, but when the herpes virus of the squirrel monkey is injected into the spider monkey it produces malignant lymphomas. Other nonhuman primates, and rabbits, are also at risk (155). Because of these and other potentially dangerous viruses, the autopsy of a monkey is now carried out with surgical precautions.

It has been difficult to prove that viruses cause tumors in humans. A virus that is oncogenic for humans is not necessarily oncogenic for another host. Furthermore, viruses in general are very choosy about the cells they infect; and some human cells are very difficult to grow *in vitro*. We also know from experiment that a virus-induced malignant tumor may be apparently virus-free when biopsied (225). However, epidemiological studies have provided powerful evidence of guilt by association, and there is no longer any doubt that some human tumors are produced by viruses. This is extremely important with regard to therapy and prevention: viruses produce antigens, virus-induced tumors carry virus-related antigens, and vaccination against such tumors becomes a distinct possibility—now a reality.

There are, in all, seven classes of tumor viruses (Table 28.1) (225): six classes of DNA viruses (they produce most of the tumors) and one class of RNA viruses (retroviruses). Overall they account for about 20 percent of the human "tumor burden"; this percentage becomes especially significant considering that vaccination against these viruses may some day—perhaps soon—prevent many if not all of the related tumors.

What Happens to a Virus-Infected Cell?

Permissive versus nonpermissive cells. The first step in understanding infection by viruses is that the effect on the cell may vary between the two extremes of lysis and transformation (Figure 28.45). In either case the virus integrates itself with the genome of the cell. If the cell permits viral replication, it is overwhelmed by viral particles and dies. At the other extreme, the cell does not permit the virus to complete its cycle of replication; the frustrated virus (one or a few particles suffice) steers the cell toward transformation. Intermediate situations exist. DNA viruses can follow either path; RNA viruses tend to produce nonlytic infection.

Changes in protein synthesis. As may be expected, virus-infected cells produce not only the virus-encoded proteins, but also the proteins encoded by their own genome, which is disturbed by the presence of the virus. There is evidence here for a stepwise process whereby some of the new cellular proteins induce immortalization and then transformation. Not only the quantity but also the quality of the cellular proteins is changed: some of the new proteins reflect the derepression of genes that had been repressed since fetal life (**oncofetal antigens**). As for the virus-encoded proteins, they can be expressed on the cell surface and thereby expose the cell to an immune response. Malignant tumors produced by the same virus tend to express the same

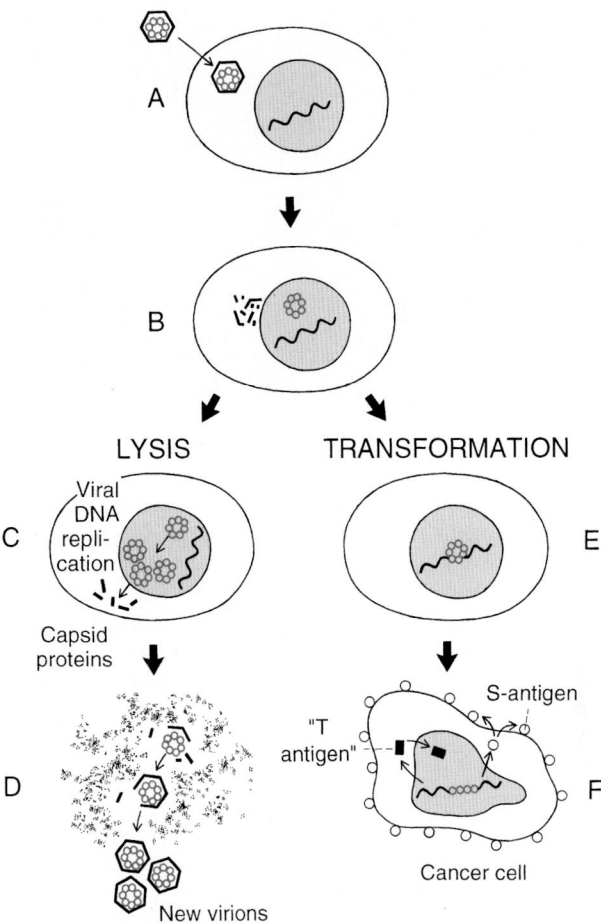

FIGURE 28.45   Diagram of the interaction between an oncogenic DNA virus (Papova virus) and a susceptible cell. The virion penetrates into the cell, is uncoated, and penetrates into the nucleus. There it can either induce the production of new viruses and lead to cell lysis, or become integrated into the host DNA and lead to "transformation"; the transformed cell produces new antigens. S antigen = tumor specific transplantation antigen. (Adapted from information appearing in the New England Journal of Medicine [5].)

surface antigens, whereas malignant tumors produced by chemical carcinogens tend to express their own specific antigens.

DNA Oncogenic Viruses

The six classes of DNA tumor viruses include a great deal of human and other animal pathology (see Figure 28.46; Table 28.1). The name *Hepadna* for one group is not a misprint but a combination of hepa(tic) DNA. Nor are the *Papova* groups of Russian origin; the word stands for PApilloma, POlyoma, and simian VAcuolating virus 40 (PA + PO + VA). Adenoviruses

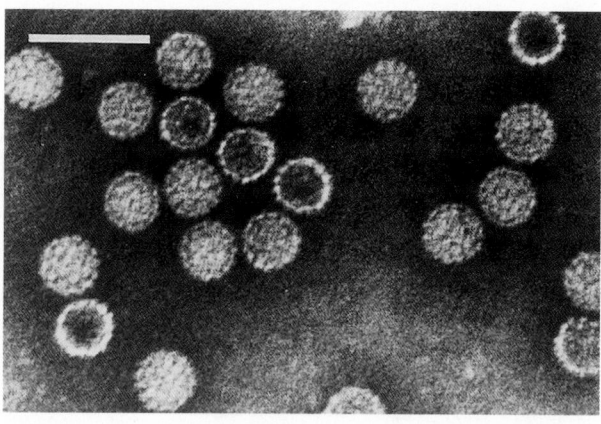

FIGURE 28.46 Electron micrograph of simian virus SV40, an oncogenic DNA virus. This virus was discovered in 1960 in cultures of monkey kidney cells used in the production of polio vaccine and was inadvertently inoculated into thousands of people before its presence became known. (Reproduced with permission from [217a].) Although it can be oncogenic experimentally, no harm was done. Negative staining. **Bar** = 0.1 μm. (Courtesy of Dr. G. Th. Diamandopoulos, Harvard Medical School, Boston, MA.)

are so named because they were first isolated from human pharyngeal tonsils or adenoids. The herpes group inherited its ancient name from the slow advance, "creeping", of some infectious herpetic lesions (*hérpein* is Greek for creeping); the *pox* group from the skin pocks.

Hepadna group. The hepatitis B virus (HBV) is a classic case of guilt by association; it is endemic in the same parts of Asia and Africa where hepatoma is also the most common form of human cancer (71). Related viruses have been found in ducks, woodchucks, and ground squirrels, which also suffer from hepatomas; yet nobody has succeeded, so far, in proving experimentally that HBV produces hepatomas. In humans, HBV is commonly transmitted by close personal contact, from mother to infant, and by blood transfusions and intravenous injections (not by fecal contamination as is the case for hepatitis A virus). The result of infection is a chronic hepatitis that may progress to hepatoma (73). Viral DNA has been found integrated with the DNA of liver cells in neoplastic as well as in nonneoplastic tissue. Current thinking is that some factor other than the

Table 28.1 Families of Tumor Viruses: Natural Cancers

Virus Group	Examples	Host	Disease
Hepadna	Hepatitis B	Human, woodchuck, duck	Primary hepatocellular carcinoma (PHC)
	Ground squirrel	Squirrel	PHC
Papilloma (Papova A)	Shope papilloma	Rabbit	Benign papilloma
	Canine papilloma	Dog	Papillomas
	Equine papilloma	Horse	Papillomas
	Human papilloma	Human	Papillomas, cervical carcinoma
Papova B	Polyoma	Mouse	Unknown
	SV40	Monkey	Unknown
	Human papova	Human	Unknown
Adenovirus	Human adeno-12-31	Human	Unknown
	Ovine adeno-	Sheep	Adenoma
Herpes	Marek's disease	Chicken	Lymphosarcoma
	Pig herpes	Guinea pig	Leukemia
	Cattle herpes	Cattle	Lymphoma
	Epstein-Barr	Human	Burkitt's lymphoma; nasopharyngeal carcinoma
Pox	Shope fibroma	Rabbit	Benign fibroma
	Yaba	Monkey	Benign histiocytoma
	Molluscum contagiosum	Human	Benign molluscum bodies
Retrovirus			
Type B	Mouse mammary tumor	Mouse	Mammary adenocarcinoma
Type C	Leukemia-sarcoma complex	Reptiles, fish, birds rodents, cattle, cats, dogs, primates	Leukemia—lymphosarcoma types of diseases
Type D	Human T-cell leukemia (HTLV)	Human	Leukemia—lymphoma

Table adapted from (225).

virus intervenes in the pathogenesis of HBV-associated hepatomas, possibly a toxic agent capable of inducing liver cell necrosis, followed by regeneration. A prime candidate is aflatoxin, common in the endemic areas. (p. 845).

The natural history of HBV infection suggested that it could be an almost ideal model for testing the possibility of preventing both HBV hepatitis and the related cancer. In 1984, a universal vaccination program was started in Taiwan; the first results are very encouraging: between 1990 and 1994, the incidence of hepatoma in children between 6 and 14 had dropped to one-half (42). By 2000, it was found that boys benefit from the vaccination much more than girls (43). Good news keeps coming (234a).

Papova A group. Papilloma viruses are proven guilty: human papilloma virus (HPV) DNA is found in 90 percent of squamous carcinomas of the cervix, vulva, penis, and anus. Over 100 types of papilloma virus (HPV) are known. They pose a major technical problem: it has not yet been possible to propagate them *in vitro*. However, they do grow in epithelia, transplanted to nude mice (Figures 28.47, 28.48) (60a). It is a virus of this group that produces Shope's rabbit papillomas. Certain types have been associated with simple warts, laryngeal papillomas, and urogenital cancers. In general, viral DNA and viral antigens are found more often in benign growths.

Nonprogressive and progressive lesions of the cervix are associated with different types of HPV, which suggests that some types of HPV are more oncogenic than others.

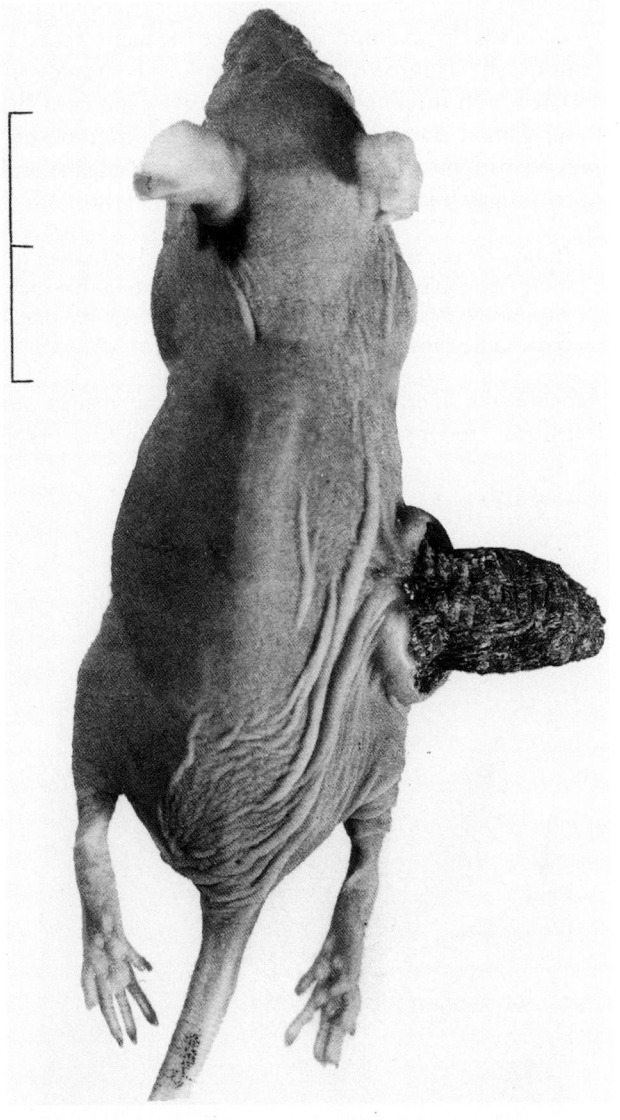

FIGURE 28.47 Nude mouse bearing a Shope (rabbit) papilloma. A domestic rabbit was infected experimentally, and three months later the papilloma was grafted to the mouse. **Scale** in centimeters. (Reproduced with permission from [138], copyright 1980 Cold Spring Harbor Laboratory.)

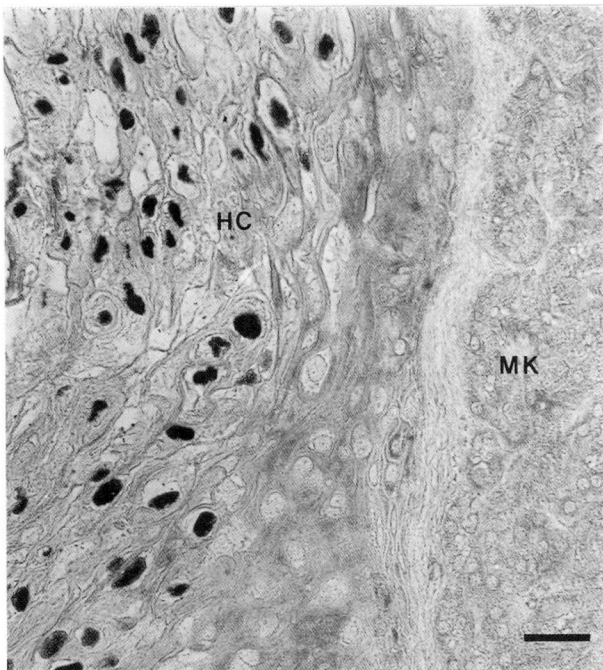

FIGURE 28.48 Although papilloma viruses cannot be grown *in vitro,* they can be used to transform human cervical epithelium (**HC**) implanted between the capsule of mouse kidney (**MK**). Prior to implantation, the chips of cervix were exposed to a cell-free extract of vulvar condylomata (benign growths related to HPV infection). The black nuclei (immuno-peroxidase stain) are producing virus antigen (HPV-II). **Bar** = 25 μm. (Courtesy of Dr. J.W. Kreider, Pennsylvania State University, Hershey, PA.)

Nonprogressive lesions of the cervix include benign outgrowths called condylomata acuminata, flat warts, and some of the epithelial "dysplasias" that are now called **c**ervical **i**ntraepithelial **n**eoplasia (CIN), Types 1 and 2 (p. 900). All are usually associated with HPV-6, 11, 31, 35, and 42. Progressive forms of CIN-I and CIN-II, as well as CIN-III, and cervical carcinomas are usually positive for HPV-16, 18, and 33 (71). Perhaps a better understanding of these HPV infections will some day help clarify the true meaning of the controversial term *dysplasia.*

Warts are another misdeed of HPV. One mysterious aspect of warts should be recorded here: their apparent ability to come or go in response to psychologic signals. For a viral infection this is certainly peculiar; it recalls the tendency of herpes blisters ("fever blisters" or "cold sores") to develop in relation to periods of stress. Anyone interested should read the wonderful essay by Lewis Thomas (243).

Laryngeal papillomas (Figures 28.49, 28.50) tend to develop in children whose mothers suffered from genital warts at the time of delivery. When removed, the papillomas tend to recur; and although they may regress at puberty, they may also progress to carcinomas. Radiation and heavy smoking may be cocarcinogens (225). The virus remains latent in the deeper layers of the epithelium and proliferates in the more mature squamous epithelial cells, which are, in technical terms, more permissive (186). The result is a clear perinuclear halo that gives these cells an empty look; hence the name *koilocyte* (empty cell) (Figure 28.51). HPV type 16 is strongly associated with severe atypias and invasive cancers of the lower genital tract (101) (Figure 28.52). Immunosuppressed patients are at risk for a higher incidence and faster progression of HPV-induced tumors (186).

> Papova viruses type B have not been related to human tumors (see Table 28.2), but it is worth recording that these viruses are related to the monkey-derived SV40, oncogenic in newborn rodents and rabbits.

Adenoviruses. Derived from humans, these viruses can transform rodent fibroblasts in culture. One type

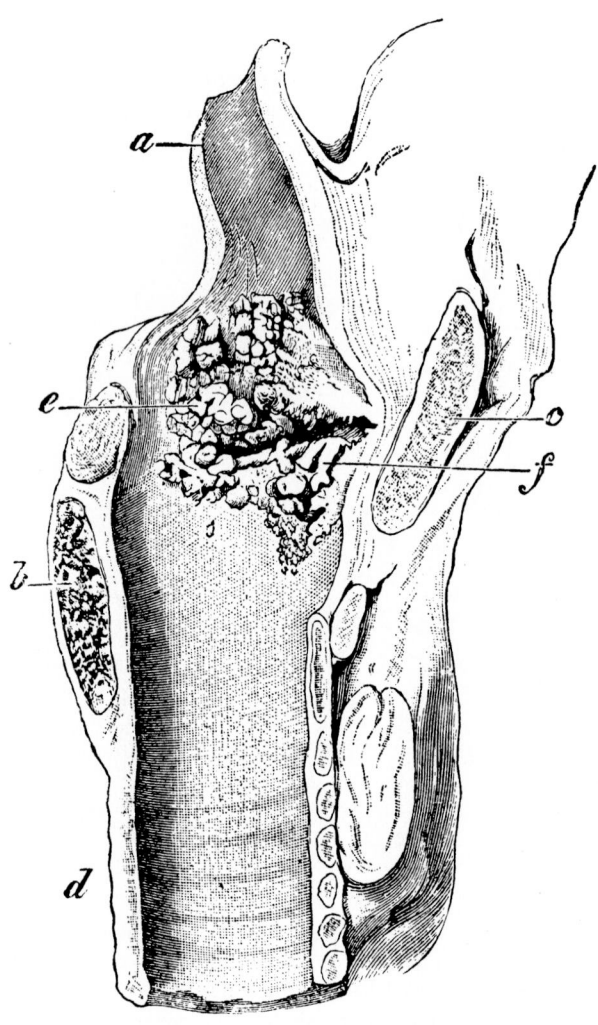

FIGURE 28.49 Papilloma of the larynx illustrated in 1908. **a:** Epiglottis. **b:** Cricoid cartilage. **c:** Thyroid cartilage. **d:** Trachea. **e, f:** Papillary growths now known to be of viral origin. (Reproduced from [290].)

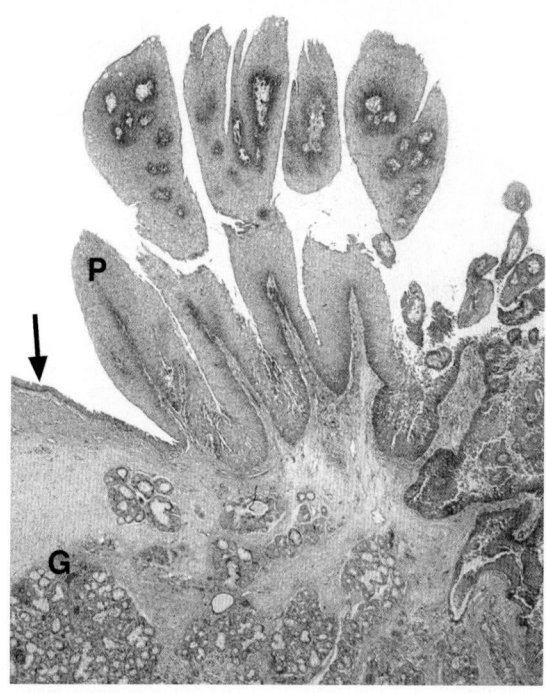

FIGURE 28.50 Part of a laryngeal papilloma, benign at this stage. **Arrow:** Normal mucosal epithelium. **P:** Papillae. **G:** Normal mucous glands. (25x)

produces fibroadenomas of the mammary glands in rats (67). No adenovirus is known to be carcinogenic in man.

Herpes viruses. All herpes viruses look alike, but they differ greatly in their natural histories. They have been linked with several human tumors, especially Burkitt's lymphoma, nasopharyngeal carcinoma, and Kaposi's sarcoma. We would like to say that these viruses *cause* the associated tumors but we would be somewhat forcing the facts. Tumors, as we have said, rarely have a single cause.

Kaposi's sarcoma was known as a sporadic tumor long before the AIDS epidemic. It consists of bluish-red plaques or nodules that appear simultaneously on the skin and mucosae with an overwhelming preference for homosexual males (Figure 28.53). The multiple location is generally interpreted as a multicentric origin (as opposed to metastatization); widespread involvement of internal organs may occur. The histologic appearance recalls a highly vascular granulation tissue, except for some atypia (Figure 28.54). The cell of origin is probably endothelium (139).

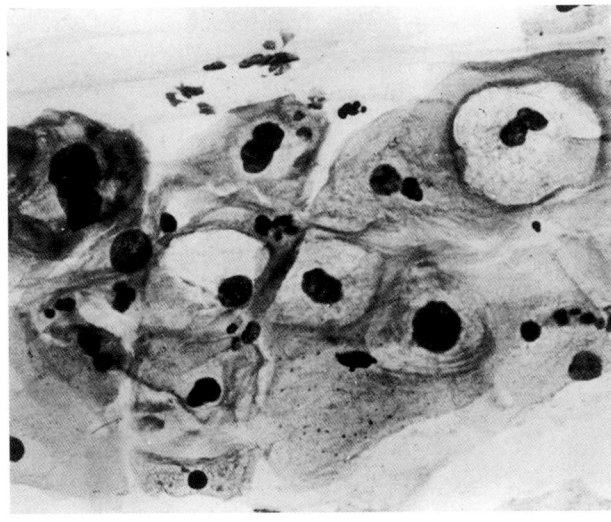

FIGURE 28.51   Typical koilocytes in a pap smear; squamous epithelial cells with a clear halo around the nucleus, indicative of infection with papilloma virus. (Courtesy of Dr. L. Koss, Albert Einstein College of Medicine, New York.)

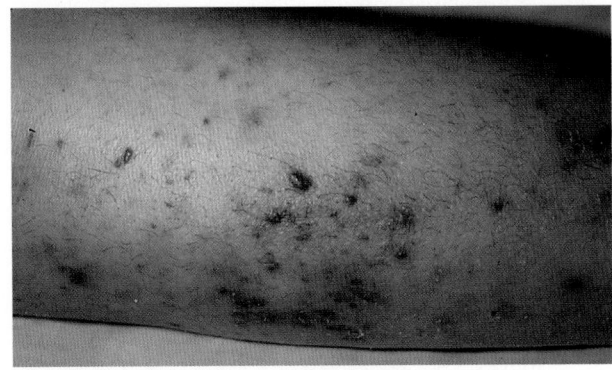

FIGURE 28.53   Typical multiple foci of Kaposi's sarcoma of the skin. (Reproduced with permission from [16], Copyright © 2001 by Dermatopathology Interactive Atlas.)

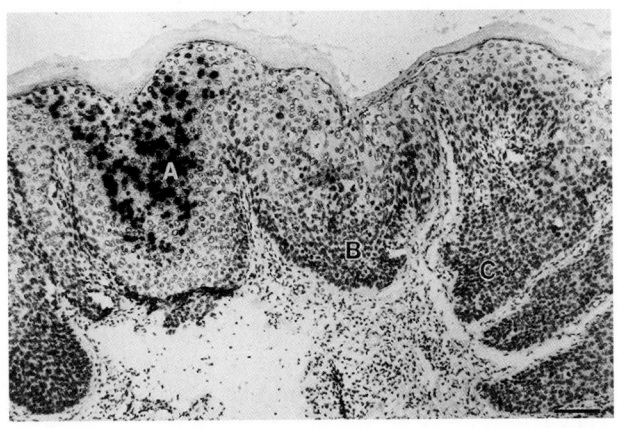

FIGURE 28.52   Biopsy of the vulva showing intraepithelial neoplasia stage II (**B**) and III (**C**) associated with human papilloma virus infection (HPV-16 demonstrated by *in situ* hybridization [**A**]). As often happens, the virus is most abundant *near* the neoplasia, but in some cases virus-positive cells can be found also within the neoplasia. **Bar** = 100 μm. (Reproduced by permission from [101], © American Society for Investigative Pathology.)

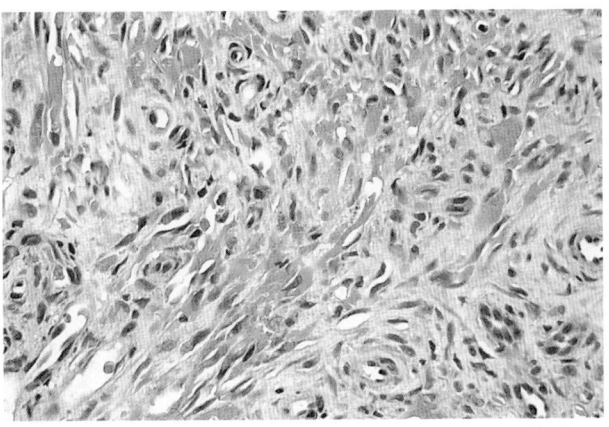

FIGURE 28.54   Biopsy of Kaposi's sarcoma. The picture is altogether not very different from granulation tissue. It shows elongated cells and poorly formed vascular spaces; some red blood cells appear to be extravasated. These features explain the red color seen clinically. A few lymphocytes are also present (90x). (Reproduced with permission from [16], Copyright © 2001 by Dermatopathology Interactive Atlas.)

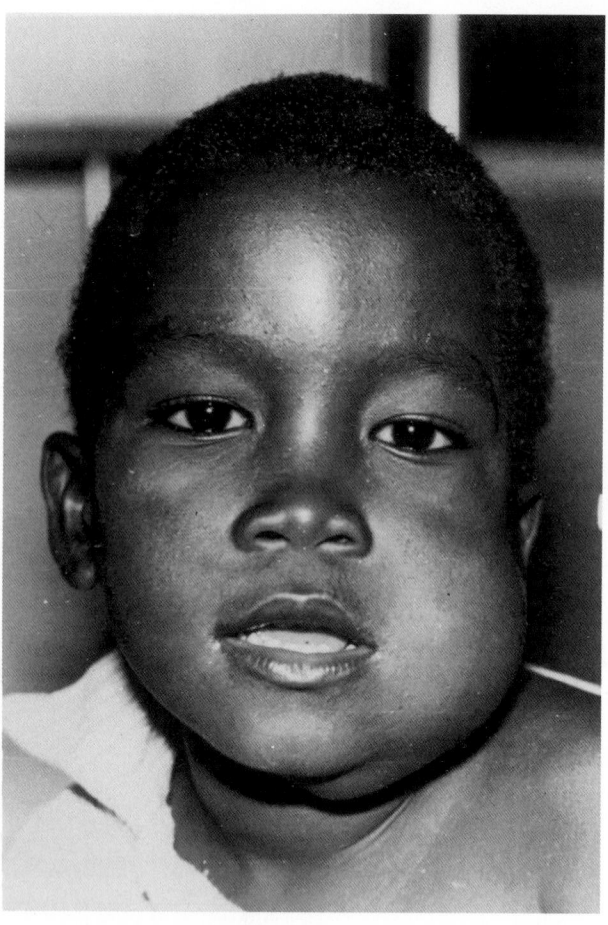

FIGURE 28.55   Typical presentation of Burkitt's tumor, affecting the upper jaw of a young man in Uganda. (Courtesy of Dr. D. P. Burkitt, Bisley, United Kingdom.)

The Epstein-Barr virus. The story of "EBV" is linked to that of Burkitt's lymphoma, the tumor that was discovered in 1958 by Denis Burkitt while working in Kampala, Uganda (35). It usually appeared as a large mass in the upper or lower jaw (Figure 28.55). Sporadic cases were later found to occur in the rest of the world (58). Shortly after Burkitt's observation, Epstein and Barr were able to grow a virus from cultures of these tumor cells. Then—surprise—it turned out that this virus is also the most common cause of **infectious mononucleosis** (209).

Almost everyone is infected by EBV by the age of 20 (209, 225) by a contagion that is mostly harmless. So here we have the case of a virus showing a full range of effects, from no disease at all to an infectious fever to cancer. The virus selects to parasitize B lymphocytes and the epithelium of the upper pharynx. To penetrate cells it borrows the receptor for the complement component C3. Thereafter it may or may not cause a clinical infection; when it does it is infectious mononucleosis. During this episode the patient's blood contains large, atypical but not malignant, B lymphocytes, and viral DNA may remain embedded in the host DNA for life. *In vitro,* EBV can immortalize a variety of cells, human and other.

So, can we really say that the EB virus causes Burkitt's lymphoma? The geographic distribution of the virus certainly does not explain the tumor distribution. It is true that Burkitt tumors in Africa almost invariably contain EBV genome and that all African patients have antibodies against EBV virus, but the sporadic cases occurring in the United States and England are usually EBV negative (they are recognized by their clinical, histologic, and cytogenetic features). Clearly some other factor must be involved. Dr. Burkitt drove all over Africa, painstakingly listing all the cases and noting the local conditions. His result: the distribution of Burkitt lymphoma in Africa coincides with that of malaria. Malaria may act as a constant stimulus for B-cell proliferation (necessary for producing antibodies against the malarial parasite) while also inducing some T-cell immunosuppression (71).

Cytogenetics provided a unifying clue for all cases of Burkitt's lymphoma. Wherever in the world they may occur, they show chromosomal translocations known to activate the oncogene c-*myc* (Figure 28.56). Evidently there is more than one pathway to that chromosomal disturbance. The contribution of EBV may be to immortalize the B cells, which would prolong the time during which a genetic accident could occur, whereby their immunoglobulin genes would be rearranged in such a way as to activate the c-*myc* gene, as required to produce Burkitt's lymphoma (71).

Nasopharyngeal carcinoma, another malignancy associated with EBV, occurs endemically in southern China, in Africa, and among the arctic Eskimos (58). It always contains DNA of the EBV, but the peculiar geographic distribution of this carcinoma suggests that some unknown environmental factor (or factors) must be involved. Some possibilities are volatile nitrosamines inhaled during food preparation, or phorbol esters (the classic cell activators, p. 61) inhaled from local *Euphorbiaceae* or present in cooking oils (71).

Considering the extraordinary range of pathology that EBV produces (gastric cancer is another candidate [114]) it is legitimate to wonder why more people are not affected. We should presumably thank the assiduous NK cells and the specific anti-EBV lymphocytes (cytotoxic T-cells), which are constantly engaged in wiping out virus-infected cells (209).

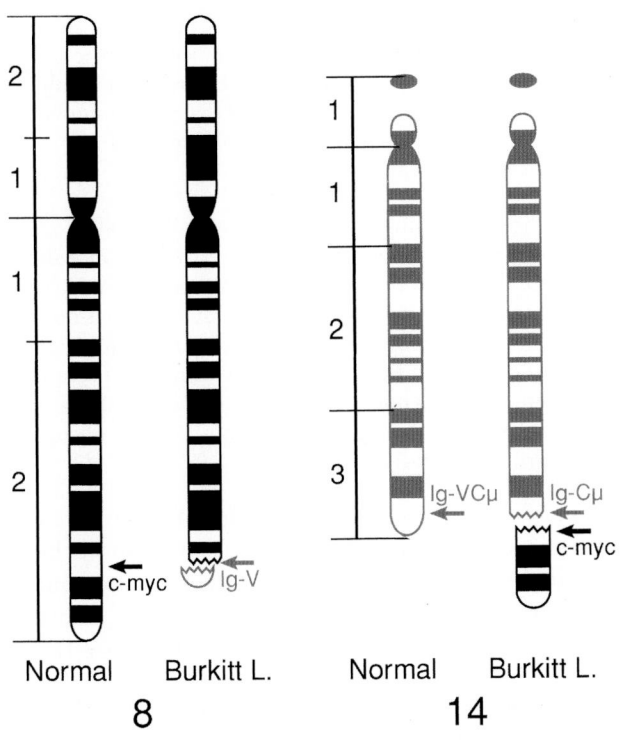

FIGURE 28.56 The typical chromosome translocations in Burkitt's lymphoma. Ig-V and Ig-Cμ represent heavy-chain immunoglobulin variable (**V**) and constant μ (**Cμ**) genes. The defective chromosome 8 loses a fragment carrying c-*myc* and acquires a small fragment carrying Ig-V. The defective chromosome 14 acquires the larger piece lost by chromosome 8, whereby c-*myc* finds itself located near Ig-Cμ. (Reprinted with permission from [289]. Copyright 1983 by the American Association for the Advancement of Science.)

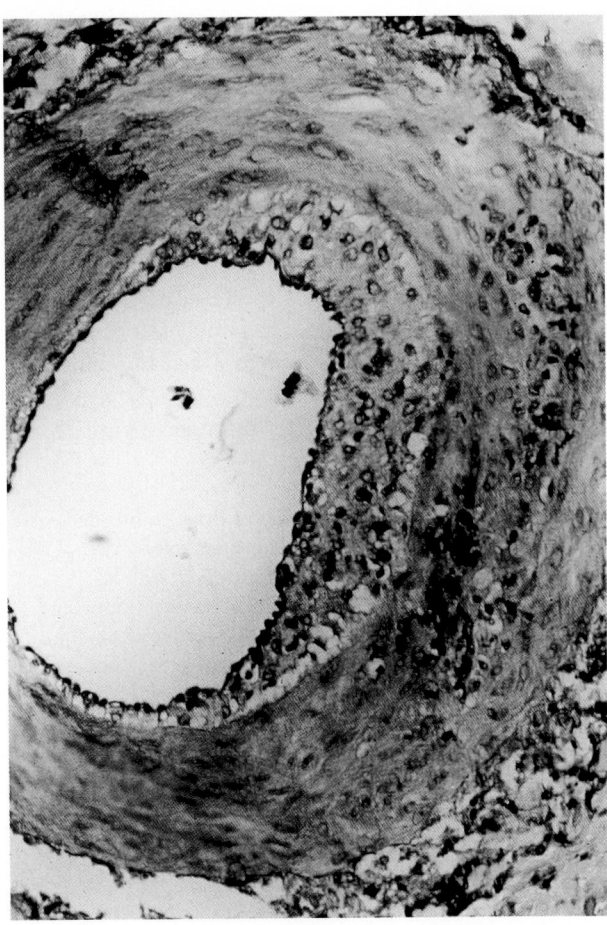

FIGURE 28.57 A strange association: in chickens, the virus of Marek's disease produces lymphomas as well as this atherosclerosis-like intimal thickening in the coronary arteries. (Courtesy of C. G. Fabricant, Cornell University, Ithaca, NY.)

Marek's disease is an unusual effect of a herpes virus in chickens, unusual because it produces arterial lesions recalling atherosclerosis (Figure 28.57) (69). It is also a malignant lymphoma against which the chickens can be vaccinated using an attenuated strain. Unlike human lymphomas, Marek's disease is highly contagious among chickens.

Another herpes virus induces *Lucké's adenocarcinoma* in leopard frogs, a tumor that became justly famous for proving that it is possible, believe it or not, to obtain a tadpole from a carcinoma (p. 925).

How do DNA viruses produce tumors? DNA viruses do not carry any "stolen," cellular, growth-related oncogenes as the retroviruses do; they produce tumor growth in other ways. Some carry genes that transform cells despite their apparent lack of homology with a known, normal cellular gene; they do so by coding for "transforming proteins." Others act indirectly by derepressing genes that normally inhibit cell growth.

An example: consider a DNA virus with a circular genome, such as polyoma or SV40. The genome includes early and late sequences (so named by the order of transcription). The early genes are essential for transformation; the late genes relate to virus replication. Now, assume that the viral DNA integrates itself with a chromosome in such a way that the late sequence is interrupted; the virus is not able to replicate. However, the early sequence is intact, it is transcribed, and the transforming proteins is produced (265).

RNA Oncogenic Viruses.

The unique survival strategy of these viruses has already been described (p. 860), namely the ability to transcribe their RNA backwards into DNA by means of their special enzyme, reverse transcriptase (hence the collective name *retroviruses* for this group). The DNA copy of the retroviral genome inserted into the host DNA is called a ***provirus.*** We have also outlined the manner in which retroviruses steal cellular genes (proto-oncogenes) and turn them into oncogenes. In this section we will provide a few more details on the retroviral family.

Many retroviruses replicate in cell cultures without causing any visible damage to the cells (191), others cause nonneoplastic disease, and a few cause tumors. To this day, only one retrovirus is definitely associated with human neoplasia, namely human T-cell lymphotropic virus Type 1 (HTVL-I).

The RNA genome of the retroviruses (Figure 28.58) comes in three variants:

- One variant consists basically of three coding sequences called *gag, pol,* and *env,* flanked by two sequences called ***long terminal repeats*** (LTRs), which are not transcribed. LTRs are very important because they can enhance the transcription of adjacent genes and even of some distant genes. The *gag* sequence codes for viral structural proteins, the *pol* for reverse transcriptase, and the *env* for glycoproteins on the lipid *env*elope of the virus.
- Another variant of retroviral genome has its prototype in the Rous sarcoma virus. Note in Figure 28.58 that it includes—besides *gag, pol,* and *env*—the v-*src* sequence, which is the oncogene.

- Last, some retroviruses have paid for acquiring an oncogene (v-*onc*) by losing some of their own genetic material; these retroviruses can reproduce only in association with a helper virus that supplies missing proteins, which are necessary for assembling mature virus particles.

Oncogene-containing retroviruses are also called acute transforming viruses because they act with incredible speed. They can produce a leukemia or a sarcoma in a matter of days or weeks (225). Retroviruses that do not contain oncogenes are called slow transforming retroviruses. They induce leukemias within one to several months. Lacking oncogenes, they can only transform cells by integrating their provirus near a cellular oncogene (insertional mutagenesis).

The three celebrities among the oncogenic retroviruses are the Rous sarcoma virus, which we have already described, Bittner's milk factor, now called MMTV (mouse mammary tumor virus), and the human T-cell lymphotropic virus Type 1 (HTLV-I).

Mouse mammary tumor virus. The MMTV (p. 859) has a number of fascinating features that are not directly applicable to humans so far as we know at present, but which sound like lessons for us to consider.

- The virus is present not only in the milk during lactation but also in the germ line (as provirus), so the

FIGURE 28.58 The genome of HIV, typical of retroviruses: the three genes code for group-specific antigen (*gag*), envelope (*env*), and polymerase (reverse transcriptase) (*pol*). (Courtesy of Dr. S. Lu, University of Massachusetts Medical School, Worcester, MA.)

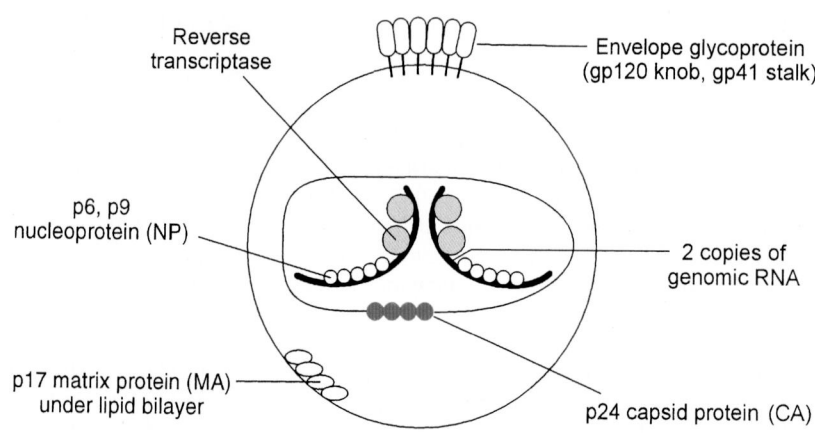

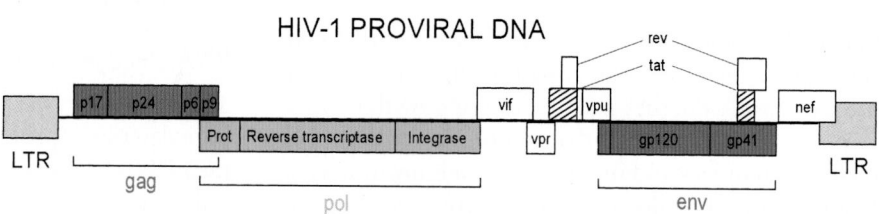

tendency to produce tumors can be acquired not only horizontally (by suckling) but also vertically (by inheritance) (125).

- The virus itself contains no oncogenes, but both of its LTRs are two or three times as large as usual for retroviruses, and contain a sequence that is sensitive to glucocorticoids, which increase transcription of the provirus (238). This fact reminds us that oncogenesis by this particular virus depends heavily on the hormonal status of its victim (p. 858); indeed several hormones affect mammary tumors in mice (153).

- In mice that develop mammary carcinomas, a large number of cells produce MMTV, and the provirus inserts itself, apparently at random, into their genome. However, only a few cells become transformed, which suggests that transformation requires insertion in some specific site or sites (225).

Human T-cell lymphotropic virus-I. The HTLV-I is a relative of the AIDS virus and is associated with a form of leukemia that occurs endemically in southern Japan, in areas where 26 percent of the population is seropositive for HTLV-I (129), in the Caribbean region, southeastern United States, and sporadically elsewhere. Epidemiologic data suggest that it is not very contagious, but health care personnel are advised to approach it with precautions similar to those used for hepatitis B. Normal T-cells cocultivated with infected leukemic cells do acquire the infection (129).

> A related virus, HTLV-II, has been isolated from a patient suffering from the so-called hairy cell leukemia. The AIDS virus, once called HTLV-III and now renamed HIV, belongs to the same group. All three viruses affect helper lymphocytes (T_H4): viruses are choosy.

HTLV-I contains no oncogene homologous to a human proto-oncogene, but it does contain a region called *tat* that may be a key to its ability to transform cells. The name *tat* stands for trans-activation of transcription, meaning that the product of that gene activates genes on other chromosomes. The protein coded by *tat* induces the infected cell to produce both interleukin-2 (IL-2) (which normally has the function of expanding T-cell clones) and IL-2 receptor. This means that the virus-infected T-cells would be set up for autocrine stimulation (157).

Here is a surprise: transgenic mice expressing the *tat* gene develop neurofibromatosis, not leukemia (Figure 28.59) and thereby became a model for studying that disease.

> *Neurofibromatosis* is a group of human neoplastic syndromes with a fairly high incidence (1 in 3000). Tumors

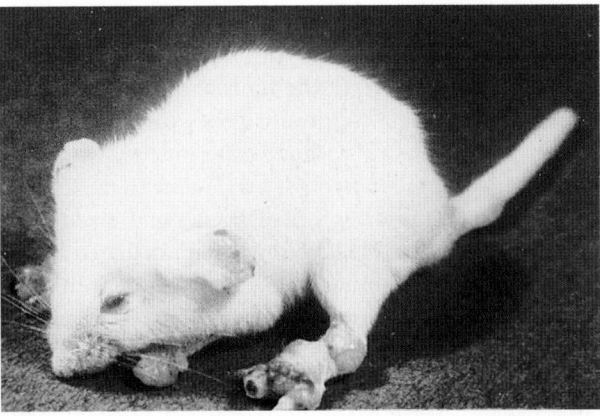

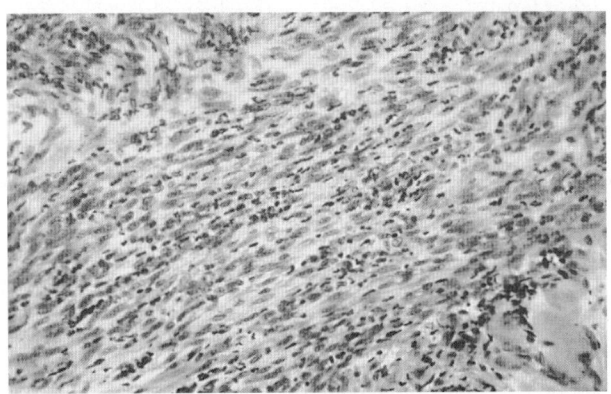

FIGURE 28.59 *Top:* This transgenic mouse is a model of human neurofibromatosis. It received the *tat* gene from human T-cell lymphotropic virus Type 1 (HTLV-I) suspected to cause adult T-cell leukemia. *Tat* also appears to activate certain cellular genes important for cell growth; indeed it produced multiple neurofibromas arising from nerve sheaths. *Bottom:* Histologic aspect of one such tumor (370x). (*Top:* Reprinted with permission from [115]. *Bottom:* Reprinted with permission from [175]. Both with Copyright 1987 by the American Association for the Advancement of Science.)

develop by the hundreds along nerve trunks. All the components of the nerve are represented in the tumors, which are initially benign but may progress to malignancy. The classic form of neurofibromatosis, called Recklinghausen's disease, is characterized by multiple neuromas, pigmented spots on the skin (*café au lait* spots), and pigmented hamartomas of the iris.

The Discovery of Suppressor Genes

Having summarized—ever so briefly—the discovery of the oncogenes, we should give equal time to another story, just as exciting, which led to the discovery of a different set of genes, the *suppressor genes* (sometimes called, not so properly, *anti-oncogenes*). The two stories have almost nothing in common. The quest for the oncogenes, as we saw, came to fruition in 1976, in the laboratory of Varmus and Bishop. That was a most sophisticated exercise, at the limit of available molecular technology. The suppressor genes came about in a totally different way, without experiments, without a laboratory, *by pure thinking*—a style dear to the ancient Greeks. Dr. Knudson is a pediatrician and a geneticist in Houston, Texas. He had long been fascinated by the behavior of a rare tumor, the retinoblastoma, that develops from the outer layer of the retina and usually grows within the eye. It has two clinical forms. It can appear *in children,* in which case it is clearly hereditary and usually develops in both eyes. (Children rarely complain of poor vision, so the first observable sign may be an abnormal reflection in the pupil [Figure 28.60]). The *adult variety* is usually sporadic, unilateral, and lacks a familial component. In 1971 Dr. Knudson realized that there was a message in this dual presentation of retinoblastoma, and concluded

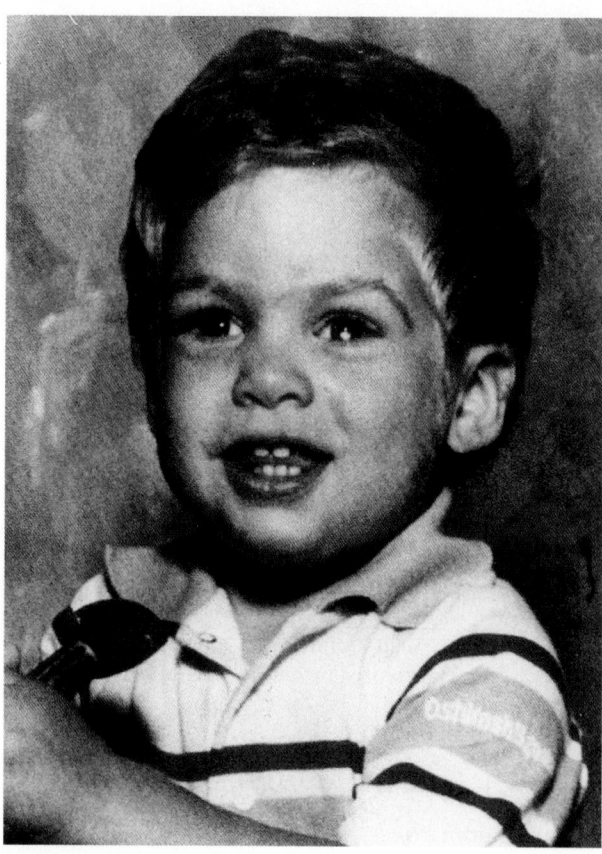

FIGURE 28.60   Child with the "cat's eye reflex" (*leukokoria*) due to a retinoblastoma. (Reproduced with permission from [61], copyright J. B. Lippincott, 1989.)

that it could be explained by assuming that a gene in a retinal cell was being knocked out by a "two-hit" mechanism (136). Soon the details were worked out, and we can now present the new concept as follows.

Retinoblastoma in both its forms is the result of two successive mutations: the first mutation affects one locus on one chromosome (i.e., one allele), and the second mutation affects the same locus on the other allele (Figure 28.61). The settings of this double accident will be different in the two forms of retinoblastoma.

Hereditary retinoblastoma. In this condition the first mutation is present in the sperm or ovum <u>before</u> fertilization; the individual therefore is born with a defective chromosome that is present in all cells. The mutant gene, present in only one allele, is recessive; therefore no disease develops. The genetic disturbance turned out to be the loss of a gene, now called *Rb* (for retinoblastoma). *A tumor develops only if the other allele (i.e., the other Rb gene) is lost.* A likely time for this accident to occur is during the development of the retina when mitoses are still occurring; there are about 10^6–10^7 retinoblasts, which might allow for three chances of mutation (39). The mutation may hit a single cell or sometimes a few cells, giving rise to multiple tumors.

Sporadic retinoblastoma. Two mutations must occur by chance, in the same cell, during extrauterine life to cause this cancer. This would have to be exceedingly rare, and indeed sporadic retinoblastoma is a very rare tumor (1 in 30,000 individuals); when it does occur, it is mostly unilateral and single (38).

> Here we should clarify a potential source of confusion. The lack of a single *Rb* gene has no somatic effect, so the gene is acting as recessive; when both *Rb* genes are missing a tumor develops, so the lack of both genes (which are recessive at the cellular level) becomes dominant by pedigree analysis (40, 87).

Knudson's "hypothesis" turned out to be a major discovery: it revealed a new category of tumor-producing genes. A retinoblastoma developed *if a gene was knocked out* (in both alleles), so we must conclude that those genes—in their normal turned-on condition—*prevent* a tumor from developing, whereas the oncogenes *produce* a tumor if they are turned on. The *Rb* gene quickly became the prototype of a large family of **tumor suppressor genes;** a family that includes such *prima donnas* as the powerful *p53* gene, nicknamed custodian of the genome, and the two suppressor genes of female breast cancer, *BRCA-1* and *BRCA-2.*

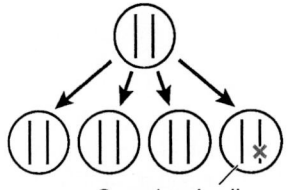
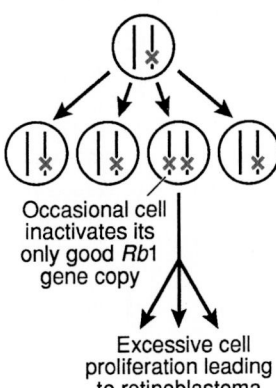
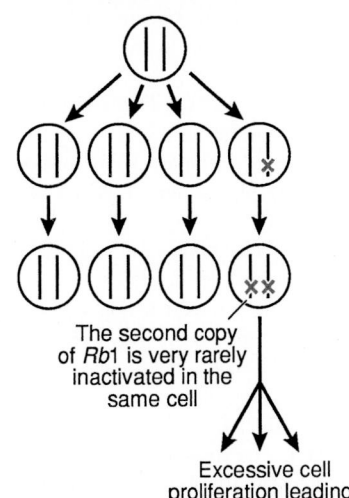

NORMAL HEALTHY INDIVIDUAL

Occasional cell inactivates one of its two good *Rb*1 genes

Result: No tumor

HEREDITARY RETINOBLASTOMA

Occasional cell inactivates its only good *Rb*1 gene copy

Excessive cell proliferation leading to retinoblastoma

Result: Most people with inherited gene develop tumor

NONHEREDITARY RETINOBLASTOMA

The second copy of *Rb*1 is very rarely inactivated in the same cell

Excessive cell proliferation leading to retinoblastoma

Result: Only about 1 in 30,000 normal people develop tumor

FIGURE 28.61   Genetic mechanisms underlying retinoblastoma. Patients with this type of tumor fall into two categories, hereditary and nonhereditary. The key to understanding this mechanism is that the recessive *Rb* gene inhibits cell growth; therefore, the loss of *both* Rb genes unleashes cell proliferation. (Reproduced with permission from [136].)

NOTE: The fact that there are different types of tumor-related genes—such as oncogenes, suppressor genes, repair genes—does not mean that there are corresponding types of tumors. In the course of progression, each tumor accumulates defective genes of all kinds.

TO SUM UP: The topic of tumors before 1976 seemed so hopeless that leading scientists were jumping ship. Viruses had offered hope, but it was obvious that most tumors were unrelated to viruses. Today, the field of tumors is one of the most studied and best understood in all of biology. The key to this astonishing progress was hidden in virus-induced tumors—although it remained true that most tumors are not caused by viruses. So, in the end, everybody in both camps can say "I told you so."

References

1. Abbas JS, Beecham JE. Burn wound carcinoma: case report and review of the literature. Burns 1988;14:222–224.
2. Abelson PH. Diet and cancer in humans and rodents. Science 1992;255:141.
3. Albert RE, Omran AR. Follow-up study of patients treated by X-ray epilation for tinea capitis. I. Population characteristics, posttreatment illnesses, and mortality experience. Arch Environ Health 1968;17:899–918.
4. Alberts B, Bray D, Lewis J, et al. Molecular biology of the cell, 2nd ed. New York: Garland Publishing, 1989.
5. Allen DW, Cole P. Viruses and human cancer. N Engl J Med 1972;286:70–82.
6. Ames BN. Dietary carcinogens and anticarcinogens. Science 1983;221:1256–1264.
7. Armstrong B, Doll R. Environmental factors and cancer incidence and mortality in different countries, with special reference to dietary practices. Int J Cancer 1975;15:617–631.
8. Aron NK, Tajuri S. Postburn scar carcinoma. Burns 1989;15:121–124.

9. Autrup H, Seremet T, Wakhisi J, Wasunna A. Aflatoxin exposure measured by urinary excretion of aflatoxin B_1-guanine adduct and hepatitis B virus infection in areas with different liver cancer incidence in Kenya. Cancer Res 1987;47: 3430–3433.

10. Balter M. Chernobyl's Thyroid Cancer Toll. Science 1995;270:1758–1759.

11. Bates RR, Klein M. Importance of a smooth surface in carcinogenesis by plastic film. J Natl Cancer Inst 1966;37: 145–151.

12. Bayon H. Epithelial proliferation induced by the injection of gasworks tar. Lancet 1912;2:1579.

13. Becker EL. The cytotoxic action of neutrophils on mammalian cells in vitro. Prog Allergy 1988;40:183–208.

14. Berenblum I. The epidemiology of cancer. In: Florey HW, ed. General pathology, 4th ed. Philadelphia: WB Saunders, 1970a, pp. 720–734.

15. Berenblum I. The study of tumours in animals. In: Florey HW, ed. General pathology, 4th ed. Philadelphia: WB Saunders, 1970b, pp. 744–780.

15a. Bhatia S, Sklar C. Second cancers in survivors of childhood cancer. Nat Rev Cancer 2002;2:124–132.

16. Bhawan J, Sau P, Byers R. Dermatopathology interactive atlas. Developed by Web Cottage Solutions: Delhi, India, 2001.

17. Billings PC, Morrow AR, Ryan CA, Kennedy AR. Inhibition of radiation-induced transformation of C3H/10T1/2 cells by carboxypeptidase inhibitor 1 and inhibitor II from potatoes. Carcinogenesis 1989;10:687–691.

18. Bischoff F, Bryson G. Carcinogenesis through solid state surfaces. Prog Exp Tumor Res 1964;5:85–133.

19. Bishop JM. Oncogenes. Sci Am 1982;246:80–92.

20. Bishop JM. Oncogenes and proto-oncogenes. Hosp Pract 1983;18:67–74.

21. Bishop JM. The molecular genetics of cancer. Science 1987; 235:305–311.

22. Biskind GS, Biskind MS. Experimental ovarian tumors in rats. Am J Clin Pathol 1949;19:501–521.

23. Biskind MS, Biskind GS. Development of tumors in the rat ovary after transplantation into the spleen. Proc Soc Exp Biol Med 1944;55:176–179.

24. Bittner JJ. The milk-influence of breast tumors in mice. Science 1942;95:462–463.

25. Bittner JJ. The causes and control of mammary cancer in mice. Harvey Lect 1947;42:221–246.

26. Blot WJ, Harrington JM, Toledo A, et al. Lung cancer after employment in shipyards during World War II. N Engl J Med 1978;299:620–624.

27. Boutwell RK. Some biological aspects of skin carcinogenesis. Prog Exp Tumor Res 1964;4:207–250.

28. Boyd NF. The epidemiology of cancer: principles and methods. In: Tannock IF, Hill RP, eds. The basic science of oncology. New York: Pergamon Press, 1987, pp. 7–23.

29. Brand KG, Buoen LC, Johnson KH, Brand I. Etiological factors, stages, and the role of the foreign body in foreign body tumorigenesis: a review. Cancer Res 1975;35: 279–286.

30. Braun AC. The story of cancer. On its nature, causes, and control. Reading, MA: Addison-Wesley, 1977.

31. Bronchud MH, Foote M, Peters WP, Robinson MO (eds). Principles of molecular oncology. Totowa, NJ: Humana Press Inc., 2000.

32. Brunekreef B, Boleij JSM. Long-term average suspended particulate concentrations in smokers' homes. Int Arch Occup Environ Health 1982;50:299–302.

33. Bulatao-Jayme J, Almero EM, Castro MCA, Jardeleza MTR, Salamat LA. A case-control dietary study of primary liver cancer risk from aflatoxin exposure. Int J Epidemiol 1982;11: 112–119.

34. Burck KB, Liu ET, Larrick JW, eds. Oncogenes. New York: Springer-Verlag, 1988.

35. Burkitt D. A sarcoma involving the jaws in African children. Br J Surg 1958;46:218–223.

36. Burkitt DP. Epidemiology of cancer of the colon and rectum. Cancer 1971;28:3–13.

37. Burns FJ. Cancer risk associated with therapeutic irradiation of skin. Arch Dermatol 1989;125:979–981.

38. Butlin HT. Three lectures on cancer of the scrotum in chimney-sweeps and others. Br Med J 1892;1:1341–1346;2: 1–6, 66–71.

39. Caggana M, Kennedy AR. c-fos mRNA levels are reduced in the presence of antipain and Bowman-Birk inhibitor. Carcinogenesis 1989;10:2145–2148.

40. Calabresi P. Leukemia after cytotoxic chemotherapy—a pyrrhic victory? N Engl J Med 1983;309:1118–1119.

41. Campbell WC. The worm and the tumor: reflections on Fibiger's Nobel prize. Perspect Biol Med 1997;40:498–504.

42. Chang MH, Chen CJ, Lai MS, et al. Universal hepatitis B vaccination in Taiwan and the incidence of hepatocellular carcinoma in children. Taiwan childhood hepatoma study group. N Engl J Med 1997;336:1855–1859.

43. Chang MH, Shau WY, Chen CJ, et al. Hepatitis B vaccination and hepatocellular carcinoma rates in boys and girls. JAMA 2000;284:3040–3042.

44. Cheever AW. Schistosomiasis and neoplasia. J Natl Cancer Inst 1978;61:13–18.

45. Clark C. Radium Girls. Women and industrial health reform, 1910–1935. Chapel Hill, NC: The University of North Carolina press, 1997.

46. Cohen SM, Purtilo DT, Ellwein LB. Pivotal role of increased cell proliferation in human carcinogenesis. Mod Pathol 1991; 4:371–382.

47. Cole P, Rodu B. Analytic epidemiology: cancer causes. In: Cancer. Principles & Practice of Oncology, 6th ed. Philadelphia: Lippincott Williams & Wilkins. 1998, pp. 241–252.

48. The Committee for the compilation of materials on damage caused by the atomic bombs in Hiroshima and Nagasaki. Hiroshima and Nagasaki. The Physical, Medical, and Social Effects of the Atomic Bombings. New York: Basic Books Inc., 1981.

49. Connolly JG, White EP. Malignant cells in the urine of men exposed to beta-naphthylamine. Can Med Assoc J 1969;100: 879–882.

50. Cook JW, Haslewood GAD, Hewett CL, et al. Chemical compounds as carcinogenic agents. Am J Cancer 1937;29: 219–259.

51. Cooper A. Observations on the structure and diseases of the testis, 2nd ed. (Cooper BB, ed). London: John Churchill, 1841.

52. Cooper GM. Cellular transforming genes. Science 1982;218: 801–806.

53. Cooper GM. Oncogenes, 2nd ed. Sudbury, MA: Jones and Bartlett Publishers, 1990.

54. Creech JL Jr, Johnson MN. Angiosarcoma of liver in the manufacture of polyvinyl chloride. J Occupat Med 1974; 16:150–151.

55. Csíkos M, Horváth Ö, Petri A, Petri I, Imre J. Late malignant transformation of chronic corrosive oesophageal strictures. Langenbecks Arch Chir 1985;365:231–238.

56. Cummings CW. The hypocrisy of US tobacco policy. Nature Med 1995;989–990.

57. Das M, Bickers DR, Mukhtar H. Protection against chemically induced skin tumorigenesis in SENCAR mice by tannic acid. Int J Cancer 1989;43:468–470.

58. de-Thé G. Epidemiology of Epstein-Barr virus and associated diseases in man. In: Roizman B, ed. The herpesviruses, vol 1. New York: Plenum Press, 1982, pp. 25–103.

59. Doll R, Morgan LG, Speizer FE. Cancers of the lung and nasal sinuses in nickel workers. Br J Cancer 1970;24: 623–632.

60. Doll R, Peto R. The causes of cancer. Oxford: Oxford University Press, 1981.

60a. Dollard SC, Chow LT, Kreider JW, et al. Characterization of an HPV type 11 isolate propagated in human foreskin implants in nude mice. Virology 1989;171:294–297.

61. Donaldson SS, Egbert PR. Retinoblastoma. In: Pizzo PA, Poplack DG, eds. Principles and practice of pediatric oncology. Philadelphia: JB Lippincott, 1989, pp.555–568.

62. Edmondson HA, Henderson B, Benton B. Liver-cell adenomas associated with use of oral contraceptives. N Engl J Med 1976;294:470–472.

63. Edwards MJ, Hirsch RM, Broadwater JR, Netscher DT, Ames FC. Squamous cell carcinoma arising in previously burned or irradiated skin. Arch Surg 1989;124:115–117.

64. Ellermann V, Bang O. Experimentelle Leukämie bei Hühnern. Zentralbl Bakteriol 1908;46:595–609.

65. El-Torky M, Giltman LI, Dabbous M. Collagens in scar carcinoma of the lung. Am J Pathol 1985;121:322–326.

66. Environmental Studies Board, Commission on Natural Resources, National Research Council. Causes and effects of stratospheric ozone reduction: an update. Washington, DC: National Academy Press, 1982.

67. Escobar MR. Oncogenic viruses. In: Sirica AE, ed. The pathobiology of neoplasia. New York: Plenum Press, 1989, pp. 81–109.

68. Eun HC, Kim JA, Lee YS. Squamous cell carcinoma in a frost-bite scar. Clin Exp Dermatol 1986;11:517–520.

69. Fabricant CG, Fabricant J, Minick CR, Litrenta MM. Herpesvirus-induced atherosclerosis. In: Essex M, Todaro G, zur Hausen H, eds. Viruses in naturally occurring cancers. Book B. Cold Spring Harbor conferences on cell proliferation, vol 7. Cold Spring Harbor: Cold Spring Harbor Laboratory, 1980, pp. 1251–1258.

70. Farber E. Chemical carcinogenesis. A biologic perspective. Am J Pathol 1982;106:271–296.

71. Farrell PJ, Tidy J. Viruses and human cancer. In: Anthony PP, Macsween RNM, eds. Recent advances in histopathology, no. 14. Edinburgh: Churchill Livingstone, 1989, pp. 23–41.

72. Favus MJ, Schneider AB, Stachura ME, et al. Thyroid cancer occurring as a late consequence of head-and-neck irradiation. Evaluation of 1056 patients. N Engl J Med 1976;294: 1019–1025.

73. Feitelson MA, Duan L-X. Hepatitis B virus x antigen in the pathogenesis of chronic infections and the development of hepatocellular carcinoma. Am J Pathol 1997;150: 1141–1157.

74. Feramisco JR, Gross M, Kamata T, Rosenberg M, Sweet RW. Microinjection of the oncogene form of the human H-ras (T-24) protein results in rapid proliferation of quiescent cells. Cell 1984;38:109–117.

75. Ferbeyre G, Lowe SW. The price of tumour suppression? Nature 2002;415:26–27.

76. Fibiger J. Untersuchungen über eine Nematode (Spiroptera sp.n.) und deren Fähigkeit, papillomatöse und carcinomatöse Geschwulstbildungen im Magen der Ratte hervorzurufen. Z Krebsforsch 1913;13:217–280.

77. Fieser LF, Fieser M, Hershberg EB, et al. Carcinogenic activity of the cholanthrenes and of other 1:2-benzanthracene derivatives. Am J Cancer 1937;29:260–268.

78. Fisher B, Fisher ER. Experimental evidence in support of the dormant tumor cell. Science 1959;130:918–919.

79. Fisher B, Fisher ER, Feduska N. Trauma and the localization of tumor cells. Cancer 1967;20:23–30.

80. Fleming MD, Hunt JL, Purdue GF, Sandstad J. Marjolin's ulcer: a review and reevaluation of a difficult problem. J Burn Care Rehabil 1990;11:460–469.

81. Floyd RA. Role of oxygen free radicals in carcinogenesis and brain ischemia. FASEB J 1990;4:2587–2597.

82. Foulds L. Neoplastic development, vol 2. London: Academic Press, 1975.

83. Fox JG, Wang TC. Helicobacter pylori—not a good bug after all. N Engl J Med 2001;345:829–831.

84. Fubini B, Bolis V, Giamello E, Volante M. Chemical Functionalities at the broken fibre surface relatable to free radicals production. In: Brown RC, Hoskins JA, Johnson NF, (eds). Mechanisms in fibre carcinogenesis. New York: Plenum Press, 1991, pp. 415–432.

85. Furth J. Thyroid-pituitary tumorigenesis. J Natl Cancer Inst 1954;15:687–691.

86. Furth J. Pituitary cybernetics and neoplasia. Harvey Lect 1969;63:47–71.

87. Furth J. Hormones as etiological agents in neoplasia. In: Becker FF, ed. Cancer: a comprehensive treatise, vol 1. New York: Plenum Press, 1975, pp. 75–120.

88. Furth J, Clifton KH. Experimental pituitary tumours. In: Harris GW, Donovan BT, eds. The pituitary gland, vol 2. Berkeley, CA: University of California Press, 1966, pp. 460–497.

89. Gardner WU, Pfeiffer CA, Trentin JJ. Hormonal factors in experimental carcinogenesis. In: Homburger F, ed. The physiopathology of cancer, 2nd ed. New York: Hoeber-Harper, 1959, pp. 152–237.

90. Garner RC, Martin CN, Clayson DB. Cacinogenic aromatic amines and related compounds. In: Searle CE, ed. Chemical carcinogens, 2nd ed, vol 1. Washington, DC: American Chemical Society, 1984, pp. 175–276.

91. Gentile JM. Schistosome related cancers: a possible role for genotoxins. Environ Mutagen 1985;7:775–785.

92. Gilchrest BA, Eller MS, Geller AC, Yaar M. The pathogenesis of melanoma induced by ultraviolet radiation. N Engl J Med 1999;340:1341–1348.

93. Grasso P. Carcinogens in food. In: Searle CE, ed. Chemical carcinogens, 2nd ed, vol 2. Washington, DC: American Chemical Society, 1984, pp. 1203–1239.

94. Greaves P, Martin J-M, Rabemampianina Y. Malignant fibrous histiocytoma in rats at sites of implanted Millipore filters. Am J Pathol 1985;120:207–214.

95. Green JA. Morphology, secretion, and transplantability of ten mouse ovarian neoplasms induced by intrasplenic ovarian grafting. Cancer Res 1957;17:86–91.

96. Greenwald P. Dietary carcinogens. In: Cancer. Principles & practice of oncology, 6th ed. Philadelphia: Lippincott Williams & Wilkins. 2001, pp. 595–600.

97. Gregg A. For future doctors. Chicago: University of Chicago Press, 1957.

98. Gross L. "Spontaneous" leukemia developing in C3H mice following inoculation, in infancy, with AK-leukemic extracts, or AK-embryos. Proc Soc Exp Biol Med 1951;76:27–32.

99. Gross L. Oncogenic viruses, vol 1, 3rd ed. Oxford: Pergamon Press, 1983.

100. Grote SJ, Revell SH. Correlation of chromosome damage and colony-forming ability in Syrian hamster cells in culture irradiated in G_1. Curr Top Radiat Res Q 1972;7:303–309.

101. Gupta J, Pilotti S, Rilke F, Shah K. Association of human papillomavirus type 16 with neoplastic lesions of the vulva and other genital sites by in situ hybridization. Am J Pathol 1987;127:206–215.

102. Habs M, Schmähl D. Diet and cancer. J Cancer Res Clin Oncol 1980;96:1–10.

103. Hammond JS, Thomsen S, Ward CG. Scar carcinoma arising acutely in a skin graft donor site. J Trauma 1987;27:681–683.

104. Hansen B. Skorstensfejerfagets Historie og Traditioner. Tønder, Denmark: Skorstensfejersvendenes Fagforbund i Danmark, 1984.

105. Hatch E, Herbst A, Hoover R, et al. Incidence of squamous neoplasia of the cervix and vagina in des-exposed daughters. Ann Epidemiol 2000;10:467.

106. Hatch EE, Herbst AL, Hoover RN, et al. Incidence of squamous neoplasia of the cervix and vagina in women exposed prenatally to diethylstilbestrol (United States). Cancer Causes Control 2001;12:837–845.

107. Hayman J, Huygens H. Angiosarcoma developing around a foreign body. J Clin Pathol 1983;36:515–518.

108. Henderson BE, Ross R, Bernstein L. Estrogens as a cause of human cancer: the Richard and Hinda Rosenthal Foundation award lecture. Cancer Res 1988;48:246–253.

109. Henderson JS. Peyton Rous (1879–1970). Reprinted from Year Book of the American Philosophical Society, 1971:168–179.

110. Herbst AL, Scully RE. Adenocarcinoma of the vagina in adolescence. A report of 7 cases including 6 clear-cell carcinomas (so-called mesonephromas). Cancer 1970;25:745–757.

111. Herbst AL, Scully RE, Robboy SJ, Welch WR, Cole P. Abnormal development of the human genital tract following prenatal exposure to diethylstilbestrol. In: Hiatt HH, Watson JD, Winsten JA, eds. Origins of human cancer. Book A. Incidence of cancer in humans. Cold Spring Harbor: Cold Spring Harbor Laboratory, 1977, pp. 399–412.

112. Herbst AL, Ulfelder H, Poskanzer DC. Adenocarcinoma of the vagina. Association of maternal stilbestrol therapy with tumor appearance in young women. N Engl J Med 1971;284:878–881.

113. Herlyn M, Satyamoorthy K. Molecular biology of cutaneous melanoma. In: Cancer. Principles & practice of oncology, 6th ed. Philadelphia: Lippincott Williams & Wilkins. 2001, pp. 2003–2012.

114. Herrera-Goepfert R, Reyes E, Hernández-Avila M, et al. Epstein-Barr virus-associated gastric carcinoma in Mexico: analysis of 135 consecutive gastrectomies in two hospitals. Mod Pathol 1999;12:873–878.

115. Hinrichs SH, Nerenberg M, Reynolds RK, Khoury G, Jay G. A transgenic mouse model for human neurofibromatosis. Science 1987;237:1340–1343.

116. Hirohata T. Radiation carcinogenesis. Semin Oncol 1976;3:25–34.

117. Hirono I. Natural carcinogenic products of plant origin. Crit Rev Toxicol 1981;8:235–277.

118. Hitchcock CR, Bell ET. Studies on the nematode parasite, *Gongylonema neoplasticum* (*Spiroptera neoplasticum*), and avitaminosis A in the forestomach of rats: comparison with Fibiger's results. J Natl Cancer Inst 1952;12:1345–1387.

119. Houghton A, Munster EW, Viola MV. Increased incidence of malignant melanoma after peaks of sunspot activity. Lancet 1978;1:759–760.

120. Huebner RJ, Todaro GJ. Oncogenes of RNA tumor viruses as determinants of cancer. Proc Natl Acad Sci 1969;64:1087–1094.

121. Huepner WC. Occupational tumors and allied diseases. Springfield, IL: Charles C. Thomas, 1942.

122. Hunter D. The diseases of occupations. London: The English Universities Press Ltd., 1969.

123. Hunter T. The proteins of oncogenes. Sci Am 1984;251:70–79.

124. Hursting SD, Perkins SN, Phang JM. Calorie restriction delays spontaneous tumorigenesis in p53-knockout transgenic mice. Proc Natl Acad Sci USA 1994;91:7036–7040.

125. Hynes NE, Groner B, Michalides R. Mouse mammary tumor virus: transcriptional control and involvement in tumorigenesis. Adv Cancer Res 1984;41:155–184.

126. Inoshita T, Youngberg GA. Malignant fibrous histiocytoma arising in previous surgical sites. Report of two cases. Cancer 1984;53:176–183.

127. Inskip PD, Tarone RE, Hatch EE, et al. Cellular-telephone use and brain tumors. N Engl J Med 2001;344:79–86.

128. Issenberg P. Nitrite, nitrosamines, and cancer. Fed Proc 1976;35:1322–1326.

129. Jandl JH. Blood. Boston: Little, Brown, 1987.

130. Kalil M, Hildebrandt AC. Pathology and distribution of plant tumors. In: Kaiser HE, ed. Neoplasms—comparative pathology of growth in animals, plants, and man. Baltimore: Williams & Wilkins, 1981, pp. 813–821.

131. Kanaar P, Oort J. Fibrosarcomas developing in scar-tissue. Dermatologica 1969;138:312–319.

132. Kee M. Cancer causation in booklet form. Nature 1983; 303:648.

133. Kennaway E. The identification of a carcinogenic compound in coal-tar. Br Med J 1955;2:749–752.

134. Kennedy AR. The conditions for the modification of radiation transformation in vitro by a tumor promoter and protease inhibitors. Carcinogenesis 1985;6:1441–1445.

135. Kirkpatrik CJ, Alves A, Köhler H, et al. Biomaterial-induced sarcoma. A novel model to study preneoplastic change. Am J Pathol 2000;156:1455–1467.

136. Knudson AG Jr. Mutation and cancer: statistical study of retinoblastoma. Proc Natl Acad Sci USA 1971;68:820–823.

137. Kohn HI, Fry RJM. Radiation carcinogenesis. N Engl J Med 1984;310:504–511.

138. Kreider JW. Neoplastic progression of the Shope rabbit papilloma. In: Essex M, Todaro G, zur Hausen H, eds. Viruses in naturally occurring cancers. Book A. Cold Spring Harbor conferences on cell proliferation, vol 7. Cold Spring Harbor: Cold Spring Harbor Laboratory, 1980, pp. 283–299.

139. Kwan TH, Hood AF. Associated cutaneous diseases. In: Nash G, Said JW, eds. Pathology of AIDS and HIV infection. Philadelphia: WB Saunders, 1992, pp. 148–173.

140. Land H, Parada LF, Weinberg RA. Cellular oncogenes and multistep carcinogenesis. Science 1983;222:771–778.

141. Laqueur GL, Spatz M. Toxicology of cycasin. Cancer Res 1968;28:2262–2267.

142. Lifeso RM, Rooney RJ, El-Shaker M. Post-traumatic squamous-cell carcinoma. J Bone Joint Surg 1990;72–A:12–18.

143. Lijinsky W. The significance of N-nitroso compounds as environmental carcinogens. J Environ Sci Health 1986;C4: 1–45.

144. Linet MS, Hatch EE, Kleinerman RA, et al. Residential exposure to magnetic fields and acute lymphoblastic leukemia in children. N Engl J Med 1997;337:1–7.

145. Lingeman CH. The vinyl chloride story. Bull Soc Pharmacol Environ Pathol 1976;4:9–15.

146. Little JB. Influence of noncarcinogenic secondary factors on radiation carcinogenesis. Radiat Res 1981;87:240–250.

147. Lowy DR, Schiller JT. Preventive cancer vaccines. In: Cancer. Principles & practice of oncology, 6th ed. Philadelphia: Lippincott Williams & Wilkins. 2001, pp. 3189–3217.

148. Lucké B. A neoplastic disease of the kidney of the frog, *Rana pipiens.* Am J Cancer 1934;20:352–379.

149. Lyon JL. Radiation exposure and cancer. Hosp Pract 1984; 19:159–173.

150. MacMahon HE, Murphy AS, Bates MI. Endothelial-cell sarcoma of liver following thorotrast injections. Am J Pathol 1947;23:585–611.

151. Marx J. Oncogenes reach a milestone. Science 1994;266: 1942–1944.

152. Maugh TH 2nd. New link between ozone and cancer. Science 1982;216:396–397.

153. McGrath CM, Jones RF. Hormonal induction of mammary tumor viruses and its implications for carcinogenesis. Cancer Res 1978;38:4112–4125.

154. McLean AEM, Magee PN. Increased renal carcinogenesis by dimethyl nitrosamine in protein deficient rats. Br J Exp Pathol 1970;51:587–590.

155. Meléndez LV, Hunt RD, Daniel MD, et al. Herpesviruses saimiri and ateles—their role in malignant lymphomas of monkeys. Fed Proc 1972;31:1643–1650.

156. Melnick S, Cole P, Anderson D, Herbst A. Rates and risks of diethylstilbestrol-related clear-cell adenocarcinoma of the vagina and cervix. An update. N Engl J Med 1987;316: 514–516.

157. Michalopoulos GK. Growth factors and neoplasia. In:Sirica AE, ed. The pathobiology of neoplasia. New York: Plenum Press, 1989, pp. 345–370.

158. Miki Y, Swensen J, Shattuck-Eldens D, Futreal PA, et al. A strong candidate for the breast and ovarian cancer susceptibility gene BRCA 1. Science 1994;266:66–71.

159. Miller AB. An overview of hormone-associated cancers. Cancer Res 1978;38:3985–3990.

160. Miller EC. Some current perspectives on chemical carcinogenesis in humans and experimental animals: presidential address. Cancer Res 1978;38:1479–1496.

161. Miller EC, Miller JA. Searches for ultimate chemical carcinogens and their reactions with cellular macro-molecules. Cancer 1981;47:2327–2345.

162. Miller JA. Carcinogenesis by chemicals: an overview—GHA Clowes memorial lecture. Cancer Res 1970;30:559–576.

163. Miller JA, Miller EC. Ultimate chemical carcinogens as reactive mutagenic electrophiles. In: Hiatt HH, Watson JD, Winsten JA, eds. Origin of human cancer. Book B. Mechanisms of carcinogenesis. Cold Spring Harbor conferences on cell proliferation, vol 4. Cold Spring Harbor: Cold Spring Harbor Laboratory, 1977, pp. 605–627.

164. Mills PK, Beeson WL, Phillips RL, Fraser GE. Cancer incidence among California Seventh-Day Adventists. Am J Clin Nutrit 1994;59(5 Suppl):1136S–1142S.

165. Mirvish SS. Formation of N-nitroso compounds: chemistry, kinetics, and in vivo occurrence. Toxicol Appl Pharmacol 1975;31:325–351.

166. Mirvish SS. The etiology of gastric cancer. Intragastric nitrosamide formation and other theories. J Natl Cancer Inst 1983;71:629–647.

167. Modal B, Baidatz D, Mart H, Steinitz R, Levin SG. Radiation-induced head and neck tumours. Lancet 1974;1: 277–279.

168. Møller P, Wallin H, Holst E, Knudsen LE. Sunlight-induced DNA damage in human mononuclear cells. FASEB J 2002; 16:45–53.

169. Mondal S, Heidelberger C. Transformation of C3H/10T1/2 CL8 mouse embryo fibroblasts by ultraviolet irradiation and a phorbol ester. Nature 1976;260:710–711.

170. Montesano R, Pepper MS, Möhle-Steinlein U, et al. Increased proteolytic activity is responsible for the aberrant morphogenetic behavior of endothelial cells expressing the middle T oncogene. Cell 1990;62:435–445.

171. Moore RD, Pearson TA. Moderate alcohol consumption and coronary artery disease. Medicine 1986;65:242–267.

172. Mossman BT, Bignon J, Corn M, Seaton A, Gee JBL. Asbestos: scientific developments and implications for public policy. Science 1990;247:294–301.

173. Murthy SM, Goldschmidt RA, Rao LM, et al. The influence of surgical trauma on experimental metastasis. Cancer 1989; 64:2035–2044.

174. National Council on Radiation Protection and Measurements: NCRP report no. 93. Bethesda, MD, 1987.

175. Nerenberg M, Hinrichs SH, Reynolds RK, Khoury G, Jay G. The *tat* gene of human T-lymphotropic virus type 1 induces mesenchymal tumors in transgenic mice. Science 1987;237:1324–1329.

176. Newcomb PA, Mandelson MT. A record-based evaluation of induced abortion and breast cancer risk (United States). Cancer Causes Control 2000;11:777–781.

177. Noodleman FR, Pollack SV. Trauma as a possible etiologic factor in basal cell carcinoma. J Dermatol Surg Oncol 1986;12:841–846.

178. Noonan FP, Recio JA, Takayama H, et al. Neonatal sunburn and melanoma in mice. Nature 2001;413:271–272.

179. Oberling C. The riddle of cancer. Translated by Woglom WH, rev ed. New Haven, CT: Yale University Press, 1952.

179a. Oliveira MJ, Van Damme J, Lauwaet T, et al. Beta-casein-derived peptides, produced by bacteria, stimulate cancer cell invasion and motility. EMBO J 2003;22:6161–6173.

180. Oppenheimer BS, Oppenheimer ET, Stout AP. Sarcomas induced in rats by implanting cellophane. Proc Soc Exp Biol Med 1948;67:33–34.

181. Oppenheimer BS, Oppenheimer ET, Stout AP, Willhite M, Danishefsky I. The latent period in carcinogenesis by plastics in rats and its relation to the presarcomatous stage. Cancer 1958;11:204–213.

182. Parsonnet J. *Helicobacter pylori* in the stomach—A paradox unmasked. N Engl J Med 1996;335:278–280.

183. Pederson-Bjergaard J, Ersboll J, Hansen VL, et al. Carcinoma of the urinary bladder after treatment with cyclophosphamide for non-Hodgkin's lymphoma. N Engl J Med 1988;318:1028–1032.

184. Perrin F. Joliot-Curie, Irène. In: Gillispie CG, ed. Dictionary of scientific biography, vol 7/8. New York: Charles Scribner's Sons, 1980, pp. 157–159.

185. Persing DH, Prendergast FG. Infection, immunity, and cancer. Arch Pathol Lab Med 1999;123:1015–1022.

186. Pfister H. Human papillomaviruses and genital cancer. Adv Cancer Res 1987;48:113–147.

187. Philips FS, Sternberg SS. The lethal actions of anti-tumor agents in proliferating cell systems in vivo. Am J Pathol 1975;81:205–218.

188. Phillips RL. Role of life-style and dietary habits in risk of cancer among Seventh-Day Adventists. Cancer Res 1975;35:3513–3522.

189. Pirchan A, Sikl H. Cancer of the lung in the miners of Jáchymov (Joachimstal). Report of cases observed in 1929–1930. Am J Cancer 1932;16:681–722.

190. Pisani P, Maxwell Parkin DM, Muñoz N, Ferlay J. Cancer and infection: estimates of the attributable fraction in 1990. Cancer Epidemiol Biomarkers Prev 1997;6:387–400.

191. Pitot HC. Fundamentals on oncology, 3rd ed. New York: Marcel Dekker, 1986.

192. Pollack ES, Nomura AMY, Heilbrun LK, Stemmermann GN, Green SB. Prospective study of alcohol consumption and cancer. N Engl J Med 1984;310:617–621.

193. Pope III CA, Burnett RT, Thun MJ, et al. Lung cancer, cardiopulmonary mortality, and long-term exposure to fine particulate air pollution. JAMA 2002;287:1132–1141.

194. Popper H. The heuristic importance of environmental pathology. Lesions from the vinyl chloride problem. Arch Pathol 1975;99:69–71.

195. Popper H, Thomas LB, Telles NC, Falk H, Selikoff IJ. Development of hepatic angiosarcoma in man induced by vinyl chloride, thorotrast, and arsenic. Am J Pathol 1978;92:349–376.

196. Pott P. Chirurgical observations. London: TJ Carnegy, 1775. Reprinted in Natl Cancer Inst Monogr 1963;10:7–13.

197. Potter JD. Fiber and colorectal cancer—where to now? N Engl J Med 1999;340:223–224.

198. Potter M. Percivall Pott's contribution to cancer research. London: TJ Carnegy, 1775. Reprinted in Natl Cancer Inst Monogr 1963;10:1–5.

199. Preston-Martin S. Prior X-ray therapy for acne related to tumors of the parotid gland. Arch Dermatol 1989;125:921–924.

200. Preston-Martin S, Pike MC, Ross RK, Jones PA, Henderson BE. Increased cell division as a cause of human cancer. Cancer Res 1990;50:7415–7421.

201. Preussmann R, Eisenbrand G. N-nitroso carcinogens in the environment. In: Searle CE, ed. Chemical carcinogens, 2nd ed, vol 2. Washington, DC: American Chemical Society, 1984, pp. 829–868.

202. Puck TT. Radiation and the human cell. Sci Am 1960;202:142–153.

203. Pullman B, Pullman A. Nucleophilicity of DNA. Relation to chemical carcinogenesis. In: Pullman B, Ts'o POP, Gelboin H, eds. Carcinogenesis: fundamental mechanisms and environmental effects. Dordrecht: D. Reidel Publishing, 1980, pp. 55–66.

204. Ramazzini B. De Morbis Artificum Diatriba, 1700.

205. Rauth AM. Radiation carcinogenesis. In: Tannock IF, Hill RP, eds. The basic science of oncology. New York: Pergamon Press, 1987, pp. 106–124.

206. Redmond DE Jr. Tobacco and cancer: the first clinical report, 1761. N Engl J Med 1970;282:18–23.

207. Rehn L. Blasengeschwülste bei Fuchsin-Arbeitern. Arch Klin Chir 1895;50:588–600.

208. Reznikoff CA, Bertram JS, Brankow DW, Heidelberger C. Quantitative and qualitative studies of chemical transformation of cloned C3H mouse embryo cells sensitive to postconfluence inhibition of cell division. Cancer Res 1973;33:3239–3249.

209. Richtsmeir WJ, Wittels EG, Mazur EM. Epstein-Barr virus-associated malignancies. Crit Rev Clin Lab Sci 1987;25:105–136.

210. Rinsky RA, Young RJ, Smith AB. Leukemia in benzene workers. Am J Indust Med 1981;2:217–245.

211. Rogers AE, Longnecker MP. Dietary and nutritional influences on cancer: a review of epidemiologic and experimental data. Lab Invest 1988;59:729–759.

212. Rohrschneider LR. Adhesion plaques of Rous sarcoma virus-transformed cells contain the src gene product. Proc Natl Acad Sci USA 1980;77:3514–3518.

213. Rous P. Transmission of a malignant new growth by means of a cell-free filtrate. JAMA 1911;56:198.

214. Rous P. A sarcoma of the fowl transmissible by an agent separable from the tumor cells. J Exp Med 1911;13:397–411.

215. Rous P, Beard JW. The progression to carcinoma of virus-induced rabbit papillomas (Shope). J Exp Med 1935;62:523–548.

216. Rous P, Kidd JG. A comparison of virus-induced rabbit tumors with the tumors of unknown cause elicited by tarring. J Exp Med 1939;69:399–424.

217. Rous P, Kidd JG. Conditional neoplasms and subthreshold neoplastic states. A study of the tar tumor of rabbits. J Exp Med 1941;73:365–389.

217a. Ruddon RW. Cancer biology, 2nd ed. New York: Oxford University Press, 1987.

218. Russell DS, Rubinstein LJ. Pathology of tumours of the nervous system, 5th ed. Baltimore: Williams & Wilkins, 1988.

219. Sarma DP, Weilbaecher TG. Carcinoma arising in burn scar. J Surg Oncol 1985;29:89–90.

220. Sauter C. Why the color white is vital for the leukocyte. N Engl J Med 1989;321:1479–1480.

221. Scapa E, Eshchar J. Chemical burns of the upper gastrointestinal tract. Burns 1985;11:269–273.

221a. Schottenfeld D, Fraumeni JF Jr, eds. Cancer epidemiology and prevention. 2nd ed., New York: Oxford University Press, 1996.

222. Schuh AC, Keating SJ, Monteclaro FS, Vogt PK, Breitman ML. Obligatory wounding requirement for tumorigenesis in v-jun transgenic mice. Nature 190;346:756–760.

223. Scott D, Zampetti-Bosseler F. The relationship between cell killing, chromosome aberrations, spindle defects and mitotic delay in mouse lymphoma cells of differential sensitivity to X-rays. Int J Radiat Biol 1980;37:33–47.

224. Sell S, Pierce GB. Maturation arrest of stem cell differentiation is a common pathway for the cellular origin of teratocarcinomas and epithelial cancers. Lab Invest 1994;70:6–22.

225. Sheinin R, Mak TW, Clark SP. Viruses and cancer. In: Tannock IF, Hill RP, eds. The basic science of oncology. New York: Pergamon Press, 1987, pp. 52–71.

226. Shih C, Shilo B-Z, Goldfarb MP, Dannenberg A, Weinberg RA. Passage of phenotypes of chemically transformed cells via transfection of DNA and chromatin. Proc Natl Acad Sci USA 1979;76:5714–5718.

227. Shimkin MB. Contrary to nature. DHEW publ no. (NIH) 76–720. Washington, DC: US Department of Health, Education, and Welfare, 1977.

228. Shimkin MB, Triolo VA. History of chemical carcinogenesis: some prospective remarks. Prog Exp Tumor Res 1969;11:1–20.

229. Shope RE. Infectious papillomatosis of rabbits. J Exp Med 1933;58:607–624.

230. Skibber JM, Minsky BD, Hoff PM. Cancer of the colon. In: Cancer. Principles & practice of oncology, 6th ed. Philadelphia: Lippincott Williams & Wilkins. 2001, pp. 1216–1271.

231. Smith EF, Townsend CO. A plant-tumor of bacterial origin. Science 1907;25:671–673.

232. Southam AH, Wilson SR. Cancer of the scrotum: the etiology, clinical features, and treatment of the disease. Br Med J 1922;2:971–973.

233. Steffen C. Marjolin's ulcer. Report of two cases and evidence that Marjolin did not describe cancer arising in scars of burns. Am J Dermatopathol 1984;6:187–193.

234. Stehelin D. Dix ans de recherches sur les oncogènes. Les Cahiers de la Fondation, no. 2. Fondation Louis Jeantet de Médecine, 1987, pp. 41–53.

234a. Stewart BW, Kleihues P. (eds). World cancer report. Lyon: IARC Press, 2003.

235. Strohsnitter WC, Noller KL, Hoover RN, et al. Cancer risk in men exposed in utero to diethylstilbestrol. J Natl Cancer Inst 2001;93:545–551.

236. Sunderman FW Jr. Mechanisms of nickel carcinogenesis. Scand J Work Environ Health 1989;15:1–12.

237. Sunderman FW Jr, Morgan LG, Andersen A, Ashley D, Forouhar FA. Histopathology of sinonasal and lung cancers in nickel refinery workers. Ann Clin Lab Sci 1989;19:44–50.

238. Sutherland DJ. Hormones and cancer. In: Tannock IF, Hill RP, eds. The basic science of oncology. New York: Pergamon Press, 1987, pp. 204–222.

239. Swan SH. Intrauterine exposure to diethylstilbestrol: long term effects in humans. APMIS 2000;108:793–804.

240. Tannenbaum SR, Fett D, Young VR, Land PD, Bruce WR. Nitrite and nitrate are formed by endogenous synthesis in the human intestine. Science 1978;200:1487–1489.

241. Temin HM. Possible implications for medicine of RNA-directed DNA synthesis. Triangle 1972;11:37–42.

242. Temin HM. On the origin of the genes for neoplasia. GHA Clowes memorial lecture. Cancer Res 1974;34:2835–2841.

243. Thomas L. On warts. In: Thomas L, ed. The medusa and the snail: more notes of a biology watcher. New York: Viking Press, 1979.

244. Thompson NL, Mead JE, Braun L, et al. Sequential proto-oncogene expression during rat liver regeneration. Cancer Res 1986;46:3111–3117.

245. Thrasher JP, Ichinose H, Pitot HC. Osteogenic sarcoma of the canine esophagus associated with *Spirocerca lupi* infection. Am J Vet Res 1963;24:808–818.

246. Trichopoulos D, Adami H-O. Cellular telephones and brain tumors. N Engl J Med 2001;344:133–134.

247. Troll W, Kennedy AR, (eds). Protease inhibitors as cancer chemopreventive agents. New York: Plenum Press, 1993.

248. Trowell HC, Burkitt DP. Western diseases: their emergence and prevention. Cambridge, MA: Harvard University Press, 1981.

249. Trowell H, Burkitt D, Heaton K, eds. Dietary fibre, fibre-depleted foods and disease. London: Academic Press, 1985.

250. Tucker MA, Coleman CN, Cox RS, Varghese A, Rosenberg SA. Risk of second cancers after treatment for Hodgkin's disease. N Engl J Med 1988;318:76–81.

251. Tucker MA, D'Angio GJ, Boice JD Jr, et al. Bone sarcomas linked to radiotherapy and chemotherapy in children. N Engl J Med 1987;317:588–593.

252. Tuyns AJ, Péquignot G, Jensen OM. Le cancer de l'oesophage en Ille-et-Vilaine en fonction des niveaux de consommation d'alcool et de tabac. Des risques qui se multiplient. Bull Cancer 1977;64:45–60.

253. Tyner SD, Venkatachalam S, Choi J, et al. p53 mutant mice that display early ageing-associated phenotypes. Nature 2002;415:45–53.

254. Uemura N, Okamoto S, Yamamoto S, et al. *Helicobacter pylori* infection and the development of gastric cancer. N Engl J Med 2001;345:784–789.

255. Ullrich RL. Etiology of cancer: physical factors. In: Cancer. Principles & practice of oncology, 6th ed. Philadelphia: Lippincott Williams & Wilkins. 2001, pp. 195–206.

256. Upton AC. Physical carcinogenesis: radiation—history and sources. In: Becker FF, ed. Cancer: a comprehensive treatise, vol 1, 2nd ed. New York: Plenum Press, 1982, pp. 551–567.

257. Van Duuren BL, Melchionne S. Mouse skin application in chemical carcinogenesis. Prog Exp Tumor Res 1983;26: 154–168.

258. van Kaick G, Bahner ML, Liebermann D, Lührs H, Wesch H. Thorotrast-induzierte Tumoren der Leber. Radiologe 1999;39:643–651.

259. Velentgas P, Daling JR. Risk factors for breast cancer in younger women. Monogr Natl Cancer Inst 1994;16:15–22.

260. Wanless IR, Medline A. Role of estrogens as promoters of hepatic neoplasia. Lab Invest 1982;46:313–320.

261. Wargotz ES, Sidawy MK, Jannotta FS. Thorotrast-associated gliosarcoma. Including comments on Thorotrast use and review of sequelae with particular reference to lesions of the central nervous system. Cancer 1988;62:58–66.

262. Warner KE. Selling smoke: cigarette advertising and public health. Washington, DC: American Public Health Association, 1986.

263. Warner KE. The tobacco subsidy: does it matter? J Natl Cancer Inst 1988;80:81–83.

264. Warren S. Effects of radiation on normal tissues. Arch Pathol 1942;34:443–450. Reprinted in CA 1980;30:350–355.

264a. Waterhouse J, Muir C, Shanmugarathnam K, Powell J, eds. Cancer incidence in five continents, vol 4. IARC Scientific Publications No. 42. Lyon: International Agency for Research on Cancer, 1982.

265. Watson JD, Hopkins NA, Roberts JW, Steitz JA, Weiner AM. Molecular biology of the gene, 4th ed. Menlo Park: Benjamin/Cummings Publishing, 1987, pp. 1016.

266. Weinberg RA. Oncogenes of spontaneous and chemically induced tumors. Adv Cancer Res 1982;36:149–163.

267. Weinberg RA. Oncogenes, antioncogenes, and the molecular bases of multistep carcinogenesis. Cancer Res 1989;49: 3713–3721.

268. Weinberg RA. One renegade cell. How cancer begins. New York: Basic Books, Inc., 1998.

269. Weinberg RA. Racing to the beginning of the road. The search for the origin of cancer. New York: W. H. Freeman and Company, 1998.

270. Weisburger JH, Williams GM. Metabolism of chemical carcinogens. In: Becker FF, ed. Cancer. A comprehensive treatise, vol 1. New York: Plenum Press, 1975, pp. 185–234.

271. Weisse AB. Barry Marshall and the resurrection of Johannes Fibiger. Hosp Pract 1996;31:105–112, 116.

272. Weitberg AB, Weitzman SA, Destrempes M, Latt SA, Stossel TP. Stimulated human phagocytes produce cytogenetic changes in cultured mammalian cells. N Engl J Med 1983; 308:26–30.

273. Weitzman SA, Stossel TP. Mutation caused by human phagocytes. Science 1981;212:546–547.

274. Weitzman SA, Stossel TP. Effects of oxygen radical scavengers and antioxidants on phagocyte-induced mutagenesis. J Immunol 1982;128:2770–2772.

275. Weitzman SA, Weitberg AB, Clark EP, Stossel TP. Phagocytes as carcinogens: malignant transformation produced by human neutrophils. Science 1985;227:1231–1233.

276. Willett W. The search for the causes of breast and colon cancer. Nature 1989;338:389–393.

277. Williams GM, Weisburger JH. Chemical carcinogens. In: Klaassen CD, Amdur MO, Doull J, eds. Casarett and Doull's toxicology. New York: Macmillan, 1986, pp. 99–173.

278. Wittes RE. Vitamin C and cancer. N Engl J Med 1985;312: 178–179.

279. Woglom WH. Experimental tar cancer. Arch Pathol 1926; 2:533–576, 709–752.

280. Womach J. CRS report for Congress. Tobacco programs of the US Department of Agriculture: their operation and cost (89–193 ENR). Washington, DC: The Library of Congress, Congressional Research Service, 1989.

281. Wong RS, Passaro E Jr. Growth factors, oncogenes and the autocrine hypothesis. Surg Gynecol Obstet 1989;168: 468–473.

282. Wood EM, Larson CP. Hepatic carcinoma in rainbow trout. Arch Pathol 1961;71:471–479.

283. Wright WC. Diseases of workers. (A translation of B. Ramazzini's De Morbis Artificum Diatriba, 1700). Chicago: The University of Chicago Press, 1940.

284. Wullems GJ, Schilperoort RA. Plant protoplast transformation by Agrobacterium in relation to plant biotechnology. In: Fowke LC, Constabel F, eds. Plant protoplasts. Boca Raton, FL: CRC Press, 1985, pp. 205–229.

285. Wynder EL, Graham EA. Tobacco smoking as a possible etiologic factor in bronchiogenic carcinoma. A study of six hundred and eighty-four proved cases. JAMA 1950;143: 329–336.

286. Wynder EL, Hoffmann D. Tobacco. In: Schottenfeld D, Fraumeni JF Jr, eds. Cancer epidemiology and prevention. Philadelphia: WB Saunders, 1982, pp. 277–292.

287. Yano E, Urano N, Evans PH. Reactive oxygen metabolite production induced by mineral fibres. In: Brown RC, Hoskins JA, Johnson NF, (eds). Mechanisms in fibre carcinogenesis. New York: Plenum Press, 1991, pp. 433–438.

288. Yavelow J, Finlay TH, Kennedy AR, Troll W. Bowman-Birk soybean protease inhibitor as an anticarcinogen. Cancer Res 1983;(suppl)43:2454s–2459s.

289. Yunis JJ. The chromosomal basis of human neoplasia. Science 1983;221:227–236.

290. Ziegler E. General pathology. New York: William Wood and Company, 1908.

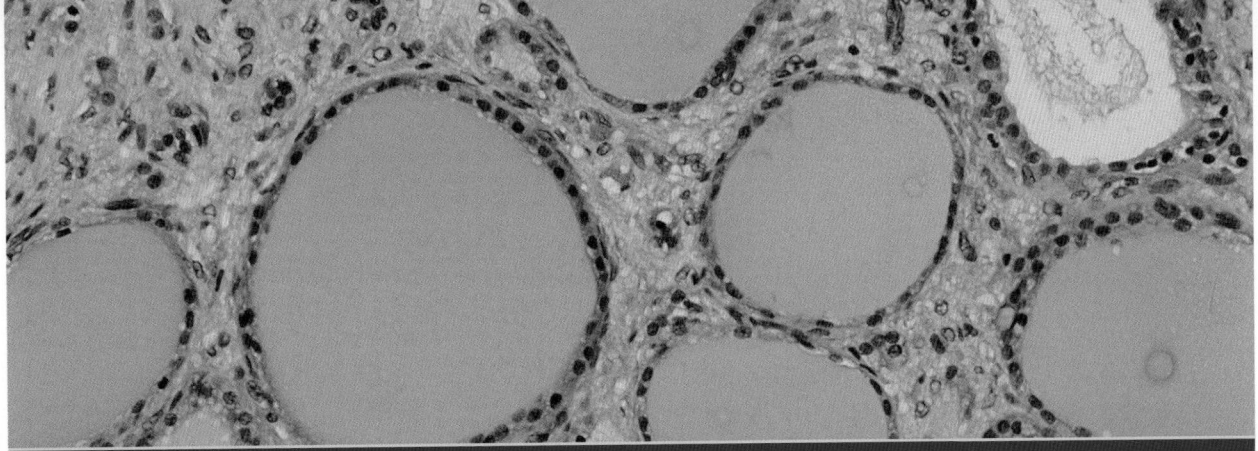

The Human Genome Project taught us recently that we have about 30,000 genes. Of these, it is estimated that about 200 are involved in producing tumors (13). This does not mean, of course, that Nature equipped us with a set of genes programmed to generate cancer: what we mean here is that *these genes can be misled* into producing cancer. But how and why?

From Genes to Tumor

If we examine the normal tasks of these cancer-related genes (102), we find that they fall into three groups: (a) **oncogenes,** which code for proteins that favor cell proliferation; (b) **suppressor genes,** which code for proteins that suppress cell proliferation; and (c) **repair genes,** which code for enzymes in charge of correcting any damage in the DNA. All the cells in the body depend on the careful work of these repair genes, which are especially important for cells that are constantly exposed to genotoxic agents, such as the keratinocytes exposed to ultraviolet light.

The oncogenes and suppressor genes are directly in charge of cell proliferation; they supervise checkpoints at given phases of the cell cyle, and control cell numbers by balancing cell birth and cell death (apoptosis). It has become customary to explain the malfunctions of these two sets of genes with an automobile metaphor. The oncogenes correspond to the accelerator: if it is jammed, the car will speed out of control. The suppressor genes correspond to the brakes: if they cease to function the car will again speed out of control. Both oncogenes and suppressor genes can be visualized as "keepers of the cell cycle," which explains why they are known collectively as **gatekeeper genes** (102). Correspondingly, cancer can be considered as a disease of the cell cycle. It is therefore "in the genes"—which leads us to the following critical question.

Is Cancer Inherited?

This question calls for two answers. *At the level of cells,* cancer is definitely inherited; cancer cells beget cancer cells, with rare exceptions (p. 950). *At the level of people,* every type of cancer *can* be in the genes: what is inherited is not the cancer itself, but the predisposition to develop a given type of tumor (Figure 29.1). However, this familial predisposition is uncommon; it is involved in no more than a fraction of cancers: 0.1 to 10 percent, depending on the site (43, 75). An optimist might add that even in families with dominantly inherited cancer, not all the gene carriers develop it, and

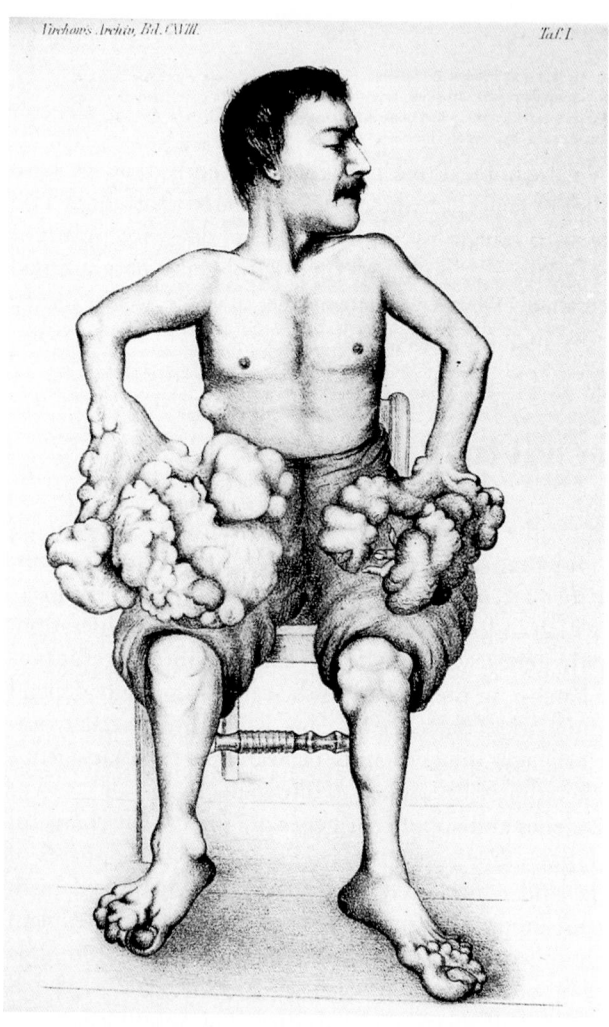

FIGURE 29.1   Extreme case of enchondromatosis (a congenital neoplastic disease) reported in 1889 by Kast and von Recklinghausen. This patient began to notice swellings on his fingers at age 3; at age 34 he requested that his right hand be amputated because its weight had become intolerable. The tumors originate in relation to metaphyseal cartilage, occasionally also along the ribs. To this day there is no cure. (Reproduced from [104].)

50 percent of family members do not carry the defective geen at all (58).

Many cases of cancer, perhaps most, seem to occur randomly in a given population ("sporadic" cancer). However, a closer look does show a tendency to familial clustering (98). It is difficult to extricate the effects of genes from those of chance and environment; but overall, siblings of a patient with a given cancer have a two- to threefold increased risk of developing the same kind of cancer (31, 75). For cancer of the lung, the risk incurred by first-degree relatives is even higher; it is ninefold for female relatives over 40 years of age (68).

For most of the common cancers there are *cancer families* in which cancer of one particular organ occurs with a higher incidence and at a younger age (40). This reminds us of the strains of commercially available mice that are guaranteed to develop a given percentage of tumors of a given organ at a given age. These strains tell us that cancer genes are there; in mice they are revealed by inbreeding.

Cancer family syndromes.   In rare cases, different cancers cluster in a single family and at early age. Typical is the **Li-Fraumeni syndrome,** in which kindred develop a spectrum of tumors including sarcomas, osteosarcomas, breast cancer, brain tumors, leukemia and adrenocortical carcinomas (35). Among the carriers, 50 percent develop a tumor by the age of 35; a second primary tumor may develop in a field of therapeutic irradiation. We shall return to this syndrome shortly.

Multiple primary cancers sometimes develop at different times in different organs of a patient. Some of these cancers are due to chance, but statistics show that many are not, which points again to a genetic influence (15, 60). For example, patients with chronic lymphocytic leukemia (CLL) are at higher risk of developing another cancer (e.g., lung cancer and melanoma [16a]). In reported autopsy series, the number of cancer patients with undetected "second primaries" is on the order of 2–6 percent; the percentage rises with age (16.5 percent in men over 80) (89, 90).

Unfortunately, second cancers can be the result of cancer therapy (6b). X-rays increase the relative risk by 2 or 3; some alkylating agents can raise it to more than 100. The relative risk is strongly dependent on the age at diagnosis and treatment of the first cancer: for breast cancer the risk after irradiation of the chest is very high before 30, low or non-existent after 45. Second cancers due to radiation are mostly acute leukemia, chronic myelocytic leukemia, cancer of the breast, lung, thyroid, and skin (non-melanoma) (62).

The Mormons of Utah are interesting from the point of view of cancer genetics and epidemiology because they represent a relatively well-defined, stable population that has abstained from alcohol, tobacco, tea, and coffee for nearly a century, thereby eliminating some major environmental factors. Cancer rates in general are 15–17 percent lower than in the rest of the United States, and several cancers (prostate, lip, melanoma, and uterus) show a definite familial clustering (16, 94).

It would be comforting to know of some way—other than eliminating every vice—to reduce our cancer prospects. At one point it seemed that allergic individuals had that privilege, but the evidence was largely shot down (41).

The study of twins has long been the gold standard for weighing the role of genetics versus the environment. Scandinavia has produced the best studies. The latest, on nearly 45,000 couples of twins (54), comes down rather clearly in favor of the environment: we have to say *rather,* because for several sites the contribution of heritable factors, although below 50 percent, is significant: prostate, 42 percent; colon and rectum, 35 percent; and breast, 27 percent. For identical twins, the absolute concordance is overall less than 15 percent; in other words, if a twin develops a cancer, the probability of the other twin will develop the same cancer is very small, especially among fraternal twins. Cases of identical cancers in twins are occasionally published (57, 63).

Cancer phenotypes. Because there are so many kinds of tumors, many cancer-prone phenotypes can be expected. A fair complexion can be considered as a phenotype that predisposes to melanoma. Less obvious phenotypes concern the individual's enzymatic makeup: there can be inborn differences in the enzymes that activate or detoxify carcinogens, as well as differences in rates of DNA repair. For example, the "poor acetylator" phenotype predisposes dye-stuff workers to bladder cancer (33).

> Another example: certain individuals respond to polycyclic hydrocarbons in smoke by producing an inducible form of cytochrome P-450 (p. 142) called P-450 IA. This isoenzyme transforms the hydrocarbons into oxygenated intermediates that bind to DNA. Individuals with this trait appear to be prone to adenocarcinoma of the lung (3).

These and many other findings have opened the new field of **ecogenetics,** which studies the interaction of genes with the environment (6, 58, 76) (not to be confused with *epigenetics,* the study of gene-regulating activities that do not involve changes in the DNA code, e.g., gene regulation by chromatin [70]).

In summary, there is strong evidence for a genetic component in many forms of cancer, and even for cancer of the lung, which is typically environmental; but the mode of inheritance is little understood. Purtilo and co-workers have listed over 240 genetic conditions that predispose to cancer (76).

We now turn to those rare forms of cancer that are definitely based on heredity, this will give us an opportunity to see how the "cancer genes" work.

Syndromes due to Defects of Suppressor Genes

Defects of the Rb gene. A great deal has been learned about the suppressor genes since Dr. Knudson came up with the two-hit hypothesis to explain the development of retinoblastoma. The Rb gene has remained the prototype suppressor, as deserved. We also know that the *Rb* gene is one of the "gatekeepers": under normal conditions it is called upon to stop the cell from cycling, to check whether there is need to repair a fault in the DNA. *Rb* does so by encoding for a 105-kDa phosphoprotein (*p105*) that binds to DNA, a logical way to interfere with the cycling process. Thus, *Rb* contributes to maintain genomic integrity (91). Regarding the development of retinal tumors, the rules were laid out in the previous chapter: two hits on the same retinal cell are needed to start the tumor.

This part of the mechanism is quite straightforward. We must now explain another worry of parents from retinoblastoma families. Why is it that a symptomless child should be more prone to develop tumors other than a neuroblastoma, such as sarcomas and osteosarcomas? The mechanism should be obvious: since every cell of that child contains an inactivated *Rb* gene, it is already half-way along the path to cancer. A second hit on a bone cell or fibroblast (e.g., in the course of radiotherapy) can remove the second "brake" an allow tumor growth. Patients with *non-hereditary* (sporadic) retinoblastoma do not have this problem (101). This rule holds for defects of other suppressor genes.

Defects of the p53 gene. While the *Rb* gene was the first suppressor to be recognized, it was somewhat eclipsed by the discovery of the omnipotent p53, which was declared *Molecule of the Year* for 1996 (80), heralded as custodian of the genome, and adopted as the subject of hundreds of papers every month (34, 97, 109).

Visualize the normal *p53* gene (with its homologues *p63* and *p73* [52a]) buried in the nuclear DNA of its cell but connected through the DNA with a complex network to dozens of other genes, an arrangement that has been compared with the Internet (103).

Under normal conditions *p53* is turned off, but if the cell is stressed or damaged, for example, by hypoxia or by ultraviolet rays, it immediately increases its output, the p53 protein: a transcription factor that binds to DNA and activates or represses the connected genes. A key function of *p53* (much as for *Rb*) is to prevent the cell from undergoing mitosis before any DNA damage is repaired. The gene does this by acting as gatekeeper at two points in the cell cycle, as shown in Figure 29.2. If the damaged DNA is repaired, the cell is allowed to proceed through mitosis; if not, the cell is led to kill itself (*p53* gene included) by apoptosis. When activated, the *p53* gene—well connected as it is—takes on another duty consistent with its main task: it inhibits angiogenesis, another way to keep a tumor in check.

All this helps us understand why the *p53* gene is found to have been disabled in more than half of all human cancers: it is so powerful, as custodian of the genome, that as long as it functions it can block the way to further progression. Because it reaches out so far, the *p53* gene—when disabled—cannot be expected to produce a single, well-defined clinical picture as is the case for the *Rb* gene. However, it seems most befitting that the loss of this powerful gene be responsible for most cases of the multifarious **Li-Fraumeni syndrome** described above (p. 886) (53, 90). The intricate molecular steps from cellular stress to *p53* activation, and from activated *p53* to apoptosis, are just beginning to be worked out (52a, 68a, 70a).

Defects of other suppressor genes. Several other tumors fit into the general model of the retinoblastoma two-hit model, although not as clearly. One of these is **nephroblastoma** or **Wilms' tumor** of the kidney (p. 903), which has an incidence of about 1 in 8000 births.

NOTE: The comparison with retinoblastoma is not perfect, because recent studies of multifocal nephroblastomas suggest that an additional, nonhereditary mechanism is involved—which has important implications for genetic counseling (11).

This bizarre tumor (Figure 29.3) is often discovered when a parent notices a lump in the child's groin while

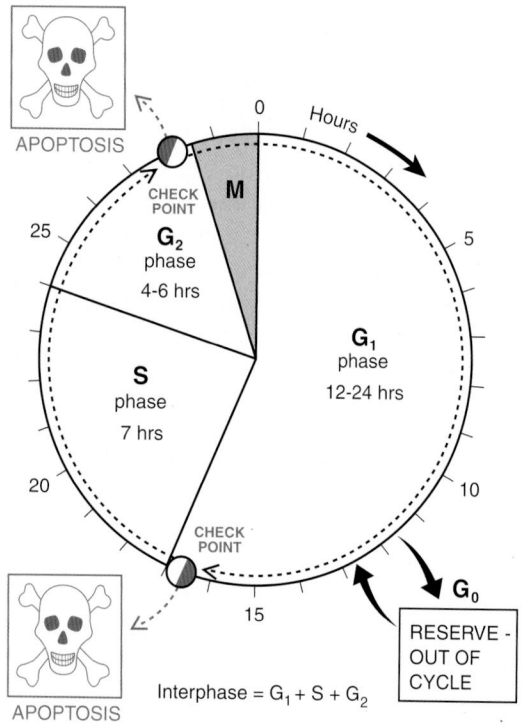

FIGURE 29.2 The cell cycle, shown here as requiring about 30 hours. This duration applies to most normal human cells but may not be applicable to abnormal cells. The G_1-phase corresponds to synthesis of enzymes and of "luxury proteins," the S-phase to replication of chromosomes (DNA and associated proteins), and the G_2-phase to synthesis of proteins for the spindle and mitotic apparatus. *Right bottom:* Cells may escape into G_0 and become quiescent or "out of cycle." *Left, top and bottom:* Two of several checkpoints where *p53* decides whether the cell should be allowed to complete the cycle, or forced to drop out and perform apoptosis. (Adapted with permission from [87].)

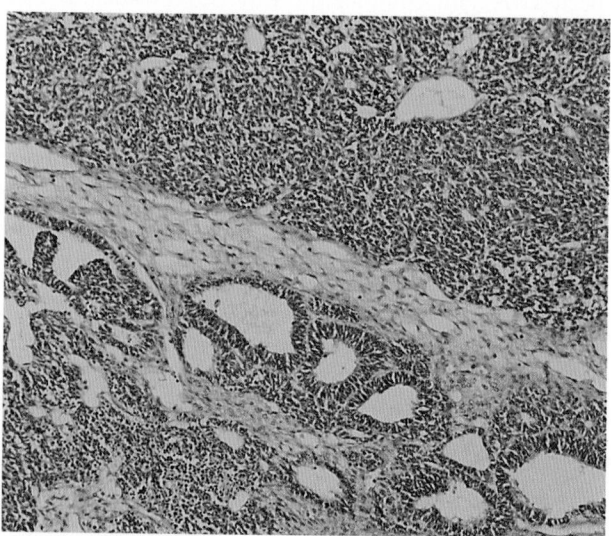

FIGURE 29.3 Nephroblastoma (Wilms' tumor) in a 4-year-old boy. *Top:* Undifferentiated part of the tumor, resembling renal blastema (see Figure 29.28). *Bottom:* Cystic or tubular spaces in a more differentiated part of the tumor. (80x)

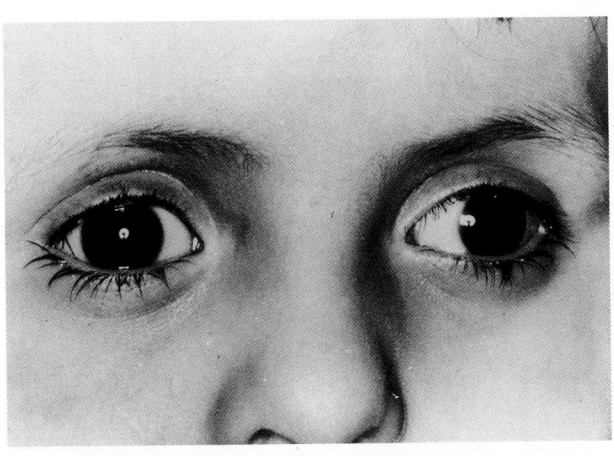

FIGURE 29.4 *Aniridia:* congenital lack of the iris, a malformation that can be associated with Wilms' tumor. This defect was congenitally present in identical twins. Wilms' tumor developed in only one; the other twin apparently escaped the second step, which was presumably due to some environmental factor. (Reproduced from [59] by permission of Pediatrics vol. 8, p. 153, copyright 1986.)

changing diapers. Some of the children affected by this tumor are born without irises (Figure 29.4) (59), a defect that is correlated with a deletion on chromosome 13 (44).

Several genes are involved (29, 35) but a key nephroblastoma gene was located on chromosome 11. This may not be a critical bit of information to remember, but it leads to a beautiful experiment of therapy *in vitro.* A line of cells from Wilms' tumor is grown *in vitro,* and some of the cells are provided by microsurgery with a normal human chromosome 11. A new line of cells derived from these modified cells is incapable of producing tumors when injected into nude mice. Chromosomes X and 13, injected into cells of the original line as controls, have no such effect (107). A similar feat was performed with the *Rb* gene (31). This is true gene therapy *in vitro;* unfortunately it is a long way from therapy *in vivo.*

Altogether, about 40 dominantly inherited syndromes predispose to cancer, and many of these are thought to occur by the Knudson suppressor-gene mechanism; the list includes breast, lung, and colon cancers in adults (44, 86). The most notorious member of this group is **familial polyposis of the colon.**

Carriers of the mutant gene APC (for *adenomatous polyposis coli*) inherit the predisposition to develop myriads of polyps in the colon. (The normal function of the APC gene is complex and not fully understood, but it is involved in the regulation of beta-catenin, an important cytoskeletal protein [26]). The polyps are not present at birth, but they may be growing by

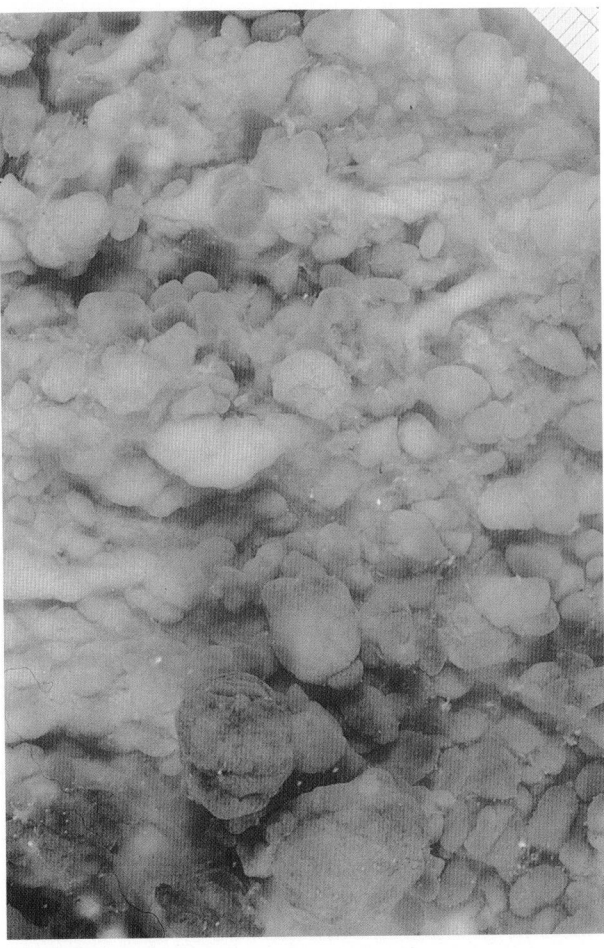

FIGURE 29.5 Familial polyposis coli. Close-up view of the mucosa of the colon surgically removed from a 21-year-old woman. The cobblestone appearance is due to myriads of polyps of various sizes with little or no normal mucosa in between. **Scale** in millimeters.

the hundreds by late adolescence and soon become uncountable, a sight difficult to believe (Figures 29.5, 29.6). At age 40 one or more carcinomas may be present in 80 percent of the patients. The only known therapy is early, preventive, total colectomy.

Syndromes due to Defects of Repair Genes

These genes, recall, are in charge of manufacturing enzymes for the repair of DNA. Although they do not control cell growth directly, they relate to cell growth by default: if they allow errors in the DNA to go uncorrected, they contribute to genomic instability (51). The classic example, **xeroderma pigmentosum,** deserves special mention because it is a miserable disease. Imagine a child with a scaly, dry skin (*xero*derma means dry skin), broken by basal and squamous cell carcinomas that erupt on the face and all areas exposed to sunlight.

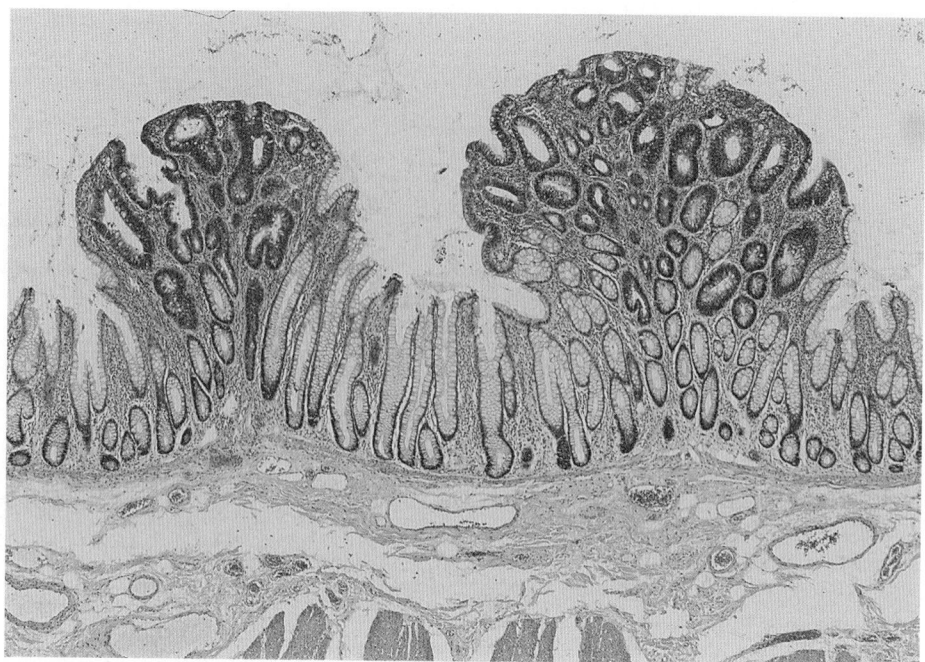

FIGURE 29.6 Two adenomatous polyps arising from the colonic mucosa in a case of polyposis coli. Note the differences between the glands in the mucosa and the glands in the polyps. (30x)

We chose a relatively mild example for Figure 29.7. It is an experiment of Nature: these patients lack an endonuclease that repairs DNA damaged by ultraviolet light (52). Therapy, alas, has little to offer.

Chromosomal Disorders

Sporadic chromosomal disorders are thought to arise by an error during meiosis in the ovum or sperm, whereby the number of chromosomes is unbalanced in all cells of the embryo. *This meiotic instability may be at the root of later mitotic instability,* which increases the risk of neoplasia. Typical examples are Down syndrome (47 chromosomes, the excess being due to three chromosomes 21, *trisomy 21*) and Klinefelter's syndrome (again 47 chromosomes: the males are XXY). Patients with Down syndrome have a 20-fold risk of developing leukemia, and males with Klinefelter's syndrome have a two- to three-fold increased risk of developing breast cancer (58).

Genes and Tumor Progression

The terse statement that "tumors tend to go from bad to worse" was as good a definition of tumor progression as could be given in 1941 (p. 779). Thirty-five years later came the oncogene revolution, and progression had to be revisited in that context.

A quick reminder: by *progression* is meant the third stage of carcinogenesis as conceived in the initiation-promotion-progression model. It is irreversible, and its characteristics include increasing growth rate, invasion and metastasis (73a).

Progression is based on the step by step involvement of a series of genes, and the rule is that *the three main types of genes can all be at fault:* if the first hit falls on a proto-oncogene, further hits may occur in suppressor genes or on DNA repair genes. Exactly how this sequence is selected is not clear; indeed it would be difficult—in 2003—to improve on Nowell's insightful statement of 1976: the mechanism of progression "is not entirely random." Yet, our understanding of progression has improved, in that there are several published examples of progression from normal to precancerous to malignant growth, *correlating the gross and microscopic aspect with genetic changes.* Such studies have been published for the colon (Figure 29.8) (27), for the pancreas (Figure 29.9) (108) and for the breast (Table 29.1). However, it should be understood that none of the genetic changes found during the progression of a given type of tumor is present in *all* the tumors of that type. These studies are important for showing what trends may be expected. They also confirm that the progression from normal to benign to malignant growth requires *six or seven steps,* a paradigm that probably has wide validity.

Another interesting trend: the activation of proto-oncogenes tends to produce leukemias and lymphomas, whereas the loss or inactivation of tumor suppressor genes is linked to carcinomas and other solid tumors (37).

The Genome During Tumor Progression

It is generally accepted that at an early stage of carcinogenesis **the entire tumor genome has become**

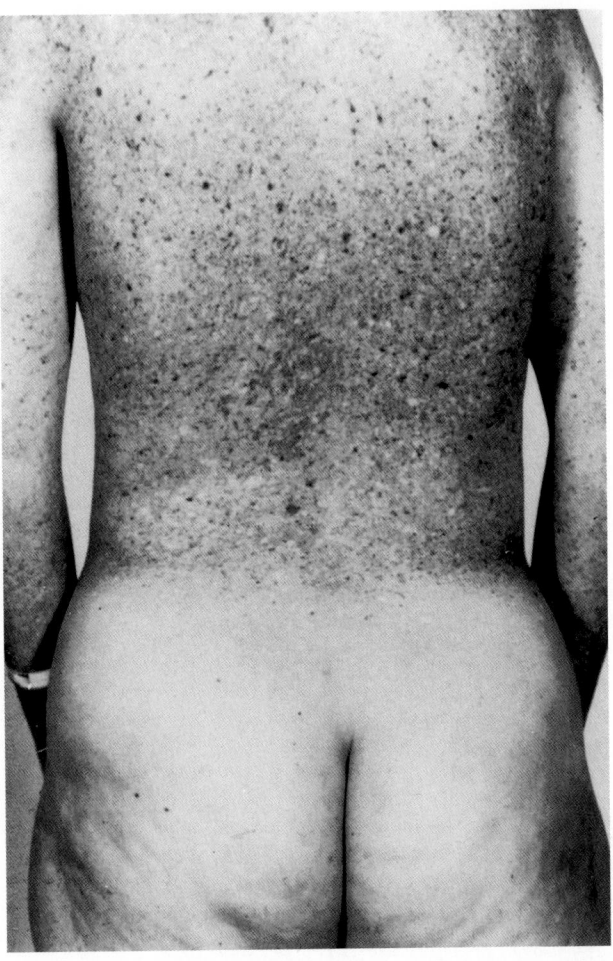

FIGURE 29.7 A patient with xeroderma pigmentosum. The areas of the skin exposed to light show hypo- and hyperpigmented spots, as well as other lesions. (Reproduced by permission from [10], © by The US & Canadian Academy of Pathology, Inc.)

unstable, as postulated by Nowell (p. 781) (65). This biological change is reflected in the microscopically visible **karyotypic instability,** which can be considered as *the main cytological marker of the progression stage;* the number of chromosomes can vary up to near-tetraploid (73a). There are also defects in the mitotic apparatus, in telomere behavior and centrosome structure, and in DNA methylation (see below) and the cells are extremely resistant to apoptosis (73a).

But then, why does the genome become unstable? Two of the 1976 pioneers, Bishop and Weinberg, give the following reasons: the genes for repairing DNA are damaged, and the equipment for deleting mutated cells is also damaged. In essence, misinformed cells are generating more misinformation. The errors can occur by disruption of the DNA at the level of the nucleotides,

of the genes, or of the chromosomes; the resulting damage is especially critical if it hits the mitotic apparatus, including the **centrosomes.** These long-neglected, minuscule organelles have just been brought into the limelight of cancer research (62a).

> They nucleate the microtubules and organize the mitotic spindle: therefore they carry a great deal of responsibility for the function—and malfunction—of mitosis, for genetic instability, and for progression (71, 72, 91a). They are also involved in determining the shape and polarity of cancer cells. Centrosome defects are common in prostate cancer (72).

Abnormal Patterns of DNA Methylation

This is another aspect of DNA pathology that is experiencing belated recognition (6a, 23a, 32a, 36a, 73a), especially in relation to tumor progression. Methylation is a normal process, whereby a methyl group is added to cytosine. Hypermethylation tends to occur on DNA of the promoter region of genes, especially of suppressor genes; the effect is gene silencing. Functionally, therefore, **hypermethylation is the equivalent of a mutation—except that it is reversible.** A concept that promises important developments.

Last, a chromosomal change typical of the progression stage is **gene amplification.** Chemotherapy provides, paradoxically, one of the best examples of iatrogenic tumor progression, whereby gene amplification leads to drug resistance (p. 961). The correlation between drug resistance and progression is self-evident: a dose of drug insufficient to kill off all the cells of a tumor will kill selectively the most sensitive cells, and spare the most resistant, whereby the tumor becomes more malignant. This effect is most obvious when using single drugs, hence the clinical practice of using several drugs at a time.

Some cells amplify their drug resistance genes so enormously that a branch of the affected chromosome becomes visibly abnormal (Figure 29.10) (85).

> Could **cell fusion** play a role in tumor progression? We are referring to fusion of neoplastic with non-neoplastic host cells. This type of intercellular marriage usually results in "taming" of malignancy (p. 929), but under given conditions it may increase it (21a). We understand that this somewhat heretical concept is undergoing a revival (69a).

Hypoxia, Apoptosis and Tumor Progression

Hypoxia is related to tumor progression by two experimentally proven facts: (1) hypoxia induces the

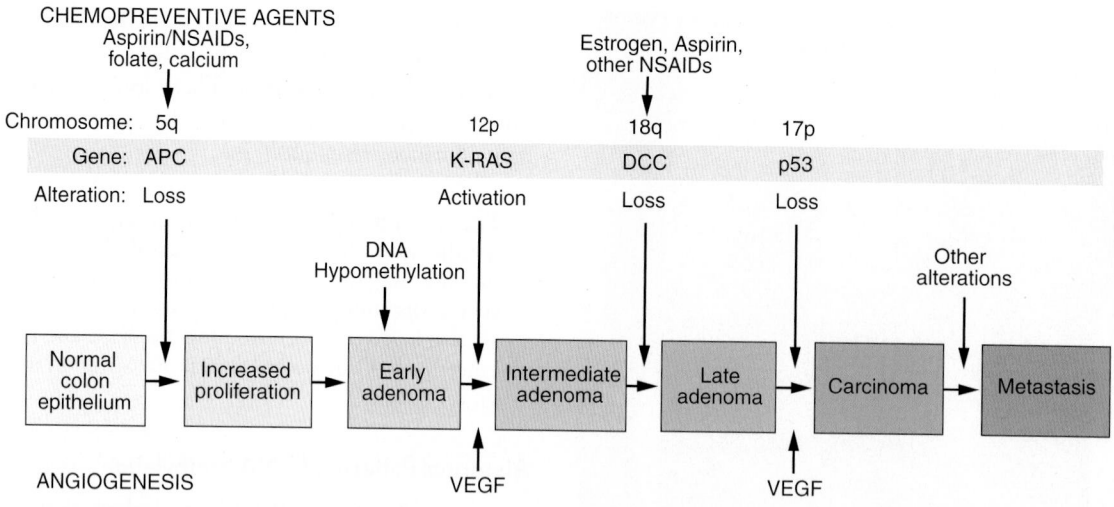

FIGURE 29.8 Progression of sporadic colorectal cancer. (Reprinted and adapted with permission from [27]. Data on angiogenesis by permission of Rak J, Filmus J, Kerbel RS. Reciprocal paracrine interactions between tumour cells and endothelial cells: the "angiogenesis progression" hypothesis. Eur J Cancer 1996;32A:2432–4250, Copyright 1996, with permission from Elsevier Science. Data on chemoprevention from [39].)

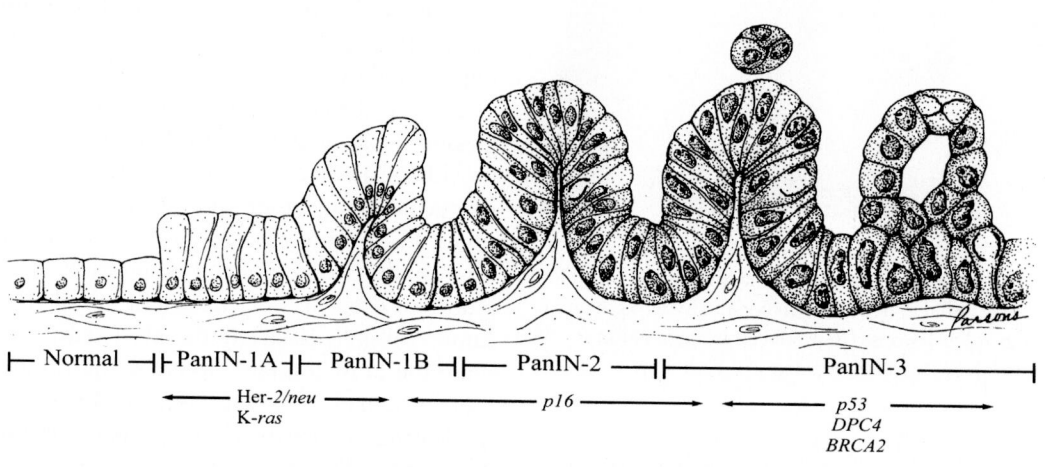

FIGURE 29.9 Progression model for the intraepithelial changes leading to pancreatic adenocarcinoma (PanIN is equivalent to CIN, Cervical Intraepithelial Neoplasia). Steps: flat duct lesion, papillary duct lesion, atypical and severely atypical duct lesion; the latter corresponds to carcinoma *in situ*. The approximate timing of genetic alterations is indicated. (Reproduced by permission from [108]. Artwork by J. L. Parsons.)

expression of *p53*, whereby mutations of this protective, anti-tumor gene are more likely to occur; (2) these pathologic, *p53*-mutant cells, when "short of air," are more reluctant to commit suicide by apoptosis; this gives them a survival advantage in hypoxic tissues (Figure 29.11).

An optimist might rejoice prematurely, by arguing as follows: if p53 acts as a brake against the birth and progression of tumors, it should be possible to plan an anti-tumor therapy based on the *p53* proteins. The

experiment was done—too many times: the first answer was YES (mice with *activated p53* genes had fewer tumors (100a), then came NO (the mice aged prematurely and died earlier (27a) then YES again (transgenic mice with an *extra dosage* of endogenous *p53* aged normally) (31a). We need a better experimental plan. An afterthought regarding apoptosis and tumors: it is tempting to call cancer a "disease of apoptosis," but the facts are too complicated to fit under this heading (pp. 216, 786) (110).

Table 29.1 Onset and Progression of Breast Cancer

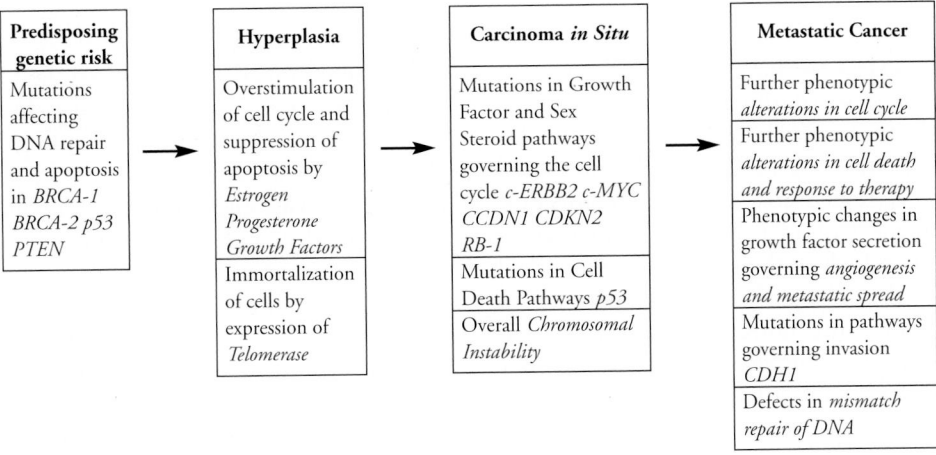

Predisposing genetic risk	Hyperplasia	Carcinoma *in Situ*	Metastatic Cancer
Mutations affecting DNA repair and apoptosis in *BRCA-1 BRCA-2 p53 PTEN*	Overstimulation of cell cycle and suppression of apoptosis by *Estrogen Progesterone Growth Factors*	Mutations in Growth Factor and Sex Steroid pathways governing the cell cycle *c-ERBB2 c-MYC CCDN1 CDKN2 RB-1*	Further phenotypic *alterations in cell cycle*
	Immortalization of cells by expression of *Telomerase*	Mutations in Cell Death Pathways *p53*	Further phenotypic *alterations in cell death and response to therapy*
		Overall *Chromosomal Instability*	Phenotypic changes in growth factor secretion governing *angiogenesis and metastatic spread*
			Mutations in pathways governing invasion *CDH1*
			Defects in *mismatch repair of DNA*

(Reproduced with permission from: Dickson, R. B., Lippman M. E. in "Cancer: Principles and Practice of Oncology." DeVita, V. T., Hellman, S., Rosenberg, S. A. (eds), Lippincott Williams & Wilkins, 2001 [22].)

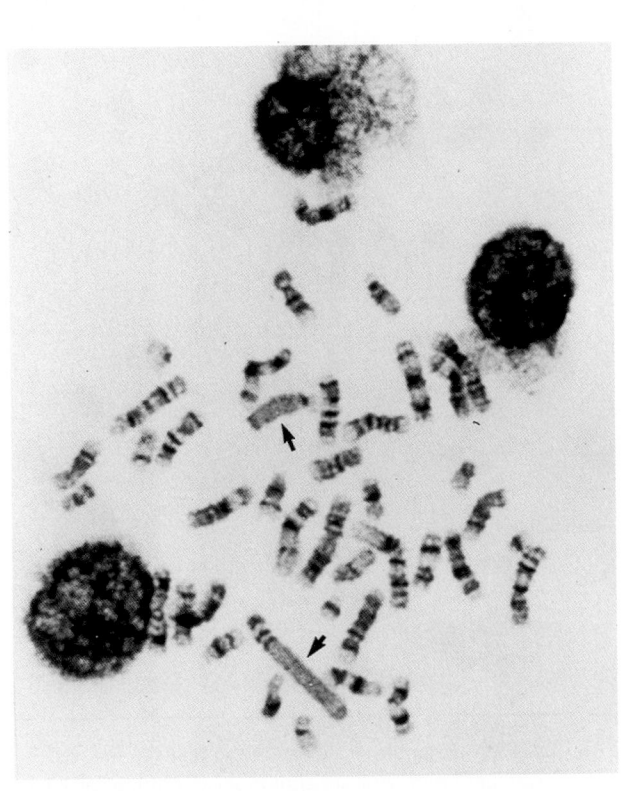

FIGURE 29.10   Typical HSRs (homogeneously stained regions, **arrows**) in a metaphase from a culture of neuroblastoma cells. Trypsin-Giemsa method. (Reprinted with permission from [8]. Copyright 1976 by the American Association for the Advancement of Science.)

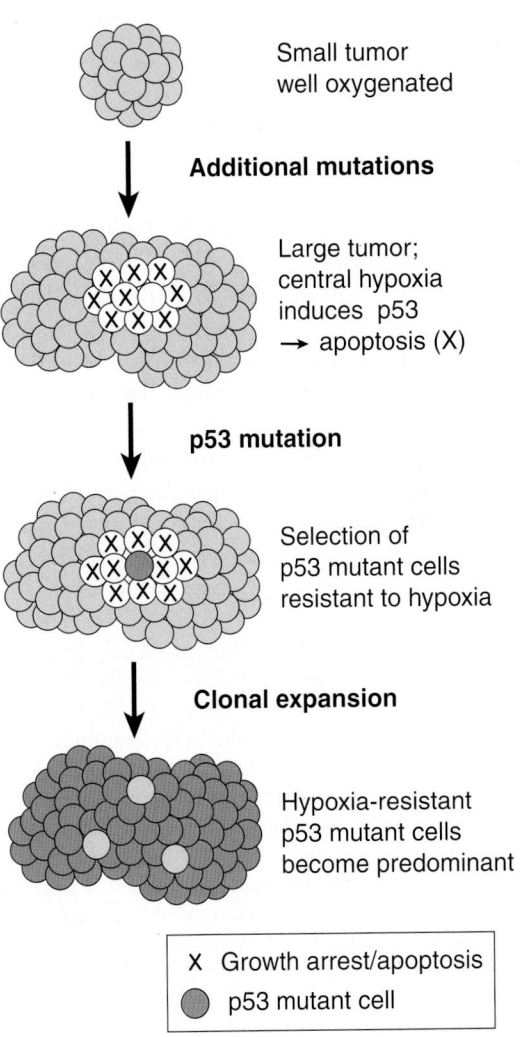

FIGURE 29.11   Role of anoxia in the progression of a tumor. See text. (Reprinted with permission from "Life (and death) in a malignant tumor," Nature 1996;379:19–20. Copyright 1996 MacMillan Magazines Limited [42].)

The Chromosomes of Tumors

In the preceding pages we have repeatedly made the point that the basic defect in tumor cells lies in one or a few genes, and the reader may have wondered: could this defect be actually *visible* by looking at chromosomes? The short answer is "sometimes," and it should not come as a disappointment. Consider that each human chromosome carries hundreds or thousands of genes packed into a little rod 3–5 μm long; the order of magnitude of a genetic defect is of course molecular: in this setting it is almost miraculous that any microscopic change may ever be seen at all. Yet the art of chromosome study, cytogenetics, has contributed a great deal to our understanding of tumors (66, 102). For example, some of the best evidence of tumor progression is the occurrence of increasingly severe karyotypic aberrations. Sometimes, as we will see, a cytogeneticist can actually glance at a map of chromosomes (the karyotype) and conclude: "This individual has developed resistance to a drug."

Karyotyping

Chromosomal abnormalities are present in most tumors (66, 77, 88, 111, 112); they can also be induced by antitumor agents (Figure 29.12) (64). Chromosomes become visible only during mitosis, and so the first limiting factor to their study is the availability of mitotic cells. This is no problem with "liquid tumors," the leukemias: The white blood cells are spun out of the blood and cultured. When they begin to divide, they are treated with a microtubular poison (e.g., colchicine), which stops mitoses in metaphase (p. 159). Then the chromosomes of every dividing cell can be spread, stained, photographed, cut out, and pasted up in an established order to the form the display known as *karyotype* (p. 171).

> It was a lunch-break that produced the first great breakthrough in cytogenetics. Because mitosis is a three-dimensional event, it is impossible on a photograph of a mitosis to distinguish individual chromosomes. Then it was found that squashing the mitotic cells produced better spreads of chromosomes, but the spreads still were not optimal. One day in the summer of 1948 a Japanese researcher prepared smears of cells (ready to be squashed), put them in fresh water, and then ran out to buy some lunch. When he returned half an hour later and squashed the cells, he saw the most beautiful chromosome spreads, without any overlapping chromosomes. Osmotic swelling of the cells in water had done the trick; the method has been used ever since (56).

Special stains, introduced in 1970, help to identify as many as 1200 bands on the 46 chromosomes which constitute the human karyotype.

An important advance has been the **FISH** technique (*fluorescence in-situ hybridization*), which extends the capacity of routine cytogenetic banding. In essence, the DNA is resolved into single strands, then hybridized with a probe carrying a reporter molecule, commonly a fluorescent dye. The preparation is then examined by fluorescence microscopy (77).

Methods continue to improve, but on the whole the procedure—as it applies to leukemias—is simple enough to be used in medical practice as a guide for therapy. The procedure for lymphomas is similar; the cells of these tumors, obtained by biopsy, are easily dissociated and suspended in fluid.

However, with other solid tumors the karyotypes are more difficult to prepare, which is why they are not known to the same depth as the karyotypes of leukemias

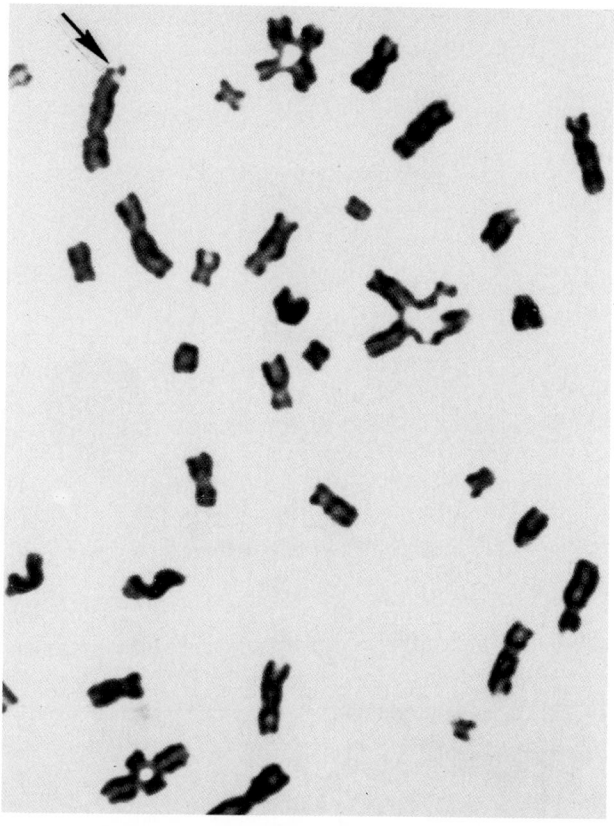

FIGURE 29.12   Example of chromosome damage induced by a drug (the antibiotic and antitumor agent mitomycin C) in a human leukocyte stimulated to divide with phytohemagglutinin. Note several abnormalities: a chromatid break (**arrow**), two typical "crosses" resulting from chromatid exchange, and a complex rearrangement. (Reproduced with permission from [64].)

and lymphomas. Tumor cells must be supplied by invasive procedures such as surgical biopsy or aspiration through a fine needle. Because not all tumor cells grow easily and because they are always admixed with normal host cells, an answer may require as long as 3 weeks.

It should be understood that karyotyping must underestimate the actual number of abnormal chromosomes. By the current methods of banding, as many as 1000 genes can be either lost or duplicated without producing a visible defect (84). And then, when an abnormality is found, the next problem is to distinguish significant nonrandom changes from random changes that occur secondarily as a result of genetic instability and progression of the tumor.

It should also be understood that almost all the chromosomal changes found in tumor cells can also be seen in abnormal but nonneoplastic cells or in cells treated *in vitro*. However, the two abnormalities known as **double minutes** and **homogeneously stained regions** (HSRs) are largely limited to tumors (5).

Types of Chromosome Changes

Visible changes of chromosomes are many (83); even circular chromosomes can occur. The changes of interest in tumors can be grouped into *balanced translocations* between one chromosome and another, *deletions* or *additions* of genetic material within chromosomes, and loss of or addition of *whole chromosomes*. The same abnormality may be found in different tumors. In general, the mechanism of these aberrations is not understood, but several chromosomes seem to be more prone to break at certain fragile sites. A few examples follow.

Balanced translocations. The prototype of balanced translocations is the tiny **Philadelphia chromosome** (Ph), an altered chromosome 22 (Figure 29.13). The Philadelphia chromosome became famous in 1960 when Nowell and Hungerford of Philadelphia recognized it as the first chromosomal abnormality consistently associated with a human malignancy: chronic myelogenous leukemia (CML). It is now clear that Ph is not quite as small as it looks; it also stains poorly. It is usually due to an exchange with chromosome 9 (Figure 29.14), with the result that part of a gene on 22 fuses with the *abl* oncogene on 9 (83). The *abl* gene has become abnormally large, and the protein that it encodes is also abnormally large. This magnified protein turns out to be a tyrosine phosphorylase that is more powerful than normal (82).

The Philadelphia chromosome is not present in the somatic cells of the patient; but it is found in all the

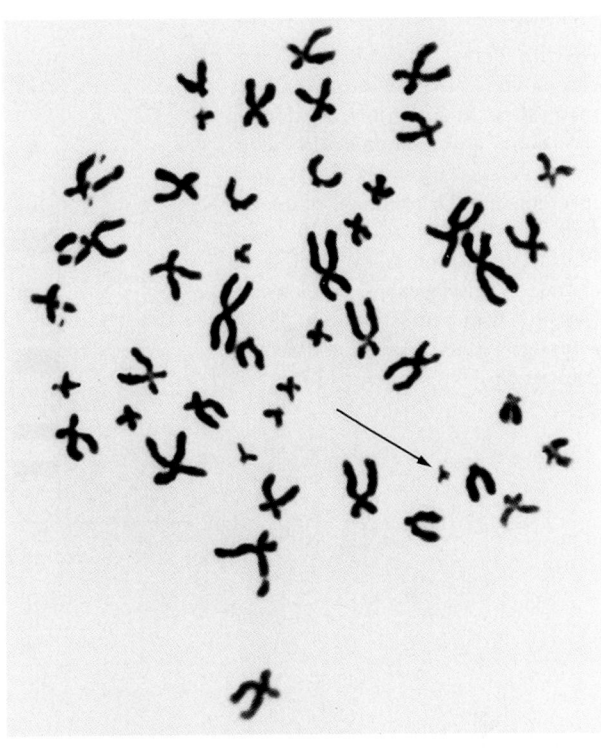

FIGURE 29.13 Metaphase showing a Philadelphia chromosome (**arrow**), which is to this day the most characteristic and consistent karyotypic change in human cancer. (Reproduced with permission from [87].)

myeloid cells (which include the erythrocyte, granulocyte, and megakaryocyte series), indicating that a clone deriving from a pluripotent stem cell has overcome the entire bone marrow. Interestingly, the Philadelphia chromosome is absent in 10 percent of the patients with CML, and their prognosis is worse.

Another translocation is typical of Burkitt's tumor, a B-cell lymphoma (p. 872). In these tumor cells, chromosome 8 loses a fragment containing the proto-oncogene *c-myc;* and this fragment relocates to chromosomes 2, 14, or 22 (see Figure 28.56). It so happens that these three chromosomes contain genes that code for immunoglobulin light or heavy chains, and it seems that *c-myc* becomes inappropriately expressed by being misplaced near these genes (14).

Deletions. The loss of genetic material is associated with some cancers; in fact, visible deletions helped develop the concept of cancer suppressor genes. Suppose that one allele undergoes a recessive mutation whereby it becomes carcinogenic; This mutation then remains latent until the other allele is lost. Deletions of this type occur, for example, in retinoblastoma

FIGURE 29.14 The normal human chromosome 9 (**A**) and three mishaps it may suffer: **B:** interstitial deletion in the short arm, common in acute lymphoblastic leukemia; **C:** paracentric inversion, and **D:** reciprocal translocation, which gives rise to the tiny Philadelphia chromosome typical of chronic myelogenous leukemia. (Adapted with permission from [83a]. Copyright 1993, American Medical Association. All rights reserved.)

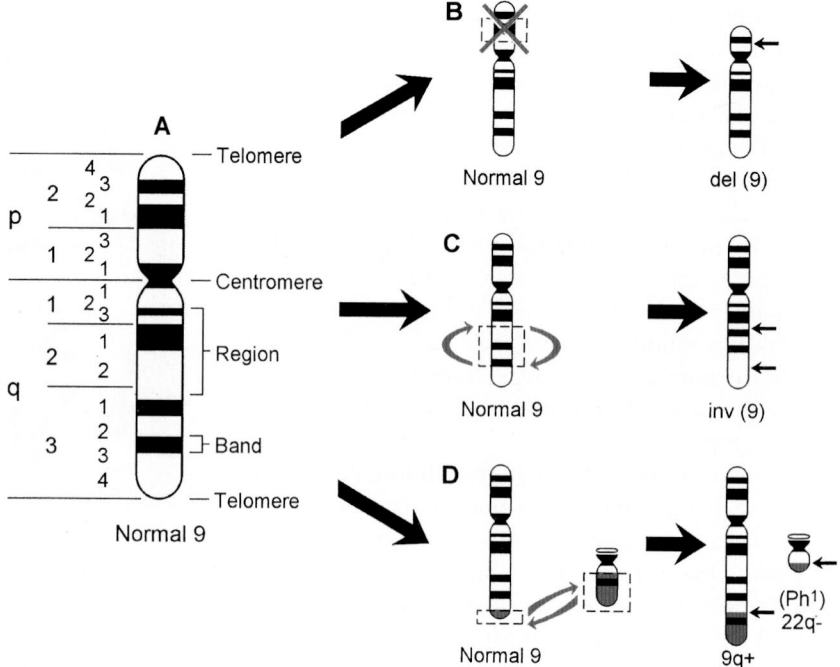

(chromosome 13, band q14) and Wilms' tumor (chromosome 11, band p13). Other deletions are known in solid tumors.

Additions. Added genetic material is visible microscopically in two forms: **homogeneously staining regions** (**HSRs**) (Figures 29.10, 29.15), which are added stretches of poorly stainable chromatin along the chromosome (8), and **double minutes** (**DMs**) (pronounced, of course, "double mynutes") (Figure 29.16), which are tiny paired fragments of chromatin that could be misunderstood as debris between the chromosomes. The homogeneously stained regions and the double minutes are thought to represent two aspects of the same phenomenon (5, 7).

Double minutes were first discovered by studying a series of cell lines that had undergone a stepwise selection for resistance to an anticancer drug, methotrexate (85). In some cases double minutes have been shown to represent multiple copies of oncogenes that code for enzymes involved in the metabolism of the drug; this means that the presence of double minutes (or of a single HSR) on a patient's karyotype enables one to venture the guess that the patient has become resistant to some drug.

The story of double minutes and HSRs is intellectually satisfying, but it has its share of mystery: why are both changes present in the cells of neuroblastoma (7)?

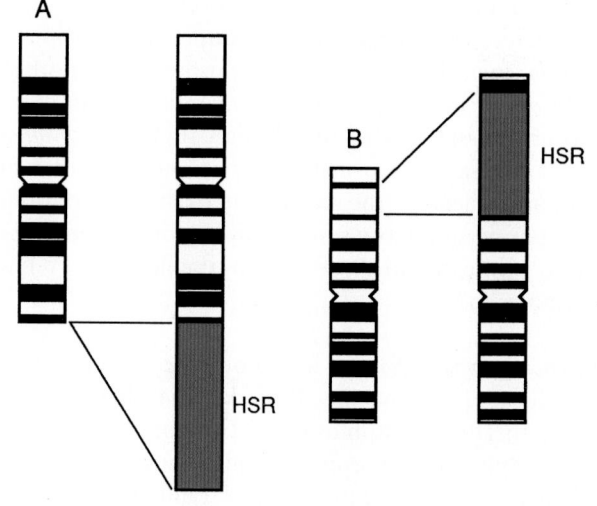

FIGURE 29.15 **A:** Normal chromosome 2 of a chinese hamster cell line. Next to it is a similar chromosome with a homogeneously stained region (HSR) from a drug-resistant cell line (resistant to antifolate). This cell line is characterized by excessive production of the enzyme dihydrofolate reductase; the gene amplification underlying the overproduction of this enzyme gives rise to the HSR. **B:** Normal human chromosome 1, and next to it a similar chromosome from a human neuroblastoma cell line, carrying an HSR. The significance of this gene expansion in neuroblastoma is not yet understood. (Adapted with permission from [8]. Copyright 1976 by the American Association for the Advancement of Science.)

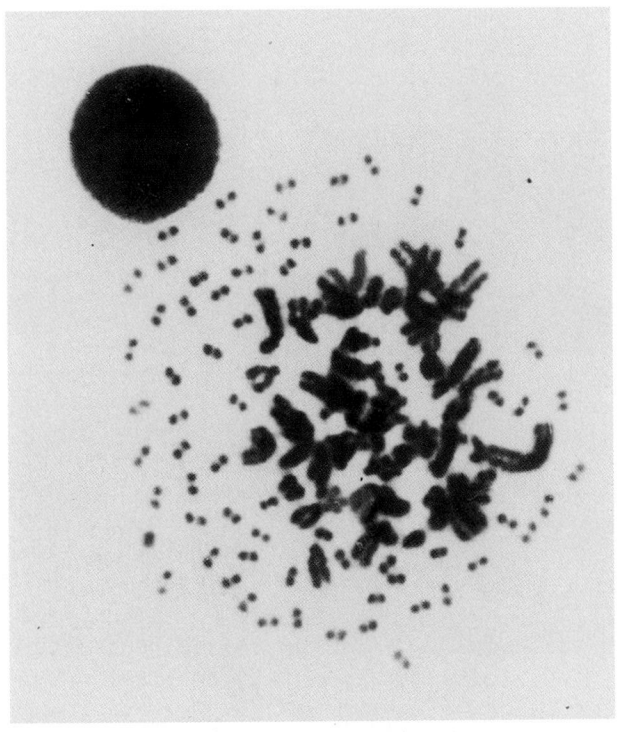

FIGURE 29.16   Double minutes in a metaphase of a cultured neuroblastoma cell. Double minutes represent the same phenomenon of gene amplification as the homogeneously stained regions (HSRs). (Reproduced with permission from [87].)

Gene amplification is also found in association with tumor progression. This has been demonstrated for N-*myc* gene and neuroblastoma, *ras* and prostatic cancer, and *neu* for breast cancer (14). Gene amplification is very rare in normal biology, but for unknown reasons it becomes an important mechanism in the accelerated evolution of tumors toward ever greater malignancy (85).

Loss or addition of whole chromosomes. Almost all meningiomas have only a single chromosome 22. Much more frequent is the addition of chromosomes, either a complete duplication of the genome (*polyploidy*) or an irregular increase of genetic material (*aneuploidy*). This topic is significant because of its prognostic value.

Polyploidy occurs in many normal tissues, where it may have survival value (p. 41). In tumors, aneuploidy and polyploidy become, by and large, a visible aspect of progression (20). For example, in a study of mammary carcinomas, most primary tumors were diploid, whereas most cells from metastatic effusions were aneuploid (95). It is still not clear why aneuploidy should correlate with a worse prognosis, but this is the case for many tumors, such as cancer of the breast or prostate (30). There are the usual exceptions: in large-cell lymphomas, aneuploidy and prognosis are not related.

Why does a defective karyotype progress toward increasing disorder? Nowell proposed that tumor cells are genetically more unstable than normal cells. This concept has much to support it. It is generally assumed that few cancer patients have preexisting genetic instabilities. Perhaps a destabilizing mutation occurs early in tumor development and precipitates a cascade of increasing chromosomal instability (66). Mutations of the all-important *p53* gene are now thought to play a role in tumor progression (p. 945).

Chromosomal fragility syndromes do exist, especially in children, but they are rare. They are due to inborn abnormalities of DNA repair or related defects (e.g., Bloom's syndrome, Fanconi's anemia, ataxia telangiectasia, xeroderma pigmentosum). These syndromes are associated with increased risk of cancer development.

We have only scratched the surface of this field; its importance is reflected in the fact that every large hospital must have a cytogenetics laboratory.

We will now turn to the structural changes that may precede cancer.

Precancerous Lesions

Many cancers, perhaps most, do not develop from normal tissues but from precursor lesions. Overwhelming proof that premalignant lesions exist comes from experimental studies and from firm medical facts about human cancer. Experience shows that such lesions may or may not progress to cancer; the frequency of malignant transformation varies a great deal.

Besides their scientific interest, precancerous lesions are important clinically. If we knew how to identify them all, we would have made one great step toward the control of cancer. Unfortunately they are often difficult to recognize. By definition we would expect them to be pretumoral, that is, small and barely visible. For this reason, we know more about precancerous lesions of the skin and of accessible mucosae, such as the mouth and the female cervix. Virtually nothing is known about premalignant changes of sarcomas and of brain tumors, which develop out of sight (36).

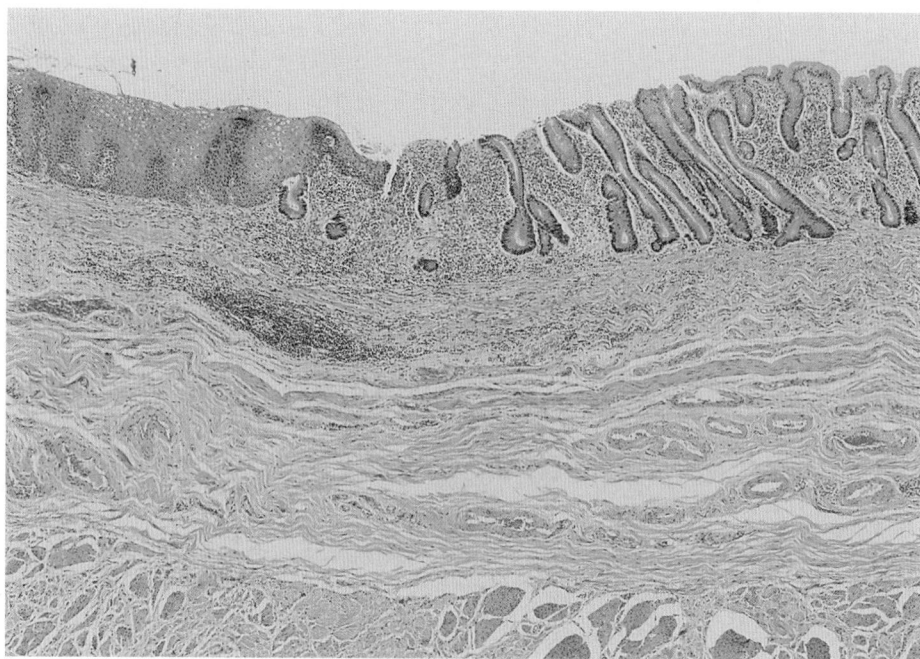

Known precancerous lesions include some forms of metaplasia, dysplasia and carcinoma *in situ,* some benign tumors and sundry lesions.

Metaplasia as a Precancerous Lesion

For reasons unknown, virtually all epithelial metaplasias can be precancerous whereas connective tissue metaplasias are generally "safe." Metaplasia implies the expression of a different set of genes, but the study of DNA in metaplastic cells is just beginning (69). A notorious example of metaplasia with high precancerous potential is represented by the islands of gastric and intestinal epithelium that develop at the distal end of the esophagus, "Barrett's epithelium" (Figure 29.17). Chromosomal changes do develop in this area, but apparently in a random fashion (105); metaplasia itself is not a clonal event. Another example is leukoplakia of the tongue (see Figures 2.58, 2.59); optical measurement of nuclear DNA in the metaplastic epithelium showed that tertaploidy and especially aneuploidy correlated with poor prognosis (100). Metaplasia of the exocervix (Figure 29.18) is not as threatening as oral leukoplakia—but we cannot say why.

Dysplasia and Carcinoma *In Situ*

Dysplasia is an imprecise but practical term: pathologists use it when they have to give a name to cellular changes that are too irregular to be called hyperplasia and not irregular enough to be called neoplasia (Figure 29.19). This is a compromise and an admission

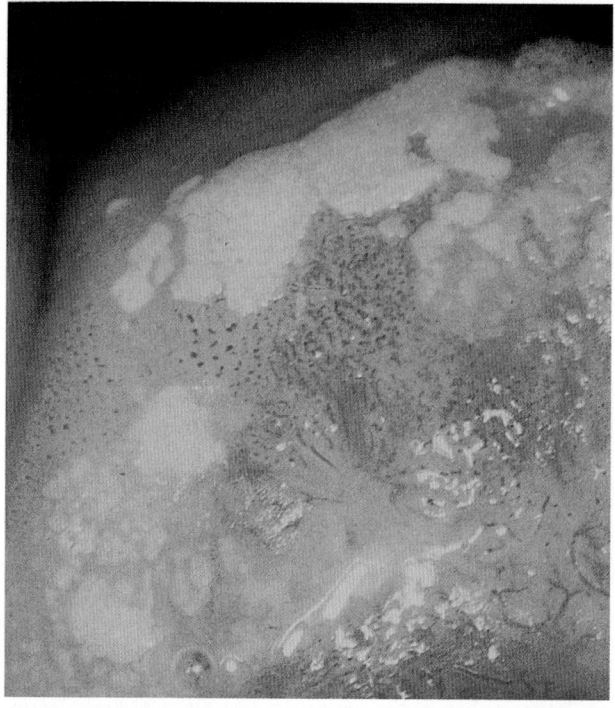

FIGURE 29.18 Human exocervix as photographed through a colposcope. The white patches represent leukoplakia (the whiteness is enhanced by painting with dilute acetic acid, an old empirical procedure); the punctate pattern corresponds to dilated and twisted capillaries, typical of carcinoma *in situ.* (Reprinted from [19], Copyright, 1981, with permission from Elsevier.)

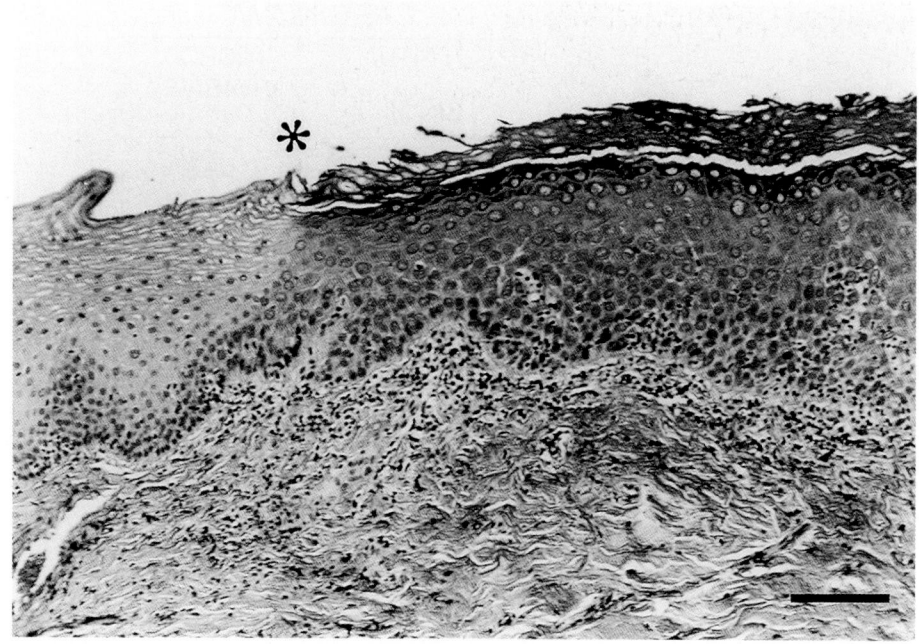

FIGURE 29.19 An example of subtle dysplasia in the mouth. Normal squamous stratified, nonkeratinized epithelium is shown at left. To the right of the **asterisk** is a fairly abrupt shift to dysplasia. The nuclei are enlarged, and the pattern of differentiation has changed; immature cells reach higher up in the epithelium and then abruptly keratinize. This dysplasia may progress to a malignancy. **Bar** = 50 μm. (Reproduced by permission from [50], © by The US & Canadian Academy of Pathology, Inc.)

of ignorance, but there is an excuse; according to the current theories of carcinogenesis, some in-between changes of this kind *should* exist. Dysplasia in surface epithelia blends into a change that is definitely neoplastic: carcinoma *in situ* (Figure 29.20).

Carcinoma in situ is Latin for "carcinoma in (its) place," whereby we mean that a covering epithelium has become replaced by a layer of cancer cells, but all boundaries are respected. The thickness of this layer is about the same as that of the epithelium, there is no outgrowth, and the basement membrane is not trespassed (Figure 29.21). If the boundaries break down, the diagnosis changes to invasive carcinoma. In the uterine cervix, the neoplastic epithelium maintains its constant cycle of division, upward migration, and finally shedding; this is what made the Pap smear possible. If there is a carcinoma *in situ* of the cervix, the Pap smear shows that epithelial cells that sloughed off from the surface failed to mature into the normal, flat, eosinophilic cell with a shriveled, pycnotic nucleus; they retained the structure and basophilia of basal cells. The difference is very obvious (Figure 29.22).

Carcinoma *in situ* occurs not only on the skin and cervix, but on any epithelial surface, including internal organs such as the urinary bladder, the gall bladder, and even the seminiferous tubules of the testis (32). One form of carcinoma *in situ* of the epidermis is known as Bowen's disease (Figure 29.23). To the naked eye, carcinoma *in situ* is a subtle change. On the skin, Bowen's disease appears as a reddened, scaly, or crusty

area; in the cervix, if it is examined with a magnifying colposcope, a patch of carcinoma *in situ* appears dotted with capillary loops that are more widely spaced than in normal tissue and of larger caliber (Figure 29.24) (19). The enlarged capillaries may represent an early form of microvascular response to angiogenesis factors.

An old trick for visualizing a patch of carcinoma *in situ* on the exocervix is to swab the area with iodine; this is a clever bit of histochemistry *in vivo*. The normal squamous cells of the cervix contain glycogen, which is stained mahogany-brown by the iodine; but the epithelial cells of a carcinoma *in situ* have lost the ability of produce glycogen, so the carcinoma remains unstained.

Carcinoma *in situ* may or may not progress to invasiveness. When it does, the time required can be estimated: in the cervix the incidence of carcinoma *in situ* peaks around the age of 30, whereas invasive carcinoma of the cervix peaks around 45; so the progression, when it does occur, takes about 15 years (Figure 29.25). This progression in the bladder, stomach, and lung is usually faster. In the bladder, for example, the rate of recurrence and progression to invasiveness is 80 percent during a period of 5 years (46).

Dysplasia and carcinoma in situ: diagnostic dilemmas. Nobody doubts that carcinoma *in situ* is a true carcinoma capable of aggressive evolution, but the significance of "dysplasia" has generated a lot of heat in the world of gynecology. As the situation now stands, follow-up studies on biopsies of the cervix show that *both dysplasia and carcinoma* in situ

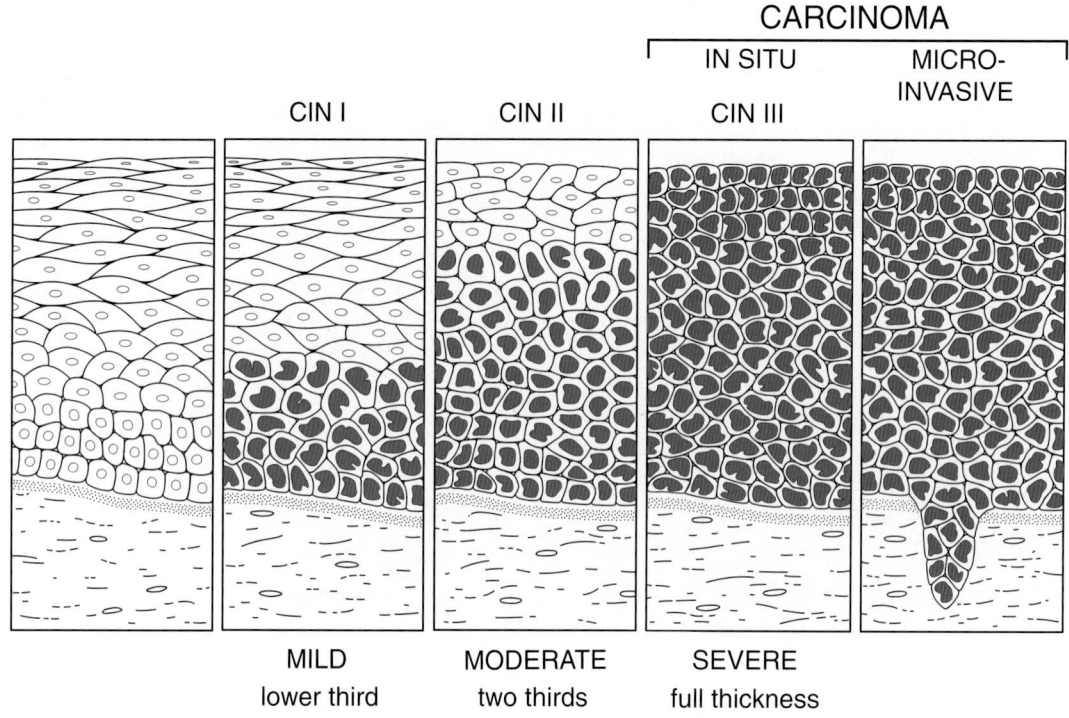

FIGURE 29.20   Epithelium of the cervix: progression from normal through dysplasia to microinvasive neoplasia (the recommended nomenclature refers to **CIN, cervical intraepithelial neoplasia**). *Two parallel changes are taking place:* (a) the modified basal cells occupy an increasing portion of the epithelium, and (b) they progressively fail to differentiate into squamous cells.

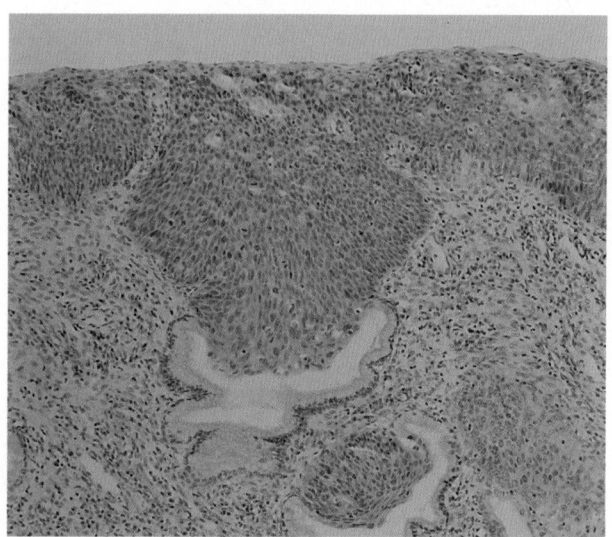

FIGURE 29.21   *Center:* Carcinoma *in situ* of the cervix, creeping into a gland. This is not yet considered to be "invasion." (90x)

can unpredictably persist, regress, or progress to invasive cancer; but in any given case it is impossible to tell what the course will be. The situation varies somewhat from organ to organ (46, 48, 49). For the human cervix, the "CIN" terminology is explained in Figure 29.20.

This debate is especially critical for the pathology of an organ in which both lesions are common, the uterine cervix (actually the part most at risk is the junction between the endocervix and the exocervix, the segment exposed to the vagina). The epithelium of the exocervix can show a series of alterations that can be lined up—on paper—as a progression in the classic sense of going from bad to worse: normal cytology → hyperplasia → dysplasia (mild) → dysplasia (severe) → carcinoma *in situ* → invasive carcinoma. It is obvious that some premalignant changes must regress because they are much more common than invasive carcinomas. The debate arises because the degree of clinical risk does not correlate with this morphologic progression (47, 48). Attempts to differentiate cervical lesions by quantitating the nuclear DNA or by "typing" any concurrent papilloma viruses have not helped. For many years it was hoped that the risk of developing an invasive carcinoma would increase as the morphologic progression seems to suggest: but some gynecologists who tailored their therapy on this concept found themselves in hot water (48, 49). *Carcinoma* in situ *may regress, and mild dysplasia may progress.*

In 1989 the problem was tackled by a committee of experts at the National Cancer Institute (61). The result was a compromise labeled the Bethesda System. Only two categories of epithelial changes are recognized: **squamous intraepithelial lesion (SIL)**; low-grade SIL (for all changes up to the old "mild dysplasia") and high-grade SIL for all the more severe changes up to carcinoma *in situ*.

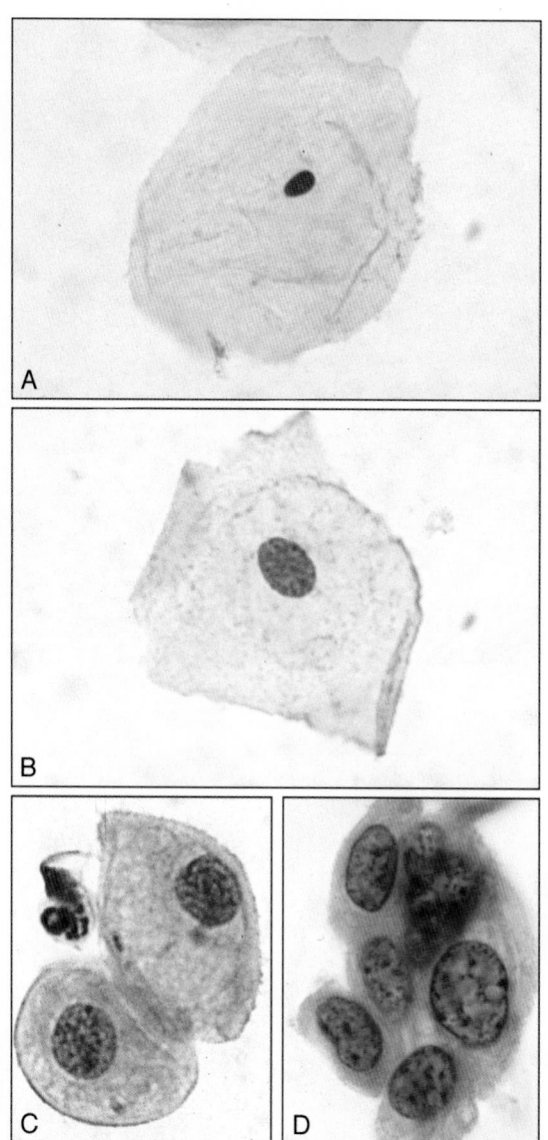

FIGURE 29.22 **A–C:** Normal cervical cells (**A** = superficial, **B** = intermediate, **C** = parabasal). As the parabasal cells mature, the chromatin becomes hyperchromatic (inactive). **D** = clump of cells from a squamous cell carcinoma *in situ*. Note increased nuclear-cytoplasmic ratio, variations in nuclear size (reflecting aneuploidy) and shape. (Pap smears, Papanicolaou stain; all cells at the same enlargement.) (Courtesy of Dr. A. Fischer, University of Massachusetts Medical School, Worcester, MA.)

NOTE: The SIL terminology is used for cytologic smears only. For histologic sections pathologists use the CIN terminology (pp. 870, 900).

This may solve the practical problem, but we are still in the dark about the biological significance of the various epithelial changes. Are they all, or part, viral? What happens to the DNA in SIL or in dysplastic nuclei?

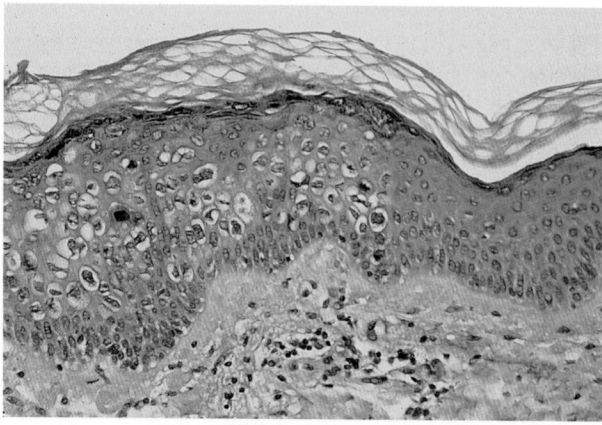

FIGURE 29.23 Bowen's disease on the skin of the calf. The epidermis at the extreme right is normal; to the left it is thickened. Note several atypical epithelial cells and the lack of differentiation from the bottom to the top layers. This pattern represents a carcinoma *in situ*. A red, scaly patch had been present for 45 months. (150x)

There is a huge literature on these precursor lesions, but the relationship between oncogene expression and preneoplasia is not understood (92).

Intramucosal or *superficial carcinomas* of the stomach are not the same as carcinoma *in situ*. This is the name given to carcinomas that have involved only the mucosal layer. The prognosis of these early carcinomas is much more favorable, even though gastric carcinomas are usually among the most lethal; but unfortunately they give no sign of their existence unless they are accompanied by an ulcer.

A sarcoma *in situ* parallel to carcinoma *in situ* cannot exist because it would lack the boundary of a basement membrane to serve as a definition of invasiveness. However, the concept has been proposed, especially to define early malignant changes in chondromas (78).

Benign Tumors as Precursors of Cancer

This title will be confusing for anyone who thinks that some tumors are benign, others malignant. Keep in mind the following points:

- Experimentally, it is proven beyond question that a benign growth, given enough time, can progress to carcinoma; this applies to both chemical and viral carcinogenesis.
- A similar progression is well established for a number of human tumors including gastrointestinal polyps, papillomas of the larynx, large congenital nevi, and pigmented moles.
- Some human tumors appear to remain stable in a benign condition (e.g., leiomyomas of the uterus), but

FIGURE 29.24   Carcinoma *in situ* of the exocervix. *Top:* A close-up view of the exocervix through an enlarging colposcope: the irregular coarse dots represent dilated capillary loops reaching toward the surface. **Bar** = 1 mm. *Center:* Vascular preparation of the mucosa after the capillaries have been demonstrated by the reaction for alkaline phosphatase (black). The wide capillary loops reaching close to the surface and running partly along it correspond exactly to the top print. *Bottom:* Typical histologic image of carcinoma *in situ*. (Reproduced with permission from [45].)

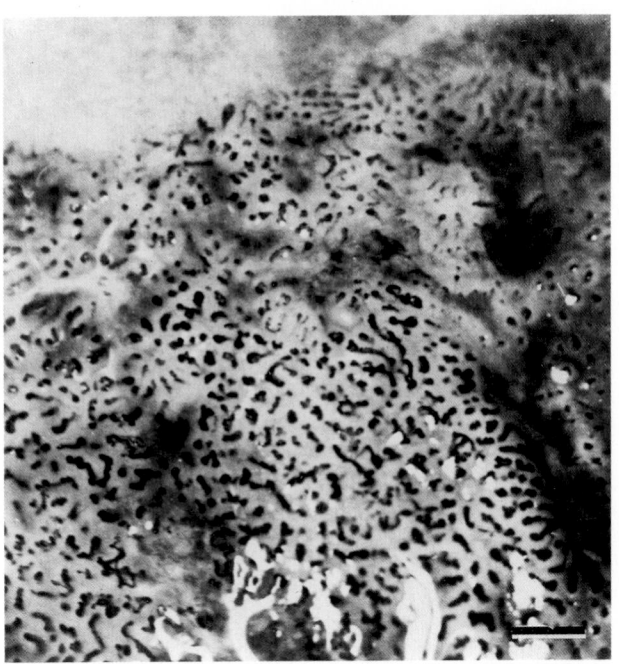

occasional leiomyomas do progress to leiomyosarcomas, indicating that they too can progress.

- Progression from benign to malignant in renal cell tumors is tacitly assumed by pathologists. Today, for lack of better criteria, kidney tumors less than 3 cm in diameter are arbitrarily called adenomas; above 3 they are called carcinomas (Figure 29.26) (99).
- In the field of hematology, the so-called **benign monoclonal gammopathy** remains benign in about 90 percent of patients; in the remaining 10 percent it progresses to multiple myeloma or other malignancies (38, 50a).

Even the typically benign fibroadenoma of the breast is known occasionally to lapse into carcinoma. Indeed, it may be impossible to find a human benign tumor that never progresses to malignancy. Benign tumors, once again, are so defined by a clinical necessity, not by a biological scheme.

Sundry Precancerous Lesions

Cellular abnormalities that precede cancer. Histologically, in the many models of experimental carcinogenesis, a variety of preneoplastic focal changes have been found and labeled hyperplasia, atypical metaplasia, dysplasia and the like; but none of these changes comes near to being specific (93). For example, during carcinogenesis in rat liver (see Figure 28.17) before malignant tumors develop, many microscopic foci of abnormal liver cells can be seen with ordinary stains (Figure 29.27) and even better with histochemical stains for enzymes (Figure 29.28) (24, 25, 73). Up to a point these hepatocyte nodules (92) are reversible, and there is good evidence that they can progress to malignancy. Similar nodules can be found in humans (2). The epidermal changes that precede cancer during the phase of promotion with TPA have been described on p. 780.

Embryonal rests. This ancient theory is undergoing a partial revival. In its original form it maintained that tumors arise from microscopic embryonic rests that

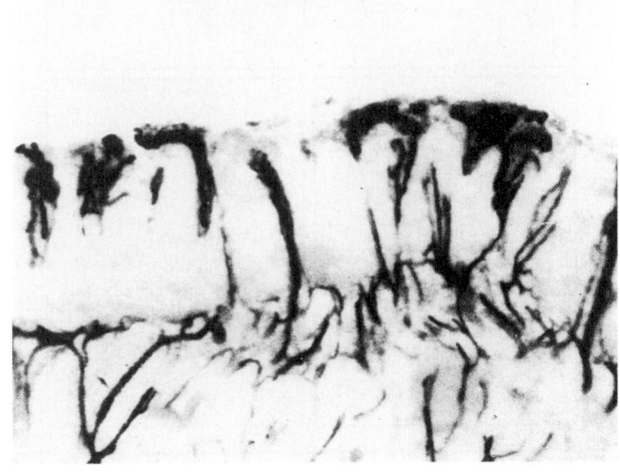

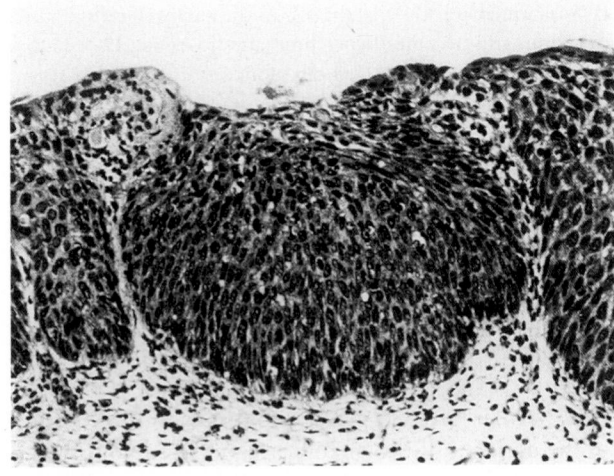

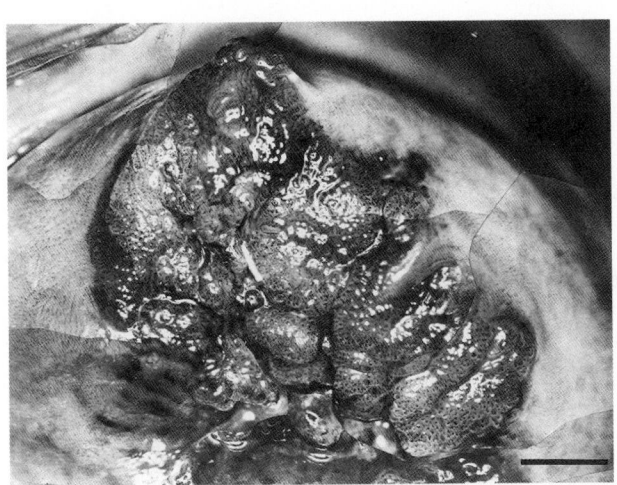

FIGURE 29.25 Invasive squamous cell carcinoma of the cervix; a composite photograph taken through the colposcope. The nodular surface is characteristic of this malignant tumor. The dark dots on its surface represent dilated capillaries, typical of malignant growth. **Bar** = 2 μm. (Reproduced with permission from [45].)

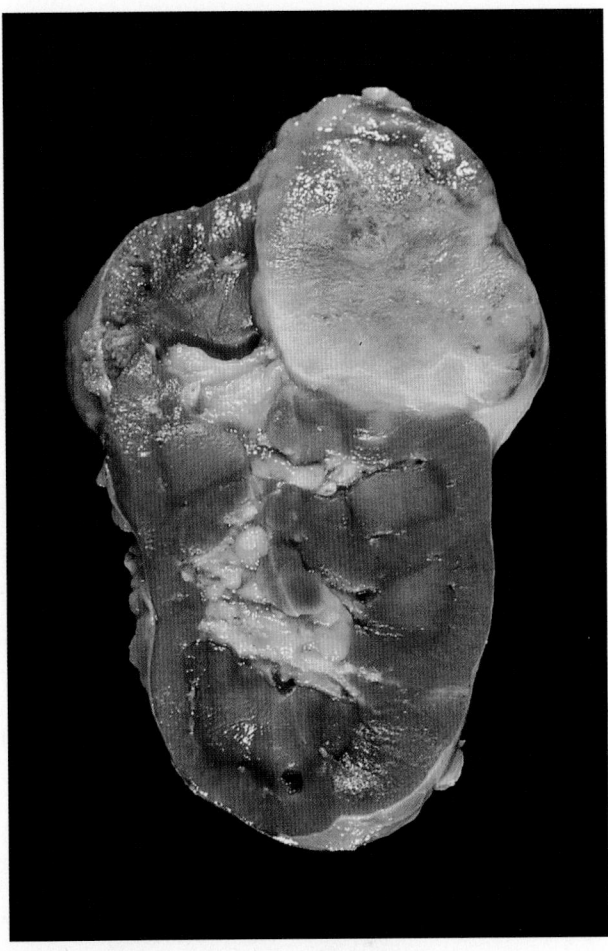

FIGURE 29.26 Carcinoma of the kidney. This tumor had infiltrated the retroperitoneum and the pericolic fat. It measured 4–5 cm in diameter. Had it been discovered when it measured 2 or 3 cm in diameter, it would have been labeled a benign adenoma. (Courtesy of Dr. B. Björnsson, University of Massachusetts Medical School, Worcester, MA.)

somehow wake up and turn into cancer. The idea, born in the early 1800s (67), had its roots in easily observable facts. For example, ordinary moles can turn into cancer (23), and some tumors—the teratomas—definitely look like embryology gone astray. By 1889 it also had the support of experiments that sound extremely modern. Read the following from Cohnheim's *Lectures on General Pathology;* he is describing experiments performed originally by Zahn:

> ". . . pieces of tissues taken from rabbits already born [and introduced into the anterior chamber of adult rabbits] became completely resorbed or greatly shrunken . . . while pieces taken from a foetus still unborn not only lived on in the new foreign organism, but almost always grew there in a very surprising way. Pieces of fetal cartilage grew to 200–300 times the original size" (18).

As we will see, the accepted method for producing mouse teratocarcinomas is to implant a mouse embryo into another mouse's testis (p. 930).

The trouble with the embryonal hypothesis was that embryonic remains were hard to find. Embryology is not known to be a sloppy process; however, microscopic clusters of cells representing embryonic leftovers can be found in a few organs. A perfect example is the nephroblastoma, also called Wilms' tumor, which we have already met in relation to suppressor genes. Almost half of the kidneys removed for nephroblastoma contain microscopic clusters of mesonephric tissue

that are thought to be the precursors of the tumor (see Figures 29.3, 29.29) (12, 74, 81). Cohnheim would have been gratified.

Nests of embryonic epithelium are common around the teeth. These are residues of the embryonic enamel organ (p. 449); in response to infection they proliferate, generating dental cysts and very rarely carcinomas. These are not to be confused with tumors that recapitulate the enamel organ, which arise at the base of the skull (adamantinomas).

Chronic inflammatory lesions. These lesions are not to be dismissed as potential precursors of cancer: at least 15 percent of malignancies worldwide can be attributed to infection (19a).

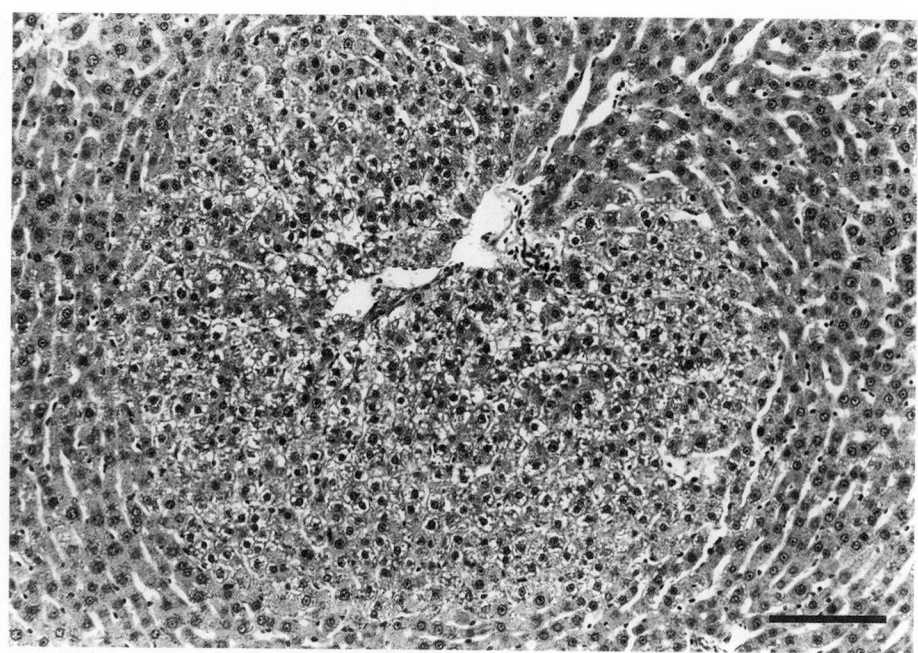

FIGURE 29.27   One of many hyperplastic (precancerous?) nodules that appeared in the liver of a rat, in the course of experimental carcinogenesis as described in Figure 29.25. **Bar** = 100 μm. (Reproduced by permission from [106], © by The US & Canadian Academy of Pathology, Inc.)

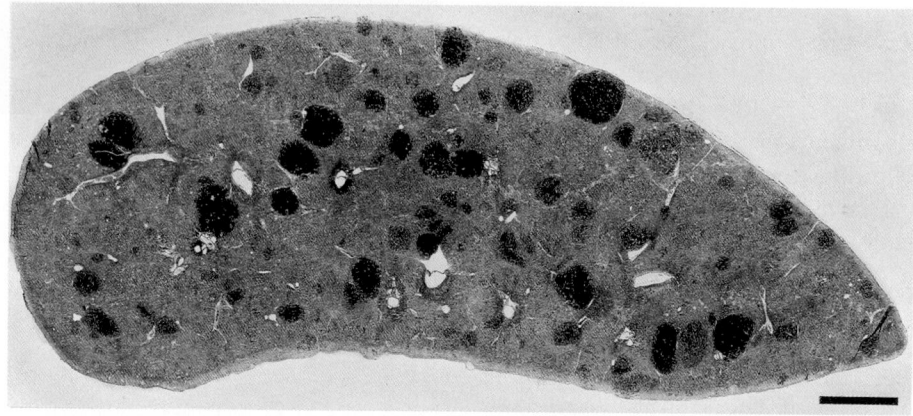

FIGURE 29.28   Multiple foci of liver hyperplasia demonstrated histochemically with a reaction for γ-glutamyl transferase. This rat was submitted to a complex regimen including a single carcinogenic dose of diethylnitrosamine and partial hepatectomy to simulate rapid growth. These nodules appear to be precursor lesions for at least some hepatocellular carcinomas. **Bar** = 500 μm. (Reproduced by permission from [96], © American Society for Investigative Pathology.)

Scars from a single trauma are rarely involved (p. 853), but ongoing chronic inflammation is another matter, especially when it leads to constant epithelial damage and regeneration. The likely mechanism, sustained cell proliferation, will be discussed on p. 951.

Many years of inflammation—usually decades—are necessary for generating cancer from inflammation in humans; fortunately, skin cancer on chronic inflammation and ulcers has become rare because there are

effective means for treating infections. However, 23 adenocarcinomas on ileostomies have been recorded; they developed within 3–38 years (55). Also, before the discovery of streptomycin, ulcerating tuberculosis of the face (*tuberculous lupus*) was incurable, and squamous cell carcinoma was a complication almost taken for granted (17). Another complication that is rarely if ever seen today is squamous cell carcinoma developing in "sinuses"—infected passages that chronically drain pus

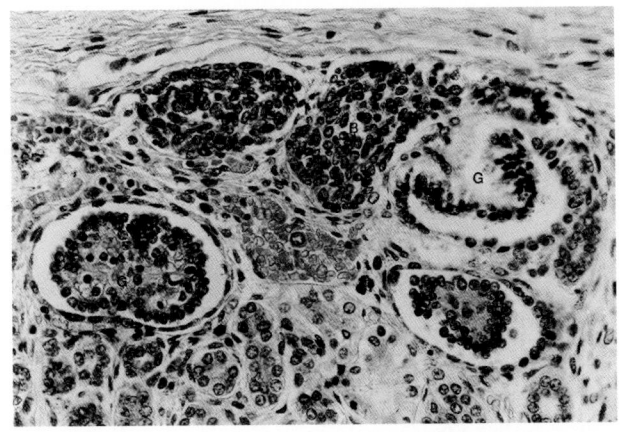

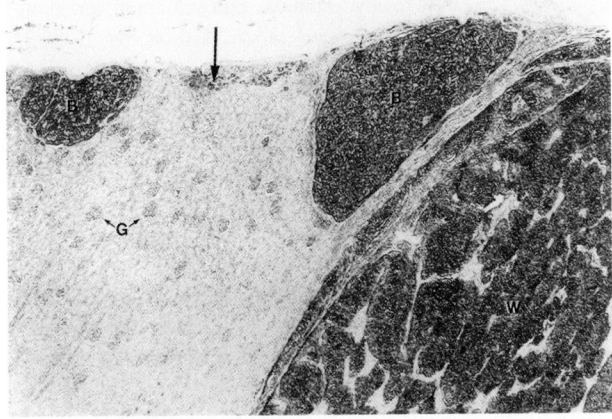

FIGURE 29.29 *Top:* The best example of embryonal rest as a potential cause for a tumor: *nodular renal blastema* (metanephric) (two nodules, top center) in a one-day old infant who died of sepsis. Normally this embryonic tissue regresses and disappears at 34–35 weeks of gestational age; however, some nodules persist and are found in one of every 200–400 pediatric autopsies. In this case they were multiple and bilateral in otherwise normal kidneys. (Courtesy of Dr. K. E. Bove, Children's Hospital Medical Center, Cincinnati, OH). *Bottom:* Association of a 1.5 Wilms' tumorlet (bottom right) with two smaller nodules of renal blastema, and a metanephric hamartoma (**arrow**). From the kidney of a 41-month old girl; another 9 × 8 cm Wilms' tumor was removed from the same kidney, and a 1 cm Wilms' tumorlet was removed from the contralateral kidney. **G** = glomeruli. (Reproduced with permission from [12].)

from infected bones (osteomyelitis). Inflammation in internal organs is another matter. A number of internal diseases are due to chronic nonbacterial inflammation that persists for years and years. For example, liver cirrhosis (alcoholic, viral, or other) has a strong inflammatory component, and it is a well-established precursor of hepatoma. Chronic gastritis due to infection with *Helicobacter pylori* (4) can be a prelude to gastric carcinoma; **ulcerative colitis** (cause unknown) carries a heavy risk of colon cancer. In the same category we can list carcinomas arising in strictures of the esophagus caused by swallowing caustics. These cancers develop 30–45 years later, presumably on chronic erosions (21). Notice, however, that in all these classic examples the role of chronic inflammation as regards neoplasia is indirect: it provides an unstable support for the epithelium, and *eventually it is the chronically regenerating epithelium that lapses into carcinoma.* One again, we find that granulation tissue is highly resistant to malignant transformation.

Patients tend to blame themselves for their sickness, even if it is a tumor ("What did I do to deserve this?") (1). From what we have said about cancer, a certain number of people can indeed blame themselves (especially smokers), but some of the blame must go to the genes, and some to chance.

References

1. Angell M. Disease as a reflection of the psyche. N Engl J Med 1985;312:1570–1572.
2. Anthony PP. Precursor lesions for liver cancer in humans. Cancer Res 1976;36:2579–2583.
3. Anttila S, Hietanen E, Vainio H, et al. Smoking and peripheral type of cancer are related to high levels of pulmonary cytochrome P450IA in lung cancer patients. Int J Cancer 1991;47:681–685.
4. Asaka M, Kudo M, Kato M, Sugiyama T, Takeda H. Review article: long-term Helicobacter pylori infection—from gastritis to gastric cancer. Aliment Pharmacol Ther 1998;12(Suppl. 1):9–15.
5. Balaban-Malenbaum G, Gilbert F. Relationship between homogeneously staining regions and double minute chromosomes in human neuroblastoma cell lines. Prog Cancer Res Ther 1980;12:97–107.
6. Bale AE, Brown SJ. Etiology of cancer: cancer genetics. In: Cancer. Principles and practice of oncology, 6th ed. Philadelphia: Lippincott Williams & Wilkins, 2001, pp. 207–217.
6a. Baylin SB, Herman JG, Graff JR, Vertino PM, Issa J-P. Alterations in DNA methylation: a fundamental aspect of neoplasia. Adv Cancer Res 1998;11:150–196.
6b. Bhatia S, Sklar C. Second cancers in survivors of childhood cancer. Nat Rev Cancer 2002;2:124–132.
7. Biedler JL, Ross RA, Shanske S, Spengler BA. Human neuroblastoma cytogenetics: search for significance of homogeneously staining regions and double minute chromosomes. Prog Cancer Res Ther 1980;12:81–96.
8. Biedler JL, Spengler BA. Metaphase chromosome anomaly: association with drug resistance and cell-specific products. Science 1976;191:185–187.
9. Bishop JM, Weinberg RA (eds). Scientific American molecular oncology. New York: Scientific American, Inc., 1996.
10. Bohr VA, Evans MK, Fornace AJ Jr. DNA repair and its pathogenetic implications. Lab Invest 1989;61:143–161.
11. Bonaïti-Pellié C, Chompret A, Tournade MF, et al. Excess of multifocal tumors in nephroblastoma: implications for

mechanisms of tumor development and genetic counseling. Hum Genet 1993;91:373–376.

12. Bove KE, McAdams AJ. The nephroblastomatosis complex and its relationship to Wilms' tumor: A clinicopathologic treatise. In: Rosenberg HS, Bolande RP, eds. Perspectives in pediatric pathology, vol 3. Chicago: Year Book Medical Publishers Inc., 1976, pp. 185–223.

13. Bronchud MH, Foote M, Peters WP, Robinson MO (eds). Principles of molecular oncology. Totowa, NJ: Humana Press, 2000.

14. Burck KB, Liu ET, Larrick JW. Oncogenes: an introduction to the concept of cancer genes. New York: Springer-Verlag, 1988, pp. 109, 118.

15. Cahan WG. International workshop on multiple primary cancers. Introductory remarks. Cancer 1977;40:1785–1789.

16. Cannon L, Bishop DT, Skolnick M, et al. Genetic epidemiology of prostate cancer in the Utah Mormon genealogy. In: Bodmer WF, ed. Inheritance of susceptibility to cancer in man. Oxford: Oxford University Press, 1982, pp. 47–69.

16a. Cheson BD. The chronic lymphocytic leukemias. In: Cancer. Principles and practice of oncology, 6th ed. Philadelphia: Lippincott Williams & Wilkins, 2001, pp. 2447–2465.

17. Clemmesen J. On the etiology of some human cancers. J Natl Cancer Inst 1951;12:1–21.

18. Cohnheim J. Lectures on general pathology. Sect II. London: The New Sydenham Society, 1889.

19. Coppleson M, Pixley EC. Colposcopy of cervix. In: Coppleson M, ed. Gynecologic oncology, vol 1. Edinburgh: Churchill Livingstone, 1981, pp. 205–224.

19a. Coussens LM, Werb Z. Inflammation and cancer. Nature 2002;420:860–867.

20. Cram LS, Bartholdi MF, Ray FA, Travis GL, Kraemer PM. Spontaneous neoplastic evolution of Chinese hamster cells in culture: multistep progression of karyotype. Cancer Res 1983;43:4828–4837.

21. Csikos M, Horváth Ö, Petri A, Petri I, Imre J. Late malignant transformation of chronic corrosive oesophageal strictures. Langenbecks Arch Chir 1985;365:231–238.

21a. De Baetselier P. Neoplastic progression by somatic cell fusion. In: Liotta LA, ed. Influence of tumor development on the host. Dordrecht: Kluwer Academic Publishers, 1989;88:112–120.

22. Dickson RB, Lippman ME. Molecular biology of breast cancer. In: Cancer. Principles and practice of oncology, 6th ed. Philadelphia: Lippincott Williams & Wilkins, 2001, pp. 1633–1651.

23. Durante F. Nesso fisio-patologico tra la struttura dei nei materni e la genesi di alcuni tumori maligni. Arch Mem Osservaz Chir Pratica 1874;11:217–226.

23a. Eden A, Gaudet F, Waghmare A, Jaenisch R. Chromosomal instability and tumors promoted by DNA hypomethylation. Science 2003;300:455.

24. Enomoto K, Farber E. Kinetics of phenotypic maturation of remodeling of hyperplastic nodules during liver carcinogenesis. Cancer Res 1982;42:2330–2335.

25. Farber E. Cellular biochemistry of the stepwise development of cancer with chemicals: GHA Clowes memorial lecture. Cancer Res 1984;44:5463–5474.

26. Fearon ER. Molecular biology of gastrointestinal cancers. In: Cancer, Principles & practice of oncology, 6th ed. Philadelphia: Lippincott Williams & Wilkins, 2001, pp. 1037–1051.

27. Fearon ER, Vogelstein B. A genetic model for colorectal tumorigenesis. Cell 1990;61:759–767.

27a. Ferbeyre G, Lowe SW. The price of tumor suppression? Nature 2002;415:26–27.

28. Fialkow PJ, Singer JW. Chronic leukemias. In: DeVita VT Jr., Hellman S, Rosenberg SA, eds. Cancer. Principles & practice of oncology, 3rd ed. Philadelphia: JB Lippincott, 1989, pp. 1836–1852.

29. Francke U. A gene for Wilms tumour? Nature 1990;343:692–694.

30. Frankfurt OS, Chin JL, Englander LS, et al. Relationship between DNA ploidy, glandular differentiation, and tumor spread in human prostate cancer. Cancer Res 1985;45:1418–1423.

31. Friend S. The genetic basis of cancer. In: Cossman J, ed. Molecular genetics in cancer diagnosis. New York: Elsevier, 1990, pp. 19–28.

31a. García-Cao I, García-Cao M, Martín-Caballero J, et al. "Super p53" mice exhibit enhanced DNA damage response, are tumor resistant and age normally. Eur Mol Biol Org J 2002;21:6225–6235.

32. Giwercman A, Hopman AHN, Ramaekers FCS, Skakkebaek NE. Carcinoma *in situ* of the testis. Detection of malignant germ cells in seminal fluid by means of *in situ* hybridization. Am J Pathol 1990;136:497–502.

32a. Goffin J, Eisenhauer E. DNA methyltransferase inhibitors—state of the art. Ann Oncol 2002;13:1699–1716.

33. Harris CC. Interindividual variation among humans in carcinogen metabolism, DNA adduct formation and DNA repair. Carcinogenesis 1989;10:1563–1566.

34. Harris CC. p53 tumor suppressor gene: from the basic research laboratory to the clinic-an abridged historical perspective. Carcinogenesis 1996;17:1187–1198.

35. Helman LJ, Malkin, D. Molecular biology of childhood cancers. In: Cancer. Principles and practice of oncology, 6th ed. Philadelphia: Lippincott Williams & Wilkins, 2001, pp. 2161–2169.

36. Henson DE, Albores-Saavedra J. The pathology of incipient neoplasia. Philadelphia: WB Saunders, 1986.

36a. Herman JG, Baylin SB. Gene silencing in cancer in association with promoter hypermethylation. N Engl J Med 2003;349:2042–2054.

37. Inskip PD. Second cancers following radiotherapy. In: Neugut Al, Meadows AT, Robinson E (eds). Multiple primary cancers. Philadelphia: Lippincott Williams & Wilkins, 1999, pp. 91–135.

38. Jandl EH. Blood. Boston: Little, Brown, 1987.

39. Jänne PA, Mayer RJ. Primary care: chemoprevention of colorectal cancer. N Engl J Med 2000;342:1960–1968.

40. King M-C. Genetic analysis of cancer in families. Cancer Surv 1990;9:417–433.

41. Kinlen LJ. Immunologic factors. In: Schottenfeld D, Fraumeni JF Jr, eds. Cancer epidemiology and prevention. Philadelphia: WB Saunders, 1982, pp. 494–505.

42. Kinzler KW, Vogelstein B. Life (and death) in a malignant tumour. Nature 1996;379:19–20.

43. Knudson AG Jr. Genetic predisposition to cancer. In: Hiatt HH, Watson JD, Winsten JA, eds. Origins of human cancer. Book A. Cold Spring Harbor conferences on cell proliferation, vol 4. Cold Spring Harbor: Cold Spring Harbor Laboratory, 1977, pp. 45–52.

44. Knudson AG Jr. Hereditary cancers: clues to mechanisms of carcinogenesis. Br J Cancer 1989;59:661–666.

45. Kolstad P, Stafl A. Atlas of colposcopy. Baltimore: University Park Press, 1972.

46. Koss LG. Precancerous lesions. In: Fraumeni JF Jr, ed. Persons at high risk of cancer. New York: Academic Press, 1975, pp. 85–102.

47. Koss LG. Dysplasia. A real concept or a misnomer? Obstetr Gynecol 1978;51:374–379.

48. Koss LG. From koilocytosis to molecular biology: the impact of cytology on concepts of early human cancer. Mod Pathol 1989a;2:526–535.

49. Koss LG. The Papanicolaou test for cervical cancer detection. A triumph and a tragedy. JAMA 1989b;261:737–743.

50. Krutchkoff DJ, Eisenberg E, Anderson C. Dysplasia of oral mucosa: a unified approach to proper evaluation. Mod Pathol 1991;4:113–119.

50a. Kyle RA, Therneau TM, Rajkumar SV, et al. A long-term study of prognosis in monoclonal gammopathy of undetermined significance. N Engl J Med 2002;346:564–569.

51. Lambert WC. Genetic diseases associated with DNA and chromosomal instability. Dermatol Clin 1987;5:85–108.

52. Lehmann AR. Xeroderma pigmentosum, Cockayne syndrome and ataxia-telangiectasia: disorders relating DNA repair to carcinogenesis. In: Bodmer WF, ed. Inheritance of susceptibility to cancer in man. Oxford: Oxford University Press, 1982, pp. 93–118.

52a. Levrero M, De Laurenzi V, Costanzo a, et al. The p53/p63/p73 family of transcription factors: overlapping and distinct functions. J Cell Sci 2000;113, 1661–1670.

53. Li FP, Fraumeni JF Jr, Mulvihill JJ, et al. A cancer family syndrome in twenty-four kindreds. Cancer Res 1988;48: 5358–5362.

54. Lichtenstein P, Holm NV, Verkasalo PK, et al. Environmental and heritable factors in the causation of cancer. N Engl J Med 2000;343:78–85.

55. Listinsky CM, Halpern NB, Workman RB, Herrera GA. Ultrastructural and immunocytochemical features of a case of neuroendocrine carcinoma developing in a prior ileostomy site. Ultrastruct Pathol 1994;18:503–509.

56. Makino S. My life in cytology. In: German J, ed. Chromosome mutation and neoplasia. New York: Alan R. Liss, 1983, pp. xxvii–xxxiii.

57. Matsukura N, Onda M, Tokunaga A, et al. Simultaneous gastric cancer in monozygotic twins. Cancer 1988;62:2430–2435.

58. Meisner LF. Genetic factors in human cancer. In: Kahn SB, Love RR, Sherman C Jr, Chakravorty R, eds. Concepts in cancer medicine. New York: Grune & Stratton, 1983, pp. 165–176.

59. Miller RW. Genes, syndromes, and cancer. Pediatr Rev 1986; 8:153–158.

60. Moertel CG. Multiple primary malignant neoplasms. Historical perspectives. Cancer 1977;40:1786–1792.

61. National Cancer Institute Workshop. The 1988 Bethesda system for reporting cervical/vaginal cytological diagnoses. JAMA 1989;262:931–934.

62. Neugut Al, Meadows AT, Robinson E (eds). Multiple primary cancers. Philadelphia: Lippincott Williams & Wilkins, 1999.

62a. Nigg EA. Centrosome aberrations: a cause or consequence of cancer progression? Nat Rev Cancer 2002;2:1–11.

63. Nores JM, Dalayeun J, Chebat J, Dieudonné P, Nenna AD. Concurrent anaplastic bronchial cancer in identical twin brothers. Respiration 1989;55:56–59.

64. Nowell PC. Mitotic inhibition and chromosome damage by mitomycin in human leukocyte cultures. Exp Cell Res 1964;33:445–449.

65. Nowell PC. The clonal evolution of tumor cell populations. Science 1976;194:23–28.

66. Nowell PC, Croce CM. Chromosomal approaches to oncogenes and oncogenesis. FASEB J 1988;2:3054–3060.

67. Oberling C. The riddle of cancer. New Haven, CT: Yale University Press, 1952.

68. Ooi WL, Elston RC, Chen VW, Bailey-Wilson JE, Rothschild H. Increased familial risk for lung cancer. J Natl Cancer Inst 1986;76:217–222.

68a. Oren M, Damalas A, Gottlieb T, et al: Regulation of *p53*: intricate loops and delicate balances. Biochem Pharmacol 2002:64,865–871.

69. Ortiz-Hidalgo C, De La Vega G, Aguirre-García J. The histopathology and biologic prognostic factors of Barrett's esophagus. A review. J Clin Gastroenterol 1998;26:324–333.

69a. Pawelek JM. Tumour cell hybridization and metastasis revisited. Melanoma Res 2000;10:1–8.

70. Pennisi E. Behind the scenes of gene expression. Science 2001;293:1064–1067.

70a. Pietenpol JA, Stewart ZA. Cell cycle checkpoint signaling: Cell cycle arrest and signaling. Toxicol 2002:181–182, 475–481.

71. Pihan GA, Doxsey SJ. The mitotic machinery as a source of genetic instability in cancer. Sem Cancer Biol 1999;9:289–302.

72. Pihan GA, Purohit A, Wallace J, et al. Centrosome defects can account for cellular and genetic changes that characterize prostate cancer progression. Cancer Res 2001;61: 2212–2219.

73. Pitot HC. The natural history of neoplasia. Am J Pathol 1977; 89:401–412.

73a. Pitot HC. Fundamentals of oncology, 4th ed. New York: Marcel Dekker, Inc., 2002.

74. Pochedly C. Persistent renal blastema: a seed of Wilms' tumor? Hosp Pract 1981;16:83–96.

75. Ponder BAJ. Inherited cancer syndromes. In: Carney D, Sikora K, eds. Genes and cancer. Chichester: John Wiley & Sons, 1990, pp. 99–106.

76. Purtilo DT, Paquin L, Gindhart T. Genetics of neoplasia—impact of ecogenetics on oncogenesis. Am J Pathol 1978; 91:609–688.

77. Qumsiyeh MB, Li P. Molecular biology of cancer: cytogenetics. In: Cancer. Principles and practice of oncology, 6th ed. Philadelphia: Lippincott Williams & Wilkins, 2001, pp. 77–90.

78. Ragsdale BD, Sweet DE. Bone. In: Henson DE, Albores-Saavedra J, eds. The pathology of incipient neoplasia. Philadelphia: WB Saunders, 1986, pp. 381–423.

79. Rak J, Filmus J, Kerbel RS. Reciprocal paracrine interactions between tumour cells and endothelial cells: the "angiogenesis progression" hypothesis. Eur J Cancer 1996;32A:2438–2450.

80. Ross DW. Introduction to oncogenes and molecular cancer medicine. New York: Springer-Verlag, 1998.

81. Roth J, Blaha I, Bitter-Suermann D, Heitz PU. Blastemal cells of nephroblastomatosis complex share an onco-developmental antigen with embryonic kidney and Wilms' tumor. An immunohistochemical study on polysialic acid distribution. Am J Pathol 1988;133:596–608.

82. Rowley JD. The Philadelphia chromosome translocation. A paradigm for understanding leukemia. Cancer 1990; 65:2178–2184.

83. Rowley JD. Chromosome translocations: dangerous liaisons revisited. Nat Rev/Cancer 2001;1:245–250.

83a. Rowley JD, Aster JC, Sklar J. The impact of new DNA diagnostic technology on the management of cancer patients. Survey of diagnostic techniques. Arch Pathol Lab Med 1993;117:1104–1109.

84. Ruddon RW. Cancer biology, 2nd ed. New York: Oxford University Press, 1987.

85. Sager R, Gadi IK, Stephens L, Grabowy CT. Gene amplification: an example of accelerated evolution in tumorigenic cells. Proc Natl Acad Sci USA 1985;82:7015–7019.

86. Sager R. Tumor suppressor genes: the puzzle and the promise. Science 1989;246:1406–1412.

87. Sandberg AA. The chromosomes in human cancer and leukemia. 2nd ed. New York: Elsevier Science Publishing Co., 1990.

88. Sandberg AA. The chromosomes in human cancer and leukemia, 2nd ed. New York: Elsevier, 1990.

89. Schottenfeld D. Multiple primary cancers. In: Schottenfeld D, Fraumeni JF Jr, eds. Cancer epidemiology and prevention. Philadelphia: WB Saunders, 1982, pp. 1025–1035.

90. Schottenfeld D, Fraumeni Jr. JF (eds). Cancer Epidemiology and Prevention, 2nd ed. New York: Oxford University Press, 1996.

91. Shackelford RE, Kaufmann WK, Paules RS. Cell cycle control, checkpoint mechanisms, and genotoxic stress. Environ Health Perspect 1999;107(Suppl 1):5–24.

91a. Shono M, Sato N, Mizumoto K, et al. Stepwise progression of centrosome defects associated with local tumor growth and metastatic process of human pancreatic carcinoma cells transplanted orthotopically into nude mice. Lab Invest 2001; 81:945–952.

92. Sirica AE. Preneoplasia and precancerous lesions. In: Sirica AE, ed. The pathobiology of neoplasia. New York: Plenum Press, 1989, pp. 199–215.

93. Sirica AE, ed. The pathobiology of neoplasia. New York: Plenum Press, 1989.

94. Skolnick M, Bishop DT, Carmelli D, et al. A population-based assessment of familial cancer risk in Utah Mormon genealogies. In: Arrighi FE, Rao PN, Stubblefield E, eds. Genes, chromosomes, and neoplasia. New York: Raven Press, 1981, pp. 477–500.

95. Smith HS, Liotta LA, Hancock MC, Wolman SR, Hackett AJ. Invasiveness and ploidy of human mammary carcinomas in short-term culture. Proc Natl Acad Sci USA 1985; 82:1805–1809.

96. Solt DB, Medline A, Farber E. Rapid emergence of carcinogen-induced hyperplastic lesions in a new model for the sequential analysis of liver carcinogenesis. Am J Pathol 1977; 88:595–618.

97. Soussi T. The p53 tumor suppressor gene: from molecular biology to clinical investigation. Ann N.Y. Acad Sci 2000; 910:121–137.

98. Strong LC, Amos Cl. Inherited susceptibility. In: Schottenfeld D, Fraumeni Jr. JF (eds). Cancer epidemiology and prevention, 2nd ed. New York: Oxford University Press, 1996, pp. 559–583.

99. Stuart AE, Smith AN, Samuel E, eds. Applied surgical pathology. Oxford: Blackwell Scientific Publications, 1975.

100. Sudbø J, Kildal W, Risberg B. DNA content as a prognostic marker in patients with oral leukoplakia. N Engl J Med 2001;344:1270–1278.

100a. Tyner SD, Venkatachalam S, Choi J, et al. p53 mutant mice that display early ageing-associated phenotypes. Nature 2002;415:45–53.

101. Van Leeuwen FE, Travis LB. Second cancers. In: Cancer. Principles and practice of oncology, 6th ed. Philadelphia: Lippincott Williams & Wilkins, 2001, pp. 2939–2964.

102. Vogelstein B, Kinzler KW (eds). The genetic basis of human cancer. New York: McGraw-Hill, 1998.

103. Volgelstein B, Lane D, Levine AJ. Surfing the p53 network. Nature 2000;408:307–310.

104. von Recklinghausen FD. Ein Fall von Enchondrom mit ungewöhnlicher Multiplication. Virchows Arch Pathol Anat Physiol Klin Med 1889;118:1–18.

105. Walch AK, Zitzelsberger HF, Bruch J, et al. Chromosomal imbalances in Barrett's adenocarcinoma and the metaplasia-dysplasia-carcinoma sequence. Am J Pathol 2000;156: 555–566.

106. Wanless IR, Medline A. Role of estrogens as promoters of hepatic neoplasia. Lab Invest 1982;46:313–320.

107. Weissman BE, Saxon PJ, Pasquale SR, et al. Introduction of a normal human chromosome 11 into a Wilms' tumor cell line controls its tumorigenic expression. Science 1987;236: 175–180.

108. Wilentz RE, Iacobuzio-Donahue CA, Argani P, et al. Loss of expression of Dpc4 in pancreatic intraepithelial neoplasia: evidence that DPC4 inactivation occurs late in neoplastic progression. Cancer Res 2000;60:2002–2006.

109. Woods DB, Vousden KH. Regulation of p53 function. Exp Cell Res 2001;264:56–66.

110. Wyllie AH. The genetic regulation of apoptosis. Curr Opin Genet Dev 1995;5:97–104.

111. Yunis JJ. The chromosomal basis of human neoplasia. Science 1983;221:227–236.

112. Yunis JJ, Brunning RD, Howe RB, Lobell M. High-resolution chromosomes as an independent prognostic indicator in adult acute nonlymphocytic leukemia. N Engl J Med 1984; 311:812–818.

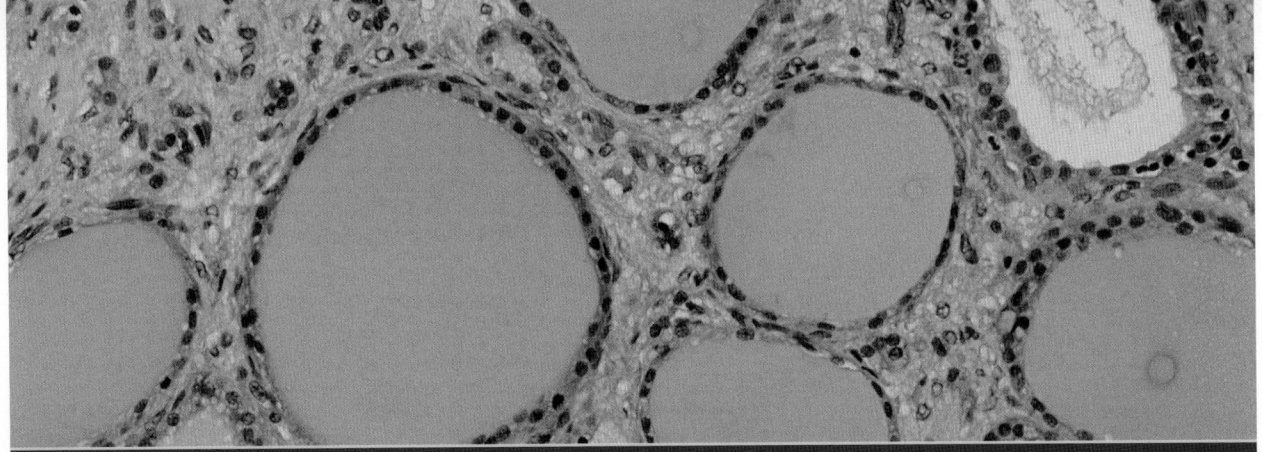

ANTITUMOR DEFENSES

For better or for worse, this will be a short chapter: we do have defenses against tumors, but how good are they? Of the 6 million humans who will develop a tumor worldwide this year, 3 million will die of it.

We can count on two very different lines of defense. The first is preventive and operates at the level of genes and cells: specialized genes hold the brakes on cell proliferation, and repair genes correct mistakes in the DNA. Overall this is a very effective protection, as we have seen.

The second line of defense, the immune system, operates at the level of the whole individual. It is planned to defend us—primarily—from the attack of microscopic creatures that are chemically different from us. There are hints that it can also attack and destroy tumor cells, but unfortunately the chemical difference between normal and tumor cells is minimal. At the beginning of this section we drew up a long list of differences between normal cells and tumor cells; yet, when we come down to the molecular level, the differences tend to vanish. So, does the immune system really protect us against tumors, and if it does, how efficient is it?

Overall, it is fair to say that the immune response against tumors is not impressive. It can be forced to perform some spectacular rejections, but mostly in mice. As a research field the topic is difficult. Correspondingly, the enthusiasm of the scientific community has waxed and waned (Figure 30.1). A review in 1998 advises us that "The Glass Is Half Full" (79); and in 2002 others agree (18a).

The Immune Response against Tumors

Tumors behave in some respects like parasites; it was natural to wonder, about a century ago, whether they elicited bodily responses similar to those induced by infection. The fact that tumor

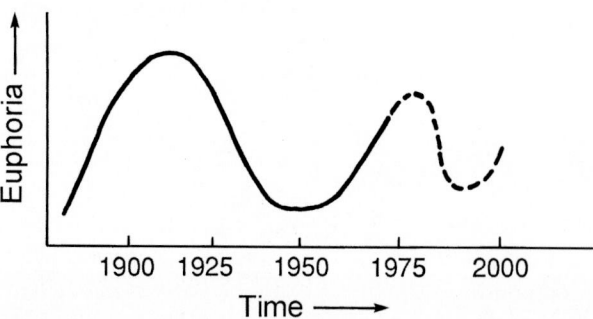

FIGURE 30.1   The changing fortunes of tumor immunology: original 1970 data of Prehn, extended by Kreider and Bartlett in 1986 (47a). In 2003 the shape of the curve depends on who draws it (immunologists, oncologists, patients). Overall it is slowly rising. (From [47a], copyright © 1986 Alan R. Liss. Reprinted by permission of Wiley-Liss, Inc., a subsidiary of John Wiley & Sons, Inc.)

grafts to laboratory animals are rejected was already familiar to Metchnikoff and Ehrlich, the founders of immunology, and predictably their explanations were miles apart (83): Ehrlich thought that tumors, like bacteria, needed special nutrients, whereas for Metchnikoff tumor growth was maintained by bacterial products absorbed from the colon. In retrospect, the behavior of tumor grafts could not be understood until the general laws of grafting had been worked out, as Peter Medawar did starting around 1944. Also, inbred strains of mice were needed, and the first were produced in the 1940s by Ludvik Gross, the discoverer of the mouse leukemia virus. Regarding tumors, these inbred mice (*syngeneic* mice, i.e., with the same genes) led to an important observation. It was possible to immunize an inbred mouse against a tumor generated in another mouse; the immunization was so specific that the mouse would reject a tumor from another individual of the same strain, even though it would accept a skin graft from the same (syngeneic) individual. This experiment showed that *tumors could develop their own specific antigens;* today they are called **tumor-specific antigens (TSA).**

The next surprise came from the Karolinska Institute in Stockholm. Gross and others in the United States had shown that the polyoma virus produced tumors if injected into immature mice (33). Now it was discovered that grafted polyoma tumors would not grow in mice that had been immunized against the virus. This seemed to open the door to immunization against tumors, or at least against virus-induced tumors (the latter proved to be correct).

After these encouraging highlights we can list some further discoveries, the first one disappointing:

- *Spontaneous tumors (as opposed to experimentally induced tumors) are in general poorly antigenic.* The reason is not clear; perhaps they are self-selected as such, because they grow more successfully.
- *When multiple tumors are produced in the same animal by a carcinogen, each tumor is antigenically different.* The reason: unlike viruses, carcinogens induce random mutations. This complicates the task of the immune response (if any), because it has to deal with each tumor as a separate set of antigens.
- If experimental tumors are listed from the most to the least antigenic, they rank as follows (48):

1. Virus induced
2. Ultraviolet-light induced
3. Chemical carcinogen induced
4. Spontaneous

Note that the tumors induced by UV light are among the most antigenic; this may explain why skin cancers in humans, as a group, have an excellent prognosis.

- Another class of tumor antigens was recognized: the so-called *tumor-associated antigens (TAAs).* Unlike the TSAs just described, these antigens correspond to proteins normally present also in adult and/or in fetal cells (the latter are called **oncofetal antigens**) and happen to be overexpressed or newly expressed in tumor cells. The first one was isolated in 1991 (55) and its gene was named MAGE-1 (for **M**elanoma-**A**ssociated **GE**ne).

Since then, MAGE-2 and -3 were added; all three turned out to be normally expressed in the testis. Their proteins are found in melanomas as well as in cancers of the breast, gliomas, and other tumors (53).

Warning: not all tumor "antigens" play a role as antigens. The antigenic properties of the so-called oncofetal antigens is weak and probably irrelevant; we prefer the term **oncofetal proteins.** As a matter of fact, one of the best known TAA's, alpha-fetoprotein, is immunosuppressive (50). So why is it called an oncofetal antigen? Simply because immunologists, faced with a protein, call it an antigen by reflex, just as molecular biologists would call it a gene product (Figure 30.2).

So far we have listed many facts about tumor antigens; what about the immune response to these antigens? The

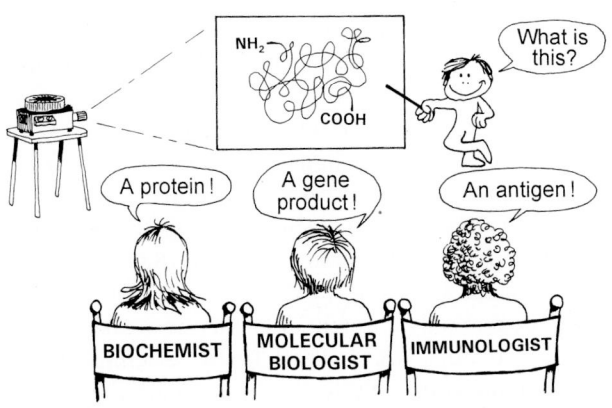

FIGURE 30.2 A protein may be called by various names, depending on the background of the observer. (Courtesy of Dr. H. F. Cuénoud, University of Massachusetts Medical School, Worcester, MA.)

main point is that *the immune response to tumor antigens is overwhelmingly cell-mediated:* antibodies seem to play no significant role. The tumors are attacked by cytotoxic T (CD8$^+$) cells and by NK cells, rarely by helper T cells (CD4$^+$). Antitumor *antibodies* exist but cannot be counted on as a natural defense; HOWEVER, *engineered* antitumor antibodies have recently appeared on the scene as a major therapeutic weapon (see Chapter 34): 400 are in clinical trials (84a).

In vitro it is possible to kill tumor cells with antibody and complement (36) but *in vivo* mammalian cells are very resistant to lysis by complement, because they express several protective proteins (10).

The target keeps changing. One of the difficulties that plague the field of tumor immunology is that the antigenic identity of the tumor keeps changing. The tumor, as if it had a perverse will of its own, can evade immune attack by several mechanisms: (a) *By producing cells that are less antigenic.* This change may occur quite simply by natural selection, the less antigenic clones being more apt to survive. (b) *By failing to express MHC class I,* which could happen by the same mechanism. (c) *By ceasing to produce a given antigen.* (d) *By shedding soluble antigens,* which float away and distract both antibodies and T cells before they make contact with the tumor cells. (e) *By growing faster,* perhaps as a result of stimulation by antibodies. (f) Or *by becoming so large that the immune system is overwhelmed,* resulting in immunosuppression (patients with a malignant tumor are often immunosuppressed). Last, there also is the possibility that (g) *the host becomes tolerant instead of immune.*

An optimistic view: immunosurveillance. Despite all these difficulties, some of the top thinkers in biology and medicine proposed a theory whereby the immune system is actively involved in protecting the host ever since birth, or earlier.

As far back as 1909, Paul Ehrlich, who discovered mast cells and originated the concept of receptors, was sure that aberrant fetal cells, ready to produce cancers, were continuously nipped off by the immune system (45). A similar concept was proposed in 1959 by the late Dr. Lewis Thomas during his distinguished career as a pathologist (before achieving fame as a writer). Shortly thereafter the concept acquired a name, *immunosurveillance,* and rose to near-dogma through the writings of Australian Nobel laureate Sir MacFarlane Burnet (13): "One can . . . picture a form of surveillance by which the body is continually patrolled, as it were, for the appearance of aberrant protein. . . ."

The strongest support for the notion of immunosurveillance comes from the established fact that genetically immunodeficient or therapeutically immunosuppressed individuals are prone to develop malignancies, mostly lymphomas (67). In three studies of patients who were immunosuppressed for kidney grafts, the risk of developing a lymphoma was increased 100, 150, and 350 times (51). However, there are also some troubling facts:

- Why are the tumors arising in the immune system itself?
- Why do they occur only in a minority of immunosuppressed individuals?
- Why is there no increase in the more common forms of tumors such as lung, breast, and colon cancers? True, there is some increase in skin and lip cancers, but it is only 3–4 percent (51).
- Why, in normal individuals, is there no greater incidence of malignancies at immunologically privileged sites such as the central nervous system? (Privileged sites are tissues in which allografts are protected against rejection, perhaps because they lack lymphatic drainage; for example, the brain and the anterior chamber of the eye.) Similar questions are raised by studies of nude mice, which are born without hair and without a thymus, and are thereby deprived of T cells: they show no increase in spontaneous tumors (perhaps they are protected by their NK cells, of which they have more than normal).

For all these and other reasons, it is now believed that the concept of immunosurveillance—while still alive—should be accepted with some restrictions (48).

NOTE: While the experts debate to what extent immunosurveillance really functions as a tumor watchdog, there is little doubt that it can do so indirectly, by protecting against *viruses* that cause tumors. In other words, the immune system can protect against tumors by eliminating their cause, rather than the tumor itself (46, 48). This line of reasoning is suggested, for example, by the congenital immunodeficiency named Duncan's disease or XLP (X-linked lymphoproliferative disease) (67), in which immunodeficiency paves the way to a virus-induced lymphoma (p. 605).

Inflammation in Tumors: What Does It Mean?

Inflammation, albeit mild, is an almost constant feature of malignant tumors (Figure 30.3). It can be strong enough to be noticed clinically: when a malignant tumor spreads to a serosal surface such as the pleura, fluid accumulates in the serosal cavity. These so-called *malignant effusions* (78) are essentially inflammatory exudates; they do contain tumor cells, but most of the cells floating within them are leukocytes (37). Some degree of inflammation can also be found in benign tumors (2, 6). Why is inflammation present? Does it represent an immune response? Is it helpful? As usual when dealing with tumors, the answers are liable to vary from one tumor to another. Here are some facts about the cells involved.

Macrophages are always present in tumors as part of the stroma (20). In some tumors as many as 80 percent

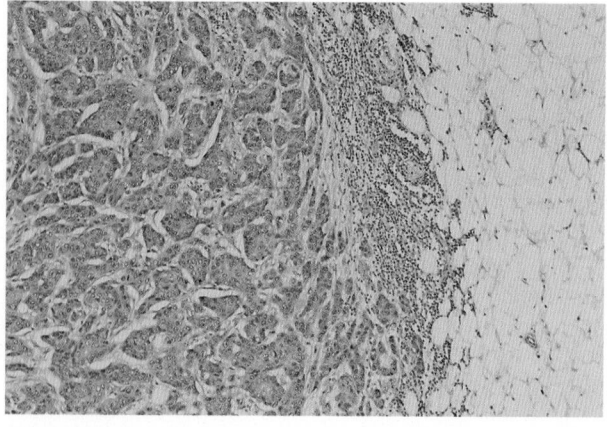

FIGURE 30.3   Disappointing lymphocytes. *Lower left*: A carcinoma of the breast, infiltrating a mass of adipose tisse (*top right*). Between the two, a substantial layer of lymphocytes has developed, but it does not appear to be holding back the invasion. (60x)

of the cells are macrophages (76) and make up 65 percent of the tumor volume (88). Why should these mighty creatures elect to go and live in the abnormal environment of a tumor? They responded to the call of duty. Some types of malignant cells grown *in vitro* secrete monocyte chemoattractant protein-1, MCP-1 (30, 88); the amount secreted correlates with the intensity of the macrophage infiltrate (88). What the macrophages are doing in the tumor is not so clear. They are certainly a potential factory of cytokines and other mediators (see Table 9.3); by selecting appropriate items from this list, we can make the case—arbitrarily—for macrophages as lifesavers or killers (52).

Mediators that should be helpful include *interferon*, which does "interfere" with the growth of some tumors (1); another is *interleukin 12*, whose antitumor and antimetastatic virtues we will describe shortly, and of course *tumor necrosis factor*, too unreliable to deserve its name. The tumor-killing capability of activated macrophages is beyond doubt (14, 32, 66, 76); if we choose the right model, the tumor-killing capacity of TNF can also be spectacular, even to the naked eye (see Figures 9.40, 9.41, 24.40) but it works much better in mice than in people.

Humans tolerate only 2 percent of the intravenous dose of TNF that can be given to mice. Dramatic tumor regressions have been obtained in patients by local injection of TNF in high doses, or by isolated limb or liver perfusion (41).

The macrophages can actually help the tumor by inducing *angiogenesis*. Much of the tumor tissue is anoxic, and anoxia induces angiogenesis factors in many and perhaps all types of cells, including tumor cells (p. 776). They secrete *growth factors* which can favor tumor cells (76). And then, by secreting enough *cachectin* (another name for TNF) they can induce cachexia and deliver the finishing blow to the host (p. 829): a drastic way to get rid of a tumor.

Lymphocytes should be in the forefront of antitumor defenses, because T and B lymphocytes alone have the privilege of specific ammunition. It is clear that antibodies are not involved in tumor rejection, so the T cells should be having their field day, especially against tumors with well-defined antigens. In fact, this is not the case; they do appear on the scene, both within and/or around the tumor (47), but they seem to behave more as spectators than as participants: they keep their distance from tumor cells—they certainly do not swarm all over them as if to kill them. For the pathologist who hopes to associate tumor inflammation with

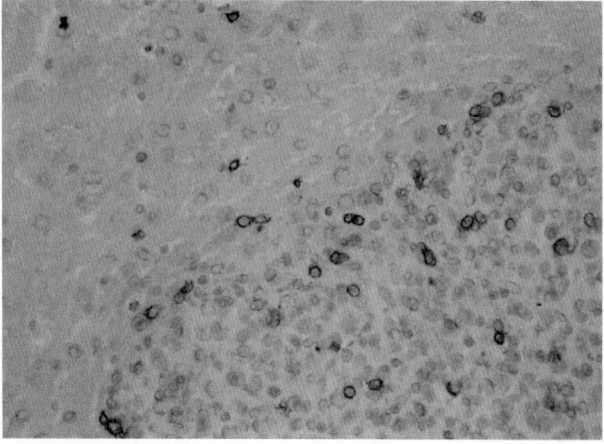

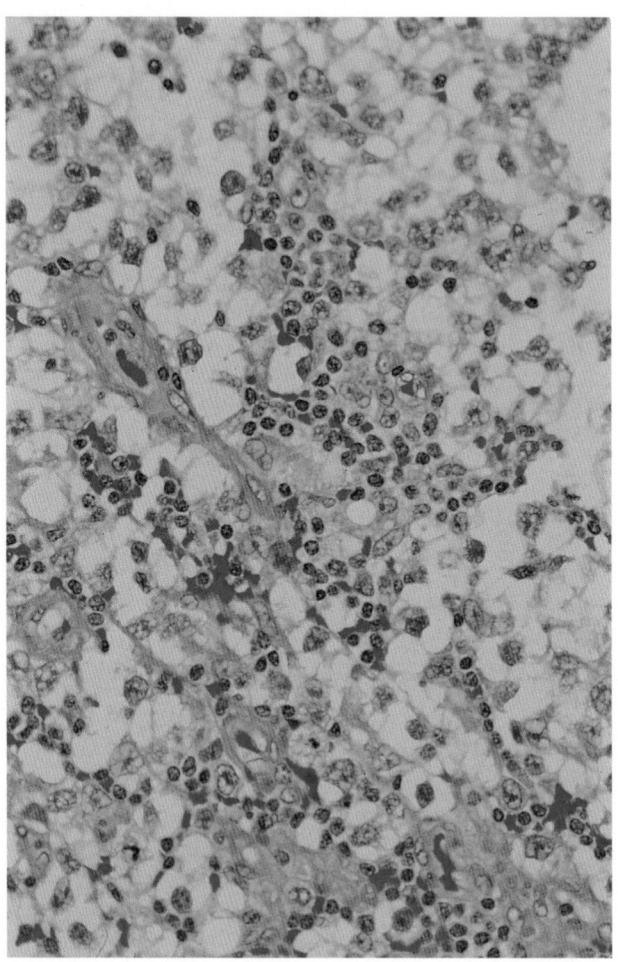

FIGURE 30.4 Histologic aspect of a seminoma. The large clear cells represent the tumor; between them are clusters of lymphocytes, often seen in seminomas, presumably as a response to tumor antigens. (350x)

FIGURE 30.5 The (sometimes) gallant NK cells. *Top left*: Rat liver. *Bottom right*: Mammary adenocarcinoma. The dark brown cells are NK cells; they did gather in the tumor, but it turned out to be NK resistant. (Experiment, antibody, and slide courtesy of Dr. J. C. Hiserodt, Pittsburg, PA.)

good news, the inflammatory infiltrates—mainly of lymphocytes—are frustrating.

Massive lymphocytic infiltration is typical of seminomas (Figure 30.4) to the point that in bygone years these tumors were said to consist of "two types of cells." The current explanation has little to do with defense: the lymphocytes are responding to sperm-related antigens that the body does not usually "see" and that are produced or expressed by the tumor cells.

Everyone agrees that medullary carcinoma of the breast, which is consistently infiltrated with lymphocytes, has a relatively good prognosis (7); a positive correlation between inflammatory response and prognosis has been found for colon carcinomas (6) and for lung carcinomas (86). For other tumors a clear-cut correlation is not apparent (2, 7). In the rabbit, Shope

papillomas that regress are massively infiltrated with lymphocytes (61); and in human malignant tumors, the largest numbers of macrophages are found in renal cell carcinomas, melanomas, and carcinomas of the colon—the malignancies that are most susceptible to immunotherapy (63). The bottom line, it seems, is that the tumor-infiltrating lymphocytes *could* perform some defensive functions, because if they are extracted, multiplied by culture, and reinjected, they demonstrably help in the fight against the tumor (p. 915).

Natural killer (NK) cells are well equipped, especially in the liver (85) but they are obviously unable to destroy an established tumor (Figure 30.5). Perhaps they are defending us from newly-born, microscopic tumors. **Neutrophils** do take part in the fight against some tumors, by killing tumor cells and by secreting cytokines, but their role is usually peripheral (18, 60).

Overall, then, it seems that in tumors something is holding back the T cells. A very significant experiment: killer CD8$^+$ T lymphocytes from a given tumor can lyse the tumor cells *in vitro* but not *in vivo* (24). This type of evidence has suggested that *in tumor-bearing patients the immune system is dysfunctional* (24, 68). It is unable to respond properly to tumor antigens at first, and later to other antigens, possibly because the cytolytic attack of killer T cells is inhibited by material diffusing out of the tumor. The mechanism of *this dysfunction is different from that of the immunosuppression induced e.g., by high doses of corticosteroids.* If all this is true, it may soon be possible to give the T cells the necessary boost.

Links between Inflammation and Tumors

It is all too natural to think of inflammation and tumors as totally different, almost incompatible processes, one defensive, one offensive, run by totally separate mechanisms. In fact, they have a number of links. We have repeatedly mentioned that chronic inflammation may give birth to tumors, by stimulating cell replication or by causing free radical damage to DNA. We have also mentioned that some cancer cells are capable of chemotaxis. But who would ever have guessed that the classic anti-inflammatory agent, *aspirin, inhibits not only inflammation but also cancer of the colon?* It has been proved in humans (27).

> The mechanism (80) was worked out in APC mice, a model for human familial **a**denomatous **p**olyposis of the **c**olon. In these mice, prostaglandin E$_2$, PGE$_2$, an inflammatory mediator, is markedly elevated in both adenomas and in colon cancers. Hypothesis: the prostaglandin is driving the tumors. Proof: in APC mice, which are also lacking an enzyme that produces PGE$_2$ (cyclooxygenase 2 [COX-2]), the number and size of the polyps are greatly reduced. Further proof: the same effect is obtained in knockout mice lacking a cell-surface receptor for PGE$_2$, called EP2. (Inhibiting the isoenzyme COX-1 has no effect.)

Another set of anti-inflammatory agents, the NSAIDs (**N**onsteroidal **a**nti-**i**nflammatory **d**rugs) also protect against colon cancer (58); *in vitro,* arachidonic acid stimulates cancer cell growth (26), whereas inhibitors of 5-lipoxygenase inhibit it (5).

Then there is a cytokine called MIF, migration inhibitory factor, one of the first cytokines discovered, which has the main function of preventing macrophages from running away. MIF also inhibits the function of the p53 protein by suppressing the transcription of the gene (15, 17, 40). To inhibit p53, the custodian of the genome, means allowing DNA mistakes to go uncorrected, and therefore to step from inflammation into cancer.

After all, it is not too surprising to find that cancer cells and inflammatory cells have similarities. Both infiltrate, both use chemotaxis (pp. 403, 816) and diapedesis, both secrete powerful molecules. Both are hunter and hunted.

Nonspecific Antitumor Defenses

The few facts that we can offer are tantalizing. Most of them concern regressions of tumors in the course of infections.

- It is an open secret among experimental oncologists that when an infectious disease breaks out in a mouse colony, the experiment has to be called off because many tumors will not take; even stress can make a difference (11).
- Infection of the pleura, resulting in empyema after resection of a lung for cancer, has improved survival (75).
- Infections can cause remissions of leukemia in children (9).
- The remission of leukemias during infection has led to another discovery: if human lung tissue is exposed *in vitro* to endotoxin, to mimic infection, it produces a factor that causes leukemia cells to differentiate (87).
- Experimental granulomas in mice produce a "mouse granuloma protein" (MGP) that—injected into other mice—protects them against a lethal infection with *Listeria monocytogenes*. A similar protein was found in human urine (HGP); mouse macrophages incubated with HGP become cytotoxic against the highly malignant Lewis carcinoma (25).

Some but not all of these effects may have been due to macrophages producing cytokines such as tumor necrosis factor. This is probably what happened in the patients treated for cancer at the turn of the century with "Coley's toxins" (p. 365). There is room here for more work.

Allografts of tumors in humans. The reader will probably assume that tumor grafts from one human to another have never been tried, because they would run against ethical as well as immunological barriers. Well, this type of experiment has been done many times, and some grafts have taken. Ludvik Gross has collected a rather disturbing series (33). A few examples: One carcinoma was accidentally grafted from the mother's ulcerated breast cancer to her suckling infant's lip. As late as 1958, before ethical guidelines were established, experiments, on "volunteers" (some with cancer, some healthy) showed that tumor implants usually regressed in 4–6 weeks; but one cancer patient developed metastases even after excision of the graft. One autologous implant remained dormant for 18 months. In 1965, a surgeon transplanted melanoma tissue from a woman to her 80-year-old mother, in the hope of producing

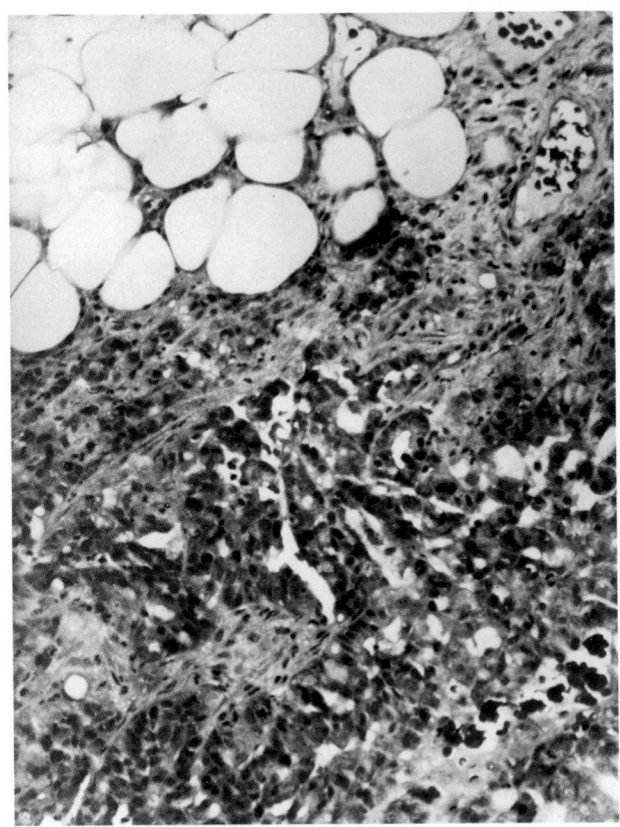

FIGURE 30.6 Needle-stick tumor. A 19-year-old healthy laboratory worker accidentally injected her finger while transplanting a line of cells derived from a human colon carcinoma. Nineteen days later a nodule measuring $9 \times 4 \times 4$ mm was excised. It contained this typical adenocarcinoma. Four years later the patient was in good health. Allogeneic transplants sometimes do take. (Courtesy of Dr. M. E. Sanders, National Cancer Institute, Bethesda, MD.)

antibodies as an aid to therapy; the daughter died, and so did the mother, with widespread metastatic melanoma despite excision of the implantation site (77). Several (immunosuppressed!) recipients of kidney transplants have died of metastases from primary or secondary tumors hidden in the donated kidney. One was a melanoma. In a recent laboratory accident, a technician injected her own finger with a suspension of cells from a line of human adenocarcinoma of the colon. Three weeks later a nodule was excised that showed a carcinoma with no inflammatory response (Figure 30.6) (34). Four years later the lady was in fine shape and considered cured.

Therapeutic Boosting of Natural Antitumor Defenses

Although surgery, radiation, and chemotherapy remain the main weapons in the fight against cancer, many attempts have been and are being made to recruit the collaboration of the immune system. We cannot even list them; the current literature is enormous (54, 70).

Nonspecific stimulation of the immune system. This approach is based on the above-mentioned occasional regressions of cancer in relation to infection. In fact, the earliest example on record of this treatment is "Coley's toxin," illustrated in Figure 9.39.

In modern times, various bacterial preparations such as BCG, an attenuated strain of *Mycobacterium tuberculosis*, were given systemically or locally in the tumor. After many trials with mixed results the method was abandoned, with the exception of intravesical injections for the treatment of superficial bladder cancer (35, 69). We have reason to suspect that the violent, painful cystitis produced by this method simply causes the whole bladder mucosa to be shed, including the cancer. A more effective manner of boosting the immune system

is the injection of interleukin-2 (IL-2), which is now approved for treating melanoma and renal cell carcinoma (70).

Lymphokine activation of killer cells. The principle is to expand and activate a patient's population of cytotoxic cells by means of IL-2 (71, 72).

Several variants were tried: (a) Lymphokine-activated cells (LAK cells) were obtained from the patient's blood, treated *in vitro* for 2–3 days with IL-2 and then reinfused. These were mainly NK cells and cytotoxic T cells. (b) Tissue-infiltrating lymphocytes (TILs) obtained from the patient's tumor were prepared in the same manner. They gave the best results (Figure 30.7) (73). This imaginative approach (*adoptive cellular immunotherapy*) has serious side effects, but the latest version is safer (18b).

Tested on patients with advanced metastatic disease, the LAK and TIL methods triggered striking regressions in some melanomas and renal cell carcinomas. One serious

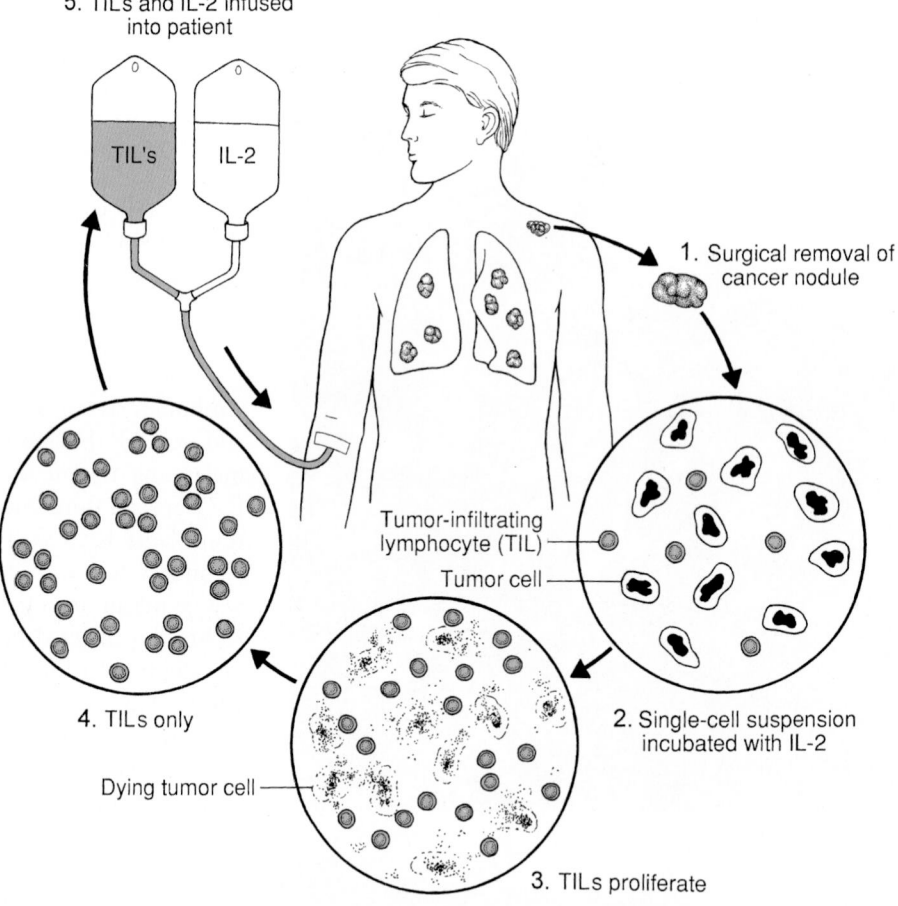

FIGURE 30.7 **1–5:** Use of tumor-infiltrating lymphocytes (TIL) as antitumor therapy. (Adapted with permission from [71]. Original illustration by C. Donner.)

5. TILs and IL-2 infused into patient

TIL's   IL-2

1. Surgical removal of cancer nodule

Tumor-infiltrating lymphocyte (TIL)

Tumor cell

2. Single-cell suspension incubated with IL-2

Dying tumor cell

4. TILs only

3. TILs proliferate

side effect is edema due to a diffuse vascular leak syndrome (74); rats and mice treated with IL-2 developed the same syndrome (Figure 30.8) (6), and infiltrates of lymphocytes and eosinophils appeared throughout the body (Figure 30.9). The vascular leakage is attributed to activation of venular endothelium by IL-2 and IL-2–generated cytokines (4, 16). A major threat is pulmonary edema: the LAK and TIL cells, being activated, are stiffer; therefore they tend to become trapped in the capillaries of the lung rather than reaching their intended target, the tumor (43).

Cancer vaccines: preventive. Because 15 percent of cancers worldwide are due to infectious agents, preventive vaccination against the infectious agent should save many lives. The three main candidates (54) are *hepatitis B virus,* for which the first data have shown that vaccination is indeed effective in preventing liver carcinoma (p. 868); *human papillomavirus type 16,* present in 50 percent of cervical cancers. In 2002, a study on 2392 young women followed for a median of 17 months showed 100 percent efficacy: 0 cases of intraepithelial neoplasia in the vaccinated group, 9 cases in the placebo group (46a); and *Helicobacter pylori,* which can be subdued by antibiotics, but

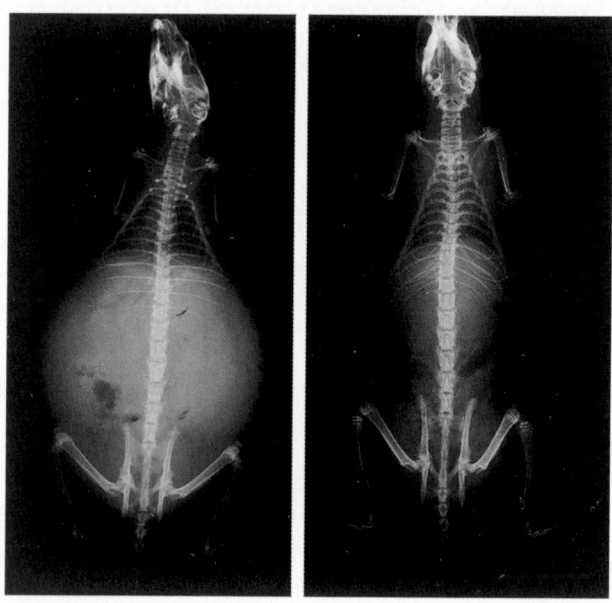

FIGURE 30.8   Ascites as part of the vascular-leak syndrome induced by recombinant interleukin-2. *Left,* a rat treated with IL-2 twice a day for 14 days; *right,* the control. (Reproduced by permission from [3], © by The US & Canadian Academy of Pathology, Inc.)

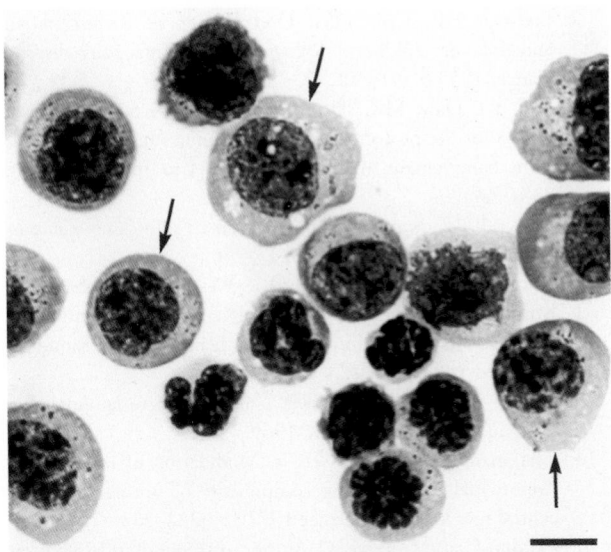

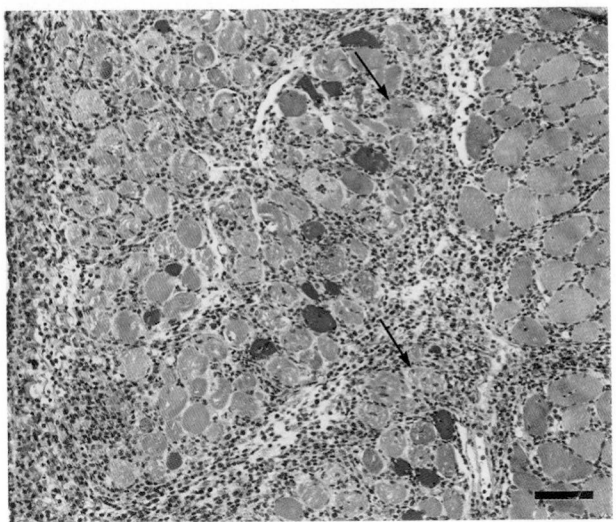

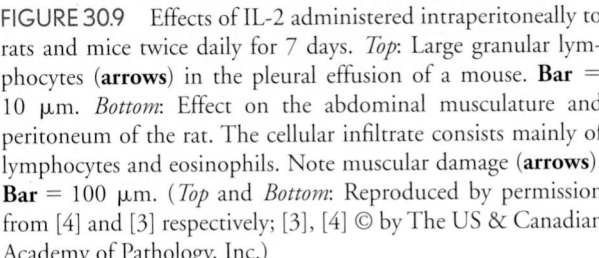

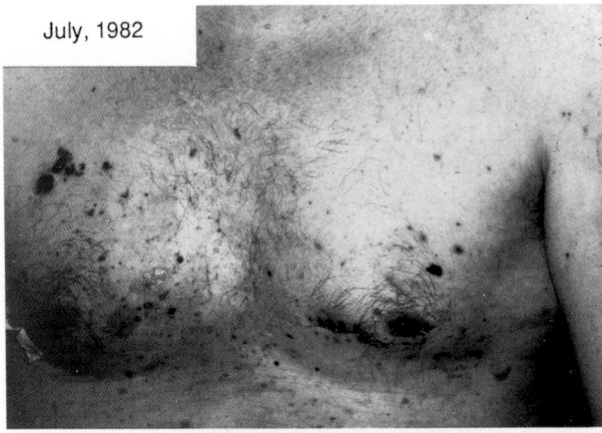

July, 1982

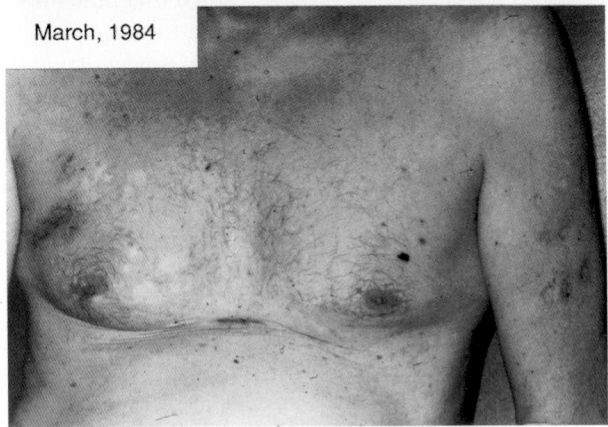

March, 1984

FIGURE 30.10 Regression of metastases from malignant melanoma after a double treatment: cyclophosphamide, to suppress the T-suppressor cells, which inhibit the antitumor response (59) and autologous vaccine against melanoma. (The residual pigmented lesion on the left breast is a benign and probably dysplastic nevus.) (Reproduced with permission from [8].)

FIGURE 30.9 Effects of IL-2 administered intraperitoneally to rats and mice twice daily for 7 days. *Top*: Large granular lymphocytes (**arrows**) in the pleural effusion of a mouse. **Bar** = 10 μm. *Bottom*: Effect on the abdominal musculature and peritoneum of the rat. The cellular infiltrate consists mainly of lymphocytes and eosinophils. Note muscular damage (**arrows**). **Bar** = 100 μm. (*Top* and *Bottom*: Reproduced by permission from [4] and [3] respectively; [3], [4] © by The US & Canadian Academy of Pathology, Inc.)

antibiotic resistance can develop; vaccines are being tested. Cats can be vaccinated against leukemia retrovirus since 1985 (39).

Cancer vaccines: therapeutic (42, 70). In this situation we are dealing with patients who already have a cancer; in theory, a vaccine should boost their defenses against it (84a). Vaccines have been prepared with dozens of antigens (proteins), including MAGE-1 and MAGE-2, prostate-specific antigen, mutated p53, mutated *ras*, and so on. Some striking temporary regressions were obtained (Figure 30.10) but no vaccine proved to be the magic bullet. Another method has been to harvest cells from the patient's tumor, irradiate them to prevent multiplication, and reinject them with an adjuvant—or with dendritic cells—to improve the response. Yet another approach: transfect the tumor cells *in vitro* so that they generate cytokines or other helpful molecules.

Many other biological treatments are being tried in mice and a few also in people. Interferons have been rather disappointing (19, 38, 62) except interferon-alpha-2a for treating life-threatening hemangiomas in infants (21). Macrophages activated with liposomes have eradicated experimental metastases (22, 23). Antitumor-antibodies coupled with drugs or radioactive nuclides hold some promise due to their theoretically unbeatable specificity (64); however, they also run into a formidable series of obstacles: (1) only a fraction of the injected antibody reaches its target because the endothelial barrier stands between the antibody and the tumor; (2) injected antibodies are antigenic; and (3) the antibodies are quickly removed by the system of mononuclear phagocytes.

TO SUM UP: Natural antitumor defenses do exist, they can be boosted, and there is reason to hope that it will be possible to boost them even further. As expected, we have learned that built-in antitumor defenses differ from one tumor to another; the likelihood of finding a single magic bullet against all tumors is as great as that of finding a single antibiotic against all infections. We have also learned that tumors have unexpected links with inflammation.

References

1. Abersold P. Antiproliferative effects of interferon. In: Ransom JH, Ortaldo JR, eds. Leukolysins and cancer. Clifton, NJ: Human Press, 1987, pp. 101–117.

2. An T, Sood U, Pietruk T, Cummings G, Hashimoto K, Crissman JD. *In situ* quantitation of inflammatory mononuclear cells in ductal infiltrating breast carcinoma. Relation to prognostic parameters. Am J Pathol 1987;128:52–60.

3. Anderson TD, Hayes TJ. Toxicity of human recombinant interleukin-2 in rats. Pathologic changes are characterized by marked lymphocytic and eosinophilic proliferation and multisystem involvement. Lab Invest 1989;60:331–346.

4. Anderson TD, Hayes TJ, Gately MK, Bontempo JM, Stern LL, Truitt GA. Toxicity of human recombinant interleukin-2 in the mouse is mediated by interleukin-activated lymphocytes. Separation of efficacy and toxicity by selective lymphocyte subset depletion. Lab Invest 1988;59:598–612.

5. Avis IM, Jett M, Boyle T, et al. Growth control of lung cancer by interruption of 5-lipoxygenase-mediated growth factor signaling. J Clin Invest 1996;97:806–813.

6. Banner BF, Sonmez-Alpan E, Yousem SA. An immunophenotypic study of the inflammatory cell populations in colon adenomas and carcinomas. Mod Pathol 1993;6:295–301.

7. Ben-Ezra J, Sheibani K. Antigenic phenotype of the lymphocytic component of medullary carcinoma of the breast. Cancer 1987;59:2037–2041.

8. Berd D, Maguire HC Jr, Mastrangelo MJ. Induction of cell-mediated immunity to autologous melanoma cells and regression of metastases after treatment with a melanoma cell vaccine preceded by cyclophosphamide. Cancer Res 1986;46:2572–2577.

9. Bierman HR, Crile DM, Dod KS, et al. Remissions in leukemia of childhood following acute infectious disease. Cancer 1953;6:591–605.

10. Blok VT, Daha MR, Tijsma OMH, et al. A possible role of CD46 for the protection in vivo of human renal tumor cells from complement-mediated damage. Lab Invest 2000;80:335–344.

11. Boutwell RK. Some biological aspects of skin carcinogenesis. Prog Exp Tumor Res 1964;4:207–250.

12. Brunda MJ, Luistro L, Warner RR, Wright RB, Hubbard BR, Murphy M, Wolf SF, Gately MK. Antitumor and antimetastatic activity of interleukin 12 against murine tumors. J Exp Med 1993;178:1223–1230.

13. Burnet FM. Self and not-self. Carleton, Victoria, Australia: Melbourne University Press, 1969.

14. Chapman HA Jr, Hibbs JB Jr. Modulation of macrophage tumoricidal capability by components of normal serum: a central role for lipid. Science 1977;197:282–285.

15. Cordon-Cardo C, Prives C. At the crossroads of inflammation and tumorigenesis. J Exp Med 1999;190:1367–1370.

16. Cotran RS, Pober JS, Gimbrone MA Jr, et al. Endothelial activation during interleukin 2 immunotherapy. A possible mechanism for the vascular leak syndrome. J Immunol 1987;139:1883–1888.

17. Coussens LM, Werb Z. Inflammatory cells and cancer: Think different! J Exp Med 2001;193:F23–F26.

18. Di Carlo E, Forni G, Lollini PL, et al. The intriguing role of polymorphonuclear neutrophils in antitumor reactions. Blood 2001;97:339–345.

18a. Dranoff G. Tumour immunology. Immune recognition and tumor protection. Curr Opin Immunol 2002;14:161–164.

18b. Dudley ME, Wunderlich JR, Robbins PF, et al. Cancer regression and autoimmunity in patients after clonal repopulation with antitumor lymphocytes. Science 2002;298:850–854.

19. Eron LJ, Judson F, Tucker S, et al. Interferon therapy for condylomata acuminata. N Engl J Med 1986;315:1059–1064.

20. Evans R. Tumor macrophages in host immunity to malignancies. In: Fink MA, ed. The macrophage in neoplasia. New York: Academic Press, 1976, pp. 27–42.

21. Ezekowitz RAB, Mulliken JB, Folkman J. Interferon alfa-2a therapy for life-threatening hemangiomas of infancy. N Engl J Med 1992;326:1456–1463.

22. Fidler IJ. Macrophage therapy of cancer metastasis. Ciba Found Symp 1988;141:211–222.

23. Fidler IJ, Schroit AJ. Recognition and destruction of neoplastic cells by activated macrophages: discrimination of altered self. Biochim Biophys Acta 1988;948:151–173.

24. Finke J, Ferrone S, Frey A, Mufson A, Ochoa A. Where have all the T-cells gone? Mechanisms of immune evasion by tumors. Immunol Today 1999;20:158–160.

25. Fontan E, Saklani H, Fauve RM. Macrophage-induced cytotoxicity and anti-metastatic activity of a 43-kDa human urinary protein against the Lewis tumor. Int J Cancer 1993;53:131–136.

26. Ghosh J, Myers CE. Arachidonic acid stimulates prostate cancer cell growth: Critical role of 5-lipoxygenase. Biochem Biophys Res Commun 1997;235:418–423.

27. Giovannucci E, Egan KM, Hunter DJ, et al. Aspirin and the risk of colorectal cancer in women. N Engl J Med 1995;333: 609–614.

28. Graeber TG, Peterson JF, Tsai M, Monica K, Fornace Jr AJ, Giaccia AJ. Hypoxia induces accumulation of p53 protein, but activation of a G_1-phase checkpoint by low-oxygen conditions is independent of p53 status. Mol Cell Biol 1994;14:6264–6277.

29. Graeber TG, Osmanian C, Jacks T, Housman DE, Koch CJ, Lowe SW, Giaccia AJ. Hypoxia-mediated selection of cells with diminished apoptotic potential in solid tumours. Nature 1996;379:88–91.

30. Graves DT, Jiang YL, Williamson MJ, Valente AJ. Identification of monocyte chemotactic activity produced by malignant cells. Science 1989;245:1490–1493.

31. Greenblatt MS, Bennett WP, Hollstein M, Harris CC. Mutations in the p53 tumor suppressor gene: clues to cancer etiology and molecular pathogenesis. Cancer Res 1994;54: 4855–4878.

32. Griffith TS, Wiley SR, Kubin MZ, et al. Monocyte-mediated tumoricidal activity via the tumor necrosis factor-related cytokin, TRAIL. J Exp Med 1999;189:1343–1353.

33. Gross L. Oncogenic viruses, vol 2, 3rd ed. Oxford: Pergamon Press, 1983.

34. Gugel EA, Sanders ME. Needle-stick transmission of human colonic adenocarcinoma. N Engl J Med 1986;315:1487.

35. Guinan P, Crispen R, Rubenstein M. BCG in management of superficial bladder cancer. Urology 1987;30:515–519.

36. Hakulinen J, Meri S. Complement-mediated killing of microtumors *in vitro*. Am J Pathol 1998;153:845–855.

37. Haskill S, Bécker S, Fowler W, Walton L. Mononuclear-cell infiltration in ovarian cancer. I. Inflammatory-cell infiltrates from tumour and ascites material. Br J Cancer 1982;45: 728–736.

38. Healy GB, Gelver RD, Trowbridge AL, Grundfast KM, Ruben RJ, Price KN. Treatment of recurrent respiratory papillomatosis with human leukocyte interferon. Results of a multicenter randomized clinical trial. N Engl J Med 1988;319: 401–407.

39. Hilleman MR. Overview of viruses, cancer, and vaccines in concept and in reality. Recent Results Cancer Res 1998;154: 345–362.

40. Hudson JD, Shoaibi MA, Maestro R, et al. A proinflammatory cytokine inhibits p53 tumor suppressor activity. J Exp Med 1999;190:1375–1382.

41. Hwu P. Gene therapy. In: Cancer. Principles & practice of oncology. Philadelphia: Lippincott Williams & Wilkins. 2001, pp. 3161–3180.

42. Jaffee EM. Progress toward cancer vaccines. Hosp Prac 2000; 35:49–65.

43. Jain RK. Delivery of molecules, particles and cells to solid tumors (Whitaker Lecture). Annal of Biomed 1996;24: 457–473.

44. Kerr JFR, Winterford CM. Apoptosis. Cancer 1994;73: 2013–2026.

45. Klein G. Tumor immunology. Transplant Proc 1973;5:31–41.

46. Klein G. Immune and non-immune control of neoplastic development: contrasting effects of host and tumor evolution. Cancer 1980;45:2486–2499.

46a. Koutsky LA, Ault KA, Wheeler CM, et al. A controlled trial of a human papillomavirus type 16 vaccine. N Engl J Med 2002;347:1645–1651.

47. Kradin RL, Bhan AK. Tumor infiltrating lymphocytes. Lab Invest 1993;69:635–638.

47a. Kreider DW, Bartlett GL. Is there a host response to metastasis? Prog Clin Biol Res 1986;212:61–75.

48. Kripe ML. Immunoregulation of carcinogenesis: past, present and future. J Natl Cancer Inst 1988;80:722–727.

49. Lane DP, Lu X, Hupp T, Hall PA. The role of the p53 protein in the apoptotic response. Phil Trans R Soc Lond B 1994;345: 277–280.

50. Lester EP, Miller JB, Yachnin S. Human alpha-fetoprotein as a modulator of human lymphocyte transformation: correlation of biological potency with electrophoretic variants. Proc Natl Acad Sci USA 1976;73:4645–4648.

51. Liebelt AG. Malignant neoplasms in organ transplant recipients. In: Levine AS, ed. Etiology of cancer in man. Dordrecht: Kluwer Academic Publishers, 1989, pp. 136–167.

52. Lin EY, Nguyen AV, Russell RG, Pollard JW. Colony-stimulating factor 1 promotes progression of mammary tumors to malignancy. J Exp Med 2001;193:727–739.

53. Lotze MT, Dallal RM, Kirkwood JM, Flickinger JC. Cutaneous melanoma. In: Cancer. Principles & practice of oncology. Philadelphia: Lippincott Williams & Wilkins. 2001, pp. 2012–2069.

54. Lowy DR, Schiller JT. Preventive cancer vaccines. Cancer. Principles & practice of oncology. Philadelphia: Lippincott Williams & Wilkins. 2001, pp. 3189–3195.

55. Lynch SA, Houghton AN. Cancer Immunology. Curr Opin Oncol 1993;5:145–150.

56. Mandelboim O, Vadai E, Fridkin M, Katz-Hillel A, Feldman M, Berke G, Eisenbach L. Regression of Established Murine Carcinoma Metastases Following Vaccination with Tumor-Associated Antigen Peptides. Nature Med 1995;1:1179–1183.

57. Marx J. Oncogenes Reach a Milestone. Science 1994;266: 1942–1944.

58. Marx J. Anti-inflammatories inhibit cancer growth-but how? Science 2001;291:581–582.

59. Marx JL. Cancer vaccines show promise at last. Science 1989;245:813–815.

60. Musiani P, Allione A, Modica A, et al. Role of neutrophils and lymphocytes in inhibition of a mouse mammary adenocarcinoma engineered to release IL-2, IL-4, IL-7, IL-10, IFN-α, IFN-γ, and TNF-α. Lab Invest 1996;74:146–157.

61. Okabayashi M, Angell MG, Budgeon LR, Kreider JW. Shope papilloma cell and leukocyte proliferation in regressing and progressing lesions. Am J Pathol 1993;142:489–496.

62. Oldham RK. Biologicals for cancer treatment: interferons. Hosp Pract 1985;20:71–91.

63. Perussia B. Tumor infiltrating cells. Lab Invest 1992;67: 155–157.

64. Pimm MV. Drug-monoclonal antibody conjugates for cancer therapy: potentials and limitations. CRC Crit Rev Ther Drug Carrier Systems 1988;5:189–227.

65. Porter PL, Gown AM, Kramp SG, Coltrera MD. Widespread p53 Overexpression in Human Malignant Tumors. Am J Pathol 1992;140:145–153.

66. Poste G. The tumoricidal properties of inflammatory tissue macrophages and multinucleate giant cells. Am J Pathol 1979;96:595–610.

67. Purtilo DT. Defective immune surveillane in viral carcinogenesis. Lab Invest 1984;51:373–385.

68. Radoja S, Frey AB. Cancer-induced defective cytotoxic T lymphocyte effector function: Another mechanism how antigenic tumors escape immune-mediated killing. Mol Med 2000;6:465–479.

69. Raghavan D, Shipley WU, Garnick MB, Russell PJ, Richie JP. Biology and management of bladder cancer. N Engl J Med 1990;322:1129–1138.

70. Restifo NP, Sznol M, Overwijk WW. Therapeutic cancer vaccines. Cancer. Principles & practice of oncology. Philadelphia: Lippincott Williams & Wilkins. 2001, pp. 3195–3217.

71. Rosenberg SA. Adoptive immunotherapy for cancer. Sci Am 1990;262:62–69.

72. Rosenberg SA, Lotze MT, Muul LM, et al. A progress report on the treatment of 157 patients with advanced cancer using lymphokine-activated killer cells and interleukin-2 or high-dose interleukin-2 alone. N Engl J Med 1987;316:889–897.

73. Rosenberg SA, Spiess P, Lafreniere R. A new approach to the adoptive immunotherapy of cancer with tumor-infiltrating lymphocytes. Science 1986;233:1318–1321.

74. Rosenstein M, Ettinghausen SE, Rosenberg SA. Extravasation of intravascular fluid mediated by the systemic administration of recombinant interleukin 2. J Immunol 1986;137:1735–1742.

75. Ruckdeschel JC, Codish SD, Stranahan A, McKneally MF. Postoperative empyema improves survival in lung cancer. Documentation and analysis of a natural experiment. N Engl J Med 1972;287:1013–1017.

76. Russell SW, Gillespie GY, Pace JL. Evidence for mononuclear phagocytes in solid neoplasms and appraisal of their non-specific cytotoxic capabilities. Contemp Top Immunobiol 1980;10:143–166.

77. Scanlon EF, Hawkins RA, Fox WW, Smith WS. Fatal homotransplanted melanoma. A case report. Cancer 1965;18:782–789.

78. Schrump DS, Nguyen DM. Malignant pleural and pericardial effusions. In: Cancer. Principles & practice of oncology. Philadelphia: Lippincott Williams & Wilkins. 2001, pp. 2729–2744.

79. Sogn JA. Tumor Immunology: The glass is half full. Immunity 1998;9:757–763.

80. Sonoshita M, Takaku K, Sasaki N, et al. Acceleration of intestinal polyposis through prostaglandin receptor EP2 in $Apc^{\Delta 716}$ knockout mice. Nature Med 2001;7:1048–1051.

81. Strominger JL. Peptide vaccination against cancer? Nature Med 1995;1:1140.

82. Symonds H, Krall L, Remington L, Saenz-Robies M, Lowe S, Jacks T, Van Dyke T. Dependent apoptosis supresses tumor growth and progression in vivo. Cell 1994;78:703–711.

83. Tauber AI, Chernyak L. Metchnikoff and the origins of immunology. From metaphor to theory. New York: Oxford University Press, 1991.

84. Wahl AF, Donaldson KL, Fairchild C, Lee FYF, Foster SA, Demers GW, Galloway DA. Loss of normal p53 function confers sensitization to Taxol by increasing G2/M arrest and apoptosis. Nature Med 1996;2:72–79.

84a. Waldmann TA. Immunotherapy: past, present and future. Nat Med 2003;9:269–277.

85. Wiltrout RH. Regulation and antimetastatic functions of liver-associated natural killer cells. Immunol Rev 2000;174:63–76.

86. Yesner R. A pathologist's view of tumor dormancy. In: Stewart THM, Wheelock EF, eds. Cellular immune mechanisms and tumor dormancy. Boca Raton, FL: CRC Press, 1992.

87. Yunis AA, Arimura GK, Wu F-M, Wu M-C. Differentiation of cultured promyelocytic leukemia cells (HL-60) induced by endotoxin-treated human lung conditioned medium. Leukemia Res 1987;11:673–679.

88. Zhang L, Khayat A, Cheng H, Graves DT. The pattern of monocyte recruitment in tumors is modulated by MCP-1 expression and influences the rate of tumor growth. Lab Invest 1997;76:579–590.

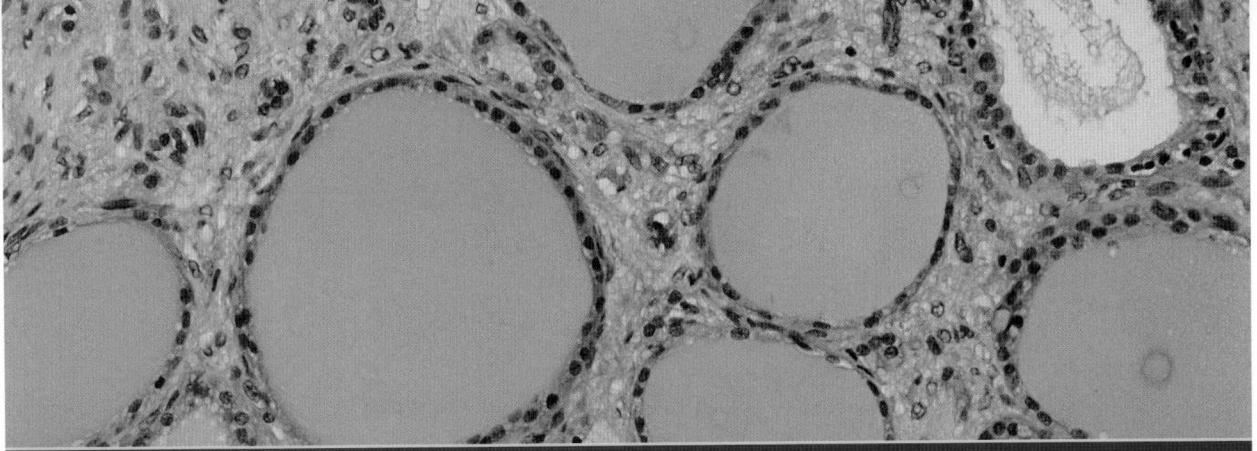

CHAPTER 31

THE REVERSIBILITY OF TUMORS

- Spontaneous Regression of Tumors
- Tumor Regression in the Laboratory

For the reader weary of invasion, metastasis, and other nefarious events, this chapter offers some measure of relief. Yes, there is a great deal to say about the reversibility of tumors; in fact this chapter includes experiments as thrilling as any reported in this book. They should demolish the notion that tumors are invincible monsters.

By regression of a tumor we mean shrinkage, which may or may not lead to total disappearance. Some regressions are temporary. Complete regression has been observed in the laboratory and in medical practice. The most intriguing regressions are those that occur in the absence of therapy; they are called spontaneous. However, it is well to remember that the label *spontaneous* is applied to biological events of which we do not know the cause.

Spontaneous Regression of Tumors

There is one tumor that regresses spontaneously in most patients (80–90 percent): the hemangioma of infants, which occurs in 2.6 percent of newborns. It usually appears within 2–4 weeks of birth, grows very fast, begins to regress, and is gone by age 10, usually leaving a scar (Figure 31.1) (35, 36). Most cases are managed without treatment other than a great deal of time spent reassuring parents (3). Unfortunately, 100 percent reassurance is not appropriate because a minority of hemangiomas, unpredictably, do not regress. Nor is the mechanism of regression understood, except that it is not thrombosis or infarction; the endothelial channels just seem to fade away. Herein lies a great challenge.

Anecdotal records of malignant tumors that disappeared without treatment are available at least since 1900, but histologic control was skimpy before 1950. The collected series of 176 regressions published between 1900 and 1966 includes transient regressions (8, 9, 13, 37, 38). Most of the cases listed

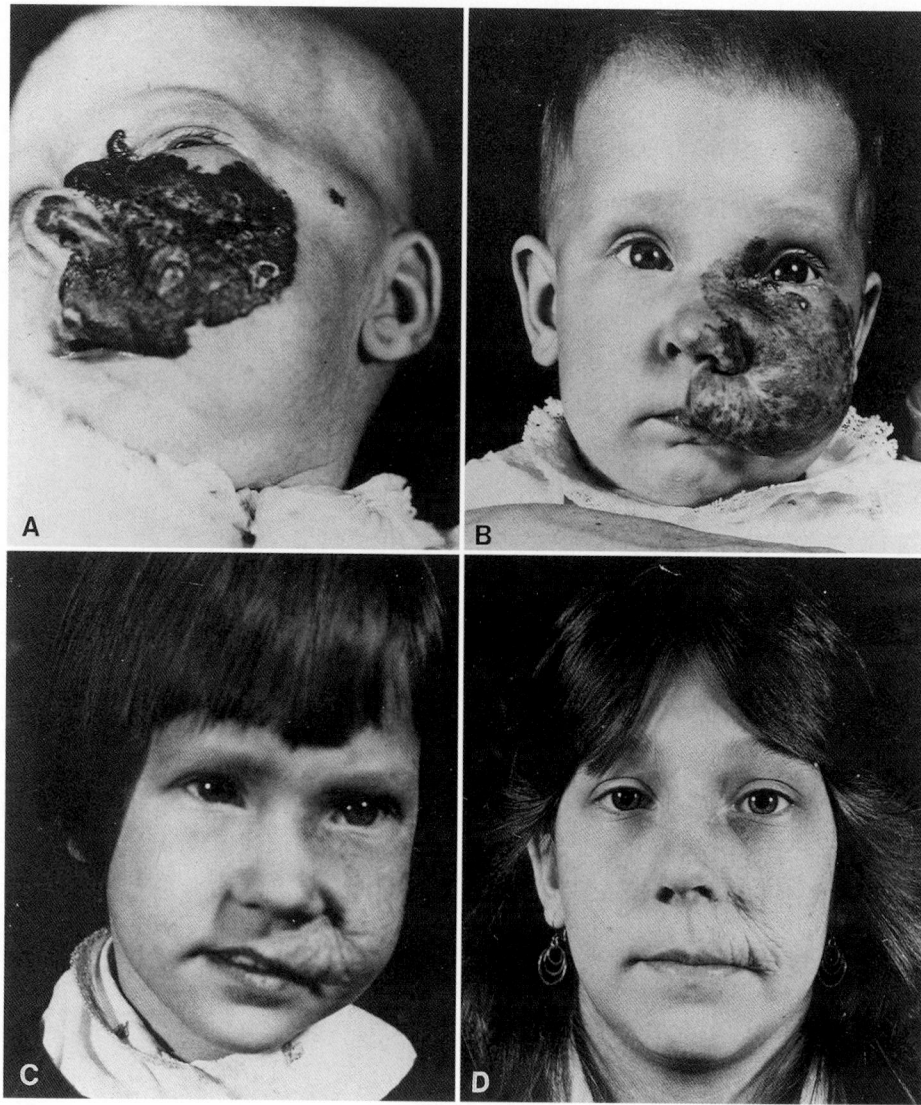

concern renal cell carcinoma (33), neuroblastoma (31), melanoma (19), choriocarcinoma (19), and carcinoma of the bladder (13). In 41 cases, metastases regressed after resection of the primary. Documented malignant tumors that disappeared are just a few.

An example: two patients underwent palliative operations for carcinoma of the stomach without resection; the tumor masses disappeared and the patients were well 10 and 11 years later (8). Considering that gastric cancer allows a 5-year survival of 5–17 percent, the reported survival itself is remarkable; as to the disappearance of the tumors, it is close to miraculous.

Currently, a review of the literature shows that spontaneous or unexplained regressions are reported—worldwide—every year, but not for all types of malignancies; the most liable to regress spontaneously include the four listed above: neuroblastoma, renal

cell carcinoma, melanoma, choriocarcinoma, and hepatoma. Although every one of these cases has something baffling about it, several distinct mechanisms of regression are hinted (4, 39).

Neuroblastomas in infants can change from malignant to benign, metastases included. Neuroblastomas can develop anywhere in the sympathetic nervous system, but usually in the adrenal, and many have metastasized by the time they are diagnosed. Neuroblasts as seen by electron microscopy contain typical neurosecretory granules (p. 958). By light microscopy they are dull-looking small round cells; but they become much more interesting when they mature into neurons with axons and dendrites (Figure 31.2). The fully differentiated tumors are called *ganglioneuromas.* This type of regression obviously amounts to differentiation. It can occur spontaneously in children; parts of tumor tissue left behind by the surgeon rarely cause a relapse.

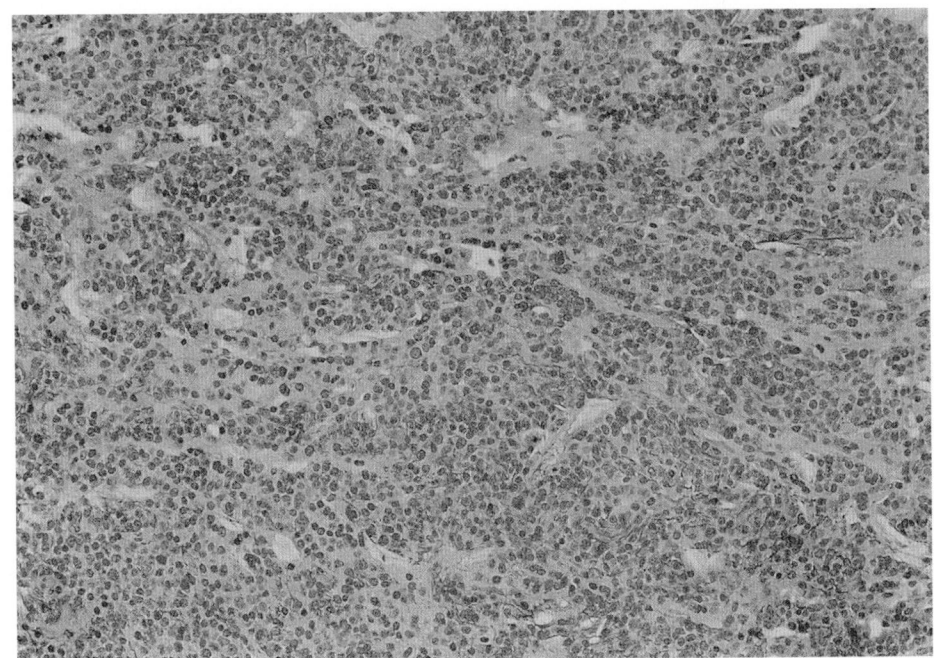

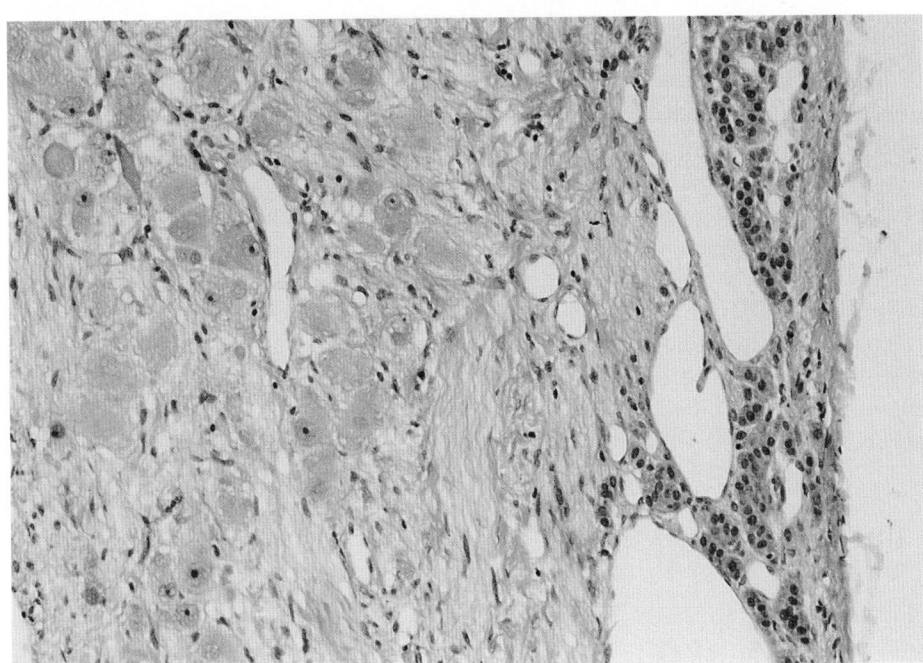

FIGURE 31.2   Nearly a miracle: spontaneous differentiation of a malignant neuroblastoma of the adrenal into a benign ganglioneuroma. *Top:* Biopsy of a neuroblastoma of the adrenal in a little girl age 8. *Bottom:* The same tumor 4 years later. The bulk is represented by mature neurons (the huge cells at left). What is left of the stretched-out, atrophic, paper-thin adrenal in the capsule of the tumor is seen at right. (180x)

However, the prognosis remains poor because the tumor is often diagnosed too late (48). This fascinating—and frustrating—behavior of neuroblastomas has inspired a great deal of research.

Interestingly, the first known case of regressed neuroblastoma, published in 1927 (10), concerned a child who had been treated with the "toxins" of the now-famous Dr. Coley mentioned on p. 365. From what we know now, that particular tumor might have regressed anyway.

Microscopic nodules of neuroblasts are present in all human fetuses (at 18–20 weeks) then disappear; how this relates to the regression of neuroblastoma is not known.

The mechanism of regression in this case is actually not regressive at all—it is DIFFERENTIATION, a theme that will continue to recur in our discussion of tumors.

Two other mechanisms have been suggested to explain the regression of neuroblastomas: **hypomethylation of the DNA** and **diminished activity of telomerase** (39).

Melanoma deserves special mention because, despite its fearful reputation, which is well deserved, it displays ambivalent behavior. The primary tumor can regress partially or even completely; this explains the occasional finding of metastatic melanoma in the absence of a primary melanoma (which went unnoticed and then disappeared). In a review of 5000 cases of melanoma, regression of metastases occurred in 2.2 cases per 1000 (37). Some of the events preceding the regression of metastases are intriguing:

- Pregnancy (an immunosuppressive condition)
- An abscess near the tumor
- A bite by a rabid dog followed by 14 injections of antirabies vaccine
- Blood transfusion from a patient who had shown regression of skin metastases from a melanoma (8)
- Consumption of a lot of garlic (37) (for another reference to garlic and tumors see p. 846)

Overall, regression of melanoma suggests an immunologic mechanism, a concept that is being exploited for therapy (p. 917). In a study of 36 cases, the only histologic difference with non-regressing melanomas was a greater number of T-helper cells (CD4$^+$) (57). This suggests that cytokine-secreting cells, rather than killer cells, are doing the job.

Retinoblastoma occasionally heals by turning its cells into the corresponding mature cell type: it becomes a *retinoma* or *retinocytoma* (50). This is, once again, the pattern followed by the neuroblastoma: DIFFERENTIATION. But retinoblastoma has yet another possibility: the eye receives blood from a single artery; by compressing it, the tumor has caused INFARCTION of the eye, tumor included.

Hepatoma is also known to regress: up to the year 2000, 11 cases were reported in the English literature (58). In one, INFARCTION was involved, due to thrombosis of a portal branch (58). In fact, hepatoma is one of the few tumors for which embolic therapy is currently being attempted.

Metastases of renal cell carcinoma are known to regress (33 cases between 1969 and 1995 [26, 66]). Many regressions were associated with removal, irradiation or embolization of the primary site. In such cases, we can hypothesize—according to Folkman's theory of angiogenic/angiostatic balance (14)—that the metastases were being maintained by angiogenic factor(s) supplied by the primary.

Regressing Lymphomas and *Helicobacter pylori*. This is the latest and perhaps most surprising addition to tumor regressions. *Helicobacter pylori* is associated not only with gastric carcinoma but also with low-grade gastric lymphoma. Several patients with such lymphomas have been treated *with antibiotics* and were cured (34, 60, 65).

There is more. A 69-year-old man presented with a lymphoma developing in Hashimoto thyroiditis, plus gastric cancer with *H. pylori* infection. Gastrectomy was followed by shrinkage of the lymphoma; *H. pylori* eradication therapy caused the lymphoma to disappear (1a). Perhaps another case of the "Folkman angiogenesis imbalance" just mentioned?

We mention these selected cases to remind the reader that such "miracles" do happen. The trouble is that even when a mechanism is hinted, we do not (yet) know how to trigger it.

Tumor Regression in the Laboratory

The first steps along this trail take us back to the Rockefeller Institute in 1940. Rous and Kidd, who had tarred many a rabbit, wrote that tar carcinomas were preceded by warty growths that had the histological appearance of tumors, including local invasiveness, but vanished if tarring was discontinued. Rous and Kidd concluded that these tumors, which they called papillomas or "carcinomatoids," had not yet acquired the capacity for independent growth; they disappeared "when no longer aided."

Judging from the published illustrations, the disappearance was accomplished by epithelial differentiation into keratinized masses (Figure 31.3). This important observation was not followed up for decades; tumors that do not kill, like all good news, make no headlines. There seems to be something dull about benign tumors. As Rous put it, "cancers outdo them in material interest" (51).

Then several astonishing experiments proved that established malignant tumors could be reversed. We will list six, the first one from the plant kingdom.

The crown gall. As mentioned on p. 857 the crown gall is a malignant tumor of plants. It is created by a bacterium that operates along the classic principles of genetic engineering. The plant must be wounded and then infected with *Agrobacterium*. If we choose the right experimental conditions, it is possible to produce

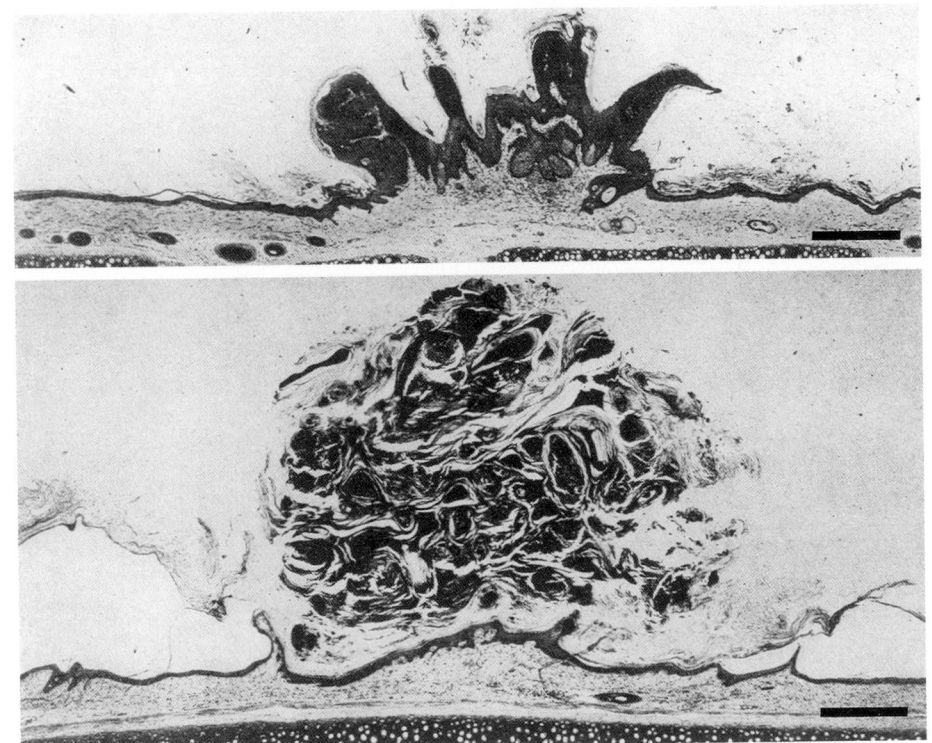

FIGURE 31.3 Histology of papillomas produced with tar in the rabbit ear; original illustrations published by Rous and Kidd in 1941. *Top:* Growing papilloma. *Bottom:* "Superficial carcinomatoid in the process of retrogression." Tarring had been stopped 24 days previously; the cells then turned into "normal" differentiated keratinized cells, indicating a reversion of the neoplasm to normal. Rous and Kidd called these tumors "conditional neoplasms." **Bars** = 500 μm. (Reproduced from the **Journal of Experimental Medicine,** 1941;73:365–390, by copyright permission of The Rockefeller University Press [51].)

a type of tumor appropriately called a *teratoma,* a chaotic mass of partly developed tissues and organs. It is a fully malignant tumor, capable of growing (like other malignant crown gall tumors) on a simple culture medium that would not support the growth of normal cells (5, 6). Now, if we graft a fragment of teratoma onto the tip of the stem of a normal, severed tobacco plant, the graft will grow; but it will be partially tamed into a less abnormal tissue. Graft this tissue onto a second stem, and then again onto a third one; now the tumor growth will gradually develop into a normal plant that will flower and go to seed. The seeds will produce normal tobacco plants (Figure 31.4).

From these and other experiments, Armin Braun concluded that the original tumor was probably not caused by damage to the DNA (such as by mutation) but by altered expression of the genome. Another way to interpret these results would be that the environment of a growing normal tissue was able to control the cellular misbehavior encoded in a faulty DNA. This theme will recur.

A tadpole grown from a tumor. Let us proceed to frogs. In the northern United States, roughly 5 percent of common leopard frogs (*Rana pipiens*) suffer from a virus-induced tumor of the kidney known as *Lucké adenocarcinoma* (Figure 31.5) (27–29, 31, 33). In 1960, King and McKinnell (and later others) obtained fresh eggs

from leopard frogs, fertilized them, then removed their nucleus and replaced it with a nucleus from a malignant cell of a Lucké adenocarcinoma (Figure 31.6). A few of the eggs did develop. What did they produce? More adenocarcinomas? Tadpoles loaded with tumors? Neither. They produced tadpoles (Figure 31.7) (29, 30). These miraculous creatures did not live beyond 10–14 days, perhaps because their foster nucleus had lost the next part of the program, but they certainly made history.

This experiment was criticized because—in theory— some of the original nuclear material could have been inadvertently left behind. This objection was met by using triploid tumors and diploid eggs; the result: triploid tadpoles (28).

The method for producing triploid tadpoles is most imaginative: a bout of very high hydrostatic pressure on the fertilized egg prevents the extrusion of the second polar body (11).

Conclusion: The malignant nucleus was tamed by the cytoplasm of the fertilized egg. Therefore, in triggering neoplasia, the cytoplasm can be as important as the nucleus. The cytoplasm could exert its influence by modifying gene expression. By definition, this type of nongenetic influence is called epigenetic.

A mouse grown from a tumor. A parallel experiment has been done with mouse teratocarcinomas.

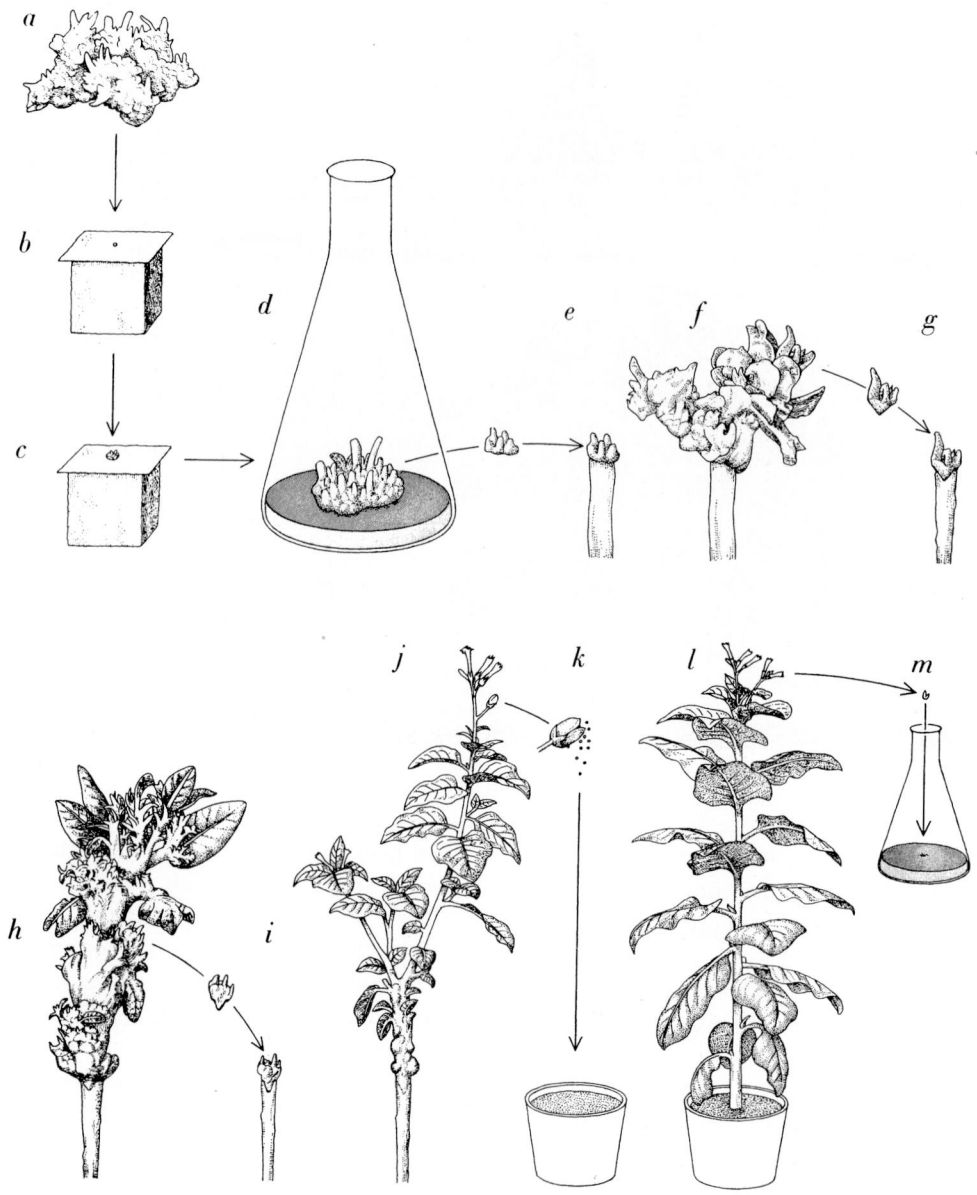

FIGURE 31.4   Reversal of malignant growth in plants. Teratoma from a tobacco plant (**a**) provides a single tumor cell (**b**) that is grown *in vitro* (**c**); in (**d**) the tissue is grown in a basic culture medium where it forms typical teratoma buds and leaves. One of the buds is then grafted onto the cut stem of a normal tobacco plant (**e**) and allowed to develop (**f**). A bud from this abnormal growth is grafted to a second normal plant (**g**) and allowed to develop again (**h**). A bud from the second plant grafted onto a third host (**i**) gradually becomes normal; it flowers (**j**) and goes to seed (**k**). Tobacco plants raised from this seed (**l**) are completely normal. Their cells do not grow on the basic medium (**m**). (Reproduced with permission from [5].)

We should first describe these complex tumors as they appear in mice. They contain 8–14 different mature cell types as well as undifferentiated malignant cells known as embryonal carcinoma cells (Figure 31.8) (23, 42, 47). There are two amazing features about these tumors: they can be produced by implanting a mouse embryo in the testis of another mouse (56), and then they can be maintained as an ascites tumor by passing them from one mouse peritoneum to another. As the malignant cells grow freely in the serosal cavity, they produce small cystic structures that look very much like rudimentary embryos and are called ***embryoid bodies*** (Figures 31.9, 31.10).

With considerable patience and skill, R. L. Brinster in Philadelphia, in 1974, injected teratocarcinoma cells into early mouse embryos (blastocysts) obtained from

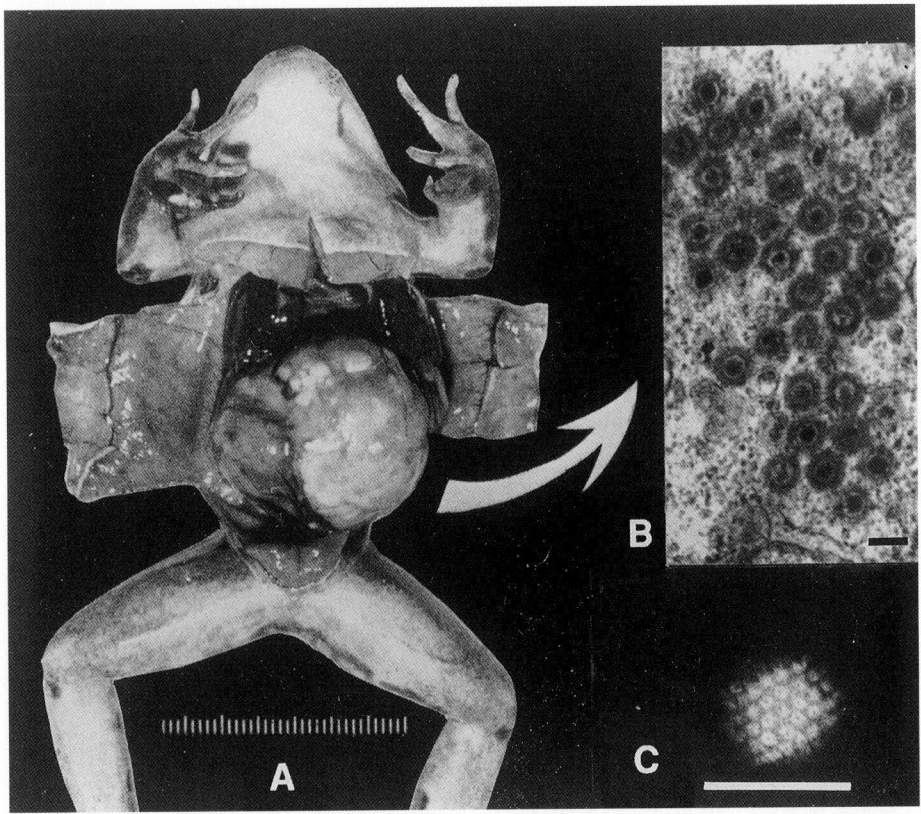

FIGURE 31.5 **A:** Frog bearing a large malignant tumor of the kidney (Lucké renal adenocarcinoma). **B:** Electron micrograph showing virus particles (herpes type) in the cytoplasm of a cell from this tumor. **Bar** = 0.2 μm. **C:** Electron micrograph of a negatively stained virus particle showing detail of the capsomere. **Bar** = 0.2 μm. (Reproduced from [33].)

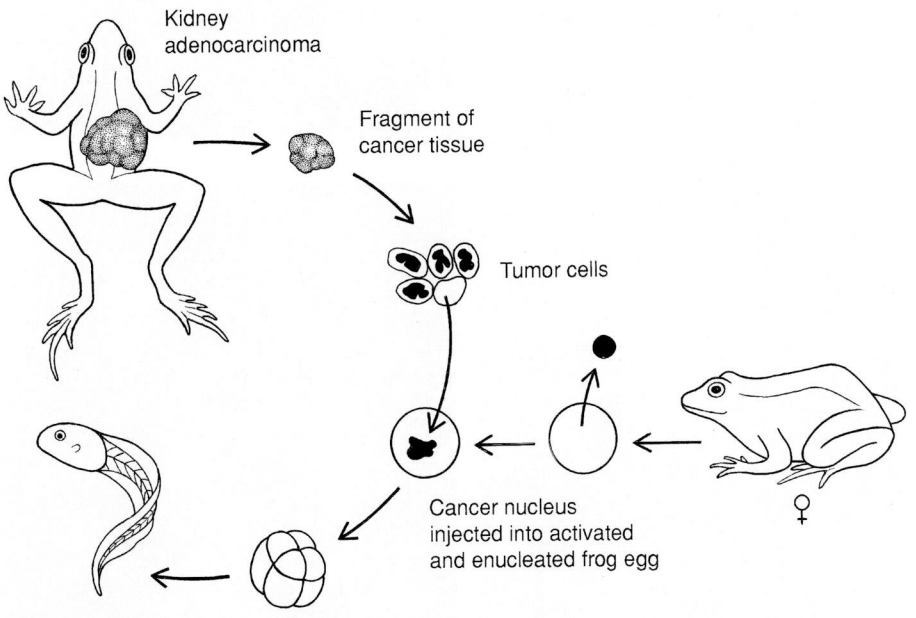

FIGURE 31.6 Diagram of an experiment showing that a tadpole can be born of a frog egg in which the nucleus had been replaced by a nucleus from a malignant frog tumor (*adenocarcinoma of Lucké*). (Adapted with permission from [6].)

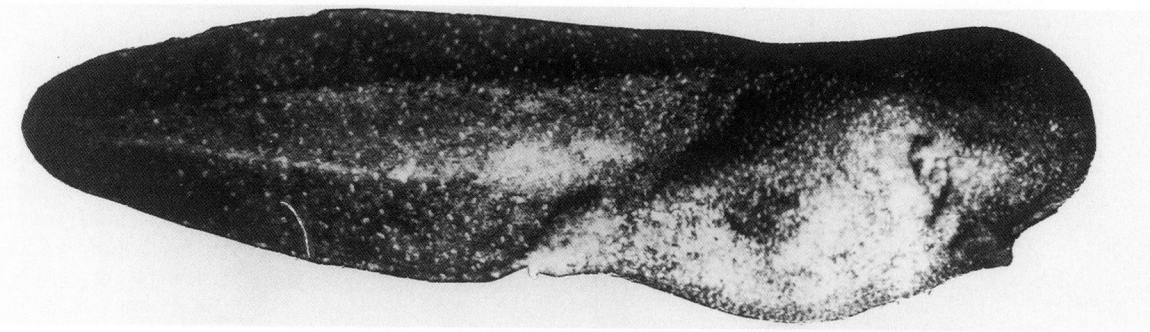

FIGURE 31.7 Historic tadpole produced by the experiment shown in Figure 31.6. Such tadpoles do not survive to become frogs, but they do live up to 10–14 days. (Reproduced by permission from [29], copyright 1972 Munksgaard International Publishers Ltd, Copenhagen, Denmark.)

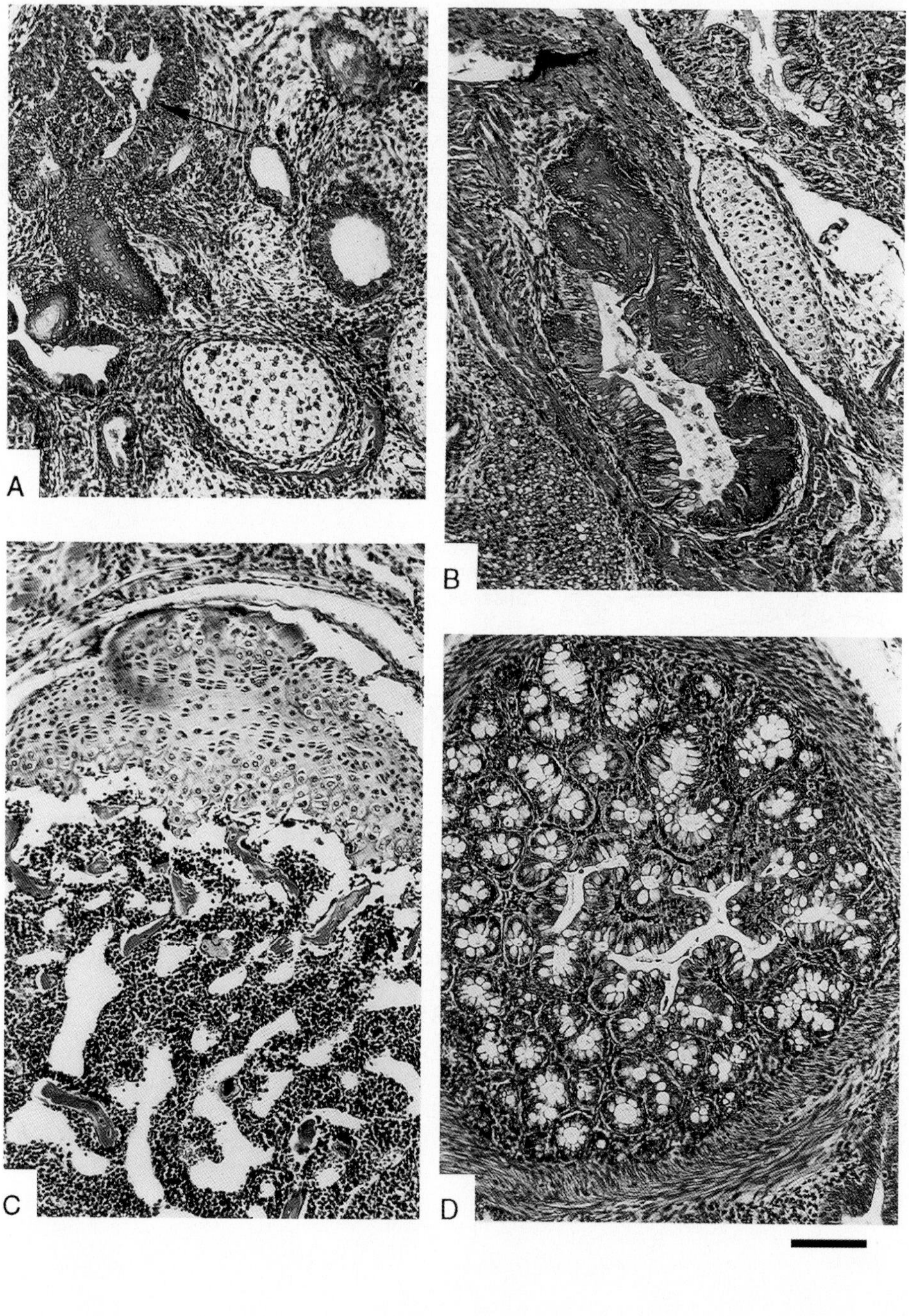

FIGURE 31.8 Examples of differentiation found in a testicular teratocarcinoma of the mouse: **A:** Undifferentiated embryonal carcinoma (**arrow**) and cartilage. **B:** Cartilage, squamous and disorganized glandular epithelium. **C:** Cartilaginous cap with endochondral ossification including bone and bone marrow. **D:** Glands surrounded by muscle, found in masses of neural tissue. **Bar** = 100 μm. (From [44a]. Copyright © 1959 American Cancer Society. Reprinted by permission of Wiley-Liss, Inc. a subsidiary of John Wiley & Sons, Inc.)

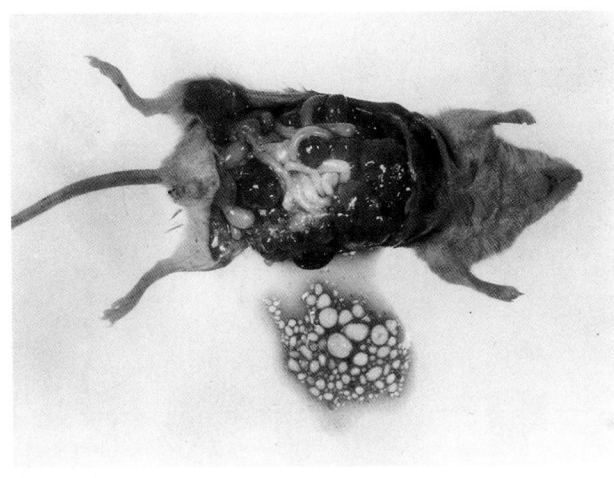

FIGURE 31.9 Mouse injected intraperitoneally 4 weeks previously with cells of a teratocarcinoma; this tumor forms large vesicular embryoid bodies, which grow freely in the peritoneum. A mass of these bodies is shown next to the animal. (Reproduced with permission from [43].)

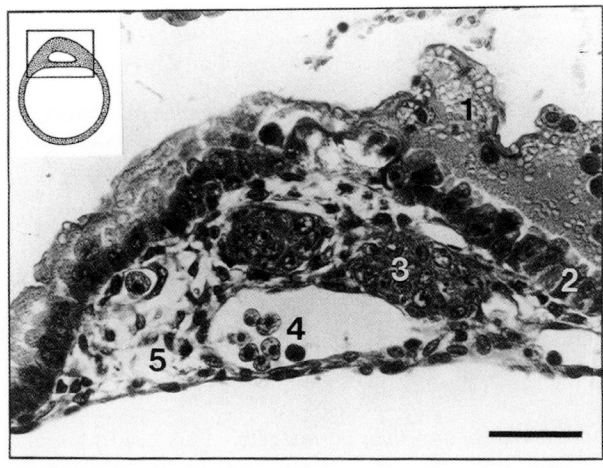

FIGURE 31.10 From a cystic embryoid body of a mouse teratocarcinoma. *Inset:* Scheme of an embryoid body; the rectangle shows the topography of the micrograph. **1:** Precipitated ascites fluid. **2:** Endoderm covering the embryoid body. **3:** Clumps of teratocarcinoma. **4:** Sinus containing hematopoietic cells. **5:** Mesenchyme. **Bar** = 50 μm. (Reproduced by permission from [45], © by The US & Canadian Academy of Pathology, Inc.)

pregnant white mice (7). Then he reintroduced the blastocysts into the uterus of pseudopregnant foster mothers (i.e., mice mated with a vasectomized male) and waited. The result: 137 normal mice, including one obvious chimera with stripes of dark hairs that could only have derived from the tumor; the pattern recalled the zebra-like allophenic mice derived from the fusion

of two embryos (p. 773). In essence, the tumor had fathered part of a mouse. We would like to say "half of a mouse," but the level of chimerism is low (40) and can regress with time (59).

Several other groups confirmed these experiments (44) using sophisticated genetic markers for identifying tumor-derived cells while maintaining the principle of deriving the original teratoma from dark-haired mice and using blastocysts of white mice (32, 40, 41, 44, 59). The experimental plan is summarized in Figure 31.11 (32). It turned out that some chimeric mice were born with teratocarcinomas or developed these or other malignant tumors in later life (40, 41).

From his pioneer experiments, Brinster concluded that "the embryo environment can bring under control the autonomous proliferation of the malignant cells" (7). G. B. Pierce went one step further and proposed that *tumors can be "reversed" by differentiation,* a concept of tremendous importance (p. 949)

Suppression of malignancy by cell fusion. It must have been extremely exciting to do this experiment for the first time: fuse a normal cell with a cancer cell, and see what happens. Remember Professor John Harris of Oxford who was playing with cell fusion in the 1960s (p. 464)? He was the first (61).

Harris found that if a malignant cell is fused with a normal fibroblast of the same species, the resulting cell does not generate tumors as long as certain critical chromosomes are not eliminated (16, 17, 22, 62–64). This led him to conclude in 1969 that malignancy can behave as a recessive trait: cells, he said, contain genes that suppress cancer, and he actually called them *suppressor genes*—but the world of science was fascinated by the newly discovered oncogenes, so nobody listened. Besides, the technique of cell fusion did not lend itself for further progress. And then, quite independently, Knudson published in 1971 his own clinical definition of suppressor genes: a classic example of converging discoveries.

Hybridomas (24) may be an exception to the recessiveness of malignancy. They are crosses between myelomas and normal lymphocytes, yet behave like tumors (p. 464). The reason is not clear, but hybridomas do show chromosomal losses, and it may also be that fusion of a malignant cell with a fibroblast may not be equivalent to fusion with a lymphocyte (17).

Following this line of experimentation: we note that fusion of a malignant cell with another type of malignant cell usually produces a malignant cell, but carcinoma–sarcoma and carcinoma–melanoma hybrids are nontumorigenic, which is interpreted as indicating that the ability to form tumors—in these types of cells—is governed by different loci (54).

FIGURE 31.11 Summary of an experiment showing that malignant cells from a teratoma can be coaxed into taking part in the growth and development of a normal animal. First, a teratoma is produced by implanting a 6-day embryo (from a couple of black mice) under the testicular capsule of a mouse. The teratoma is then grown as an ascites tumor in the peritoneum where it produces vast numbers of embryoid bodies. The inner core of an embryoid body is implanted in the blastocyst obtained from two white parents. The blastocyst is then transferred to the uterus of a pseudopregnant foster mother where it gives rise to a normal mouse with a striped coat, showing that it is a mosaic. (Adapted with permission from Mintz B, Illmensee K. Proc Natl Acad Sci USA 1975;72:3585–2589.)

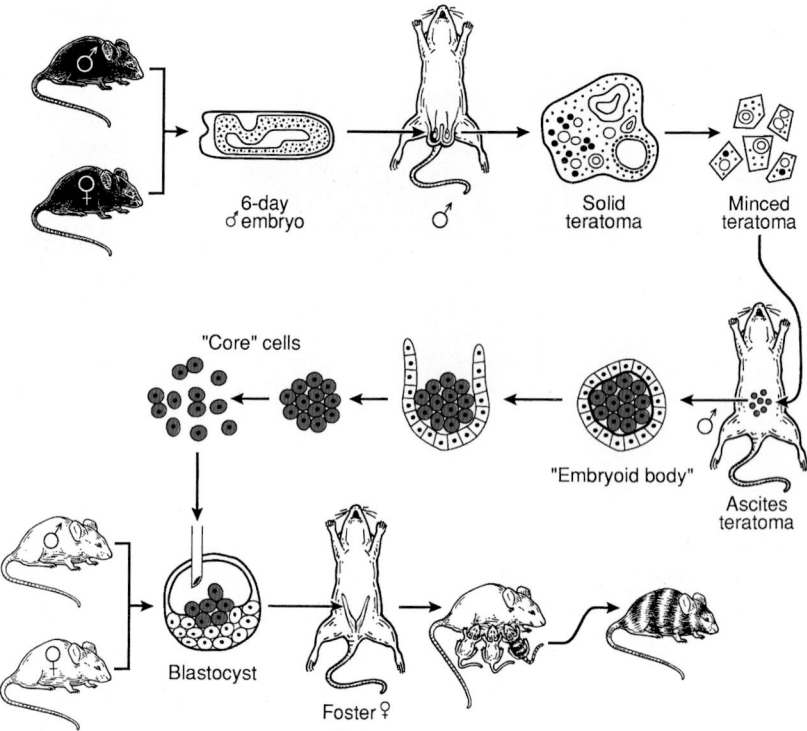

The taming of malignancy by cell fusion *in vitro* is great news. Could this ever happen in real life, inside a tumor? Could tumor cells ever "mate" with normal cells? As Harris put it, the cells of the body do not normally engage in sex (15), but evidence of such a fusion (albeit as a rare event) was published by reputable groups (2, 25, 62). The type of host cell most likely to mate with a tumor cell seemed to be the macrophage.

These results have been criticized (49), but we believe that they are full of promise. In fact we have seen one tumor in which macrophages appeared to have "tamed" the cells of a carcinoma by fusing with them, as both cell types spread over cholesterol crystals (21). *There is reason to daydream about the possibility of taming tumor cells by forcing them to fuse with host cells.* The daydream is tempered by a sobering thought: what if the hybrids lost the critical chromosomes and became even more malignant? Experimentally this is possible (7a, 12, 41a).

Cybrids are the result of fusion of any whole cell and the enucleated cytoplasm (cytoplast) of another. Tests with cybrids have shown once again that the cytoplasm of a normal cell can suppress malignancy (18, 19). The mechanism is not yet known; mitochondrial genetic material is one possibility. In one report, mouse leukemia cytoplasts, fused with human T and B cells, immortalized them without making them malignant (1).

Suppression of malignancy by introduction of genes. As mentioned earlier, some tumors—such as Wilms' tumor of the kidney (nephroblastoma), retinoblastoma, and some osteosarcomas—are brought about by the loss of a suppressor gene (p. 888). It stands to reason that if one of these malignant cell types is supplied with the missing suppressor gene, it should revert to its nonmalignant state. This is precisely what happens in elegant experiments that are feasible, alas, only *in vitro* (p. 889).

Suppression of growth by normal cells. This heading seems to contradict the obvious fact that malignancy begins among normal cells, but it is possible to demonstrate *in vitro* that a monolayer of fibroblasts stops the growth of certain malignant cells in contact with it (53). Normal human myoepithelial cells suppress tumor invasion and metastasis (55). If all normal tissues could be induced to behave this way, there would be no tumors. Could this inspire another approach to tumor therapy?

Suppression of growth by differentiation. This was a grand idea, which took 20 or 30 years to catch on (20, 52). It has the additional virtue of being simple, and it works, at least for some tumors (p. 949).

At this point we hope the reader has acquired a new way to look at malignant cells. The beast can be tamed *in vitro,* and sometimes *in vivo.*

References

1. Abken H, Jungfer H, Albert WHW, Willecke K. Immortalization of human lymphocytes by fusion with cytoplasts of transformed mouse L cells. J Cell Biol 1986;103:795–805.

1a. Arima N, Tsudo M. Extragastric mucosa-associated lymphoid-tissue lymphoma showing the regression by Helicobacter pylori eradication therapy. Br J Haematol 2003;120:790–792.

2. Ber R, Wiener F, Fenyö E-M. Proof of in vivo fusion of murine tumor cells with host cells by universal fusers: brief communication. J Natl Cancer Inst 1978;60:931–933.

3. Bingham HG. Predicting the course of a congenital hemangioma. Plast Reconst Surg 1979;63:161–166.

4. Bodey B, Bodey B Jr, Siegel SE, Kaiser HE. The spontaneous regression of neoplasms in mammals: possible mechanisms and their application in immunotherapy. In vivo 1998;12:107–122.

5. Braun AC. The reversal of tumor growth. Sci Am 1965;213:75–83.

6. Braun AC. The story of cancer. On its nature, causes, and control. Reading, MA: Addison-Wesley, 1977.

7. Brinster RL. The effect of cells transferred into the mouse blastocyst on subsequent development. J Exp Med 1974;140:1049–1056.

7a. Chakraborty AK, de Freitas Sousa J, Espreafico EM, Pawelek JM. Human monocyte x mouse melanoma fusion hybrids express human gene. Gene 2001;275:103–106.

8. Cole WH. Spontaneous regression of cancer: the metabolic triumph of the host? Ann NY Acad Sci 1974;230:111–141.

9. Cole WH. Opening address: spontaneous regression of cancer and the importance of finding its cause. Natl Cancer Inst Monogr 1976;44:5–9.

10. Cushing H, Wolbach SB. The transformation of a malignant paravertebral sympathicoblastoma into a benign ganglioneuroma. Am J Pathol 1927;3:203–216.

11. Dasgupta S. Induction of triploidy by hydrostatic pressure in the leopard frog, Rana pipiens. J Exp Zool 1962;151:105–121.

12. De Baetselier P. Neoplastic progression by somatic cell fusion. In: Liotta LA, ed. Influence of tumor development on the host. Dordrecht: Kluwer Academic Publishers, 1989, pp. 112–120.

13. Everson TC, Cole WH. Spontaneous regression of malignant melanoma. In: Spontaneous regression of cancer. Philadelphia: WB Saunders, 1966, p. 560.

14. Hanahan D, Folkman J. Patterns and emerging mechanisms of the angiogenic switch during tumorigenesis. Cell 1996;86:353–364.

15. Harris H. The Croonian lecture, 1971. Cell fusion and the analysis of malignancy. J Natl Cancer Inst 1972;48:851–864.

16. Harris H. The genetic analysis of malignancy. J Cell Sci Suppl 1986;4:431–444.

17. Harris H. The analysis of malignancy by cell fusion: the position in 1988. Cancer Res 1988;48:3302–3306.

18. Israel BA, Schaeffer WI. Cytoplasmic suppression of malignancy. In Vitro Cell Dev Biol 1987;23:627–632.

19. Iwakura Y, Nozaki M, Asano M, et al. Pleiotropic phenotypic expression in cybrids derived from mouse teratocarcinoma cells fused with ray myoblast cytoplasts. Cell 1985;43:777–791.

20. Jimenez JJ, Yunis AA. Tumor cell rejection through terminal cell differentiation. Science 1987;238:1278–1280.

21. Kerschmann RL, Woda BA, Majno G. The fusion of tumor cells with host cells; reflections on an ovarian tumor: Persp Biol Med 1995;38:467–475.

22. Klein G, Bregula U, Wiener F, Harris H. The analysis of malignancy by cell fusion. I. Hybrids between tumour cells and L cell derivatives. J Cell Sci 1971;8:659–672.

23. Kleinsmith LJ, Pierce GB. Multipotentiality of single embryonal carcinoma cells. Cancer Res 1964;24:1544–1551.

24. Köhler G, Milstein C. Derivation of specific antibody-producing tissue culture and tumor lines by cell fusion. Eur J Immunol 1976;6:511–519.

25. Lala PK, Santer V, Rahil KS. Spontaneous fusion between Ehrlich ascites tumor cells and host cells in vivo: kinetics of hybridization, and concurrent changes in the histocompatibility profile of the tumor after propagation in different host strains. Eur J Cancer 1980;16:487–510.

26. Lokich J. Spontaneous regression of metastatic renal cancer. Case report and literature review. Am J Clin Oncol (CCT) 1997;20:416–418.

27. Lucké B. A neoplastic disease of the kidney of the frog, Rana pipiens. Am J Cancer 1934;20:352–379.

28. McKinnell RG. Lucké renal adenocarcinoma: epidemiological aspects. In: Mizell M, ed. Biology of amphibian tumors. Recent Results in Cancer Research, Special Supplement. New York: Springer-Verlag, 1969, pp. 254–260.

29. McKinnell RG. Nuclear transfer in Xenopus and Rana compared. In: Harris R, Allin P, Viza D, eds. Cell Differentiation. Copenhagen: Munksgaard, 1972, pp. 61–64.

30. McKinnell RG, Parchment RE, Perantoni AO, Pierce GB. The biological basis of cancer. Cambridge: Cambridge University Press, 1999.

31. McKinnell RG, Steven LM Jr, Labat DD. Frog renal tumors are composed of stroma, vascular elements and epithelial cells: what type nucleus programs for tadpoles with the cloning procedure? In: Müller-Bérat N, Rosenfeld C, Tarin D, Viza D, eds. Progress in differentiation research. Amsterdam: North Holland Publishing Company, 1976, pp. 319–330.

32. Mintz B, Illmensee K. Normal genetically mosaic mice produced from malignant teratocarcinoma cells. Proc Natl Acad Sci USA 1975;72:3585–3589.

33. Mizell M. Lucké frog carcinoma herpes virus: transmission and expression during early development. In: Klein G., ed. Advances in viral oncology, vol 5. New York: Raven Press, 1985, pp. 129–146.

34. Montalban C, Manzanai A, Boixeda D, Redondo C, Bellas C. Treatment of low-grade gastric MALT lymphoma with Helicobacter pylori eradication. Lancet 1995;345:798–799.

35. Mulliken JB. Cutaneous vascular lesions of children. In: Serafin D, Georgiade N, eds. Pediatric plastic surgery. St. Louis: CV Mosby, 1984, pp. 137–154.

36. Mulliken JB, Murray JE. Natural history of vascular birthmarks. In: Williams HB, ed. Symposium on vascular malformations and melanotic lesions, vol 22. St. Louis: The CV Mosby Company, 1983, pp. 58–73.

37. Nathanson L. Spontaneous regression of malignant melanoma: a review of the literature on incidence, clinical features,

and possible mechanisms. Natl Cancer Inst Monogr 1976;44: 67–76.

38. National Cancer Institute. Conference on spontaneous regression of cancer. Bethesda, MD: US Department of Health, Education and Welfare, NIH publ no. 76–1038, 1976.

39. Papac RJ. Spontaneous regression of cancer. Cancer Treat Rev 1996;22:395–423.

40. Papaioannou VE, Gardner RL, McBurney MW, Babinet C, Evans MJ. Participation of cultured teratocarcinoma cells in mouse embryogenesis. J Embryol Exp Morphol 1978;44: 93–104.

41. Papaioannou VE, McBurney MW, Gardner RL, Evans MJ. Fate of teratocarcinoma cells injected into early mouse embryos. Nature 1975;258:70–73.

41a. Pawelek JM. Tumour cell hybridization and metastasis revisited. Melanoma Res 2000;10:1–8.

42. Pierce GB. Teratocarcinoma: model for a developmental concept of cancer. Curr Top Dev Biol 1967;2:223–246.

43. Pierce GB Jr. Teratocarcinomas, a problem in developmental biology. In: National Cancer Institute of Canada. Canadian cancer conference. Proceedings of the Canadian cancer research conference, vol 4. Toronto: University of Toronto Press, 1961, pp. 119–137.

44. Pierce GB, Arechaga J, Jones A, Lewellyn A, Wells RS. The fate of embryonal-carcinoma cells in mouse blastocysts. Differentiation 1987;33:247–253.

44a. Pierce GB, Dixon FJ Jr. Testicular teratomas. I. Demonstration of teratogenesis by metamorphosis of multipotential cells. Cancer 1959;12:573–583.

45. Pierce GB Jr, Dixon FJ Jr, Verney EL. Teratocarcinogenic and tissue-forming potentials of the cell types comprising neoplastic embryoid bodies. Lab Invest 1960;9:583–602.

46. Pierce GB, Shikes R, Fink LM. Cancer. A problem of developmental biology. Englewood Cliffs, NJ: Prentice-Hall, 1978.

47. Pierce GB, Wallace C. Differentiation of malignant to benign cells. Cancer Res 1971;31:127–134.

48. Pizzo PA, Horowitz ME, Poplack DG, Hays DM, Kun LE. Solid tumors of childhood. In: Devita VT Jr, Hellman S, Rosenberg SA, eds. Cancer: Principles and practice of oncology, 3rd ed. Philadelphia: JB Lippincott, 1989, pp. 1612–1670.

49. Ringertz NR, Savage RE. Cell hybrids. New York: Academic Press, 1976.

50. Rootman J, Carruthers JDA, Miller RR. Retinoblastoma. Perspect Pediatr Pathol 1987;10:208–258.

51. Rous P, Kidd JG. Conditional neoplasms and subthreshold neoplastic states. A study of the tar tumors of rabbits. J Exp Med 1941;73:365–390.

52. Sachs L. Growth, differentiation and the reversal of malignancy. Sci Am 1986;254:40–47.

53. Sager R. Genetic suppression of tumor formation: a new frontier in cancer research. Cancer Res 1986;46:1573–1580.

54. Stanbridge EJ, Der CJ, Doersen C-J, et al. Human cell hybrids: analysis of transformation and tumorigenicity. Science 1982; 215:252–259.

55. Sternlicht MD, Kedeshian P, Shao Z-M, Safarians S, Barsky S. The human myoepithelial cell is a natural tumor suppressor. Clin Cancer Res 1997;3:1949–1958.

56. Stevens LC. The development of transplantable teratocarcinomas from intratesticular grafts of pre- and post-implantation mouse embryos. Dev Biol 1970;21:364–382.

57. Tefany FJ, Barnetson RS, Halliday GM, McCarthy SW, McCarthy WH. Immunocytochemical analysis of the cellular infiltrate in primary regressing and non-regressing malignant melanoma. J Invest Dermatol 1991;97:197–202.

58. Uenishi T, Hirohashi K, Tanaka H, Ikebe T, Kinoshita H. Spontaneous regression of a large hepatocellular carcinoma with portal vein tumor thrombi: Report of a case. Surg Today Jpn J Surg 2000;30:82–85.

59. Webb CG, Gootwine E, Sachs L. Developmental potential of myeloid leukemia cells injected into midgestation embryos. Dev Biol 1984;101:221–224.

60. Weber DM, Dimopoulos MA, Anandu DP, Pugh WC, Steinbach G. Regression of gastric lymphoma of mucosa-associated lymphoid tissue with antibiotic therapy for *Helicobacter pylori*. Gastroenterology 1994;107:1835–1838.

61. Weinberg RA. Racing to the beginning of the road. The search for the origin of cancer. New York: W.H. Freeman and Company, 1996.

62. Wiener F, Fenyö EM, Klein G. Tumor-host cell hybrids in radiochimeras. Proc Natl Acad Sci USA 1974;71:148–152.

63. Wiener F, Fenyö EM, Klein G, Harris H. Fusion of tumour cells with host cells. Nature [New Biol] 1972;238:155–159.

64. Wiener F, Klein G, Harris H. The analysis of malignancy by cell fusion. III. Hybrids between diploid fibroblasts and other tumour cells. J Cell Sci 1971;8:681–692.

65. Wotherspoon AC, Doglioni C, Diss TC, et al. Regression of primary low grade B-cell gastric lymphoma of mucosa-associated lymphoid tissue after eradication of *Helicobacter pylori*. Lancet 1993;342:575–577.

66. Young RC. Metastatic renal-cell carcinoma: what causes occasional dramatic regressions? N Engl J Med 1998;338: 1305–1306.

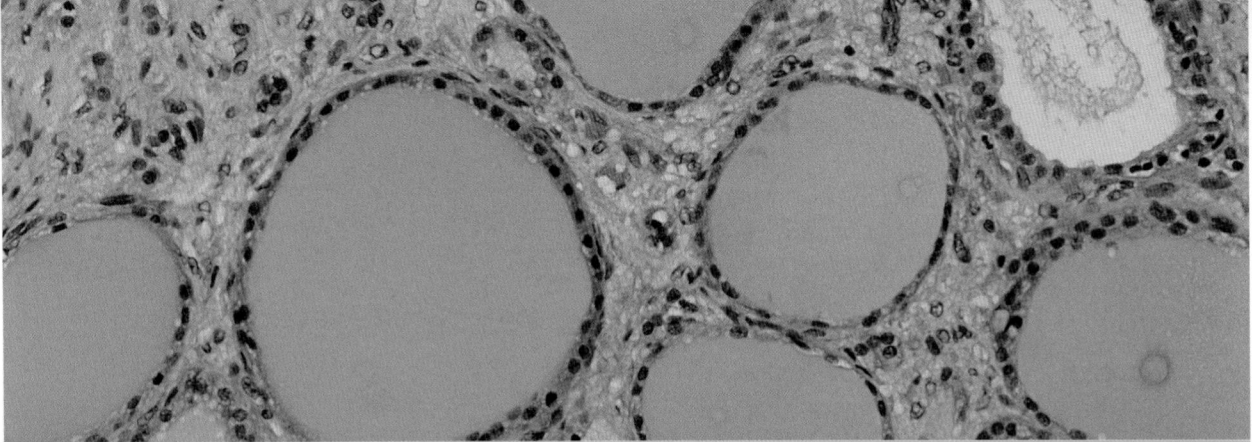

EPIDEMIOLOGY OF HUMAN CANCER

Cancer is a global problem, and with reference to the globe, it is also a spotty problem. Why do the "spots" occur? In each case, is it a matter of genes, parasites, chemicals, lifestyle, age or some other factor? The answer must come from those specialized detectives called epidemiologists. By definition, the task of epidemiology is to explain why a particular patient developed a particular disease at a particular time and place (6). Its ultimate goal is to find all causes of all diseases and to suggest preventive measures for every one. We have already presented some specific causes of cancer (chemical, physical, viral, and genetic); now we will present an overall view of these agents as they cluster in relation to geography and other factors (33).

The two basic rules of cancer epidemiology (as firm as any rules can be in the world of cancer) are that *all types of cancer can occur everywhere,* and that *the incidence of each type varies from place to place.* The lowest incidence of a particular cancer observed anywhere on the globe is taken to represent the "baseline" for that cancer, which is due to shared genetic and/or environmental factors. Any higher incidence is interpreted as reflecting some special local cause, usually environmental. This rule has been exploited for detecting causes in high-incidence populations.

> We should recall here that ***incidence*** is the number of new cases in a population during a given period. ***Prevalence*** is the number of existing cases at a given time.

Demographics of Cancer

Assuming that human cancer has many causes (genetic, occupational, dietary, and so on), which cause is, overall, the most important? The answer varies somewhat from country to country.

The USA does not have a nationwide tumor registry. The main source of statistical data is the SEER (Surveillance, Epidemiology and End Results) program, an ongoing, contract-supported program of the National Cancer Institute, which funds and coordinates the collection of cancer data in population-based cancer registries located throughout the USA. For the latest (2003) data worldwide, the WHO Cancer Report is an excellent source (36a).

Because we are writing in the United States, we will speak for this country, assuming it to be typical of industrialized nations. The startling answer again is that 80–90 percent of all cancers are due to avoidable causes, beginning with tobacco (p. 842). This message, conveyed by the indispensable monograph by Doll and Peto, tells a great deal about human behavior (14).

NOTE: In common parlance, the expression "environmental factors" means simply pollution by man-made chemicals; but when Doll and Peto refer to **environmental causes,** they include **lifestyle, diet, reproductive activities,** and other factors **determined by personal behavior.** This inclusive definition is important because it covers all of the causes of cancer that are avoidable—at least in theory.

United States. In the United States cancer is the number 2 killer; it is responsible for almost one fourth of all deaths (Figure 32.1). Cancer maps, with shades of color reflecting mortality rates, have been very useful for tracking down known and unsuspected risks. One such map for the United States, which has a lot of color along the East Coast, helped identify the danger of exposure to asbestos in shipyards during World War II (4). We have chosen three maps to illustrate the wide geographical differences in the distribution of cancer (Figures 32.2–32.4). Similar maps produced in China were the stimulus for important studies of cancer of the esophagus and of the liver, prevalent in some areas (15).

International differences. Almost every country has its own special cancer story to tell. Some of the major international differences: Cancer of the breast is high in the United States, lowest in Japan and Senegal (Figure 32.5). Cancer of the colon follows a similar trend; it tends to parallel the degree of economic development (9) as well as the consumption of red meat and animal fat (41). However, the position of Japan at the low end of the scale suggests that other factors must be

FIFTEEN LEADING CAUSES OF DEATH, US, 1998		
RANK	CAUSE OF DEATH	PERCENT OF TOTAL DEATHS
	All Causes	100.0
1	Heart Diseases	31.0
2	Cancer	23.2
3	Cerebrovascular Diseases	6.8
4	Chronic Obstructive Pulmonary Diseases	4.8
5	Accidents	4.2
6	Pneumonia & Infuenza	3.9
7	Diabetes Mellitus	2.8
8	Suicide	1.3
9	Nephritis	1.1
10	Cirrhosis of Liver	1.1
11	Septicemia	1.0
12	Alzheimer's disease	1.0
13	Homicide	0.8
14	Atherosclerosis	0.7
15	HIV Infection	0.6
	Other & Ill-defined	15.8

FIGURE 32.1 The 15 most frequent causes of death in the United States. (Adapted with permission from [18].)

involved (see Figure 28.11). Cancer of the stomach is almost epidemic in parts of China (43) and in Japan, but it is rare and decreasing in the United States. Cancer of the liver is the third most common form of cancer in China, after stomach and esophagus; but it is vanishingly rare in Canada (Figure 32.6).

Ethnic differences. Are these geographic differences due to genetic causes? Let us look at migrant groups. Many data show that migrants tend to acquire the cancer rates of the host country (14). *The shift occurs over decades or generations,* depending in part on the extent of adherence to traditional lifestyles (17, 37). For example, African Americans have cancer rates quite unlike those of their distant West African ancestors, and similar, although not identical, to those of European Americans (14). Japanese women living in Hawaii lose some of their "resistance" to breast cancer, thus the incidence among them is intermediate between that of women in Japan and of white women in the United States. Clearly, a major factor in these international differences is environmental and probably dietary.

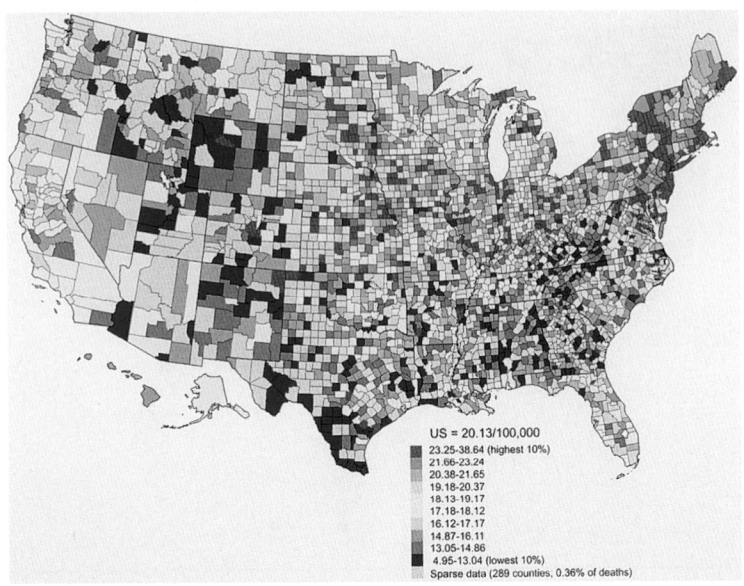

FIGURE 32.2   Mortality rates for **colon cancer** in **white males,** 1970–1994. The mortality rates are highest in the northeast quadrant of the United States, in part due to increased risks of urban populations with high socioeconomic levels. **Red areas:** Highest rate (i.e., in the highest decile). **Blue areas:** Lower rate than average for the United States. (Mortality rates by county; reproduced from Devesa SS, et al. Atlas of cancer mortality in the US 1950–1994, 1999 [13].)

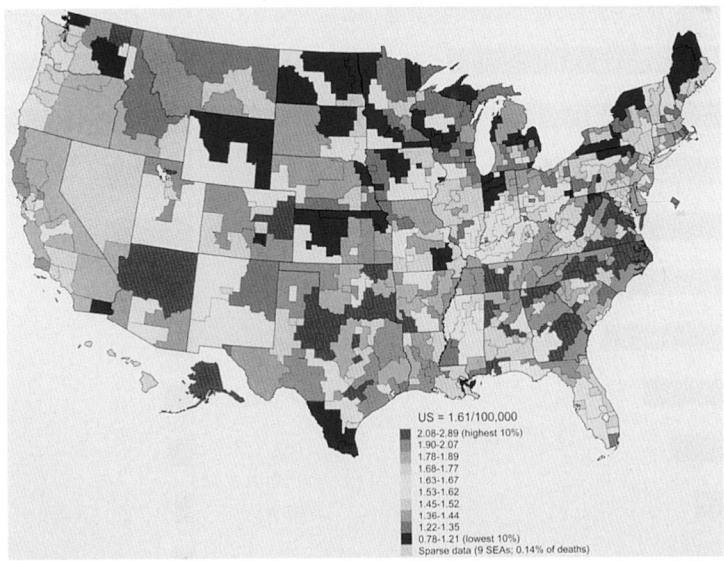

FIGURE 32.3   Mortality rates for **melanoma of the skin** in **white females,** 1970–1994. The southern band of high mortality is also present in the corresponding chart for white males. This latitudinal gradient is attributed to UV radiation from sunlight. **Red areas:** Highest rate (i.e., in the highest decile). **Blue areas:** Lower rate than average for the United States. (Mortality rates by state economic area; reproduced from Devesa SS, et al. Atlas of cancer mortality in the US 1950–1994, 1999 [13].)

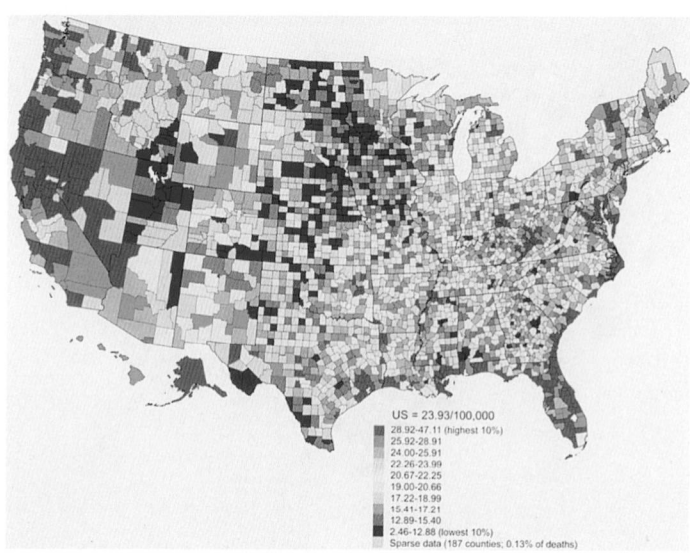

FIGURE 32.4 Mortality rates for cancer of the **lung, bronchi, trachea and pleura** in **white females,** 1970–1994. The elevated rates seen along the Atlantic and Pacific coasts are consistent with variations in smoking patterns of the last 10–30 years. **Red areas:** Highest rate (i.e., in the highest decile). **Blue areas:** Lower rate than average for the United States. (Mortality rates by county; reproduced from Devesa SS, et al. Atlas of cancer mortality in the US 1950–1994, 1999 [13].)

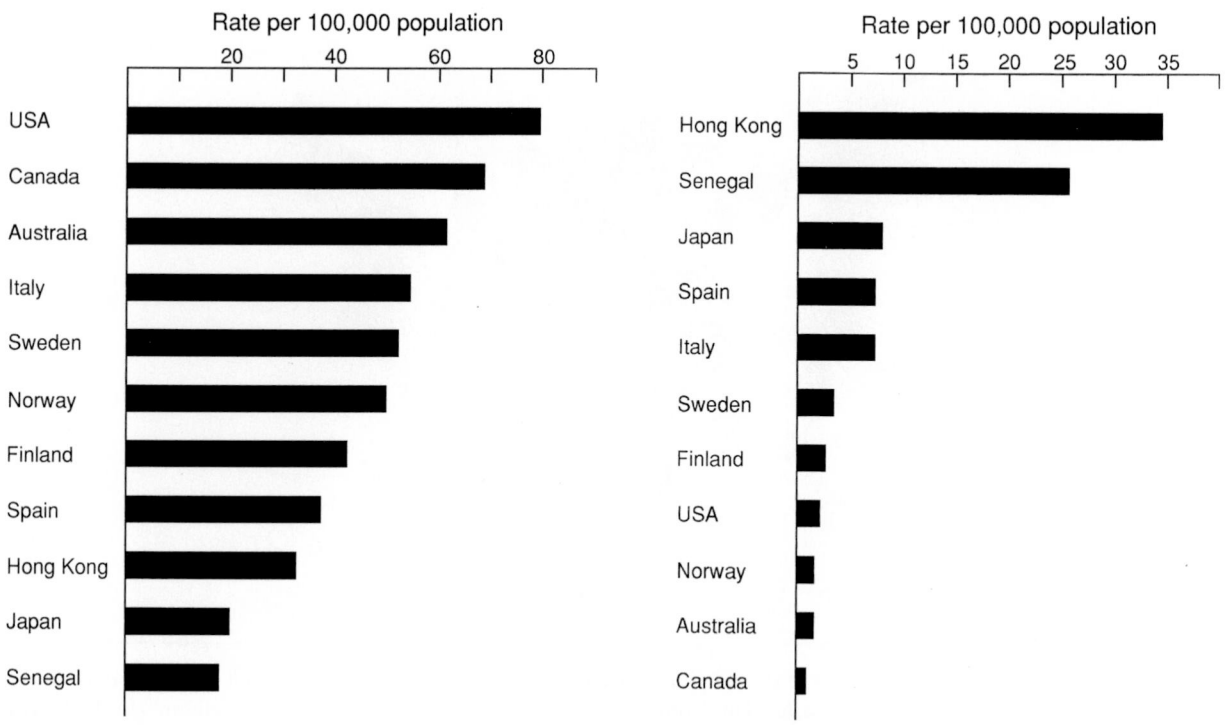

FIGURE 32.5 International variation in the incidence of breast cancer. (Adapted from [40].)

FIGURE 32.6 International variation in the incidence of liver cancer. (Adapted from [40].)

Cancer of the liver is probably related to hepatitis B and aflatoxin; cancer of the stomach may be related to diet, to infection with *Helicobacter pylori,* or to methods of food preservation. The most striking of all international differences (14) is probably genetic; a dermatologist practicing in India may not see a single cancer of the skin in a whole year, whereas a dermatologist in the Caucasian world sees basal cell carcinomas almost daily.

Ethnic differences also exist within the USA. Despite tribal variations, the overall incidence of cancer tends to be lower among Native Americans (29). For the years 1988–1992, cancer deaths per 100,000 were lowest for Native Americans and highest for African Americans (123 versus 319); for the same period, men and women compared as follows (31):

Black males 319   Black females . . . 168
White males 213   White females . . . 143

Role of gender. The death rates just given indicate that males, who (globally speaking) tend to acquire more of everything, also have considerably more cancer than females. When males and females are compared for cancers at various sites (Figure 32.7), the top concern is the same for both: cancer of the lung, showing that

smoking women have done a good job in catching up with the men (25 versus 31 percent).

Role of age. Overall, the incidence of cancer begins to rise steadily after the age of 25–30 (Figures 32.8, 32.9). This does not mean that aging itself is carcinogenic. The passage of years simply allows time for the carcinogens to act, and they act slowly (this is why prehistoric people, with a lifespan of about 35 years, had little to worry about cancer). Perhaps it is for this reason that *epithelial cancers are rare in childhood.* However, there are—of course—childhood tumors; note that they too have a second peak with advancing age (Figures 32.10, 32.11). A typical old-age cancer is carcinoma of the prostate, the most prevalent cancer in men (8). About 75 percent of the cases world-wide occur in men aged 65 or older. It begins as a slow-growing cancer, which remains latent for ~20 years and typically develops an aggressive behavior in the 7th decade (36a).

Trends over time. Mortality trends for several tumors are shown in Figures 32.12, 32.13, and 32.14. Figure 32.12 shows the steep, constant rise of mortality by **melanoma,** due in large part to a behavioral factor, which is apparently very difficult to overcome. The same figure shows also a spectacular ethnic effect: dark

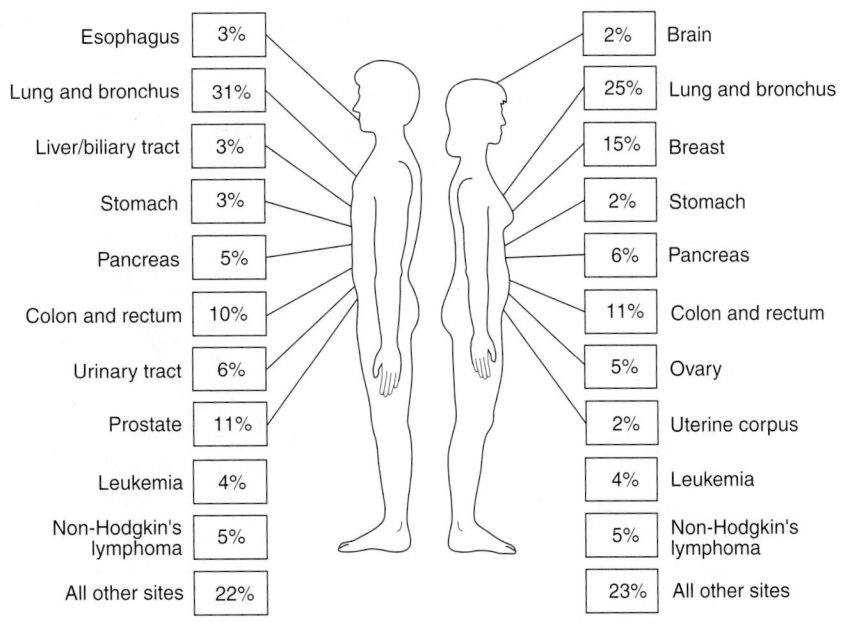

Esophagus	3%		2%	Brain
Lung and bronchus	31%		25%	Lung and bronchus
Liver/biliary tract	3%		15%	Breast
Stomach	3%		2%	Stomach
Pancreas	5%		6%	Pancreas
Colon and rectum	10%		11%	Colon and rectum
Urinary tract	6%		5%	Ovary
Prostate	11%		2%	Uterine corpus
Leukemia	4%		4%	Leukemia
Non-Hodgkin's lymphoma	5%		5%	Non-Hodgkin's lymphoma
All other sites	22%		23%	All other sites

FIGURE 32.7   Cancer deaths by site and gender: 2001 estimates. Carcinomas *in situ* are excluded except for urinary bladder. (Reproduced with permission from [18].)

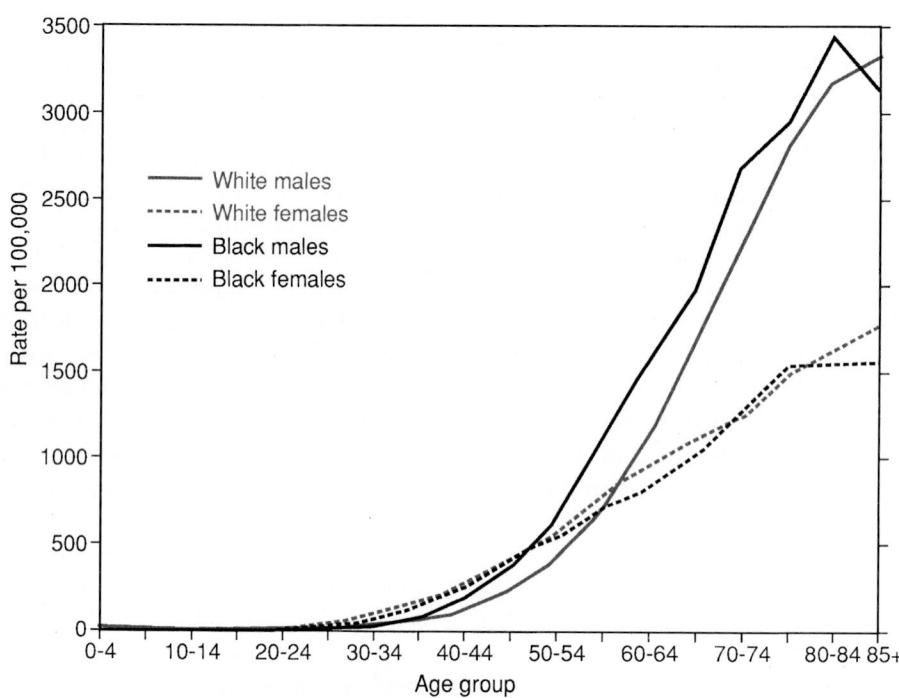

FIGURE 32.8   Incidence of malignant tumors by race, gender, and age for the period 1973–1977. (Adapted with permission from [44].)

FIGURE 32.9   Age-related incidence of selected carcinomas in the female. (Adapted with permission from [17], copyright by J.B. Lippincott, 1989.)

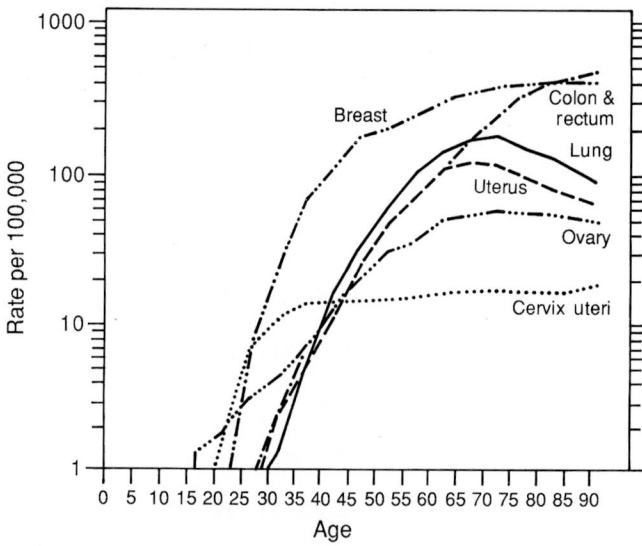

skin is a highly effective (although not 100 percent safe) insurance against melanoma. Figures 32.13 and 32.14 compare the progressive changes in male and female mortality by seven important tumors. Both show a dramatic rise for lung tumors, which requires no comment, except to point out that in the late 1960s the line of mortality by lung cancer for women crossed the line of breast cancer.

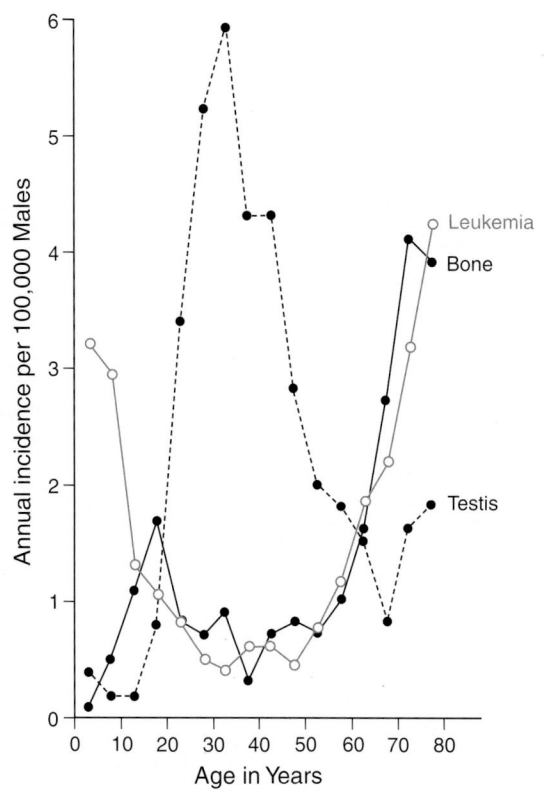

FIGURE 32.10   Peak incidence of three cancers in youth; note the secondary rise of all three in old age. (Adapted with permission from [26].)

Figures 32.13 and 32.14 also show two dramatic decreases. The sharpest is for **cancer of the stomach,** noteworthy because it is unrelated to any active preventive measure. In the USA cancer of the stomach is uncommon; at the opposite extreme is Japan (23, 36a) where the incidence in the 1960s was so high that it was tackled aggressively much like an epidemic, with mobile units equipped with X-ray machines. The incidence is dropping, but why was it so high? *Helicobacter pylori*—which colonizes about half of humanity (3a)—is a major cause, but there are many others: insufficient consumption of fruit and vegetables, poor refrigeration, high consumption of salt, nitrites, and smoked fish; bacterial factors (virulence) are also important (24a, 24b). Oddly enough, *H. pylori reduces* the risk for esophageal carcinomas (24b).

The other mortality curve that shows a steady downward trend in the USA concerns **cancer of the uterus,** but it is just as difficult to explain. Pap smears come immediately to mind, but the drop began well before the current preventive campaign (32). A similar phenomenon was the sharp decline of tuberculosis in Europe, which began long before the advent of antibiotics.

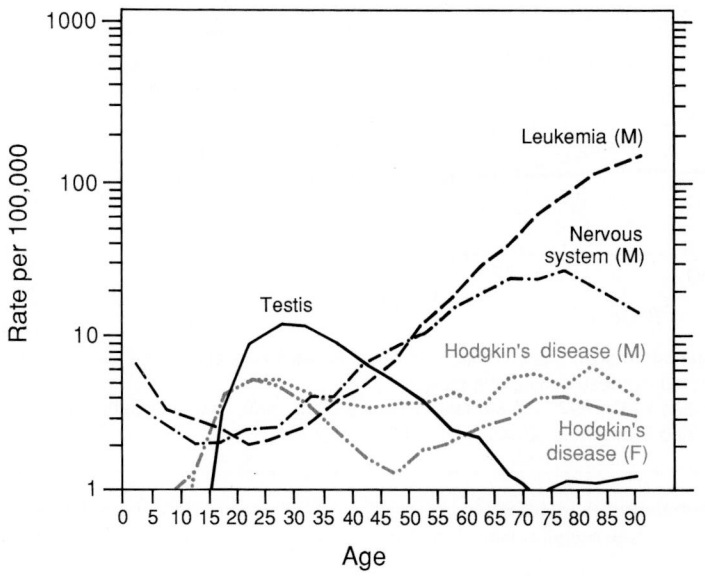

FIGURE 32.11   Age-related incidence of selected nonepithelial cancer in males and females. Note that the curves tend to be biphasic. (Adapted with permission from [17], copyright by J.B. Lippincott, 1989.)

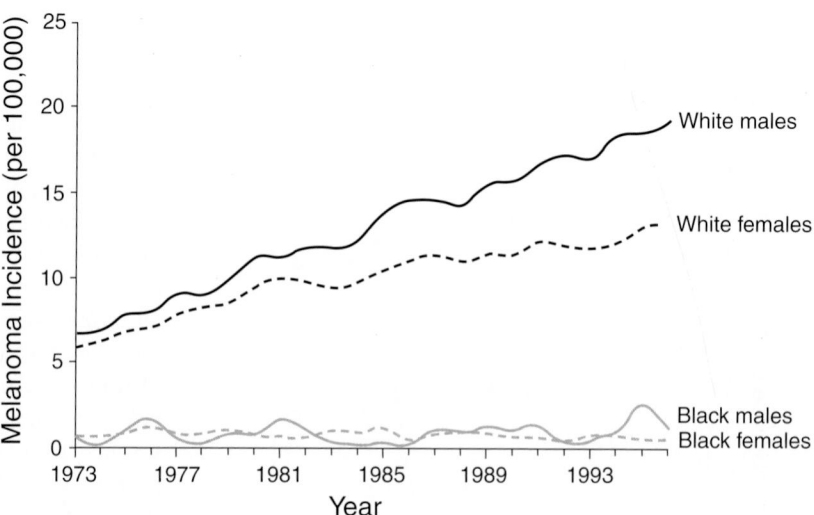

FIGURE 32.12 Age-adjusted incidence of melanoma in the United States from 1973 to 1996. The incidence has increased for the white population (rising faster in male than female) without affecting the black population. (Reproduced with permission from: Lotze, MT et al. in "Cancer: Principles and Practice of Oncology", 6th ed. DeVita VT, Hellman S, Rosenberg SA, (eds); Lippincott Williams & Wilkins, 2001 [25].)

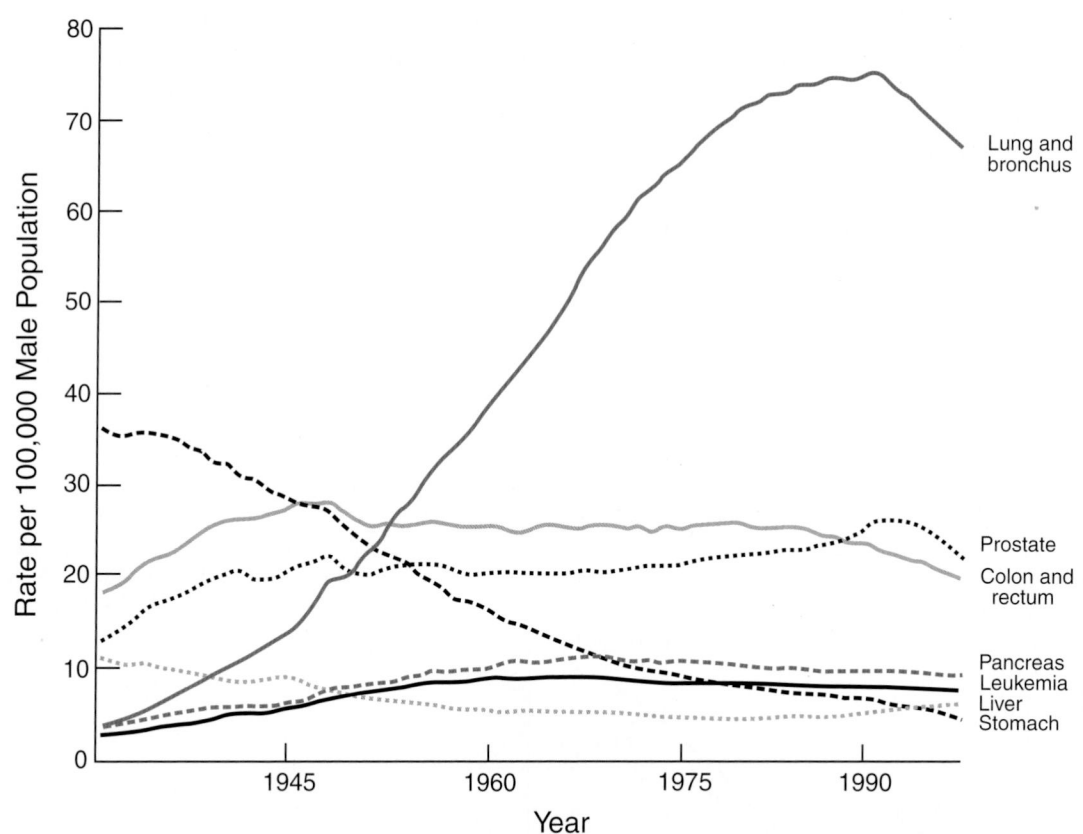

Note: Due to changes in ICD coding, numerator information has changed over time. Rates for cancers of the liver, lung & bronchus, and colon & rectum are affected by these coding changes.
Data Source: US Mortality Public Use Data Tapes 1960-1997, US Mortality Volumes 1930-1959, National Center for Health Statistics, Centers for Disease Control and Prevention, 2000.

FIGURE 32.13 Cancer death rates by sites for the male population, United States 1930–1997. (Rates are for 100,000 and are age-adjusted to the 1970 US standard population.) (Reproduced with permission from [18].)

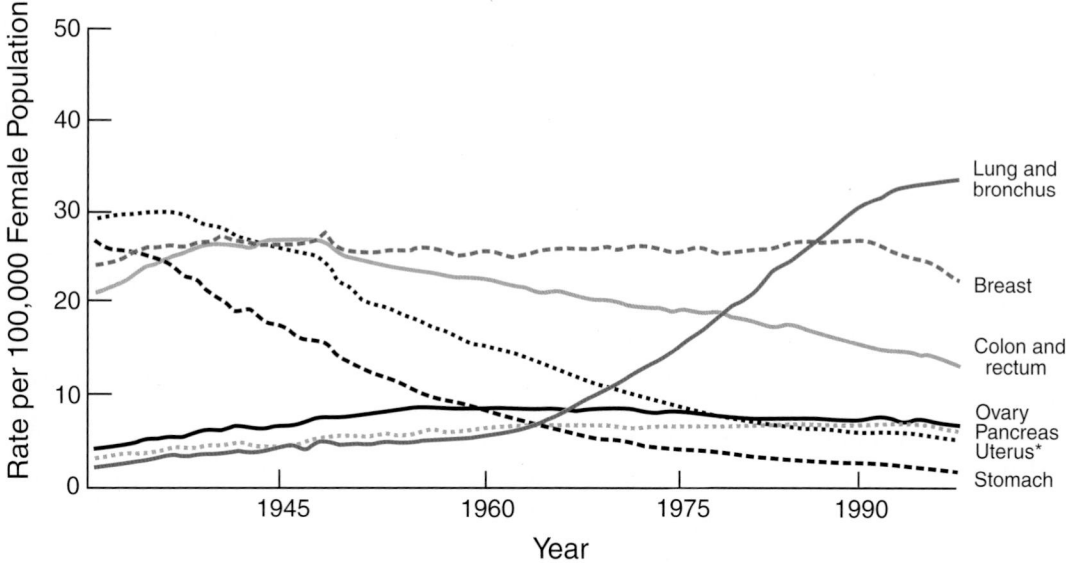

*Uterus cancer death rates are for uterine cervix and uterine corpus combined.
Note: Due to changes in ICD coding, numerator information has changed over time. Rates for cancers of the uterus, ovary, lung & bronchus, and colon & rectum are affected by these coding changes.
Data Source: US Mortality Public Use Data Tapes 1960-1997, US Mortality Volumes 1930-1959, National Center for Health Statistics, Centers for Disease Control and Prevention, 2000.

FIGURE 32.14   Cancer death rates by sites for the female population, United States 1930–1997. (Rates are for 100,000 and are age-adjusted to the 1970 US standard population.) (Reproduced with permission from [18].)

Lifestyle and the Avoidability of Cancer

The critical point of Doll and Peto in their fact-filled monograph is that most cancer is self-inflicted and therefore avoidable (14). This news has not been welcomed by everyone. In facing cancer, that seemingly blind killer, we have an innate reflex to place the blame somewhere else—on industrial pollution, on sundry fumes that we are forced to breathe. The figures speak otherwise. Cancer from pollution certainly exists (see below), and environmental pollution is certainly beginning to spell doom for the planet—but not by cancer. The environment can kill in many other and more efficient ways than by cancer: climates can change, crops can shrivel up, cattle and people can starve.

Tobacco and alcohol. Tobacco, as we have seen (p. 842), kills enough people every year to equal the deaths from a major war: about 1 million, of which an estimated 350,000 die in the United States, accounting for about one-sixth of deaths from all causes (12). Tobacco kills by producing emphysema, vascular disease, and cancer in the lungs and a variety of other organs: mouth,

pharynx, larynx, esophagus, bladder, pancreas, and cervix; the latter can even be caused by passive smoking (36).

This list of organs suggests a preference for squamous stratified epithelia, but smokers are also at some risk for leukemia (1). Regarding the bladder, the presence of carcinogens in the urine creates a situation comparable to that of tar products being painted on mouse skin. Smoke contains even the archetype carcinogen, benzo[a]pyrene; and smokers, as well as passive smokers, have a lung-specific carcinogen in their urine (24). Passive smoking was recently shown to be a major risk factor for lung cancer in women "never-smokers" (2). Experimentally, condensate of cigarette smoke behaves as a typical initiator; nicotine behaves as a promoter (1). The only good news about cigarettes is that filters help a little—and giving up the habit does decrease the risk of cancer.

Note that tobacco, like coca, was discovered by Native Americans; in their original setting, which was partly ritual, both drugs were harmless and even useful.

Alcohol as a risk factor for cancer was already discussed (p. 842).

Diet. Diet contributes to cancer in many ways, some proved, some hypothetical (14). Most obvious is the absorption of carcinogens, such as aflatoxins from spoiled foods (p. 845). There seems to be a correlation between the consumption of meat and cancer of the colon; between smoked fish (in Iceland) and cancer of the stomach; between salted fish and nasopharyngeal carcinoma (45). Broiling, smoking, and frying in fats that have been used over and over again produce a variety of carcinogens, including benzo[*a*]pyrene (32) (p. 840). The possible role of nitrites as food additives was mentioned on p. 845.

Overweight and obesity. Until recently both these afflictions were known to threaten life by plenty of complications (diabetes, hypertension, arthritis, etc. [pp. 91, 589]) but cancer was low on the list. No longer: in 2003 a prospective study on 900,000 individuals in the USA showed that the death rate by cancer (all cancers combined) was 52 percent higher for men and 62 percent higher for women (9a) and could account for 90,000 deaths per year (as compared with 350,000 for tobacco). Hopefully this bad news will add new motivation for losing weight.

> The definition of overweight was based on body-mass index (the weight in kilograms divided by the square of the height in meters); normal vs overweight vs obesity = 18.5–24.9 versus 25–29.9 versus 30.0 or higher. Biological mechanisms proposed vary and include sex steroids, insulin and insulin-like growth factors.

There are established pathways from obesity to cancer of the uterus. It is known that this form of cancer can be induced by excess estrogen, be it medically prescribed or endogenous: After menopause, the level of estrogens in the blood is directly proportional to the degree of adiposity because fat cells synthesize it from adrenal hormones (14).

Sexual development and behavior. The dangers here are of two kinds: from inside (hormones) and from outside (viruses). Mammary cancer can be produced in mice with estrogens (32); correspondingly, in humans, some of the risk factors suggest a longer exposure to hormonal stimulation: early menarche, delayed first pregnancy, and late menopause (but NOT induced abortion, p. 847). Pregnancy and childbirth (but not lactation) have a protective effect (14). Cancers of the endometrium, ovary, and breast are more frequent in women that have borne no children. Men share none of

these problems, but an undescended testicle has a greater risk of developing cancer, for reasons that are unclear, but which may include hormones.

A safe way for women to reduce the risk of breast cancer by 37 percent is regular exercise: best results in lean women under 45 (38).

Regarding sexual behavior, viral cacinogenesis is all too well represented: the second most common cancer in women worldwide is **cervical cancer,** and virtually all cases test positive for human papilloma virus, usually Type 16 (39). This type of cancer may soon be 100 percent preventable by vaccination (p. 916). Another correlation is appearing between genital warts (*condylomata acuminata*) and anal cancer (35). Some cases of Kaposi's sarcoma should be included in this category of virus-induced tumors spread by sexual behavior (34).

Occupation. Of all cancers in developed countries, 4 to 5 percent are attributed to occupational exposures (14, 36a). Not a large percentage, perhaps, but exposures of this kind are immediately preventable, as opposed to "lifestyle" exposures such as smoking and alcohol abuse. Furthermore, we should keep in mind this statement from an authoritative textbook of epidemiology: *"no workplace has been shown conclusively not to be associated with an increased risk of cancer"* (27) (emphasis ours).

Geophysical factors. Ionizing radiations and UV light were estimated to cause about 3 percent of cancer deaths (14); by comparison medical treatments cause about 1 percent (half of this due to radiation), or possibly 2 percent if current estimates of the effect of chronic medication are confirmed.

Exposure to radon accounts for about half of the radiation exposure of the general population, and may cause up to 24,000 deaths per year in the USA (5).

Pollution. About 2 percent of cancer deaths are due to pollution (14), but this low figure is probably too low (30) and misleading: by contaminating the environment, humans are spreading cancer (and other diseases) to species that account for over 99.99 percent of the animal world. Fish have been particularly hard hit, especially the bottom-feeding species (Figure 32.15) (19, 20, 22). In some parts of the United States, cancer in fresh and salt-water fish occurs at rates that are 100 and possibly 1000 times higher than expected (7). The reader may recall the outbreak of liver cancer in rainbow trout, due to food pellets containing fungus-contaminated peanuts (p. 845); that episode alerted the federal Food and Drug Administration to the carcinogenic potential of aflatoxin and probably saved many

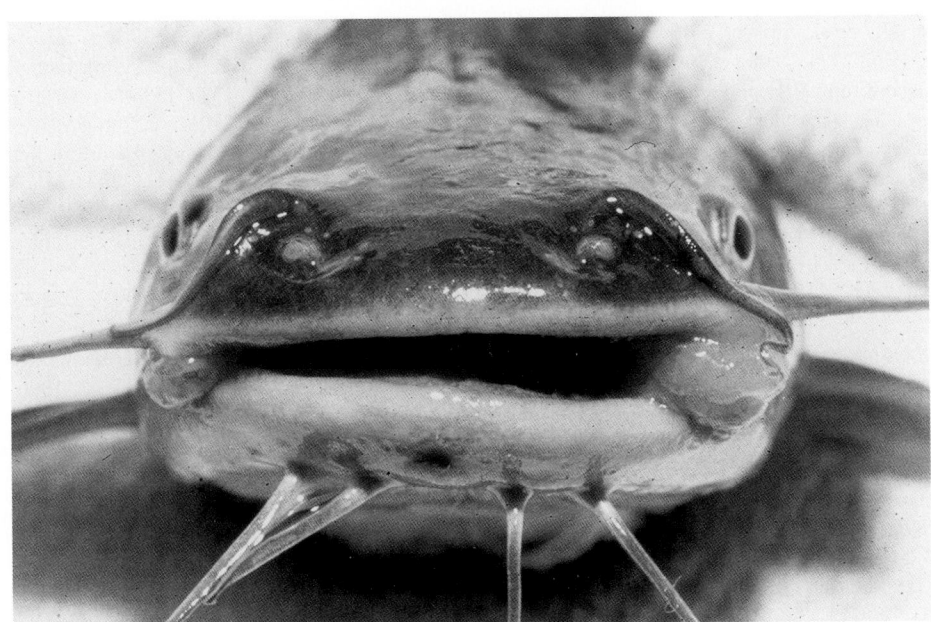

FIGURE 32.15 Fish tumors attributed to pollution: a black bullhead with a papilloma at both corners of the mouth. (Courtesy of J. M. Grizzle, Department of Fisheries and Allied Aquacultures, Alabama Agricultural Experiment Station, Auburn University, Alabama.)

human lives (21). As a matter of fact, fish populations have been considered sentinels of carcinogens in the environment (3, 10, 42, 46).

TO SUM UP: Much of human cancer is potentially avoidable, but reality indicates that human behavior is extremely difficult to change: witness the current war on drugs. For some cancers, such as hepatoma in Asia and Africa, the environmental causes are apparent but—in practice—difficult to eliminate. However, the first step is to know the facts.

References

1. Baron JA, Rohan TE. The causes of cancer. In: Schottenfeld D, Fraumeni JF Jr (eds). Cancer epidemiology and prevention. New York: Oxford University Press. 1996, pp. 269–289.

2. Bennett WP, Alavanja MCR, Blomeke B, et al. Environmental tobacco smoke, genetic susceptibility, and risk of lung cancer in never-smoking women. J Natl Cancer Inst 1999;91: 2009–2014.

3. Bickham JW, Sandhu S, Hebert PDN, Chikhi L, Athwal R. Effects of chemical contaminants on genetic diversity in natural populations: implications for biomonitoring and ecotoxicology. Mutat Res 2000;463:33–51.

3a. Bjorkholm B, Falk P, Engstrand L, Nyron O, Helicobacter pylori: resurrection of the cancer link. J Intern Med 2003;253: 102–119.

4. Blot WJ, Mason TJ, Hoover R, Fraumeni JF Jr. Cancer by county: etiologic implications. In: Hiatt HH, Watson JD, Winsten JA, eds. Origins of human cancer. Book A. Cold Spring Harbor: Cold Spring Harbor Laboratory, 1977, pp. 21–32.

5. Boice JD Jr, Land CE, Preston DL. The causes of cancer. In: Schottenfeld D, Fraumeni JF Jr (eds). Cancer epidemiology and prevention. New York: Oxford University Press, 1996, pp. 319–354.

6. Boyd NF. The epidemiology of cancer: principles and methods. In: Tannock IF, Hill RP, eds. The basic science of oncology. New York: Pergamon Press, 1987, pp. 7–23.

7. Breaux JB. Hearing before the Subcommittee on Fisheries and Wildlife Conservation and the Environment of the Committee on Merchant Marine and Fisheries, 98th Congress, 1st Session, 1983.

8. Breslow N, Chan CW, Dhom G, et al. Latent carcinoma of prostate at autopsy in seven areas. Int J Cancer 1977;20: 680–688.

9. Burkitt DP. Epidemiology of cancer of the colon and rectum. Cancer 1971;28:3–13.

9a. Calle EE, Rodriguez C, Walker-Thurmond K, Thun MJ. Overweight, obesity and mortality from cancer in a prospectively studied cohort of U.S. adults. N Engl J Med 2003; 348:1625–1638.

10. Couch JA. The fishy side. In: Hoover KL. Use of small fish species in carcinogenicity testing. Natl Cancer Inst Monogr 65. NIH publ no. 84–2653. Bethesda, MD: National Institutes of Health, 1984, pp. 229–235.

11. Covacci A, Telford JL, Del Giudice G, Parsonnet J, Rappuoli R. Helicobacter pylori virulence and genetic geography. Science 1999;284:1328–1333.

12. Davis RM. Current trends in cigarette advertising and marketing. N Engl J Med 1987;316:725–732.

13. Devesa SS, Grauman DJ, Blot WJ, et al. Atlas of cancer mortality in the United States, 1950–1994. National Institutes of Health, National Cancer Institute, NIH publication No. 99-4564, 1999. (http://www.nci.gov/atlasplus)

14. Doll R, Peto R. The causes of cancer: quantitative estimates of avoidable risks of cancer in the United States today. J Natl Cancer Inst 1981;66:1192–1308.

15. Editorial Committee for the Atlas of Cancer Mortality in the People's Republic of China. Atlas of cancer mortality in the People's Republic of China. Shanghai: China Map Press, 1979.

16. Fraumeni JF Jr, Blot WJ. Lung and pleura. In: Schottenfeld D, Fraumeni JF Jr, eds. Cancer epidemiology and prevention. Philadelphia: WB Saunders, 1982, pp. 564–582.

17. Fraumeni JF Jr, Hoover RN, Devesa SS, Kinlen LJ. Epidemiology of cancer. In: DeVita VT Jr, Hellman S, Rosenberg SA, eds. Cancer: Principles and practice of oncology, 3rd ed. Philadelphia: JB Lippincott, 1989, pp. 196–235.

18. Greenlee RT, Hill-Harmon MB, Murray T, Thun M. Cancer statistics, 2001. CA Cancer J Clin 2001;51:15–36 and Erratum. CA Cancer J Clin 2001;51:144.

19. Grizzle JM, Melius P, Strength DR. Papillomas on fish exposed to chlorinated wastewater effluent. J Natl Cancer Inst. 1984;73:1133–1142.

20. Grizzle JM, Schwedler TE, Scott AL. Papillomas of black bullheads, Ictalurus melas (Rafinesque), living in a chlorinated sewage pond. J Fish Dis 1981;4:345–351.

21. Harshbarger J. Hearing before the Subcommittee on Fisheries and Wildlife Conservation and the Environment of the Committee on Merchant Marine and Fisheries, 98th Congress, 1st Session, 1983.

22. Harshbarger JC, Clark JB. Epizootiology of neoplasms in bony fish of North America. Sci Total Environ 1990;94:1–32.

23. Haruma K. Trend toward a reduced prevalence of Helicobacter pylori infection, chronic gastritis, and gastric cancer in Japan. Gastroenterol Clin North Am 2000;29:623–631.

24. Hecht SS, Carmella SG, Murphy SE, Akerkar S, Brunnemann KD, Hoffmann D. A tobacco-specific lung carcinogen in the urine of men exposed to cigarette smoke. N Engl J Med 1993;329:1543–1546.

24a. Kelley JR, Duggan JM. Gastric cancer epidemiology and risk factors. J Clin Epidemiol 2003;56:1–9.

24b. Kikuchi S. Epidemiology of Helicobacter pylori and gastric cancer. Gastric Cancer 2002;5:6–15.

25. Lotze MT, Dallal RM, Kirkwood JM, Flickinger JC. Cutaneous melanoma. In: DeVita VT Jr, Hellman S, Rosenberg SA (eds). Cancer. Principles and practice of Oncology, 6th ed. Philadelphia: Lippincott Williams & Wilkins. 2001, pp. 2012–2069.

26. Miller DG. On the nature of susceptibility to cancer. The presidential address. Cancer 1980;46:1307–1318.

27. Monson RR. The causes of cancer. In: Schottenfeld D, Fraumeni JF Jr (eds). Cancer epidemiology and prevention. New York: Oxford University Press. 1996, pp. 373–405.

28. National Cancer Institute. Cancer statistics review 1973–1986. Washington, DC: US Department of Health and Human Services, National Institutes of Health, 1989.

29. Nutting PA, Freeman WL, Risser DR, et al. Cancer incidence among American Indians and Alaska Natives, 1980 through 1987. Am J Public Health 1993;83:1589–1598.

30. Pope III CA, Burnett RT, Thun MJ, et al. Lung cancer, cardiopulmonary mortality, and long-term exposure to fine particulate air pollution. JAMA 2002;287:1132–1141.

31. Ries LAG, Eisner MP, Kosary CL, et al. (eds). SEER Cancer Statistics Review, 1973–1998, National Cancer Institute. Bethesda, MD, 2001.

32. Ruddon RW. Cancer biology, 2nd ed. New York: Oxford University Press, 1987.

33. Schottenfeld D, Fraumeni JF Jr (eds). Cancer epidemiology and prevention. New York: Oxford University Press, 1996.

34. Schulz TF. Kaposi's sarcoma-associated herpesvirus (human herpesvirus-8). J Gen Virol 1998;79:1573–1591.

35. Shank B, Cohen AM, Kelsen D. Cancer of the anal region. In: DeVita VT Jr, Hellman S, Rosenberg SA, eds. Cancer: Principles and practice of oncology, 3rd ed. Philadelphia: JB Lippincott, 1989, pp. 965–978.

36. Slattery ML, Robison LM, Schuman KL, et al. Cigarette smoking and exposure to passive smoke are risk factors for cervical cancer. JAMA 1989;261:1593–1598.

36a. Stewart BW, Kleihues P (eds). World cancer report. Lyon: IARC Press, 2003.

37. Thomas DB, Karagas MR. Cancer in first and second generation Americans. Cancer Res 1987;47:5771–5776.

38. Thune I, Brenn T, Lund E, Gaard M. Physical activity and the risk of breast cancer. N Engl J Med 1997;336:1269–1275.

39. Walboomers JMM, Jacobs MV, Manos MM, et al. Human papillomavirus is a necessary cause of invasive cervical cancer worldwide. J Pathol 1999;189:12–19.

40. Waterhouse J, Shanmugaratnam K, Muir C, Powell J, eds. Cancer incidence in five continents, Vol IV. Lyon: International Agency for Research on Cancer, 1982.

41. Willett WC, Stampfer MJ, Colditz GA, Rosner BA, Speizer FE. Relation of meat, fat, and fiber intake to the risk of colon cancer in a prospective study among women. N Engl J Med 1990;323:1664–1672.

42. Williams DE, Lech JJ, Buhler DR. Xenobiotics and xenoestrogens in fish: modulation of cytochrome P450 and carcinogenesis. Mutat Res 1998;399:179–192.

43. You W-C, Blot WJ, Chang Y-S, et al. Diet and high risk of stomach cancer in Shandong, China. Cancer Res 1988;48:3518–3523.

44. Young JL, Pollack ES. The incidence of cancer in the United States. In: Schottenfeld D, Fraumeni JF Jr, eds. Cancer epidemiology and prevention. Philadelphia: WB Saunders, 1982, pp. 138–165.

45. Yu MC, Ho JHC, Shiu-Hung L, Henderson BE. Cantonese-style salted fish as a cause of nasopharyngeal carcinoma: report of a case-control study in Hong Kong. Cancer Res 1986;46:956–961.

46. Zelikoff JT. Biomarkers of immunotoxicity in fish and other non-mammalian sentinel species: predictive value for mammals? Toxicology 1998;129:63–71.

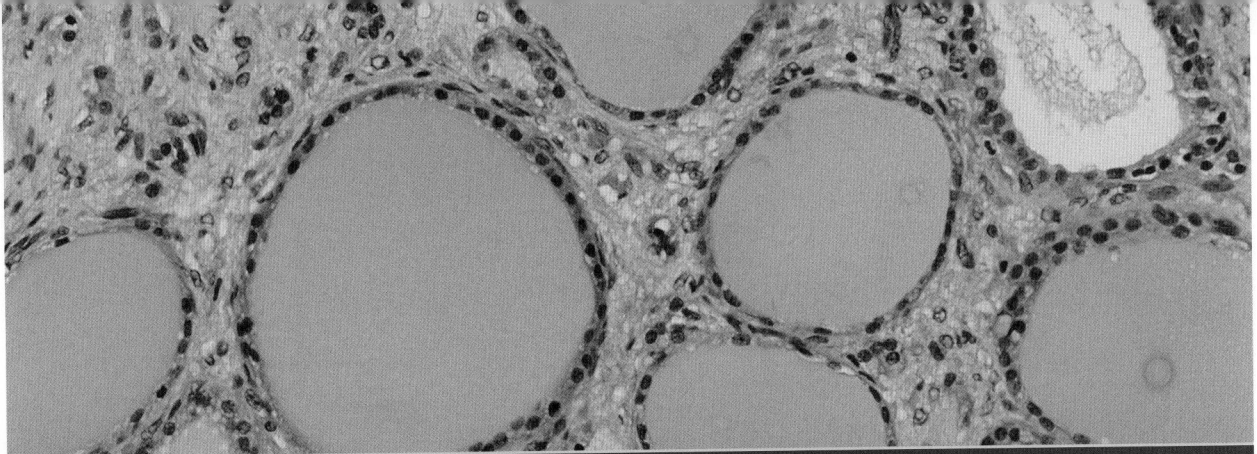

We opened our discussion of tumors with this dictionary-type definition: *a tumor is a purposeless growth of tissue that tends to be atypical, autonomous, and aggressive.* Now, many pages later, we still have question marks; we still must contend with ambiguous-looking lesions that we call ambiguous names such as *dysplasia, adenosis,* or *epulis* (Figure 33.1). However, we can supplement our working definition with a few addenda that address the nature of tumors more deeply.

DNA Damage: Not the Only Path to a Tumor

"All tumors have in common a disturbance of their DNA." So we wrote in the first edition, and we added with a comment "This is a solid fact." Eight years later the fact is still solid, but there are other facts to complete and complicate the picture. Here is one: some genes can be silenced without disturbing their primary nucleotide sequence. It is an interesting exercise to look at Figure 33.2 which shows 5 possible ways to produce mutations by disturbing the double helix, and try and work out a sixth pathway to a tumor and yet leave the double helix intact. The answer is hypermethylation (p. 891).

Two Tumors May Never Be Identical

Unlike real parasites, tumor cells die with their victim, usually after years of "progression." By that time their genetic makeup must be extremely varied and unique, beyond the range of current understanding. For example: the most common cancer-related genetic change known is a mutation of *p53,* the suppressor gene

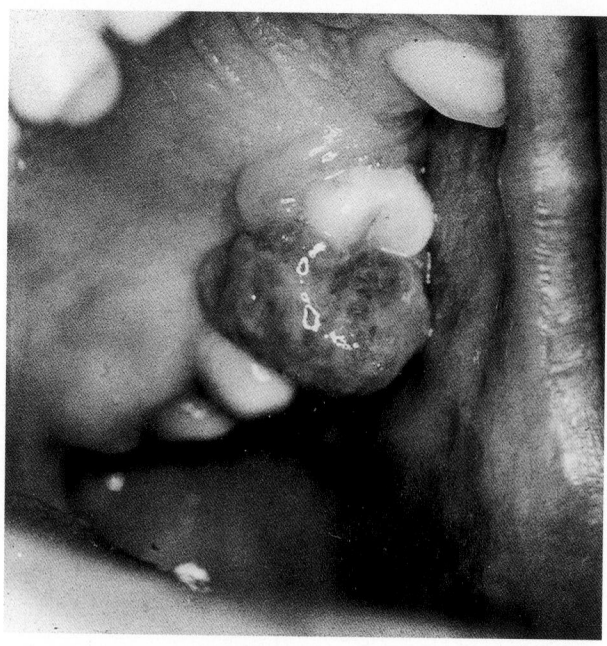

FIGURE 33.1　A pseudotumor: A pregnancy epulis, which is a highly vascularized growth resembling granulation tissue; it tends to regress after the pregnancy. (Courtesy of Dr. G. Fiore-Donno, School of Dentistry, Geneva, Switzerland.)

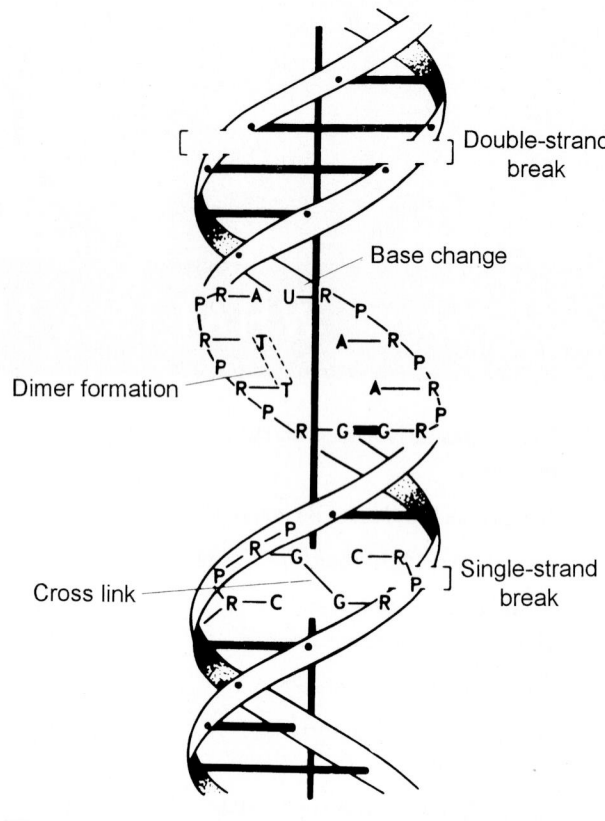

FIGURE 33.2　Schematic of a double-stranded DNA helix, showing the nature of five lesions that can damage or alter the helical structure. (Reproduced from [20].)

discovered in 1979. By 1991, **280** base substitution mutations of this gene alone were known (21), and 9 years later "The First **10,000**" were celebrated (17). Today, the widely accepted model of Vogelstein et al. for tumor progression includes 6–7 stages (see Figure 29.8), yet other reputable groups find that the number of mutations per cell, in cancer, is on the order of 11,000 or even 100,000 (39). *It may turn out some day that the molecular defect for a particular histologic type of tumor is never exactly the same.* We can only conclude, as William Boyd did in 1966, that "neoplasia is a process of infinite variety" (3).

Tumors Have More Than One Cause

We made the point earlier that every disease has more than one cause (p. 837). Seen in this light, the causation of tumors is a chain with many links, as many as 15 in the example of Figure 33.3; and each link offers a different opportunity for therapy.

Most Tumors Are the Result of Successive Genetic Changes

This means that the actual "time of birth" of a tumor may be difficult to pinpoint. Carcinomas of the colon are a well-documented example of this step-wise genesis (Figure 29.8); so are some melanomas (Figure 33.4) (23). And then, once malignancy is achieved, genetic changes continue under the guise of tumor progression; so the very nature of the tumor continues to change. This concept is best illustrated by a cartoon that has enjoyed decades of popularity in the oncological world (Figure 33.5). This progression may not be inevitable, as the natural history of moles abundantly proves.

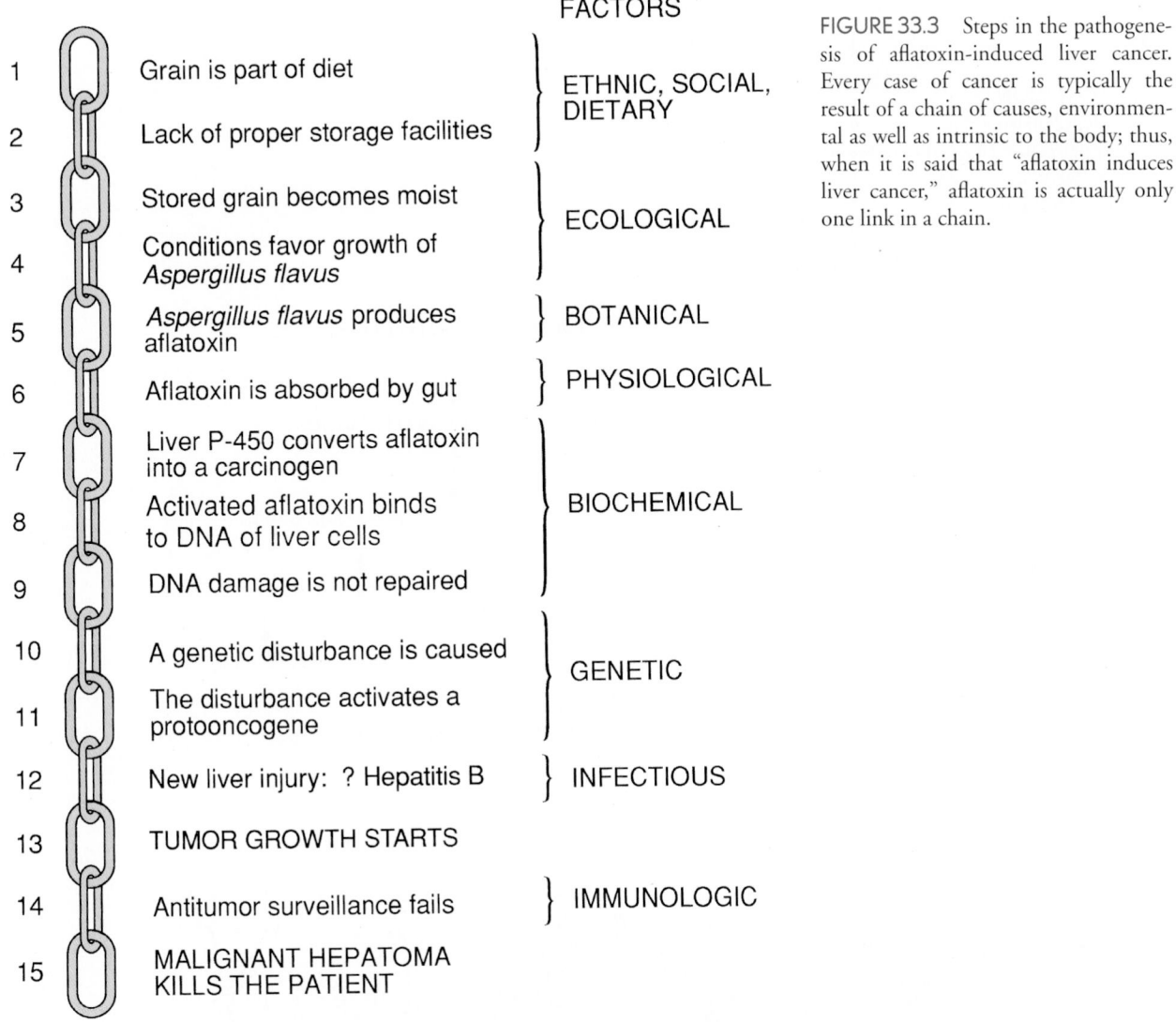

		FACTORS
1	Grain is part of diet	ETHNIC, SOCIAL, DIETARY
2	Lack of proper storage facilities	
3	Stored grain becomes moist	ECOLOGICAL
4	Conditions favor growth of *Aspergillus flavus*	
5	*Aspergillus flavus* produces aflatoxin	BOTANICAL
6	Aflatoxin is absorbed by gut	PHYSIOLOGICAL
7	Liver P-450 converts aflatoxin into a carcinogen	BIOCHEMICAL
8	Activated aflatoxin binds to DNA of liver cells	
9	DNA damage is not repaired	
10	A genetic disturbance is caused	GENETIC
11	The disturbance activates a protooncogene	
12	New liver injury: ? Hepatitis B	INFECTIOUS
13	TUMOR GROWTH STARTS	
14	Antitumor surveillance fails	IMMUNOLOGIC
15	MALIGNANT HEPATOMA KILLS THE PATIENT	

FIGURE 33.3 Steps in the pathogenesis of aflatoxin-induced liver cancer. Every case of cancer is typically the result of a chain of causes, environmental as well as intrinsic to the body; thus, when it is said that "aflatoxin induces liver cancer," aflatoxin is actually only one link in a chain.

Tumors Are Not Irreversible

The evidence has already been presented. Most significant are the experiments in which malignant cells appear to be tamed by their environment, and malignant nuclei by a normal cytoplasm. This line of research has produced a new way to look at tumors, which we will consider next.

The Key Defect of Tumors May Not Be Proliferation

Here is an exercise in "thinking differently." The notion being proposed is that proliferation, the obvious feature of tumors, may not be the basic problem. The ambitious reader may want to pause here and try to guess what else might be going on, besides proliferation.

The answer: a tumor could be a mass of undifferentiated stem cells that continue to multiply because they are prevented from reaching their goal—**differentiation.** Barry Pierce of Denver, Colorado has been the champion of this concept since 1961 (26, 34). The concept

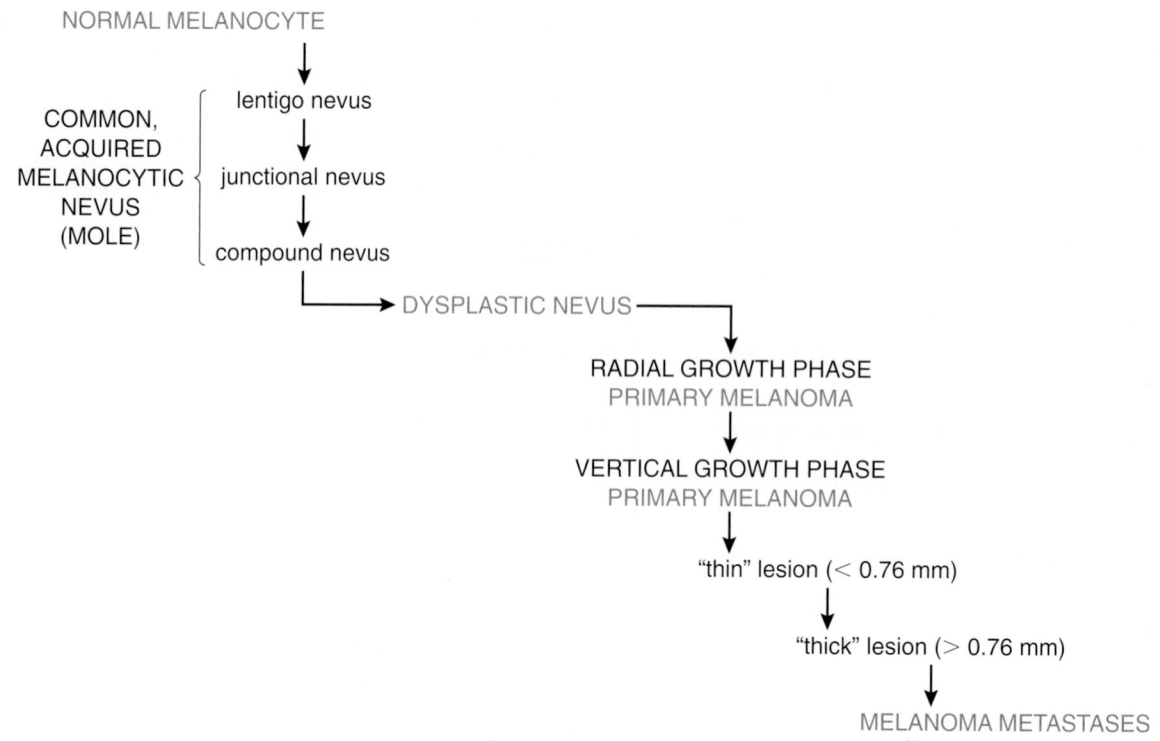

FIGURE 33.4 Stages of progression of melanocytic neoplasia in humans. Needless to say, this progression is a rare event. (Adapted with permission from [23].)

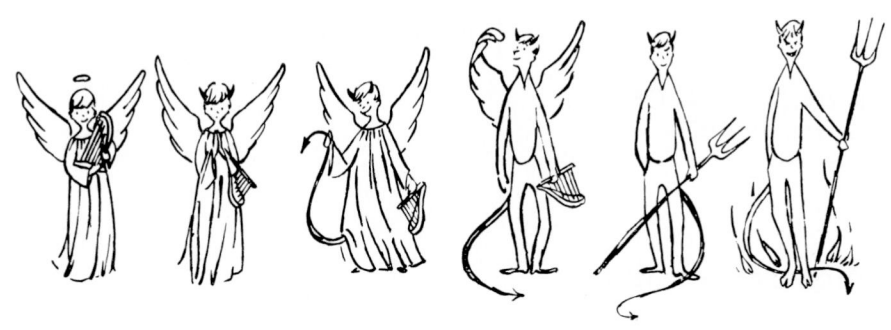

FIGURE 33.5 Cartoon from 1952 suggesting that malignant transformation may occur by stages. Today this concept is generally accepted. The number of steps is thought to be on the order of 6–7. (Drawn by Dr. H. Grady and published by Dr. A. T. Hertig.) (Reproduced with permission from [19].)

has enormous practical implications because it offers a handle for therapy. It would be difficult to correct a defect in the DNA; it is much simpler to find substances that encourage differentiation.

Pierce's arguments are compelling. Consider, for example, the teratocarcinoma of the mouse mentioned earlier (p. 925). All of its fourteen fully differentiated, apparently normal tissues plus the malignant components can be derived from a single malignant cell injected into the peritoneum of a normal mouse (24). This means that the original malignant cell, much like an embryonic cell, contained and used the genetic program for differentiating into many harmless adult tissues (29, 30). A similar argument can be made for

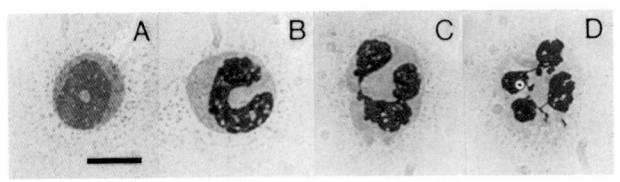

FIGURE 33.6 Differentiation of mouse leukemic cells *in vitro* induced by a protein secreted by normal mouse fibroblasts. **A:** Immature "blast cell." **B, C, D:** Stages of differentiation to mature granulocyte. **Bar** = 10 μm. (Reprinted with permission from Nature [10]. Copyright 1972 Macmillan Magazines Limited.)

squamous cell carcinomas: the famous pearls of these tumors (Figure 26.41) are made of keratinized, fully differentiated tumor cells. This tells us, once again, that the progeny of a malignant stem cell is able to march along the entire path of differentiation and die upon arrival, as all keratinocytes do. Why would it not be possible, some day, to coax all stem cells along this path?

Experimental differentiation of tumor cells *in vitro* (called *reverse transformation*) is easily obtained; the bulk of the data comes from neuroblastoma and myeloid leukemia (Figure 33.6) (13). The maturation *in vitro* of leukemic cells has become commonplace; human leukemic cells can be artificially matured *in vitro* (10) to the point of recovering their defensive functions (Figure 33.7) (7, 12). Such miraculous effects can be produced by a surprising variety of agents: hormones, regulatory peptides, cytotoxic drugs, retinoids (41), phorbol esters, vitamin D (46), dimethylsulfoxide (DMSO) and other polar compounds (7), short-chain fatty acids, cyclic AMP (32), some steroids, purines, actinomycin D, recombinant granulocyte colony-stimulating factor (35), even X-rays (7, 16), and nondescript "differentiation factors" obtained, for instance, from endotoxin-treated human lung (46). This last experiment, by the way, was suggested by a case of leukemia that went into remission after a bout of pneumonia.

Retinoids deserve special mention (43). These are a family of compounds, natural or synthetic, related to vitamin A (retinol). Beta-carotene is a dietary precursor of vitamin A: one molecule yields two molecules of the vitamin. The first faint connection between retinoids and cancer surfaced in 1925 (37, 44) when Wolbach and Howe discovered that vitamin A *deficiency* in rats caused squamous metaplasia of various epithelia, sometimes to the point of suggesting "the acquisition of neoplastic properties." The reader may recall these experiments from the section on metaplasia (p. 56)

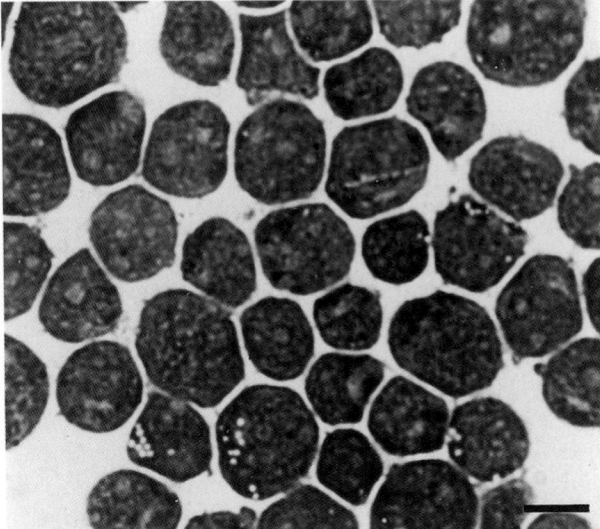

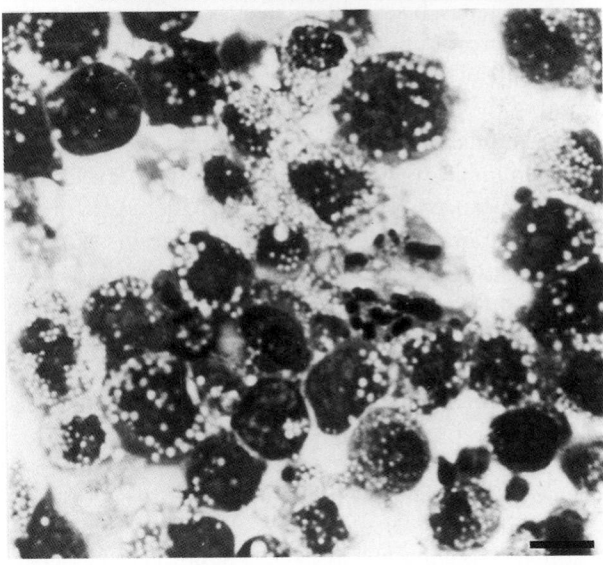

FIGURE 33.7 Differentiation of malignant cells *in vitro*. *Top:* Cells from a human promyelocytic leukemia, incubated for 24 hours with latex particles, fail to ingest them: they are too undifferentiated to perform that function. *Bottom:* The same experiment repeated with leukemia cells exposed for 5–7 days to a "differentiating medium"; most cells are now able to take up the beads. The medium was obtained by incubating bits of human lung tissue with endotoxin. For the fascinating rationale of this experiment see text. **Bars** = 5 μm. (Reproduced with permission from [46].)

where we also mentioned the classic *in vitro* studies of Cambridge by Dame Honor B. Fell and E. Mellanby, who confirmed the role of vitamin A in differentiation with almost mirror-image results (37): an excess of vitamin A suppressed normal keratinization and caused stratified epithelia to become mucociliary.

A study of neuroblastoma cells treated with retinoic acid showed that the expression of N-*myc,* often overexpressed in this tumor, is down regulated within 1 hour (40).

The final connection between vitamin A and malignancy was made in 1955 when Ilse Lasnitzki (also in the laboratory of Dame Honor B. Fell) showed that vitamin A could suppress the changes induced in mouse prostate by a carcinogen (25). Eventually the retinoids became the focus of intense interest as potential anticancer agents. In high doses they are toxic, hence the search for other derivatives. In the meantime a long list of promising results has piled up. For example, it has been possible to obtain terminal differentiation of mouse teratocarcinoma cells *in vitro* (36, 37), and even *in vivo* by injecting a vitamin A analog directly into the tumor. In treated experimental animals, inhibition has been obtained against cancers of the bladder, breast, and skin (15). Notice also the striking antiproliferative effects of a retinoid on the mammary gland of the rat (Figure 33.8) (27). Over a dozen studies in humans have shown an inverse relationship between intake of vitamin A or beta-carotene and incidence of cancer, with a 2 to 2.5 higher risk for the low-intake group. A number of possible mechanisms have been suggested.

Full differentiation of teratocarcinomas has been observed also in humans. After cytotoxic therapy, lung metastases of teratocarcinomas sometimes fail to regress; biopsy shows fully matured tissues of the types usually found in teratomas (4, 31).

> Neuroblastoma-differentiating agents (except the retinoids) have been used successfully, but their actual contribution is difficult to assess because other chemotherapy is given at the same time.

Now if we plug the concept of cancer as a disease of differentiation into the scheme of malignant transformation, we can conclude that cells turn malignant in different ways (33). For example, they might

- Constitutively produce their own growth factor
- Lose the ability to produce differentiation factor
- Lose the ability to respond to differentiation factor

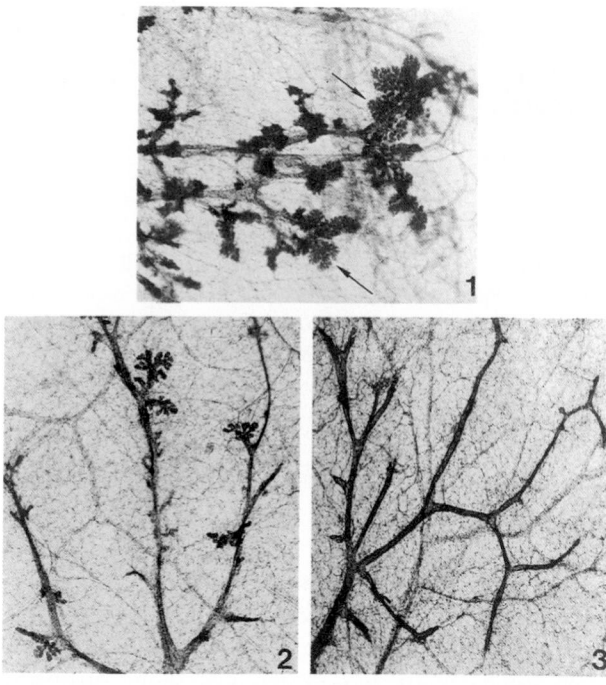

FIGURE 33.8   Antiproliferative effect of a retinoid. **1:** Whole mount of a normal rat mammary gland. **Arrow:** marked proliferation of end-buds. **2:** Mammary gland from a rat maintained on a low dose of retinoid for 182 days. Notice the reduced end-bud proliferation. **3:** Effect of high doses of retinoid after 182 days: almost total absence of end-bud proliferation. **Bar =** 500 μm. (Reproduced with permission from [27].)

As G. B. Pierce proposed in the 1960s, some tumor cells tend to differentiate on their own, and some malignant cells can be forced to differentiate. The good news is that "contrary to dogma, **cancer cells do not always beget cancer cells**" (31).

> The concept of "therapy by differentiation" has achieved some striking successes, mainly against acute promyelocytic leukemia using all-*trans* retinoic acid and lately also intravenous arsenic trioxide, a Chinese contribution (43).

Tumors Can Arise without the Help of Mutagens

The chapter on carcinogenesis left us with a paradox: the list of carcinogens includes hormones and other agents that cannot be construed as genotoxic, that is, capable of damaging DNA. Estrogens, for example, induce endometrial hyperplasia and can eventually lead to endometrial carcinoma. In this case, the initiation–promotion dogma offers little help. The hormone can only act as a promoter; to postulate that there "must be" an unknown initiator is not satisfactory.

A way out, proposed by S. M. Cohen and co-workers (6), is to remember that every time a cell goes through mitosis there is a small chance for a genetic error, and sometimes that error is of the kind that triggers cancer. A biological model, simulated by computer modeling techniques, showed that carcinogenesis by nongenotoxic compounds can be accounted for by increases in cell proliferation (5, 14). The model assumes two irreversible genetic events, initiation and transformation (meaning malignant change) (Figure 33.9). In essence, *it proposes cell proliferation as prelude to cancer,* a view supported by the well-established fact that most precancerous states imply accelerated cell division. Genotoxic agents are also partly dependent on this scheme.

> More support for this view comes from transgenic mice carrying a gene derived from the hepatitis B virus. These mice develop chronic hepatitis accompanied by constant regeneration. Eventually hepatomas appear (8).

Superficially, the new scheme resembles the initiation–promotion pattern (p. 779); it does overlap it but differs because it requires no mutagen. It also eliminates a disturbing feature of the old initiation–promotion paradigm: namely, the fact that most carcinogens are initiators as well as promoters.

Another satisfying aspect of Cohen's concept is that it explains why some carcinogens score negative when tested by mutagenicity tests (there are over 200 such tests)(42).

> The saccharin-conscious reader will be interested to know that sodium saccharin was the nongenotoxic agent used to model the new theory. **Saccharin** is an established carcinogen for rats only, especially for males. The urine of rats given huge doses of saccharin in the diet produces silicate-containing crystals that act as microabrasives and induce mild, chronic, regenerative proliferation (9). Mice, in which these silicates do not form, are resistant to the tumorigenic effect of saccharin. Humans also are unlikely to be affected.

In summary, the two theories are not mutually exclusive. The old initiation-promotion scheme is well adapted to explain certain models; the new scheme is broader and includes non-genotoxic agents.

Stem Cells in Tumors

How do **stem cells** fit in these theories of carcinogenesis? The presence of stem cells in tumors has long been assumed (Figure 33.9) and is becoming a science of its own. A critical step was accomplished by studying *acute myeloid leukemia* (AML) in which stem cells have special surface markers (27a). The analysis of AML showed that cancer cells can be divided in hierarchies of malignant stem cells, with extensive proliferative potential, to

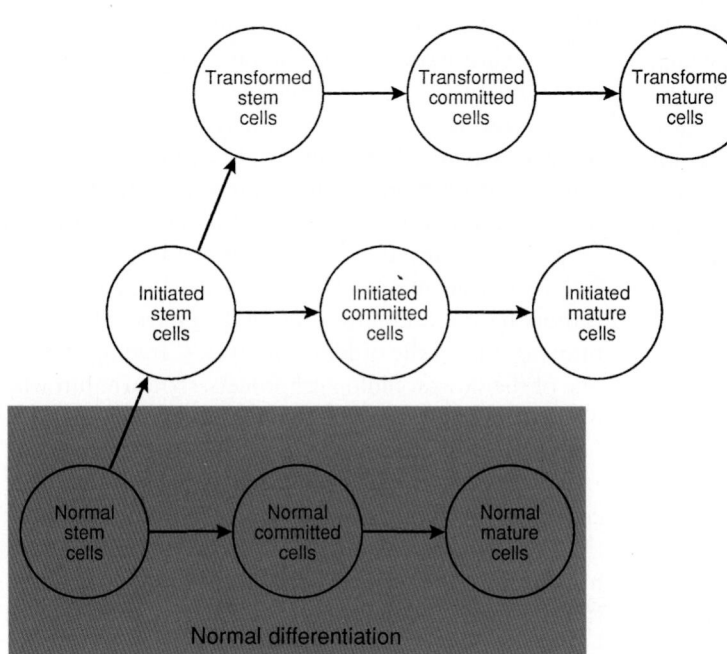

FIGURE 33.9 Biological model of carcinogenesis originally proposed by Greenfield and co-workers in 1984. The bottom row of circles represents the normal differentiation of a tissue. Ascending along the left side are two stages of carcinogenesis: initiation and transformation. This model assumes that cancer develops from normal cells through two irreversible genetic events. In this context, an agent can induce cancer in only two ways: by causing genetic damage or by increasing cell proliferation; the latter increases the number of opportunities for spontaneous genetic damage. (Adapted from [14] by permission of Oxford University Press.)

differentiated cancer cells with limited proliferative potential. Breast cancer, among others, fits into this scheme. This type of work requires the refined technology of proteomics, whose ultimate goal is to identify the estimated 10,000 proteins present in every cell (25a). The drive to find markers for each cell subtype is based, of course, on the hope of applications to highly specific therapy.

What Is a Benign Tumor?

We know ever so little about benign tumors. As we mentioned earlier (pp. 737, 770), cancer experts virtually ignore them. In the current scheme of progression there is a "benign" stage on the way to malignancy, and yet there are sleepy tumors such as lipomas that remain clinically unchanged for decades.

We submitted questions about benign tumors to several authorities in the field of experimental carcinogenesis. They seemed to agree that benign tumors are a mixed lot, and probably include:

- *Slowly growing malignant tumors that have not yet expressed their metastatic potential.* Thyroid adenomas might fit into this category.

- *Terminally differentiated tumors that were potentially malignant;* this would be in line with Pierce's theory.

- *Nodules of preneoplastic cells in an early stage of progression,* similar to the clusters of abnormal cells seen in the liver during multistage hepatic carcinogenesis (see Figures 29.27, 29.28).

In daily life the distinction between benign and malignant tumors is an oversimplification (11) made necessary by the clinical need to define those lumps that have a better prognosis and thereby to reassure the patients. Biologically, however, benign tumors are not a distinct entity.

Why Tumors?

Cells engage in so many activities. Is proliferation the only one that can run amok? Could any other cell function become aggressive? We can briefly speculate. The only other activity that could enable a cell to upset the economy of the body is secretion, e.g., of a hormone or cytokine. However, a single hypersecreting cell would have no impact; it would need clonal expansion, which means, once again, proliferation. So we must look for a pathologic condition in which hypersecretion prevails, with minimal proliferation; something akin to a "tumor of secretion." We know only one possible candidate: the **benign monoclonal gammopathy of unknown significance (MGUS)** (22, 24a) mentioned earlier (p. 902).

> About 5 percent of adults show this phenomenon: a plasma abnormality consisting of a monoclonal secretion of immunoglobulins, with no evidence of myeloma. Presumably these individuals harbor, somewhere in the bone marrow, a small clone of hypersecreting plasma cells, which some day may progress to myeloma.

Earlier we found that MGUS was interesting as an example of progression from benign to malignant in humans. Now we propose that "MGUS" might also come as close as possible to a "tumor of secretion."

We close with a thought borrowed from the *Encyclopedia of Medical Ignorance* (28). Much of our scientific knowledge about tumors comes from mouse tumors, yet mouse tumors are in some ways very different from ours, and we are so different from mice. We are about 3000 times larger and live 30–50 times longer. Mice have a metabolic rate 7 times faster than ours, and process some carcinogens differently (32a). Mice tend to generate mesenchymal cancers (lymphomas, sarcomas); humans tend to generate epithelial tumors. Most mouse cells express constitutive telomerase, and mouse chromosomes have telomeres much longer than ours. In a lifetime, human cells undergo 10^5 times more mitoses (10^{16} versus 10^{11}) (32a). Mouse tumors have a doubling time of 1–6 days, whereas in humans it is on the order of months. Carcinogenesis is one of the slowest biological processes known, but why is it so much faster in rodents? Richard Peto noted that our *lifelong risk of cancer is about the same as the lifelong risk for a mouse.* He calculated that human epithelial cells must be about a billion times more cancer-proof than mouse epithelial cells, and he points out that human cells in culture are extremely difficult to transform, whereas rodent cells comply quite easily. We will leave explanations to the experts (17a) and merely point out how grateful we should be that rodent time runs faster. If it ran like ours, we would have to wait 20–25 years for a carcinogen to show its effect, rodents would be presumably free of tumors, and cancer research would be free of grants.

So—What Is a Tumor?

Up to this point we evaded the difficult question "What is a tumor?" by breaking it up into small pieces that we found most significant. Here we bow out and listen to a team of tumor experts; our readers should recall Dr. R. A. Weinberg as the author of two books on the 1976 revolution (p. 861). The report "The Hallmarks of Cancer" (17a) (confirmed in 2002 as *Rules for Making Human Tumor Cells* [16a]) suggests that "the vast catalog of cancer cell genotypes is a manifestation of six essential alterations in cell physiology." These are:

- Self-sufficiency in growth signals
- Insensitivity to antigrowth signals
- Evasion of apoptosis
- Limitless replicative potential
- Sustained angiogenesis
- Tissue invasion and metastasis.

We will close with this authoritative summary. Classifications of scientific facts tend to have a short life—but they help crystallize thoughts.

References

1. Boveri T. Zur Frage der Entstehung maligner Tumoren. Jena: Gustav Fischer, 1914.
2. Boveri T. The origin of malignant tumors. Baltimore: Williams & Wilkins, 1929.
3. Boyd W. The spontaneous regression of cancer. Springfield, IL: Charles C. Thomas, 1966.
4. Carr BI, Gilchrist KW, Carbone PP. The variable transformation in metastases from testicular germ cell tumors: the need for selective biopsy. J Urol 1981;126:52–54.
5. Cohen SM, Ellwein LB. Cell proliferation in carcinogenesis. Science 1990;249:1007–1011.
6. Cohen SM, Purtilo DT, Ellwein LB. Pivotal role of increased cell proliferation in human carcinogenesis. Mod Pathol 1991; 4:371–382.
7. Collins SJ, Ruscetti FW, Gallagher RE, Gallo RC. Terminal differentiation of human promyelocytic leukemia cells induced by dimethyl sulfoxide and other polar compounds. Proc Natl Acad Sci USA 1978;75:2458–2462.
8. Dunsford HA, Sell S, Chisari FV. Hepatocarcinogenesis due to chronic liver cell injury in hepatitis B virus transgenic mice. Cancer Res 1990;50:3400–3407.
9. Ellwein LB, Cohen SM. The health risks of saccharin revisited. Crit Rev Toxicol 1990;20:311–326.
10. Fibach E, Landau T, Sachs L. Normal differentiation of myeloid leukaemic cells induced by a differentiation-inducing protein. Nature New Biol 1972;237:276–278.
11. Foulds L. Neoplastic development, vol 1. London: Academic Press, 1969.
12. Frankel SR, Warrell RP Jr. Retinoids in leukemia and myelodysplastic syndromes. In: Hong WK, Lotan R, eds.

Retinoids in oncology. New York: Marcel Dekker, 1993: 147–168.
13. Freshney RI. Induction of differentiation in neoplastic cells. Anticancer Res 1985;5:111–130.
14. Greenfield RE, Ellwein LB, Cohen SM. A general probabilistic model of carcinogenesis: analysis of experimental urinary bladder cancer. Carcinogenesis 1984;5:437–445.
15. Greenwald P. Principles of cancer prevention: diet and nutrition. In: DeVita VT Jr, Hellman S, Rosenberg SA, eds. Cancer: principles and practice of oncology, 3rd ed. Philadelphia: JB Lippincott, 1989:167–195.
16. Guimaraes JETE, Francis GE, Berney JJ, Wing MA, Hoffbrand AV. Differentiation of human acute myeloid leukaemia cells in response to exogenous and endogenous stimuli: different patterns of response suggested by a bioassay system. Leukemia 1985;9:869–878.
16a. Hahn WC, Weinberg RA. Rules for making human tumor cells. N Engl J Med 2002;347:1593–1603.
17. Hainaut P, Hollstein M. p53 and human cancer: the first ten thousand mutations. Adv Cancer Res 2000;77:81–137.
17a. Hanahan D, Weinberg RA. The hallmarks of cancer. Cell 2000;100:57–70.
18. Hansemann D. Ueber asymmetrische Zelltheilung in Epithelkrebsen und deren biologische Bedeutung. Virchows Arch Pathol Anat Physiol Klin Med 1890;119:299–326.
19. Hertig AT, Younge PA. A debate: what is cancer in situ of the cervix? Is it the preinvasive form of true carcinoma? Am J Obstet Gynecol 1952;64:807–815.
20. Hewitt RR, Harless J, Lloyd RS, Love J, Robberson DL. Molecular test systems for identification of DNA-reactive

agents. In: Griffin AC, Shaw CR, eds. Carcinogens: identification and mechanisms of action. New York: Raven Press, 1979:107–120.

21. Hollstein M, Sidransky D, Vogelstein B, Harris CC. p53 mutations in human cancers. Science 1991;253:49–53.

22. Jandl JH. Blood. Boston: Little, Brown, 1987.

23. Kerbel RS. Growth dominance of the metastatic cancer cell: cellular and molecular aspects. Adv Cancer Res 1990;55:87–132.

24. Kleinsmith LJ, Pierce GB Jr. Multipotentiality of single embryonal carcinoma cells. Cancer Res 1964;24:1544–1551.

24a. Kyle RA, Therneau TM, Rajkumar SV, et al. A long-term study of prognosis in monoclonal gammopathy of undetermined significance. N Engl J Med 2002;346:564–569.

25. Lasnitzki I. The influence of a hypervitaminosis on the effect of 20-methylcholanthrene on mouse prostate glands grown *in vitro*. Br J Cancer 1955;9:434–441.

25a. Liang P, Pardee AB. Analysing differential gene expression in cancer. Nat Rev Cancer 2003;3:869–876.

26. McKinnell RG, Parchment RE, Perantoni AO, Pierce GB (eds). The biological basis of cancer. Cambridge: Cambridge University Press, 1999.

27. Moon RC, Thompson HJ, Becci PJ, et al. N-(4-hydroxyphenyl)retinamide, a new retinoid for prevention of breast cancer in the rat. Cancer Res 1979;39:1339–1346.

27a. Pardal R, Clarke MF, Morrison SJ. Applying the principles of stem-cell biology to cancer. Nat Rev Cancer 2003;3:895–902.

28. Peto R. The need for ignorance in cancer research. In: Duncan R, Weston-Smith M, eds. The encyclopaedia of medical ignorance. Oxford: Pergamon Press, 1984:129–133.

29. Pierce GB. Teratocarcinoma: a model for a developmental concept of cancer. Curr Top Dev Biol 1967;2:223–246.

30. Pierce GB, Shikes R, Fink LM. Cancer: a problem of developmental biology. Englewood Cliffs, NJ: Prentice-Hall, 1978.

31. Pierce GB, Speers WC. Tumors as caricatures of the process of tissue renewal: prospects for therapy by directing differentiation. Cancer Res 1988;48:1996–2004.

32. Puck TT. Cyclic AMP, the microtubule-microfilament system, and cancer. Proc Natl Acad Sci USA 1977;74:4491–4495.

32a. Rangarajan A, Weinberg RA. Comparative biology of mouse versus human cells: modelling human cancer in mice. Nat Rev Cancer 2003;3:952–959.

33. Sachs L. Origin and reversibility of malignancy. Carcinog Compr Surv 1985;10:23–33.

34. Sell S, Pierce GB. Maturation arrest of stem cell differentiation is a common pathway for the cellular origin of teratocarcinomas and epithelial cancers. Lab Invest 1994;70:6–22.

35. Souza LM, Boone TC, Gabrilove J, et al. Recombinant human granulocyte colony-stimulating factor: effects on normal and leukemic myeloid cells. Science 1986;232:61–65.

36. Speers WC. Conversion of malignant murine embryonal carcinomas to benign teratomas by chemical induction of differentiation *in vivo*. Cancer Res 1982;42:1843–1849.

37. Sporn MB. Retinoids and suppression of carcinogenesis. Hosp Pract 1983;18:83–98.

38. Stanbridge EJ. The reemergence of tumor suppression. Cancer Cells 1989;1:31–33.

39. Stoler DL, Chen N, Basik M, et al. The onset and extent of genomic instability in sporadic colorectal tumor progression. Proc Natl Acad Sci USA 1999;96:15121–15126.

40. Thiele CJ, Israel MA. Regulation of N-myc expression is a critical event controlling the ability of human neuroblasts to differentiate. Exp Cell Biol 1988;56:321–333.

41. Tsokos M, Kyritsis AP, Chader GJ, Triche TJ. Differentiation of human retinoblastoma *in vitro* into cell types with characteristics observed in embryonal or mature retina. Am J Pathol 1986;123:542–552.

42. Wagner BM. The mutagen-carcinogen controversy. Mod Pathol 1990;3:555–556.

43. Warrell RP Jr. Differentiation agents. In: Cancer. Principles & practice of oncology, 6th ed. Philadelphia: Lippincott Williams & Wilkins, 2001, pp. 489–494.

44. Wolbach SB, Howe PR. Tissue changes following deprivation of fat-soluble A vitamin. J Exp Med 1925;42:753–777.

45. Wolf U. Theodor Boveri and his book "On the Problem of the Origin of Malignant Tumors." In: German J, ed. Chromosomes and cancer. New York: John Wiley & Sons, 1974: 3–20.

46. Yunis AA, Arimura GK, Wu F-M, Wu M-C. Differentiation of cultured promyelocytic leukemia cells (HL-60) induced by endotoxin-treated human lung conditioned medium. Leukemia Res 1987;11:673–679.

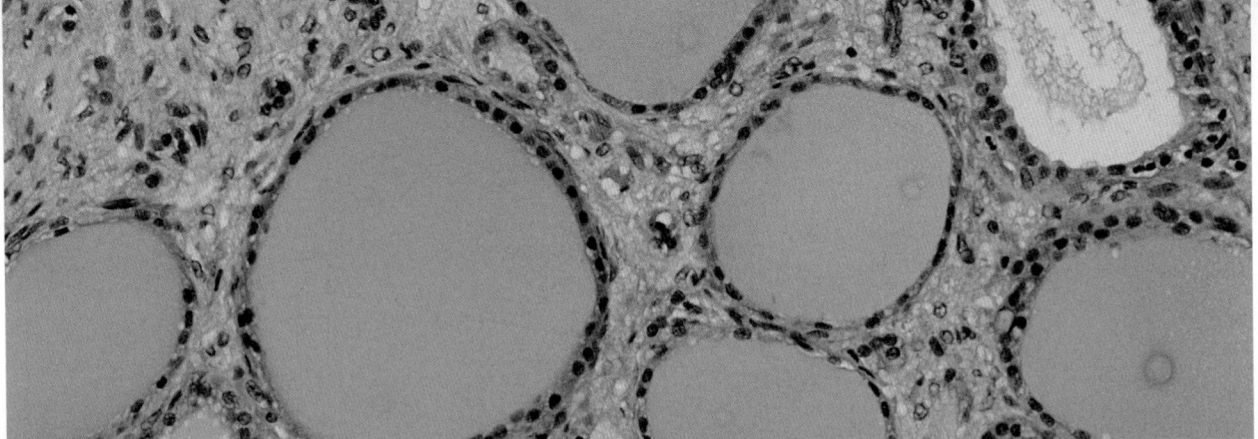

CHAPTER 34

TUMORS AS A CLINICAL PROBLEM

- Concepts of Tumor Diagnosis
- Concepts of Tumor Prognosis
- Concepts of Tumor Therapy

Most solid tumors are recognized at first as abnormal lumps or masses—with the naked eye, by palpation, or by radiologic or endoscopic means. The next step in diagnosis is microscopic. As a rule, no treatment should be undertaken unless the nature of the mass is known (it might not be a tumor at all). Skin tumors are a partial exception: many are so obvious that they can be excised first, then examined microscopically.

Concepts of Tumor Diagnosis

The first major challenge, in tumor diagnosis, is to recognize that a tumor indeed exists. As we just mentioned, for superficial tumors this is fairly simple; for deep-seated tumors it is another matter. The ideal solution would be to have a blood test that would tell us "malignant tumor present." Unfortunately, there seems to be no metabolic abnormality common to all malignant tumor cells, so the quest for a general tumor test is probably hopeless. One is announced every year or so and then fades away. However, some types of tumor cells do produce molecules that can be used as biochemical indicators that a certain type of tumor is present. The molecules that are found in the blood or urine are called **clinical tumor markers;** those identified in microscopic preparations are called **histochemical tumor markers.**

Clinical Tumor Markers

Clinical tumor markers are molecules of many kinds (4, 28, 63) but usually proteins secreted by known cell types, and found in the blood and/or urine. They are present under normal conditions at a baseline level, and when elevated they are indicative of a tumor. None is absolutely specific (35a), but overall they are very helpful (Table 34.1). Four common examples are listed on the next page.

Table 34.1 Circulating Tumor Markers

Marker	Tumor(s)
Human chorionic gonadotropin	Gestational trophoblastic
	Germ cell
	Urothelial
	Gastrointestinal
α-Fetoprotein	Germ cell
	Hepatocellular
Lactate dehydrogenase	Germ cell
Placental alkaline phosphatase	Germ cell
	Lymphoma
Prostate-specific antigen	Prostate
Carcinoembryonic antigen	Gastrointestinal (colorectal)
	Breast
Neuron-specific enolase	Small cell lung cancer
	Neuroendocrine
CA125	Ovarian
CA19.9	Pancreas
	Gastrointestinal
	Ovarian

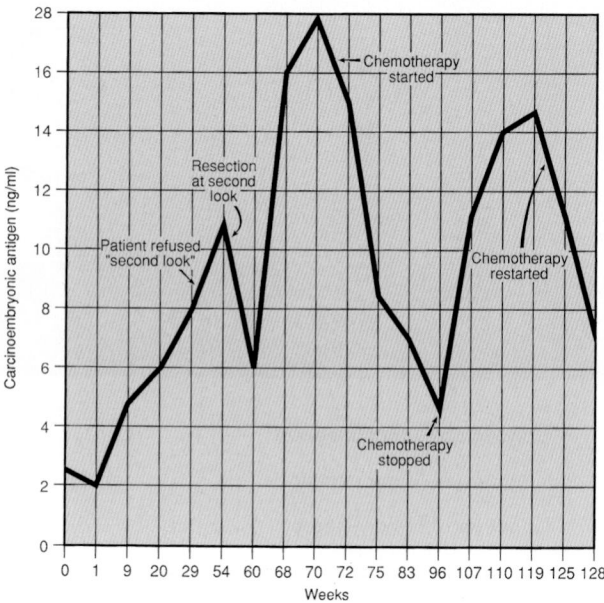

FIGURE 34.1   Demonstration that the plasma level of carcinoembryonic antigen (CEA) can be used to monitor the size of the tumor mass, in this case a colon cancer. (Adapted with permission from [58].)

The Bence-Jones protein. This protein, found in the urine (p. 288), is mentioned here first because it is historically the oldest tumor marker. Dr. Bence-Jones discovered it in 1846. It betrays the presence of multiple myeloma.

Prostate-specific antigen. PSA is a glycoprotein specific for prostatic epithelium. It is present in the blood and in seminal fluid (10, 57): its level in the blood is about doubled if the prostate is forcefully massaged (not a recommended practice). It also tends to increase in prostatic hypertrophy. PSA is the most sensitive marker for the progression of prostatic cancer and its response to therapy (11). PSA is a normal product of the adult prostate, and it continues to be produced by its malignant counterpart. Rather different is the situation of the so-called *oncofetal proteins,* such as carcinoembryonic antigen and alpha-fetoprotein, which are not significantly expressed in the adult but become derepressed in some tumors.

Carcinoembryonic antigen. CEA is the product of a gene that is active mainly in the normal fetus. It is the most reliable clinical marker for colorectal cancer (52). CEA is a high-molecular-weight, cell-surface glycoprotein that was described in 1965 as typical of fetal colon and of carcinomas of adult colons (51). It is not suitable for screening purposes because it also appears in the blood of patients with other carcinomas (e.g., pancreas up to 90 percent and lung up to 70 percent; compared with colon and rectum, 60–90 percent). Interestingly, the CEA gene undergoes some degree of derepression in a number of nonmalignant diseases: alcoholic cirrhosis,

gastric ulcer, bronchitis, and others (37). In practice, the rise and fall of CEA levels can be used cautiously to monitor the success of treatment, as well as recurrences (Figure 34.1) (39, 58).

Alpha-fetoprotein. AFP was discovered by G. I. Abelev in Moscow in 1963, in newborn or pregnant mice and in mice bearing liver carcinoma. Shortly thereafter it was discovered in the blood of a patient with liver carcinoma (50).

AFP is normally synthesized by the liver, yolk sac, and gastrointestinal epithelia, with a peak in early fetal life. It is clinically useful as a marker for liver cell carcinoma and germ cell tumors (except seminomas). Its behavior is similar to that of CEA. It can also be present in carcinomas of the pancreas and stomach, as well as in nonneoplastic conditions, including pregnancy; and it can be used to monitor therapy and recurrence. Blood levels can rise from less than 20 ng/ml in normal adults to 100,000 and even 10,000,000 ng/ml (37).

The reader may have been surprised to see that none of the examples given represent a known oncogene, such as the notorious *p53*. After all, the genesis of a tumor is supposed to imply the overexpression of several normal genes and/or the expression of mutated genes: it should be possible to find, in the blood and in the tumor, (a) an excess of normal gene products, such as growth factors; (b) abnormal forms of normal gene products; and (c) antibodies to these abnormal proteins. In fact, *all these products can be found in the blood of cancer patients,* but there are two problems: the laboratory methods are still cumbersome and expensive, and then, every tumor is the result of mutations in several genes—6 or 7, perhaps many more—and the lists of genes involved in different tumors overlap. In practice, this means that a clinician cannot hope to find, in the blood or urine, a single protein indicative of a single tumor, such as one enzyme, phospholipase, can correspond to a single condition, acute pancreatitis.

For example: increased levels of mutant p53 protein were found in the serum of 20 percent of patients with hepatoma, 30 percent of patients with cirrhosis, 8 percent with breast cancer, 13 percent with lung cancer, 18 percent with Hodgkin's lymphoma, 38 percent with colon adenomas, 64 percent with colon carcinomas; antibodies against *p53* were found in 9 percent of patients with breast cancers, 13 percent with lung cancer, 25 percent with hepatoma, 2 percent with prostate cancer, 28 percent with bladder cancer, and so on (8, 9).

Yet, protein technology is advancing fast. The microarray approach may soon be providing us with a "multigene formula" for each tumor.

Histochemical Tumor Markers

Depending on the degree of urgency, microscopic sections can be prepared during surgery (the tissue is frozen and cut as such) or within 1–2 days after embedding in paraffin, a method that produces better sections. **Histochemistry** and especially **immunohistochemistry** are essential for diagnosing many tumors.

The latter technique is based on the use of commercial antibodies, mostly against markers (proteins) of a particular kind of tumor, often referred to not very accurately as **oncoproteins.** Hundreds are available. Antibodies are also used to identify normal cellular components, e.g., cyclins (26). They are usually visualized by an enzymatic reaction based on the use of peroxidase. An example: chromogranins are invaluable markers for neuroendocrine tumors (Figure 34.2) (1).

Diagnostic antibodies are prepared by injecting suspensions of human tumors into animals. When antibodies form they are tested on sections from a variety of human tumors with the hope that they will bind only and specifically to some component of the original tumor. Catalogs of new antibodies continue to appear.

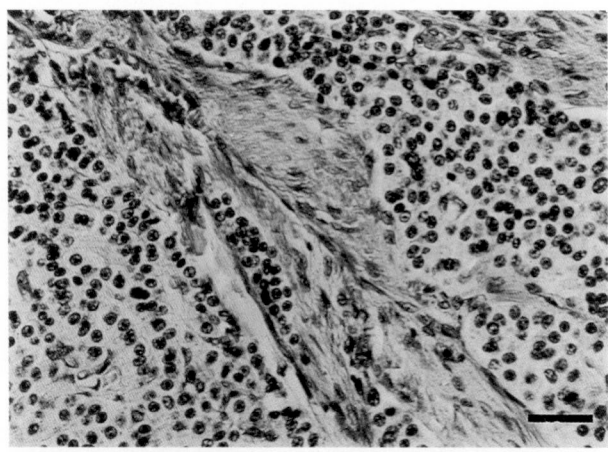

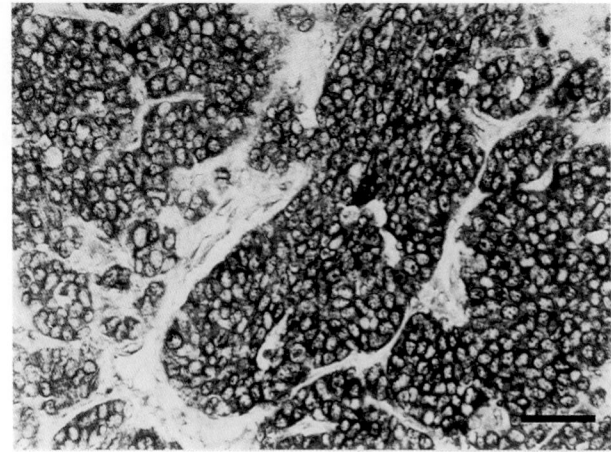

FIGURE 34.2   *Top:* Histological aspect of a bronchial carcinoid. This particular carcinoid produced *synaptophysin,* a protein originally found in presynaptic vesicles of bovine neurons. *Bottom:* Positive reaction of the tumor cells after treatment with an immunohistochemical stain for synaptophysin. **Bars** = 25 μm. (Courtesy of Dr. E. Gould, Rush Medical College, Chicago.)

NOTE: Some people erroneously refer to the commercial antibodies as "markers." The marker is the molecule to which the antibody binds.

Diagnostic antibodies enable us to establish, for example, that a given metastatic adenocarcinoma originated in the prostate. Faced with a poorly differentiated tumor, the pathologist may have to answer an even more basic question: is this an epithelial or a mesenchymal tumor? Because epithelial cells contain filaments of cytokeratin (p. 158), an antikeratin antibody should give the answer. Keratin, incidentally, comes in 20 varieties, and it is one of the five types of intermediate filaments; of these, vimentin is supposed to predominate in connective tissue cells, and desmin in smooth muscle cells (p. 158).

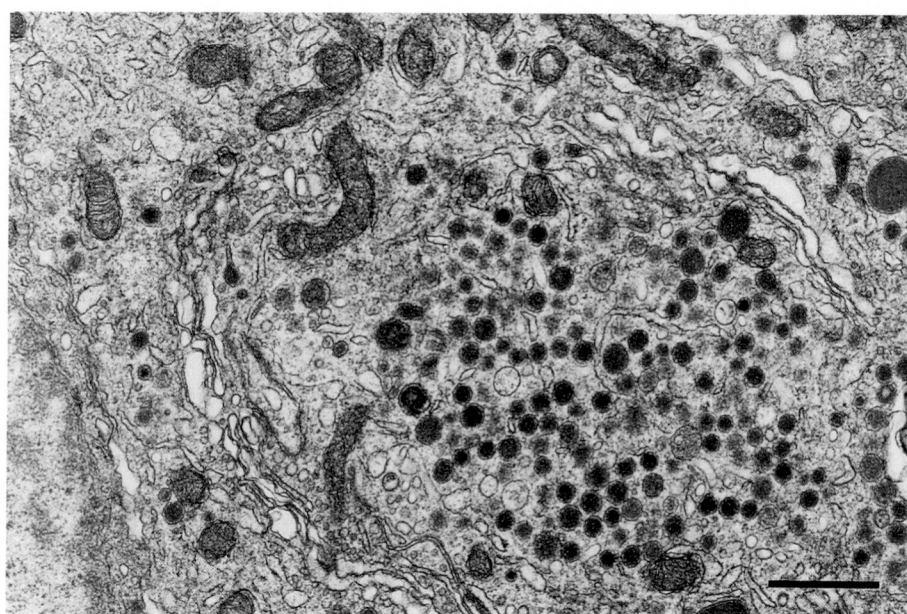

FIGURE 34.3   From a human bronchial carcinoid: part of a tumor cell showing the typical neuroendocrine granules of different size and structure. Carcinoids are tumors of the so-called *dispersed neuroendocrine system,* consisting of cells found in the nervous system, endocrine organs, gastrointestinal and bronchopulmonary tracts, and skin. Their cells produce a variety of neuroamines and neuropeptides. **Bar** = 1 μm. (Courtesy of Dr. V. E. Gould, Rush Medical College, Chicago, IL.)

These basic correlations are statistically valid, but there are pitfalls. Individual tumors can be capricious (23); for example, malignant smooth muscle cells can stray close enough to epithelium to express keratin (24). All cells have all the genes, and tumor cells master the art of derepression.

Fluorescence *in situ* hybridization (usually referred to as the **FISH** technique) detects specific nucleic acid sequences of DNA in chromosomes and of RNA in cells.

Electron Microscopy

The electron microscope has made one important negative contribution to cancer diagnosis: there is no ultrastructural feature typical of cancer. It is still unequaled for revealing fine details of cell structure, e.g., in neuroendocrine tumors (Figure 34.3), and remains essential as a research tool. In a hospital environment, however, it is considered slow and expensive, and therefore liable to become an administrator's target.

Molecular Technology

Molecular (i.e., DNA related) technology has become essential for the diagnosis, prognosis and management of many tumors, especially leukemias and lymphomas, because in these malignancies isolated cells are more easily available. **Microarray methodology** is making inroads (9a) (p. 175), but for diagnostic purposes it remains a rare adjunct to microscopic examination (21a).

Concepts of Tumor Prognosis

Prognosis—the art of predicting the outcome of disease—has been a major concern ever since the times of Hippocrates, side by side with diagnosis. It is still an art. For each tumor, it requires synthesis of clinical and laboratory data. The fullest approach to prognosis requires two steps: grading and staging. Grading is based on microscopic study; staging on clinical criteria.

Grading

Grading evaluates the aggressiveness *from histologic features* such as cellular atypia, architectural atypia, number of mitoses, degree of differentiation and invasiveness. Again, special criteria are set for each organ. Carcinoma of the prostate, for example, is graded according to the Gleason system (p. 767) (22). Grading can be only indicative because it is fraught with difficulties; atypia can vary in different parts of the tumor. It is partly subjective, and may not always correlate with the aggressive behavior of a tumor. For these reasons, the help of other techniques has been sought. In breast cancer, for example, the presence of abundant estrogen receptors in the cancer cells correlates with a long disease-free interval; antibodies to such receptors can provide a striking histochemical picture (Figure 34.4).

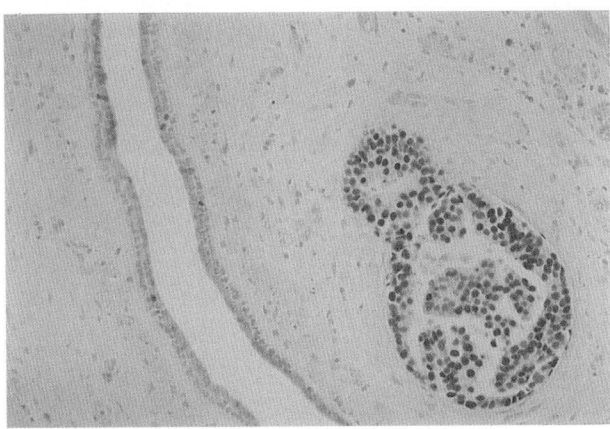

FIGURE 34.4 Human breast, showing estrogen receptors by immunohistochemistry (reaction product = brown). *Left:* Normal duct; very few cells are positive. *Right:* Intraductal atypical hyperplasia; many cells are positive. (Courtesy of Dr. M. E. Bur, Baystate Medical Center, Springfield, MA.)

Estrogen receptors can also be quantitated by a more cumbersome biochemical test (19), but the homogenizing biochemist can never quite know what is in the mixture—live carcinoma, necrotic carcinoma, normal glands, or connective tissue.

Aneuploidy can be measured by flow cytometry. It tends to correlate with poor prognosis (33, 34, 49) but the correlation is not ironclad: it works well for cancers of the bladder and prostate, questionably for breast and colon, and not at all for stomach and thyroid (33).

We should add here that **aneuploidy** is currently the basis of an alternative theory of carcinogenesis (18b) but it has not yet achieved broad recognition.

A promising approach to detect aneuploidy is to construct panels of immunohistochemical markers, as was done for stage I lung cancer (17).

Five molecular markers were associated with the risk of recurrence and death, representing: apoptosis (p53), angiogenesis (factor VIII), growth regulation (*erb*-b2), adhesion (CD44), and cell cycle regulation (Rb recessive oncogene).

DNA testing will surely become a major adjunct to immunohistochemistry in determining prognosis (41).

Staging

The staging step addresses the question: *to what extent has the tumor spread at the time of diagnosis?* It stands to reason that it should take into account the size and infiltration of the original tumor, its spread (if any) to the regional lymph nodes, and the presence or absence of metastases. All these data can be expressed by a sort of shorthand system proposed by the *Union Internationale Contre le Cancer* (UICC) (56); it is also called the TNM system because it considers features of the primary *tumor,* involved lymph *nodes,* and distant *metastases.* Special criteria are set for each organ, especially in reference to the assessment of local invasion; to cover all organs an atlas is necessary (55). Proper staging is important for choosing the proper treatment.

In particular: the T of TNM can be T0 (no evidence of primary), TIS (primary *in situ*), or T1 to T4 according to size; N can vary from N0 to N3; and M can be M0 or M1. A particular cancer of the colon, for example, could be T2N1M0. Obviously, this type of staging requires surgery followed by pathologic examination.

Staging: biopsy of the sentinel lymph node. This is a technique currently being developed; the purpose is to avoid unnecessary surgery, especially the complete dissection of the axillary lymph nodes for breast cancer, which is a very traumatic procedure.

The basic assumption is that *the lymph (and metastatic cells) from a primary tumor flow mainly to one or few nodes,* which can be considered as the early warning system. Surgery should therefore concentrate on the sentinel node, instead of dissecting the whole axilla. To identify the sentinel node, several protocols are being tested. Basically, a radioactive colloid tracer and a blue dye are injected around the primary tumor; 5–10 minutes later an incision (guided by the radioactivity) is made over the node area. A blue node is assumed to be the "sentinel," excised, and thoroughly investigated histologically; if it is free of metastases, no axillary dissection is performed. The procedure requires a team approach and it is not easy, but it reduces postoperative complications without loss of accuracy regarding the staging process (6, 32).

Concepts of Tumor Therapy

Therapy is not the subject of this book, but the reader might be interested in seeing how certain features of tumor biology have been exploited as Achilles' heels to attack tumors.

Prevention, of course, remains the best therapy. We have already stated that about 80 percent of cancers are self-inflicted and theoretically preventable. The next best approach would be chemoprevention (18a, 58a, 65).

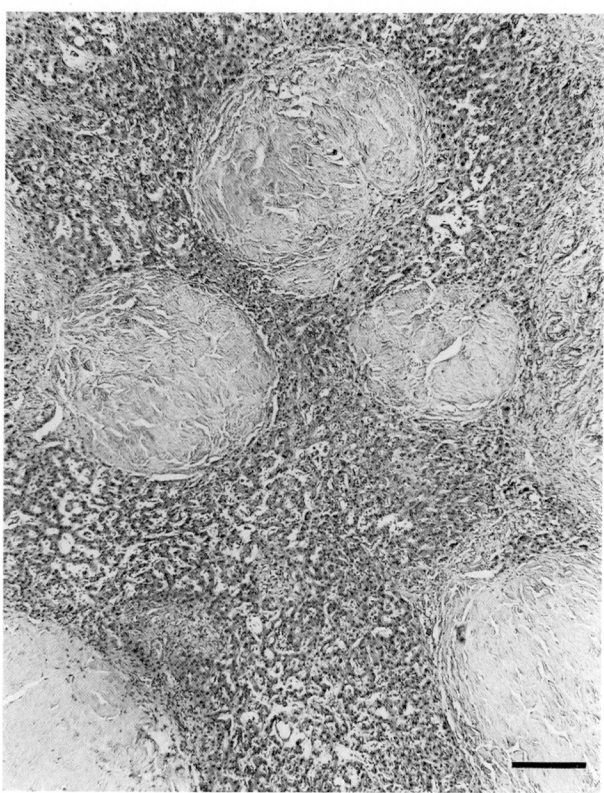

FIGURE 34.5   Nodular hyalin scars in a liver several years after successful irradiation for Hodgkin's disease. Such scars are typical residues of irradiated neoplasms, especially in Hodgkin's disease. **Bar** = 250 μm. (Reproduced with permission from [21]. Photomicrograph courtesy of Dr. Fajardo, Stanford School of Medicine, Palo Alto, CA.)

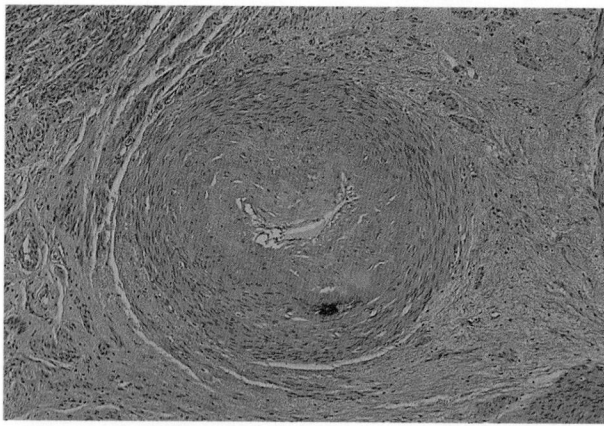

FIGURE 34.6   Radiation injury of an artery near an irradiated endometrial carcinoma. The thickened intima restricts the lumen. (The dark spot is a calcification of the internal elastic lamina.) (60x)

Compounds of different classes have been shown to be experimentally effective (18a, 58a). Some compounds are being tested on a large scale, and some are quite simple, such as aspirin or calcium supplements for colon cancer (3, 31).

Surgery and radiotherapy are now the most successful therapeutic approaches to localized disease, and chemotherapy is appropriate for systemic disease. Radio- and chemotherapy share the disturbing feature that they can also produce tumors, because both aim at the DNA of the tumor but cannot avoid also hitting the DNA of normal cells. When they do destroy a tumor, what is left behind is a scar (Figure 34.5), and irradiated tissues tend to develop fibrosis as well as vascular changes that reduce blood flow (Figure 34.6).

Chemotherapy against tumors, as well as against bacteria, is a sophisticated process with a mathematical background of its own. Its beginnings were worked out in the early 1960s by Skipper and co-workers, using a

nonviral mouse leukemia called L1210, characterized by a logarithmic cellular growth (27, 53, 54). Here are some of the results:

- *A single leukemic cell can be lethal;* unfortunately this is bound to remain true.
- *The percentage of leukemic cells killed by a given dose of a drug is constant.* For example, suppose that a certain dose given to a mouse with a leukemic burden of 10^4 cells reduces the burden to an average of 1 leukemic cell per animal (99.99 percent kill). Many of the surviving mice (actually 40 percent according to a Poisson distribution) will have zero leukemic cells. If that same dose is given to a mouse with 10^6 cells, it will knock the leukemic population down to 10^2 cells, but no mouse will have zero cells. This is the fractional kill or fixed-log kill hypothesis.
- *The fraction of leukemic cells killed is directly related to the drug level.* Therefore, if the dose must be repeated, it is more effective to use a short-term–high-dose schedule of therapy than long-term–low-dose schedule.
- *The net cell-kill per cycle of drug is the initial cell-kill minus the regrowth of the cells before the next cycle.* Therefore, successive drug cycles must be close enough to remain ahead of the regrowth (Figure 34.7) (48).

Some of these data have been confirmed in other experimental tumors and in humans (27), but the theory of Skipper and others has been criticized because it is based on an animal model of leukemia characterized by logarithmic growth. Human tumors follow a

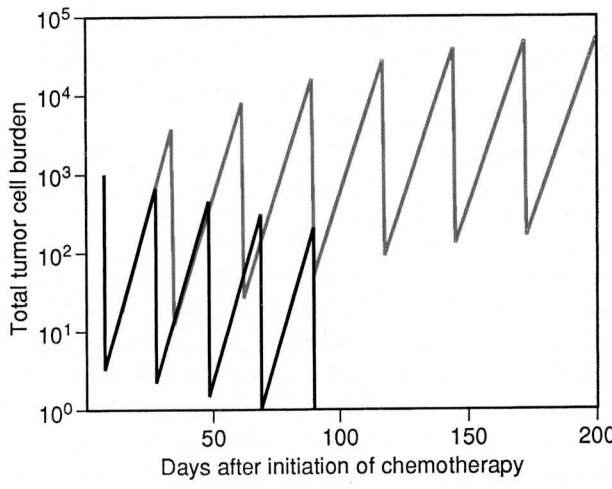

FIGURE 34.7   Effect of the treatment schedule on the outcome of chemotherapy for microscopic tumor residues after primary surgery. Each perpendicular line on the tumor growth curve indicates a tumor cell kill of 99.7 percent following a course of chemotherapy. According to the schedule, treatment at 3-week intervals (**black line**) results in a cure after five courses; a cure would not be achieved with a 4-week interval (**red line**) regardless of the number of courses. (Adapted from [48] with permission from Elsevier Science Publishing.)

Point	% maximum size	% maximum growth fraction	% maximum growth rate
1	0.5	50	7
2	10	20	64
3	37	8	100
4	85	1	38
5	97	0.3	8
6	99	0.05	1

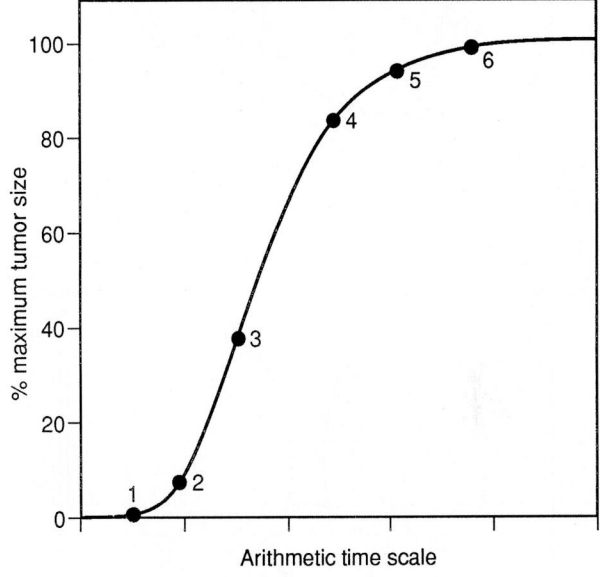

FIGURE 34.8   Theoretical Gompertzian curve of tumor growth: relationship between tumor size, growth fraction, and growth rate. (Reproduced with permission from [40].)

Gompertzian growth curve (p. 783); this means that a drug cannot be equally effective all along the growth curve. It should be less effective on very small and very large tumors, and maximally effective on tumors that have reached about 37 percent of their final size (Figure 34.8) (40).

The number of malignant cells in human tumors is enormous, and chemotherapy is hampered by three major obstacles:

- The safety margin between toxicity for the tumor and toxicity for the patient (chemotherapeutic index) is narrow.
- Metastatic cells hide behind endothelial barriers that are impassable for drugs, such as the blood–brain and the blood–skin barriers (p. 319).
- Tumor cells, especially in metastases, can be or can become insensitive to drugs. This is a major issue.

The Phenomenon of Drug Resistance

Like mythical cats, tumor cells have at least nine ways to survive cytotoxic drugs. They can adapt their metabolism to inactivate a drug or reduce its activation; they can modify, reduce, or overproduce target proteins, alter transport mechanisms, and even improve DNA repair (7, 13). Similar responses are known also in bacteria; they are attributed to mutations followed by

selective growth. Most important is a mechanism whereby tumor cells respond to a drug by becoming resistant to that and to other unrelated drugs: the phenomenon of **multidrug resistance.** An intriguing detail: normal tissues *never* develop chemoresistance—so we are told (13).

One way tumor cells perform this feat is to increase the expression of a group of genes called *mdr* (for *multidrug resistance*). These genes encode glycoproteins embedded in the tumor cell plasma membrane (P-glycoproteins) that pump out certain cytotoxic, lipophilic molecules (Figure 34.9) (42). A P-glycoprotein is present in the plasma membrane of normal cells exposed to toxic agents, such as in the liver, kidney, and colon; the list includes the placenta and adrenal where it may be related to hormone secretion. Homologous proteins exist in bacteria. Transfection of an *mdr* gene to cultured cells makes them multidrug resistant.

We have mentioned that many multiresistant cells have distinctive chromosomal features: double minute chromosomes and homogeneous staining regions (HSRs)

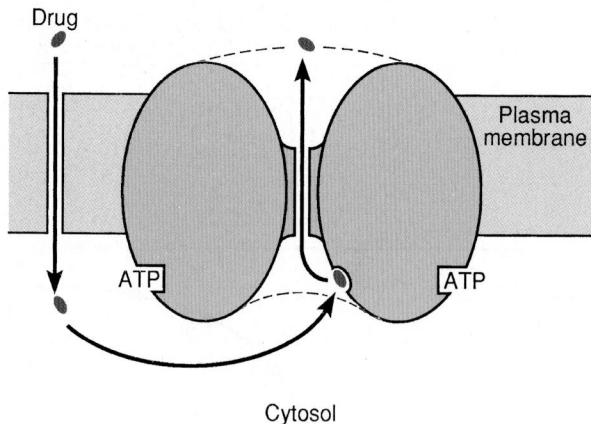

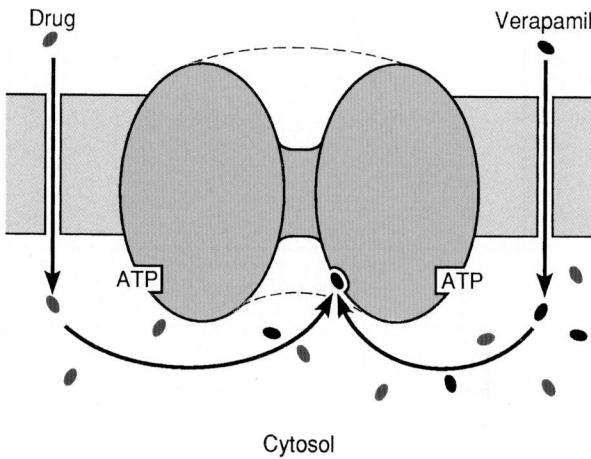

FIGURE 34.9   Artist's view of the multidrug-resistance protein involved in transporting cytotoxic drugs out of cells (P-glycoprotein). It is represented here as doughnut-shaped. *Top:* A toxic molecule (*left*) penetrating across the plasma membrane is pumped out the center of the doughnut, by an ATP-dependent mechanism. *Bottom:* A second drug (e.g., Verapamil) can interfere with the extrusion process by competing with the toxic drug and blocking the pump. (Adapted with permission from [42], copyright by J.B. Lippincott, 1988.)

(p. 896). Both contain enormous amplifications of an *mdr* gene (20). The P-glycoproteins are a functional part of the endothelial barriers and of cells in the "altered nodules" of livers treated with carcinogens (p. 902). Only molecular biology could reveal a link between such disparate cell types.

Overcoming Drug Resistance

Kill-and-rescue. A rather frightening device for taming a drug-resistant tumor is to give the patient a *lethal* dose of chemotherapy (lethal for the tumor *and* for the

patient) and then rescue the patient by reinjecting his or her own blood-derived hemopoietic stem cells harvested before the treatment, after mobilization with growth factors (16). A problem: the stem cells may be contaminated with tumor cells. A bonus: if allogeneic stem cells are used, they may unleash a helpful graft-versus-leukemia reaction (p. 579) (12).

Debulking. A tumor that cannot be entirely removed by surgery is sometimes treated by partial removal or "debulking" (**cytoreduction** is a more palatable term). There is a biological justification for this seemingly hopeless procedure: if the bulk of a tumor is reduced, the part that is left behind is said to undergo a burst of mitoses (as if it were moving back along its Gompertzian curve) (p. 783) and to thereby become more susceptible to chemotherapy (18, 61, 62).

Other Approaches to Tumor Therapy

Oncologists have come up with some highly imaginative antitumor tactics and strategies. The reader may have anticipated one or two. **Antiangiogenic therapy** was discussed earlier (p. 778) as well as the use of **antitumor vaccines,** both preventive and therapeutic (p. 916). **Hypermethylation** (p. 891) is under study for possible applications to prognosis and/or therapy. Some examples follow: we will list selected facts of tumor biology and the therapy that they inspired.

Fact: Some tumors, notably acute lymphoblastic leukemia, require the amino acid L-asparagine, having lost the ability to synthesize it (60). **Therapy:** Treat the patient with bacterial asparaginase. It works, to a point. Some remissions occur, but there are toxic and immunologic side effects.

Fact: Cancer cells can be tamed, as we have seen (p. 949) by being forced to differentiate. **Therapy:** Treatment with differentiating agents such as retinoids (p. 950). This therapy is currently used for acute promyelocytic leukemia (64). Retinoids are effective also in preventing the progression of leukoplakia to carcinoma of the mouth (46).

Fact: Viruses can infect cells and kill them. Is it possible to find specific "oncolytic" viruses? **Therapy** (potential): Engineer an "oncolytic virus."

Alas, oncolytic viruses do exist in the literature, but their name oversells their properties. An engineered herpes virus injected into xenografts of human brain tumors caused some regressions (44), but a natural antiviral reaction was only one of the problems (29).

Fact: Experience with bone marrow allografts has shown that a very disturbing *graft-versus-host disease*

(GVH) can follow; however, if the host is leukemic, a helpful *graft-versus-leukemia reaction* can develop (p. 579). **Therapy:** Could a *graft-versus-tumor reaction* be generated? This concept was tested with moderate success; for example, in a 50-year-old man with pulmonary metastases of a renal cell carcinoma, the primary tumor was removed, and an allogeneic blood stem cell graft was given. The pulmonary metastases disappeared in 110 days and had not returned after 2 years (12a). GVH disease also developed. Regression after removal of the primary tumor can occur (p. 924).

Fact: Many tumors are based on the malfunction of a gene, which produces a defective protein. It should be possible to target this protein and/or the cell that produces it, with an antibody. **Therapy:** Indeed: we will close this incomplete list of antitumor approaches with a sketch of the first design drug of this kind, **Herceptin** (35, 48a).

Her-2 is the name of an oncogene (human epidermal growth factor receptor-2, also called *neu* or *erb-b*) that codes for a cell surface receptor that straddles the cell membrane; a normal breast epithelial cell carries 20,000–100,000 copies of this protein, but in 25–30 percent of breast cancers the cells carry 1–2 million copies (Figure 34.10). The Her-2/neu protein is a tyrosine kinase; when the outer portion is phosphorylated, the intracellular portion orders the cell to divide. Therapeutic strategy: flood the cancer cells with antibody that binds to the exposed part of the protein and inactivates it. The strategy works, but only for those cancers in which *Her-2/neu* is overexpressed, and only if the overexpression is due to gene amplification, not to excessive transcription of the gene. (Last-minute news: In some patients the drug is cardiotoxic [5].)

Gleevec is another pioneer "design-drug"; the architecture of this molecule was aimed at deactivating the specific Bcr-Abl protein of the Philadelphia chromosome, thereby preventing it from stimulating the overproduction of myeloid cells of chronic myeloid leukemia.

Fact: Antibodies are very specific but may not succeed in killing the tumor cells; they act by secreting ozone (p. 539) and by directing complement and leukocytes, through the mechanisms called antibody-dependent complement-mediated cytotoxicity (p. 536) and ADCC (antibody-dependent cell-mediated cytotoxicity [p. 536]). **Therapy:** The antibodies can be made more powerful by conjugating them with toxins, radionuclides, or even cytokines. These *armed antibodies,* of course, act also nonspecifically on bystander cells (11a).

We have barely touched on the possible approaches to tumor therapy. Perhaps someone will also try—some day—a method that works *in vitro:* the forced marriage (fusion) of tumor cells with normal cells of the host (p. 929).

Survival Trends

For most cancers, survival—measured after 5 years—depends on the stage of the disease at the time of diagnosis, as shown in Figure 34.11; the same figure shows that race, most regrettably, still makes a difference in the United States. Infection remains a major

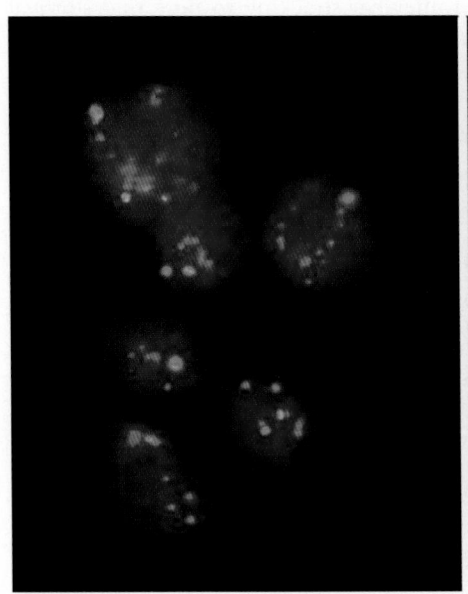
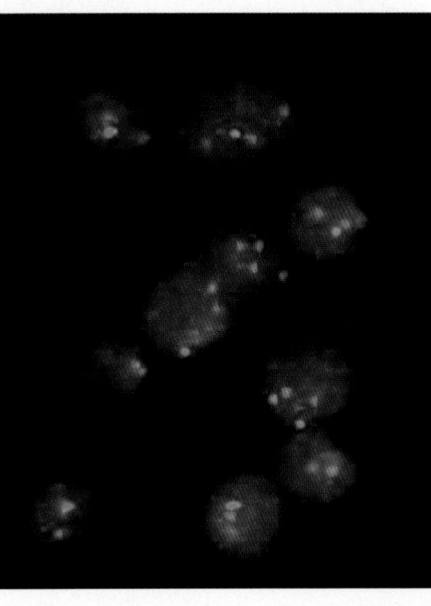

FIGURE 34.10 Amplification of the *Her2/neu* gene in breast carcinoma. Fluorescence *in situ* hybridization of breast carcinoma cells stained with *Her2/neu* (orange) and chromosome 17 centromeric (green) DNA probes. *Left:* Increased orange/green signal ratio (gene/chromosome) in a tumor with amplified *Her2/neu* compared with the normal ratio seen in a tumor without amplification (*right*). (Courtesy of Dr. G. Pihan, University of Massachusetts Medical School, Worcester, MA.)

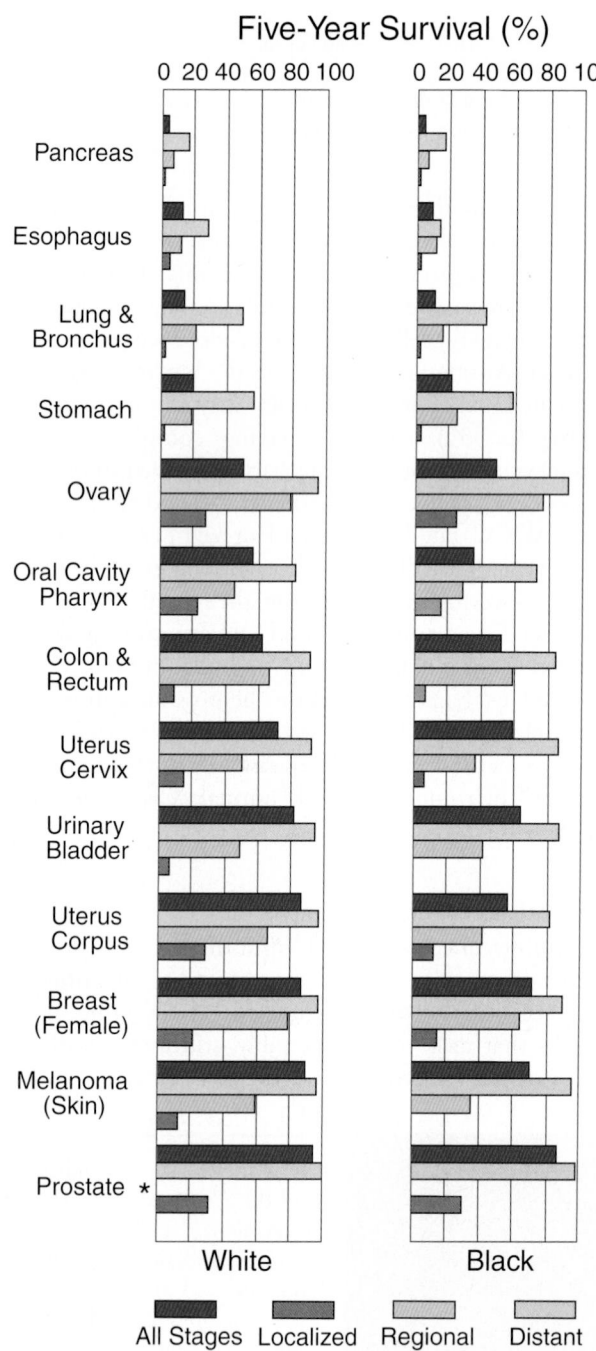

Five-Year Survival (%)

Pancreas
Esophagus
Lung & Bronchus
Stomach
Ovary
Oral Cavity Pharynx
Colon & Rectum
Uterus Cervix
Urinary Bladder
Uterus Corpus
Breast (Female)
Melanoma (Skin)
Prostate *

White   Black

All Stages   Localized   Regional   Distant

FIGURE 34.11   Five-year survival rates for 13 carcinomas by race and stage (USA, 1989–1996). In the United States, survival is influenced by race and by stage at diagnosis: the prognosis is much better if the tumor is still localized. (Adapted with permission from [25].)

complication of advanced cancer because bodily defenses are depressed by so many factors, including chemotherapy (Figure 34.12). There have been notable improvements—for whites and blacks—in the probability of survival from most common cancers and

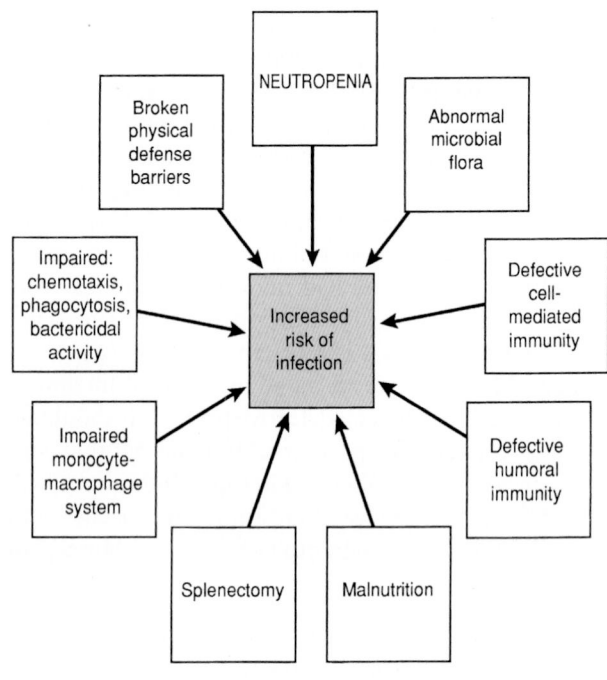

FIGURE 34.12   Mechanisms of increased susceptibility to infection in cancer patients. The single most important is neutropenia, usually defined as granulocyte count of 500/mm³ or less. (Adapted with permission from [43]. Original illustration by A. Miller.)

from all cancers combined; survival has *not* significantly improved for cancers of the uterine, cervix, larynx, and oral cavity in the past 25 years (25). Acute lymphoblastic leukemia—the most common form of malignancy in children—was virtually hopeless in the 1960s; by 2000 the 4-year survival rate was 80 percent (68). Overall, it is somewhat shocking to note that survival for some forms of cancer edges toward "worse" (Figure 34.13).

Who Is Winning the War on Cancer?

There are many ways to look at the big picture: overall cancer incidence, mortality rates, survival trends by gender, age, ethnic background, type of cancer, and so on. Figure 34.13 portrays the change in mortality over 16 years (1973–1989). A 1997 review based largely on these data is entitled "Cancer Undefeated" (2), and it is followed by a commentary entitled "Winning the War on Cancer" (36). Fishing in the sea of available facts, we choose to retain the following:

1. The overall incidence of cancer—after decades of slow rise—began to plateau around 1990 for both males and females, and the incidence for lung, breast, and prostate cancer has been declining ever since (14, 15). These statements concern the "war"

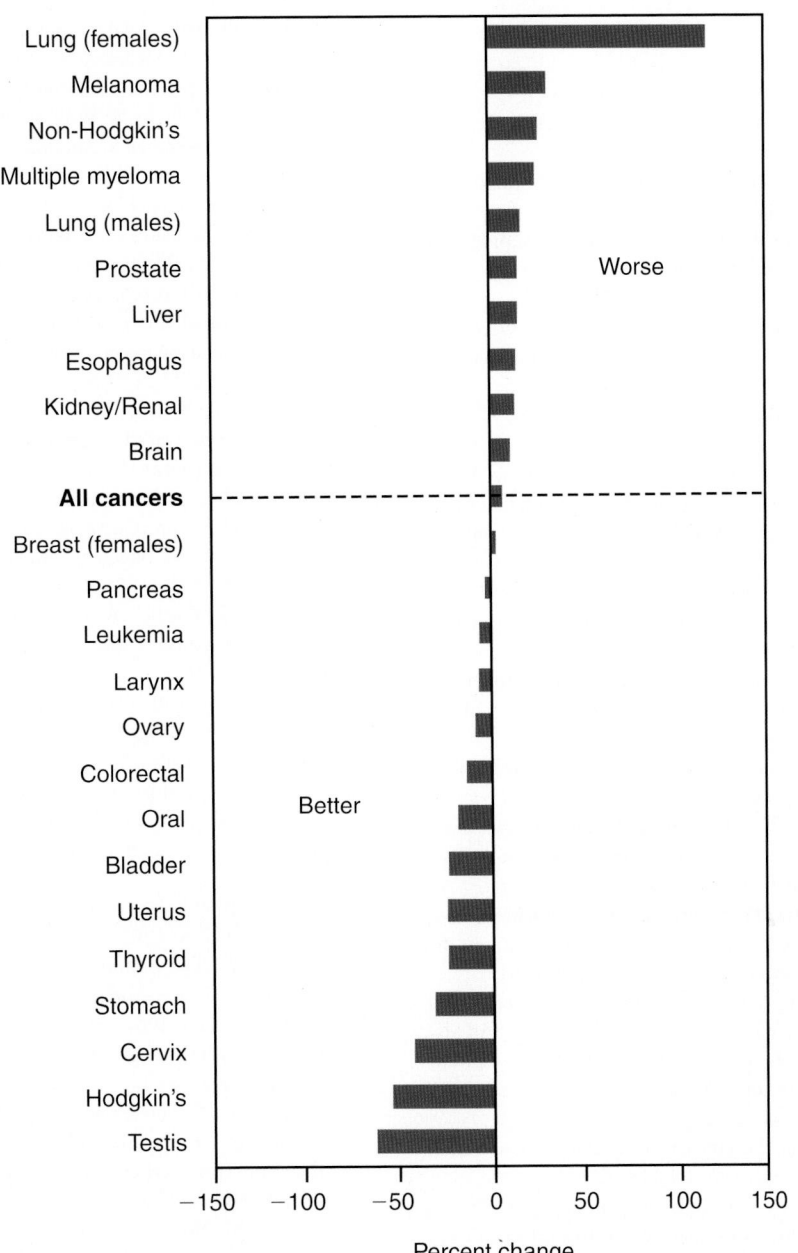

FIGURE 34.13   Changes in cancer mortality trends over 16 years (1973–1989) for all races, males and females. (Reproduced from Cancer Stat Rev: 1973–1989, 1992 [38].)

at large; it is important to also focus on individual successful battles.

2. Several cancers considered fatal during the past 2–3 decades are now curable in the majority of cases: such is the case for advanced testicular cancer, Hodgkin's disease, childhood leukemia, and non-Hodgkin's lymphoma.

3. Cancer of the stomach, worldwide the second most frequent, is now recognized to often be caused by *Helicobacter pylori* and therefore preventable with antibiotics.

4. The battle against the so-called environmental cancers (mainly due to tobacco and herpes viruses) has saved many lives and can save many more, as long as humans are susceptible to the call of reason.

5. It is true that the Revolution of 1976 (66, 67)—which created a new basic science of tumors—has not yet affected the statistics, but new "designer" drugs have appeared at the bedside, and the second part of the revolution will manifest itself in statistics before long.

References

1. Angeletti RH. Chromogranins and neuroendocrine secretion. Lab Invest 1986;55:387–390.

2. Bailar III JC, Gornik HL. Cancer undefeated. N Engl J Med 1997;336:1569–1574.

3. Baron JA, Beach M, Mandel JS, et al. Calcium supplements for the prevention of colorectal adenomas. N Engl J Med 1999;340:101–107.

4. Beastall GH, Cook B, Rustin GJS, Jennings J. A review of the role of established tumour markers. Ann Clin Biochem 1991;28:5–18.

5. Behr TM, Béhé M. Trastuzumab and breast cancer. N Engl J Med 2001;345:995–996.

6. Borgstein PJ, Pijpers R, Comans EF, et al. Sentinel lymph node biopsy in breast cancer: guidelines and pitfalls of lymphoscintigraphy and gamma probe detection. J Am Coll Surg 1998;186:275–283.

7. Bradshaw DM, Arceci RJ. Clinical relevance of transmembrane drug efflux as a mechanism of multidrug resistance. J Clin Oncol 1998;16:3674–3690.

8. Brandt-Rauf PW. Biomarkers of gene expression: growth factors and oncoproteins. Environ Health Perspect 1997; 105(Suppl 4):807–816.

9. Brandt-Rauf PW, Pincus MR. Molecular markers of carcinogenesis. Pharmacol Ther 1998;77:135–148.

9a. Camp RL, Chung GG, Rimm DL. Automated subcellular localization and quantification of protein expression in tissue microarrays. Nat Med 2002;8:1323–1327.

10. Catalona WJ, Smith DS, Ratliff TL, et al. Measurement of prostate-specific antigen in serum as a screening test for prostate cancer. N Engl J Med 1991;324:1156–1161.

11. Carroll PR, Lee KL, Fuks ZY, Kantoff PW. Cancer of the prostate. In: DeVita VT Jr, Hellman S, Rosenberg SA (eds). Cancer: Principles & practice of oncology, 6th edition. Philadelphia: Lippincott, Williams & Wilkins, 2001, pp. 1418–1479.

11a. Carter P. Improving the efficacy of antibody-based cancer therapies. Nat Rev Cancer 2001;1:118–129.

12. Childs RW. Allogeneic stem cell transplantation. In: DeVita VT Jr, Hellman S, Rosenberg SA (eds). Cancer: Principles & practice of oncology, 6th edition. Philadelphia: Lippincott, Williams & Wilkins, 2001, pp. 2779–2798.

12a. Childs R, Chernoff A, Contentin N, et al. Regression of metastatic renal-cell carcinoma after nonmyeloablative allogeneic peripheral-blood stem-cell transplantation. N Engl J Med 200;343:750–758.

13. Chu E, DeVita VT Jr. Principles of cancer management: chemotherapy. In: DeVita VT Jr, Hellman S, Rosenberg SA (eds). Cancer: Principles & practice of oncology, 6th edition. Philadelphia: Lippincott, Williams & Wilkins, 2001, pp. 289–306.

14. Cole P, Rodu B. Descriptive epidemiology: cancer statistics. In: DeVita VT Jr, Hellman S, Rosenberg SA (eds). Cancer: Principles & practice of oncology, 6th edition. Philadelphia: Lippincott, Williams & Wilkins, 2001, pp. 228–241.

15. Cole P, Rodu B. Analytic epidemiology: cancer causes. In: DeVita VT Jr, Hellman S, Rosenberg SA (eds). Cancer: Principles & practice of oncology, 6th edition. Philadelphia: Lippincott, Williams & Wilkins, 2001, pp. 241–252.

16. Cooper DL, Seropian S. Autologous stem cell transplantation. In: DeVita VT Jr, Hellman S, Rosenberg SA (eds). Cancer: Principles & practice of oncology, 6th edition. Philadelphia: Lippincott, Williams & Wilkins, 2001, pp. 2767–2778.

17. D'Amico TA, Massey M, Herndon II JE, Moore M-B, Harpole DH Jr. A biologic risk model for stage I lung cancer: immunohistochemical analysis of 408 patients with the use of ten molecular markers. J Thorac Cardiovasc Surg 1999; 117;746–743.

18. Dauplat J, Le Bouëdec G, Pomel C, Scherer C. Cytoreductive surgery for advanced stages of ovarian cancer. Semin Surg Oncol 2000;19:42–48.

18a. DeVita VT Jr, Hellman S, Rosenberg SA. Cancer prevention: diet and chemopreventive agents. Ch. 23 in: Cancer: principles & practice of oncology, 6rd ed. Philadelphia: Lippincott Williams & Wilkins, 2001, pp. 561–615.

18b. Duesberg P, Rasnick A. Aneuploidy, the somatic mutation that makes cancer a species of its own. Cell Motil Cytoskel 2000;47:81–107.

19. El-Badawy N, Cohen C, DeRose PB, Sgoutas D. Immunohistochemical estrogen receptor assay: quantitation by image analysis. Mod Pathol 1991;4:305–309.

20. Fairchild CR, Goldsmith ME, Cowan KH. Molecular biology of antineoplastic drug resistance. In: Cossman J, ed. Molecular genetics in cancer diagnosis. New York: Elsevier, 1990: 113–141.

21. Fajardo LF. Pathology of radiation injury. New York: Masson Publishing USA, 1982.

21a. Fischer AH. The evolution of tumor biology: seeking a balance between gene expression profiling and morphology studies. J Mol Diagn 2002;4:65.

22. Gleason DF. Histologic grading and clinical staging of prostatic carcinoma. In: Tannenbaum M, ed. Urologic pathology: the prostate. Philadelphia: Lea & Febiger, 1977:171–197.

23. Gould VE. Histogenesis and differentiation: a reevaluation of these concepts as criteria for the classification of tumors. Hum Pathol 1986;17:212–215.

24. Gown AM, Boyd HC, Chang Y, Ferguson M, Reichler B, Tippens D. Smooth muscle cells can express cytokeratins of "simple" epithelium. Immunocytochemical and biochemical studies in vitro and in vivo. Am J Pathol 1988;132: 223–232.

25. Greenlee RT, Hill-Harmon MB, Murray T, Thun M. Cancer statistics, 2001. CA Cancer J Clin 2001;51:15–36.

26. Hall PA, Woods AL. Immunohistochemical markers of cellular proliferation: achievements, problems and prospects. Cell Tissue Kinet 1990;23:505–522.

26a. Herman JG, Baylin SB. Gene silencing in cancer in association with promoter hypermethylation. New Engl J Med 2003; 349:2042–2054.

27. Hill BT. The relevance of certain concepts of cell cycle kinetics. Biochim Biophys Acta 1978;516:389–417.

28. Horwich A, Ross G. Circulating tumor markers. In: Bronchud MH, Foote MA, Peters WP, Robinson MO (eds).

Principles of molecular oncology. Totowa, NJ: Humana Press, 2000, pp. 111–124.

29. Ikeda K, Ichikawa T, Wakimoto H, et al. Oncolytic virus therapy of multiple tumors in the brain requires suppression of innate and elicited antiviral responses. Nat Med 1999;5: 881–887.

30. Jain RK. Normalizing tumor vasculature with anti-angiogenic therapy: a new paradigm for combination therapy. Nat Med 2001;7:987–989.

31. Jänne PA, Mayer RJ. Chemoprevention of colorectal cancer. N Engl J Med 2000;342:1960–1968.

32. Kelemen PR. Comprehensive review of sentinel lymphadenectomy in breast cancer. Clin Breast Cancer 2000;1: 111–125.

33. Koss LG, Czerniak B, Herz F, Wersto RP. Flow cytometric measurements of DNA and other cell components in human tumors: a critical appraisal. Hum Pathol 1989;20: 528–548.

34. Lee AKC, Dugan J, Hamilton WM, et al. Quantitative DNA analysis in breast carcinomas: a comparison between image analysis and flow cytometry. Mod Pathol 1991;4:178–182.

35. Lewis R. Herceptin earns recognition in breast cancer arsenal. Scientist 2001;15:10–12.

35a. Liotta LA, Ferrari M, Petricoin E. Written in blood. Nature 2003;425:905.

36. Mayer RJ, Schnipper LE. Winning the war on cancer. N Engl J Med 1997;337:935.

37. McIntire KR. Tumor markers: how useful are they? Hosp Pract 1984;19:55–68.

38. Miller BA, Ries LAG, Hankey BF, Kosary CL, Edwards BK (eds.) Cancer statistics review 1973–1989. Bethesda, MD: National Cancer Institute, US Department of Health and Human Services (NIH publication No. 92-2789), 1992.

39. Moertel CG, Fleming TR, Macdonald JS, Haller DG, Laurie JA, Tangen C. An evaluation of the carcinoembryonic antigen (CEA) test for monitoring patients with resected colon cancer. JAMA 1993;270:943–947.

40. Norton L, Simon R. Tumor size, sensitivity to therapy, and design of treatment schedules. Cancer Treat Rep 1977;61: 1307–1317.

41. Offit K. Genetic prognostic markers for colorectal cancer. N Engl J Med 2000;342:124–125.

42. Pastan IH, Gottesman MM. Molecular biology of multidrug resistance in human cells. In: DeVita VT Jr, Hellman S, Rosenberg SA, eds. Important advances in oncology 1988. Philadelphia: JB Lippincott, 1988:3–16.

43. Pizzo PA. Combating infections in neutropenic patients. Hosp Pract 1989;24:93–95.

44. Pyles RB, Warnick RE, Chalk CL, Szanti BE, Parysek LM. A novel multiply-mutated HSV-1 strain for the treatment of human brain tumors. Hum Gene Ther 1997;8:533–544.

45. Restifo NP, Sznol M, Overwijk WW. Therapeutic cancer vaccines. In: DeVita VT Jr, Hellman S, Rosenberg SA (eds). Cancer: Principles & practice of oncology, 6th edition. Philadelphia: Lippincott, Williams & Wilkins, 2001, pp. 3195–3217.

46. Richtsmeier WJ. Biologic modifiers and chemoprevention of cancer of the oral cavity. N Engl J Med 1993;328:58–59.

47. Rowley JD, Aster JC, Sklar J. The impact of new DNA diagnostic technology on the management of cancer patients. Arch Pathol Lab Med 1993;117:1104–1109.

48. Salmon SE. Kinetic rationale for adjuvant chemotherapy of cancer. In: Salmon SE, Jones SE, eds. Adjuvant therapy of cancer. Amsterdam: North Holland Publishing, 1977: 15–27.

48a. Schnitt SJ. Breast cancer in the 21st century: Neu opportunities and Neu challenges. Mod Pathol 2001;14:213–218.

49. Seckinger D, Sugarbaker E, Frankfurt O. DNA content in human cancer. Application in pathology and clinical medicine. Arch Pathol Lab Med 1989;113:619–626.

50. Sell S. Alphafetoprotein. In: Sell S, ed. Cancer markers. Clifton, NJ: Humana Press, 1980:249–293.

51. Shively JE, Todd CW. Carcinoembryonic antigen A: chemistry and biology. In: Sell S, ed. Cancer markers. Clifton, NJ: Humana Press, 1980:295–314.

52. Skibber JM, Minsky, BB, Hoff, PM. Cancer of the colon. In: DeVita VT Jr, Hellman S, Rosenberg SA (eds). Cancer: Principles & practice of oncology, 6th edition. Philadelphia: Lippincott, Williams & Wilkins, 2001, pp. 1216–1271.

53. Skipper HE. Kinetic considerations associated with therapy of solid tumors. In: The Twenty-First Annual Symposium on Fundamental Cancer Research, 1967, for the University of Texas MD Anderson Hospital and Tumor Institute at Houston. The proliferation and spread of neoplastic cells. Baltimore: Williams & Wilkins, 1968:213–233.

54. Skipper HE, Schabel FM Jr, Wilcox WS. Experimental evaluation of potential anticancer agents. XIII. On the criteria and kinetics associated with "curability" of experimental leukemia. Cancer Chemother Rep 1964;35:1–111.

55. Sobin LH, Wittekind C (eds). TNM classification of malignant tumors. 6th ed. New York: Wiley, 2002.

56. Spiessl B, Beahrs OH, Hermanek P, et al., eds. TNM atlas: illustrated guide to the TNM/pTNM classification of malignant tumours, 3rd ed. Berlin: Springer-Verlag, 1990.

57. Stamey TA, Yang N, Hay AR, McNeal JE, Freiha FS, Redwine E. Prostate-specific antigen as a serum marker for adenocarcinoma of the prostate. N Engl J Med 1987;317:909–916.

58. Steele G Jr, Zamcheck N, Wilson R, et al. Results of CEA-initiated second-look surgery for recurrent colorectal cancer. Am J Surg 1980;139:544–548.

58a. Stewart BW, Kleihues P (eds). World cancer report. Lyon; IARC Press, 2003.

59. Teicher B (ed). Antiangiogenic agents in cancer therapy. Totowa, NJ: Humana Press, 1999.

60. Uren JR, Handschumacher RE. Enzyme therapy. In: Becker FF, ed. Cancer: a comprehensive treatise, vol 5: chemotherapy. New York: Plenum Press, 1977:457–487.

61. van der Burg MEL, van Lent M, Buyse M, et al. The effect of debulking surgery after induction chemotherapy on the prognosis in advanced epithelial ovarian cancer. N Engl J Med 1995;332:629–634.

62. Vergote I, de Wever I, Tjalma W, et al. Interval debulking surgery: an alternative for primary surgical debulking? Semin Surg Oncol 2000;19:49–53.

63. Virji MA, Mercer DW, Herberman RB. Tumor markers in cancer diagnosis and prognosis. CA 1988;38:104–126.

63a. Waldmann TA. Immunotherapy: past, present and future. Nat Med 2003;9:269–277.

64. Warrell RP. Retinoic acid and acute promyelocytic leukemia. Biologic Therapy Cancer 1991;1:1–12.

65. Wattenberg LW. Chemoprevention of cancer. Cancer Res 1985;45:1–8.

66. Weinberg RA. Racing to the beginning of the road: the search for the origin of cancer. New York: W.H. Freeman and Company, 1996.

67. Weinberg RA. One renegade cell: how cancer begins. New York: Basic Books, 1998.

68. Weinstein HJ, Tarbell NJ. Leukemias and lymphomas of childhood. In: DeVita VT Jr, Hellman S, Rosenberg SA (eds). Cancer: Principles & practice of oncology, 6th edition. Philadelphia: Lippincott, Williams & Wilkins, 2001, pp. 2235–2256.

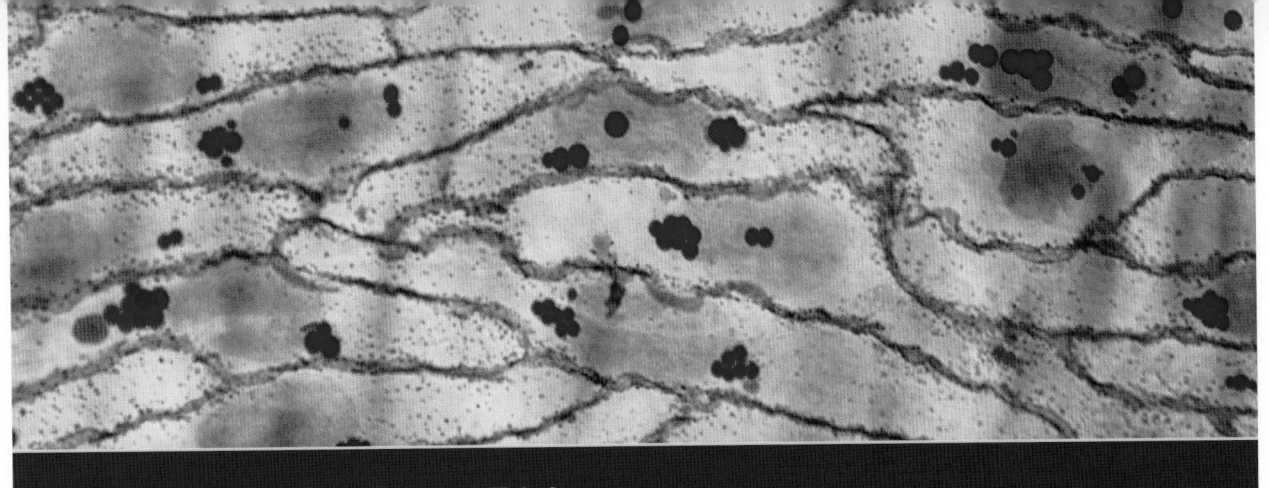

FAREWELL

Here end our travels through the vast lands of *Cells, Tissues, and Disease*. Looking back along our trail, we hope that—as your guides—we stopped in the right places, and gave you the correct explanations. Our plan has been to thread selected facts on a unifying theme: the cell, which we like to call the elementary patient.

We tried to keep the book as readable and well illustrated as possible. For some it will be too short, for some too long. We did the best we could, with an eye on consistency. Your comments would be extremely welcome.

Ten or twenty years from now someone may write a mirror image of this story, not from the cell up, but from the cell down; perhaps *Cells, Molecules (or proteins? atoms?/electrons?), and Disease.* We would love to read that book, but it will not replace the kind of book that you are holding in your hand. To understand disease, it will always be essential to understand the microscopic world of cells and tissues.

Index

Note: Page numbers followed by f and t refer to figures and tables, respectively.